DIAGNOSTIC PATHOLOGY

PEDIATRIC NEOPLASMS

AMIRSYS®

DIAGNOSTIC PATHOLOGY

PEDIATRIC NEOPLASMS

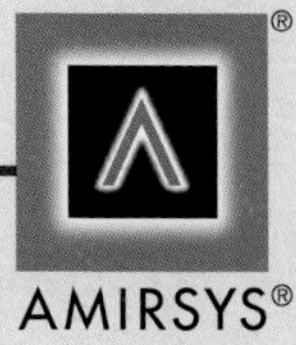

Angelica R. Putnam, MD
Assistant Professor
University of Utah School of Medicine
Pathologist
Primary Children's Medical Center
Salt Lake City, UT

Alexandros D. Polydorides, MD, PhD
Assistant Professor of Pathology
Mount Sinai School of Medicine
Attending Pathologist
Mount Sinai Medical Center
New York, NY

Jessica M. Comstock, MD
Assistant Professor
Division of Pediatric Pathology
University of Utah Hospital
Salt Lake City, UT

Silvia Skripenova, MD
Pathologist
Spectrum Medical Group
Department of Pathology
Maine Medical Center
Portland, ME

Brian J. Hall, MD
Resident
Department of Pathology
University of Utah Hospital
Salt Lake City, UT

Sarah Culkin Mengshol, MD
Pediatric and Perinatal Pathologist
Unipath, PC
Presbyterian St. Luke's Medical Center
Denver, CO

Bahig M. Shehata, MD
Professor of Pathology and Pediatrics
Emory University School of Medicine
Children's Healthcare of Atlanta
Atlanta, GA

Jeremy C. Wallentine, MD
Pathologist
Intermountain Healthcare and Utah Pathology Services, Inc.
LDS Hospital
Salt Lake City, UT

Larissa V. Furtado, MD
Co-Chief Resident of Anatomic and Clinical Pathology
Department of Pathology
University of Utah Hospital
Salt Lake City, UT

Karen S. Thompson, MD
Associate Professor of Pathology
John A. Burns School of Medicine, University of Hawaii
Pan Pacific Pathologists/Clinical Laboratories of Hawaii
Kapiolani Medical Center for Women and Children
Honolulu, HI

Aliya N. Husain, MD
Professor of Pathology
University of Chicago
Chicago, IL

Kelley E. Capocelli, MD
Assistant Professor Pathology
University of Colorado Denver
Pediatric Pathology and Transfusion Medicine
Children's Hospital Colorado
Denver, CO

Scott R. Owens, MD
Assistant Professor of Pathology
Medical Director of Professional Practice Evaluation
University of Michigan
Ann Arbor, MI

Anna P. Matynia, MD
Resident
Department of Pathology
University of Utah Hospital
Salt Lake City, UT

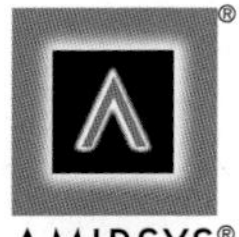

AMIRSYS®
Names you know. Content you trust.®

First Edition

Published in Salt Lake City, Utah

Printed in Canada by Friesens, Altona, Manitoba, Canada

ISBN: 978-1-931884-54-9

Notice and Disclaimer

Library of Congress Cataloging-in-Publication Data

Diagnostic pathology. Pediatric neoplasms / [edited by] Angelica R. Putnam, Jeremy C. Wallentine. -- 1st ed.
p. ; cm.
Pediatric neoplasms
Includes bibliographical references and index.
ISBN 978-1-931884-54-9
I. Putnam, Angelica R. II. Wallentine, Jeremy C. III. Title: Pediatric neoplasms.
[DNLM: 1. Neoplasms--pathology. 2. Child. 3. Neoplasms--diagnosis. QZ 275]

618.92'994--dc23

2011044434

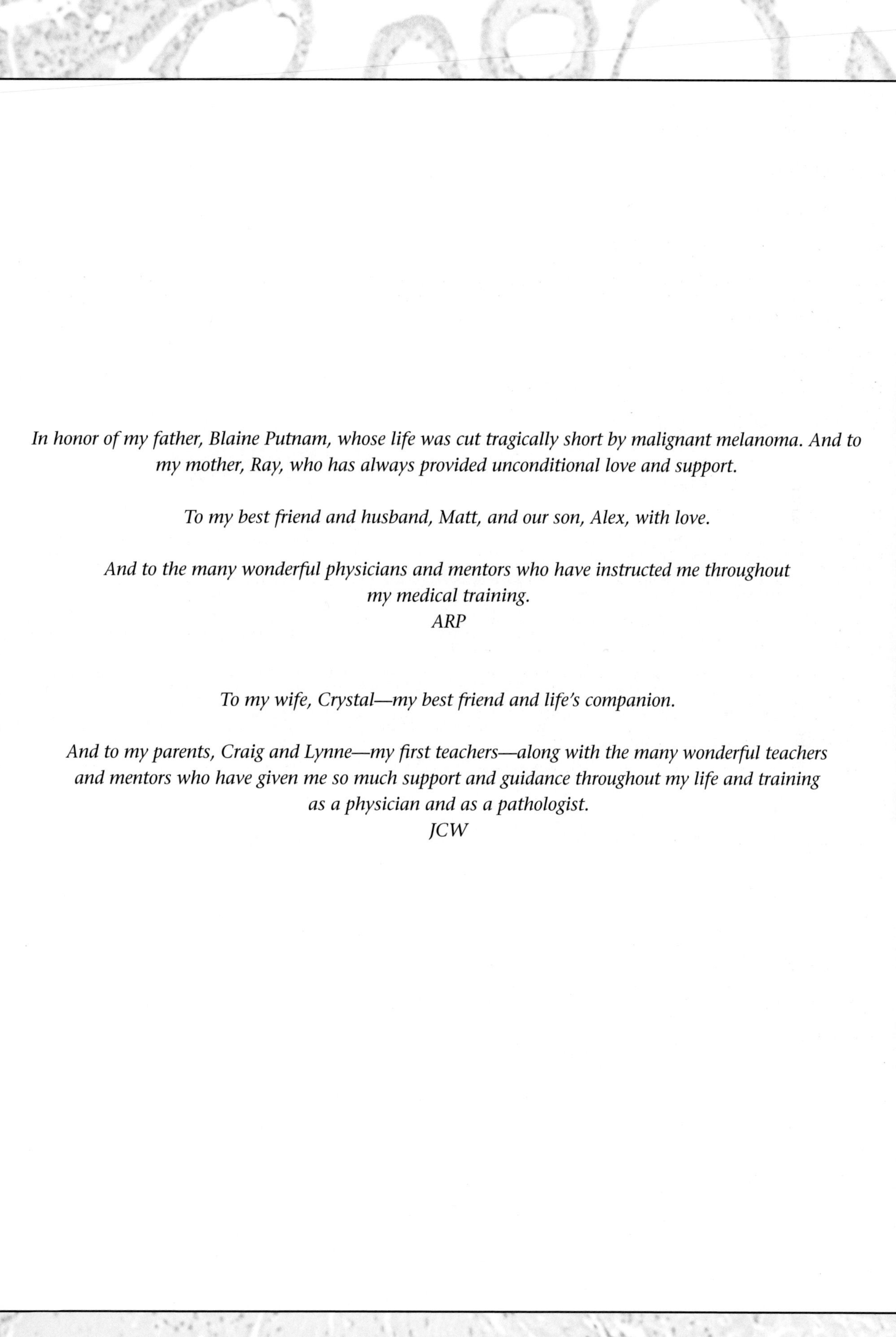

In honor of my father, Blaine Putnam, whose life was cut tragically short by malignant melanoma. And to my mother, Ray, who has always provided unconditional love and support.

To my best friend and husband, Matt, and our son, Alex, with love.

And to the many wonderful physicians and mentors who have instructed me throughout my medical training.
ARP

To my wife, Crystal—my best friend and life's companion.

And to my parents, Craig and Lynne—my first teachers—along with the many wonderful teachers and mentors who have given me so much support and guidance throughout my life and training as a physician and as a pathologist.
JCW

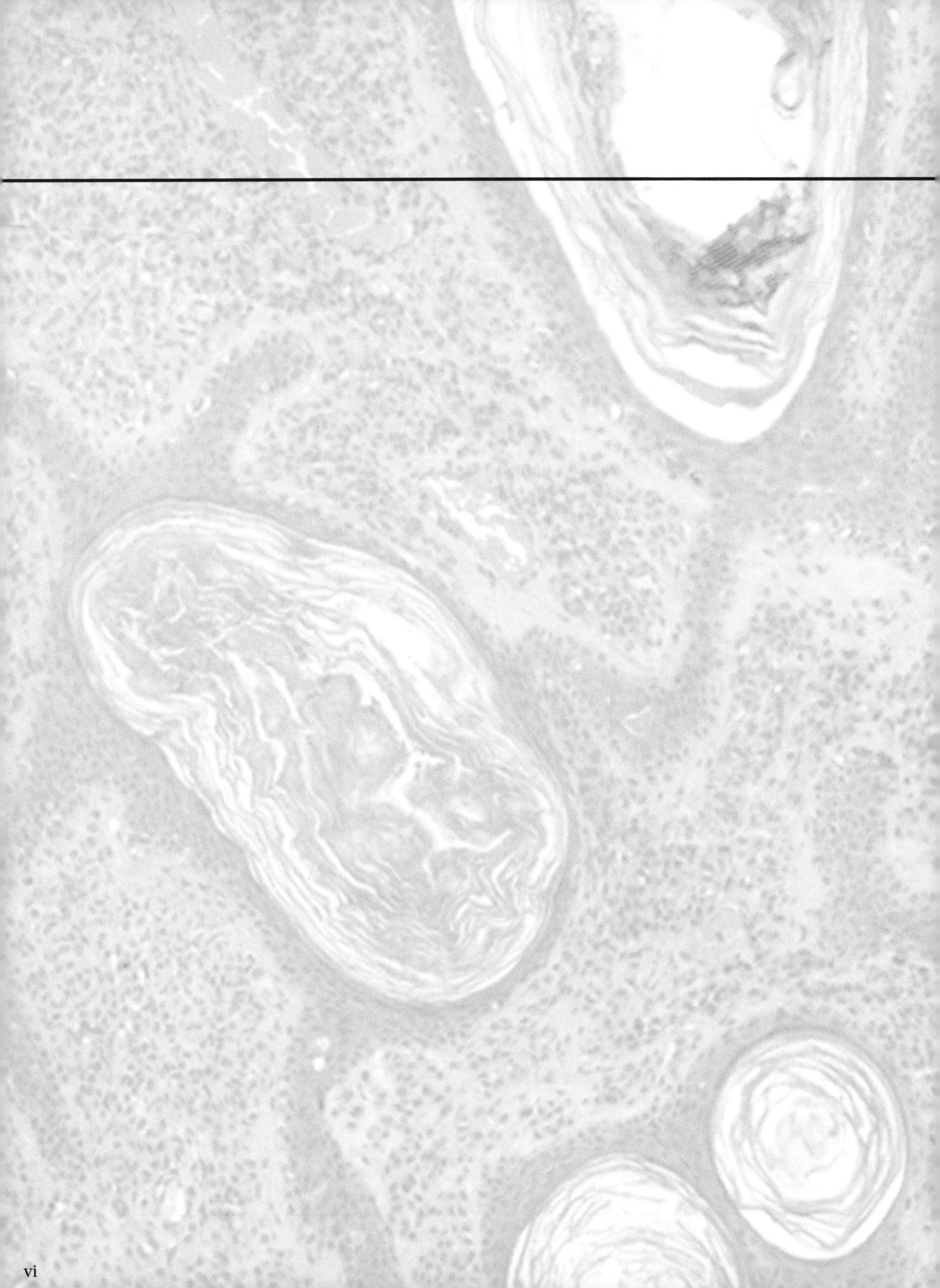

CONTRIBUTORS

Cyril Fisher, MD, DSc, FRCPath
Consultant Histopathologist
Royal Marsden NHS Foundation Trust
Professor of Tumor Pathology
Institute of Cancer Research
University of London
London, United Kingdom

Brenda L. Nelson, DDS, MS
Head of Anatomic Pathology
Naval Medical Center San Diego
San Diego, CA

Carlos E. Bueso-Ramos, MD, PhD
Professor
Department of Hematopathology
The University of Texas M. D. Anderson Cancer Center
Houston, TX

David G. Hicks, MD
Professor of Pathology and Laboratory Medicine
Director of Surgical Pathology Unit
University of Rochester Medical Center
Rochester, NY

Pei Lin, MD
Associate Professor
Department of Hematopathology
The University of Texas M. D. Anderson Cancer Center
Houston, TX

Keyur Patel, MD, PhD
Assistant Professor
Department of Hematopathology
The University of Texas M. D. Anderson Cancer Center
Houston, TX

Saul Suster, MD
Professor and Chairman
Department of Pathology and Laboratory Medicine
Medical College of Wisconsin
Milwaukee, WI

Francisco Vega, MD, PhD
Assistant Professor
Department of Hematopathology
The University of Texas M. D. Anderson Cancer Center
Houston, TX

Qian-Yun Zhang, MD, PhD
Associate Professor of Pathology
University of New Mexico Health Sciences Center
Albequerque, NM

Elizabeth A. Montgomery, MD
Professor of Pathology, Oncology, and Orthopedic Surgery
John Hopkins Medical Institutions
Baltimore, MD

Vania Nosé, MD, PhD
Professor of Pathology and Endocrinology
Vice Chair and Director of Anatomic Pathology
Chief of Endocrine Pathology Service
University of Miami Miller School of Medicine
Miami, FL

David Czuchlewski, MD
Assistant Professor of Pathology
University of New Mexico Health Sciences Center
Albequerque, NM

Susan C. Lester, MD, PhD
Chief, Breast Pathology Services
Brigham and Women's Hospital
Assistant Professor, Harvard Medical School
Staff Pathologist, Dana Farber Cancer Institute
Boston, MA

G. Petur Nielsen, MD
Associate Professor
Harvard Medical School
Director of Bone and Soft Tissue Pathology
Director of Electron Microscopy Unit
Massachusetts General Hospital
Boston, MA

Andrew E. Rosenberg, MD
Professor
Department of Pathology
University of Miami Miller School of Medicine
Miami, FL

Satish K. Tickoo, MD
Attending Pathologist
Department of Pathology
Memorial Sloan-Kettering Cancer Center
New York, NY

Sa A. Wang, MD
Associate Professor
Department of Hematopathology
The University of Texas M. D. Anderson Cancer Center
Houston, TX

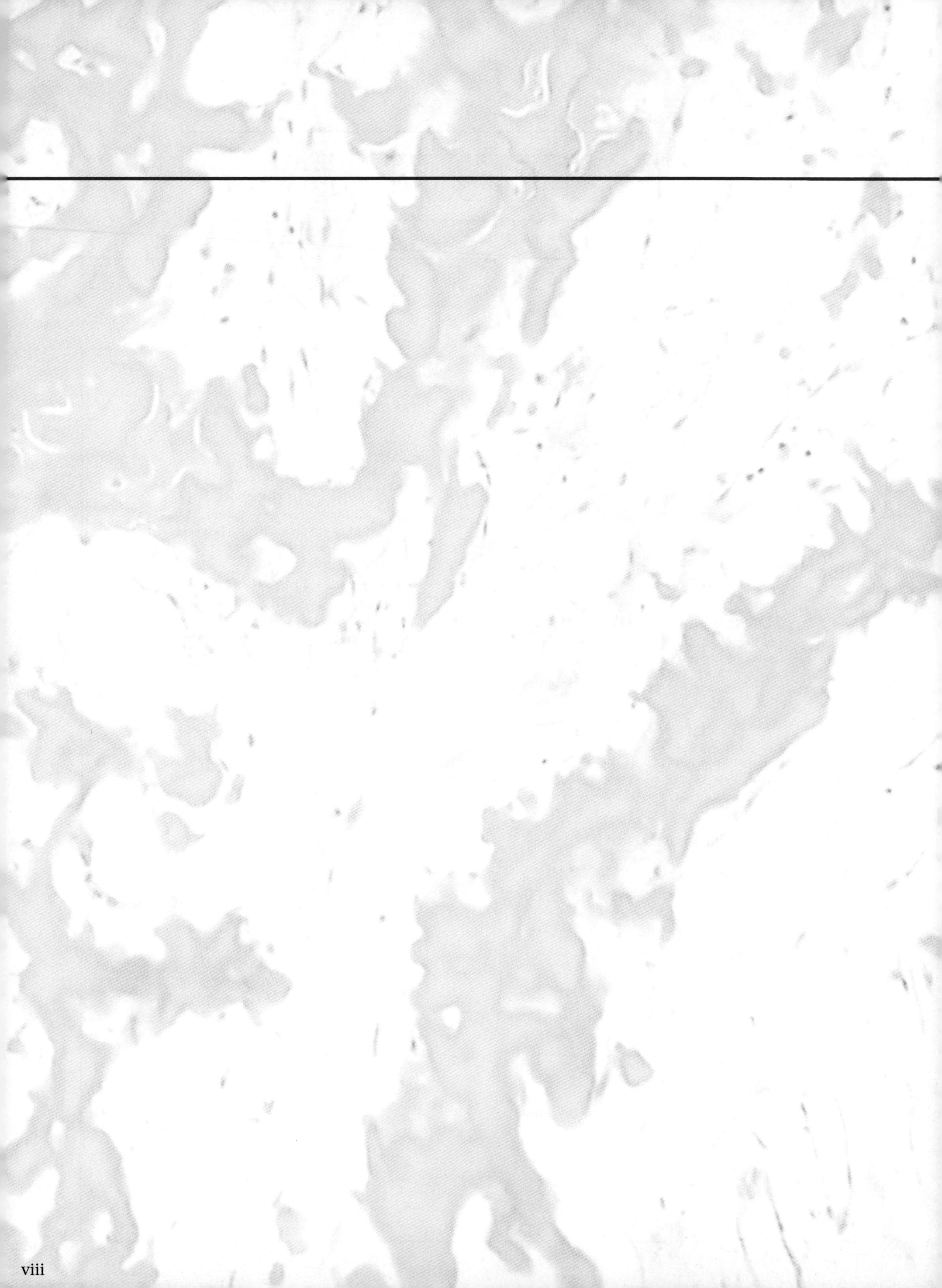

DIAGNOSTIC PATHOLOGY

PEDIATRIC NEOPLASMS

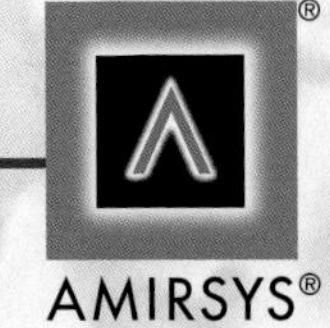

Amirsys, creators of the highly acclaimed radiology series Diagnostic Imaging, proudly introduces its new Diagnostic Pathology series, designed as easy-to-use reference texts for the busy practicing surgical pathologist. Written by world-renowned experts, the series will consist of 15 titles in all the crucial diagnostic areas of surgical pathology.

The most recent book in this series, *Diagnostic Pathology: Pediatric Neoplasms*, contains approximately 900 pages of comprehensive, yet concise, descriptions of more than 200 specific diagnoses. Amirsys's pioneering bulleted format distills pertinent information to the essentials. Each chapter has the same organization providing an easy-to-read reference for making rapid, efficient, and accurate diagnoses in a busy surgical pathology practice. A highlighted Key Facts box provides the essential features of each diagnosis. Detailed sections on Terminology, Etiology/Pathogenesis, Clinical Issues, Macroscopic and Microscopic Findings, and the all important Differential Diagnoses follow so you can find the information you need in the exact same place every time.

Most importantly, every diagnosis features numerous high-quality images, including gross pathology, H&E and immunohistochemical stains, correlative radiographic images, and richly colored graphics, all of which are fully annotated to maximize their illustrative potential.

We believe that this lavishly illustrated series, with its up-to-date information and practical focus, will become the core of your reference collection. Enjoy!

Elizabeth H. Hammond, MD
Executive Editor, Pathology
Amirsys, Inc.

Paula J. Woodward, MD
President
Amirsys Publishing, Inc.

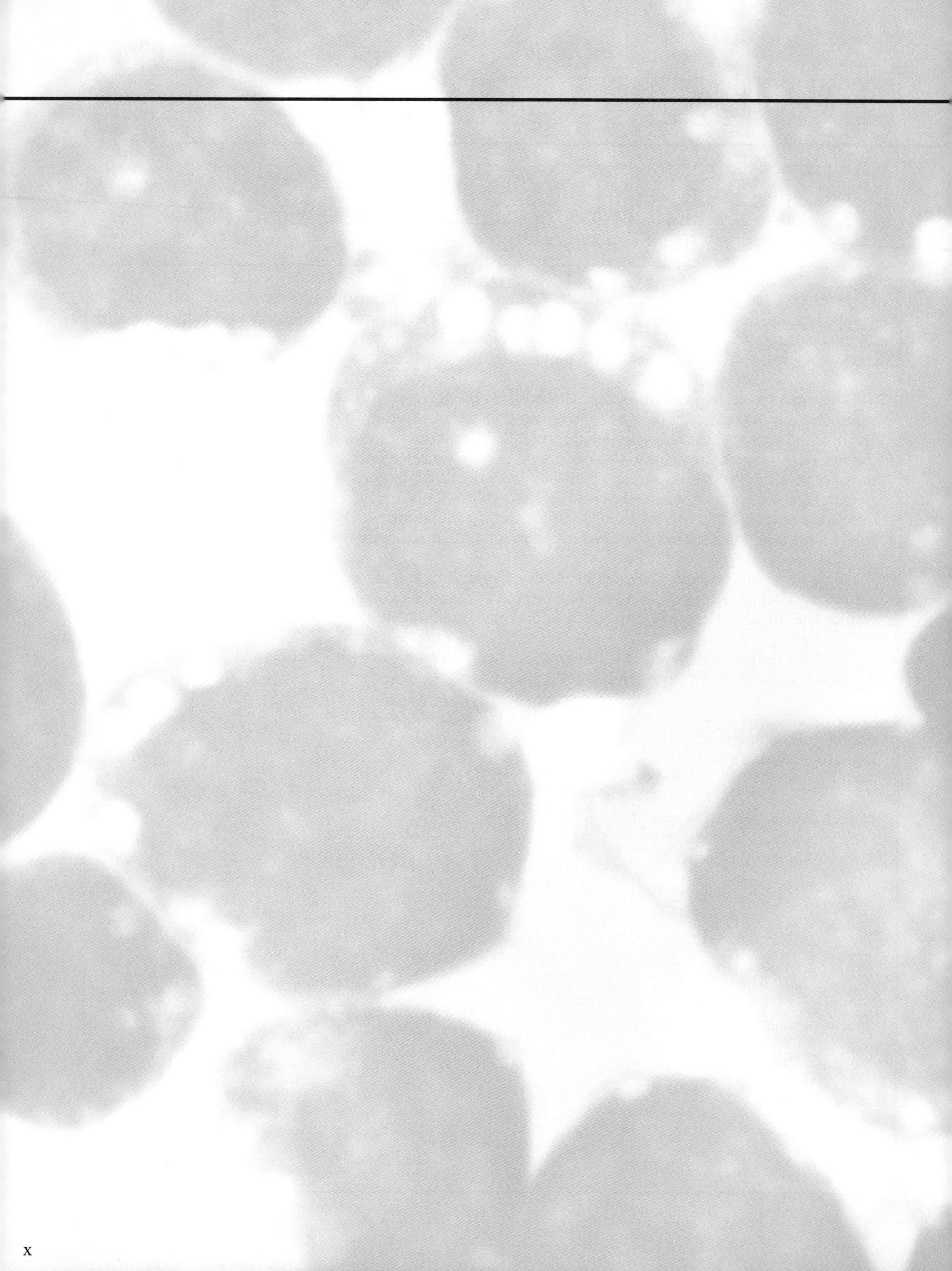

PREFACE

Our goal when we set off on this journey was to create a comprehensive, user-friendly resource for the adult and pediatric surgical pathologist alike that would address the vast majority of the neoplastic processes encountered in the pediatric population. Pediatric pathology often poses a challenge to the general surgical pathologist. Although there are numerous entities that overlap both pediatric and adult age groups, there are of course entities unique to this population that, when encountered, create great anxiety to the pathologist who largely sees adult material.

A combination of succinct, bulleted text along with rich and diverse clinical, radiographic, gross, and microscopic images will help the pathologist to arrive at the correct diagnosis, consider key differential diagnostic possibilities, and select the most helpful ancillary techniques. Each chapter also contains a highlighted box of key facts for ease of use. In addition, there are rich medical illustrations throughout this book that further enhance its value. We also believe that the format of this book will make it an invaluable resource for residents and fellows as they strive to master such a large body of information.

The book has been organized and arranged according to organ systems that, in the end, provide a comprehensive overview of the diverse field of pediatric pathology. However, as the field of pediatric and adult pathology continues to evolve in the era of personalized medicine, it is likely that the list of ancillary studies that provide diagnostic, prognostic, and therapeutic information will continue to expand. The Amirsys eBook version of this book, therefore, will be a key tool in staying informed and on top of this expanding area of information. The Amirsys eBook Advantage™ license included with each printed copy of this book provides a more accessible and portable body of information that can be updated as the information changes and expands.

On behalf of all of the authors and contributors of this book, we hope that *Diagnostic Pathology: Pediatric Neoplasms* will prove to be a favorite reference to which pathologists turn to again and again in their daily practice.

Angelica R. Putnam, MD
Assistant Professor
University of Utah School of Medicine
Pathologist
Primary Children's Medical Center
Salt Lake City, UT

Jeremy C. Wallentine, MD
Pathologist
Intermountain Healthcare and Utah Pathology Services, Inc.
LDS Hospital
Salt Lake City, UT

ACKNOWLEDGMENTS

Text Editing
Ashley R. Renlund, MA
Arthur G. Gelsinger, MA
Matthew R. Connelly, MA
Lorna Morring, MS
Rebecca L. Hutchinson, BA
Angela M. Green, BA
Katherine Riser, MA

Image Editing
Jeffrey J. Marmorstone, BS
Lisa A. Magar, BS

Medical Text Editing
Portia A. Krieger, MD
Staci Bryson, MD

Illustrations
Laura C. Sesto, MA
Richard Coombs, MS
Lane R. Bennion, MS

Art Direction and Design
Laura C. Sesto, MA
Mirjam Ravneng, BA

Assistant Editor
Dave L. Chance, MA

Publishing Lead
Kellie J. Heap, BA

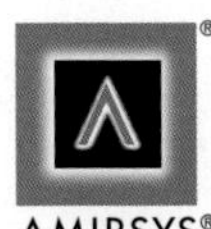

AMIRSYS®
Names you know. Content you trust.®

SECTIONS

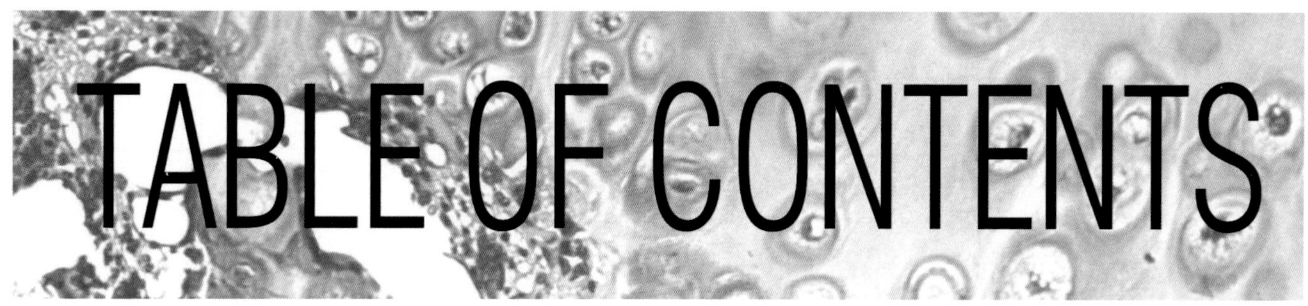

SECTION 1
Skin

Neoplasm, Benign

Neoplasm, Borderline

Neoplasm, Malignant Primary

Protocol for the Examination of Specimens from Patients with Melanoma of the Skin

SECTION 2
Soft Tissue

Neoplasm, Benign

Neoplasm, Borderline

Neoplasm, Malignant Primary

Protocol for the Examination of Specimens from Patients with Tumors of Soft Tissue

Protocol for the Examination of Specimens from Patients with Rhabdomyosarcoma

SECTION 3
Joint

Neoplasm, Benign

SECTION 4
Bone

Neoplasm, Benign

Neoplasm, Malignant Primary

Protocol for the Examination of Specimens from Patients with Bone Tumors

Protocol for the Examination of Specimens from Patients with Primitive Neuroectodermal Tumor/Ewing Sarcoma

SECTION 5 Breast

Neoplasm, Benign

Neoplasm, Borderline

Neoplasm, Malignant Primary

SECTION 6 Central Nervous System

Neoplasm, Benign

Neoplasm, Malignant Primary

Protocol for the Examination of Specimens from Patients with Tumors of the Brain/Spinal Cord

SECTION 7 Endocrine

Neoplasm, Benign

Neoplasm, Malignant Primary

Protocol for the Examination of Specimens from Patients with Tumors of the Thyroid Gland

Protocol for the Examination of Specimens from Patients with Carcinoma of the Adrenal Gland

Protocol for the Examination of Specimens from Patients with Neuroblastoma

SECTION 8 Head and Neck

Neoplasm, Benign

Neoplasm, Malignant Primary

Protocol for the Examination of Specimens from Patients with Retinoblastoma

Protocol for the Examination of Specimens from Patients with Carcinomas of the Salivary Glands

SECTION 9 Respiratory

Neoplasm, Benign

SECTION 10 Mediastinum

Neoplasm, Benign

Neoplasm, Malignant Primary

Neoplasm, Malignant Primary

Protocol for the Examination of Specimens from Patients with Wilms Tumors

Protocol for the Examination of Specimens from Patients with Malignant Germ Cell and Sex Cord-Stromal Tumors of the Testis

Protocol for the Examination of Specimens from Patients with Carcinoma of the Ovary

SECTION 15 Hematopoietic

Neoplasm, Borderline

Neoplasm, Malignant Primary

Protocol for the Examination of Specimens from Patients with Hematopoietic Neoplasms Involving Bone Marrow

Protocol for the Examination of Specimens from Patients with Hodgkin Lymphoma

Protocol for the Examination of Specimens from Patients with Non-Hodgkin Lymphoma

SECTION 16
Reference

Antibody Index

Molecular Factors Index

DIAGNOSTIC PATHOLOGY
PEDIATRIC NEOPLASMS

AMIRSYS®

Skin

Neoplasm, Benign

Neoplasm, Borderline

Neoplasm, Malignant Primary

Protocol for the Examination of Specimens from Patients with Melanoma of the Skin

MELANOCYTIC NEVUS

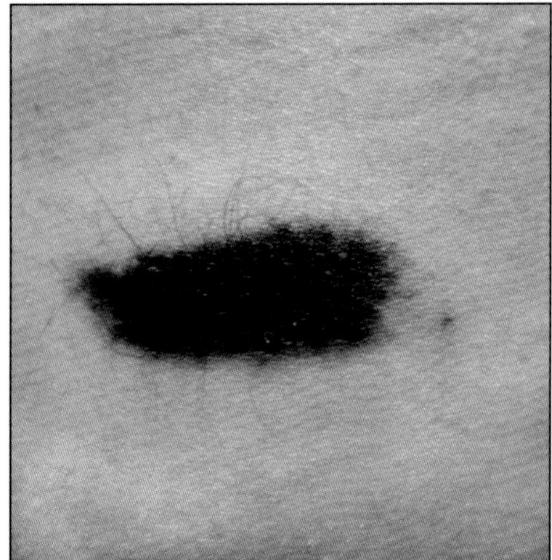

A congenital nevus with deeply brown pigmented hairy jagged edges is shown. Although malignant potential is debatable, an excision may be indicated to exclude a deep melanoma. (Courtesy S. Vanderhooft, MD.)

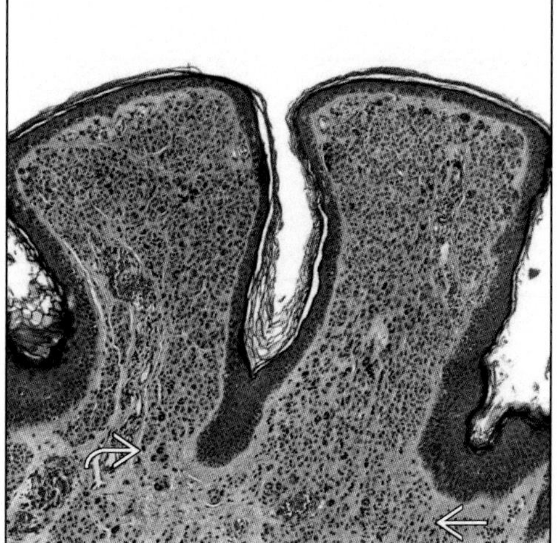

This is a predominantly intradermal nevus with congenital features. Note the scattered giant cells ➡ and that the lesion seems to "mature" with depth ➡. (Courtesy C. Cockerell, MD.)

TERMINOLOGY

Abbreviations

- Melanocytic nevus (MN)

Synonyms

- Benign melanocytic nevus, common mole, banal nevi, nevocellular nevus, pigmented nevus

Definitions

- Localized benign neoplasms composed of melanocytes

CLINICAL ISSUES

Epidemiology

- Incidence
  - Congenital
    - 1-2% of newborn infants
  - Acquired
    - Very high prevalence
- Age
  - Congenital
    - By definition present at or soon after birth
  - Acquired
    - Incidence increases through 1st 3 decades of life
    - Incidence peaks in 4th and 5th decades
    - Low incidence in elderly patients
- Gender
  - No clear predilection; M = F
- Ethnicity
  - Much more common in light-skinned individuals

Presentation

- Congenital melanocytic nevi (CMN)
  - Tan to dark brown well-circumscribed papule or plaque
  - Usually solitary
  - Giant congenital nevi defined as measuring ≥ 20 cm
    - Increased risk for development of melanoma (up to 5-7%) at site of giant CMN
- Acquired nevi
  - Typically < 1 cm
  - Can be pigmented (typically brown or black) or nonpigmented
    - Pigmented, flat or slightly elevated non-hairy nevi are usually junctional nevi
    - Nonpigmented, elevated, hairy nevi are usually intradermal nevi
  - Undergo progressive maturation with increasing age
  - Initially present as flat macular lesions
  - With maturation, junctional activity ceases
    - Lesions then become predominantly dermal
    - Most nevi are intradermal by early adult life
  - With increasing age, numbers typically decrease

Treatment

- Surgical approaches
  - Surgical excision is best method of removal
  - Shave excision also acceptable and probably more common
    - Can cause sampling error if whole lesion is not captured
  - Punch biopsy is best avoided
- Adjuvant therapy
  - Monsel solution sometimes used to decrease bleeding after biopsy
    - Can cause histologic artifact: "Monsel solution granuloma"
    - Causes a granulomatous reaction, ferrugination of collagen and elastic fibers, and deposition of slightly refractile, gray-brown substance strongly positive with Perls stain
    - May make interpretation of re-biopsy difficult
  - 10% aluminum chloride more commonly used now to avoid this histologic artifact

Prognosis

- Generally excellent
  - Rare chance of development into melanoma

MELANOCYTIC NEVUS

Key Facts

Clinical Issues

- Increased risk for development of melanoma (up to 5-7%) at site of giant CMN
- Most nevi are intradermal by early adult life
  - Junctional nevus arising in an elderly patient should be viewed with caution
- Rare chance of development into melanoma
  - Exact frequency of transformation into malignant melanoma unknown

Microscopic Pathology

- Symmetry
- Circumscription
- Maturation
- Well-nested melanocytes at dermo-epidermal junction
- No pigment in deep melanocytic nests of dermis (excluding blue nevi)
- No deep mitoses
- Acral melanocytic nevi
  - Sections cut perpendicular to dermatoglyphics will aid in recognizing symmetry and circumscription in these often difficult lesions

Diagnostic Checklist

- Understanding the histology of nevi of special sites and acral nevi is of paramount importance
- Proper recognition of Spitz nevi and subtypes can simplify difficult lesions
- Difficult lesions (especially if there is not concordance among pathologists in the group) should be referred to experts

---

    - Exact frequency of transformation into malignant melanoma unknown, but higher risk (up to 5-7%) in giant CMN

MICROSCOPIC PATHOLOGY

Histologic Features

- Symmetry
- Circumscription
  - Lesion starts in a nest (or theque) and ends in a nest
- Well-nested melanocytes at dermo-epidermal (DE) junction
- Maturation
  - Refers to dermal component (if present)
  - Melanocytes become smaller toward base of lesion
  - Melanocytes "disperse" and become less nested with more single cells at base of lesion
  - Type A cells epithelioid and at DE junction
  - Type B melanocytes lymphocytic with less cytoplasm, darker nuclei, and in mid-dermis
  - Type C melanocytes more spindled and in deep dermis
  - Blue nevi are an exception and typically do not mature
- No pigment in deep dermal melanocytic nests
  - Blue nevi are also an exception to this rule
- No deep mitoses
- Neurotized or spindled and s-shaped melanocytes that resemble nerve may be seen
- Melanocytic "giant" cells can be seen and are actually more common in benign melanocytic nevi
  - Atypical giant cells more often in melanoma
- Nuclear pseudoinclusions often present in melanocytes
  - Can occur in both malignant melanoma and benign melanocytic nevi
  - Feature most useful to differentiate melanocytic from nonmelanocytic tumors

Subtypes

- CMN
  - Type 1 or superficial congenital nevus
    - Most common, usually single lesion
    - Involves only 1 anatomic region
    - Cords, strands, nests, and single cells between collagen bundles in dermis and epidermis
    - Melanocytes do not infiltrate into deep fat and hypodermis
    - Melanoma rarely develops from it
  - Type 2 or deep congenital nevus
    - Much less common
    - Often multiple lesions with 1 larger "garment-like" lesion
    - Cords, strands, nests, sheets, and single cells between collagen bundles in dermis, epidermis, and deep subcutaneous structures
- Nevus of Ota/Ito
  - Blue patch present on face (Ota) or shoulder (Ito)
  - More common in Asians
  - Pigmentation often present at birth
    - Lesions may not become apparent until later
  - Histology
    - Dendritic spindle-shaped melanocytes scattered throughout dermis
    - Melanocytes often pigmented
    - Melanocytes often in upper 1/3 of dermis
- Mongolian spot
  - Related to nevus of Ota/Ito
  - Slate-colored patches usually in sacral region
  - Clinically may be mistaken as a sign of child abuse
  - More common in Asians
  - Present at birth or soon after
  - Histology
    - Widely scattered pigmented melanocytes in deep dermis (lower 1/2 vs. nevus of Ota/Ito)
    - Cells often spindle-shaped
- Halo nevus
  - Typically occurs in older children or young adults, on trunk
  - So named for clinical appearance of white halo around nevus
  - Histologically shows dense lichenoid infiltrate that may obscure melanocytes
    - Lesion otherwise shows benign features

MELANOCYTIC NEVUS

        - S100 stain can be helpful to identify melanocytes
    - Clinical diagnosis only because some nevi may show similar histology without "halo" appearance clinically
- Junctional lentiginous nevus
    - Proliferation of nests of melanocytes along sides and bases of rete ridges
    - Lacks dermal component
- Intradermal nevus
    - Melanocytic nests localized to dermis
    - Technically should not have epidermal involvement, but can be present focally
        - For this reason many prefer term "predominantly intradermal nevus"
- Compound nevus
    - Melanocytic nests involving both dermo-epidermal junction and dermis
- "Neural" or neurotized nevus
    - Lesions in which melanocytes may take on a neural appearance
    - Can mimic neurofibroma
    - Often only a focal change surrounded by more conventional melanocytes
- "Ancient" nevus
    - Nests surrounded by degenerated, hyalinized stroma
    - May have focal atypia that can resemble melanoma
    - Besides focal areas of cytologic atypia, same general features of a benign nevus
- Recurrent nevus (persistent nevus, pseudomelanoma)
    - Often resembles melanoma and is a major diagnostic pitfall for all pathologists
    - Nevus that has recurred after a previous excision
    - Melanocytes may be confluent, poorly nested, &/or irregularly nested
    - Key is identifying a scar below the lesion or soliciting clinical history of a previous biopsy
    - May see residual bland nevus underneath scar
- Spitz nevus (spindle and epithelioid cell nevus)
    - Benign nevi originally called "benign juvenile melanoma" by Dr. Sophie Spitz
    - Most commonly pink papule on face or scalp of child
    - Can occur in all ages
    - Histology
        - Symmetrical, well-nested proliferation of large spindled and epithelioid melanocytes
        - Sharp circumscription
        - Maturation with depth
        - Pagetoid spread of cells may be present in center of the lesion but should not be seen in the periphery
        - Kamino bodies often present
        - Cells have "2-tone" cytoplasm
    - Multiple variants including desmoplastic, halo, plexiform, atypical, and malignant or metastasizing (controversial)
- Pigmented spindle cell nevus (PSCN) of Reed
    - Considered by some to be a variant of Spitz nevus
    - Tight fascicles of heavily pigmented spindle cells with sharp circumscription
- Dysplastic or Clark nevus
    - May have cytologic atypia, which is graded at some institutions
    - Shoulder phenomenon in lesion
        - Epidermal component (nests or single melanocytes) extends beyond dermal component
        - Usually for 3 or more rete ridges
    - Concentric or lamellar fibroplasia just below nests in papillary dermis
        - Characteristic collagen deposition and eosinophilic fibrosis in superficial papillary dermis
    - Bridging of melanocytic nests
        - Melanocytic nests at bases of adjacent rete ridges touch
    - Single melanocytes may predominate at 1 edge
- Nevus of special site
    - Nevi in certain regions that show unusual histopathologic features
        - Includes anogenital, acral, ear, breast, scalp, flexural, umbilicus, ankle, and conjunctival areas
        - Nevi in pregnant patients can also show atypical features like increased basal melanocytes and increased mitotic activity
    - Unusual histologic features can include
        - Enlargement of junctional nests
        - Variability in size, shape, and position of nests
        - Pagetoid spread of melanocytes
        - Poor circumscription
        - Shouldering
        - Elongation and bridging of rete ridges
- Acral melanocytic nevus
    - Up to 1/3 will have pagetoid spread in center
    - Should not have pagetoid spread in periphery
    - Sections cut perpendicular to dermatoglyphics will aid in recognizing symmetry and circumscription in these often difficult lesions
- Balloon cell nevus
    - Large ballooned melanocytes with pale granular cytoplasm and central nucleus
    - Can be confused with other pale cell tumors such as renal cell carcinoma
        - Often more typical melanocytic nests also present
    - Ballooned change actually a degenerative feature
- Blue nevus
    - Spindle-shaped dendritic melanocytes in dermis
    - Often heavily pigmented with melanin
        - Often melanophages phagocytizing melanin
    - Exception to rules of no deep pigment in nests and no maturation with depth
    - Sclerosis of collagen common
    - Often combined with other melanocytic nevi
    - Deep penetrating nevus
        - Melanocytes have small hyperchromatic nuclei with a smudge chromatin pattern and inconspicuous nucleoli
        - Sharply demarcated nodule
        - Vertical orientation
        - Extends into fat
        - Can have nuclear pleomorphism
    - Epithelioid blue nevus
        - Melanocytes dispersed as single cells in collagen bundles (occasional fascicles)

- Intensely pigmented globular and fusiform melanocytes
- Sclerotic stroma lacking
- Associated with Carney complex
- Has tendency to be multiple
- In some cases referred to as superficial variant of deep penetrating nevus
- Considered by some to be low-grade melanoma (nodal metastases common but course is indolent)
- Cellular blue nevus
  - Densely packed, fusiform dendritic melanocytes with islands of plump epithelioid spindle cells (biphasic appearance)
  - Often little pigment
- Combined nevus
  - Combination of 2 or more populations of melanocytic nevi
  - Often contains an ordinary melanocytic nevus and a blue nevus variant
    - However, any combination can be present
- Speckled lentiginous nevus (nevus spilus)
  - Congenital light brown macules with small dark hyperpigmented speckles
  - Mainly clinical diagnosis
  - Lesions present at birth or in childhood
  - Histology shows features of lentigo or lentiginous nevus admixed with junctional or even small compound nests of melanocytes

DIFFERENTIAL DIAGNOSIS

Melanoma

- Asymmetrical
- Poorly circumscribed
- Pagetoid spread of single cells above dermo-epidermal junction
  - Especially at periphery of lesion
- Cytologic atypia and mitoses
- Lack of maturation

Simple Lentigo (Lentigo Simplex)

- Common brown macule of children or young adults
- Basal hyperpigmentation (may be variable)
- Unrelated to sun (no solar elastosis)
- Usually increased single melanocytes in basal layer
- Regular elongation of rete ridges
- No nests of melanocytes

Melanotic Macule

- May be labial, genital, areolar, conjunctival, or of nail bed or nail matrix
- Previously regarded as variant of simple lentigo
- Broad rete ridges with basal hyperpigmentation and slight increase in single melanocytes

Solar Lentigo

- Abnormal pigment retention of keratinocytes (keratinocytic lesion vs. simple lentigo)
- Uncommon in children (related to sun exposure, peak age 30-50)
  - May be seen in xeroderma pigmentosum
- Elongated, bulbous rete ridges with basal hyperpigmentation
  - Phenomenon often described as having appearance of "dirty feet" or "dirty socks"
- No nests of melanocytes but may have slight increase in single melanocytes

Café au Lait Spot or Macule (CALM)

- Common light brown round or oval macule
- Can be associated with neurofibromatosis type 1 (especially if 6 or more and all > 0.5 cm)
- Increased melanin in basal layer
- No elongation of rete ridges; no nests of melanocytes
- Normal number of "more active" melanocytes

Ephelis (Freckle)

- Very common red-brown macular lesions, often in fair-skinned patients
- Increased melanin in basal layer
- No elongation of rete ridges; no nests of melanocytes

DIAGNOSTIC CHECKLIST

Pathologic Interpretation Pearls

- Understanding histology of nevi of special sites and acral nevi is of paramount importance
- Proper recognition of Spitz nevi and subtypes can simplify difficult lesions
- Difficult lesions should be referred to experts

SELECTED REFERENCES

1. Murali R et al: Blue nevi and related lesions: a review highlighting atypical and newly described variants, distinguishing features and diagnostic pitfalls. Adv Anat Pathol. 16(6):365-82, 2009
2. Requena C et al: Spitz nevus: a clinicopathological study of 349 cases. Am J Dermatopathol. 31(2):107-16, 2009
3. Sinha S et al: Nevus of Ota in children. Cutis. 82(1):25-9, 2008
4. Tannous ZS et al: Congenital melanocytic nevi: clinical and histopathologic features, risk of melanoma, and clinical management. J Am Acad Dermatol. 52(2):197-203, 2005
5. Hurwitz RM et al: Superficial congenital compound melanocytic nevus. Another pitfall in the diagnosis of malignant melanoma. Dermatol Surg. 23(10):897-900, 1997
6. Boyd AS et al: Acral melanocytic neoplasms: a histologic analysis of 158 lesions. J Am Acad Dermatol. 31(5 Pt 1):740-5, 1994
7. Ackerman AB et al: Naming acquired melanocytic nevi. Common and dysplastic, normal and atypical, or Unna, Miescher, Spitz, and Clark? Am J Dermatopathol. 14(5):447-53, 1992
8. Clemmensen OJ et al: The histology of "congenital features" in early acquired melanocytic nevi. J Am Acad Dermatol. 19(4):742-6, 1988
9. Silvers DN et al: Melanocytic nevi in neonates. J Am Acad Dermatol. 4(2):166-75, 1981

Clinical and Morphologic Features

(Left) *In this well-demarcated steel blue nevus, the bluish tint comes from the deep-seated but benign nevus cells. (Courtesy K. Harris, MD.)* ***(Right)*** *A blue nevus shows heavily pigmented, spindled and dendritic melanocytes ⇨ traversing thickened collagen bundles ➡ in the dermis. Melanin is present deep in this lesion and is the one exception to the rule that benign nevi typically lack deep pigment. (Courtesy T. McCalmont, MD.)*

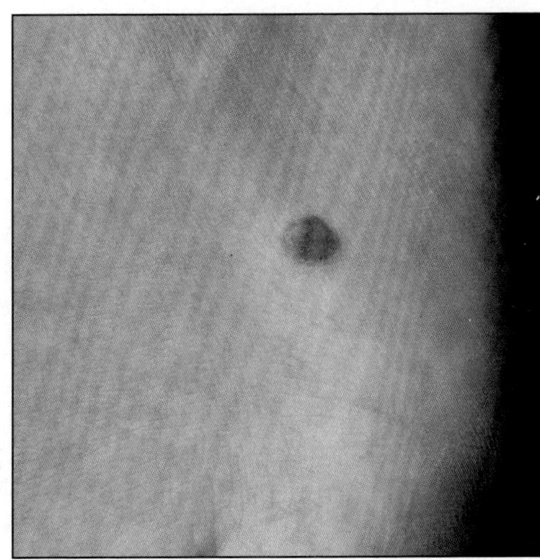

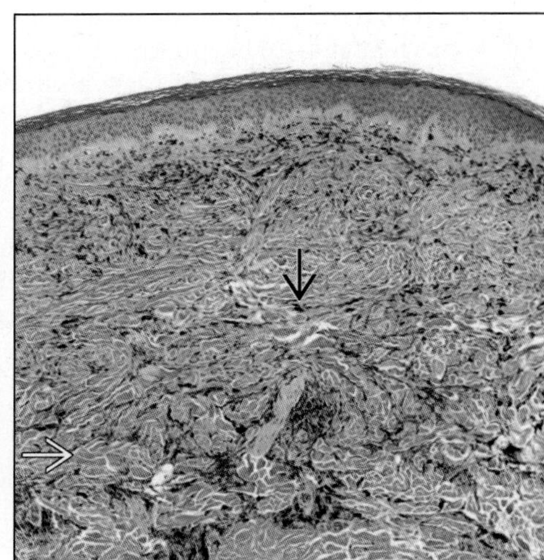

(Left) *This is a combined nevus. Most combined nevi are a combination of an ordinary nevus and a blue nevus variant.* ***(Right)*** *The histology of a combined nevus shows blue nevus cells that are spindled, heavily pigmented melanocytes outlined with melanin ⇨ admixed with a dermal nevus showing more typical melanocytic nests ↪. (Courtesy A. Bowen, MD.)*

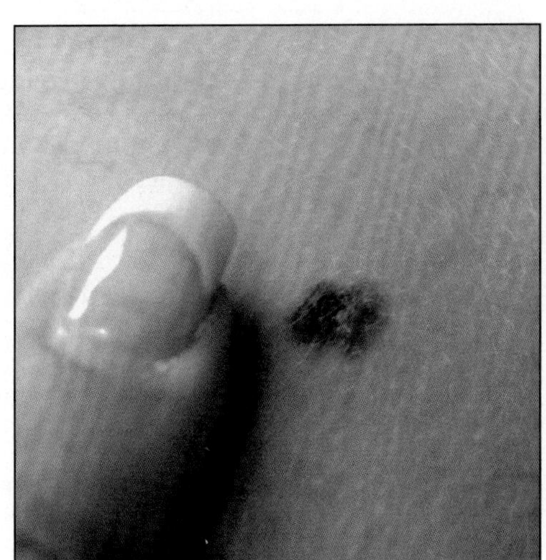

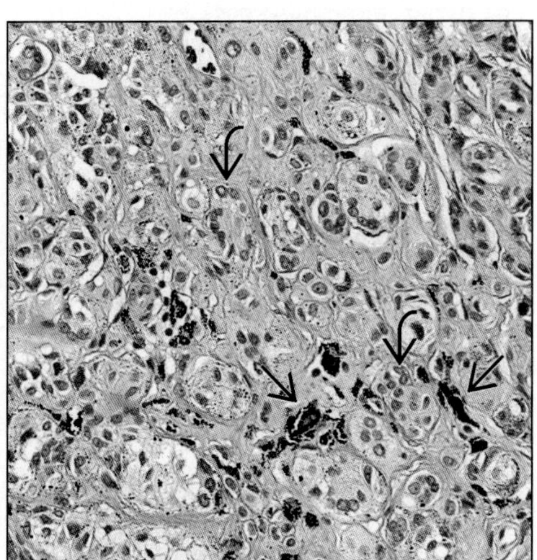

(Left) *This Spitz nevus ➡ (a subtype of MN) is dome-shaped, well demarcated, and brown-orange in color. These tumors are benign but can be very difficult to distinguish from a spitzoid malignant melanoma.* ***(Right)*** *The histology of a Spitz nevus shows prominent globoid, dull pink Kamino bodies ⇨ as well as spindled and epithelioid melanocytes ➡. (Courtesy C. Cockerell, MD.)*

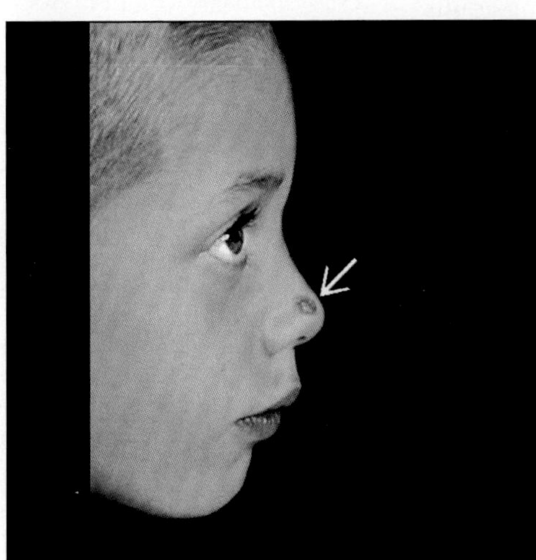

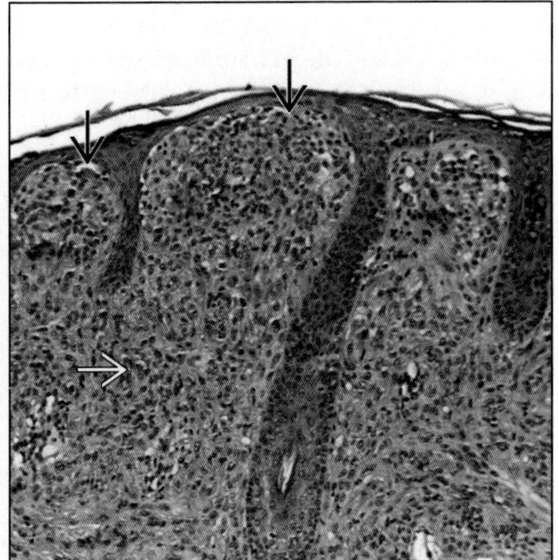

MELANOCYTIC NEVUS

Clinical and Variant Microscopic Features

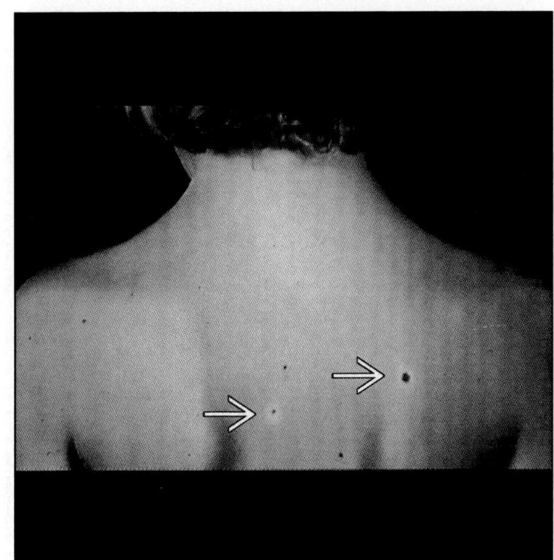

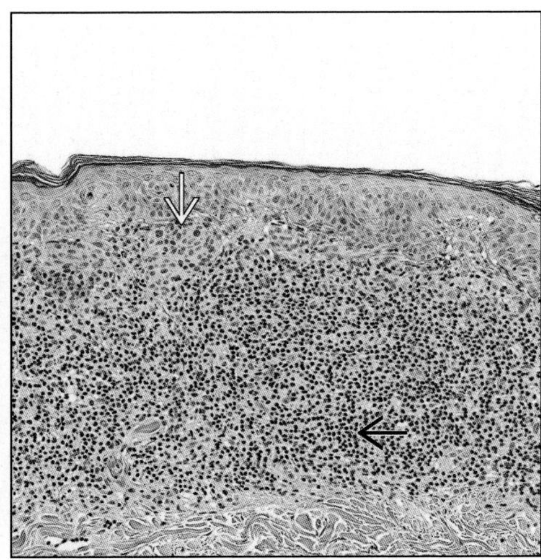

(Left) *Two halo nevi ➡ seen on the back of a young girl are oval, well demarcated, and depigmented. These areas do not indicate malignancy. With time, the white area may replace the nevus entirely and then it too may fade.* ***(Right)*** *The histology of a halo nevus shows a dense lymphoid infiltrate ⇨. It can sometimes be hard to see the melanocytes ➡ in these lesions. This should be signed out as consistent with halo nevus as it is truly a clinical diagnosis. (Courtesy R. Harris, MD.)*

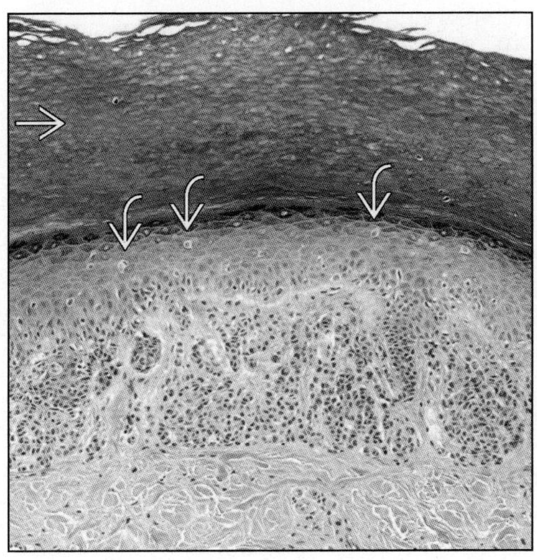

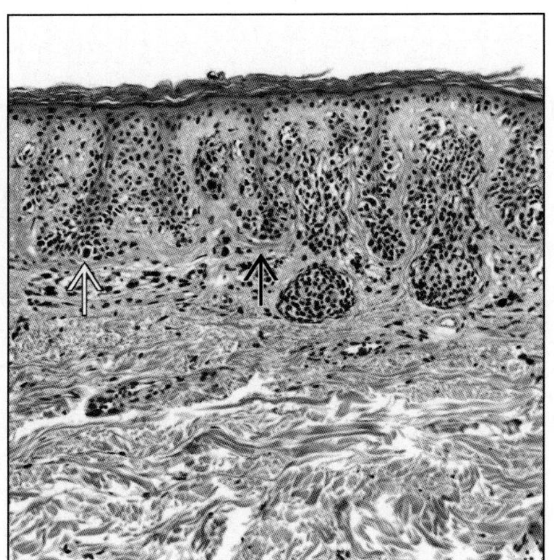

(Left) *Acral melanocytic nevi show hyperkeratosis ➡ characteristic of acral skin and pagetoid spread of single melanocytes ➡ in the center of the lesion, which is allowable at this special site. Pagetoid spread should not be present at the periphery, however. (Courtesy B. Ruben, MD.)* ***(Right)*** *Dysplastic nevi show characteristic prominent eosinophilic lamellar fibroplasia in the superficial papillary dermis ⇨ and some mild cytologic atypia ➡. (Courtesy G. Fraga, MD.)*

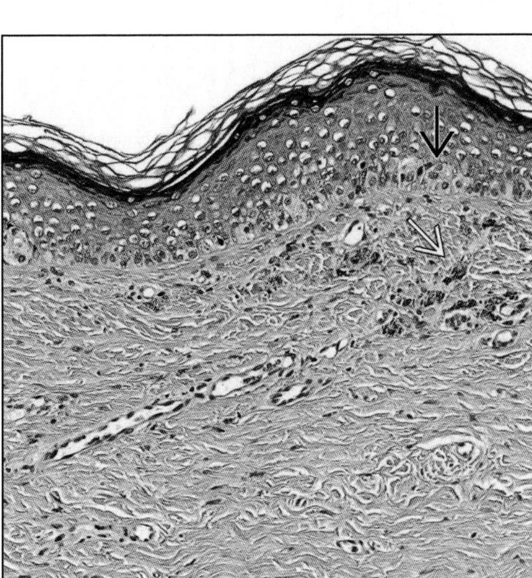

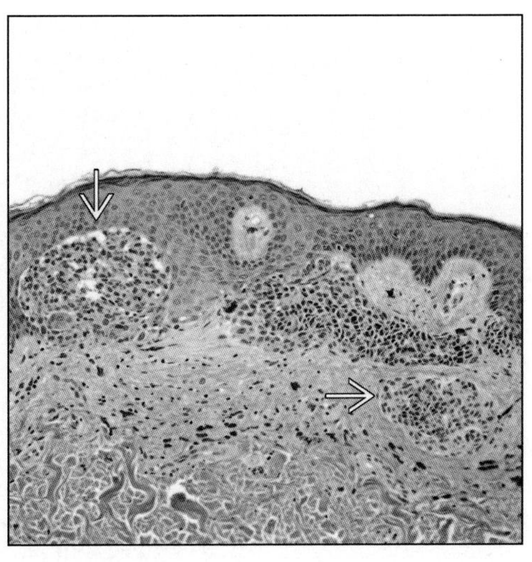

(Left) *Recurrent nevus or pseudomelanoma shows a predominance of single melanocytes at the basal layer ⇨ and prominent pigmented melanophages in the dermis ➡. A scar with vertically oriented vessels was evident deeper in this biopsy. (Courtesy S. Florell, MD.)* ***(Right)*** *This is a special site nevus from the vulva. These lesions can show an increase in the number of melanocytes ➡, larger melanocytes, asymmetry, pagetoid spread, or loss of cohesion. (Courtesy G. Fraga, MD.)*

SPITZ NEVUS

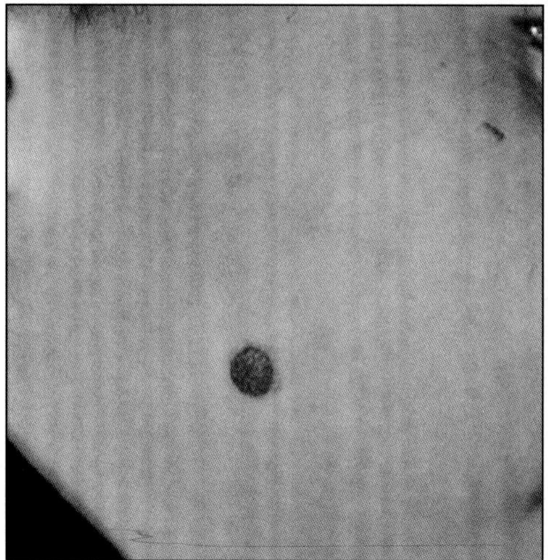

A pink papule on the face of a child is shown, typical of a Spitz nevus. (Courtesy S. Vanderhooft, MD.)

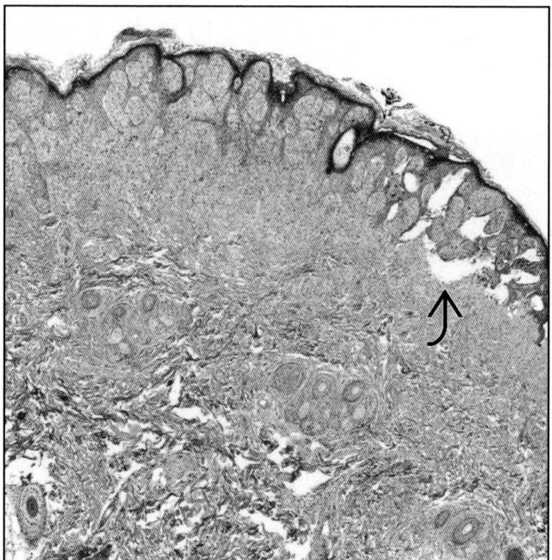

Hematoxylin & eosin at low power shows nests of spindled and epithelioid melanocytes at the dermal-epidermal junction and in the dermis. Note the symmetry and the clefting at the right ➔.

TERMINOLOGY

Synonyms

- Spindle and epithelioid cell nevus
- Spindle cell nevus
- Epithelioid cell nevus
- Nevus of large spindle &/or epithelioid cells
- Benign juvenile melanoma

CLINICAL ISSUES

Site

- Extremities, especially thigh
- Trunk
- Head and neck

Presentation

- Most common in children and young adults
  - 0.5-1% of all nevi in children and adolescents
  - May occur at all ages
- Solitary
  - Can be clustered or disseminated

Treatment

- Excision

Prognosis

- Benign
- Low recurrence rate, even after incomplete excision

MACROSCOPIC FEATURES

General Features

- Dome-shaped dermal nodule
- Pink or flesh-colored
- Often misdiagnosed clinically as hemangioma or pyogenic granuloma

Size

- Usually < 1 cm

MICROSCOPIC PATHOLOGY

Histologic Features

- Junctional, compound, and dermal forms
  - Most common type is compound with highly prominent dermal component
- Symmetric
  - Usually no lateral extension of junctional nests beyond dermal component
- Varying proportions of spindled and epithelioid melanocytes
  - Spindle cells much more common
  - Spindle cells only in ~ 45% of Spitz nevi
  - Spindle and epithelioid cells in ~ 35%
  - Epithelioid cells only in ~ 20%
  - Epithelioid cells usually dispersed individually throughout lesion
- Spindle cells are arranged in fascicles perpendicular to epidermis
- Kamino bodies
  - Eosinophilic globules at dermal-epidermal junction
  - Important diagnostic clue but may need step sections to find
  - PAS and trichrome positive
- Melanocytes "mature" by becoming smaller from superficial to deep
  - Deep melanocytes resemble ordinary nevus cells
  - Important clue for differentiating from melanoma
- Artifactual clefting of junctional nests from overlying epidermis
  - Commonly seen but may be present only focally
- Melanocytes taper to narrow point in deep dermis, forming upside-down triangle
- Small clusters of melanocytes can be seen in epidermis
  - Very rarely can see pagetoid spread of single melanocytes

SPITZ NEVUS

Key Facts

Clinical Issues

- Benign
- Most common in children and young adults
- Common site: Extremities, especially thigh
- Pink or flesh-colored, dome-shaped dermal nodule

Microscopic Pathology

- Junctional, compound, and dermal forms
  - Most common type is compound with highly prominent dermal component
- Symmetric
- Varying proportions of spindled and epithelioid melanocytes
  - Spindle cells much more common
  - Epithelioid cells usually dispersed individually throughout lesion
- Melanocytes "mature" by becoming smaller from superficial to deep
- Kamino bodies: Eosinophilic globules at dermal-epidermal junction
- Artifactual clefting of papillary dermal nests from overlying epidermis
- Can show atypical features
- Overall background of benignity

Top Differential Diagnoses

- More suspicious for malignant melanoma if
  - Patient > 10 years of age
  - Lesion > 1 cm
  - Ulceration present
  - Subcutis involvement

- Other unique features
  - Vascular and sometimes edematous stroma
  - Pseudoepitheliomatous hyperplasia
  - Giant nevus cells may be present and may be multinucleated
  - Lymphocytic infiltration sometimes seen
- Can show atypical features
  - Extreme cellular pleomorphism
  - Large, irregular nuclei
  - Prominent eosinophilic nucleoli
  - Nuclear pseudoinclusions
  - Typical mitoses
- Overall background of benignity
- **Atypical Spitz nevus**
  - Uncertain malignant potential
  - In continuum between typical Spitz nevus and Spitzoid melanoma
- **Halo Spitz nevus**
  - Nevus with depigmented rim
  - Heavy lymphocytic infiltrate with sparing of adjacent basal melanocytes
  - Often seen in combined Spitz and melanocytic nevus

Predominant Pattern/Injury Type

- Nested

Predominant Cell/Compartment Type

- Spindle and epithelioid

DIFFERENTIAL DIAGNOSIS

Malignant Melanoma

- Will show more coarse anaplastic nuclear features
- No "maturation" of melanocytes
- Asymmetry
- Marginal or atypical mitoses
- More suspicious for melanoma if
  - Patient > 10 years of age
  - Lesion > 1 cm
  - Ulceration present
  - Subcutis involvement

Melanocytic Nevus

- Will not have Kamino bodies or characteristic clefting

SELECTED REFERENCES

1. Pellacani G et al: Spitz nevi: In vivo confocal microscopic features, dermatoscopic aspects, histopathologic correlates, and diagnostic significance. J Am Acad Dermatol. 60(2):236-47, 2009
2. Requena C et al: Spitz nevus: a clinicopathological study of 349 cases. Am J Dermatopathol. 31(2):107-16, 2009
3. Situm M et al: Nevus Spitz--everlasting diagnostic difficulties--the review. Coll Antropol. 32 Suppl 2:171-6, 2008
4. Massi G: Melanocytic nevi simulant of melanoma with medicolegal relevance. Virchows Arch. 451(3):623-47, 2007
5. Schaffer JV: Pigmented lesions in children: when to worry. Curr Opin Pediatr. 19(4):430-40, 2007
6. Sulit DJ et al: Classic and atypical Spitz nevi: review of the literature. Cutis. 79(2):141-6, 2007
7. Mones JM et al: "Atypical" Spitz's nevus, "malignant" Spitz's nevus, and "metastasizing" Spitz's nevus: a critique in historical perspective of three concepts flawed fatally. Am J Dermatopathol. 26(4):310-33, 2004
8. Mooi WJ: Spitz nevus and its histologic simulators. Adv Anat Pathol. 9(4):209-21, 2002
9. Paniago-Pereira C et al: Nevus of large spindle and/ or epithelioid cells (Spitz's nevus). Arch Dermatol. 114(12):1811-23, 1978
10. Weedon D et al: Spindle and epithelioid cell nevi in children and adults. A review of 211 cases of the Spitz nevus. Cancer. 40(1):217-25, 1977
11. Allen AC et al: Histogenesis and clinicopathologic correlation of nevi and malignant melanomas; current status. AMA Arch Derm Syphilol. 69(2):150-71, 1954

SPITZ NEVUS

Microscopic Features

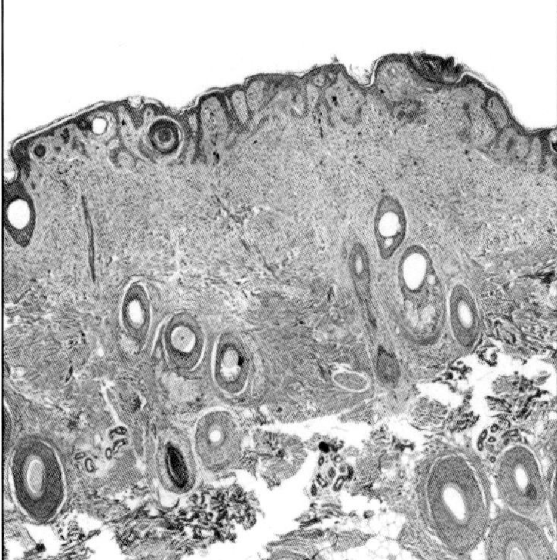

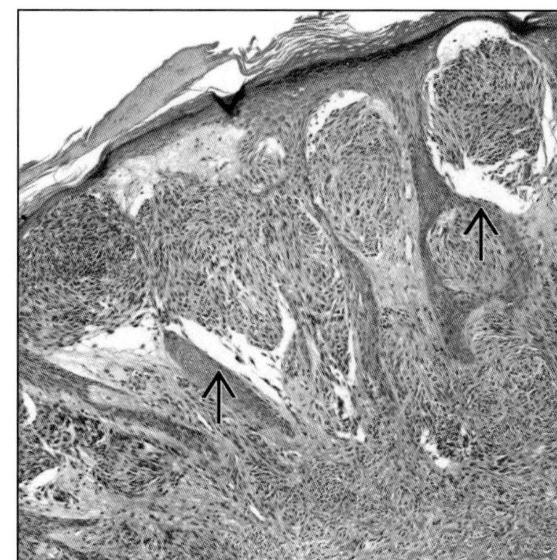

(Left) *Hematoxylin & eosin at low power shows spindled and epithelioid melanocytes, mostly in the dermis but also at the dermal-epidermal junction. Note the symmetry of this lesion and the vague "upside-down triangle" pattern.* ***(Right)*** *Hematoxylin & eosin at medium power shows the characteristic artifactual clefting that occurs between nests of spindled melanocytes and the overlying epidermis* →.

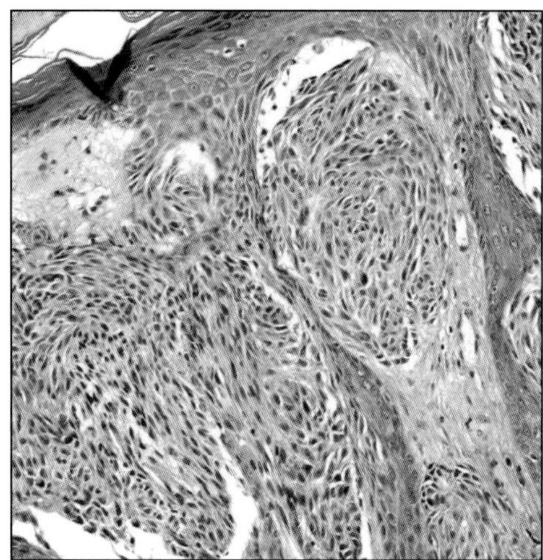

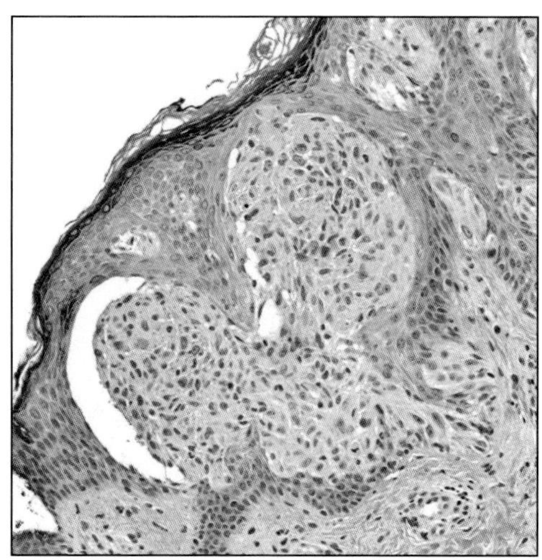

(Left) *Hematoxylin & eosin at high power shows the "vertical" arrangement of spindled melanocytes typically seen in Spitz nevus, along with the artifactual clefting of the melanocytic nests from the overlying epidermis.* ***(Right)*** *Hematoxylin & eosin at high power shows nests of predominantly epithelioid melanocytes in this Spitz nevus. Typical artifactual clefting is also seen at the left.*

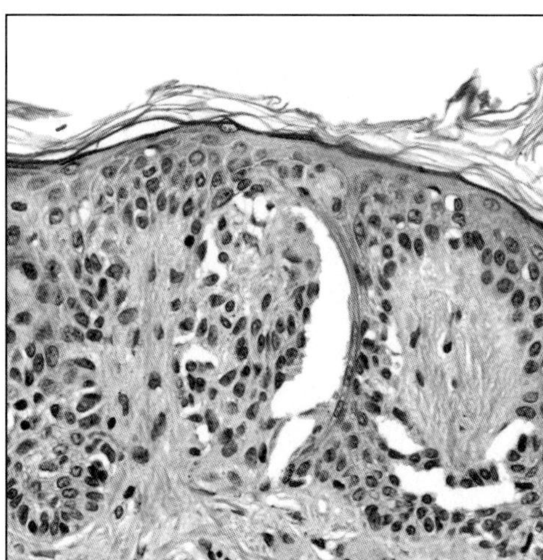

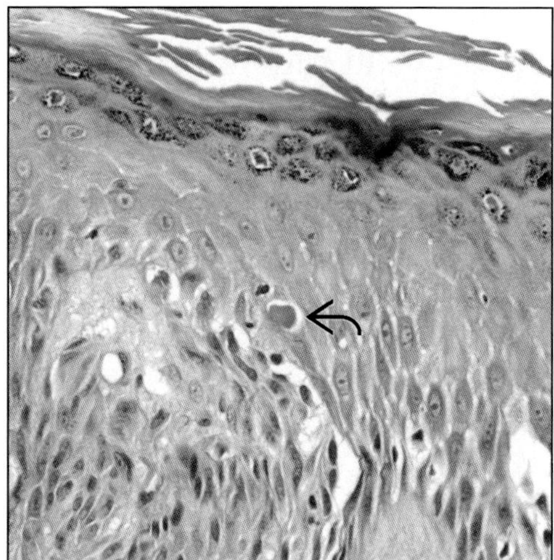

(Left) *Hematoxylin & eosin at high power shows a nest of melanocytes with a small artifactual cleft. While clefting is typical of a Spitz nevus, it is not always seen, or may only be present in focal areas.* ***(Right)*** *Hematoxylin & eosin at high power shows a Kamino body* ↗*, an eosinophilic globule found at the dermal-epidermal junction. These are typical of Spitz nevi but may be difficult to find.*

Microscopic Features

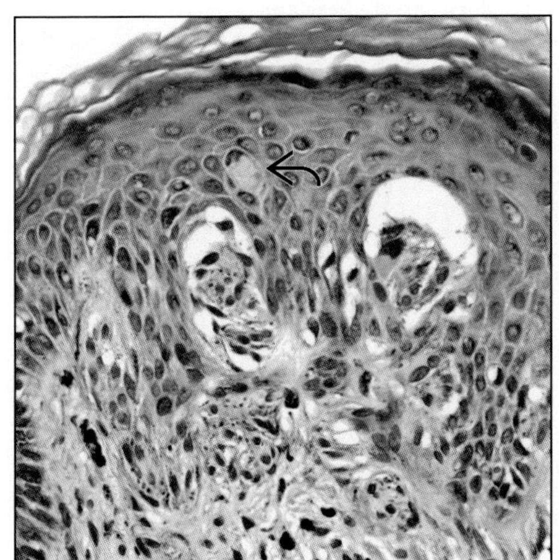
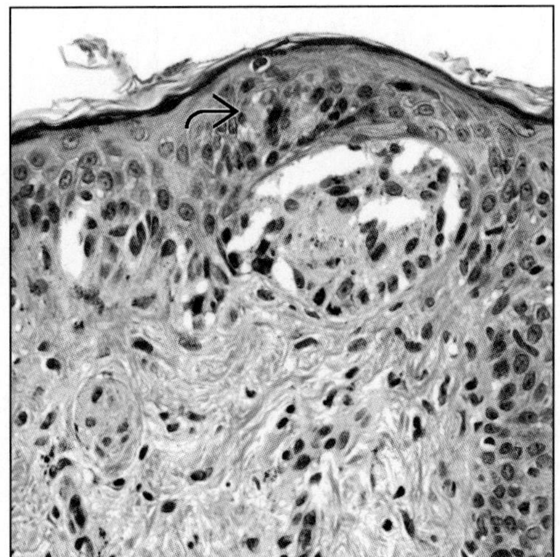

(Left) *Hematoxylin & eosin at high power shows small nests of epithelioid to spindled melanocytes with overlying artifactual clefting and a nearby Kamino body* ➩. ***(Right)*** *Hematoxylin & eosin at high power shows small nests of epithelioid melanocytes with clefting and a Kamino body* ➩. *Kamino bodies sometimes require step-sections to find.*

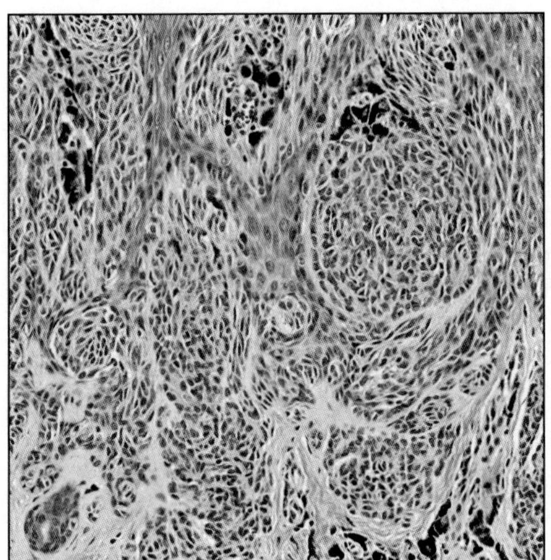
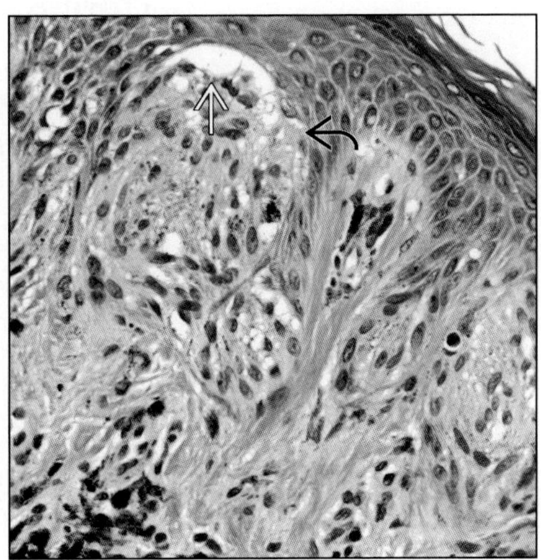

(Left) *Hematoxylin & eosin at medium power shows nests of spindled melanocytes at the dermal-epidermal junction (top), which become smaller as they go deeper into the dermis. This is the "maturation" of melanocytes that is an important feature in distinguishing from melanoma.* ***(Right)*** *Hematoxylin & eosin at high power shows small nests of epithelioid melanocytes with a small overlying cleft* ➔ *and a Kamino body* ➩.

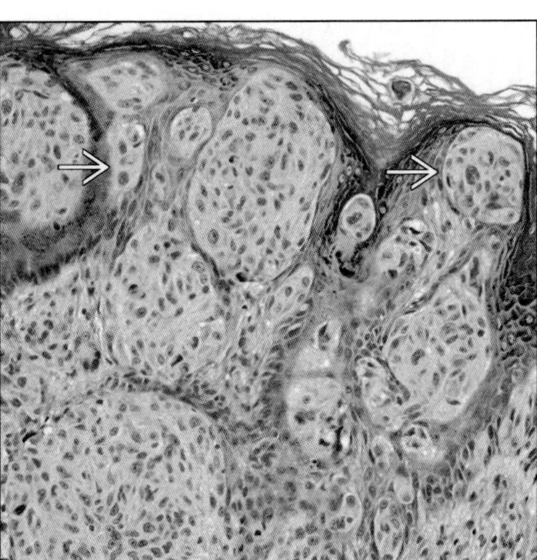
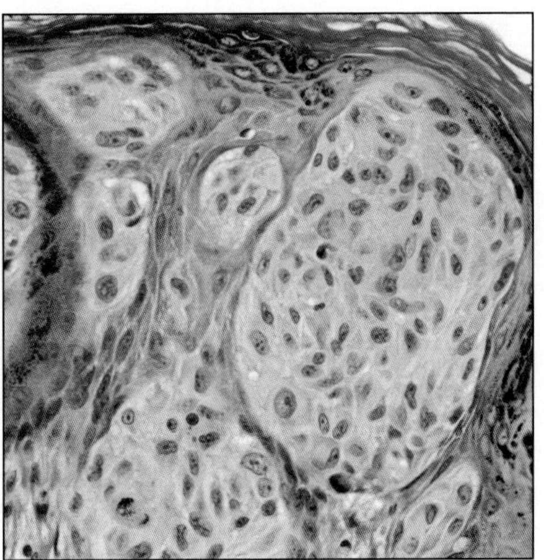

(Left) *Hematoxylin & eosin at medium power shows nests of epithelioid melanocytes at the dermal-epidermal junction and within the epidermis (transepidermal elimination)* ➔. *While nests of nevus cells within the epidermis are acceptable, individual cells would make the lesion suspicious for melanoma.* ***(Right)*** *Hematoxylin & eosin at high power shows epithelioid melanocytes at the dermal-epidermal junction and within the epidermis.*

BLUE NEVUS

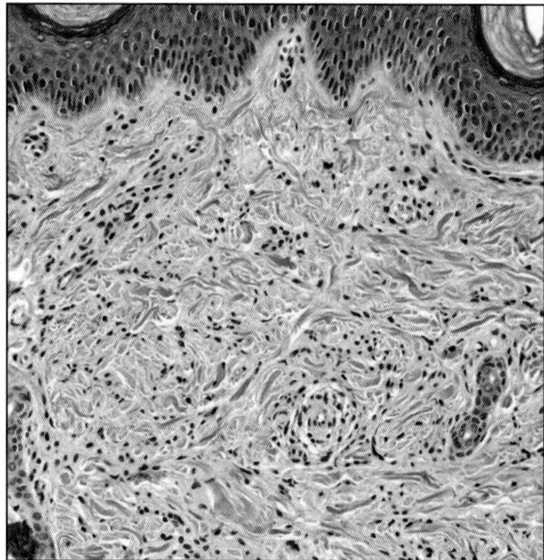

Hematoxylin & eosin at medium power shows a common blue nevus characterized by dendritic, dusty-gray melanocytes dissecting through collagen bundles in the reticular dermis.

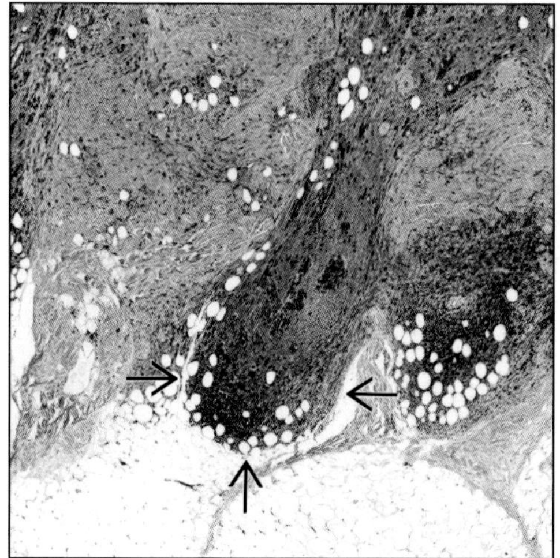

Hematoxylin & eosin at low power shows a cellular blue nevus with characteristic nodular downgrowth into the subcutaneous fat ⇒.

TERMINOLOGY

Synonyms

- Tièche nevus

Definitions

- Common blue-black papule or nodule characterized by heavy pigmentation and spindled dendritic melanocytes within dermis

CLINICAL ISSUES

Site

- **Common blue nevus**
  - Most commonly found on extremities
    - Especially dorsum of hands and feet
- **Cellular blue nevus**
  - Buttocks
  - Low back
  - Scalp
  - Extremities
- **Epithelioid blue nevus**
  - Similar to common blue nevus

Presentation

- **Common blue nevus**
  - Slate-blue to blue-black macule or papule
  - Small (< 1 cm)
  - Acquired lesion; therefore, more common in adults
- **Cellular blue nevus**
  - Bluish dermal nodule or plaque
  - Large (> 1.5 cm)
- **Epithelioid blue nevus**
  - Clinically resembles common blue nevus
  - Tends to be multiple
  - Associated with Carney complex

Treatment

- Simple excision

Prognosis

- Benign
- Only rarely recurs

MICROSCOPIC PATHOLOGY

Histologic Features

- **Common blue nevus**
  - Elongated, delicate, sometimes branching melanocytes dissect through dermal collagen in reticular dermis
  - Melanocytes are often periadnexal
  - Variable numbers of melanophages
  - Pigment can be so heavy as to obscure melanocytes, although some are amelanotic
  - May have dermal fibrosis (sclerosing blue nevus)
  - May have overlying melanocytic or Spitz nevus
- **Cellular blue nevus**
  - Well-circumscribed cellular lesion
  - Fascicles of dendritic melanocytes, plump spindled cells, and epithelioid cells
  - Usually little pigment but can be heavily pigmented
  - Melanophages present between cellular islands
  - Tumor bulges into subcutaneous fat in characteristic nodular downgrowth
  - Can have cytologic atypia and typical mitoses
  - May have stromal desmoplasia (desmoplastic blue nevus)
- **Epithelioid blue nevus**
  - Intensely pigmented globular and fusiform cells mixed with spindle cells
  - Melanocytes scattered singly among collagen bundles, with occasional fascicles
  - Often part of combined nevus
- **Malignant blue nevus**
  - Very rare
  - Usually middle-aged to elderly, but childhood cases reported
  - Poorly circumscribed nodule

BLUE NEVUS

Key Facts

Clinical Issues

- Common blue nevus is small slate-blue to blue-black macule on extremities
- Cellular blue nevus is larger nodule on buttocks, low back, scalp, or extremities
- Epithelioid blue nevus tends to be multiple and is associated with Carney complex

Microscopic Pathology

- Common blue nevus
  - Elongated melanocytes among dermal collagen in mid and upper dermis
  - Variable numbers of melanophages
- Cellular blue nevus
  - Tumor bulges into subcutaneous fat in characteristic nodular downgrowth
- Epithelioid blue nevus
  - Often part of combined nevus

  - Cytologic features of malignancy, including atypical mitoses

ANCILLARY TESTS

Immunohistochemistry

- Melanocytes in all blue nevi stain positively for
  - S100
  - Melan-A
  - HMB-45

DIFFERENTIAL DIAGNOSIS

Dermatofibroma

- In the differential for cellular blue nevus, along with other spindle cell tumors
- Close examination of cellular blue nevus would show dermal melanocytes
  - Immunohistochemistry can help highlight melanocytes

Deep Penetrating Nevus

- Epithelioid blue nevus has melanocytes singly dispersed

Blue Nevus-like Metastatic Melanoma

- Very rare; need history of previous melanoma in same anatomic region
- Melanoma would have atypical melanocytes and mitoses
- Melanoma may have inflammatory reaction that blue nevus would not

SELECTED REFERENCES

1. Martin RC et al: So-called "malignant blue nevus": a clinicopathologic study of 23 patients. Cancer. 115(13):2949-55, 2009
2. Piana S et al: Cellular blue nevus with satellitosis: a possible diagnostic pitfall. Am J Dermatopathol. 31(4):401-2, 2009
3. Cerroni L et al: "Ancient" blue nevi (cellular blue nevi with degenerative stromal changes). Am J Dermatopathol. 30(1):1-5, 2008
4. Bogart MM et al: Blue nevi: a case report and review of the literature. Cutis. 80(1):42-4, 2007
5. King R et al: Primary invasive melanoma and basal cell carcinoma (collision tumor) with blue nevus-like cutaneous metastases. J Cutan Pathol. 34(8):629-33, 2007
6. Mones JM et al: "Atypical" blue nevus, "malignant" blue nevus, and "metastasizing" blue nevus: a critique in historical perspective of three concepts flawed fatally. Am J Dermatopathol. 26(5):407-30, 2004
7. Carney JA et al: Epithelioid blue nevus and psammomatous melanotic schwannoma: the unusual pigmented skin tumors of the Carney complex. Semin Diagn Pathol. 15(3):216-24, 1998

IMAGE GALLERY

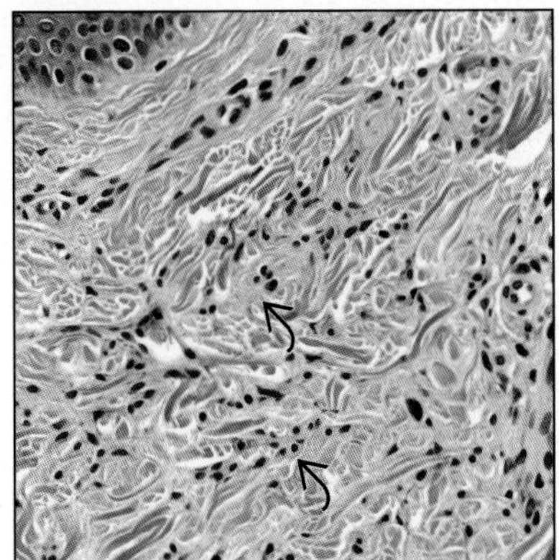

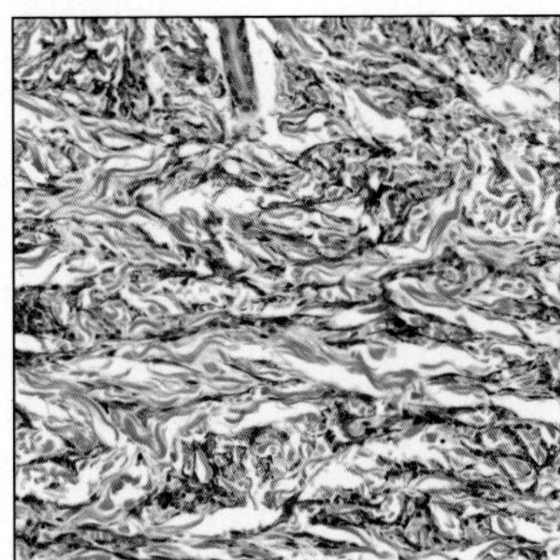

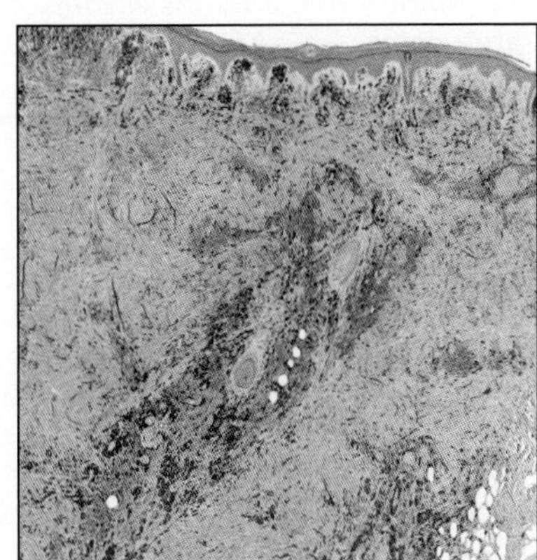

*(**Left**) High power shows dendritic melanocytes with dusty gray cytoplasm ⮳ dissecting through collagen bundles in this common blue nevus. A small amount of pigment is present. (**Center**) Some common blue nevi are heavily pigmented. (**Right**) Low power of this cellular blue nevus highlights the periadnexal distribution of the melanocytes and melanophages. Individual melanocytes can still be seen dissecting through the collagen bundles away from the larger nests.*

EPIDERMAL NEVUS

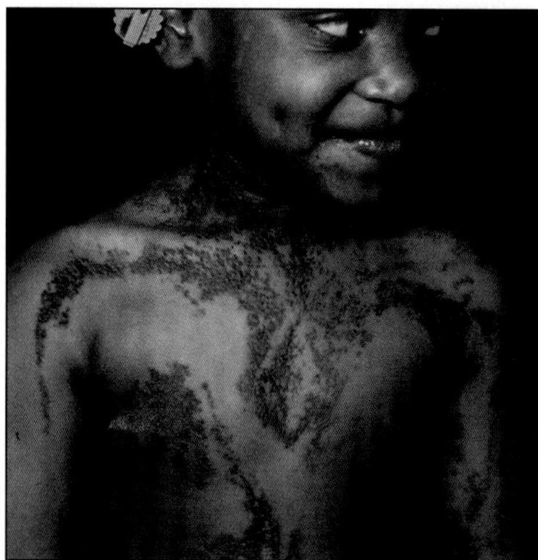

Whorls of keratotic, hyperpigmented, verrucous skin indicate systematized epidermal nevus. Note that lesions follow lines of Blaschko. A single lesion or linear epidermal nevus is actually the more common clinical presentation.

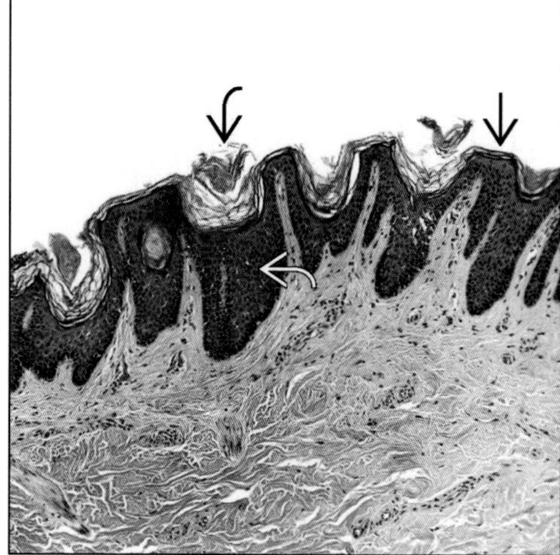

Epidermal nevus demonstrates broad and flat papillomatosis ➔, hyperkeratosis ➔, acanthosis ➔, and mild dermal inflammation. (Courtesy C. Cockerell, MD.)

TERMINOLOGY

Abbreviations

- Epidermal nevus (EN)
- Inflammatory linear verrucous epidermal nevus (ILVEN) syndrome
  - Most consider ILVEN a distinct subgroup

Definitions

- Congenital hamartoma of proliferating epidermis
- Linear epidermal nevus or nevus unius lateralis occurs on 1 side of body
- Systematized epidermal nevi or ichthyosis hystrix are less common, appear on 1 or both sides of body, and are multiple in number
- There are distinct syndromes called "epidermal nevus syndromes"
  - Include linear sebaceous, linear nevus comedonicus (NC), linear epidermal nevus (LEN), and ILVEN
  - Somewhat poorly defined and confusing

ETIOLOGY/PATHOGENESIS

Developmental Anomaly

- Malformation of epidermis with excess of keratinocytes

CLINICAL ISSUES

Epidemiology

- Incidence
  - 1 in 1,000 live births
- Age
  - Presents at birth or early childhood
- Gender
  - Generally 1:1
    - Exception is ILVEN (M:F = 1:4)

Site

- Usually on extremities, trunk, or neck
- ILVEN: Lower extremities along lines of Blaschko

Presentation

- Tan to brown verrucous linear plaques noted at birth or early childhood

Treatment

- Mainly only used for cosmetic purposes
  - Can include laser therapy or surgical excision

Prognosis

- Generally excellent
- Epidermal nevi do persist indefinitely
- Rarely, various tumors reported arising in EN
  - Include basal cell carcinoma (BCC), squamous cell carcinoma (SCC), and keratoacanthoma (KA)

Disease Associations

- Estimated 1/3 will have other organ systems involved
  - Several syndromes are associated with EN
    - CHILD, Proteus, sebaceous nevus, nevus comedonicus, phakomatosis pigmentokeratotica, Becker nevus, and Schimmelpenning syndromes
  - Associated neurological, ocular, and skeletal abnormalities
    - Epilepsy, learning disabilities, rickets, arrhythmias, cataracts, kyphoscoliosis, limb hypertrophy
  - Cutaneous hemangiomas may also be present
  - Morbidity and mortality are related to associated abnormalities and not EN itself

MICROSCOPIC PATHOLOGY

Histologic Features

- At least 10 histologic patterns have been described
- More than 1 pattern can be present in a single lesion
- 3 features present in most lesions

Key Facts

Terminology

- Congenital hamartoma of proliferating epidermis

Clinical Issues

- Several associated syndromes with neurological, ocular, and skeletal abnormalities
- Also distinct epidermal nevus syndromes
  - Linear sebaceous, linear nevus comedonicus (NC), linear epidermal nevus (LEN), and ILVEN

Microscopic Pathology

- At least 10 histologic patterns have been described
- More than 1 pattern can be present in a single lesion
- 3 features present in most lesions
  - Hyperkeratosis, papillomatosis, acanthosis
- ILVEN considered a distinct subgroup
  - Psoriasiform epidermal hyperplasia with alternating ortho- and parakeratosis

---

  - Hyperkeratosis, papillomatosis that is usually flat and broad, acanthosis
- Often hypergranulosis, basal layer hyperpigmentation

Subtypes

- ILVEN
  - Linear persistent pruritic plaque usually on lower extremities
  - Histology
    - Psoriasiform epidermal hyperplasia
    - Alternating areas of orthokeratosis and parakeratosis
    - Parakeratotic areas often have hypogranulosis
    - Orthokeratotic areas often have hypergranulosis
    - Zones of parakeratosis broader than in psoriasis
    - Mild perivascular infiltrate in the upper dermis
- Linear sebaceous nevus (organoid nevus syndrome)
  - Sebaceous nevi and cerebral anomalies
- Linear nevus comedonicus (NC)
  - Cataracts may be prominent feature
- Linear epidermal nevus (LEN) syndrome
  - Nervous, ophthalmologic, &/or skeletal findings often also present
  - Mental retardation, seizures, and movement disorders

DIFFERENTIAL DIAGNOSIS

Seborrheic Keratosis

- May look histologically identical to EN
- Not seen in children (adult onset)

Lichen Striatus

- Not present at birth (usually)
- Less hyperkeratosis and acanthosis
- Spongiosis, dyskeratosis, and more lichenoid and perifollicular inflammation

Acanthosis Nigricans (AN)

- Characteristic clinical location (axilla and neck) and appearance (symmetric, pigmented, velvety plaques)
- Despite the name, there is only mild to minimal acanthosis (sometimes absent)

Psoriasis

- Zones of parakeratosis less broad
- No alternating orthokeratosis and parakeratosis

Confluent and Reticulated Papillomatosis of Gougerot and Carteaud (CRP)

- Considered a variant of AN by some or closely related
- Undulating hyperkeratosis and acanthosis in between (in the valleys of) papillomatous areas

SELECTED REFERENCES

1. Happle R: Gustav Schimmelpenning and the syndrome bearing his name. Dermatology. 209(2):84-7, 2004
2. Vidaurri-de la Cruz H et al: Epidermal nevus syndromes: clinical findings in 35 patients. Pediatr Dermatol. 21(4):432-9, 2004
3. Mall V et al: CNS lipoma in patients with epidermal nevus syndrome. Neuropediatrics. 31(4):175-9, 2000

DIFFERENTIAL DIAGNOSIS

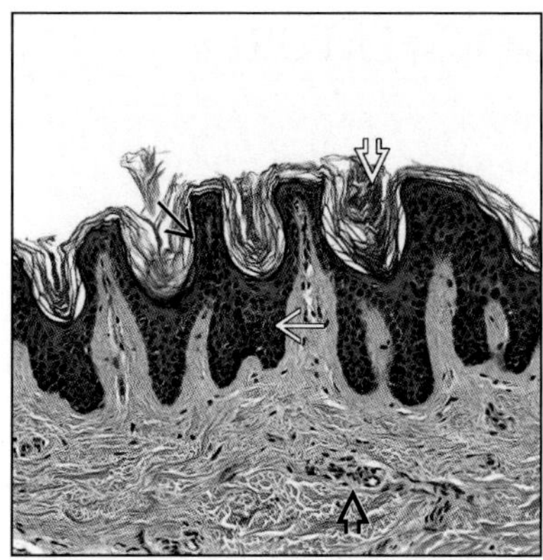

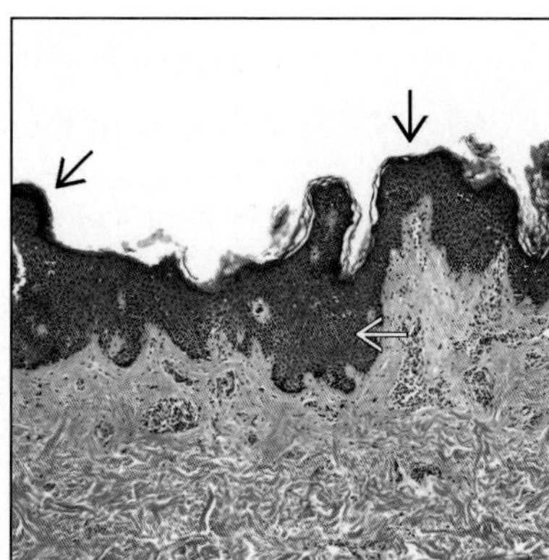

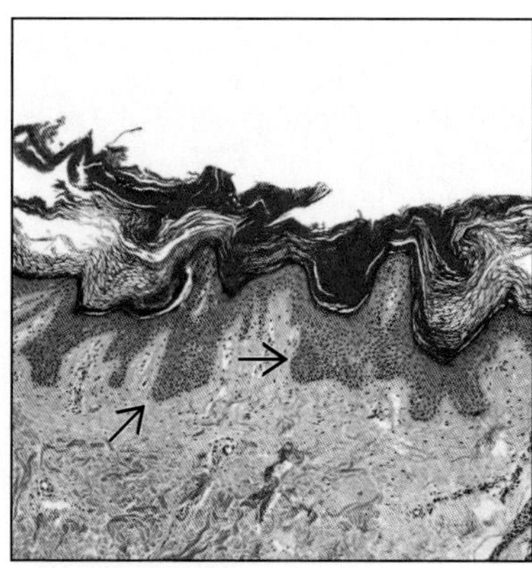

(Left) *Epidermal nevus shows papillomatosis ⇒, acanthosis ➡, hyperkeratosis ➡, and perivascular lymphocytes ⇒. (Courtesy C. Cockerell, MD.)* ***(Center)*** *Confluent and reticulated papillomatosis is shown. Note the acanthosis ➡ present in the valley between papillomatosis ⇒. (Courtesy G. Fraga, MD.)* ***(Right)*** *Acanthosis nigricans is shown. This lesion can look very similar to epidermal nevus, although there is usually no dermal inflammation and milder acanthosis ⇒. (Courtesy G. Fraga, MD.)*

VERRUCA VULGARIS

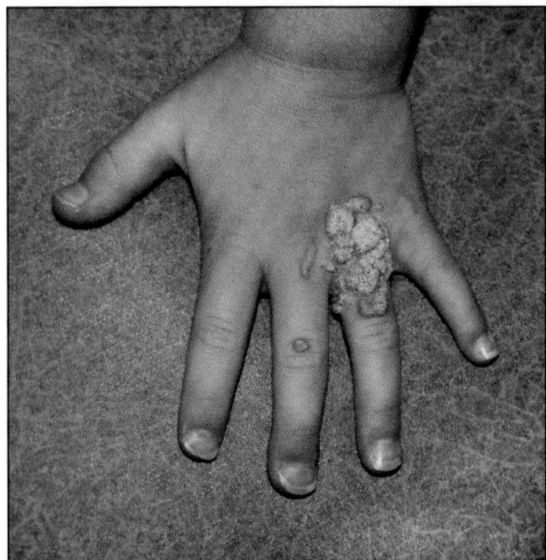

Verrucae vulgaris occur predominantly on dorsal surface of the hands. Multiple, rough-surfaced papules are pictured here. Multiple single lesions may coalesce into larger plaque-like lesions. (Courtesy S. Vanderhooft, MD.)

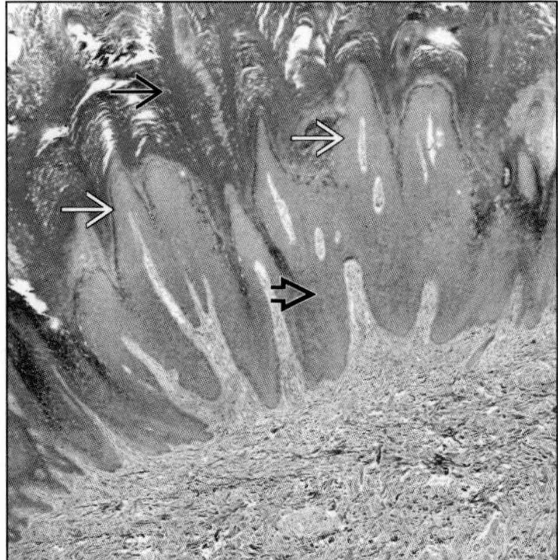

Note the hyperkeratosis ⇒, acanthosis ⇒, and marked papillomatosis ➡ (sometimes described as "church spire" papillomatosis) in this verruca vulgaris. Most lesions show few or no dermal changes.

TERMINOLOGY

Synonyms

- Common wart

Definitions

- Common viral infection of the skin and mucosa caused by human papillomavirus

ETIOLOGY/PATHOGENESIS

Infectious Agents

- Associated with HPV-2
  - Also induced by HPV-1, HPV-4, HPV-7
    - Extensive verrucae can be seen in immunodeficiency syndromes
    - HPV-75, HPV-76, HPV-77 are seen in immunosuppressed patients regardless of age
- Transmission via
  - Skin-to-skin contact
  - Fomites
    - Recently shed viruses can survive in a warm, moist environment
    - Locker room floors, showers, etc.
- Entry site
  - Subclinical abrasion
  - Area of recent trauma
- Incubation period
  - 1-6 months
- Majority of lesions involute spontaneously within 2 years

CLINICAL ISSUES

Presentation

- Seen predominantly in children and adolescents
  - Incidence is estimated at 10%
- Can be solitary or multiple
- Found on exposed parts of skin
  - Most frequently
    - Finger
    - Dorsal surface of hands
    - Subungual or periungual
  - Filiform warts are typically seen on lips, nose, or eyelids
- Koebner phenomenon
  - New wart that forms at the site of trauma
  - Linear group of warts develop along a path of excoriation

Treatment

- Watchful waiting
- Topical salicylic acid
- Cryotherapy
- Manual paring or filing
- Oral or topical immunotherapy

Prognosis

- Frequently self-involute over years
- Inadvertent autoinoculation
- Immunity to warts is not well understood
  - Inducing inflammation around 1 wart can induce others to regress

MACROSCOPIC FEATURES

General Features

- Rough-surfaced papules
- Flesh-colored
- Variable size
- Exophytic
- Filiform
  - Warts appear as spiny projection from the skin surface with a narrow stalk

VERRUCA VULGARIS

Key Facts

Terminology

- Common viral infection of the skin and mucosa caused by human papillomavirus

Etiology/Pathogenesis

- Transmission via fomites or skin-to-skin contact
- Majority of lesions involute spontaneously within 2 years

Microscopic Pathology

- Marked hyperkeratosis and acanthosis
- Elongated rete ridges
- Columns of parakeratosis are directly above the papillomatous projections
- Granular layer is lacking at the tips of the papillomas but is thickened in other areas
- Dilated vessels extend into core of papillomatous projections

MICROSCOPIC PATHOLOGY

Histologic Features

- Marked hyperkeratosis and acanthosis
- Elongated rete ridges
  - Rete ridges turn inward at edge of lesion
- Variable papillomatosis
  - Epidermis can have a serrated appearance
  - Also described as "church spire" papillomatosis
  - Columns of parakeratosis are directly above the papillomatous projections
  - Hemosiderin and extravasated red blood cells may be seen in stratum corneum
  - Granular layer is lacking at the tips of papillomas but is thickened in other areas
  - Keratohyaline granules are present in granular layer
- Koilocytes
  - Not present in older lesions
- Nuclei may be vacuolated
- Dilated vessels extend into core of papillomatous projections
- Few other dermal changes
  - Lymphocytic infiltrate can be seen in upper dermis

DIFFERENTIAL DIAGNOSIS

Epidermal Nevus

- Present since birth or early childhood
- Hamartomatous verrucous epidermal growth

Nevus Sebaceous of Jadassohn

- Associated with underlying malformed adnexal structures

Verruca Plana

- Has plate-like configuration

Verruca Plantaris

- Plantar form
- Invaginated rather than exophytic

Condyloma Acuminatum

- Irregularly acanthotic sessile growth
- Perineal region

SELECTED REFERENCES

1. Bruggink SC et al: Cryotherapy with liquid nitrogen versus topical salicylic acid application for cutaneous warts in primary care: randomized controlled trial. CMAJ. 182(15):1624-30, 2010
2. Faghihi G et al: A double-blind, randomized trial of local formic acid puncture technique in the treatment of common warts. Skinmed. 8(2):70-1, 2010
3. Syrjänen S: Current concepts on human papillomavirus infections in children. APMIS. 118(6-7):494-509, 2010

IMAGE GALLERY

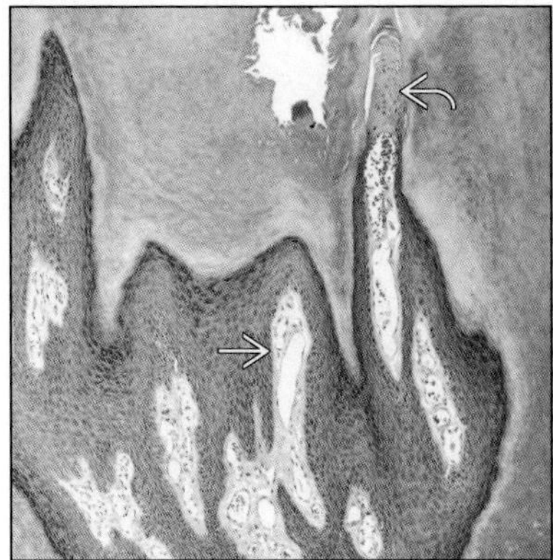

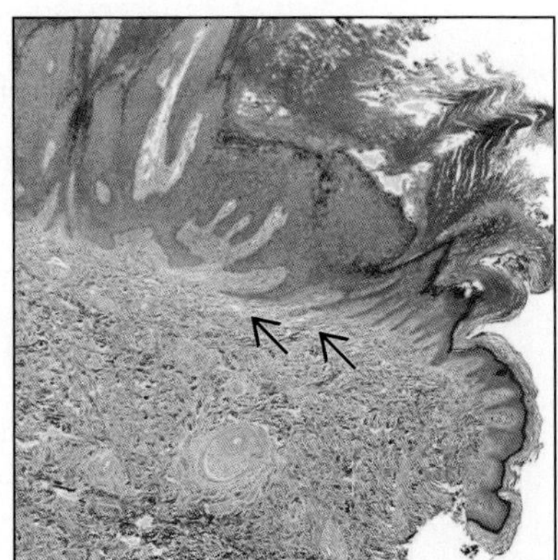

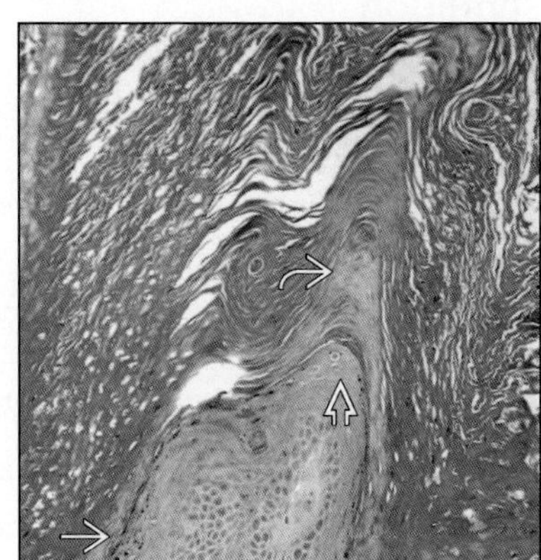

(Left) *Most warts show few changes in the dermis; however, dilated vessels ➔ do extend into the cores of the papillomatous projections. Note the parakeratosis ➔.* ***(Center)*** *This common wart shows acanthosis and papillomatosis. Note the inward turning ➔ of the elongated rete ridges at the edge of the lesion. This is a characteristic finding.* ***(Right)*** *Columns of parakeratosis ➔ overlie the tips of the papillomatous projections. The granular layer is lacking in this area ➔ but is prominent elsewhere ➔.*

EPIDERMODYSPLASIA VERRUCIFORMIS

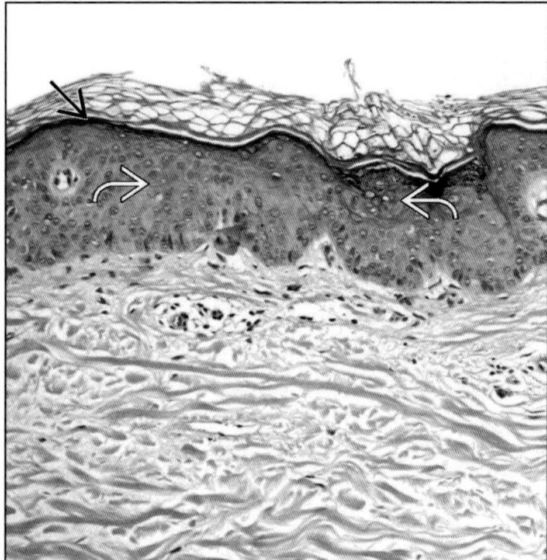

EDV is characterized by irregular epidermal acanthosis associated with an intraepidermal proliferation of enlarged, bluish-gray staining keratinocytes ➨. Note the overlying hypergranulosis ➔.

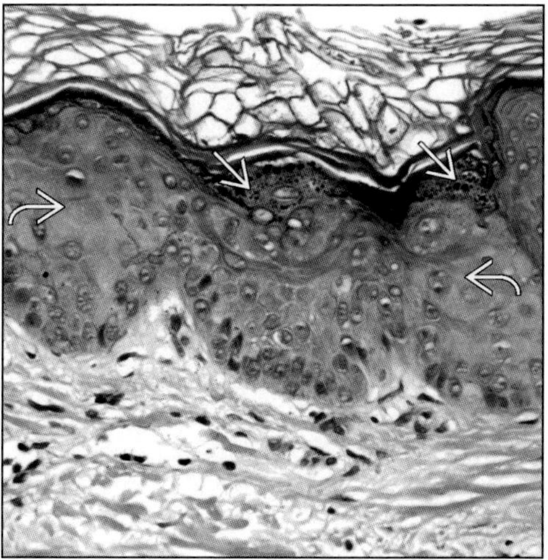

Higher magnification of EDV shows a proliferation of enlarged, bluish-gray staining keratinocytes ➨ with prominent keratohyaline granules ➔.

TERMINOLOGY

Abbreviations

- Epidermodysplasia verruciformis (EDV)

Definitions

- HPV-related intraepidermal proliferation of enlarged, often bluish-gray staining keratinocytes

ETIOLOGY/PATHOGENESIS

Infectious Agents

- HPV infection is established as etiologic agent
- Subtypes implicated include HPV-3, -5, -8, -9, -10, -12

Genetic Condition

- Majority of cases are familial (genodermatosis)
- Inherited mutations in *EVER1/TMC6* or *EVER2/TMC8* lead to susceptibility to infections with HPV
  - Increased risk for development of in situ and invasive squamous cell carcinoma (SCC)

CLINICAL ISSUES

Presentation

- Scaly papules or plaques

Treatment

- Options, risks, complications
  - As most cases are benign, aggressive treatment not usually indicated
  - Radiotherapy reported to increase risk for malignant transformation and should be avoided
- Surgical approaches
  - Excision may be considered in patients considered at higher risk for SCC
- Drugs
  - Topical antivirals (similar to those used for verruca vulgaris) may be used
  - Liquid nitrogen (cryotherapy) is usually effective

Prognosis

- Risk for malignant transformation increased in genetic forms
- Up to 25-50% of patients may eventually develop in situ or invasive SCC

MICROSCOPIC PATHOLOGY

Histologic Features

- Epidermal acanthosis with expansion of epidermis by enlarged, mildly atypical-appearing cells
- Cells typically show abundant bluish-gray staining cytoplasm
- Nuclei can be hyperchromatic or cleared out with small nucleoli
  - Perinuclear haloes usually prominent
- Mitotic figures are rare
- High-grade atypia usually not present
  - If full thickness frank atypia present, should be diagnosed as SCCis (Bowen disease), which can arise in EDV

Cytologic Features

- Enlarged squamous cells with abundant bluish-gray cytoplasm
- Nuclear clearing may be seen in some cells

Predominant Pattern/Injury Type

- Epithelial proliferation of atypical enlarged squamous cells

DIFFERENTIAL DIAGNOSIS

Verruca Plana

- Clinically shows overlapping features with EDV

EPIDERMODYSPLASIA VERRUCIFORMIS

Key Facts

Terminology
- Epidermodysplasia verruciformis (EDV)
- HPV-related intraepidermal proliferation of enlarged, often bluish-gray staining keratinocytes

Etiology/Pathogenesis
- Subtypes implicated include HPV-3, -5, -8, -9, -10, -12
- Majority of cases are familial (genodermatosis)
  - Increased risk for development of in situ and invasive SCC

Microscopic Pathology
- Epidermal acanthosis with proliferation of enlarged cells with abundant bluish-gray staining cytoplasm
- Perinuclear haloes usually prominent

Top Differential Diagnoses
- Verruca plana
- Actinic keratosis (AK)
- Bowen disease/squamous cell carcinoma in situ
- EDV acanthoma

- Histologically shows epidermal acanthosis with hypergranulosis and overlying orthokeratosis or hyperkeratosis
- Superficial koilocytic cells with nuclear hyperchromasia and prominent perinuclear haloes
- Lacks prominent bluish-gray staining cells of EDV

Actinic Keratosis (AK)
- Basilar keratinocytes show nuclear enlargement and atypia
- Basilar budding and overlying parakeratosis usually present
- Mitotic figures usually easily identified
- No bluish-gray staining cells as in EDV

Bowen Disease/Squamous Cell Carcinoma In Situ (SCCis)
- Full thickness epidermal atypia with enlarged squamous cells
- Numerous mitotic figures usually present
- No bluish-gray staining cells as in EDV

EDV Acanthoma
- Rarely, histologic changes typical of EDV can be seen as a single lesion
- May be the only finding or may be associated with another benign lesion, including nevus, seborrheic keratosis, or acantholytic acanthoma
- If patient has only 1 lesion, it may be referred to as "EDV acanthoma"

DIAGNOSTIC CHECKLIST

Pathologic Interpretation Pearls
- Intraepidermal proliferation of enlarged, often bluish-gray staining keratinocytes with perinuclear haloes

SELECTED REFERENCES

1. Kim T et al: Development of aggressive squamous cell carcinoma in epidermodysplasia verruciformis associated with human papillomavirus type 22b. Dermatology. 220(4):326-8, 2010
2. Dell'Oste V et al: High beta-HPV DNA loads and strong seroreactivity are present in epidermodysplasia verruciformis. J Invest Dermatol. 129(4):1026-34, 2009
3. Rogers HD et al: Acquired epidermodysplasia verruciformis. J Am Acad Dermatol. 60(2):315-20, 2009
4. Mitsuishi T et al: Epidermodysplasia verruciformis with keratoacanthoma, Bowen's disease and squamous cell carcinoma: isolation of high-risk types of HPV 5 and unknown type of human papillomavirus. J Eur Acad Dermatol Venereol. 22(9):1126-7, 2008
5. Ko CJ et al: Changes of epidermodysplasia verruciformis in benign skin lesions: the EV acanthoma. J Cutan Pathol. 34(1):44-8, 2007
6. Cassarino DS et al: Cutaneous squamous cell carcinoma: a comprehensive clinicopathologic classification. Part one. J Cutan Pathol. 33(3):191-206, 2006
7. Orth G: Genetics of epidermodysplasia verruciformis: Insights into host defense against papillomaviruses. Semin Immunol. 18(6):362-74, 2006

IMAGE GALLERY

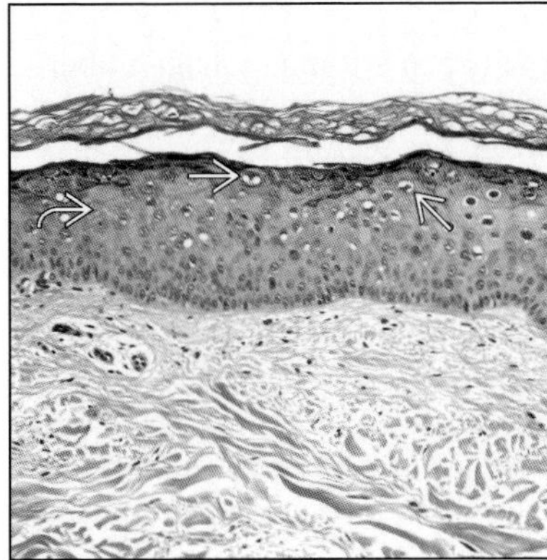

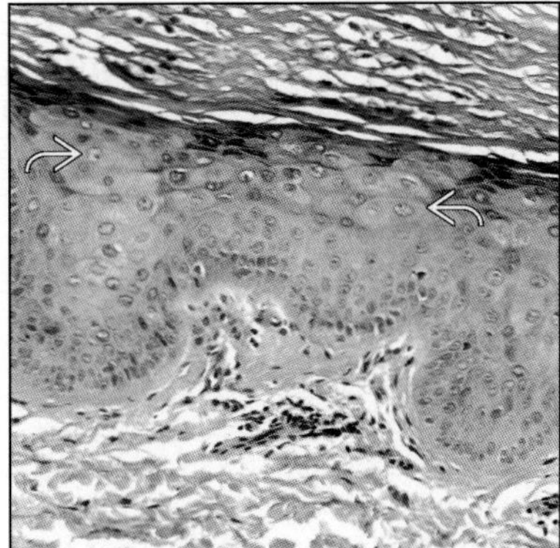

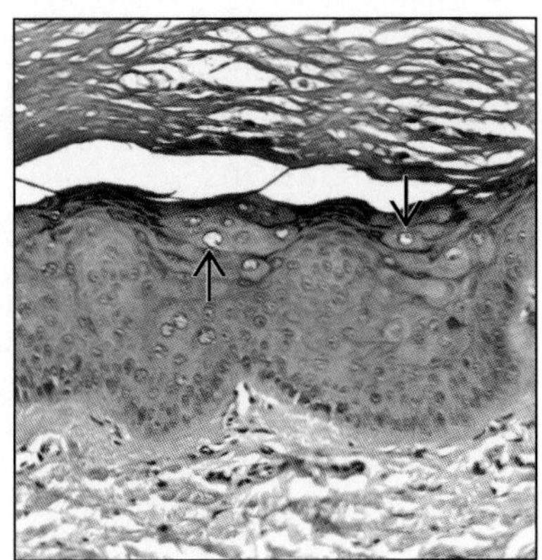

(Left) *EDV shows epidermal acanthosis and a proliferation of enlarged keratinocytes ➡ involving the upper levels of the epidermis. Note the perinuclear haloes in many of the keratinocytes ➡.* ***(Center)*** *Higher magnification of EDV shows a proliferation of enlarged bluish-gray keratinocytes ➡ involving the mid to upper layers of the epidermis. There is dense overlying hyperkeratosis and parakeratosis.* ***(Right)*** *Some of the cells show prominent nuclear clearing ➡.*

TRICHOEPITHELIOMA

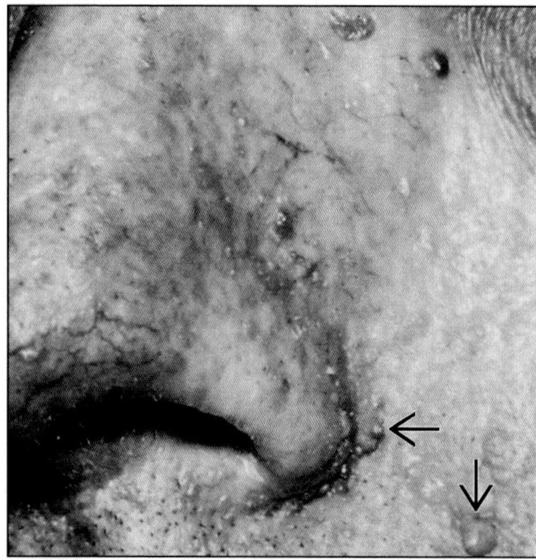

Multiple trichoepitheliomas (epithelioma adenoides cysticum) are scattered over the central face and nasolabial area presenting as flesh-colored, 1-4 mm papules.

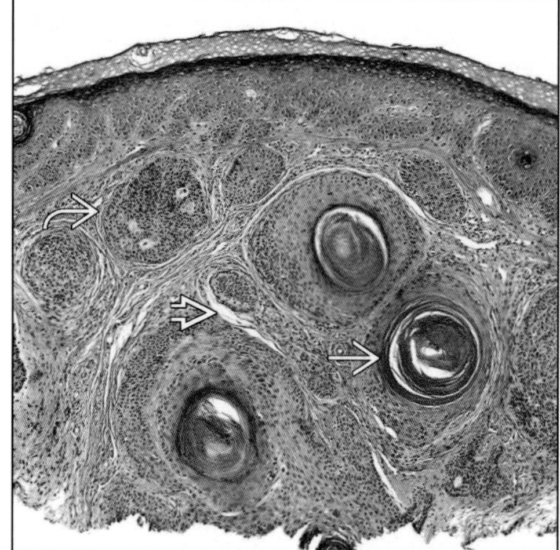

In this trichoepithelioma, note the proliferation of islands of basaloid cells with prominent horn cysts and clefts between collagen bundles but no retraction artifact as in BCC.

TERMINOLOGY

Abbreviations

- Trichoepithelioma (TE)

Synonyms

- Trichoblastoma (considered a separate entity by some)

Definitions

- Poorly differentiated hamartoma of hair germ

CLINICAL ISSUES

Presentation

- May be multiple or solitary
  - Solitary trichoepithelioma is the classical type
    - Typically ≤ 0.5 cm skin-colored papules
    - Predilection for the face but can be seen elsewhere
    - Large or giant solitary trichoepitheliomas are referred to as trichoblastomas by many
  - When multiple, can be through autosomal dominant inheritance (multiple familial trichoepithelioma) or epithelioma adenoides cysticum
    - Multiple small skin-colored papules in a symmetric distribution, typically on the face
    - Onset during puberty
    - Lessened expressivity and penetrance in males

Disease Associations

- Brooke-Spiegler syndrome (familial cylindromatosis or turban tumor syndrome)
  - Autosomal dominant syndrome with multiple cylindromas, spiradenomas, multiple trichoepitheliomas, and milia
  - Variable clinical presentation
    - Patients may present with only multiple cylindromas or multiple trichoepitheliomas
  - Characteristic confluent growth of large cylindromas on the scalp ("turban tumor")
  - Characteristic centrofacial location
  - Various mutations in the *CYLD* tumor suppressor gene (chromosome 16q)
- Rombo syndrome
  - Very rare, possible autosomal dominant inheritance
  - Multiple trichoepitheliomas, vermiculate atrophy, milia, hypotrichosis, peripheral vasodilation, vellus hair cysts, basal cell carcinomas, and cyanosis

MICROSCOPIC PATHOLOGY

Histologic Features

- Same histological features whether solitary, multiple, or syndromic
- Dermal lobular arrays of uniform islands of basaloid cells separated by concentric collagen and fibroblasts
- Can have finger-like projections of the tumor islands with cribriform or "Swiss cheese" pattern
- Papillary mesenchymal bodies are typically prominent
  - Fibroblastic aggregations that represent abortive attempts to form the papillary mesenchyme responsible for hair induction
  - Helpful feature when differentiating from basal cell carcinoma (BCC)
- Mucin can be present in cribriform tumor islands but never in stroma (vs. BCC)
- Clefts may occur between stromal collagen fibers, but there is no retraction artifact between tumor epithelium and stroma as seen in BCC
- Horns cysts and calcifications are common

Subtypes

- Desmoplastic trichoepithelioma (DTE)
  - Most commonly found on the face of women
  - Firm cutaneous or subcutaneous nodule clinically
  - Red desmoplastic stroma and tumor islands can have a "paisley-tie" or tadpole-shaped pattern
  - Horn cysts and calcifications are common as in TE

TRICHOEPITHELIOMA

Key Facts

Clinical Issues

- When TEs are multiple and inherited, called multiple familial trichoepithelioma or epithelioma adenoides cysticum
- Disease associations
  - Brooke-Spiegler and Rombo syndrome

Microscopic Pathology

- Same histological features whether solitary, multiple, or syndromic
- Lobular arrays of uniform islands of basaloid cells in the dermis separated by concentric collagen and many fibroblasts
- Papillary mesenchymal bodies typically prominent
- Can have finger-like projections of tumor islands with cribriform or "Swiss cheese" pattern
- Clefts may occur between collagen fibers in the stroma but not between tumor epithelium and stroma (i.e., no retraction artifact as in BCC)

DIFFERENTIAL DIAGNOSIS

Trichoblastoma

- Trichoepithelioma is considered by some to simply be a distinctive type or variant of trichoblastoma
- Since clinical presentation and behavior of trichoblastomas and TEs are similar and there is often histologic overlap, the pedantic differences of these tumors will not be discussed

Basal Cell Carcinoma (BCC)

- Myxoid stroma with metachromatic mucin (TE has mucin in tumor islands but not in stroma)
- Horn cysts and calcification are rarer than in TEs
- Retraction artifact vs. only clefting between collagen fibers in TEs
- Immunohistochemistry
  - Bcl-2 and BER-EP4 staining is strong and diffuse in BCC vs. Bcl-2 staining in periphery of tumor islands of TEs and ± staining for BER-EP4
  - CD34 is typically negative in the immediate tumor stroma but strongly positive in surrounding stroma (vs. diffuse positivity in all stromal cells of TEs)
- Typically lack papillary mesenchymal bodies

Microcystic Adnexal Carcinoma (MAC)

- Distinguish from DTE
- Calcification is rarer; lymphoid aggregates and perineural extension are often present
- Clinically, MACs appear as plaques, and DTEs appear as firm nodules
- p63 staining may be useful; scattered p63(+) cells at periphery of tumor nests in MAC vs. diffuse staining pattern in DTE and sclerosing BCC

Morpheaform BCC

- Horn cysts and calcification are rarer, and retraction artifact is typically present
- Clinically, morpheaform BCCs have a scar-like appearance, and DTEs are firm nodules
- Morpheaform BCC is typically androgen receptor (AR) (+) and CK20(-); DTE is typically AR(-), CK20(+)

Syringoma

- Calcification and horn cysts rarer in syringomas
- Clinically appear as small papules around eyelids vs. DTEs (firm nodules)
- Syringomas are typically smaller and more well demarcated vs. DTEs (broader lesions)

SELECTED REFERENCES

1. Mamelak AJ et al: Desmoplastic trichoepithelioma. J Am Acad Dermatol. 62(1):102-6, 2010
2. Johnson H et al: Trichoepithelioma. Dermatol Online J. 14(10):5, 2008
3. Bettencourt MS et al: Trichoepithelioma: a 19-year clinicopathologic re-evaluation. J Cutan Pathol. 26(8):398-404, 1999
4. Poniecka AW et al: An immunohistochemical study of basal cell carcinoma and trichoepithelioma. Am J Dermatopathol. 21(4):332-6, 1999

IMAGE GALLERY

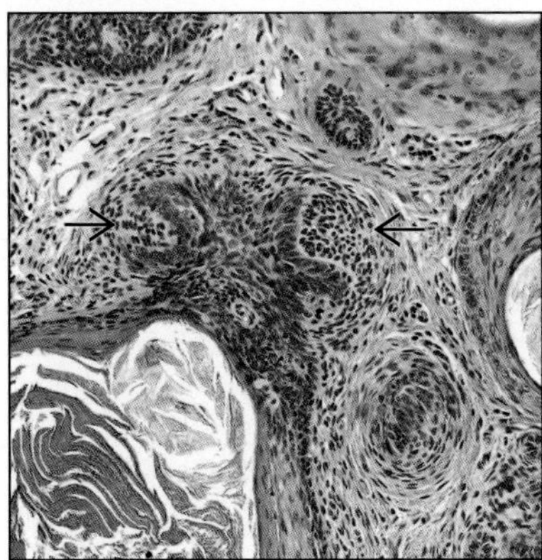

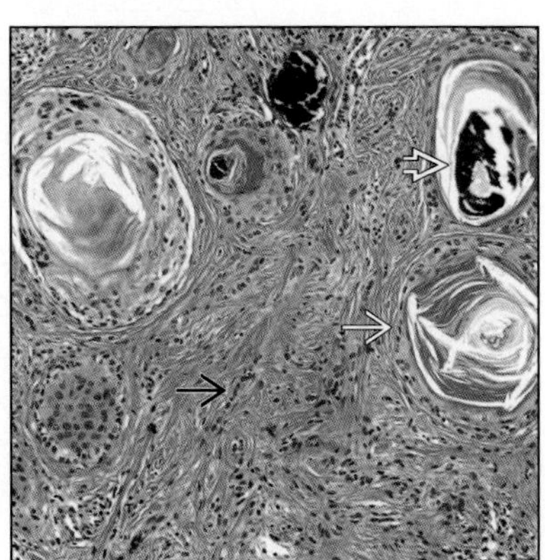

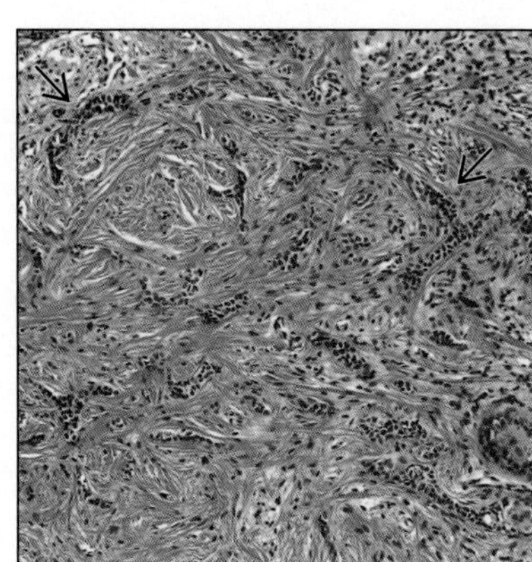

(Left) *High-power view of a trichoepithelioma demonstrates characteristic papillary mesenchymal bodies ➔. (Courtesy A. Bowen, MD.)* ***(Center)*** *Desmoplastic trichoepithelioma (DTE) is seen with areas mimicking a morpheaform BCC ➔. The horn cysts ➔ and calcifications ➔ are good clues to this being a benign trichoepithelioma. (Courtesy G. Fraga, MD.)* ***(Right)*** *Another area of a DTE shows areas ➔ mimicking a desmoplastic BCC. (Courtesy G. Fraga, MD.)*

ORGANOID NEVUS

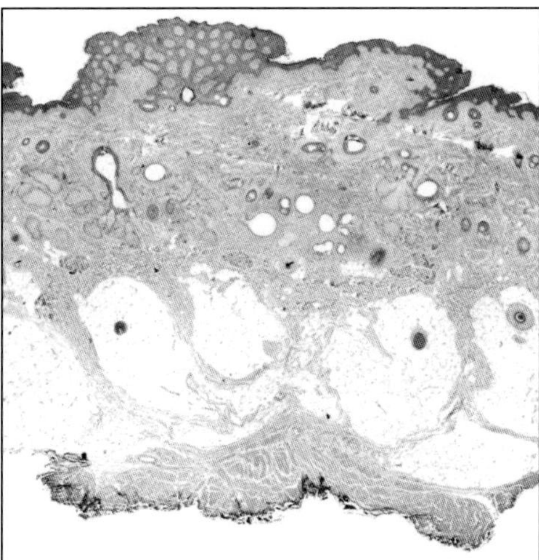

This low-power view of an organoid nevus shows a mildly acanthotic epidermis overlying a dermis that contains a collection of abnormally formed pilosebaceous units.

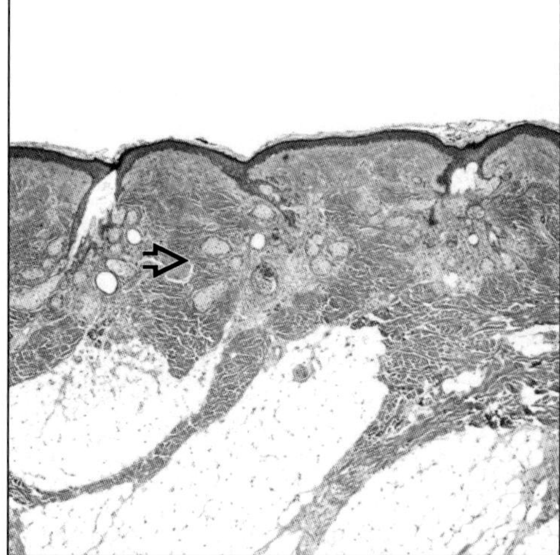

This organoid nevus from a young child shows no acanthosis or papillomatosis of the epithelium. There are immature and abnormally formed pilosebaceous units ➩.

TERMINOLOGY

Synonyms

- Nevus sebaceus of Jadassohn
- Sebaceous nevus

Definitions

- Complex hamartoma of epidermis and adnexal structures
- Many consider this a variant of epidermal nevus

CLINICAL ISSUES

Epidemiology

- Incidence
  - < 0.5% of newborns
  - Familial forms have been reported
- Age
  - Birth or early childhood
- Gender
  - Equal predilection
- Ethnicity
  - Equal predilection

Site

- Scalp
- Forehead
- Face
- Neck
- Trunk (much less common)

Presentation

- In infants and young children, hairless velvety to smooth plaque
- After puberty, lesion becomes more verrucoid

Treatment

- Complete excision
  - Ideally excised before puberty when risk of malignant change increases
  - Must take into account cosmetic factor
- Topical ablation not recommended but can be done in certain cases

Prognosis

- Tumors arise in up to 30% of organoid nevi in adults
  - Basal cell carcinoma
  - Trichoblastoma
  - Hidradenoma
- **Nevus sebaceous syndrome**
  - Associated with defects of
    - Central nervous system (mental retardation, seizures)
    - Skeletal system (rickets, spina bifida)
    - Eyes (nystagmus, ptosis)

IMAGE FINDINGS

General Features

- Can be seen on prenatal ultrasound
  - Echogenic soft tissue structures external to the cranium

MACROSCOPIC FEATURES

General Features

- Yellow or waxy color
- Surface varies from smooth to wart-like
- Up to 10 cm

MICROSCOPIC PATHOLOGY

Histologic Features

- Varies with age
- Infants and young children
  - Immature and abnormally formed pilosebaceous units
  - Pilosebaceous units may be reduced in number

ORGANOID NEVUS

Key Facts

Terminology
- Sebaceous nevus
- Complex hamartoma of epidermis and adnexal structures

Clinical Issues
- Most common sites include scalp, face

Macroscopic Features
- Yellow or waxy color

Microscopic Pathology
- Varies with age
- Immature and abnormally formed pilosebaceous units

Top Differential Diagnoses
- Epidermal nevus
- Seborrheic keratosis

  - Only mild acanthosis and mild papillomatosis
- After puberty
  - Enlargement of sebaceous glands, which sit high in the dermis
  - Hair follicles are vellus
  - Epidermis is more acanthotic and papillomatous
- Dermis is often thickened
- Mild lymphoplasmacytic infiltrate

DIFFERENTIAL DIAGNOSIS

Epidermal Nevus
- Underlying adnexal structures are normal
- Some consider sebaceous nevus to be a variant of epidermal nevus

Seborrheic Keratosis
- Older patients
- No papillomatosis
- Underlying adnexal structures are normal

Wart
- Generally smaller than sebaceous nevus
- Underlying adnexal structures are normal

Aplasia Cutis Congenita
- Thin dermis with absent adnexal structures

SELECTED REFERENCES

1. Malhotra P et al: Squamous cell carcinoma, syringocystadenoma papilliferum and apocrine adenoma arising in a nevus sebaceus of Jadassohn. Indian J Pathol Microbiol. 54(1):225-6, 2011
2. Kurokawa I et al: Immunohistochemical study of cytokeratin expression in nevus sebaceous. Int J Dermatol. 49(4):402-5, 2010
3. Eisen DB et al: Sebaceous lesions and their associated syndromes: part I. J Am Acad Dermatol. 61(4):549-60; quiz 561-2, 2009
4. Eisen DB et al: Sebaceous lesions and their associated syndromes: part II. J Am Acad Dermatol. 61(4):563-78; quiz 579-80, 2009
5. Menascu S et al: Linear nevus sebaceous syndrome: case reports and review of the literature. Pediatr Neurol. 38(3):207-10, 2008
6. Santibanez-Gallerani A et al: Should nevus sebaceus of Jadassohn in children be excised? A study of 757 cases, and literature review. J Craniofac Surg. 14(5):658-60, 2003
7. Laino L et al: Familial occurrence of nevus sebaceus of Jadassohn: another case of paradominant inheritance? Eur J Dermatol. 11(2):97-8, 2001

IMAGE GALLERY

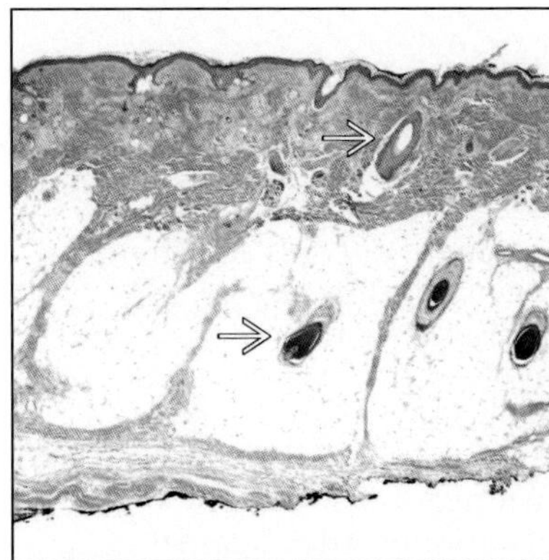

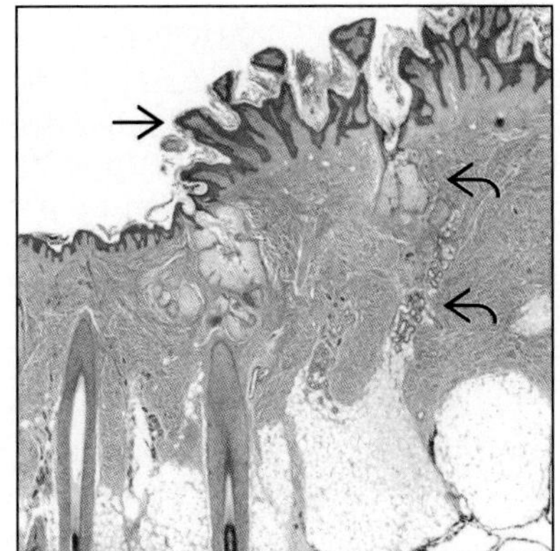

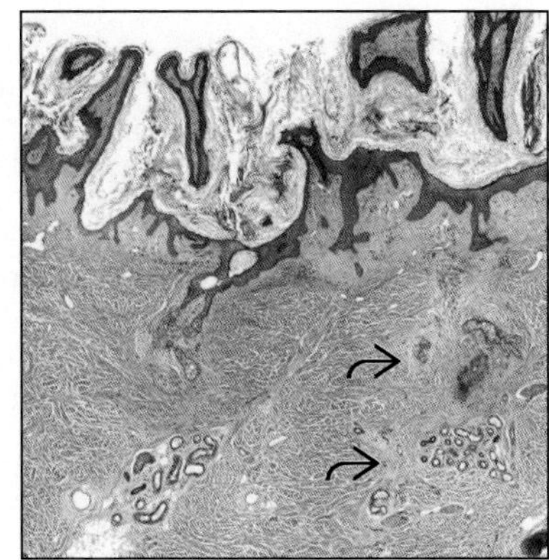

(Left) *This low-power view shows the border between organoid nevus (left) and normal skin (right). Looking for normal hair follicles ➡ is an easy way to determine margins.* ***(Center)*** *Organoid nevus in older children often has more acanthosis and papillomatosis ➡, similar to epithelioid nevus. Look for abnormal pilosebaceous units ➡ to diagnose organoid nevus.* ***(Right)*** *Papillomatous epithelium overlies abnormal pilosebaceous units ➡ in this organoid nevus.*

TRICHILEMMOMA

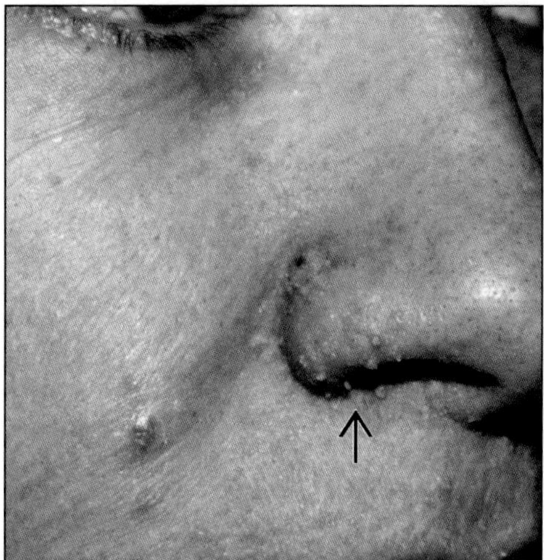

Multiple trichilemmomas ⇒ are seen on the nose of a patient with Cowden syndrome. (Courtesy D. Kaplan, MD.)

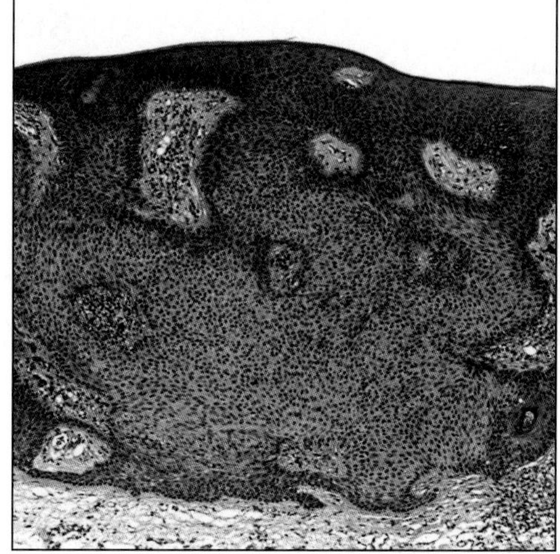

Trichilemmoma shows a lobule of clear glycogenated cells that is attached to the epidermis. (Courtesy C. Cockerell, MD.)

TERMINOLOGY

Synonyms

- Tricholemmomas, trichilemmal verruca (preferred terminology by some)

Definitions

- Benign neoplasm with differentiation toward the pilosebaceous follicular epithelium

ETIOLOGY/PATHOGENESIS

Unclear Pathogenesis

- Thought to be related to outer sheath of pilosebaceous unit (trichilemma)
- May differentiate toward infundibular keratinization and proliferation of outer root sheath

CLINICAL ISSUES

Epidemiology

- Age
  - Usually adults except when multiple (seen in Cowden syndrome)

Site

- Almost always on the face, especially the nose and upper lip
  - Rare case reports of nonfacial localization

Presentation

- Small solitary or multiple flesh-colored papular lesions on the face
- Clinically can mimic basal cell carcinomas or warts
  - Reason for importance of histologic examination of these lesions

Treatment

- Often none needed due to benign nature and common location on face

Prognosis

- Generally excellent

Disease Associations

- When multiple, can be a marker of Cowden syndrome
  - Autosomal dominant disease associated with multiple trichilemmomas on face, multiple papules on oral mucosa, and visceral malignancies

MICROSCOPIC PATHOLOGY

Histologic Features

- Lobular acanthosis with anastomosing clear glycogen-rich cells
  - Pushing, downward-growing lobule
- Peripheral nuclear palisading at edge of clear cells
  - Resembles the outer root sheath of hair follicle (trichilemma)
- Thickened basement membrane outlining the lobules
  - Basement membrane is PAS(+), diastase resistant
- Hyperkeratosis, sometimes prominent granular layer

Subtypes

- Desmoplastic trichilemmoma (DT)
  - Similar histologic features as trichilemmoma at periphery
  - Central prominent desmoplastic stroma
    - More random pattern of cords and strands separated by dense hyaline stroma
    - Can mimic invasive carcinoma
- Keratinizing trichilemmoma
  - Pseudocystic architecture
  - Abundant central keratinization
  - Squamous eddy formation
- Other entities can also show trichilemmal differentiation including

TRICHILEMMOMA

Key Facts

Terminology

- Benign neoplasm with differentiation toward pilosebaceous follicular epithelium

Clinical Issues

- Small solitary or multiple flesh-colored papular lesions on the face
- When multiple, can be a marker of Cowden syndrome

Microscopic Pathology

- Lobular acanthosis with anastomosing of clear glycogen-rich cells
  - Pushing, downward-growing lobule
- Peripheral nuclear palisading at the edge of clear cells
- Thickened PAS(+), diastase-resistant basement membrane outlining lobules

---

  - Warts, basal cell carcinomas (BCCs), squamous cell carcinomas (SCCs), inverted follicular keratoses (IFKs) and seborrheic keratoses (SKs)

DIFFERENTIAL DIAGNOSIS

Malignant Trichilemmoma (Trichilemmocarcinoma)

- Small number of cases
- Existence questioned (thought by some to be clear cell variant of SCC)
- High mitotic rate, moderate to marked cytologic atypia
- Lacks desmoplastic stromal reaction
- Peripheral invasive lobules and central area of well-differentiated cells (opposite of DT)

Clear Cell Acanthoma (Pale Cell Acanthoma)

- Usually on the leg
- Sharp demarcation of clear keratinocytes from normal epidermis
- Psoriasiform silhouette

Inverted Follicular Keratosis (IFK)

- Downward-growing seborrheic keratosis
- Cells not as clear
- More frequent squamous eddies

Tumor of Follicular Infundibulum (TFI)

- Plate-like pattern (vs. lobular) with interconnecting epithelial cords
- Thin strands of clear cells vs. lobules
  - Extend parallel to epidermis with bridging between adjacent follicles

Verruca

- Trichilemmomas are considered by some to be verrucae with trichilemmal differentiation or "trichilemmal verrucae"
  - Several studies seem to refute this idea
- Fewer clear cells
- More hypergranulosis and koilocytosis

Clear Cell Bowen Disease

- Rare histopathologic subtype of Bowen disease
- Atypical epidermal keratinocytes
- Extremely acanthotic epidermis
- No cytoplasmic glycogen present
- Lacks lobular architecture

SELECTED REFERENCES

1. Tellechea O et al: Desmoplastic trichilemmoma. Am J Dermatopathol. 14(2):107-4, 1992
2. Leonardi CL et al: Trichilemmomas are not associated with human papillomavirus DNA. J Cutan Pathol. 18(3):193-7, 1991
3. Salem OS et al: Cowden's disease (multiple hamartoma and neoplasia syndrome). A case report and review of the English literature. J Am Acad Dermatol. 8(5):686-96, 1983

IMAGE GALLERY

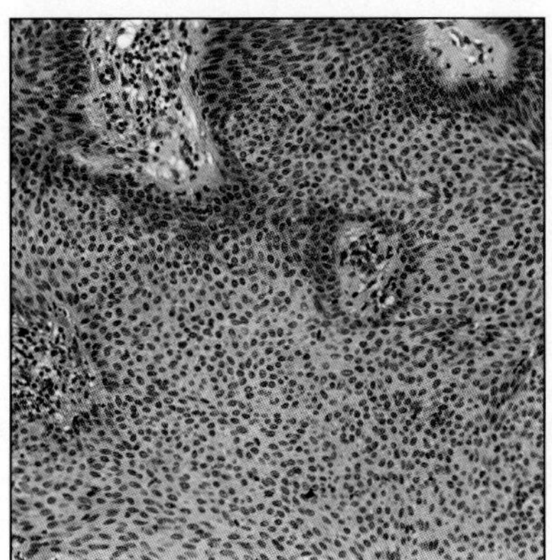

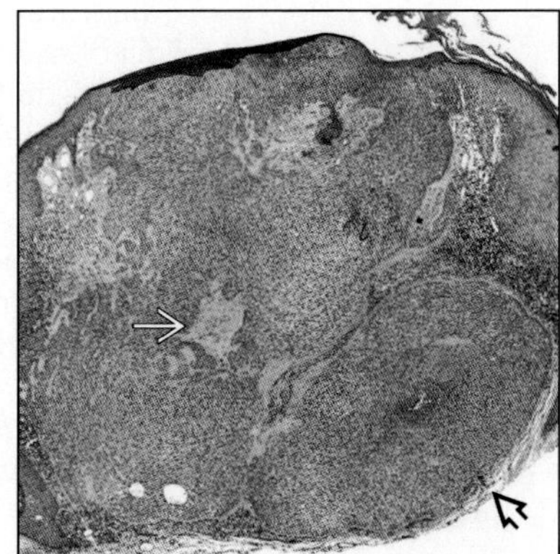

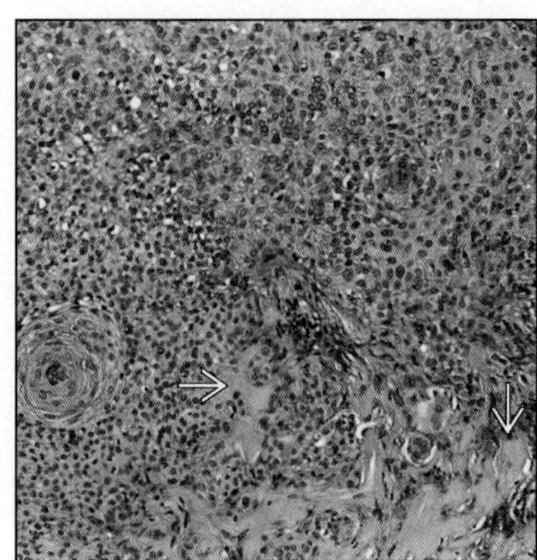

(Left) *High-power view of a trichilemmoma shows the clear glycogenated cells.* ***(Center)*** *Low-power view shows a desmoplastic trichilemmoma with entrapped sclerotic collagen ➡ and the similar lobules of clear glycogenated cells ⇨ that are seen with regular trichilemmomas.* ***(Right)*** *Close-up view of a lobule from a desmoplastic trichilemmoma shows sclerotic collagen ➡. (Courtesy C. Cockerell, MD.)*

PILOMATRICOMA

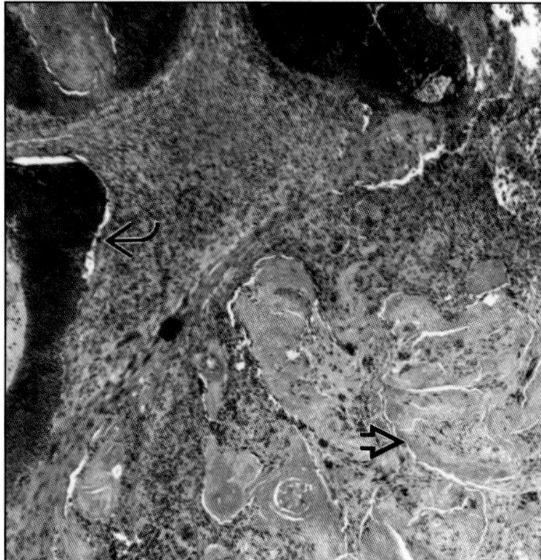

Hematoxylin & eosin shows a lesion with islands of basaloid cells ⮫, anucleate shadow cells ⮚, and intervening stroma.

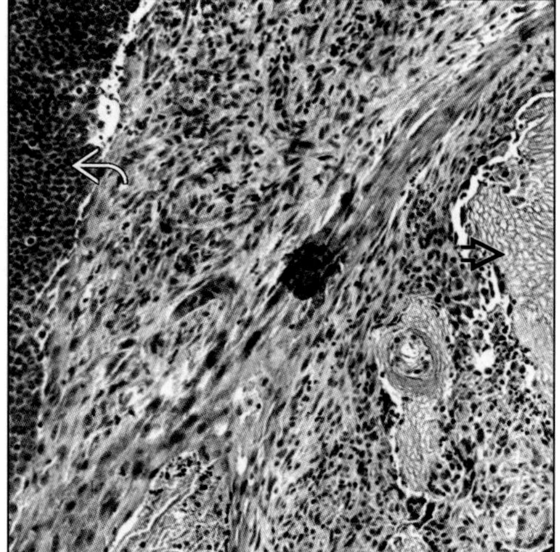

Hematoxylin & eosin shows a higher power view of basaloid cells ⮫ and anucleate shadow cells ⮚. Intervening stroma is spindled with mixed inflammatory cells.

TERMINOLOGY

Synonyms

- Pilomatrixoma
- Calcifying epithelioma of Malherbe
- Trichomatricoma

Definitions

- Benign dermal or subcutaneous tumor showing differentiation toward matrix of hair follicle

ETIOLOGY/PATHOGENESIS

Pathogenesis

- Benign neoplasm arising from hair matrix

Molecular

- Associated with mutations in β-catenin gene

CLINICAL ISSUES

Epidemiology

- Age
  - > 60% identified within 1st 2 decades
  - 2nd peak after 5th decade

Site

- Head, neck, and upper extremities
- Usually solitary

Presentation

- Firm nodule, 0.5-3.0 cm
  - Usually deep and slow growing
  - May feel cystic
  - Hemorrhage may cause rapid growth
  - Superficial erosion or perforation through skin with transepidermal elimination possible
- Multiple lesions associated with Myotonic dystrophy, Turner syndrome, Gardner syndrome

Treatment

- Surgical approaches
  - Simple surgical excision curative

Prognosis

- Rare recurrence even with incomplete excision
- No definitive reports of malignant transformation to pilomatrical carcinoma reported

MACROSCOPIC FEATURES

General Features

- Variegated chalky, gray-brown to yellow-white tissue
  - May have visible melanin pigment
- Nodules of calcification and ossification possible

MICROSCOPIC PATHOLOGY

Histologic Features

- Involves lower dermis and upper subcutis
- Sheets of basaloid epithelial cells, eosinophilic shadow cells, and keratin
  - Intervening spindled stroma with foreign body giant cells and chronic inflammation
  - Calcification within shadow cells occurs in > 60%
  - Foci of osteoid, hemosiderin, melanin, amyloid, and extramedullary hematopoiesis possible
  - Mitotic activity present, usually in basaloid cells
- Epithelial subtypes
  - Basaloid cells: Monomorphous population of small cells with minimal cytoplasm, uniform hyperchromatic nuclei, and small nucleoli
  - Shadow or ghost cells: Eosinophilic cells with more cytoplasm, distinct borders, but no nuclear staining
  - Transition from basal to shadow cells can be abrupt or can have intervening transitional cells
  - Variable ratio between cell types depending on age of lesion

PILOMATRICOMA

Key Facts

Terminology
- Calcifying epithelioma of Malherbe
- Benign dermal or subcutaneous tumor showing differentiation toward matrix of hair follicle

Clinical Issues
- > 60% identified within 1st 2 decades
- Head, neck, and upper extremities
- Most will not recur even with incomplete excision

Macroscopic Features
- Variegated chalky, gray-brown to yellow-white tissue

Microscopic Pathology
- Sheets of basaloid epithelial cells, eosinophilic shadow cells, and keratin
- Calcification within shadow cells occurs in > 60%
- Foci of osteoid, hemosiderin, melanin, amyloid, and extramedullary hematopoiesis possible

Predominant Pattern/Injury Type
- Biphasic

Predominant Cell/Compartment Type
- Epithelial, biphasic or mixed

DIFFERENTIAL DIAGNOSIS

Pilomatrical Carcinoma
- Presents in older adults
- Cytologic atypia, necrosis, high mitotic activity
- Locally aggressive behavior with infiltrating borders, ulceration
- Lymphovascular invasion (rare)

Aggressive Variant of Pilomatricoma
- Detached nests of tumor cells invade adjacent soft tissues
- Higher rate of local recurrence

Basal Cell Carcinoma
- Small sampling of basaloid cells may be misinterpreted
  - Frequent misdiagnosis on aspiration cytology
  - Adequate sampling required for correct diagnosis
- Age and presentation help with differentiation

Neuroendocrine Carcinoma
- Neuroendocrine immunohistochemical markers
- Lacks anucleate shadow cells

Metastatic Carcinoma
- Presentation, medical history, immunohistochemical stains

DIAGNOSTIC CHECKLIST

Clinically Relevant Pathologic Features
- Rare recurrence even with positive margins

Pathologic Interpretation Pearls
- Combination of basaloid cells, anucleate shadow cells, keratin, foreign body giant cells
  - Ratio of basaloid cells to shadow cells depends on age of lesion
- Pitfalls include diagnosis on cytology/fine-needle aspiration; requires adequate sampling

SELECTED REFERENCES

1. Zamanian A et al: Clinical and histopathologic study of pilomatricoma in Iran between 1992 and 2005. Pediatr Dermatol. 25(2):268-9, 2008
2. Hardisson D et al: Pilomatrix carcinoma: a clinicopathologic study of six cases and review of the literature. Am J Dermatopathol. 23(5):394-401, 2001
3. Viero RM et al: Fine needle aspiration (FNA) cytology of pilomatrixoma: report of 14 cases and review of the literature. Cytopathology. 10(4):263-9, 1999
4. Taaffe A et al: Pilomatricoma (Malherbe). A clinical and histopathologic survey of 78 cases. Int J Dermatol. 27(7):477-80, 1988

IMAGE GALLERY

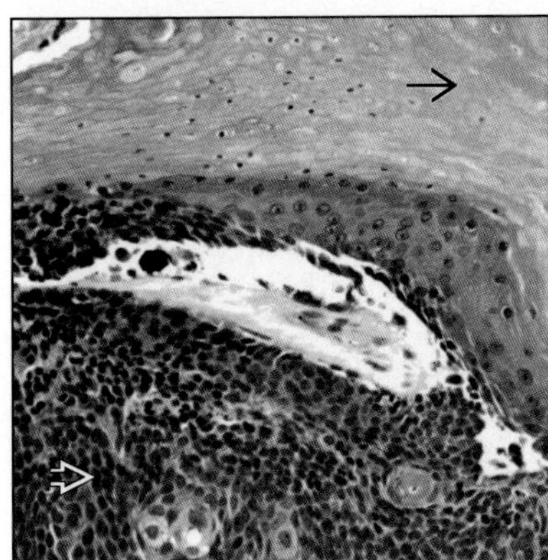

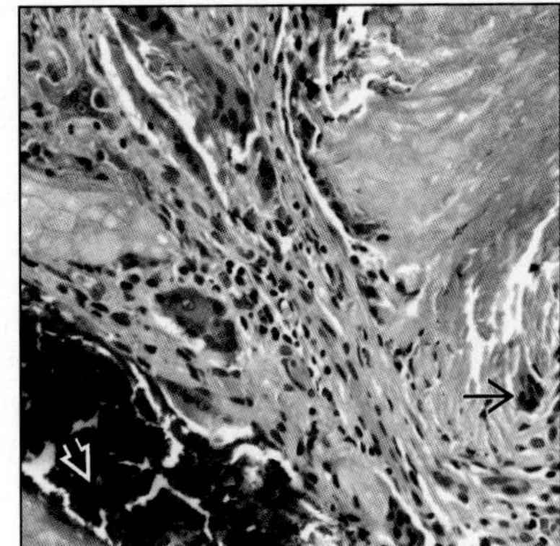

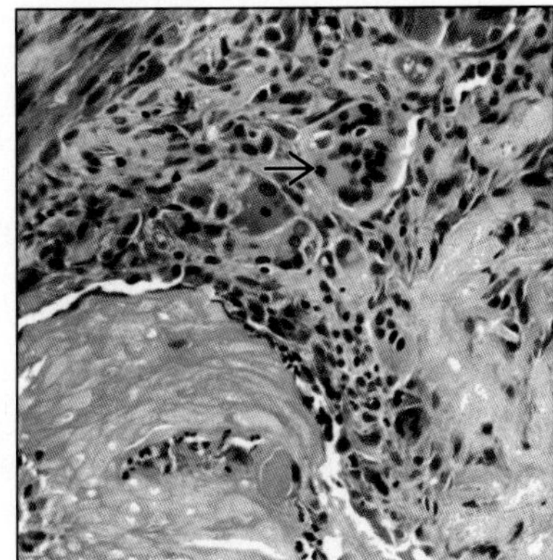

(Left) *Hematoxylin & eosin shows a gradual transition from dark blue ⇨ basaloid cells to anucleate shadow cells →. This transition may not always be identified.* ***(Center)*** *Hematoxylin & eosin shows foci of calcification ⇨ within islands of shadow cells. Loose keratin and a giant cell → are present at the edge of the nested shadow cells.* ***(Right)*** *Hematoxylin & eosin shows a spindled stroma surrounding islands of shadow cells. Multinucleate giant cells → and chronic inflammation are present within the stroma.*

SYRINGOMA

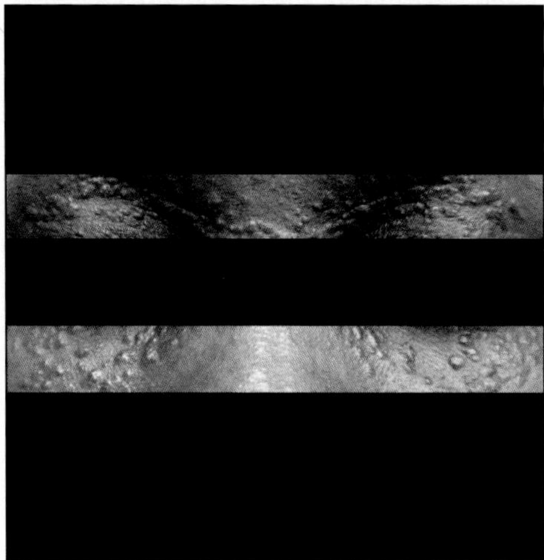

Typical appearance of syringomas as multiple small flesh-colored papules surrounding the eyelids on an adolescent African-American female. (Courtesy J. Endo, MD.)

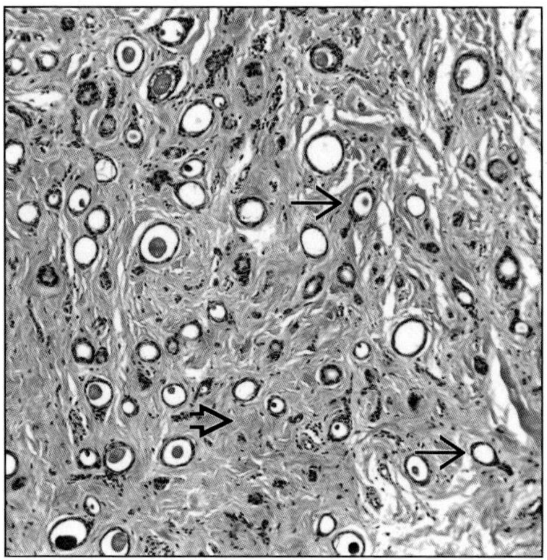

Typical cuboidal lined ducts are seen with a "paisley-tie" or "tadpole" appearance →. Note the dense sclerotic stroma surrounding the ducts ⇒.

TERMINOLOGY

Definitions

- Benign tumor of the eccrine sweat gland

CLINICAL ISSUES

Epidemiology

- Incidence
  - Affects approximately 0.6% of the population
- Age
  - Often occurs at puberty or later in life
- Gender
  - Predominantly women
- Ethnicity
  - Especially common in Asian women

Presentation

- Presents as multiple 1-2 mm flesh- or yellow-colored papules but can also be solitary
- Most often on lower eyelid or malar area
- Less frequently involves genitalia (can cause marked pruritus)
- Eruptive syringomas appear to be more common in patients with Down syndrome

Treatment

- Options, risks, complications
  - Scar
- Surgical approaches
  - Electrodissection, CO2 laser ablation, excision
- Drugs
  - Topical or systemic retinoids

Prognosis

- Generally excellent
- Treatment usually considered only for cosmetic reasons

MICROSCOPIC PATHOLOGY

Histologic Features

- Proliferation of multiple small ducts lined by 2 layers of epithelium
- Ducts often referred to as being tadpole-shaped or having a "paisley-tie" pattern
- Dense red sclerotic or fibrotic stroma
- Horn cysts sometimes
- Nests and strands of cells may be present having a basaloid appearance
- Milia may coexist
- Some ducts are dilated with eosinophilic material

Subtypes

- Clear cell syringoma
  - Ducts lined by larger, epithelioid clear cells having pale cytoplasm
    - Cells contain abundant glycogen (PAS positive)
  - Otherwise similar histologic features as syringoma
  - Commonly associated with diabetes mellitus
- Eruptive syringoma
  - Small hyperpigmented papules
  - Typically on chest, back, or penis of dark-skinned patients
  - May be associated with Down syndrome

ANCILLARY TESTS

Immunohistochemistry

- Tumor cells express CK10 in intermediate cells
- Luminal cells stain positive with CK6, CK10, and CEA (CEA is negative in desmoplastic trichoepithelioma)
- EMA stains in peripheral cells of the duct
- Progesterone receptors expressed in most syringomas
  - Supports hypothesis that these lesions are under hormonal control

SYRINGOMA

Key Facts

Clinical Issues

- Presents as multiple 1-2 mm flesh- or yellow-colored papules but can also be solitary
- Most often on lower eyelid or malar area

Microscopic Pathology

- Proliferation of multiple small ducts lined by 2 layers of epithelium
- Ducts often referred to as being tadpole-shaped or having "paisley-tie" pattern
- Dense red sclerotic or fibrotic stroma
- Nests and strands of cells may be present having basaloid appearance

Top Differential Diagnoses

- Microcystic adnexal carcinoma
- Morpheaform or sclerosing basal cell carcinoma
- Desmoplastic trichoepithelioma

DIFFERENTIAL DIAGNOSIS

Microcystic Adnexal Carcinoma (MAC)

- Uncommon in children
- Larger size, infiltrative growth pattern
- Perineural extension and invasion commonly
- Commonly appears as a plaque on upper lip, chin, or cheek
- May also show mild cytologic atypia and occasional mitoses
- Lymphoid aggregates commonly present

Morpheaform or Sclerosing Basal Cell Carcinoma (BCC)

- BCCs are exceedingly rare in pediatric patients and are usually associated with a genetic defect such as
  - Xeroderma pigmentosum, basal cell nevus syndrome, or nevus sebaceous
- Thickened or skin-colored scar clinically
- More atypia
- Ductal spaces uncommon
- Epidermal attachment
- Poorly circumscribed

Desmoplastic Trichoepithelioma

- Clinically presents as a firm nodule vs. small papules
- Broader lesion
- More horned cysts
- No sweat ducts
- Calcification common
- Fails to stain with carcinoembryonic antigen (CEA)
  - Syringoma typically positive for CEA staining in luminal cells
- Keratinous material within tubular lumina vs. syringoma (basophilic material in tubular lumina)
- Less commonly shows tadpole-like configuration of tubular structures

Metastatic Adenocarcinoma

- Not typically seen in pediatric patients
- Larger cells, more cytologic atypia
- No sweat ducts

SELECTED REFERENCES

1. Petersson F et al: Eruptive syringoma of the penis. A report of 2 cases and a review of the literature. Am J Dermatopathol. 31(5):436-8, 2009
2. Lee JH et al: Syringoma: a clinicopathologic and immunohistologic study and results of treatment. Yonsei Med J. 48(1):35-40, 2007
3. Patrizi A et al: Syringoma: a review of twenty-nine cases. Acta Derm Venereol. 78(6):460-2, 1998
4. Urban CD et al: Eruptive syringomas in Down's syndrome. Arch Dermatol. 117(6):374-5, 1981

IMAGE GALLERY

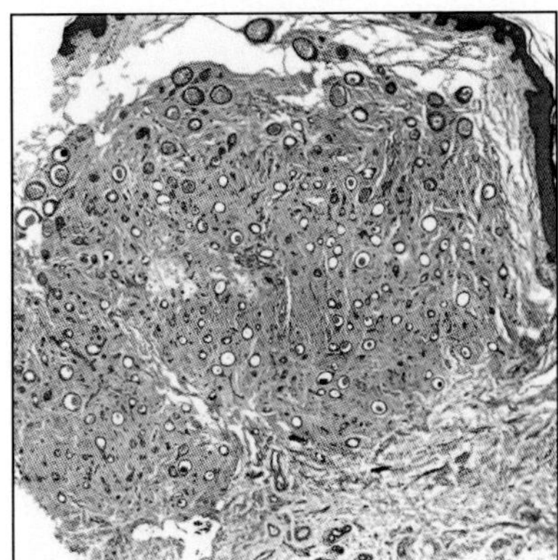

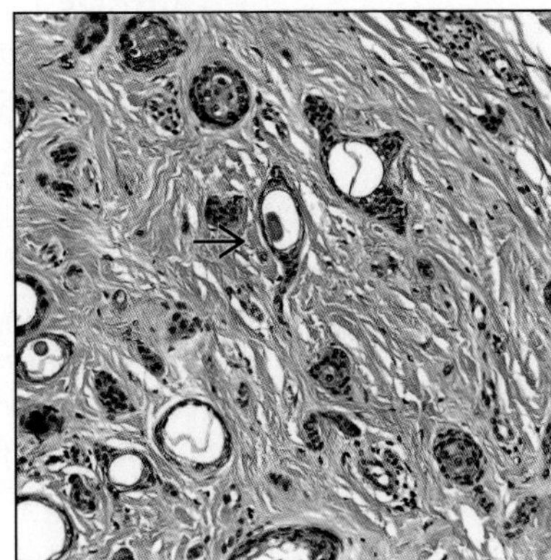

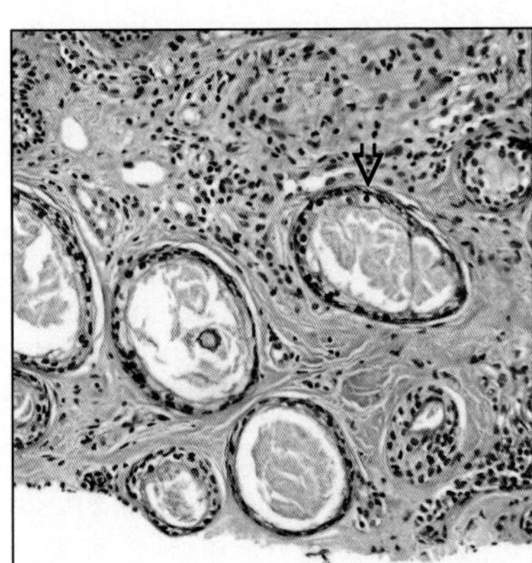

(Left) *Low-power view of syringoma (40x) shows how well circumscribed the lesion is. "Paisley-tie" and tadpole-like configuration of the ducts can be appreciated even at this power. (Courtesy C. Cockerell, MD.)* ***(Center)*** *High-power view shows the characteristic tadpole-shaped or "paisley-tie" patterned ducts ➔.* ***(Right)*** *In this clear cell syringoma, note how there are larger, epithelioid clear cells ➔ that have pale cytoplasm. (Courtesy G. Fraga, MD.)*

LANGERHANS CELL HISTIOCYTOSIS

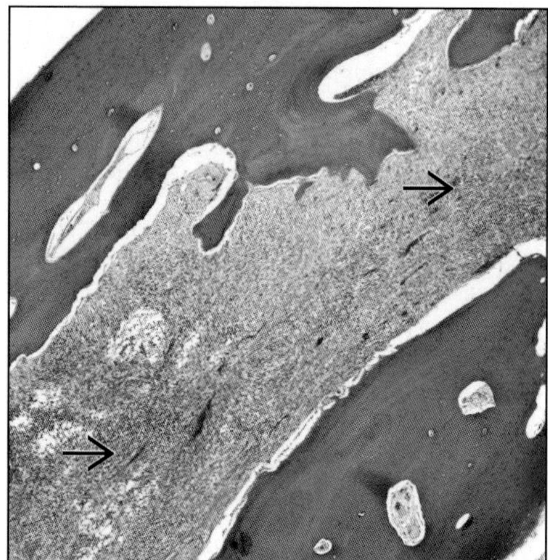

This low-power view of skull shows Langerhans cell histiocytosis infiltrating through and replacing the marrow space ➡. The skull is a common place for LCH to occur.

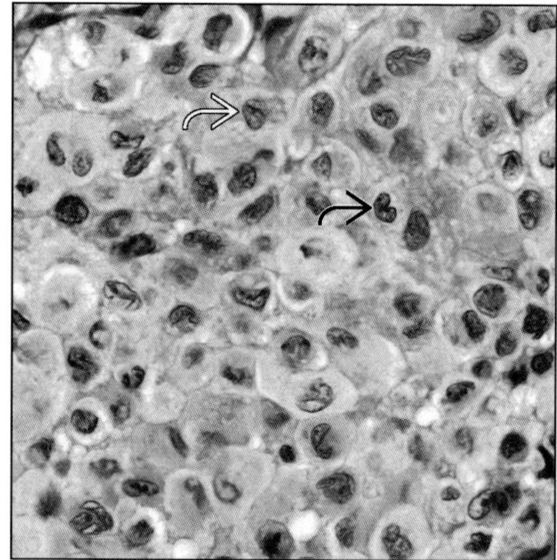

This high-power view shows the characteristic features of a Langerhans cell: Folded ➡ or grooved ➡ nuclei and abundant pink cytoplasm.

TERMINOLOGY

Abbreviations

- Langerhans cell histiocytosis (LCH)

Synonyms

- Histiocytosis X
- Eosinophilic granuloma

Definitions

- Clonal proliferation of Langerhans cells

CLINICAL ISSUES

Epidemiology

- Age
  - 1st 3 decades of life
- Gender
  - Male to female ratio = 2:1

Site

- Skin
  - Erythematous, crusted, vesiculopustular rash, or
  - Salmon-colored macular-papular rash
- Bone and bone marrow
  - Skull, pelvis, long bones, vertebrae
- Lung
- Lymph nodes
- Liver
- Thymus
- GI tract
- CNS
  - Primary in dura, leptomeninges, or parenchyma
  - May be secondary to skull or vertebral involvement
  - Parasellar and cavernous sinus regions common

Presentation

- Newborns and infants usually present with limited skin or bone lesions
- Generalized disease is more common in young children
- Rash may precede systemic findings by several months
- **Eosinophilic granuloma**
  - Single or multiple lesions restricted to bone
- **Hand-Schüller-Christian disease**
  - Multiple organ involvement
  - Diabetes insipidus
  - Exophthalmos
- **Letterer-Siwe disease**
  - Disseminated disease with skin, lymph node, visceral, and marrow involvement
  - Aggressive; many die within 1 year due to extensive lung involvement

Natural History

- May spontaneously resolve or progress

Treatment

- Surgical approaches
  - Bone lesions usually managed with curettage
- Drugs
  - Chemotherapy for disseminated disease
- Radiation
  - Low-dose radiation for difficult-to-resect lesions

Prognosis

- Poor prognosis associated with
  - Hepatosplenomegaly
  - Thrombocytopenia
  - Young age at diagnosis
  - Lesions in 3 bones or more

IMAGE FINDINGS

Radiographic Findings

- Bone lesions generally well defined and lytic

Key Facts

Terminology
- LCH is also known as
  - Histiocytosis X
  - Eosinophilic granuloma
- LCH: Clonal proliferation of Langerhans cells

Clinical Issues
- Common sites include skin, bone and bone marrow, and lung
- Male to female ratio = 2:1
- **Eosinophilic granuloma** is restricted to bone
- **Hand-Schüller-Christian disease** has multiple organ involvement and diabetes insipidus
- **Letterer-Siwe disease** aggressive with multisystem involvement

Image Findings
- Bone lesions generally well defined and lytic

Microscopic Pathology
- Langerhans cell
  - Abundant eosinophilic cytoplasm
  - Coffee bean-shaped nucleus
- Large numbers of eosinophils and other inflammatory cells

Ancillary Tests
- CD1a immunostaining
- Birbeck granules seen on EM

MICROSCOPIC PATHOLOGY

Histologic Features
- Langerhans cell
  - Abundant eosinophilic cytoplasm
  - Coffee bean-shaped nucleus
    - Lobulated nucleus with central groove
  - Small nucleolus
- Large numbers of eosinophils
  - Other inflammatory cells also seen, including multinucleated giant cells
- Necrosis is common
- Mitoses common but usually not atypical
- Bone marrow aspirates
  - Langerhans cells may be single or in small groups intermixed with hematopoietic precursors
- Skin
  - Langerhans cells infiltrate subcutis and dermis, and extend through epidermis to stratum corneum
- Lymph nodes
  - Architecture generally preserved
  - Germinal centers may be hypoplastic
  - Sinuses are distended by Langerhans cells
- Liver
  - Portal or parenchymal nodules, or diffusely infiltrates sinusoids
  - Langerhans cells can be hard to identify in advanced disease
  - May result in sclerosing cholangitis
    - 15% of all sclerosing cholangitis in children caused by LCH
- Disease passes through various stages
  - Necrosis and increasing fibrosis seen in older lesions

ANCILLARY TESTS

Immunohistochemistry
- CD1a is very specific for Langerhans cells
- S100 is not specific but does stain Langerhans cells

Electron Microscopy
- Birbeck granules
  - Tubular pentalaminar membrane-bound cytoplasmic bodies, often with terminal oval protrusion
  - Tennis racket-shaped

DIFFERENTIAL DIAGNOSIS

Osteomyelitis, Granuloma
- Histiocytic cells are CD1a(-)

Hodgkin and Non-Hodgkin Lymphoma
- Cells lack characteristic nuclear features
- Neoplastic cells are CD1a(-)

Rosai-Dorfman Disease
- Histiocytes are CD1a(-)
- LCH does not display emperipolesis

SELECTED REFERENCES

1. Ezra N et al: CD30 positive anaplastic large-cell lymphoma mimicking Langerhans cell histiocytosis. J Cutan Pathol. 37(7):787-92, 2010
2. Degar BA et al: Langerhans cell histiocytosis: malignancy or inflammatory disorder doing a great job of imitating one? Dis Model Mech. 2(9-10):436-9, 2009
3. Gavhed D et al: Biomarkers in the cerebrospinal fluid and neurodegeneration in Langerhans cell histiocytosis. Pediatr Blood Cancer. 53(7):1264-70, 2009
4. Imashuku S et al: Langerhans cell histiocytosis with multifocal bone lesions: comparative clinical features between single and multi-systems. Int J Hematol. 90(4):506-12, 2009
5. Jaffe R: Is there a role for histopathology in predicting the clinical outcome in congenital and infant Langerhans cell disease? Pediatr Blood Cancer. 53(6):924-5, 2009

LANGERHANS CELL HISTIOCYTOSIS

Microscopic Features

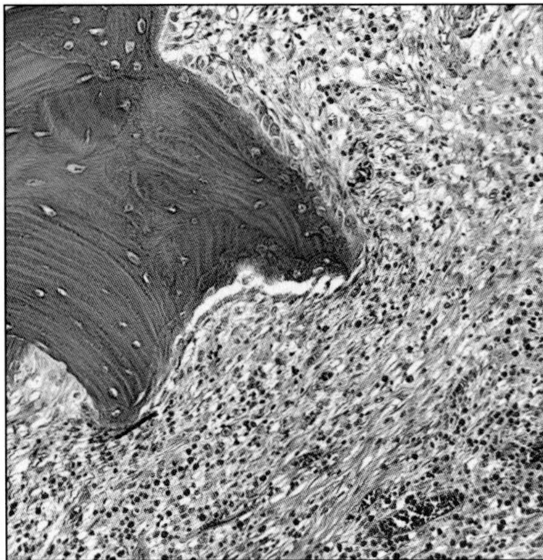

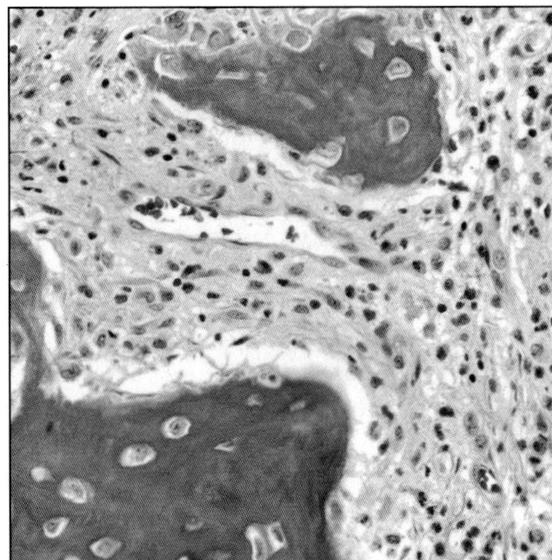

(Left) *The histology of Langerhans cell histiocytosis in bone can vary widely. In this example, there is fibrosis and less cellularity; Langerhans cells can be hard to find without the aid of immunostains.* ***(Right)*** *High-power view of this case of Langerhans cell histiocytosis in bone shows less cellularity and a fibrous stroma with scattered eosinophils. Langerhans cells can be difficult to identify, making immunostains, especially CD1a, very helpful.*

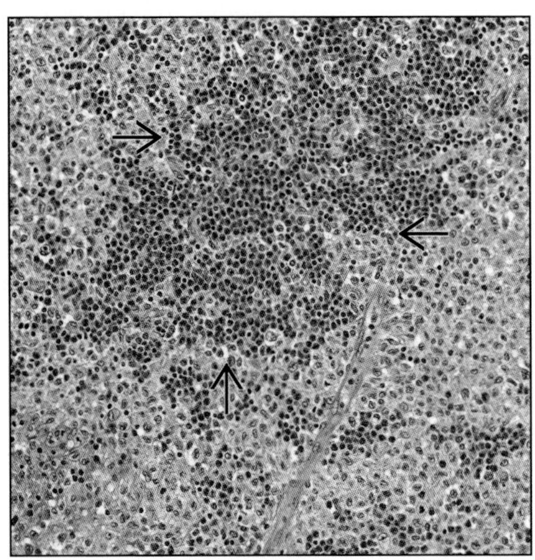

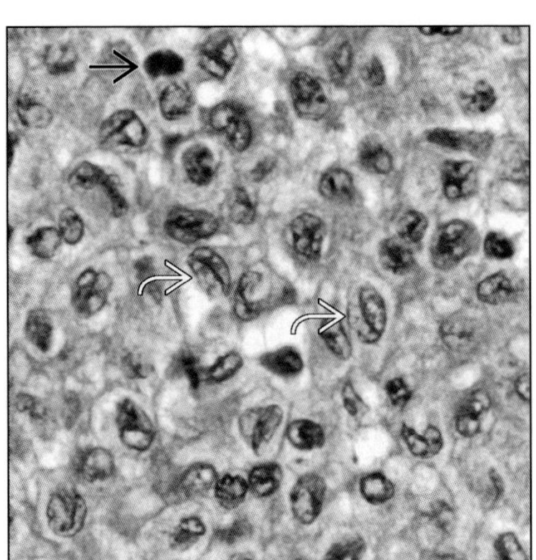

(Left) *Low-power view of Langerhans cell histiocytosis shows a collection of eosinophils ⇒ representing an eosinophilic granuloma. Eosinophilic granuloma is another term for Langerhans cell histiocytosis used to describe nodules restricted to bone.* ***(Right)*** *High-power view highlights the typical nuclear features of Langerhans cells. The nuclei are folded, show long grooves ➦, and often resemble coffee beans. An eosinophil is seen ⇒.*

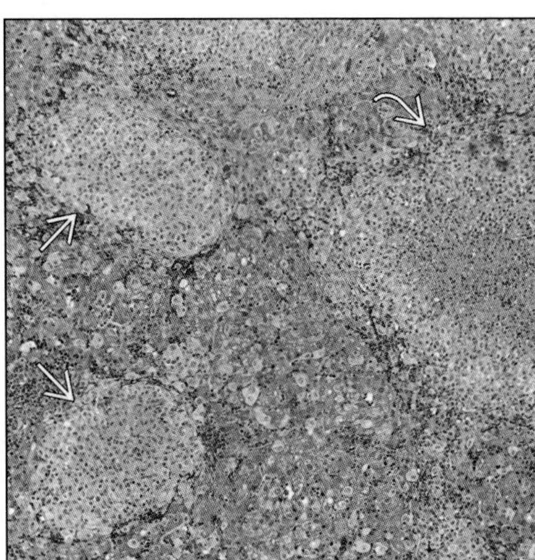

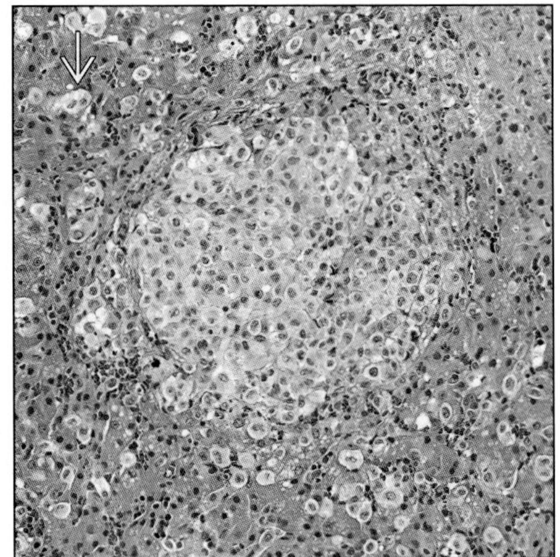

(Left) *This low-power example of Langerhans cell histiocytosis in the liver shows multiple scattered nodules ➡. The large nodule on the right ➦ has a necrotic center; necrosis is common in Langerhans cell histiocytosis.* ***(Right)*** *Medium-power view of this nodule of Langerhans cell histiocytosis in the liver shows the typical nuclear features and very few eosinophils. Single Langerhans cells ➡ are also scattered throughout the liver parenchyma.*

Additional Features

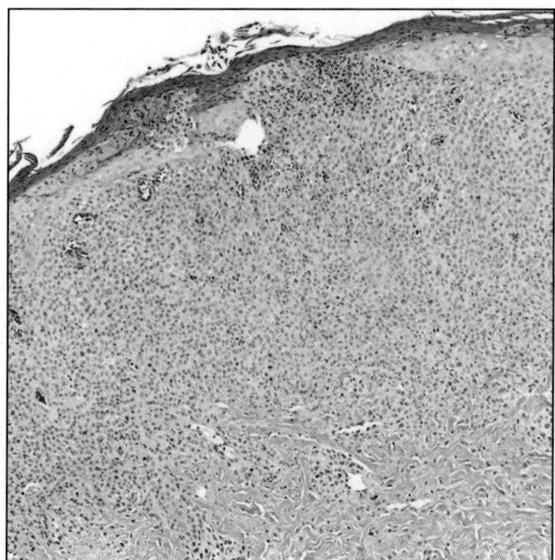

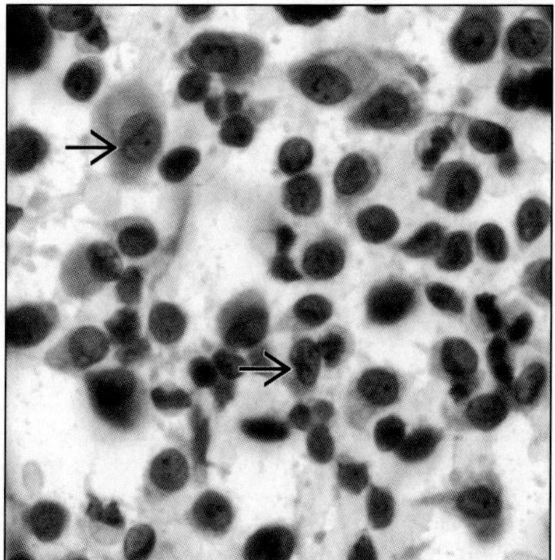

(Left) *Cutaneous involvement of Langerhans cell histiocytosis, as seen here, can often resemble a melanocytic nevus from a low-power view. The correct diagnosis is easily made by looking for the characteristic nuclear features, and with immunohistochemical stains if necessary.* ***(Right)*** *Touch preps made at the time of frozen section can be very helpful. The characteristic Langerhans cell features are easily identified, with grooved nuclei ➔ and abundant pink cytoplasm.*

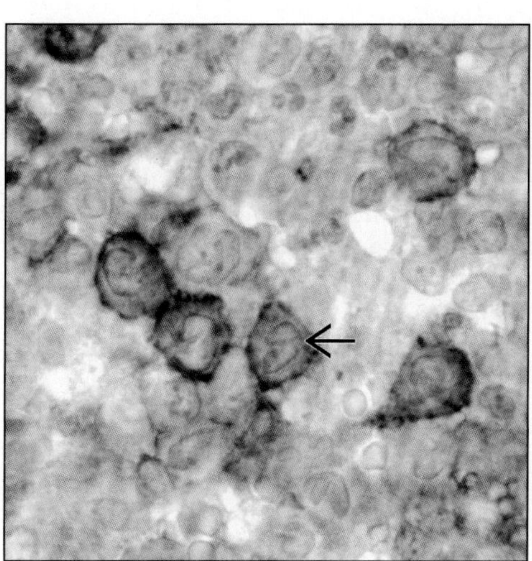

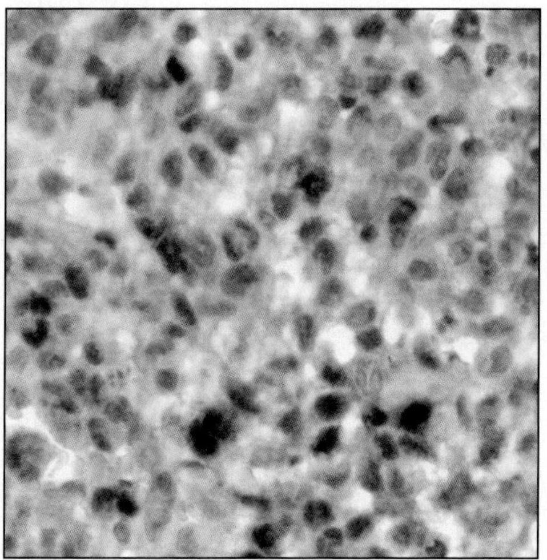

(Left) *Langerhans cells show positive membranous and cytoplasmic immunoreactivity for CD1a. Grooved nuclei ➔ can be seen within the positive-staining cells. CD1a is very specific for Langerhans cells, and is tremendously useful in cases where the cellularity is low.* ***(Right)*** *Langerhans cells show positive nuclear immunoreactivity for S100. While S100 is not as specific as CD1a for Langerhans cells, it still can be quite useful.*

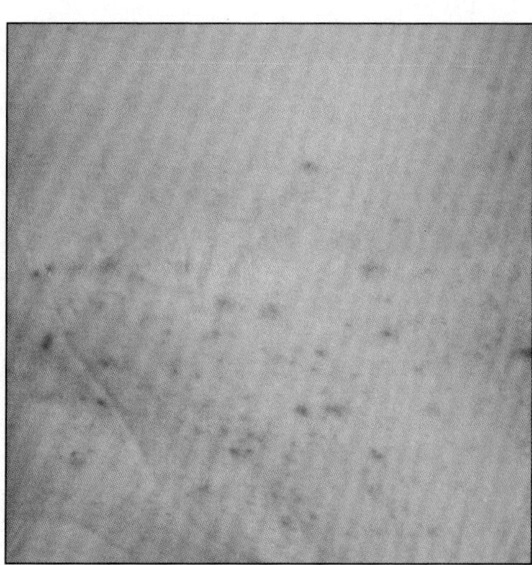

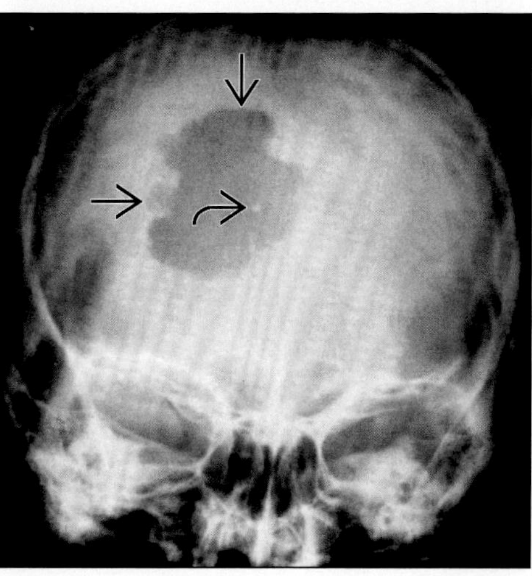

(Left) *This example of Langerhans cell histiocytosis of the skin presented as a seborrheic-like erythematous rash with petechiae on the abdomen of a 23-month-old child. (Courtesy S. Vanderhooft, MD.)* ***(Right)*** *This radiograph of the skull shows the typical appearance of Langerhans cell histiocytosis in bone ➔. The lesion is lytic with scalloped edges and sharp borders, with a radiodense focus ↗ that is commonly seen in skull lesions.*

PYOGENIC GRANULOMA

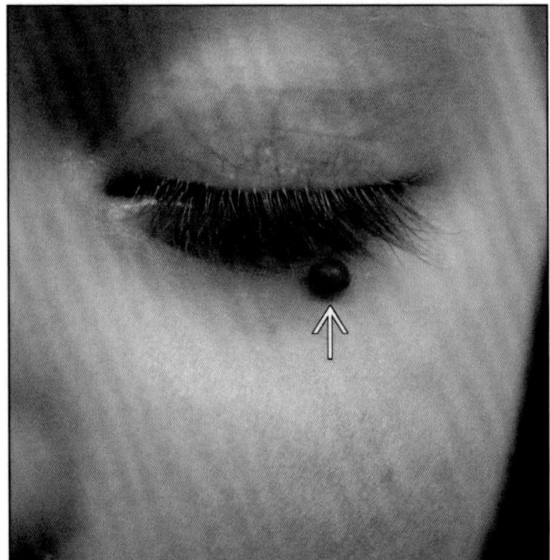

Clinical photograph shows a small pyogenic granuloma ➔ on the left lower eyelid of a young child. (Courtesy S. Vanderhooft, MD.)

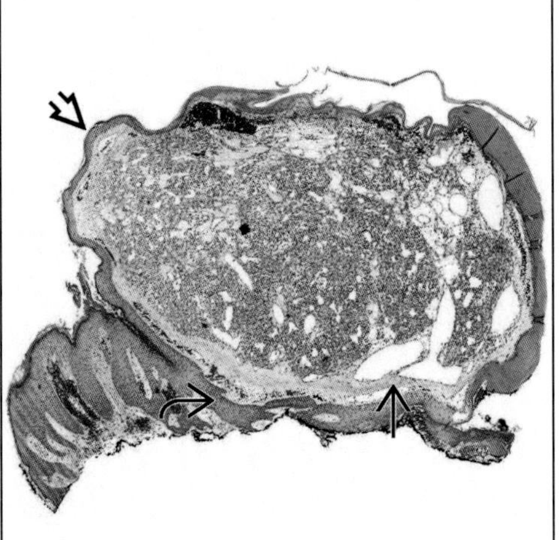

Pyogenic granuloma from low power shows a lobular proliferation of capillaries with scattered large feeder vessels ➔, an overlying attenuated epithelium ➔, and epidermal collarette ➔.

TERMINOLOGY

Synonyms

- Lobular capillary hemangioma
- Granulation tissue-type hemangioma

Definitions

- Benign acquired vascular lesion of skin and mucous membranes

ETIOLOGY/PATHOGENESIS

Reactive

- Thought to represent reactive neoplastic process
- Arises in response to various stimuli
  - Chronic irritation and traumatic injury
  - Hormones and drugs
- Unrelated to infection

CLINICAL ISSUES

Epidemiology

- Age
  - Common in all age groups
    - Most common in 2nd decade
- Gender
  - M < F
    - Likely due to vascular effects of female hormones
    - More common in males in younger age groups
    - Equal distribution among older age groups

Site

- Mucous membranes
  - Gingiva (75% of all cases)
- Skin
  - Trunk, upper extremities, and head
- Intravenous
  - **Intravenous pyogenic granuloma**
  - Most common in head, neck, and upper extremity

Presentation

- Polypoid red mass with surface ulceration
  - Sessile lesions more likely with recurrences
- Rapid growth
  - Reach maximal size within weeks to several months
- Considerable hemorrhage with minor trauma
- Correlation with pregnancy
  - **Granuloma gravidarum**
    - Arise from foci of gingival injury
    - Related to effects of altered growth factor and hormone levels during pregnancy
    - Generally arise in 1st trimester

Natural History

- 3 distinct phases
  - Cellular phase
    - Cellular compact lobules with indistinct lumina
  - Capillary phase
    - Vascular lobules with intraluminal red blood cells
  - Involutionary phase
    - Intra- and perilobular fibrosis

Treatment

- Surgical approaches
  - Complete surgical excision

Prognosis

- Excellent
- Recurrence rate of ~ 16%
  - Solitary or multiple (satellitosis)
  - Likely related to incomplete excision
- Often regress spontaneously

MACROSCOPIC FEATURES

Size

- 2 mm to 2 cm in diameter

Gross Features

- Erythematous lobulated surface

PYOGENIC GRANULOMA

Key Facts

Terminology
- Benign acquired vascular lesion of skin and mucous membranes

Etiology/Pathogenesis
- Arises in response to various stimuli
- Unrelated to infection

Clinical Issues
- Common in all age groups
- Mucous membranes
  - Gingiva (75% of all cases)
- Rapid growth
- Excellent prognosis
- Often regress spontaneously

Microscopic Pathology
- Lobular proliferation of capillary-sized blood vessels surround central branching vessel
- Thinned epidermis with frequent surface ulceration

- Surface ulceration
- Red hemorrhagic cut surface

MICROSCOPIC PATHOLOGY

Microscopic Features
- Lobular proliferation of capillary-sized blood vessels surround central branching vessel
  - Lined by bland endothelial cells
  - Perithelial or pericytic cells may surround vessels
  - Clusters of endothelial cells with indistinct lumina
  - Lobules surrounded by thin layer of collagen
- Thinned epidermis with frequent surface ulceration
- Superficial neutrophilic infiltrates
- Collarette of thickened epidermis
  - Acanthosis and hyperkeratosis along periphery
- Marked stromal edema
  - Irregular distribution of variably sized blood vessels
- Mitotic activity may be brisk

DIFFERENTIAL DIAGNOSIS

Kaposi Sarcoma
- Proliferation of dysplastic spindle cells
- Slit-like vascular spaces
- Intracellular and extracellular hyaline globules
- Infectious etiology (HHV8)

Infantile (Capillary) Hemangioma
- Typically appear in neonatal period
- Lack inflammatory cell infiltrate
- GLUT1(+)

Peripheral Giant Cell Granuloma
- Blue to purple exophytic lesion of gingiva
- May show bone resorption
- Presence of multinucleated giant cells
- Lacks distinct vascular component

Well-Differentiated Angiosarcoma
- Anastomosing network of irregular vessels that infiltrate soft tissue
- Lacks lobular growth pattern
- Lacks cytologically bland endothelial cells

SELECTED REFERENCES

1. Fortna RR et al: A case of lobular capillary hemangioma (pyogenic granuloma), localized to the subcutaneous tissue, and a review of the literature. Am J Dermatopathol. 29(4):408-11, 2007
2. Jafarzadeh H et al: Oral pyogenic granuloma: a review. J Oral Sci. 48(4):167-75, 2006
3. Toida M et al: Lobular capillary hemangioma of the oral mucosa: clinicopathological study of 43 cases with a special reference to immunohistochemical characterization of the vascular elements. Pathol Int. 53(1):1-7, 2003

IMAGE GALLERY

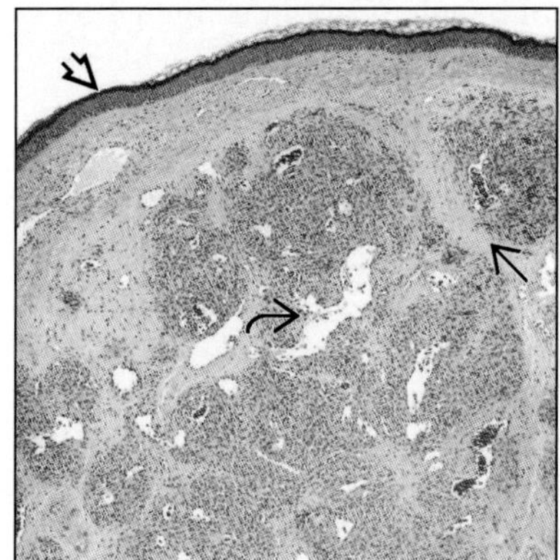

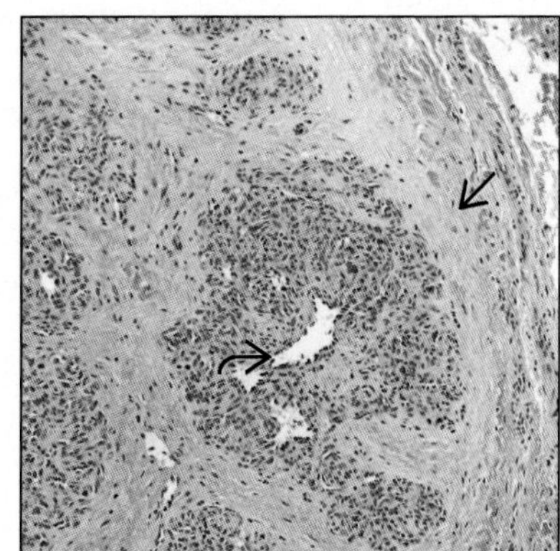

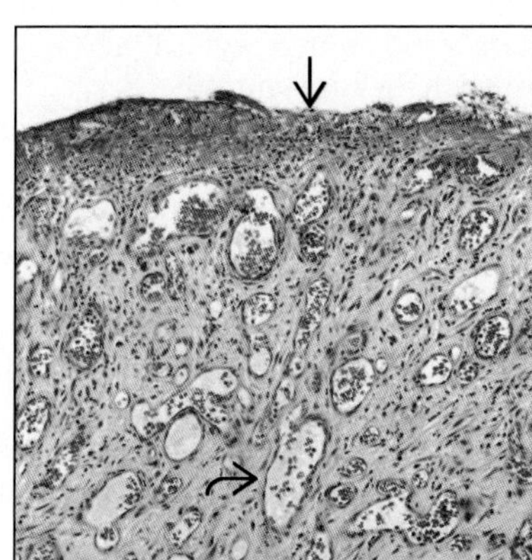

(Left) *A lobular proliferation of small capillaries surrounded by dense collagen ⇒, scattered dilated feeder vessels ⇒, and an attenuated epithelium ⇒ is shown in this pyogenic granuloma.* ***(Center)*** *Dense collagen ⇒ surrounding a lobule with a central feeder vessel ⇒ is shown.* ***(Right)*** *Surface ulceration ⇒, stromal edema with an irregular distribution of variably sized vessels ⇒, and a brisk neutrophilic infiltrate is shown in this pyogenic granuloma.*

DYSPLASTIC NEVUS

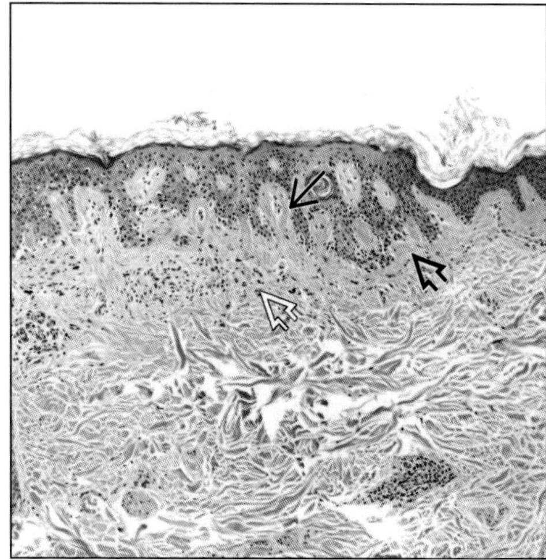

The "shoulder phenomenon" occurs when the junctional component ⇨ extends beyond the dermal component ➡. Fibroplasia involves the papillary dermis ⇨.

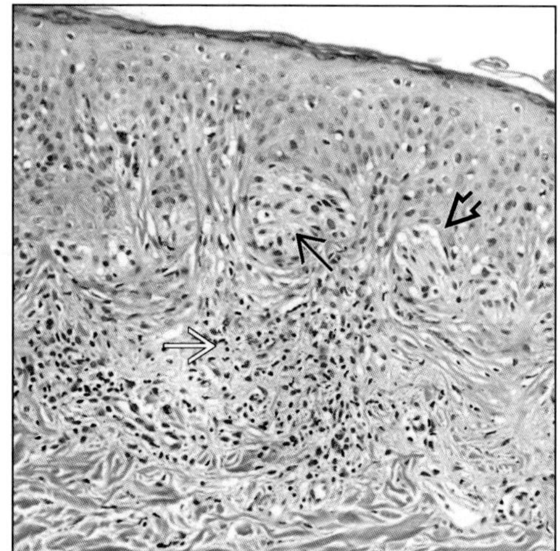

Lentiginous hyperplasia may occur as a proliferation of single cells or as nests along the basal layer ⇨. These cells may show shrinkage artifact ⇨. Note the superficial lymphocytic infiltrate ➡.

TERMINOLOGY

Synonyms

- Atypical nevus
- Clark nevus

Definitions

- Clinically distinct nevus with cytological and architectural abnormalities
  - Typically a compound nevus with peripheral lentiginous and junctional activity
  - Random cytological atypia in epidermal component

CLINICAL ISSUES

Presentation

- Acquired nevus
  - May arise de novo or in association with preexisting nevus
  - Typically not seen until puberty
  - Incidence is higher in patients from melanoma-prone families
  - Atypical nevi may occur at any site
- "Cheetah phenotype"
  - Individuals with numerous (usually > 100) small, darkly pigmented atypical nevi
- Dysplastic nevus syndrome
  - Autosomal dominant hereditary cancer predisposition syndrome
  - Atypical nevi develop in 2nd and 3rd decades of life
  - Multiple, even hundreds of dysplastic nevi are present
  - Large variability in size of nevi
  - At risk for developing 1 or more primary melanomas
  - Required for diagnosis
    - Multiple dysplastic nevi
    - 2 or more family members with malignant melanoma
  - Chromosomal associations
    - Deletion of chromosome 11
    - Deletion of 17p13
  - Originally called B-K mole syndrome and familial atypical multiple mole-melanoma (FAMMM) syndrome
- Incidence of dysplastic nevi in pediatric population is extremely low

Prognosis

- Children with atypical nevi are at risk for developing malignant melanoma
  - Lifetime risk of 10%

MACROSCOPIC FEATURES

General Features

- Shares features with malignant melanoma
  - Raised pigmented lesion
  - Marked lesion-to-lesion variability
  - Irregular color
  - Irregular texture
  - Irregular borders
  - Larger size
    - Typically measure 6-15 mm in greatest dimension
- May have cobblestone appearance
- Small, dark central papule surrounded by lighter color periphery
  - "Fried egg" appearance

MICROSCOPIC PATHOLOGY

Histologic Features

- Proliferation of nevomelanocytes
  - Irregular nests
  - Lentiginous proliferation
  - Individual cells show atypia
    - Atypia is random and ranges from mild to severe
    - Enlarged hyperchromatic nuclei
    - May have prominent nucleoli

DYSPLASTIC NEVUS

Key Facts

Clinical Issues

- Acquired nevus
- Typically not seen until puberty
- Atypical nevi may occur at any site
- Children with atypical nevi are at risk for developing malignant melanoma

Microscopic Pathology

- Lentiginous melanocytic hyperplasia
- Atypia is random and ranges from mild to severe
- Junctional component extends beyond dermal component (shoulder phenomenon)
- Lamellar and concentric fibroplasia of papillary dermis
- Bridging of adjacent tips of rete ridges by melanocytes

Diagnostic Checklist

- Evaluation of surgical margins for complete excision is important

- Lentiginous melanocytic hyperplasia
  - Proliferation of nevomelanocytes, singly or in nest along basal layer
  - Present throughout lesion
  - Extends laterally beyond dermal component (if present) to produce a "shoulder area"
  - Nevomelanocytes
    - May show shrinkage artifact
    - Spindled or cuboidal cells
    - Scant cytoplasm
    - Dusty pigment
- Dermal component
  - Centrally located
  - Epithelioid cells
  - Does not show much evidence of maturation
- Mild hyperplasia of epidermal rete
- Lamellar and concentric fibroplasia of papillary dermis
- Bridging of adjacent tips of rete ridges by melanocytes
- Patchy lymphocytic infiltrate in underlying superficial dermis
  - May contain melanophages

DIFFERENTIAL DIAGNOSIS

Malignant Melanoma

- Consists largely of anaplastic cells
- Dyscohesive infiltration of epidermis by atypical nevomelanocytes

DIAGNOSTIC CHECKLIST

Pathologic Interpretation Pearls

- Evaluation of surgical margins for complete excision is important
- Dyscohesive infiltration of epidermis by atypical nevomelanocytes suggests malignant melanoma
  - This feature should not be seen in dysplastic nevi

SELECTED REFERENCES

1. Decarlo K et al: Oncogenic BRAF-positive dysplastic nevi and the tumor suppressor IGFBP7--challenging the concept of dysplastic nevi as precursor lesions? Hum Pathol. 41(6):886-94, 2010
2. Elder DE: Dysplastic naevi: an update. Histopathology. 56(1):112-20, 2010
3. Gupta M et al: Morphologic features and natural history of scalp nevi in children. Arch Dermatol. 146(5):506-11, 2010
4. Koller J: [Pigment nevi in children.] Hautarzt. 61(5):443-51; quiz 452, 2010

IMAGE GALLERY

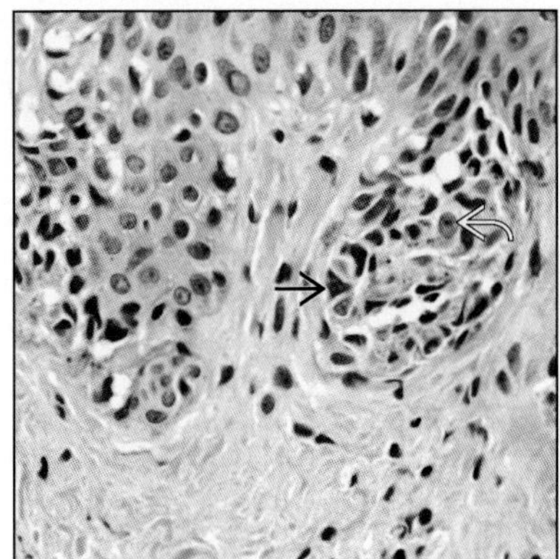

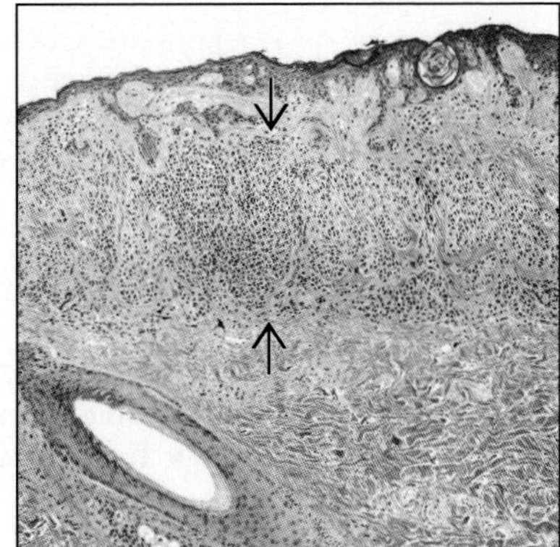

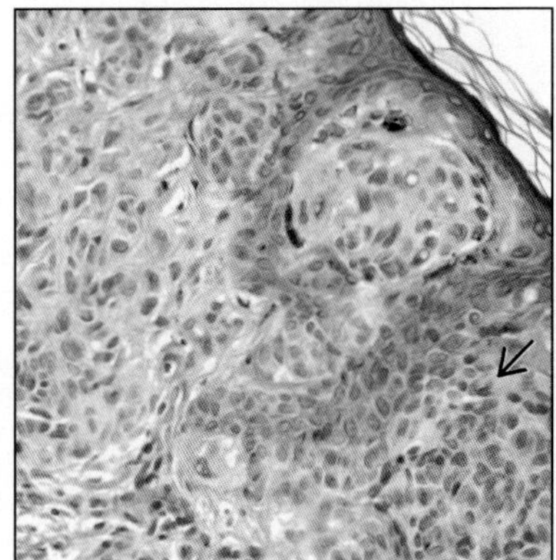

(Left) *Note the random, mild cytological atypia. These features include enlarged hyperchromatic nuclei ⇒ and small nucleoli ⇒.* ***(Center)*** *The dermal component ⇒ is located centrally within the lesion, consists of epithelioid cells, and shows little maturation.* ***(Right)*** *The dermal component consists of epithelioid cells with faint, dusty pigment ⇒.*

MALIGNANT MELANOMA

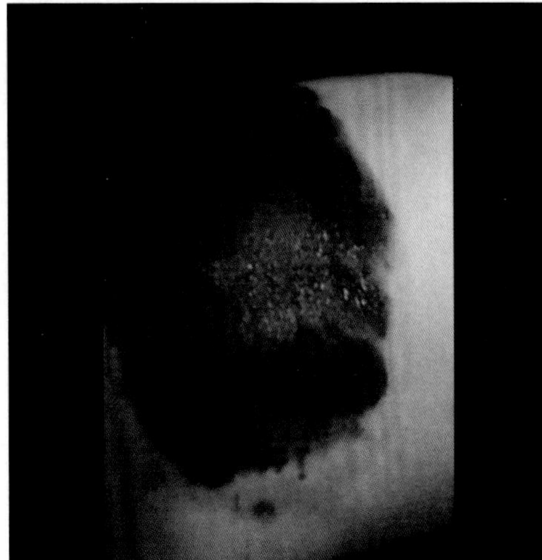

This is a giant congential pigmented nevus on the back of a newborn, in which a melanoma that was ultimately fatal developed.

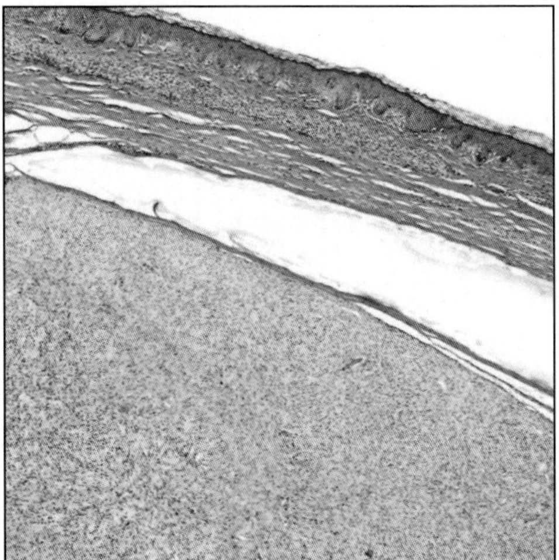

This is a section of a malignant melanoma arising within a giant congenital melanocytic nevus. This cellular nodule is a sharply demarcated, expansile growth. Cytologic atypia and mitoses were present on higher power.

TERMINOLOGY

Abbreviations

- Malignant melanoma (MM)

Definitions

- Malignant cutaneous melanocytic neoplasm

CLINICAL ISSUES

Epidemiology

- Incidence
  - Accounts for 1-3% of all childhood malignancies
  - 7x more frequent in 2nd decade than 1st decade of life
  - < 1% of all melanomas occur in prepubertal children (< 14 years old)
  - On the rise in children and teenagers
  - Accounts for < 0.5% of all melanomas
- Age
  - Prepubescent melanoma
    - Develop transplacentally, de novo, within a congenital melanocytic nevus (CMN) or in association with another cutaneous lesion
    - Congenital and infantile melanomas are rare
  - Postpubescent melanoma
    - > 14 years of age
    - Clinical features and prognosis tend to resemble adult counterparts
- Gender
  - Slight female predominance

Site

- Can occur anywhere on the skin
  - Rarely mucous membranes and meninges

Presentation

- 50% arise in association within preexisting lesion
  - 30% arise within a giant CMN (> 20 cm)
    - 50-70% will arise before puberty
    - Tend to arise within the dermis
    - Worse prognosis
  - 20% in association with other cutaneous lesions
    - Small to medium-sized CMNs
    - Acquired melanocytic nevi
    - More likely to occur after puberty
- 50% arise de novo
- May arise with neurocutaneous melanosis
  - Rare but carries high risk of malignant transformation in children
  - Median age is 3 years old
  - Up to 2/3 of patients may develop primary intracranial melanomas
- Signs and symptoms may include
  - Rapid increase in size of lesion, hemorrhage, ulceration, change in color, loss of previously regular borders, pruritus, lymphadenopathy
- Important clinical signs ("ABCD")
  - Asymmetry
  - Border irregularity
  - Color/pigmentation irregularities
  - Diameter of 6 mm or greater
- "ABCD" changes of adult melanomas may be absent in pediatric patients
- **Risk factors**
  - Fair skin
  - Giant CMN (bathing trunk nevus)
    - Risk correlates with size, depth, and number of melanocytes
    - Occurs in 1 in 20,000 newborns
    - ≥ 20 cm in largest diameter
    - Up to 5-7% risk of malignant transformation
  - Dysplastic nevus syndrome
  - Numerous acquired melanocytic nevi
    - Independent risk factor
  - Sporadic atypical nevi
    - Independent risk factor
  - Xeroderma pigmentosum
  - Albinism
  - Immunosuppression

Key Facts

Clinical Issues
- Knowledge of clinical dimensions is of maximum importance
  - Ensure viewing entirety or most of the lesion before making a benign diagnosis
  - Can be difficult, especially in cases of giant congenital melanocytic nevus (CMN)

Microscopic Pathology
- Asymmetry of lesion
  - Probably most powerful criterion for diagnosing melanoma
- Lack of circumscription
- Pagetoid spread of single melanocytes above basal layer, especially at periphery of lesion
- Lack of maturation
- Lack of dispersion
- Deep dermal mitoses
- Pigment deep in lesion
- Solitary epidermal melanocytes predominating over nests

Reporting Considerations
- Breslow thickness, not histologic subtype, is most important prognostic parameter
- Presence or absence of ulceration changes stage

Malpractice Considerations
- Expert consultation recommended before diagnosing melanoma in any pediatric patient
- Due to wide range of histologic features and subtypes of melanomas
  - Diagnosis of melanoma should be considered when encountering any unusual cutaneous malignancy

---

- Family history of melanoma (familial melanoma)
  - Occur at younger age
  - Often multifocal
  - Germline mutations of *CDKN2A* tumor suppressor gene

Treatment
- Options, risks, complications
  - Surgical resection with standard margins
    - Treatment of choice in primary diseases
    - Potentially curative
    - May also include sentinel lymph node biopsy or regional lymphadenectomy
    - Both the National Comprehensive Cancer Network (NCCN) and the American Academy of Dermatology (AAD) publish online guidelines for surgical margins
  - Chemotherapy of minimal benefit
  - Experimental immunotherapy of unproven benefit
  - Treatment protocols based on adult population

Prognosis
- Most important prognostic factors
  - Depth of invasion
    - Measured by Breslow thickness
  - Stage at diagnosis
    - Stage IV 5-year survival rate (34%)
    - Stage I-II 5-year survival rate (90%)
- Other poor prognostic indicators
  - Previous nonmelanocytic malignancies, nodular histologic type, fusiform or spitzoid cytology, vertical growth phase
  - High dermal mitotic activity, ulceration, vascular invasion, age > 10 years, and presence of metastases at diagnosis
- Overall 5-year survival (79%)
- Survival characteristics similar to adult population

MICROSCOPIC PATHOLOGY

Histologic Features
- Size usually > 7 mm
- May or may not have ulceration
- Asymmetry
  - Probably the most powerful histologic criterion
  - Nests showing
    - Variability in size and shape
    - Haphazard interval and array
  - Haphazard arrangement of solitary epidermal melanocytes
- Solitary epidermal melanocytes predominate over nests
- Poor circumscription
  - Lesion does not start or end in a nest
  - Difficult to discern where lesion starts and stops
  - Single melanocytes predominate at edge of lesion
- Pagetoid spread of melanocytes
  - Ascent of single melanocytes above dermoepidermal (DE) junction
  - Can also be present in Spitz nevi (sometimes full nests) and acral nevi
  - Should not be in periphery of Spitz or acral nevi
- Lack of maturation
  - Deeper melanocytes as large as superficial ones
- Deep dermal mitoses
- Pigment present deep in lesion
- Atypical melanocytes
  - Atypical features not always present
  - May have marked nuclear pleomorphism
  - Melanocytes may be small and spindled or epithelioid
- Confluence of melanocytes
- Melanomas arising in giant CMN
  - When arising in type 1 CMN, usually arises at DE junction
  - When arising in type 2 CMN, usually arises in dermal component
- Inflammatory infiltrate can be helpful especially if asymmetrical
  - Often seen surrounding invasive component

Cytologic Features
- High nuclear to cytoplasmic ratio
- Prominent nucleoli, often "cherry red"

- Marked nuclear pleomorphism
- Hyperchromasia
- Dusty melanin

Classification of Pediatric Melanoma

- Classified according to mode of occurrence and histology
    - Transplacental melanoma
    - Transformation from giant CMN
    - In association with congenital predisposing conditions
    - Development from healthy skin
    - Development from preexisting nevus

Histologic Subtypes

- **Superficial spreading melanoma**
    - Most common subtype
    - Found on non-sun-exposed skin
    - Characteristic radial (lateral) growth phase
    - Asymmetrical proliferation of atypical nondendritic epithelioid melanocytes
        - Cells often pleomorphic with prominent nucleoli, fine melanin pigmentation, and scattered mitotic figures
    - Pagetoid spread of single melanocytes common
    - Epidermal acanthosis with effacement of rete ridges
    - FISH and CGH studies less sensitive
- **Acral lentiginous melanoma**
    - Found on palms and soles ("acral" skin)
    - More common in Asian and black populations
    - Acanthosis and elongation of epidermal ridges infiltrated by atypical melanocytes
        - Often pleomorphism, hyperchromasia, conspicuous nucleoli, and mitoses
        - Fixation retraction artifact
    - Scattered foci of junctional nests
    - Lichenoid chronic inflammatory infiltrate
    - FISH and CGH studies more sensitive
- **Nodular melanoma**
    - Large nodules of oval to round epithelioid melanocytes
    - May be symmetrical in all directions
    - Lacks intraepidermal melanocytic proliferation
    - FISH and CGH studies more sensitive
    - No maturation
- **Desmoplastic melanoma**
    - Dense desmoplastic stroma
    - p16 staining can be helpful in differentiating from desmoplastic Spitz nevus
        - p16 staining often lost in desmoplastic melanomas
    - S100 only reliable immunostain (may be absent)
        - Often HMB-45 and mart-1 negative
- **Spindle cell melanoma**
    - Spindled cytology
    - S100 only reliable immunostain (may be absent)
        - Often HMB-45 and mart-1 negative
- Other rare melanoma variants
    - Neurotropic, amelanotic, balloon cell, pedunculated, nevoid, spitzoid, small cell, and myxoid

ANCILLARY TESTS

Immunohistochemistry

- S100 positive, considered the most sensitive stain
- HMB-45 and Melan-A (MART-1) positive, more specific but less sensitive
- MITF, SOX10, and tyrosinase positive

In Situ Hybridization

- FISH assays targeting most common chromosomal aberrations can be helpful
    - Probes vary from institution to institution but 6p25, 6q23, Cep6, and 11q13 are often used

Array CGH

- Can be a very helpful adjunctive test, especially for difficult cases
- > 96% of malignant melanomas demonstrate chromosomal aberrations
    - Most common are gains of chromosome 1q, 6p, 7p, 7q, 8q, 17q, and 20q or losses of 6q, 9p, 9q, 10q, 10p, and 11q
- Benign proliferations in CMNs can show chromosomal aberrations
    - However, these differ from aberrations found in melanomas arising in CMNs, which are similar to melanomas arising de novo

DIFFERENTIAL DIAGNOSIS

Benign Proliferative Nodule in Giant CMNs

- Area of higher cell density and nuclear enlargement with higher mitotic activity in CMN
- Can also be hamartoma arising in giant CMN
    - Nonmelanocytic cells such as smooth muscle, nerve, or sebaceous cells normally also present
- Typically become softer in time, stop growing, and subsequently become smaller or regress completely

Spitz Nevus

- Preferentially involves head and neck of children
- Usually < 1 cm in diameter
- Characterized by large spindled or epithelioid cells
- Features to support diagnosis of Spitz nevi
    - Symmetry, maturation with depth, wedge-shaped silhouette
    - Melanocytic nests clutched by rete ridges or showing pagetoid spread
    - Clefts around melanocytic nests
    - Evidence of dull pink globules often situated above tips of dermal papillae ("Kamino bodies")

Melanocytic Nevus

- Symmetrical and well-circumscribed nests of melanocytes
- Typically lacks cytologic atypia and pagetoid spread
    - Pagetoid spread can be seen in middle of Spitz and acral nevi
- Lacks deep mitoses
- Melanocytes mature with depth
- Usually lacks lymphocytes

- Exceptions include irritated nevi, Spitz nevus, halo nevus, and dysplastic nevus
- **Deep penetrating nevus**
  - Rare variant reported most often in 3rd decade
  - Typically wedge-shaped, heavily pigmented, and often sharply demarcated
  - Can have cellular atypia, pleomorphism, and a deep infiltrating growth pattern, but typically rare to no mitoses

Dysplastic Nevus

- Pigmented papules, macules, and plaques
- Clinical features may resemble melanoma
- Features to support diagnosis of dysplastic nevus
  - Elongated clubbed rete ridges and bridging melanocytic nests
  - Concentric or lamellar fibroplasia in papillary dermis
  - Melanocytic maturation, well nested at dermoepidermal junction, no deep mitoses, and no pigment deep in lesion

Blue Nevus

- Proliferation of heavily pigmented melanocytes with dendritic processes dissecting through collagen fibers
- **Cellular blue nevi**
  - Still composed of dendritic melanocytes but often islands of epithelioid or spindle cells as well
  - Often depigmented (vs. typical blue nevi)
  - Nodular downgrowth (vs. infiltrative) into subcutaneous fat
- **Malignant blue nevus:** Very rare but has been reported in children
  - Infiltrating growth pattern vs. typical blue nevus
  - Atypical mitoses, pleomorphism, and often necrosis

Spindle Cell Malignancies

- Cutaneous leiomyosarcoma
  - Extremely rare in children
  - Positive for smooth muscle markers (SMA, MSA, desmin, or h-caldesmon)
  - Typically S100 negative, rare positive cases
- Malignant peripheral nerve sheath tumor (MPNST)
  - Can be focally positive for S100 vs. the diffuse and strong positivity usually seen in melanoma
  - Can be a very difficult differential diagnosis
  - By definition must arise from a nerve
- Spindle cell squamous cell carcinoma (SCC)
  - SCC may be seen in children with xeroderma pigmentosa and dystrophic epidermolysis bullosa
  - Rare variant but can cause diagnostic confusion
  - Usually cytokeratin positive
- Atypical fibroxanthoma (not seen in children)
- Dermatofibrosarcoma protuberans (DFSP)
  - Densely cellular proliferation of dark spindle cells that deeply infiltrate fat in storiform pattern
  - CD34 extensively positive in almost all tumors
  - Negative for S100 and other melanoma markers
  - Can be pigmented "Bednar tumor"

MALPRACTICE CONSIDERATIONS

Misdiagnosis

- Common
- Up to 40% of pediatric melanomas may initially be misdiagnosed
- Up to 60% of patients < 20 years experience delay in treatment

Points of Diagnostic Confusion

- Similar histologic presentations as Spitz nevi
- Atypia in proliferative nodules of giant CMN
- Multiple histologic variants that mimic other entities
  - Small cell, desmoplastic, balloon cell, spitzoid, rhabdoid, myxoid, signet ring cell, and others

Uncertainty

- Not uncommon in these difficult lesions and challenging patient population
- Consultation encouraged of any suspicious lesion
  - Expert review of cases often needed and improves patient care
- Often only true measure of malignancy in pediatric population is death or distant metastasis

STAGING

AJCC

- Staging does not differ from that for adults
- **Breslow thickness**
  - Measurement in mm from top of granular layer to the deepest point of invasion
  - Extension along adnexal structures is not measured
  - Considered most important prognostic indicator and more accurate than Clark levels
- Ulceration and mitotic index may increase stage and result in lymph node dissection

SELECTED REFERENCES

1. Phadke PA et al: Proliferative nodules arising within congenital melanocytic nevi: a histologic, immunohistochemical, and molecular analyses of 43 cases. Am J Surg Pathol. 35(5):656-69, 2011
2. Berk DR et al: Melanoma and melanocytic tumors of uncertain malignant potential in children, adolescents and young adults--the Stanford experience 1995-2008. Pediatr Dermatol. 27(3):244-54, 2010
3. Ducharme EE et al: Pediatric malignant melanoma: an update on epidemiology, detection, and prevention. Cutis. 84(4):192-8, 2009
4. Jen M et al: Childhood melanoma. Clin Dermatol. 27(6):529-36, 2009
5. Downard CD et al: Melanoma in children and adolescents. Surg Oncol. 16(3):215-20, 2007
6. Krengel S et al: Melanoma risk in congenital melanocytic naevi: a systematic review. Br J Dermatol. 155(1):1-8, 2006
7. Ferrari A et al: Does melanoma behave differently in younger children than in adults? A retrospective study of 33 cases of childhood melanoma from a single institution. Pediatrics. 115(3):649-54, 2005

MALIGNANT MELANOMA

Clinical and Microscopic Features

(Left) Clinical photograph shows a large melanoma with variegated color, jagged border, and irregular surface, all of which are concerning clinical signs. *(Right)* H&E shows melanoma from the back of a 16-year-old female. Note that single cells predominate ➔, and there are single cells advancing up through the epidermis (pagetoid spread) ➔. (Courtesy C. Cockerell, MD.)

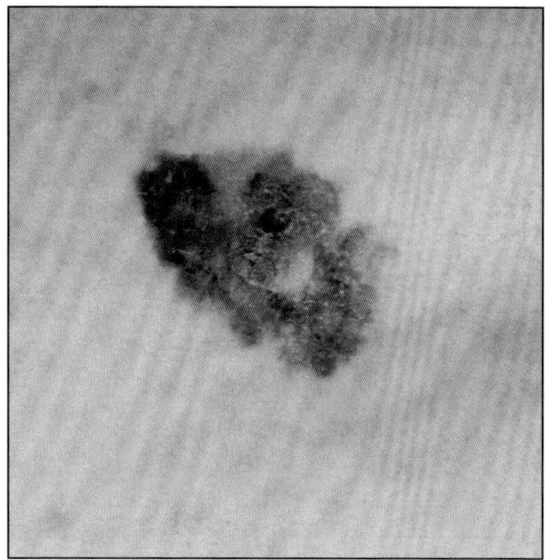

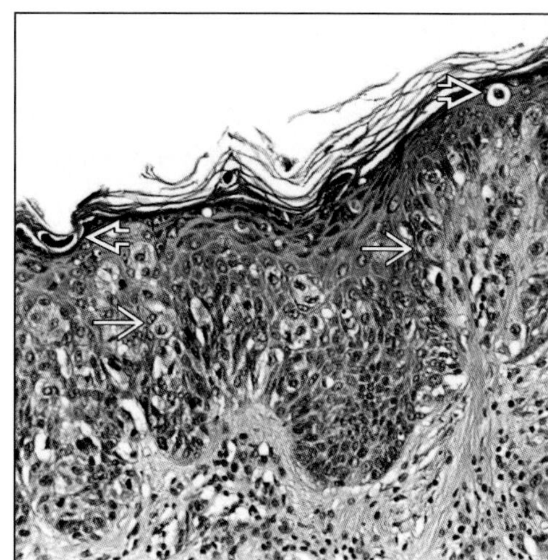

(Left) This nodular melanoma presents as a dark brown asymmetric nodule with leakage of pigment around the edge of the lesion ➔. *(Right)* Nodular melanoma demonstrates characteristic pedunculated shape. These are usually sharply circumscribed and contain nests of oval to round atypical epithelioid melanocytes growing throughout the dermis. Lack of maturation (uniform cells throughout) and large irregular nests are other helpful features. (Courtesy G. Fraga, MD.)

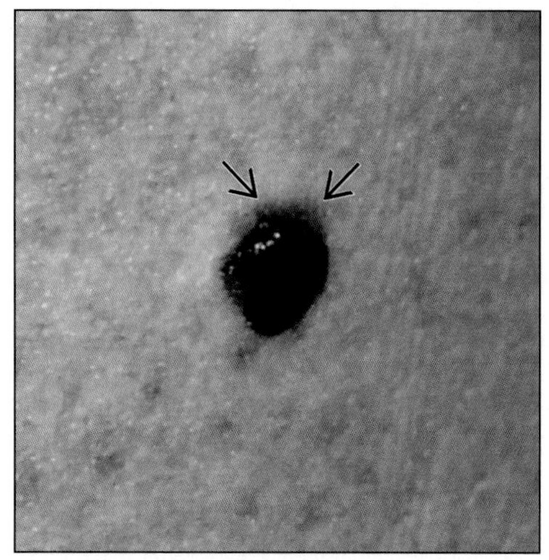

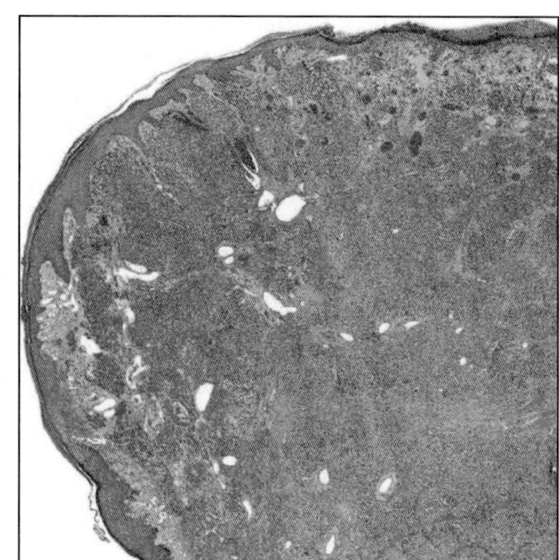

(Left) This preauricular superficial spreading melanoma is larger than 6 mm with an irregular border, asymmetry, and a pseudopod of different color on the superior edge ➔. *(Right)* Superficial spreading melanoma shows prominent pagetoid spread ➔ and obvious nuclear hyperchromasia ➔, pleomorphism, and cytologic atypia. (Courtesy G. Fraga, MD.)

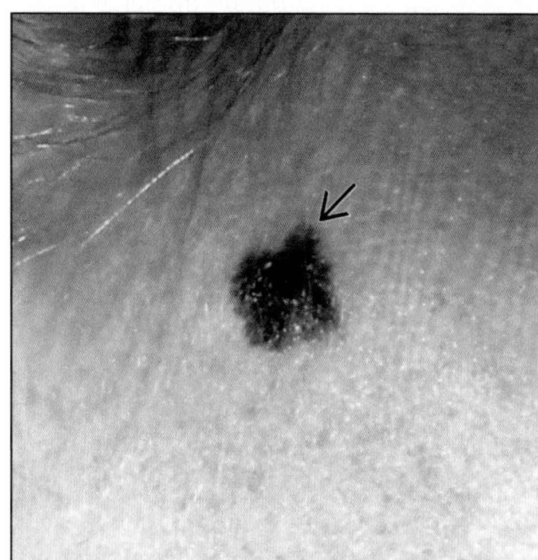

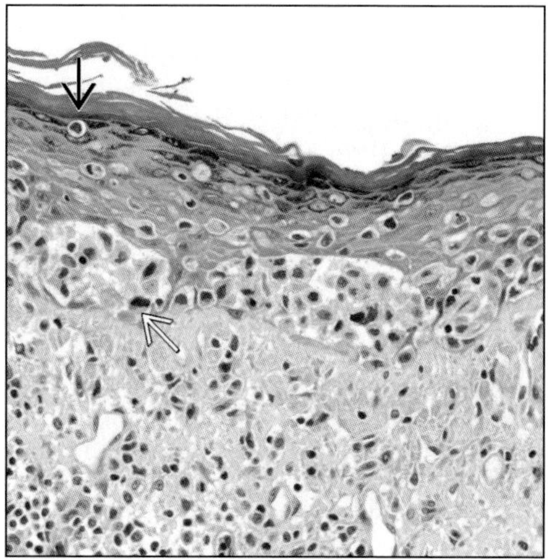

Clinical and Microscopic Features

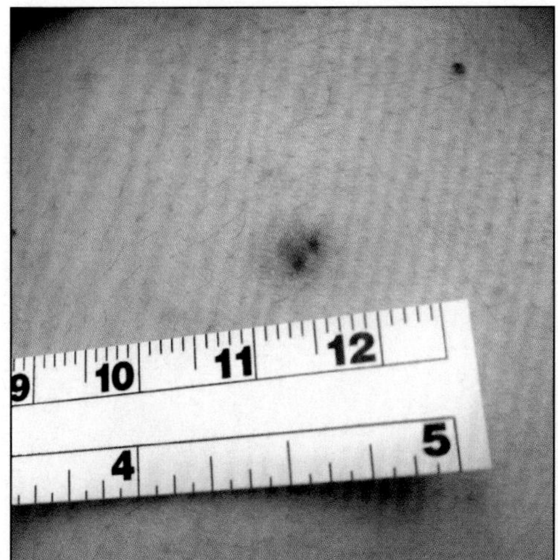

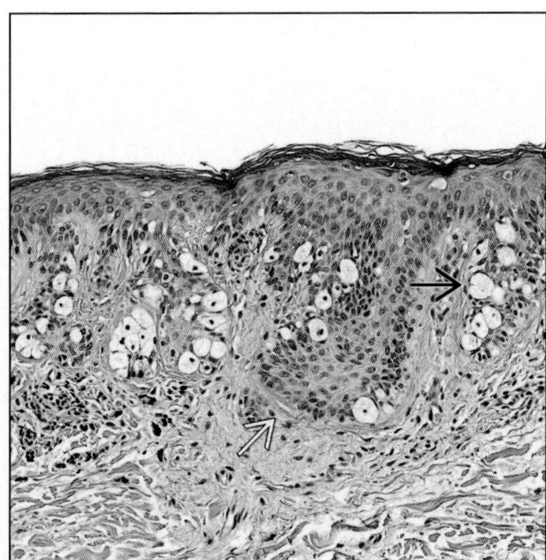

(Left) *This multicolored, irregularly bordered, asymmetric dysplastic nevus clinically mimics melanoma, as it is notoriously known to do. Biopsy is often helpful to clarify this clinical differential.* ***(Right)*** *Dysplastic nevus with balloon cell features demonstrates ballooning of some of the melanocytes ⇒ as well as the characteristic eosinophilic fibroplasia ➡ of this dysplastic nevus. Balloon cells are a completely benign degenerative feature seen in some nevi.*

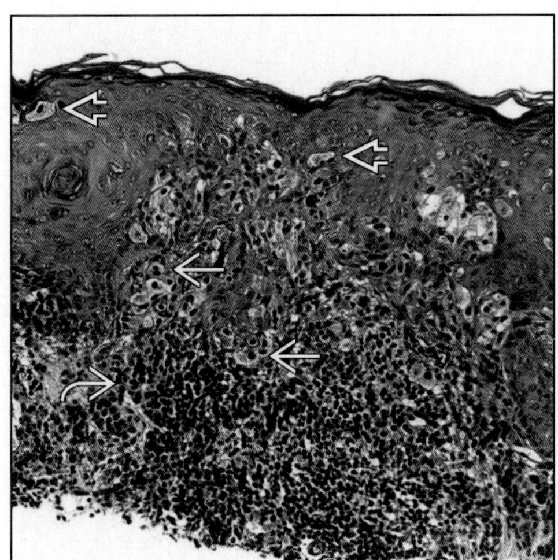

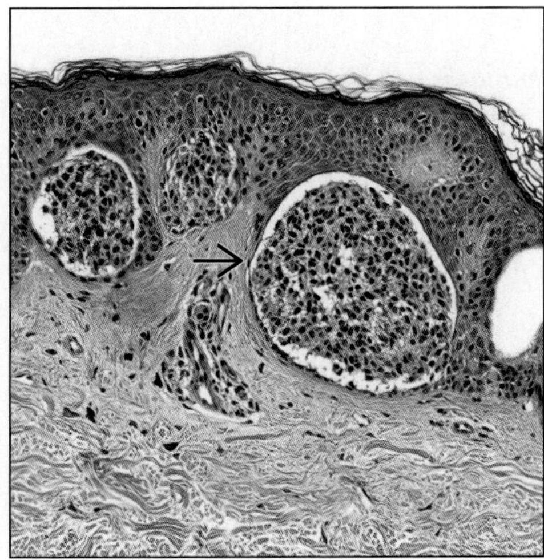

(Left) *This melanoma arose in association with a nevus ➡ from the back of a 13-year-old girl. Note the prominent pagetoid spread ➡ of atypical melanocytes with dusty melanin in the epidermis and the predominance of single cells ➡ in the melanoma. (Courtesy L. Karai, MD.)* ***(Right)*** *This is a junctional nevus for comparison. Note how well nested ⇒ these melanocytes are, and nests predominate over single cells. (Courtesy T. McCalmont, MD.)*

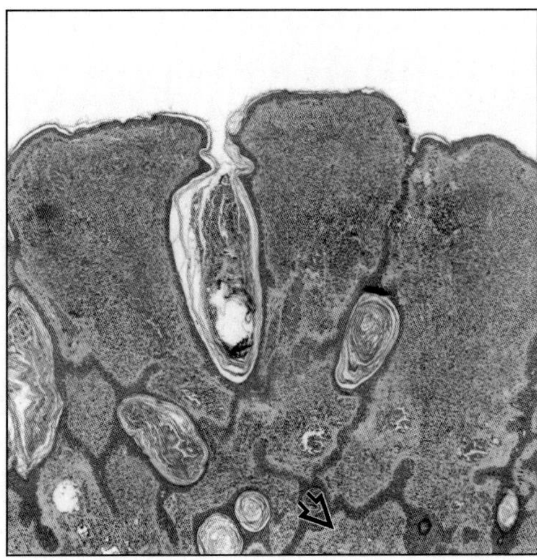

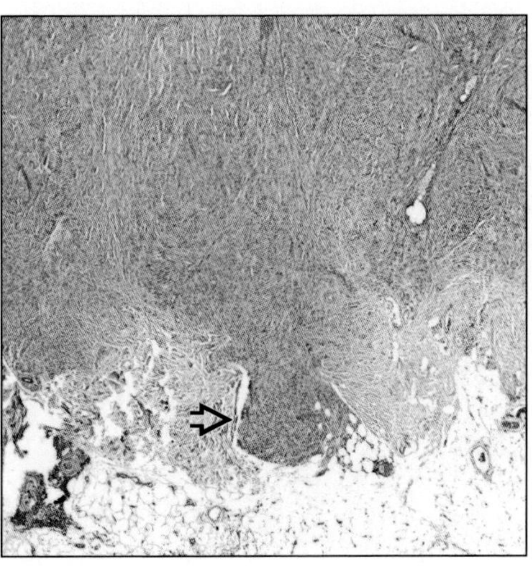

(Left) *This is a compound nevus. Note how the lesion is symmetric and that the melanocytes seem to "mature" and disperse at the base ⇒. (Courtesy P. LeBoit, MD.)* ***(Right)*** *This is a large melanoma with "spitzoid" morphology on a pediatric patient who developed bulky metastases. In benign lesions, melanocytes should mature and disperse into single melanocytes toward the base. This tongue of melanocytes ⇒ at the base makes the diagnosis. (Courtesy D. Elston, MD.)*

PROTOCOL FOR MELANOMA SPECIMENS

Melanoma of the Skin

Biopsy, Excision, Re-excision

Procedure (select all that apply)

___ Biopsy, shave
___ Biopsy, punch
___ Biopsy, incisional
___ Excision
___ Re-excision
___ Lymphadenectomy, sentinel node(s)
___ Lymphadenectomy, regional nodes (specify): ____________________________
___ Other (specify): ____________________________
___ Not specified

Specimen Laterality

___ Right
___ Left
___ Midline
___ Not specified

Tumor Site

Specify, if known: ____________________________
___ Not specified

Tumor Size (required only if tumor is grossly present)

Greatest dimension: _________ cm
*Additional dimensions: _________ x _________ cm
___ Indeterminate

Macroscopic Satellite Nodule(s) (required for excision specimens only)

___ Not identified
___ Present
___ Indeterminate

****Macroscopic Pigmentation***

*___ Not identified
*___ Present, diffuse
*___ Present, patchy/focal
*___ Indeterminate

Histologic Type

Malignant melanoma
___ Melanoma, not otherwise specified
___ Superficial spreading melanoma
___ Nodular melanoma
___ Lentigo maligna melanoma
___ Acral-lentiginous melanoma
___ Desmoplastic &/or desmoplastic neurotropic melanoma
___ Melanoma arising from blue nevus
___ Melanoma arising in a giant congenital nevus
___ Melanoma of childhood
___ Nevoid melanoma
___ Persistent melanoma
___ Other (specify): ____________________________

Maximum Tumor Thickness

Specify: __________ mm
At least _________ mm
___ Indeterminate

PROTOCOL FOR MELANOMA SPECIMENS

*Anatomic Level

*___ I (melanoma in situ)
*___ II (melanoma present in, but does not fill and expand, papillary dermis)
*___ III (melanoma fills and expands papillary dermis)
*___ IV (melanoma invades reticular dermis)
*___ V (melanoma invades subcutaneum)

Ulceration

___ Present
___ Not identified
___ Indeterminate

Margins (select all that apply)

Peripheral margins

___ Cannot be assessed
___ Uninvolved by invasive melanoma
Distance of invasive melanoma from closest peripheral margin: ________ mm (required for excisions only)
Specify location(s), if possible: ________________________
___ Involved by invasive melanoma
Specify location(s), if possible: ________________________
___ Uninvolved by melanoma in situ
Distance of melanoma in situ from closest margin: ________ mm (required for excisions only)
Specify location(s), if possible: ________________________
___ Involved by melanoma in situ
Specify location(s), if possible: ________________________

Deep margin

___ Cannot be assessed
___ Uninvolved by invasive melanoma
Distance of invasive melanoma from margin: ________ mm (required for excisions only)
Specify location(s), if possible: ________________________
___ Involved by invasive melanoma
Specify location(s), if possible: ________________________

Mitotic Index

___ < 1 mm^2
Specify number/mm^2: ________

Microsatellitosis

___ Not identified
___ Present
___ Indeterminate

Lymphovascular Invasion

___ Not identified
___ Present
___ Indeterminate

*Perineural Invasion

*___ Not identified
*___ Present
*___ Indeterminate

*Tumor-infiltrating Lymphocytes

*___ Not identified
*___ Present, nonbrisk
*___ Present, brisk

*Tumor Regression

*___ Not identified

PROTOCOL FOR MELANOMA SPECIMENS

*___ Present, involving < 75% of lesion

*___ Present, involving ≥ of lesion

*___ Indeterminate

*Growth Phase (select all that apply)

*___ Radial

*___ Vertical

*___ Indeterminate

Lymph Nodes (required only if lymph nodes are present in the specimen) (select all that apply)

Number of sentinel nodes examined: ________

Total number of nodes examined (sentinel and nonsentinel): ________

Number of lymph nodes with metastases: ________

*Extranodal tumor extension

*___ Present

*___ Not identified

*___ Indeterminate

*Size of largest metastatic focus: ________ (mm) (for sentinel node)

*Location of metastatic tumor (for sentinel node)

*___ Subcapsular

*___ Intramedullary

*___ Subcapsular and intramedullary

Pathologic Staging (pTNM)

TNM descriptors (required only if applicable) (select all that apply)

___ m (multiple

___ r (recurrent)

___ y (post treatment)

Primary tumor (pT)

___ pTX: Primary tumor cannot be assessed (e.g., shave biopsy or regressed melanoma)

___ pT0: No evidence of primary tumor

___ pTis: Melanoma in situ (i.e., not an invasive tumor: Anatomic level 1)

pT1: Melanoma ≤ 1 mm in thickness, ± ulceration

___ pT1a: Melanoma ≤ 1.0 mm in thickness, no ulceratin, < 1 mitosis/mm²

___ pT1b: Melanoma ≤ 1.0 mm in thickness with ulceration &/or ≥ 1 mitosis/mm²

pT2: Melanoma 1.01-2.0 mm in thickness, ± ulceration

___ pT2a: Melanoma 1.01-2.0 mm in thickness, no ulceration

___ pT2b: Melanoma 1.01-2.0 mm in thickness, with ulceration

pT3: Melanoma 2.01-4.0 mm in thickness, ± ulceration

___ pT3a: Melanoma 2.01-4.0 mm in thickness, no ulceration

___ pT3b: Melanoma 2.01-4.0 mm in thickness, with ulceration

pT4: Melanoma > 4.0 mm in thickness, ± ulceration

___ pT4a: Melanoma > 4.0 mm in thickness, no ulceration

___ pT4b: Melanoma > 4.0 mm in thickness, with ulceration

Regional lymph nodes (pN)

___ pNX: Regional lymph nodes cannot be assessed

___ pN0: No regional lymph node metastasis

pN1: Metastasis in 1 regional lymph node

___ pN1a: Clinically occult (microscopic) metastasis

___ pN1b: Clinically apparent (macroscopic metastasis

pN2: Metastasis in 2-3 regional lymph nodes or in intralymphatic regional metastasis without nodal metastasis

___ pN2a: Clinically occult (microscopic) metastasis

___ pN2b: Clinically apparent (macroscopic) metastasis

___ pN2c: Satellite or in-transit metastasis without nodal metastasis

___ pN3: Metastasis in ≥ 4 regional lymph nodes, or matted metastatic nodes, or in-transit metastasis or satellite(s) with metastasis in regional node(s)

___ No nodes submitted or found

Number of lymph nodes identified: _________

Number containining metastasis identified macroscopically: ________

Number containing metastases identified microscopically: ________

Matted nodes

___ Present

___ Not identified

Distant metastasis (pM)

___ Not applicable

___ pM1: Distant metastasis (documented in this specimen)

*___ pM1a: Metastasis in skin, subcutaneous tissues, or distant lymph nodes

*___ pM1b: Metastasis to lung

*___ pM1c: Metastasis to all other visceral sites or distant metastasis at any site associated with an elevated serum lactic dehydrogenase (LDH)

*Specify site, if known: ___________________________

***Additional Pathologic Findings (select all that apply)**

*___ Nevus remnant

*___ Other (specify): ___________________________

*Adapted with permission from College of American Pathologists, "Protocol for the Examination of Specimens from Patients wtih Melanoma of the Skin." Posting date: November 2011, www.cap.org *Data elements with asterisks are not required. These elements may be clinically important but are not yet validated or regularly used in patient management.*

Soft Tissue

Neoplasm, Benign

Neoplasm, Borderline

Neoplasm, Malignant Primary

Protocol for the Examination of Specimens from Patients with Tumors of Soft Tissue

Protocol for the Examination of Specimens from Patients with Tumors of Rhabdomyosarcoma

HEMANGIOMA OF INFANCY

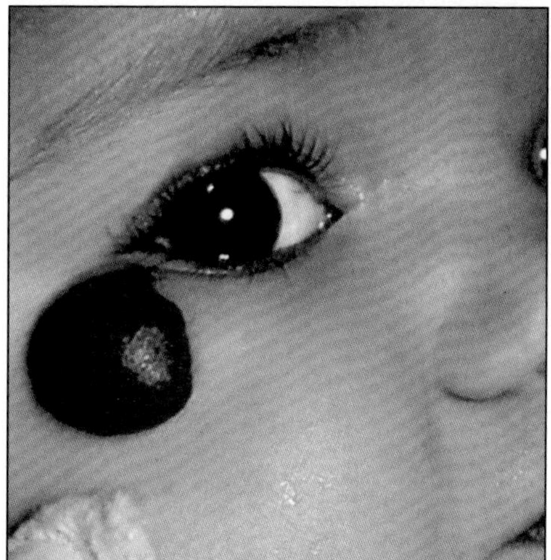

Clinical photograph of a female infant with a medium-sized hemangioma is shown. Many of these lesions are located in the head and neck region. (Courtesy J. Hall, MD.)

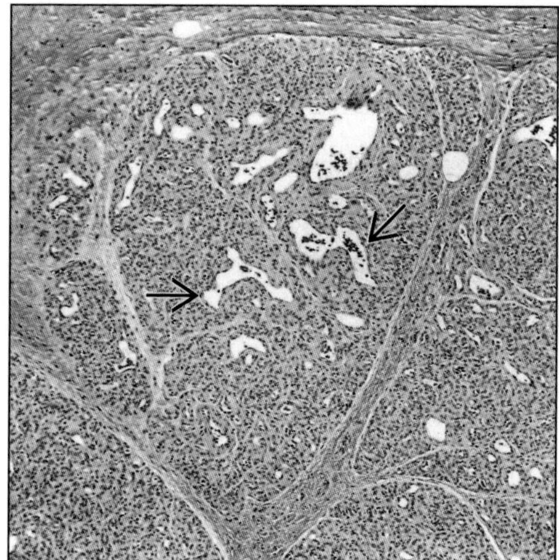

Multiple lobules composed of tightly packed small capillaries separated by fibroconnective tissue are shown in this hemangioma of infancy. Note the scattered centrally located "feeding" vessels ⇒.

TERMINOLOGY

Synonyms

- Juvenile hemangioma
- Cellular hemangioma of infancy
- Strawberry nevus/hemangioma

Definitions

- Vascular neoplasm of infancy with characteristic onset, rapid growth, and spontaneous involution

CLINICAL ISSUES

Epidemiology

- Incidence
  - Most common tumor of infancy
  - Affects ~ 4% of children
- Gender
  - M < F
- Ethnicity
  - Caucasians more frequently affected

Site

- Skin and subcutis
  - Head and neck (60%)
  - Extremities, trunk, and genitals
- Viscera

Presentation

- Appear within a few weeks after birth
  - Blanched telangiectatic area

Natural History

- Rapidly enlarge over several months
  - Maximum size usually achieved by 6-12 months
- Regress over several years
  - 75-90% involute by age 7 years

Treatment

- Options, risks, complications
  - Corticosteroids
  - Pulse dye laser
  - Surgical excision
  - Watchful waiting
    - Small innocuous lesions
  - Interferon-α
    - Restricted to life-threatening lesions
  - Topical imiquimod

Prognosis

- Excellent
- All spontaneously regress

MACROSCOPIC FEATURES

General Features

- Crimson-colored multinodular mass

MICROSCOPIC PATHOLOGY

Histologic Features

- Multiple lobules composed of tightly packed small to moderate-sized capillaries
- Early lesions
  - Plump endothelial cells that line small vascular spaces
  - Inconspicuous vascular lumens
  - Distinct lobules separated by normal stroma
  - Moderate mitotic activity and scattered mast cells
- Mature lesions
  - Small vessels lined by flattened endothelial cells
  - Zonal maturation begins at periphery
- Regressing lesions
  - Progressive and diffuse interstitial fibrosis
  - Increased apoptotic bodies and mast cells
- End-stage lesion
  - Scattered residual vessels
  - Fibrofatty background

HEMANGIOMA OF INFANCY

Key Facts

Terminology
- Vascular neoplasm of infancy

Clinical Issues
- Most common tumor of infancy
- Appear within 1st few weeks of life
- Rapidly enlarge over several months
- All spontaneously regress

Microscopic Pathology
- Multiple lobules composed of tightly packed small to moderate-sized capillaries

Ancillary Tests
- GLUT1 is most useful marker for diagnosis

Top Differential Diagnoses
- Pyogenic granuloma
- Vascular malformation

Immunohistochemistry

Antibody	Reactivity	Staining Pattern	Comment
VEGF	Positive	Cytoplasmic	Intense staining in early lesions
CD31	Positive	Cell membrane	Lost after fully involuted
CD34	Positive	Cell membrane	Lost after fully involuted
Actin-sm	Positive	Cytoplasmic	
FVIIIRAg	Positive	Cell membrane & cytoplasm	Lost after fully involuted
GLUT1	Positive	Cell membrane	Not expressed in other vascular neoplasms
IGF-2	Positive	Cell membrane	Not expressed in other vascular neoplasms

Predominant Pattern/Injury Type
- Vascular
- Lobular

Predominant Cell/Compartment Type
- Endothelial cell
- Pericytic cell

DIFFERENTIAL DIAGNOSIS

Pyogenic Granuloma
- Polypoid red mass surrounded by epidermal collarette
- Nodules of small capillaries subserved by "feeder" vessel

Kaposiform Hemangioendothelioma
- Infiltrating sheets of slender spindled endothelial cells

Tufted Angioma
- Small capillaries in "cannonball" pattern

Granulation Tissue
- Fibroblastic cells, collagenous matrix with small capillaries and inflammatory cells

Vascular Malformation
- Dilated vessels within papillary and reticular dermis

SELECTED REFERENCES

1. North PE et al: Vascular tumors of infancy and childhood: beyond capillary hemangioma. Cardiovasc Pathol. 15(6):303-17, 2006
2. North PE et al: GLUT1: a newly discovered immunohistochemical marker for juvenile hemangiomas. Hum Pathol. 31(1):11-22, 2000

IMAGE GALLERY

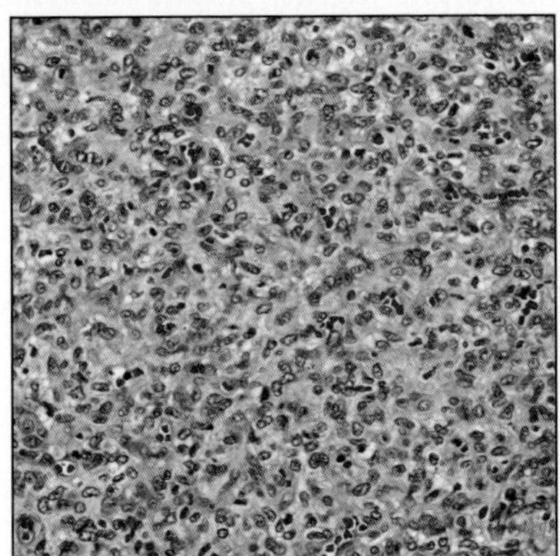

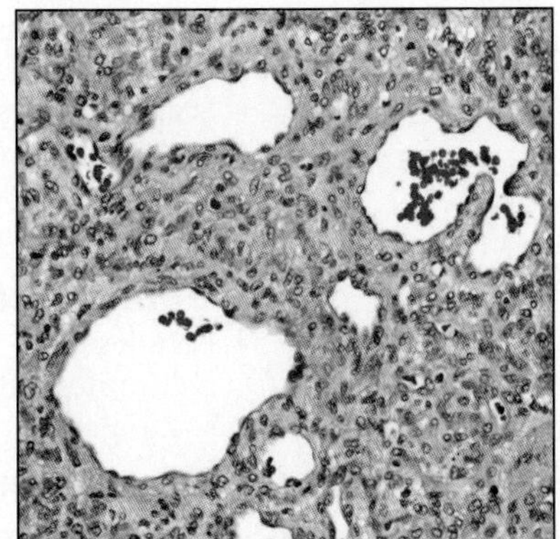

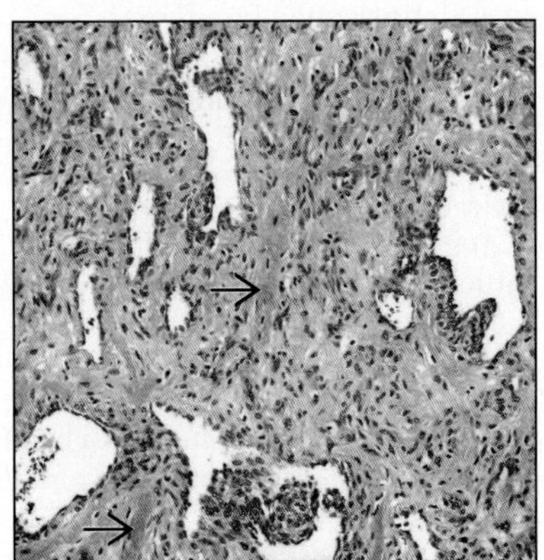

(Left) *Hemangioma of infancy is shown at high power. Early lesions, as illustrated, are composed of plump endothelial cells with inconspicuous vascular lumens. Numerous mitoses may also be present.* ***(Center)*** *The central "feeding" vessels with dilated lumens lined by flattened endothelial cells are shown.* ***(Right)*** *An older, involuting lesion composed of scattered dilated vessels in a background of progressive and diffuse interstitial fibrosis ⇒ is shown.*

TUFTED ANGIOMA

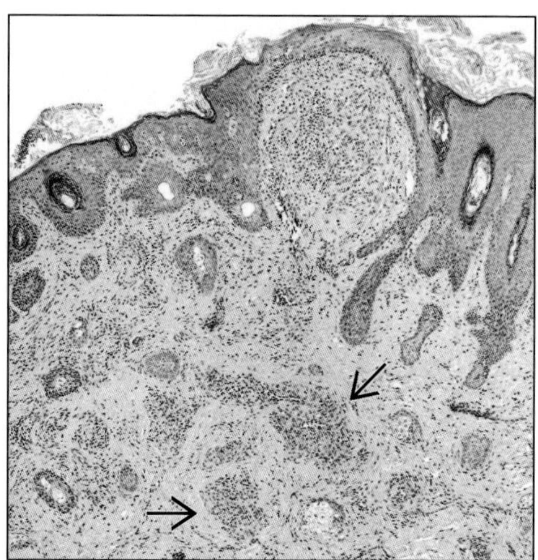

Note the discrete, irregularly shaped lobules →, composed of tightly packed spindle cells randomly distributed throughout the dermis.

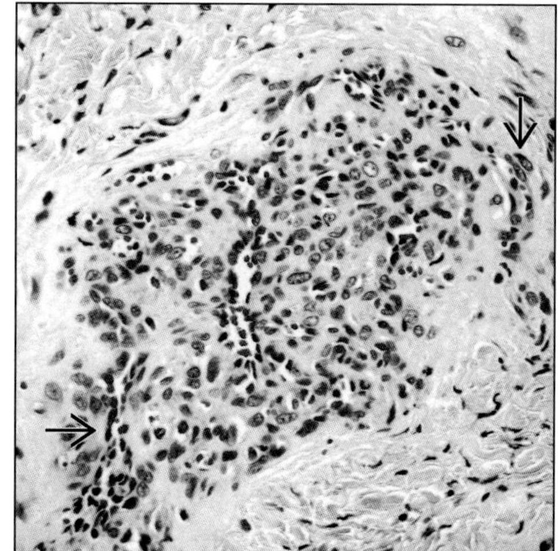

A single discrete lobule composed of tightly packed endothelial and perithelial cells with slit-like vascular channels → is shown. Note the bland appearance and lack of mitotic activity.

TERMINOLOGY

Synonyms

- Angioblastoma of Nakagawa

Definitions

- Rare, slow-growing vascular tumor of childhood

CLINICAL ISSUES

Epidemiology

- Age
  - Most arise before 5 years (congenital in up to 15%)
- Gender
  - Affects both genders equally

Site

- Upper torso and neck

Presentation

- Erythematous to red-brown indurated nodular plaques
- Slow, indolent growth over few months to years
- Often stabilize after growth period
- Tender to palpation
  - May develop paroxysmal episodes of pain
- Hypertrichosis may be present
- May develop Kasabach-Merritt syndrome
  - Consumption coagulopathy

Laboratory Tests

- Obtain complete blood count
  - Evaluation of thrombocytopenia
  - Rule out Kasabach-Merritt syndrome

Treatment

- Options, risks, complications
  - No single treatment shown to be effective
  - Spontaneous regression occasionally occurs
  - Complete excision
    - Smaller lesions more amenable to excision
    - Larger lesions often show recurrences
  - Steroid injections
  - Systemic corticosteroids and INF-α
    - Reported to induce shrinkage
  - Systemic chemotherapy
    - Cases associated with Kasabach-Merritt syndrome

Prognosis

- Malignant change not reported
- Guarded prognosis when associated with Kasabach-Merritt syndrome

MACROSCOPIC FEATURES

General Features

- Ill-defined violaceous plaque
- Gray-white to red cut surface

Size

- Variable, most 2-5 cm

MICROSCOPIC PATHOLOGY

Histologic Features

- Multiple discrete lobules of tightly packed capillaries in "cannonball" distribution
  - Randomly distributed throughout dermis
- Scattered tufts of capillaries and endothelial cells
- Tightly packed vessels with slit-like lumens
- Background of normal collagen
- May extend deep to involve fascia and muscle

Predominant Pattern/Injury Type

- Lobules
  - "Cannonball" distribution of tightly packed capillaries

Predominant Cell/Compartment Type

- Endothelial cell
- Perithelial cell

TUFTED ANGIOMA

Key Facts

Terminology
- Rare, slow-growing vascular tumor of childhood

Clinical Issues
- Most arise before 5 years of age
- Erythematous to red-brown indurated nodular plaques
- Slow, indolent growth over few months to years
- Obtain complete blood count
  - Rule out Kasabach-Merritt syndrome
- No single treatment shown to be effective

Microscopic Pathology
- Multiple, discrete lobules of tightly packed capillaries in "cannonball" distribution
- Randomly distributed throughout dermis

Top Differential Diagnoses
- Kaposiform hemangioendothelioma
- Hemangioma of infancy (juvenile hemangioma)

ANCILLARY TESTS

Immunohistochemistry
- Endothelial cells stain positive for CD34 and CD31
- Muscle-specific actin (HHF-35 actin) staining is minimal

DIFFERENTIAL DIAGNOSIS

Kaposiform Hemangioendothelioma
- Infiltrating sheets of spindle cells
- May show histologic overlap with tufted angioma
- Paucity of muscle-specific actin(+) cells
- CD31 & CD34 positivity in endothelial luminal cells only
- Frequently associated with Kasabach-Merritt syndrome

Vascular Malformation
- Dilated vessels lined by endothelial cells

Hemangioma of Infancy (Juvenile Hemangioma)
- Crimson-colored nodule
- Spontaneous involution
- Plump endothelial cells lining vascular spaces
- GLUT1(+)

Pyogenic Granuloma
- Red, firm papule with ulceration and bleeding
- Angiomatous lobules in superficial dermis

Hemangiopericytoma
- Packed spindle cells surround branching capillaries
- Lacks distinct lobular architecture
- CD34(+) and CD99(+)

Kaposi Sarcoma
- Marked spindle cell and vascular proliferation
- Extravasated erythrocytes and hyaline globules
- High mitotic activity and HHV8(+)

Angiosarcoma
- Irregular endothelial-lined spaces
- Cytologic atypia and hyperchromasia
- High mitotic activity
- CD31(+) and CD34(+)

SELECTED REFERENCES

1. Herron MD et al: Tufted angiomas: variability of the clinical morphology. Pediatr Dermatol. 19(5):394-401, 2002
2. Alvarez-Mendoza A et al: Histopathology of vascular lesions found in Kasabach-Merritt syndrome: review based on 13 cases. Pediatr Dev Pathol. 3(6):556-60, 2000
3. Jones EW et al: Tufted angioma (angioblastoma). A benign progressive angioma, not to be confused with Kaposi's sarcoma or low-grade angiosarcoma. J Am Acad Dermatol. 20(2 Pt 1):214-25, 1989
4. Padilla RS et al: Acquired "tufted" angioma (progressive capillary hemangioma). A distinctive clinicopathologic entity related to lobular capillary hemangioma. Am J Dermatopathol. 9(4):292-300, 1987

IMAGE GALLERY

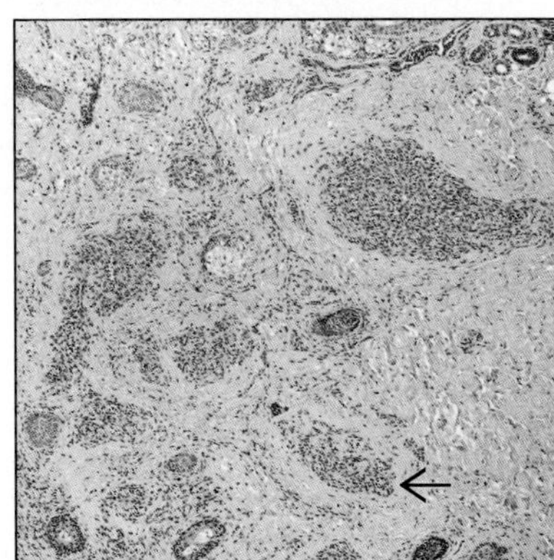

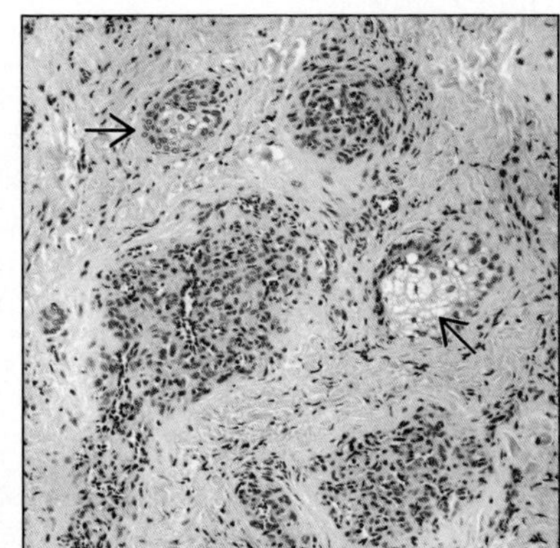

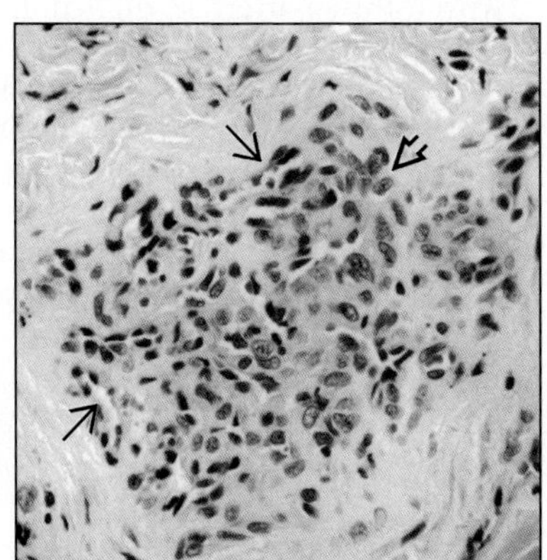

(Left) Note the irregular and randomly distributed lobules ("cannonballs") ⇒ set within a normal-appearing dermis in the background. *(Center)* Medium-power image depicts several discrete round to oval lobules composed of tightly packed endothelial cells. Note the scattered adnexal structures ⇒ and the normal-appearing dermis in the background. *(Right)* A discrete round lobule (cannonball") composed of tightly packed plump to flattened endothelial and perithelial cells ⇨ and small slit-like vascular spaces ⇒ is shown.

HEMANGIOPERICYTOMA

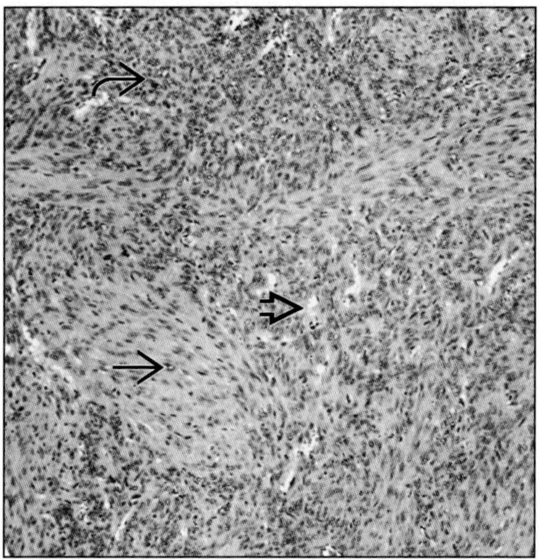

Infantile hemangiopericytoma is characterized by varying proportions of spindle cells ⇒ and primitive-appearing rounded cells ⇗ surrounding irregularly distributed, irregularly shaped vascular spaces ⇒.

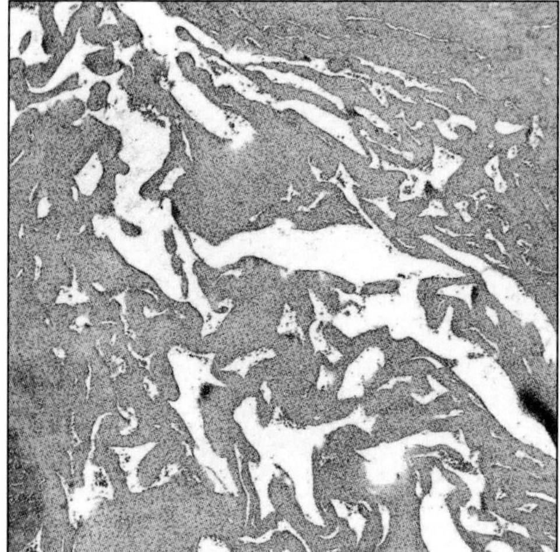

Adult-type hemangiopericytoma may also present in childhood and demonstrates oval to slightly spindled tumor cells with round to oval nuclei surrounding irregularly shaped, "staghorn" vessels.

TERMINOLOGY

Abbreviations

- Infantile hemangiopericytoma (IHPC)
- Adult-type hemangiopericytoma (AHPC)

Synonyms

- IHPC
  - Infantile variant of hemangiopericytoma
  - Congenital hemangiopericytoma

Definitions

- Hemangiopericytoma (HPC) in childhood includes 2 distinct entities
  - Infantile hemangiopericytoma (IHPC)
    - Multilobular perivascular neoplasm of infancy characterized by irregularly branching, thin-walled vascular spaces surrounded by immature-appearing and spindled neoplastic cells
    - Clinicopathologic features distinct from adult-type HPC
    - Currently considered to be at the primitive end of the spectrum of infantile myofibromatosis
  - Adult-type hemangiopericytoma (AHPC)
    - Tumor composed of oval to slightly spindled cells with diffuse pattern of dilated, branching, thin-walled vessels
    - Many tumors previously called HPC now classified as cellular form of solitary fibrous tumor (SFT)
    - Tumors previously called HPC with myoid differentiation now classified as myopericytoma
    - Number of non-HPC tumors have hemangiopericytomatous vascular pattern

CLINICAL ISSUES

Epidemiology

- Incidence
  - IHPC: Uncommonly diagnosed
  - AHPC: Rare in infancy and childhood
- Age
  - IHPC: Presents at birth or during 1st year of life
  - AHPC: Most pediatric cases present at > 5 years of age
- Gender
  - IHPC: Slight predilection for boys
  - AHPC: No gender predilection

Site

- IHPC
  - Subcutis and oral cavity most commonly
  - Deep soft tissues, rarely
    - Muscle, mediastinum, and abdomen reported
    - Tend to occur in older children
  - Visceral locations possible
- AHPC
  - Extremities, head and neck, trunk, abdomen, retroperitoneum
  - Most are deep-seated

Presentation

- Painful or painless slow-growing mass
- Hypoglycemia
  - Occasional, via secretion of insulin-like growth factor
- IHPC: Can be multilobulated or multicentric

Treatment

- Surgical approaches
  - Complete surgical excision
  - Rare recurrences with incomplete excision
  - Effectiveness of chemotherapy and radiation therapy in pediatric patients remains to be established

Prognosis

- IHPC
  - Behavior more indolent than that of AHPC
    - May be due to ability of IHPC to differentiate into more mature tissue

Key Facts

Terminology
- HPC in childhood includes 2 distinct entities
  - IHPC: Currently considered to be at primitive end of spectrum of infantile myofibromatosis
  - AHPC: Diagnosis is now rarely made; HPC describes a group of neoplasms that share a common growth pattern

Clinical Issues
- IHPC: Behavior more indolent than AHPC with very low incidence of recurrence or metastases
- IHPC: May be multilobulated or multicentric

Macroscopic Features
- Well circumscribed

Microscopic Pathology
- IHPC
  - Irregular distribution of thin-walled vessels
  - Round, primitive-appearing tumor cells surround vascular spaces and variable amounts of spindle cells
  - Intravascular and perivascular satellite nodules: Feature unique to IHPC
- AHPC
  - Monotonous appearance with moderate to high cellularity
  - Numerous thin-walled, branching, "staghorn" vessels
- Morphology does not correlate well with prognosis

Top Differential Diagnoses
- Solitary fibrous tumor, synovial sarcoma, mesenchymal chondrosarcoma, infantile fibrosarcoma

  - Very low incidence of recurrence
  - Very low metastatic potential
  - Spontaneous regression reported
- AHPC
  - Favorable clinical behavior
  - Reported incidence of metastasis in childhood varies

MACROSCOPIC FEATURES

General Features
- Well circumscribed
- Gray-white to red-brown cut surface
- ± hemorrhage, cystic change, and necrosis

MICROSCOPIC PATHOLOGY

Histologic Features
- IHPC
  - Irregular distribution of thin-walled vessels
    - More irregular than that of AHPC
    - Bland endothelial lining
    - Endovascular endothelial proliferation
  - Round primitive-appearing tumor cells surround vascular spaces
    - Indistinct cytoplasmic borders
  - Variable amounts of spindle cells resembling smooth muscle cells
  - Intravascular and perivascular satellite nodules
    - Located away from main mass
    - Feature unique to IHPC
  - May show prominent collagenous matrix
  - Increased mitotic activity, vascular invasion, and focal necrosis
    - Does not portend a poor prognosis in IHPC
  - Areas may resemble AHPC and infantile myofibromatosis
- AHPC
  - Monotonous appearance with moderate to high cellularity
  - Perivascular hyalinization common
  - Numerous ramifying, thin-walled, branching vessels of various calibers
  - Monomorphic, round to oval tumor cell nuclei
  - Although morphology does not correlate well with prognosis, the most important histologic predictors of a poor outcome include
    - Increased cellularity, mitotic index > 4 per HPF, lack of alternating sclerotic hypocellular areas

ANCILLARY TESTS

Cytogenetics
- IHPC: No specific abnormalities described
- AHPC: Rearrangements of chromosome 12 reported

Electron Microscopy
- AHPC and IHPC
  - EM shows varying features of pericytic, fibroblastic, &/or myofibroblastic differentiation
  - Basal lamina surround vascular-pericyte units
  - Plasmalemmal pinocytosis
  - Weibel-Palade bodies consistently absent

DIFFERENTIAL DIAGNOSIS

Infantile Myofibroma/Myofibromatosis
- Multilobulated spindle cell neoplasm with biphasic pattern
- Considered by many to be synonymous with IHPC

Solitary Fibrous Tumor
- Spindle cell neoplasm with "patternless" pattern with variable cellularity and stromal collagenization; can show HPC-like vascular pattern
- Does not express myoid immunohistochemical markers
- Many tumors previously called hemangiopericytoma are now classified as cellular SFT

Infantile Fibrosarcoma
- Poorly circumscribed, infiltrative
- Most with t(12;15)(p13;q26) translocation

HEMANGIOPERICYTOMA

Comparative Immunohistochemistry				
Antibody	IHPC/IM	Solitary Fibrous Tumor	AHPC	Myopericytoma
Actin-sm	Positive (75%)	Negative (14%)	Positive (98%)	Positive (98%)
Actin-HHF-35	Positive (78%)	Negative (7%)	Positive (100%)	Positive (100%)
HCAD	Negative (0%)	Negative (0%)	Positive (91%)	Positive (91%)
Desmin	Equivocal (42%)	Negative (6%)	Negative (0%)	Usually negative (15%)
Bcl-2	Usually negative (21%)	Positive (97%)	Positive (100%)	
CD34	Usually negative (21%)	Positive (94%)	Positive (71%)	
Calponin	Positive (92%)	Usually negative (25%)	Usually negative (20%)	
β-catenin-nuclear	Negative (0%)	Equivocal (60%)	Equivocal (40%)	
Collagen IV	Usually negative (10%)	Usually negative (10%)	Positive (100%)	

This table compares the immunohistochemical profiles of infantile myofibromatosis (IM) (considered by many to be synonymous with infantile hemangiopericytoma [IHPC]), solitary fibrous tumor, adult hemangiopericytoma (AHPC), and myopericytoma. Actin-sm = smooth muscle actin, actin-HHF-35 = skeletal muscle actin, HCAD = caldesmon.

Glomangioma

- Tumor of round to oval nonspindled cells with abundant eosinophilic cytoplasm arranged in eccentric fashion around vessels
- In contrast to HPC, tumor cells have distinct cell border and tumor lacks HPC-like vascular pattern

Angioleiomyoma

- Unlike HPC, angioleiomyoma is usually desmin positive

Myopericytoma

- Characterized by proliferation of bland round to ovoid cells arranged in concentric perivascular pattern
  - Tumor cells resemble glomus cells but are larger with more abundant cytoplasm and lack a clearly demarcated cell border
- Hemangiopericytomatous vascular pattern common
- Tumors previously called HPC with myoid differentiation now classified as myopericytoma

Synovial Sarcoma

- Highly cellular spindle cell fascicles with epithelial &/or glandular differentiation seen in biphasic form
- EMA &/or keratin usually positive

Mesenchymal Chondrosarcoma

- Small round blue cells in hemangiopericytomatous pattern intimately associated with islands of low-grade cartilage
- S100(+)

DIAGNOSTIC CHECKLIST

Pathologic Interpretation Pearls

- HPC-like vascular pattern is not specific; therefore broad differential must be considered

SELECTED REFERENCES

1. Wilson T et al: Intranasal myopericytoma. A tumour with perivascular myoid differentiation: the changing nomenclature for haemangiopericytoma. J Laryngol Otol. 121(8):786-9, 2007
2. Dray MS et al: Myopericytoma: a unifying term for a spectrum of tumours that show overlapping features with myofibroma. A review of 14 cases. J Clin Pathol. 59(1):67-73, 2006
3. Gengler C et al: Solitary fibrous tumour and haemangiopericytoma: evolution of a concept. Histopathology. 48(1):63-74, 2006
4. Mentzel T et al: Myopericytoma of skin and soft tissues: clinicopathologic and immunohistochemical study of 54 cases. Am J Surg Pathol. 30(1):104-13, 2006
5. Ferrari A et al: Hemangiopericytoma in pediatric ages: a report from the Italian and German Soft Tissue Sarcoma Cooperative Group. Cancer. 92(10):2692-8, 2001
6. Rodriguez-Galindo C et al: Hemangiopericytoma in children and infants. Cancer. 88(1):198-204, 2000
7. Granter SR et al: Myofibromatosis in adults, glomangiopericytoma, and myopericytoma: a spectrum of tumors showing perivascular myoid differentiation. Am J Surg Pathol. 22(5):513-25, 1998
8. Magid MS et al: Infantile myofibromatosis with hemangiopericytoma-like features of the tongue: a case study including ultrastructure. Pediatr Pathol Lab Med. 17(2):303-13, 1997
9. Nappi O et al: Hemangiopericytoma: histopathological pattern or clinicopathologic entity? Semin Diagn Pathol. 12(3):221-32, 1995
10. Mentzel T et al: Infantile hemangiopericytoma versus infantile myofibromatosis. Study of a series suggesting a continuous spectrum of infantile myofibroblastic lesions. Am J Surg Pathol. 18(9):922-30, 1994
11. Henn W et al: Recurrent t(12;19)(q13;q13.3) in intracranial and extracranial hemangiopericytoma. Cancer Genet Cytogenet. 71(2):151-4, 1993
12. Enzinger FM et al: Hemangiopericytoma. An analysis of 106 cases. Hum Pathol. 7(1):61-82, 1976

HEMANGIOPERICYTOMA

Microscopic Features and Differential Diagnosis

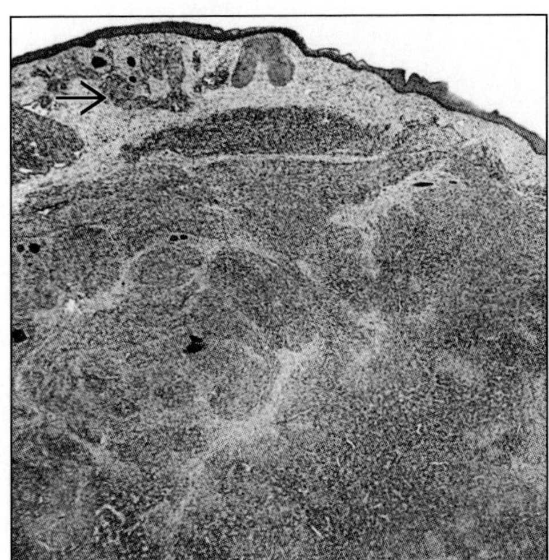

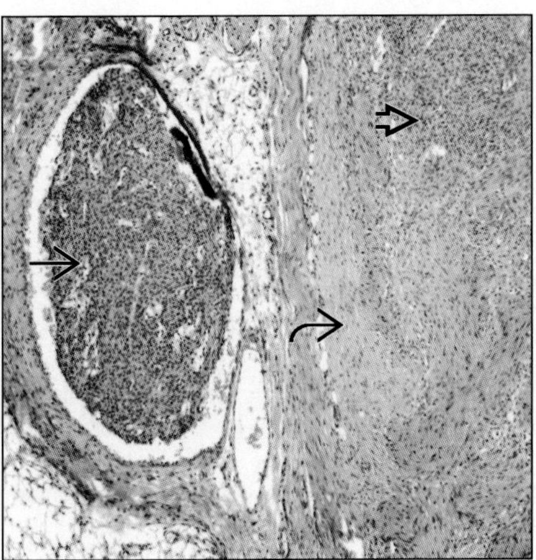

(Left) *IHPC is typically multinodular with satellite nodules* → *and endovascular growth. IHPC usually presents in the subcutis, as illustrated here, in comparison to its adult-type counterpart, which tends to be more deep-seated.* ***(Right)*** *A satellite nodule is seen at a higher power in this IHPC* →. *Areas of spindle cells* ↪ *admixed with primitive rounded cells* ⇨ *are characteristic.*

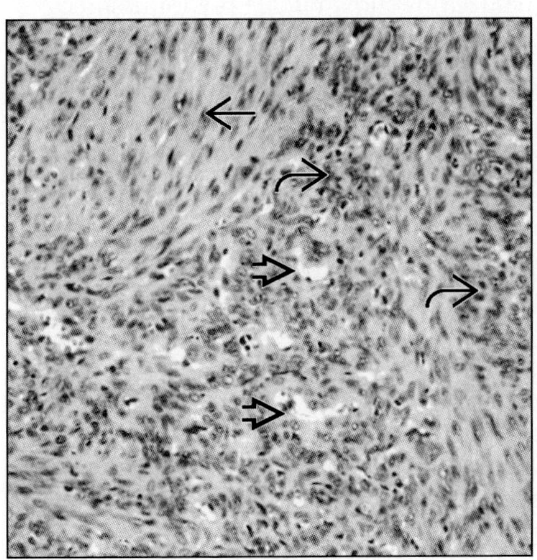

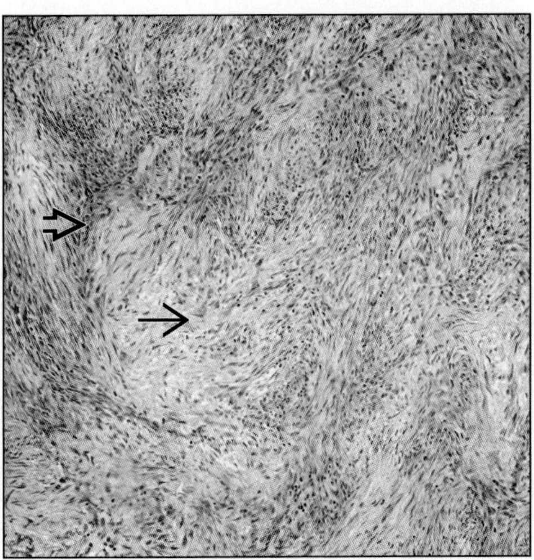

(Left) *IHPC is thought by many to be at the primitive end of the spectrum of myofibroma/ myofibromatosis. A typical IHPC is shown with spindle cells that resemble smooth muscle cells* → *and more primitive rounded cells* ↪ *with an associated HPC-like vascular pattern* ⇨. ***(Right)*** *A typical myofibroma demonstrates a biphasic pattern of more mature, paler myofibroblasts* → *centrally within the fascicle and more primitive, darker cells at the periphery* ⇨.

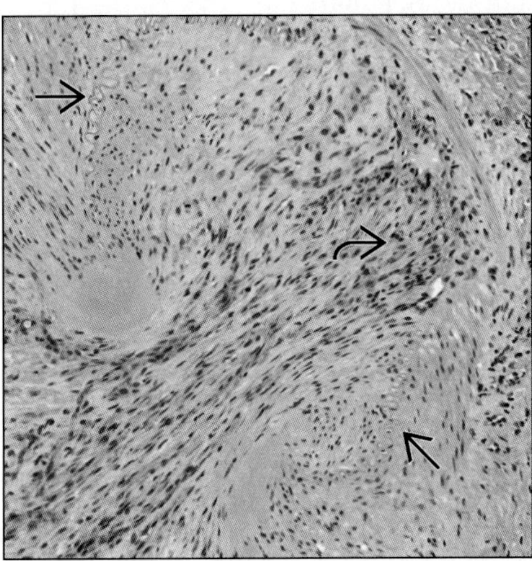

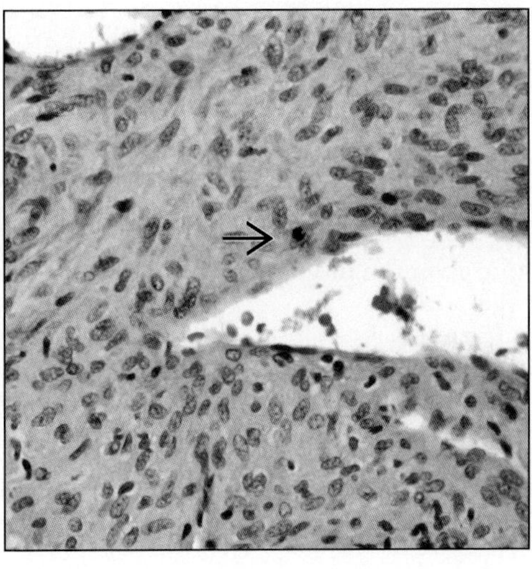

(Left) *IHPC and myofibroma are known for their propensity for endovascular growth. An IHPC is shown here extending into a vessel. The vascular elastic lamina is designated* →. *IHPC have a very favorable prognosis despite endovascular spread and mitotic figures* ↪. ***(Right)*** *AHPCs are composed of monotonous ovoid to slightly spindled cells with round to oval nuclei in a perivascular growth pattern. Mitotic figures may be seen* → *but do not correlate well with recurrence.*

GLOMUS TUMOR

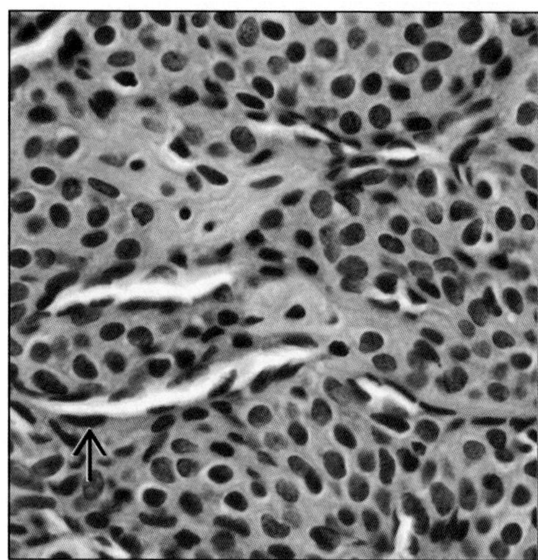

High-power view shows the solid, "classic" type of a glomus tumor. Uniform, round cells arranged in sheets and small clusters surround small scattered vessels lined by flat endothelial cells ➔.

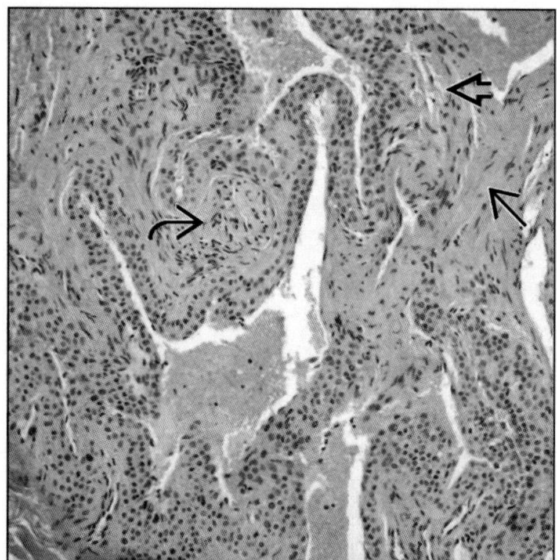

Hematoxylin & eosin shows a glomangioma. Note the dilated vascular channels, entrapped nerve ➔, smooth muscle component ➔, and focal myxoid change ➔.

TERMINOLOGY

Definitions

- Benign tumor of soft tissue composed of cells that resemble modified smooth muscle cells of normal glomus body
  - Glomus body
    - Neuromyoarterial body found within reticular dermis
    - Functions as specialized form of arteriovenous anastomosis
    - Involved in thermoregulation
  - Common subcategories
    - Solid "classic" glomus tumor
    - Glomangioma
    - Glomangiomyoma
  - Subcategory dependent on proportion of glomus cells, vasculature, and smooth muscle

CLINICAL ISSUES

Epidemiology

- Incidence
  - Approximately 1-2% of all soft tissue neoplasms
- Age
  - Tumor of young adults (20-40 years of age)
    - 70% occur by age 30
  - Multiple glomus tumors more common in younger age groups (15-20 years of age)
    - More often hereditary and painless
  - Glomangiomas occur more often in childhood
  - Familial glomangiomas
    - Often congenital
    - Autosomal dominant inheritance
    - Incomplete penetrance
    - Due to truncating mutations in glomulin gene (chromosome 1p21-22)
- Gender
  - Equally distributed
    - Subungual lesions show female predominance

Site

- Found in areas rich in glomus bodies
- Upper and lower extremities
  - Subungual region of digit most common site
  - Deep dermis of palm, wrist, forearm, and foot
- Described in almost every location

Presentation

- Subcutaneous nodules
  - Solitary or multiple
  - Small, blue-red-purple
- Painful or painless mass
  - Pain radiates away from site of lesion
    - Elicited by exposure to cold
    - Exacerbated with blunt palpation
    - Out of proportion to size of tumor
- Ridging &/or discoloration of nail bed
- Glomangiomatosis
  - Diffusely infiltrating lesions
  - More prevalent in childhood
  - More often painless
- Duration of symptoms between 7-11 years
  - Related to delay in diagnosis

Treatment

- Surgical approaches
  - Simple local excision
- Other approaches
  - Sclerotherapy and laser ablation for recurrences and multiple glomangiomata

Prognosis

- Excellent prognosis with complete surgical excision
- 10% risk of local recurrence
  - More likely with multiple lesions

GLOMUS TUMOR

Key Facts

Terminology
- Benign tumor of soft tissue composed of cells that resemble modified smooth muscle cells of normal glomus body

Clinical Issues
- Approximately 1-2% of all soft tissue neoplasms
- Tumor of young adults (20-40 years of age)
- Upper and lower extremities
- Subungual region of finger most common site
- Painful or painless mass
- 10% risk of local recurrence

Macroscopic Features
- Well-circumscribed, small, blue-red nodules
- Rarely exceeds 1 cm

Microscopic Pathology
- Solid glomus tumor
  - Small, convoluted, capillary-sized vessels surrounded by clusters of glomus cells
- Glomangioma
  - Dilated veins surrounded by clusters of glomus cells
- Glomangiomyoma
  - Components of solid glomus tumor or glomangioma with distinctive smooth muscle component

Top Differential Diagnoses
- Nodular hidradenoma
- Intradermal nevi
- Myopericytoma
- Hemangioma

IMAGE FINDINGS

Radiographic Findings
- Subungual glomus tumors
  - Scalloped osteolytic defect of terminal phalynx with sclerotic border

MR Findings
- Sensitive imaging modality for diagnosis of glomus tumors
- Decreased signal intensity on T1-weighted images
- Increased signal intensity on T2-weighted images
- Negative MR result should not impede surgical excision

MACROSCOPIC FEATURES

General Features
- Well-circumscribed, small, blue-red nodules
- Bulging and unencapsulated

Size
- Rarely exceed 1 cm
- > 2 cm suggests malignant potential

MICROSCOPIC PATHOLOGY

Histologic Features
- Composed of 3 components
  - Glomus cells
  - Vasculature
  - Smooth muscle cells
- Stroma
  - Variable amounts of fibrosis, hyaline, and myxoid change
- Solid glomus tumor
  - Small, convoluted, capillary-sized vessels surrounded by clusters of glomus cells
  - Glomus cells form nests, small clusters, and sheets
  - Capillary-sized channels lined by endothelial cells
- Glomangioma
  - Dilated veins surrounded by clusters of glomus cells
  - Dual layer of glomus cells often surrounds vascular spaces
  - Nests and clusters of glomus cells often seen along periphery
  - Vasculature channels lined by endothelial cells
- Glomangiomyoma
  - Components of solid glomus tumor or glomangioma with distinctive smooth muscle component
  - Resembles cavernous hemangioma
- Glomangiomatosis
  - Diffuse &/or infiltrative vessels of varying size
  - Accompanied by mature fat
  - Clusters of glomus cells surround vessels
  - May resemble angiomatosis
- Glomangiopericytoma
  - Sheets of glomus cells
  - Hemangiopericytoma-like vasculature
- Malignant glomus tumor (glomangiosarcoma)
  - Moderate to high nuclear grade
  - Elevated mitotic activity (≥ 5/50 HPF)
  - Atypical mitotic figures
  - Tumor size > 2 cm
  - Deep location
  - May resemble leiomyosarcoma or round cell sarcoma
  - Benign component not required for diagnosis
  - Exceedingly rare
  - Metastases in 38%
- Glomus tumor of uncertain malignant potential (atypical glomus tumor)
  - Lack complete criteria for malignant glomus tumor
  - High mitotic activity
- Symplastic glomus tumor
  - Display marked nuclear atypia
  - Absence of other malignant features
  - Thought to be degenerative phenomenon

Predominant Pattern/Injury Type
- Solid

GLOMUS TUMOR

Immunohistochemistry

Antibody	Reactivity	Staining Pattern	Comment
Actin-sm	Positive	Cytoplasmic	
Vimentin	Positive	Cytoplasmic	
Laminin	Positive	Cell membrane	Highlight basal lamina
Collagen IV	Positive	Cell membrane	Highlight basal lamina
HCAD	Positive	Cytoplasmic	
Desmin	Negative		Usually negative
S100	Negative		Usually negative
AE1/AE3	Negative		

 - 75% of all glomus tumors (solid, "classic" glomus tumor)
- Mixed
  - 20% show mixture of glomus cells and dilated vasculature (glomangioma)
  - 5% show a mixture of glomus cells, dilated vasculature, and smooth muscle (glomangiomyoma)

Predominant Cell/Compartment Type

- Glomus cell
  - Centrally placed, uniformly round, "punched out " nuclei
  - Eosinophilic to amphophilic cytoplasm
  - Distinct cell borders
  - Cell borders highlighted by reticulin

DIFFERENTIAL DIAGNOSIS

Nodular Hidradenoma

- Cytokeratin, EMA, and CEA positive
- Ductular differentiation and epithelial mucin production
- Lack of intimately associated and distinct glomus cells around vessels

Intradermal Nevi

- S100, melan-A, and HMB-45 positive
- Symmetric proliferation of round, bland melanocytes
- Maturation with increasing depth

Myopericytoma

- Larger, less-rounded cells with ill-defined borders
- Concentric plump spindle cells surround open vessels
- Distinction in cases with histologic overlap may not be possible

Myofibromatosis

- Biphasic growth pattern
  - Spindle cells arranged in fascicles and whorls
  - Primitive spindle cells with hemangiopericytomatous vasculature

Angioleiomyoma

- Monomorphic, spindle-shaped, smooth muscle cells associated with vascular channels
- Desmin positive

Hemangioma

- Predilection for head and neck
- Rapid enlargement with spontaneous regression
- Flattened endothelial cells
- Multilobular arrangement
- CD31 and factor VIII associated antigen positive

Arteriovenous Malformation

- Composed of veins and arteries of variable size and number
- Elastic stain to highlight arteries
- Predilection for head and neck

SELECTED REFERENCES

1. Gombos Z et al: Glomus tumor. Arch Pathol Lab Med. 132(9):1448-52, 2008
2. Schiefer TK et al: Extradigital glomus tumors: a 20-year experience. Mayo Clin Proc. 81(10):1337-44, 2006
3. Brouillard P et al: Mutations in a novel factor, glomulin, are responsible for glomuvenous malformations ("glomangiomas"). Am J Hum Genet. 70(4):866-74, 2002
4. Folpe AL et al: Atypical and malignant glomus tumors: analysis of 52 cases, with a proposal for the reclassification of glomus tumors. Am J Surg Pathol. 25(1):1-12, 2001
5. Drapé JL et al: Standard and high resolution magnetic resonance imaging of glomus tumors of toes and fingertips. J Am Acad Dermatol. 35(4):550-5, 1996
6. Gould EP: Sclerotherapy for multiple glomangiomata. J Dermatol Surg Oncol. 17(4):351-2, 1991
7. Maxwell GP et al: Multiple digital glomus tumors. J Hand Surg [Am]. 4(4):363-7, 1979
8. Carroll RE et al: Glomus tumors of the hand: review of the literature and report on twenty-eight cases. J Bone Joint Surg Am. 54(4):691-703, 1972
9. Kohout E et al: The glomus tumor in children. Cancer. 14:555-66, 1961
10. Soule EH et al: Scientific exhibits: primary tumors of the soft tissues of the extremities exclusive of epithelial tumors; an analysis of five hundred consecutive cases. AMA Arch Surg. 70(3):462-74, 1955

GLOMUS TUMOR

Microscopic Features and Ancillary Techniques

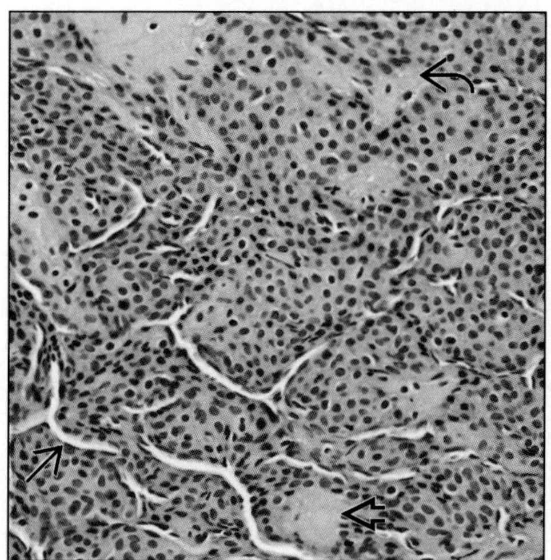

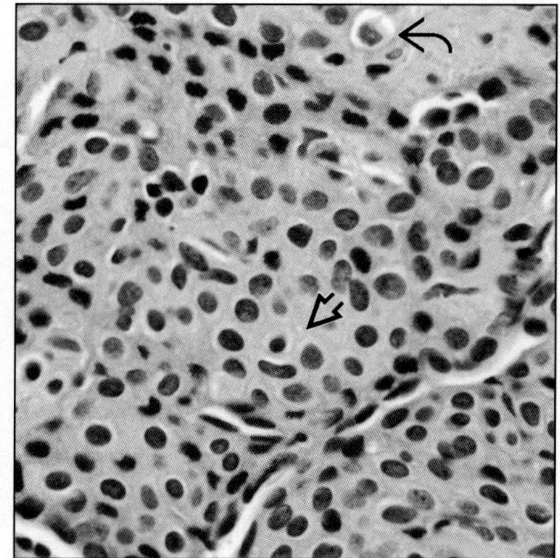

(Left) Medium-power view of a solid glomus tumor shows uniform, round cells with eosinophilic cytoplasm arranged in sheets interspersed with small vessels →. Oncocytic change and hyalinization ⇨ may be prominent features. Focal myxoid change ↷ is also present. **(Right)** High-power view of a solid glomus tumor shows the punched out appearance of the round nuclei ↷, pale eosinophilic cytoplasm, and prominent cell borders ⇨.

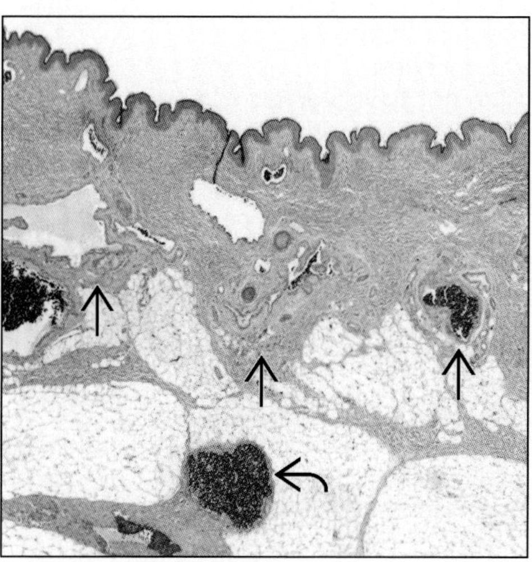

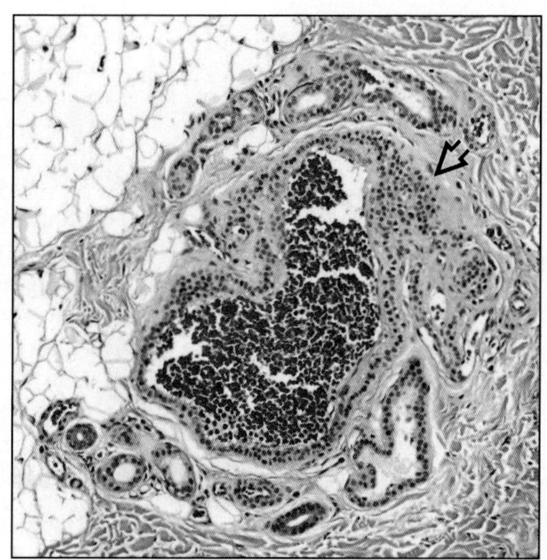

(Left) Hematoxylin & eosin from low power shows numerous glomangiomata within the dermis and extending into the subcutaneous adipose tissue →. Several of the dilated vessels are filled with abundant red blood cells ↷. **(Right)** Hematoxylin & eosin from high power shows a glomangioma. The focal clusters ⇨ of round glomus cells within and along the periphery of the dilated vessel help distinguish it from a cavernous hemangioma.

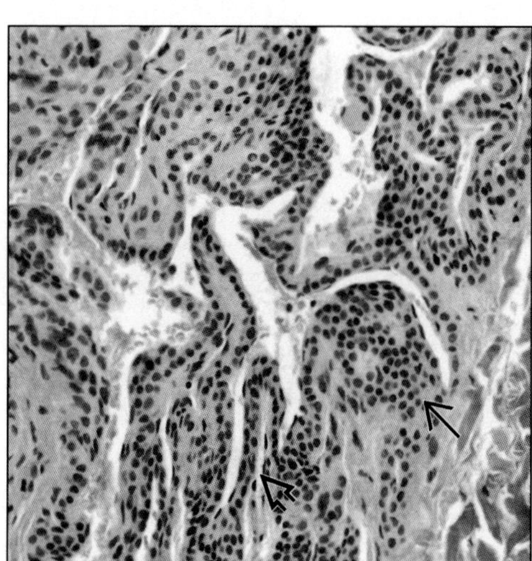

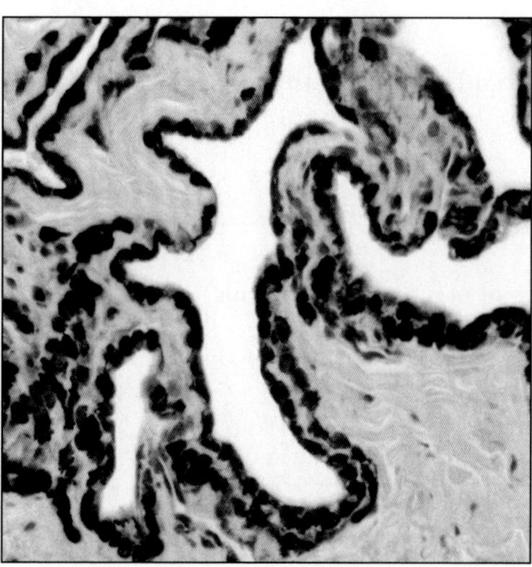

(Left) Hematoxylin & eosin from medium power shows a glomangioma. Note the frequent bi-layer arrangement ⇨ of the uniformly round glomus cells and the focal clustering of glomus cells along the periphery →. These features help distinguish this tumor from adnexal neoplasms. **(Right)** Smooth muscle actin shows strong cytoplasmic staining of the glomus cells that invest the dilated vessels of this glomangioma.

INTRAVASCULAR PAPILLARY ENDOTHELIAL HYPERPLASIA

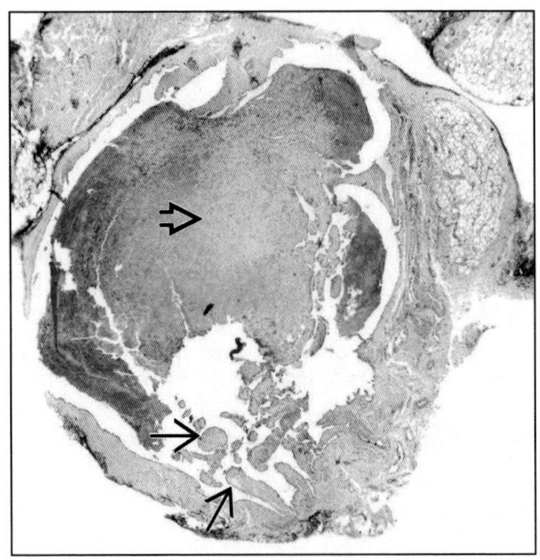

An organizing thrombus within a vessel ➯ shows an associated papillary endothelial proliferation ➔.

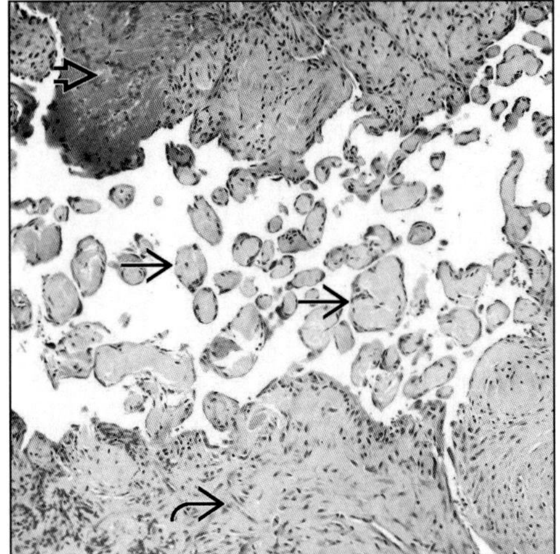

IPEH is characterized by the formation of hyalinized papillary cores lined by a single layer of endothelium ➔ in close association with fibrin thrombi ➯ and organizing thrombi ➔.

TERMINOLOGY

Abbreviations

- Intravascular papillary endothelial hyperplasia (IPEH)

Synonyms

- Vegetant intravascular hemangioendothelioma
- Masson angioma
- Masson pseudoangiosarcoma (extravascular form)

Definitions

- Benign reactive lesion characterized by papillary endothelial proliferation associated with thrombus formation
- Subtypes
  - Primary or intravascular form (56%)
    - Originates within dilated blood vessels
  - Secondary or mixed form (40%)
    - Arises within aneurysms, hemangiomas, or arteriovenous malformations
  - Extravascular form (4%)
    - Occurs within hematomas
    - Diagnosis of this form should be made with caution

ETIOLOGY/PATHOGENESIS

Pathogenesis

- Thought to be a peculiar type of organizing thrombus with exuberant endothelial hyperplasia
  - May be stimulated by autocrine loop of endothelial basic fibroblast growth factor (bFGF) secretion
- Association with trauma is debated

CLINICAL ISSUES

Site

- Can occur at any location throughout body
- Primary form occurs most commonly on fingers, head and neck, elbow, and hand
  - Subcutaneous location
- Mixed lesions do not have a preferred site
  - Approximately 1/2 arise in intramuscular location

Presentation

- Demographics depend upon subtype
  - Typically presents in middle age
  - Secondary or mixed form tends to occur in younger patients
- Slow-growing mass with blue or red skin discoloration overlying lesion
  - Most often solitary but may be multiple
- Appearance and symptoms are nonspecific, so biopsy is required for diagnosis

Treatment

- Surgical excision

Prognosis

- Excellent
- Recurrence is rare with adequate excision

IMAGE FINDINGS

MR Findings

- Nodular soft tissue mass accompanied by low signal intensity, indicating thrombi and surrounding hemorrhage

MACROSCOPIC FEATURES

General Features

- Dark red, multicystic
- Surrounded by fibrous pseudocapsule comprised of residual vessel wall tissue

Size

- Small, most 0.2-2 cm

INTRAVASCULAR PAPILLARY ENDOTHELIAL HYPERPLASIA

Key Facts

Terminology
- Benign papillary endothelial proliferation associated with thrombus formation within a vessel

Macroscopic Features
- Small, dark red, multicystic lesions
- Well circumscribed, surrounded by pseudocapsule comprised of residual vessel wall tissue

Microscopic Pathology
- Collagenized papillae extending into lumen of vessel lined by a single layer of endothelium lacking significant atypia

Top Differential Diagnoses
- Angiosarcoma
  - Pleomorphism, high mitotic rate, rarely confined within vascular lumen

MICROSCOPIC PATHOLOGY

Histologic Features
- Well circumscribed
- Numerous delicate papillae extend into lumen of vessel to form anastomosing vascular pattern
  - Collagenized papillae are lined by a single layer of plump endothelium
- Papillary growth is intimately associated with thrombus formation
  - Thrombi can be of various stages of organization
  - Thrombi appear to serve as matrix for development of papillary endothelial proliferation
- No significant mitoses
- Lesion may spill into surrounding soft tissue with vessel rupture

Cytologic Features
- Endothelial cells lining papillae are plump but lack significant atypia

DIFFERENTIAL DIAGNOSIS

Angiosarcoma
- Pleomorphism, high mitotic rate
- Rarely is angiosarcoma confined within vascular lumen
- Frank tissue necrosis present

DIAGNOSTIC CHECKLIST

Pathologic Interpretation Pearls
- Hyalinized papillary cores lined by single layer of non-atypical endothelium in association with fibrin thrombi and organizing thrombi

SELECTED REFERENCES

1. Campos MS et al: Intravascular papillary endothelial hyperplasia: report of 4 cases with immunohistochemical findings. Med Oral Patol Oral Cir Bucal. 14(10):e506-9, 2009
2. Juan YH et al: Intravascular papillary endothelial hyperplasia of the calf in an infant: MR features with histological correlation. Pediatr Radiol. 39(3):282-5, 2009
3. Korkolis DP et al: Intravascular papillary endothelial hyperplasia (Masson's hemangioma) presenting as a soft-tissue sarcoma. Anticancer Res. 25(2B):1409-12, 2005
4. Pins MR et al: Florid extravascular papillary endothelial hyperplasia (Masson's pseudoangiosarcoma) presenting as a soft-tissue sarcoma. Arch Pathol Lab Med. 117(3):259-63, 1993
5. Hashimoto H et al: Intravascular papillary endothelial hyperplasia. A clinicopathologic study of 91 cases. Am J Dermatopathol. 5(6):539-46, 1983
6. Cozzutto C et al: Intravascular endothelial proliferations in children. Am J Clin Pathol. 71(3):247-52, 1979
7. Barr RJ et al: Intravascular papillary endothelial hyperplasia. A benign lesion mimicking angiosarcoma. Arch Dermatol. 114(5):723-6, 1978
8. Clearkin KP et al: Intravascular papillary endothelial hyperplasia. Arch Pathol Lab Med. 100(8):441-4, 1976

IMAGE GALLERY

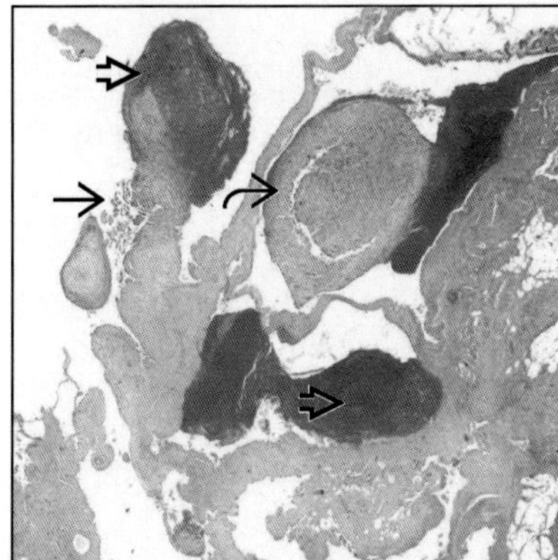

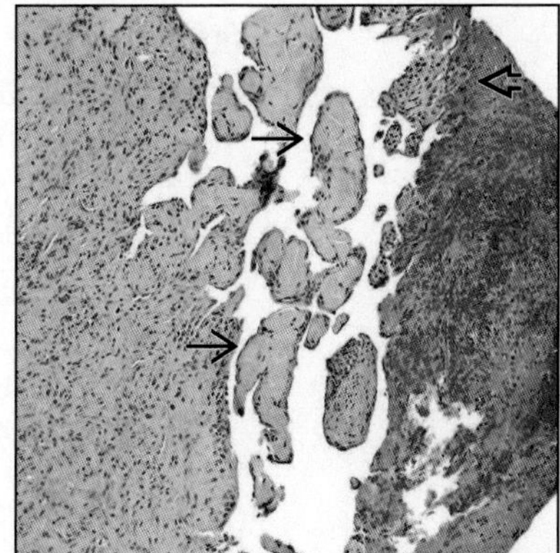

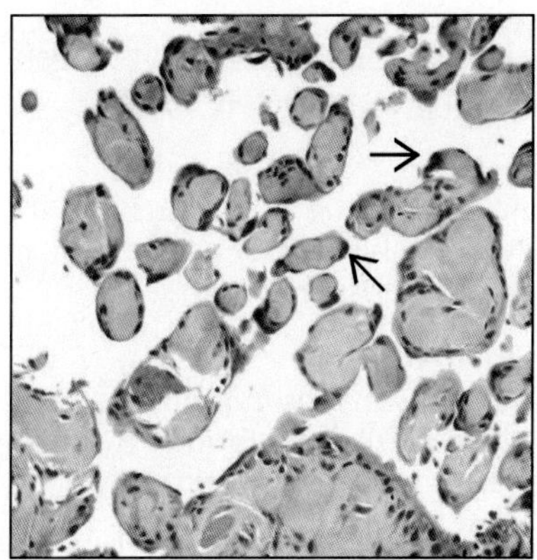

(Left) *Fibrin thrombi ⮚, an organizing thrombus ⮫, and a focus of IPEH → can be seen in this low-power view of a dilated vessel.* ***(Center)*** *Early stages of IPEH are characterized by a thrombus with an ingrowth of endothelial cells ⮚. The endothelium then subdivides the thrombus, resulting in endothelial-lined papillae →.* ***(Right)*** *Papillary cores are lined by a single layer of plump endothelium lacking significant atypia →.*

SPINDLE CELL HEMANGIOMA

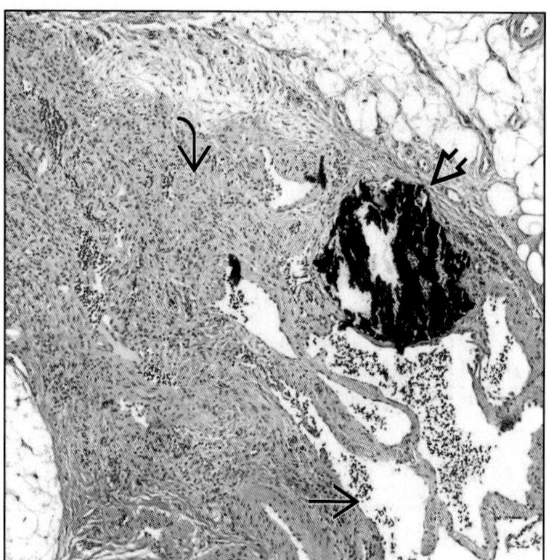

Low-power view of a spindle cell hemangioma shows the open cavernous vessels ➔ adjacent to the spindle cell component ➔. Note the prominent phlebolith ➔ within the dilated vessel.

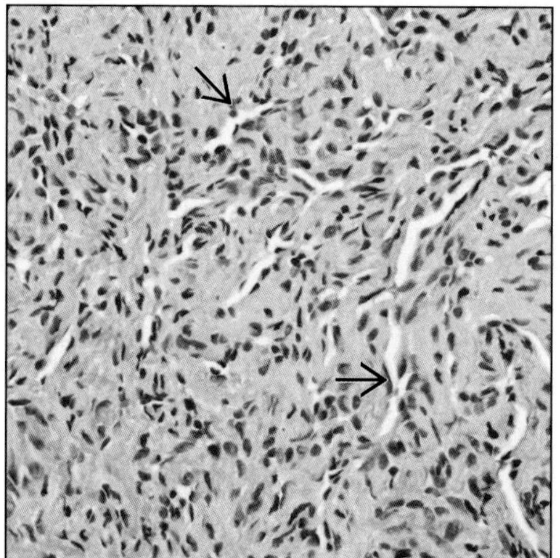

High-power view shows a spindle cell hemangioma. Note the numerous collapsed, slit-like vascular spaces ➔ which, when prominent, can be confused with Kaposi sarcoma.

TERMINOLOGY

Synonyms

- Spindle cell hemangiomatosis
  - Term proposed for multifocal lesions
- Spindle cell hemangioendothelioma
  - Initially considered low-grade angiosarcoma

Definitions

- Benign vascular lesion characterized by cavernous blood vessels and spindle cell areas

ETIOLOGY/PATHOGENESIS

Neoplastic vs. Reactive

- Exact pathogenesis controversial
  - Most appear to favor neoplastic process
  - Reactive process also favored
    - Thought to be related to presence of malformed vasculature

CLINICAL ISSUES

Epidemiology

- Age
  - Affects all ages (mean = 34 years)
  - Often presents before age 25

Site

- Subcutis of distal extremities
  - Tend to cluster in single general area
- Deeper soft tissues (rare)

Presentation

- Most frequently asymptomatic
- Little to no discoloration of overlying skin
- Single or multiple nodules
  - Intravascular > 50%
- May be associated with
  - Maffucci syndrome, Klippel-Trenaunay syndrome, early onset varicose veins, lymphedema, and epithelioid hemangioendothelioma

Treatment

- Complete surgical excision

Prognosis

- Overall prognosis is excellent
- Frequent recurrences (60%)
  - Likely represent contiguous or multifocal intravascular growth
- No evidence of distant or regional metastases
- Report of radiation-induced malignant transformation

MACROSCOPIC FEATURES

Gross Features

- Discrete red to red-brown nodules
- Thrombi or phleboliths may be present

Size

- Ranges from < 1 cm to 4 cm in diameter

MICROSCOPIC PATHOLOGY

Microscopic Features

- 2 components in variable amounts
  - Thin-walled cavernous blood vessels lined by attenuated endothelial cells
    - Space may be empty or filled with erythrocytes, thrombi, or phleboliths
    - Intimal redundancies and herniations common
    - May resemble cavernous hemangioma and angiomatosis
  - Cellular bland spindled zones
    - Consist of collapsed cavernous vessels separated by fibroblastic stromal cells
    - Distinct vacuolated epithelioid cells often present

SPINDLE CELL HEMANGIOMA

Key Facts

Terminology

- Benign vascular lesion characterized by cavernous blood vessels and spindle cell areas

Clinical Issues

- Affects all ages (mean = 34 years)
- Subcutis of distal extremities
- Most frequently asymptomatic
- Frequent recurrences (60%)
- No evidence of distant or regional metastases

Macroscopic Features

- Discrete red to red-brown nodules

Microscopic Pathology

- Thin-walled cavernous blood vessels lined by attenuated endothelial cells
  - May resemble cavernous hemangioma
- Cellular bland spindled zones
  - May resemble Kaposi sarcoma or epithelioid hemangioendothelioma

    - May resemble Kaposi sarcoma or epithelioid hemangioendothelioma

    - Lack significant nuclear atypia or mitotic activity
- Malformed, variably sized vessels at periphery

ANCILLARY TESTS

Immunohistochemistry

- Reactivity for CD31, factor VIII, and other endothelial markers

DIFFERENTIAL DIAGNOSIS

Angiosarcoma

- Rudimentary intercommunicating vascular channels infiltrating soft tissues
- High-grade nuclei with frequent mitoses
  - Differentiating from low-grade angiosarcomas may be difficult
- Lacks 2 distinct components of spindle cell hemangioma

Kaposi Sarcoma

- Slit-like vascular spaces lined by atypical endothelial cells with frequent mitoses
- Rarely contain cavernous vessels
- Lacks distinct epithelioid endothelial cells

Cavernous Hemangioma

- Predominantly located in upper body
- Large and poorly circumscribed
- Large, dilated vessels lined by flat endothelial cells
- Lack spindle cell component of spindle cell hemangioma

Epithelioid Hemangioendothelioma

- Angiocentric solitary tumor of superficial or deep soft tissue
- Round to spindled endothelial cells with intracytoplasmic lumina
- Typically lack large dilated vessels
- More likely to show cytologic atypia

Angiomatosis

- Affects large segments of body in contiguous fashion
- Clusters of variably sized vessels scattered throughout soft tissue with abundant mature adipose tissue

SELECTED REFERENCES

1. Perkins P et al: Spindle cell hemangioendothelioma. An analysis of 78 cases with reassessment of its pathogenesis and biologic behavior. Am J Surg Pathol. 20(10):1196-204, 1996
2. Fletcher CD et al: Spindle cell haemangioendothelioma: a clinicopathological and immunohistochemical study indicative of a non-neoplastic lesion. Histopathology. 18(4):291-301, 1991
3. Weiss SW et al: Spindle cell hemangioendothelioma. A low-grade angiosarcoma resembling a cavernous hemangioma and Kaposi's sarcoma. Am J Surg Pathol. 10(8):521-30, 1986

IMAGE GALLERY

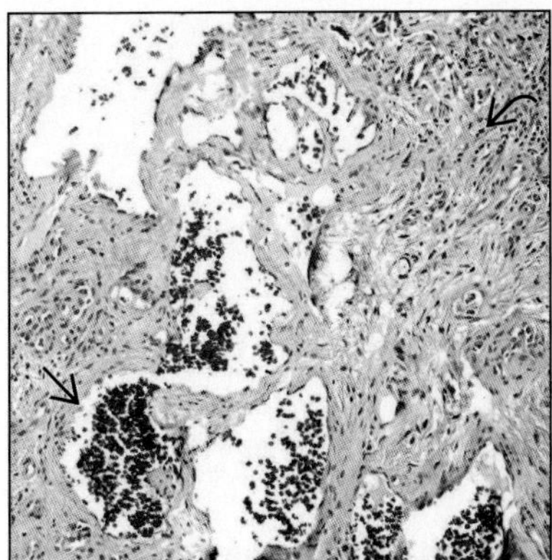

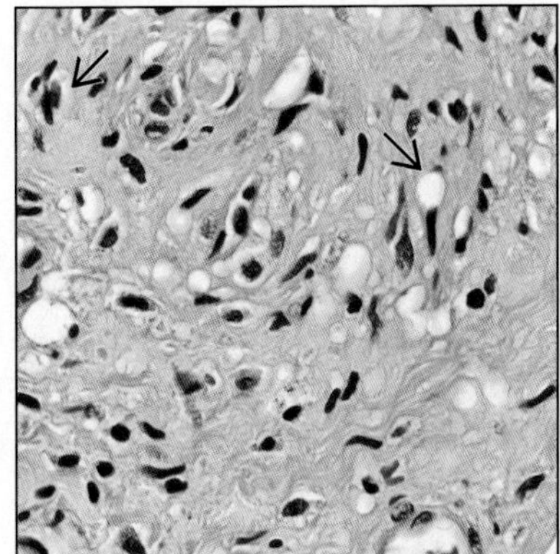

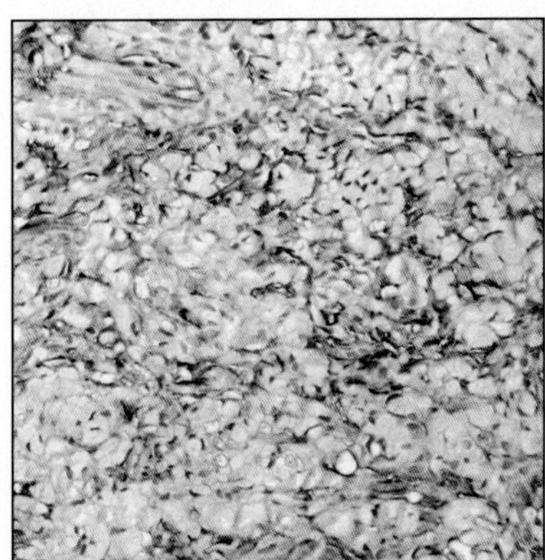

(Left) *Spindle cell hemangioma from medium power demonstrates the cavernous ⇒ and spindle cell ⇒ components.* ***(Center)*** *Spindle cell hemangioma seen at high power shows a spindle cell component. Note the numerous epithelioid cells with intracytoplasmic vacuoles ⇒ reminiscent of an epithelioid hemangioendothelioma.* ***(Right)*** *Strong CD31 membranous reactivity highlights the numerous collapsed slit-like vascular spaces that form the spindle cell component of this spindle cell hemangioma.*

ANGIOMATOSIS

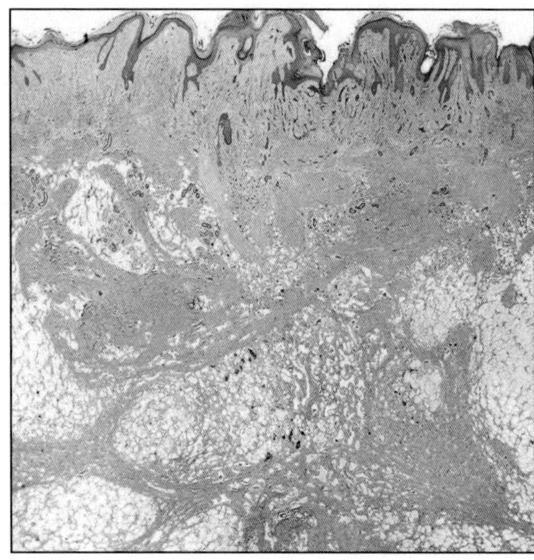

In this example of angiomatosis, a diffuse vascular proliferation involving the upper dermis and extending down into the subcutaneous adipose tissue is seen.

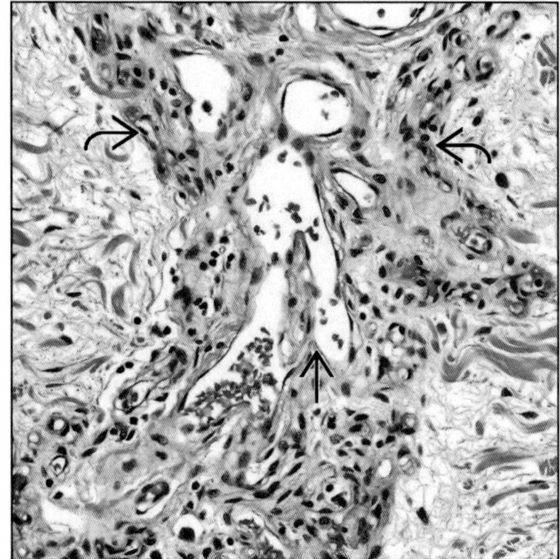

A large cavernous vessel with an irregular wall ➔ is surrounded by numerous, small to medium-sized capillaries ➔.

TERMINOLOGY

Synonyms

- Diffuse hemangioma
- Vascular malformation
- Infiltrating angiolipoma

Definitions

- Diffuse, benign, vascular lesion of soft tissue affecting large segments of body or multiple tissue planes in contiguous fashion

ETIOLOGY/PATHOGENESIS

Developmental Anomaly

- Likely represents congenital malformation
  - Thought to arise in early intrauterine life during limb-bud formation

CLINICAL ISSUES

Epidemiology

- Age
  - Most present in early childhood
  - 2/3 develop by 2nd decade of life
- Gender
  - Females affected slightly more than males

Site

- Lower extremities (> 50%)
- Chest wall, abdomen, and upper extremities may also be affected

Presentation

- Diffuse and persistent swelling
- Pain and discoloration
- Swelling worsened by strenuous exercise

Treatment

- Conservative but complete excision

Prognosis

- Benign lesion with frequent recurrences and persistent disease
  - Majority will develop recurrences (60-90%)
  - Multiple recurrences (40%)
  - Likely reflects incomplete excision
- Metastases or malignant transformation not reported

IMAGE FINDINGS

CT Findings

- Ill-defined, nonhomogeneous mass
- Serpiginous densities in low-density areas
  - Correspond to tortuous vessels

MACROSCOPIC FEATURES

General Features

- Ill-defined mass

Size

- 3-26 cm

Gross Features

- Variable coloration
- Most have predominantly fatty appearance

MICROSCOPIC PATHOLOGY

Predominant Pattern/Injury Type

- Vascular malformation

Predominant Cell/Compartment Type

- Vascular
- Adipose

ANGIOMATOSIS

Key Facts

Terminology
- Diffuse, benign, vascular lesion of soft tissue affecting large segments of body or multiple tissue planes in contiguous fashion

Clinical Issues
- Most present in early childhood
- Lower extremities (> 50%)
- Benign lesion with frequent recurrences and persistent disease

Macroscopic Features
- Predominantly fatty appearance

Microscopic Pathology
- Haphazard arrangement of venous-, cavernous-, and capillary-sized vessels
  - Most common and most characteristic pattern

Diagnostic Checklist
- Clinicopathologic diagnosis

Microscopic Features
- 2 common patterns
  - Haphazard arrangement of venous-, cavernous-, and capillary-sized vessels
    - Irregular and thick to attenuated walls with herniations and intimal redundancies
    - Clusters of capillary vessels within or adjacent to vein walls
    - Large amounts of mature adipose tissue
    - Most common and most characteristic pattern
  - Infiltrating capillary hemangioma
    - Nodules of tumor infiltrate into soft tissue
    - Large amounts of mature adipose tissue
    - Previously referred to as infiltrating angiolipoma
- May involve multiple tissue planes (vertical involvement)
  - Skin, subcutis, muscle, and bone
- May involve only single tissue type
  - Multiple muscles
- Lacks distinct lobular pattern
- Osseous involvement can occur

DIFFERENTIAL DIAGNOSIS

Glomangiomatosis
- Diffusely infiltrating
- Well-formed vessels of varying size surrounded by clusters of glomus cells
- Often accompanied by mature adipose tissue
- May be associated with pain

Infantile Hemangioma (Capillary Hemangioma)
- Distinct lobular pattern
- Lacks extensive involvement
- GLUT1 positive

Intramuscular Hemangioma
- Homogeneous groups of capillary-sized vessels
- Lack mixture of vessel sizes
- Lack soft tissue involvement
- May require clinical correlation to make distinction

DIAGNOSTIC CHECKLIST

Clinically Relevant Pathologic Features
- Clinicopathologic diagnosis
  - Requires the above benign microscopic features
  - Must affect large segments of body in contiguous fashion

SELECTED REFERENCES

1. Rao VK et al: Angiomatosis of soft tissue. An analysis of the histologic features and clinical outcome in 51 cases. Am J Surg Pathol. 16(8):764-71, 1992
2. Howat AJ et al: Angiomatosis: a vascular malformation of infancy and childhood. Report of 17 cases. Pathology. 19(4):377-82, 1987
3. Koblenzer PJ et al: Angiomatosis (hamartomatous hem-lymphangiomatosis). Report of a case with diffuse involvement. Pediatrics. 28:65-76, 1961

IMAGE GALLERY

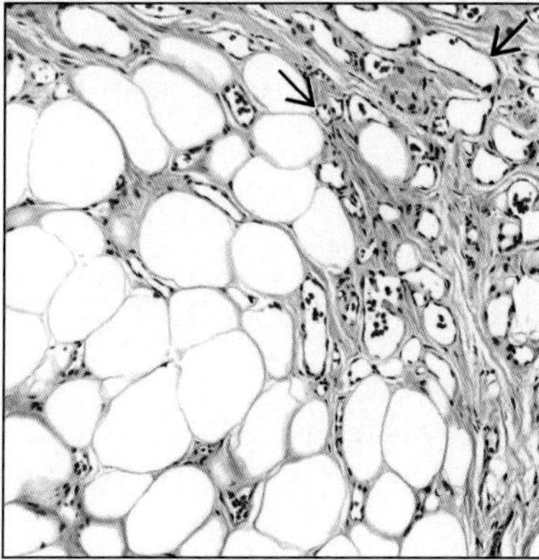

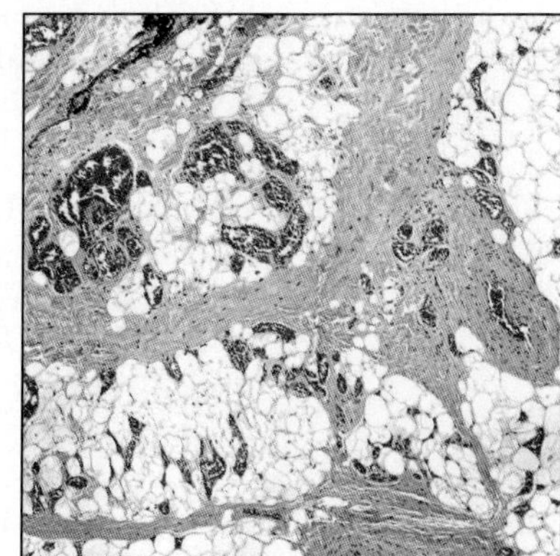

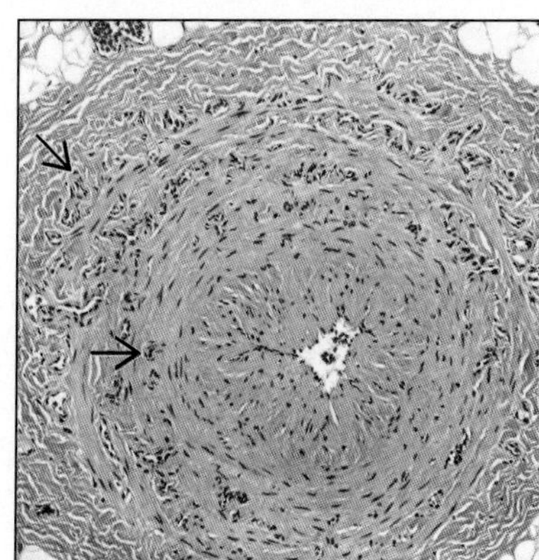

*(**Left**) Numerous small and dilated capillaries ⇒ are shown infiltrating the fibrous connective tissue and extending down into the adjacent adipose tissue. (**Center**) Scattered vessels of varying size and wall thickness are seen within the fibrous connective tissue and lobules of mature adipose tissue. (**Right**) Numerous small capillaries ⇒ are distributed within and adjacent to this thick-walled artery.*

FIBROLIPOMATOUS HAMARTOMA OF NERVE

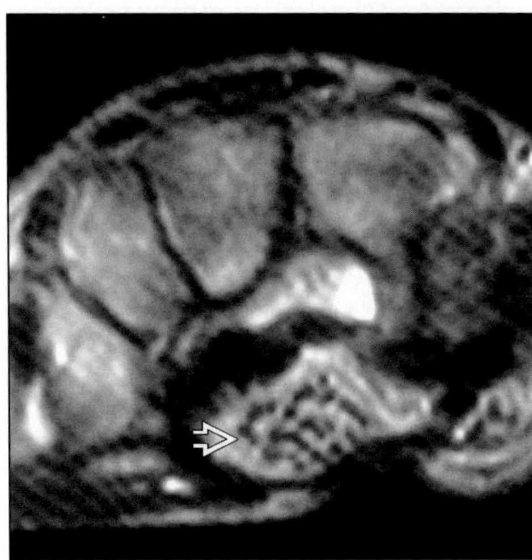

MR image shows fat signal in stroma between nerve fascicles ➩.

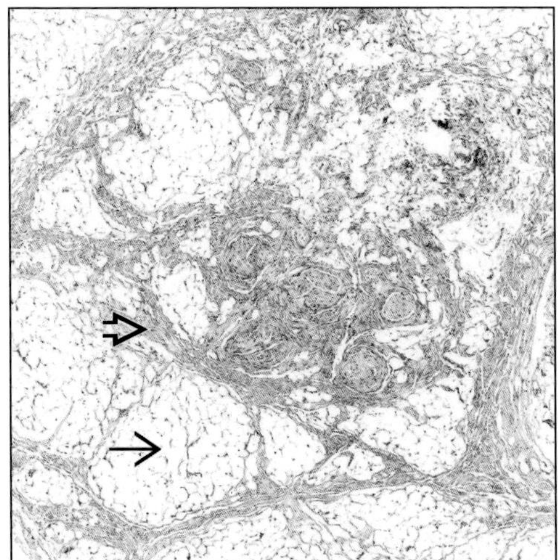

Hematoxylin & eosin shows accumulation of mature adipose tissue ➔ with hypocellular fibrous septa ➩ around and between nerve bundles.

TERMINOLOGY

Synonyms

- Neural lipofibromatous hamartoma
- Neurolipomatosis

Definitions

- Increased fibrofatty tissue infiltrating and surrounding nerves

CLINICAL ISSUES

Epidemiology

- Age
  - Predominantly in children
    - Lesions most often present at birth or early childhood
  - Some cases seen in young adults, up to 30 years of age

Site

- Affects palmar surface of hand, wrist, forearm
- Median nerve and branches most commonly affected
- Rarely involves ulnar or radial nerve
- Involves left arm more often than right arm
- Very rarely involves sciatic, peroneal, or cranial nerve

Presentation

- Subcutaneous mass
  - Slow growing
  - Leads to compression neuropathy
    - Paresthesia
    - Increasing pain
- Macrodactyly (digital gigantism, macrodystrophia lipomatosa)
  - In 27% of cases
  - Can be congenital and progressive
  - Increased growth of bone and soft tissue of affected digit

Treatment

- Options, risks, complications
  - Complete excision contraindicated because of nerve damage
- Surgical approaches
  - Biopsy confirms diagnosis
  - Debulking or carpal tunnel release for symptomatic control
  - Removal of deformed digit

Prognosis

- Usually stabilizes if incompletely excised

IMAGE FINDINGS

MR Findings

- Fusiform enlargement of affected nerve segment
  - Secondary to fatty infiltration
- "Telephone cable" sign

MACROSCOPIC FEATURES

General Features

- Sausage-shaped mass
- Yellow-white tissue
- Surrounds and expands nerve
- Can extend into adjacent soft tissue of hand and wrist

Size

- Variable, up to 10 cm length of nerve involved

MICROSCOPIC PATHOLOGY

Histologic Features

- Adipose tissue and fibrous tissue
  - Infiltrate around and between nerve branches and along perineurium
- Epineurial and perineurial fibrous thickening

FIBROLIPOMATOUS HAMARTOMA OF NERVE

Key Facts

Terminology
- Increased fibrofatty tissue infiltrating and surrounding nerves

Clinical Issues
- Median nerve most commonly affected
- Predominantly in children, including congenitally
- Macrodactyly
- Complete excision contraindicated because of nerve damage

Macroscopic Features
- Sausage-shaped mass
- Can extend into adjacent soft tissue of hand and wrist

Microscopic Pathology
- Adipose tissue and fibrous tissue
- Perineurium can become hyperplastic
- Nerve bundles become separated

- Perineurium can become hyperplastic
  - Concentric layers
  - "Onion bulb" intraneural hyperplasia
- Nerve bundles become separated
- Nerves can become atrophic in longstanding cases
- Rare metaplastic bone formation

DIFFERENTIAL DIAGNOSIS

Lipoma of Nerve
- Circumscribed
- Confined within nerve

Neurofibroma
- Proliferation of neural elements
- No fatty component

Neuroma
- Increased number of nerve bundles
- No fatty component

Lipomatosis
- Histologically similar
- Usually skin and subcutis
- Spares nerves

Other Causes of Macrodactyly
- Neurofibromatosis type 1
- Ollier disease
- Maffucci syndrome
- Klippel-Trenaunay syndrome
- Congenital lymphedema
- Proteus syndrome
  - Mutations in *PTEN* tumor suppressor gene
  - Localized gigantism and lipomatous masses

SELECTED REFERENCES

1. Bisceglia M et al: Neural lipofibromatous hamartoma: a report of two cases and review of the literature. Adv Anat Pathol. 14(1):46-52, 2007
2. Razzaghi A et al: Lipofibromatous hamartoma: review of early diagnosis and treatment. Can J Surg. 48(5):394-9, 2005
3. Al-Qattan MM: Lipofibromatous hamartoma of the median nerve and its associated conditions. J Hand Surg [Br]. 26(4):368-72, 2001
4. Marom EM et al: Fibrolipomatous hamartoma: pathognomonic on MR imaging. Skeletal Radiol. 28(5):260-4, 1999
5. Berti E et al: Fibrolipomatous hamartoma of a cranial nerve. Histopathology. 24(4):391-2, 1994
6. Amadio PC et al: Lipofibromatous hamartoma of nerve. J Hand Surg [Am]. 13(1):67-75, 1988
7. Dell PC: Macrodactyly. Hand Clin. 1(3):511-24, 1985
8. Silverman TA et al: Fibrolipomatous hamartoma of nerve. A clinicopathologic analysis of 26 cases. Am J Surg Pathol. 9(1):7-14, 1985

IMAGE GALLERY

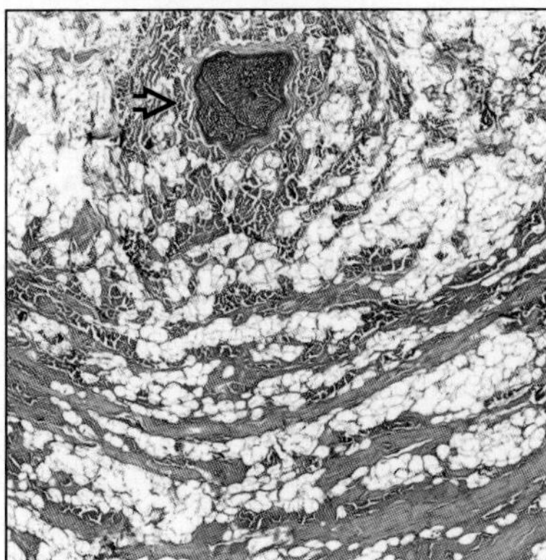

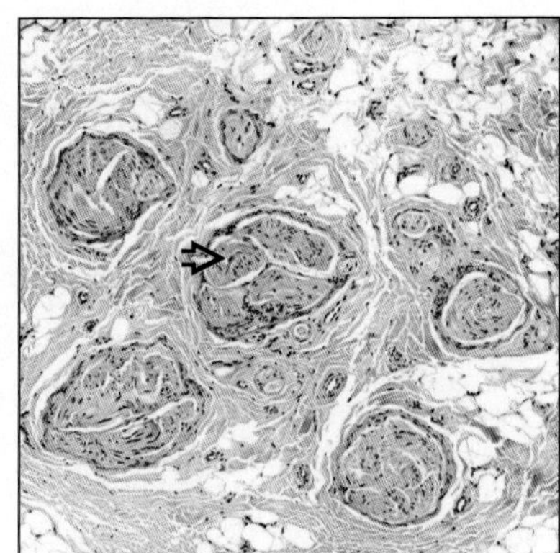

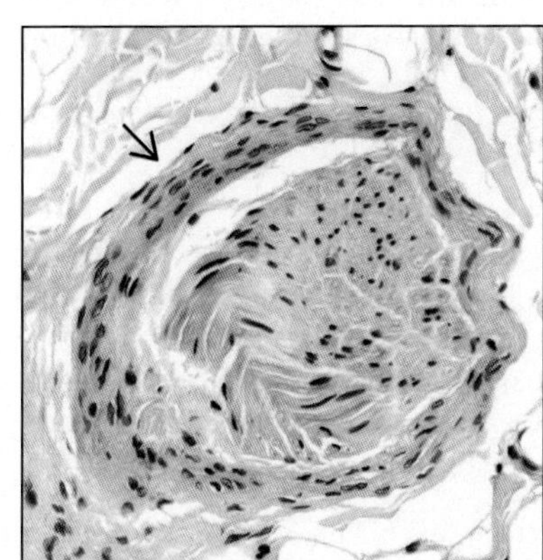

(Left) *Hematoxylin & eosin shows fibrous bands and adipose tissue in subcutis adjacent to nerve ⇨. Note prominent extension of lesional tissue beyond nerve.* ***(Center)*** *Hematoxylin & eosin shows nerve bundles ⇨ separated by fibrous tissue within fat.* ***(Right)*** *Hematoxylin & eosin shows perineurial cell hyperplasia with several layers of elongated spindle cells →. These demonstrate immunoreactivity for epithelial membrane antigen (EMA).*

HETEROTOPIC NEUROGLIAL TISSUE

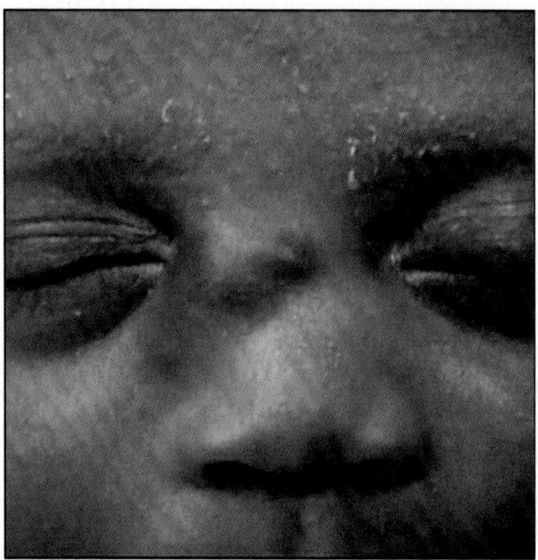

Clinical photograph shows heterotopic neuroglial tissue presenting as subcutaneous nodule at the base of the nose in an infant. These can also occur as intranasal polyps.

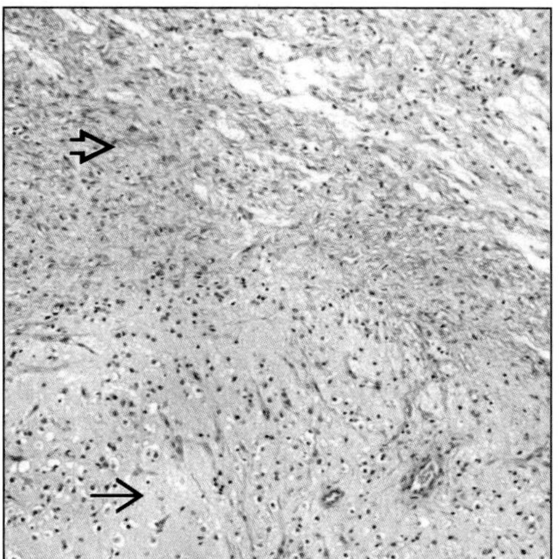

Hematoxylin & eosin shows neuroglial tissue lobules ➔ intimately admixed with dense collagen bands ➔ of surrounding fibrous connective tissue.

TERMINOLOGY

Abbreviations

- Heterotopic neuroglial tissue (HNT)

Synonyms

- Nasal "glioma"
- Nasal glial/cerebral heterotopia
- Glial hamartoma/choristoma
- Heterotopic glial/brain tissue

Definitions

- Ectopic deposits of mature nonneoplastic neuroglial tissue outside the central nervous system

ETIOLOGY/PATHOGENESIS

Developmental Anomaly

- Entrapped neuroectoderm during development
  - Biologically benign malformation process
  - Nasal "glioma" is a misnomer
- Anterior encephalocele variant (disconnected)
  - Rarely attached to olfactory bulb or frontal lobe
    - Contiguously or through simple fibrous tract
- Distant locations suggest different pathogenesis
  - Differentiated pluripotential embryonic stem cells

CLINICAL ISSUES

Epidemiology

- Incidence
  - Rare: 1 in 20,000-40,000 live births
- Age
  - Congenital; generally presents within 1st year of life
  - Rare cases presenting in adulthood

Site

- Extranasal (60%): Midline or parasagittal subcutaneous tissue at base of nose
- Intranasal (30%): Polyp or mass
- Also described in orbit, scalp, occipital bone, oral cavity, tongue, pharynx, intrapulmonary

Presentation

- Asymptomatic
  - Especially when small (< 1 cm)
- Extranasal: Cosmetic complaint, visible protuberance
- Intranasal: Stuffiness, allergy symptoms, respiratory distress/obstruction (if large)
- CSF rhinorrhea, meningitis
  - If brain communication (through cribriform plate)

Treatment

- Options, risks, complications
  - Recurrence after incomplete excision: Rare (< 10%)
    - Residual tissue may continue to grow
- Surgical approaches
  - Simple, complete excision
  - Guided by brain communication, relationship to facial nerve, cosmetic considerations

Prognosis

- Neoplastic transformation vanishingly rare
- Oligodendroglioma reported in nasopharyngeal HNT

IMAGE FINDINGS

MR Findings

- Identifies intracranial communication, bone defect

MACROSCOPIC FEATURES

General Features

- Firm or partially cystic mass
- Covered by normal mucosa or skin

Size

- Generally < 10 cm (mean: 2-3 cm)

HETEROTOPIC NEUROGLIAL TISSUE

Key Facts

Terminology
- Ectopic deposits of mature nonneoplastic neuroglial tissue outside the central nervous system

Etiology/Pathogenesis
- Entrapped neuroectoderm or encephalocele variant
- Nasal "glioma" is a misnomer

Clinical Issues
- Congenital, generally presents within 1st year of life
- Most commonly extranasal or intranasal
- Simple complete excision; recurrence rare

Microscopic Pathology
- Predominantly mature, GFAP(+) astrocytes
- Occasional neurons (Nissl substance, axons)
- Dense fibrovascular connective tissue

Diagnostic Checklist
- High index of suspicion (infant, nasal area, mass)

MICROSCOPIC PATHOLOGY

Histologic Features
- Neuroglial lobules amidst fibrovascular bands
  - Intimate but disorganized mixture
  - Masson trichrome stain highlights juxtaposition
- Neuroglial component: Predominantly mature glia
  - Large, GFAP(+) astrocytes; can mimic neurons
    - May be gemistocytic or show reactive gliosis
  - Fibrillar matrix (neuropil)
- Neurons occasionally found
  - Cytoplasmic Nissl substance, arborizing axons
  - Silver stain-positive
- Ependymal structures, choroid plexus, pigmented retinal epithelium also described
- Dense fibrovascular connective tissue
  - Dark pink-staining collagen stroma
  - Microcalcifications, inflammation may be present

DIFFERENTIAL DIAGNOSIS

Astrocytoma
- Eroding through cribriform plate into nasal cavity
- More cellular and pleomorphic than HNT

Encephalocele
- Usually cystic, with meningeal coverings
- Always communicates with intracranial space
- Histologically indistinguishable from HNT

Teratoma
- All 3 germ layers (endoderm, mesoderm, ectoderm)

DIAGNOSTIC CHECKLIST

Clinically Relevant Pathologic Features
- No syndromic associations reported
- Biopsy or fine needle aspiration contraindicated
  - Possible brain communication increases risk of meningitis or removal of functional brain tissue
- May represent variant of sequestered encephalocele
  - Distinction largely academic
  - Brain communication determines surgical approach
    - Best resolved through imaging

Pathologic Interpretation Pearls
- Failure to recognize neuroglial tissue → erroneous diagnosis of "fibroconnective tissue"
  - High index of suspicion (infant, nasal area, mass)
  - Masson trichrome, GFAP stains may help

SELECTED REFERENCES

1. Husein OF et al: Neuroglial heterotopia causing neonatal airway obstruction: presentation, management, and literature review. Eur J Pediatr. 167(12):1351-5, 2008
2. Penner CR et al: Nasal glial heterotopia: a clinicopathologic and immunophenotypic analysis of 10 cases with a review of the literature. Ann Diagn Pathol. 7(6):354-9, 2003

IMAGE GALLERY

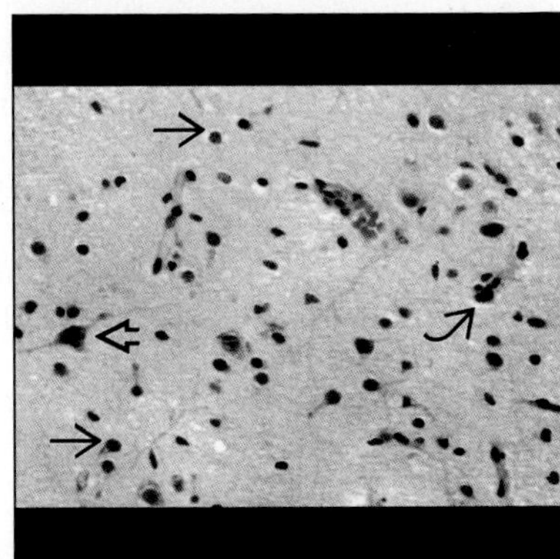

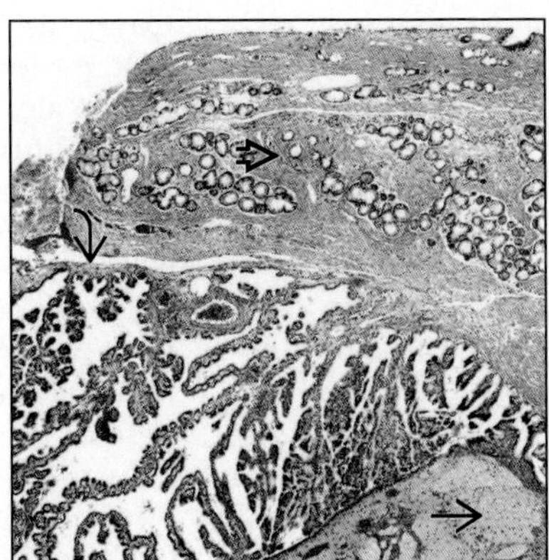

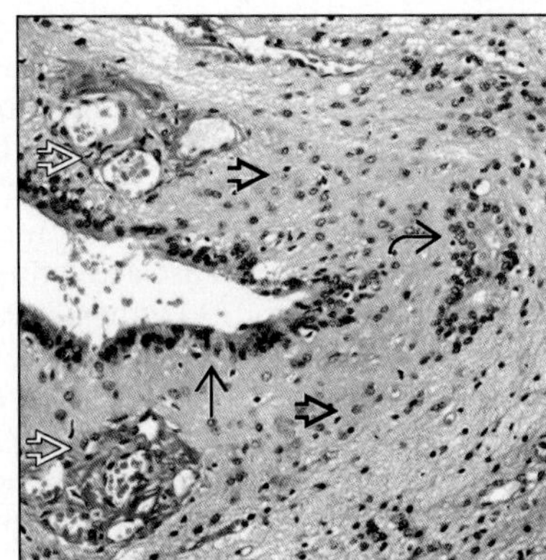

(Left) *High-magnification view shows heterotopic neuroglial tissue with numerous enlarged astrocytes ⇒ in a fibrillar matrix (neuropil), a neuron ⇨, and microcalcifications ⇗.* ***(Center)*** *Respiratory mucosa of nasopharynx is shown with submucosal seromucinous glands ⇨ and heterotopic neuroglial tissue lying below it ⇒, with choroid plexus ⇗.* ***(Right)*** *Heterotopic glial tissue is seen with neuroglial component ⇨, ependymal cells lining a central canal-type structure ⇒, & true ependymal rosettes ⇗. Disorganized fibrovascular bundles ➡ can also be seen.*

NEUROFIBROMA

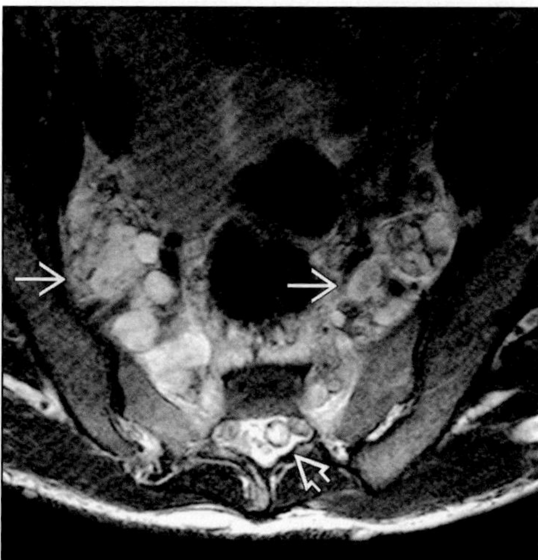

Axial T2WI MR shows bilateral plexiform neurofibromas ➡ involving the sacral plexus with the characteristic "bag of worms" appearance. There is intraspinal extension ➡.

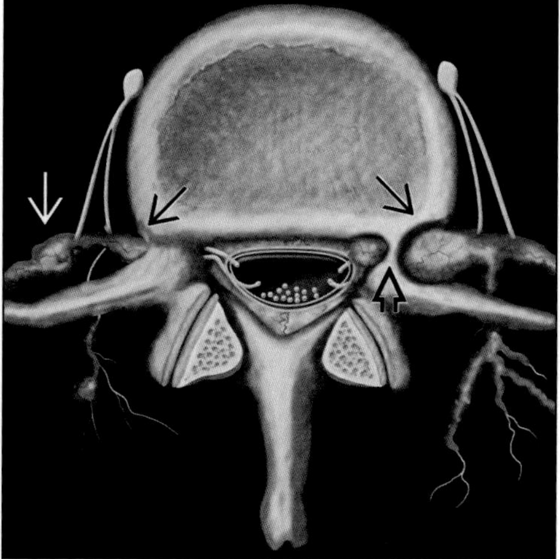

Graphic shows plexiform neurofibromas ➡ of bilateral spinal roots with a "braided rope" ➡ and "dumbbell" ➡ appearance (intra- and extradural tumor portions).

TERMINOLOGY

Abbreviations

- Neurofibroma (NF)
- Neurofibromatosis type 1 (NF1)

Synonyms

- Elephantiasis neuromatosa = massive soft tissue NF
- Von Recklinghausen disease = NF1

Definitions

- Common peripheral nerve sheath (WHO grade I) tumor of Schwann cells, fibroblasts, perineurial-like cells, and residual nerves in myxoid/collagen matrix
- Subtypes (anatomic location, macroscopic appearance)
  - Cutaneous: Localized or diffuse
  - Intraneural: Localized or plexiform
  - Soft tissue or visceral NF: "Gigantism," "elephantiasis"
- Sporadic (most) or in NF1 (multiple, large, plexiform)

ETIOLOGY/PATHOGENESIS

Histogenesis

- Close relationship to parent nerve (gave rise to tumor)
  - Thought to arise from peripheral nerve sheaths
    - Endoneurium or connective tissue
- Mixed, heterogeneous cell composition
  - Initially suggested hyperplastic nature
- 2-hit hypothesis in NF1 genetic syndrome
  - Germline mutation in *NF1* (chromosome 17q11.2)
    - Neurofibromin: GTPase-activating protein
    - Tumor suppressor: Downregulates Ras, cAMP
  - Somatic mutation in *NF1* gives rise to NF
- Evidence supporting neoplastic nature of NF
  - Sporadic NF histologically resemble NF1-associated
  - Monoclonality (X chromosome inactivation studies)
  - Lesional Schwann cells carry *NF1* gene deletion
  - Malignant transformation in NF
    - Additional loss of tumor suppressors (e.g., *TP53*)

CLINICAL ISSUES

Epidemiology

- Incidence
  - Most common tumor of peripheral nerve
  - NF1 incidence: 1 in 2,500-4,000 births
- Age
  - Solitary, sporadic lesions: 20-30 years old
  - Multiple (in setting of NF1): Puberty
  - Plexiform NF may be congenital

Site

- Localized cutaneous NF
  - Most common type by presentation/site
  - Nodular or polypoid, usually well circumscribed
  - Freely movable, soft, round lesions that elevate skin
  - Generally not associated with recognizable nerve
    - Presumably arise from smaller peripheral nerves
  - Matrix tends to be more dense, with collagen fibers
- Diffuse cutaneous NF
  - Often large, plaque-like; affects head and neck
  - Relatively uncommon, 10% associated with NF1
  - Ill-defined, yellow-white, fatty cut surface
  - Extraneural infiltration of dermis, subcutis
  - Entrap (not displace) dermal vessels, nerves, adnexa
  - Spread along subcutaneous connective tissue septa
- Localized intraneural NF
  - In larger, more deeply seated single nerves
  - Sensorimotor or autonomic peripheral nerves
  - Spinal nerve roots (cervical, brachial, lumbosacral)
  - Rare intradural cranial nerves (unlike schwannoma)
  - Well-circumscribed, fusiform nerve enlargement
  - Endoneurial growth, enveloped by peri/epineurium
- Plexiform NF
  - Elongated, multinodular lesions
    - Involving multiple nerve fascicles or branches
  - On branching nerves (e.g., trunks of brachial plexus)

NEUROFIBROMA

Key Facts

Terminology
- Common peripheral nerve sheath tumor (grade I)
- Schwann cells, fibroblasts, perineurial-like cells, and residual nerve axons in myxoid/collagen matrix
- Most are sporadic; NF1: Multiple, large, or plexiform

Clinical Issues
- Localized cutaneous NF most common subtype
  - Circumscribed, nodular, no recognizable nerve
- Diffuse cutaneous NF: Relatively uncommon
  - Large, plaque-like; infiltrate dermis, subcutis
- Localized intraneural NF: Larger, deeper nerves
  - Fusiform endoneurial growth, within perineurium
- Plexiform NF: Multiple nerve fascicles or branches
  - "Bag of worms" (branching) or "braided rope"
- Massive soft tissue NF: Pelvis, shoulder, limb
  - Widespread infiltration of fat, muscle ("gigantism")

Macroscopic Features
- Soft, translucent, gelatinous; may be firm, opaque
- Lack degeneration (hemorrhage, cystic change)

Microscopic Pathology
- Bundles of spindle cells; angulated or curved nuclei
  - Partially S100, GFAP, EMA/MUC1 positive
- Loose, myxoid (mucopolysaccharide-rich) matrix
- Variable stromal coarse collagen ("shredded carrots")
- Residual, central, neurofilament-positive axon fibers
- Delicate microvasculature, occasional mast cells
- Atypical NF: No prognostic significance
  - Scattered large cells with degenerative atypia

Diagnostic Checklist
- Transformation (MPNST): 2-10% of plexiform NF
  - ↑ cellularity, atypia, hyperchromasia, mitoses

    - Intertwined tangles, "bag of worms" appearance
  - Nonbranching nerves (e.g., sciatic nerve fascicles)
    - Thick, "braided rope" appearance
  - Generally affect nerves with smaller diameter
    - Residual axons more central in nerve fascicle
- (Massive) soft tissue NF
  - Tend to be very large, diffuse, and plexiform
  - Widespread infiltration of adipose tissue and muscle
  - Pendulous folds of neurofibromatous tissue
    - Marked enlargement of single anatomic region
    - Pelvis, shoulder, limb ("localized gigantism")
  - Visceral NF: Mesenteric, liver, genitourinary tract
    - Rare cardiac and laryngeal cases reported

Presentation
- Most are solitary, sporadic
- Superficial cutaneous or localized intraneural NF
  - Painless, palpable, asymptomatic mass
- Deep intraneural tumors
  - Pain, dysthesia in nerve distribution
- Intraspinal (nerve root) NF
  - Spinal cord compression

Natural History
- Hormonal influence may affect growth of NF
  - Increased rates seen in puberty, pregnancy
- Malignant transformation
  - Malignant peripheral nerve sheath tumor (MPNST)
  - Rare in cutaneous (0.001%)
  - More common in plexiform NF (2-10%)
  - Clinical suspicion for malignant transformation
    - Rapid enlargement of preexisting NF
    - Pain, change in neurological symptoms
  - More in older patients (prone to NF recurrence)

Treatment
- Surgical approaches
  - Complete resection
    - Attainable in superficial cutaneous lesions
  - Decompression of spinal cord if symptomatic

Prognosis
- Recurrence rare, even after partial removal
- Location, multiplicity (NF1) create medical problems
  - Surgical resection not always feasible
- Overall life expectancy shortened

IMAGE FINDINGS

MR Findings
- Irregular or bright on T2WI MR
- Gadolinium-enhancing on T1WI
- "Target" sign: Reduced signal in intraneural NF
  - Less mucinous residual nerve center
- "Dumbbell tumors": Paraspinal lesions
  - Intradural and extradural portions form "dumbbell"

MACROSCOPIC FEATURES

General Features
- Soft to firm, translucent to opaque, gray to tan surface
- Glistening/gelatinous (mucin) to firm/fibrous (collagen)
- Relatively well circumscribed but not encapsulated
  - Intraneural NF may be covered by epineurium
- Lack degeneration (hemorrhage, cystic change)

Size
- Localized cutaneous lesions: Up to 2 cm
- May reach much larger size (massive soft tissue NF)

MICROSCOPIC PATHOLOGY

Histologic Features
- Irregular bundles/fascicles of spindle/wavy cells
- Ovoid to spindle nuclei, thin cell processes
- Perineurial-like cells with angulated or curved nuclei
- Loose, myxoid (mucopolysaccharide-rich) matrix
  - Alcian blue positive
- Variable amounts of stromal coarse collagen bundles
  - Trichrome positive; "shredded carrot" appearance
- Residual axons (myelinated or unmyelinated)
  - Single nerve fibers, through central tumor bulk

NEUROFIBROMA

- Occasional mast cells, pigmented Schwann cells
- Delicate, inconspicuous microvasculature
- Only rare mitoses

Predominant Pattern/Injury Type

- Neoplastic

Predominant Cell/Compartment Type

- Nervous, Schwannian
- Nervous, perineural
- Mesenchymal, fibroblast
- Nervous, neural

Histologic Variants

- Cellular NF
  - Patchy or more widespread hypercellularity
  - Mildly enlarged nuclei, p53 immunoreactivity
  - Occasional mitotic figures but still low proliferation
  - Probably represent MPNST precursors
- Atypical NF
  - Scattered large cells with degenerative atypia
    - Bizarre, smudgy, hyperchromatic nuclei
  - Little or no increase in proliferative activity
  - No prognostic significance

ANCILLARY TESTS

Immunohistochemistry

- Partially immunoreactive for S100, GFAP
  - In Schwann cells; less than schwannoma
- Fibroblasts: Positive for vimentin
- Perineurial cells: Occasionally positive for EMA/MUC1
- Nerve axons: Scattered positive neurofilament protein
- Variable staining for collagen IV, CD34

Cytogenetics

- Clonal karyotypic abnormalities (banding studies)
  - But fewer than in schwannoma, MPNST
  - 1/3 of NF have been found to be aneuploid

Electron Microscopy

- Heterogeneous mixture of cell types
- Schwann cells: Surrounded by continuous basal lamina, processes envelop axons or collagen bundles
- Perineurial cells: Long attenuated cell processes, numerous surface pinocytic vesicles, incomplete (interrupted) pericellular basal lamina
- Fibroblasts: Abundant rough endoplasmic reticulum, lack basal lamina

DIFFERENTIAL DIAGNOSIS

(Plexiform) Schwannoma

- Solitary, encapsulated, more globular
- Eccentric to nerve: Peripheral displaced residual axons
  - Lack diffuse extraneural component
- More cystic, with lipid accumulation (yellow surfaces)
  - Less solid, lack gray mucinous areas
- Uniformly composed of S100(+) Schwann cells
  - Verocay bodies, biphasic Antoni A and B areas
- Vessel hyalinization, perivascular hemosiderin
- Often intradural or involving extremities

Perineurioma

- Concentric, "onion bulb" or whorled proliferations
  - Centered around nerve fibers
- Diffusely, strongly positive for EMA

Ganglioneuroma

- Large neoplastic neurons (ganglion cells)
  - Pleomorphic, binucleated
  - With cytoplasmic vacuoles, prominent nucleoli
- Lack stromal mucin
- Have abundant unmyelinated axons

Malignant Peripheral Nerve Sheath Tumor

- Especially relevant for cellular NF
- Storiform or "herringbone" growth pattern
- Pleomorphism, nuclear enlargement, necrosis
- High mitotic activity (> 4/10 HPF)

Plexiform Fibrohistiocytic Tumors

- Especially relevant for plexiform NF
- Female predilection
- Small firm texture, not "bag of worms"
- Lack association with nerve
- Composed of myofibroblasts, epithelioid/giant cells
- Actin-HHF-35(+), CD68(+), S100(-)

DIAGNOSTIC CHECKLIST

Clinically Relevant Pathologic Features

- Almost pathognomonic for NF1
  - Multiple intraneural or cutaneous involvement
  - Plexiform architecture
  - Large (massive) soft tissue lesions
- Cutaneous NF associated with NF1
  - Overlying café au lait spots (pigmented macules)

Pathologic Interpretation Pearls

- Histologic features: Transformation to MPNST
  - ↑ cellularity, atypia, hyperchromasia, mitoses
  - Nuclear enlargement (3x size of normal NF nuclei)
  - Changes can be focal only (sample extensively)
    - May be masked in massive soft tissue NF
  - Precise cut-off from cellular/atypical NF is subjective
- Large diffuse NF tend to have plexiform elements
  - Whorled structures resembling Meissner corpuscles
    - Wagner-Meissner-like bodies
  - May overtake dorsal root or sympathetic ganglia
    - Do not confuse for ganglioneuroma
- Cutaneous NF may be separated from epidermis by uninvolved grenz zone

SELECTED REFERENCES

1. Skovronsky DM et al: Pathologic classification of peripheral nerve tumors. Neurosurg Clin N Am. 15(2):157-66, 2004
2. Ferner RE et al: Neurofibroma and schwannoma. Curr Opin Neurol. 15(6):679-84, 2002
3. Woodruff JM: Pathology of tumors of the peripheral nerve sheath in type 1 neurofibromatosis. Am J Med Genet. 89(1):23-30, 1999

NEUROFIBROMA

Microscopic Features

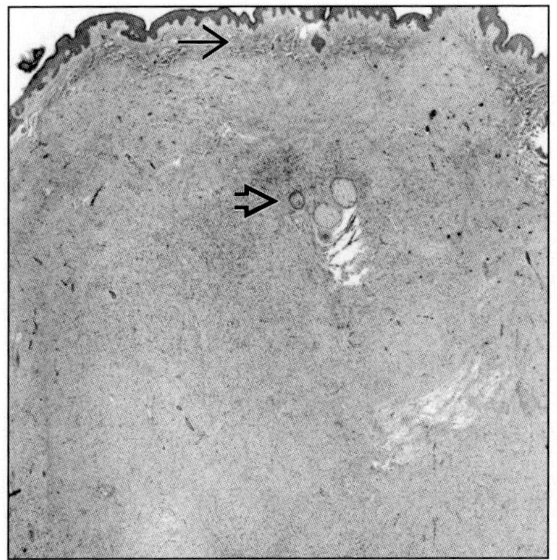

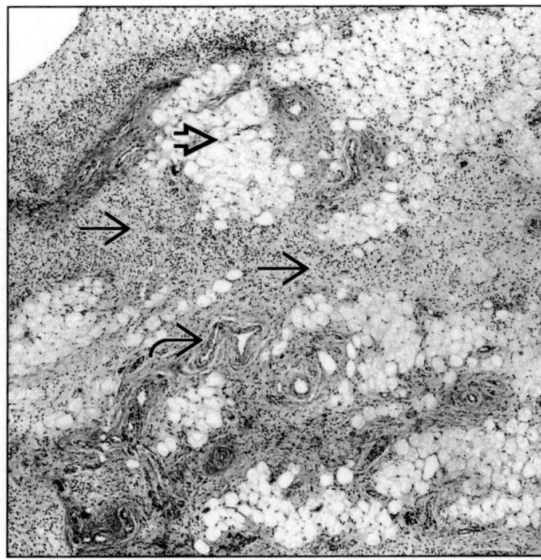

(Left) *Low-power view of localized cutaneous NF with uninvolved Grenz zone* ⇒ *between tumor and epidermis. These NF are usually nodular, not associated with a recognizable nerve, have a denser collagenous matrix, and may trap adnexal structures* ⇨*, although the latter more commonly occurs in diffuse NF.* ***(Right)*** *Low-power view shows diffuse cutaneous NF* ⇒ *with extraneural infiltration of subcutaneous adipose* ⇨ *and connective tissue with trapped vessels* ↗*.*

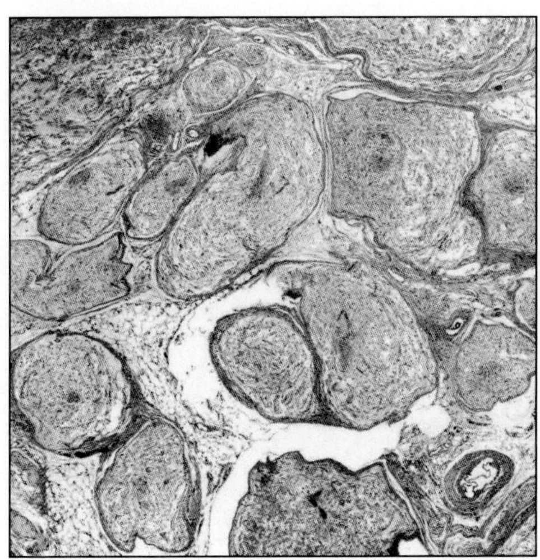

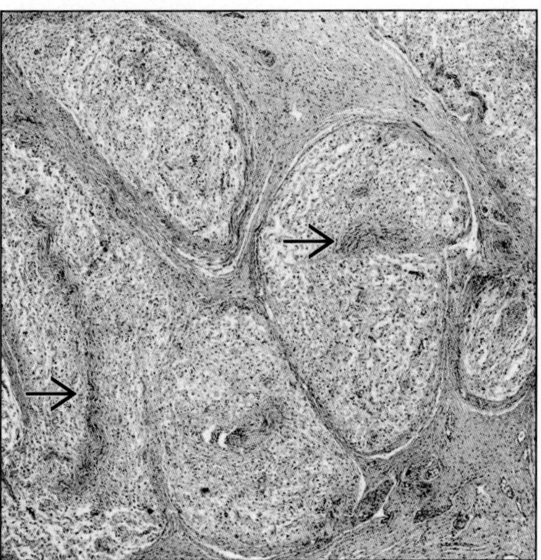

(Left) *Low-power view shows plexiform NF with multiple nerve fascicles being expanded by the tumor, leading to a multinodular appearance, which grossly resembles a "bag of worms."* ***(Right)*** *Higher power view of plexiform NF shows each nerve fascicle or branch expanded by a myxoid matrix-containing neoplasm, which surrounds the centrally located, aggregated residual nerve axon fibers* ⇒*.*

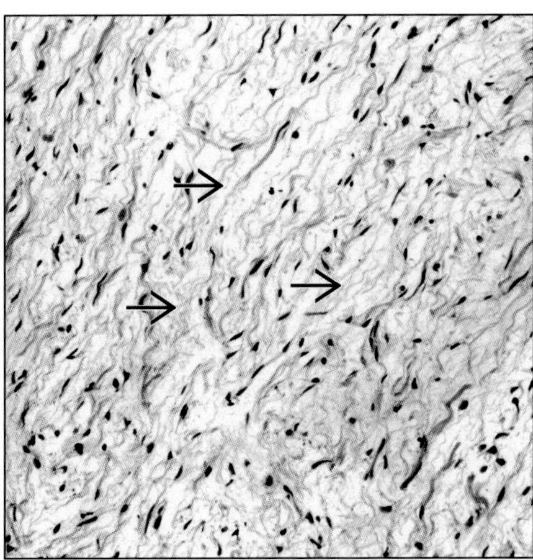

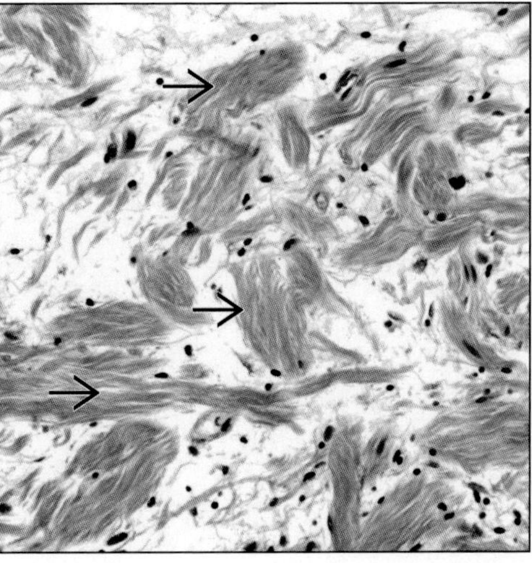

(Left) *High-power view of NF shows the classic hypocellular appearance of spindle and wavy cells with angulated or ovoid nuclei and thin cell processes amidst a loose myxoid matrix* ⇒*.* ***(Right)*** *High-power view shows accumulation of coarse stromal collagen bundles* ⇒*, which usually occurs in localized NF and gives the appearance of "shredded carrots."*

NEUROFIBROMA

Microscopic Features

(Left) High-power view of the characteristic delicate microvasculature ⇒ is commonly seen amidst the myxoid matrix background of NF. *(Right)* Medium-power view shows localized intraneural NF of the spinal nerve root, involving the dorsal root ganglion and trapping ganglion cells ⇒, which are otherwise cytologically normal. These elements can lead to a misdiagnosis of ganglioneuroma. Delicate blood vessels ⇨ can also be seen.

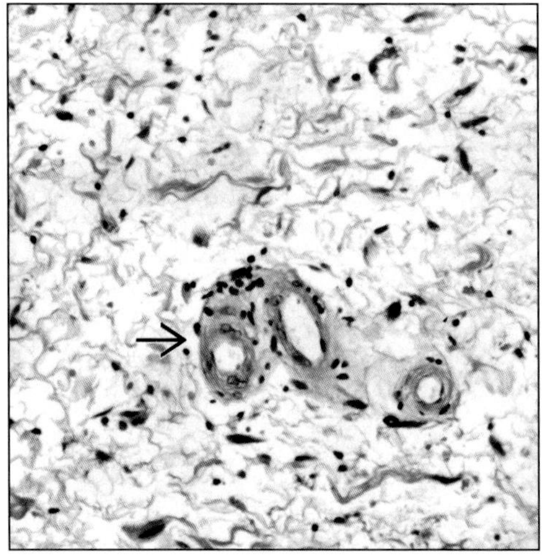

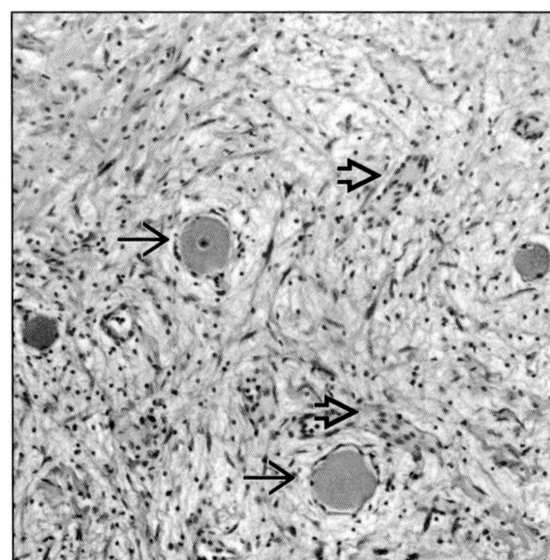

(Left) High-power view of NF shows mast cells ⇒, which are commonly seen "floating" in the myxoid matrix in small numbers. *(Right)* High-power view shows whorled structures ⇒ resembling Meissner or pacinian corpuscles. Also termed pseudo-meissnerian corpuscles or Wagner-Meissner-like bodies, these are commonly found in large diffuse or massive soft tissue NF.

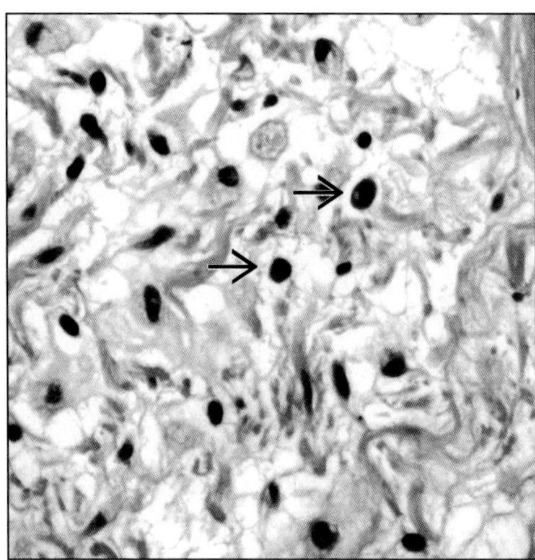

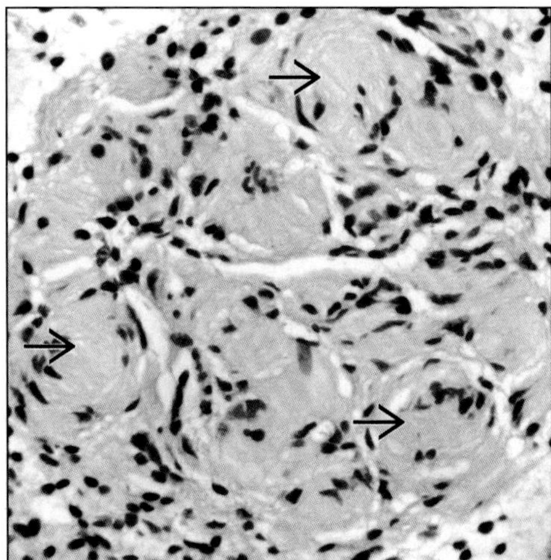

(Left) High-power view of "atypical NF" shows occasional large cells, most likely Schwann cells, with smudgy, hyperchromatic nuclei ⇒. In the absence of increased proliferative activity, this is thought to represent degenerative atypia and has no prognostic significance. *(Right)* High-power view shows patchy hypercellularity and mildly enlarged nuclei ⇨. Termed "cellular NF," these are thought to be precursors to MPNST, the precise cut-off from which is rather subjective.

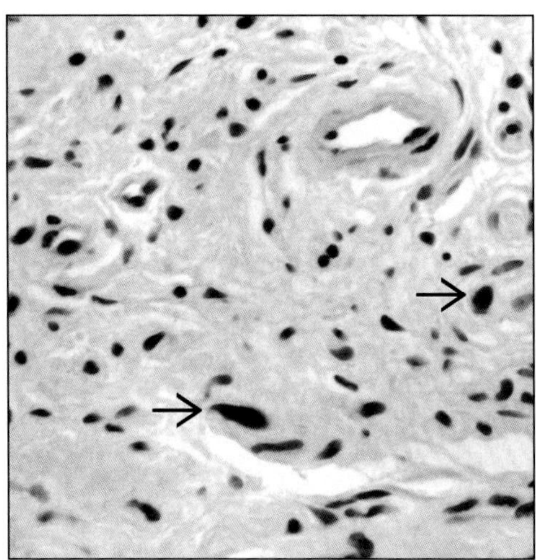

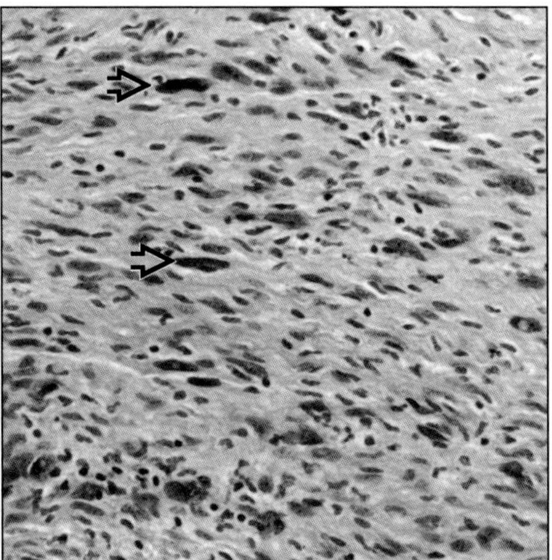

Ancillary Techniques

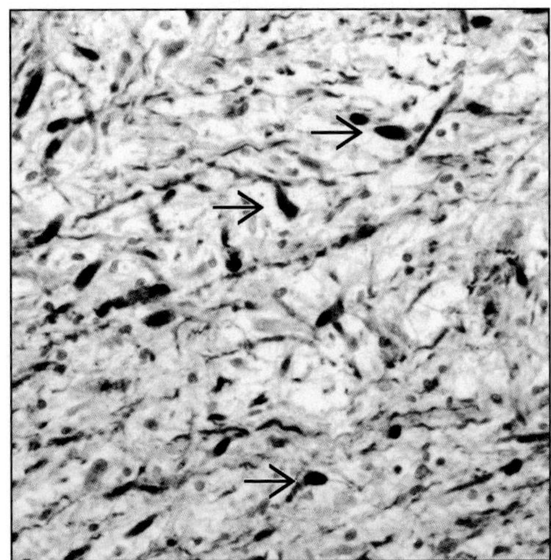

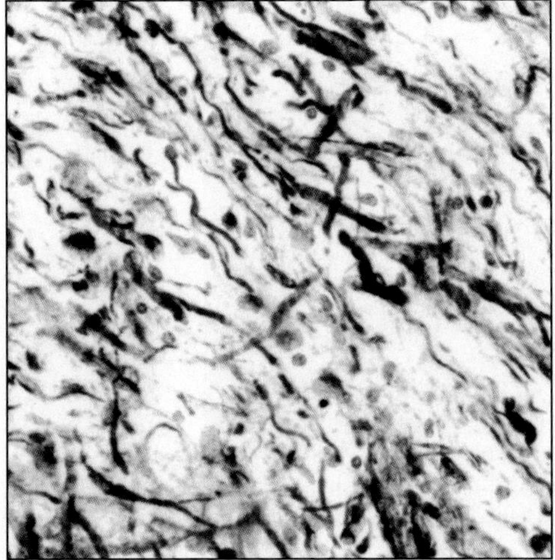

(Left) *High-power view of immunohistochemical staining with antibodies against the S100 protein shows that only the ovoid Schwann cells are positive, highlighting their cell processes ➔. In contrast to schwannoma, there are many tumor cells that are not staining.* ***(Right)*** *High-power view of immunohistochemical staining with antibodies against vimentin shows strong positivity in fibroblasts.*

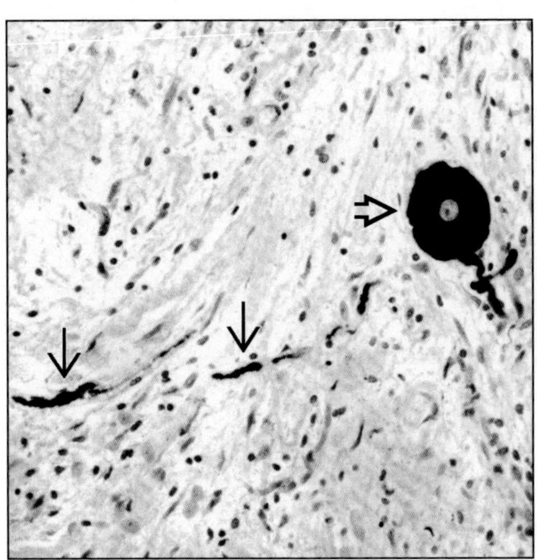

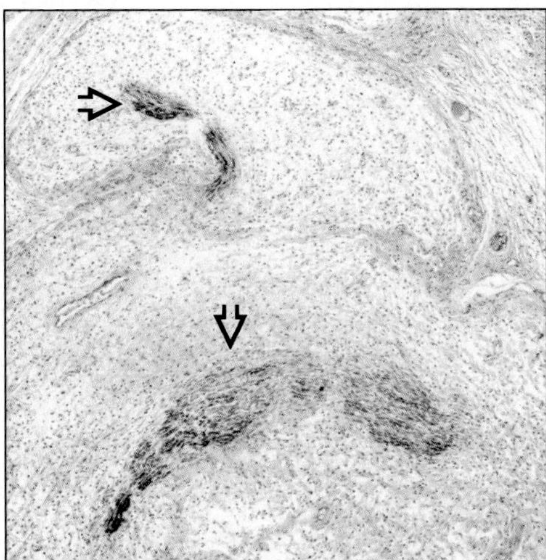

(Left) *High-power view of immunohistochemical staining with antibodies against neurofilament protein highlights cell bodies ➲ of residual ganglion cells and their axonal processes ➔.* ***(Right)*** *High-power view of immunohistochemical staining with antibodies against neurofilament protein shows the centrally located fibers ➲ of residual nerves in a plexiform NF.*

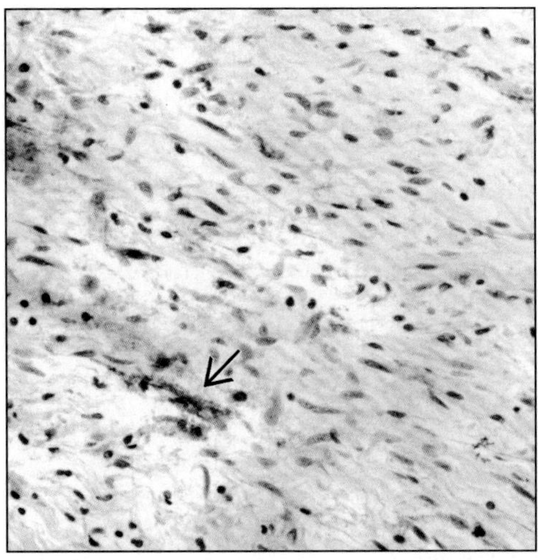

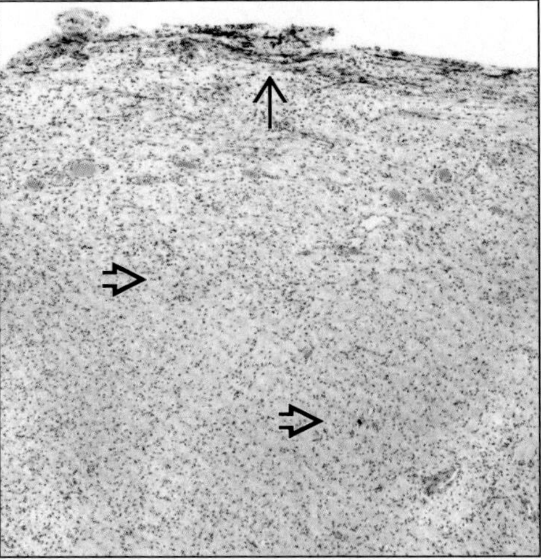

(Left) *High-power view of immunohistochemical staining with antibodies against EMA/MUC1 shows scattered positivity in perineurial-like cells ➔.* ***(Right)*** *Medium-power view of immunohistochemical staining with antibodies against EMA shows the epineurium ➔ still enveloping a localized intraneural NF, manifested by well-circumscribed fusiform nerve enlargement ➲.*

SCHWANNOMA

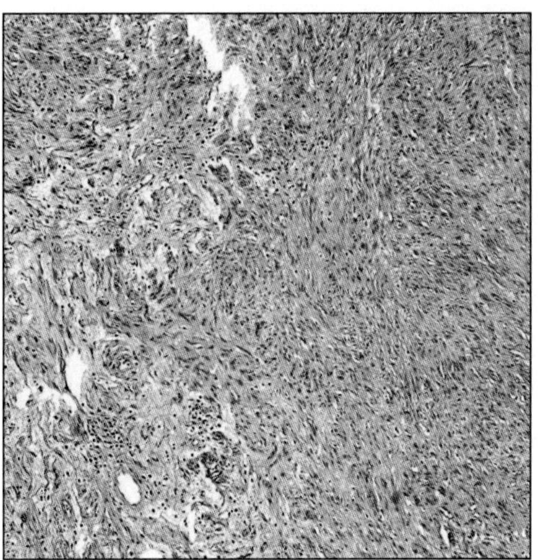

Hematoxylin & eosin at low power shows the more cellular Antoni A (right) and less cellular Antoni B (left) areas of a typical schwannoma.

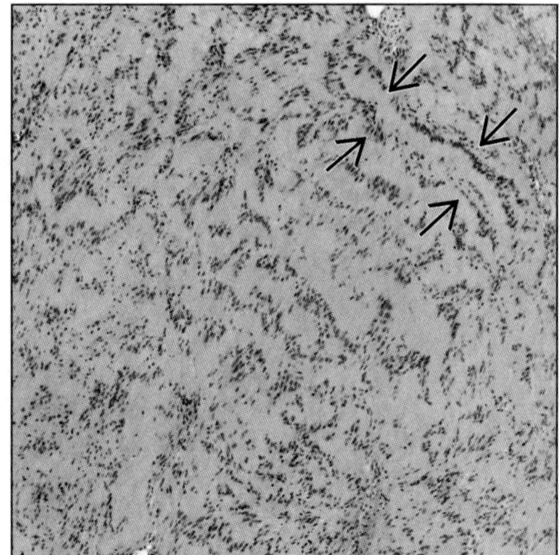

Hematoxylin & eosin at low power shows numerous Verocay bodies ⇒ within an Antoni A area of a typical schwannoma. Verocay bodies can be quite variable in number from case to case.

TERMINOLOGY

Synonyms

- Neurilemoma

Definitions

- Encapsulated nerve sheath tumor consisting of cellular component and loose myxoid component
  - Stains intensely with S100 protein

CLINICAL ISSUES

Presentation

- Occurs in all ages
  - Most common between 20-50 years
- Slowly growing
- Pain unusual unless large
- Common locations
  - Head and neck
    - Schwannoma of 8th cranial nerve termed **acoustic neuroma**
  - Flexor surfaces of extremities
  - Posterior mediastinum
  - Retroperitoneum
- 90% sporadic, 3% with NF2, 2% with schwannomatosis, 5% with multiple meningiomas
  - Neurofibromatosis type 2
    - Autosomal dominant disease
    - Bilateral vestibular schwannomas
    - Patients also get meningiomas, ependymomas, gliomas
  - Schwannomatosis
    - Autosomal dominant with reduced penetrance
    - Not associated with NF1 or NF2
    - Multiple, painful schwannomas

Treatment

- Simple excision

Prognosis

- Benign
- Very rare malignant transformation

MACROSCOPIC FEATURES

General Features

- Encapsulated
- Small tumors may be fusiform and obliterate nerve of origin
- Large tumors are eccentric masses that splay nerve fibers

Size

- Usually < 5 cm
- Mediastinal and retroperitoneal tumors may be quite large

Cut Surface

- Pink, white, or yellow
- Large tumors may show cystic degeneration or calcification

MICROSCOPIC PATHOLOGY

Histologic Features

- Alternating Antoni A and Antoni B areas
  - Relative amounts of 2 components varies
- Antoni A
  - Compact spindle cells in short bundles
  - May have nuclear palisading, Verocay bodies, or whorls
- Antoni B
  - Spindle or oval cells haphazardly arranged in myxoid matrix
  - Microcystic change, inflammatory cells, delicate collagen are common
  - Large irregular vessels

Key Facts

Terminology
- Encapsulated nerve sheath tumor consisting of cellular component and loose myxoid component

Clinical Issues
- Most common between 20-50 years
- Benign
- 90% sporadic, 3% with NF2, 2% with schwannomatosis, 5% with multiple meningiomas
- Very rare malignant transformation

Macroscopic Features
- Encapsulated
- Usually < 5 cm, although mediastinal and retroperitoneal tumors may be quite large

Microscopic Pathology
- Alternating Antoni A and Antoni B areas
  - Antoni A (cellular)
  - Antoni B (loose, myxoid)
- Subtypes include
  - Ancient schwannoma
  - Cellular schwannoma
  - Plexiform schwannoma
  - Epithelioid schwannoma

Ancillary Tests
- Strongly S100 positive

Top Differential Diagnoses
- Neurofibroma
- Well-differentiated leiomyosarcoma
- Malignant peripheral nerve sheath tumor

Predominant Pattern/Injury Type
- Biphasic
  - Antoni A (cellular)
  - Antoni B (loose, myxoid)

Predominant Cell/Compartment Type
- Spindle

Subtypes
- Ancient schwannoma
  - Large tumors, usually deep
  - Degenerative changes
    - Marked nuclear atypia without mitoses, cyst formation, hemorrhage, hyalinization
- Cellular schwannoma
  - Usually retroperitoneum or posterior mediastinum
  - Predominantly Antoni A areas without Verocay bodies; may have long, sweeping fascicles
  - < 4 mitoses per 10 HPF
  - May have focal necrosis
- Plexiform schwannoma
  - Rare; usually in skin, rarely deep
  - Plexiform or nodular pattern
  - More cellular, as in cellular schwannomas
- Epithelioid schwannoma
  - Rare
  - Small rounded Schwann cells arranged singly, in small aggregates or cords
  - Collagenous or myxoid stroma
  - Areas of conventional schwannoma may be present
  - Occasional atypical cells without mitoses

Psammomatous Melanotic Schwannoma
- Although similarly named, generally **not** considered subtype of schwannoma
- Associated with Carney complex
  - Myxomas, spotty pigmentation, and endocrine overactivity
- Often multiple tumors
- Usually seen in adults
- Microscopic features
  - Heavily pigmented
  - Spindled to polygonal cells that can form syncytia
  - Vague palisading or whorling may be seen
  - Psammoma bodies usually present but may need extensive sampling
  - S100 and HMB-45 positive

ANCILLARY TESTS

Immunohistochemistry
- All types are strongly S100(+)

DIFFERENTIAL DIAGNOSIS

Neurofibroma
- Has less intense S100 staining than schwannoma
- Usually has myxoid background
- Unencapsulated

Well-differentiated Leiomyosarcoma
- Only rarely shows S100 staining
- Positive for smooth muscle markers

Malignant Peripheral Nerve Sheath Tumor
- Increased mitotic rate
- Only focal and limited S100 staining
- Can be difficult to differentiate from cellular schwannoma

Fibroblastic Meningioma
- Meningioma will be EMA(+)

SELECTED REFERENCES

1. MacCollin M et al: Diagnostic criteria for schwannomatosis. Neurology. 64(11):1838-45, 2005
2. Wilkes D et al: Clinical phenotypes and molecular genetic mechanisms of Carney complex. Lancet Oncol. 6(7):501-8, 2005
3. Kurtkaya-Yapicier O et al: The pathobiologic spectrum of Schwannomas. Histol Histopathol. 18(3):925-34, 2003
4. Uppal S et al: Neurofibromatosis type 2. Int J Clin Pract. 57(8):698-703, 2003

SCHWANNOMA

Microscopic Features

(Left) Hematoxylin & eosin shows the thick capsule ⇒ that is characteristic of schwannoma. ***(Right)*** Hematoxylin & eosin shows Verocay bodies ⇒ in an Antoni A area. Verocay bodies are made up of palisading cells separated by a hypocellular hyalinized area in between.

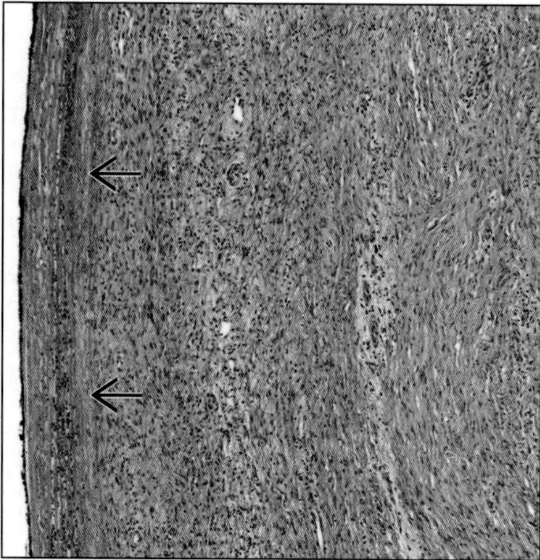

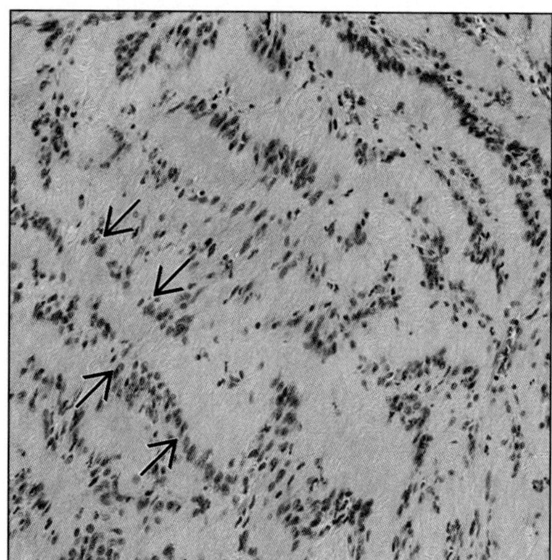

(Left) Hematoxylin & eosin shows a cellular Antoni A area with a prominent, hyalinized vessel ⇒. This type of hyalinized vessel is commonly seen in schwannoma. ***(Right)*** Hematoxylin & eosin shows spindled cells in a loose, myxoid pattern (Antoni B area) with prominent, hyalinized vessels ⇒.

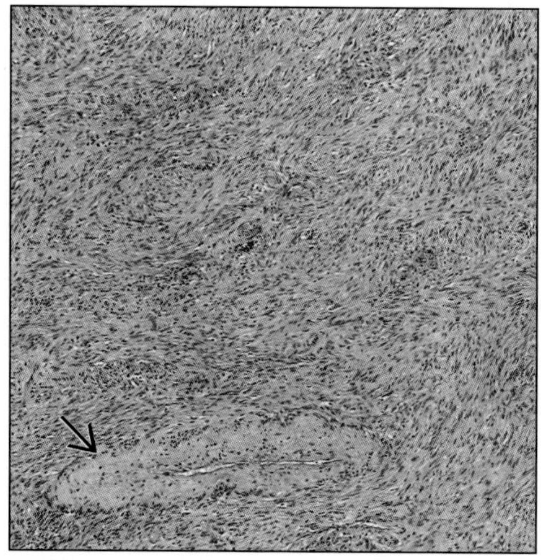

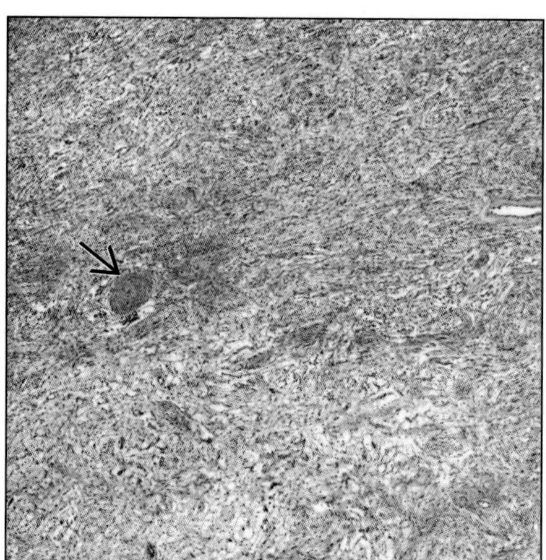

(Left) Hematoxylin & eosin shows a medium-power view of an Antoni B area with hyalinized vessels ⇒. ***(Right)*** Hematoxylin & eosin shows a high-power view of an Antoni B area with spindled, wavy cells in a myxoid background.

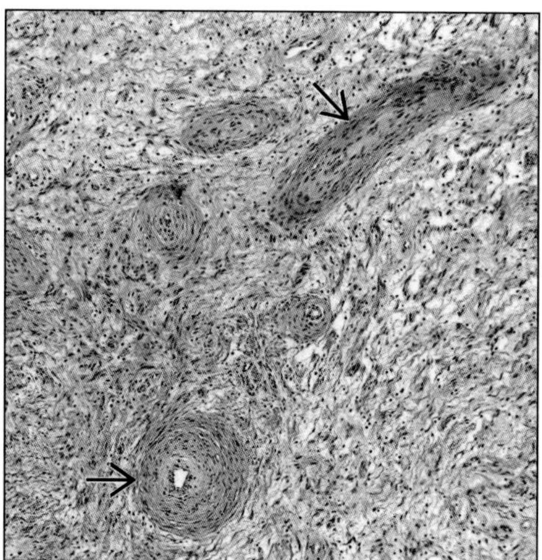

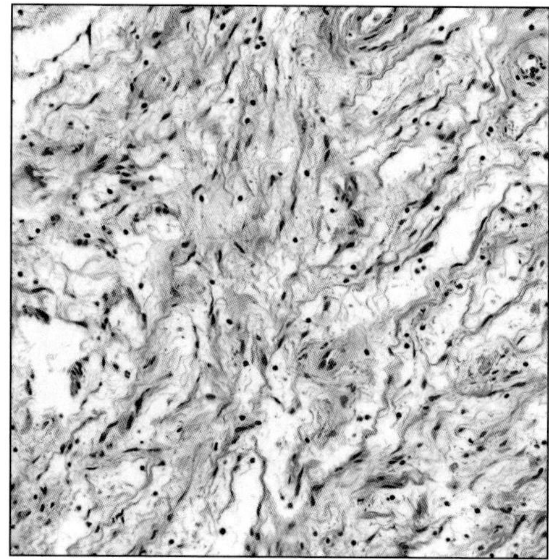

Microscopic Features and Ancillary Techniques

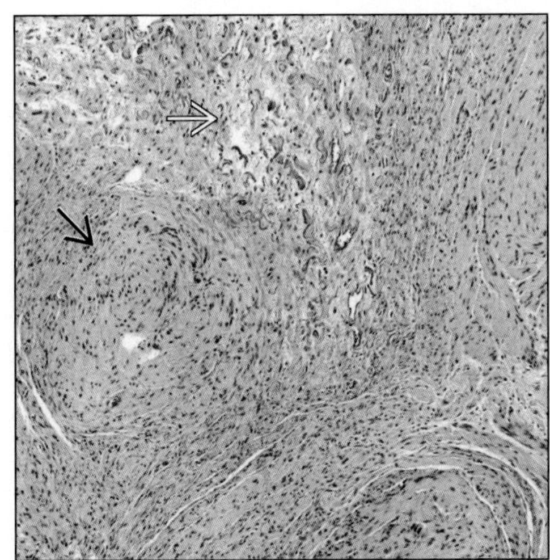

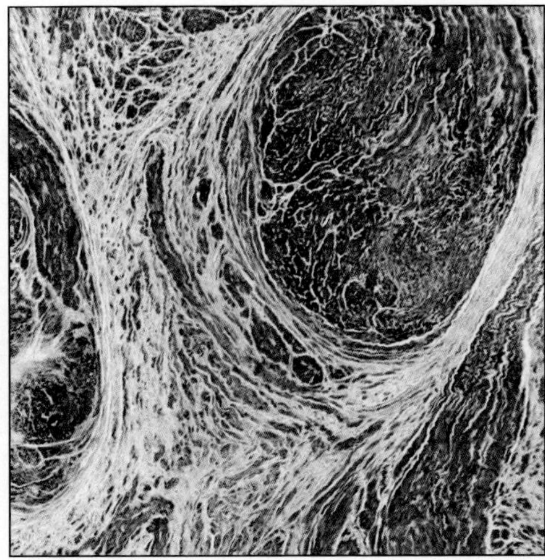

(Left) *Hematoxylin & eosin shows cellular areas of spindle cells (Antoni A)* ⇨ *in a nodular or plexiform growth pattern, with intervening loose, myxoid stroma (Antoni B)* ➡. *This is typical of a plexiform schwannoma.* ***(Right)*** *Positive S100 shows strong cytoplasmic staining in all subtypes of schwannoma.*

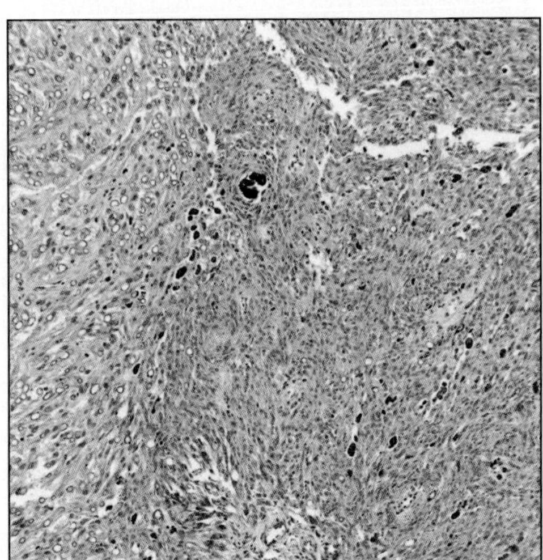

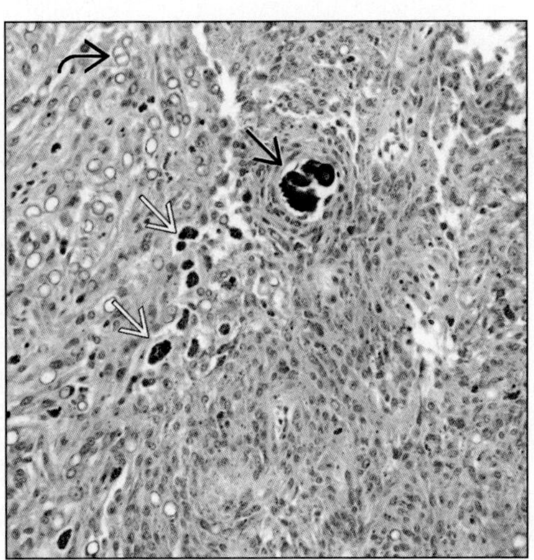

(Left) *Hematoxylin & eosin shows a psammomatous melanotic schwannoma. A cellular, Antoni A-type area is seen on the right, and a more loose, Antoni B-type area is seen on the left.* ***(Right)*** *Hematoxylin & eosin shows a higher power view of a psammomatous melanotic schwannoma. Characteristic clear pseudonuclear inclusions* ↪ *are seen in the loose Antoni B areas, as well as a psammoma body* ⇨, *and cells containing melanin pigment* ➡.

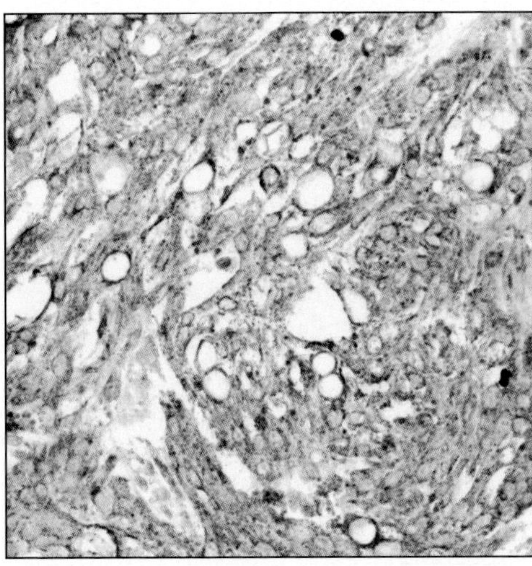

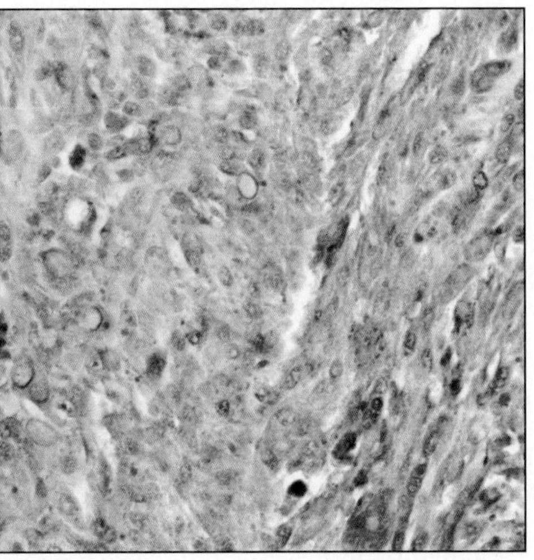

(Left) *HMB-45 shows strong cytoplasmic staining in this psammomatous melanotic schwannoma.* ***(Right)*** *S100 shows strong staining in this psammomatous melanotic schwannoma, similar to that typical of all schwannoma subtypes.*

NEUROTHEKEOMA

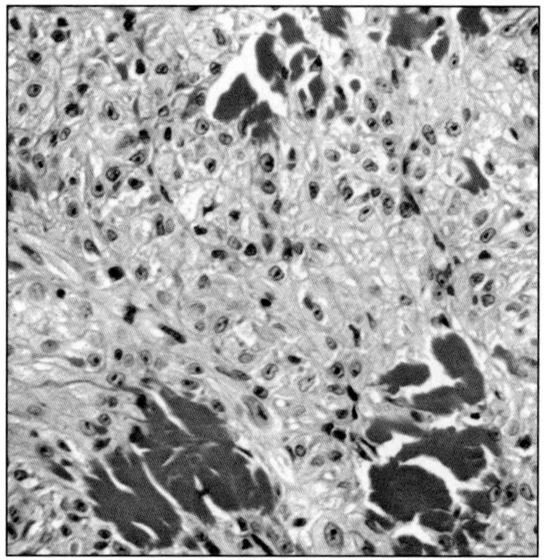

High-power view of cellular NTK is shown with compact nests and organoid fascicles of plump epithelioid and vaguely nevoid tumor cells with no myxoid matrix.

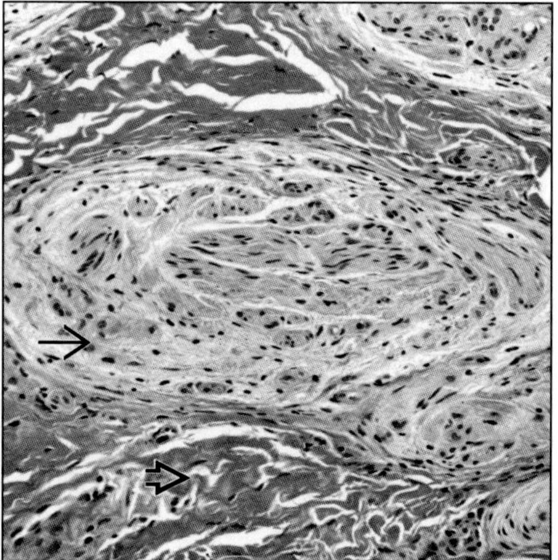

High-power view shows perineural appearance in NSM: Plexiform, concentric growth in a fibromyxoid stroma ➡, surrounded by dense collagen bands ⇨.

TERMINOLOGY

Abbreviations

- Neurothekeoma (NTK)
- Nerve sheath myxoma (NSM)

Synonyms

- NTK: Cellular NTK, classic (cutaneous) NTK
- NSM: Dermal NSM, cutaneous lobular neuromyxoma
- Pacinian or bizarre cutaneous neurofibroma

Definitions

- Heterogeneous group of benign tumors of putative peripheral nerve sheath origin with predilection for superficial dermis of head, neck, and extremities

ETIOLOGY/PATHOGENESIS

Differentiation and Histogenesis

- Varying morphologic patterns may encompass many separate entities historically termed "neurothekeoma"
- Mixed tumors, similar features suggest continuum
- Divergent differentiation suggests distinct entities

Nerve Sheath Myxoma

- Described as myxoid/hypocellular NTK, mature NSM
  - Many do not support grouping with neurothekeoma
- Histologically predominantly myxoid pattern
- Schwannian or perineural differentiation
  - Usually diffusely positive for S100 &/or GFAP
  - Limited reactivity for EMA/MUC1, collagen type IV, CD57
  - Usually negative for NK1/C3, actin-sm

(Cellular) Neurothekeoma

- Described as mixed/intermediate NTK, immature NSM
  - Nerve sheath differentiation has not been shown
- Histologically predominantly cellular pattern
- More primitive (myo)fibroblast-like morphology
  - Positive for PGP9.5, FXIIIA, CD63, NSE
  - Negative or only weakly reactive for S100, EMA/MUC1
  - May be actin-sm positive (not desmin)

CLINICAL ISSUES

Epidemiology

- Incidence
  - Rare tumors, a few hundred cases reported
- Age
  - NTK: Peak in 2nd or 3rd decade (mean: 22-24 years)
    - ~ 25% seen in children/infants (< 10 years old)
  - NSM: Peak in 4th decade (mean: 36-38 years)
- Gender
  - NTK: M < F (1:2); NSM: M = F

Site

- Superficial and mid dermis; rarely deeper soft tissue
- NTK: Face, scalp, upper extremities (shoulders, arms)
  - Intracranial, intraspinal, oral cavity cases reported
- NSM: Predilection for extremities (fingers, knees)

Presentation

- Solitary, slow growing, painless swelling

Treatment

- Simple, complete surgical excision

Prognosis

- Benign: No metastases or aggressive local growth
- Recurrences rare (< 3%); due to incomplete removal
- Atypical features described in ~ 10% of NTK
  - Size > 2 cm, growth into fat or muscle, infiltrating margins, vascular invasion, > 5 mitoses/HPF, atypia
  - Still, no adverse outcome (metastases, recurrence)

MACROSCOPIC FEATURES

General Features

- Dome-shaped papules or nodules

NEUROTHEKEOMA

Key Facts

Terminology
- Heterogeneous, benign tumors of superficial dermis

Clinical Issues
- NTK: M < F (1:2), mean: 22-24 years (25% children)
- NSM: M = F, mean: 36-38 years
- NTK: Face, scalp, upper extremities (shoulders, arms)
- NSM: Predilection for extremities (fingers, knees)
- Solitary, slow growing, painless swelling
- Benign: No metastases or aggressive local growth
- Recurrences rare (< 3%); due to incomplete removal

Microscopic Pathology
- Myxoid pattern (NSM)
  - Plexiform arrangement, prominent myxoid matrix
  - Broadly separated cells, whorl around vessels
  - Schwannian/perineural: S100, GFAP positive
- Cellular pattern (NTK)
  - Compact nests of epithelioid, vaguely nevoid cells
  - Myofibroblast-like; smooth muscle actin positive
  - PGP9.5, CD63 positive; S100 negative

Top Differential Diagnoses
- Plexiform fibrous histiocytoma
  - Biphasic, many giant cells, scant myxoid matrix
- Dermal Spitz nevus, malignant melanoma
  - Junctional component, S100/HMB-45 positive

Diagnostic Checklist
- Some studies: High recurrence rates for NSM (~ 50%)
- Lack epidermal or junctional component
- "Grenz zone" (sparing) between tumor and epidermis
- Mixed: Heterogeneous myxoid and cellular areas
  - Difficult to categorize; ~ 10% of NTK are myxoid

- Nonpigmented or tan-red, sometimes translucent
- Variably firm, rarely ulcerated, frequently myxoid

Size
- 0.3-6.0 cm in diameter (90% < 2 cm)

MICROSCOPIC PATHOLOGY

Myxoid Pattern (NSM)
- Micronodular, multilobular expansile mass in dermis
  - Distinct plexiform, compartmentalized arrangement
  - Separated by thin bands of dense fibrous tissue
- Prominent myxoid or fibromyxoid stroma (matrix)
  - Rich in hyaluronic acid, mucopolysaccharides
- Loose, broadly separated, syncytial-like aggregates
  - Bland spindle, stellate, or fusiform cells
  - Small, angulated nuclei, inconspicuous nucleoli
  - Pale cytoplasm with fibrillary extensions
  - Resemble perineurial cells (whorl around vessels)
- Inconspicuous nuclear atypia and mitotic figures
- Lymphoid aggregates, multinucleated giant cells seen

Cellular Pattern (NTK) (Histiocytic or Epithelioid)
- Organoid fascicles and compact nests in dermis
  - Less concentric than NSM; like melanocytic thekes
  - May have dense, sheet-like growth, solid aggregates
- May have poorly defined margins, dissecting growth
- Closely spaced, epithelioid, vaguely nevoid cells
  - Plump, polygonal, or bluntly fusiform spindle cells
  - Appear histiocytic (plenty eosinophilic cytoplasm)
- Many have mild to moderate cytologic atypia
  - Polymorphic, hyperchromatic nuclei, many mitoses

DIFFERENTIAL DIAGNOSIS

Plexiform Fibrous Histiocytoma
- Biphasic, many giant cells, scant myxoid matrix
- More aggressive: Recur, metastasize

Dermal Spitz Nevus or Malignant Melanoma
- Junctional component, S100/HMB-45(+)

Epithelioid Cutaneous (Pilar) Leiomyoma
- Elongated nuclei, eosinophilic cells, desmin(+)

Superficial (Cutaneous) (Angio) Myxoma
- Pleomorphic cells, smudgy chromatin, CD34(+)

Myxoid Schwannoma
- Nuclear palisading, Verocay bodies
- Possibly related to NSM

DIAGNOSTIC CHECKLIST

Clinically Relevant Pathologic Features
- Not associated with neurofibromatosis
- Some studies: High recurrence rates for NSM (~ 50%)
  - Margin of normal tissue advised during excision

Pathologic Interpretation Pearls
- Axons not a usual component of any variant
- Lack epidermal or junctional component
- "Grenz zone" of sparing between tumor and epidermis
- Best to separately diagnose NTK vs. NSM
- Mixed/intermediate histologic pattern
  - Heterogeneous: Myxoid and highly cellular areas
  - ~ 10% of NTK may have diffusely myxoid stroma
    - Difficult to categorize, overlap with NSM
  - Integrate clinicopathologic data, immunophenotype
- "Myxoid neurothekeoma"
  - Used to describe both NSM, myxoid variant of NTK
  - Unclear whether separate, distinguishable entities

SELECTED REFERENCES

1. Fetsch JF et al: Neurothekeoma: an analysis of 178 tumors with detailed immunohistochemical data and long-term patient follow-up information. Am J Surg Pathol. 31(7):1103-14, 2007
2. Hornick JL et al: Cellular neurothekeoma: detailed characterization in a series of 133 cases. Am J Surg Pathol. 31(3):329-40, 2007

Microscopic Features of Cellular Neurothekeoma

*(**Left**) Low-power view shows cellular NTK located in the shoulder. The tumor occupies the deep dermis and has poorly defined margins, deeply infiltrating into the underlying skeletal muscle →. (**Right**) High-power view of cellular NTK shows closely spaced, epithelioid tumor cells with moderate cytologic atypia and pleomorphic, slightly hyperchromatic nuclei ⇨. Mitotic figures → are easily found.*

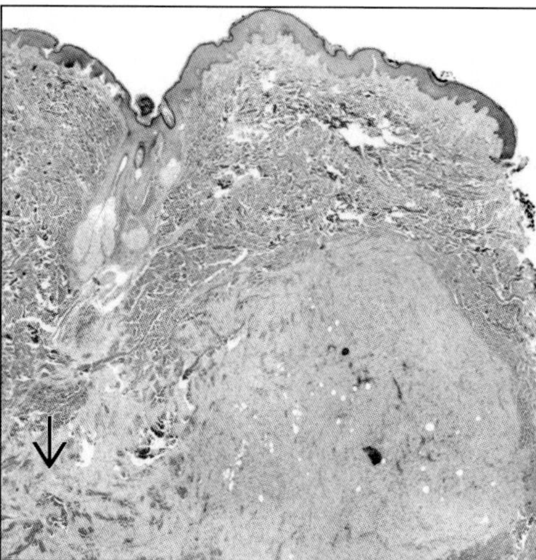

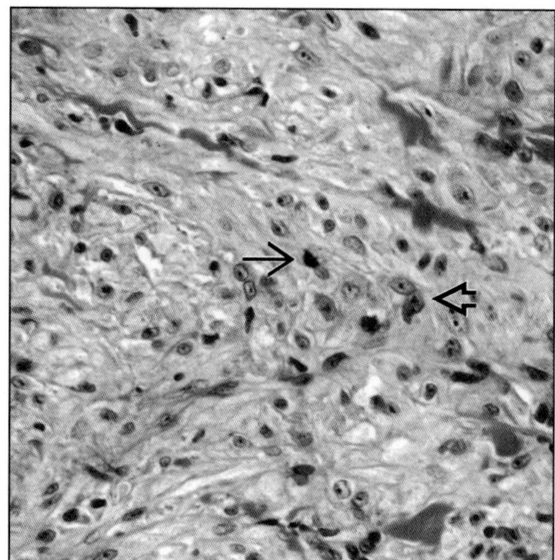

*(**Left**) High-power view of cellular NTK is shown immunohistochemically stained with antibodies against PGP9.5 protein. Tumor cells are diffusely and strongly positive, supporting the diagnosis of NTK. (**Right**) High-power view of cellular NTK is immunohistochemically stained with antibodies against smooth muscle actin. Tumor cells are focally positive →, supporting the diagnosis of NTK.*

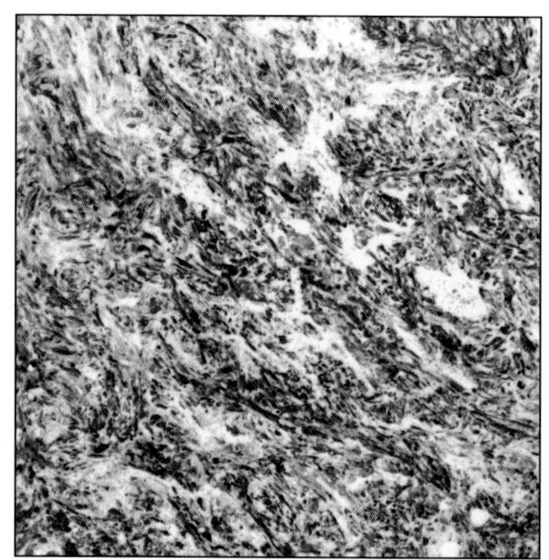

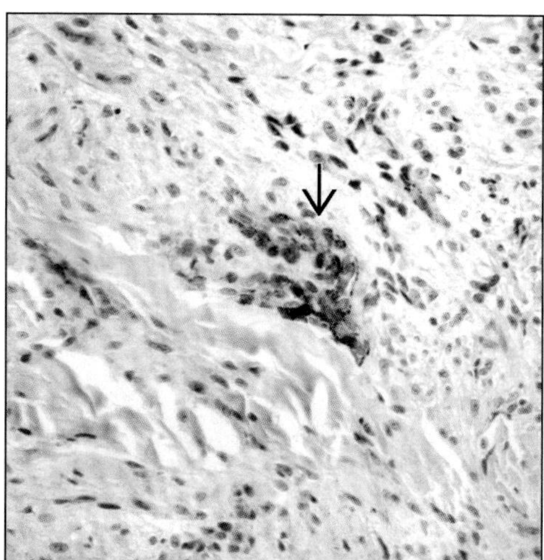

*(**Left**) High-power view shows a lesion from the upper lip. Tumor cells form vague nodules ⇨, surrounded by dense fibrous bands →, in this cellular NTK with extensive secondary fibrosis. (**Right**) High-power view of cellular NTK is immunohistochemically stained with antibodies against PGP9.5 protein. Tumor cells are focally positive →, supporting the diagnosis of NTK.*

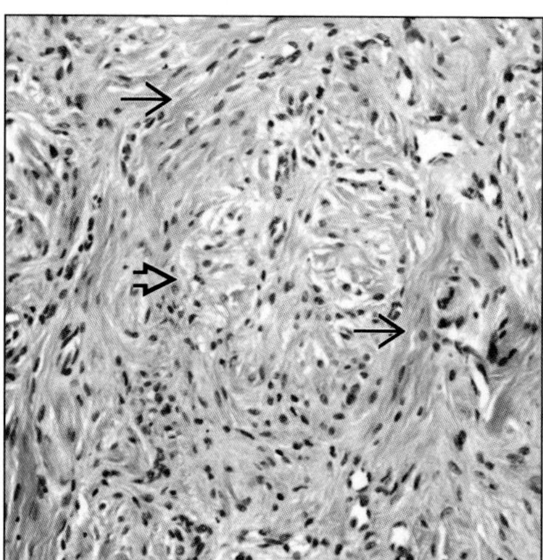

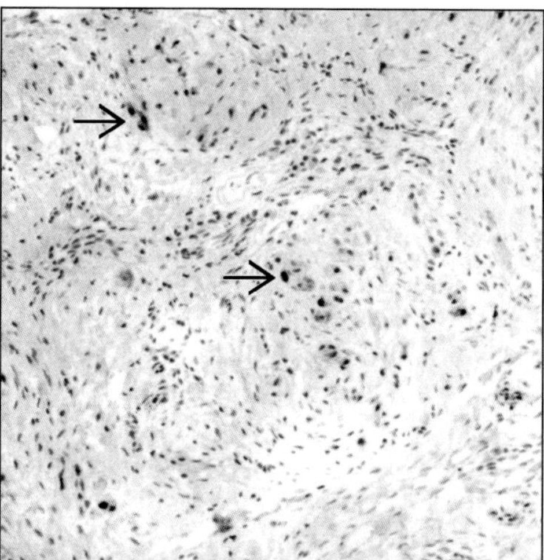

Microscopic Features of Nerve Sheath Myxoma

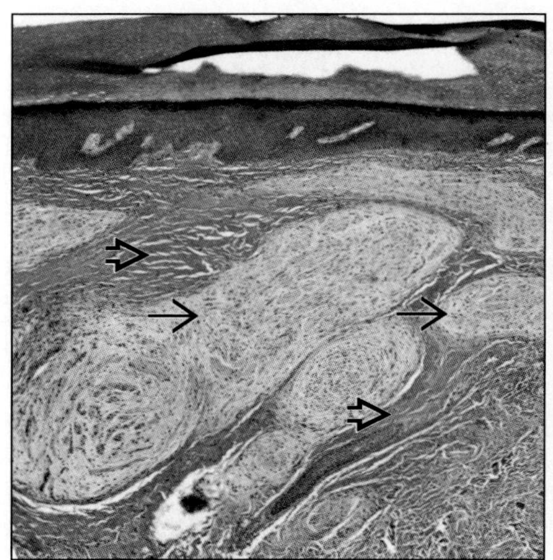

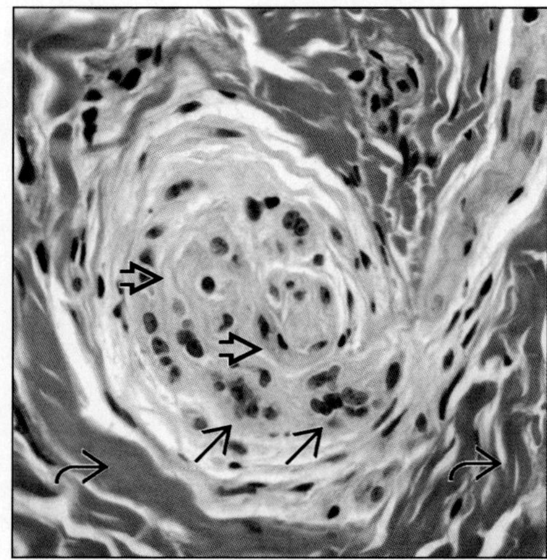

(Left) *Low-power view of NSM is seen located on the finger. Located in the superficial dermis with no epidermal component, the tumor has a multinodular appearance with lobules ➔ separated by bands of dense fibrous tissue ➲.* ***(Right)*** *High-power view of NSM is shown with syncytial-like aggregates ➔ of bland fusiform to spindle cells that resemble perineurial cells with fibrillary cytoplasmic extensions forming whorls ➲. Note the surrounding dense fibrous tissue ↗.*

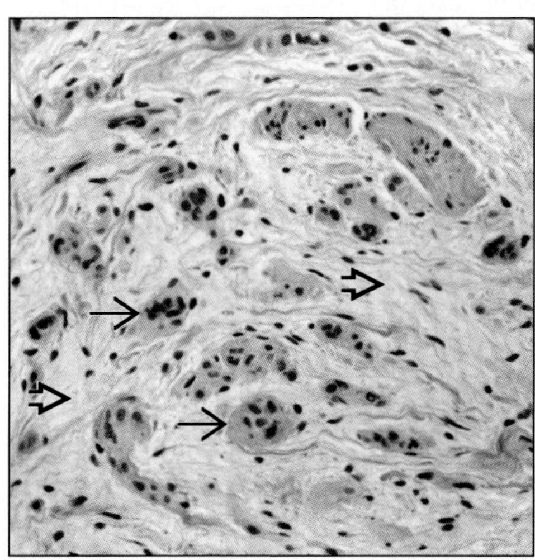

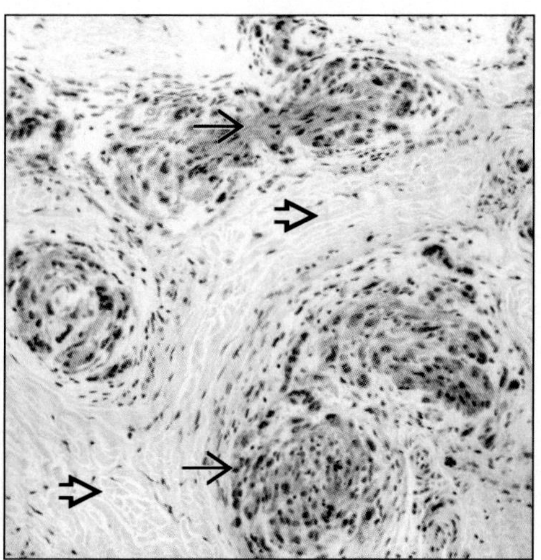

(Left) *High-power view of NSM shows nests of multinucleated giant cells ➔ amidst abundant hypocellular myxoid stroma ➲.* ***(Right)*** *High-power view shows NSM immunohistochemically stained with antibodies against S100 protein. The lobules of tumor cells are positive ➔, while the myxoid matrix is negative ➲.*

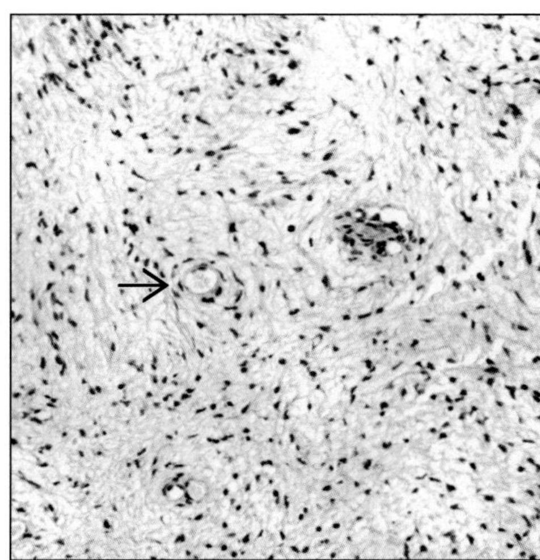

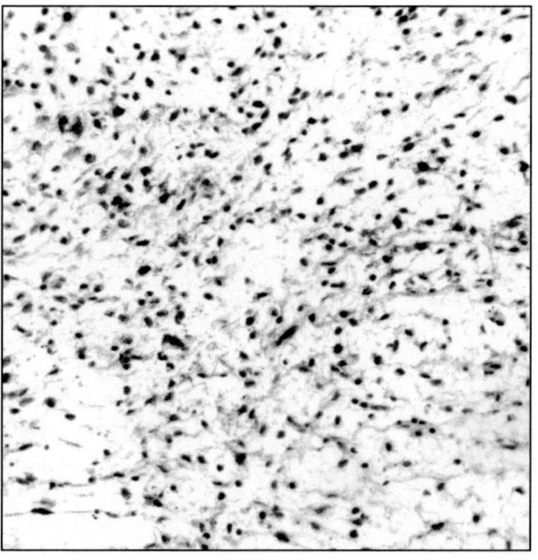

(Left) *High-power view shows a highly myxoid NSM with tumor cells having a more stellate appearance but still forming whorls around vessels ➔. The differential diagnosis with myxoid schwannoma is difficult, but this NSM lacks highly cellular (Antoni A) areas or nuclear palisading (Verocay bodies).* ***(Right)*** *High-power view shows NSM immunohistochemically stained with antibodies against EMA protein. Focal scattered positivity confirms this lesion is a NSM rather than a myxoid schwannoma.*

MELANOTIC NEUROECTODERMAL TUMOR OF INFANCY

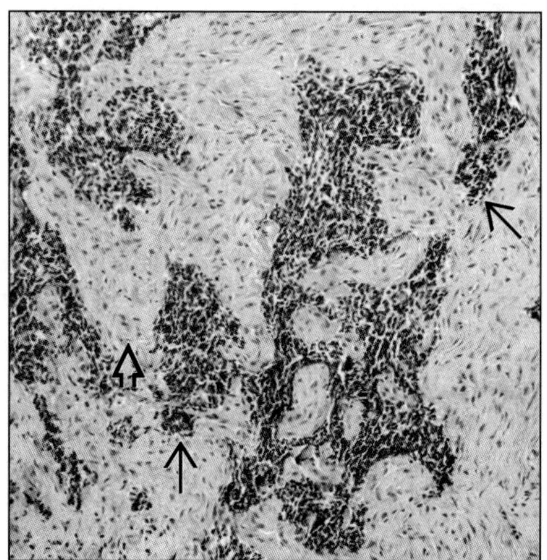

The neuroblastic small cells ➔ separated by a fibrocollagenous stroma ➲ demonstrate an alveolar pattern of growth in this MNTI.

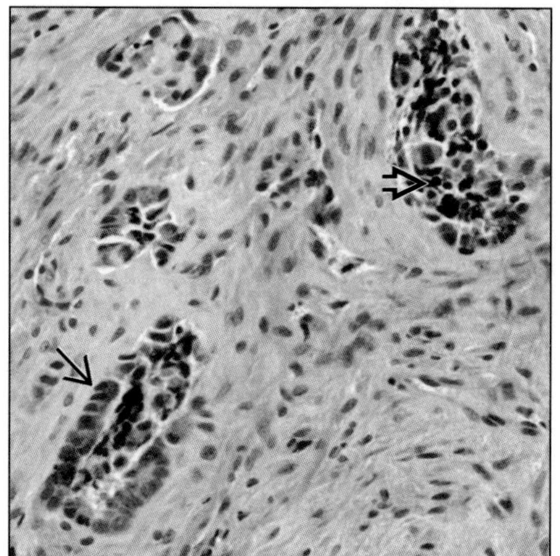

Epithelial cells with abundant eosinophilic cytoplasm and melanin pigment ➔ form glandular structures with scattered small neuroblastic cells ➲ in this MNTI.

TERMINOLOGY

Abbreviations

- Melanotic neuroectodermal tumor of infancy (MNTI)

Synonyms

- Retinal anlage tumor
- Melanotic progonoma
- Melanotic ameloblastoma

Definitions

- Rare, fast-growing, pigmented neoplasm of likely neural crest origin

ETIOLOGY/PATHOGENESIS

Disputed Histogenesis

- Current studies support neural crest (neuroectodermal) origin

CLINICAL ISSUES

Epidemiology

- Age
  - Most present in 1st year of life (> 90%)

Site

- Most involve craniofacial sites
  - Upper and lower jaw
    - Maxilla: 69%
    - Mandible: 6%
  - Skull: 11%
- Unusual sites
  - Epididymis, mediastinum, brain, shoulder, and skin

Presentation

- Rapidly enlarging, firm, expansile mass
- Erosion into adjacent bone
- Nontender
- Intact overlying mucosa
- Bluish discoloration

Laboratory Tests

- Elevated urinary vanillylmandelic acid may be present

Treatment

- Complete local excision
  - Local recurrence rate: 10-15%
  - Usually recurs in 1st postoperative year

Prognosis

- Benign to intermediate clinical course
  - Recurrence rate: 10-15%
  - Metastatic spread in < 5%

IMAGE FINDINGS

General Features

- Well-demarcated radiolucent lesion
- Capacity for local destruction

MACROSCOPIC FEATURES

Gross Features

- Firm
- Well circumscribed
- Gray to blue-black cut surface

MICROSCOPIC PATHOLOGY

Predominant Pattern/Injury Type

- Glandular/alveolar
  - Spaces lined by cuboidal pigmented epithelial cells
  - Small neuroblastic cells found within spaces
- Solid
  - Background of fibrocollagenous stroma

Key Facts

Terminology
- Rare, fast-growing, pigmented neoplasm of likely neural crest origin

Clinical Issues
- Most present in 1st year of life
- Commonly involve craniofacial sites
  - Maxilla: 69%
- Rapidly enlarging expansile mass
- Elevated urinary vanillylmandelic acid may be present

Microscopic Pathology
- 3 distinct components
  - Clusters of small round neuroblastic cells
  - Primitive gland-like structures
  - Fibrocollagenous stroma

Top Differential Diagnoses
- Neuroblastoma
  - Sheets and lobules of small round hyperchromatic cells
- Alveolar rhabdomyosarcoma
  - Aggregates and nests of poorly differentiated small hyperchromatic cells
  - Characteristic immunohistochemical and cytogenetic findings
- Primitive neuroectodermal tumor
  - Sheets of small-medium round blue cells
  - Characteristic t(11;22)
- Congenital epulis
  - Characteristic location in labial aspect of dental ridge
  - Protruding round or ovoid nodule

Immunohistochemistry

Antibody	Reactivity	Staining Pattern	Comment
AE1/AE3	Positive	Cell membrane & cytoplasm	Epithelial cells
HMB-45	Positive	Cytoplasmic	Epithelial cells
NSE	Positive	Cytoplasmic	Frequently expressed by neuroblastic cells and epithelial cells
Synaptophysin	Positive	Cytoplasmic	Neuroblastic cells and variably expressed in epithelial cells
CD57	Positive	Cell membrane & cytoplasm	Neuroblastic cells and epithelial cells

Predominant Cell/Compartment Type
- Dual population of cells
  - Flat to cuboidal pigmented epithelial cells
  - Small neuroblastic cells
  - Fibrocollagenous stroma

Microscopic Features
- 3 distinct components
  - Primitive gland-like structures
    - Larger cells with round vesicular nuclei
    - Abundant cytoplasm with melanin granules
    - Alveolar or glandular arrangements
    - May contain neuroblastic cells within gland space
  - Clusters of small round neuroblastic cells
    - Small round hyperchromatic nuclei
    - Scant cytoplasm
    - Arranged in small islands and cords
    - Crush artifact frequently encountered
    - May be found independent from gland-like structures
  - Fibrocollagenous stroma

DIFFERENTIAL DIAGNOSIS

Neuroblastoma
- Predominantly located in retroperitoneum
- Sheets and lobules of small round hyperchromatic cells
- Homer Wright rosettes

Alveolar Rhabdomyosarcoma
- More commonly located in extremities
- Aggregates and nests of poorly differentiated small hyperchromatic cells
- Separated by fibrous septae
- Characteristic immunohistochemical and cytogenetic findings

Primitive Neuroectodermal Tumor
- Sheets of small-medium round blue cells
- Frequent mitoses and foci of necrosis
- Characteristic t(11;22)

Congenital Epulis
- Characteristic location in labial aspect of dental ridge
- Protruding round or ovoid nodule
- Microscopically resembles adult granular cell tumor
  - Polygonal cells with abundant eosinophilic cytoplasm
  - Lack pseudoepitheliomatous hyperplasia

SELECTED REFERENCES

1. Chaudhary A et al: Melanotic neuroectodermal tumor of infancy: 2 decades of clinical experience with 18 patients. J Oral Maxillofac Surg. 67(1):47-51, 2009
2. Selim H et al: Melanotic neuroectodermal tumor of infancy: review of literature and case report. J Pediatr Surg. 43(6):E25-9, 2008
3. George JC et al: Melanotic neuroectodermal tumor of infancy. AJNR Am J Neuroradiol. 16(6):1273-5, 1995
4. Borello ED et al: Melanotic neuroectodermal tumor of infancy--a neoplasm of neural crese origin. Report of a case associated with high urinary excretion of vanilmandelic acid. Cancer. 19(2):196-206, 1966

MELANOTIC NEUROECTODERMAL TUMOR OF INFANCY

Clinical, Radiologic, and Microscopic Features

*(**Left**) Clinical photograph shows a huge mass extending toward parietal squama superiorly ➔ and in upper neck inferiorly ↷ behind displaced left ear ⇨. The overlying skin looks normal. (**Right**) Axial bone CT shows the most common appearance, location, and age for melanotic neuroectodermal tumor: Maxillary expansion with osteolysis ➔ and adjacent soft tissue changes ↷ in an infant.*

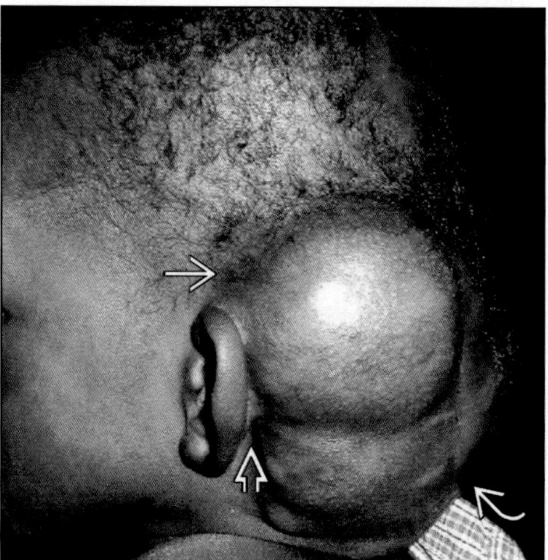

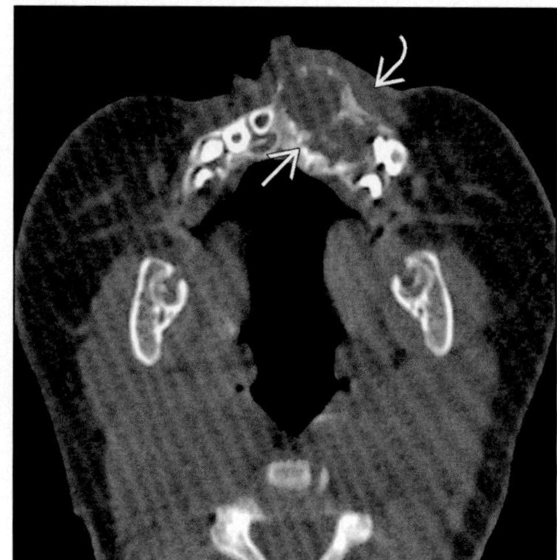

*(**Left**) Pigmented epithelial cells ➔ with focal small neuroblastic cells in a dense fibrous stroma are shown infiltrating the bony trabeculae. (**Right**) Higher power view shows a MNTI infiltrating bone. Note the small scattered pigmented epithelial cells, some of which show glandular formations ⇨.*

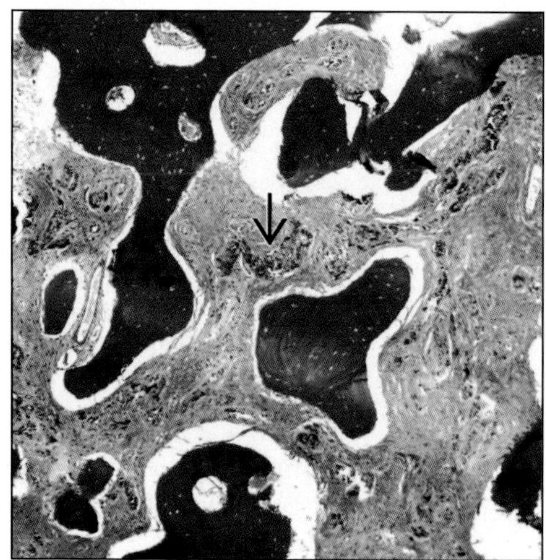

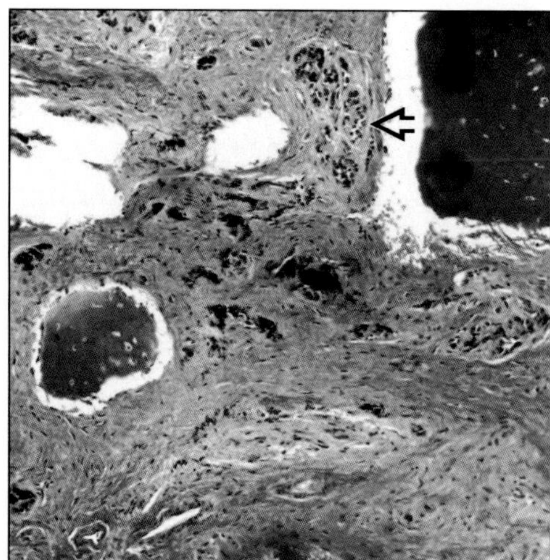

*(**Left**) A mixture of pigmented epithelial cells ↷ and small neuroblastic cells ➔ separated by dense fibrocollagenous stroma show an alveolar pattern of growth in this MNTI. Note the crush artifact in the small hyperchromatic small cells ⇨. (**Right**) Dense fibrous stroma is shown with scattered small neuroblastic cells arranged individually and in cords ➔ in this MNTI. Note the lack of a prominent epithelial component in this field.*

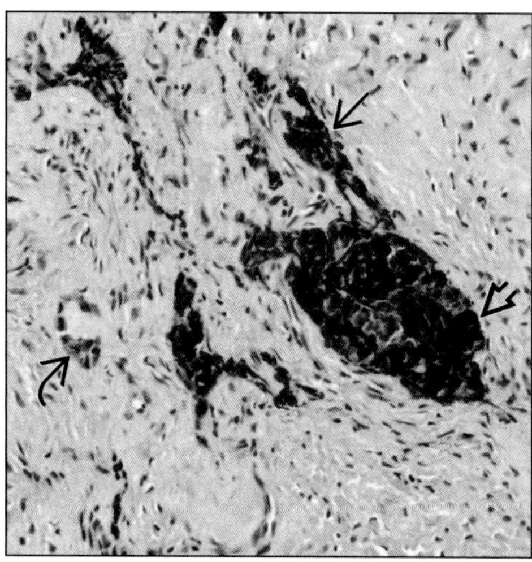

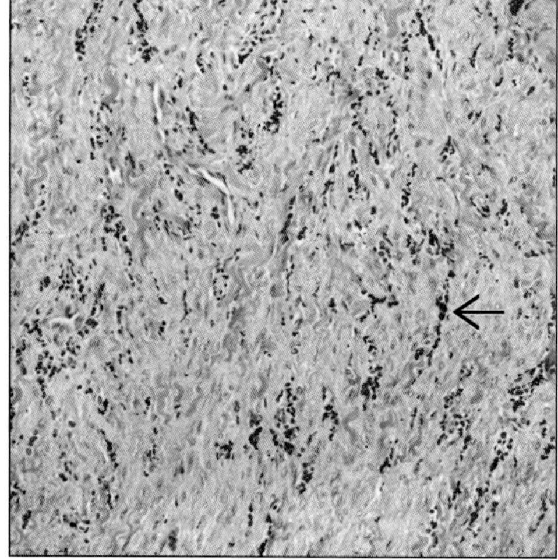

Microscopic Features and Ancillary Techniques

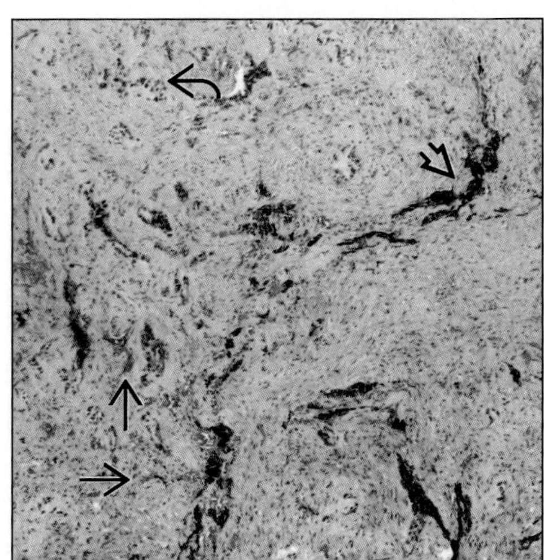

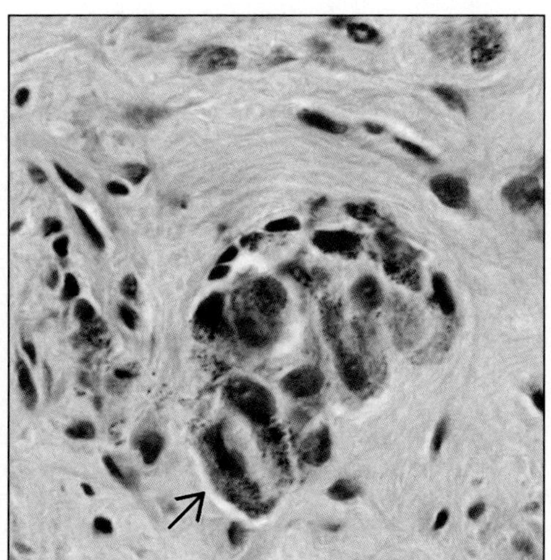

(Left) *Scattered nests of small neuroblastic cells* ⇨ *show crush artifact and pigmented epithelial cells* ⇨*. Note the numerous vessels* ⇨ *in the well-vascularized fibrocollagenous stroma that is a frequent feature of MNTI.* ***(Right)*** *High-power view of this MNTI highlights the prominent melanin granules in the abundant eosinophilic cytoplasm of these epithelial cells* ⇨*. The small neuroblastic cells may or may not be associated with the epithelial cells.*

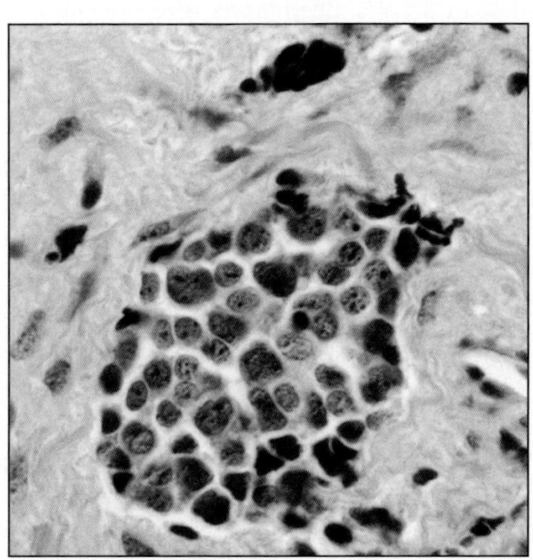

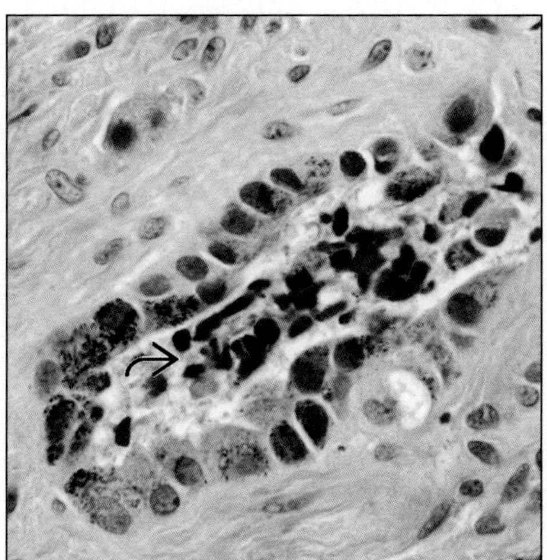

(Left) *High-power view of this nest of small neuroblastic round cells highlights the scant amount of cytoplasm and the small nucleoli with dispersed "salt and pepper" chromatin. Mitotic figures are rarely observed.* ***(Right)*** *High-power view highlights the presence of the small neuroblastic cells* ⇨ *within the lumen of this glandular structure.*

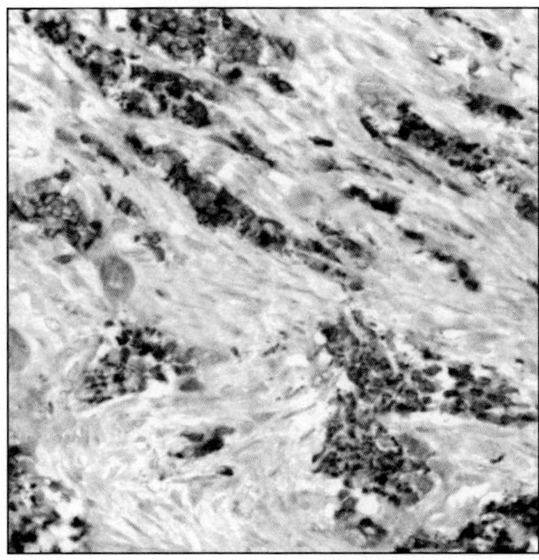

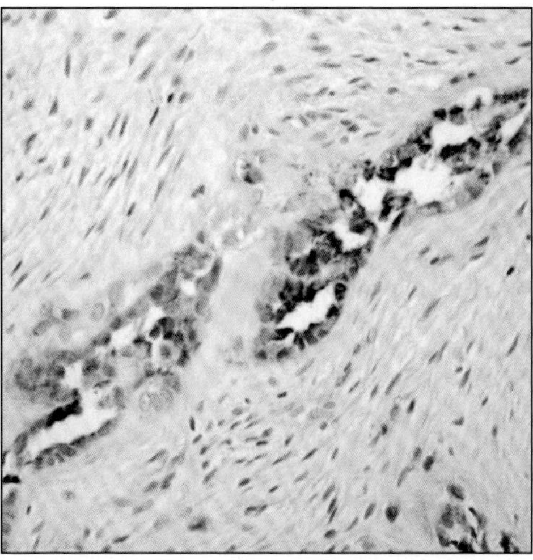

(Left) *Immunohistochemical staining for synaptophysin shows strong cytoplasmic reactivity in both the epithelial and small neuroblastic cellular components.* ***(Right)*** *Immunohistochemical reactivity for HMB-45 is observed in the cytoplasm of the epithelial cells.*

NODULAR FASCIITIS

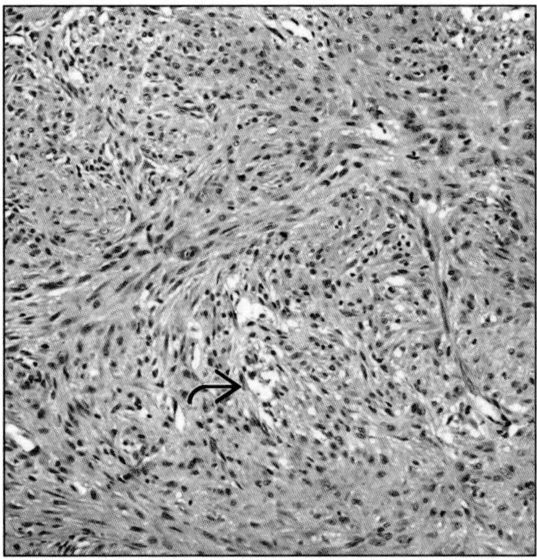

Hematoxylin & eosin of nodular fasciitis shows bland spindle cells lacking hyperchromasia and atypia arranged in short fascicles with scattered microcysts ⮫ and chronic inflammatory cells.

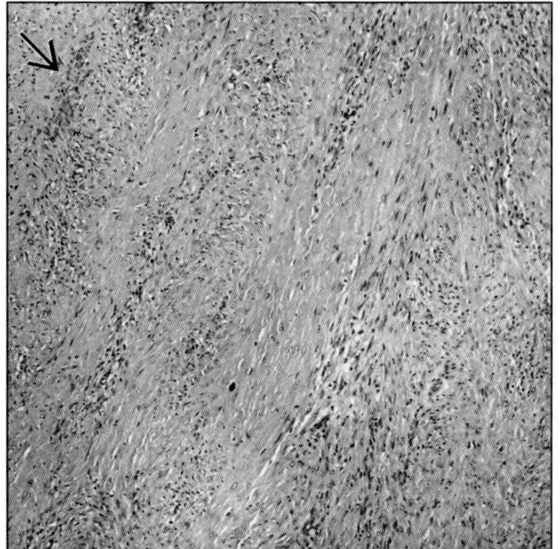

Low-power view shows nodular fasciitis with varying cellularity ranging from cellular to less cellular hyalinized zones. Extravasated red blood cells ⇒ are another common feature of this lesion.

TERMINOLOGY

Synonyms

- Pseudosarcomatous fasciitis

Definitions

- Benign, reactive, self-limiting proliferation of myofibroblastic and fibroblastic cells
  - Variants show overlapping histologic features and include
    - Intravascular fasciitis
    - Cranial fasciitis
    - Ossifying fasciitis

CLINICAL ISSUES

Epidemiology

- Age
  - All ages affected
    - Most commonly affects young adults, 20-40 years of age
- Gender
  - Affects males and females equally

Presentation

- Rapidly growing mass
  - Preoperative duration of 1-2 weeks to several months
  - Previous injury or trauma to site reported in 10-15%
- Painful or painless mass
  - Approximately 50% of cases present with pain and tenderness
- Upper extremity involvement most common
  - Other common sites include
    - Chest wall
    - Back
  - Trunk involvement common in children
- Most arise in subcutis
  - May also arise in dermis, deep fascia, and skeletal muscle
- Cranial involvement (cranial fasciitis)
  - Most present in 1st 2 years of life
  - Male predominance
  - Arise from deep fascial layers of scalp or underlying periosteum
  - Involves soft tissue of scalp and underlying skull
    - Erosion of outer skull table
    - Rarely involves inner skull table
- Intravascular involvement (intravascular fasciitis)
  - Involves small to medium-sized veins and arteries
    - Intraluminal, intramural, and extramural involvement
  - Most patients < 30 years of age
- Joint and oral cavity involvement reported
- Paresthesia and numbness rarely encountered

Treatment

- Surgical approaches
  - Complete surgical excision

Prognosis

- Excellent
- Rarely recur, even following incomplete excision
  - Recurrences should prompt careful evaluation of original diagnosis
  - Recurrences reported in children
- Metastases do not occur

MACROSCOPIC FEATURES

General Features

- Circumscribed to infiltrative
- Nonencapsulated nodular mass
- Variable myxoid to fibrous cut surface
- Lacks visible gross hemorrhage
- Focal cystic change

NODULAR FASCIITIS

Key Facts

Terminology
- Benign, reactive, self-limiting proliferation of myofibroblastic and fibroblastic cells

Clinical Issues
- Rapidly growing mass
- Most commonly affects young adults 20-40 years of age
- Upper extremity involvement most common
- Cranial involvement (cranial fasciitis)
- Intravascular involvement (intravascular fasciitis)
- Excellent prognosis
  - Rarely recur even following incomplete excision
  - Recurrences should prompt careful evaluation of original diagnosis
  - Metastases do not occur

Macroscopic Features
- Nonencapsulated nodular mass
- Variable myxoid to fibrous cut surface
- Typically measure < 2 cm in diameter

Microscopic Pathology
- Predominance of plump immature-appearing myofibroblasts arranged in short fascicles
- Partial, loose, feathery, tissue culture-like pattern
- Hyalinization prominent in older lesions
- Extravasation of red blood cells
- Microcystic degeneration
- Chronic inflammatory cells
- Mitotically active
  - Atypical mitoses should not be present
- Nuclei lack hyperchromasia and atypia

Size
- Typically < 2-3 cm in diameter
  - > 3-5 cm in diameter should prompt careful evaluation
- Intramuscular lesions typically larger than those of subcutaneous tissue

MICROSCOPIC PATHOLOGY

Predominant Pattern/Injury Type
- Fibrous
  - Variable amounts of collagen
  - Degree of collagenization related to duration of lesion
  - More frequently seen in older lesions
- Cellular
  - Plump myofibroblasts without nuclear atypia or hyperchromasia
- Fibromyxoid
  - Loose areas with feathery, tissue culture-like appearance
  - More frequently seen in early lesions
- Microcysts
- Nonencapsulated
- Infiltrative
  - Fascial and intramuscular lesions
- Circumscribed
  - Subcutaneous lesions

Predominant Cell/Compartment Type
- Fibroblast
- Myofibroblast
  - Resemble immature fibroblasts seen in tissue culture
  - Bipolar, oval to stellate nuclei
  - Small, round, basophilic nucleoli

Microscopic Features
- Predominance of plump immature-appearing myofibroblasts arranged in short fascicles
  - Focally storiform
  - Lack of significant collagen in younger lesions
- Partial, loose, feathery, tissue culture-like pattern
  - Rich in mucopolysaccharides
  - Prominent in early lesions
- Variable cellularity
- Hyalinization prominent in older lesions
- Extravasation of red blood cells
- Microcystic degeneration
- Chronic inflammatory cells
- Osteoclast-like giant cells
- Osseous metaplasia
  - Feature of ossifying fasciitis
  - Frequently observed in cranial fasciitis
- Mitotically active
  - Atypical mitoses should not be present
- Nuclei lack hyperchromasia and atypia

ANCILLARY TESTS

Flow Cytometry
- High proliferative index
- Diploidy in majority of cases

Cytogenetics
- Rare case reports of clonal cytogenetic abnormalities
  - Translocations involving chromosome 15
    - Translocations (2;15), (3;15), and (15;15) reported
  - Marker chromosomes and loss of chromosomes 2 and 13 also reported
  - 3q21 rearrangements

DIFFERENTIAL DIAGNOSIS

Myxoma
- Homogeneous lesions
- Lack regional heterogeneity
- Paucicellular

Benign Fibrous Histiocytoma
- Dermal based
- Polymorphous proliferation of spindle-round cells
  - Hyperchromatic, blunt-rounded nuclei

NODULAR FASCIITIS

- More consistent storiform pattern
- Peripheral dense hyalinized collagen fibers observed in both lesions
- Factor XIIIa positive
- Variable and focal smooth muscle actin reactivity

Fibromatosis

- Large, infiltrative, fibrous lesion
- Usually situated in deep soft tissues
- Spindle-shaped fibroblasts arranged in long sweeping fascicles
- Abundant collagen
- Fewer observed mitotic figures
- Nuclear expression of β-catenin is characteristic
  - Absent in nodular fasciitis

Fibrosarcoma

- Present as solitary palpable mass
- Typically larger in size (3-8 cm in diameter)
- Deep soft tissue of lower extremities most common
- Malignant cytologic features
  - Low-grade tumors have uniform and orderly cellular appearance
- Distinct fascicular herringbone pattern
- Atypical mitoses
- Variable necrosis

Myxoid Fibrosarcoma

- Slowly enlarging painless mass
- Admixture of heavily collagenized, hypocellular, and cellular myxoid nodules
- Fascicular to whorling pattern of growth
- Bland to malignant cytologic features
- Elongated curvilinear capillaries
- Atypical mitoses
- Focal smooth muscle actin and muscle-specific actin reactivity

Proliferative Fasciitis

- Myofibroblastic and fibroblastic proliferation
- Characteristic large basophilic ganglion-like cells
  - 1-2 vesicular nuclei with prominent nucleoli
  - Abundant basophilic granular cytoplasm
- Typically lack multinucleated giant cells
- Immunohistochemical profile similar to nodular fasciitis

DIAGNOSTIC CHECKLIST

Clinically Relevant Pathologic Features

- Mitotic rate
  - High
  - Lack atypical mitoses
- Nuclear features
  - Bland, plump to stellate
  - Lack atypia and hyperchromasia

Pathologic Interpretation Pearls

- Broad morphologic spectrum
  - Loose fibromyxoid, cellular and fibrous
- Histologic features may correlate with duration
- Mitotically active

MALPRACTICE CONSIDERATIONS

Diagnosis

- Frequently misdiagnosed as sarcoma
- Recognition of bland cytologic features, lack of atypical mitoses, architecture, and reactive nature to avoid misdiagnosis
- Size > 3-5 cm in diameter should prompt careful evaluation

Prognosis

- Rarely recur even following incomplete surgical excision
  - Recurrences should prompt careful evaluation of original diagnosis
  - Recurrences observed more frequently in children

SELECTED REFERENCES

1. Dauendorffer JN et al: [Nodular fasciitis of childhood: a clinicopathological analysis of 10 cases] Ann Dermatol Venereol. 135(8-9):553-8, 2008
2. Rosenberg AE: Pseudosarcomas of soft tissue. Arch Pathol Lab Med. 132(4):579-86, 2008
3. Bhattacharya B et al: Nuclear beta-catenin expression distinguishes deep fibromatosis from other benign and malignant fibroblastic and myofibroblastic lesions. Am J Surg Pathol. 29(5):653-9, 2005
4. Velagaleti GV et al: Cytogenetic findings in a case of nodular fasciitis of subclavicular region. Cancer Genet Cytogenet. 141(2):160-3, 2003
5. Birdsall SH et al: Cytogenetic findings in a case of nodular fasciitis of the breast. Cancer Genet Cytogenet. 81(2):166-8, 1995
6. Sawyer JR et al: Clonal chromosome aberrations in a case of nodular fasciitis. Cancer Genet Cytogenet. 76(2):154-6, 1994
7. Montgomery EA et al: Nodular fasciitis. Its morphologic spectrum and immunohistochemical profile. Am J Surg Pathol. 15(10):942-8, 1991
8. Shimizu S et al: Nodular fasciitis: an analysis of 250 patients. Pathology. 16(2):161-6, 1984
9. Bernstein KE et al: Nodular (pseudosarcomatous) fasciitis, a nonrecurrent lesion: clinicopathologic study of 134 cases. Cancer. 49(8):1668-78, 1982
10. Patchefsky AS et al: Intravascular fasciitis: a report of 17 cases. Am J Surg Pathol. 5(1):29-36, 1981
11. Lauer DH et al: Cranial fasciitis of childhood. Cancer. 45(2):401-6, 1980
12. Wirman JA: Nodular fasciitis, a lesion of myofibroblasts: an ultrastructural study. Cancer. 38(6):2378-89, 1976
13. Allen PW: Nodular fasciitis. Pathology. 4(1):9-26, 1972
14. Price EB Jr et al: Nodular fasciitis: a clinicopathologic analysis of 65 cases. Am J Clin Pathol. 35:122-36, 1961

Microscopic Features and Ancillary Techniques

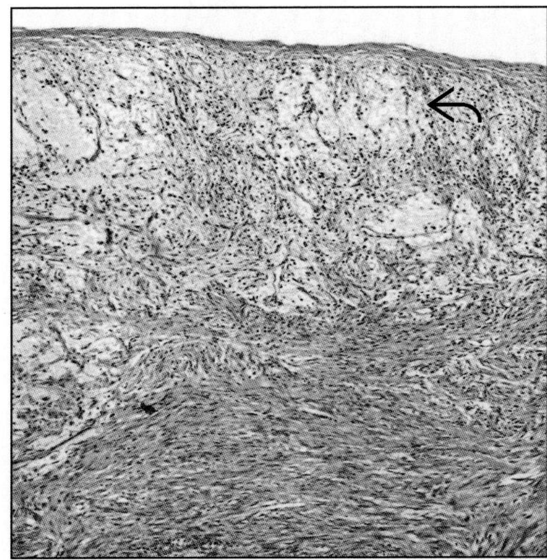

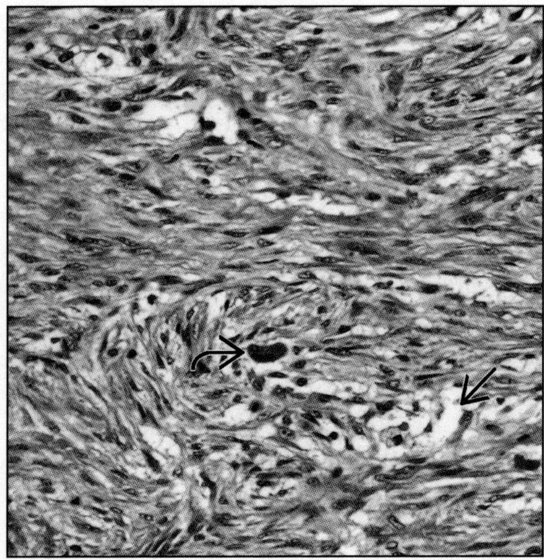

(Left) *Hematoxylin & eosin from low power shows histologic features typical of nodular fasciitis. Loose fibromyxoid areas ↪ rich in mucopolysaccharides are seen along the periphery. Fibroblasts suspended in the myxoid matrix impart a tissue-culture appearance. More densely cellular areas are seen centrally.* ***(Right)*** *Nodular fasciitis from high power shows a multinucleated giant cell ↪ surrounded by numerous microcysts → and bland spindle cells.*

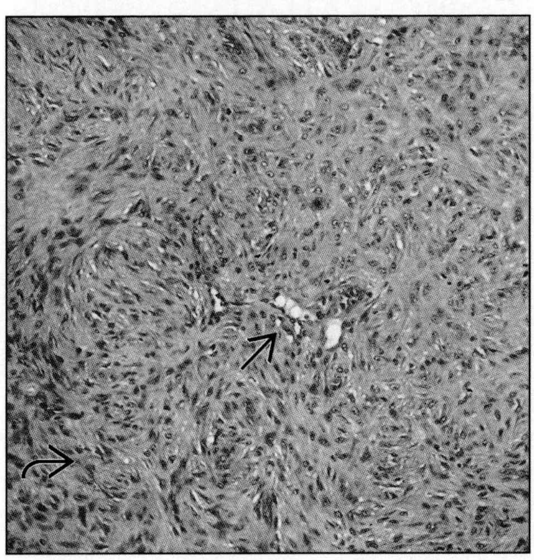

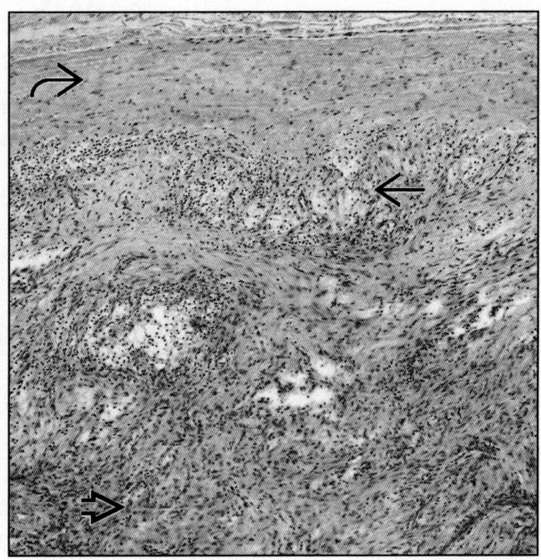

(Left) *Cranial fasciitis from medium power shows histologic features that are indistinguishable from nodular fasciitis. Note the extravasated red blood cells ↪, microcysts →, and short fascicles composed of bland, plump spindle cells.* ***(Right)*** *An example of intravascular fasciitis shows an intraluminal proliferation of spindle cells with prominent zonation. Note the more loose, fibromyxoid areas → adjacent to the vessel wall ↪ and increased cellularity centrally ⇨.*

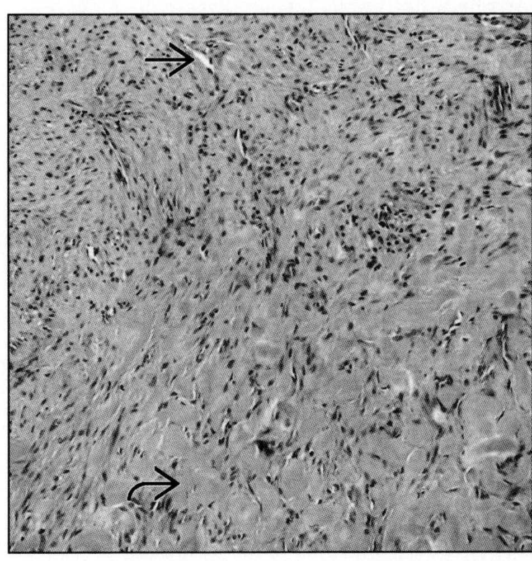

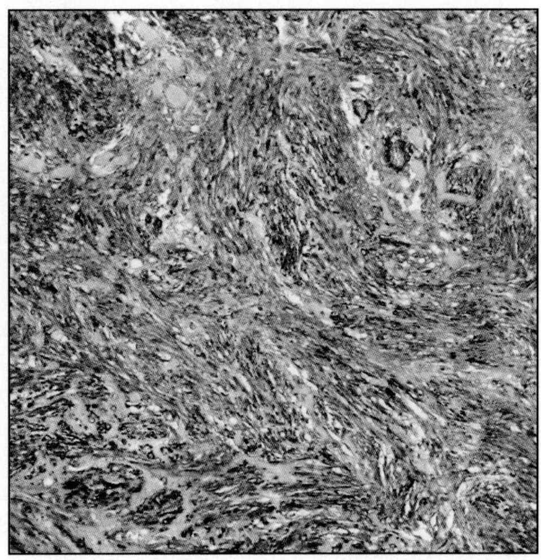

(Left) *Nodular fasciitis from medium power shows dense keloid-like collagen ↪ adjacent to more typical cellular areas arranged in short fascicles. Scattered chronic inflammatory cells and slit-like vascular spaces → are also shown. Confusion with angiosarcoma and Kaposi sarcoma may occur when these slit-like vascular spaces predominate.* ***(Right)*** *Actin-sm stained section of nodular fasciitis shows diffuse immunoreactivity in a cytoplasmic distribution.*

PROLIFERATIVE FASCIITIS/MYOSITIS

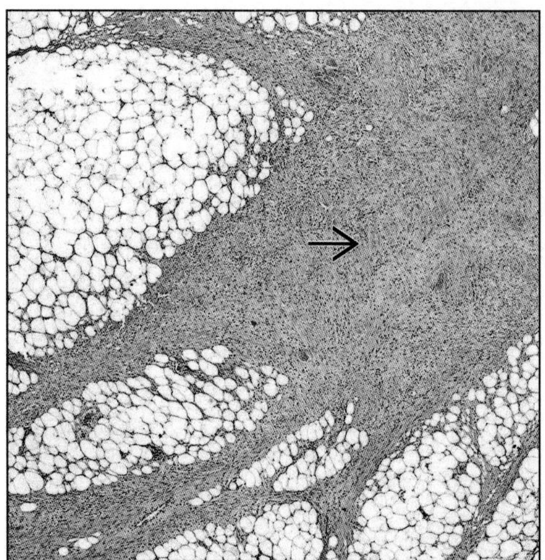

This case shows proliferative fasciitis at low magnification. Note the tracking along fibrous septa with somewhat less cellularity in the center ⇒, where there is often keloid-like collagen.

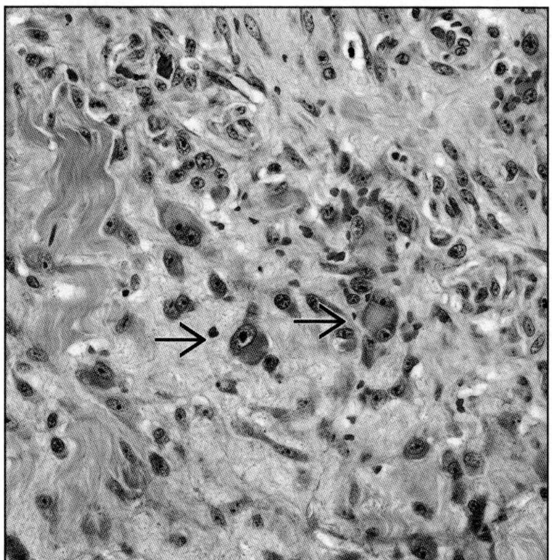

High-power magnification shows the so-called ganglion-like cells ⇒ of proliferative fasciitis. These are fibroblasts, but their nuclear and cytoplasmic features are reminiscent of ganglion cells.

TERMINOLOGY

Definitions

- Tumefactive subcutaneous (fasciitis) or intramuscular (myositis) proliferation featuring ganglion-like fibroblasts in a background of myofibroblasts and fibroblasts similar to those in nodular fasciitis

CLINICAL ISSUES

Epidemiology

- Incidence
  - Rare
    - Less common than nodular fasciitis
- Age
  - Middle-aged and older adults
    - Rare in children
- Gender
  - No predominance

Site

- Proliferative fasciitis: Upper extremity (forearm) > lower extremity > trunk
- Proliferative myositis: Trunk > shoulder girdle > upper arm > thigh

Presentation

- Rapidly growing mass
- Painless mass
  - More likely to be painful than nodular fasciitis
- Usually no history of trauma

Treatment

- Simple excision

Prognosis

- Benign lesions
  - Usually no recurrence even with incomplete excision

MACROSCOPIC FEATURES

General Features

- Poorly circumscribed mass extending along connective tissue septa

Size

- Usually 2-3 cm
  - Rare lesions up to ~ 5 cm

MICROSCOPIC PATHOLOGY

Histologic Features

- Mostly plump stellate to spindled fibroblasts and myofibroblasts
- Extravasated erythrocytes
- Background lymphocytes
- Large ganglion-like fibroblasts
  - Macronucleoli, abundant amphophilic cytoplasm
  - Not true ganglion cells: No Nissl substance
- Mitotic activity common
- Pediatric examples
  - Predominance of ganglion-like cells
  - Exuberant mitotic activity
  - Frequently misinterpreted as sarcomas
- Immunohistochemical profile
  - Ganglion-like cells: Vimentin(+), CD68 (variable), actin(-), desmin(-), myogenin(-), MYOD1(-), synaptophysin(-), S100(-), keratins(-), CD34(-)
  - Background fibroblasts and myofibroblasts: Vimentin(+), smooth muscle actin (usually [+]), muscle specific actin (usually [+]), desmin (usually [-]), myogenin(-), MYOD1(-), S100(-), keratins(-), CD68 (variable), CD34(-)
- Rare reports of abnormal karyotypes
  - No consistent abnormality reported
  - Diploid on flow cytometry
  - Few reports available

PROLIFERATIVE FASCIITIS/MYOSITIS

Key Facts

Terminology
- Tumefactive subcutaneous (fasciitis) or intramuscular (myositis) proliferation featuring ganglion-like fibroblasts in a background of myofibroblasts and fibroblasts similar to those in nodular fasciitis

Macroscopic Features
- Usually 2-3 cm

Microscopic Pathology
- Mostly plump stellate to spindled fibroblasts and myofibroblasts
- Large ganglion-like fibroblasts
- Macronucleoli, abundant amphophilic cytoplasm
- Mitotic activity common
- Pediatric examples have exuberant mitotic activity, which can lead to misinterpretation as sarcomas

DIFFERENTIAL DIAGNOSIS

Nodular Fasciitis
- Usually in young adults
- 2-3 cm mass
- Loose storiform pattern
- Stellate myofibroblasts
  - Lacks ganglion-like cells
- Background lymphocytes, extravasated erythrocytes
- Benign outcome even if incompletely excised

Dermatofibroma/Fibrous Histiocytoma
- Usually in adults
- Storiform pattern
- Background histiocytes, hemosiderin, plasma cells common
- CD68(+), FXIIIA(+), S100(-), actin (variable), CD34(-)
- Benign

Embryonal Rhabdomyosarcoma
- Usually involve genital region or head and neck of infants and young children
- Enhanced cellularity beneath mucous membranes (cambium layer)
- Atypical nuclei
- Often lack prominent nucleoli
- Display skeletal muscle differentiation on immunolabeling
  - Desmin(+), myogenin(+), MYOD1(+)

Pleomorphic Rhabdomyosarcoma
- Highly aggressive lesions of adults, often in deep soft tissue of thigh
- Markedly pleomorphic cells
- Skeletal muscle differentiation on immunolabeling
  - Desmin(+), myogenin(+), MYOD1(+)
- Poor 5-year survival

High-Grade Undifferentiated Pleomorphic Sarcoma/Malignant Fibrous Histiocytoma
- Large mass of deep soft tissues: Buttocks and thighs common
- Pleomorphic spindle cells
- Immunoprofile: CD68 (variable), actin (variable), desmin (variable), myogenin(-), MYOD1(-), CD34 (variable), keratins (usually [-]), S100(-)

SELECTED REFERENCES

1. McComb EN et al: Chromosomal anomalies in a case of proliferative myositis. Cancer Genet Cytogenet. 98(2):142-4, 1997
2. Dembinski A et al: Trisomy 2 in proliferative fasciitis. Cancer Genet Cytogenet. 60(1):27-30, 1992
3. Meis JM et al: Proliferative fasciitis and myositis of childhood. Am J Surg Pathol. 16(4):364-72, 1992
4. Chung EB et al: Proliferative fasciitis. Cancer. 36(4):1450-8, 1975

IMAGE GALLERY

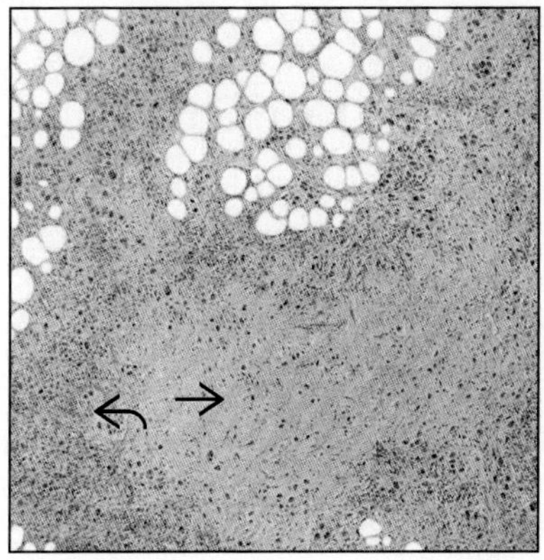

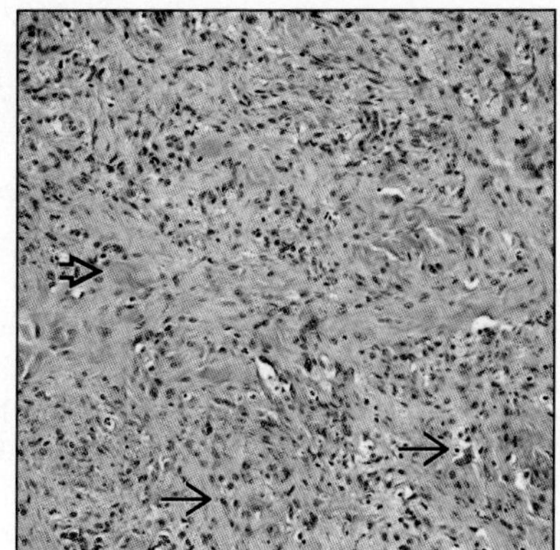

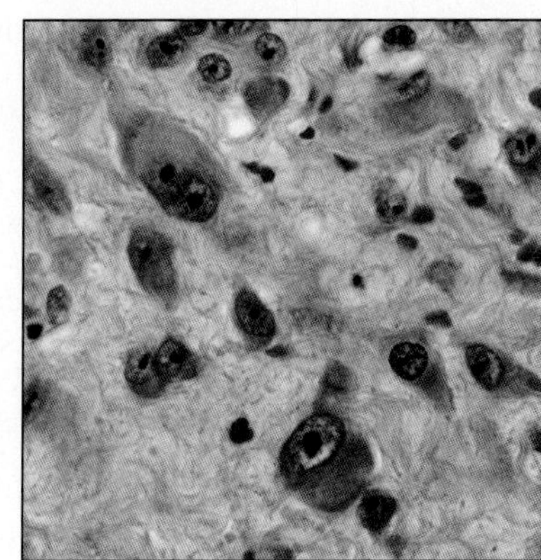

(Left) *Low-power view shows a tumefactive example of proliferative fasciitis. The central portion ⇒ is less cellular than the periphery ⇒, which can resemble nodular fasciitis.* ***(Center)*** *Low-power view shows a nodular fasciitis-like component with keloid-like collagen ⇒ and many background lymphocytes ⇒.* ***(Right)*** *High-power view shows ganglion-like cells. This field also shows extravasated erythrocytes, a feature shared with nodular fasciitis.*

MYOSITIS OSSIFICANS

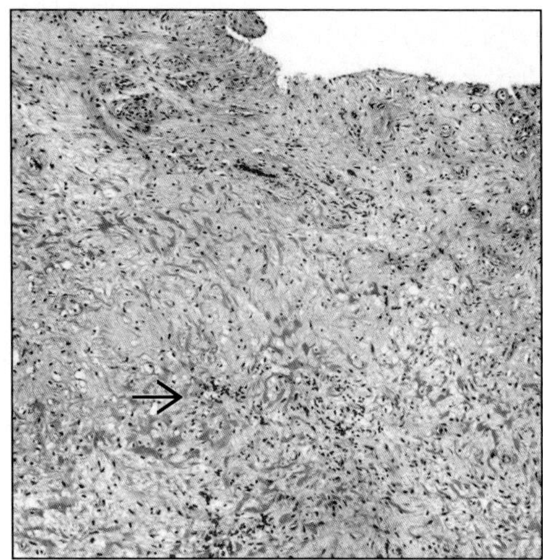

A loose, vascular fibroblastic/myofibroblastic proliferation is seen centrally. This area can have mild pleomorphism, prominent mitotic activity, focal hemorrhage ⇒, and entrapped muscle fibers.

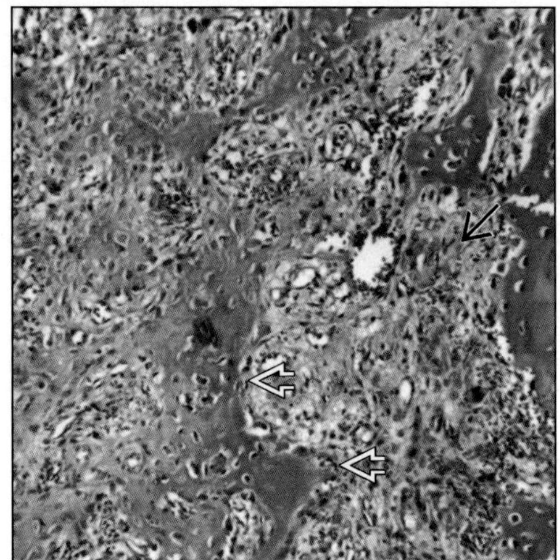

The intermediate zone shows a transition from fibroblastic/myofibroblastic spindled cells ⇒ to osteoblast-lined trabeculae of osteoid ➡.

TERMINOLOGY

Abbreviations

- Myositis ossificans (MO)

Synonyms

- Nonneoplastic heterotopic ossification
- Pseudomalignant osseous tumors of soft tissues
- Extraosseous localized, nonneoplastic bone and cartilage formation

Definitions

- Benign ossifying process, most often found in musculature, but may occur in other tissues
  - Panniculitis ossificans: Ossifying process of subcutaneous fat
    - Typically seen in upper extremities in women
  - Fasciitis ossificans: Ossifying process of tendon
- Technically, MO is a misnomer, as it may occur outside of musculature, can be devoid of bone, and lacks significant inflammation

CLINICAL ISSUES

Site

- Musculature or soft tissue of extremities, but may occur anywhere

Presentation

- Typically seen in young males
- Initial complaint of pain, followed by diffuse, doughy soft tissue swelling
- After 2-3 weeks, swelling becomes indurated, circumscribed, and firm to stoney on palpation
- Patients may or may not have history of trauma
- Rapidly growing lesions may be mistaken for neoplasm
- 3-6 cm on average
- Lesion is likely not MO if surgeon has difficultly removing it

Treatment

- Rest, immobilization, anti-inflammatory medication
- Surgical excision if lesion is irritating nerve or interfering with joint mobility

Prognosis

- Excellent
- If incompletely excised, during early phase of growth, lesion may continue to grow for limited time

IMAGE FINDINGS

Radiographic Findings

- Roentgenograms are usually negative during 1st 2-3 weeks, or may show slight increase in soft tissue density
- Peripheral mineralization with central lucency is seen after 3rd week

MACROSCOPIC FEATURES

General Features

- Solitary and well circumscribed
  - White, soft, hemorrhagic, or gelatinous center
  - Rough, tan-gray, granular surface

MICROSCOPIC PATHOLOGY

Histologic Features

- MO has characteristic zonal pattern, reflecting cellular maturation
  - Seen in lesions older than 3 weeks duration
- Central zone: Vascular fibroblastic/myofibroblastic spindled cell population
  - Close resemblance to granulation tissue or nodular fasciitis
  - Mild cellular pleomorphism and prominent mitotic figures can be seen

MYOSITIS OSSIFICANS

Key Facts

Terminology
- Calcification of muscle or soft tissue

Clinical Issues
- Typically seen in young males
- Patients may or may not have history of trauma
- Rapidly growing lesion, which may be mistaken for neoplasm

Image Findings
- Peripheral mineralization with central lucency seen after 3rd week

Macroscopic Features
- Solitary and well circumscribed

Microscopic Pathology
- MO has characteristic zonal pattern, reflecting cellular maturation

- Intermediate zone: Spindle-shaped cells transition to trabeculae of osteoid rimmed by plump osteoblasts
- Peripheral zone: Osteoid calcifies and evolves into mature lamellar bone
- Loose myxoid or fibrous tissue separates lesion from surrounding muscle
- In panniculitis ossificans, zonal pattern can be more difficult to distinguish
- Older lesions can be indistinguishable from osteoma

Predominant Pattern/Injury Type
- Zoneation phenomenon

DIFFERENTIAL DIAGNOSIS

Myositis Ossificans Progressiva
- Also referred to as fibrodysplasia ossificans progressiva
- Inherited in autosomal dominant pattern
- Ossification can occur without injury
- Typically grows in predictable pattern

Extraosseous Osteosarcomas
- Occur rarely in young people
- Greater cellular atypia and disorderly growth with infiltrative border
- Osteoid is lace-like rather than trabecular
- Osteoid is located centrally within lesion

DIAGNOSTIC CHECKLIST

Pathologic Interpretation Pearls
- Distinguishing between traumatic and nontraumatic MO is of little value as both forms are histologically identical and are most likely secondary to injury
- Diagnosis during early stage disease can be difficult
  - Immature and highly cellular areas can mimic extraskeletal osteosarcoma, especially on biopsy
- Late stage lesions consisting predominantly of mature lamellar bone can mimic osteoma

SELECTED REFERENCES

1. Conner GA et al: Myositis ossificans: a case report of multiple recurrences following third molar extractions and review of the literature. J Oral Maxillofac Surg. 67(4):920-6, 2009
2. Macarenco AC et al: Cutaneous myositis ossificans: an appropriate descriptor for fibro-osseous lesion of the external auditory canal. Am J Dermatopathol. 31(2):170-2, 2009
3. Micheli A et al: Myositis ossificans circumscripta: a paediatric case and review of the literature. Eur J Pediatr. 168(5):523-9, 2009
4. Morrison JE et al: Massive ventral hernia with extensive heterotopic ossification: the honeycomb-abdomen. J Trauma. 66(4):1234-7, 2009
5. Rosa M et al: Myositis ossificans traumatica of the abdominal wall. Can J Surg. 52(2):E33-4, 2009
6. Kaplan FS et al: Early diagnosis of fibrodysplasia ossificans progressiva. Pediatrics. 121(5):e1295-300, 2008

IMAGE GALLERY

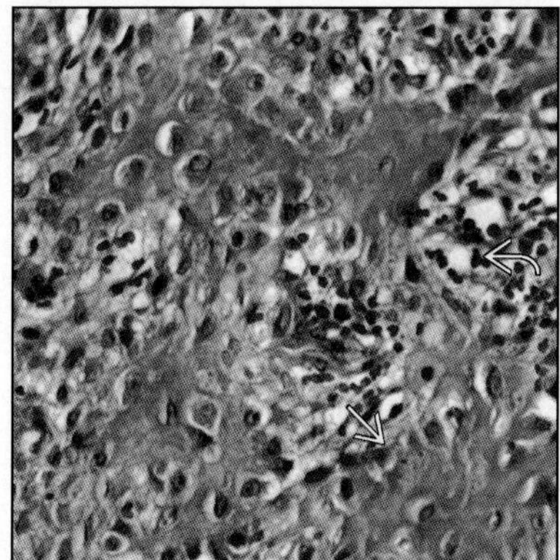

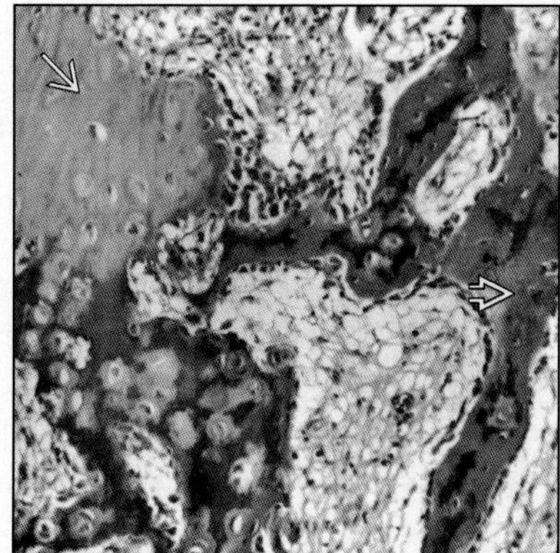

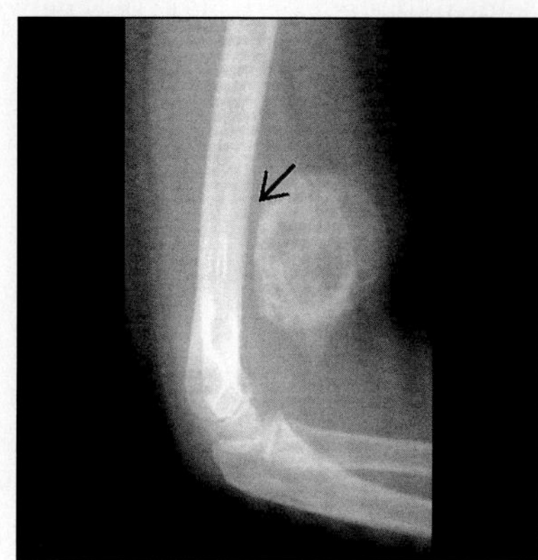

(Left) *Osteoblast-lined osteoid ➡ forming ill-defined trabeculae are surrounded by a spindled cell population with thin-walled vascular channels ➡.* ***(Center)*** *At the periphery of the lesion, osteoid ➡ calcifies and becomes mature lamellar bone ➡.* ***(Right)*** *Radiograph of the upper arm shows a well-defined soft tissue mass that is most densely calcified at its periphery. Note the radiolucent area between the mass and humerus ➡, which helps to distinguish MO from an osteochondroma.*

FIBRODYSPLASIA OSSIFICANS PROGRESSIVA

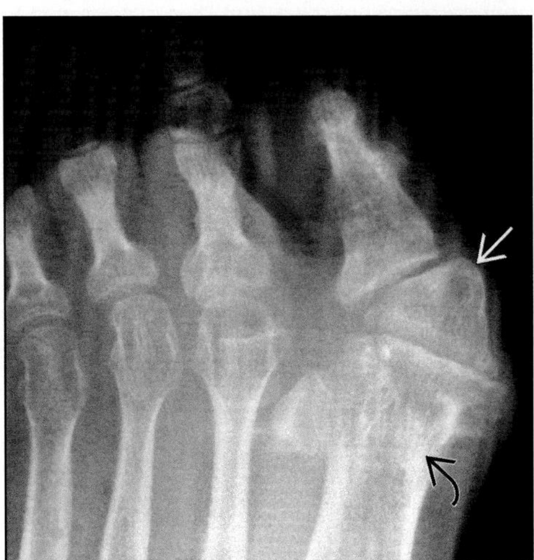

Plain radiograph of the left foot demonstrates a shortened 1st metatarsal ➩ as well as a large free osseous body ➡ that have resulted in marked hallux valgus. These features are characteristic of FOP.

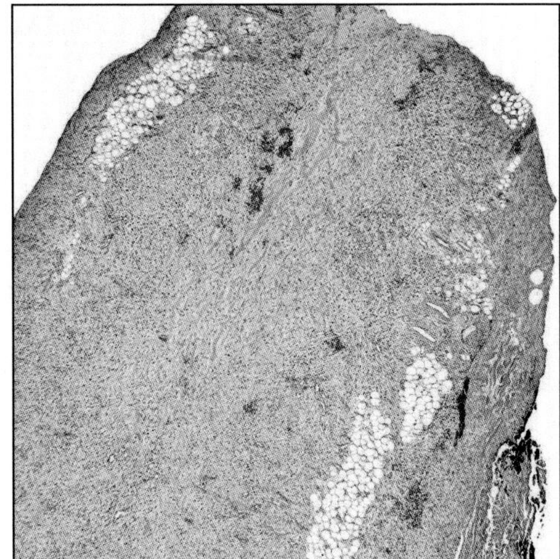

The appearance of the lesions in fibrodysplasia ossificans progressiva is related to the duration of the lesions. This lesion was early, and it appears similar to nodular fasciitis.

TERMINOLOGY

Abbreviations

- Fibrodysplasia ossificans progressiva (FOP, FDOP)

Synonyms

- Myositis ossificans progressiva, stone man disease

Definitions

- Rare disabling genetic disorder of progressive heterotopic ossification

ETIOLOGY/PATHOGENESIS

Genetics

- Heterozygous activating mutation of gene encoding activin receptor A type 1/activin-like kinase 2 (*ACVR1/ ALK2*)
  - Bone morphogenic protein (BMP) type 1 receptor

CLINICAL ISSUES

Epidemiology

- Incidence
  - Approximately 1 in 2,000,000 persons
- Age
  - Childhood onset
- Gender
  - No predilection
- Ethnicity
  - No predilection

Presentation

- Hallux valgus
- Short 1st metatarsals
- Rapidly changing swellings in neck or back
- Minor trauma results in progressive heterotopic ossification
  - Ideally, diagnosis should be made by clinical presentation and imaging study findings
    - Metatarsal changes occur early
  - Biopsy contraindicated since it will exacerbate lesions, cause new lesions

Treatment

- None exists
  - Supportive care

Prognosis

- Progressive from childhood
- Most patients wheelchair bound by 3rd decade
- Median lifespan: 56 years
  - Most common cause of death: Cardiorespiratory failure from thoracic insufficiency syndrome
    - Costovertebral malformations
    - Orthotopic ankylosis of costovertebral joints
    - Fusion of ribs
    - Ossification of intercostal muscles, paravertebral muscles, and aponeuroses
    - Progressive spinal deformity (kyphoscoliosis or thoracic lordosis): Surgical correction contraindicated

IMAGE FINDINGS

General Features

- Characteristic appearance of 1st metatarsals on plain radiographs
- MR highlights lesions in muscles of back and neck

MICROSCOPIC PATHOLOGY

Histologic Features

- Early lesions are nodular fasciitis-like
  - Disorganized collagen
  - Large myofibroblastic cells
  - Extravasated erythrocytes

FIBRODYSPLASIA OSSIFICANS PROGRESSIVA

Key Facts

Terminology
- Rare disabling genetic disorder of progressive heterotopic ossification

Etiology/Pathogenesis
- Heterozygous activating mutation of gene encoding activin receptor A type 1/activin-like kinase 2 (*ACVR1/ALK2*)

Clinical Issues
- Approximately 1 in 2,000,000 persons
- Childhood onset
- No treatment exists

Microscopic Pathology
- Early lesions are nodular fasciitis-like
- Progressive ossification similar to that of myositis ossificans

- Mitotic activity
- Progressive ossification similar to that of myositis ossificans
  - Less prominent zonation than in myositis
- Histologic material should not be generally available since biopsy is deleterious for patient

DIFFERENTIAL DIAGNOSIS

Myositis Ossificans
- Presents in individuals in their 30s
- Arises in extremities
  - Elbow, thigh, buttock, shoulder
  - 2-5 cm, well marginated
- No associated skeletal anomalies
- Zonated lesions with cellular central portion and peripheral ossification
  - Central portion consisting of short fascicles of myofibroblastic cells
  - Numerous mitoses
  - Vascular stroma, numerous mitoses
  - Peripheral portion with trabeculae of woven bone rimmed by osteoblasts
    - Older lesions show mature bone
- Benign and nonprogressive

Extraskeletal Osteosarcoma
- Large lesions of deep soft tissue
  - Common in deep soft tissues of thigh
- Older adults
- Marked cytologic atypia
- Irregularly distributed zones of osteoid rimmed by cytologically malignant cells
- Dismal outcome: Death due to widely metastatic disease

Nodular Fasciitis
- Lesions of young adults
- Classically involves forearm
  - Head and neck also common site
- 2-3 cm
- Loose storiform pattern
- Myofibroblasts, myxoid matrix
- Keloid-like collagen, extravasated erythrocytes, lymphocytes
- Benign and nonprogressive

SELECTED REFERENCES

1. Kaplan FS et al: Early mortality and cardiorespiratory failure in patients with fibrodysplasia ossificans progressiva. J Bone Joint Surg Am. 92(3):686-91, 2010
2. Shore EM et al: A recurrent mutation in the BMP type I receptor ACVR1 causes inherited and sporadic fibrodysplasia ossificans progressiva. Nat Genet. 38(5):525-7, 2006
3. Maxwell WA et al: Histochemical and ultrastructural studies in fibrodysplasia ossificans progressiva (myositis ossificans progressiva). Am J Pathol. 87(3):483-98, 1977

IMAGE GALLERY

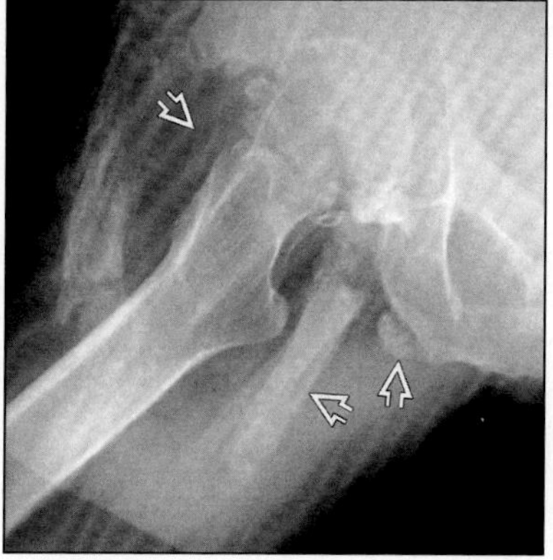

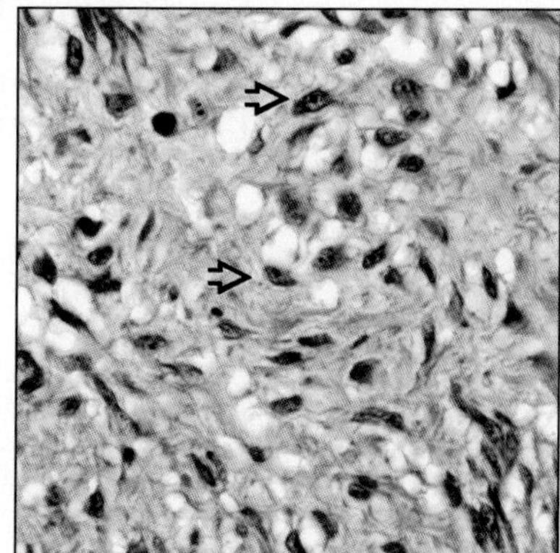

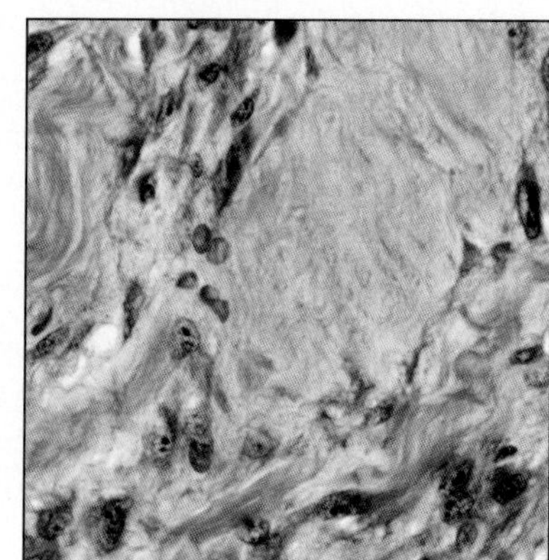

(Left) *Radiograph of the right hip demonstrates severe destructive skeletal changes as well as prominent soft tissue ossification ⇒. Generally, biopsy is not recommended of these lesions since surgical manipulation results in additional lesions.* ***(Center)*** *This fibrodysplasia ossificans progressiva lesion is composed of reactive-appearing myofibroblasts ⇒.* ***(Right)*** *H&E shows a collagenized area in fibrodysplasia ossificans progressiva.*

FIBROUS UMBILICAL POLYP

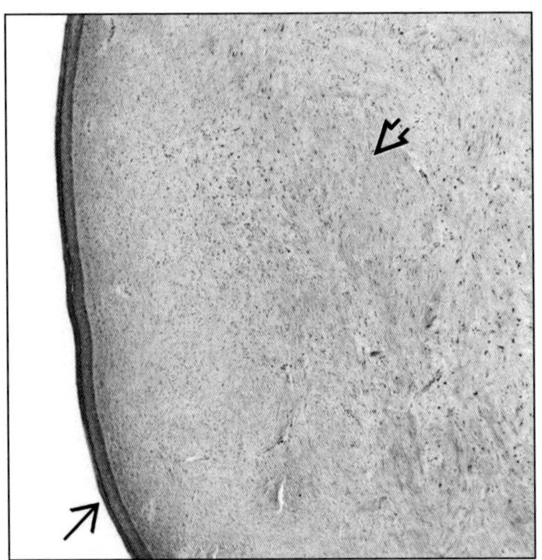

Hematoxylin & eosin shows a nonencapsulated, well-circumscribed fibrous umbilical polyp composed of keratinized squamous epithelium ➔ and fibrous stroma ➢ with no adnexal structures.

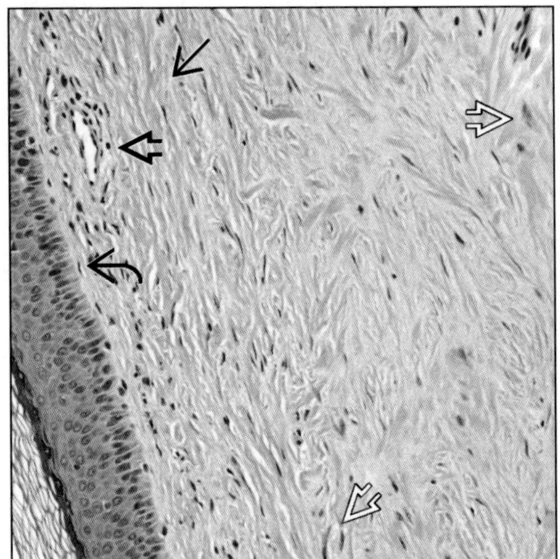

Hematoxylin & eosin shows keratinized squamous epithelium with loss of rete ridges ➔ and stroma composed of collagen ➔, fibroblasts ➢, and sparse vascularity ➢.

TERMINOLOGY

Definitions

- Benign nodular proliferation of fibrous tissue in umbilical region with no associated inflammation

ETIOLOGY/PATHOGENESIS

Etiology

- Exact mechanism of pathogenesis is still uncertain
  - Umbilical susceptibility to fibrogenic stimuli at young age has been proposed

CLINICAL ISSUES

Epidemiology

- Incidence
  - Unclear; formal case series have not been published
- Age
  - Most commonly occurs from 3-18 months
- Gender
  - Marked male predominance (15:1 ratio)

Site

- Umbilical region

Presentation

- Polypoid mass in umbilical region

Treatment

- General approaches
  - Conservative treatment
  - Complete local excision

Prognosis

- Good prognosis
  - Absence of local recurrence

MACROSCOPIC FEATURES

General Features

- Well-circumscribed, polypoid lesion

Size

- Size varies approximately from 0.4-1.2 cm

MICROSCOPIC PATHOLOGY

Histologic Features

- Nonencapsulated, well-circumscribed dermal proliferation of moderately cellular fibrous tissue
  - Plump to elongated fibroblastic cells
  - Abundant amphophilic cytoplasm
  - Plump/vesicular nuclei with small nucleoli
  - Occasional cell atypia (enlarged nuclei) or ganglion-cell like morphology
  - Scant to moderate collagen
  - Sparse vascularity
  - Lack inflammatory component
- Loss of rete ridges and basket-weave hyperkeratosis in overlying epidermis
  - Absence of adnexal structures

Predominant Pattern/Injury Type

- Fibrous

Predominant Cell/Compartment Type

- Fibroblast

DIFFERENTIAL DIAGNOSIS

Keloid

- Thick bundles of hyaline collagen

Umbilical Granuloma

- Characterized by granulomatous inflammation

FIBROUS UMBILICAL POLYP

Key Facts

Terminology
- Benign nodular proliferation of fibrous tissue in umbilical region with no associated inflammation

Etiology/Pathogenesis
- Exact mechanism of pathogenesis is still uncertain

Clinical Issues
- Most commonly occurs from 3-18 months
- Marked male predominance (15:1 ratio)

Microscopic Pathology
- Nonencapsulated, well-circumscribed dermal proliferation of moderately cellular fibrous tissue
- Scant to moderate collagen
- Sparse vascularity
- **Inflammation is not present**
- Loss of rete ridges and basket-weave hyperkeratosis in overlying epidermis

Immunohistochemistry

Antibody	Reactivity	Staining Pattern	Comment
Actin-sm	Positive	Cytoplasmic	May be focal
Desmin	Positive	Cytoplasmic	Rare
EMA	Negative		
CD34	Negative		
S100	Negative		

Granulation Tissue
- Richly vascularized fibrous connective tissue
- Prominent inflammatory component

Umbilical Polyp
- Result of incomplete regression of omphalomesenteric duct or urachal remnants
- Red, moist umbilical mass
- Occasionally bleeds or is exudative
- Often found in older children and adults
- Contains ectopic epithelium

Nodular Fasciitis
- Most commonly involve upper extremity, trunk, head and neck
- Greater cellularity; storiform pattern
- Inflammatory cells and mitoses

Desmoid Fibromatosis
- Head and neck are most commonly involved sites
- Broad age range
- Large size and infiltrative pattern

DIAGNOSTIC CHECKLIST

Pathologic Interpretation Pearls
- **Not all umbilical polyps represent fibrous umbilical polyps**
  - Fibrous umbilical polyps
    - Most commonly occurs from 3-18 months
    - Male predominance
    - Lack epithelial and smooth muscle components
    - Lack inflammatory component
    - Dermal fibrous proliferation

SELECTED REFERENCES

1. Vargas SO: Fibrous umbilical polyp: a distinct fasciitis-like proliferation of early childhood with a marked male predominance. Am J Surg Pathol. 25(11):1438-42, 2001
2. Larralde de Luna M et al: Umbilical polyps. Pediatr Dermatol. 4(4):341-3, 1987

IMAGE GALLERY

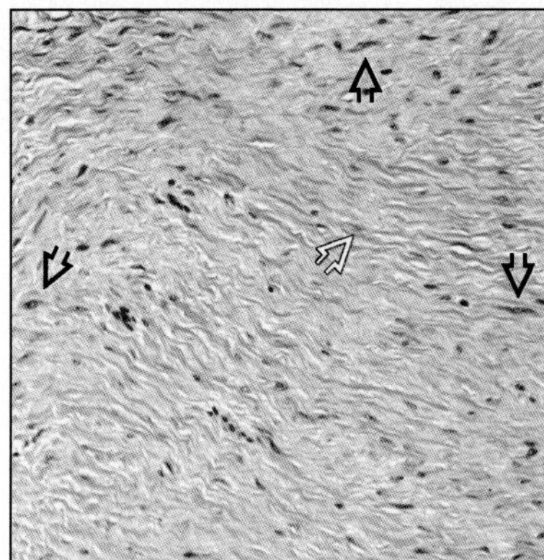

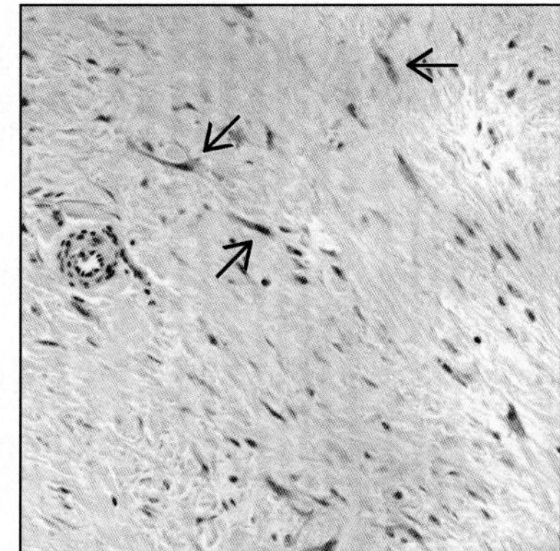

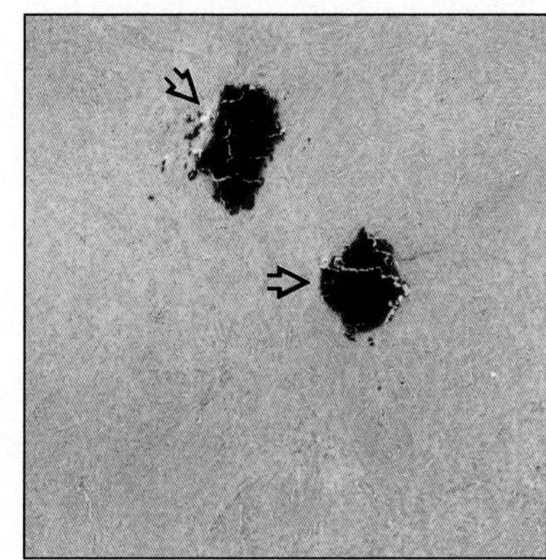

(Left) *Fibrous umbilical polyp at high power shows a cellular stroma composed of plump, elongated fibroblastic cells with amphophilic cytoplasm ⮚ admixed with collagen ⮚. Note the absence of inflammatory cells.* ***(Center)*** *Fibrous umbilical polyp at high power shows ganglion-like cells with enlarged nuclei ⮚.* ***(Right)*** *Fibrous umbilical polyp at low power shows a hypovascular stroma with focal dystrophic calcification ⮚.*

GARDNER FIBROMA

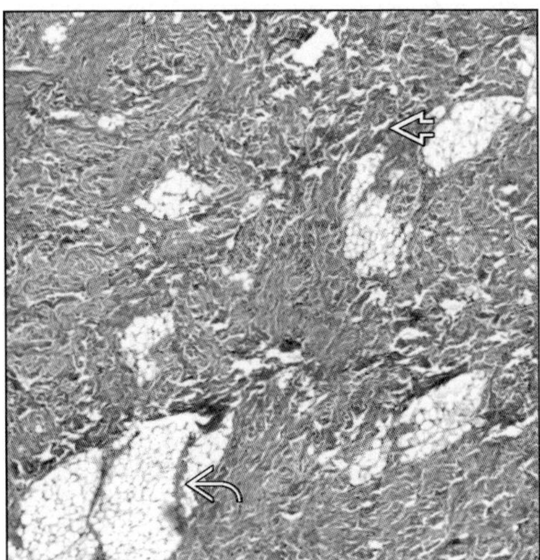

Low-power view of a Gardner fibroma shows bundles of coarse collagen separated by irregular cracking artifact ➡. Note the infiltrative growth pattern and entrapment of subcutaneous fat ➡.

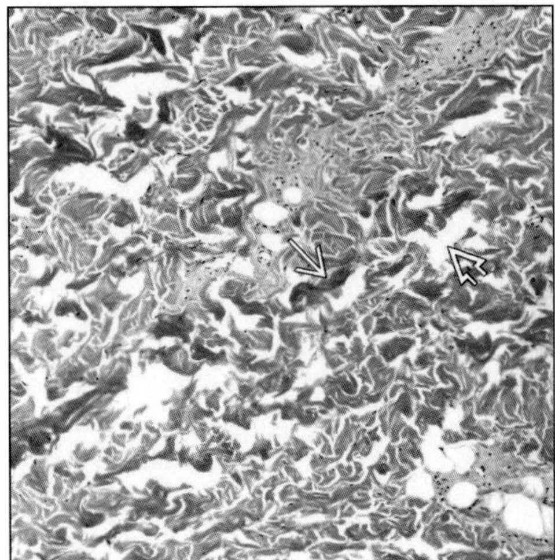

High-power view of a Gardner fibroma demonstrates that the lesion is composed of formless sheets of dense, haphazardly arranged collagen bands ➡ separated by clear clefts ➡.

TERMINOLOGY

Abbreviations

- Gardner fibroma (GAF)

Definitions

- Benign, patternless fibrocollagenous proliferation involving soft tissue, with predilection for children and young adults

ETIOLOGY/PATHOGENESIS

Etiology/Pathogenesis

- Etiology of these tumors is unclear

CLINICAL ISSUES

Epidemiology

- Incidence
  - Rare
- Age
  - Most commonly occurs in 1st 2 decades of life
- Gender
  - Males and females are equally affected

Site

- Superficial and deep soft tissues of
  - Paraspinal region
  - Back
  - Head and neck
  - Extremities
  - Chest wall

Presentation

- Superficial or deep soft tissue mass
- **GAF may be initial presentation** in children with *APC* mutations

Natural History

- May occur sporadically
- Synchronous and metachronous association with desmoid tumors
- Propensity for locally infiltrative growth and recurrence

Treatment

- Complete surgical excision is treatment of choice

Prognosis

- May recur locally if incompletely resected

Genetics

- Associated with de novo *APC* mutations and with familial adenomatous polyposis (FAP) syndrome
  - Unclear whether all Gardner fibromas harbor *APC* mutations
- May be associated with Gardner syndrome
  - Autosomal dominant
  - Considered a phenotypical variant of FAP
  - Characterized by
    - Multiple adenomatous polyps in any part of digestive tract, with colorectal predominance and potential for malignant transformation
    - Osteomas
    - Epidermoid and dermoid cysts
    - Soft tissue tumors
  - Symptoms are usually evident by 2nd and 3rd decades of life
  - Extracolonic symptoms (e.g., osteomas, dermoid cysts) are related with mutations located between the 1395 and 1578 codons of *APC*

MACROSCOPIC FEATURES

General Features

- Poorly circumscribed, plaque-like appearance
- White, rubbery cut surface
- Often solitary

GARDNER FIBROMA

Key Facts

Terminology
- Benign, patternless fibrocollagenous proliferation involving soft tissue, with predilection for children and young adults

Etiology/Pathogenesis
- Associated with de novo *APC* mutations and with familial adenomatous polyposis (FAP) syndrome
  - Unclear whether *APC* mutations are present in all Gardner fibromas

Clinical Issues
- Most commonly occurs in 1st 2 decades of life
- GAF may be initial presentation in children with *APC* mutations
- Synchronous and metachronous association with desmoid tumors

Macroscopic Features
- Poorly circumscribed, plaque-like appearance

Immunohistochemistry

Antibody	Reactivity	Staining Pattern	Comment
β-catenin-nuclear	Positive	Nuclear	Not all cases exhibit positive β-catenin stain
CD34	Positive	Cell membrane	Positive in ~ 70-80% of cases

MICROSCOPIC PATHOLOGY

Histologic Features
- Composed of thick, haphazardly arranged collagen bundles and scanty bland fibroblasts
  - Fibroblasts are often spindle shaped with inconspicuous nuclei, without atypia
- Clear clefts separate collagen bundles
  - "Cracked collagen bundles"
- Infiltrative growth pattern
- Occasional entrapment of fat, blood vessels, and peripheral nerves
- Sparse mast cells may be scattered within lesion

DIFFERENTIAL DIAGNOSIS

Nuchal-type Fibroma
- Most commonly occurs in middle-aged men
- Frequently associated with diabetes mellitus but not with FAP
- Lobular arrangement of collagen bundles

Desmoid Tumor
- Fascicular architecture
- Lacks clear clefts between collagen bands

Elastofibroma
- Most commonly occurs in elderly females
- Associated with repetitive trauma
- Elastic fiber fragments dispersed in myxocollagenous stroma: Hallmark of this lesion
- Lacks clear clefts in stroma

Scar Tissue
- Does not exhibit infiltrative growth pattern
- Lacks clear clefts between collagen bundles

SELECTED REFERENCES

1. Levesque S et al: Neonatal Gardner fibroma: a sentinel presentation of severe familial adenomatous polyposis. Pediatrics. 126(6):e1599-602, 2010
2. Coffin CM et al: Gardner fibroma: a clinicopathologic and immunohistochemical analysis of 45 patients with 57 fibromas. Am J Surg Pathol. 31(3):410-6, 2007
3. Wehrli BM et al: Gardner-associated fibromas (GAF) in young patients: a distinct fibrous lesion that identifies unsuspected Gardner syndrome and risk for fibromatosis. Am J Surg Pathol. 25(5):645-51, 2001

IMAGE GALLERY

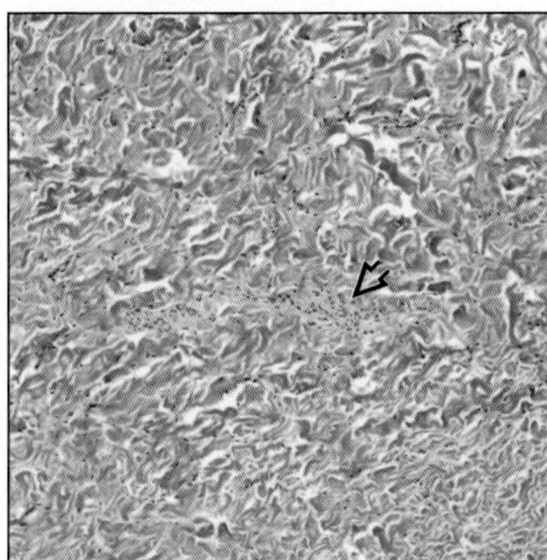

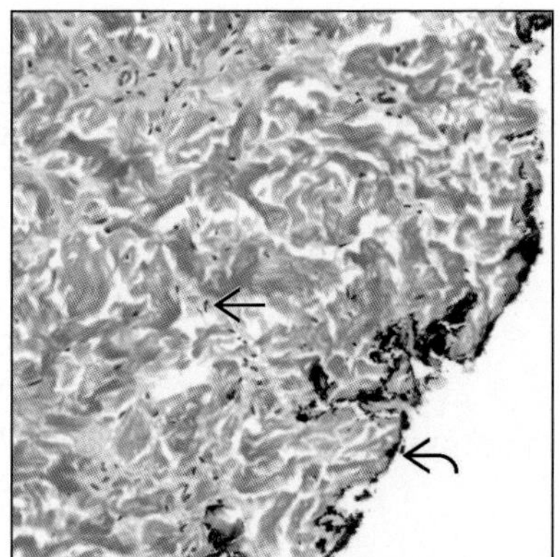

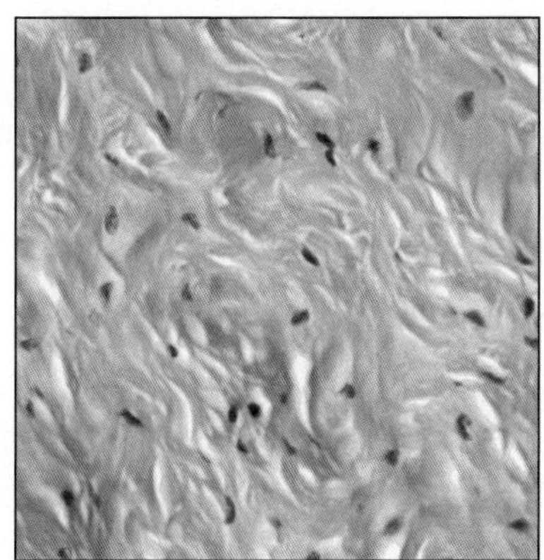

(Left) *This Gardner fibroma diffusely infiltrates the dermis and entraps a blood vessel ⇒.* ***(Center)*** *Hematoxylin & eosin shows a Gardner fibroma composed of thick collagen bundles without a patterned arrangement. Sparse fibroblasts → are embedded in the collagenous proliferation. The lesion shows an infiltrative growth pattern and extends to the inked margin ↩.* ***(Right)*** *High-power view of a Gardner fibroma shows bland spindle-shaped fibroblasts without atypia.*

FIBROUS HAMARTOMA OF INFANCY

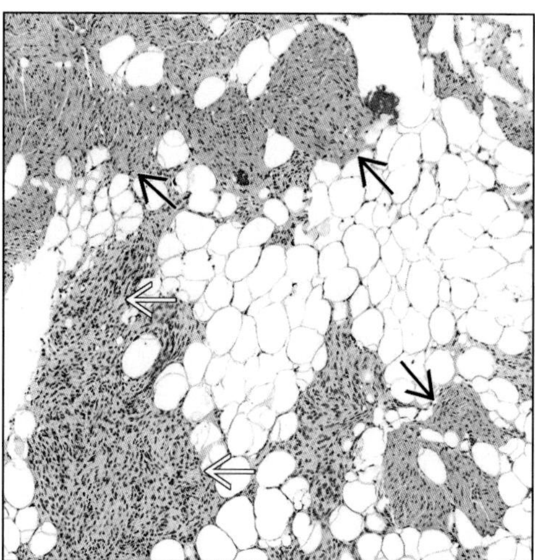

The triphasic pattern of FHI is easily seen here, with the fibrous component on the top and bottom right ⇒, immature mesenchymal component on the left ➡, and intervening adipose tissue.

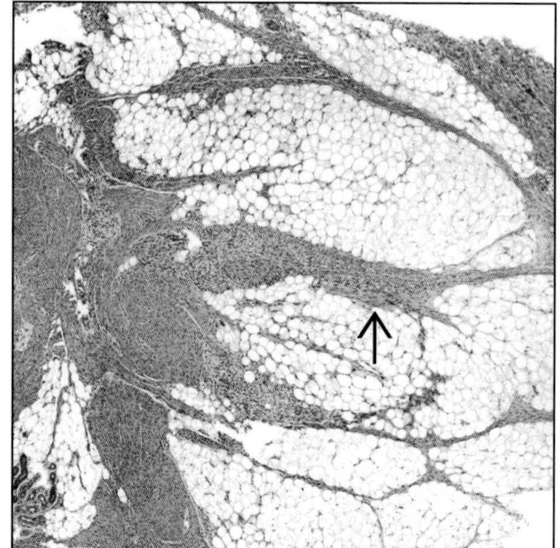

This low-power view shows the infiltrative nature of FHI ⇒. The adipose tissue seen here is likely part of the lesion, and it can be very difficult to determine negative surgical margins.

TERMINOLOGY

Abbreviations

- Fibrous hamartoma of infancy (FHI)

Synonyms

- Subdermal fibrous tumor of infancy

ETIOLOGY/PATHOGENESIS

Unknown

- Hamartomatous process favored over true neoplasm or reactive process
- Only rarely related to trauma

CLINICAL ISSUES

Epidemiology

- Age
  - Usually presents before 2 years of age
    - 15-25% present at birth
    - Only rarely in older children
- Gender
  - Seen more often in boys

Site

- Most common
  - Axillary fold, arm, thigh, inguinal area, shoulder, back
- Unusual
  - Hands and feet, head and neck

Presentation

- Rapidly growing mass in subcutis
  - Usually freely mobile
  - Occasionally involves underlying fascia or muscle
- Usually solitary
- No familial tendencies

Natural History

- Will not spontaneously regress

Treatment

- Complete surgical resection

Prognosis

- Benign
- Surgical resection is curative
  - May locally recur if not completely excised

MACROSCOPIC FEATURES

General Features

- Poorly circumscribed

Size

- Generally 3-5 cm
- Can be up to 15 cm

Gross Appearance

- Varies according to relative amounts of adipose and fibrous tissue
- Generally, gray-white rubbery cut surface with flecks of yellow

MICROSCOPIC PATHOLOGY

Histologic Features

- Triphasic
- Fibrous component
  - Orderly interlacing fascicles of fibroblasts
  - Straight to wavy nuclei
  - Collagenous stroma
- Immature mesenchymal cells
  - Sheets of undifferentiated spindled, stellate, or oval cells
  - Basophilic matrix
  - Often surround small veins

FIBROUS HAMARTOMA OF INFANCY

Key Facts

Clinical Issues
- Presents before 2 years of age
- Rapidly growing mass in subcutis
- Most commonly found in axillary fold
- Usually solitary

Macroscopic Features
- Poorly circumscribed

Microscopic Pathology
- Triphasic
  - Fibrous component, immature mesenchymal cells, mature adipose tissue

Top Differential Diagnoses
- Infantile fibromatosis, diffuse myofibromatosis, calcifying aponeurotic fibroma

- Mature adipose tissue
  - Amount varies
  - No clear delineation between fat of tumor and fat of surrounding normal tissue
- Occasionally, areas similar to neurofibroma can be seen

Predominant Pattern/Injury Type
- Organoid

ANCILLARY TESTS

Immunohistochemistry
- Vimentin is positive throughout lesion
- Fibrous areas positive for actin, sometimes desmin

DIFFERENTIAL DIAGNOSIS

Infantile Fibromatosis
- Arises primarily in muscle
- Lacks organoid pattern

Diffuse Myofibromatosis
- Contains hemangiopericytoma-like vessels

Calcifying Aponeurotic Fibroma
- Early phase may have no calcifications
- Should have cartilaginous component
- Older age group

Other Fibroblastic Proliferations
- Rarely can resemble
  - Neurofibroma
  - Giant cell fibroblastoma
  - Fibrolipoma
  - Desmoid tumor
  - Embryonal rhabdomyosarcoma, spindle cell form

SELECTED REFERENCES

1. Han HJ et al: A large infiltrating fibrous hamartoma of infancy in the abdominal wall with rare associated tuberous sclerosis. Pediatr Radiol. 39(7):743-6, 2009
2. Gupta R et al: Cytologic diagnosis of fibrous hamartoma of infancy: a case report of a rare soft tissue lesion. Acta Cytol. 52(2):201-3, 2008
3. Grynspan D et al: Cutaneous changes in fibrous hamartoma of infancy. J Cutan Pathol. 34(1):39-43, 2007
4. Rougemont AL et al: A complex translocation (6;12;8)(q25;q24.3;q13) in a fibrous hamartoma of infancy. Cancer Genet Cytogenet. 171(2):115-8, 2006
5. Dickey GE et al: Fibrous hamartoma of infancy: current review. Pediatr Dev Pathol. 2(3):236-43, 1999
6. Efem SE et al: Clinicopathological features of untreated fibrous hamartoma of infancy. J Clin Pathol. 46(6):522-4, 1993
7. Groisman G et al: Fibrous hamartoma of infancy: an immunohistochemical and ultrastructural study. Hum Pathol. 22(9):914-8, 1991
8. Enzinger FM: Fibrous hamartoma of infancy. Cancer. 18:241-8, 1965
9. Reye RD: A consideration of certain subdermal fibromatous tumours of infancy. J Pathol Bacteriol. 72(1):149-54, 1956

IMAGE GALLERY

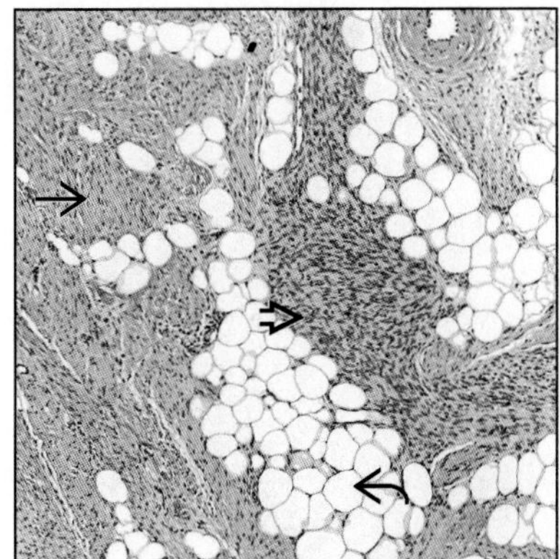
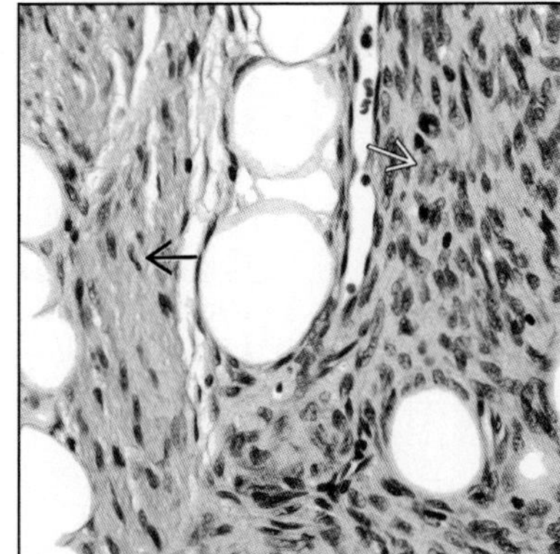
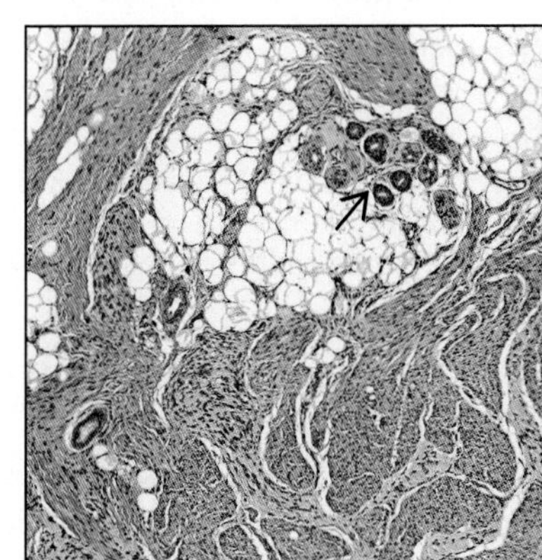

(Left) *The triphasic pattern of FHI is easily seen here. Note the fibrous component ⇒, immature mesenchymal component ⇒, and intervening adipose tissue ⇒.* ***(Center)*** *The fibrous component of FHI ⇒ is composed of fascicles of thin spindled cells with somewhat wavy nuclei in a pink, collagenous background. The immature mesenchymal component ➡ is composed of more plump cells in a basophilic matrix.* ***(Right)*** *This FHI has trapped dermal appendages ⇒.*

INCLUSION BODY FIBROMATOSIS

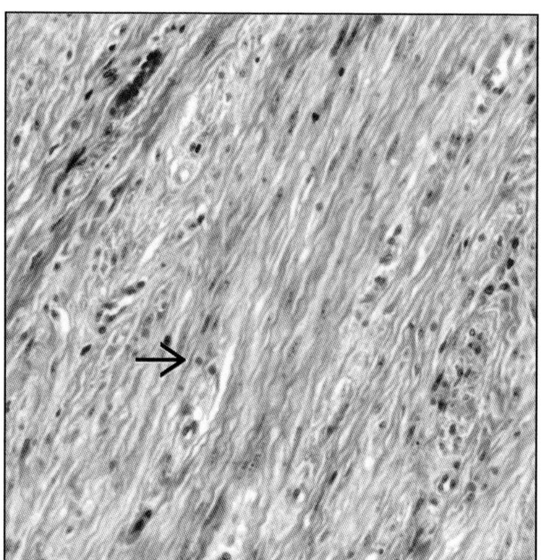

Hematoxylin & eosin at medium power shows intersecting fascicles of myofibroblasts, dense extracellular collagen, and scattered intracytoplasmic eosinophilic spherical inclusions ➔.

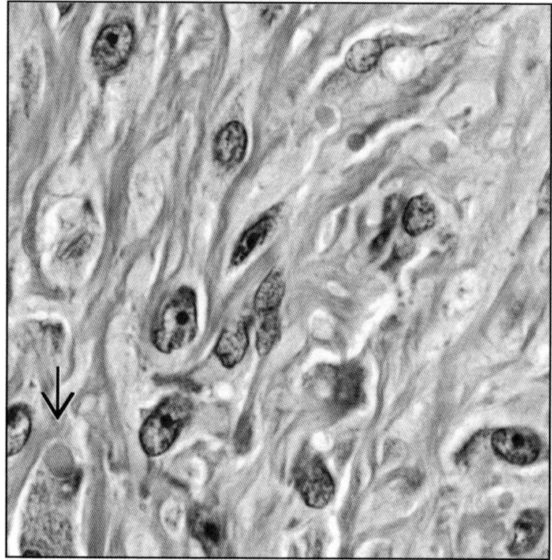

Hematoxylin & eosin at high power shows plump, bland-appearing myofibroblasts with scattered intracytoplasmic eosinophilic inclusions ➔.

TERMINOLOGY

Synonyms

- Infantile digital fibromatosis
- Digital fibrous tumor of childhood
- Infantile digital fibroma
- Reye tumor

Definitions

- Nodular proliferation of benign fibroblastic and myofibroblastic cells with characteristic intracytoplasmic eosinophilic spherical inclusions

CLINICAL ISSUES

Epidemiology

- Age
  - Present in 1st 3 years of life
    - ~ 1/3 are congenital

Site

- Typically located over dorsal or lateral aspect of digits
- Principle involvement of 2nd-5th digits
  - Thumb and great toe typically spared
- Extradigital presentation in soft tissue is rare

Presentation

- Broad-based or dome-shaped nodule
- Nontender
- Overlying skin is firm, stretched, and erythematous
- Up to 2 cm in diameter
- Functional impairment or deformity may be present

Natural History

- 12% of cases spontaneously involute over 2-3 years

Treatment

- Options, risks, complications
  - Observation recommended in absence of deformity and impairment
    - Spontaneous involution reported
- Surgical approaches
  - Complete surgical excision
    - 60-75% of cases recur upon excision
    - Lower recurrence rates reported with wider surgical excisions
  - Surgical excision recommended with
    - Functional impairment
    - Continued growth
    - Cosmetic concerns
  - Removal by Mohs micrographic surgery without recurrence reported

Prognosis

- Excellent overall prognosis
- Tendency for local recurrence
  - 60-75% of cases
- No evidence of
  - Aggressive behavior
  - Metastatic potential
  - Malignant transformation

MACROSCOPIC FEATURES

General Features

- Nodular firm mass covered by intact skin

Size

- Rarely exceeds 2 cm in diameter
  - Range of 0.3-3.5 cm reported in large series
  - Median size = 1 cm

Gross Features

- Solid, gray-white, cut surface
- Lacks hemorrhage
- Lacks necrosis

INCLUSION BODY FIBROMATOSIS

Key Facts

Terminology
- Nodular proliferation of benign fibroblastic and myofibroblastic cells with characteristic intracytoplasmic eosinophilic spherical inclusions

Clinical Issues
- Broad-based or dome-shaped, nontender nodule over dorsal or lateral aspect of digits
- Present in 1st 3 years of life
  - ~ 1/3 are congenital
- Extradigital presentation in soft tissue is rare
- Excellent overall prognosis
- Tendency for local recurrence (60-75% of cases)
- No evidence of aggressive behavior, metastatic potential, or malignant transformation
- Observation recommended in absence of deformity and impairment

Macroscopic Features
- Nodular firm mass covered by intact skin
- Rarely exceeds 2 cm in diameter

Microscopic Pathology
- Sheets and fascicles of uniform myofibroblastic cells with intracytoplasmic eosinophilic spherical inclusions
- Inclusions often perinuclear and stain bright red with Masson trichrome
- Dense collagenous stroma
- Overlying epidermis is often acanthotic with loss of rete ridges

Ancillary Tests
- Masson trichrome
  - Inclusions stain bright red

MICROSCOPIC PATHOLOGY

Predominant Pattern/Injury Type
- Fascicular
- Whorled
- Fibrous
- Diffuse
- Infiltrative
  - Entrapped adnexal structures and periadnexal fat

Predominant Cell/Compartment Type
- Myofibroblast

Microscopic Features
- Sheets and fascicles of uniform myofibroblastic cells
  - Fascicles often oriented perpendicular to skin surface
- Intracytoplasmic eosinophilic spherical inclusions
  - Inclusions often perinuclear in location
  - Variable size (3-15 μm) and lack of refringence help distinguish inclusions from erythrocytes
  - Composed of dense microfilaments
  - Stain bright red with Masson trichrome
  - Presence is characteristic but not required for diagnosis
- Dense collagenous stroma
- Overlying epidermis is often acanthotic with loss of rete ridges
  - Epidermal ulceration is rare
- Mitotic figures vary from rare to absent
- Rare, multinucleated giant cells

ANCILLARY TESTS

Histochemistry
- Masson trichrome
  - Reactivity: Positive
  - Staining pattern
    - Cytoplasmic inclusion
    - Inclusions stain bright red

DIFFERENTIAL DIAGNOSIS

Myofibroma
- Most cases present at birth or within 1st 2 years of life
- Frequently located in subcutaneous tissue of head and neck
- Nodular to multinodular proliferation of myofibroblasts surrounding vessels
- Variable zonal appearance
  - Hemangiopericytoma-like to hyalinized spindle cells
- Lack cytoplasmic inclusions

Fibroma of Tendon Sheath
- Frequently occurs in upper extremities and fingers
- Most commonly affect adults 20-50 years of age
- Histologic features may overlap with infantile digital fibromatosis
- Elongated cleft-like spaces along periphery are characteristic
- Lack cytoplasmic inclusions
- Desmin negative

Fibrous Hamartoma of Infancy
- Poorly circumscribed soft tissue mass
- Most commonly affects axillary folds, upper and lower extremities
- Admixture of mature adipose tissue, fibrous bands, and primitive mesenchymal cells
- Fibrous component lacks cytoplasmic inclusions

Palmar/Plantar Fibromatosis
- Fibroblastic proliferation of palmar and plantar soft tissues
- More frequently affects adults
- Associated with aponeurosis and subcutaneous fat
- Do not involve digits
- Lack cytoplasmic inclusions

Juvenile/Infantile Fibromatosis (Lipofibromatosis)
- Deep-seated, solitary, poorly circumscribed mass
- Most present in 1st 8 years of life

INCLUSION BODY FIBROMATOSIS

Immunohistochemistry

Antibody	Reactivity	Staining Pattern	Comment
Actin-sm	Positive	Cytoplasmic	Tram track pattern, increased reactivity with antigen retrieval
Calponin	Positive	Cytoplasmic	Diffuse pattern, strong reactivity
Desmin	Positive	Cytoplasmic	Diffuse pattern
CD99	Positive	Cell membrane	Variable reactivity
Vimentin	Positive	Cytoplasmic	Moderate reactivity

- Typically originate in skeletal muscle
- Most commonly affects
  - Head and neck
  - Shoulder
  - Upper arm
  - Thigh
- Rapid growth
- Wide spectrum of morphologic appearances
- Variable amounts of lipocytic elements (lipofibromatosis)
- Lack cytoplasmic inclusions
- Variable expression of smooth muscle actin, muscle-specific actin, and desmin

Calcifying Aponeurotic Fibroma

- Small tumor of palms, soles, and extremities of children
- Propensity for local recurrence
- Arises near tendons and aponeuroses
- Characteristic nodular deposits of calcification
- Lacks cytoplasmic inclusions
- Desmin negative

DIAGNOSTIC CHECKLIST

Clinically Relevant Pathologic Features

- Age distribution
  - Most present in 1st 3 years of life
  - 1/3 present at birth

Pathologic Interpretation Pearls

- Location
  - 2nd-5th digits
- Bland, dermal-based myofibroblastic proliferation
- Infiltration of adnexal structures and periadnexal fat
- Fascicles arranged perpendicular to skin surface
- Presence of cytoplasmic eosinophilic inclusions

MALPRACTICE CONSIDERATIONS

Management

- Tendency for local recurrence
  - 60-75% of cases
- Lower recurrence rates reported with wider surgical excisions
- No evidence of aggressive behavior, metastatic potential, or malignant transformation
- Margins often difficult to accurately evaluate
- Observation following initial biopsy diagnosis is recommended by most experts

SELECTED REFERENCES

1. Laskin WB et al: Infantile digital fibroma/fibromatosis: a clinicopathologic and immunohistochemical study of 69 tumors from 57 patients with long-term follow-up. Am J Surg Pathol. 33(1):1-13, 2009
2. Netscher DT et al: Non-malignant fibrosing tumors in the pediatric hand: a clinicopathologic case review. Hand (N Y). 4(1):2-11, 2009
3. Niamba P et al: Further documentation of spontaneous regression of infantile digital fibromatosis. Pediatr Dermatol. 24(3):280-4, 2007
4. Albertini JG et al: Infantile digital fibroma treated with mohs micrographic surgery. Dermatol Surg. 28(10):959-61, 2002
5. Kang SK et al: A case of congenital infantile digital fibromatosis. Pediatr Dermatol. 19(5):462-3, 2002
6. Kanwar AJ et al: Congenital infantile digital fibromatosis. Pediatr Dermatol. 19(4):370-1, 2002
7. Kawaguchi M et al: A case of infantile digital fibromatosis with spontaneous regression. J Dermatol. 25(8):523-6, 1998
8. Burgert S et al: Recurring digital fibroma of childhood. J Hand Surg [Br]. 21(3):400-2, 1996
9. Coffin CM et al: Fibroblastic-myofibroblastic tumors in children and adolescents: a clinicopathologic study of 108 examples in 103 patients. Pediatr Pathol. 11(4):569-88, 1991
10. Choi KC et al: Infantile digital fibromatosis. Immunohistochemical and immunoelectron microscopic studies. J Cutan Pathol. 17(4):225-32, 1990
11. Mukai M et al: Infantile digital fibromatosis. An electron microscopic and immunohistochemical study. Acta Pathol Jpn. 36(11):1605-15, 1986
12. Chung EB: Pitfalls in diagnosing benign soft tissue tumors in infancy and childhood. Pathol Annu. 20 Pt 2:323-86, 1985
13. Bhawan J et al: A myofibroblastic tumor. Infantile digital fibroma (recurrent digital fibrous tumor of childhood). Am J Pathol. 94(1):19-36, 1979
14. Beckett JH et al: Recurring digital fibrous tumors of childhood: a review. Pediatrics. 59(3):401-6, 1977
15. Bloem JJ et al: Recurring digital fibroma of infancy. J Bone Joint Surg Br. 56-B(4):746-51, 1974
16. Allen PW: Recurring digital fibrous tumours of childhood. Pathology. 4(3):215-23, 1972

Clinical and Microscopic Features

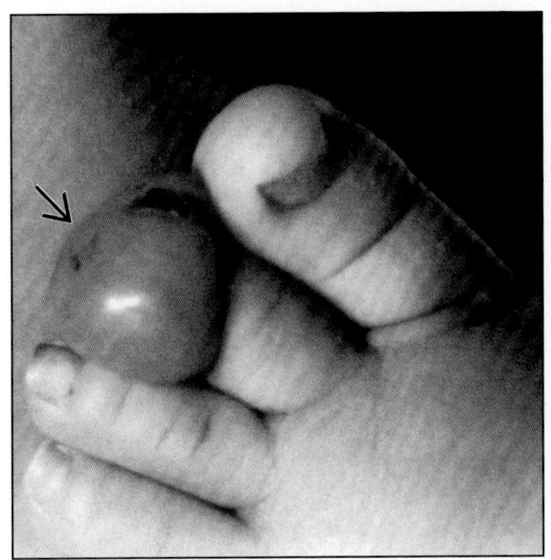

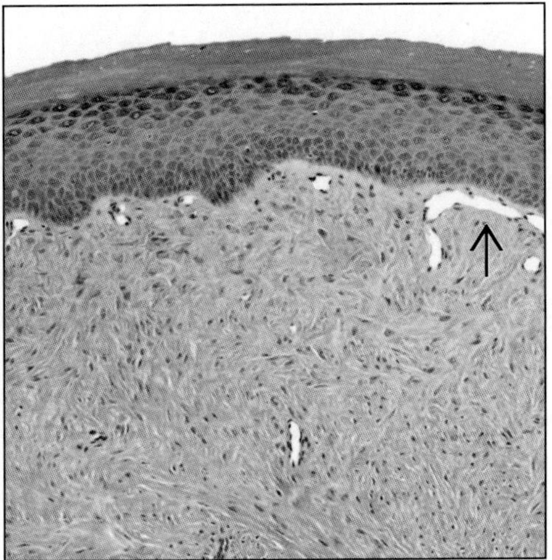

(Left) *Infantile digital fibromatosis is shown. A single nodule ➔ overlies the distal interphalangeal joint of the left foot. Note the taut and stretched overlying skin and lack of ulceration. (Courtesy R. Flinner, MD.)* ***(Right)*** *Hematoxylin & eosin at low power shows a dermal-based spindle cell proliferation with moderate acanthosis and flattening of the rete ridges. The dilated vessels ➔ shown here are often present in the superficial aspects of this lesion.*

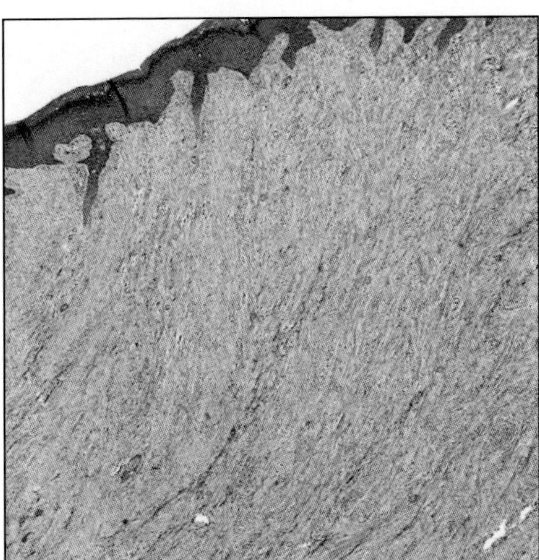

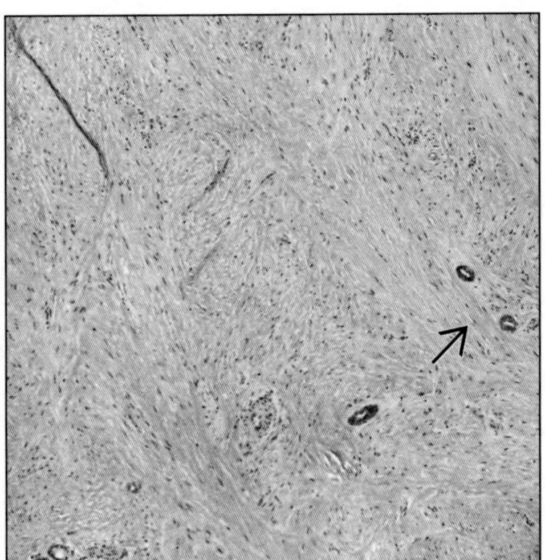

(Left) *Hematoxylin & eosin shows fascicles of bland spindle cells radiating perpendicular to the overlying skin surface.* ***(Right)*** *Hematoxylin & eosin shows bland spindle cells arranged in fascicles with scattered entrapped adnexal structures ➔.*

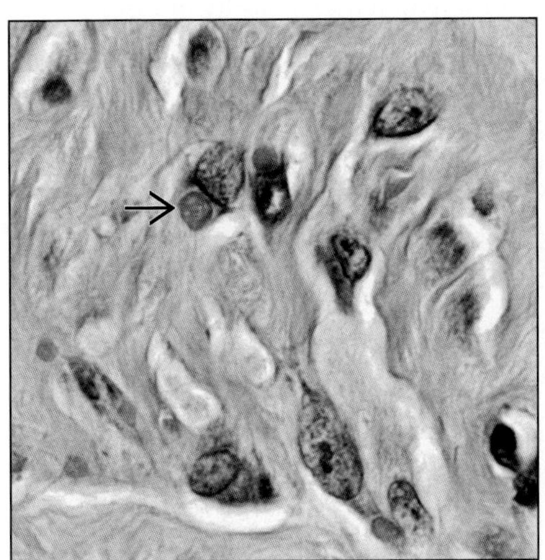

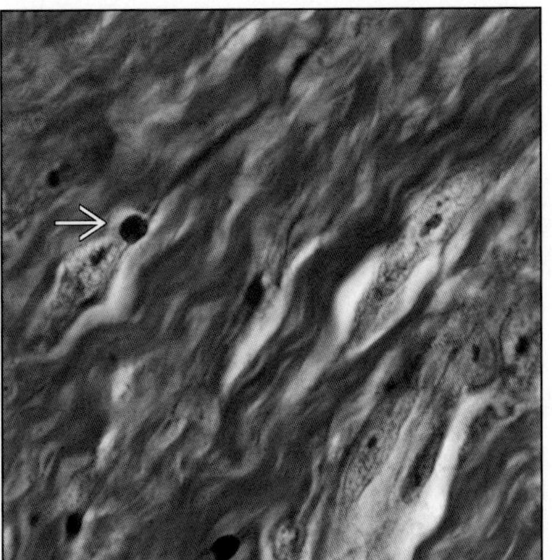

(Left) *Hematoxylin & eosin at high power highlights the numerous cytoplasmic/ perinuclear eosinophilic spherical inclusions ➔ characteristic of infantile digital fibromatosis.* ***(Right)*** *Masson trichrome highlights the dense collagenous stroma that surrounds the plump myofibroblasts. Several cytoplasmic/ perinuclear spherical inclusions ➔ show the bright red staining pattern typical of this stain.*

FIBROMATOSIS COLLI

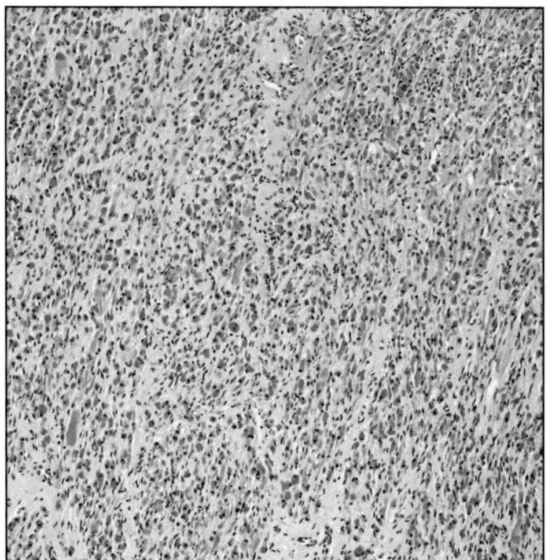

Hematoxylin & eosin shows diffuse fibrosis separating muscle fibers and imparting a fine checkerboard-like pattern in this biopsy specimen from the sternomastoid muscle.

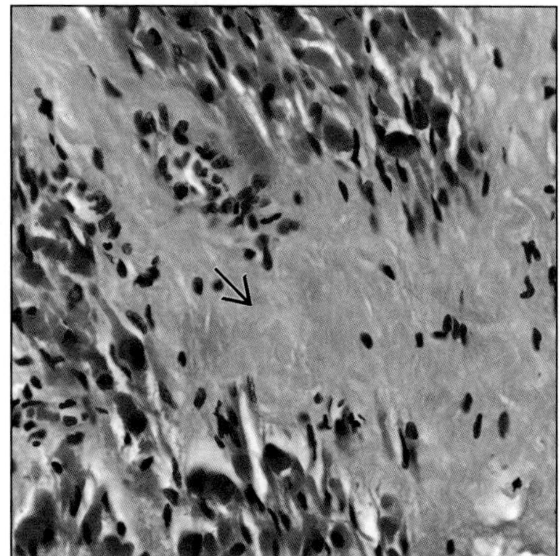

Hematoxylin & eosin shows hypocellular, finely fibrillary collagen forming a focus of confluent fibrosis ⇒ in this late-stage example of fibromatosis colli.

TERMINOLOGY

Synonyms

- Sternomastoid tumor
- Congenital muscular torticollis
  - Clinical condition with several associated factors
  - Only up to 1/3 have fibromatosis colli

Definitions

- Benign fibrous growth of sternocleidomastoid muscle

ETIOLOGY/PATHOGENESIS

Developmental Anomaly

- Most cases develop spontaneously
  - Presumed relation to intrauterine trauma
- Rarely familial

Environmental Exposure

- Obstetric trauma has been proposed as causal factor
  - Breech or forceps delivery
- Associated with muscular torticollis
  - Synchronous or delayed
- Associated with congenital dislocation of hip, anomalies of foot

CLINICAL ISSUES

Epidemiology

- Incidence
  - Rare, < 1% of newborns
  - Although rare, it is one of the more common fibrous tumors of childhood
- Age
  - Congenital or within 1st 6 months
- Gender
  - Equal incidence

Site

- Lower 1/3 of sternomastoid muscle
- Rarely in trapezius muscle

Presentation

- Painless mass
- Unilateral, with predilection for right side
- Grows rapidly at first, then stops and persists
- Mass is mobile and does not involve the skin
- Head will rotate and tilt toward affected side

Natural History

- 90% of cases eventually regress by age of 1-2 years
- Approximately 10% persist
  - Cervicofacial asymmetry

Treatment

- Options, risks, complications
  - Physiotherapy with stretching in early stages
- Surgical approaches
  - No intervention required in majority of cases
  - Surgery can be required for persistent cases

Prognosis

- Excellent in most cases
- Worse in patients older than 1 year
  - Fibrosis leads to shortening of muscle and deformity

MACROSCOPIC FEATURES

General Features

- Firm, white, fibrous lesion involving part of the muscle
- Infiltrative border within the muscle
- Does not extend into adjacent soft tissue

Size

- Average: 1-3 cm in diameter

FIBROMATOSIS COLLI

Key Facts

Terminology
- Fibrosing lesion of infants involving muscles of head and neck

Etiology/Pathogenesis
- Rarely familial
- Obstetric trauma has been proposed as causal factor
  - Breech or forceps delivery
- Found in up to 1/3 of cases of congenital torticollis

Clinical Issues
- Majority in lower 1/3 of sternomastoid muscle
- Grows rapidly at first, then stops and persists
- Most cases eventually regress

Microscopic Pathology
- Variably cellular fibroblastic infiltrate between skeletal muscle bundles
- Early stage more cellular, followed by scarring
- Muscle fibers swell, then atrophy

MICROSCOPIC PATHOLOGY

Histologic Features
- Variably cellular fibroblastic infiltrate between skeletal muscle bundles
  - No significant nuclear hyperchromasia
  - No pleomorphism
  - Lacks significant mitotic activity
- Early stage is proliferative and more cellular
- Fibrosis in later stages
  - Infiltrates between muscle fibers in fine checkerboard-like pattern
  - Eventual confluent scarring
- Muscle fibers swell, then atrophy
  - Occasional fiber regeneration
  - Loss of cross-striations
  - Proliferation of sarcolemmal nuclei
- Minimal inflammation, no necrosis or atypia

ANCILLARY TESTS

Immunohistochemistry
- Infiltrating fibroblasts are SMA(+) in early stages
- Lesional cells are β-catenin(-)

DIFFERENTIAL DIAGNOSIS

Nodular Fasciitis
- More circumscribed
- Does not infiltrate between muscle bundles
- Myxoid and storiform areas
- Extravasated red blood cells, lymphocytes

Fibromatosis
- Discrete mass
- Parallel-aligned myofibroblasts
- Mast cells
- β-catenin immunoreactivity in nuclei

SELECTED REFERENCES

1. Lowry KC et al: The presentation and management of fibromatosis colli. Ear Nose Throat J. 89(9):E4-8, 2010
2. Smiti S et al: Case report: fibromatosis colli in a neonate. Indian J Radiol Imaging. 20(1):45-6, 2010
3. Thway K et al: Beta-catenin expression in pediatric fibroblastic and myofibroblastic lesions: a study of 100 cases. Pediatr Dev Pathol. 12(4):292-6, 2009
4. Tatli B et al: Congenital muscular torticollis: evaluation and classification. Pediatr Neurol. 34(1):41-4, 2006
5. Cheng JC et al: The clinical presentation and outcome of treatment of congenital muscular torticollis in infants--a study of 1,086 cases. J Pediatr Surg. 35(7):1091-6, 2000
6. Ho BC et al: Epidemiology, presentation and management of congenital muscular torticollis. Singapore Med J. 40(11):675-9, 1999
7. Lawrence WT et al: Congenital muscular torticollis: a spectrum of pathology. Ann Plast Surg. 23(6):523-30, 1989

IMAGE GALLERY

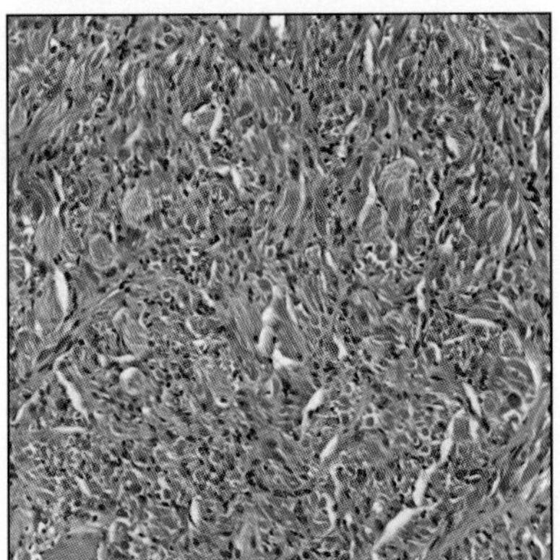

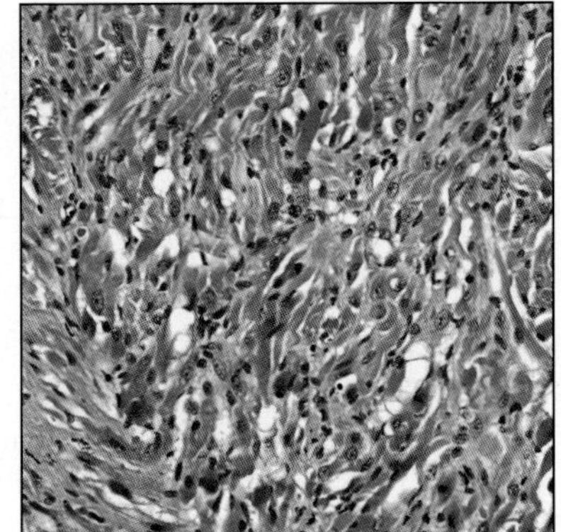

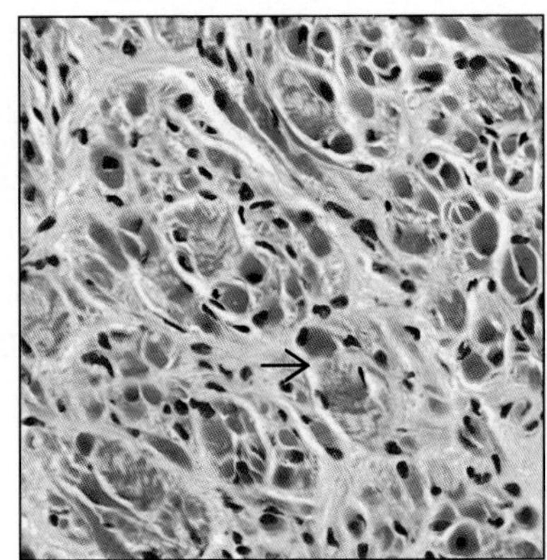

*(**Left**) Hematoxylin & eosin shows early-stage fibromatosis colli with cellular infiltrate between muscle fibers. The infiltrate includes cellular fibrous tissue and inflammatory cells. The muscle fibers undergo swelling, then atrophy. (**Center**) Hematoxylin & eosin shows early fibrosis with atrophy of skeletal muscle fibers. Fatty replacement of atrophied muscle is not a feature of this condition. (**Right**) Hematoxylin & eosin shows late-stage fibrosis with reduction in size of muscle fibers. The skeletal muscle is dissected by the fibrous tissue into small groups of fibers ⇒.*

DESMOID FIBROMATOSIS

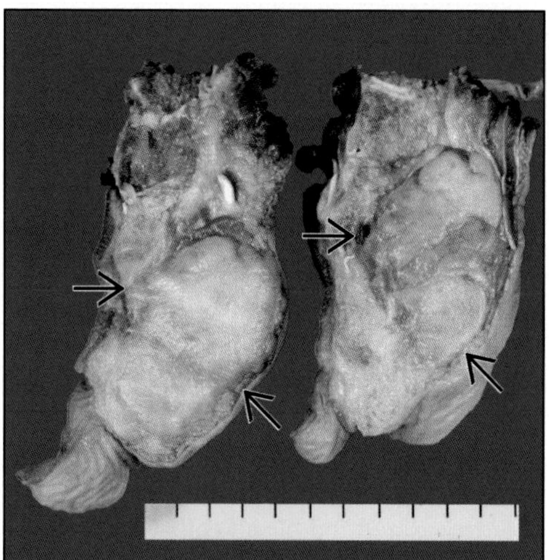

Cut section of a distal foot reveals a firm to hard gray-pink mass corresponding to a desmoid tumor ➔. The mass infiltrates extensively around, but not into, the surrounding metatarsal bones.

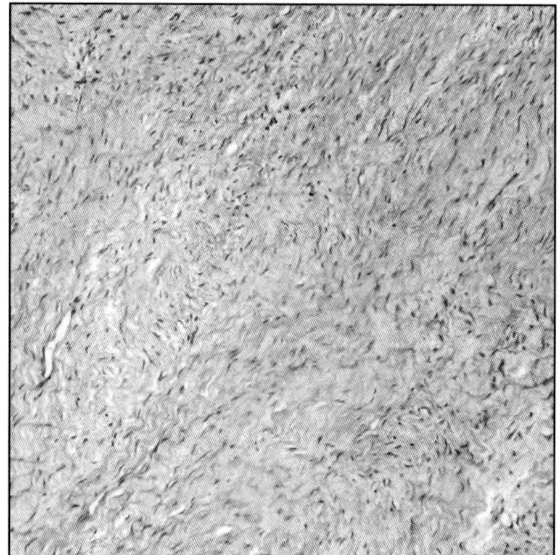

H&E stained section reveals sweeping fascicles of spindle cells with elongated nuclei. The stroma varies from myxoid to collagenous. Nuclear features are bland, and mitoses are scarce.

TERMINOLOGY

Abbreviations

- Desmoid fibromatosis (DF)

Synonyms

- Aggressive fibromatosis (AF)
- Abdominal fibromatosis
- Intraabdominal fibromatosis
- Extraabdominal fibromatosis
- Deep fibromatosis

Definitions

- Soft tissue tumor arising principally from the connective tissue of muscle and overlying fascia
- Clonal neoplasm that consists of elongated fibroblastic and myofibroblastic cells
- Although nonmetastasizing, has significant potential for local invasion and recurrence

ETIOLOGY/PATHOGENESIS

Molecular

- Likely related to somatic mutations of adenomatous polyposis coli (*APC*) and β-catenin genes
  - Both are components of the Wnt signaling pathway

Other

- Most likely multifactorial including genetic predisposition, endocrine factors, and trauma
  - Associations with surgical trauma have been reported in Gardner fibromatoses

CLINICAL ISSUES

Epidemiology

- Incidence
  - Peak incidence during 2nd and 3rd decades; 5% of patients are ≤ 10 years old
  - Incidence of DF in childhood is estimated at 2-4 new diagnoses per 1,000,000 per year
- Gender
  - Childhood DF has slight male predominance
  - Women more commonly affected in adulthood

Site

- Extraabdominal: Predilection for shoulder, chest wall, back, thigh, head and neck
- Abdominal: Abdominal wall, especially rectus and internal oblique muscles and fascia
- Intraabdominal: Pelvis, mesentery, fibromatosis of Gardner syndrome

Presentation

- Most common location for DF in the pediatric age group is extraabdominal
- Abdominal tumors in young women often occur during or following pregnancy
- Can be a component of Gardner syndrome
  - Autosomal dominant syndrome comprised of desmoid tumors, familial adenomatous polyposis, osteomas, and epidermal or sebaceous cysts
  - Gardner syndrome patients harbor germline mutations in *APC* gene
  - Gardner fibromatoses tend to be mesenteric and are more likely to be multicentric
- Incidence of fibromatosis is much higher in families with familial DF and Gardner syndrome

Treatment

- Primary surgery unless there is risk of significant mutilation or impairment
- Role of adjuvant radiotherapy &/or chemotherapy in childhood DF has not been established to date

Prognosis

- Recurrence rate of 50% reported in children with DF
  - Abdominal tumors tend to have lower recurrence rate and are less aggressive than extraabdominal tumors

DESMOID FIBROMATOSIS

Key Facts

Terminology
- Abdominal fibromatosis, intraabdominal fibromatosis, extraabdominal fibromatosis, deep fibromatosis
- Soft tissue tumor arising principally from connective tissue of muscle and overlying fascia
- Clonal neoplasm that consists of elongated, fibroblastic and myofibroblastic cells
- Although nonmetastasizing, has significant potential for local invasion and recurrence

Clinical Issues
- Extraabdominal: Predilection for shoulder, chest wall, back, thigh, head and neck
- Abdominal: Abdominal wall, especially rectus and internal oblique muscles and fascia
- Intraabdominal: Pelvis, mesentery, fibromatosis of Gardner syndrome

Microscopic Pathology
- Poorly circumscribed and infiltrative
- Sweeping fascicles of uniform, bland, elongated spindled fibroblasts interspersed with collagen
- Nuclei lack atypia or hyperchromasia; mitoses are rare

Ancillary Tests
- Positive nuclear staining for β-catenin

Top Differential Diagnoses
- Myofibroma/myofibromatosis
- Low-grade fibromyxoid sarcoma
- Superficial fibromatosis (plantar, palmar, penile)

- Recurrence rate is considerably higher in Gardner syndrome
  - Risk of desmoid tumors in familial polyposis patients reported to be 852x that of the general population
- Mortality is rare

MACROSCOPIC FEATURES

General Features
- Most tumors are 5-10 cm in greatest dimension
- Most are solitary; 5% are multicentric
- Firm, gritty cut surface that is white-tan and trabeculated

MICROSCOPIC PATHOLOGY

Histologic Features
- Poorly circumscribed and infiltrative, usually into adjacent skeletal muscle
- Sweeping fascicles of uniform, bland, elongated spindled fibroblasts interspersed with collagen deposition
  - Fibroblasts may be stellate shaped in some areas
  - Collagen deposition is usually abundant, and may be keloid-like
  - Myxoid areas can be seen, and are usually prominent in mesenteric DF
- Nuclei lack atypia or hyperchromasia
  - Small, delicate micronuclei
- Characteristic prominent vasculature
- Mitoses are rare
- Fibromatosis associated with Gardner syndrome
  - Histology very similar to sporadic cases
  - These lesions engulf surrounding fat and normal structures in contrast to tentacle-like extensions of sporadic DF
  - Does not tend to have long sweeping fascicles

ANCILLARY TESTS

Immunohistochemistry
- Positive nuclear staining for β-catenin can be helpful in distinguishing DF from other fibroblastic and myofibroblastic tumors
  - Nuclear positivity is thought to be supportive of but not definitive for DF diagnosis
  - Negativity does not preclude a diagnosis of DF

Molecular Genetics
- β-catenin gene mutations reported in ≤ 74% of sporadic deep fibromatoses and in virtually 100% of Gardner-associated fibromatoses
- Somatic *APC* gene mutations (chromosome 5q22) have been reported in 21% of sporadic cases of adult DF

Electron Microscopy
- Prominent rough endoplasmic reticulum
- Mature collagen fibers in extracellular space

DIFFERENTIAL DIAGNOSIS

Myofibroma/Myofibromatosis
- Characteristic zonation pattern
- Negative nuclear staining for β-catenin
- Positive for vimentin, smooth muscle actin, and muscle specific actin

Solitary Fibrous Tumor
- Patternless pattern of spindle cells
- CD34(+)

Low-Grade Fibromyxoid Sarcoma
- Fibrous hypocellular areas adjacent to cellular myxoid areas with spindle cells arranged in a swirling pattern around blood vessels
- Collagenous rosette formation
- Negative nuclear staining with β-catenin
- Typically occurs in young to middle-aged adults, but can occur in children

DESMOID FIBROMATOSIS

Comparative Immunohistochemistry of Desmoid Tumor and Other Deep-seated Fibromatoses

Stain	Desmoid Fibromatosis	Fibroblastic/ Myofibroblastic Tumors	GIST	Solitary Fibrous Tumor
β-catenin-nuclear	+	-	-	-/+
Desmin	-/+	-	-	-
C-Kit	-/+	-	+	-
CD34	-	-	+	+

GIST = gastrointestinal stromal tumor.

Gastrointestinal Stromal Tumor (GIST)

- Usually involves muscularis propria of stomach
- Spindled or epithelioid tumor cells
- Most are positive for C-Kit and CD34

Leiomyosarcoma

- Perpendicularly oriented fascicles of spindle cells
- Atypical blunt-ended nuclei with paranuclear vacuoles and increased mitoses
- Negative for β-catenin, positive for desmin
- Rare in children

Myxofibrosarcoma

- Nuclear atypia present
- Usually presents in extremities of elderly patients

Fibrosarcoma

- Cellular herringbone fascicular pattern

Nodular Fasciitis

- Loose storiform pattern with scattered inflammatory cells, osteoclast-type giant cells, and extravasated erythrocytes
- Myxoid areas and scattered keloid-like collagen
- Negative nuclear staining with β-catenin

Inflammatory Myofibroblastic Tumor

- Abundant chronic inflammatory infiltrate
- ALK(+) in 60% of cases

Sclerosing Mesenteritis

- Affects small bowel mesentery most commonly, usually as an isolated large mass
- Consists of fibrous bands infiltrating and encasing fat lobules with associated mixed inflammatory cells
- Negative nuclear staining for β-catenin

Superficial Fibromatosis (Plantar, Palmar, Penile)

- Palmar and penile fibromatoses are unusual in childhood
- Very similar to deep fibromatoses histologically, but the location is superficial
- Some degree of nuclear accumulation of β-catenin present on immunohistochemistry, but negative for detectable *APC* or *β-catenin* mutations

SELECTED REFERENCES

1. Wu C et al: Aggressive fibromatosis (desmoid tumor) is derived from mesenchymal progenitor cells. Cancer Res. 70(19):7690-8, 2010
2. Lips DJ et al: The role of APC and beta-catenin in the aetiology of aggressive fibromatosis (desmoid tumors). Eur J Surg Oncol. 35(1):3-10, 2009
3. Thway K et al: Beta-catenin expression in pediatric fibroblastic and myofibroblastic lesions: a study of 100 cases. Pediatr Dev Pathol. 12(4):292-6, 2009
4. Miyaki M et al: Difference in characteristics of APC mutations between colonic and extracolonic tumors of FAP patients: variations with phenotype. Int J Cancer. 122(11):2491-7, 2008
5. Carlson JW et al: Immunohistochemistry for beta-catenin in the differential diagnosis of spindle cell lesions: analysis of a series and review of the literature. Histopathology. 51(4):509-14, 2007
6. Jilong Y et al: Analysis of APC/beta-catenin genes mutations and Wnt signalling pathway in desmoid-type fibromatosis. Pathology. 39(3):319-25, 2007
7. Owens CL et al: Deep fibromatosis (desmoid tumor): cytopathologic characteristics, clinicoradiologic features, and immunohistochemical findings on fine-needle aspiration. Cancer. 111(3):166-72, 2007
8. Bhattacharya B et al: Nuclear beta-catenin expression distinguishes deep fibromatosis from other benign and malignant fibroblastic and myofibroblastic lesions. Am J Surg Pathol. 29(5):653-9, 2005
9. Buitendijk S et al: Pediatric aggressive fibromatosis: a retrospective analysis of 13 patients and review of literature. Cancer. 104(5):1090-9, 2005
10. Fetsch JF et al: Palmar-plantar fibromatosis in children and preadolescents: a clinicopathologic study of 56 cases with newly recognized demographics and extended follow-up information. Am J Surg Pathol. 29(8):1095-105, 2005
11. Montgomery E et al: Beta-catenin immunohistochemistry separates mesenteric fibromatosis from gastrointestinal stromal tumor and sclerosing mesenteritis. Am J Surg Pathol. 26(10):1296-301, 2002
12. Montgomery E et al: Superficial fibromatoses are genetically distinct from deep fibromatoses. Mod Pathol. 14(7):695-701, 2001
13. Wehrli BM et al: Gardner-associated fibromas (GAF) in young patients: a distinct fibrous lesion that identifies unsuspected Gardner syndrome and risk for fibromatosis. Am J Surg Pathol. 25(5):645-51, 2001
14. Coffin CM et al: Fibroblastic-myofibroblastic tumors in children and adolescents: a clinicopathologic study of 108 examples in 103 patients. Pediatr Pathol. 11(4):569-88, 1991

Radiologic and Microscopic Features

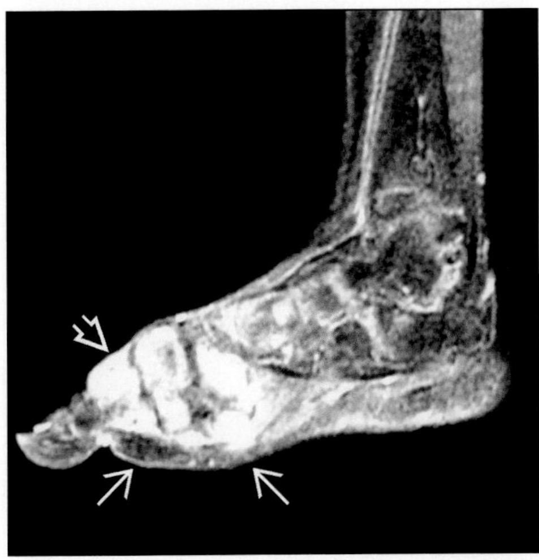

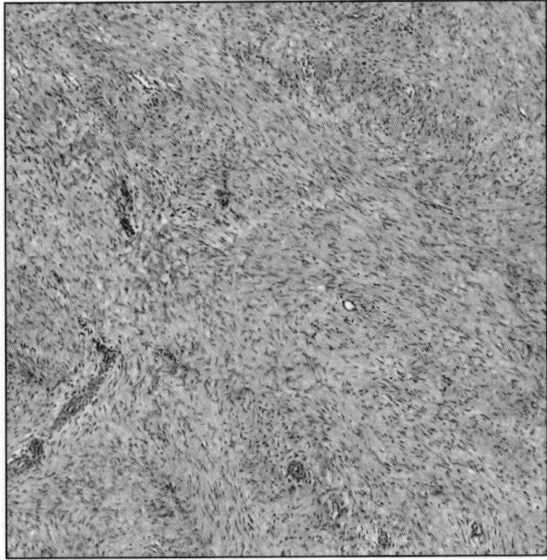

(Left) *Magnetic resonance imaging (MRI) reveals a lobulated soft tissue mass ➡ extending from the plantar soft tissues between the metatarsal bones to involve the dorsal subcutaneous tissues of the foot superiorly ➡.* ***(Right)*** *This low-power view reveals a spindle cell lesion of moderate cellularity in a fascicular arrangement. The background shows variable collagenization. No atypia or mitoses are noted. Stroma may be predominantly collagenous or predominantly myxoid.*

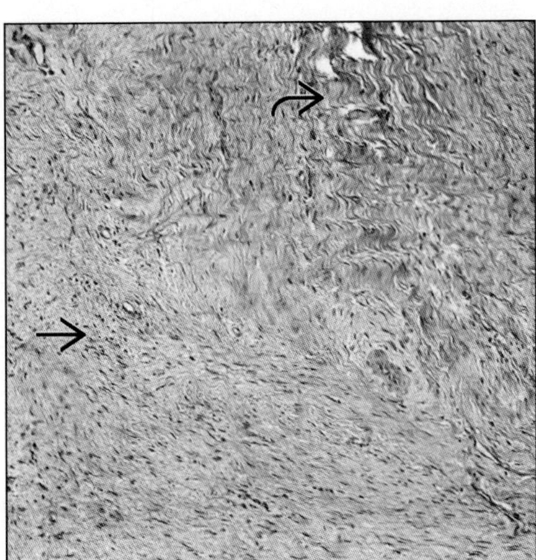

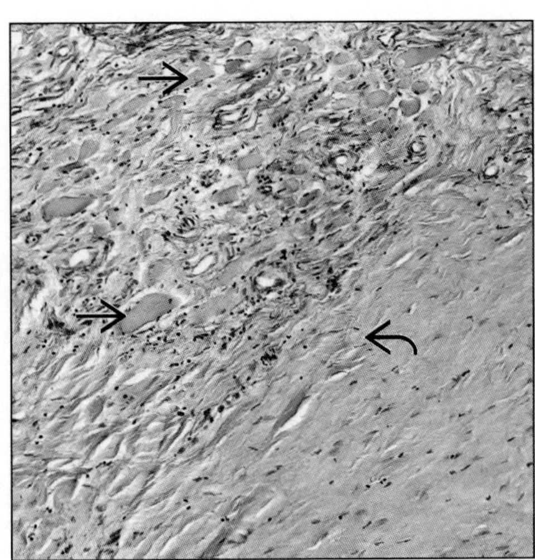

(Left) *This image highlights a loosely cellular, myxoid area ➡ adjacent to an area with a dense, collagenous stroma ➡. Thick, keloid-like collagen can be present in some cases.* ***(Right)*** *Desmoid fibromatosis is an invasive lesion that extends into adjacent soft tissues. This image depicts a densely collagenous desmoid tumor invading adjacent skeletal muscle ➡. Note residual skeletal muscle fibers ➡. Degenerative changes are noted in the skeletal muscle.*

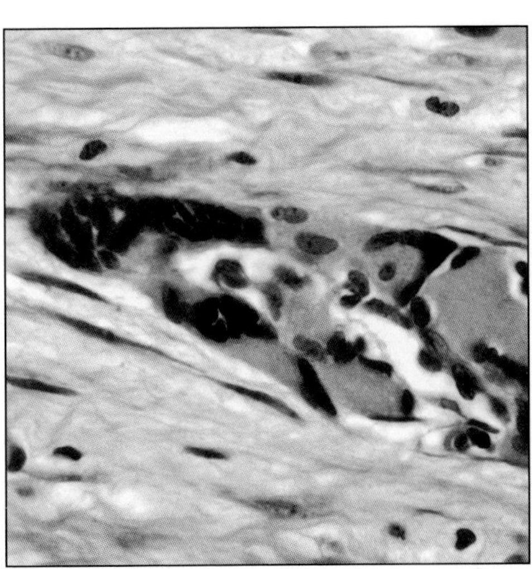

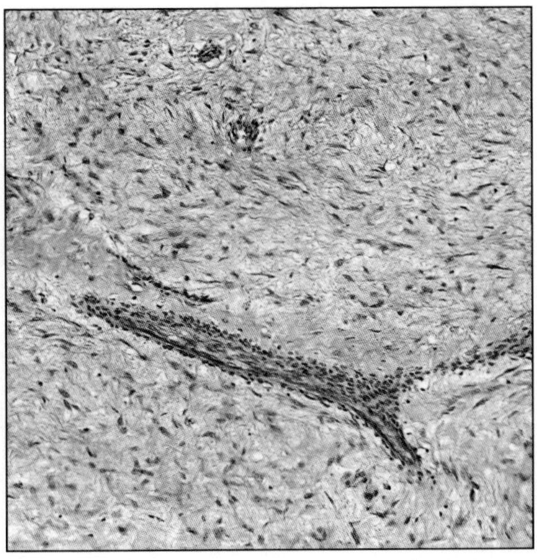

(Left) *Entrapped degenerating skeletal muscle fibers within a deep fibromatosis may present as clusters of multinucleated giant cells. (Courtesy E. Montgomery, MD.)* ***(Right)*** *Prominent vasculature is a characteristic finding in desmoid fibromatosis.*

DESMOID FIBROMATOSIS

Microscopic and Radiologic Features

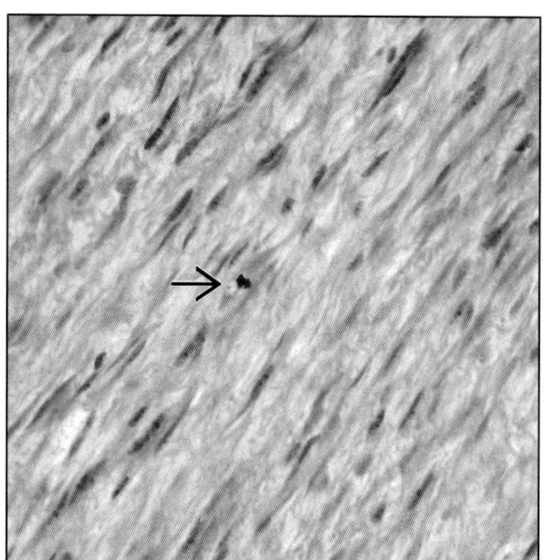
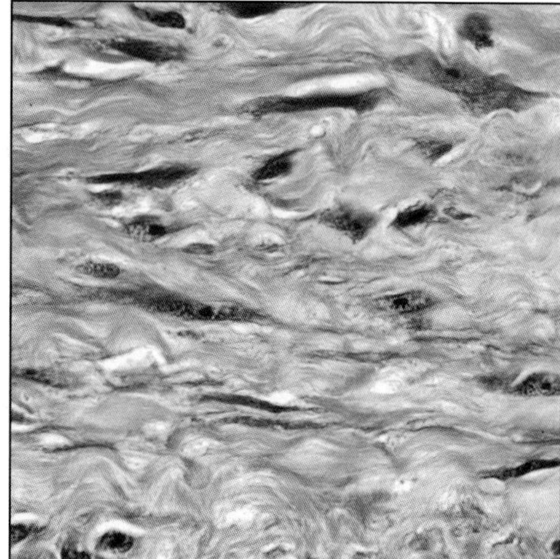

(Left) *Mitotic figures are usually rare in desmoid fibromatosis, although numerous mitoses may be seen in some cases. When present, mitoses are typical in appearance ⇒.* ***(Right)*** *High magnification of desmoid fibromatosis shows nuclei with a single inconspicuous nucleolus and bipolar or stellate cytoplasm. (Courtesy E. Montgomery, MD.)*

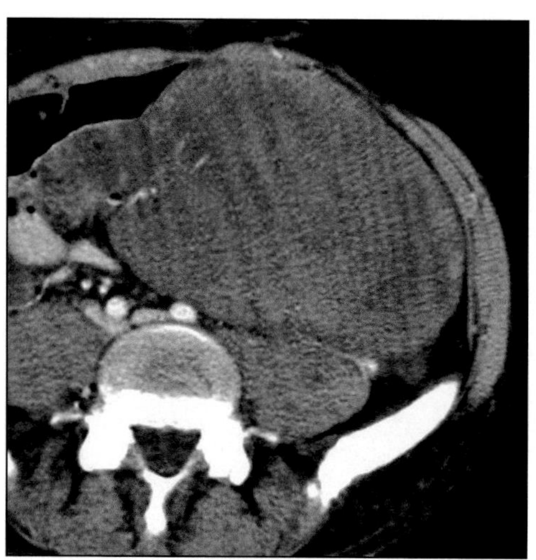
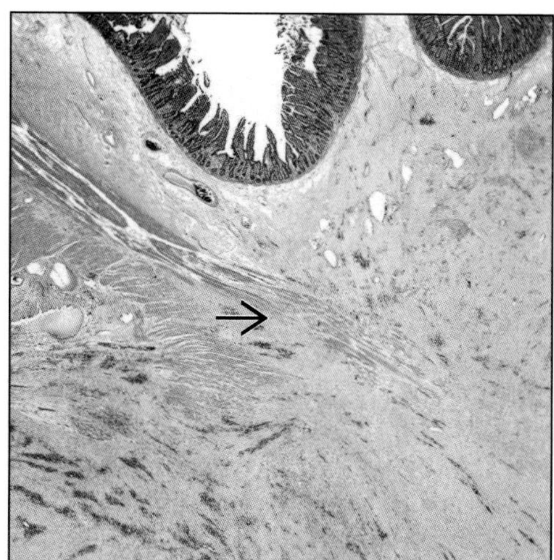

(Left) *Axial CECT 20 months following a colectomy for Gardner syndrome shows rapid growth of a mesenteric mass (desmoid tumor).* ***(Right)*** *Low-power magnification reveals a mesenteric fibromatosis occurring in the small intestine. The tumor originates in the mesentery and has infiltrated the adjacent muscularis propria of the small bowel ⇒. (Courtesy E. Montgomery, MD.)*

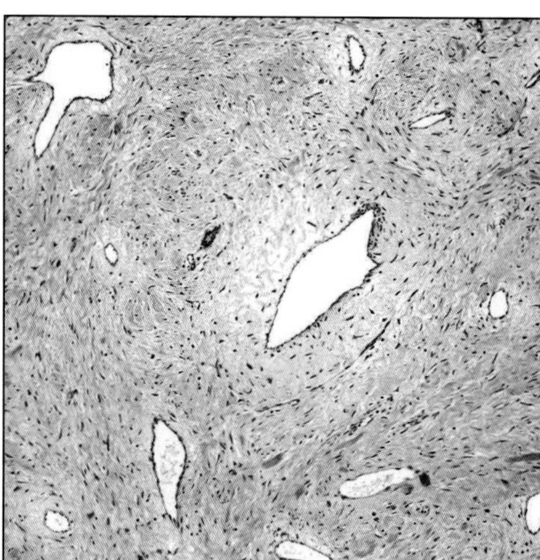
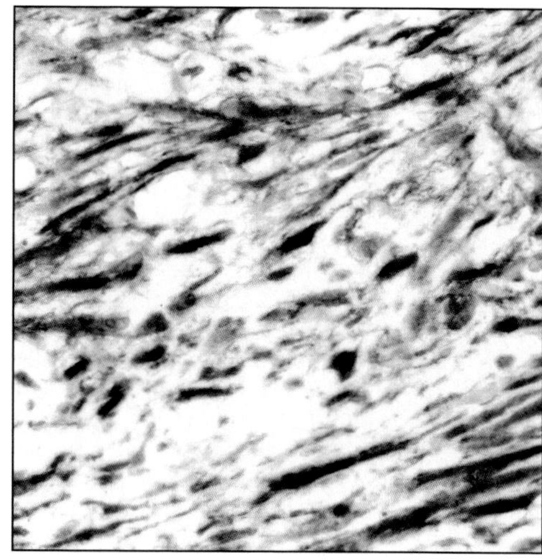

(Left) *H&E stained section of a mesenteric fibromatosis shows the dilated vessels and myxoid matrix that are most characteristic of fibromas in this location. (Courtesy E. Montgomery, MD.)* ***(Right)*** *β-catenin stain demonstrates nuclear staining in a desmoid fibromatosis. This finding reflects the presence of APC or β-catenin mutations. (Courtesy E. Montgomery, MD.)*

Microscopic Features and Differential Diagnosis

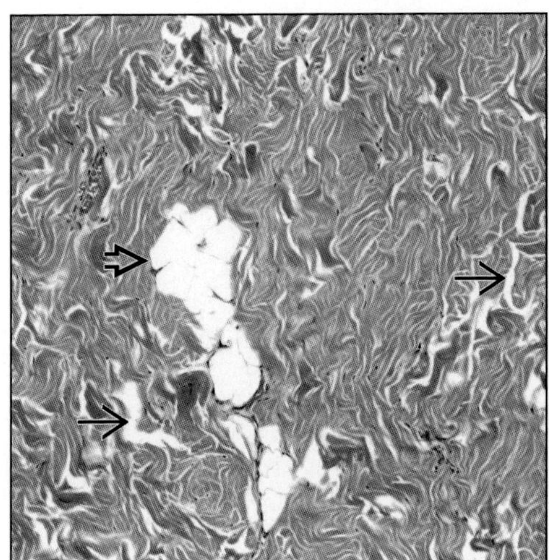

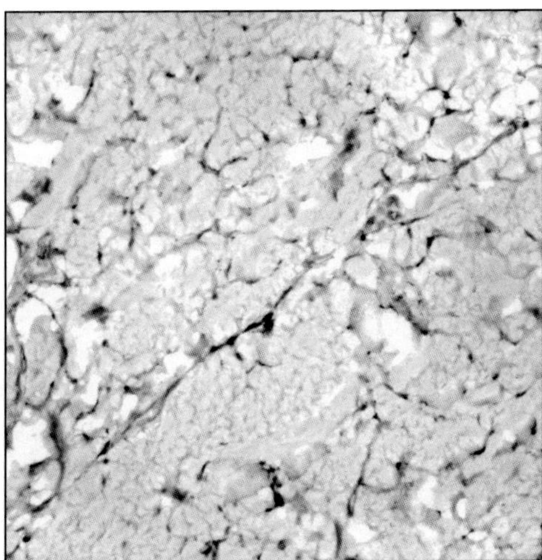

(Left) *This H&E stained section depicts a mesenteric fibromatosis associated with Gardner syndrome. These tumors tend to infiltrate and entrap mesenteric fat ⇨. The background is hypocellular, composed of thick, haphazardly arranged collagen bands separated by clear clefts →. Nuclear features are bland.* ***(Right)*** *CD34 shows cell membrane positivity in 70-80% of Gardner fibromas. (Courtesy E. Montgomery, MD.)*

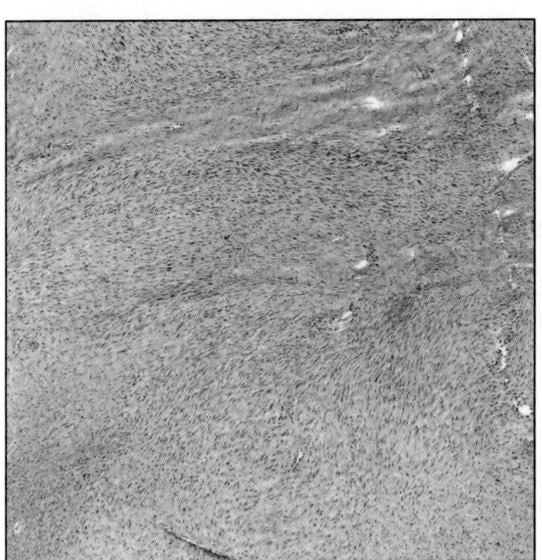

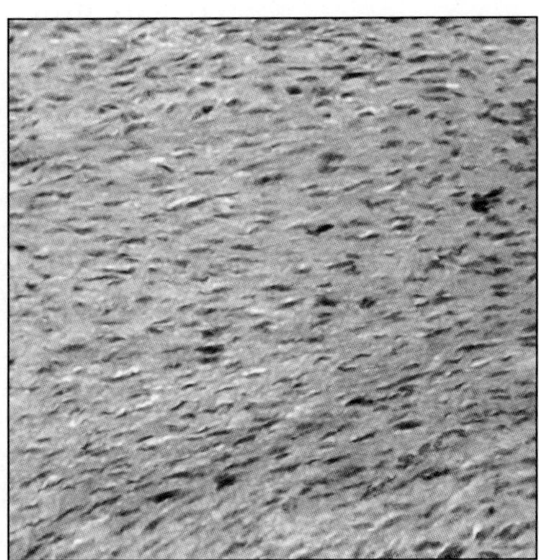

(Left) *Superficial fibromatoses, such as plantar fibromatosis as pictured here, are histologically very similar to desmoid fibromatosis. This low-power view demonstrates sweeping fascicles of bland spindle cells within a variably collagenous stroma. Clinical and radiographic information is extremely helpful in differentiating the 2 lesions.* ***(Right)*** *Like desmoid fibromatoses, superficial fibromatoses also show bland, elongated nuclei and sparse typical mitotic figures.*

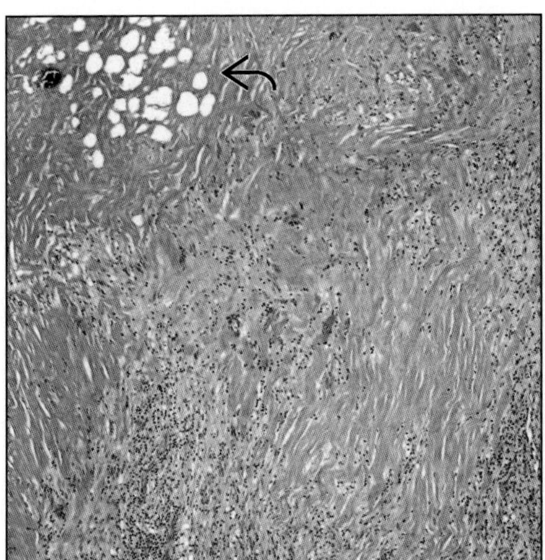

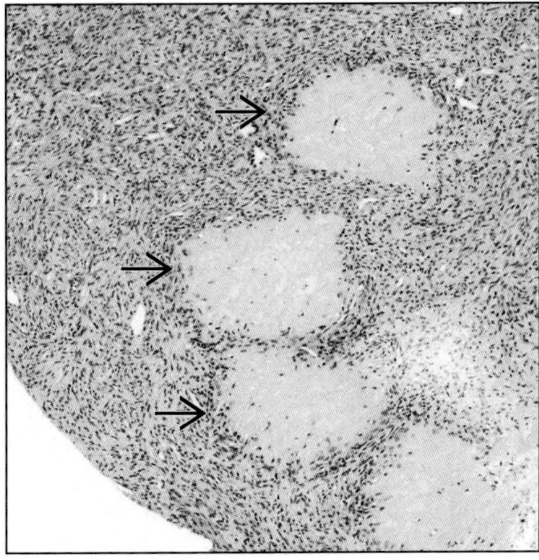

(Left) *Sclerosing mesenteritis is included in the differential for DF. The tumor is densely sclerotic with a marked lymphoplasmacytic infiltrate. Fat necrosis is seen ↶. (Courtesy E. Montgomery, MD.)* ***(Right)*** *Low-grade fibromyxoid sarcoma, like DF, is composed of bland spindle cells within an alternating collagenous and myxoid matrix. Mitoses are rare. Cells can be arranged in whorls or fascicles, and prominent collagenous rosette formations are present →. (Courtesy K. Thway, MBBS.)*

CALCIFYING APONEUROTIC FIBROMA

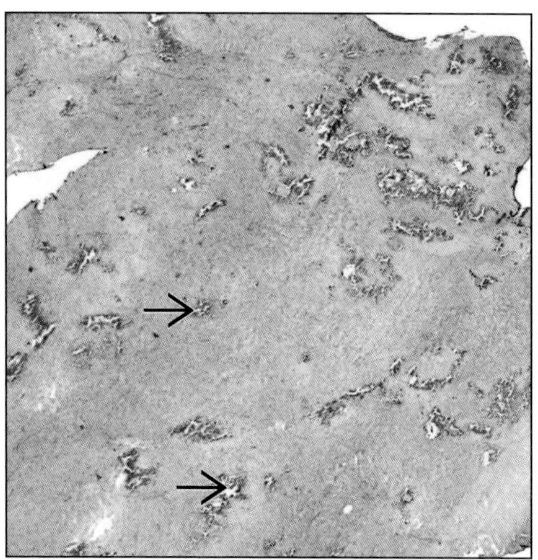

Low-power view of a calcifying aponeurotic fibroma. Numerous calcifications ⇒ are surrounded by a pale chondroid-like matrix. (Courtesy C. M. Coffin, MD.)

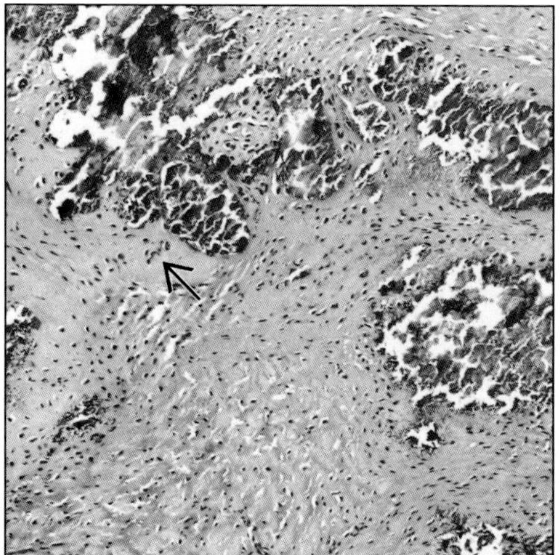

High-power view shows the nodular deposits of calcification surrounded by palisades of rounded chondrocyte-like cells set in a pale chondroid matrix ⇒. (Courtesy C. M. Coffin, MD.)

TERMINOLOGY

Synonyms

- Keasbey tumor
- Juvenile aponeurotic fibroma
- Aponeurotic fibroma
- Calcifying fibroma

Definitions

- Lesion consisting of spindled fibroblasts, epithelioid mesenchymal cells, and chondroid foci ± mineralization
  - Typically arises in hands and feet of children in 1st decade

CLINICAL ISSUES

Epidemiology

- Incidence
  - Rare: < 150 examples available in Armed Forces Institute of Pathology repository
- Age
  - Median age: 11-12 years
    - Most arise in 1st decade of life
  - Adult examples known
- Gender
  - Male predominance

Presentation

- Slow growing
- Painless infiltrative mass
- Typically involving hands or feet
  - Usually involves palms and fingers
    - Dorsum of hand is rare
  - Other involved anatomic sites
    - Back
    - Knee
    - Thigh
    - Forearm

Treatment

- Conservative excision if typical histology
  - Re-excision of recurrences
  - Morbid operations discouraged

Prognosis

- Prone to local recurrences
  - About 40% reported to recur
    - Highly infiltrative
- Rare case reports of metastases
  - Review of illustrations from 1 case suggests lesion was not calcifying aponeurotic fibroma

MACROSCOPIC FEATURES

General Features

- Ill-defined
- Firm or rubbery
- Can have gritty areas

MICROSCOPIC PATHOLOGY

Histologic Features

- Fibrous growth with multiple extensions into surrounding tissue
- Centrally located zones of cartilage formation and stippled calcification
  - Associated osteoclast-like giant cells may be present
  - Calcifications range from fine granules to large masses
  - Chondrocyte-like cells can be arranged in linear columns radiating from pockets of calcification
  - True ossification uncommon
- Mitoses scarce
- Calcification increases with age
  - Lesions from infants and small children may lack calcification
- Aneuploidy reported

CALCIFYING APONEUROTIC FIBROMA

Key Facts

Terminology
- Lesion consisting of spindled fibroblasts, epithelioid mesenchymal cells, and chondroid foci ± mineralization
  - Typically arises in hands and feet of children in 1st decade

Clinical Issues
- Male predominance
- Median age: 11 years; most arise in 1st decade of life
- Prone to local recurrences
- Painless infiltrative mass, typically involving hands or feet

Microscopic Pathology
- Fibrous growth with multiple extensions into surrounding tissue
- Centrally located zones of cartilage formation and stippled calcification
- Mitoses scarce

- No characteristic translocation/fusion product

DIFFERENTIAL DIAGNOSIS

Infantile Fibromatosis
- Usually involves proximal extremities or head and neck
- Rarely involves distal extremities
- Elongated fibroblasts with myxoid background
- Seldom calcified or ossified
- Lack giant cells

Synovial Sarcoma
- Usually deep soft tissue of more proximal extremity
- Cellular
- Display focal keratin labeling
- Characteristic t(X;18) with associated rearrangements of *SYT* gene
- Can be calcified, but calcified areas usually lack chondroid rim

Palmar and Plantar Fibromatosis
- Multinodular
- Sweeping cellular fascicles of fibroblasts
  - Plantar fibromatosis often has brisk mitotic activity
- Cartilage and calcification rare
- Giant cells can be seen (especially in plantar fibromatosis)
- Not common in children

Chondroma
- Well-circumscribed lobulated mass
- Usually affects older adults
- Usually involves hands
- Lack spindle cell fibromatosis-like component
- Greater extent of chondroid differentiation

SELECTED REFERENCES

1. Kacerovska D et al: Cutaneous and superficial soft tissue lesions associated with Albright hereditary osteodystrophy: clinicopathological and molecular genetic study of 4 cases, including a novel mutation of the GNAS gene. Am J Dermatopathol. 30(5):417-24, 2008
2. Fetsch JF et al: Calcifying aponeurotic fibroma: a clinicopathologic study of 22 cases arising in uncommon sites. Hum Pathol. 29(12):1504-10, 1998
3. Marty-Double C et al: Juvenile fibromatosis resembling aponeurotic fibroma and congenital multiple fibromatosis. One case with pleuropulmonary involvement. Cancer. 61(1):146-52, 1988
4. Allen PW et al: Juvenile aponeurotic fibroma. Cancer. 26(4):857-67, 1970
5. Lichenstein L et al: The cartilage analogue of fibromatosis. A reinterpretation of the condition called "juvenile aponeurotic fibroma." Cancer. 17:810-6, 1964
6. Keasbey L: Juvenile aponeurotic fibroma (calcifying fibroma); a distinctive tumor arising in the palms and soles of young children. Cancer. 6(2):338-46, 1953

IMAGE GALLERY

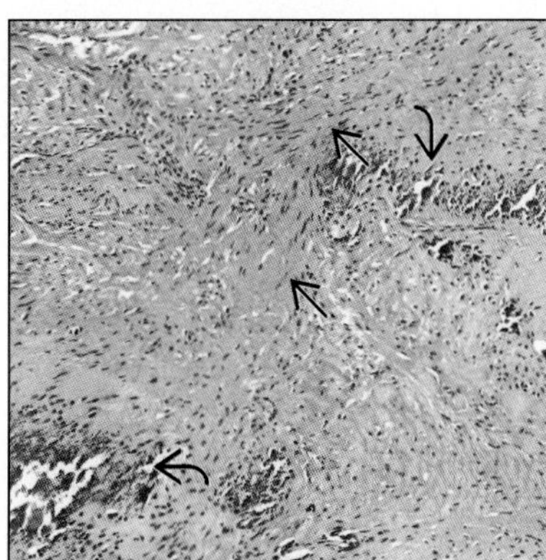

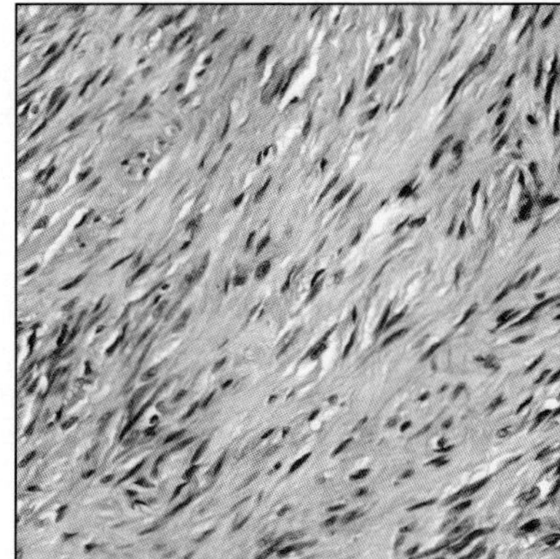

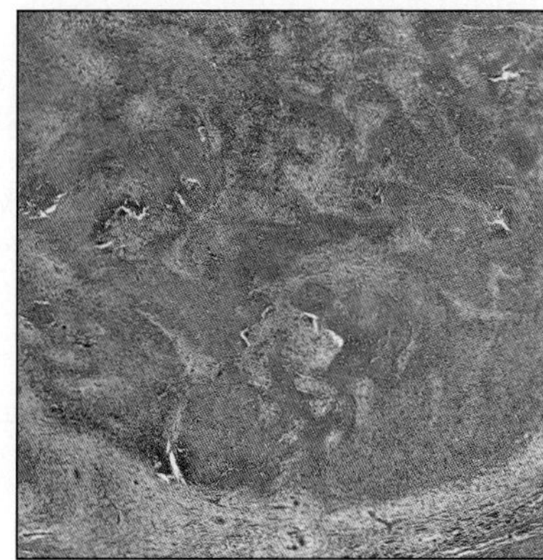

(Left) *Medium-power view of a calcifying aponeurotic fibroma shows fascicular areas ⇒ adjacent to the nodules of calcification ⇒ that are reminiscent of fibromatosis. (Courtesy C. M. Coffin, MD.)* ***(Center)*** *Hematoxylin & eosin shows a predominantly fascicular portion of a calcifying aponeurotic fibroma reminiscent of a fibromatosis.* ***(Right)*** *Hematoxylin & eosin shows an adult lesion that has an overall lobulated appearance. This lesion also featured zones of ossification.*

INFLAMMATORY MYOFIBROBLASTIC TUMOR

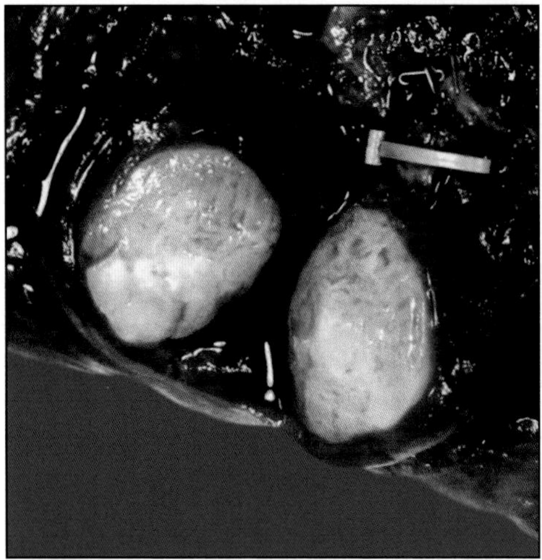

Bisected inflammatory myofibroblastic tumor of the lung is seen as a well-circumscribed mass with a tan, fleshy to gelatinous cut surface. A central tan-yellow hyalinized area with a histiocytic infiltrate is seen.

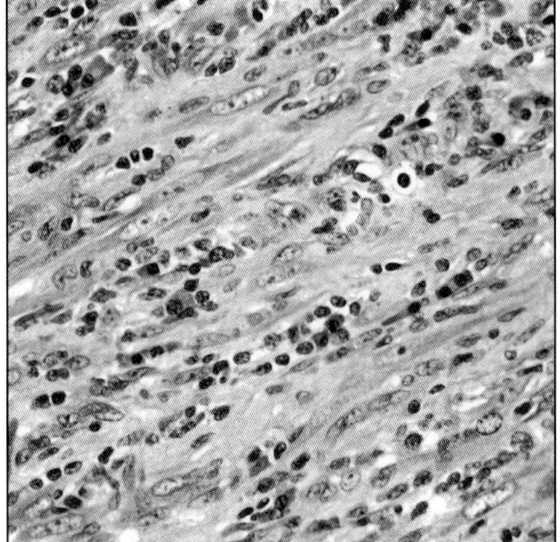

Inflammatory myofibroblastic tumors are composed of spindle-shaped myofibroblasts within a variably collagenous background interspersed with an inflammatory infiltrate of varying density.

TERMINOLOGY

Abbreviations

- Inflammatory myofibroblastic tumor (IMT)

Synonyms

- Inflammatory pseudotumor, plasma cell granuloma, plasma cell pseudotumor, pseudosarcomatous myofibroblastic lesion

Definitions

- Lesion of myofibroblastic spindle cells with inflammatory infiltrate of plasma cells, lymphocytes, and eosinophils
  - Intermediate biological potential
  - Unknown etiology
- Term inflammatory pseudotumor has been used to describe multiple different entities, thus its use is discouraged

ETIOLOGY/PATHOGENESIS

Anaplastic Lymphoma Kinase (ALK) Mutations

- Many IMTs have clonal rearrangement of *ALK* gene thought to be a key event in its pathogenesis, which supports current view of this tumor as true neoplasm
- Mutation results in expression and activation of *ALK* gene
- Various fusion partners have been described, which explains the different patterns of ALK protein immunoreactivity

CLINICAL ISSUES

Epidemiology

- Age
  - Occurs most commonly in children and young adults; average age: 10 years
- Gender
  - Slight female predominance

Presentation

- Visceral and soft tissue tumor
  - Most common sites
    - Lung, mesentery, omentum, and gastrointestinal tract
  - Other sites
    - Soft tissue and bladder
- Presenting symptoms related to anatomic location of tumor
  - Pulmonary IMT can present with chest pain and dyspnea
  - Abdominal IMT can present with gastrointestinal obstruction
  - May also be asymptomatic with discovery as incidental finding during work-up for unrelated disease or symptom
- Clinical syndrome in 1/3 of patients
  - B symptoms
    - Fever, growth failure, malaise, weight loss
  - Anemia
  - Thrombocytosis
  - Polyclonal hyperglobulinemia
  - Elevated erythrocyte sedimentation rate (ESR)
- Syndrome resolves with excision of mass

Treatment

- Complete surgical resection is preferred treatment modality
- Chemotherapy, steroids, and nonsteroidal anti-inflammatory drugs (NSAIDs) have been tried as adjunctive therapies with variable success
  - May be tried in aggressive or metastatic disease

Prognosis

- Difficult to predict based on histopathology alone
- Vast majority behave in benign fashion

INFLAMMATORY MYOFIBROBLASTIC TUMOR

Key Facts

Terminology

- Tumor of myofibroblastic spindle cells with inflammatory infiltrate of plasma cells, lymphocytes, and eosinophils
- Intermediate biological potential: Propensity to recur, but metastases are rare

Clinical Issues

- Most common sites include lung, mesentery, and omentum
- 1/3 of patients present with clinical syndrome including
  - Fever, malaise, growth failure, weight loss, anemia, thrombocytosis, polyclonal hyperglobulinemia, elevated ESR
- Prognosis is difficult to predict based on histopathology alone
- Increased aggressive potential: Aneuploidy, p53 positivity, cytologic atypia

Microscopic Pathology

- 3 histologic patterns
  - Loosely arranged plump myofibroblasts
  - Compact spindle cells in fascicles
  - Low cellularity scar-like pattern
- Immunohistochemical positivity for ALK not specific for IMT but positive in 50% of cases

Ancillary Tests

- 50-70% of IMTs are positive for *ALK* gene rearrangements involving 2p23

- Increased aggressive potential associated with the following
  - Aneuploidy
  - Expression of p53
  - Cytologic atypia
- Recurrence rates
  - *ALK* gene rearrangements associated with younger age and higher recurrence rates
  - Pulmonary tumors confined to lung (1.5%)
  - Extrapulmonary tumors confined to a single organ (8%)
  - IMTs found outside a single organ at presentation (35%)
  - Abdominal IMTs (33%)
- Metastases are rare

IMAGE FINDINGS

Radiographic Findings

- Lobulated solid mass with or without calcifications

MACROSCOPIC FEATURES

General Features

- Circumscribed, solitary or multinodular mass
- Firm, rubbery, tan-yellow, white or gray fleshy cut surface
- Focal hemorrhage, necrosis, and calcifications in some cases
- 6 cm in average diameter, reported range 1-22 cm
  - Most tumors are 5-10 cm in diameter

MICROSCOPIC PATHOLOGY

Histologic Features

- 3 histologic patterns, all of which may intermingle within a single tumor
  - Loosely arranged plump myofibroblasts, "nodular fasciitis-like"
    - Edematous myxoid background
    - Mixed infiltrate of plasma cells, lymphocytes, and eosinophils
    - Ganglion-like myofibroblasts
    - Numerous blood vessels
    - Extravasated red blood cells infrequently seen
  - Compact spindle cells with storiform or fascicular growth pattern
    - Variable myxoid and collagenized regions
    - Mixed infiltrate of plasma cells, lymphocytes, and eosinophils
    - Small aggregates of plasma cells or lymphoid nodules
    - Ganglion-like myofibroblasts
  - Low cellularity scar-like pattern
    - Plate-like collagen
    - Sparse inflammation with plasma cells and eosinophils
    - Osseous metaplasia or calcifications may be present
- Collections of foam cells are seen in some cases
- Mitoses may be present but are not atypical
- Many tumors have large amounts of plasma cells (thus old name of plasma cell granuloma) and lymphocytes
- Histologic evolution to a higher grade
  - Does not necessarily predict aggressive behavior or metastases
    - Highly atypical polygonal cells
    - Oval vesicular nuclei with prominent nucleoli
    - Variable mitoses, some of which may be atypical
    - Large ganglion-like cells
    - Reed-Sternberg-like cells
    - Associated with p53 immunoreactivity

ANCILLARY TESTS

Molecular Genetics

- 50-70% of IMTs are positive for *ALK* gene rearrangements involving chromosome 2p23
  - ALK immunohistochemistry correlates well with presence of *ALK* gene rearrangement
  - Associated with better prognosis

INFLAMMATORY MYOFIBROBLASTIC TUMOR

Immunohistochemistry

Antibody	Reactivity	Staining Pattern	Comment
Vimentin	Positive	Cytoplasmic	Strong diffuse staining
Actin-sm	Positive	Cytoplasmic	Focal to diffuse staining
Desmin	Positive	Cytoplasmic	
ALK1	Positive	Cytoplasmic	Positive in 50% of cases but not specific for IMT
p53	Positive	Nuclear	Positivity associated with recurrence and malignant transformation
Myogenin	Negative		
Myoglobin	Negative		
S100	Negative		
CD117	Negative		

DIFFERENTIAL DIAGNOSIS

Nodular Fasciitis

- History of rapidly growing lesion, present for only 1-2 weeks
- Practically always solitary
- Most common in adults 20-40 years of age
- Majority of lesions are subcutaneous or intermuscular in location
- Most are well-circumscribed lesions ≤ 2 cm in size
- Composed of spindle cells within variably myxoid and hyalinized background with scattered lymphoid and histiocytic cells
  - Extravasated red blood cells are characteristic finding

Inflammatory Leiomyosarcoma

- More nuclear atypia than IMT
- Located in deep soft tissues of older adults
- Behaves as a high-grade sarcoma
- ALK(-), no characteristic molecular alterations

Desmoid Fibromatosis

- Not well circumscribed, infiltrative
- Lacks inflammatory infiltrate
- Immunohistochemistry
  - Actin(+), desmin(-), β-catenin(+)
- β-catenin or *APC* mutations

Inflammatory Fibrosarcoma

- Overlapping features make distinction difficult
- Current view is that, at least in children, these 2 lesions are the same

Nodular Sclerosing Hodgkin Disease

- Reed-Sternberg cells are CD15 and CD30 positive; both are negative in IMT

Gastrointestinal Stromal Tumor

- Usually arises from muscularis propria of stomach
- Composed of uniform spindle-shaped or epithelioid cells
- No significant inflammatory infiltrate
- Immunohistochemistry
  - CD34(+), CD117(+), DOG1(+), S100(-)
- *KIT* or *PDGFRA* mutations present

Non-Hodgkin Lymphoma

- Monotonous clonal proliferation of lymphoid cells
- Seldom spindled
- Differentiate with panel of immunohistochemical lymphoid markers
- Malignant, prognosis depends upon subtype

Extranodal Rosai-Dorfman Disease

- Spindled histiocytes within lymphoplasmacytic background
- Emperipoleses
- Immunohistochemistry
  - S100(+), CD68(+), ALK(-), CD1a(-)
- Most with indolent behavior

DIAGNOSTIC CHECKLIST

Pathologic Interpretation Pearls

- Immunohistochemical positivity for ALK not specific for IMT
  - Positive in 50% of cases
  - Correlates with presence of *ALK* rearrangements
  - *ALK* rearrangements detectable by FISH
- Tumor protein p53 positivity associated with recurrence and malignant transformation

SELECTED REFERENCES

1. Coffin CM et al: Inflammatory myofibroblastic tumor: comparison of clinicopathologic, histologic, and immunohistochemical features including ALK expression in atypical and aggressive cases. Am J Surg Pathol. 31(4):509-20, 2007
2. Kovach SJ et al: Inflammatory myofibroblastic tumors. J Surg Oncol. 94(5):385-91, 2006
3. Janik JS et al: Recurrent inflammatory pseudotumors in children. J Pediatr Surg. 38(10):1491-5, 2003
4. Cook JR et al: Anaplastic lymphoma kinase (ALK) expression in the inflammatory myofibroblastic tumor: a comparative immunohistochemical study. Am J Surg Pathol. 25(11):1364-71, 2001
5. Coffin CM et al: Extrapulmonary inflammatory myofibroblastic tumor (inflammatory pseudotumor). A clinicopathologic and immunohistochemical study of 84 cases. Am J Surg Pathol. 19(8):859-72, 1995

Gross, Radiologic, and Microscopic Features

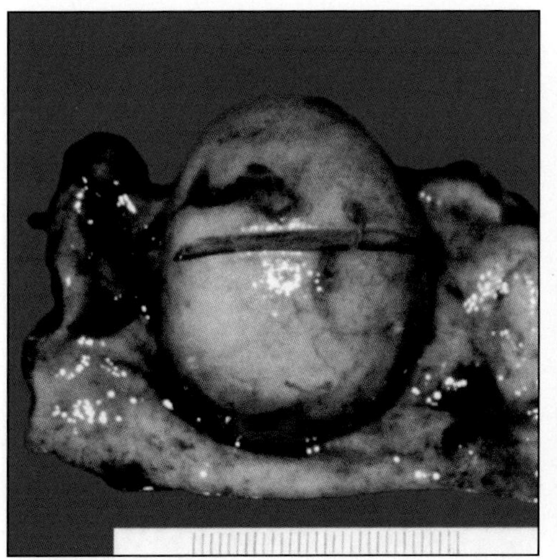

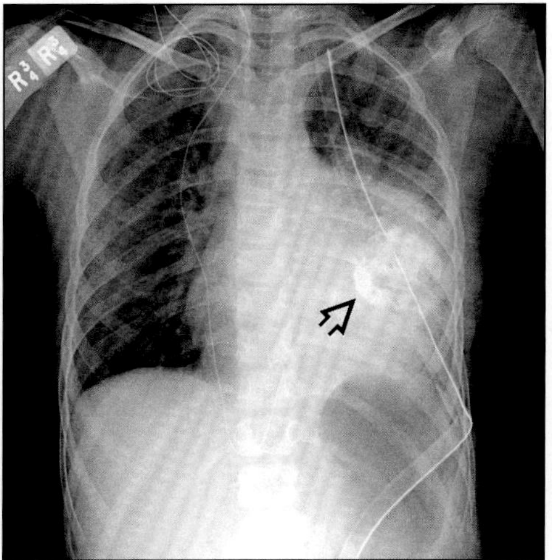

(Left) *Gross photograph depicts an IMT of the small bowel. The circumscribed mass is covered by mucosa and projects into the bowel lumen. Other common locations of IMT include the lungs, mesentery, omentum, bladder, and soft tissue.* ***(Right)*** *Chest x-ray in this 7 year old shows a large mass in the lower lobe of the left lung that extends into the mediastinum. A large area of calcification ⇨ is present within the tumor. Further evaluation of this mass showed it to be an IMT.*

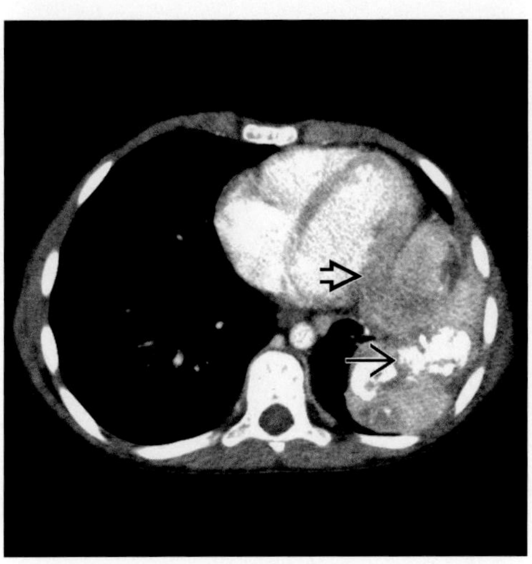

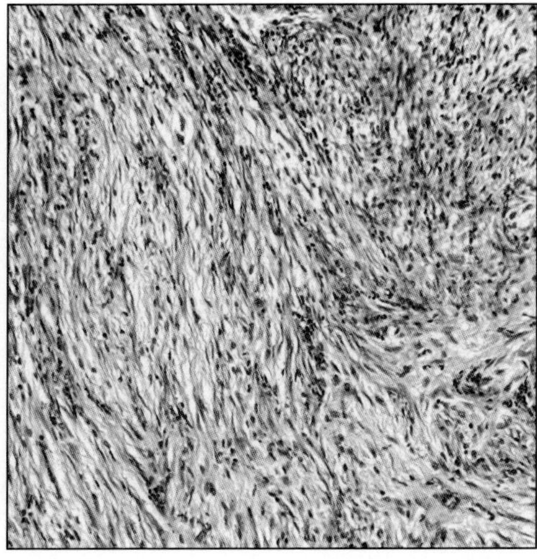

(Left) *CT scan shows a heterogeneous mass almost filling the left lower chest. This tumor was resected in a 2-stage operation but had positive margins due to mediastinal extension ⇨. Note the presence of intratumoral calcifications →.* ***(Right)*** *Section of a nodular-fasciitis-like IMT is shown. Loosely arranged spindle cells, stellate to plump, are present within an edematous myxoid background stroma with scattered inflammatory cells.*

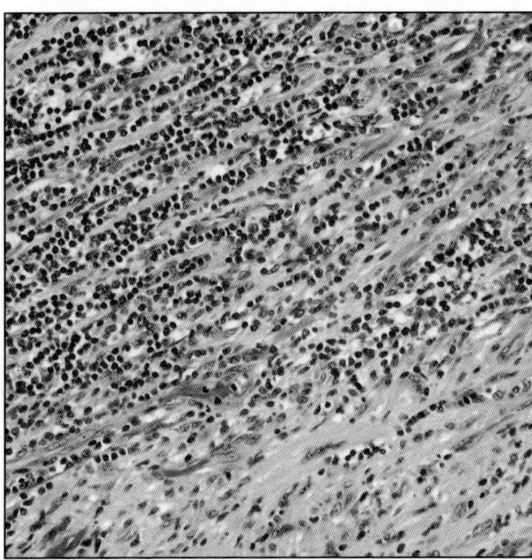

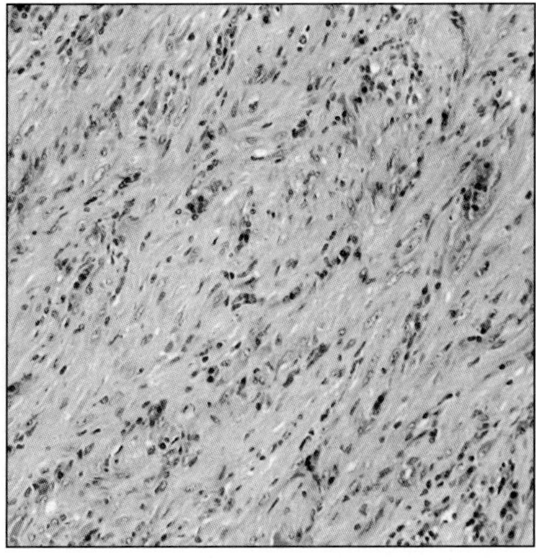

(Left) *The 2nd histologic type of IMT is composed of densely packed myofibroblastic spindle cells in a fascicular pattern. A dense lymphoplasmacytic infiltrate is interspersed between the stromal cells.* ***(Right)*** *A hyalinized hypocellular stroma characterizes the 3rd histologic type of IMT. Desmoid fibromatosis is a major differential diagnosis of this histologic type. All 3 histologic patterns may be closely intermixed within the same tumor.*

INFLAMMATORY MYOFIBROBLASTIC TUMOR

Microscopic Features

*(**Left**) Medium-power photomicrograph of an inflammatory myofibroblastic tumor demonstrates a heavy plasmacytic infiltrate ⇒ interspersed between the myofibroblastic stromal cells. (**Right**) High magnification of an inflammatory myofibroblastic tumor shows myofibroblastic nuclei with prominent nucleoli ⇒. The cells are spindled with eosinophilic to amphophilic cytoplasm. Mitotic figures may be present but are usually nonatypical.*

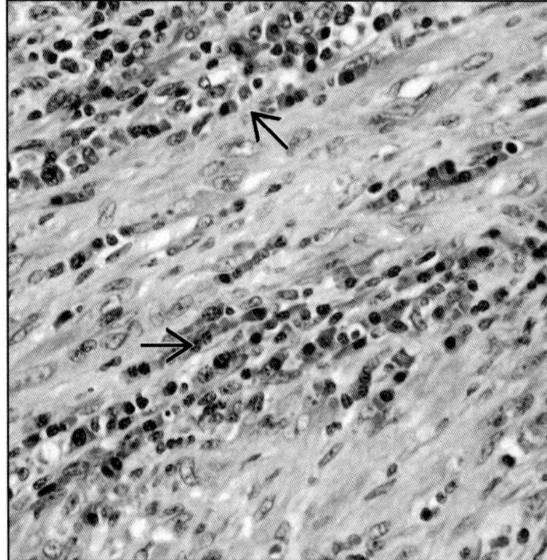

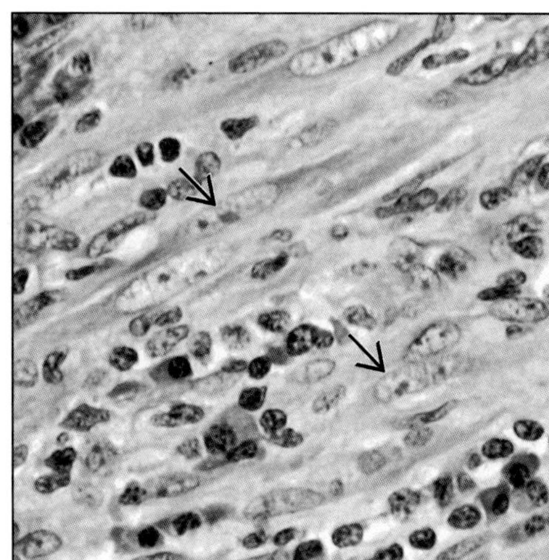

*(**Left**) Spindle cells intermixed with chronic inflammation of variable density are shown in this IMT. Small blood vessels are spaced uniformly, giving a granulation tissue appearance. (**Right**) Areas of necrosis ⇒ are present in this case of IMT of the lung in a 14-year-old girl who presented with an unresectable mass in the lower lobe extending into the mediastinum. The necrosis is bland (not granulomatous) and may indicate a worse prognosis.*

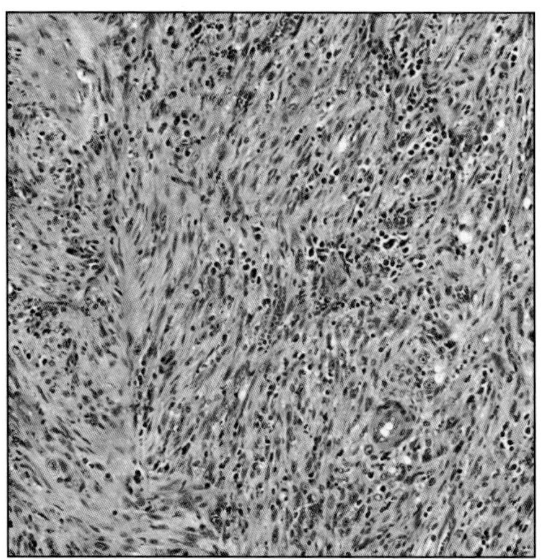

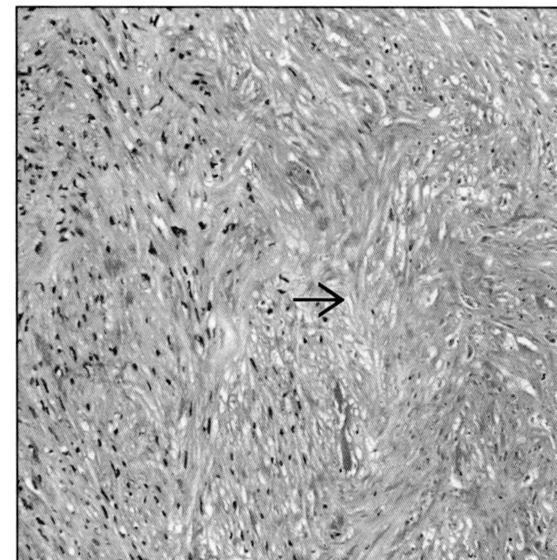

*(**Left**) High-power view in a case of IMT of the lung shows plump spindle cells with vesicular nuclei ⇗ and prominent nucleoli. This field has relatively fewer inflammatory cells (mostly lymphocytes and plasma cells). (**Right**) Occasional atypical cells ⇒ are present in this case of IMT, which was invading the mediastinum, but no atypical mitoses are seen. The atypical cells are large, single, or multinucleated with prominent nucleoli. Many chronic inflammatory cells are also present.*

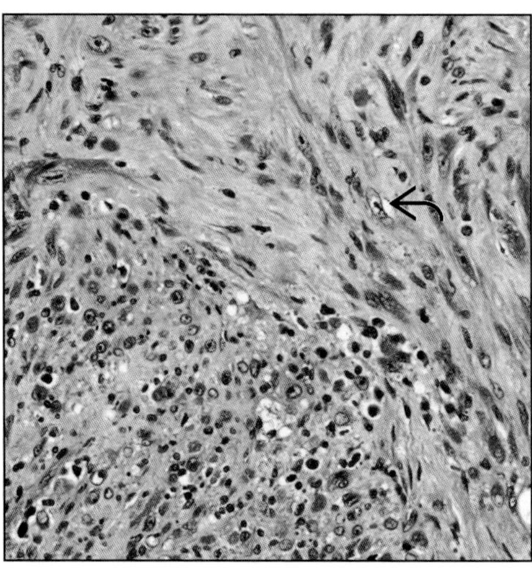

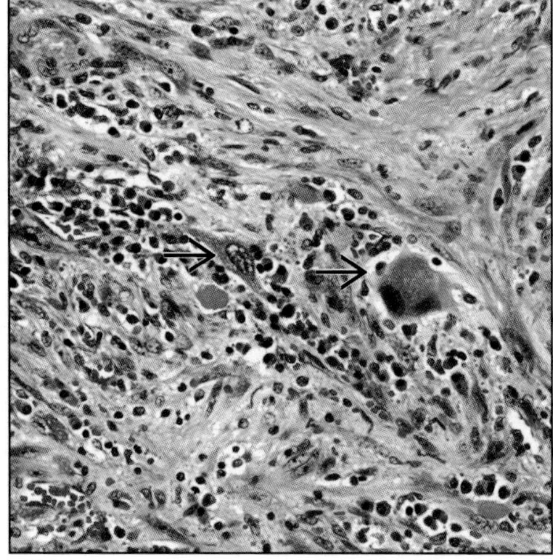

Microscopic and Immunohistochemical Features

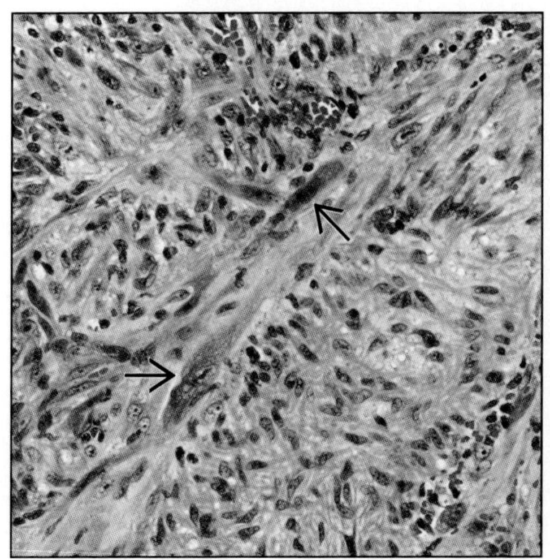

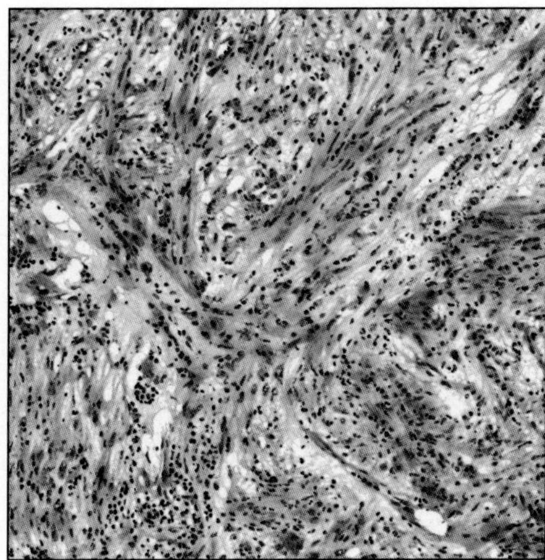

(Left) *High-power view in a case of IMT shows atypical spindle cells ➙, which may indicate a more aggressive course. This field has only sparse inflammatory cells.* ***(Right)*** *Frozen section of this pulmonary mass from a 7 year old shows the characteristic features of IMT, allowing for an intraoperative diagnosis to be made. Spindle cells admixed with chronic inflammatory cells are clearly recognizable. There is no atypia, and the underlying lung architecture is obliterated.*

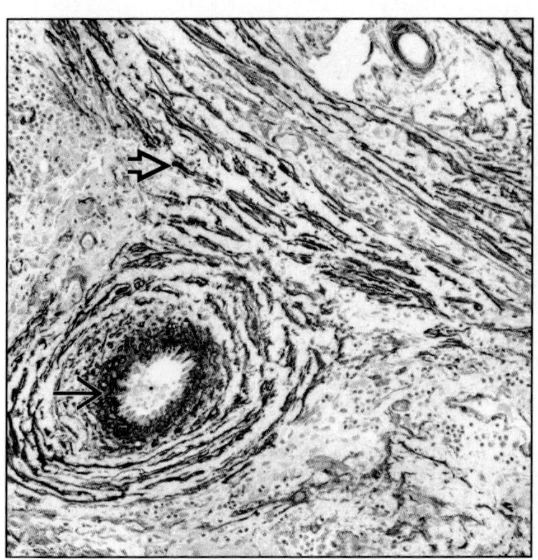

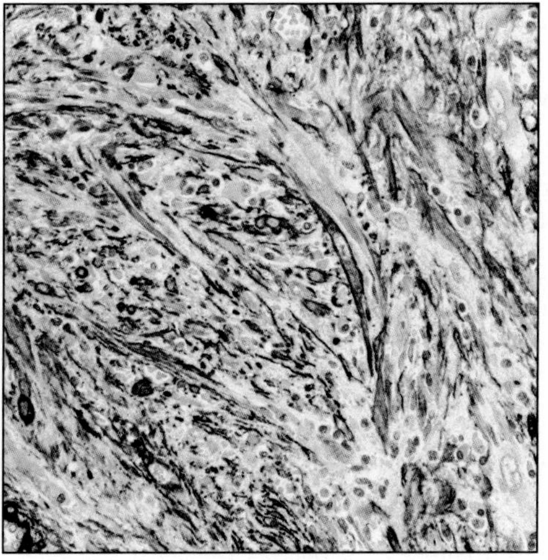

(Left) *In this case of IMT, immunohistochemical stain for smooth muscle actin is positive (cytoplasmic staining pattern) in the spindle cells ⇨, which are myofibroblasts. Note positive staining of vascular smooth muscle ➙, which serves as a good internal control.* ***(Right)*** *IMT of the lung at high power shows positive IHC staining with smooth muscle actin in most of the spindle cells (cytoplasmic staining) in this field; however, staining can be variable.*

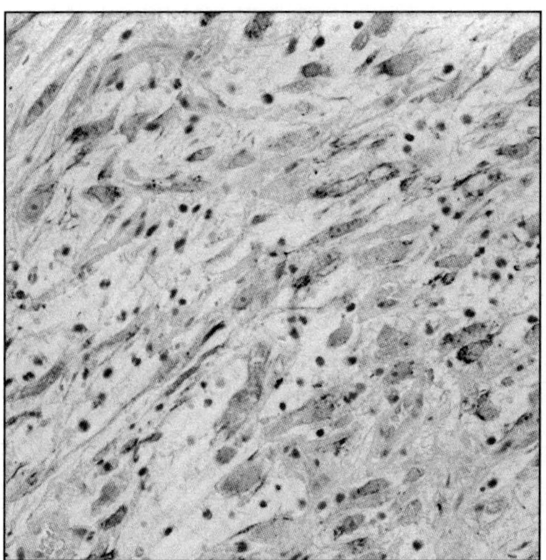

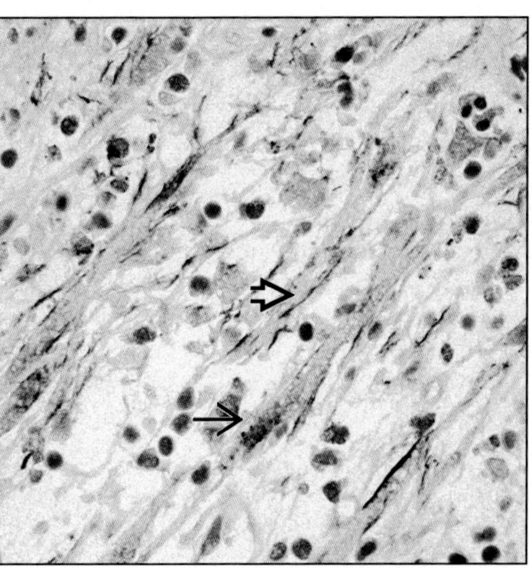

(Left) *IHC stain for ALK1 shows granular positivity in the cytoplasm of the spindle cells in this case of IMT. The staining tends to be variable with some fields being completely negative. Likewise, the intensity of staining is also variable.* ***(Right)*** *ALK1 staining of the spindle cells can be granular ➙, membranous ⇨, or both, as seen in this high-power photomicrograph of IMT. The admixed chronic inflammatory cells are negative.*

INFANTILE/JUVENILE HYALINE FIBROMATOSIS

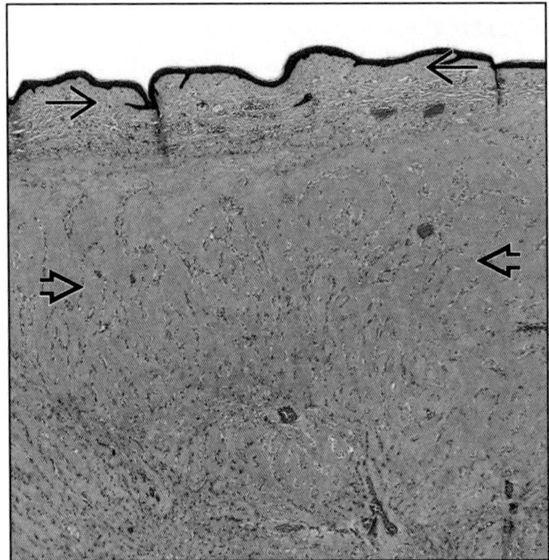

Hematoxylin & eosin shows juvenile hyaline fibromatosis of the face in the deep dermis ⇨. There is a tumor-free (grenz) zone → between the epidermis and the lesional tissue.

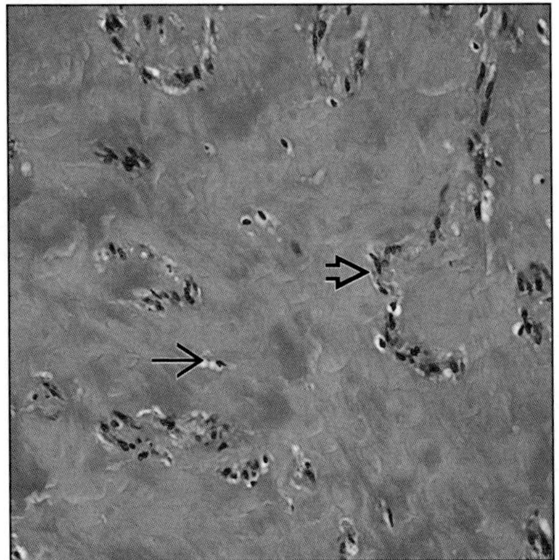

Higher magnification shows scattered lesional cells in homogeneous-appearing dense eosinophilic stroma. The cells are small and uniform, arranged in short curved cords ⇨. Some nuclei appear in spaces →.

TERMINOLOGY

Abbreviations

- Juvenile hyaline fibromatosis (JHF)

Synonyms

- Related disorder: Infantile systemic hyalinosis (ISH)
  - Suggested synonym: Hyaline fibromatosis syndrome

Definitions

- Rare autosomal recessive disorder (often found in consanguineous populations) characterized by multiple skin papules and early onset

ETIOLOGY/PATHOGENESIS

Genetic Disorder

- Mutations in *ANTXR2* in both juvenile hyaline fibromatosis and infantile systemic hyalinosis
- Autosomal recessive transmission

CLINICAL ISSUES

Presentation

- Juvenile hyaline fibromatosis
  - Infantile presentation of lesions of scalp, face, neck, retroauricular areas, and perineal region, and gingival hypertrophy
  - Joint contractures and motion limitation
  - Osteolytic lesions, mainly in phalanges and distal portions of long bones; cortical defects in subset of patients
- Infantile systemic hyalinosis
  - More severe end of clinical spectrum of mutations in *ANTXR2*
    - Hyaline changes are seen in multiple viscera as well as in skin
    - More prominent than those described in JHF
    - Affected individuals usually die in first years of life as result of complications of visceral involvement
  - Infiltration of intestines leads to malabsorption

MACROSCOPIC FEATURES

Skin and Gingival Lesions

- Plaques and papules of skin
- Larger lesions form soft tissue masses
- Gingival hyperplasia

Systemic Lesions

- Infiltration of small bowel and colon, forming masses

MICROSCOPIC PATHOLOGY

Histologic Features

- Histologic findings in both JHF and ISH are indistinguishable
  - Round to spindle cell proliferation composed of bland fibroblasts often lying in clear spaces and simulating chondrocyte lacunae
  - No significant cellular pleomorphism or mitoses
  - Homogeneous, hyalinized, dense eosinophilic intercellular matrix
  - PAS positive; diastase-resistant stromal material
  - Displaces normal components of dermis and lamina propria of gingival and intestinal mucosa
  - Early lesions can lack classic hyalinized stroma

DIFFERENTIAL DIAGNOSIS

Fibrodysplasia (Myositis) Ossificans Progressiva

- Rare, autosomal dominant disease
  - Characterized by soft tissue ossification at multiple sites and skeletal abnormalities of digits and cervical spine

INFANTILE/JUVENILE HYALINE FIBROMATOSIS

Key Facts

Terminology
- Related disorder: Infantile systemic hyalinosis (ISH)
- Juvenile hyaline fibromatosis (JHF)

Clinical Issues
- Autosomal recessive transmission
- Infantile presentation of lesions of scalp, face, neck, retroauricular areas
  - Gingival hypertrophy
- Cutaneous papules and plaques

Microscopic Pathology
- Uniform round to spindle cells
  - Some in clear spaces
- No significant cellular pleomorphism
- No mitoses or necrosis
- Homogeneous, hyalinized, pale, eosinophilic intercellular matrix
  - PAS positive; diastase resistant
- Blood vessels sparse

  - Short great toes
- No gender predominance
- Trauma (accidental or surgical) results in painful soft tissue lesions
  - Progressive ossification of lesions over 2-3 months
- Lesions appear similar to those of myositis ossificans
  - Mitotically active myofibroblasts
  - Variable ossification depending on age of lesions

Infantile Myofibromatosis
- Multiple lesions presenting in infancy
  - Can involve bones, soft tissues, and viscera
    - Pulmonary involvement is poor prognostic feature
- Biphasic lobulated lesions
  - Central myoid nodules composed of short oval to spindle-shaped cells
  - Peripheral hemangiopericytoma-like zones

Desmoid-type Fibromatosis
- Large masses of deep soft tissues, usually solitary
- Cellular fascicular lesions
- Associated with familial adenomatous polyposis (FAP)
- Nuclear immunoreactivity for β-catenin (deep examples)

Calcifying Aponeurotic Fibroma
- Distal extremities of infants and children
- Solitary lesions
- Stippled calcifications and fibrous areas

Nuchal Fibrocartilaginous Tumor
- Solitary lesion of adults
- Associated with prior neck injury
- Posterior aspect of base of neck
  - Junction of nuchal ligament and deep cervical fascia
- Fibrocartilaginous tissue forming mass

SELECTED REFERENCES

1. Nofal A et al: Juvenile hyaline fibromatosis and infantile systemic hyalinosis: a unifying term and a proposed grading system. J Am Acad Dermatol. 61(4):695-700, 2009
2. Tanaka K et al: Abnormal collagen deposition in fibromas from patient with juvenile hyaline fibromatosis. J Dermatol Sci. 55(3):197-200, 2009
3. Al-Malik MI et al: Gingival hyperplasia in hyaline fibromatosis--a report of two cases. J Int Acad Periodontol. 9(2):42-8, 2007
4. Antaya RJ et al: Juvenile hyaline fibromatosis and infantile systemic hyalinosis overlap associated with a novel mutation in capillary morphogenesis protein-2 gene. Am J Dermatopathol. 29(1):99-103, 2007
5. Anadolu RY et al: Juvenile non-hyaline fibromatosis: juvenile hyaline fibromatosis without prominent hyaline changes. J Cutan Pathol. 32(3):235-9, 2005
6. Hanks S et al: Mutations in the gene encoding capillary morphogenesis protein 2 cause juvenile hyaline fibromatosis and infantile systemic hyalinosis. Am J Hum Genet. 73(4):791-800, 2003
7. Rahman N et al: The gene for juvenile hyaline fibromatosis maps to chromosome 4q21. Am J Hum Genet. 71(4):975-80, 2002

IMAGE GALLERY

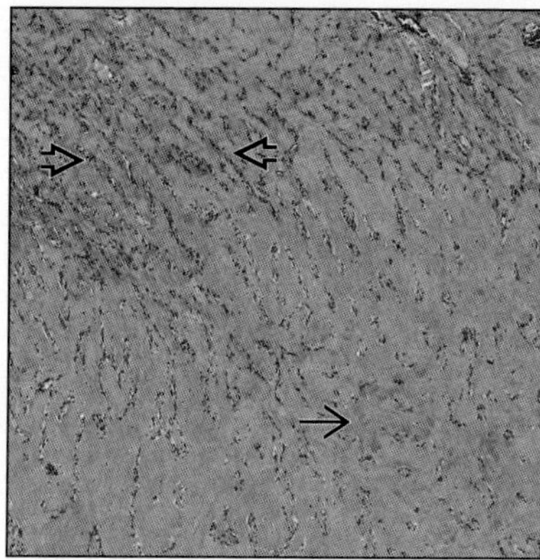

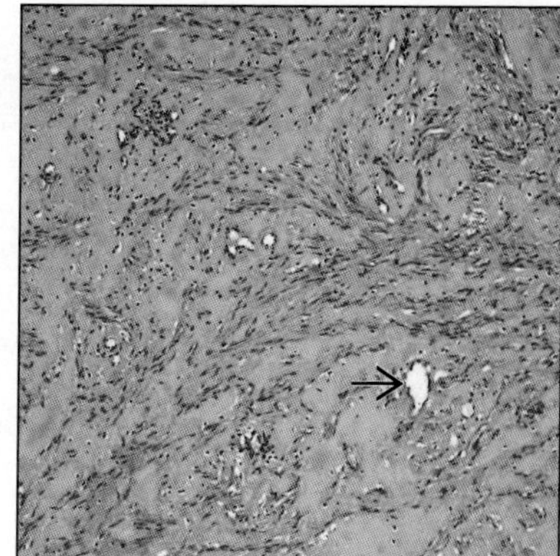

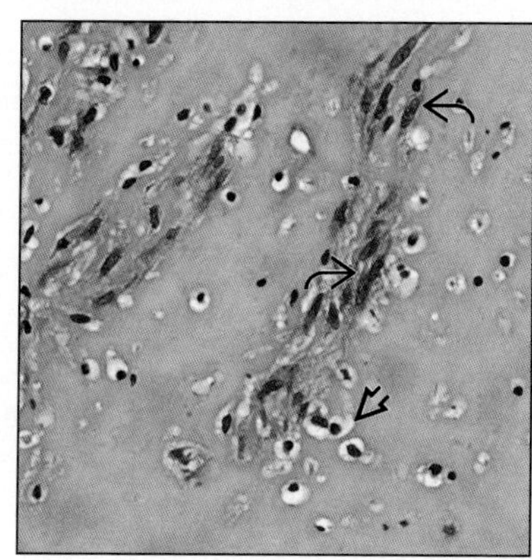

(Left) *Low-magnification H&E stain shows cords of cells within characteristic sclerotic stroma. The cords show a vaguely parallel alignment ⊳. Some parts of the tumor → are less cellular.* ***(Center)*** *A cellular example of JHF with branching cords of spindle cells. Note the occasional thin-walled, dilated blood vessel →.* ***(Right)*** *High magnification shows numerous cells with clear cytoplasm ⊳ resembling chondrocytes, and small clusters of spindle cells ↷. Note the absence of pleomorphism and mitotic activity.*

CALCIFYING FIBROUS TUMOR

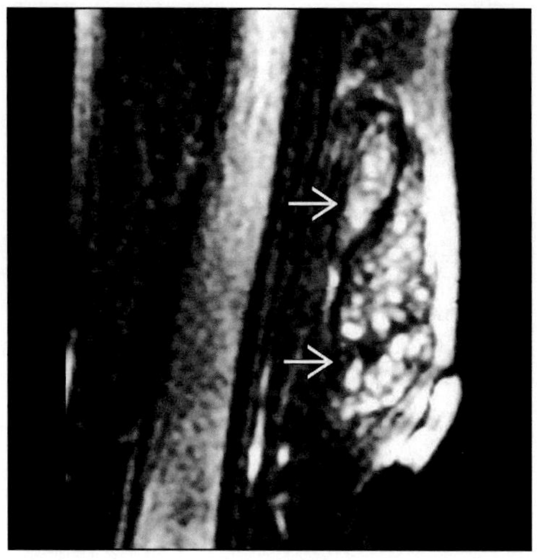

MR shows a soft tissue mass ➔ in the arm of a child consistent with a calcifying fibrous tumor.

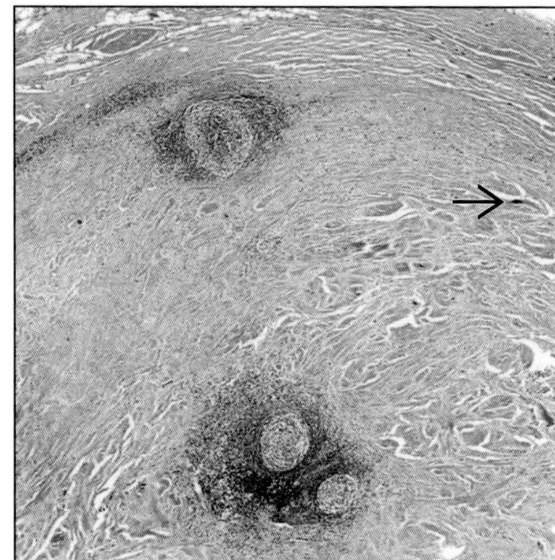

Hematoxylin & eosin shows a calcifying fibrous tumor. At this low magnification, there are lymphoid aggregates, a hypocellular spindle cell population, and calcifications ➔.

TERMINOLOGY

Abbreviations

- Calcifying fibrous tumor (CFT)

Synonyms

- Calcifying fibrous pseudotumor
- Childhood fibrous tumor with psammoma bodies

Definitions

- Rare benign hypocellular fibrous lesion
- Composed of fibroblasts, dense collagen, psammomatous and dystrophic calcifications, and lymphoplasmacytic inflammation with lymphoid aggregates
  - May reflect end stage of another lesion
  - Appears unrelated to inflammatory myofibroblastic tumor based on immunophenotyping

CLINICAL ISSUES

Epidemiology

- Age
  - Median age at resection = 18.5 years
    - Lesions often present for many years prior to excision

Presentation

- Soft tissue examples
  - Painless soft tissue mass in children and young adults
    - Most in extremities and trunk
    - Usually deep
    - No gender predilection
- Visceral examples
  - Described in pleura, peritoneum, mediastinum, paratesticular, adrenal, heart, lung
    - Most reported in adults with rare pediatric examples
    - Multiplicity not uncommon; reported in both pleura and peritoneum
    - No gender predilection
    - Familial peritoneal example reported (sisters, multifocal lesions)
- Rare cases associated with
  - Castleman disease
  - Inflammatory myofibroblastic tumor
  - Sclerosing angiomatoid nodular transformation of spleen

Treatment

- Excision

Prognosis

- Excellent

MACROSCOPIC FEATURES

General Features

- Well marginated
- Unencapsulated, firm, white mass
- Sometimes gritty on sectioning

Size

- Median size = 5 cm

MICROSCOPIC PATHOLOGY

Microscopic Features

- Well-marginated, unencapsulated borders
- Hypocellular hyalinized sclerotic tissue with fibroblastic bland nuclei
- Variable inflammatory infiltrate consisting of lymphocytes, plasma cells, and lymphoid aggregates
- Scattered psammomatous and dystrophic calcifications

CALCIFYING FIBROUS TUMOR

Key Facts

Terminology

- Benign hypocellular fibrous lesion
- Composed of fibroblasts, dense collagen, psammomatous and dystrophic calcifications, & lymphoplasmacytic inflammation with lymphoid aggregates
  - Possibly end stage of another lesion; appears unrelated to inflammatory myofibroblastic tumor

Clinical Issues

- Painless soft tissue mass in children and young adults
- Visceral examples: Pleura, peritoneum, mediastinum, paratesticular, adrenal, heart, lung
- Multiplicity not uncommon: Pleura and peritoneum
- Rare cases associated with Castleman disease, inflammatory myofibroblastic tumor, and sclerosing angiomatoid nodular transformation of spleen

Immunohistochemistry

Antibody	Reactivity	Staining Pattern	Comment
CD34	Positive	Cytoplasmic	About 2/3 of cases
α-1-antichymotrypsin	Positive	Cytoplasmic	Focal (rare cells)
Desmin	Positive	Cytoplasmic	Focal (rare cells)
ALK1	Negative		
S100	Negative		

DIFFERENTIAL DIAGNOSIS

Inflammatory Myofibroblastic Tumor

- Cellular lesions with more abundant inflammation
- Larger, more atypical myofibroblasts
- ALK expression in subset of cases

Gastrointestinal Stromal Tumor

- Cellular lesions with minimal inflammation
- CD117 expression (CFT is CD117[-])

Fibromatosis

- Cellular lesions without inflammation or calcifications
- Typically CD34(-)
- Display nuclear β-catenin labeling (CFT is β-catenin[-])

Fibroma of Tendon Sheath

- Variable cellularity
- Lacks inflammation and calcifications

SELECTED REFERENCES

1. Chen KT: Familial peritoneal multifocal calcifying fibrous tumor. Am J Clin Pathol. 119(6):811-5, 2003
2. Nascimento AF et al: Calcifying fibrous 'pseudotumor': clinicopathologic study of 15 cases and analysis of its relationship to inflammatory myofibroblastic tumor. Int J Surg Pathol. 10(3):189-96, 2002
3. Van Dorpe J et al: Is calcifying fibrous pseudotumor a late sclerosing stage of inflammatory myofibroblastic tumor? Am J Surg Pathol. 23(3):329-35, 1999
4. Pinkard NB et al: Calcifying fibrous pseudotumor of pleura. A report of three cases of a newly described entity involving the pleura. Am J Clin Pathol. 105(2):189-94, 1996
5. Fetsch JF et al: Calcifying fibrous pseudotumor. Am J Surg Pathol. 17(5):502-8, 1993

IMAGE GALLERY

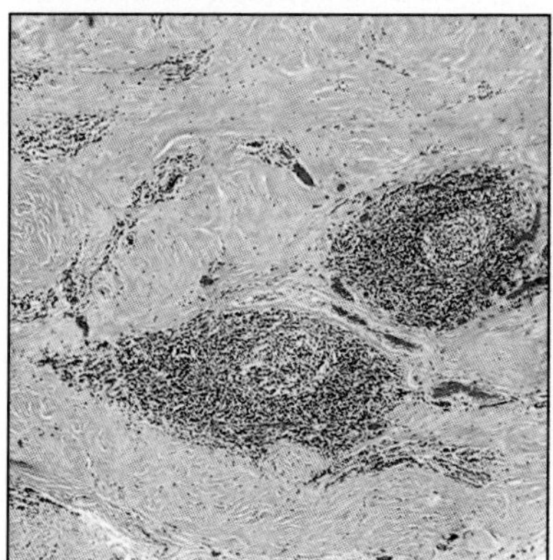

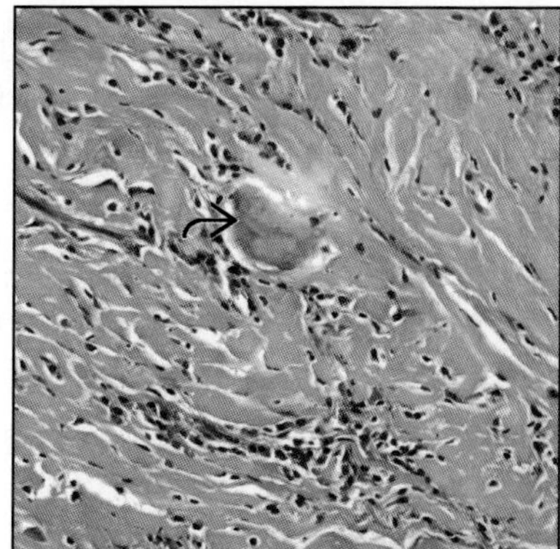

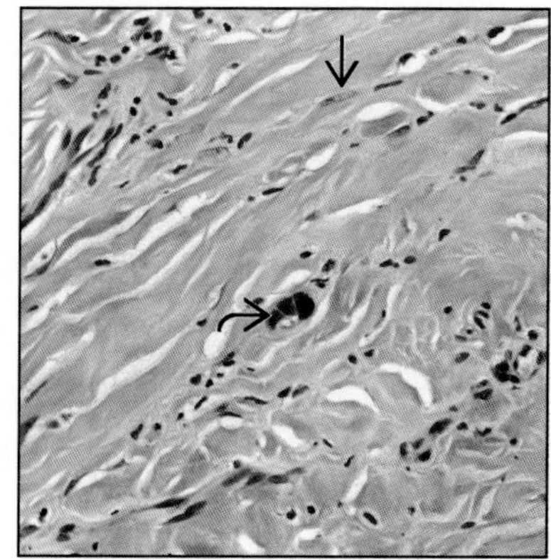

(Left) *Low cellularity, lymphoid aggregates, and background lymphocytes and plasma cells are seen in this CFT.* ***(Center)*** *CFT at high magnification shows single calcification ⇗, scattered inflammatory cells, and dense hypocellular collagen. Calcifications can be either dystrophic or psammomatous. (Courtesy C. M. Coffin, MD.)* ***(Right)*** *Hematoxylin & eosin shows the bland appearance of the proliferating fibroblasts ⇒ in a CFT. Scattered inflammatory cells and a single calcification ⇗ are present in the background. (Courtesy C. M. Coffin, MD.)*

FIBROUS HISTIOCYTOMA

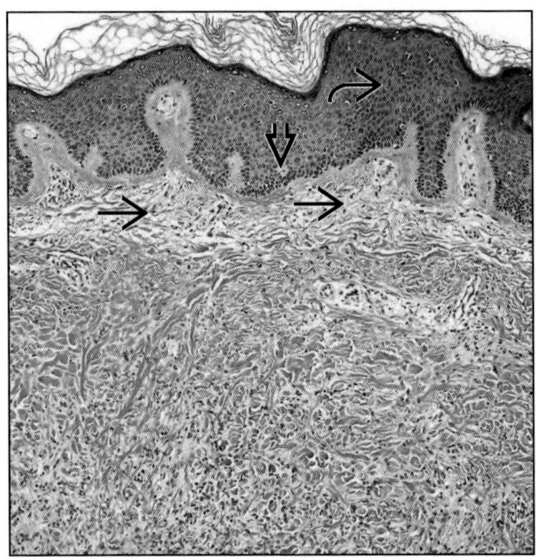

A typical benign fibrous histiocytoma of the skin is shown at low power. A grenz zone is noted ➔, as well as epidermal hyperplasia ➔ and hyperpigmentation ➔. (Courtesy D. Cassarino, MD, PhD.)

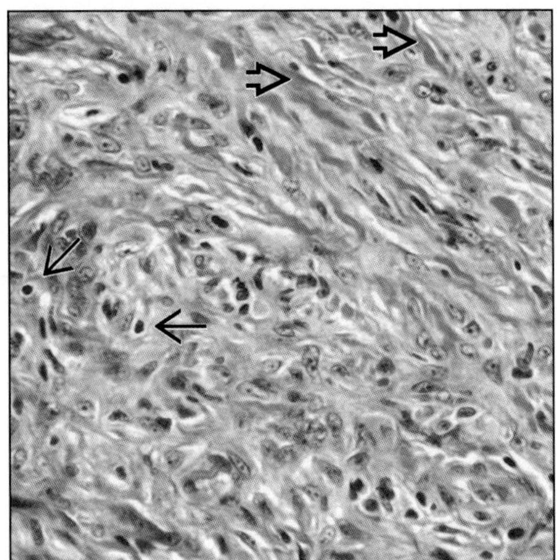

Plump histiocytic spindle cells are seen dissecting between collagen bundles ➔. Nuclear features are bland. Admixed lymphocytes are present ➔.

TERMINOLOGY

Abbreviations

- Fibrous histiocytoma (FH)

Synonyms

- Dermatofibroma (DF)
- Benign fibrous histiocytoma
- FH variants
  - Cellular FH: 5% of FH
  - Aneurysmal FH: < 2% of FH
  - Other histologic variants described in the literature
    - Epithelioid, lipidized, palisading, atypical, atrophic, myxoid, granular cell, keloidal, clear cell, lichenoid, balloon cell, signet ring cell
  - Deep FH: < 1% of FH

Definitions

- Common, benign proliferation of intradermal mesenchymal cells

ETIOLOGY/PATHOGENESIS

Unknown

- Originally thought to be derived from "fibrohistiocytes"
- Further studies showed no convincing evidence of a true histiocytic nature
- Line of differentiation is currently uncertain
- Evidence for both reactive and neoplastic processes

CLINICAL ISSUES

Site

- Most common on extremities overall
  - More common on trunk and head and neck area in infants
  - Almost any site may be involved

Presentation

- Wide age range
  - Most 20-60 years
  - Comprised 8.9% of infantile soft tissue tumors in a large series
- Slowly growing solitary nodule
  - Most are dermal lesions < 1 cm in size
  - Presence of central dimple on lateral compression is a useful diagnostic sign
  - Overlying skin often darkly pigmented and scaly
- Deep FH
  - Subset arising in subcutaneous or deep soft tissues
  - Larger than superficial counterparts, median size: 3 cm

Prognosis

- Excellent in vast majority of cases
  - FH: < 2% recurrence with incomplete excision
  - Deep FH: 22% recurrence rate reported
    - Similar recurrence rates reported for cellular, aneurysmal, and atypical variants of cutaneous FH
  - Metastasizing "benign" FH is a rare entity
    - Mostly occurs in cellular, atypical, or aneurysmal variants

MACROSCOPIC FEATURES

General Features

- FH
  - Circumscribed solid yellow-tan cut surface
- Deep FH
  - Well circumscribed
  - Yellow-tan firm cut surface
  - Cystic degeneration may be noted in larger lesions

FIBROUS HISTIOCYTOMA

Key Facts

Terminology

- Dermatofibroma
- Benign fibrous histiocytoma
- Common, benign proliferation of intradermal mesenchymal cells

Clinical Issues

- Most common on extremities
- Wide age range, most 20-60 years
- Small, slowly growing solitary cutaneous nodule
- Excellent prognosis in vast majority of cases

Microscopic Pathology

- Bland, plump, ovoid to spindle cells with a storiform or short fascicular growth pattern
- Tightly to loosely arranged, with admixed inflammatory cells
- Peripheral collagen entrapment seen in cutaneous lesions
- Grenz zone
- Basilar epidermal hyperplasia overlying dermatofibroma

Ancillary Tests

- FXIIIA(+), KI-M1P(+), α-1-antitrypsin(+), CD163(+), smooth muscle actin(+)
- CD68 often (+); highlights histiocytic cells
- CD34 is typically negative but has been reported to be positive in up to 40% of deep FH

Top Differential Diagnoses

- Dermatofibrosarcoma protuberans (DFSP)
- Solitary fibrous tumor

MICROSCOPIC PATHOLOGY

Histologic Features

- Bland, plump, ovoid to spindle cells with a storiform or short fascicular growth pattern
  - Tightly to loosely arranged, with admixed inflammatory cells
  - Spindle cells with indistinct, pale eosinophilic cytoplasm
    - Bland nuclei with vesicular chromatin and a single nucleolus
  - Inflammatory cells may include
    - Lymphocytes, histiocytes, "foam cells," or giant cells (osteoclast-type or Touton)
    - Peripheral lymphocytic infiltrates sometimes noted
    - Siderophages
- Peripheral collagen entrapment seen in cutaneous lesions
- Variable cellularity and collagenization
- Myxoid stromal areas may be evident focally
- Hemorrhage can be present in larger lesions
- Grenz zone (tumor spares band of superficial dermis)
- Focal extension into superficial subcutaneous tissue not infrequently seen
- Features of overlying skin
  - Basilar epidermal hyperplasia overlying dermatofibroma
  - Hyperpigmentation of basal keratinocytes
  - Proliferation of hair follicle-like structures may be confused with basal cell carcinoma

Fibrous Histiocytoma Subtypes

- Cellular variant
  - High cellularity with short fascicular and focal storiform growth
  - Extends into deep reticular dermis with lace-like extension along septa into superficial subcutaneous fat
  - Normal mitoses are common, up to 10 mitoses/10 HPF
  - Central necrosis sometimes noted
- Epithelioid variant
  - Commonly an exophytic, well-demarcated proliferation
    - Located in papillary and superficial reticular dermis
    - Surrounded by an epidermal collarette
  - At least 50% of tumor composed of rounded epithelioid cells
    - Abundant eosinophilic cytoplasm
    - Round to oval nuclei with small eosinophilic nucleoli
  - Grenz zone may be lacking
- Aneurysmal variant
  - Contains blood-filled cystic spaces, nonendothelial-lined
  - Diffuse hemosiderin deposition
  - Prominent erythrocyte extravasation between spindle cells
- Atypical FH
  - Pleomorphic histiocyte-like and spindled fibroblast-like cells in a common FH background
    - Admixed with multinucleated giant cells
    - Nuclei of pleomorphic cells are large and hyperchromatic with prominent nucleoli
    - Pleomorphism may be focal or widespread
  - Mitoses are usually present, 3/10 HPF, with occasional atypical mitoses
  - Geographic necrosis and infiltrative growth may be present
- Deep FH
  - Thick fibrous pseudocapsule often surrounds tumor
  - Most located entirely within subcutis
    - Focal extension to the dermis may be seen
  - Branched, staghorn hemangiopericytoma-like vessels in 40% of cases
  - More prominent storiform pattern than dermal type

FIBROUS HISTIOCYTOMA

Immunohistochemical Stain Comparison: FH, DFSP, SFT

Stain	FH	DFSP	SFT
CD34	7% positive, superficial type; up to 40% positive, deep FH	87% positive	94% positive
Podoplanin (membrane/cytoplasm)	100% positive	0% positive	0% positive
α-1-antitrypsin (cytoplasm)	75% positive	0% positive	0% positive
Bcl-2 (cytoplasm)	0% positive	54% positive	95% positive
KI-M1P (cytoplasm)	92% positive	0% positive	N/A
FXIIIA (cytoplasm)	67% positive	15% positive	81% positive

FH = fibrous histiocytoma; DFSP = dermatofibrosarcoma protuberans; SFT = solitary fibrous tumor.

ANCILLARY TESTS

Immunohistochemistry

- FXIIIA(+), KI-M1P(+), α-1-antitrypsin(+), CD163(+), smooth muscle actin(+)
- CD68 often (+); highlights histiocytic cells
- CD34 is typically negative but has been reported to be positive in up to 40% of deep FH
- Smooth muscle actin: Focally positive in 60% of cellular variant

DIFFERENTIAL DIAGNOSIS

Dermatofibrosarcoma Protuberans (DFSP)

- Locally aggressive tumor of dermal origin
- Infiltration through subcutaneous adipose tissue ("honeycombing")
- Small, slender nuclei in contrast to plump, ovoid to spindle-shaped FH nuclei
- Sprinkling of lymphocytes not generally seen

Solitary Fibrous Tumor

- Usually deep seated
- "Patternless architecture" contrasts with storiform pattern of FH
- CD34 not always helpful, as many deep FH are CD34(+)

Soft Tissue Perineurioma

- Storiform pattern of spindled cells
- Whorled architecture and bipolar cytoplasmic processes help to differentiate it from FH
- EMA(+)

Giant Cell Tumor of Tendon Sheath

- Well-circumscribed nodule, most on digits
- May have numerous foam cells, Touton and osteoclast-type giant cells
- Prominent stromal hyalinization
- Composed of sheets of histiocytoid cells, no storiform pattern

Juvenile Xanthogranuloma

- Proliferation of histiocytes with eosinophilic cytoplasm admixed with spindle cells, foamy macrophages, and Touton giant cells

Kaposi Sarcoma

- Differential consideration for aneurysmal FH
- Multifocal disorder
- Lymphomatoid and angiomatoid features
- CD34(+)

Angiomatoid Fibrous Histiocytoma (AFH)

- Differential consideration for aneurysmal FH
- Extremities of younger patients, deeper seated than aneurysmal FH
- Associated with systemic symptoms
- Monomorphic cells surrounded by prominent inflammatory infiltrate with germinal centers
- Tumor cells show desmin positivity

Reticulohistiocytoma

- Differential consideration for epithelioid FH
- Large mononuclear and multinucleated giant cells with glassy cytoplasm
- Admixed with lymphocytes and neutrophils

SELECTED REFERENCES

1. Luzar B et al: Cutaneous fibrohistiocytic tumours - an update. Histopathology. 56(1):148-65, 2010
2. Gleason BC et al: Deep "benign" fibrous histiocytoma: clinicopathologic analysis of 69 cases of a rare tumor indicating occasional metastatic potential. Am J Surg Pathol. 32(3):354-62, 2008
3. Sachdev R et al: Expression of CD163 in dermatofibroma, cellular fibrous histiocytoma, and dermatofibrosarcoma protuberans: comparison with CD68, CD34, and Factor XIIIa. J Cutan Pathol. 33(5):353-60, 2006
4. Li N et al: Differential expression of HMGA1 and HMGA2 in dermatofibroma and dermatofibrosarcoma protuberans: potential diagnostic applications, and comparison with histologic findings, CD34, and factor XIIIa immunoreactivity. Am J Dermatopathol. 26(4):267-72, 2004
5. Weinrach DM et al: Immunohistochemical expression of matrix metalloproteinases 1, 2, 9, and 14 in dermatofibrosarcoma protuberans and common fibrous histiocytoma (dermatofibroma). Arch Pathol Lab Med. 128(10):1136-41, 2004
6. Hui P et al: Clonal analysis of cutaneous fibrous histiocytoma (dermatofibroma). J Cutan Pathol. 29(7):385-9, 2002
7. Chen TC et al: Dermatofibroma is a clonal proliferative disease. J Cutan Pathol. 27(1):36-9, 2000
8. Zelger BW et al: Aneurysmal and haemangiopericytoma-like fibrous histiocytoma. J Clin Pathol. 49(4):313-8, 1996
9. Coffin CM et al: Soft tissue tumors in first year of life: a report of 190 cases. Pediatr Pathol. 10(4):509-26, 1990

Microscopic Features

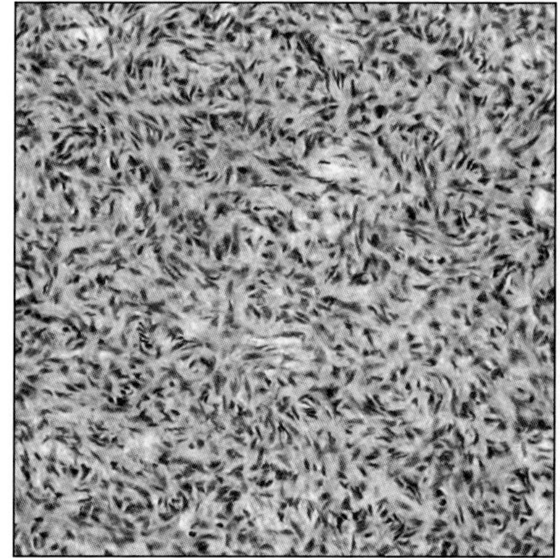

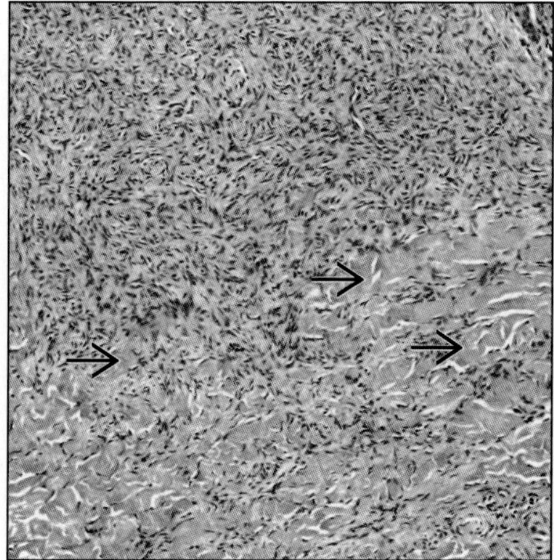

(Left) *A storiform pattern as seen here characterizes FH. These tumors can be variably cellular and variably collagenous.* ***(Right)*** *Medium-power magnification highlights collagen entrapment of tumor cells at the periphery of the lesion →, a typical feature of FH/dermatofibroma.*

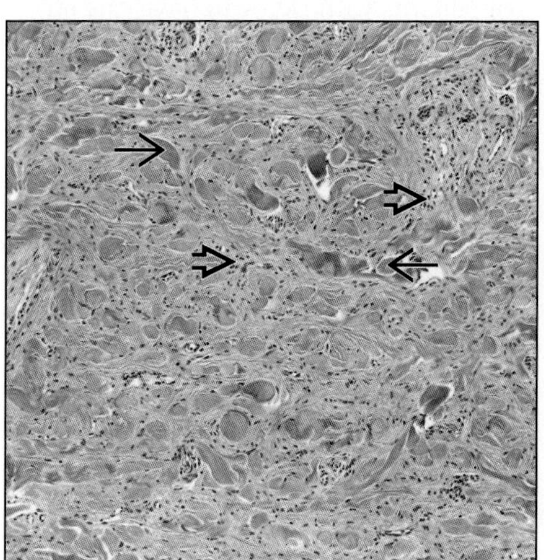

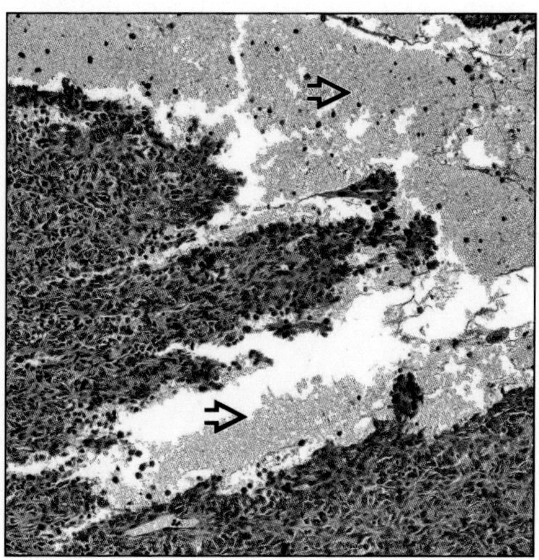

(Left) *Many histologic variants of FH exist. This keloidal FH demonstrates thick, glassy keloid-like collagen fibers → with interspersed fibrohistiocytic tumor cells ⇒. (Courtesy D. Cassarino, MD, PhD.)* ***(Right)*** *An example of aneurysmal FH is shown here. Large, irregular blood-filled spaces ⇒ characterize this variant. (Courtesy D. Cassarino, MD, PhD.)*

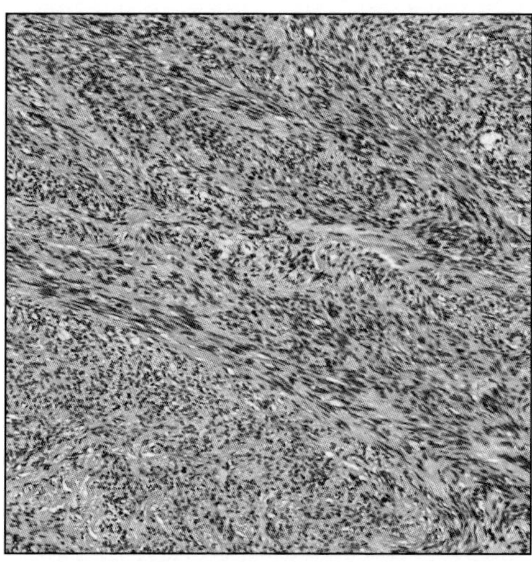

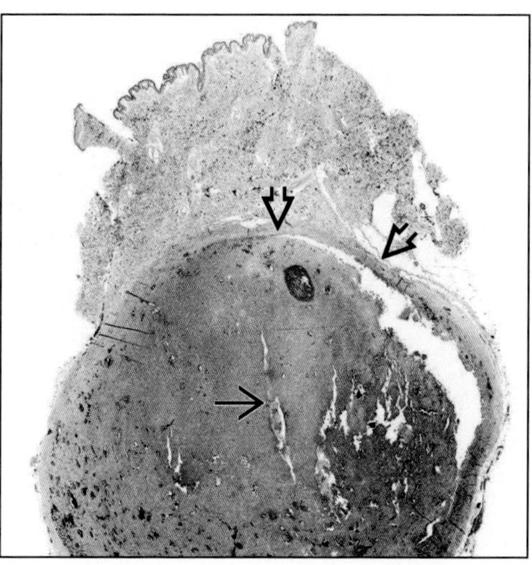

(Left) *This image exhibits the fascicular growth pattern of a cellular FH. Nuclear atypia and increased mitoses may be seen in this FH variant. The grenz zone may be lost in cellular FH, and the tumor cells sometimes infiltrate into superficial subcutaneous fat. (Courtesy D. Cassarino, MD, PhD.)* ***(Right)*** *Low-power view of a deep FH reveals pseudoencapsulation ⇒ and a subcutaneous location. A hemangiopericytomatous vascular pattern → is often seen. (Courtesy E. Montgomery, MD.)*

JUVENILE XANTHOGRANULOMA

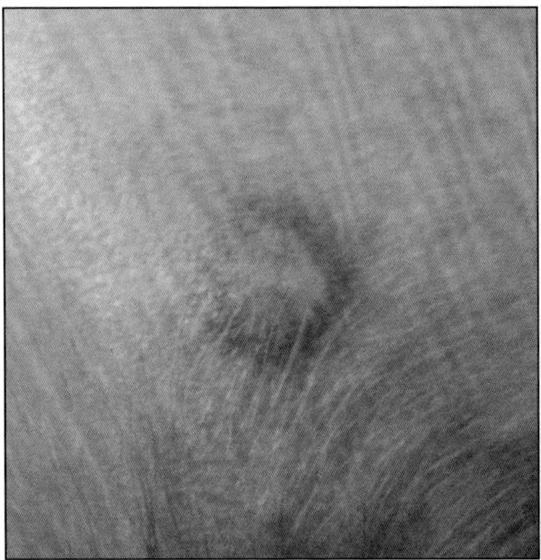

This red to yellow nodule on the scalp of an infant is a typical appearance of JXG. (Courtesy S. Vanderhooft, MD.)

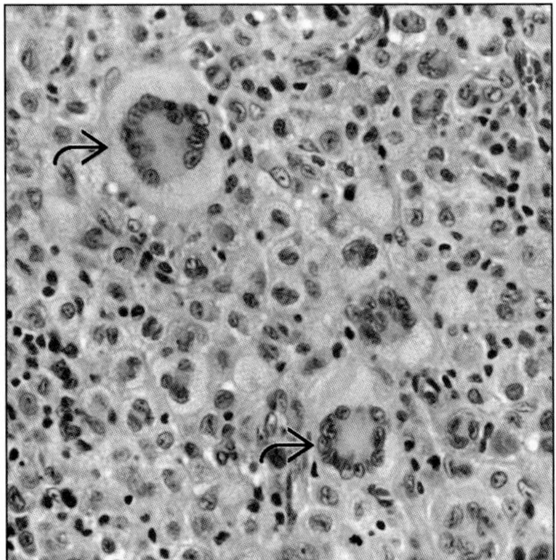

Touton giant cells ➔ are multinucleated, with the nuclei arranged like a wreath or horseshoe. Finding these cells is diagnostic of JXG, but they may not always be present.

TERMINOLOGY

Abbreviations

- Juvenile xanthogranuloma (JXG)

Synonyms

- Nevoxanthoendothelioma
- Nevoxanthogranuloma

Definitions

- Benign cutaneous histiocytosis

CLINICAL ISSUES

Site

- Head and neck
- Trunk
- Proximal limbs
- Small percentage have ocular involvement
- Visceral involvement is very rare

Presentation

- Young children, typically within 6-9 months of life
  - Can be seen in adolescence or adulthood
  - Adult cases usually termed "xanthogranuloma"
- Slightly more common in males
- Solitary or multiple
- Yellow to red to brown plaques or nodules
- 1-10 mm, sometimes larger

Natural History

- Spontaneous involution can occur months or years later
  - Adult lesions usually persist

Prognosis

- Benign
- No recurrence after excision

Associations

- Neurofibromatosis (NF1)
  - About 20% of patients with JXG will have café au lait spots
- Juvenile myelomonocytic leukemia
  - Prevalence especially high in patients with both JXG and NF1
- Niemann-Pick disease
- Urticaria pigmentosa

MICROSCOPIC PATHOLOGY

Histologic Features

- Nodular
- Poorly demarcated
- Dense infiltrate of homogeneous histiocytes within dermis
  - Rarely can have deep extension
- Cells are polygonal to spindle-shaped with indistinct cytoplasmic borders
  - Eosinophilic or amphophilic cytoplasm
  - May have fine vacuoles
- Foamy histiocytes in mature lesions
  - Can form aggregates
  - Some lesions can be fully xanthomized
- Touton giant cells
  - Wreath-like nuclei
  - Diagnostic feature, but may not be present in early lesions
- Mitoses rare
- Scattered lymphocytes and neutrophils, sometimes plasma cells and eosinophils
- Inconspicuous vascularity
- Older lesions can be fibrotic
- Overlying epidermis thin with attenuated and elongated rete ridges

ANCILLARY TESTS

Immunohistochemistry

- Histiocytes are positive for CD68

JUVENILE XANTHOGRANULOMA

Key Facts

Terminology
- Juvenile xanthogranuloma (JXG)

Clinical Issues
- Head and neck
- Trunk
- Young children, but can be seen in adolescence or adulthood
- Benign

Microscopic Pathology
- Touton giant cells
  - Wreath-like nuclei

Ancillary Tests
- Histiocytes are positive for CD68
- Histiocytes are negative for CD1a and S100

Top Differential Diagnoses
- Langerhans cell histiocytosis

- Histiocytes are negative for CD1a and S100
  - Important in differential of Langerhans cell histiocytosis (CD1a positive)

Electron Microscopy
- Lipid vacuoles
- Cholesterol clefts
- No Birbeck granules

DIFFERENTIAL DIAGNOSIS

Langerhans Cell Histiocytosis
- JXG cells will not have nuclear grooves like in LCH
- CD1a is negative in JXG
- No Touton giant cells are seen in LCH

Dermatofibroma
- Usually has dense collagenous stroma
- Overlying epidermis is hyperplastic

Xanthomas of Hyperlipidemia
- Foamy histiocytes tend to be more uniformly distributed

Reticulohistiocytoma
- Multinucleated giants cells have eosinophilic cytoplasm
- Matrix is reticulin-rich

SELECTED REFERENCES

1. Fassina A et al: Fine-needle cytology of cutaneous juvenile xanthogranuloma and langerhans cell histiocytosis. Cancer Cytopathol. 119(2):134-40, 2011
2. Raygada M et al: Juvenile xanthogranuloma in a child with previously unsuspected neurofibromatosis type 1 and juvenile myelomonocytic leukemia. Pediatr Blood Cancer. 54(1):173-5, 2010
3. Kolivras A et al: Congenital disseminated juvenile xanthogranuloma with unusual skin presentation and renal involvement. J Cutan Pathol. 36(6):684-8, 2009
4. Sun LP et al: Intracranial solitary juvenile xanthogranuloma in an infant. World J Pediatr. 5(1):71-3, 2009
5. Yamamoto Y et al: A case of S-100-positive juvenile xanthogranuloma: a longitudinal observation. Pediatr Dermatol. 26(4):475-6, 2009
6. Chantorn R et al: Severe congenital systemic juvenile xanthogranuloma in monozygotic twins. Pediatr Dermatol. 25(4):470-3, 2008
7. Haughton AM et al: Disseminated juvenile xanthogranulomatosis in a newborn resulting in liver transplantation. J Am Acad Dermatol. 58(2 Suppl):S12-5, 2008
8. Barroca H et al: Deep-seated congenital juvenile xanthogranuloma: report of a case with emphasis on cytologic features. Acta Cytol. 51(3):473-6, 2007
9. Weitzner S et al: Juvenile xanthogranuloma (nevoxanthoendothelioma). Arch Dermatol. 87:644-8, 1963

IMAGE GALLERY

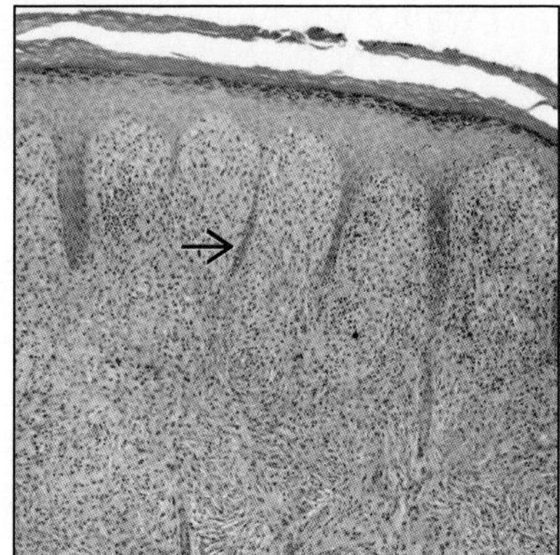
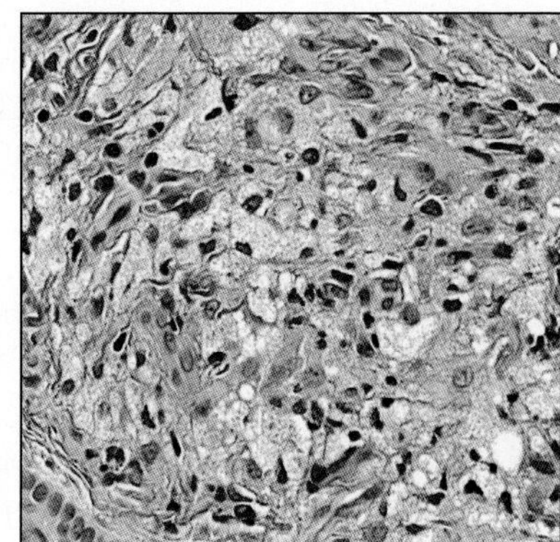
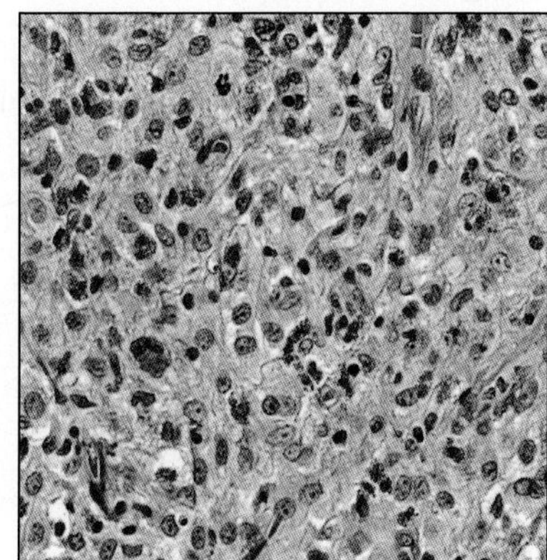

(Left) *Low-power view of this JXG shows the overlying epidermis to have thin and elongated rete ridges* ⇒*.* ***(Center)*** *High-power view shows a cluster of foamy histiocytes typically seen in a JXG.* ***(Right)*** *High-power view shows the mixed inflammation that can be present within a JXG. Scattered lymphocytes and neutrophils are common. The eosinophils seen here would raise the possibility of a Langerhans cell histiocytoma; immunostaining would help make the correct diagnosis.*

GIANT CELL FIBROBLASTOMA/DERMATOFIBROSARCOMA PROTUBERANS

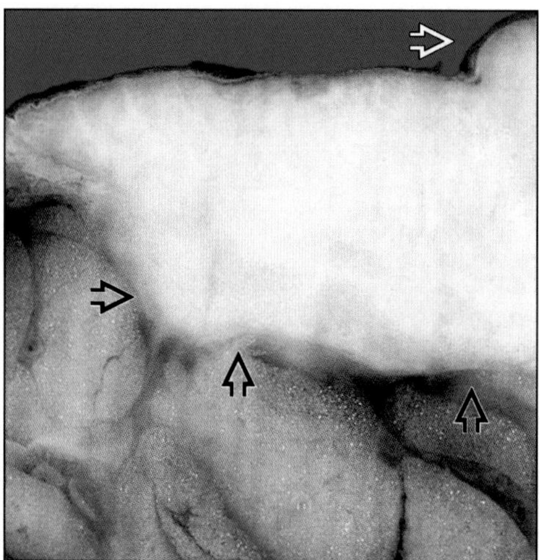

This gross photograph of DFSP shows its exophytic nature ⇨, as well as its propensity to infiltrate subcutaneous fat ⇨. (Courtesy T. Mentzel, MD.)

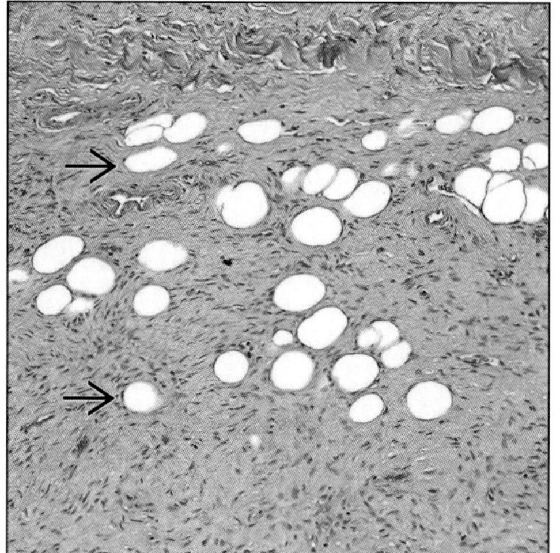

DFSP is a spindle cell lesion composed of fibrohistiocytic cells in a storiform arrangement that dissects between individual subcutaneous adipocytes →.

TERMINOLOGY

Abbreviations

- Giant cell fibroblastoma (GCF)
- Dermatofibrosarcoma protuberans (DFSP)

Definitions

- DFSP: Rare cutaneous tumor of fibrohistiocytic origin
  - Characterized by intermediate malignancy occurring predominantly in adults
  - Can progress to fibrosarcomatous DFSP
- Bednar tumor, a.k.a. pigmented DFSP, is a histologic variant that occurs in 5% of DFSP
- GCF: Tumor involving dermis and subcutis occurring in a younger population
  - Related to DFSP morphologically and immunohistochemically
  - Currently thought to be part of the spectrum of DFSP rather than a "juvenile" form of DFSP

ETIOLOGY/PATHOGENESIS

Etiology

- Cause unknown
- Trauma has been implicated

Pathogenesis

- DFSP and GCF: Chromosomal abnormalities involving chromosomes 17 and 22
  - These genetic aberrations fuse *COL1A1* with *PDGF-β* inducing tumor formation

CLINICAL ISSUES

Epidemiology

- Incidence
  - DFSP: 0.5-5 cases per 1 million persons per year
- Age
  - DFSP most frequent in adults between 2nd and 5th decade
  - DFSP thought to be rare in children, but more pediatric and congenital cases reported in recent years
    - About 170 pediatric cases reported, including 30 congenital cases
  - GCF: Median age 6 years, with majority < 10 years
- Gender
  - DFSP: Equal or male predilection reported
  - GCF: Male predominance
- Ethnicity
  - DFSP more common in those of African descent than in Caucasians

Site

- DFSP can occur at any site
  - Adults: DFSP occurs most commonly on the trunk, proximal extremities, and head and neck regions
  - Children: DFSP tends to arise in acral areas
- GCF occurs predominantly on the back and trunk

Presentation

- DFSP
  - Raised, indurated asymptomatic plaque that is red, blue, or brown-colored
  - Children: Often atrophic, nonprotuberant lesion
  - May resemble a vascular lesion, resulting in diagnostic delay in pediatric patients
  - Irregular protuberant swellings may be present with ulceration
- GCF
  - May or may not be protuberant
  - Polypoid lesions can be seen
- Hybrid DFSP and GCF exist

Treatment

- Wide excision recommended
  - Finger-like projections of tumor into surrounding tissues may not be grossly evident

GIANT CELL FIBROBLASTOMA/DERMATOFIBROSARCOMA PROTUBERANS

Key Facts

Terminology
- DFSP: Cutaneous tumor of fibrohistiocytic origin
  - Characterized by intermediate malignancy
  - Can progress to fibrosarcomatous DFSP
- GCF: Tumor involving dermis and subcutis occurring in a younger population
  - Currently thought to be part of the spectrum of DFSP rather than a "juvenile" form of DFSP

Clinical Issues
- DFSP: Progressive local growth, 20-50% recurrence rate
- GCF: Benign behavior with 50% recurrence rate

Microscopic Pathology
- **DFSP**
  - Fascicles of fibroblast-like storiform spindle cells
  - "Honeycombing" around adipocytes
  - Adnexal sparing
  - Fibrosarcomatous transformation: Herringbone pattern, atypia, mitoses
- **GCF**
  - Parallel fascicles of wavy uniform spindled cells
  - Angiectoid pseudovascular spaces lined by pleomorphic giant cells
  - Honeycomb growth pattern, adnexal sparing

Ancillary Tests
- CD34(+) in both DFSP and GCF
- Cytogenetics: t(17;22)(q22;q13) or ring chromosome

Top Differential Diagnoses
- Benign fibrous histiocytoma
- Diffuse neurofibroma

- Mohs micrographic surgery shows promising results in children
- Radiation and chemotherapy debated for recurrent disease in children

Prognosis
- DFSP is characterized by progressive local growth and propensity for local recurrence
  - Recurrence rate: 20-50%
  - Higher recurrence rate for head and neck tumors
- Metastases have been reported in DFSP
  - Especially for those with fibrosarcomatous transformation
  - Metastases extremely rare in children
- Prognostic factors for recurrence
  - Fibrosarcomatous transformation
  - Positive resection margins
  - Increased cellularity
  - High mitotic rate
- GCF has benign behavior with recurrence reported in about 1/2 of cases
  - Metastasis has not been reported

MACROSCOPIC FEATURES

General Features
- DFSP: Firm, infiltrative
- DFSP punch biopsies tend to be firm and cylindrical, due to subcutaneous penetration

Size
- DFSP in children usually ranges from 1-5 cm
- GCF in children usually ranges from 1-7 cm

MICROSCOPIC PATHOLOGY

Histologic Features
- **DFSP**
  - Fascicles of slender fibroblast-like monomorphous spindle cells in a storiform arrangement
    - Eosinophilic or amphophilic cytoplasm
    - Bland elongated nuclei
  - Subcutaneous infiltration around adipocytes, resulting in "honeycomb" pattern
  - Infiltrating "pseudopods" of tumor extending into surrounding tissue
  - Myoid whorls and giant cells may be present
  - Adnexal sparing
  - Mitoses may be seen (4/10 HPF)
  - Parallel growth patterns often seen
  - Fibrosarcomatous transformation
    - Herringbone fascicular pattern with nuclear atypia and increased mitotic figures
- **Bednar tumor**
  - DFSP with melanin pigment
- **GCF**
  - Parallel fascicles of wavy uniform spindled cells
  - Wiry collagen fibers with densely sclerosed areas
  - Scattered pleomorphic giant cells lining dilated and branching pseudovascular spaces
    - Giant cells appear multinucleated, but nuclei are actually multilobulated
  - Distinctive perivascular extravasation of lymphocytes in onionskin pattern
  - Like DFSP, can show honeycomb and parallel growth patterns, adnexal sparing, myxoid change, prominent vasculature, & myoid whorls
  - In contrast to DFSP, absence of true storiform areas without giant cells
  - Lower mitotic rate than DFSP
- **Recurrent tumors**
  - GCF has recurred as DFSP and vice versa

ANCILLARY TESTS

Immunohistochemistry
- CD34(+) in both DFSP and GCF
- FXIIIA(-) and S100(-)

Cytogenetics
- Supernumerary ring chromosome
  - Contains sequences of chromosome 17 and 22
- Reciprocal translocation: t(17;22)(q22;q13)

GIANT CELL FIBROBLASTOMA/DERMATOFIBROSARCOMA PROTUBERANS

Immunohistochemical Staining Comparison: DFSP, Fibrous Histiocytoma, and Diffuse Neurofibroma

Stain	DFSP	FH	Diffuse Neurofibroma
CD271 (membrane)	72% positive	0% positive	88% positive
Podoplanin (membrane/cytoplasm)	0% positive	100% positive	10% positive
KI-M1P (cytoplasm)	0% positive	100% positive	13% positive
CD63 (membrane)	100% positive	11% positive	17% positive
S100 (nucleus/cytoplasm)	1% positive	2% positive	77% positive
MMP-2 (cytoplasm)	22% positive	98% positive	30% positive
α-1-antitrypsin (cytoplasm)	0% positive	75% positive	0% positive
E-cadherin (membrane)	0% positive	75% positive	4% positive
CD34	87% positive	7% positive	40% positive
Collagen IV (cytoplasm)	0% positive	0% positive	85% positive

DFSP = dermatofibrosarcoma protuberans; FH = fibrous histiocytoma.

- Only reported in children: t(X;7)(q21.2;q11.2)

DIFFERENTIAL DIAGNOSIS

Benign Fibrous Histiocytoma

- Most occur on distal extremities
- Single papules or nodules
- Epidermal hyperplasia and hyperpigmentation
- Polymorphous cellular infiltrate
- May invade superficial subcutaneous fat
- Many may show focal CD34 positivity

Malignant Fibrous Histiocytoma/ Undifferentiated High-Grade Pleomorphic Sarcoma

- Much greater nuclear pleomorphism and mitotic activity than DFSP
- Deeper location than DFSP

Diffuse Neurofibroma

- Short spindle cells without storiform pattern
- Dissects around subcutaneous adipocytes
- Meissner-like corpuscles often present
- Diffuse S100 positivity

SELECTED REFERENCES

1. Kim JW et al: Congenital Bednar's tumour. Clin Exp Dermatol. 34(5):e85-7, 2009
2. Llombart B et al: Dermatofibrosarcoma protuberans: clinical, pathological, and genetic (COL1A1-PDGFB) study with therapeutic implications. Histopathology. 54(7):860-72, 2009
3. Reddy C et al: Dermatofibrosarcoma protuberans in children. J Plast Reconstr Aesthet Surg. 62(6):819-23, 2009
4. Gerlini G et al: Dermatofibrosarcoma protuberans in childhood: two case reports and review of the literature. Pediatr Hematol Oncol. 25(6):559-66, 2008
5. Macarenco RS et al: Genomic gains of COL1A1-PDFGB occur in the histologic evolution of giant cell fibroblastoma into dermatofibrosarcoma protuberans. Genes Chromosomes Cancer. 47(3):260-5, 2008
6. McAllister JC et al: CD34+ pigmented fibrous proliferations: the morphologic overlap between pigmented dermatofibromas and Bednar tumors. Am J Dermatopathol. 30(5):484-7, 2008
7. Patel KU et al: Dermatofibrosarcoma protuberans COL1A1-PDGFB fusion is identified in virtually all dermatofibrosarcoma protuberans cases when investigated by newly developed multiplex reverse transcription polymerase chain reaction and fluorescence in situ hybridization assays. Hum Pathol. 39(2):184-93, 2008
8. Jha P et al: Giant cell fibroblastoma: an update and addition of 86 new cases from the Armed Forces Institute of Pathology, in honor of Dr. Franz M. Enzinger. Ann Diagn Pathol. 11(2):81-8, 2007
9. Maire G et al: A clinical, histologic, and molecular study of 9 cases of congenital dermatofibrosarcoma protuberans. Arch Dermatol. 143(2):203-10, 2007
10. Reimann JD et al: Myxoid dermatofibrosarcoma protuberans: a rare variant analyzed in a series of 23 cases. Am J Surg Pathol. 31(9):1371-7, 2007
11. Domanski HA: FNA diagnosis of dermatofibrosarcoma protuberans. Diagn Cytopathol. 32(5):299-302, 2005
12. Gu W et al: Congenital dermatofibrosarcoma protuberans with fibrosarcomatous and myxoid change. J Clin Pathol. 58(9):984-6, 2005
13. Terrier-Lacombe MJ et al: Dermatofibrosarcoma protuberans, giant cell fibroblastoma, and hybrid lesions in children: clinicopathologic comparative analysis of 28 cases with molecular data--a study from the French Federation of Cancer Centers Sarcoma Group. Am J Surg Pathol. 27(1):27-39, 2003
14. Layfield LJ et al: Fine-needle aspiration cytology of giant cell fibroblastoma: case report and review of the literature. Diagn Cytopathol. 26(6):398-403, 2002
15. Sheng WQ et al: Expression of COL1A1-PDGFB fusion transcripts in superficial adult fibrosarcoma suggests a close relationship to dermatofibrosarcoma protuberans. J Pathol. 194(1):88-94, 2001
16. Díaz-Cascajo C et al: Giant cell fibroblastoma. New histological observations. Am J Dermatopathol. 18(4):403-8, 1996
17. Pinto A et al: Giant cell fibroblastoma in childhood immunohistochemical and ultrastructural study. Mod Pathol. 5(6):639-42, 1992
18. Shmookler BM et al: Giant cell fibroblastoma. A juvenile form of dermatofibrosarcoma protuberans. Cancer. 64(10):2154-61, 1989

Clinical and Microscopic Features

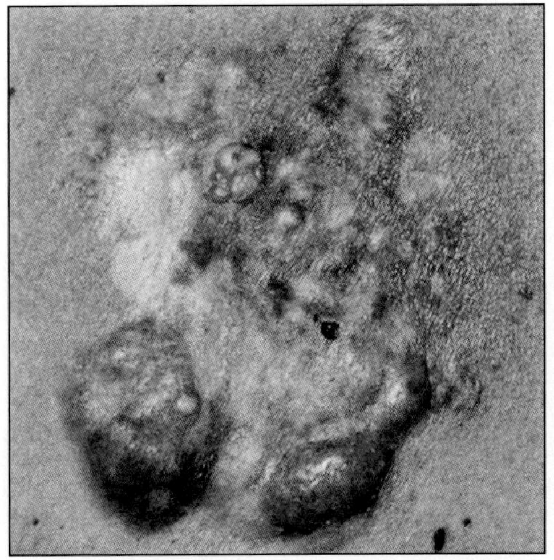

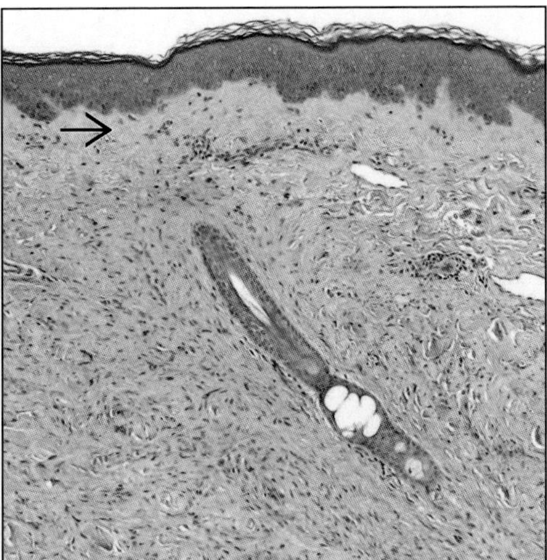

(Left) *DFSP is characterized clinically by multiple nodular exophytic dermal lesions. (Courtesy T. Mentzel, MD.)* ***(Right)*** *A grenz zone may be present in DFSP ➔. Slender spindle cells interdigitate between collagen bundles within the dermis, similar to benign fibrous histiocytoma. Unlike benign fibrous histiocytoma, epidermal hyperplasia is not usual.*

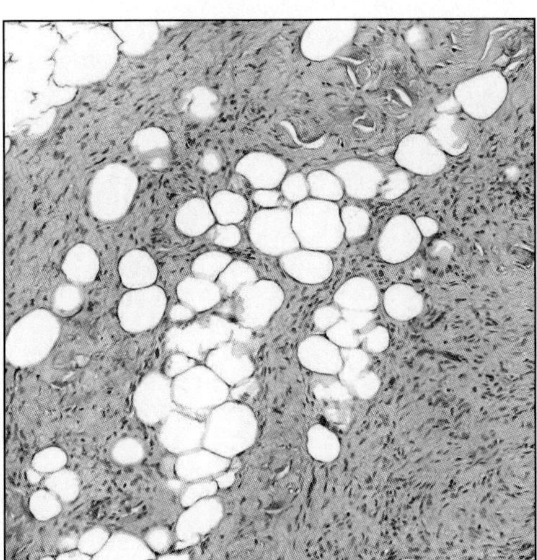

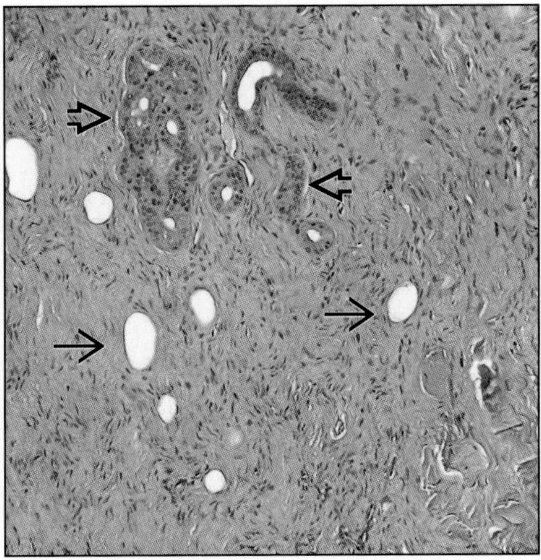

(Left) *Spindle cells in DFSP extend along subcutaneous septae to surround and encase adipocytes.* ***(Right)*** *DFSP typically surrounds adnexal structures ⇨. Entrapped adipocytes are also seen ➔.*

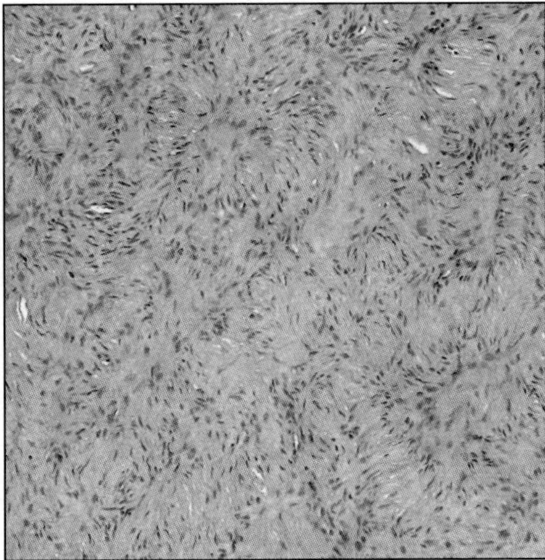

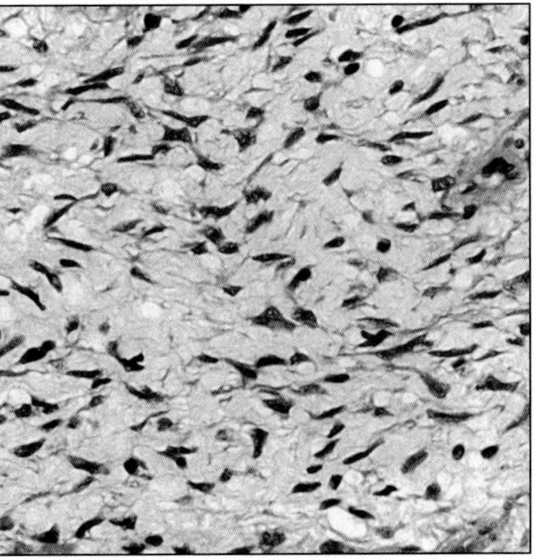

(Left) *This image highlights the interlacing short fascicles with a whorled pattern characteristic of DFSP. Nuclei are elongated with bland cytologic features.* ***(Right)*** *Sections of myxoid DFSP show stellate spindle cells within a pale, myxoid stroma. A residual storiform pattern can be appreciated but is less evident due to the wide separation of cells. (Courtesy T. Mentzel, MD.)*

GIANT CELL FIBROBLASTOMA/DERMATOFIBROSARCOMA PROTUBERANS

Microscopic Features

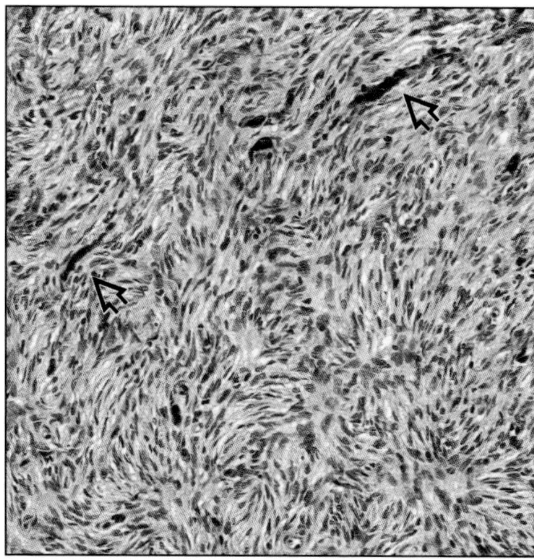

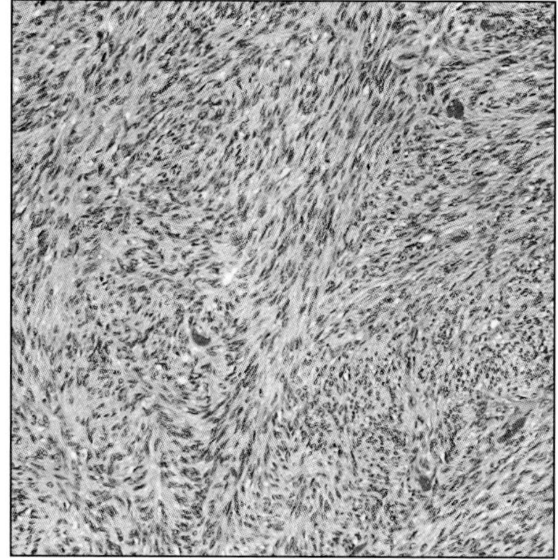

(Left) *Bednar tumors represent DFSP with hemosiderin deposition ⇨. This feature is of no prognostic significance and may be seen in fibrosarcomatous DFSP and GCF. A typical storiform pattern is noted. (Courtesy T. Mentzel, MD.)* ***(Right)*** *This microscopic image depicts an area of fibrosarcomatous transformation within a DFSP. A highly cellular "herringbone" fascicular pattern typical of fibrosarcoma is seen.*

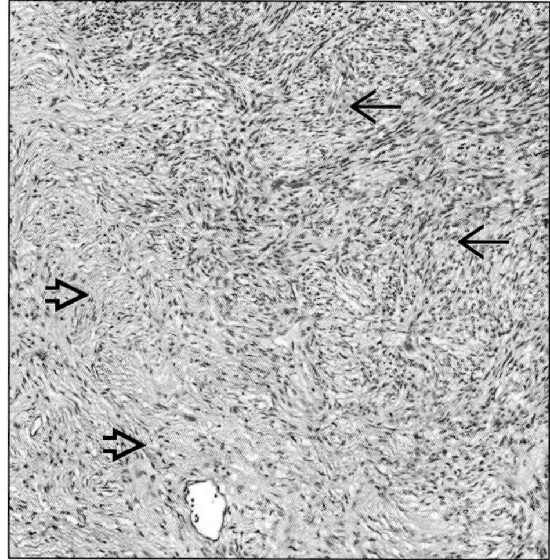

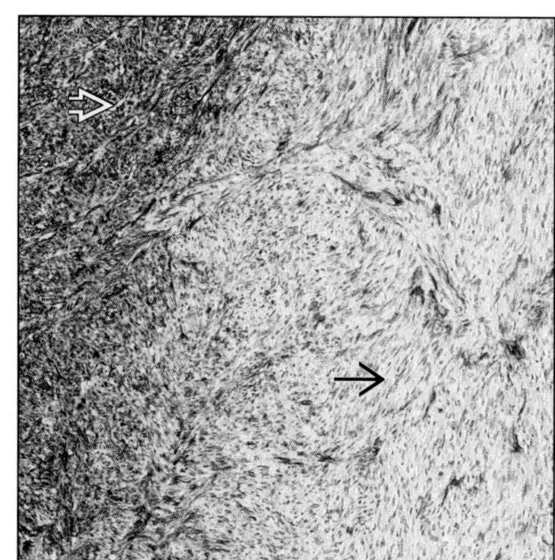

(Left) *The transition between a storiform DFSP ⇨ and an area of fibrosarcomatous transformation → is shown in this image. The fibrosarcomatous area demonstrates higher cellularity and a herringbone fascicular arrangement.* ***(Right)*** *Often CD34 staining intensity is lost in fibrosarcomatous regions of DFSP → compared with nonsarcomatous areas ➡.* *(Courtesy T. Mentzel, MD.)*

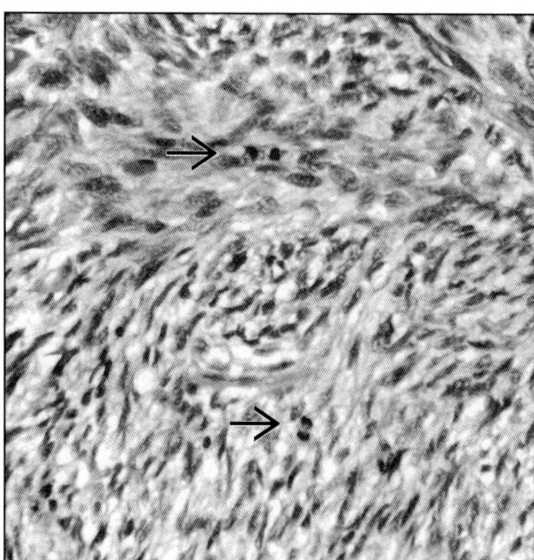

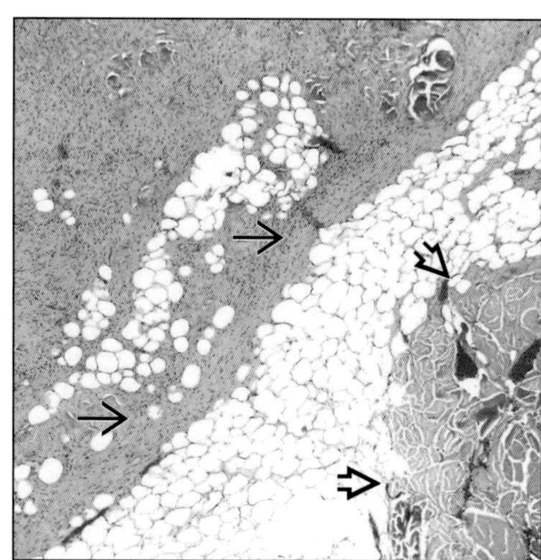

(Left) *Nuclear atypia is noted and the mitotic rate is significantly increased → in fibrosarcomatous DFSP.* ***(Right)*** *DFSP can be deeply invasive into the subcutis. The tumor in this section infiltrates through the subcutaneous adipose tissue → to approach the deep fascia ⇨.*

Microscopic Features and Differential Diagnoses

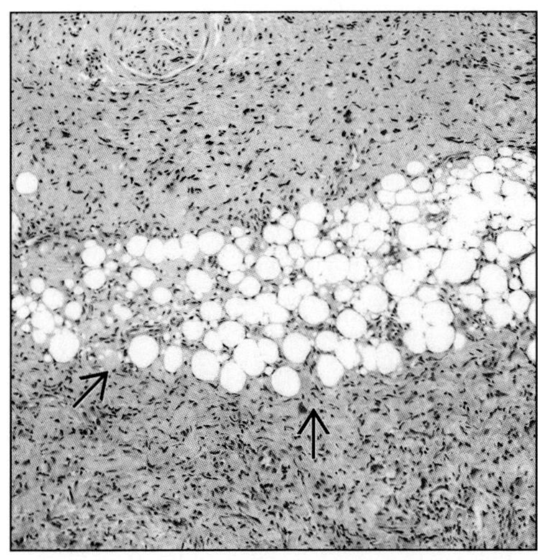

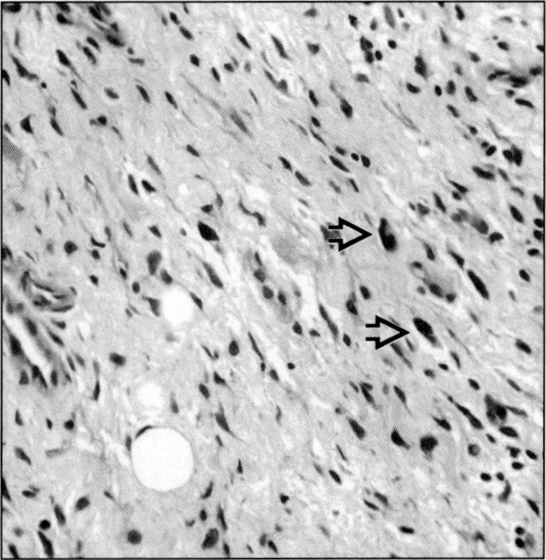

(Left) *Giant cell fibroblastoma has many similarities histologically with DFSP, including invasion into adipose tissue creating a "honeycomb" pattern* [arrow]*. GCF may resemble liposarcoma when giant cells become interspersed between lipocytes, mimicking adipocyte atypia.* ***(Right)*** *A parallel growth pattern as shown here is typical for GCF, although storiform areas can be present. Scattered giant cells characterize this tumor* [open arrow]*, seen here within a myxoid stromal background.*

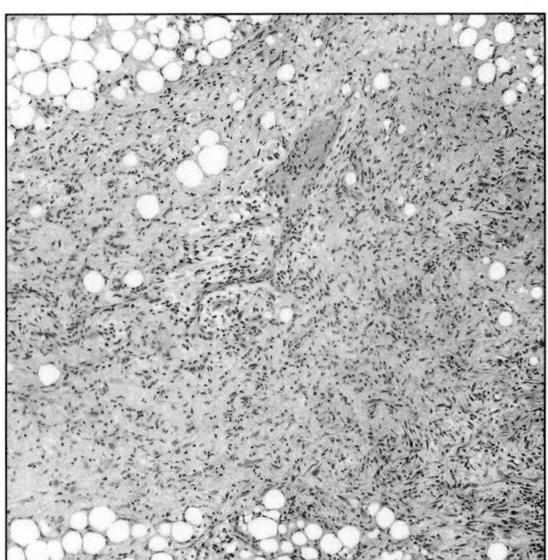

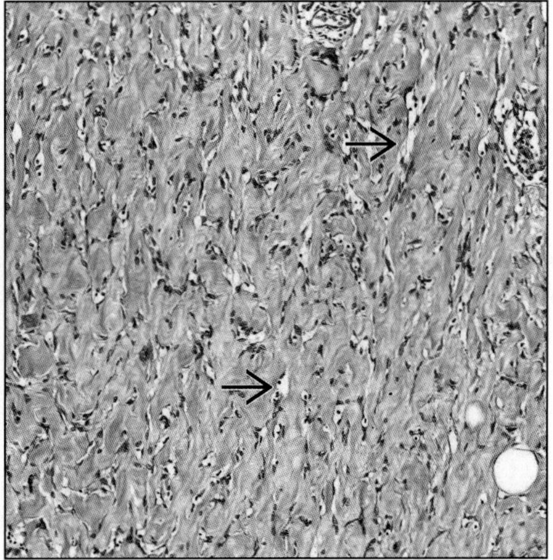

(Left) *Like DFSP, GCF extends along subcutaneous septa as seen in this section. The tumor stroma may be densely collagenous in these areas.* ***(Right)*** *A collagenized GCF is pictured here, with characteristic pseudovascular spaces* [arrow]*. These spaces are often angiectoid or sinusoidally dilated and are usually lined by multinucleated giant cells. The cells lining the pseudovascular spaces are typically dyscohesive. (Courtesy T. Mentzel, MD.)*

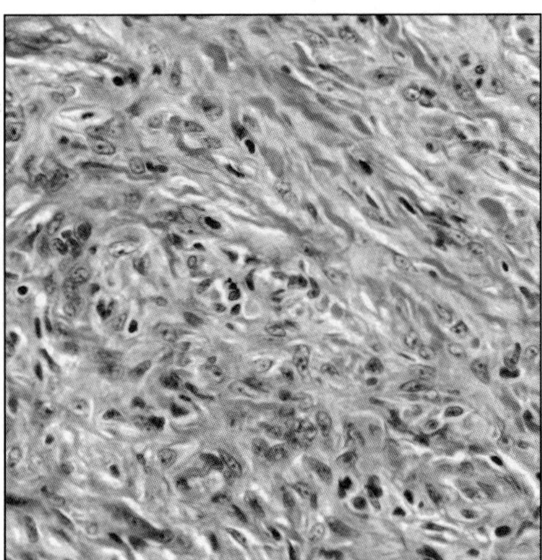

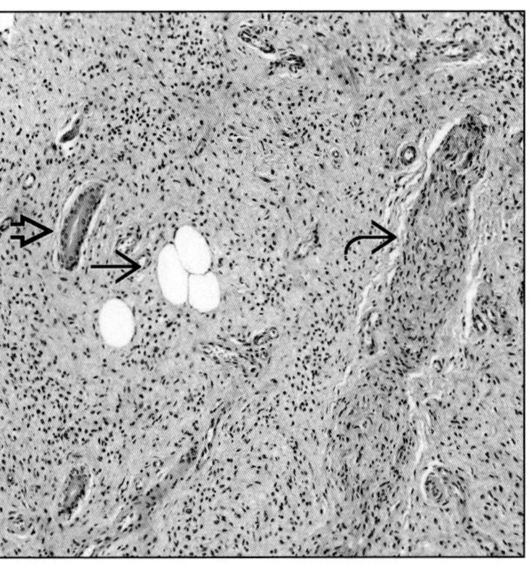

(Left) *Both benign fibrous histiocytoma and DFSP demonstrate a storiform architecture. The spindle cells in benign fibrous histiocytoma (shown here) are plumper and more polymorphous than those of DFSP.* ***(Right)*** *Diffuse neurofibromas (DNF) encase subcutaneous adipocytes* [arrow] *and spare adnexal structures* [open arrow]*, similar to DFSP. DNF is composed of short spindle cells without a storiform pattern. Meissner-like corpuscles can sometimes be seen in DNF, as well as enlarged nerves* [curved arrow]*.*

RHABDOMYOMATOUS MESENCHYMAL HAMARTOMA

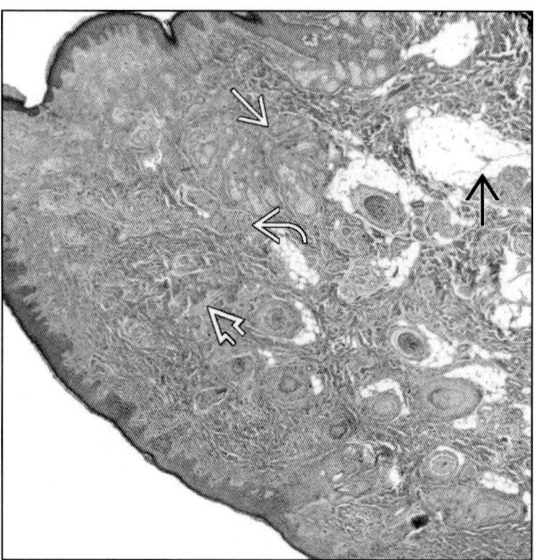

RMHS typically occurs on the face and neck of newborns. The lesion consists of a disordered collection of mature adipose tissue ⇒, skeletal muscle ⇒, adnexal elements ⇒, and nerve bundles ⇒.

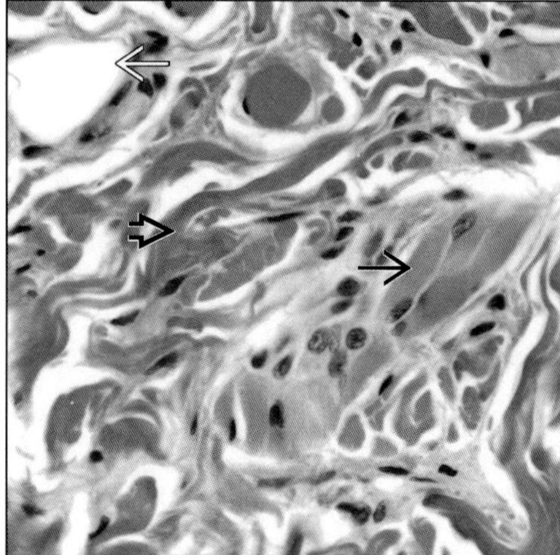

Skeletal fibers ⇒ are present in a background of collagenous stroma ⇒. Note the mature adipocyte ⇒.

TERMINOLOGY

Abbreviations

- Rhabdomyomatous mesenchymal hamartoma of skin (RMHS)

Synonyms

- Striated muscle hamartoma
- Congenital midline hamartoma
- Hamartoma of cutaneous adnexa and mesenchyme

Definitions

- Extremely rare congenital lesion of dermis and soft tissues
- Consists of a disordered collection of mature adipose tissue, skeletal muscle, adnexal elements, and nerve bundles

CLINICAL ISSUES

Presentation

- Seen in newborns, infants, and young children
- Rare case reports in adults
  - Unclear if lesions were present since birth
- Lesions typically present on face and neck of newborns
- Male predominance
- May be single or multiple
  - Most often a single lesion
- Predilection for
  - Chin
  - Periorbital
  - Periauricular
  - Anterior mid-neck
- Also reported in
  - Vagina
  - Nares
  - Oral cavity
- Some patients have associated congential anomalies
  - Dermoid cysts
  - Facial clefts
  - Amniotic bands
  - Sclerocorneas

Treatment

- Surgical approaches
  - Local excision

Prognosis

- Benign lesion

MACROSCOPIC FEATURES

General Features

- Flat, plaque-like
- Grossly polypoid
  - Attached to skin by a long stalk
- Dome-shaped papule
  - Central umbilication
- Yellow-brown, ill-defined mass
  - Within dermis and subcutaneous tissue

Size

- Varies from millimeters to 1-2 centimeters

MICROSCOPIC PATHOLOGY

Histologic Features

- Groups of well-differentiated skeletal muscle fibers
  - Unencapsulated
  - Aligned perpendicular to surface epithelium
  - In a background of collagenous stroma
- Lesion also associated with
  - Mature adipose tissue
  - Adnexal structures
  - Blood vessels
  - Peripheral nerves
  - Central calcification and ossification is rare

RHABDOMYOMATOUS MESENCHYMAL HAMARTOMA

Key Facts

Terminology
- Seen in newborns, infants, and young children
- Extremely rare congenital lesion of dermis and soft tissues

Clinical Issues
- Local excision
- Benign lesion
- Most often occurs in males
- Lesions typically present on face and neck of newborns

Microscopic Pathology
- Consists of a disordered collection of mature adipose tissue, skeletal muscle, adnexal elements, and nerve bundles
- Groups of well-differentiated skeletal muscle fibers
  - Aligned perpendicular to surface epithelium

- Overlying surface epithelium is unremarkable

DIFFERENTIAL DIAGNOSIS

Fibrous Hamartoma of Infancy (FHI)
- Small, rapidly growing mass
- Most common location is posterior axillary fold
- 3 distinct components forming organoid pattern
  - Fibrous tissue
  - Mature adipose tissue
  - Immature small, round mesenchymal cells
- FHI does not contain skeletal muscle or nerve
- RMHS does not contain an immature mesenchymal component

Nevus Lipomatosis Superficialis
- Multiple or single lesions
- Predilection for the lines of skinfold of the pelvic girdle
- Groups of ectopic adipocytes within papillary or reticular dermis
- Can see increased vascularity, scattered lymphocytes

Cutaneous Embryonal Rhabdomyosarcoma
- Superficial location
- Extremely rare
- Consists of less differentiated small round blue cells

SELECTED REFERENCES

1. Brinster NK et al: Rhabdomyomatous mesenchymal hamartoma presenting on a digit. J Cutan Pathol. 36(1):61-3, 2009
2. Han SH et al: Rhabdomyomatous mesenchymal hamartoma of the vagina. Pediatr Dermatol. 26(6):753-5, 2009
3. Williams NP et al: Rhabdomyomatous mesenchymal hamartoma: clinical overview and report of a case with spontaneous regression. West Indian Med J. 58(6):607-9, 2009
4. De la Sotta P et al: Rhabdomyomatous (mesenchymal) hamartoma of the tongue: report of a case. J Oral Pathol Med. 36(1):58-9, 2007
5. Solis-Coria A et al: Rhabdomyomatous mesenchymal hamartoma presenting as a skin tag in the sternoclavicular area. Pathol Oncol Res. 13(4):375-8, 2007
6. Chang CP et al: Rhabdomyomatous mesenchymal hamartoma: a plaque-type variant in an adult. Kaohsiung J Med Sci. 21(4):185-8, 2005
7. Magro G et al: Rhabdomyomatous mesenchymal hamartoma of oral cavity: an unusual location for such a rare lesion. Virchows Arch. 446(3):346-7, 2005
8. Takeyama J et al: Rhabdomyomatous mesenchymal hamartoma associated with nasofrontal meningocele and dermoid cyst. J Cutan Pathol. 32(4):310-3, 2005
9. Rosenberg AS et al: Rhabdomyomatous mesenchymal hamartoma: an unusual dermal entity with a report of two cases and a review of the literature. J Cutan Pathol. 29(4):238-43, 2002

IMAGE GALLERY

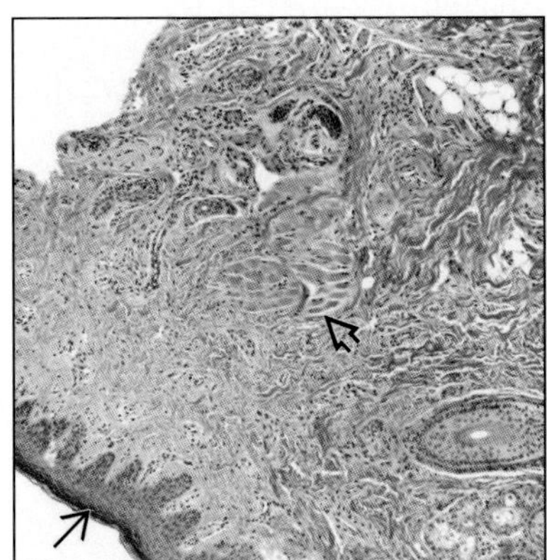

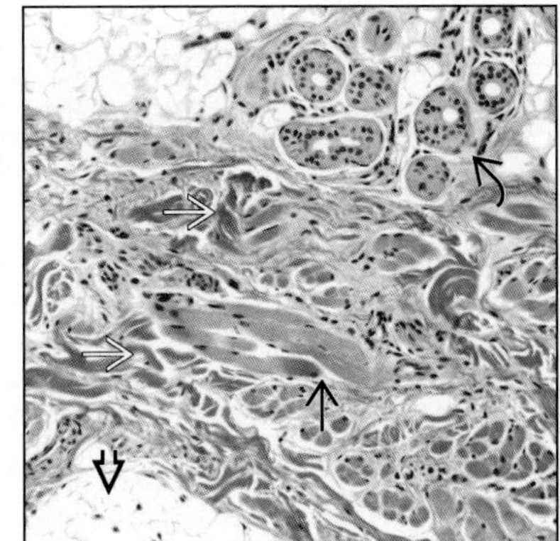

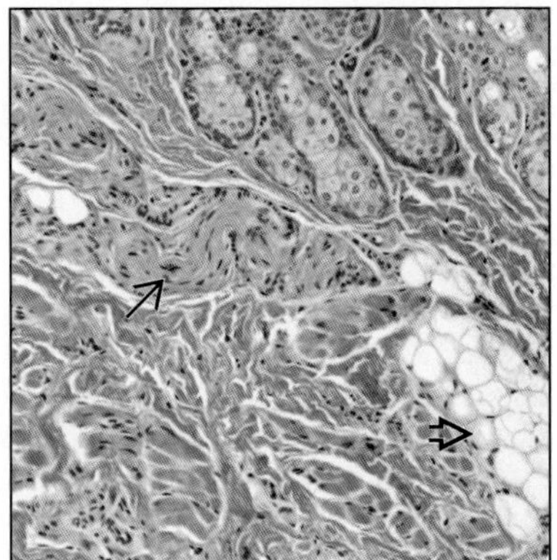

*(**Left**) Overlying surface epithelium is unremarkable ⇒. Notice that the lesion is unencapsulated. Skeletal muscle fibers, seen within the dermis, tend to be aligned perpendicular ⇒ to the surface epithelium. (**Center**) Mature-appearing skeletal muscle fibers ⇒ surrounded by a collagenous stroma ➡, adnexal structures ⇒, and mature adipocytes ⇒ are seen in this RMHS. (**Right**) Nerve ⇒ is seen adjacent to mature adipocytes ⇒.*

FETAL RHABDOMYOMA

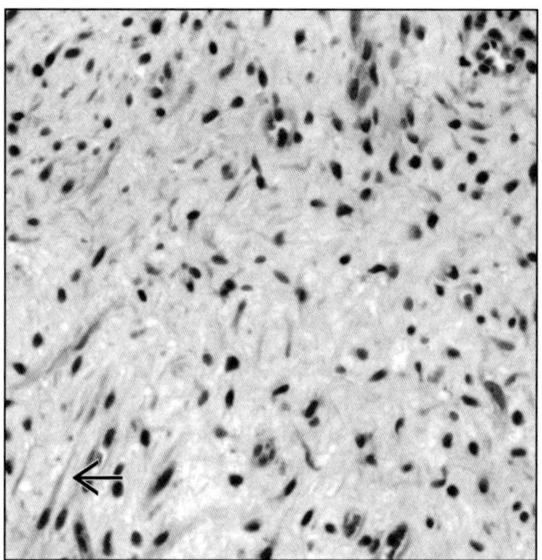

Fetal rhabdomyoma, myxoid type shows primitive round, oval and spindled cells in a myxoid background. Note the bipolar eosinophilic cytoplasmic processes ⇒.

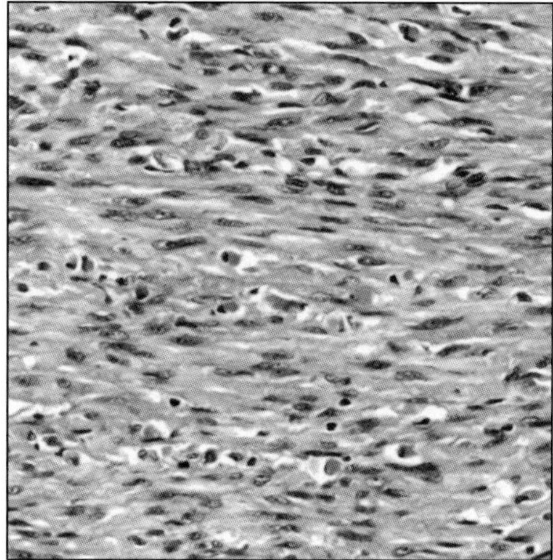

Fetal rhabdomyoma, intermediate type contains more differentiated muscle fibers with frequent cross striations and little to no myxoid stroma.

TERMINOLOGY

Abbreviations

- Fetal rhabdomyoma (FR)

Synonyms

- Myxoid type is also known as classic type
- Intermediate type is also known as cellular or juvenile type

Definitions

- Extracardiac, soft tissue, benign neoplasm with skeletal muscle differentiation
- FR is one of the subtypes of extracardiac rhabdomyomas
  - Adult type occurs in head and neck of elderly patients
  - Fetal type occurs in head and neck of children and adults
    - Myxoid or classic type is predominantly myxoid with immature skeletal differentiation
    - Cellular, juvenile or intermediate type shows high degree of cellular differentiation with little myxoid matrix
  - Genital type occurs in vagina and vulva of middle-aged women

ETIOLOGY/PATHOGENESIS

Developmental Anomaly

- Some fetal rhabdomyomas associated with nevoid basal cell syndrome
  - Autosomal dominant syndrome
  - Multiple basal cell carcinomas appear in childhood
  - Associated with abnormalities of bones, skin, nervous system, and reproductive system
  - *PTCH* mutations
    - Inhibitory receptor in sonic hedgehog signaling pathway

CLINICAL ISSUES

Epidemiology

- Incidence
  - Rare
- Age
  - Mostly in childhood; median: 4 years
    - About 1/2 are seen in 1st year of life or are congenital
    - Rare examples in adults up to 6th decade

Site

- Most often in head and neck region
  - Orbit, tongue, soft palate, pre- and postauricular, nasopharynx
- Rare sites include extremities, chest and abdominal wall, axilla, spermatic cord, perianal region, retroperitoneum

Presentation

- Myxoid (classic) type
  - Boys, in 1st year of life
  - Pre- or postauricular mass
- Intermediate (cellular, juvenile) type
  - Seen more often in adults
  - Head and neck region

Treatment

- Surgical approaches
  - Simple complete excision

Prognosis

- Excellent after complete excision
- Can recur if incompletely excised

MACROSCOPIC FEATURES

General Features

- Usually solitary; can occasionally be multinodular or multicentric

FETAL RHABDOMYOMA

Key Facts

Terminology
- Extracardiac, soft tissue, benign neoplasm with skeletal muscle differentiation
- Fetal type occurs in head and neck of children and adults
- Myxoid or classic type is predominantly myxoid with immature skeletal differentiation
- Cellular, juvenile or intermediate type shows a high degree of cellular differentiation with little myxoid matrix

Etiology/Pathogenesis
- Some fetal rhabdomyomas associated with nevoid basal cell syndrome

Clinical Issues
- About 1/2 are seen in 1st year of life or are congenital
- Excellent prognosis after complete excision
- Can recur if incompletely excised

Microscopic Pathology
- Myxoid type
  - Immature skeletal muscle fibers with a myxoid stroma
- Intermediate type
  - Differentiated muscle fibers with little or no myxoid stroma

Ancillary Tests
- Immunoreactive for
  - Desmin
  - Myogenin
  - MYOD1

- Submucosal or subcutis in location
- Mucosal lesions can be polypoid or pedunculated
- Well circumscribed
- Gray-white, mucoid cut surface

Size
- Most lesions are small (< 10 cm diameter); median: ~ 3 cm

MICROSCOPIC PATHOLOGY

Histologic Features
- Variable histologic patterns
- Myxoid type
  - Primitive oval or spindle-shaped cells
    - Indistinct cytoplasm
    - Slight nuclear hyperchromasia
  - Immature skeletal muscle fibers
    - Small, uniform nuclei
    - Unipolar or bipolar eosinophilic cytoplasmic processes
    - Similar to what is seen at approximately 10 weeks gestation
  - Myxoid stroma
  - No atypia or necrosis; mitoses usually absent
- Intermediate type
  - Little or no myxoid stroma
  - Differentiated muscle fibers
    - Spectrum of skeletal muscle differentiation
    - Strap cells, smooth muscle-like cells, and rounded rhabdomyoblasts
    - Abundant eosinophilic cytoplasm
    - Cross striations frequent
    - Vesicular nuclei
    - Mild cellular pleomorphism is OK
    - No marked atypia or necrosis; mitoses usually absent
- May see transitional forms with both myxoid and intermediate features

ANCILLARY TESTS

Immunohistochemistry
- Immunoreactive for desmin, myogenin, and MYOD1

Electron Microscopy
- Sarcomeric differentiation: Thick and thin myofilaments, Z-bands, glycogen deposits associated with filaments

DIFFERENTIAL DIAGNOSIS

Embryonal and Spindle Cell Rhabdomyosarcoma
- Typically not well circumscribed
- Tend to be deep lesions rather than superficial
- Mitotic figures, necrosis, pleomorphism easily identified

DIAGNOSTIC CHECKLIST

Pathologic Interpretation Pearls
- Knowledge of this tumor is important, as it can mimic embryonal rhabdomyosarcoma

SELECTED REFERENCES

1. Valdez TA et al: Recurrent fetal rhabdomyoma of the head and neck. Int J Pediatr Otorhinolaryngol. 70(6):1115-8, 2006
2. Watson J et al: Nevoid basal cell carcinoma syndrome and fetal rhabdomyoma: a case study. Ear Nose Throat J. 83(10):716-8, 2004
3. Kapadia SB et al: Fetal rhabdomyoma of the head and neck: a clinicopathologic and immunophenotypic study of 24 cases. Hum Pathol. 24(7):754-65, 1993

FETAL RHABDOMYOMA

Microscopic Features

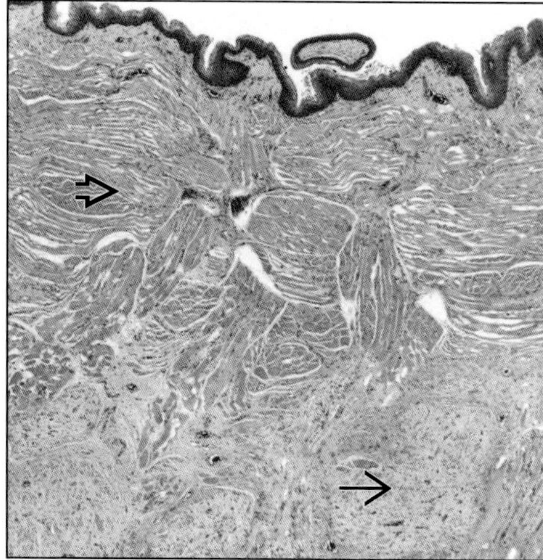

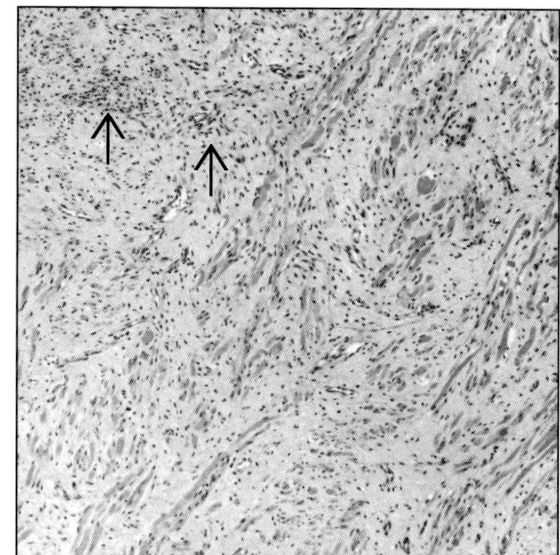

(Left) *This lesion developed in the tongue. Note the fetal rhabdomyoma (myxoid type) → deep to the normal skeletal muscle ⇨. At low power, one can appreciate the myxoid background.* ***(Right)*** *Scattered, small clusters of lymphocytes → are present in this fetal rhabdomyoma, myxoid type. Note the lack of necrosis.*

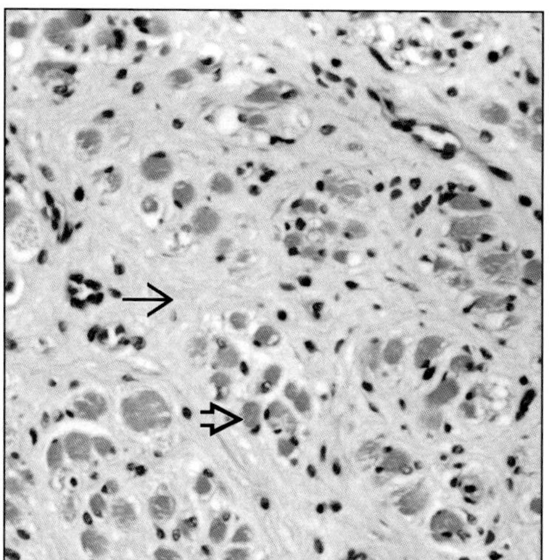

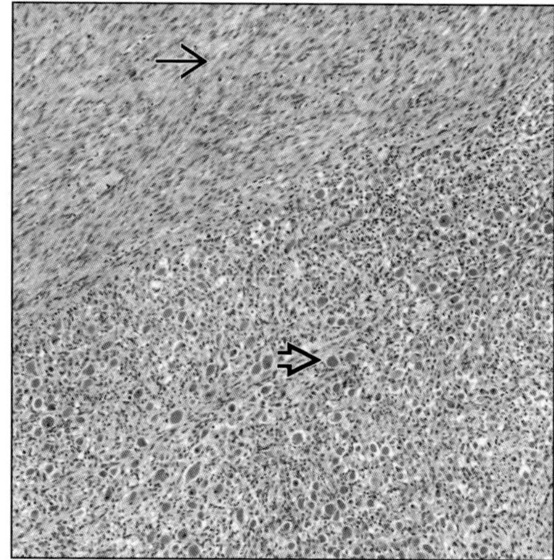

(Left) *Transitional forms between the myxoid and intermediate types are not uncommon. Mature, rhabdomyoblast-like large cells ⇨ are surrounded by myxoid stroma →.* ***(Right)*** *Fetal rhabdomyoma, intermediate type shows intersecting bundles or fascicles → of differentiated muscle fibers juxtaposed to a significant number of mature rhabdomyoblast-like large cells ⇨ with abundant eosinophilic cytoplasm. Note the lack of necrosis.*

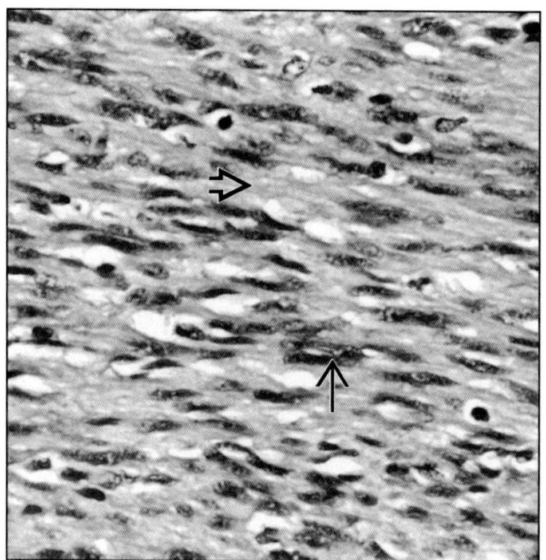

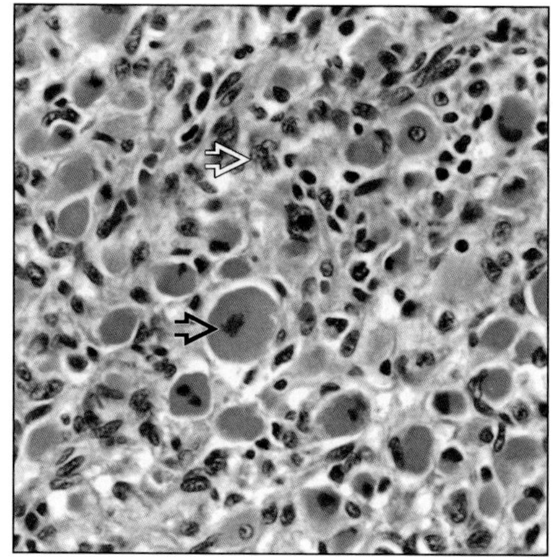

(Left) *Fetal rhabdomyoma, intermediate type shows cells that are broad and strap-like. The nuclei are vesicular → and may show mild pleomorphism, but marked nuclear atypia should not be present. The eosinophilic cytoplasm ⇨ is abundant and may contain cross striations.* ***(Right)*** *A wide spectrum of skeletal muscle differentiation can be seen within a single case of FR. Large rhabdomyoblast-like cells ⇨ are mixed with less-differentiated round to oval cells ➡.*

Microscopic and Immunohistochemical Features

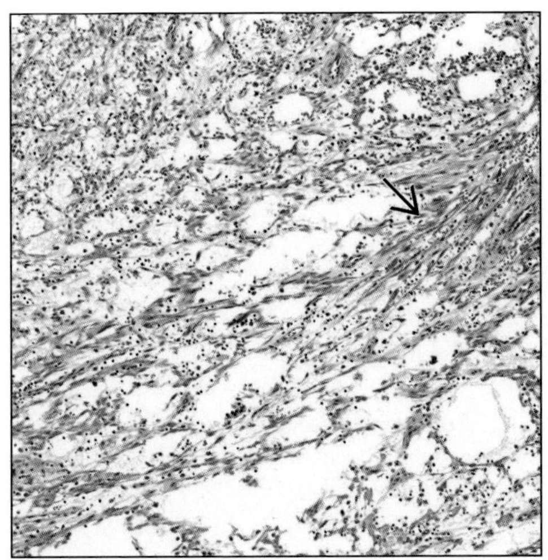

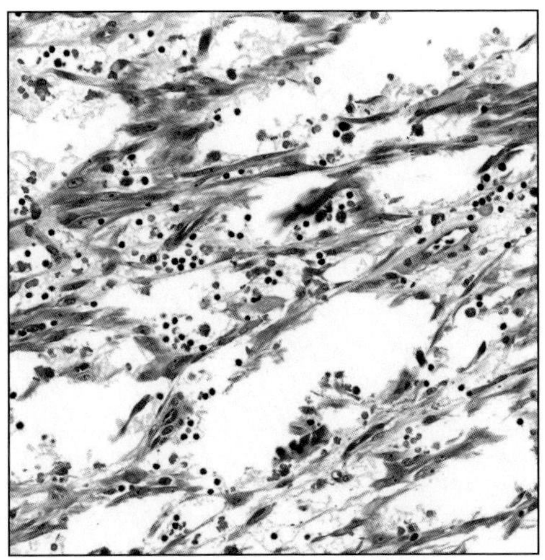

*(**Left**) Hematoxylin & eosin shows fetal rhabdomyoma of myxoid (immature) type. Slender spindle cells form loosely organized fascicles ➔ in myxoid stroma. Note the absence of pleomorphism and necrosis. (**Right**) Hematoxylin & eosin shows fetal rhabdomyoma of myxoid (immature) type, with spindle cells arranged in a vaguely fascicular pattern in myxoid stroma. Pleomorphism and necrosis are absent.*

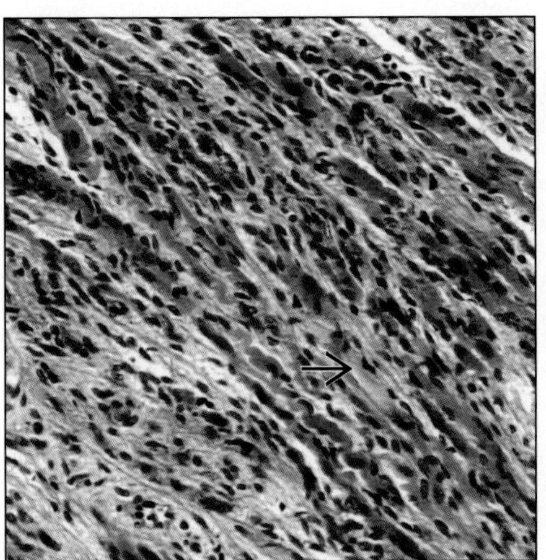

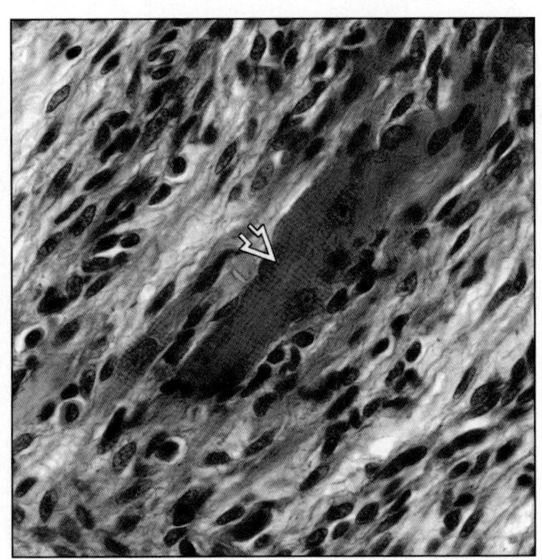

*(**Left**) Hematoxylin & eosin shows intermediate-type fetal rhabdomyoma manifesting relatively uniform spindle cells ➔, with differentiation resembling late-stage embryonic skeletal muscle development. Nuclei are uniform, and no mitotic activity is seen. (**Right**) Hematoxylin & eosin shows intermediate-type fetal rhabdomyoma at higher magnification. Note variation in cell type. Typical cross-striations ➨, characteristic of skeletal muscle differentiation, are apparent in the cytoplasm.*

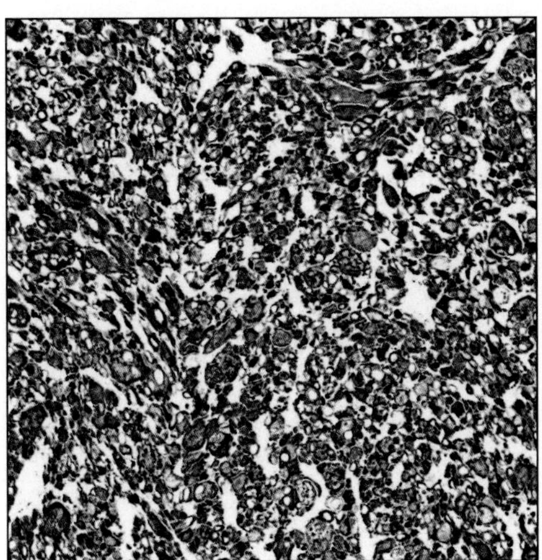

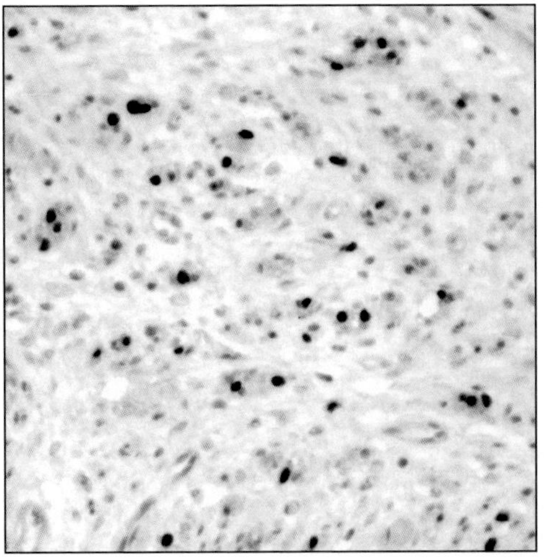

*(**Left**) Desmin stain shows strong diffuse positivity throughout the lesion. This is a diagnostic finding in rhabdomyoma and can also highlight cross-striations. (**Right**) Myogenin shows immunoreactivity in the nuclei of many of the lesional cells. This is diagnostic of skeletal muscle differentiation. Cytoplasmic staining is sometimes seen but is nonspecific and should be disregarded.*

DIFFUSE LIPOMATOSIS

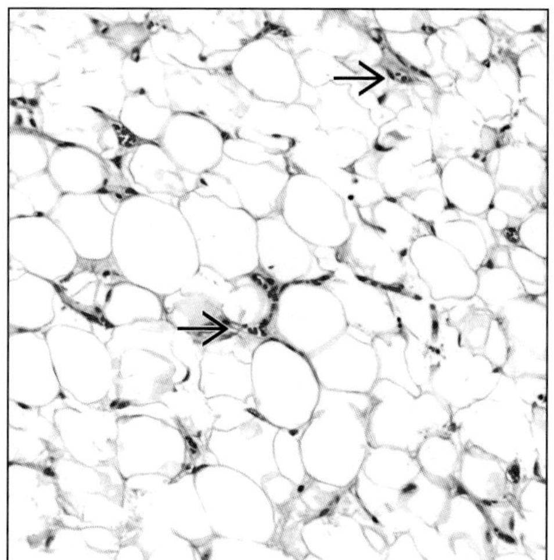

Lipomatosis is histologically indistinguishable from lipoma. It is composed of mature fat cells and is well vascularized ⇒.

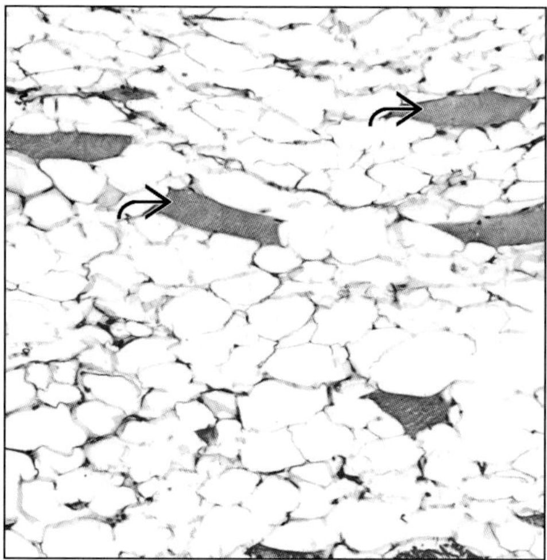

The adipose tissue overgrowth in lipomatosis frequently extends into underlying skeletal muscle ⇒ *and therefore mimics an intramuscular lipoma.*

TERMINOLOGY

Definitions

- Diffuse overgrowth of mature adipose tissue

CLINICAL ISSUES

Presentation

- Usually affects children in 1st 2 years of life
- Painful or painless mass
  - May mimic a neoplasm
    - Rapid growth
    - Large size
- Limb enlargement in extremity lesions
- May be associated with macrodactyly and gigantism
- Also seen in head, neck, abdominal cavity, and GI tract

Treatment

- Palliative surgical resection of excessive adipose tissue

Prognosis

- Tendency for recurrence due to poor circumscription

IMAGE FINDINGS

Radiographic Findings

- Abnormally large accumulations of fat with poor margination
- Signal intensity of lesion identical to normal subcutaneous tissue

MACROSCOPIC FEATURES

General Features

- Poorly marginated large accumulations of normal-appearing fatty tissue
- Subcutis and muscle are involved
- Nerves are not involved

MICROSCOPIC PATHOLOGY

Histologic Features

- Indistinguishable from lipoma
- Mature adipose tissue in sheets or lobules
- May infiltrate into skeletal muscle or underlying deeper structures

Cytologic Features

- No nuclear atypia
- No lipoblasts

DIFFERENTIAL DIAGNOSIS

Symmetric Lipomatosis

- Synonyms: Madelung disease, Launois-Bensaude syndrome
- Massive fat deposition around neck (lipoma annulare colli)
- Almost exclusively in middle-aged men
- May extend around cheek, breast, upper arm
- Mostly sporadic but may be familial
- Point mutations in mitochondrial genes reported in symmetric lipomatosis

Pelvic Lipomatosis

- Perirectal and perivesical regions involved
- Most commonly affects black men in 3rd-4th decade
- Association with cystitis cystica and cystitis glandularis

Steroid Lipomatosis

- Source may be endogenous (as in Cushing disease) or exogenous (steroid therapy)
- Unevenly distributed fatty deposits
- Face, sternum, or back involved most commonly

HIV Lipodystrophy

- Related to use of protease inhibitors

DIFFUSE LIPOMATOSIS

Key Facts

Terminology
- Diffuse overgrowth of mature adipose tissue

Clinical Issues
- Presents as painless mass or with obstructive symptoms
- Tendency for recurrence due to poor circumscription
- Usually affects children in 1st 2 years of life
- May mimic a neoplasm with rapid growth and large size

Macroscopic Features
- Poorly marginated large accumulations of normal-appearing fatty tissue

Microscopic Pathology
- Indistinguishable from lipoma
- May infiltrate into skeletal muscle or underlying deeper structures
- No nuclear atypia

- Associated with diabetes
- Increased deposition on back and abdomen

Intramuscular Lipoma (IML)
- Confined to muscle
- Nodular rather than diffuse overgrowth of adipose tissue seen in IML
- Entrapped skeletal muscle fibers present in both conditions (more in IML)

Dercum Disease
- Nodular or diffuse deposits of mature adipose tissue
- Confined to subcutaneous region
- Fatty deposits are painful and tender
- Mostly in postmenopausal women around thigh or pelvis

Atypical Lipomatous Tumor (ALT)
- Atypical stromal cells with hyperchromatic nuclei present in ALT
- Atypical multivacuolated lipoblasts present in ALT

DIAGNOSTIC CHECKLIST

Clinically Relevant Pathologic Features
- Gross appearance
  - Diffuse overgrowth of adipose tissue that, on imaging, has same signal as normal subcutaneous tissue

Pathologic Interpretation Pearls
- Morphologically normal adipose tissue that may infiltrate into underlying structures or skeletal muscle

SELECTED REFERENCES

1. Sözen S et al: The importance of re-evaluation in patients with cystitis glandularis associated with pelvic lipomatosis: a case report. Urol Oncol. 22(5):428-30, 2004
2. Klopstock T et al: Mitochondrial DNA mutations in multiple symmetric lipomatosis. Mol Cell Biochem. 174(1-2):271-5, 1997
3. Coode PE et al: Diffuse lipomatosis involving the thoracic and abdominal wall: CT features. J Comput Assist Tomogr. 15(2):341-3, 1991
4. Heyns CF: Pelvic lipomatosis: a review of its diagnosis and management. J Urol. 146(2):267-73, 1991
5. Klein FA et al: Pelvic lipomatosis: 35-year experience. J Urol. 139(5):998-1001, 1988
6. Shukla LW et al: Mediastinal lipomatosis: a complication of high dose steroid therapy in children. Pediatr Radiol. 19(1):57-8, 1988
7. Ruzicka T et al: Benign symmetric lipomatosis Launois-Bensaude. Report of ten cases and review of the literature. J Am Acad Dermatol. 17(4):663-74, 1987
8. Nixon HH et al: Congenital lipomatosis: a report of four cases. J Pediatr Surg. 6(6):742-5, 1971

IMAGE GALLERY

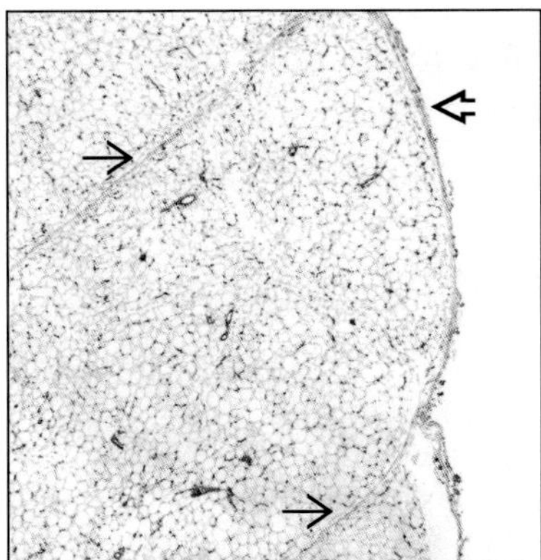

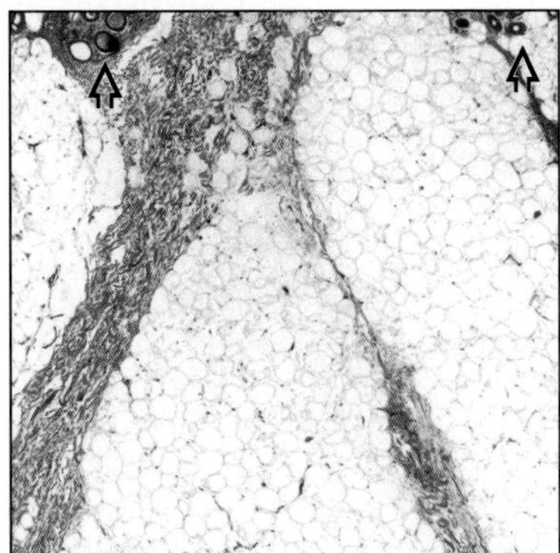

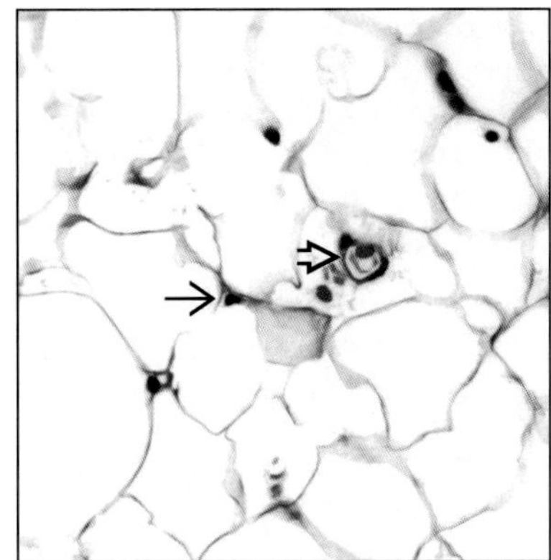

(Left) *This lesion is thinly encapsulated ⇨. Note the thin, fibrous septa →.* ***(Center)*** *Axillary lipomatosis is shown with massive accumulation of mature adipose tissue in the subcutaneous region. Note dermal appendages ⇨ at the top of the image.* ***(Right)*** *The mature adipocytes vary little in size and shape. Nuclei are small and uniform →. Note the capillary structure ⇨.*

LIPOBLASTOMA

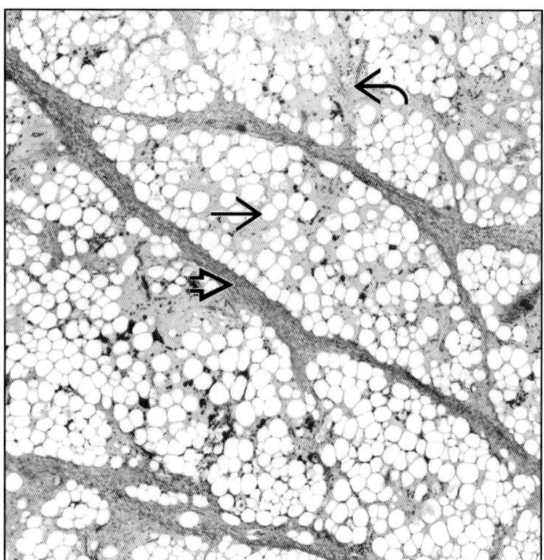

Hematoxylin & eosin at low power shows fibrous bands ⇨ separating lobules of adipose tissue → with varying maturation and myxoid change ↶.

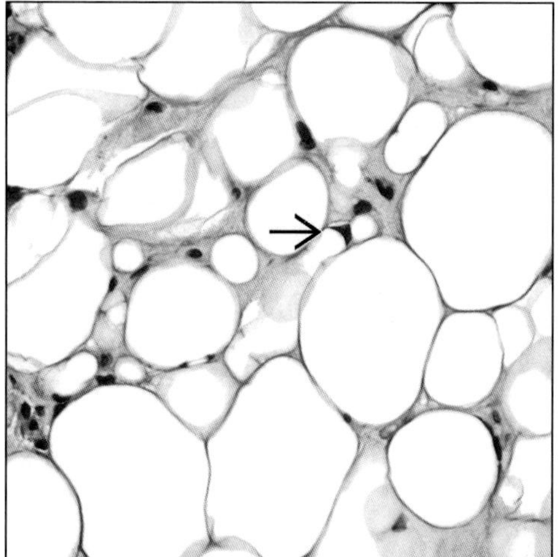

Hematoxylin & eosin at high power shows adipocytes of varying differentiation, including lipoblasts → within a myxoid background.

TERMINOLOGY

Synonyms

- Fetal lipoma
- Fetal fat tumor
- Fetocellular lipoma
- Embryonal lipoma
- Congenital lipomatoid tumor
- Lipoblastic tumor of childhood

CLINICAL ISSUES

Site

- Extremities most common
- Less common sites include
  - Head and neck
  - Trunk
  - Mediastinum
  - Retroperitoneum
  - Mesentery and omentum
  - Scrotum

Presentation

- Usually presents within 1st 3 years of life
  - Only rarely seen in adults
- More common in males
- Painless mass
- Can be slowly or rapidly growing
- Diffuse types can compress adjacent structures and compromise function

Treatment

- Surgical approaches
  - Complete local excision

Prognosis

- Excellent
- Recurrences associated with incomplete resection

IMAGE FINDINGS

General Features

- Well-delineated, soft tissue mass with density of adipose tissue
- Cannot reliably distinguish from lipoma or liposarcoma

MACROSCOPIC FEATURES

General Features

- Circumscribed vs. diffuse
  - Circumscribed type is located in superficial tissues
  - Diffuse type infiltrates underlying subcutis and muscle
    - Greater tendency for recurrence
    - Also known as lipoblastomatosis
- Although benign, may compress or interfere with adjacent structures

Size

- Usually 3-5 cm
- Very large tumors can be seen, especially in mediastinum or retroperitoneum

Cut Surface

- Yellow, creamy white, or tan
- Myxoid nodules
- Cystic spaces
- Fibrous septae may or may not be visible grossly

MICROSCOPIC PATHOLOGY

Histologic Features

- Irregular lobules of adipose tissue
- Fat cells in different stages of development
  - Primitive stellate to spindled cells
  - Multivacuolated lipoblasts and signet ring cells
  - Mature adipocytes

LIPOBLASTOMA

Key Facts

Clinical Issues

- Most common on extremities
- Presents within 1st 3 years of life
- Complete local excision is curative
  - Recurrences associated with incomplete resection
- Diffuse types can compress adjacent structures and compromise function

Macroscopic Features

- Usually 3-5 cm
- Circumscribed type is located in superficial tissues
- Diffuse type infiltrates underlying subcutis and muscle

Microscopic Pathology

- Irregular lobules of adipose tissue
- Fat cells in different stages of development
- Fibrous septae of varying thicknesses separate lobules
- Mesenchymal areas with loose myxoid appearance
- Zonal maturation
- May see 2-3 mitoses per HPF
  - No atypical mitoses

Ancillary Tests

- Rearrangement of chromosome 8q11-13 (*PLAG1* gene on 8q12)
- *PLAG1* fusion genes can be detected by FISH

Top Differential Diagnoses

- Myxoid liposarcoma
- Lipoma
- Fibrolipoma

- Fibrous septae of varying thicknesses separate lobules
  - Contain numerous capillaries and venules
  - Diffuse subtype may have less distinct lobular pattern
- Mesenchymal areas with loose myxoid appearance
  - Rich in hyaluronic acid
  - Decreases with maturation
- Zonal maturation
  - Immature cells and lipoblasts near periphery
  - Mature fat cells at center
- Lobules contain numerous blood vessels in plexiform or "chicken wire" pattern
  - More prominent in highly myxoid areas
- May see 2-3 typical mitoses per HPF
  - No atypical mitoses
- **Histologic variants**
  - Hyaline collagen deposition
  - Chondroid metaplasia
  - Extramedullary hematopoiesis
  - Chronic inflammation
- **Tumor maturation**
  - Decreased myxoid stroma
  - Thinner fibrous bands
  - Fewer lipoblasts
  - Extensively matured lipoblastoma can be difficult to differentiate from fibrolipoma

Predominant Pattern/Injury Type

- Lobulated

Predominant Cell/Compartment Type

- Adipose cell

ANCILLARY TESTS

Cytogenetics

- Rearrangement of chromosome 8q11-13
  - *PLAG1* gene found on chromosome 8q12
  - *PLAG1* fusion genes can be detected by FISH
- Polysomy 8 found in cases without *PLAG1* rearrangement
- Can be very helpful in differentiating from myxoid liposarcoma

DIFFERENTIAL DIAGNOSIS

Myxoid Liposarcoma

- Very rarely seen in children
- Focal nuclear atypia or atypical mitoses
- Characteristic t(12;16) translocation

Lipoma

- Lacks lipoblasts

Fibrolipoma

- Lacks lipoblasts

SELECTED REFERENCES

1. Antoniou D et al: A case of maturing perineal lipoblastoma in an infant. Med Princ Pract. 18(4):335-8, 2009
2. Meloni-Ehrig AM et al: A case of lipoblastoma with seven copies of chromosome 8. Cancer Genet Cytogenet. 190(1):49-51, 2009
3. Bartuma H et al: Cytogenetic and molecular cytogenetic findings in lipoblastoma. Cancer Genet Cytogenet. 183(1):60-3, 2008
4. Speer AL et al: Contemporary management of lipoblastoma. J Pediatr Surg. 43(7):1295-300, 2008
5. Moholkar S et al: Radiological-pathological correlation in lipoblastoma and lipoblastomatosis. Pediatr Radiol. 36(8):851-6, 2006
6. Miller GG et al: Tumor karyotype differentiates lipoblastoma from liposarcoma. J Pediatr Surg. 32(12):1771-2, 1997
7. Bolen JW et al: Benign lipoblastoma and myxoid liposarcoma: a comparative light- and electron-microscopic study. Am J Surg Pathol. 4(2):163-74, 1980

LIPOBLASTOMA

Microscopic Features

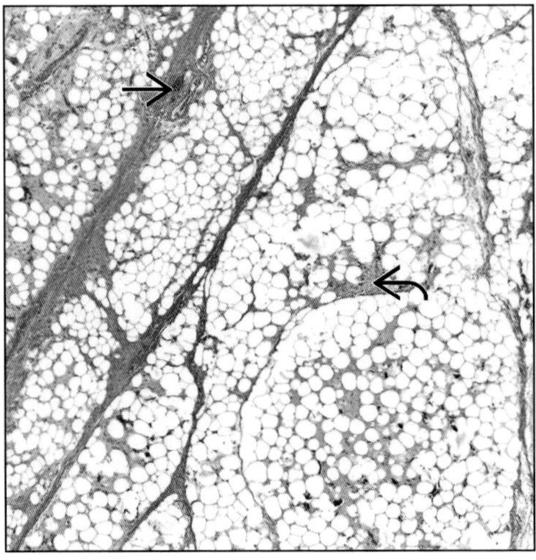

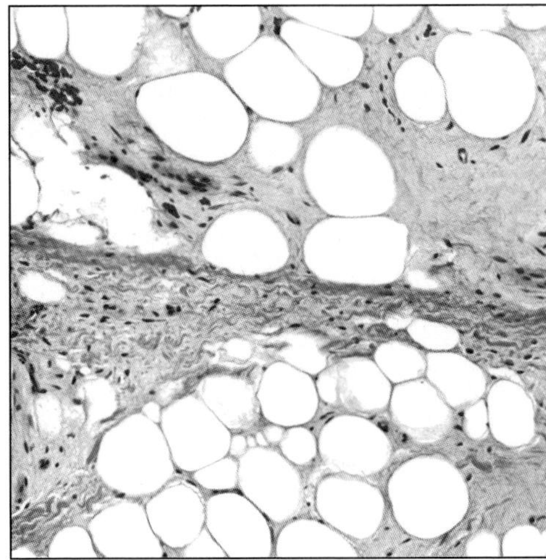

*(**Left**) Hematoxylin & eosin at low power shows fibrous bands ➔ separating lobules of adipocytes with interspersed myxoid stroma ➚. This is typical of a lipoblastoma. (**Right**) Hematoxylin & eosin at medium power shows a fibrous band separating lobules of adipose tissue and myxoid stroma. Note the variability in the adipose cells.*

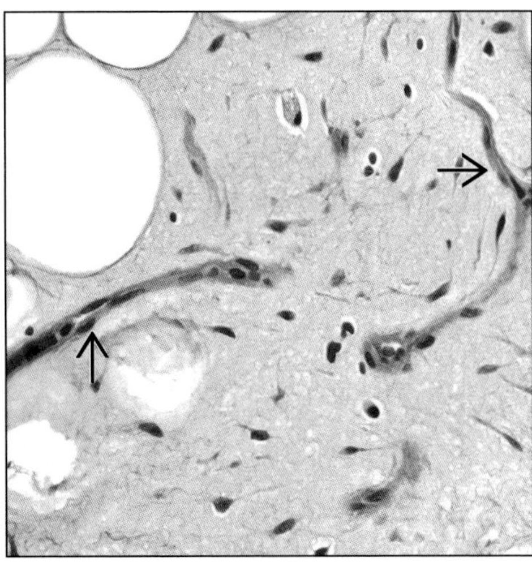

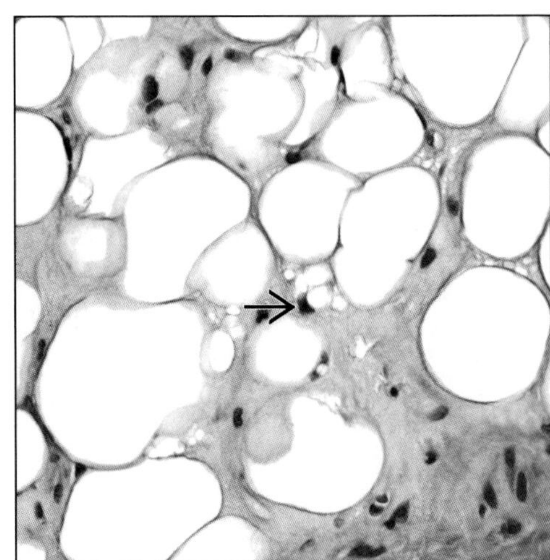

*(**Left**) Hematoxylin & eosin at high power shows a hypocellular myxoid stroma with a "chicken wire" vascular pattern ➔. These areas can be difficult to distinguish from a myxoid liposarcoma. (**Right**) Hematoxylin & eosin at high power shows a lipoblast ➔, interspersed with maturing adipocytes within a myxoid stroma. Lipoblasts are small, vacuolated cells with nuclei that are pushed to 1 side.*

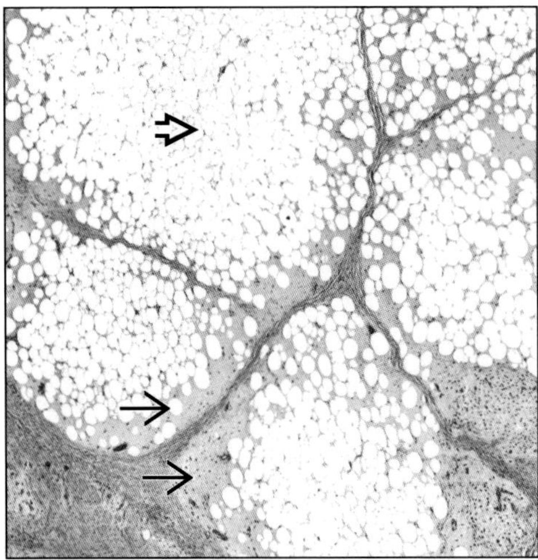

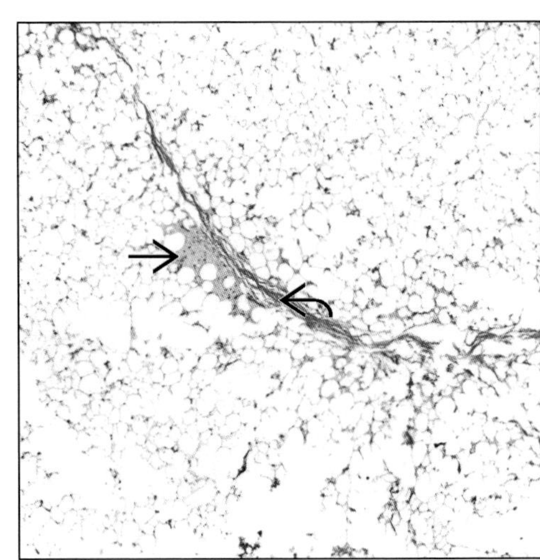

*(**Left**) Hematoxylin & eosin at lower power shows a lipoblastoma with the typical zonation pattern. Myxoid areas containing more immature adipocytes and lipoblasts are near the fibrous bands ➔, while more mature adipocytes ➲ are in the center of the lobules. (**Right**) Hematoxylin & eosin at low power shows a lipoblastoma with a relatively small amount of myxoid stroma ➔ and only thin fibrous bands ➚. Note the zonation of myxoid stroma near the fibrous bands.*

Microscopic Features and Differential Diagnosis

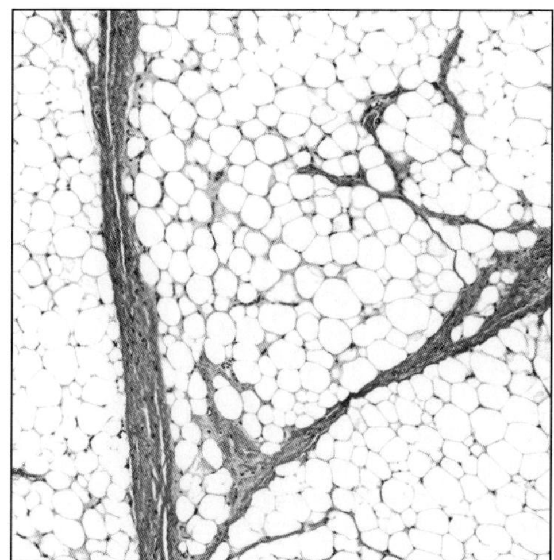

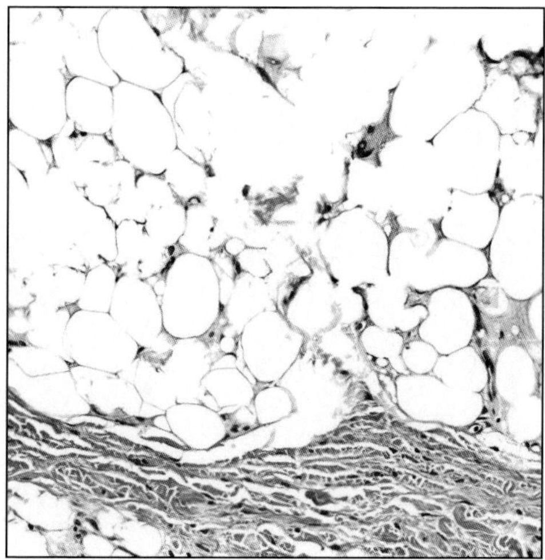

(Left) *Hematoxylin & eosin at medium power shows adipocytes of varying sizes within a small amount of myxoid stroma near a fibrous band. This zonation pattern is typical of a lipoblastoma.* ***(Right)*** *Hematoxylin & eosin at medium-high power shows varied adipocytes and probable lipoblasts within the myxoid stroma, next to a thick fibrous band.*

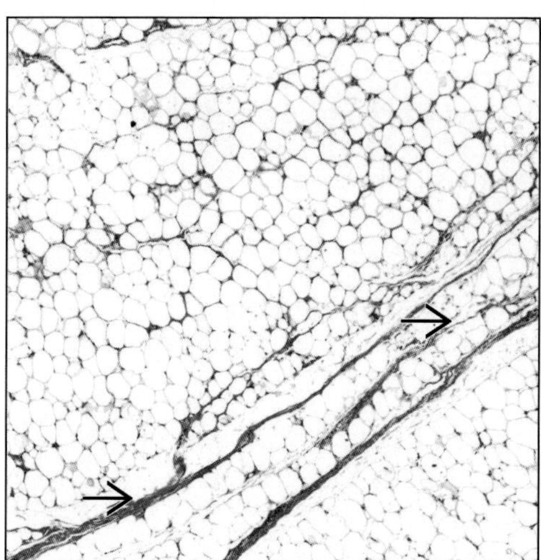

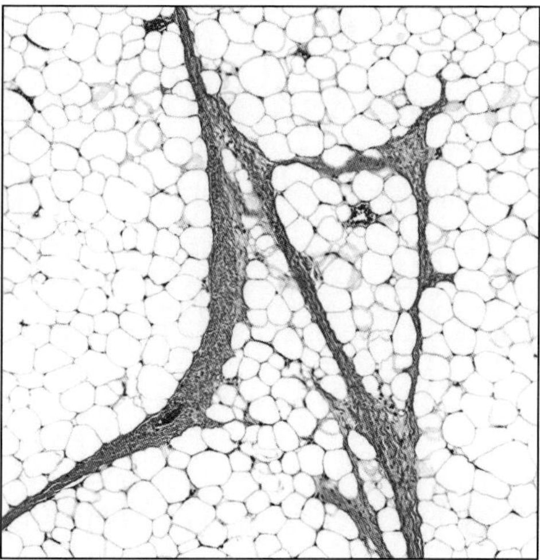

(Left) *Hematoxylin & eosin at low power shows a maturing lipoblastoma, characterized by relatively thin fibrous bands ⇨ and only small amounts of myxoid stroma. Searching through the myxoid areas will still reveal scattered lipoblasts.* ***(Right)*** *Hematoxylin & eosin at medium power shows a very mature lipoblastoma, with very little myxoid stroma and thin fibrous bands. This can be difficult to differentiate from a fibrolipoma, but a careful search will reveal lipoblasts.*

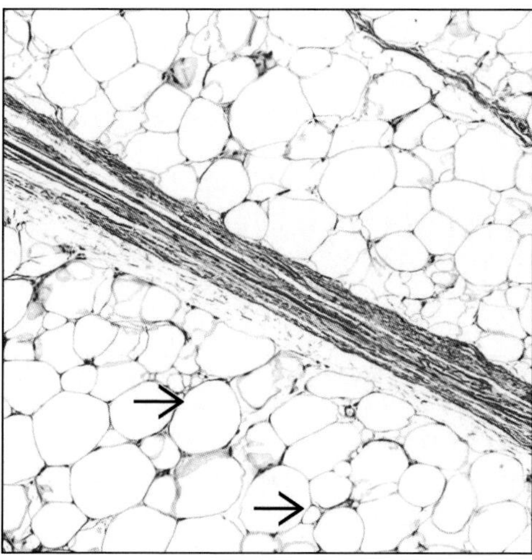

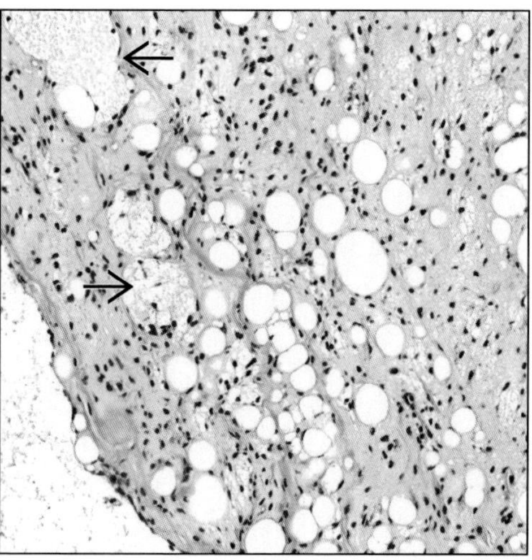

(Left) *Hematoxylin & eosin at high power shows a maturing lipoblastoma. This can be difficult to differentiate from a fibrolipoma, but here the adipocytes vary in size ⇨, and lipoblasts can still be found.* ***(Right)*** *Hematoxylin & eosin at medium power shows a myxoid liposarcoma, the main differential diagnosis of lipoblastoma. Features of myxoid liposarcoma include atypical lipoblasts, atypical mitoses, mucin pools ⇨, and a patient of older age.*

OMENTAL MESENTERIC HAMARTOMA

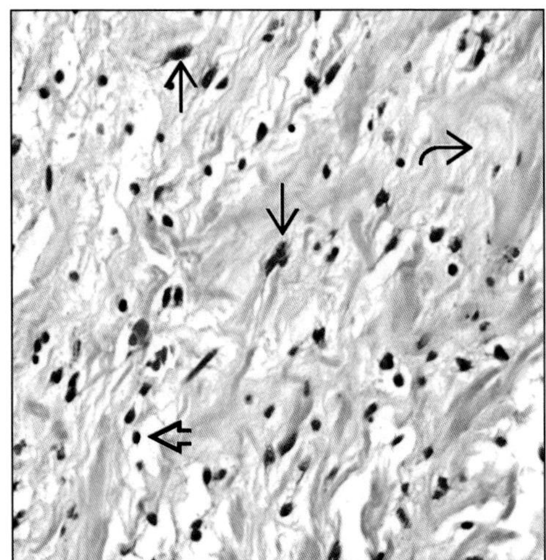

Hematoxylin & eosin shows omental mesenteric hamartoma with plump mesenchymal tumor cells ➙, lymphoplasmacytic infiltrate ➙, and abundant myxoid stroma with collagenization ➙.

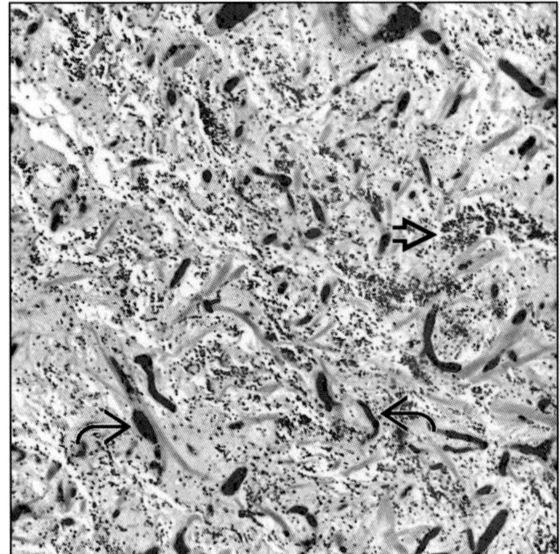

Omental mesenteric hamartoma shows collagenized myxoid stroma with many thin-walled, variably sized blood vessels ➙ and red blood cell extravasation ➙. (Courtesy B. Shehata, MD.)

TERMINOLOGY

Synonyms

- Omental-mesenteric myxoid hamartoma

Definitions

- Benign hamartomatous neoplasm that occurs in omentum and mesentery

CLINICAL ISSUES

Epidemiology

- Incidence
  - Rare
- Age
  - Affects mostly infants and neonates
- Gender
  - No sex predilection

Presentation

- Abdominal distension
- Anorexia
- Vomiting
- Palpable intraabdominal mass

Laboratory Tests

- Noncontributory

Treatment

- Surgical excision is treatment of choice
- Adjuvant therapy is not warranted

Prognosis

- Benign behavior
- No recurrences have been documented following complete surgical excision
- Because this neoplasm may mimic malignant tumor, unnecessary adjuvant chemo- or radiotherapy may lead to increased morbidity and mortality

MACROSCOPIC FEATURES

General Features

- Multiple nodules in omentum and mesentery
  - Solid, soft
  - Well circumscribed, lobulated
  - Multifocal
  - Tan-yellow-white, glistening, translucent
  - Variable size
    - Nodules can be as large as 10 cm
  - Rare instances of omental mesenteric hamartoma of mesoappendix have been reported

MICROSCOPIC PATHOLOGY

Histologic Features

- Plump mesenchymal cells
  - Amphophilic cytoplasm
  - Centrally placed, prominent nucleoli
  - Variable cellularity
- Myxoid stroma with abundant vascularization consisting mostly of capillary-sized vessels
  - Stroma may show variable collagenization
- Mixed inflammatory infiltrate composed of plasma cells, lymphocytes, and neutrophils

Predominant Pattern/Injury Type

- Primitive mesenchymal cells
- Myxoid

ANCILLARY TESTS

Immunohistochemistry

- Positive staining for vimentin and desmin

OMENTAL MESENTERIC HAMARTOMA

Key Facts

Terminology

- Omental-mesenteric myxoid hamartoma
- Benign hamartomatous neoplasm that occurs in omentum and mesentery

Clinical Issues

- Affects mostly infants and neonates

Macroscopic Features

- Multiple nodules in omentum and mesentery

Microscopic Pathology

- Plump mesenchymal cells
- Myxoid stroma with abundant vascularization consisting mostly of capillary-sized vessels
- Mixed inflammatory infiltrate composed of plasma cells, lymphocytes, and neutrophils

Ancillary Tests

- Positive staining for vimentin and desmin

DIFFERENTIAL DIAGNOSIS

Inflammatory Myofibroblastic Tumor

- Tumor cells are predominantly spindle-shaped
- Myxoid stroma and lymphoplasmacytic infiltrate is usually present
- Majority of tumors are positive for ALK staining

Myxoid Liposarcoma

- Lipoblastic differentiation
- "Chicken-wire" vasculature
- Variable mitotic activity
- Common sites include lower extremities and retroperitoneum
- Extremely rare in infants and neonates

Lipoblastomatosis

- Lipoblastic differentiation
- Usually involve extraabdominal soft tissue
- Multilobulated
- ± extramedullary hematopoiesis

Retroperitoneal/Abdominal Leiomyosarcoma

- Most commonly occur in retroperitoneum
- Rare in children
- Aggressive clinical course
- Spindled tumor cells have elongated nuclei and are arranged in fascicles that often intersect at right angles
- Pleomorphic tumor cells are often present

Omental Mesenteric Lymphangioma

- Cystic nodules
- Dilated lymphatic channels on histology

DIAGNOSTIC CHECKLIST

Pathologic Interpretation Pearls

- Multiple solid nodules in mesentery and omentum
- Plump mesenchymal cells and inflammatory cells admixed in myxoid, highly vascular stroma

SELECTED REFERENCES

1. Nagae I et al: Primary omental-mesenteric myxoid hamartoma of the mesoappendix incidentally detected after abdominal trauma in a child: report of a case. Surg Today. 35(9):792-5, 2005
2. Wootton-Gorges SL et al: Giant cystic abdominal masses in children. Pediatr Radiol. 35(12):1277-88, 2005
3. Vyas MC et al: Omento-mesentral myxoid hamartoma--a case report. Indian J Cancer. 31(3):212-4, 1994
4. Gonzalez-Crussi F et al: Primary peritoneal, omental, and mesenteric tumors in childhood. Semin Diagn Pathol. 3(2):122-37, 1986
5. Gonzalez-Crussi F et al: Omental-mesenteric myxoid hamartomas. Infantile lesions simulating malignant tumors. Am J Surg Pathol. 7(6):567-78, 1983

IMAGE GALLERY

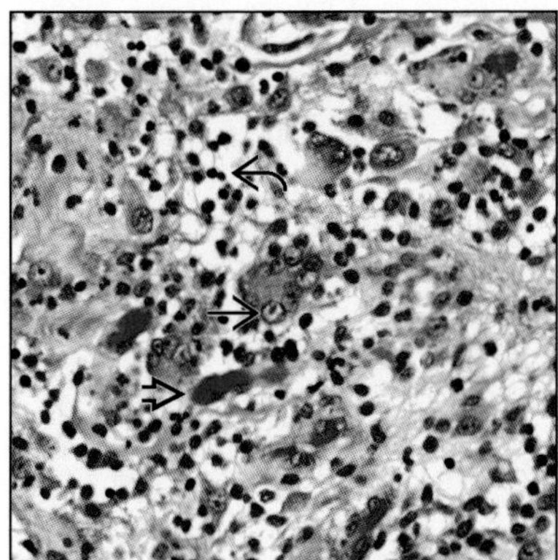

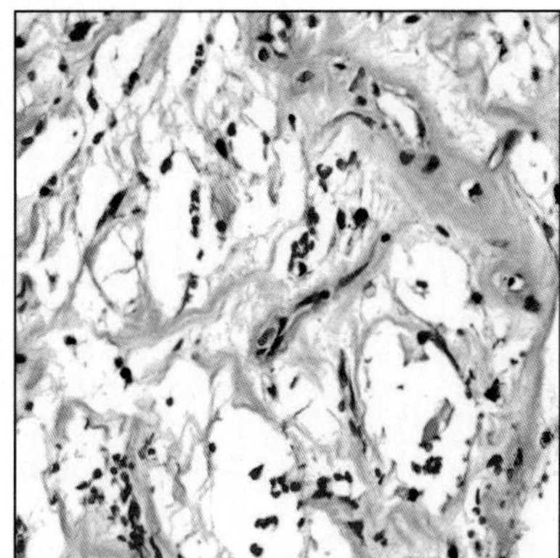

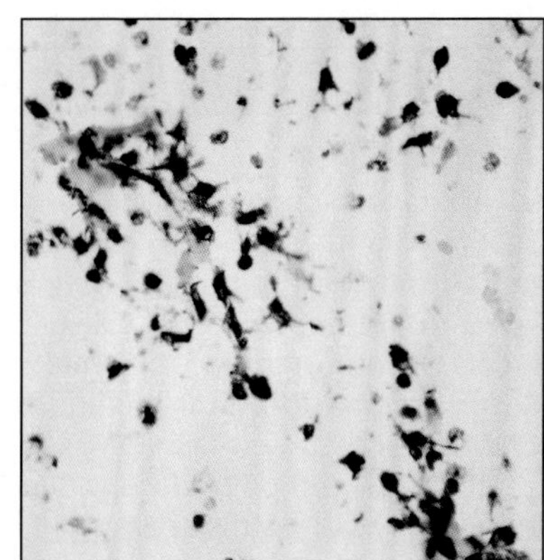

(Left) *Omental mesenteric hamartoma shows plump mesenchymal cells with prominent, centrally located nucleoli ⇒ in a background of a mixed inflammatory infiltrate → and loose myxoid stroma with numerous blood vessels ⇨.* ***(Center)*** *The neoplasm may have hypocellular areas with stromal predominance.* ***(Right)*** *Immunohistochemical staining for vimentin shows cytoplasmic and nuclear staining of mesenchymal cells. (Courtesy B. Shehata, MD.)*

PIGMENTED VILLONODULAR TENOSYNOVITIS

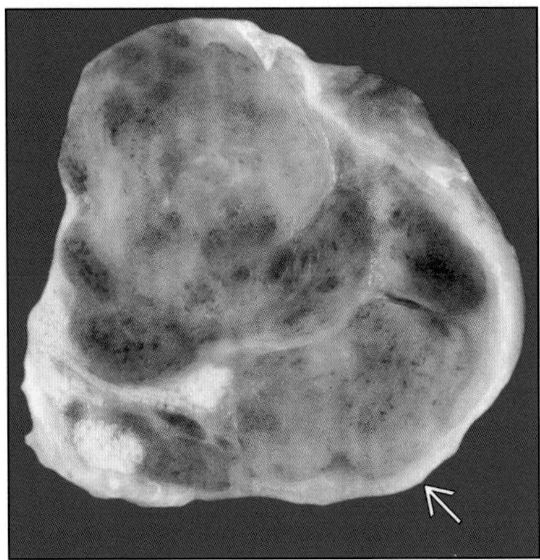

Cross section of this gross GCTTS specimen shows an encapsulated ➡ and multilobular tumor. The cut surface is tan-brown to tan-yellow. (Courtesy D. Lucas, MD.)

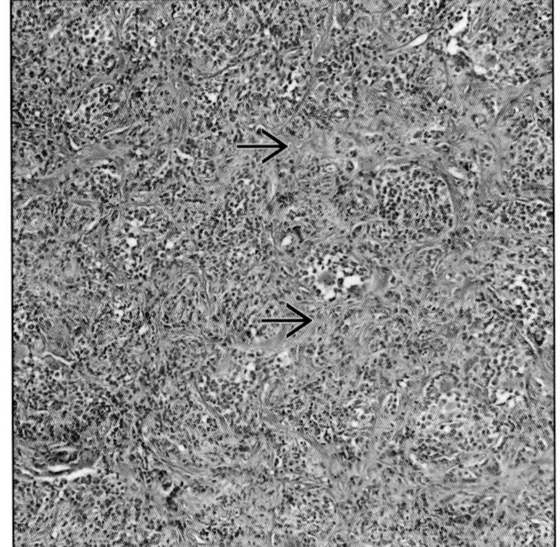

Low-power view of GCTTS reveals sheets of bland mononuclear cells separated by collagenous stroma ➡. Scattered multinucleated giant cells are interspersed between the mononuclear cells.

TERMINOLOGY

Synonyms

- Giant cell tumor of tendon sheath (GCTTS)
  - Tenosynovial giant cell tumor
  - Localized nodular tenosynovitis
- Pigmented villonodular synovitis (PVNS)
  - Fibrous histiocytoma of synovium
  - Fibrous xanthoma of synovium

Definitions

- Soft tissue tumor characterized histologically by a proliferation of synovial-type cells
  - Accompanied by multinucleated giant cells, inflammatory cells, hemosiderin-laden macrophages, and foamy macrophages
- GCTTS
  - Localized nodule in vicinity of tenosynovium
- PVNS
  - Diffuse intraarticular form
  - Locally progressive with joint damage
- Diffuse-type giant cell tumor (DTGCT)
  - Extraarticular soft tissue counterpart of PVNS
  - Some represent soft tissue extensions of PVNS
  - Locally aggressive, but nonmetastasizing

ETIOLOGY/PATHOGENESIS

Pathogenesis

- Evidence favors a neoplastic process
  - Trisomy 5 and 7 and translocations suggest clonality
- Balanced translocations of 1p13 involving *CSF1* gene
  - Leads to overexpression of CSF1, an inflammatory mediator important in inflammatory arthritis
  - Recurrent translocations include 2q35 involving *COL6A3*; t(1;2)
- GCTTS, PVNS, and DTGCT considered as different manifestations of a single disease

CLINICAL ISSUES

Site

- GCTTS
  - Hand: 77-86%
    - Thumb, followed by index finger, other fingers
  - Foot/ankle complex: 3-14%
  - Intraosseous involvement can be seen
  - Arises in subcutaneous plane adjacent to tendon sheath
- PVNS
  - Any joint may be affected, usually single joint involvement
    - Knee most common (80%)
    - Other frequently involved joints: Hip, shoulder, ankle
  - Polyarticular disease in children is associated with other congenital anomalies, suggesting a genetic basis
- DTGCT
  - Most commonly located in knee

Presentation

- GCTTS
  - 2nd most common benign tumor of hand after ganglion cysts
  - Peak incidence between 20 and 29 years with 2nd peak at 40-49 years
    - Mean age reported in pediatric population: 11 years
  - Female predominance (reported F:M ratios 2:1-3:2)
  - Longstanding painless or painful swelling
- PVNS
  - Rare in adults and children
    - Results in frequent delay of diagnosis in pediatric patients
  - Longstanding painful swelling
- DTGCT
  - Presents in younger population than localized type: < 40 years

PIGMENTED VILLONODULAR TENOSYNOVITIS

Key Facts

Terminology
- Giant cell tumor of tendon sheath (GCTTS)
- Pigmented villonodular synovitis (PVNS)
- Diffuse-type giant cell tumor (DTGCT)
- Soft tissue tumor characterized by a proliferation of synovial-type cells

Etiology/Pathogenesis
- Evidence favors a neoplastic process
- Balanced translocations of 1p13 involving *CF1* gene

Clinical Issues
- GCTTS: Most located in the hand
- PVNS and DTGCT: Knee most common location
- Recurrence rate: High for all types
- Complete excision is therapy of choice

Macroscopic Features
- GCTTS: Well circumscribed, partially encapsulated
- PVNS: Frond-like or nodular synovial hyperplasia
- DTGCT: Larger and more irregular than localized form

Microscopic Pathology
- Moderately cellular nodules and sheets of plump mononuclear histiocytic cells
- Eosinophilic cytoplasm with bland nuclei
- Foamy histiocytes, multinucleated giant cells, hemosiderin deposition

Top Differential Diagnoses
- Giant cell tumor of bone
- Giant cell tumor of soft tissue
- Malignant PVNS

Treatment
- GCTTS
  - Complete excision
- PVNS
  - Arthroscopic synovectomy
  - Followed by isotopic synoviorthesis in some cases
- DTGCT
  - Wide local excision

Prognosis
- GCTTS
  - Recurrence rate: Up to 30% for all patients
    - In pediatric patients: 0-44%
    - Recurrences usually nondestructive
  - Recurrence risk factors include
    - Osseous erosions, high mitotic rate, incomplete excision, proximity to arthritic joint
- PVNS: 20-50% recurrence rate
- DTGCT: 18-46% recurrence rate

IMAGE FINDINGS

Radiographic Findings
- GCTTS
  - Soft tissue swelling: 50-70%
  - Cortical erosion may be seen, reflective of pressure changes: 9-25%
- PVNS
  - Diffuse synovial hyperplasia with extensive effusion
  - Discrete intraarticular mass may be seen
  - Bone erosion
    - 50% of adult cases
    - 17% reported in a small series of children
- DTGCT
  - Ill-defined soft tissue masses

MACROSCOPIC FEATURES

GCTTS
- Well circumscribed, partially encapsulated
- Lobulated or multinodular mass
  - Surface grooves may be formed by overlying tendons
- Cut surface: Gray-brown to orange-yellow
  - These colors reflect amount of hemosiderin and lipid, respectively
- Size range: 0.5-2.0 cm

PVNS
- Frond-like or nodular synovial hyperplasia
  - Usually involves most of synovial surface
  - Variegated cut surface
  - Hemosiderin deposition imparts reddish or brown color to tumor
- Poorly demarcated
- Size usually > 5 cm

DTGCT
- Larger and more irregular than localized form

MICROSCOPIC PATHOLOGY

Histologic Features
- General
  - Moderately cellular nodules and sheets of plump mononuclear histiocytic cells
    - Eosinophilic cytoplasm
    - Bland reniform nuclei
  - Accumulation of foamy histiocytes
    - Cholesterol clefts may be present
  - Scattered multinucleated giant cells
    - Less prevalent in more cellular areas
    - Variable number of nuclei from 3 or 4 up to 50 per cell
  - Hemosiderin deposition
  - Variably collagenous background
  - Occasional to moderate mitotic activity
- Features specific to GCTTS
  - Encapsulated with vague nodularity
- Features specific to PVNS
  - Papillary projections of hyperplastic synovium
  - Solid areas may be present
- Features specific to DTGCT

- Infiltrative sheets of tumor cells
- Synovial-lined clefts are common
- Fewer multinucleated giant cells than localized type
- Pseudoalveolar spaces, often blood-filled

ANCILLARY TESTS

Immunohistochemistry

- GCTTS, PVNS, and DTGCT
  - CD68(+)
  - FXIIIA(+)
  - Vimentin(+)
  - S100(-)

Cytogenetics

- Gain of chromosomes 5 and 7
  - More common in PVNS and DTGCT
- Translocations of 1p13
  - Found in a minority of tumor cells (2-16%)
    - These tumor cells are surrounded by nonneoplastic macrophages that express the *CSF1* receptor, *CSF1R*
  - Recurrent translocations include: 2q35-37, 5q22-23, 11q11-12, 8q21-22

In Situ Hybridization

- High levels of CSF1 protein and RNA expression found in a majority of cases of GCTTS and PVNS
  - Most of these cases demonstrate a translocation at the 1p13 locus
  - Significant minority of cases lack this translocation

Synovial Fluid Aspiration

- Aspirated synovial fluid in PVNS is typically xanthochromic or serosanguineous

DIFFERENTIAL DIAGNOSIS

Giant Cell Tumor of Bone

- Primary tumor of bone but may invade adjacent soft tissue
- Uniform mononuclear stromal cell population
- Multinucleated giant cells are very large with numerous nuclei
  - Nuclear features of giant cells and mononuclear cells are similar
- Stroma less collagenized

Giant Cell Tumor of Soft Tissue

- Identical histologically to giant cell tumor of bone

Hemarthrosis

- In the differential for PVNS
- Villiform synovial hyperplasia with hemosiderosis
- Lacks solid areas
- History of recurrent hemarthroses
  - Trauma-related
  - Hemophilia

Malignant PVNS

- Malignant cytologic features
  - Pleomorphic spindle cells
  - High mitotic rate and necrosis
  - Association with radiation therapy

Juvenile Idiopathic Arthritis

- In the differential for PVNS
- Formerly known as juvenile rheumatoid arthritis
- Gross appearance also papillary synovial hyperplasia
  - No solid or nodular components
- Dense lymphoplasmacytic infiltrate
- Fibrinous exudate

Fibroma of Tendon Sheath

- More uniformly hyalinized stroma than GCTTS
- Cells are fibroblastic
- May represent an end stage of GCTTS

Tendinous Xanthoma

- In differential for GCTTS
- Forms in setting of hyperlipidemia
- Often multiple

SELECTED REFERENCES

1. Batra VV et al: Cytomorphologic spectrum of giant cell tumor of tendon sheath. Acta Cytol. 52(2):152-8, 2008
2. Darwish FM et al: Giant cell tumour of tendon sheath: experience with 52 cases. Singapore Med J. 49(11):879-82, 2008
3. Murphey MD et al: Pigmented villonodular synovitis: radiologic-pathologic correlation. Radiographics. 28(5):1493-518, 2008
4. Cupp JS et al: Translocation and expression of CSF1 in pigmented villonodular synovitis, tenosynovial giant cell tumor, rheumatoid arthritis and other reactive synovitides. Am J Surg Pathol. 31(6):970-6, 2007
5. Gholve PA et al: Giant cell tumor of tendon sheath: largest single series in children. J Pediatr Orthop. 27(1):67-74, 2007
6. Neubauer P et al: Pigmented villonodular synovitis in children: a report of six cases and review of the literature. Iowa Orthop J. 27:90-4, 2007
7. Nilsson M et al: Molecular cytogenetic mapping of recurrent chromosomal breakpoints in tenosynovial giant cell tumors. Virchows Arch. 441(5):475-80, 2002
8. Llauger J et al: Pigmented villonodular synovitis and giant cell tumors of the tendon sheath: radiologic and pathologic features. AJR Am J Roentgenol. 172(4):1087-91, 1999
9. Abdul-Karim FW et al: Diffuse and localized tenosynovial giant cell tumor and pigmented villonodular synovitis: a clinicopathologic and flow cytometric DNA analysis. Hum Pathol. 23(7):729-35, 1992
10. Ushijima M et al: Giant cell tumor of the tendon sheath (nodular tenosynovitis). A study of 207 cases to compare the large joint group with the common digit group. Cancer. 57(4):875-84, 1986

Clinical and Other Features

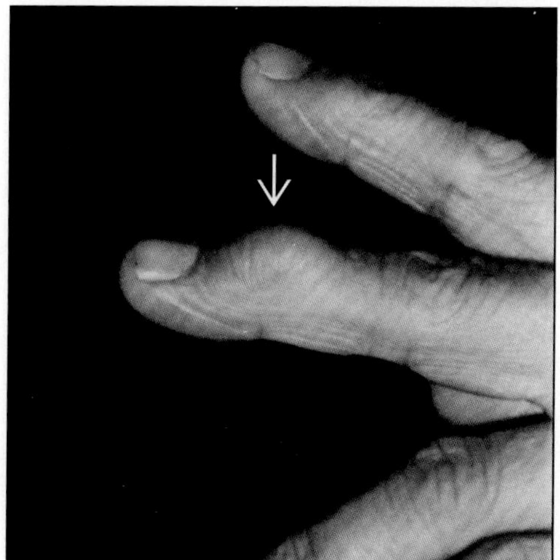

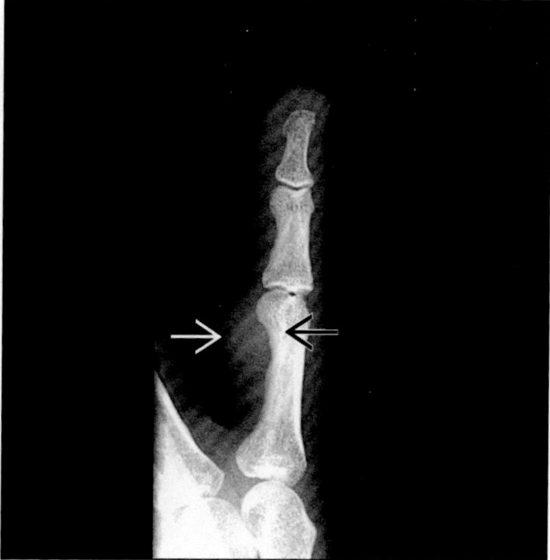

(Left) *Localized giant cell tumor of tendon sheath presents as a slowly growing painless mass →. It is most commonly located on the thumb and fingers in a periarticular location. (Courtesy D. Lucas, MD.)* ***(Right)*** *Radiographic image of localized giant cell tumor of tendon sheath shows a soft tissue mass → with adjacent bony cortical erosion secondary to pressure exerted by the mass →. (Courtesy D. Lucas, MD.)*

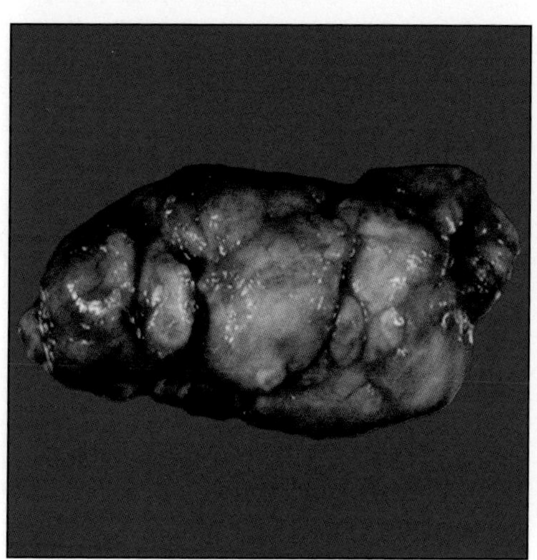

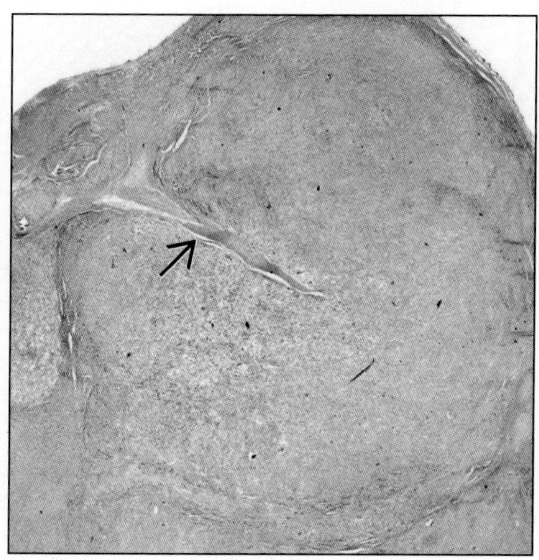

(Left) *Grossly, the external surface of the GCTTS is multilobulated and encapsulated. (Courtesy D. Lucas, MD.)* ***(Right)*** *Low-power microscopic view of GCTTS reveals an encapsulated lobular mass with interlobular clefting present →.*

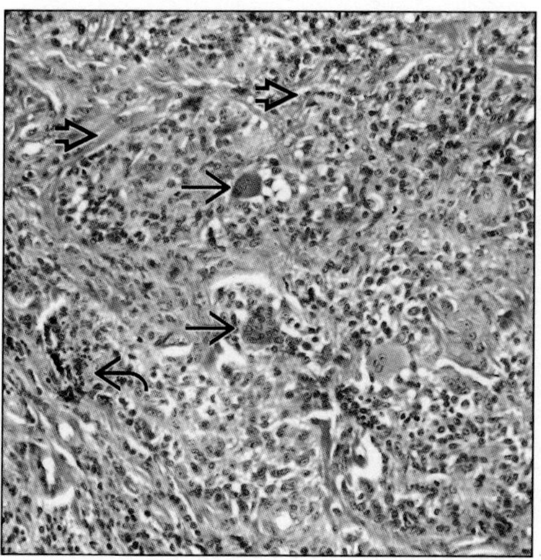

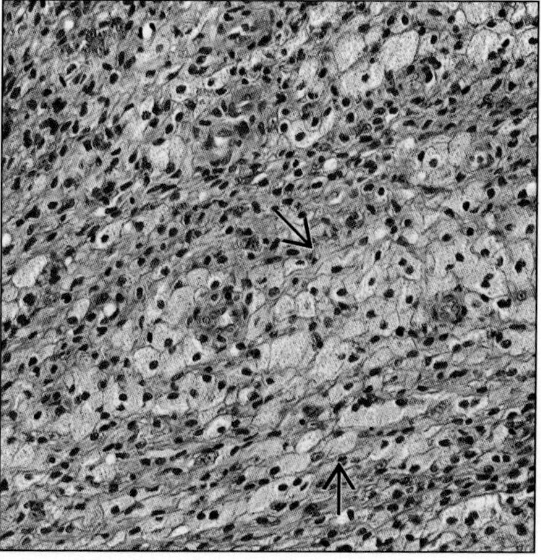

(Left) *Medium-power view shows a proliferation of bland, mononuclear cells interspersed with multinucleated giant cells → within a variably collagenous background →. Foci of hemosiderin deposition are noted →.* ***(Right)*** *Collections of foamy macrophages → are commonly seen in GCTTS, as well as in PVNS and DTGCT.*

PIGMENTED VILLONODULAR TENOSYNOVITIS

Microscopic and Other Features

(Left) Scattered multinucleated giant cells ⇒ are more numerous in GCTTS compared to the diffuse type of giant cell tumor. Multinucleated giant cells can have a few nuclei to up to 50 nuclei per cell. *(Right)* Hemosiderin deposition ⇒ is a common feature of GCTTS, PVNS, and DTGCT.

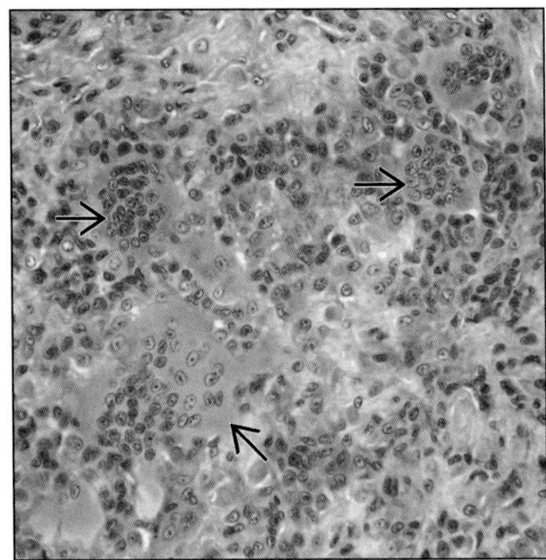

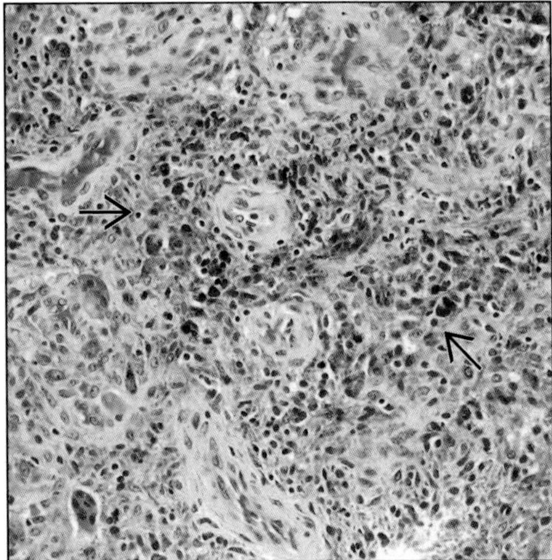

(Left) T1-weighted MR of PVNS demonstrates diffuse, infiltrative growth involving the entire surface of the synovium ⇨, with associated bony erosion by the tumor ⇒. (Courtesy D. Lucas, MD.) *(Right)* Intraoperative photograph of PVNS demonstrates the characteristic villonodular appearance of the mass, which covers the synovial surface. The brown color is indicative of hemosiderin deposition. (Courtesy D. Lucas, MD.)

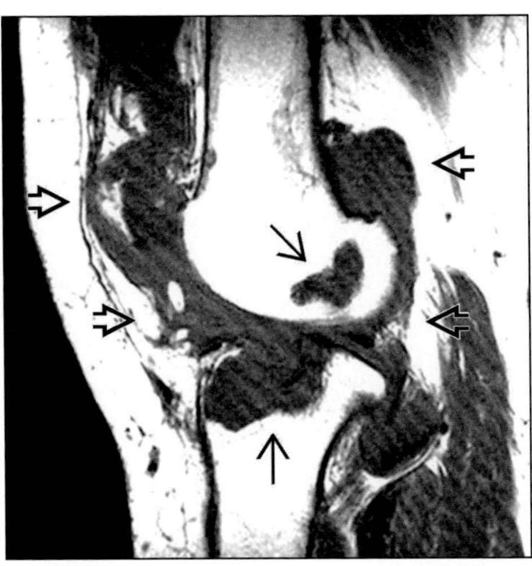

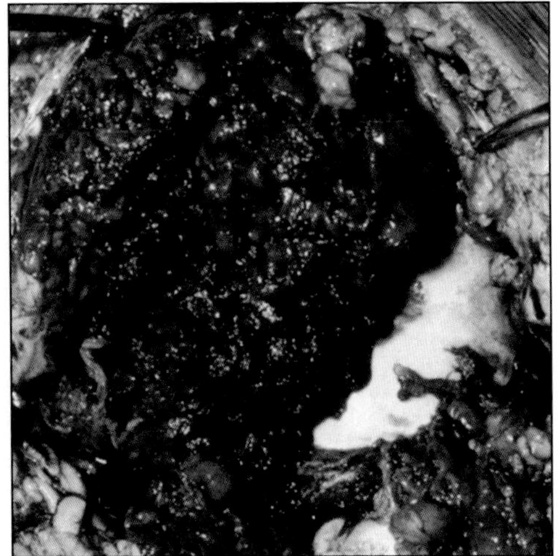

(Left) A gross PVNS synovectomy specimen demonstrates shaggy, villous protrusions. (Courtesy D. Lucas, MD.) *(Right)* H&E stained section of PVNS shows the villous structures that characterize this lesion. These structures are lined by synoviocytes, and contain cellular constituents and histologic features similar to those of GCTTS. Solid or nodular areas can be present in PVNS. (Courtesy D. Lucas, MD.)

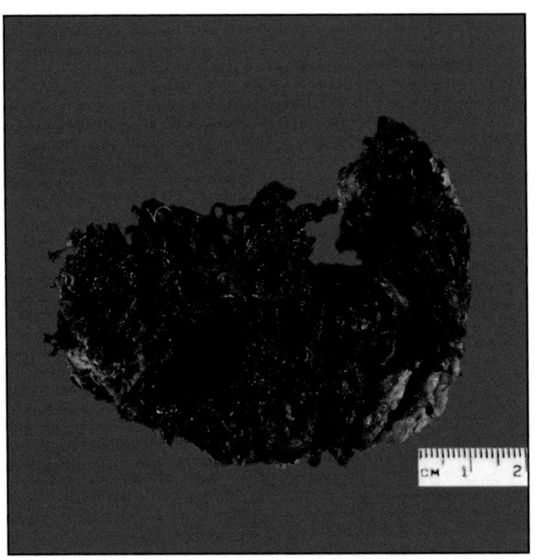

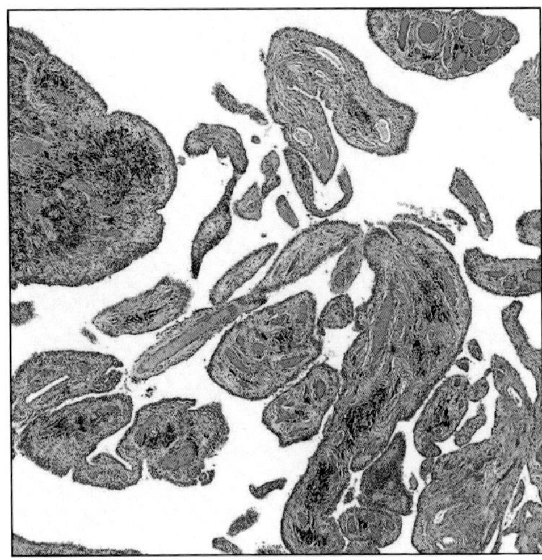

Microscopic and Radiologic Features

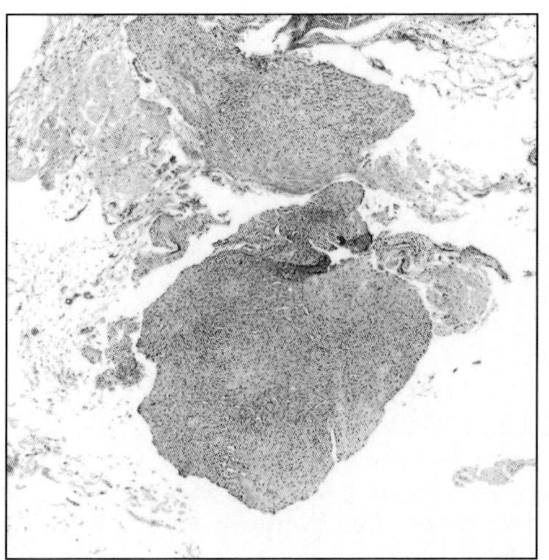

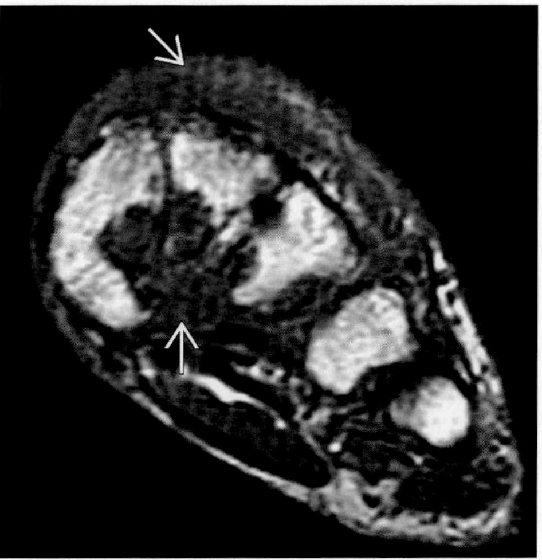

(Left) *This arthroscopic biopsy reveals detached nodular and papillary structures admixed with articular tissue components.* ***(Right)*** *The DTGCT, unlike the GCTTS, presents as a diffuse soft tissue mass ➔ that in this T1-weighted MR is seen infiltrating between metatarsal bones to involve deep and superficial soft tissue. (Courtesy D. Lucas, MD.)*

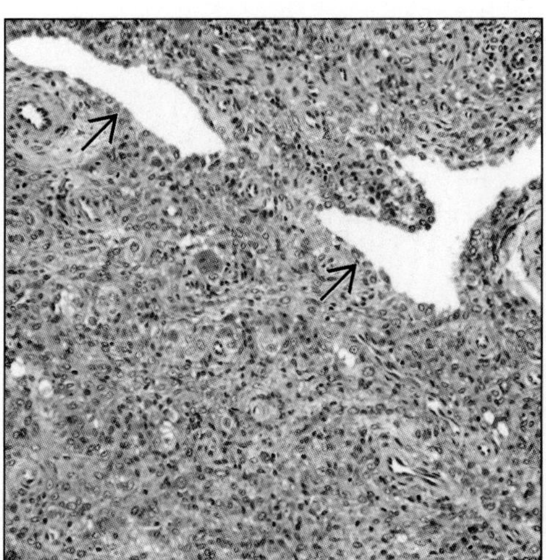

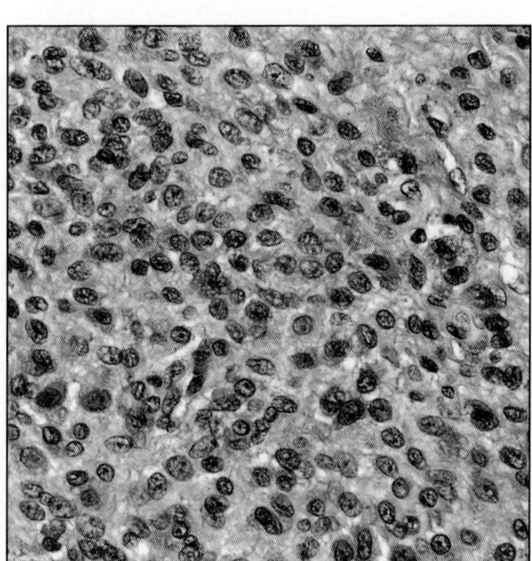

(Left) *Histologically, DTGCTs show diffuse sheets of tumor cells separated by synovial-lined cleft-like spaces ➔.* ***(Right)*** *Multinucleated giant cells tend to be less numerous in DTGCT (shown here) than in GCTTS. (Courtesy D. Lucas, MD.)*

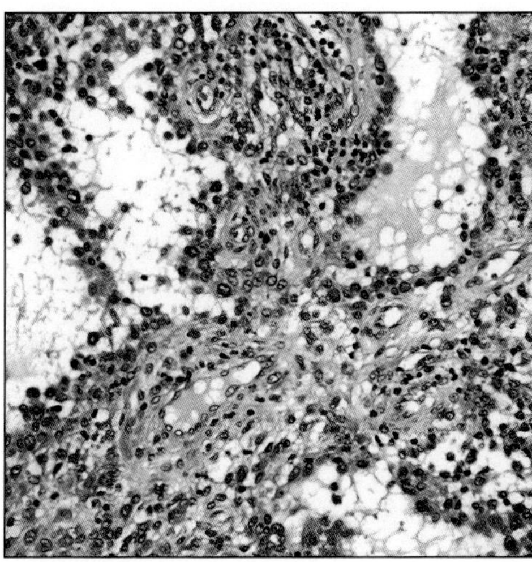

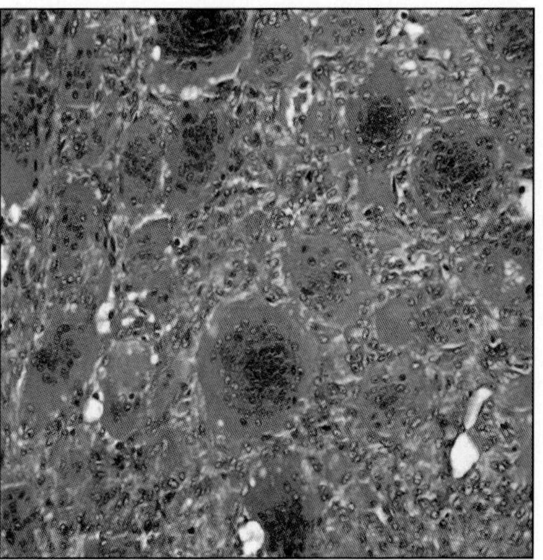

(Left) *Pseudoalveolar spaces lined by synoviocytes are a typical feature of DTGCT. (Courtesy D. Lucas, MD.)* ***(Right)*** *Giant cell tumor of bone and giant cell tumor of soft tissue are histologically identical, and are the main differential diagnoses for GCTTS, PVNS, and DTGCT. These tumors are characterized by dense sheets of very large multinucleated giant cells that may contain hundreds of nuclei, and mononuclear stomal cells whose nuclear features are similar to those of the giant cells.*

INFANTILE FIBROMATOSIS

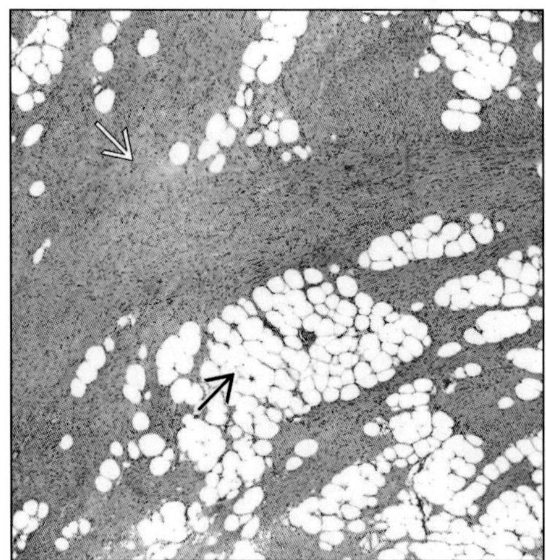

Hematoxylin & eosin shows diffuse infantile fibromatosis composed of a poorly circumscribed, infiltrating proliferation of fibroconnective tissue ➡ entrapping mature adipose cells ➡.

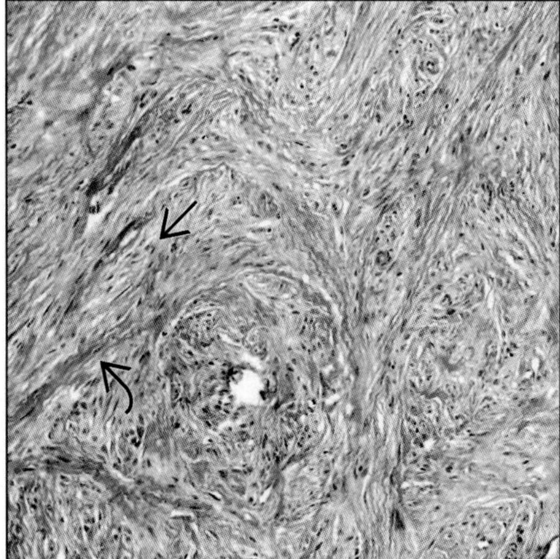

Hematoxylin & eosin shows infantile fibromatosis, desmoid type, composed of bland fibroblasts ➡ and thick keloid-like collagen fibers ➡ that display an infiltrative growth pattern.

TERMINOLOGY

Synonyms

- Lipofibromatosis

Definitions

- Benign fibrous neoplasm originating from musculoaponeurotic structures throughout body
  - Classified as
    - Diffuse (mesenchymal) type: Most common
    - Desmoid type

ETIOLOGY/PATHOGENESIS

Etiology

- Uncertain
- Trauma has been implicated as a risk factor

CLINICAL ISSUES

Epidemiology

- Incidence
  - Rare
- Age
  - Diffuse type tends to occur in infants
  - Desmoid type is most common in children older than 5 years of age
- Gender
  - Slightly more frequent in males than in females

Site

- Head and neck
  - May involve mandible, tongue, and maxilla
- Upper arm
- Shoulder
- Thigh

Presentation

- Poorly circumscribed, deep, solitary mass
  - Asymptomatic
  - Lesion may be painful

Natural History

- Does not metastasize

Treatment

- Complete surgical excision is treatment of choice

Prognosis

- Local recurrence if incompletely excised
- Status of resection margin is most important prognostic factor
- Histiologic features do not correlate with clinical course

MACROSCOPIC FEATURES

General Features

- Unencapsulated, firm, ill-defined, white-gray mass

MICROSCOPIC PATHOLOGY

Histologic Features

- Composed of fibroblasts and myofibroblasts
  - Various stages of fibroblastic differentiation
- **Diffuse (mesenchymal) type**
  - Small, round to oval fibroblasts embedded in variably myxoid stroma
  - Variable cellularity
  - Tumor cells are often interspersed with muscle and adipocytes
  - ± lymphocytic infiltrate
  - Infiltrative growth pattern
- **Desmoid type**
  - Proliferation of spindle-shaped fibroblasts and myofibroblasts
  - Variable cellularity
  - Abundant keloid-like collagen fibers

INFANTILE FIBROMATOSIS

Key Facts

Terminology

- Benign fibrous neoplasm originating from musculoaponeurotic structures throughout body
- Classified as
  - Diffuse (mesenchymal) type
  - Desmoid type

Clinical Issues

- Common sites
  - Head and neck
  - Upper arm, shoulder
  - Thigh
- Slightly more frequent in males than in females
- Complete surgical excision is treatment of choice
  - Local recurrence if incompletely excised
- Status of resection margin is a prognostic factor

Microscopic Pathology

- Composed of fibroblastic and myofibroblastic proliferation
  - Infiltrative growth pattern

Immunohistochemistry

Antibody	Reactivity	Staining Pattern	Comment
Vimentin	Positive	Cytoplasmic	
Desmin	Positive	Cytoplasmic	Staining varies according to proportion of myofibroblasts present in lesion
Actin-sm	Positive	Cytoplasmic	Variable staining pattern
CD117	Negative		

DIFFERENTIAL DIAGNOSIS

Congenital/Infantile Fibrosarcoma

- High cellularity
- Herringbone arrangement of neoplastic spindle cells
- Frequent mitotic figures
- ± hemorrhage and necrosis
- t(12;15)(p13;q25): *ETV6-NTRK3* gene fusion

Lipoblastomatosis

- Lobular pattern
- Composed primarily of lipoblasts

Fibrodysplasia Ossificans Progressiva

- Associated with congenital malformation of great toes and progressive heterotopic ossification in distinct anatomic sites
- Episodes of pain; inflammatory soft tissue swelling precedes heterotopic bone formation

Myxoid Liposarcoma

- Rare in young children
- Distinctive plexiform capillaries ("chicken-wire" pattern)
- Variable amount of lipoblasts

Fibrous Hamartoma of Infancy

- Primitive mesenchymal component is not seen in diffuse infantile fibromatosis

SELECTED REFERENCES

1. Fetsch JF et al: A clinicopathologic study of 45 pediatric soft tissue tumors with an admixture of adipose tissue and fibroblastic elements, and a proposal for classification as lipofibromatosis. Am J Surg Pathol. 24(11):1491-500, 2000
2. Coffin CM et al: Fibroblastic-myofibroblastic tumors in children and adolescents: a clinicopathologic study of 108 examples in 103 patients. Pediatr Pathol. 11(4):569-88, 1991

IMAGE GALLERY

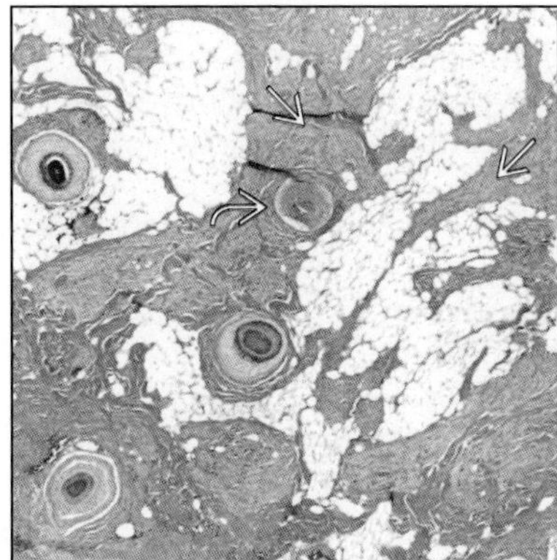

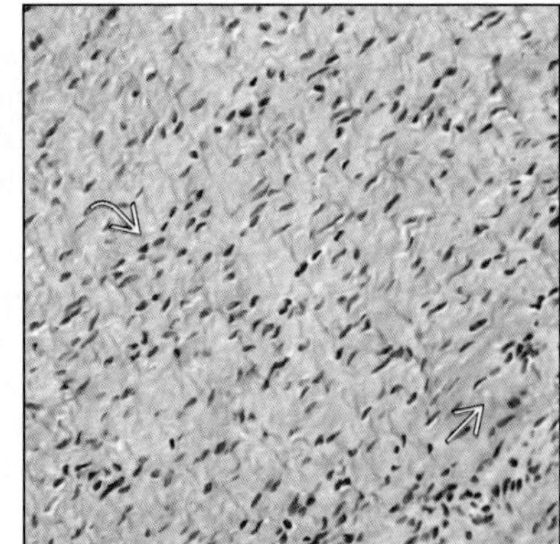

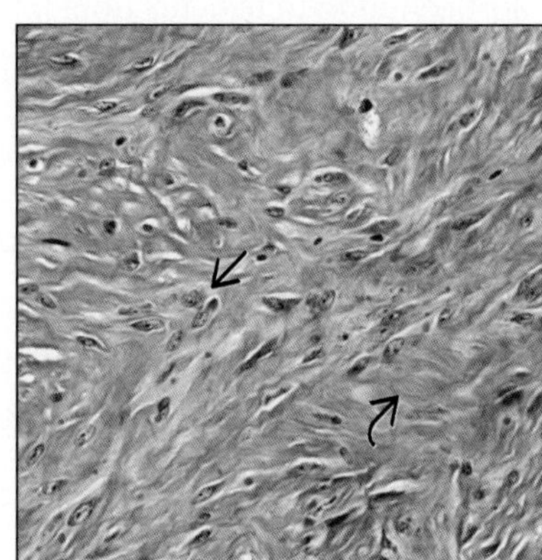

(Left) *Diffuse infantile fibromatosis is demonstrated as an infiltrating fibrous lesion involving septa of adipose tissue ➡ and focally surrounding hair follicles ➡.* ***(Center)*** *High-power view of an infantile fibromatosis, diffuse type, shows bland fibroblasts ➡ and collagen ➡ embedded in a vaguely myxoid background.* ***(Right)*** *Infantile fibromatosis, desmoid type, shows a proliferation of bland fibroblasts ➡ intermixed with dense keloid-like collagen ➡.*

MYOFIBROMA AND MYOFIBROMATOSIS

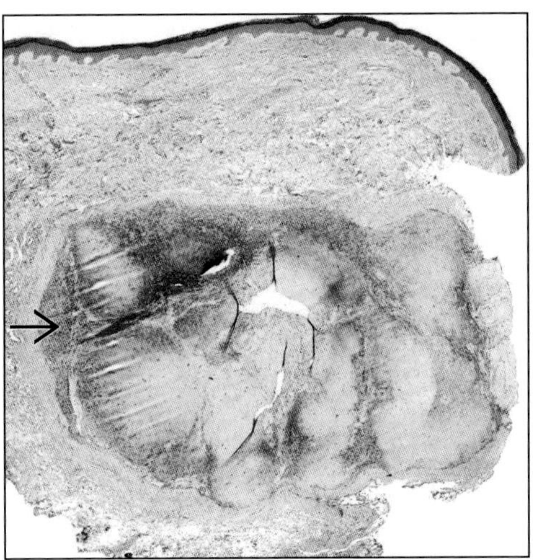

Hematoxylin & eosin shows a cutaneous myofibroma. Note the lobulated appearance at scanning magnification. In this example, the darker hemangiopericytoma-like component is peripheral ⇒.

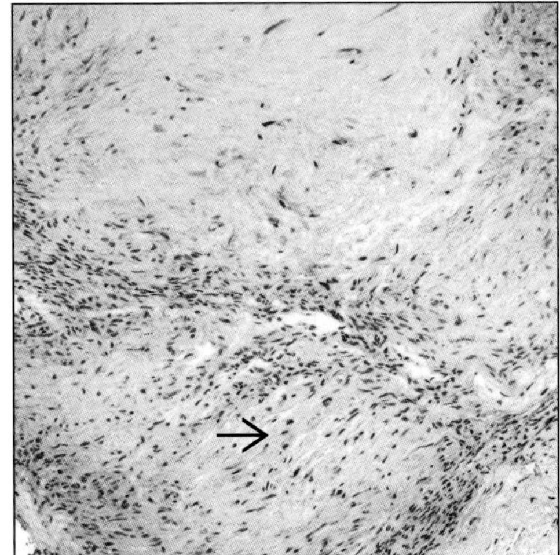

Hematoxylin & eosin shows myoid lobules separated by more cellular areas. The myoid cells have prominent cytoplasmic eosinophilia ⇒.

TERMINOLOGY

Synonyms

- Infantile myofibromatosis, congenital generalized fibromatosis
  - Continuum with lesions termed "myopericytoma, infantile hemangiopericytoma"

Definitions

- Benign neoplasms composed of lobules of myoid cells separated by vascularized zones (biphasic pattern)
  - Solitary form (myofibroma)
  - Multicentric form (myofibromatosis)

CLINICAL ISSUES

Epidemiology

- Incidence
  - Solitary form rare but more common than multicentric form
  - Multicentric form extremely rare
  - Rare familial cases
- Age
  - Wide age range (neonates to elderly)
  - Most common in patients from birth to 2 years of age
- Gender
  - Male predominance

Site

- Most solitary examples in subcutaneous tissues of head and neck
  - Trunk, extremities
  - Occasional skeletal example, especially skull
- Multicentric form usually involves soft tissue and bone
  - Usually long bones
  - Visceral sites
    - Gastrointestinal tract
    - Liver, kidney, pancreas

Presentation

- Asymptomatic skin nodules with purplish color (solitary form)
- Visceral lesions with site-specific presentations
- Bone lesions seen as multiple elongated radiolucencies in metaphysis

Treatment

- Simple excision for solitary lesions
- Selective excisions for multicentric form

Prognosis

- Excellent for solitary form
- Outcome for multicentric form is function of involved sites
  - Extensive lung involvement is poor prognostic factor

MICROSCOPIC PATHOLOGY

Histologic Features

- Most lesions well marginated
  - Can be locally infiltrative with intravascular and osseous extension and foci of necrosis
- Biphasic pattern
  - Myoid nodules separated by cellular pockets with hemangiopericytoma-like vascular pattern
  - Variable amounts of each component
  - Most cases have minimal mitotic activity
- Spindle cell areas
  - Prominent beneath ulcerated mucosal surfaces
- Myoid nodules
  - Pink cytoplasm and round to tapered nuclei
  - Myxoid change or hyalinization
- Hemangiopericytoma-like areas
  - Cellular but with minimal mitotic activity
  - Round cell similar to glomus cells

Key Facts

Terminology

- Benign neoplasms composed of lobules of myoid cells separated by vascularized zones (biphasic pattern)
  - Solitary form (myofibroma)
  - Multicentric form (myofibromatosis)
- Synonyms: Infantile myofibromatosis, congenital generalized fibromatosis
  - Continuum with lesions termed "myopericytoma, infantile hemangiopericytoma"

Clinical Issues

- Most common from birth to 2 years of age
- Most solitary examples in subcutaneous tissues of head and neck
- Simple excision for solitary lesions
- Selective excisions for multicentric form
- Extensive lung involvement is poor prognostic factor

Microscopic Pathology

- Biphasic pattern
  - Myoid nodules separated by cellular pockets with hemangiopericytoma-like vascular pattern
  - Variable amounts of each component
- Most cases have minimal mitotic activity
- Spindle cell areas
  - Prominent beneath ulcerated mucosal surfaces

Ancillary Tests

- Positive for vimentin, SMA, and MSA (actin-HHF-35)
- Usually label with α-actin and calponin but negative to focal desmin/focal caldesmon
- Negative S100 protein and keratin
- No characteristic alterations or mutation

Immunohistochemistry

Antibody	Reactivity	Staining Pattern	Comment
Actin-HHF-35	Positive	Cytoplasmic	
Actin-sm	Positive	Cytoplasmic	May be present only in the central zone
Vimentin	Positive	Cytoplasmic	All components label
S100	Negative		
CD34	Negative		Occasional focal labeling
CK-PAN	Negative		
Desmin	Equivocal	Cytoplasmic	Usually focal and weak (or negative)
Caldesmon	Equivocal	Cytoplasmic	Focal in myofibroma; more labeling in myopericytoma

ANCILLARY TESTS

Immunohistochemistry

- Positive for vimentin, smooth muscle actin, and muscle specific actin (actin-HHF-35)
- Usually label with α-actin and calponin but not desmin or caldesmon
- Negative S100 protein and keratin

Cytogenetics

- No characteristic alterations or mutation

DIFFERENTIAL DIAGNOSIS

Smooth Muscle Tumors

- Not lobulated
- Perpendicularly oriented fascicles, cigar-shaped nuclei
- Express actins, desmin, caldesmon

Fibromatosis

- Highly infiltrative growth pattern; sweeping fascicles of myofibroblasts
- Express actins, usually not desmin; nuclear β-catenin labeling
- β-catenin and *APC* mutations

Hemangiopericytoma

- No myoid areas
- Infantile form part of continuum with myofibroma

SELECTED REFERENCES

1. Dray MS et al: Myopericytoma: a unifying term for a spectrum of tumours that show overlapping features with myofibroma. A review of 14 cases. J Clin Pathol. 59(1):67-73, 2006
2. Gengler C et al: Solitary fibrous tumour and haemangiopericytoma: evolution of a concept. Histopathology. 48(1):63-74, 2006
3. Mentzel T et al: Myopericytoma of skin and soft tissues: clinicopathologic and immunohistochemical study of 54 cases. Am J Surg Pathol. 30(1):104-13, 2006
4. Montgomery E et al: Myofibromas presenting in the oral cavity: a series of 9 cases. Oral Surg Oral Med Oral Pathol Oral Radiol Endod. 89(3):343-8, 2000
5. Granter SR et al: Myofibromatosis in adults, glomangiopericytoma, and myopericytoma: a spectrum of tumors showing perivascular myoid differentiation. Am J Surg Pathol. 22(5):513-25, 1998
6. Coffin CM et al: Congenital generalized myofibromatosis: a disseminated angiocentric myofibromatosis. Pediatr Pathol Lab Med. 15(4):571-87, 1995
7. Smith KJ et al: Cutaneous myofibroma. Mod Pathol. 2(6):603-9, 1989
8. Jennings TA et al: Infantile myofibromatosis. Evidence for an autosomal-dominant disorder. Am J Surg Pathol. 8(7):529-38, 1984
9. Chung EB et al: Infantile myofibromatosis. Cancer. 48(8):1807-18, 1981

MYOFIBROMA AND MYOFIBROMATOSIS

Microscopic Features

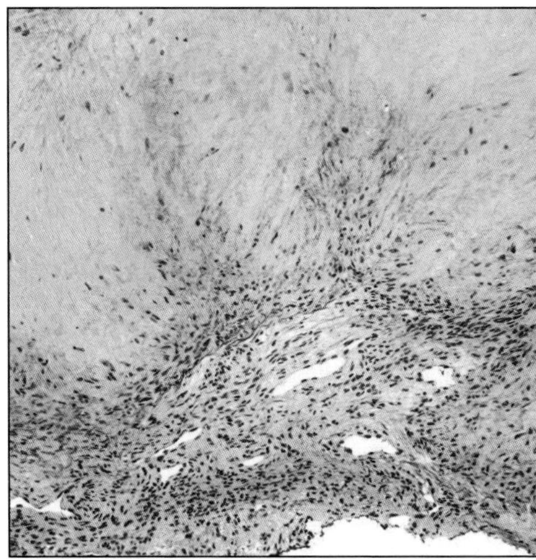

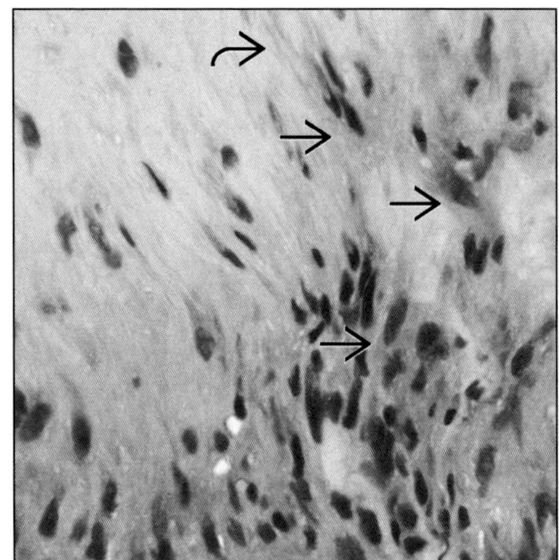

(Left) Hematoxylin & eosin shows many vessels at the periphery of a myoid nodule in a myofibroma. The stroma has a chondromyxoid appearance. **(Right)** Hematoxylin & eosin shows high magnification of the myoid cells in a myofibroma. Many of the cells have prominent cytoplasmic eosinophilia ⇒, and there are delicate amphophilic cytoplasmic processes ↗.

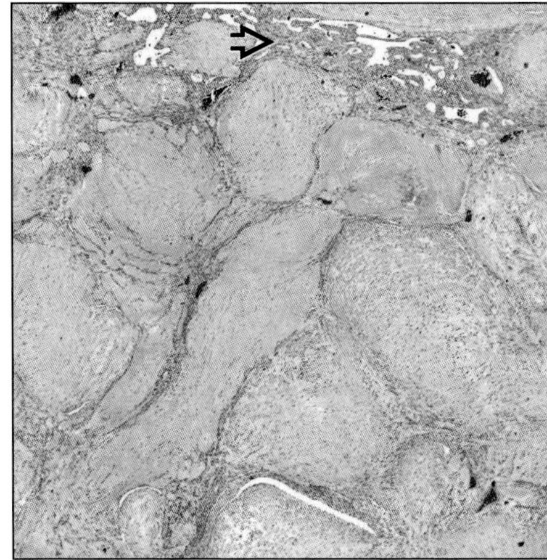

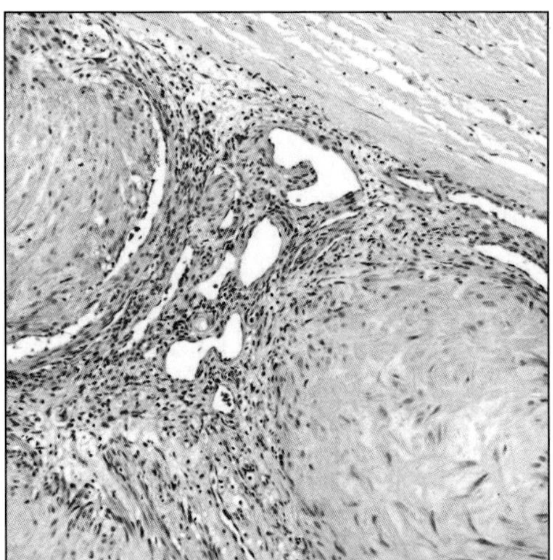

(Left) Hematoxylin & eosin shows a prominent lobular configuration in a myofibroma. Note the biphasic appearance; the upper portion of the field shows a prominent hemangiopericytomatous vascular pattern ⇨. **(Right)** Hematoxylin & eosin shows higher magnification of the hemangiopericytoma-like component of a myofibroma.

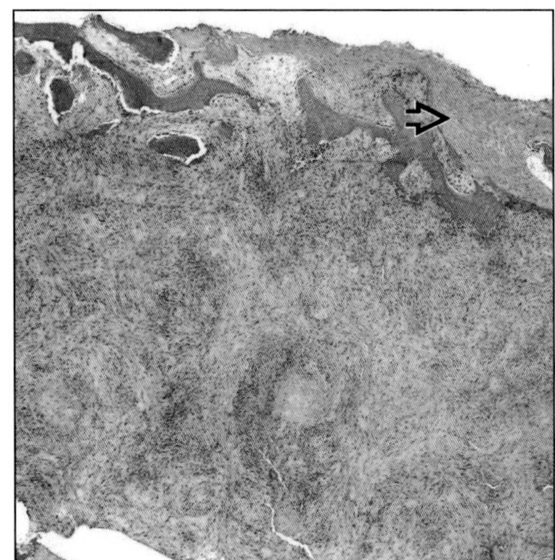

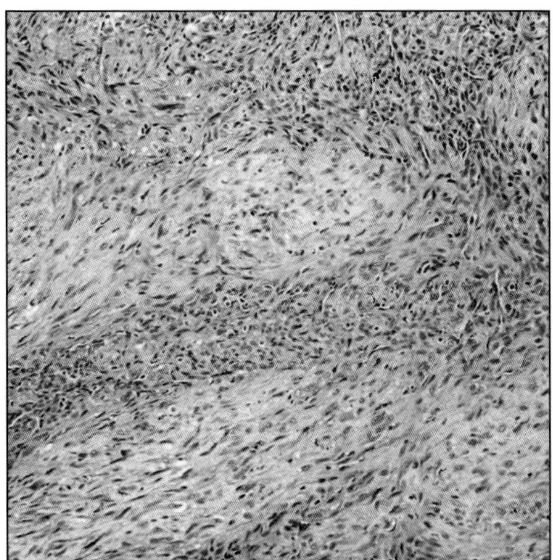

(Left) Hematoxylin & eosin shows a skeletal myofibroma. There is a vaguely lobulated appearance, and the tumor is infiltrative at the periphery. There is also focal necrosis ⇨. **(Right)** Hematoxylin & eosin shows a myofibroma of the parotid region of a child. The spindle cells are arranged in nodules.

Microscopic Features and Ancillary Techniques

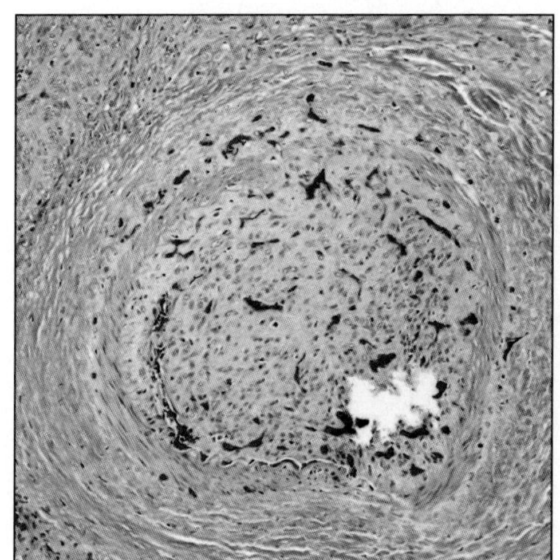

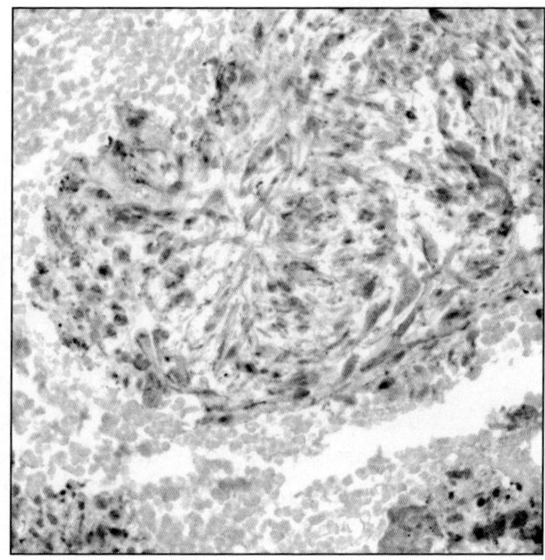

(Left) *Hematoxylin & eosin shows vascular space invasion in a myofibroma. This feature can lead to an erroneous interpretation of malignancy.* ***(Right)*** *Actin-HHF-35 (muscle specific actin) shows cytoplasmic labeling in a myofibroma.*

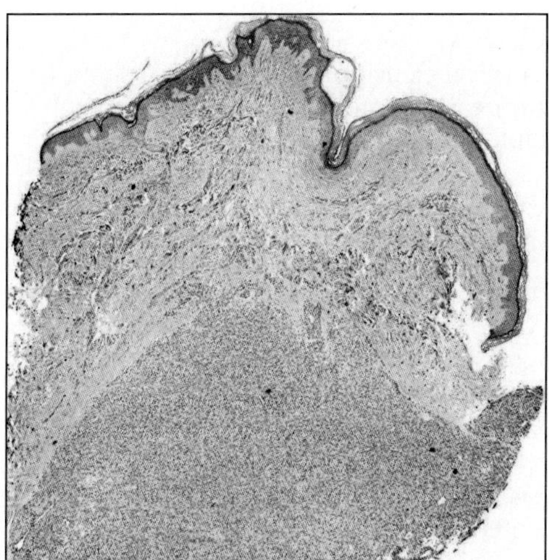

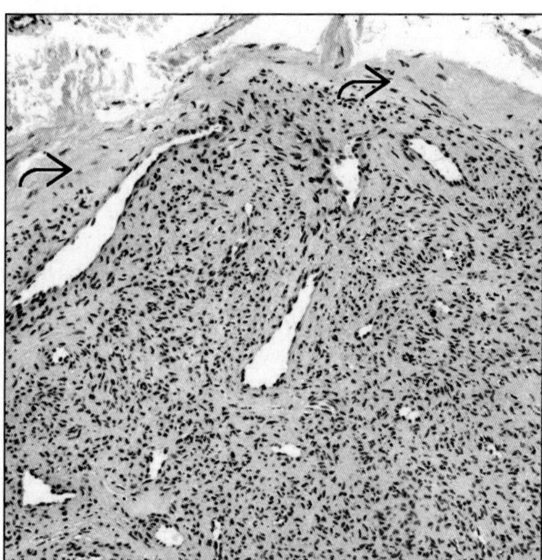

(Left) *Hematoxylin & eosin shows another lesion that has a predominance of hemangiopericytoma-like areas. This lesion would be regarded as "myopericytoma" to underscore this finding.* ***(Right)*** *Hematoxylin & eosin shows higher magnification. Subtle myoid features can be appreciated, particularly at the edge of the nodule ⤻.*

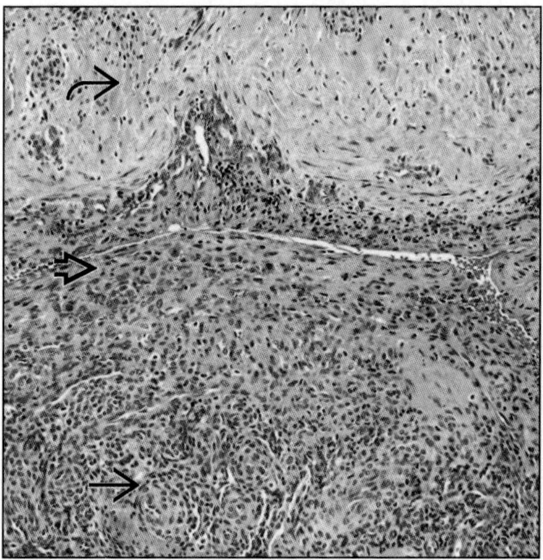

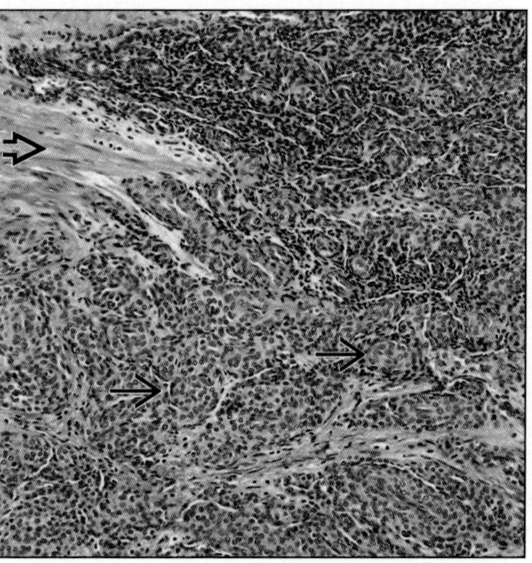

(Left) *Hematoxylin & eosin shows a lesion with myoid ⤻, whorled hemangiopericytomatous →, and glomus cell ⇨ areas. Such a lesion would be classified as a myopericytoma, a tumor within a continuum with myofibroma.* ***(Right)*** *Hematoxylin & eosin shows cellular areas that are alarming but have negligible mitotic activity. Note the myoid area ⇨ and whorled areas →.*

KAPOSIFORM HEMANGIOENDOTHELIOMA

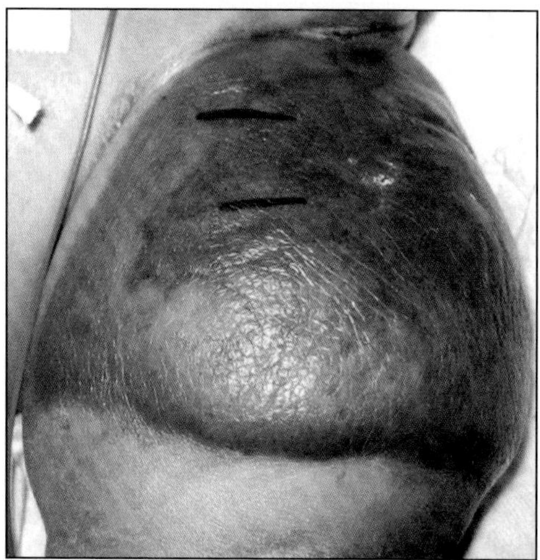

Clinical photograph shows a large inguinal KH in an infant. (Courtesy S. Billings, MD.)

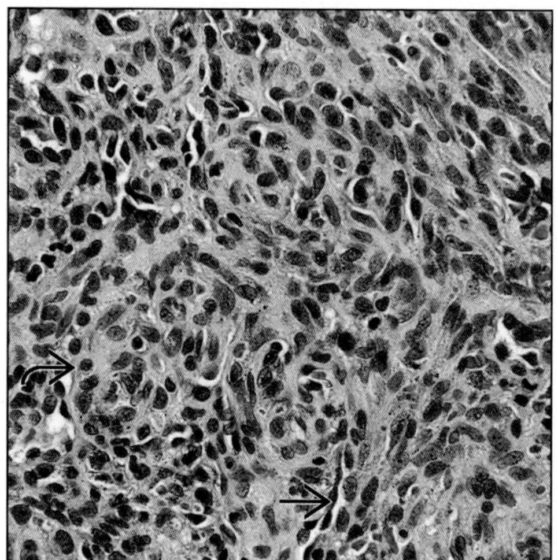

Kaposiform hemangioendothelioma at high power shows a spindle cell proliferation with slit-like vascular spaces ➔ and glomeruloid structures ➜. (Courtesy S. Billings, MD.)

TERMINOLOGY

Abbreviations
- Kaposiform hemangioendothelioma (KH)

Synonyms
- Kaposi-like infantile hemangioendothelioma
- Hemangioma with Kaposi sarcoma-like features

Definitions
- Locally aggressive vascular neoplasm occurring in infants and children characterized by Kaposi sarcoma-like spindle cell pattern of growth

CLINICAL ISSUES

Epidemiology
- Age
  - 1st decade of life; adult cases reported

Site
- Deep soft tissue
  - Retroperitoneum and peritoneum
  - Head and neck, mediastinum, trunk, and extremities also reported
- Skin

Presentation
- Superficial sites
  - Ill-defined violaceous plaques
- Deep soft tissues
  - Painful or painless mass, single or multiple
  - Locally aggressive
  - Often associated with Kasabach-Merritt phenomenon (KMP); consumptive coagulopathy
  - Most often in retroperitoneum
    - May present with ascites, intestinal obstruction, or jaundice
  - May be associated with lymphangiomatosis

Treatment
- Surgical approaches
  - Complete surgical excision when feasible
    - Retroperitoneal and mediastinal cases often unresectable
- Drugs
  - Vincristine, cyclophosphamide, methotrexate, actinomycin D, α-interferon, and steroids
  - Often used when complete excision not possible

Prognosis
- Do not regress
- Prognosis strongly influenced by
  - Site, clinical extent, and development of KMP
- 10% mortality rate
- Poor prognosis with large tumors complicated by KMP
- Lymph node metastases (rare)
- Distant metastases not reported

MACROSCOPIC FEATURES

General Features
- Superficial sites
  - Ill-defined violaceous plaques
- Deep soft tissues
  - Firm, multinodular, gray-red mass
  - Coarse interconnecting nodules
  - Often encase surrounding structures

MICROSCOPIC PATHOLOGY

Microscopic Features
- Infiltrating nodules of spindled endothelial cells
  - Form slit-like or crescentic vessels
    - Resembles Kaposi sarcoma
  - Contain hemosiderin and fragmented erythrocytes
  - Poorly canalized vessels
  - Dense hyaline fibrosis surrounds nodules

Key Facts

Terminology
- Locally aggressive vascular neoplasm occurring in infants and children

Clinical Issues
- Occur in 1st decade of life
- Retroperitoneum and peritoneum most common locations
- Often associated with KMP
- Do not regress
- Prognosis strongly influenced by
  - Site, clinical extent, and development of KMP
- 10% mortality rate
- Distant metastases not reported

Microscopic Pathology
- Infiltrating nodules of spindled endothelial cells
  - Form slit-like or crescentic vessels
- Glomeruloid nests

Top Differential Diagnoses
- Infantile hemangioma (capillary hemangioma)
  - Lacks spindle cells and glomeruloid structures
- Kaposi sarcoma
  - Lacks glomeruloid and infantile hemangioma-like components
- Tufted angioma
  - Lacks infiltrative growth of KH
- Spindle cell hemangioma
  - Cavernous vessel component not present in KH

Diagnostic Checklist
- Occur almost exclusively in children
- Strong association with KMP

Immunohistochemistry

Antibody	Reactivity	Staining Pattern	Comment
CD31	Positive	Cell membrane	
CD34	Positive	Cell membrane	
FLI-1	Positive	Nuclear	
Podoplanin	Positive	Cell membrane	Positive in peripheral lymphatic component (D2-40 epitope)
Actin-HHF-35	Positive	Cytoplasmic	Highlights scattered pericytic cells
GLUT1	Negative		Positive in infantile/juvenile hemangioma
Lewis-Y	Negative		Positive in infantile/juvenile hemangioma

- Occasional vessels with round lumina
  - Resembles infantile hemangioma
- Glomeruloid nests
  - Rounded epithelioid endothelial cells
  - Intra- and extracellular hyaline granules, stippled hemosiderin, and vacuoles
  - Platelet-rich fibrin microthrombi
- Well-formed vessels with perithelial elements

DIFFERENTIAL DIAGNOSIS

Infantile (Capillary) Hemangioma
- Distinct lobules of capillary-sized vessels
- GLUT1 and Lewis-Y positive
- Lacks spindle cells and glomeruloid structures
- Not associated with KMP

Kaposi Sarcoma
- Found in immunosuppressed patients; HHV8-positive
- Lacks glomeruloid and infantile hemangioma-like components
- Lacks dense hyaline fibrosis

Tufted Angioma
- Distinct nodules of dermis
- Histologically and immunophenotypically very similar
  - May represent part of spectrum of KH
- Contain more conventional capillary vessels
- Lacks infiltrative growth of KH

Spindle Cell Hemangioma
- Combination of cavernous vessels and spindle cells
- Cavernous vessel component not present in KH

Composite Hemangioendothelioma
- Vascular neoplasm showing varying combinations of benign, low-grade malignant and malignant vascular components that mainly affects adults
  - Components may include features of epithelioid, spindle cell, retiform, and kaposiform hemangioendotheliomas, in addition to papillary intralymphatic angioendothelioma
- Usually localized in the distal extremity of the limbs

DIAGNOSTIC CHECKLIST

Clinically Relevant Pathologic Features
- Age distribution
  - Occur almost exclusively in children
- Symptom complex
  - Strong association with KMP

SELECTED REFERENCES

1. Lyons LL et al: Kaposiform hemangioendothelioma: a study of 33 cases emphasizing its pathologic, immunophenotypic, and biologic uniqueness from juvenile hemangioma. Am J Surg Pathol. 28(5):559-68, 2004

KAPOSIFORM HEMANGIOENDOTHELIOMA

Microscopic Features

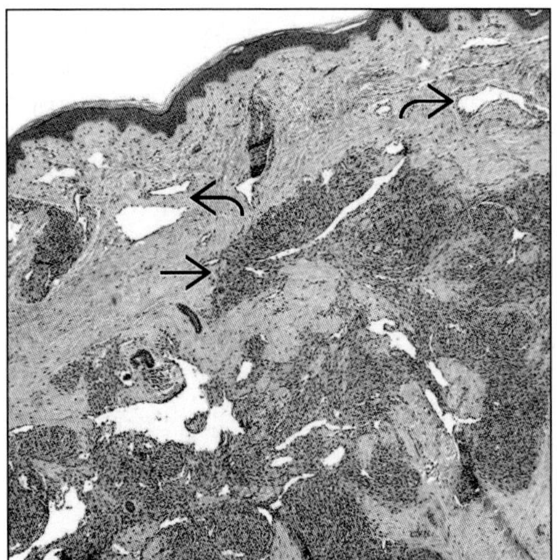

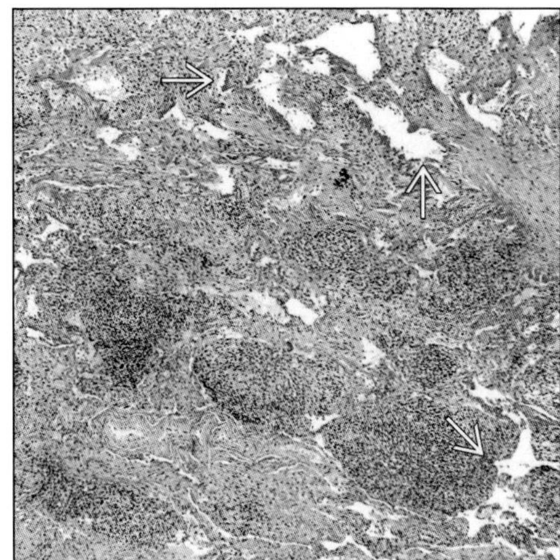

(Left) *Kaposiform hemangioendothelioma at low power shows the nodules of tumor ⇒ infiltrating into the dermis and scattered dilated lymphatic channels ⇒. (Courtesy S. Billings, MD.)* ***(Right)*** *Kaposiform hemangioendothelioma at low power shows hemangioma-like areas ⇒. (Courtesy S. Billings, MD.)*

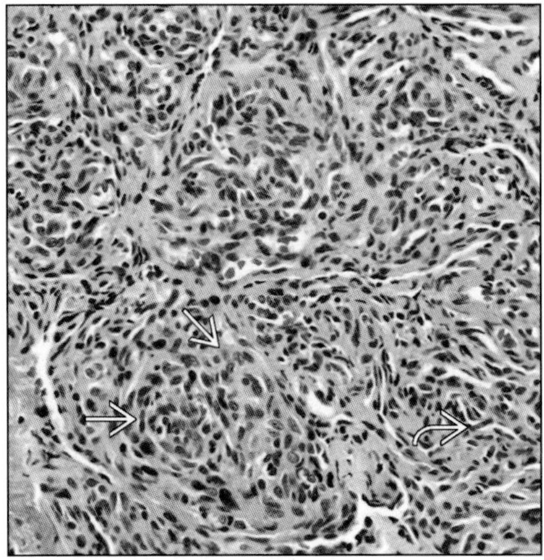

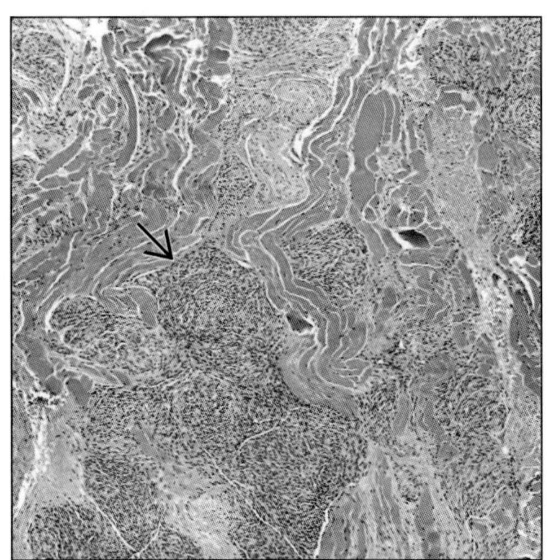

(Left) *Kaposiform hemangioendothelioma at high power shows scattered glomeruloid structures ⇒ amongst a background of slit-like vascular spaces ⇒.* ***(Right)*** *Kaposiform hemangioendothelioma at low power shows the nodules of tumor ⇒ infiltrating and dissecting into soft tissue. This infiltrative pattern is highly characteristic.*

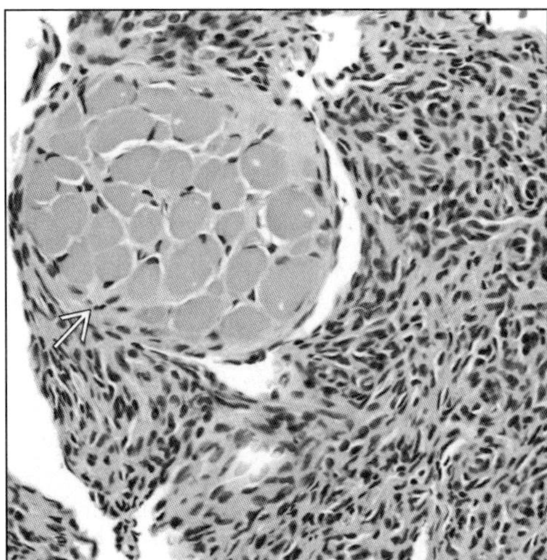

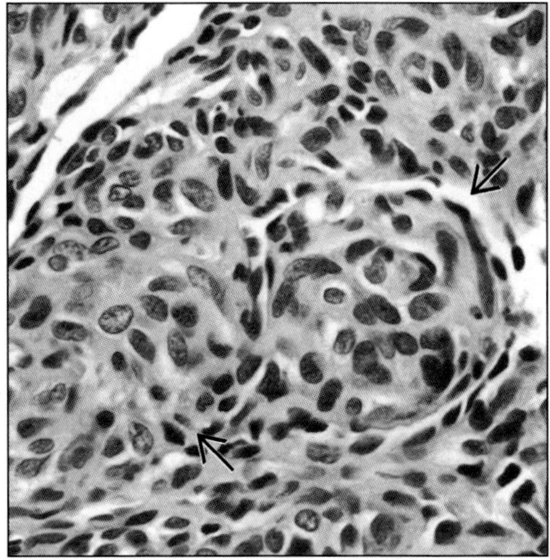

(Left) *Kaposiform hemangioendothelioma is shown surrounding a bundle of skeletal muscle ⇒.* ***(Right)*** *Kaposiform hemangioendothelioma from high power shows 2 well-defined glomeruloid structures ⇒. Their presence can be helpful in distinguishing KH from Kaposi sarcoma.*

Microscopic Features and Differential Diagnosis

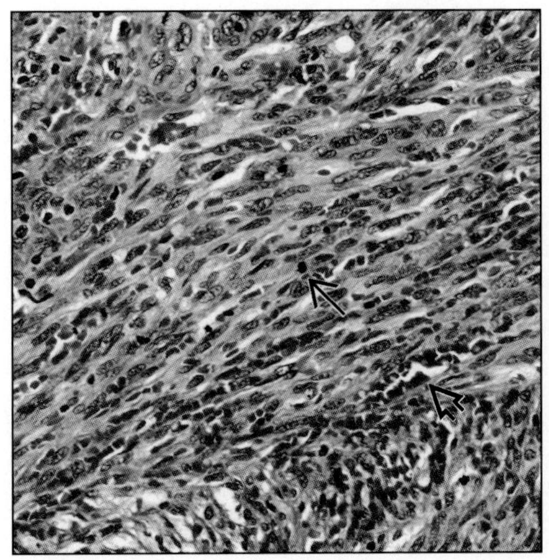

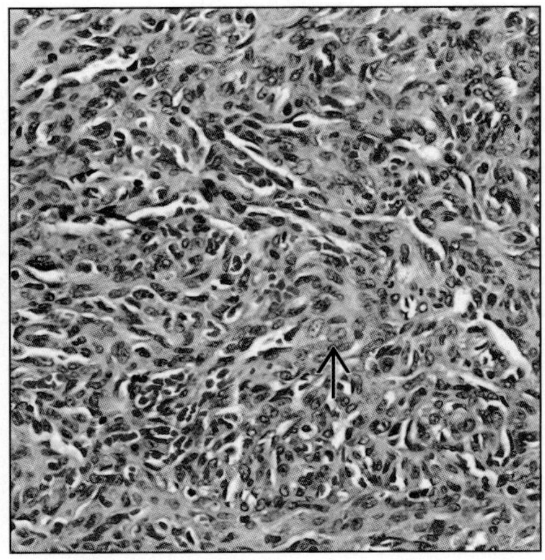

(Left) *Unlike KH, Kaposi sarcoma, as shown here, is composed entirely of a spindle cell proliferation with numerous slit-like vascular spaces ⇨. Note the more frequent mitotic figures →, slightly higher nuclear grade, and lack of epithelioid endothelial cells.* ***(Right)*** *Kaposiform hemangioendothelioma at high power shows a Kaposi sarcoma-like area. Note the scattered epithelioid endothelial cells → and lack of mitotic activity.*

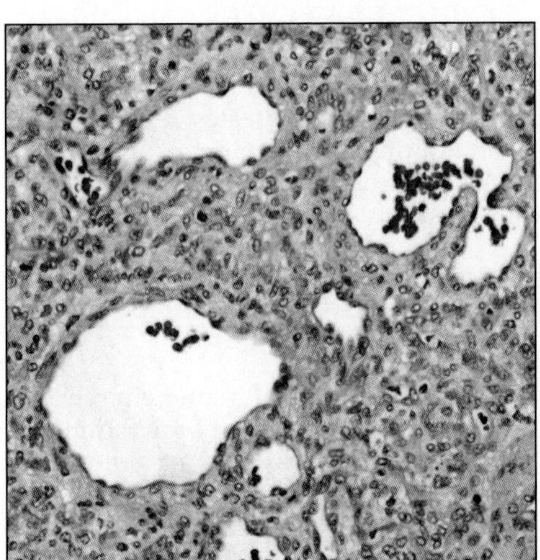

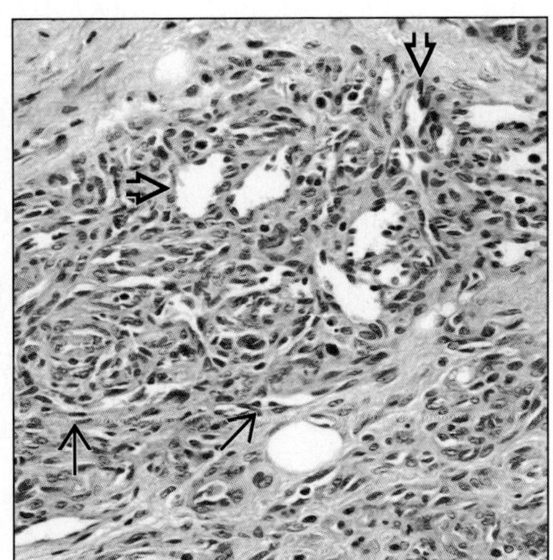

(Left) *The lack of spindle cells and glomeruloid structures, as shown in this example of an infantile (capillary) hemangioma, are helpful features when distinguishing from a KH.* ***(Right)*** *Kaposiform hemangioendothelioma at medium power shows a focal hemangioma-like area ⇨. The interspersed spindle cells forming slit-like vascular spaces → can help distinguish this lesion from an infantile (capillary) hemangioma.*

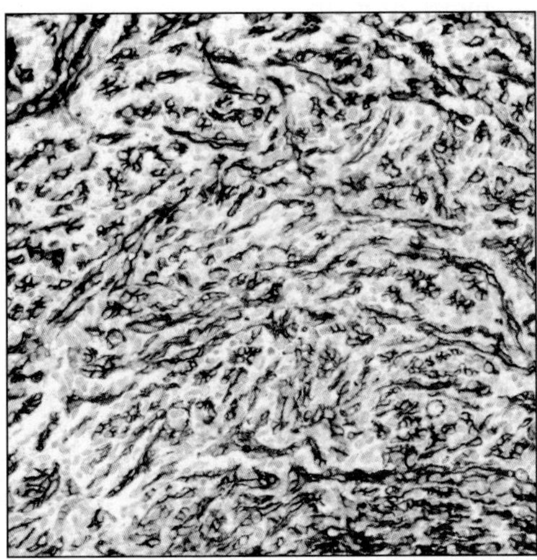

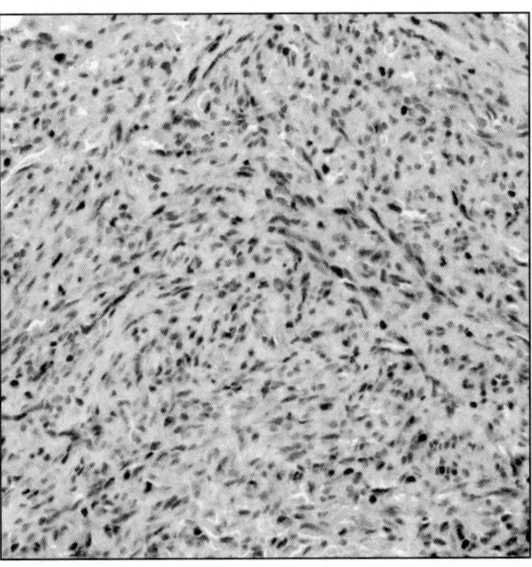

(Left) *Strong CD34 immunoreactivity is shown highlighting the neoplastic cells of this kaposiform hemangioendothelioma.* ***(Right)*** *FLI-1 immunoreactivity highlights the nuclei of the neoplastic cells in this kaposiform hemangioendothelioma.*

DESMOPLASTIC SMALL ROUND CELL TUMOR

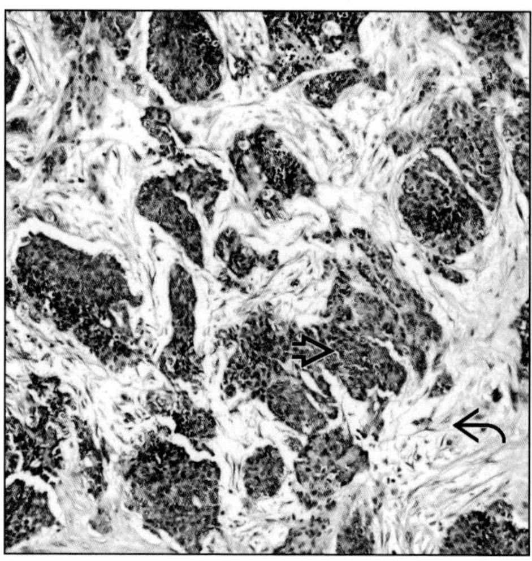

In DSRCT, islands of neoplastic cells proliferate in dense desmoplastic stroma. The tumor cells are markedly hyperchromatic ➡ in contrast to the stromal myofibroblasts ↗.

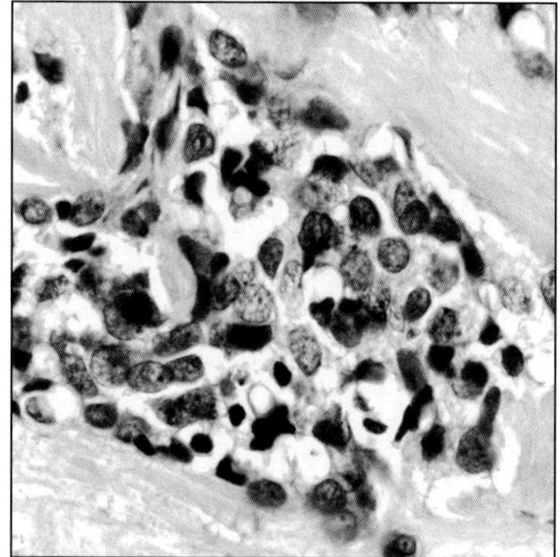

The neoplastic cells in desmoplastic round cell tumor are quite uniform, a feature of sarcomas with balanced reciprocal translocations. Nucleoli are inconspicuous, and cytoplasm is scanty.

TERMINOLOGY

Abbreviations

- Desmoplastic small round cell tumor (DSRCT)

Synonyms

- Desmoplastic small round cell tumor with divergent differentiation
- Polyphenotypic small round cell tumor
- Desmoplastic primitive neuroectodermal tumor
- Intraabdominal desmoplastic small round cell tumor

Definitions

- Primitive malignant neoplasm arising in serosal surfaces with distinctive histology composed of primitive small round blue cells embedded in abundant desmoplastic stroma

CLINICAL ISSUES

Presentation

- Male predilection
- Pain and weight loss
- Most common in children and young adults (2nd or 3rd decade; median age: 20 years)
- Most commonly present in peritoneal cavity
  - Also reported in paratesticular region, ovary, thoracic cavity, lung, central nervous system, and head and neck

Treatment

- Surgical excision
- Chemotherapy

Prognosis

- Poor prognosis
  - Nearly uniformly fatal
- Frequent local recurrence; rarely metastasizes
- Median survival is 24 months

MACROSCOPIC FEATURES

General Features

- Large, bulky tumors (> 10 cm in greatest dimension)
- May also grow in multinodular fashion
- Firm homogeneous cut surface
- Hemorrhage and necrosis

MICROSCOPIC PATHOLOGY

Histologic Features

- Nests, trabeculae, or sheets of small round blue cells embedded in abundant desmoplastic fibrous stroma
- Nests may display peripheral palisading of tumor cells
- Rosette-like structures

Cytologic Features

- Small to intermediate-sized round to oval cells with scant cytoplasm
- Round to oval, hyperchromatic nuclei
- Small nucleoli
- High mitotic rate, with atypical mitoses (translocation sarcoma)

ANCILLARY TESTS

Immunohistochemistry

- Staining pattern is polyphenotypic
- Vimentin, cytokeratin, desmin, EMA, and WT1 consistently stain tumor cells in ~ 90% of cases
- Staining pattern for desmin and vimentin is characteristically dot-like and paranuclear
- May also show focal positivity for CD56, NSE, chromogranin, synaptophysin, and S100 protein

Cytogenetics

- Shows t(11:22)(p13;q12), similar to Ewing sarcoma/PNET

DESMOPLASTIC SMALL ROUND CELL TUMOR

Key Facts

Clinical Issues
- Most common in children and young adults
  - Median age: 20 years
- Male predilection
- Large abdominal mass on chest x-rays and CT scans
- Poor prognosis
- Median survival is 24 months

Macroscopic Features
- Large, bulky tumors (> 10 cm in greatest dimension)

Microscopic Pathology
- Nests, trabeculae, or sheets of uniform small round cells embedded in abundant desmoplastic fibrous stroma
- Rosette-like structures
- Small to intermediate-sized round to oval cells with scant cytoplasm
- High mitotic index, often with atypical (abnormal) mitoses
- Immunohistochemically polyphenotypic
- Vimentin, keratin, desmin, EMA, and WT1 consistently positive in tumor cells in approximately 90% of cases
  - Staining pattern for desmin and vimentin is characteristically dot-like and paranuclear
- May also show focal positivity for CD56, NSE, chromogranin, synaptophysin, and S100 protein
- Genetically shows t(11:22)(p13;q12), similar to Ewing sarcoma/PNET
  - Differs from Ewing sarcoma as rearranged gene on chromosome 11 is *WT1* rather than *FLI1*

- Unlike Ewing sarcoma, site on chromosome 11 is *WT1* gene rather than *FLI1* gene
  - The 2 genes (*EWS* and *WT1*) are rearranged and functionally fused
  - *EWS* breakpoint in introns 7-10
  - *WT1* breakpoint between exons 7 and 8
- *EWS-WT1* chimera encodes novel transcription factor detectable by PCR as diagnostic test
- Rare hybrid tumors have *EWS-ERG* fusion

DIFFERENTIAL DIAGNOSIS

Peripheral Neuroectodermal Tumor (PNET)/ Ewing Sarcoma
- Similar cell population in both, but prominent desmoplastic stroma is not seen in PNET
- Lacks strong expression of polyphenotypic markers, such as desmin, cytokeratin, and WT1
- Strongly positive for CD99 in most cases; CD99 is seen only in 20% of cases of DSRCT
- Translocation in PNET is t(11:22)(p24;q12); translocation in DSRCT is t(11:22)(p13;q12)

Metastatic Neuroendocrine Carcinoma
- Lacks prominent desmoplastic stroma separating tumor cell nests
- Has distinctive "smudged" or "salt & pepper" chromatin pattern
- Positive for neuroendocrine markers, such as chromogranin, CD56, and synaptophysin
- Does not express EMA, desmin, or WT1

Malignant Lymphoma
- Dyscohesive pattern of growth without striking desmoplasia
- Express CD45 and variety of other lymphoid markers, e.g., CD3, CD20, CD30, CD43, but not keratin, desmin, or WT1
- Lymphoblastic lymphoma in children and adolescents shows nuclear positivity for TdT and is positive for CD99

Alveolar Rhabdomyosarcoma
- Multinucleated cells, some pleomorphism
- Diffuse positivity for desmin and myogenin

DIAGNOSTIC CHECKLIST

Clinically Relevant Pathologic Features
- Preferentially affects children and young adults, although it can affect older patients

Pathologic Interpretation Pearls
- Nests of small round blue cells surrounded by abundant desmoplastic fibrous stroma
- Primitive appearance of tumor cells
- High mitotic activity and areas of tumor cell necrosis
- Distinctive pattern of immunohistochemical staining: CK, EMA, vimentin, desmin, and WT1 positive
- Dot-like, paranuclear (Golgi zone) staining for vimentin and desmin
- Specific cytogenetic translocation: t(11:22)(p13;q12)

SELECTED REFERENCES

1. Lae ME et al: Desmoplastic small round cell tumor: a clinicopathologic, immunohistochemical, and molecular study of 32 tumors. Am J Surg Pathol. 26(7):823-35, 2002
2. Ordóñez NG: Desmoplastic small round cell tumor: I: a histopathologic study of 39 cases with emphasis on unusual histological patterns. Am J Surg Pathol. 22(11):1303-13, 1998
3. Ordóñez NG: Desmoplastic small round cell tumor: II: an ultrastructural and immunohistochemical study with emphasis on new immunohistochemical markers. Am J Surg Pathol. 22(11):1314-27, 1998
4. Ladanyi M et al: Fusion of the EWS and WT1 genes in the desmoplastic small round cell tumor. Cancer Res. 54(11):2837-40, 1994
5. Gerald WL et al: Intra-abdominal desmoplastic small round-cell tumor. Report of 19 cases of a distinctive type of high-grade polyphenotypic malignancy affecting young individuals. Am J Surg Pathol. 15(6):499-513, 1991

DESMOPLASTIC SMALL ROUND CELL TUMOR

Microscopic Features

(Left) *Well-demarcated nests of tumor cells ⇨ are surrounded by a vascular →, desmoplastic stroma.* ***(Right)*** *Sharply demarcated nests of various size and shape are surrounded by dense fibrous stroma → in this desmoplastic small round cell tumor.*

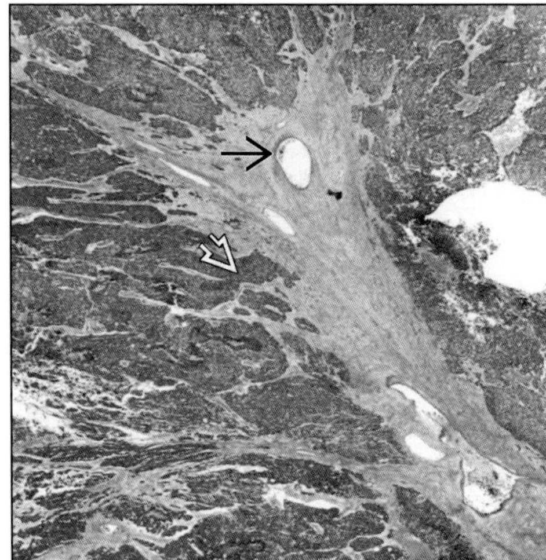

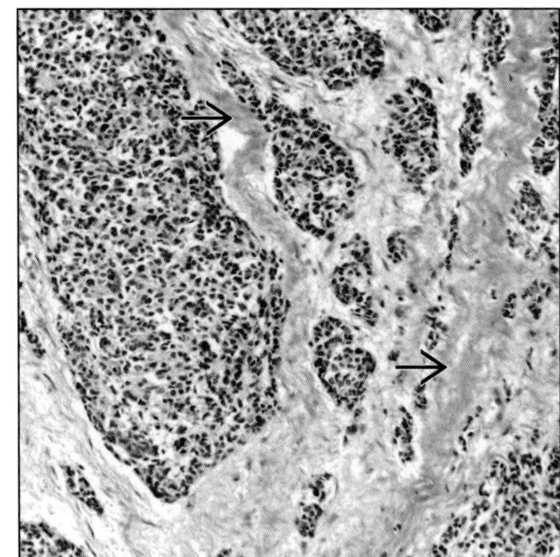

(Left) *Central necrosis → is not an uncommon finding within larger nests of tumor cells. Note the band of desmoplastic stroma ⇨.* ***(Right)*** *Sharply demarcated nests of various size and shape are surrounded by a desmoplastic stroma. Cell may also form chords, tubular-like structures →, or trabeculae with fibrous septa.*

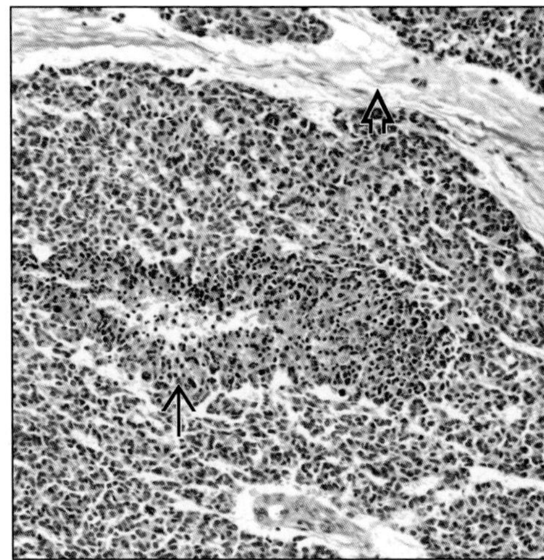

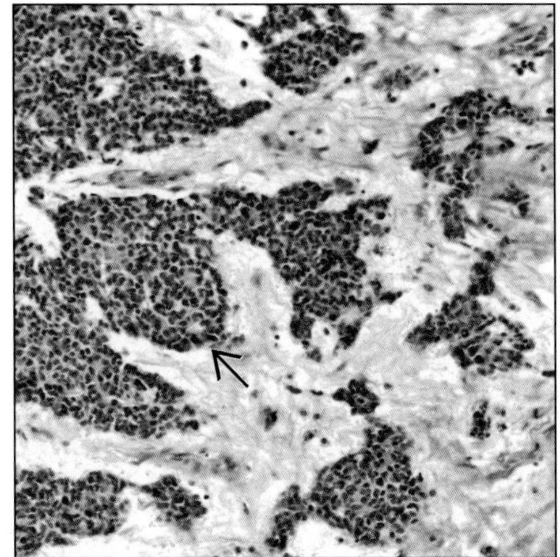

(Left) *Tumor cells are undifferentiated and somewhat monotonous in appearance. The nuclei are small and round to oval with inconspicuous nucleoli and scant eosinophilic cytoplasm. Occasionally, tumor cells may have vacuolated cytoplasm →. Foci with increased nuclear atypia may be present.* ***(Right)*** *Cords of malignant cells are surrounded by a desmoplastic stroma, mimicking lobular carcinoma of the breast. Spindle-shaped fibroblasts → and myofibroblasts can be seen in the stroma.*

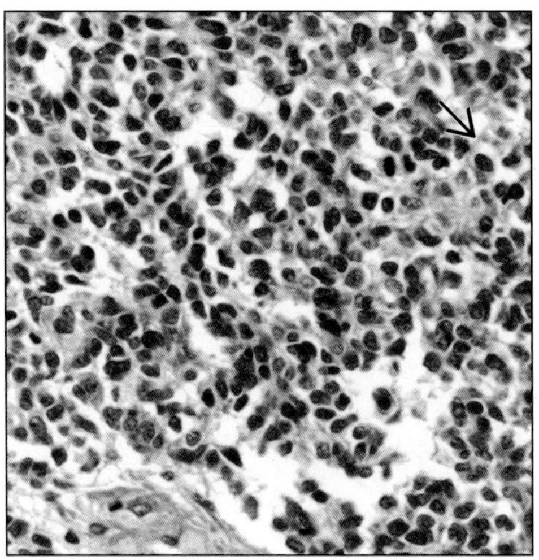

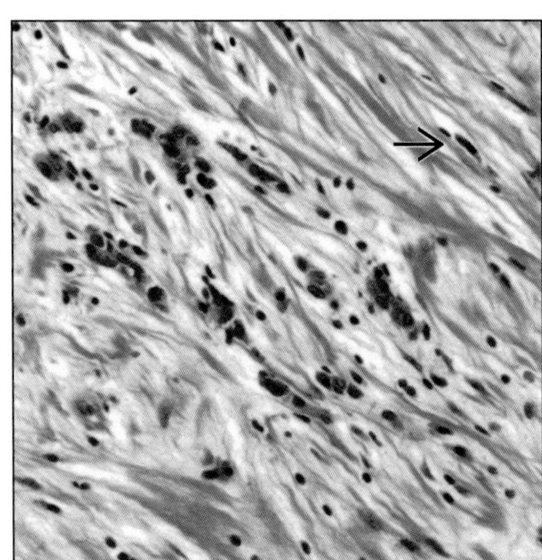

Immunohistochemical Features

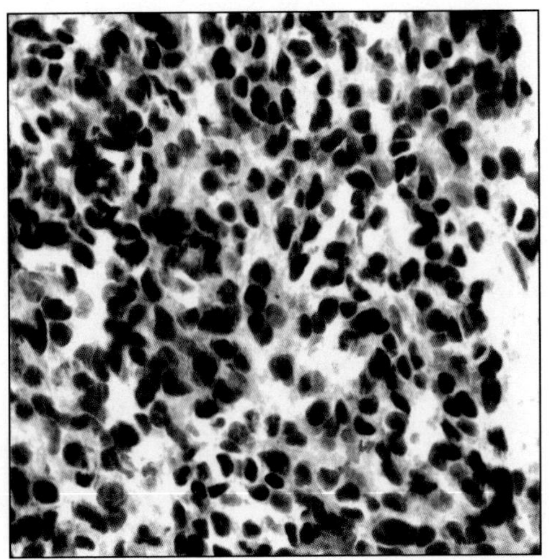

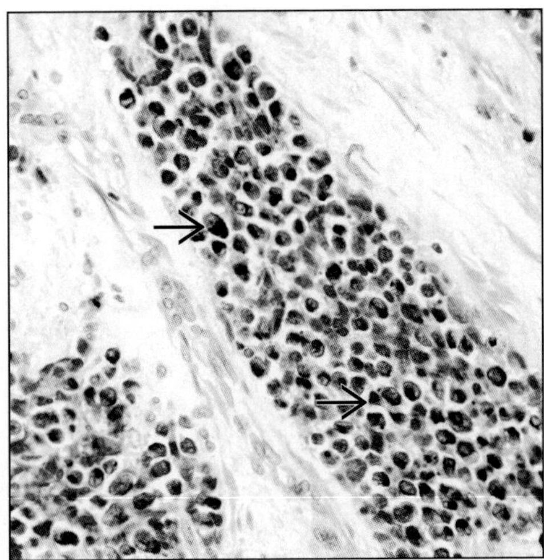

(Left) *Desmoplastic small round cell tumors display strong nuclear labeling for WT1 in most cases. This helps distinguish them from Ewing sarcoma and alveolar rhabdomyosarcoma (which can have cytoplasmic positivity).* ***(Right)*** *Immunohistochemical staining of desmoplastic small round cell tumor for vimentin shows the majority of the tumor cells are positive for this marker and display a distinctive dot-like, paranuclear (Golgi zone) staining pattern ⇒.*

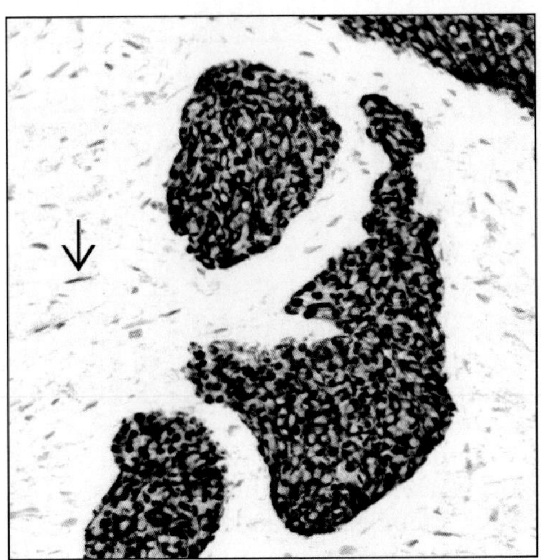

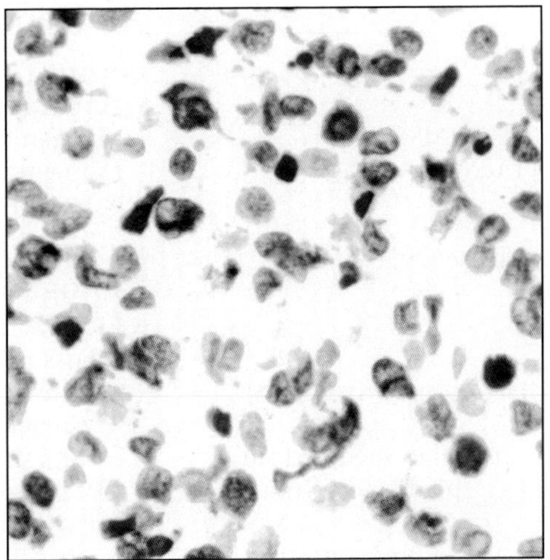

(Left) *Desmin expression is a characteristic feature of DSRCT, present in > 90% of cases. In this example, the staining is diffuse and highlights the tumor islands. The spindle cells in the stroma ⇒ are negative.* ***(Right)*** *Immunohistochemical staining of desmoplastic small round blue cell tumor of the pleura for desmin shows cytoplasmic positivity in the majority of the tumor cells. The staining pattern is dot-like and paranuclear (Golgi zone) and very distinctive for this tumor.*

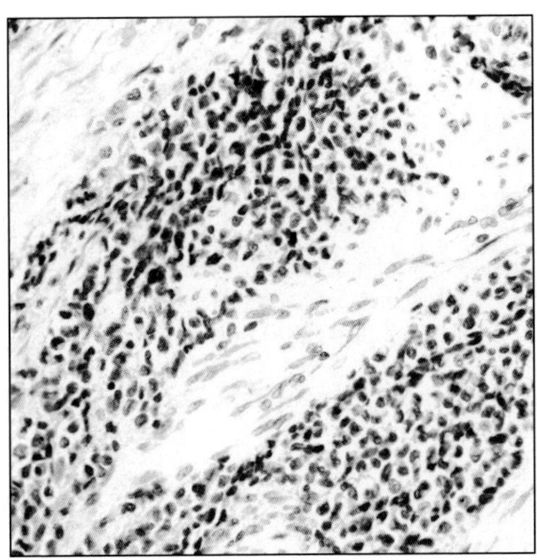

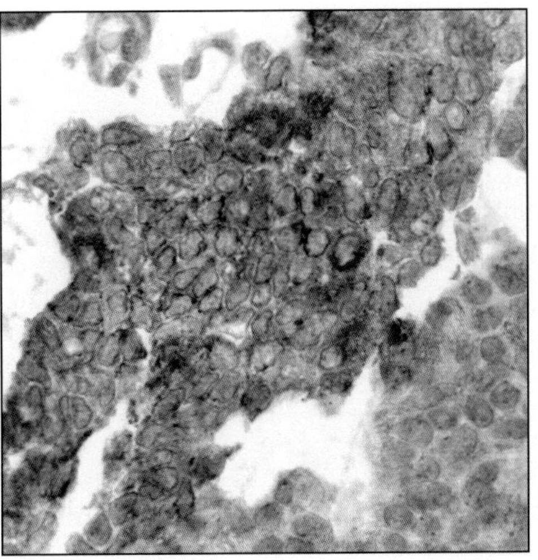

(Left) *Immunohistochemical staining of desmoplastic small round cell tumor for CD99 shows no reactivity in the tumor cells in most cases. This helps to distinguish this tumor from Ewing sarcoma and lymphoblastic lymphoma.* ***(Right)*** *CD99 is usually negative in desmoplastic round cell tumors, but weak cytoplasmic staining is seen in some cases. This differs from the strong membranous staining of Ewing sarcoma, but cytogenetic studies may be required to make the diagnosis.*

RHABDOMYOSARCOMA

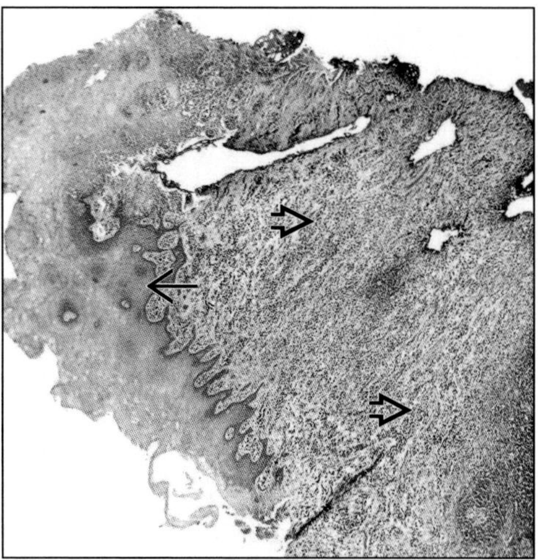

Pictured is an embryonal rhabdomyosarcoma (ERMS) of the larynx in a young child, covered by squamous mucosa →. Sheets of primitive small ovoid cells are situated within a myxoid stroma ⇒.

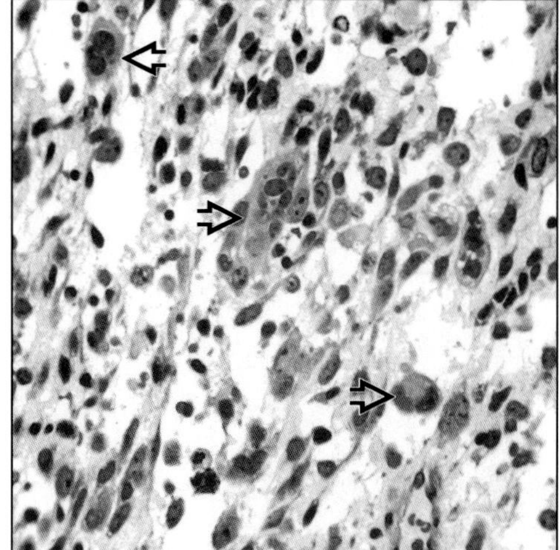

Features of skeletal muscular differentiation are evident in a number of the tumor cells in this high-power view of a paratesticular ERMS ⇒.

TERMINOLOGY

Abbreviations

- Rhabdomyosarcoma (RMS)
- Embryonal rhabdomyosarcoma (ERMS)
- Alveolar rhabdomyosarcoma (ARMS)

Definitions

- Tumor derived from primitive mesenchyme with a propensity toward myogenesis
- **Histologic subtypes**
  - Embryonic
    - Conventional, or not otherwise specified (NOS)
    - Spindle cell
    - Botryoid: Arises from an epithelial-lined surface and projects into lumen (e.g., bladder, vagina)
  - Alveolar
    - Composed of alveolar-type structures containing dyscohesive tumor cells
  - Sclerosing
    - Rare variant, newly described in adults and children
    - Abundant, hyalinizing matrix
  - Anaplastic
    - Forms of embryonal and alveolar RMS containing large, hyperchromatic nuclei and atypical mitoses
    - Embryonal forms of anaplastic RMS have more aggressive behavior
  - Pleomorphic
    - Occurs almost exclusively in older adults
- **Classification systems**
  - Several have been introduced and implemented since Horn and Enterline in 1952
  - International classification of RMS, 1998
    - Intergroup RMS Study Group (IRSG), now part of the Children's Oncology Group, currently uses this system

ETIOLOGY/PATHOGENESIS

Etiology

- Tumor derived from primitive mesenchyme
- Myogenic differentiation identified by one of the following techniques
  - Morphologic, immunohistochemical, ultrastructural, molecular

Pathogenesis

- **ERMS:** Causation thought to be epigenetic
  - Loss of heterozygosity at 11p15.5 also seen in Wilms tumors, hepatoblastomas, and Beckwith-Wiedemann syndrome
  - Alterations of imprinting may play a role
- **ARMS:** Related to *PAX/FKHR* gene fusion
  - *PAX3* and *PAX7*: Members of paired box transcription factor family
  - *FKHR*: Member of fork head transcription factor family
  - Fusion protein causes aberrant transcription with resultant myogenesis

CLINICAL ISSUES

Epidemiology

- Incidence
  - RMS comprises 60% of sarcomas reported in children and adolescents each year
  - Annual incidence: 4-7 per 1,000,000 children ≤ 15 years of age
  - Most common soft tissue malignancy of childhood and adolescence

Presentation

- **Embryonal rhabdomyosarcoma**
  - General features
    - Affects infants and young children

RHABDOMYOSARCOMA

Key Facts

Terminology

- Most common soft tissue malignancy of childhood and adolescence
- Tumor derived from primitive mesenchyme with a propensity toward myogenesis
- **Histologic subtypes**
  - Conventional ERMS: Intermediate prognosis
  - Spindle cell ERMS: Superior prognosis
  - Botryoid ERMS: Superior prognosis
  - ARMS: Poor prognosis
  - Sclerosing RMS: Superior prognosis
  - Anaplastic RMS: Poor prognosis

Clinical Issues

- EMRS
  - Affects infants and young children
  - Sites: Genitourinary tract, head and neck, abdomen
- Botryoid ERMS: Occurs in bladder, vagina
- Spindle cell ERMS: Majority in paratesticular region
- ARMS affects adolescents; occurs in extremities
- Sclerosing RMS: Most occur in extremities

Ancillary Tests

- Myogenin and MYOD1
  - Both with very high sensitivity and specificity for RMS
- t(2;13)(q35;q14) is unique to alveolar RMS
- Alternate translocation: t(1;13)(p36;q14)

Top Differential Diagnoses

- Ewing sarcoma/PNET
- Desmoplastic small cell tumor
- Pleuropulmonary blastoma

- Arises from genitourinary tract, head and neck, abdomen
- Associated with Beckwith-Wiedemann syndrome
- **Spindle cell RMS**
  - Vast majority occur in paratesticular region
- **Botryoid RMS**
  - Characteristically occurs in urinary bladder, vagina, extrahepatic bile ducts, conjunctiva
- **Alveolar rhabdomyosarcoma**
  - Affects adolescent population
  - Most often present in extremities
- **Sclerosing rhabdomyosarcoma**
  - Occurs in children, adolescents, and adults
  - Most common in head and neck region in children

Treatment

- Surgery
- Multi-agent chemotherapy ± radiotherapy

Prognosis

- Differs among histologic subtypes
  - **ERMS**
    - **Conventional type:** Intermediate prognosis: 66% 5-year survival
    - **Botryoid type:** Superior prognosis: 95% 5-year survival
    - **Spindle cell type:** Superior prognosis: 88% 5-year survival
  - **ARMS, NOS or solid variant**
    - Poor prognosis: 53% 5-year survival
    - *PAX3/FKHR* fusion positivity an adverse prognostic factor
    - Fusion-negative ARMS: Prognosis reported to be intermediate between *PAX7/FKHR*(+) and *PAX3/FKHR*(+) ARMS
  - **RMS with diffuse anaplasia**
    - Poor prognosis: 45% 5-year survival
- Staging
  - 2 systems are used, with comparable results
    - Clinical grouping system (CGS): Surgically based
    - Tumor, node, metastasis system (TNM): Site based
- Other prognostic factors
  - Tumor size, completeness of resection
  - Anatomic site
    - Orbit: Best prognosis
    - Retroperitoneum: Worst prognosis
  - Post-therapy cytodifferentiation is associated with more favorable outcome
    - Occurs most frequently in botryoid and conventional ERMS histologic types
  - Diffuse myogenin immunohistochemical expression correlates with poor prognosis

MACROSCOPIC FEATURES

General

- Poorly circumscribed tan mass
- Variably collagenous and myxoid stroma
- Hemorrhage and necrosis may be present

Botryoid ERMS

- Resembles a gelatinous "bunch of grapes" projecting into the lumen of a hollow organ
- Multinodular excrescences of various sizes

MICROSCOPIC PATHOLOGY

Embryonal Rhabdomyosarcoma

- **Conventional ERMS**
  - Variable cellularity with tumor cells separated by loose, myxoid stroma
    - Alternating zones of hypocellularity and hypercellularity
  - Recapitulates normal embryonal myogenesis histologically with all phases variably represented
    - Undifferentiated stellate mesenchymal cells with round to oval nuclei and minimal cytoplasm
    - Rhabdomyoblasts: Strap cells, tadpole cells, spider cells with eccentric round nuclei and brightly eosinophilic cytoplasm
    - Well-differentiated myofibers with cross striations
- **Spindle cell type**
  - Fascicular, spindled growth pattern

RHABDOMYOSARCOMA

- Has been described as "leiomyomatous"
  - Some with a storiform architecture
  - May be densely collagenous
- **Botryoid type**
  - Polypoid lesion
  - "Cambium layer": Subepithelial condensation of tumor cells, similar to cambium layer of plants
- **Anaplastic**
  - Defined using criteria similar to that of Wilms tumor
    - Lobulated, hyperchromatic nuclei 3x larger than neighboring nuclei
    - Obviously atypical mitotic figures
  - Focal anaplasia in RMS
    - Single or a few scattered anaplastic tumor cells
  - Diffuse anaplasia in RMS
    - Anaplastic cells aggregate in clusters or continuous sheets

Alveolar Rhabdomyosarcoma

- Tumor is arranged in alveolar-type structures
  - Fibrous septae provide a scaffolding for tumor cells contained within
  - Tumor cells are small, round, dyscohesive, and appear to float in alveolar spaces
    - Round, monomorphous lymphoma-like nuclei
    - Peripheral "cracking" artifact at border of tumor cell clusters
  - Less evident myogenic differentiation than in ERMS
- **Solid variant of ARMS**
  - Especially prevalent at tumor periphery
  - Characteristic cytologic features are a helpful feature in recognition
  - Often presents as palisading of tumor cells around fibrovascular cores
  - Usually cleft-like alveolar spaces can be seen elsewhere in the tumor

Sclerosing Rhabdomyosarcoma

- Hyalinizing matrix that entraps tumor cells
- Imparts a chondroid or osteoid appearance
- May resemble ARMS with thick fibrous septae
- Pseudovascular architecture
- Small alveolar spaces may be present

Post-therapy RMS Specimens

- Post-treatment cytodifferentiation occurs more often in botryoid or conventional ERMS than in ARMS

ANCILLARY TESTS

Immunohistochemistry

- Required in at least 20% of RMS cases for definitive diagnosis
- Myogenin and MYOD1
  - Most useful stains for confirmation of RMS
    - Both with very high sensitivity and specificity for RMS
  - ARMS vs. ERMS
    - Both stains, especially myogenin, show stronger and more diffuse positivity in ARMS than in ERMS
    - May help to differentiate the 2 RMS subtypes, especially in absence of *PAX3* or *PAX7/FKHR* fusion genes
    - Cases with diffuse myogenin positivity are more likely to be fusion-positive
    - Does not seem to be a difference in staining between classic ARMS and solid variant of ARMS
  - Sclerosing RMS
    - Stronger staining with MYOD1 than with myogenin
  - Only true intranuclear staining is specific for RMS
  - Both proteins represent transcription factors that are present in cells committed to earliest phase of myogenesis
- Desmin and muscle-specific actin (actin-HHF-35)
  - Good sensitivity, lesser specificity for RMS
- Myoglobin
  - Lacks sensitivity
  - Expressed in well-differentiated tumor cells

Cytogenetics

- **ERMS**
  - No recurrent translocations known
  - Highly variable karyotypes reported
  - Recurring allelic imbalances
    - Loss of heterozygosity (LOH) at 11p15.5
- **ARMS**
  - t(2;13)(q35;q14) is unique to alveolar RMS
    - Genetic breakpoints result in fusion protein *PAX3/FKHR*
  - Alternate translocation: t(1;13)(p36;q14), 20% of ARMS
    - Genetic breakpoints result in fusion protein *PAX7/FKHR*
  - However, at least 25% of ARMS do not demonstrate either of these translocations
- **Sclerosing RMS**
  - May resemble ARMS morphologically, but is negative for t(2;13) translocation

Molecular Genetics

- **ARMS**
  - *PAX3/FKHR* and *PAX7/FKHR* fusion genes detected by RT-PCR
    - Correspond to t(2;13) and t(1;13) translocations, respectively
    - Like the translocations, at least 25% of ARMS lack these fusion genes
    - Solid variant of ARMS more likely to be fusion-negative than classic ARMS

Electron Microscopy

- Thick and thin arrays of actin and myosin identified
  - Myosin filaments lined by free ribosomes represents the earliest stage of ultrastructural muscle differentiation
- Z-bands
  - May be present in well-differentiated RMS
- Nonspecific features
  - Submembranous filament arrays
  - Interrupted basal lamina

DIFFERENTIAL DIAGNOSIS

General Features

- RMS differential diagnosis (DDx) falls under 3 general categories
  - Other small round cell neoplasms
  - Other myogenic neoplasms
  - Other spindle cell neoplasms

Ewing Sarcoma/PNET

- May be desmin(+)
- CD99 may be positive in RMS
- Negative for myogenin and MYOD1
- FLI-1(+)

Desmoplastic Small Cell Tumor

- Occurs within abdomen
- Frequent desmin positivity
- Tumor nests may resemble alveolar pattern
- Negative myogenin stains
- Positive for *EWS-WT1* fusion gene

Lymphoma

- Included in DDx for solid variant of ARMS
- LCA positivity
- Myogenin and MYOD1 negative

Extrarenal Rhabdoid Tumor

- Hyaline inclusions composed of intermediate filaments ultrastructurally
- Cytokeratin(+), desmin(-), INI1(-)
- Chromosome 22 deletions

Monophasic Synovial Sarcoma

- Cellular tight fascicles of spindle cells with hyperchromatic nuclei
- Cytokeratin and EMA usually at least focally positive
- *SYT-SSX* fusion gene positive

Infantile Fibrosarcoma

- Short, usually ill-defined fascicles of primitive ovoid tumor cells
- Prominent lymphocytic infiltrate is typical
- Hemangiopericytomatous vascular pattern often present
- Most positive for *NTRK3-ETV6* fusion gene

Malignant Triton Tumor

- Malignant peripheral nerve sheath tumor with myogenous differentiation
- Occur sporadically and in patients with neurofibromatosis type 1
- High-grade sarcomas that rarely occur in children

Ectomesenchymoma

- Biphenotypic sarcoma, express both myogenin and neural features
- Some contain molecular gene rearrangements typical of Ewing sarcoma

Wilms Tumor with Myogenic Differentiation

- RMS may express WT1 with cytoplasmic staining
- Wilms tumor may stain positively with desmin or MYOD1
- Primary site in kidney

Pleuropulmonary Blastoma

- Occurs in peripheral lung tissue and pleura
- Presents with varying degrees of cyst formation
- Small primitive blastematous-appearing tumor cells
- May be desmin(+)

SELECTED REFERENCES

1. Davicioni E et al: Molecular classification of rhabdomyosarcoma--genotypic and phenotypic determinants of diagnosis: a report from the Children's Oncology Group. Am J Pathol. 174(2):550-64, 2009
2. Heerema-McKenney A et al: Diffuse myogenin expression by immunohistochemistry is an independent marker of poor survival in pediatric rhabdomyosarcoma: a tissue microarray study of 71 primary tumors including correlation with molecular phenotype. Am J Surg Pathol. 32(10):1513-22, 2008
3. Qualman S et al: Prevalence and clinical impact of anaplasia in childhood rhabdomyosarcoma: a report from the Soft Tissue Sarcoma Committee of the Children's Oncology Group. Cancer. 113(11):3242-7, 2008
4. Gallego Melcón S et al: Molecular biology of rhabdomyosarcoma. Clin Transl Oncol. 9(7):415-9, 2007
5. Parham DM et al: Correlation between histology and PAX/FKHR fusion status in alveolar rhabdomyosarcoma: a report from the Children's Oncology Group. Am J Surg Pathol. 31(6):895-901, 2007
6. Morotti RA et al: An immunohistochemical algorithm to facilitate diagnosis and subtyping of rhabdomyosarcoma: the Children's Oncology Group experience. Am J Surg Pathol. 30(8):962-8, 2006
7. Parham DM et al: Rhabdomyosarcomas in adults and children: an update. Arch Pathol Lab Med. 130(10):1454-65, 2006
8. Zambrano E et al: Pediatric sclerosing rhabdomyosarcoma. Int J Surg Pathol. 14(3):193-9, 2006
9. Chiles MC et al: Sclerosing rhabdomyosarcomas in children and adolescents: a clinicopathologic review of 13 cases from the Intergroup Rhabdomyosarcoma Study Group and Children's Oncology Group. Pediatr Dev Pathol. 7(6):583-94, 2004
10. Joshi D et al: Age is an independent prognostic factor in rhabdomyosarcoma: a report from the Soft Tissue Sarcoma Committee of the Children's Oncology Group. Pediatr Blood Cancer. 42(1):64-73, 2004
11. Vadgama B et al: Sclerosing rhabdomyosarcoma in childhood: case report and review of the literature. Pediatr Dev Pathol. 7(4):391-6, 2004
12. Peydró-Olaya A et al: Electron microscopy and other ancillary techniques in the diagnosis of small round cell tumors. Semin Diagn Pathol. 20(1):25-45, 2003
13. Qualman SJ et al: Protocol for the examination of specimens from patients (children and young adults) with rhabdomyosarcoma. Arch Pathol Lab Med. 127(10):1290-7, 2003
14. Sebire NJ et al: Myogenin and MyoD1 expression in paediatric rhabdomyosarcomas. J Clin Pathol. 56(6):412-6, 2003
15. Qualman SJ et al: Risk assignment in pediatric soft-tissue sarcomas: an evolving molecular classification. Curr Oncol Rep. 4(2):123-30, 2002
16. Parham DM: Pathologic classification of rhabdomyosarcomas and correlations with molecular studies. Mod Pathol. 14(5):506-14, 2001
17. Dias P et al: Strong immunostaining for myogenin in rhabdomyosarcoma is significantly associated with tumors of the alveolar subclass. Am J Pathol. 156(2):399-408, 2000

RHABDOMYOSARCOMA

International Classification of Rhabdomyosarcoma[1]

Diagnosis	Incidence	Prognosis
Embryonal, botryoid	6%	Superior
Embryonal, spindle cell	3%	Superior
Embryonal, NOS	49%	Intermediate
Alveolar, NOS or solid variant	31%	Poor
Anaplasia, diffuse[2]	2%	Poor
Undifferentiated sarcoma[3]	3%	Poor

[1]Modified from Qualman SJ et al: Intergroup Rhabdomyosarcoma Study: update for pathologists. Pediatr Dev Pathol. 1(6):550-61, 1998. [2]A further IRSG addition. [3]No longer treated as RMS by the Children's Oncology Group. NOS = not otherwise specified.

Comparison of Clinical Group and TNM Staging Systems for Rhabdomyosarcoma[1]

Stage	CGS Group and Disease Extent	TNM Site	T	N	M
I	Group A: Localized tumor, confined to site of origin, completely resected	Orbit, head and neck, genitourinary	T1 or T2, a or b	NON1 or NX	M0
	Group B: Localized tumor, infiltrating beyond site of origin, completely resected				
II	Group A: Localized tumor, gross total resection with microscopic residual disease	Bladder, prostate, extremity, cranial parameningeal, others	T1 or T2, a	NON1 or NX	M0
	Group B: Locally extensive tumor (regional lymph node involvement), completely resected				
	Group C: Locally extensive tumor (regional lymph node involvement), gross total resection, with microscopic residual disease				
III	Group A: Localized or locally extensive tumor, gross residual disease after biopsy only	Bladder, prostate	T1 or T2, a	N1	M0
	Group B: Localized or locally extensive tumor, gross residual disease after major resection (> 50% debulking)	Extremity, cranial parameningeal, others	T1 or T2, b	NON1 or NX	M0
IV	Any size tumor, with or without regional lymph node involvement, with distant metastases	All	T1 or T2, a or b	NO or N1	M1

[1]Modified from Qualman SJ et al: Intergroup Rhabdomyosarcoma Study: update for pathologists. Pediatr Dev Pathol. 1(6):550-61, 1998. T1 = confined to anatomic site of origin; T2 = extension; a: < 5 cm in diameter; b: > 5 cm in diameter; NO = not clinically involved; N1 = clinically involved; NX = clinical status unknown; M0 = no distant metastases; M1 = distant metastasis present.

Differential Staining Characteristics in RMS Histologic Types and Subtypes

Stain	ERMS	ARMS, Classic Type	ARMS, Solid Type	Sclerosing RMS
Myogenin (nuclear)	Heterogeneous, focal, or absent staining	Strong, homogeneous staining	Strong, homogeneous staining	Weaker staining than MYOD1
MYOD1 (nuclear)	Heterogeneous, focal, or absent staining	Strong, homogeneous staining	Strong, homogeneous staining	Strong, homogeneous staining
Desmin (cytoplasmic)	Positive	Positive	Positive	Positive
Actin-HHF-35 (cytoplasmic)	Positive	Positive	Positive	Positive
Myoglobin (cytoplasmic)	Expressed in well-differentiated tumor cells	Expressed in well-differentiated tumor cells		

RMS = rhabdomyosarcoma; ERMS = embryonal rhabdomyosarcoma; ARMS = alveolar rhabdomyosarcoma.

18. Pohar-Marinsek Z et al: Rhabdomyosarcoma. Cytomorphology, subtyping and differential diagnostic dilemmas. Acta Cytol. 44(4):524-32, 2000
19. Qualman SJ et al: Intergroup Rhabdomyosarcoma Study: update for pathologists. Pediatr Dev Pathol. 1(6):550-61, 1998
20. Newton WA Jr et al: Classification of rhabdomyosarcomas and related sarcomas. Pathologic aspects and proposal for a new classification--an Intergroup Rhabdomyosarcoma Study. Cancer. 76(6):1073-85, 1995
21. Kodet R et al: Childhood rhabdomyosarcoma with anaplastic (pleomorphic) features. A report of the Intergroup Rhabdomyosarcoma Study. Am J Surg Pathol. 17(5):443-53, 1993

Gross and Microscopic Features

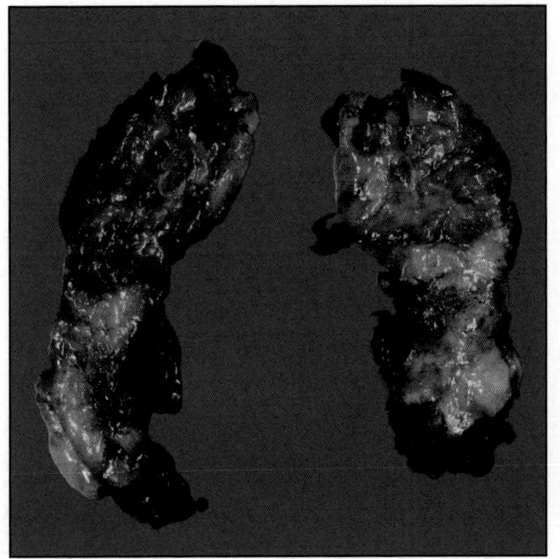

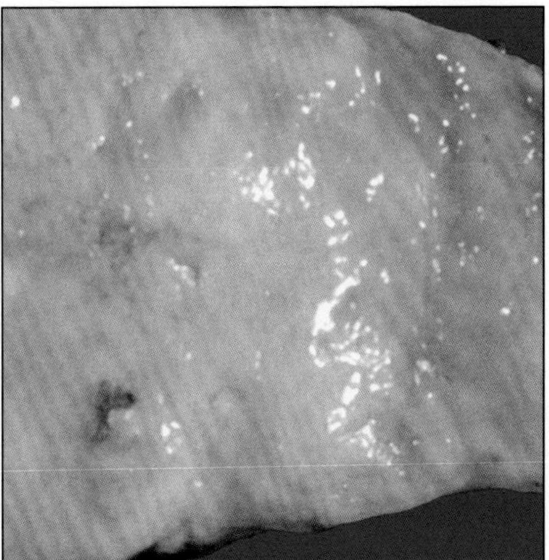

(Left) *Cut sections reveal the fleshy, tan to tan-pink cut surface of a recurrent alveolar rhabdomyosarcoma (ARMS) presenting in the thigh of a 13-year-old girl.* **(Right)** *The tan, glistening cut surface of a testicular ERMS is shown. The gross appearance of RMS varies depending upon the degree of myxoid vs. collagenous composition of the stroma.*

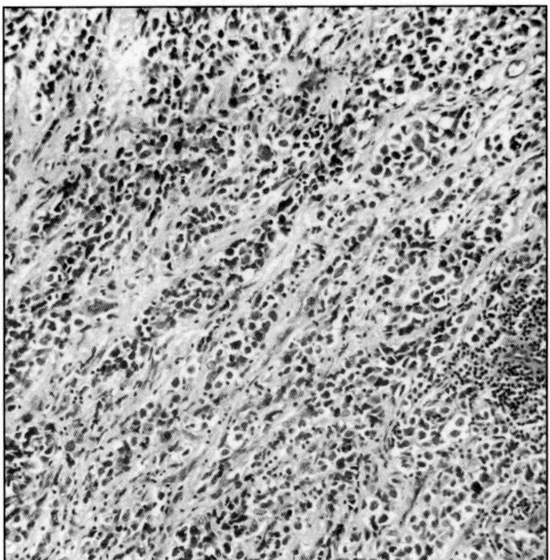

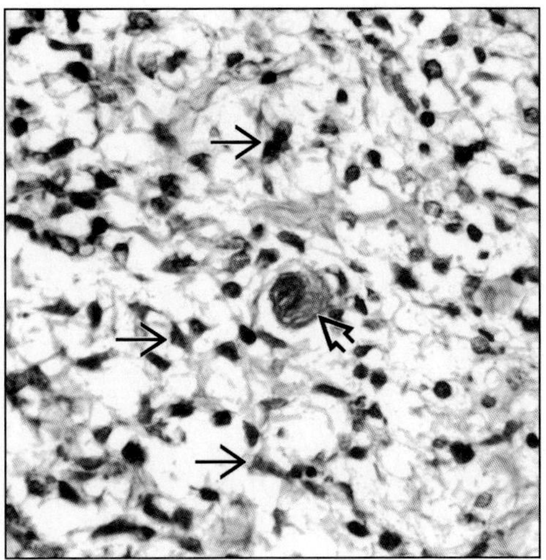

(Left) *Alternating cellular and less cellular myxoid zones are characteristic of ERMS.* **(Right)** *ERMS can demonstrate a wide spectrum of differentiation, from primitive ovoid to stellate tumor cells ⇒ to rhabdomyoblasts ⇒ with distinct features of skeletal muscle differentiation. Shown here is a rhabdomyoblast with concentrically arranged eosinophilic fibrils.*

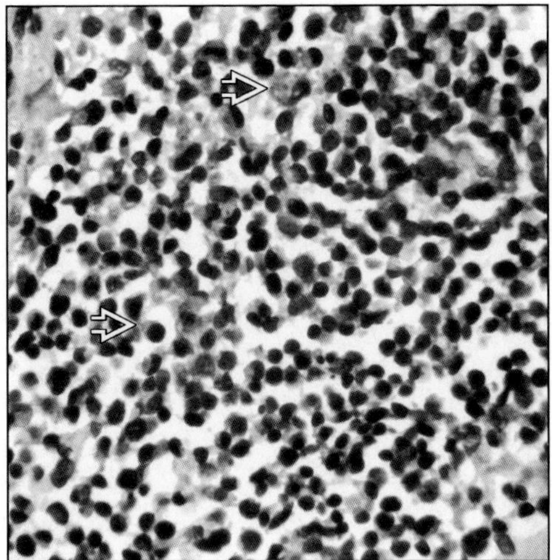

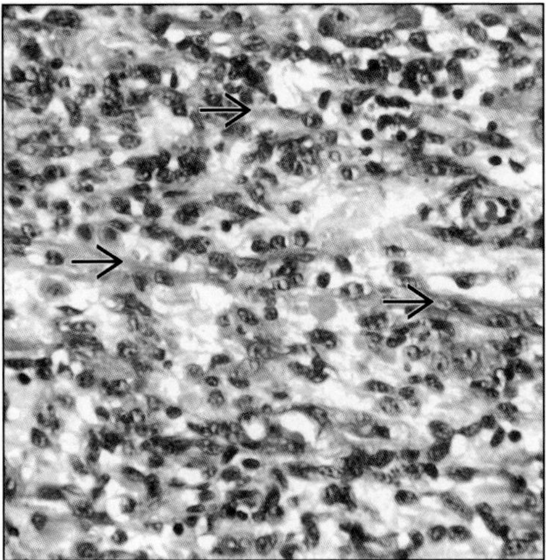

(Left) *Primitive round to oval tumor cells comprise this ERMS. Some of the cells reveal eosinophilic cytoplasm, indicative of skeletal muscle differentiation ⇒.* **(Right)** *Spindle-shaped rhabdomyoblasts are prominent in this ERMS ⇒.*

RHABDOMYOSARCOMA

Microscopic Features and Ancillary Techniques

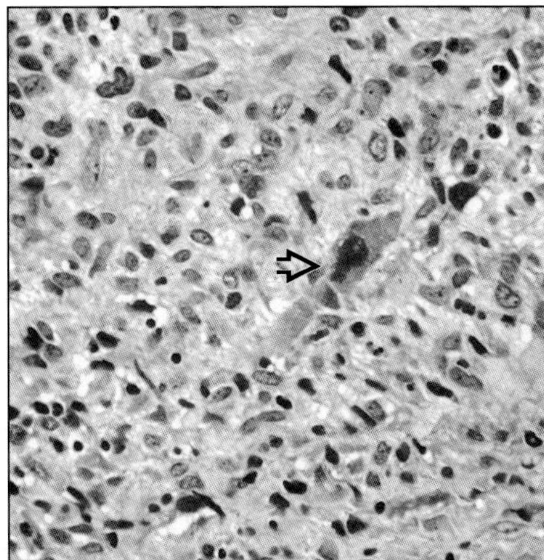

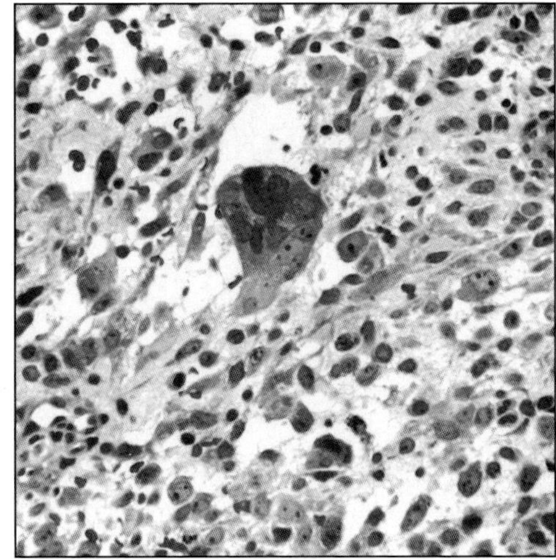

(Left) *Rhabdomyoblast morphologies may range from slender spindle cells to tadpole-shaped cells, tennis racquet-shaped cells, and strap cells (as pictured here ⇨).* ***(Right)*** *A multinucleated tumor cell is present in the center of the field in this section from a paratesticular ERMS.*

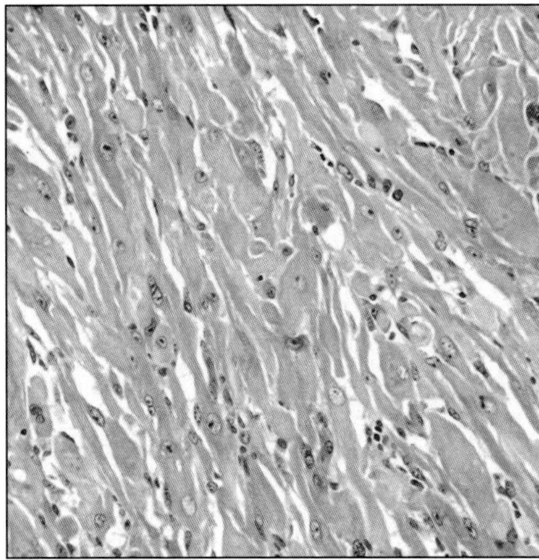

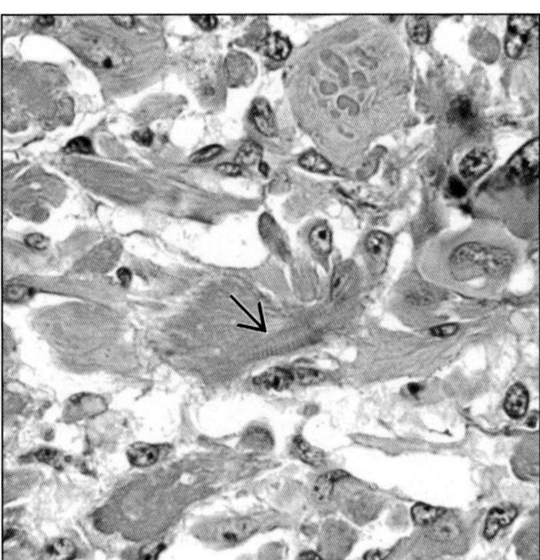

(Left) *Well-differentiated ERMS is composed almost entirely of large, differentiated spindle-shaped rhabdomyoblasts with abundant eosinophilic cytoplasm. This morphology is commonly seen in post-therapy RMS specimens, although the chest wall ERMS shown here was not previously treated.* ***(Right)*** *High-power view of a well-differentiated rhabdomyosarcoma demonstrates cytoplasmic cross striations →, which are more irregular than those seen in normal skeletal muscle.*

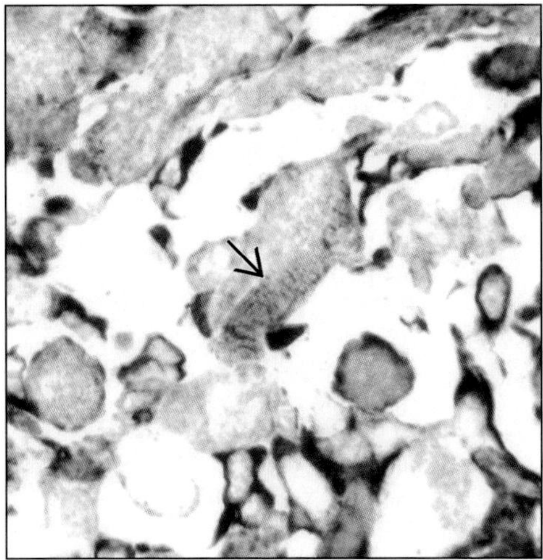

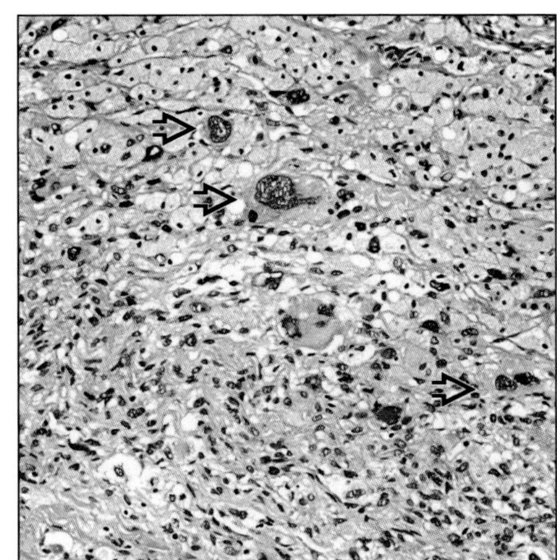

(Left) *Desmin stain is strongly positive in this well-differentiated ERMS, and cross striations are highlighted →. Myogenin and MYOD1 are often negative in well-differentiated RMS.* ***(Right)*** *Anaplastic foci within an ERMS may resemble adult-type pleomorphic RMS ⇨. Areas of typical ERMS can usually be identified in these tumors. (Courtesy K. Thway, MBBS.)*

Microscopic Features

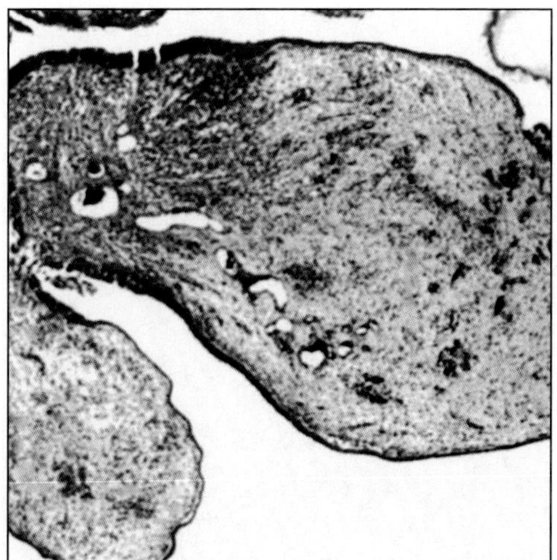

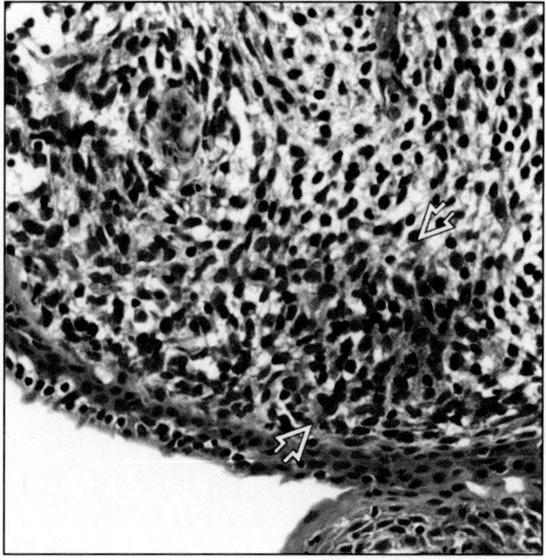

(Left) *Low-power view of a botryoid RMS demonstrates the polypoid, "grape-like" nature of the tumor.* ***(Right)*** *Botryoid RMS is characterized by subepithelial zones of hypercellularity ➡, referred to as the "cambium layer," which resemble the cambium layer of plants. (Courtesy K. Thway, MBBS.)*

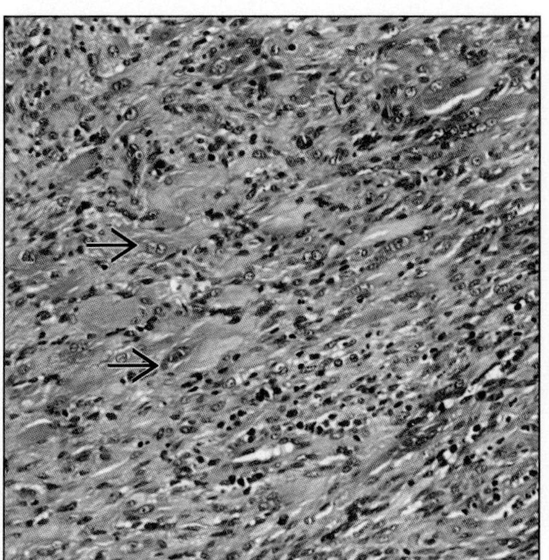

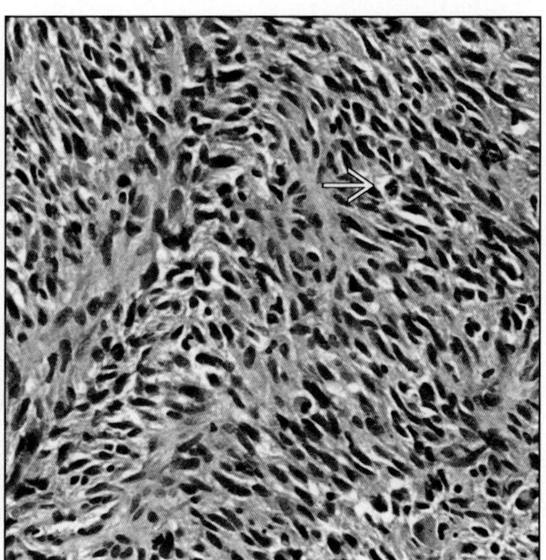

(Left) *This image reveals a spindle cell ERMS presenting in a child. Atypical spindle cells and rhabdomyoblasts ➡ are present within a collagenous background. (Courtesy K. Thway, MBBS.)* ***(Right)*** *Sections of this spindle cell RMS show cellular, tightly packed fascicles of spindle cells with elongated, hyperchromatic nuclei. A mitotic figure is seen ➡. (Courtesy K. Thway, MBBS.)*

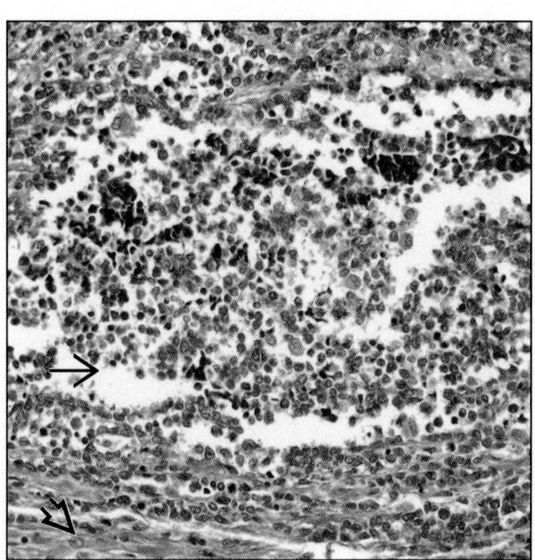

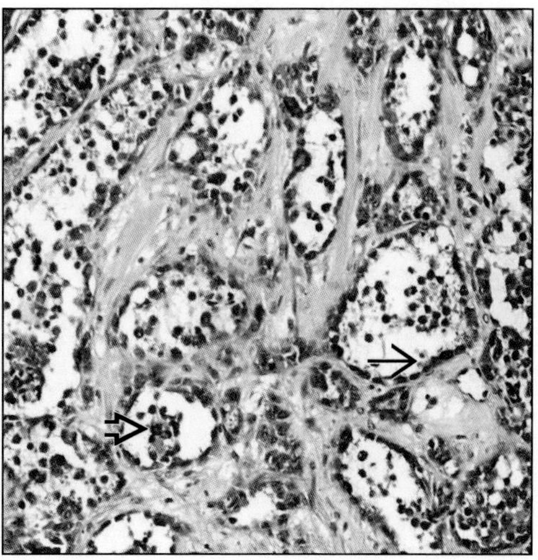

(Left) *Alveolar rhabdomyosarcoma is comprised of fibrous septae ➡ that serve as a scaffold for dyscohesive tumor cells contained within, resembling a lung alveolus. A "cracking" artifact is noted at the periphery of the tumor cell clusters ➡.* ***(Right)*** *The resemblance to lung alveoli is striking in this ARMS, where a single layer of tumor cells adheres to the fibrous septae ➡ with central "free floating" tumor cells and cell clusters ➡. (Courtesy K. Thway, MBBS.)*

RHABDOMYOSARCOMA

Microscopic Features

*(**Left**) Dense, collagenous septae characterize this ARMS. Central dyscohesion of tumor cells is evident. (**Right**) Dyscohesive small cells with round nuclei are pictured in a high-power view of an ARMS.*

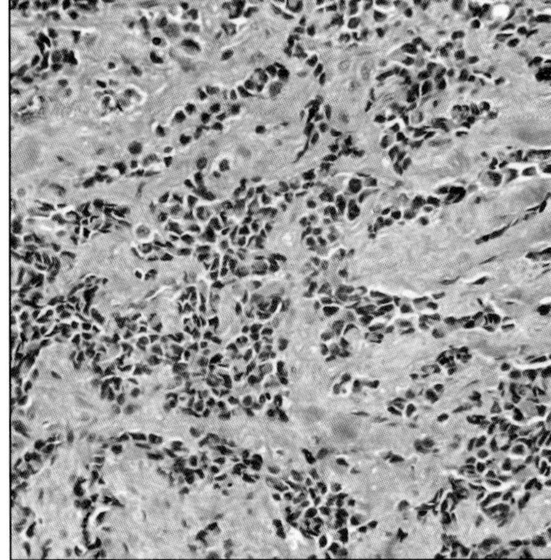

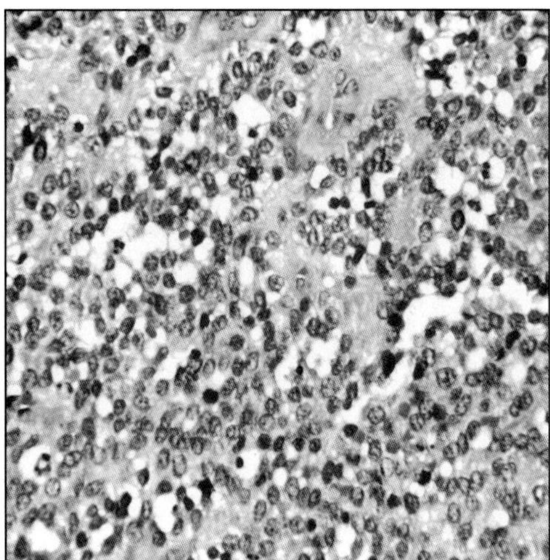

*(**Left**) Scattered rhabdomyoblasts ⇨ can be seen in ARMS. (**Right**) Alveolar architecture is often preserved in ARMS metastases, as demonstrated in this lymph node with metastatic ARMS. Tumor giant cells with a wreath-like nuclear arrangement are typically present ⇨. (Courtesy K. Thway, MBBS.)*

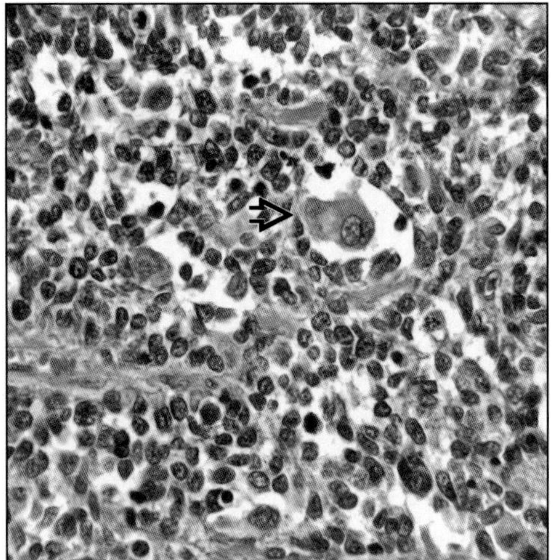

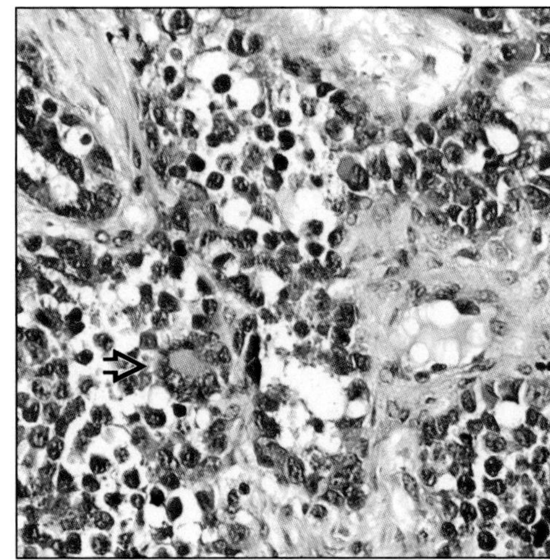

*(**Left**) The solid variant of ARMS is composed of solid sheets of round tumor cells without alveolar architecture. Foci with typical ARMS features or staining with myogenic markers may be helpful in differentiating this ARMS variant from ERMS. Distinction is important, given the significant difference in outcome between these 2 entities. (Courtesy K. Thway, MBBS.) (**Right**) A sclerosing RMS shows clusters and cords of round to spindle cells situated within a hyalinized stroma.*

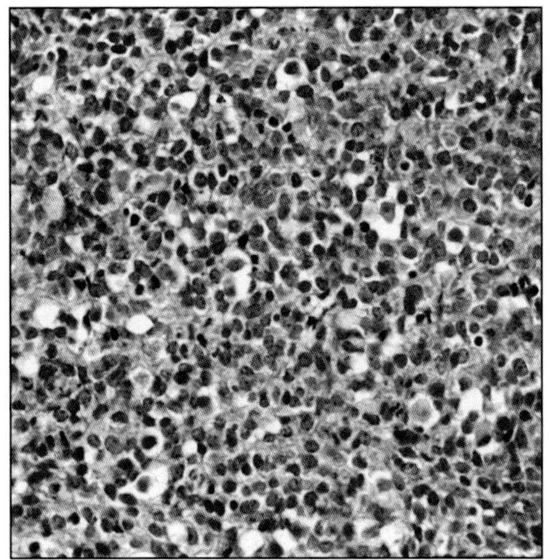

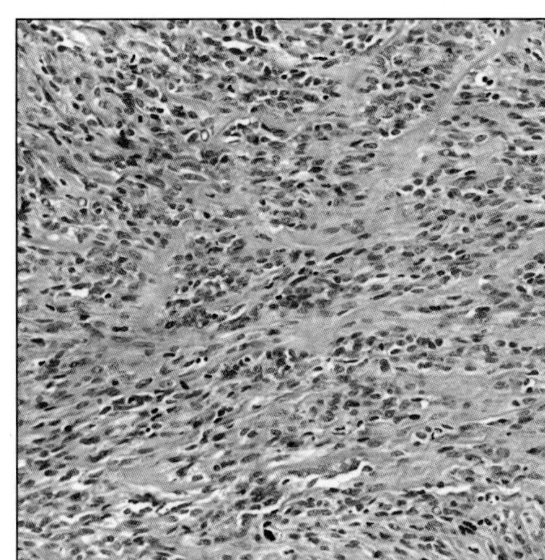

Microscopic Features and Ancillary Techniques

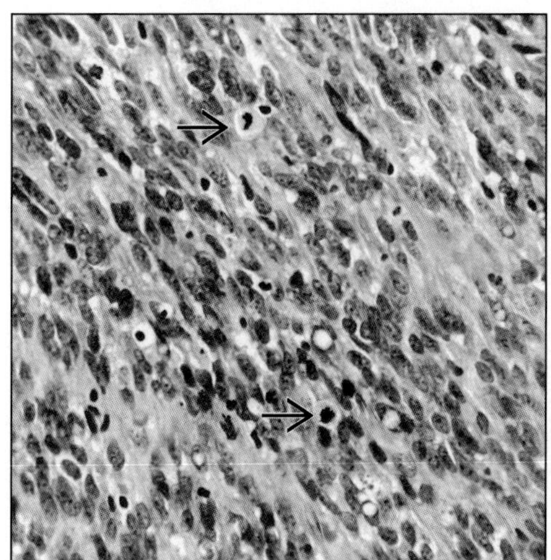

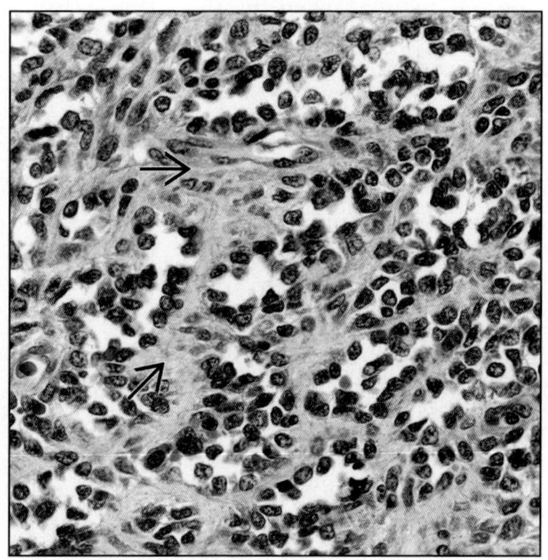

(Left) *Tumor cells with ovoid to spindle-shaped hyperchromatic nuclei are noted in this sclerosing RMS. The stroma is densely collagenous. Mitoses are prominent ➔.* ***(Right)*** *An alveolar pattern reminiscent of ARMS may be seen in sclerosing RMS, with tumor cells surrounded by fibrous, hyalinized septae ➔. The alveolar spaces in sclerosing RMS are smaller, and the tumor cells more cohesive than in ARMS. (Courtesy D. Lucas, MD.)*

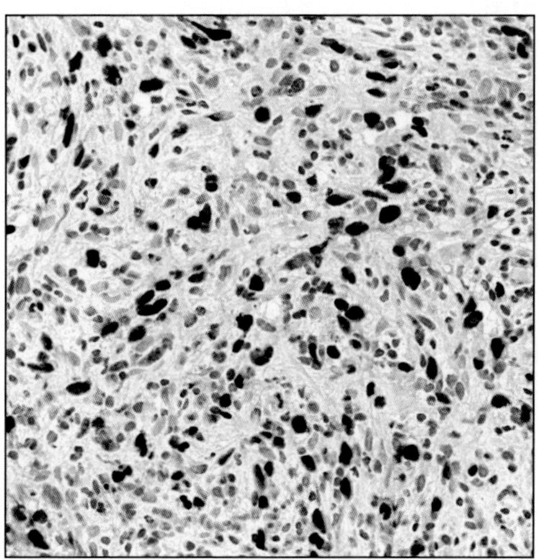

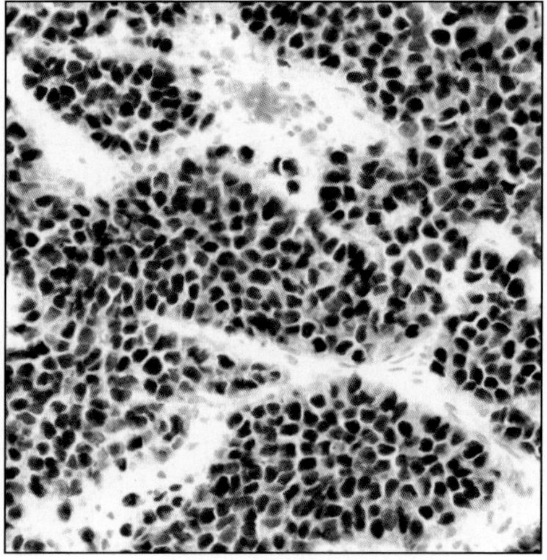

(Left) *Scattered, strong nuclear staining with myogenin is typical for ERMS. Only nuclear staining is specific for RMS. (Courtesy K. Thway, MBBS.)* ***(Right)*** *Strong nuclear staining for myogenin is also typical for ARMS, as shown here. In contrast to ERMS, myogenin staining in ARMS is diffuse and widespread. (Courtesy K. Thway, MBBS.)*

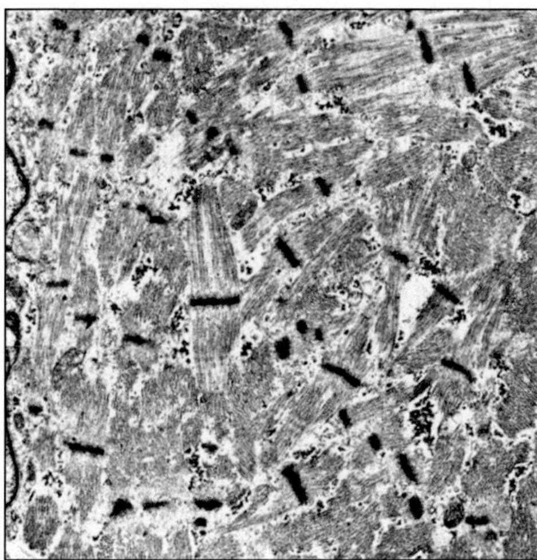

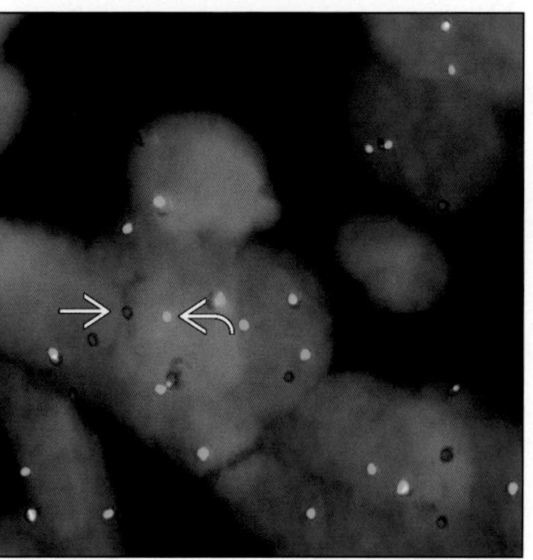

(Left) *Bundles of actin and myosin myofibrils with prominent Z-bands are evident in this EM of well-differentiated RMS. In less well-differentiated tumor cells, only scattered actin and myosin filaments may be seen.* ***(Right)*** *This fluorescence in situ hybridization (FISH) in ARMS utilizes dual color breakapart probes for the FKHR gene on chromosome 13q14 and shows split red ➔ and green ➔ signals, indicating a translocation involving FKHR. (Courtesy K. Thway, MBBS.)*

MALIGNANT PERIPHERAL NERVE SHEATH TUMOR

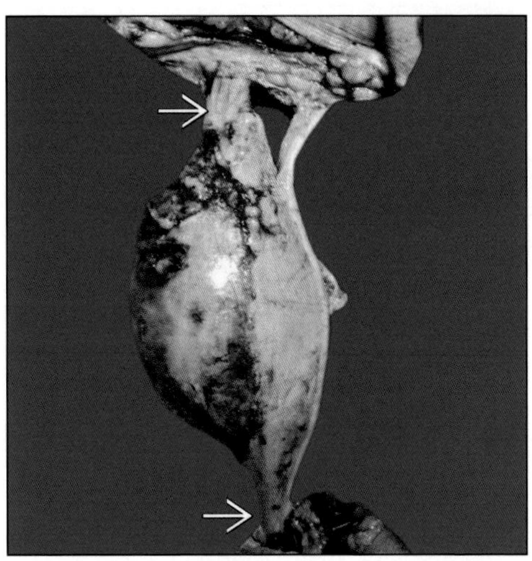

This intraoperative photograph of MPNST shows a large fusiform tumor mass arising from the femoral nerve. Note the enlarged nerve ➔ entering and exiting the tumor. (Courtesy D. Lucas, MD.)

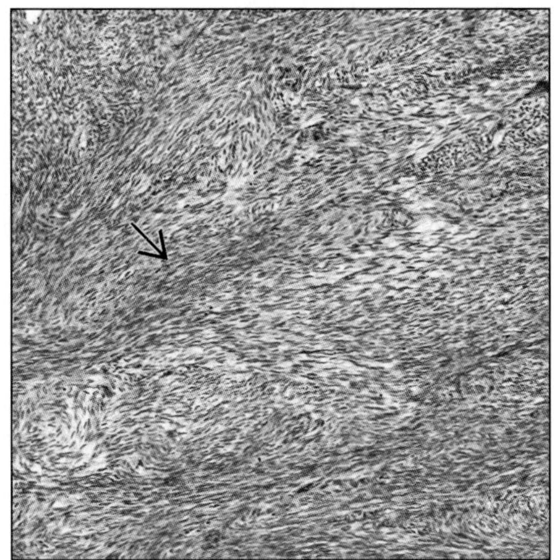

Long sweeping fascicles ➔ of spindle cells of alternating densities create a "marbled pattern," characteristic of the spindle cell type of MPNST. Spindle cell MPNST comprises 80% of these tumors.

TERMINOLOGY

Abbreviations

- Malignant peripheral nerve sheath tumor (MPNST)

Synonyms

- Neurofibrosarcoma, malignant schwannoma, neurogenic sarcoma

Definitions

- Sarcoma arising from a nerve or benign nerve sheath tumor, or showing nerve sheath cellular differentiation
  - Diagnostic criteria includes any of the following
    - Arises from a nerve or benign nerve sheath tumor
    - Shows histological evidence of nerve sheath differentiation in neurofibromatosis type 1 (NF1) patient
    - Shows histological plus immunohistochemical or ultrastructural evidence of nerve sheath differentiation in non-NF1 patient

ETIOLOGY/PATHOGENESIS

Genetic Predisposition

- 50% of cases associated with NF1
  - Lifetime incidence of MPNST: 2-16%
- 40% of cases are sporadic

Molecular Pathogenesis

- NF1 caused by germline mutation of *NF1* tumor suppressor gene mapped to 17q11.2
  - Encodes an oncosuppressor protein, neurofibromin
  - Loss of neurofibromin activity results in activation of *RAS* oncogene
  - Inactivation of a second wild-type *NF1* allele is also necessary for tumor development
- Malignant transformation in both NF1-associated and sporadic MPNST often involves *INK4A* and *P53* and their downstream pathways

Environmental

- Association with radiation therapy

CLINICAL ISSUES

Epidemiology

- Incidence
  - 10-20% of MPNSTs are diagnosed in 1st 2 decades of life
  - MPNSTs represent one of the most frequent nonrhabdomyosarcomatous pediatric sarcomas
  - Malignancy rates in children with NF1 range from 5-8%
  - Sporadic cases in children are rare
- Age
  - Presents mostly in adults (20-50 years)
    - Average age in NF1: 30 years
    - Average age in sporadic MPNST: 40 years
- Gender
  - Roughly equal male:female predominance

Site

- Common sites: Thigh, buttock, trunk, upper arm, retroperitoneum, head and neck
  - Mostly deep seated
  - Central body axis more common in NF1
- Most (70%) arise in major nerve trunks
  - Sciatic nerve most common
  - Brachial plexus, sacral plexus, paraspinal nerves
  - Nerve of origin can be identified in 70% of cases

Presentation

- Painful mass with neurologic deficit in some

Treatment

- Complete surgical resection is mainstay of treatment and a strong predictor of survival
  - However, many tumors cannot be completely resected due to local aggressiveness

MALIGNANT PERIPHERAL NERVE SHEATH TUMOR

Key Facts

Terminology
- Sarcoma arising from a nerve or benign nerve sheath tumor, or showing nerve sheath cellular differentiation

Etiology/Pathogenesis
- 50% associated with NF1

Clinical Issues
- Most (70%) arise in major nerve trunks
- Local recurrence and metastases are common
- NF1 patients have worse prognosis compared to those without NF1
  - Overall 5-year survival in children with and without NF1: 32% and 55%, respectively
- 10-20% of MPNSTs are diagnosed in 1st 2 decades of life

Microscopic Pathology
- Most are high-grade sarcomas
- Spindle cell MPNST (80%)
  - Long fascicles of closely spaced hyperchromatic spindle cells
  - Alternating cellular fascicles and hypocellular areas
  - Extensive necrosis with perivascular preservation
- Epithelioid MPNST (5%)
- Heterologous differentiation (15%)

Ancillary Tests
- S100: 50-60%

Top Differential Diagnoses
- Synovial sarcoma
- Cellular schwannoma
- Atypical neurofibroma

- Role of chemotherapy in pediatric patients is not clearly established
- Studies suggest a benefit of irradiation for microscopic residual tumor
  - Role of irradiation for macroscopic tumor is uncertain

Prognosis
- Very poor
  - Many children have advanced disease at time of presentation
  - Aggressive behavior with high rate of local recurrence and propensity to metastasize
- NF1 patients have worse prognosis compared to those without NF1
  - Overall 5-year survival in children with and without NF1: 32% and 55%, respectively
  - Probably due to higher incidence of large, central axis tumors
  - Tumors less responsive to therapy
- Better prognosis with small, completely resected tumors

IMAGE FINDINGS

General Features
- Morphology
  - Large heterogeneous mass
  - Fusiform mass within major nerve trunk

MACROSCOPIC FEATURES

General Features
- Fusiform or eccentric mass when arising in major nerve trunk
  - Nerve thickening adjacent to mass usually indicates tumor spread along epineurium and perineurium
- Coexisting neurofibroma in some
  - Solitary or plexiform
- Most > 5 cm, can be massive
- Fleshy, white-tan cut surface with hemorrhage and necrosis

MICROSCOPIC PATHOLOGY

Histologic Features
- Most are high-grade sarcomas with high mitotic rate and necrosis
  - Only about 15% are low grade
- Spindle cell MPNST (80%)
  - Long fascicles of uniform, closely spaced, hyperchromatic spindle cells resembling fibrosarcoma
    - Cellular features resemble those of normal Schwann cells
    - Tapered, wavy nuclei in well-differentiated tumors
    - Hyperchromatic nucleus with dispersed, coarse chromatin
  - Alternating cellular fascicles and hypocellular areas ("marbled" pattern)
  - Hyaline bands and nodules
  - Nerve sheath differentiation
    - Nuclear palisading uncommon (15%), usually focal
    - Tactoid differentiation with whorling or curlicue pattern
  - Extensive necrosis with perivascular preservation
  - Intraneural tumors
    - Plexiform architecture
    - Microscopic extension within nerve fascicle
  - Tumors arising from preexisting benign nerve sheath tumor
    - Neurofibroma most common, usually in NF1 patients
    - Tend to be lower grade
  - Primitive neuroepithelial differentiation with small round blue cells
    - More common feature in pediatric cases
  - Anaplastic MPNST
    - Associated with NF1
- Heterologous differentiation (15%)

MALIGNANT PERIPHERAL NERVE SHEATH TUMOR

  - Osseous and osteosarcomatous
  - Chondroid and chondrosarcomatous
  - Rhabdomyosarcomatous (triton tumor)
  - Angiosarcomatous
  - Glandular
  - Neuroepithelial (rosettes)
- Epithelioid MPNST (5%)
  - Multinodular architecture
  - Cords and clusters in some
  - Large epithelioid cells
    - Abundant eosinophilic cytoplasm
    - Large vesicular nuclei with macronucleoli
    - Clear cytoplasm can be seen
  - Often mixed with spindle cells

ANCILLARY TESTS

Immunohistochemistry

- S100(+) in about 60%, usually focal
- Nestin(+) in 50-80%

Cytogenetics

- Complex structural and numeric chromosomal abnormalities
  - Frequent loss of *NF1* at 17q11
  - Frequent loss of *P53* at 17q13

DIFFERENTIAL DIAGNOSIS

Monophasic or Poorly Differentiated Synovial Sarcoma

- Nuclei have less coarse chromatin with a lower mitotic rate
- Usually cytokeratin(+), EMA(+), and TLE1(+)
  - MPNST usually negative
- Usually S100(-)
- t(X:18) by cytogenetics
- *SYT* break apart by FISH
- *SSX-SYT* fusion by RT-PCR

Cellular Schwannoma

- Usually located in retroperitoneum, pelvis, posterior mediastinum
- Exclusively Antoni A areas; often lacks Verocay bodies
- Necrosis and mitotic figures may be present
- Lacks malignant cytologic features
- Strong, diffuse S100 staining
  - MPNST usually has only focal staining

Atypical Neurofibroma

- Large, hyperchromatic spindle cells
- Degenerated (smudged) chromatin
- Low mitotic rate
- Usually retains cytoarchitectural features of neurofibroma

Malignant Melanoma

- Rare in childhood
- Spindle cell/sarcomatoid melanoma
  - Diffusely S100(+)
  - Usually HMB-45(-) and melan-A(-)
- Epithelioid melanoma
  - Amelanotic melanoma may be indistinguishable from epithelioid MPNST
  - Usually HMB-45(+) and melan-A(+)
    - MPNST negative for these markers

Clear Cell Sarcoma

- Predilection for acral extremities
- Multinodular, vague nested architecture
- Uniform epithelioid and spindle cells with prominent nucleoli
- Diffuse S100, HMB-45, and melan-A staining in most
- t(12:22) by cytogenetics
- *EWSR1* break apart by FISH
- *EWS-ATF1* or *EWS-CREB1* by RT-PCR

Extraskeletal Ewing Sarcoma

- Small round blue cell tumor
  - Often with glycogenated (clear) cytoplasm
  - Diffusely CD99(+), usually S100(-)
    - MPNST sometimes CD99(+) but usually weak/focal and nonmembranous
  - t(11:22), t(7:22), t(21:22), or t(2:22) by cytogenetics
  - *EWSR1* break apart by FISH
  - *EWS-FLI1* or *EWS-ERG* fusion by RT-PCR

Embryonal Rhabdomyosarcoma

- Small round blue cells and spindle cells
- Scattered rhabdomyoblasts
- S100(-), desmin(+) and myogenin(+)

SELECTED REFERENCES

1. Gottfried ON et al: Neurofibromatosis type 1 and tumorigenesis: molecular mechanisms and therapeutic implications. Neurosurg Focus. 28(1):E8, 2010
2. Jagdis A et al: Prospective evaluation of TLE1 as a diagnostic immunohistochemical marker in synovial sarcoma. Am J Surg Pathol. 33(12):1743-51, 2009
3. Ferrari A et al: Soft-tissue sarcomas in children and adolescents with neurofibromatosis type 1. Cancer. 109(7):1406-12, 2007
4. Friedrich RE et al: Malignant peripheral nerve sheath tumors (MPNST) in NF1-affected children. Anticancer Res. 27(4A):1957-60, 2007
5. Carli M et al: Pediatric malignant peripheral nerve sheath tumor: the Italian and German soft tissue sarcoma cooperative group. J Clin Oncol. 23(33):8422-30, 2005
6. Birindelli S et al: Rb and TP53 pathway alterations in sporadic and NF1-related malignant peripheral nerve sheath tumors. Lab Invest. 81(6):833-44, 2001
7. Meis JM et al: Malignant peripheral nerve sheath tumors (malignant schwannomas) in children. Am J Surg Pathol. 16(7):694-707, 1992
8. Ducatman BS et al: Malignant peripheral nerve sheath tumors. A clinicopathologic study of 120 cases. Cancer. 57(10):2006-21, 1986
9. Ducatman BS et al: Malignant peripheral nerve sheath tumors in childhood. J Neurooncol. 2(3):241-8, 1984
10. Guccion JG et al: Malignant Schwannoma associated with von Recklinghausen's neurofibromatosis. Virchows Arch A Pathol Anat Histol. 383(1):43-57, 1979

Gross and Microscopic Features

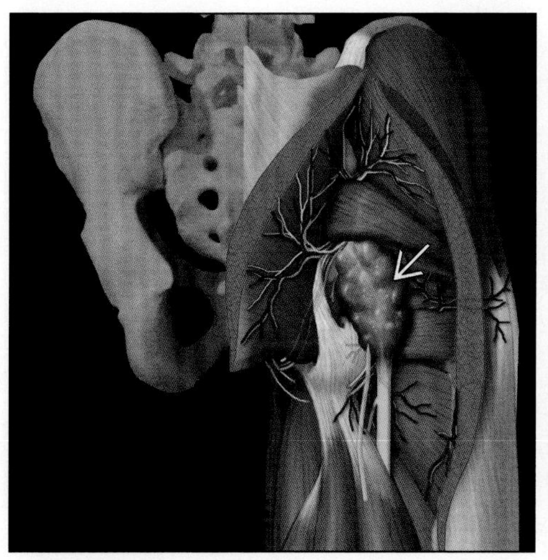

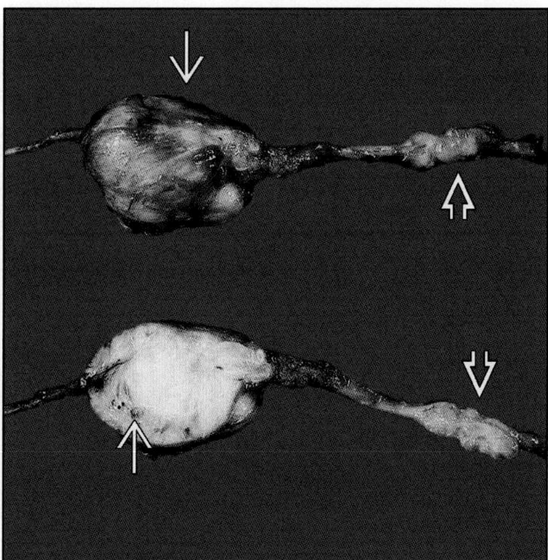

(Left) *Coronal graphic of the pelvis shows a malignant peripheral nerve sheath tumor ➡ arising from the sciatic nerve. The mass has a typical fusiform shape and is contiguous with the nerve. Origin in a large deep-seated nerve is typical.* ***(Right)*** *MPNSTs often arise from a major nerve trunk, such as this sciatic nerve tumor forming a fusiform, lobulated, intraneural mass ➡. MPNSTs can extend along the nerve to form satellite nodules ⇨. (Courtesy D. Lucas, MD.)*

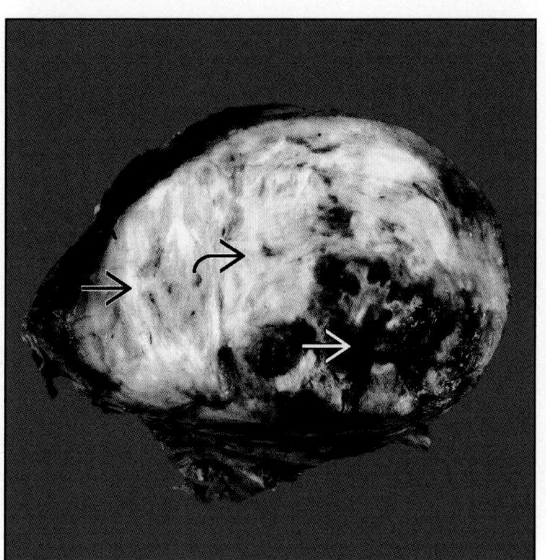

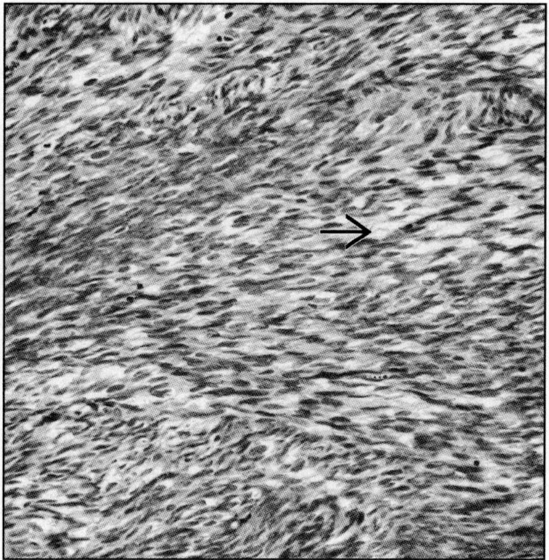

(Left) *MPNSTs tend to form circumscribed, pseudoencapsulated masses. Cut surface is variegated, including firm white-tan solid areas of viable tumor →, yellow necrotic areas ↷, and cystic hemorrhagic foci ➡. (Courtesy D. Lucas, MD.)* ***(Right)*** *Sections of spindle cell MPNST characteristically reveal densely cellular fascicles alternating with less densely cellular areas. The less cellular regions are paler, with a myxoid background →.*

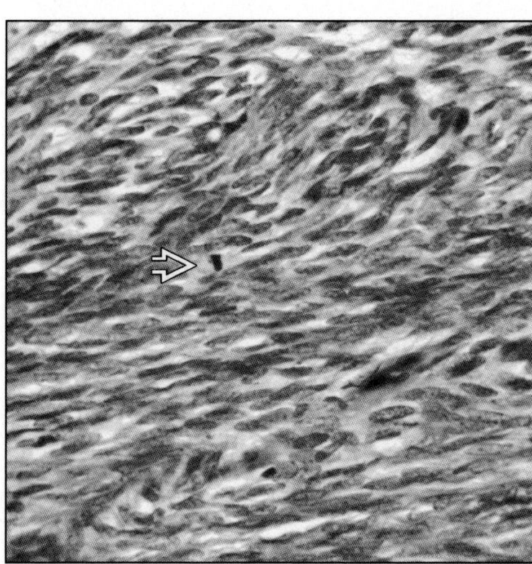

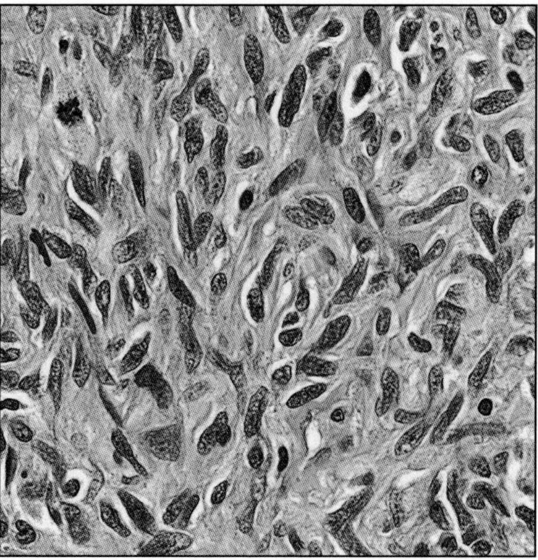

(Left) *Most MPNSTs are high grade with a brisk mitotic rate ⇨.* ***(Right)*** *Microscopically, MPNSTs are highly variable in their degree of differentiation. Well-differentiated tumors have spindle cells with tapered and wavy to buckled nuclei and indistinct cytoplasm. (Courtesy D. Lucas, MD.)*

MALIGNANT PERIPHERAL NERVE SHEATH TUMOR

Microscopic Features

(Left) *Tactoid differentiation can be present in MPNST but is uncommon. This micrograph depicts cell clusters with a vague whorling growth pattern → and hyaline matrix ↗. (Courtesy D. Lucas, MD.)* ***(Right)*** *Microscopic evidence of nerve sheath differentiation is uncommon in MPNST. Nuclear palisading with Verocay body formation → is seen in only 15% of MPNSTs, and it is usually a focal finding. (Courtesy D. Lucas, MD.)*

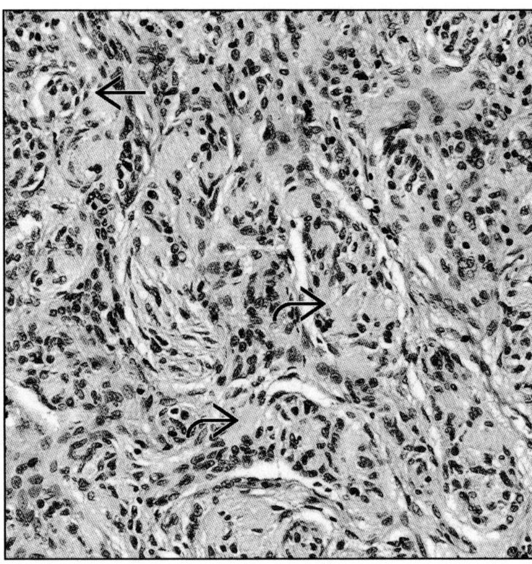

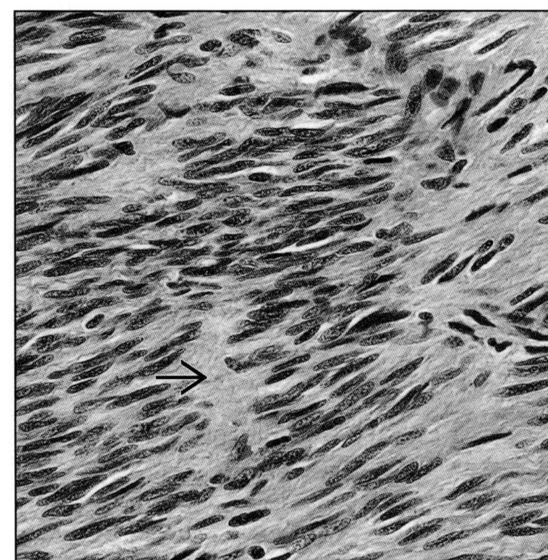

(Left) *MPNSTs that arise within large nerve trunks frequently have a plexiform architecture, which is formed by enlarged nerve fascicles → that are expanded by malignant cells. (Courtesy D. Lucas, MD.)* ***(Right)*** *Large geographic zones of necrosis → are a common and characteristic feature of high-grade MPNSTs. In this example, a cuff of viable malignant cells surrounds a blood vessel ⇨. (Courtesy D. Lucas, MD.)*

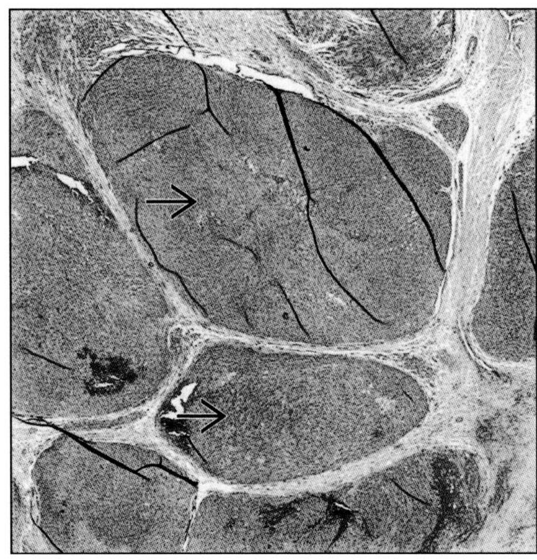

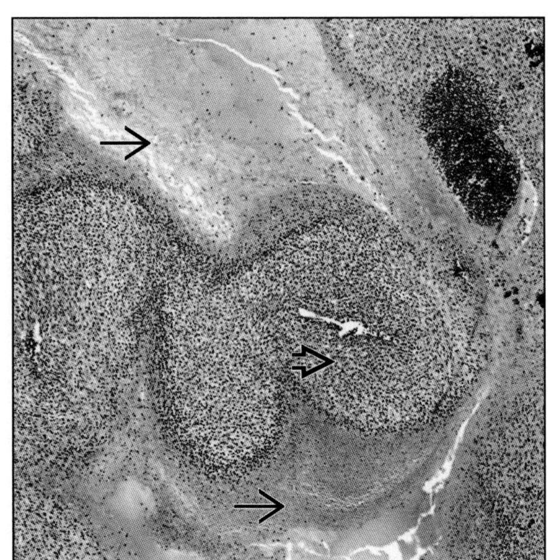

(Left) *Small round blue cell areas can be prominent in MPNST, mimicking Ewing sarcoma/PNET or poorly differentiated synovial sarcoma. This histologic pattern is more common in the pediatric population. (Courtesy D. Lucas, MD.)* ***(Right)*** *MPNST may show a pleomorphic spindle cell pattern with marked nuclear enlargement → and atypical mitotic figures ↗, mimicking pleomorphic undifferentiated sarcoma. Identifying more typical areas can help distinguish the two. (Courtesy D. Lucas, MD.)*

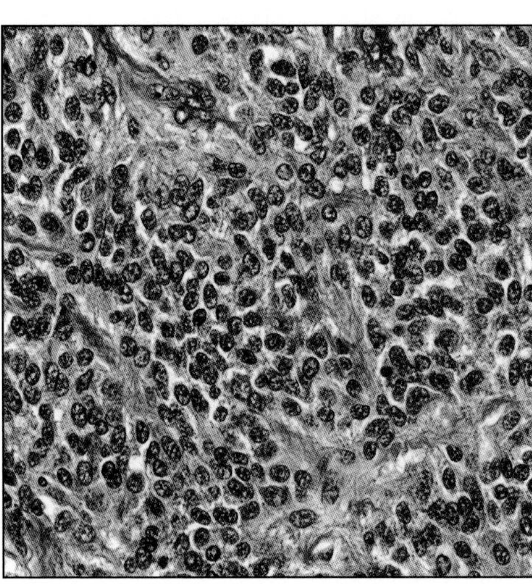

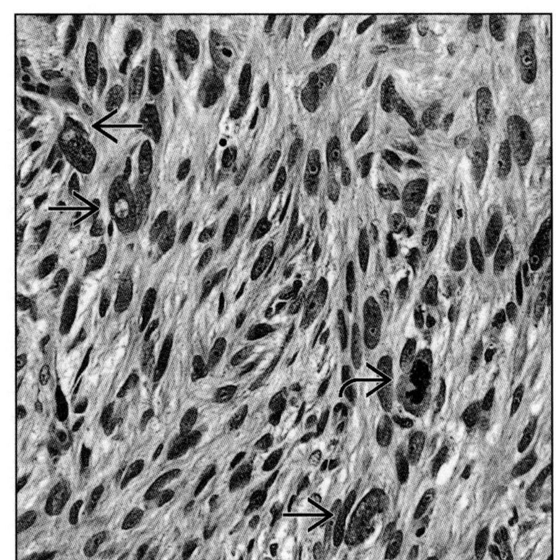

Microscopic Features and Ancillary Techniques

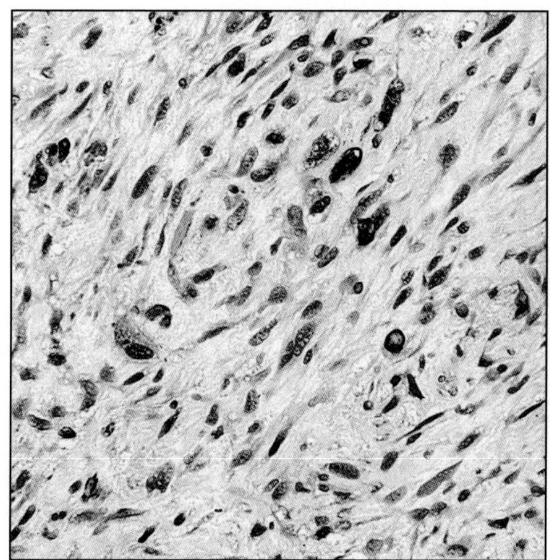

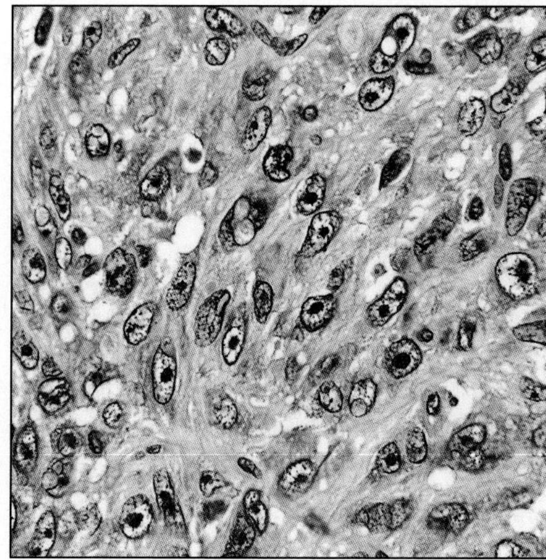

(Left) *Most MPNSTs are positive for S100, and in most cases the staining reaction is focal as shown. Well-differentiated tumors can show more diffuse staining. (Courtesy D. Lucas, MD.)* ***(Right)*** *Epithelioid MPNST is composed of large polygonal cells with abundant eosinophilic cytoplasm and vesicular nuclei with prominent nucleoli. Epithelioid MPNST is negative for HMB-45 and melan-A, which distinguishes it from malignant melanoma. (Courtesy D. Lucas, MD.)*

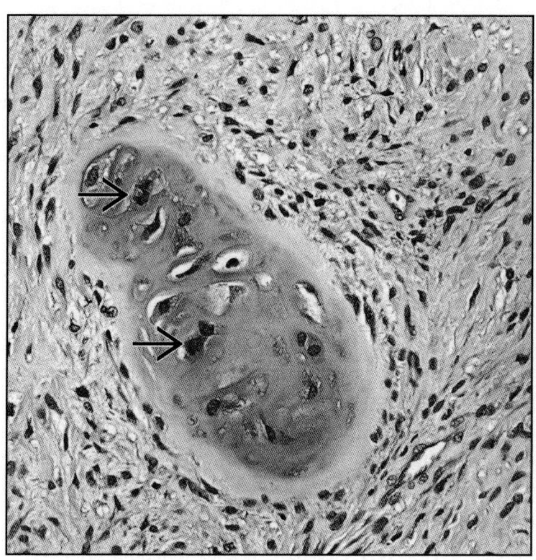

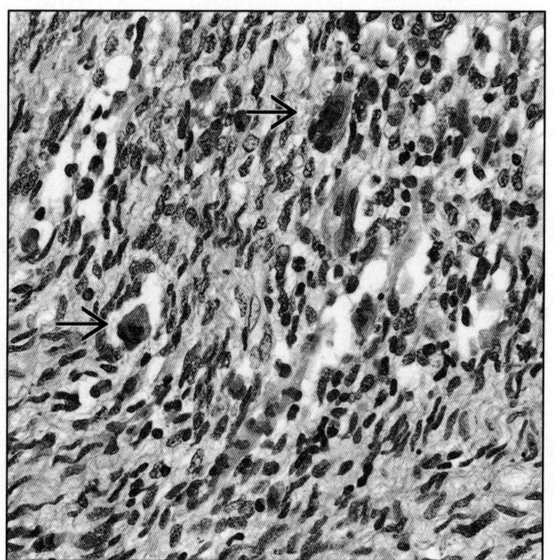

(Left) *Cartilaginous differentiation in MPNST can be benign or malignant as indicated in this case by cytologic atypia ⇒. (Courtesy D. Lucas, MD.)* ***(Right)*** *Malignant rhabdomyoblasts with deeply eosinophilic cytoplasm ⇒ are present within a spindle cell MPNST representing rhabdomyosarcomatous differentiation. Such tumors are called "triton tumors" and should be distinguished from embryonal rhabdomyosarcoma. (Courtesy D. Lucas, MD.)*

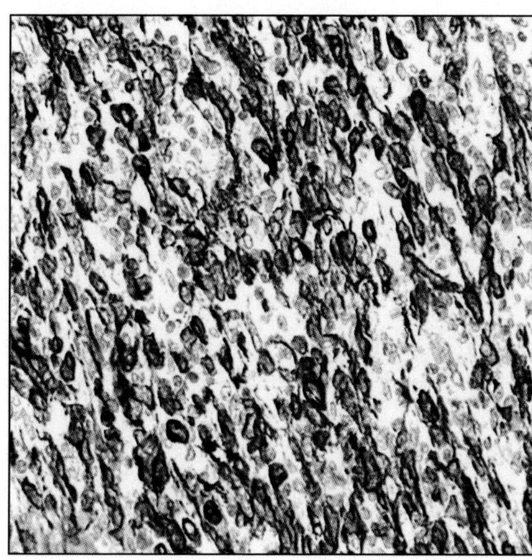

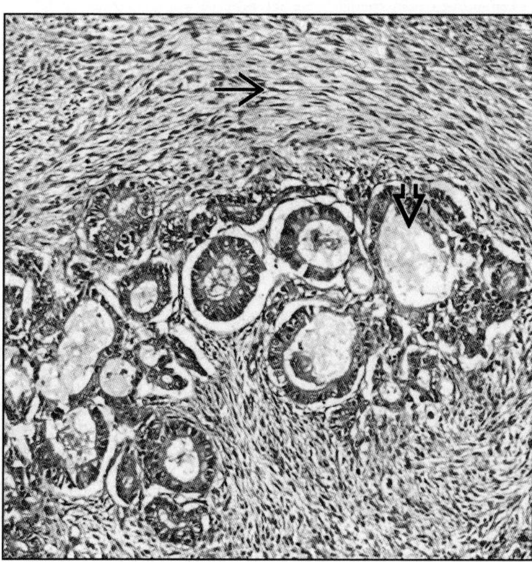

(Left) *Rhabdomyoblasts in malignant triton tumor can be distinguished from background MPNST by immunoreactivity for desmin, as shown here, and by myogenin positivity in nuclei. (Courtesy D. Lucas, MD.)* ***(Right)*** *MPNST ⇒ rarely can have heterologous glandular differentiation. The glands secrete mucin ⇒ and can have focal neuroendocrine differentiation. Biphasic synovial sarcoma is the main differential consideration. (Courtesy D. Lucas, MD.)*

INFANTILE FIBROSARCOMA

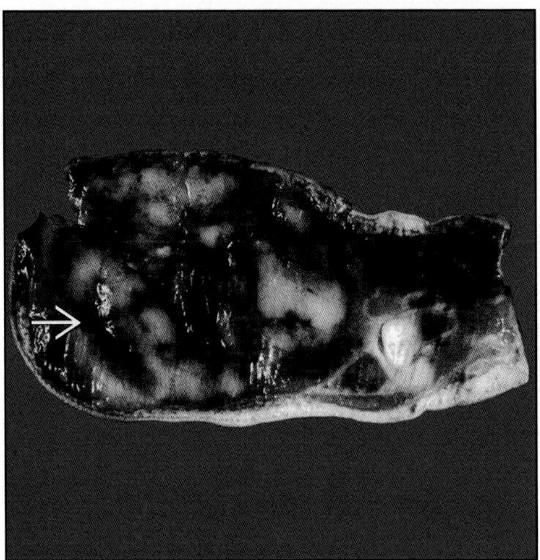

Cut section of this infantile fibrosarcoma from the arm of a 13-day-old baby reveals a large tan mass with admixed hemorrhage ➔. (Courtesy T. Mentzel, MD.)

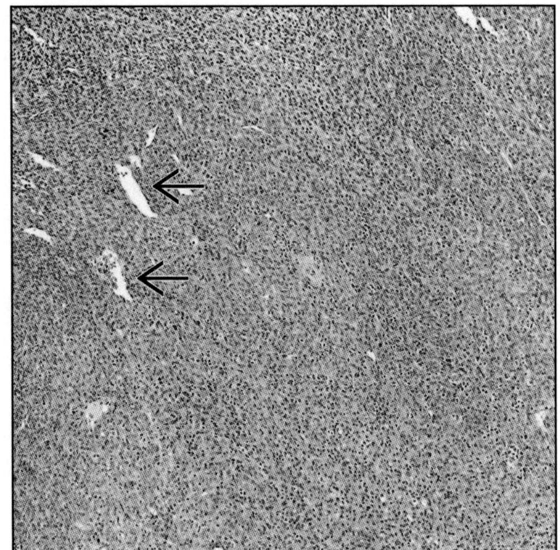

Infantile fibrosarcomas are highly cellular and composed of plump, short spindle cells. Thin-walled blood vessels ➔ are present in the background, imparting a hemangiopericytomatous appearance.

TERMINOLOGY

Abbreviations

- Infantile fibrosarcoma (IF)

Synonyms

- Congenital fibrosarcoma
- Juvenile fibrosarcoma

Definitions

- Occurs in infants and young children and represents a low-grade fibrosarcoma that carries favorable prognosis
- Harbors *ETV6-NTRK3* gene fusion
  - Identical gene fusion and histologic morphology seen in cellular congenital mesoblastic nephroma
  - IF and cellular congenital mesoblastic nephroma are thought to represent closely related or equivalent lesions

ETIOLOGY/PATHOGENESIS

Pathogenesis

- *ETV6-NTRK3* fusion gene identified in most IF
  - *ETV6*: Known oncogene
  - *NTRK3*: Tyrosine kinase that mediates growth and development
  - This chimeric protein has potent transforming activity

CLINICAL ISSUES

Epidemiology

- Incidence
  - Accounts for about 12% of mesenchymal malignancies in infants
- Age
  - Congenital or presents within 1st 2 years of life
  - Rare in children > 2 years of age
- Gender
  - Slight male predominance

Site

- Superficial and deep soft tissues of extremities are most common sites of involvement
- Less commonly occurs on trunk and in head and neck region
- Rare in retroperitoneum and in mesentery

Presentation

- Limb enlargement
- Rapidly enlarging painless mass
  - Large solitary neoplasms
  - Overlying skin may be ulcerated

Treatment

- Surgical approaches
  - Complete excision with tumor-free margins
- Adjuvant therapy
  - Chemotherapy has been proven effective

Prognosis

- Recurrence rate varies (5-50%)
- Metastases are very rare
- Mortality ranges from 5-25%
- Spontaneous regression has been reported
- Favorable prognosis
  - Considerably better prognosis than adult fibrosarcoma

IMAGE FINDINGS

General Features

- Large soft tissue mass
- Shows heterogeneous enhancement pattern
- May show osseous erosion

INFANTILE FIBROSARCOMA

Key Facts

Terminology
- Occurs in infants and young children; represents low-grade fibrosarcoma that carries favorable prognosis

Clinical Issues
- Congenital or arises in 1st 2 years of life
- Superficial and deep soft tissues of extremities are most common sites
- Large solitary neoplasms
- Recurrence rate varies (5-50%)
- Favorable prognosis
- Complete excision with tumor-free margins

Microscopic Pathology
- Cellular tumors composed of intersecting fascicles of primitive, immature tumor cells
- Usually very little cellular pleomorphism
- Numerous mitoses
- Areas of tumor necrosis &/or hemorrhage are frequent
- Often prominent vessels with hemangiopericytoma-like pattern
- Scattered lymphocytic infiltrate is typical

Ancillary Tests
- Most cases contain chromosomal translocation t(12;15)(p13;q26)
  - Corresponds to *NTRK3-ETV6* fusion

Top Differential Diagnoses
- Cellular infantile fibromatosis
  - Alternating cellular and less cellular areas
- Infantile myofibroma/myofibromatosis
  - Biphasic growth

MACROSCOPIC FEATURES

General Features
- Poorly circumscribed, lobulated soft tissue tumor
- Infiltration of adjacent tissues
- Firm gray-white cut surfaces
- Variably myxoid stroma
- Hemorrhagic and necrotic foci often present

MICROSCOPIC PATHOLOGY

Histologic Features
- Cellular neoplasm composed of intersecting fascicles of primitive, immature tumor cells
  - Fascicles often short and ill-defined
  - May impart a focal herringbone pattern resembling adult fibrosarcoma
- Primitive ovoid and spindled tumor cells
  - Usually little cellular pleomorphism
  - Numerous mitoses
- Areas of tumor necrosis &/or hemorrhage frequent
- Variably collagenous stroma
- Scattered inflammatory cells, especially lymphocytes, are characteristic
- Prominent thin-walled vessels with hemangiopericytoma-like pattern often seen

ANCILLARY TESTS

Cytogenetics
- Most cases contain chromosomal translocation t(12;15)(p13;q26)
  - Corresponds to *NTRK3-ETV6* fusion
  - Identical genetic profile is seen in cellular congenital mesoblastic nephroma
- In addition, trisomies for chromosomes 8, 11, 17, and 20 are characteristic

Electron Microscopy
- Features of fibroblasts and myofibroblasts present
- Large tumor cell nuclei
- Dilated rough endoplasmic reticulum
- Abundant lysosomes
- Cytoplasmic filaments

DIFFERENTIAL DIAGNOSIS

Cellular Infantile Fibromatosis
- Alternating cellular and less cellular areas
- Diffusely infiltrative
- Myxoid stromal changes commonly seen
- Lower proliferative activity than IF
- No metastatic potential
- Usually no tumor necrosis present
- Negative for t(12;15)(p13;q26)

Infantile Myofibroma/Myofibromatosis
- Biphasic growth
  - Mature spindled myogenic tumor cells
  - Immature ovoid tumor cells with numerous vessels showing hemangiopericytoma-like pattern
- Homogeneous expression of actins
- Composite infantile myofibromatoses have been described
  - Composite features of IF, infantile myofibromatosis, and infantile hemangiopericytoma
  - Myofibromatous features predominate
  - Studies show negativity for t(12;15)(p13;q26)

Desmoid Fibromatosis
- Mature fibroblastic bland spindled tumor cells
- Low proliferative activity
- No metastatic potential
- Nuclear expression of β-catenin
- Negative for t(12;15)(p13;q26)

Spindle Cell Rhabdomyosarcoma
- Arises predominantly in paratesticular location
- Scattered rhabdomyoblasts
- Expression of desmin, myogenin, and MYOD1
- Negative for t(12;15)(p13;q26)

INFANTILE FIBROSARCOMA

Immunohistochemistry

Antibody	Reactivity	Staining Pattern	Comment
Vimentin	Positive	Cytoplasmic	
Actin-HHF-35	Positive	Cytoplasmic	Variable expression
Actin-sm	Positive	Cytoplasmic	Variable expression
Desmin	Positive	Cytoplasmic	Variable expression
NSE	Positive	Cytoplasmic	Variable expression
Myogenin	Negative		
S100	Negative		
AE1/AE3	Negative		

Infantile Rhabdomyofibrosarcoma

- Extremely rare
- Combination of fibrosarcomatous tumor areas and scattered rhabdomyoblasts
- Focal expression of desmin and myogenin
- Poor clinical outcome
- Negative for t(12;15)(p13;q26)

Inflammatory Myofibroblastic Tumor

- Occurs most often in viscera and in deep soft tissues
- Systemic symptoms sometimes present
- Multinodular, lobular neoplasms
- Myofibroblastic tumor cells, more mature than those of IF
- Myxoid stromal changes usually evident
- Prominent inflammatory infiltrate
- Negative for t(12;15)(p13;q26)

Low-Grade Myofibroblastic Sarcoma

- Tends to occur in adults
- Diffuse infiltration of preexisting structures
- Myofibroblastic tumor cells, more mature than those of IF
- Lower proliferative activity than IF
- Tumor necrosis usually absent
- Negative for t(12;15)(p13;q26)

DIAGNOSTIC CHECKLIST

Pathologic Interpretation Pearls

- Immature-appearing plump spindled tumor cells
- Fibroblastic/myofibroblastic neoplasm
- Low degree of cytologic atypia
- Numerous mitoses
- Often areas of tumor necrosis
- Characteristic genetic changes
- Scattered lymphocytic infiltrate

SELECTED REFERENCES

1. Russell H et al: Infantile fibrosarcoma: clinical and histologic responses to cytotoxic chemotherapy. Pediatr Blood Cancer. 53(1):23-7, 2009
2. Alaggio R et al: Morphologic overlap between infantile myofibromatosis and infantile fibrosarcoma: a pitfall in diagnosis. Pediatr Dev Pathol. 11(5):355-62, 2008
3. Ferguson WS: Advances in the adjuvant treatment of infantile fibrosarcoma. Expert Rev Anticancer Ther. 3(2):185-91, 2003
4. McCahon E et al: Non-resectable congenital tumors with the ETV6-NTRK3 gene fusion are highly responsive to chemotherapy. Med Pediatr Oncol. 40(5):288-92, 2003
5. Loh ML et al: Treatment of infantile fibrosarcoma with chemotherapy and surgery: results from the Dana-Farber Cancer Institute and Children's Hospital, Boston. J Pediatr Hematol Oncol. 24(9):722-6, 2002
6. Sandberg AA et al: Updates on the cytogenetics and molecular genetics of bone and soft tissue tumors: congenital (infantile) fibrosarcoma and mesoblastic nephroma. Cancer Genet Cytogenet. 132(1):1-13, 2002
7. Adem C et al: ETV6 rearrangements in patients with infantile fibrosarcomas and congenital mesoblastic nephromas by fluorescence in situ hybridization. Mod Pathol. 14(12):1246-51, 2001
8. Cecchetto G et al: Fibrosarcoma in pediatric patients: results of the Italian Cooperative Group studies (1979-1995). J Surg Oncol. 78(4):225-31, 2001
9. Dubus P et al: The detection of Tel-TrkC chimeric transcripts is more specific than TrkC immunoreactivity for the diagnosis of congenital fibrosarcoma. J Pathol. 193(1):88-94, 2001
10. Mrad K et al: [Infantile fibrosarcoma: a clinicopathological and molecular study of five cases.] Ann Pathol. 21(5):387-92, 2001
11. Sheng WQ et al: Congenital-infantile fibrosarcoma. A clinicopathologic study of 10 cases and molecular detection of the ETV6-NTRK3 fusion transcripts using paraffin-embedded tissues. Am J Clin Pathol. 115(3):348-55, 2001
12. Argani P et al: Detection of the ETV6-NTRK3 chimeric RNA of infantile fibrosarcoma/cellular congenital mesoblastic nephroma in paraffin-embedded tissue: application to challenging pediatric renal stromal tumors. Mod Pathol. 13(1):29-36, 2000
13. Bourgeois JM et al: Molecular detection of the ETV6-NTRK3 gene fusion differentiates congenital fibrosarcoma from other childhood spindle cell tumors. Am J Surg Pathol. 24(7):937-46, 2000
14. Knezevich SR et al: A novel ETV6-NTRK3 gene fusion in congenital fibrosarcoma. Nat Genet. 18(2):184-7, 1998
15. Knezevich SR et al: ETV6-NTRK3 gene fusions and trisomy 11 establish a histogenetic link between mesoblastic nephroma and congenital fibrosarcoma. Cancer Res. 58(22):5046-8, 1998
16. Rubin BP et al: Congenital mesoblastic nephroma t(12;15) is associated with ETV6-NTRK3 gene fusion: cytogenetic and molecular relationship to congenital (infantile) fibrosarcoma. Am J Pathol. 153(5):1451-8, 1998
17. Variend S et al: Are infantile myofibromatosis, congenital fibrosarcoma and congenital haemangiopericytoma histogenetically related? Histopathology. 26(1):57-62, 1995
18. Chung EB et al: Infantile fibrosarcoma. Cancer. 38(2):729-39, 1976

Microscopic Features and Ancillary Techniques

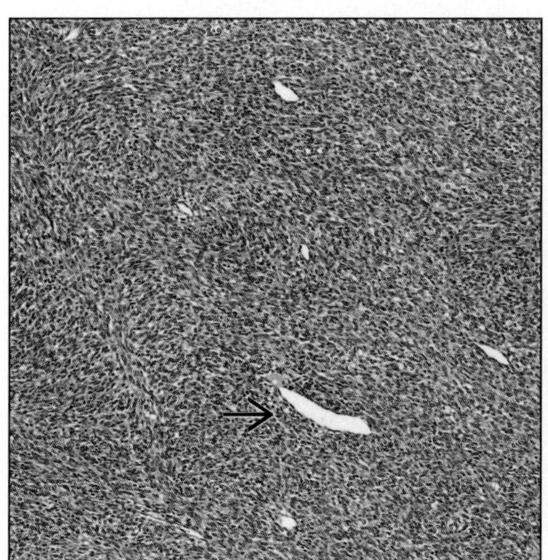

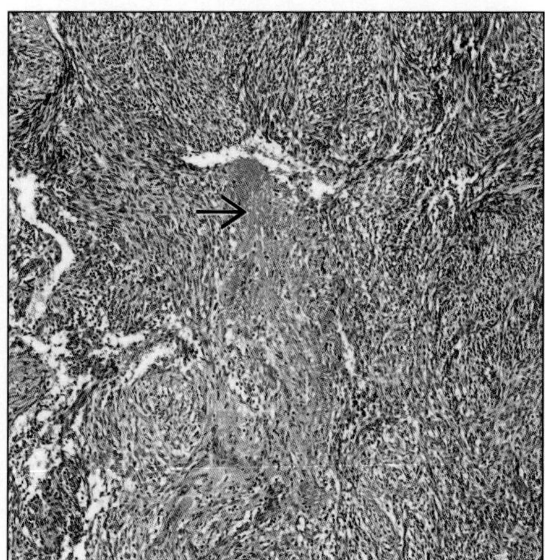

(Left) *Indistinct fascicles of short, spindled, primitive-appearing cells characterize infantile fibrosarcoma. Note the scattered thin-walled vessels ⇒. (Courtesy T. Mentzel, MD.)* ***(Right)*** *Areas of hemorrhage and tumor necrosis ⇒ are often present in infantile fibrosarcoma, as shown here. (Courtesy T. Mentzel, MD.)*

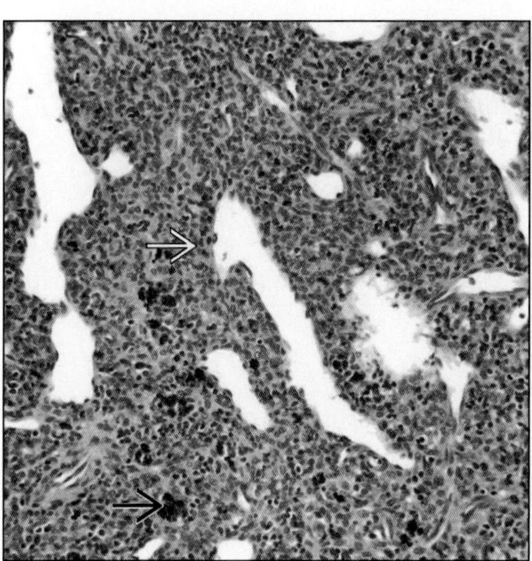

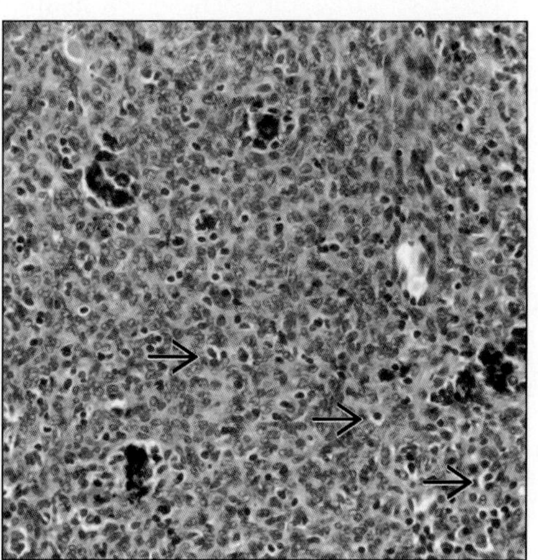

(Left) *A prominent hemangiopericytomatous vascular pattern ➡ is seen in this infantile fibrosarcoma. Hemosiderin deposition ⇒ is noted.* ***(Right)*** *Scattered chronic inflammatory cells typify infantile fibrosarcoma ⇒.*

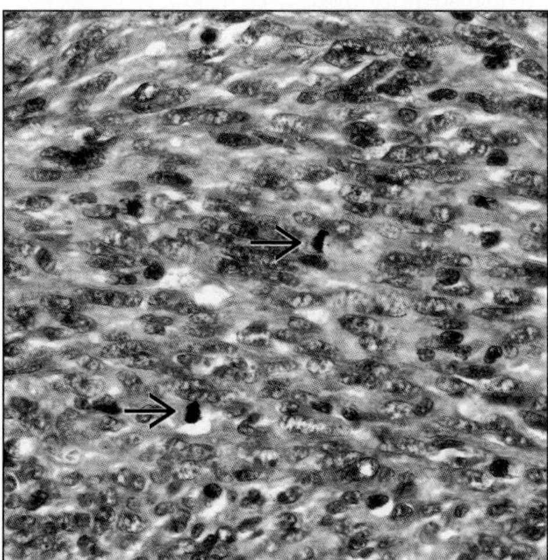

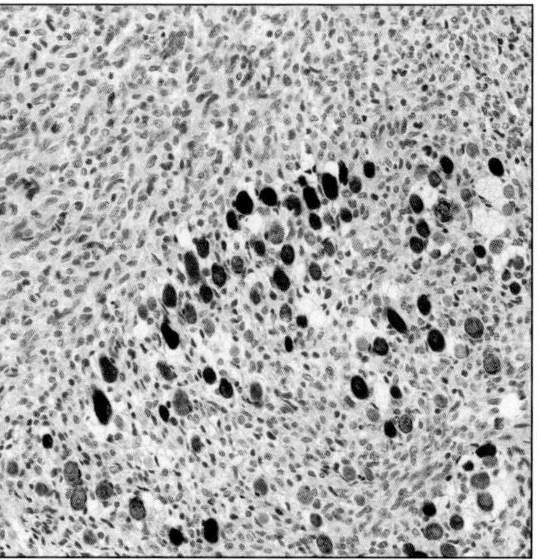

(Left) *High-power view shows immature-appearing plump spindled tumor cells with elongated hyperchromatic nuclei. Mitotic figures are brisk ⇒. (Courtesy T. Mentzel, MD.)* ***(Right)*** *Desmin immunohistochemical stain shows entrapped skeletal muscle fibers in this case of a diffusely infiltrating infantile fibrosarcoma. (Courtesy T. Mentzel, MD.)*

SYNOVIAL SARCOMA

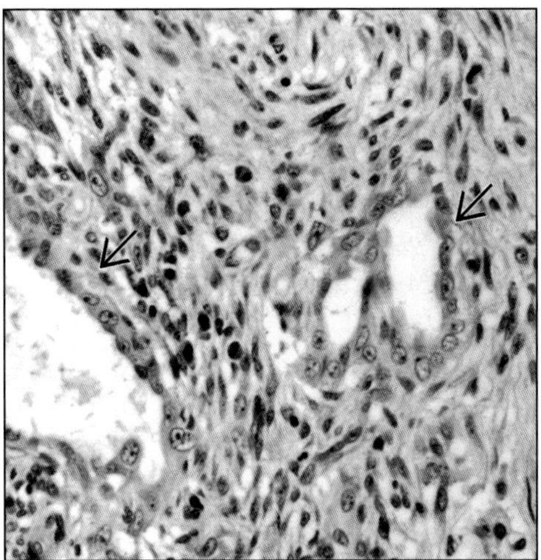

Biphasic synovial sarcoma is easily recognized by the presence of spindle cells and epithelial cells forming nests, cords, or glandular structures ⇒, as seen here.

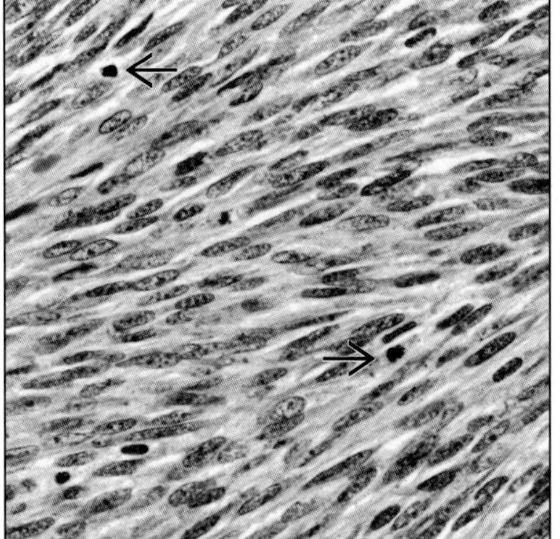

Monophasic synovial sarcoma with plump, spindle cells with uniform, oval nuclei and eosinophilic cytoplasm. Note the mitotic figures ⇒.

TERMINOLOGY

Abbreviations

- Synovial sarcoma (SS)

Synonyms

- Antiquated terminology
  - Synovial cell sarcoma
  - Malignant synovioma

Definitions

- Mesenchymal spindle cell tumor with variable epithelial differentiation, including gland formation
  - Characterized by specific chromosomal translocation t(X;18)(p11;q11)
- Name is historical accident
  - Tumor does not arise from or differentiate toward synovium

ETIOLOGY/PATHOGENESIS

Environmental Exposure

- Very rare examples develop in field of prior irradiation
- 1 case reported at site of metal prosthetic implant

Acquired Genetic Abnormality

- Translocation between chromosomes X and 18

CLINICAL ISSUES

Epidemiology

- Incidence
  - 5-10% of all soft tissue sarcomas
  - Can occur in any anatomic location; rare in joints
  - 90% in extremities
    - Most common around knee
    - In periarticular soft tissue and tendon sheaths
  - Subset in head and neck
    - Parapharynx, oral cavity, tonsil
  - Rare subsets
    - Abdominal wall
    - Retroperitoneum/omentum
    - Mediastinum
    - Intravascular, intraneural
- Age
  - Majority in young adults 15-35 years old
  - Rare over age 50
- Gender
  - More frequent in males

Presentation

- Slow growing
- Deep mass with local pressure effects
- Painful mass
  - > 1/2 of cases
- Painless mass
  - < 1/2 of cases

Natural History

- Can be present for long period: 2-20 years
- Local recurrence frequent, especially if inadequate resection
- Metastasis in 45% of cases
  - Lung (95%)
    - Late metastases can appear after many years
  - Bone (5%)
  - Lymph nodes (10%)

Treatment

- Options, risks, complications
  - Based on
    - Size, location of primary tumor, and stage
- Adjuvant therapy
  - Preoperative irradiation for large or initially unresectable primary tumor
  - Chemotherapy for disseminated disease
    - Ifosfamide or doxorubicin
    - Combination chemotherapy
- Surgical approaches
  - Local excision of primary tumor with clear margin

SYNOVIAL SARCOMA

Key Facts

Terminology

- Name is historical accident, as tumor does not arise from or differentiate toward synovium
- Mesenchymal spindle cell tumor with variable epithelial differentiation, including gland formation
  - Characterized by specific chromosomal translocation t(X;18)(p11;q11)

Clinical Issues

- Accounts for 5-10% of all soft tissue sarcomas
- Can occur in any anatomic location
- Majority in young adults 15-35 years old
- More frequent in males
- Presence of biphasic pattern does not influence behavior
- Poorly differentiated histology worsens prognosis

Image Findings

- Scattered calcifications

Microscopic Pathology

- Sheets of uniform small spindle cells with ovoid nuclei and scanty cytoplasm
  - If pleomorphic, consider other diagnoses
- Focal epithelial differentiation
  - Glandular structures
  - Solid cords or nests
- Never low-grade tumor

Ancillary Tests

- Epithelial markers focally positive
- If CD34 positive, consider other diagnoses
- Identification of t(X;18)(p11;q11) and *SS18-SSX* fusions diagnostic

    - Limb-sparing
    - Amputation rarely required
  - Excision of recurrences
    - Limb-sparing where possible
    - Radical, including amputation
  - Pulmonary metastasectomy for small numbers of metastases

Prognosis

- 5-year survival: 50-85%
- Presence of biphasic pattern does not influence behavior
- Favorable prognostic factors
  - Small tumor size (< 5 cm)
  - Young age, especially childhood
  - Calcifying/ossifying variant (not in all series)
  - Possibly tumors with *SSX2* gene rearrangement (not in all series)
- Adverse prognostic factors
  - Age > 40 years
  - Large tumor size (> 5 cm)
  - Poorly differentiated histology

IMAGE FINDINGS

General Features

- Best diagnostic clue
  - Scattered calcifications
  - Circumscribed mass
- Location
  - 1st consideration for tumors around knee
- Size
  - Variable
    - Usually > 5 cm in diameter
    - Can be very small
    - Rarely > 10 cm: Up to 15 cm described
- Morphology
  - Circumscribed

Specimen Radiographic Findings

- Small scattered calcifications

MACROSCOPIC FEATURES

General Features

- Circumscribed tan tumor mass
- Soft cut surface
- Cysts occasionally seen
  - Smooth walled
  - Contain mucoid fluid or blood
- Focal necrosis and hemorrhage in poorly differentiated tumors

Sections to Be Submitted

- Sample margins and representative sections of tumor

Size

- Wide range from minute (< 1 cm) to 15 cm diameter

MICROSCOPIC PATHOLOGY

Histologic Features

- Sheets of uniform small spindle cells with ovoid nuclei and scanty cytoplasm
- Focal epithelial differentiation
  - Glandular structures
  - Solid cords or nests
- Intercellular stroma minimal except in
  - Occasional hyalinizing monophasic SS
  - Calcifying variants
  - Recurrences after irradiation

Lymphatic/Vascular Invasion

- Rarely

Margins

- Infiltrative microscopically, pseudocapsule of adjacent tissue

Lymph Nodes

- Metastases in up to 10% of cases

Predominant Pattern/Injury Type

- Fascicular
  - Herringbone

SYNOVIAL SARCOMA

- Sheets
- Ill-defined palisading occasionally seen
- Hemangiopericytic pattern common, especially in poorly differentiated SS

Predominant Cell/Compartment Type

- Spindle and epithelioid
- Small round

Grade

- Either grade II or III; never grade I

ANCILLARY TESTS

Cytology

- Diagnosis can be made on cell-rich aspirates
  - Biphasic pattern rarely seen
  - Monophasic SS
    - Cellular clusters
    - Hyperchromatic, overlapping short ovoid nuclei
    - Inconspicuous nucleoli
    - Scanty cytoplasm
    - Mast cells, calcifications

Flow Cytometry

- Not routinely used for diagnosis or prognosis
- About 2/3 diploid, 1/3 aneuploid; some have intratumoral heterogeneity

Cytogenetics

- > 90% of SS have balanced reciprocal translocation
  - t(X;18)(p11;q11)
  - *SSX* gene on chromosome X fuses to *SS18* gene (formerly termed SYT) on chromosome 18
    - Commonly exon 10 of *SS18* gene is fused to exon 6 of *SSX* gene
  - *SSX* gene has 5 variants
    - *SSX1*, *SSX2*, and very rarely *SSX4* undergo rearrangement
  - Results in SS18-SSX fusion protein (unknown function)
- Additional rare abnormalities include t(X;20)(p11;q13)

In Situ Hybridization

- Translocated chromosomes can be identified by FISH

PCR

- Fusion transcripts can be identified by RT-PCR
- Sensitivity in paraffin material
  - Improves with laboratory's experience
  - ↓ with time since fixation and processing

Gene Expression Profiling

- Has identified unsuspected genes activated in SS
  - e.g., TLE1 (transducin-like enhancer of split)
    - In 95% of synovial sarcomas
    - Rare in other sarcoma types

Electron Microscopy

- Transmission
  - Biphasic SS
    - Glands enclosed in continuous external lamina
    - Junctional complexes, surface microvilli, tonofilaments
  - Monophasic SS
    - Cells closely packed with rare, poorly formed intercellular junctions
    - Rare intercellular spaces with few microvilli
    - Rare fragments of external lamina
    - Variable rough endoplasmic reticulum sometimes resembling fibroblast

DIFFERENTIAL DIAGNOSIS

Malignant Peripheral Nerve Sheath Tumor

- Association with neurofibromatosis type 1
- Alternating myxoid and cellular areas
- Nuclei wavy, buckled, or arrowhead-shaped
- S100 protein positive in 67% of cases
- Epithelial markers usually absent; CK19(-)

Spindle Cell Carcinoma

- Relationship to epithelial surface
- Dysplasia or in situ carcinoma in overlying epithelium
- Nuclear pleomorphism
- Cytokeratin positivity can be diffuse rather than focal

Leiomyosarcoma

- Relationship to vein
- Fascicles arranged at abrupt right angles
- Nontapered cell shape
- Elongated parallel-sided nuclei with blunt ends
- Paranuclear vacuoles
- Eosinophilic cytoplasm with longitudinal fibrils
- Can be pleomorphic
- Desmin, smooth muscle actin, h-caldesmon positive
- Cytokeratin, EMA rarely expressed

Spindle Cell Rhabdomyosarcoma

- Focal rhabdomyoblastic differentiation
- Desmin, myogenin positive

Solitary Fibrous Tumor

- Hemangiopericytic pattern usually peripheral
- So-called "patternless" pattern
  - Random orientation of cells
- Diffuse or focal collagenization
- CD34(+)

Ewing Sarcoma/PNET

- Lacks hemangiopericytic pattern
- Uniform sheets of cells without spindle cell or epithelial areas
- Nuclei rounded
  - Do not appear to overlap
- Reticulin fibers are typically
  - Absent between cells
  - Around blood vessels only
- CD99 diffusely positive with membrane staining
- LMWK sometimes positive
  - Often with paranuclear dot distribution
- CD56(-)
- Different translocations
  - t(11;22)(q24;q12) with *FLI1-EWS* fusion gene most common
  - Others fuse *EWS* with different gene partners

Immunohistochemistry

Antibody	Reactivity	Staining Pattern	Comment
EMA/MUC1	Positive	Cell membrane	In 70-100% of MSS, focal
CK-PAN	Positive	Cytoplasmic	In 90% of MSS, focal
Bcl-2	Positive	Cytoplasmic	In 98% of cases, diffuse
CD56	Positive	Cytoplasmic	In 80% of cases
CD99	Positive	Cell membrane	In 66% of cases, focal
S100	Positive	Nuclear	In 40% of cases, focal
Calretinin	Positive	Nuclear	In 40% of cases, focal
β-catenin	Positive	Nuclear	In 40% of cases, diffuse
FLI-1	Positive	Nuclear	In 22% of cases
TLE1	Positive	Nuclear	In 95% of cases
CD34	Negative		Very focally positive in < 5% of cases

Alveolar Rhabdomyosarcoma

- Solid variant can mimic poorly differentiated SS
- Immunohistochemical positivity for
  - Desmin in cytoplasm
  - Myogenin in nuclei
- Specific translocations
  - t(1;13)(p36;q14) with *PAX7-FKHR* fusion gene
  - t(2;13)(q35;q14) with *PAX3-FKHR* fusion gene

Epithelioid Sarcoma

- Classical type superficially located
- Proximal-type pleomorphic: Resembles carcinoma or melanoma
- Not biphasic; epithelioid and spindle cells merge
- Cells have more cytoplasm
- Epithelial markers diffusely positive
- CD34(+) in 50% of cases
- INI1(-) in 90% of cases
- Lacks t(X;18)

DIAGNOSTIC CHECKLIST

Clinically Relevant Pathologic Features

- Age distribution
- Organ distribution
  - Most common site is around knee
  - Can arise at any anatomical site
- Symptom time frame
  - Unusually among sarcomas, can be present for several years before presentation

Pathologic Interpretation Pearls

- Biphasic pattern distinctive
- Monophasic SS has sheets of uniform spindle cells
  - CK positivity is focal (single cells) not diffuse
  - EMA positivity is focal (single cells) not diffuse
  - CD34 almost always negative
  - Bcl-2 almost always positive
  - TLE1 very sensitive marker
- Pleomorphism very rare
- Poorly differentiated SS has nested reticulin pattern
- Genetic findings are specific and diagnostic

SELECTED REFERENCES

1. Terry J et al: TLE1 as a diagnostic immunohistochemical marker for synovial sarcoma emerging from gene expression profiling studies. Am J Surg Pathol. 31(2):240-6, 2007
2. Michal M et al: Minute synovial sarcomas of the hands and feet: a clinicopathologic study of 21 tumors less than 1 cm. Am J Surg Pathol. 30(6):721-6, 2006
3. Ferrari A et al: Synovial sarcoma: a retrospective analysis of 271 patients of all ages treated at a single institution. Cancer. 101(3):627-34, 2004
4. Guillou L et al: Histologic grade, but not SYT-SSX fusion type, is an important prognostic factor in patients with synovial sarcoma: a multicenter, retrospective analysis. J Clin Oncol. 22(20):4040-50, 2004
5. Akerman M et al: Fine-needle aspiration of synovial sarcoma: criteria for diagnosis: retrospective reexamination of 37 cases, including ancillary diagnostics. A Scandinavian Sarcoma Group study. Diagn Cytopathol. 28(5):232-8, 2003
6. Chan JA et al: Synovial sarcoma in older patients: clinicopathological analysis of 32 cases with emphasis on unusual histological features. Histopathology. 43(1):72-83, 2003
7. Coindre JM et al: Should molecular testing be required for diagnosing synovial sarcoma? A prospective study of 204 cases. Cancer. 98(12):2700-7, 2003
8. Ladanyi M et al: Impact of SYT-SSX fusion type on the clinical behavior of synovial sarcoma: a multi-institutional retrospective study of 243 patients. Cancer Res. 62(1):135-40, 2002
9. Pelmus M et al: Monophasic fibrous and poorly differentiated synovial sarcoma: immunohistochemical reassessment of 60 t(X;18)(SYT-SSX)-positive cases. Am J Surg Pathol. 26(11):1434-40, 2002
10. Spillane AJ et al: Synovial sarcoma: a clinicopathologic, staging, and prognostic assessment. J Clin Oncol. 18(22):3794-803, 2000
11. Krane JF et al: Myxoid synovial sarcoma: an underappreciated morphologic subset. Mod Pathol. 12(5):456-62, 1999
12. van de Rijn M et al: Poorly differentiated synovial sarcoma: an analysis of clinical, pathologic, and molecular genetic features. Am J Surg Pathol. 23(1):106-12, 1999
13. Fisher C: Synovial sarcoma. Ann Diagn Pathol. 2(6):401-21, 1998
14. Smith ME et al: Synovial sarcoma lack synovial differentiation. Histopathology. 26(3):279-81, 1995

SYNOVIAL SARCOMA

Gross and Microscopic Features

(Left) *This well-circumscribed tumor is located within skeletal muscle beneath the deep fascial layer ⇨. The cut surface is nodular, tan, and displays focal hemorrhage ➡.* ***(Right)*** *This monophasic synovial sarcoma shows spindle cells arranged in distinct fascicles ⇨. The cells are uniform and have a fibrosarcoma-like appearance.*

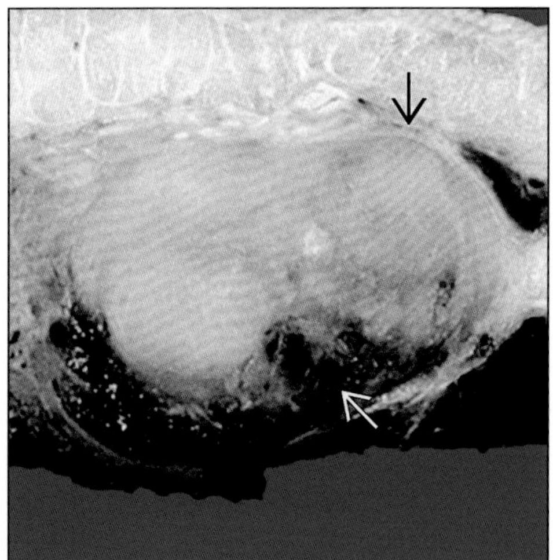

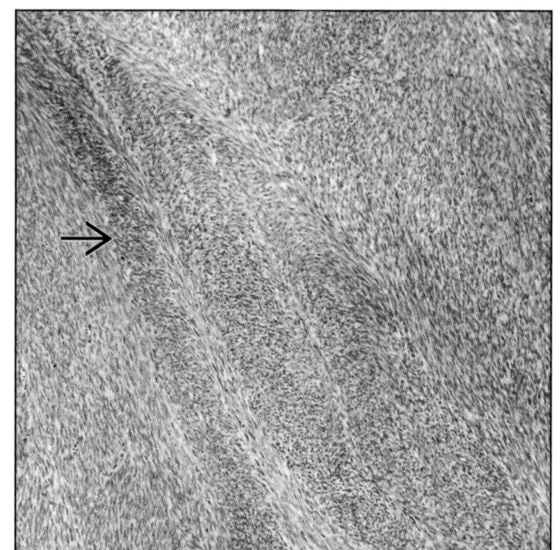

(Left) *Note the area of hyalinization ⇨. Hyalinized zones may be focal or diffuse. Extensive hyalinization can compress the spindle cells.* ***(Right)*** *This poorly differentiated synovial sarcoma has a small round cell appearance. The dilated, thin-walled vascular spaces ⇨ have a hemangiopericytomatous appearance.*

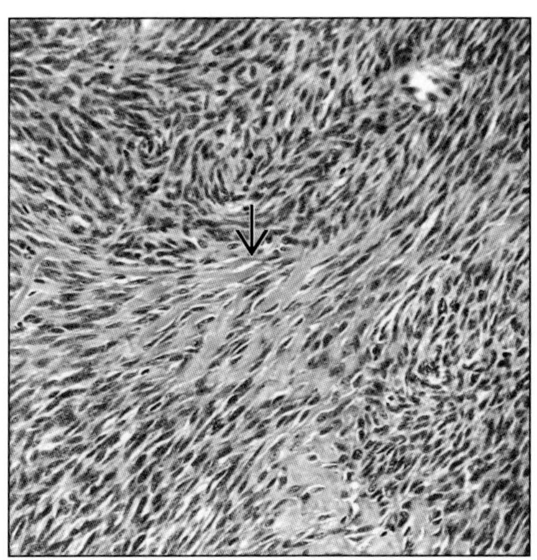

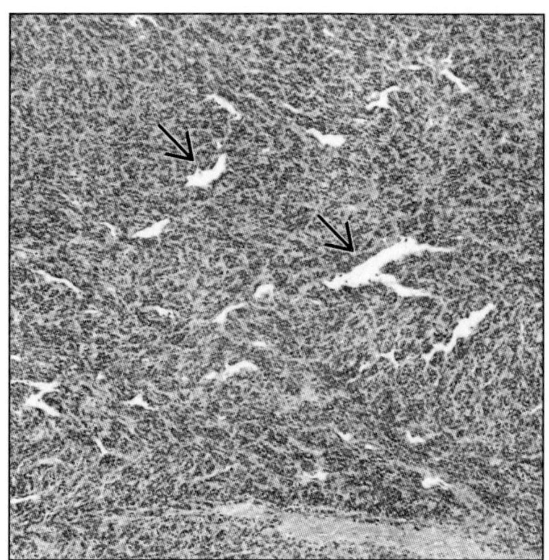

(Left) *Hematoxylin & eosin shows a biphasic synovial sarcoma in which the epithelial component forms solid nests with an occasional tiny glandular lumen ⇨.* ***(Right)*** *Hematoxylin & eosin shows a biphasic synovial sarcoma in which the epithelial component forms solid cords of cells ⇨ permeating between areas of spindle cell tumor.*

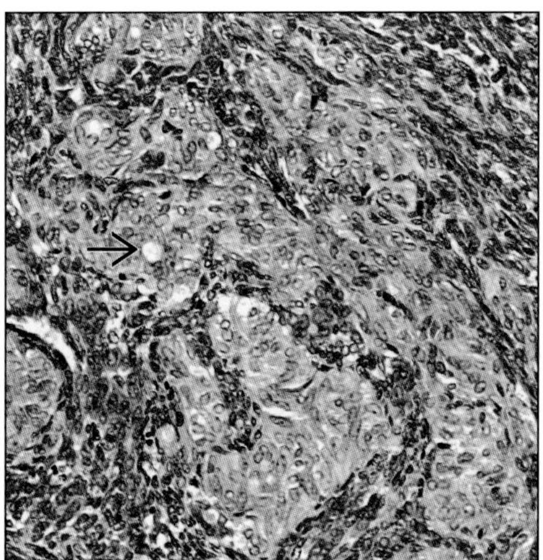

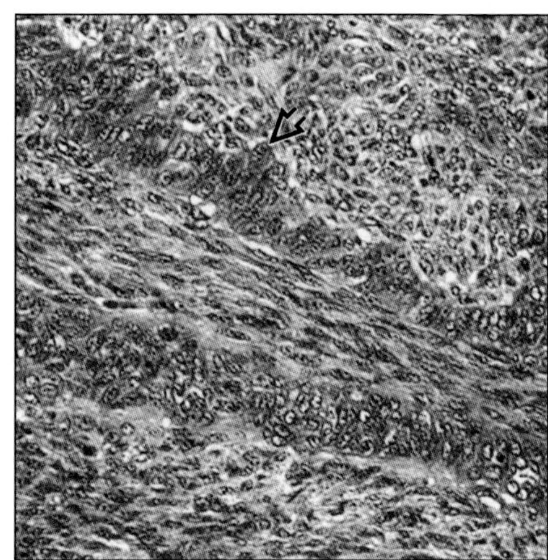

Microscopic Features and Ancillary Techniques

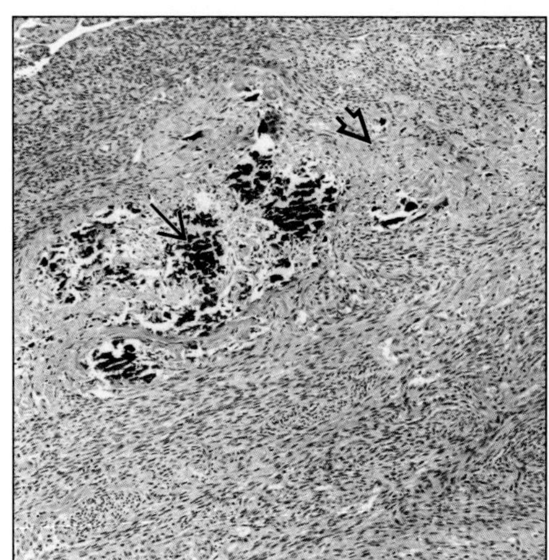

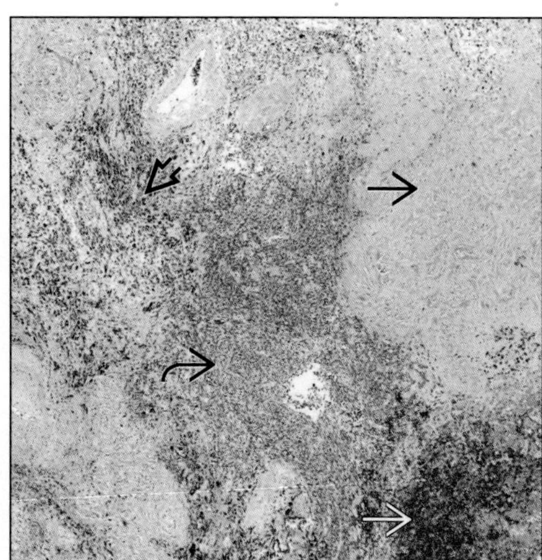

(Left) *Calcification in a case of SS ⇨ is shown. This feature is seen in approximately 20% of cases. Note the adjacent hyalinization ⇨.* ***(Right)*** *Treatment effect in SS shows large areas of necrosis ⇨, hemorrhage ➡, and hemosiderin-laden macrophages ⇨. Viable tumor is still present ↷.*

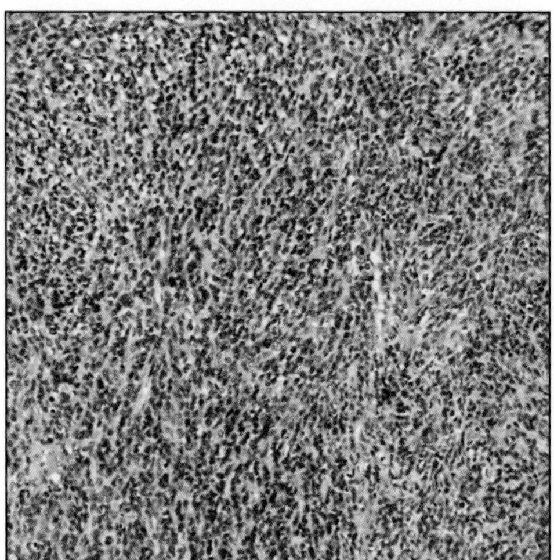

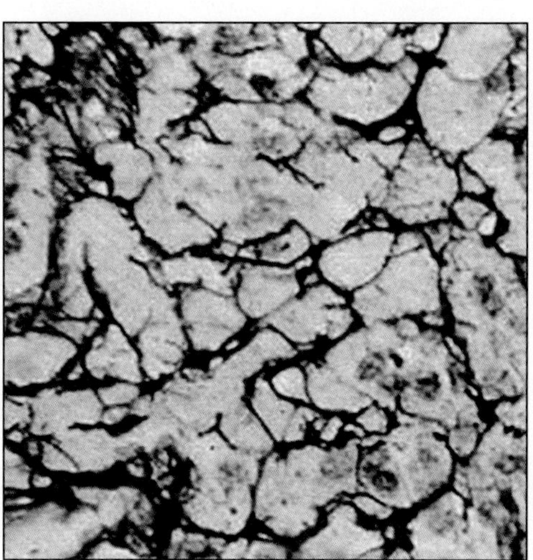

(Left) *Recognizing poorly differentiated SS is important, as it has a worse prognosis. Histologically, the nuclei are round, small, large, or epithelioid. The spindle cell variant of poorly differentiated SS has high-grade nuclear features. This field shows the small cell pattern.* ***(Right)*** *Poorly differentiated SS has a nested reticulin pattern, unlike other sarcomas that have a pericellular reticulin pattern.*

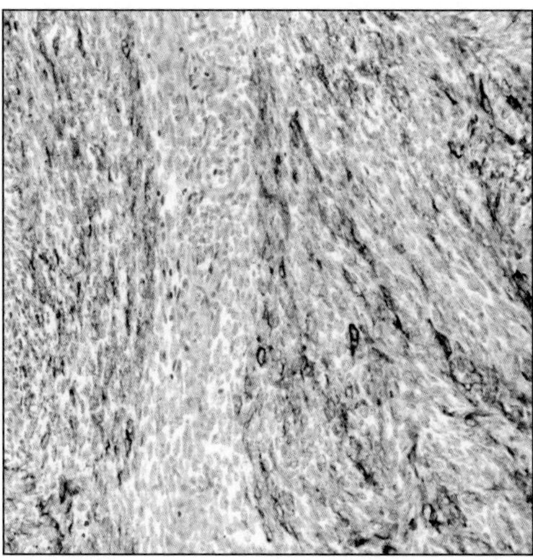

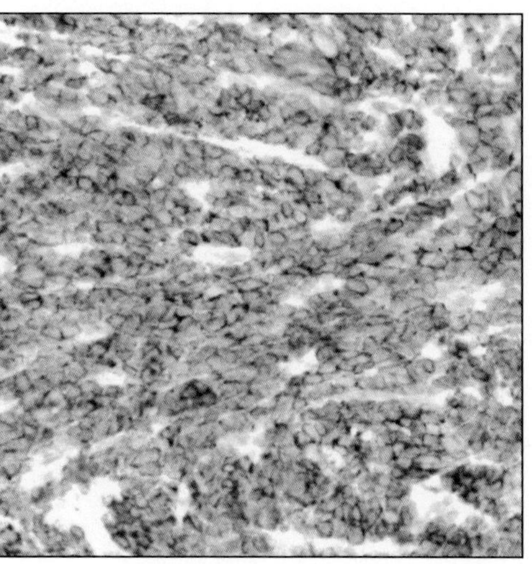

(Left) *In monophasic SS, it may be necessary to stain several sections, as only a few scattered cells may be immunoreactive for EMA (as seen here). Immunohistochemical staining with CK7 and CK19 is also helpful.* ***(Right)*** *Bcl-2 is diffusely expressed in synovial sarcoma. Although typically cytoplasmic, this field shows a more membranous staining pattern. Bcl-2 is a sensitive but not specific marker. TLE1 has recently emerged as a potentially specific marker for SS.*

PROTOCOL FOR SOFT TISSUE TUMOR SPECIMENS

Soft Tissue: Biopsy

Surgical Pathology Cancer Case Summary (Checklist)

Procedure

___ Core needle biopsy
___ Incisional biopsy
___ Other (specify): ____________________________
___ Not specified

Tumor Site

___ Specify (if known) : ____________________________
___ Not specified

Tumor Size

Greatest dimension: _________ cm
*Additional dimensions: _________ x _________ cm
___ Cannot be determined

Macroscopic Extent of Tumor (select all that apply)

___ Superficial
 ___ Dermal
 ___ Subcutaneous/suprafascial
___ Deep
 ___ Fascial
 ___ Subfascial
 ___ Intramuscular
 ___ Mediastinal
 ___ Intraabdominal
 ___ Retroperitoneal
 ___ Head and neck
 ___ Other (specify): ____________________________
___ Cannot be determined

Histologic Type (World Health Organization [WHO] Classification of Soft Tissue Tumors)

Specify: ____________________________
___ Cannot be determined

Mitotic Rate

Specify: _________ /10 high-power fields (HPF)
(1 HPF x 400 = 0.1734 mm^2; X40 objective; most proliferative area)

Necrosis

___ Not identified
___ Present
 Extent: _________ %
___ Cannot be determined

Histologic Grade (French Federation of Cancer Centers Sarcoma Group [FNCLCC])

___ Grade 1
___ Grade 2
___ Grade 3
___ Ungraded sarcoma
___ Cannot be determined

Margins (for excisional biopsy only)

___ Cannot be assessed
___ Margins negative for sarcoma
 Distance of sarcoma from closest margin: _________ cm
 Specify margin: ____________________________
 Specify other close (< 2 cm) margin(s): ____________________________

___ Margin(s) positive for sarcoma

Specify margin(s): ___________________________

*Lymph-Vascular Invasion

*___ Not identified

*___ Present

*___ Indeterminate

*Additional Pathologic Findings

*Specify: __________________________

Ancillary Studies

Immunohistochemistry

Specify: ___________________________

___ Not performed

Cytogenetics

Specify: ___________________________

___ Not performed

Molecular pathology

Specify: ___________________________

___ Not performed

Prebiopsy Treatment

___ No therapy

___ Chemotherapy performed

___ Radiation therapy performed

___ Therapy performed, type not specified

___ Unknown

Treatment Effect

___ Not identified

___ Present

*Specify percentage of viable tumor: _________ %

___ Cannot be determined

*Data elements with asterisks are not required. These elements may be clinically important but are not yet validated or regularly used in patient management. Adapted with permission from College of American Pathologists, "Protocol for the Examination of Specimens from Patients with Tumors of Soft Tissue." Web posting date February 2011, www.cap.org.

Soft Tissue: Resection

Surgical Pathology Case Summary (Checklist)

Procedure

___ Intralesional resection

___ Marginal resection

___ Wide resection

___ Radical resection

___ Other (specify): ___________________________

___ Not specified

Tumor Site

Specify (if known): ___________________________

___ Not specified

Tumor Size

Greatest dimension: _________ cm

*Additional dimensions: _________ x _________ cm

___ Cannot be determined

Macroscopic Extent of Tumor (select all that apply)

___ Superficial

___ Dermal

___ Subcutaneous/suprafascial

PROTOCOL FOR SOFT TISSUE TUMOR SPECIMENS

___ Deep
 ___ Fascial
 ___ Subfascial
 ___ Intramuscular
 ___ Mediastinal
 ___ Intraabdominal
 ___ Retroperitoneal
 ___ Head and neck
 ___ Other (specify): ___________________________
___ Cannot be determined

Histologic Type (World Health Organization [WHO] Classification of Soft Tissue Tumors)

Specify: ____________________________
___ Cannot be determined

Mitotic Rate

Specify: _________ /10 high-power fields (HPF)
(1 HPF x 400 = 0.1734 mm²; X40 objective; most proliferative area)

Necrosis

___ Not identified
___ Present
 Extent: _________ %

Histologic Grade (French Federation of Cancer Centers Sarcoma Group [FNCLCC])

___ Grade 1
___ Grade 2
___ Grade 3
___ Ungraded sarcoma
___ Cannot be determined

Margins

___ Cannot be assessed
___ Margins negative for sarcoma
 Distance of sarcoma from closest margin: _________ cm
 Specify margin: ____________________________
 Specify other close (< 2 cm) margin(s): ____________________________
___ Margin(s) positive for sarcoma
 Specify margin(s): ____________________________

**Lymph-Vascular Invasion*

*___ Not identified
*___ Present
*___ Indeterminate

Pathologic Staging (pTNM)

TNM descriptors (required only if applicable, select all that apply)
 ___ m (multiple)
 ___ r (recurrent)
 ___ y (post treatment)

Primary tumor (pT)
 ___ pTX: Primary tumor cannot be assessed
 ___ pT0: No evidence of primary tumor
 ___ pT1a: Tumor ≤ 5 cm in greatest dimension, superficial tumor
 ___ pT1b: Tumor ≤ 5 cm in greatest dimension, deep tumor
 ___ pT2a: Tumor > 5 cm in greatest dimension, superficial tumor
 ___ pT2b: Tumor > 5 cm in greatest dimension, deep tumor

Regional lymph nodes (pN)
 ___ pNx: Regional lymph nodes cannot be assessed

____ pN0: No regional lymph node metastasis

____ pN1: Regional lymph node metastasis

____ No nodes submitted or found

Number of lymph nodes examined

Specify: __________

____ Number cannot be determined (explain): ______________________________

Number of lymph nodes involved

Specify: __________

____ Number cannot be determined (explain): ______________________________

Distant metastasis (pM)

____ Not applicable

____ pM1: Distant metastasis

*Specify site(s), if known: ______________________________

*Additional Pathologic Findings

*Specify: ______________________________

Ancillary Studies

Immunohistochemistry

Specify: ______________________________

____ Not performed

Cytogenetics

Specify: ______________________________

____ Not performed

Molecular pathology

Specify: ______________________________

____ Not performed

Preresection Treatment (select all that apply)

____ No therapy

____ Chemotherapy performed

____ Radiation therapy performed

____ Therapy performed, type not specified

____ Unknown

Treatment Effect

____ Not identified

____ Present

*Specify percentage of viable tumor: __________ %

____ Cannot be determined

**Data elements with asterisks are not required. These elements may be clinically important but are not yet validated or regularly used in patient management. Adapted with permission from College of American Pathologists, "Protocol for the Examination of Specimens from Patients with Tumors of Soft Tissue." Web posting date February 2011, www.cap.org.*

PROTOCOL FOR RHABDOMYOSARCOMA SPECIMENS

Rhabdomyosarcoma and Related Neoplasms

Resection or Biopsy

Procedure

___ Biopsy
___ Excision, local
___ Excision, radical
___ Excision, compartmentectomy
___ Amputation (specify type: ___________________________)
___ Other (specify): ___________________________
___ Not specified

Specimen Laterality

___ Right
___ Left
___ Midline
___ Indeterminate
___ Not specified

Tumor Site

___ Bladder/prostate
___ Cranial parameningeal
___ Extremity
___ Genitourinary (not bladder/prostate)
___ Head and neck (excluding parameningeal)
___ Orbit
___ Other(s) (includes trunk, retroperitoneum, etc.) (specify): ___________________________

Tumor Size

Greatest dimension: _________ cm
*Additional dimensions: _________ x _________ cm
___ Cannot be determined

**Tumor Depth for Soft Tissue-Based Tumors (select all that apply)*

*___Dermal
*___Subcutaneous
*___Subfascial
*___Intramuscular
*___Intraabdominal
*___Retroperitoneal
*___Intracranial
*___Organ based
*___Other (specify): ___________________________
*___Cannot be assessed

Histologic Type

___ Embryonal, botryoid
___ Embryonal, spindle cell
___ Embryonal, not otherwise specified (NOS)
___ Alveolar
___ Mixed embryonal and alveolar rhabdomyosarcoma
(Specify percentage of each type): ___________________________
___ Rhabdoid rhabdomyosarcoma
___ Sclerosing rhabdomyosarcoma
___ Undifferentiated sarcoma
___ Ectomesenchymoma
___ Other (specify): ___________________________
___ Rhabdomyosarcoma, subtype indeterminate

PROTOCOL FOR RHABDOMYOSARCOMA SPECIMENS

Anaplasia

___ Not identified
___ Focal (single or few scattered anaplastic cells)
___ Diffuse (clusters or sheets of anaplastic cells)
___ Indeterminate
___ Cannot be assessed

Margins

___ Cannot be assessed
___ Sarcoma involvement of margins not identified
    Distance of sarcoma from closest margin: _________ mm OR _________ cm
    Specify margin: ___________________________
___ Margin(s) involved by sarcoma
    Specify margin(s): ___________________________
___ Indeterminate

Lymph Nodes

___ No regional lymph nodes sampled
___ Metastatic involvement of regional lymph nodes not identified
___ Regional lymph node metastasis present
___ No nodes submitted or found
Number of lymph nodes examined
Specify: _________
___ Number cannot be determined (explain): ___________________________
Number of lymph nodes involved
Specify: _________
___ Number cannot be determined (explain): ___________________________

Distant Metastasis

___ Not applicable
___ Distant metastasis present
    *Specify site(s), if known: ___________________________

Intergroup Rhabdomyosarcoma Study Postsurgical Clinical Grouping System†

___ Not applicable
___ Cannot be assessed
Group I
___ A: Localized tumor, confined to site of origin, completely resected
___ B: Localized tumor, infiltrating beyond site of origin, completely resected
Group II
___ A: Localized tumor, gross total resection, but with microscopic residual disease
___ B: Locally extensive tumor (spread to regional lymph nodes), completely resected
___ C: Locally extensive tumor (spread to regional lymph nodes), gross total resection, but microscopic residual disease
Group III
___ A: Localized or locally extensive tumor, gross residual disease after biopsy only
___ B: Localized or locally extensive tumor, gross residual disease after major resection (> 50% debulking)
Group IV
___ Any size primary tumor, ± regional lymph node involvement, with distant metastases,
without respect to surgical approach to primary tumor

****Modified Site, Size, Metastasis Staging for Rhabdomyosarcoma (for relevant stage) (select all that apply)††***

*___Not applicable
*___Cannot be assessed
*___Stage I (requires all of the following to be true)
    *___ Tumor involves orbit, head and neck, or genitourinary site (excluding bladder, prostate, and cranial parameningeal)
    *___ Tumor metastatic to distant site not identified
*___Stage II (requires all of the following to be true)

PROTOCOL FOR RHABDOMYOSARCOMA SPECIMENS

*___ Tumor does not involve orbit, non-parameningeal head and neck, or non-bladder/non-prostate genitourinary tract

*___ Tumor size ≤ 5 cm

*___ Tumor involvement of lymph nodes not identified

*___ Tumor metastatic to distant site not identified

*___ Stage III (select one if applicable)

*___ Tumor involves bladder or prostate and is metastatic to regional lymph nodes but distant metastases are not identified

*___ Stage IV

*___ Distant metastases present

*Additional Pathologic Findings

*Specify: ___________________________

**Data elements with asterisks are not required. These elements may be clinically important but are not yet validated or regularly used in patient management. Adapted with permission from College of American Pathologists, "Protocol for the Examination of Specimens from Patients with Rhabdomyosarcoma." Web posting date February 2011, www.cap.org. †Clinical information required to definitively assign stage group (e.g., gross residual disease or distant metastatic disease) may not be available to the pathologist. Alternatively, this protocol may not be applicable to some situations (e.g., group IIIA). If applicable, the appropriate stage group may be assigned by the pathologist. ††Clinical information required to definitively assign stage (e.g., nodal status or distant metastatic disease) may not be available to the pathologist.*

Joint

Neoplasm, Benign

SYNOVIAL LIPOMATOSIS (HOFFA DISEASE)

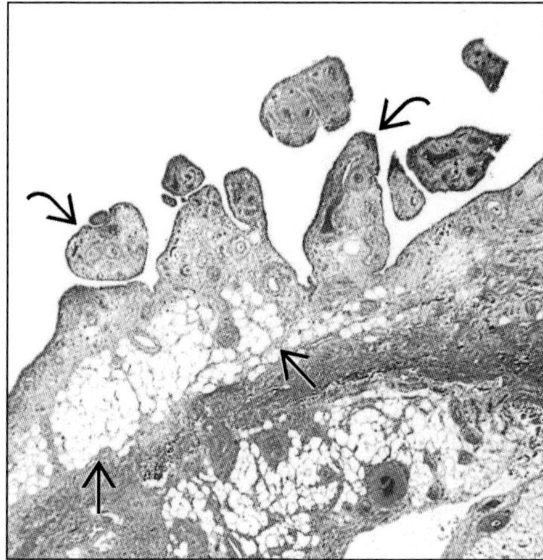

Characteristic features of synovial lipomatosis are shown, including villi/frond formation with overlying hyperplastic synovial membrane ⇗ and increased subsynovial adipose tissue ⇒.

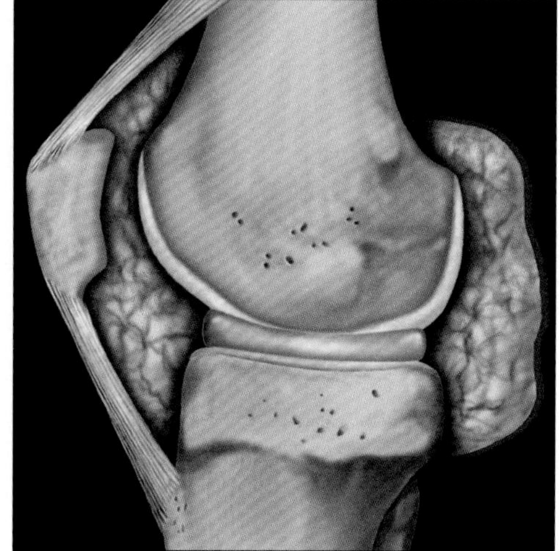

Sagittal graphic shows fatty infiltration of the synovium resulting in distention of the joint capsule.

TERMINOLOGY

Synonyms

- Lipoma arborescens
- Diffuse lipoma of joint
- Diffuse synovial lipoma
- Villous lipomatous proliferation of synovial membrane

Definitions

- Uncommon intraarticular benign lipomatous lesion characterized by extensive villous proliferation of synovial membrane and hyperplasia of subsynovial fat
- Diagnosis based on combination of location, radiologic findings, and identification of mature adipose tissue
- Term Hoffa disease refers more specifically to involvement of Hoffa fat pad of knee (infrapatellar fat pad)

ETIOLOGY/PATHOGENESIS

Unknown

- Thought of as secondary reactive process associated with
  - Chronic synovial irritation
  - Degenerative joint disease
  - Chronic rheumatoid arthritis
  - Prior trauma

CLINICAL ISSUES

Epidemiology

- Incidence
  - Rare
- Age
  - Reported in adolescents and adults (9-66 years)
- Gender
  - Males more commonly affected

Site

- Knee
  - Majority of cases
  - Most prominently in suprapatellar pouch
- Other joints can also be affected

Presentation

- Chronic refractory joint effusion
- Chronic knee or joint pain
- Gradual joint/synovial swelling and thickening
- Range of motion restriction
- Symptoms may progress over several to many years
- Symptoms may mimic ligament injury

Natural History

- Painless or painful swelling usually without complete regression

Treatment

- Surgical approaches
  - Arthroscopic synovectomy
  - Recurrent lesions may require open synovectomy
  - Recurrences following synovectomy reported

IMAGE FINDINGS

General Features

- Best diagnostic clue
  - Increased (fat) signal thickening of synovium
- Location
  - Within capsule of knee joint
    - Most prominently in suprapatellar pouch
- Size
  - Small fronds of affected synovium to large infiltrated fronds filling joint
- Morphology
  - Usually frond-like until large, then globular and rounded masses

SYNOVIAL LIPOMATOSIS (HOFFA DISEASE)

Key Facts

Terminology
- Rare intraarticular lipomatous lesion characterized by extensive villous proliferation of synovial membrane and hyperplasia of subsynovial fat

Etiology/Pathogenesis
- Thought of as secondary reactive process

Clinical Issues
- Reported in adolescents and adults (9-66 years)
- Knee most common site of involvement

Macroscopic Features
- Fatty enlargement of synovium with frond-like architecture

Microscopic Pathology
- Infiltration of subsynovial connective tissue by mature adipose tissue

Radiographic Findings
- Increased lucency in joint (fat density)

MR Findings
- T1WI: Increased signal intensity synovial masses (fat signal intensity)
- T2WI: Signal intensity decreases as with subcutaneous fat

CT Findings
- Decreased density synovial masses

Imaging Recommendations
- Best imaging tool: MR, CT

MACROSCOPIC FEATURES

General Features
- Fatty enlargement of synovium with frond-like architecture
- Fatty-appearing globules and villous projections seen at arthroscopy

MICROSCOPIC PATHOLOGY

Histologic Features
- Synovial membrane hyperplasia with villous/frond formation
- Infiltration of subsynovial connective tissue by mature adipose tissue
- Aggregates and individually scattered chronic inflammatory cells are often present

DIFFERENTIAL DIAGNOSIS

Synovial Lipoma
- Found in/on Hoffa fat pad
- Single mass

Synovial Osteochondromatosis
- Calcific masses

Synovitis and Chronic Joint Swelling
- Visualized as thickened synovium but without saturation with fat saturation techniques
- ± synovial fronds
- Acute and chronic inflammation

SELECTED REFERENCES

1. Bansal M et al: Synovial lipomatosis of the knee in an adolescent girl. Orthopedics. 31(2):185, 2008
2. Murphey MD et al: From the archives of the AFIP: benign musculoskeletal lipomatous lesions. Radiographics. 24(5):1433-66, 2004
3. Narváez J et al: Lipoma arborescens of the knee. Rev Rhum Engl Ed. 66(6):351-3, 1999
4. Kloen P et al: Lipoma arborescens of the knee. J Bone Joint Surg Br. 80(2):298-301, 1998
5. Hallel T et al: Villous lipomatous proliferation of the synovial membrane (lipoma arborescens). J Bone Joint Surg Am. 70(2):264-70, 1988

IMAGE GALLERY

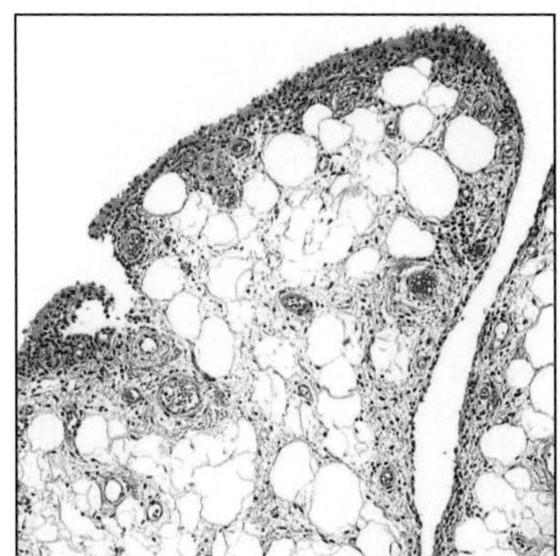

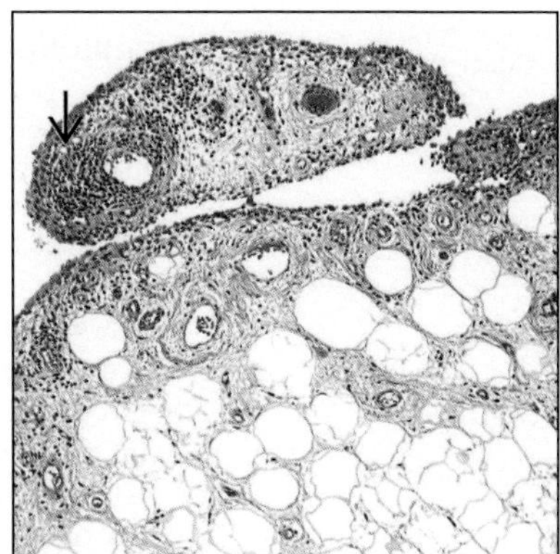

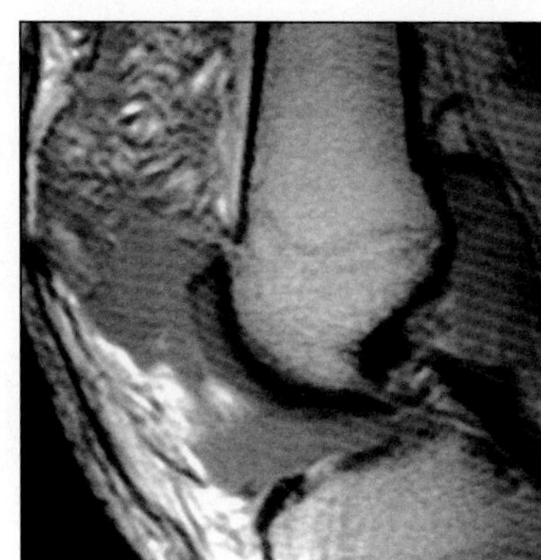

(Left) *High-power view shows increased amounts of mature adipose tissue within a villous/frond structure and synovial hyperplasia (top right).* ***(Center)*** *High-power view highlights the increased subsynovial adipose tissue (bottom) and a focal area of chronic inflammation ⇨ seen within the tip of a papillary villous structure.* ***(Right)*** *Sagittal MR shows intraarticular synovial lipomatosis occupying the suprapatellar pouch.*

OSTEOCHONDRITIS DISSECANS

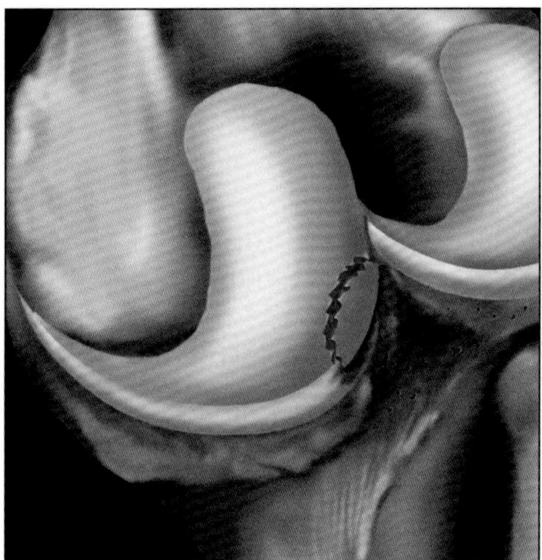

Coronal oblique graphic shows an osteochondral lesion of the lateral aspect of the medial femoral condyle. This is typical of osteochondritis dissecans.

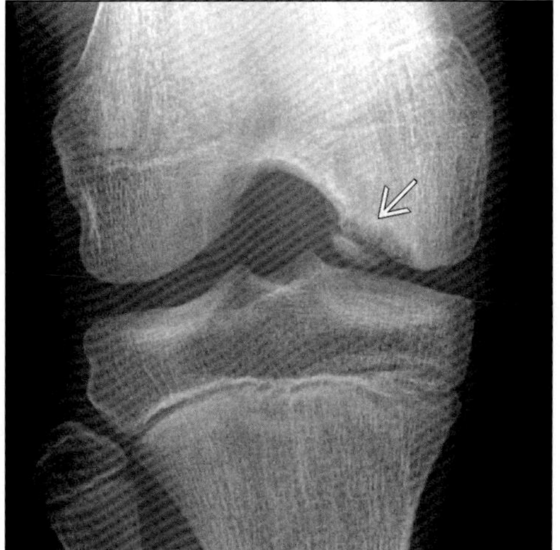

Radiograph tunnel view shows fragmentation and sclerosis of the adjacent medial femoral condyle ➔ consistent with osteochondritis dissecans. This lesion was stable on MR.

TERMINOLOGY

Abbreviations

- Osteochondritis dissecans (OCD)

Synonyms

- Osteochondral injury
- Juvenile osteochondritis dissecans (JOCD)
- "Quiet necrosis" of bone

Definitions

- Term that describes separation of an articular cartilage subchondral bone segment from remaining articular surface

ETIOLOGY/PATHOGENESIS

Uncertain

- Believed to be related to repetitive microtrauma with disruption of epiphyseal vasculature that may result in ischemic changes
- Frequently observed in athletically active individuals
- Likely begins as chronic shear stress injury within subchondral bone
- Subchondral trabecular microfractures coalesce into fracture line
- May extend to overlying cartilage if injury pattern continues without protection
- Hereditary abnormalities of ossification suggested

CLINICAL ISSUES

Epidemiology

- Age
  - Maximum incidence between ages of 10-20 years
- Gender
  - M:F = 6:1 for elbow
  - M:F = 5:3 for knee
  - M:F = 2:1 for ankle

Site

- Knee: Most frequent joint
  - Medial femoral condyle: 85%
  - Inferocentral lateral femoral condyle: 13%
  - Trochlea (femoral sulcus): 2%
  - Bilaterality reported in 30-40% of young patients
- Ankle: Talus far more common than tibial plafond
  - Posteromedial aspect of talus: 56%
  - Anterolateral aspect of talus: 44%
  - 6.5% of sprained ankles develop OCD
    - This number is likely an underestimate; MR often shows unsuspected OCD
- Elbow (capitellum): About 5% overall

Presentation

- Most common signs/symptoms
  - Pain
    - Worse with activity; improves with rest
  - Catching, grinding, and locking of joint
    - More common with loose or detached osteochondrotic lesions
  - Positive Wilson sign
    - Specific for medial femoral condyle lesions
    - Pain at 30° of flexion while holding tibia in internal rotation and slowly extending knee
  - Onset and history usually insidious
  - Symptoms preceded by trauma in 40-60% of cases

Treatment

- Dependent on following variables
  - Fragment size
  - Fragment location
  - Fragment stability
    - Stable lesions: Non-weight-bearing; muscle strengthening exercises
    - Unstable lesions: Removal of loose bodies may be required, with debridement of defect, and osteochondral grafting; in situ loose body may be pinned, drilled, &/or microfractured if overlying cartilage is mostly intact

OSTEOCHONDRITIS DISSECANS

Key Facts

Terminology
- Separation of an articular cartilage subchondral bone segment from remaining articular surface

Etiology/Pathogenesis
- Believed to be related to repetitive microtrauma with disruption of epiphyseal vasculature

Clinical Issues
- Maximum incidence between 10-20 years
- Knee: Most frequent joint
- Most common signs/symptoms
  - Catching, grinding, and locking of joint
  - Symptoms preceded by trauma in 40-60% of cases

Image Findings
- Convex articular surface with concave defect, ± osseous body
- Radiographic abnormalities occur late in process

Macroscopic Features
- Osseous bodies
  - May contain fibrous tissue or fibrocartilage
- Bony defects
  - May have intact overlying articular cartilage
  - May be firmly attached by fibrous tissue

Top Differential Diagnoses
- Pseudodefect of capitellum
- Panner disease
- Insufficiency fracture of femoral condyle
- Normal posterior femoral cortical irregularity

  - Age (skeletal immaturity and maturity)
    - Lesions in skeletally mature patients have less predictable course and may require surgery
    - Stable lesions in skeletally immature patients are generally amenable to conservative management

Prognosis
- Stable lesions treated appropriately: 50% heal with return to full function
- Instability or loose bodies may result in persistent pain & mechanical symptoms
- Even with treatment, as many as 50% of unstable lesions yield persistent pain in long term
- Unstable lesion eventually develops osteoarthritis

IMAGE FINDINGS

General Features
- Best diagnostic clue
  - Convex articular surface with concave defect, ± osseous body
- Location
  - Bilateral (20%)
  - Knee: Most frequent site
    - Lateral aspect of medial femoral condyle
    - Trochlea (femoral sulcus): Usually anterior aspect of lateral femoral condyle, close to midline; may occur medially
  - Ankle: Next most frequent site
    - Posteromedial talar dome
    - Anterolateral talar dome
  - Elbow: Anterolateral capitellum
  - Shoulder: Humeral head or glenoid
    - Do not mistake central developmental defect of glenoid
  - Wrist: Rare involvement of scaphoid
    - Distal or proximal pole
- Size
  - Ranges from small to ≥ 3 cm
- Morphology
  - Concave bed containing (at some point) osseous bodies

Radiographic Findings
- Radiographic abnormalities occur late in process
  - Radiograph shows rounded lucency in subarticular region, usually at convex surface of bone
  - If radiograph is profiled properly, concave defect at convex osseous surface is seen, often containing osseous body
    - Oblique view of capitellum or ankle is useful
    - For trochlear (femoral sulcus) OCD, axial view of patella is useful
  - Flattening of normal convexity of articular surface
  - Loose bodies may be in situ (within concave "bed" of defect) or may be displaced elsewhere within joint

MR Findings
- Earliest MR findings: Subchondral stress reaction
  - Hypointense on T1, hyperintense on fluid-sensitive sequences; enhancement with contrast
  - No fracture line
  - Intact overlying cartilage
- With progression, fracture line forms, but articular surface is intact
  - Focal T1 hypointensity may obscure fracture line
  - Focal hyperintensity on fluid-sensitive sequences may obscure fracture line
    - Central signal of body variable: Low, high, or mixture of both
- With further progression, articular surface is disrupted; can be directly seen if fluid from effusion surrounds fragment within defect
- Use of contrast
  - Enhancement of osseous fragment indicates viability but does not predict stability
  - Indirect arthrogram from IV contrast administration may produce enough fluid to demonstrate either intact or disrupted articular cartilage over defect
  - Not routinely required for evaluation of OCD

OSTEOCHONDRITIS DISSECANS

- MR used to determine stability of lesion (92% sensitive, 90% specific for differentiating unstable lesions from stable lesions)
  - Fluid-sensitive sequences: Hyperintensity at majority of peripheral rim indicates instability
    - Etiology of hyperintensity is uncertain: Granulation tissue, edematous fibrous tissue, or fluid
  - Fluid entering defect through articular cartilage defect indicates instability
  - Subchondral cysts formed at peripheral rim indicate instability
  - Focal osteochondral defect filled with joint fluid

CT Findings

- Reformats required for full evaluation
- Concave defect with sclerotic margin
- Osseous fragments seen within defect; if displaced above articular margin, lesion is unstable
- Loose bodies not adjacent to defect
- Subchondral cysts: Indicate instability of lesion

Imaging Recommendations

- Best imaging tool
  - Detection is usually by radiograph
    - May be subtle; MR often demonstrates unsuspected talar dome OCD
  - Evaluation for stability performed by MR

MACROSCOPIC FEATURES

Gross Pathologic, Surgical, & Histologic Features

- Bony defect spectrum
  - May be a true defect
  - May contain osseous bodies
  - May contain fibrous tissue or fibrocartilage
- Osseous fragments spectrum
  - May have intact overlying articular cartilage
  - May be firmly attached by fibrous tissue
  - May be partially or completely detached
- Necrotic bone, granulation tissue, synovitis

MICROSCOPIC PATHOLOGY

Histologic Features

- Basic process described as aseptic necrosis involving subchondral bone ± other secondary changes
  - Fibrous or fibrocartilaginous tissue often seen in radiolucent bed
  - Necrotic bone
  - ± inflammation

DIFFERENTIAL DIAGNOSIS

Pseudodefect of Capitellum

- Located posteriorly in capitellum
- Normal indentation at junction of cartilage-covered capitellum with noncartilaginous posterior bone

Panner Disease

- Avascular necrosis of entire capitellum
- Generally in younger patients (5-11 years)

Insufficiency Fracture of Femoral Condyle

- Formerly known as SONK (spontaneous osteonecrosis of knee)
- Location generally directly in center of weight-bearing portion of medial femoral condyle
- Occurs in older, osteoporotic age group
- Pain pattern is different; acute, severe pain occurs
- May see depressed fracture fragment, with flattening of cortex, or only marrow edema

Normal Posterior Femoral Cortical Irregularity

- Osseous irregularity & pseudodefect may occur in posterior femoral condyles (not a usual site for OCD)
- Normal overlying cartilage
- Nearly always fills in with normal bone as patient matures
- Younger patient age group (8-12 years)

SELECTED REFERENCES

1. Ramirez A et al: Juvenile osteochondritis dissecans of the knee: perifocal sclerotic rim as a prognostic factor of healing. J Pediatr Orthop. 30(2):180-5, 2010
2. Kocher MS et al: Management of osteochondritis dissecans of the knee: current concepts review. Am J Sports Med. 34(7):1181-91, 2006
3. Robertson W et al: Osteochondritis dissecans of the knee in children. Curr Opin Pediatr. 15(1):38-44, 2003
4. De Smet AA et al: Osteochondritis dissecans of the knee: value of MR imaging in determining lesion stability and the presence of articular cartilage defects. AJR Am J Roentgenol. 155(3):549-53, 1990

Radiologic and Diagrammatic Features

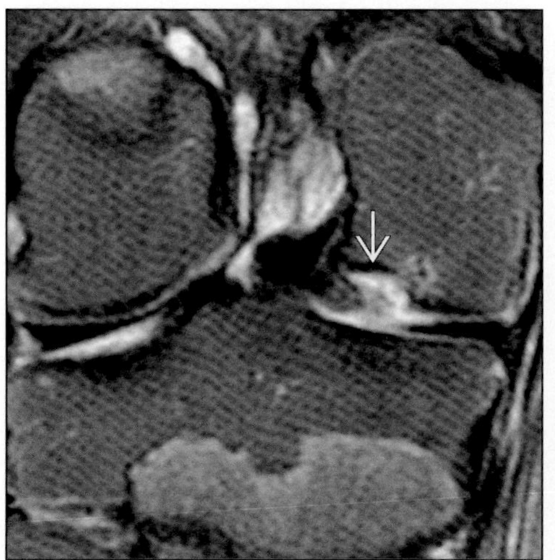

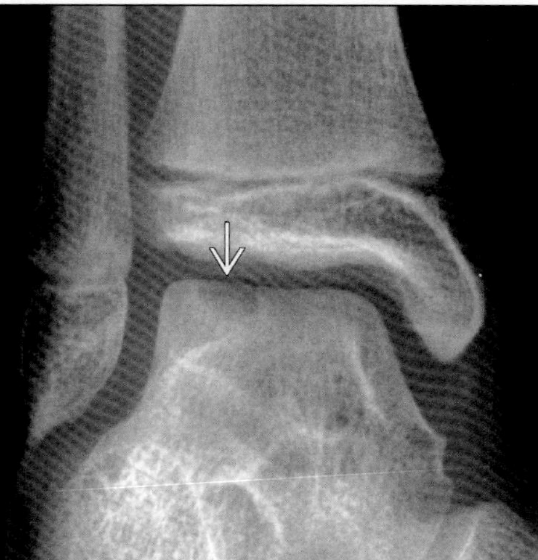

(Left) *Coronal T2WI MR shows a partially detached unstable lesion of the medial femoral condyle with an overlying cartilage breach and fluid partially surrounding the osteochondritis dissecans fragment ➡.* ***(Right)*** *Anteroposterior radiograph shows a lucent lesion in the lateral talar dome ➡ with a minimal sclerotic margin, consistent with an osteochondritis dissecans lesion.*

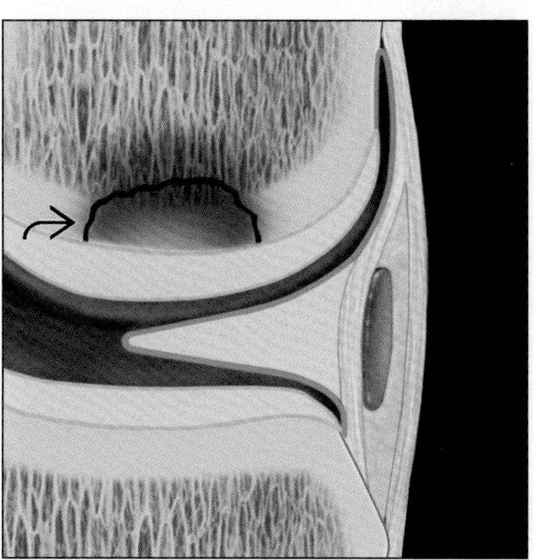

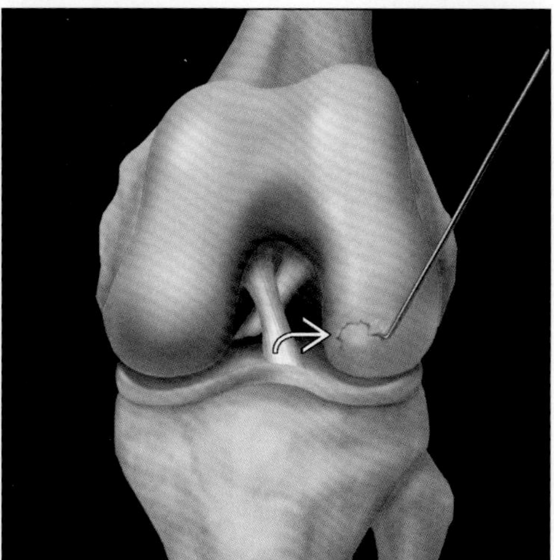

(Left) *Graphic of the left knee illustrates a stage I lesion ↪ on the femoral condyle. A stage I lesion by definition is a stable lesion that remains in continuity with host bone and is covered by intact cartilage.* ***(Right)*** *Graphic of the left knee illustrates a stage II lesion on the lateral femoral condyle ↪. A stage II lesion by definition is in partial discontinuity but stable on probing.*

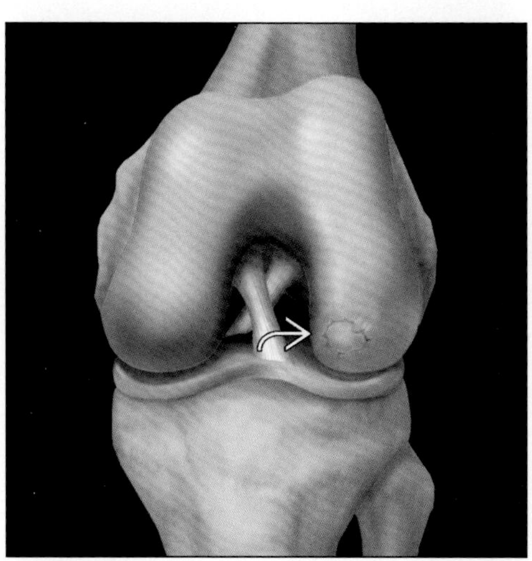

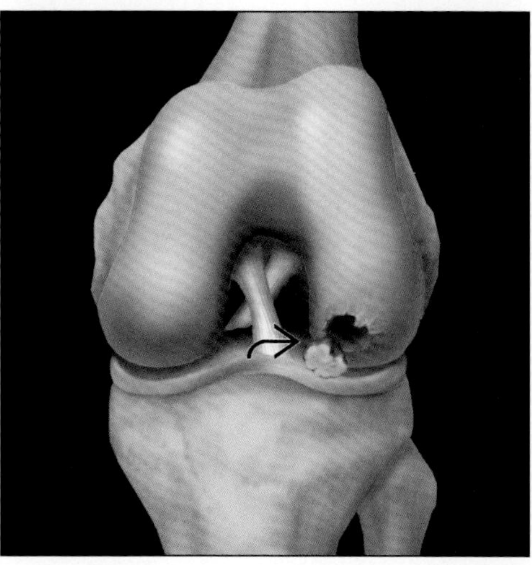

(Left) *Graphic of the left knee illustrates a stage III lesion on the lateral femoral condyle ↪. A stage III lesion by definition shows complete discontinuity of the "dead in situ" lesion, but the fragment is not dislocated.* ***(Right)*** *Graphic of the left knee illustrates a stage IV lesion on the lateral femoral condyle ↪. A stage IV lesion by definition shows a completely dislocated fragment (loose body).*

Bone

Neoplasm, Benign

Neoplasm, Malignant Primary

Protocol for the Examination of Specimens from Patients with Bone Tumors

Protocol for the Examination of Specimens from Patients with Primitive Neuroectodermal Tumor/Ewing Sarcoma

OSTEOCHONDROMA

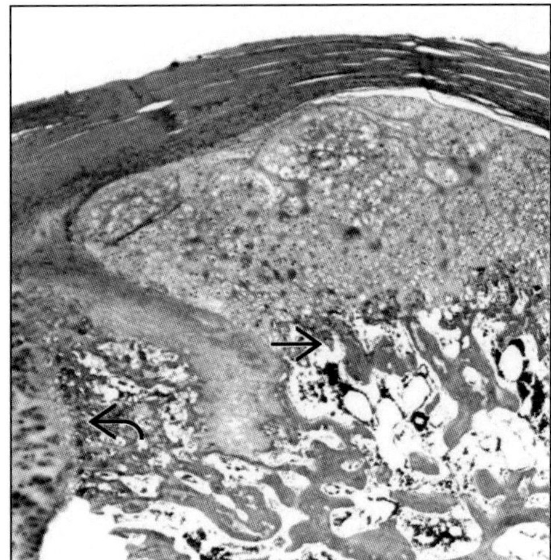

Hematoxylin & eosin shows an early osteochondroma arising adjacent to the growth plate ⇗ in the rib of a child. Bony trabeculae ⇒ of the osteochondroma are continuous with the medullary cavity.

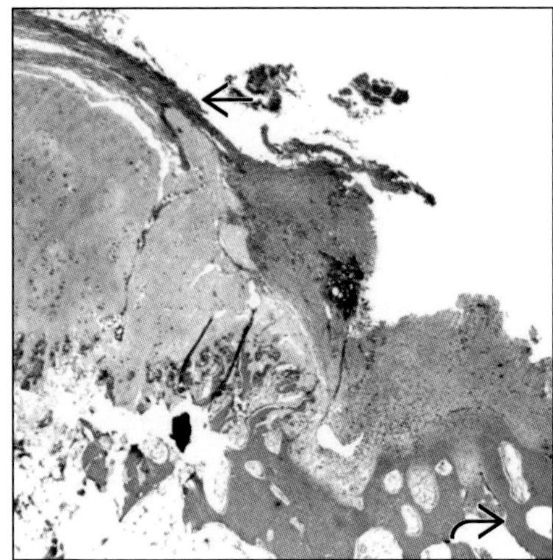

Hematoxylin & eosin shows osteochondroma arising from cortex ⇗ of parent bone. Periosteum ⇒ continues up over cartilaginous cap.

TERMINOLOGY

Abbreviations

- Hereditary multiple osteochondromas (HMO)

Synonyms

- Osteochondromatous exostosis
- Solitary osteochondroma

Definitions

- Benign bony projection with cartilaginous cap arising from cortical surface of bone and contiguous with underlying marrow cavity

ETIOLOGY/PATHOGENESIS

Developmental Anomaly

- May represent breakage, rotation, or herniation of growth plate into metaphysis

Environmental Exposure

- Reported after radiation therapy in children

Neoplastic

- Cytogenic abnormalities in hereditary multiple osteochondromas
  - May indicate neoplastic etiology in sporadic form

CLINICAL ISSUES

Epidemiology

- Incidence
  - Most common bone tumor
    - 30-35% of all benign bone tumors
    - 9-10% of all bone tumors
- Age
  - Majority detected in first 2 decades, but can present at any age
- Gender
  - Slight male predominance

Site

- Arise primarily in bones preformed by cartilage (enchondral ossification)
- Most common sites
  - Metaphysis of distal femur
  - Proximal humerus
  - Proximal tibia
- Flat bone involvement less common
  - Ilium
  - Vertebra-posterior elements
  - Scapula
- Distal extremity involvement rare unless HMO

Presentation

- Most asymptomatic
  - Incidental radiographic finding
- Symptomatic lesions
  - Dependent on size and location
    - Mass effect
    - Nerve impingement
    - Inflamed overlying bursa

Natural History

- Usually solitary
  - Up to 15% of patients will have multiple
- Majority benign
  - Low-risk malignant transformation
    - Benign osteochondroma = no risk for metastasis
- Lesions may grow until skeleton mature
  - Minimal growth after fusion of growth plate
- Differential diagnosis for multiple osteochondromas
  - Hereditary multiple osteochondromas or osteochondromatosis
  - Langer-Giedion syndrome
  - DEFECT-11 (Potocki-Shaffer) syndrome
- Hereditary multiple osteochondromas or osteochondromatosis
  - Autosomal dominant
  - 3 genetic loci identified

OSTEOCHONDROMA

Key Facts

Terminology

- Bony projection with cartilaginous cap arising from cortical surface and contiguous with underlying marrow cavity

Etiology/Pathogenesis

- May represent breakage, rotation, or herniation of growth plate into metaphysis
- Reports of cytogenetic abnormalities and aneuploidy suggest possible neoplastic nature

Clinical Issues

- Majority detected in 1st 2 decades
- Most common sites: Metaphysis of distal femur, proximal humerus, proximal tibia and fibula
- Surgical excision usually curative

Macroscopic Features

- During prosection, cut perpendicular to stalk for accurate measurement of cartilage cap
- Cartilaginous cap usually less than 1 cm

Microscopic Pathology

- Cartilaginous cap with portion of underlying bone should fit on 1 slide
- 3 histologic layers: Perichondrium, cartilaginous cap, bony trabeculae
- Medullary cavity with fat and hematopoietic marrow

Diagnostic Checklist

- Chondrocytes usually arranged in linear pattern
- Cartilaginous cap has lobulated surface but no invasion of islands of cartilage into overlying soft tissues

---

    - *EXT1:* 8q24.1
    - *EXT2:* 11p11-12
    - *EXT3:* 19p
  - Secondary chondrosarcoma more common in HMO

Treatment

- Options, risks, complications
  - Observation for asymptomatic lesions
- Surgical approaches
  - Usually curative
  - Recurrence possible with incomplete excision

Prognosis

- Malignant transformation rare
  - Less than 1% in patients with solitary lesions
  - Up to 8% of patients with HMO
  - Chondrosarcoma most common secondary malignancy
    - Rare cases of secondary osteosarcoma

IMAGE FINDINGS

General Features

- Pedunculated or sessile growth in continuity with underlying cortex and medullary cavity
  - Plain radiographs may not delineate cartilaginous cap or relationship to underlying bone
  - Overlying bursa may simulate malignancy/soft tissue involvement
  - Pedunculated lesions usually point away from adjacent joint
- Flocculent cartilage-type calcification suspicious for malignant transformation

MR Findings

- Displays continuity of marrow space into lesion
- Allows measurement of cartilaginous cap

MACROSCOPIC FEATURES

General Features

- Sessile or pedunculated bony mass
  - Periosteum continues as perichondrium
  - Bluish cartilaginous cap
  - Cancellous bone with marrow cavity underlies cap
- Cortex and medullary cavity of underlying bone continuous with lesional tissue
- Overlying bursa may be resected with osteochondroma
  - Bursa may show reactive features
    - Features consistent with synovial chondromatosis possible

Sections to Be Submitted

- Cut perpendicular to stalk for accurate measurement of cartilaginous cap
  - Measure and report thickness of cap
  - Thickness greater than 2 cm worrisome for secondary chondrosarcoma
- Surface of cartilaginous cap to underlying bone
- Cartilaginous cap with portion of underlying bone should fit on 1 slide
  - If cap too thick for 1 slide, worrisome for secondary chondrosarcoma
- Surgical resection margin if concerned for malignancy

Size

- Cartilaginous cap usually less than 1 cm

MICROSCOPIC PATHOLOGY

Histologic Features

- 3 histologic layers
  - Perichondrium: Thin eosinophilic layer continuous with periosteum of underlying bone
  - Cartilage: Chondrocytes clustered near surface but arranged in columns in deeper sections (resembles growth plate); intervening chondroid matrix
  - Bone: Enchondral ossification forms bony trabeculae
- Medullary cavity contains fat and hematopoietic marrow
- Cartilaginous cap can have lobulated surface
  - Invasion of overlying tissue by islands of cartilage absent

OSTEOCHONDROMA

Predominant Pattern/Injury Type
- Polypoid
- Sessile

Predominant Cell/Compartment Type
- Cartilaginous
- Bony trabeculae

DIFFERENTIAL DIAGNOSIS

Surface Chondrosarcoma
- No true stalk
- Lobular masses of cartilage infiltrate soft tissue

Chondrosarcoma Arising in Osteochondroma
- Clinical features
  - Multiple recurrence
  - Rapidly increasing growth
  - New onset pain
- Pathologic features
  - Cartilage cap greater than 2 cm
  - Lobules of cartilage invade surrounding soft tissue
  - Nuclear pleomorphism with hyperchromasia and binucleation
  - Loss of orderly columnar pattern of deeper chondrocytes

Parosteal Osteosarcoma
- May have peripheral zone of cartilage simulating cartilage cap
- Fibroblastic proliferations and cellular atypia present

Osteophyte
- Bony outgrowth
- Often lacks cartilage cap
- No connection to marrow cavity

Exostosis
- Common in craniofacial and jaw bones
- Often response to irritant or trauma

Subungual Exostosis
- Arise under nail
- Rapid growth
- Lacks continuity with underlying cortex and medullary cavity
- Osteochondromas rare under nail

Bizarre Parosteal Osteochondromatous Proliferation
- Disorganized mass of bone, cartilage, fibrous tissue
- No continuity with underling cortex and medullary cavity

Trevor Disease
- Nonhereditary skeletal dysplasia

DIAGNOSTIC CHECKLIST

Clinically Relevant Pathologic Features
- Gross appearance
  - Thickness of cartilage cap less than 2 cm
  - Continuity of periosteum, cortex, and medullary cavity of host bone into lesional tissue

Pathologic Interpretation Pearls
- Orderly chondrocytes
  - Linear pattern
- Chondrocytes lack pleomorphism
  - Nuclear hyperchromasia and binucleation absent
- Cartilaginous cap has lobulated surface
  - No invasion of islands of cartilage into overlying soft tissues

REPORTING CONSIDERATIONS

Key Elements to Report
- Gross measure of cartilaginous cap thickness

CODING CONSIDERATIONS

Exostosis Excision
- 88305

Decalcification
- 88311

SELECTED REFERENCES

1. Kitsoulis P et al: Osteochondromas: review of the clinical, radiological and pathological features. In Vivo. 22(5):633-46, 2008
2. Mavrogenis AF et al: Skeletal osteochondromas revisited. Orthopedics. 31(10), 2008
3. Hameetman L et al: The role of EXT1 in nonhereditary osteochondroma: identification of homozygous deletions. J Natl Cancer Inst. 99(5):396-406, 2007
4. Staals EL et al: Dedifferentiated chondrosarcomas arising in preexisting osteochondromas. J Bone Joint Surg Am. 89(5):987-93, 2007
5. Porter DE et al: Severity of disease and risk of malignant change in hereditary multiple exostoses. A genotype-phenotype study. J Bone Joint Surg Br. 86(7):1041-6, 2004
6. Murphey MD et al: Imaging of osteochondroma: variants and complications with radiologic-pathologic correlation. Radiographics. 20(5):1407-34, 2000
7. Porter DE et al: The neoplastic pathogenesis of solitary and multiple osteochondromas. J Pathol. 188(2):119-25, 1999
8. Day FN et al: Recurrent osteochondroma. J Foot Ankle Surg. 37(2):162-4; discussion 173, 1998
9. Mehta M et al: MR imaging of symptomatic osteochondromas with pathological correlation. Skeletal Radiol. 27(8):427-33, 1998
10. Wicklund CL et al: Natural history study of hereditary multiple exostoses. Am J Med Genet. 55(1):43-6, 1995
11. D'Ambrosia R et al: The formation of osteochondroma by epiphyseal cartilage transplantation. Clin Orthop Relat Res. 61:103-15, 1968

OSTEOCHONDROMA

Diagrammatic and Other Features

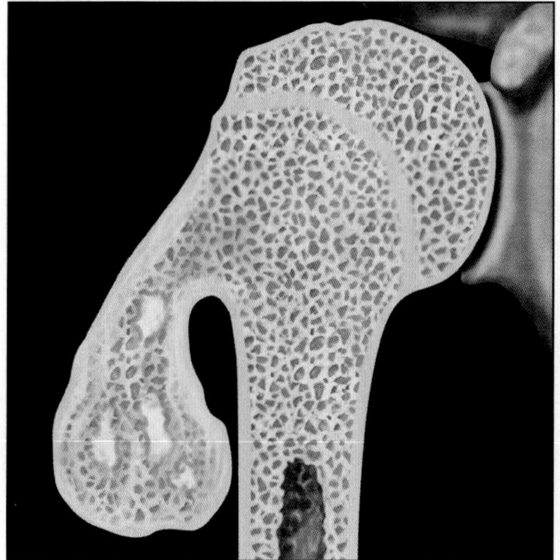

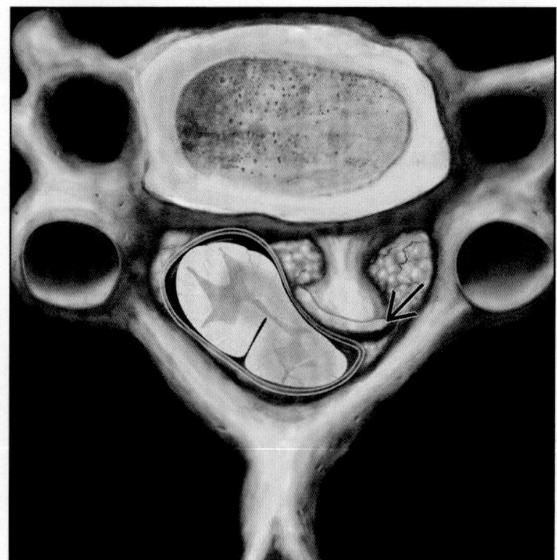

(Left) *Coronal graphic shows a pedunculated osteochondroma arising from the humeral metaphysis. Continuity of the cortex and medullary canal of host bone into the osteochondroma is shown.* ***(Right)*** *Axial graphic shows a polypoid osteochondroma protruding into central spinal canal, producing symptoms of spinal cord compression. Cartilaginous cap is demonstrated ➔.*

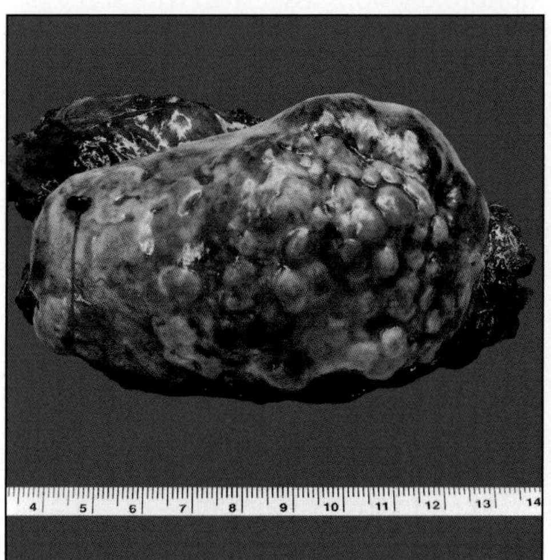

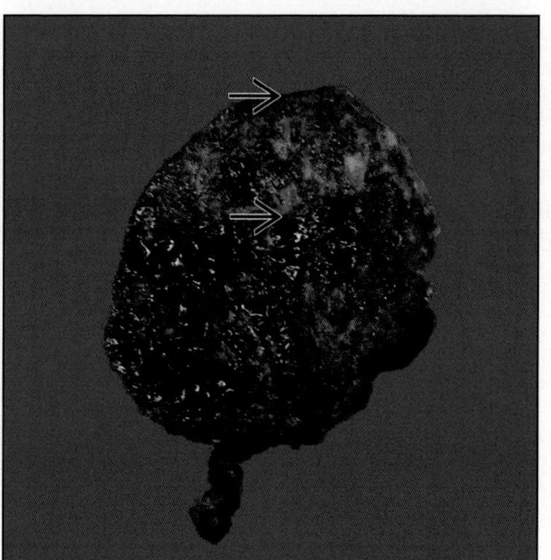

(Left) *Gross photograph shows a sessile osteochondroma which has been shaved from the underlying bone. The surface shows a lobulated cartilaginous cap.* ***(Right)*** *Gross photograph shows a cross section from the center of an osteochondroma. The cartilaginous cap must be measured at its thickest point ➔. This measurement should be documented in the pathology report.*

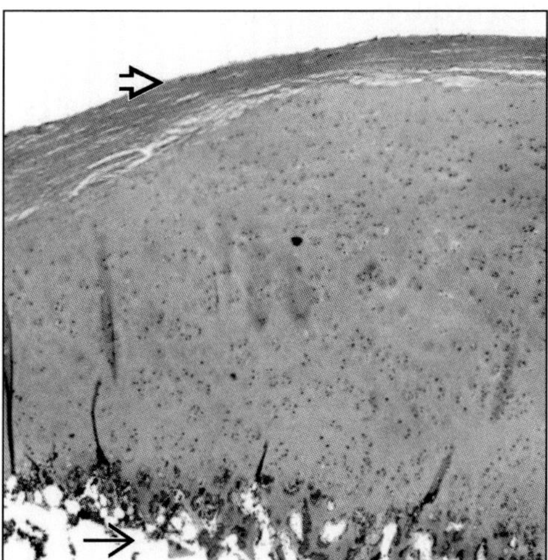

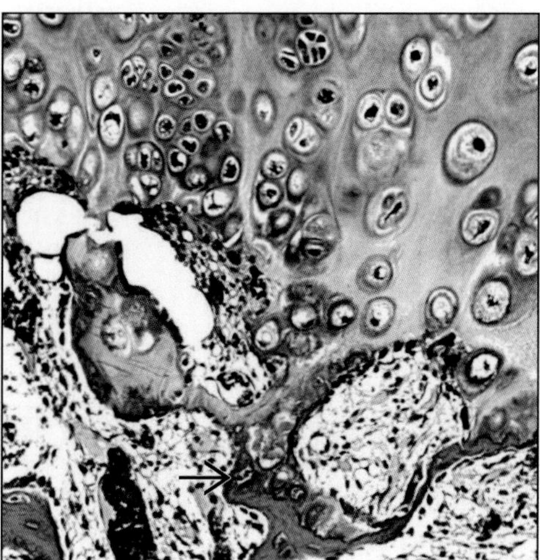

(Left) *Hematoxylin & eosin shows an intact cartilaginous cap overlying bony trabeculae ➔ formed via enchondral ossification. Periosteum ➲ continues from cortical bone to cover the cartilaginous cap.* ***(Right)*** *Hematoxylin & eosin shows orderly arrangement of chondrocytes at inferior portion of cartilage cap; underlying bony trabeculae are formed via ➔ enchondral ossification.*

ENCHONDROMA

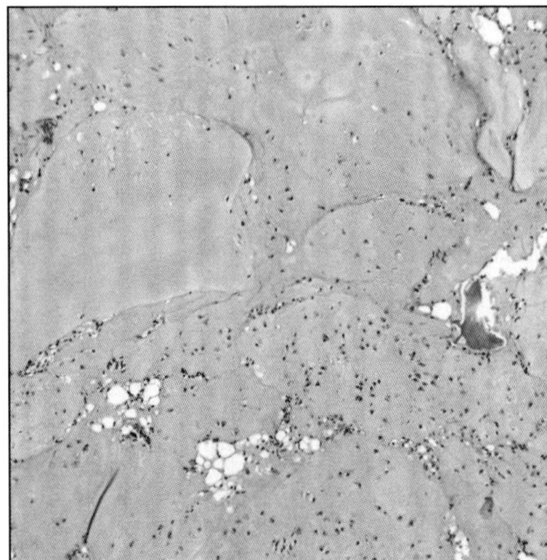

Low-power view of this enchondroma shows the somewhat lobulated architecture that is typical for this lesion.

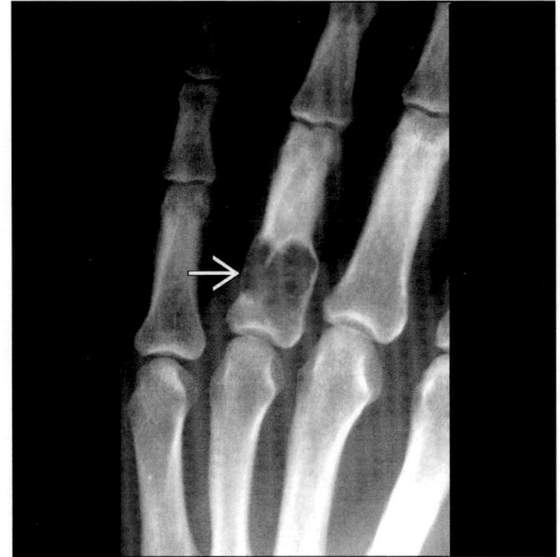

This radiograph of the hand shows a lucent lesion ➡ in the 4th proximal phalanx. The overlying cortex is scalloped and thinned. This is a typical appearance for an enchondroma.

TERMINOLOGY

Definitions

- Chondroma: Benign cartilaginous neoplasm
- Enchondroma: Chondroma within bone (intramedullary)
- Periosteal chondroma: Chondroma on surface of bone
- Soft tissue chondroma: Chondroma in soft tissue not associated with bone

CLINICAL ISSUES

Site

- Any bone formed by enchondral ossification can be involved
- Short, tubular bones of hands and feet: 60%
- Long tubular bones: 25-45%
    - Metaphysis, proximal/distal end of diaphysis
    - Femur: 17%
    - Humerus: 7%
- Pelvis: < 3%
- Spine, scapula, ribs: Rare

Presentation

- Can occur in any age
    - Most common 10-30 years
- No sex predilection
- Usually no symptoms
    - Chondroma of small bones of hands and feet can cause pathologic fractures
- Ollier disease (enchondromatosis)
    - Nonfamilial
    - Multiple chondromas of long and flat bones
        - Usually unilateral and often of only 1 limb
    - Higher incidence of malignant transformation
    - Lesions tend to regress when skeleton matures
- Maffucci syndrome
    - Nonfamilial
    - Multiple chondroid lesions associated with soft tissue hemangiomas
    - May be associated with very high incidence of malignancy in skeleton or visceral organs
- Carney triad
    - Rare condition affecting young females
    - Pulmonary chondroma, gastrointestinal stromal tumor, paraganglioma

Treatment

- Surgical approaches
    - Usually curettage
    - Resection is rare

Prognosis

- Benign
- Rarely can develop into chondrosarcoma

IMAGE FINDINGS

Radiographic Findings

- Well circumscribed
- Radiolucent
- Metaphysis or diaphysis of long bones
    - Entire shaft usually involved in small bones of hands and feet
- Does not invade cortex
    - May thin and scallop inner cortex in small bones of hands and feet
- Flecks of calcification appear as "arcs and rings"
    - Most commonly seen in long bone lesions

MACROSCOPIC FEATURES

General Features

- Pale blue color typical of cartilage

ENCHONDROMA

Key Facts

Terminology
- Chondroma: Benign cartilaginous neoplasm

Clinical Issues
- Small bones of hands and feet or larger long bones
- Usually no symptoms
- Ollier disease: Multiple enchondromas
- Maffucci syndrome: Multiple enchondromas and hemangiomas

Microscopic Pathology
- Lesions of large long bones are hypocellular with no myxoid change
- Lesions of small bones of hands and feet are hypercellular and may have mild atypia

Top Differential Diagnoses
- Chondrosarcoma

MICROSCOPIC PATHOLOGY

Histologic Features
- Of larger long bones
  - Hypocellular
  - Few, if any, doubly nucleated cells
  - No myxoid change
- Of small bones of hands and feet
  - Hypercellular
  - Frequent doubly nucleated cells
  - Myxoid change
  - Looks like grade 1 chondrosarcoma
    - Benign radiographic appearance defines chondroma
- In Ollier disease
  - Hypercellular
  - Frequently myxoid

DIFFERENTIAL DIAGNOSIS

Chondrosarcoma
- Painful lesion of large bones
- Cortical erosion seen on radiographs
- Permeates marrow space
- Marked myxoid change

DIAGNOSTIC CHECKLIST

Pathologic Interpretation Pearls
- **Must** interpret along with radiology

SELECTED REFERENCES

1. Carney JA: Carney triad: a syndrome featuring paraganglionic, adrenocortical, and possibly other endocrine tumors. J Clin Endocrinol Metab. 94(10):3656-62, 2009
2. Fahim DK et al: Periosteal chondroma of the pediatric cervical spine. J Neurosurg Pediatr. 3(2):151-6, 2009
3. Romeo S et al: Benign cartilaginous tumors of bone: from morphology to somatic and germ-line genetics. Adv Anat Pathol. 16(5):307-15, 2009
4. Cabay RJ et al: Cytologic features of primary chondroid tumors of bone in crush preparations. Diagn Cytopathol. 36(10):758-61, 2008
5. Domson GF et al: Periosteal chondroma at birth. Skeletal Radiol. 37(6):559-62, 2008
6. Ojeda-Thies C et al: Solitary epiphyseal enchondroma of the proximal femur in a 23-month-old girl. J Pediatr Orthop. 28(5):565-8, 2008
7. Walden MJ et al: Incidental enchondromas of the knee. AJR Am J Roentgenol. 190(6):1611-5, 2008
8. Müller PE et al: Malignant transformation of a benign enchondroma of the hand to secondary chondrosarcoma with isolated pulmonary metastasis. Acta Chir Belg. 104(3):341-4, 2004

IMAGE GALLERY

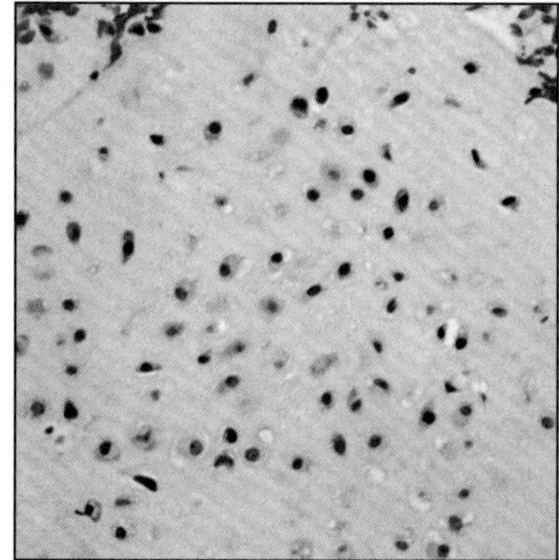

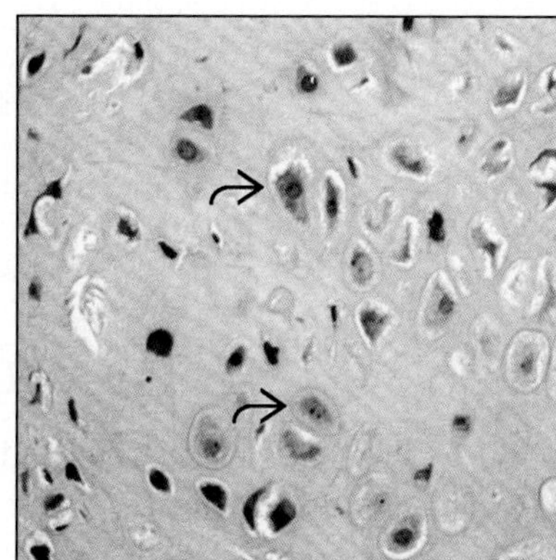

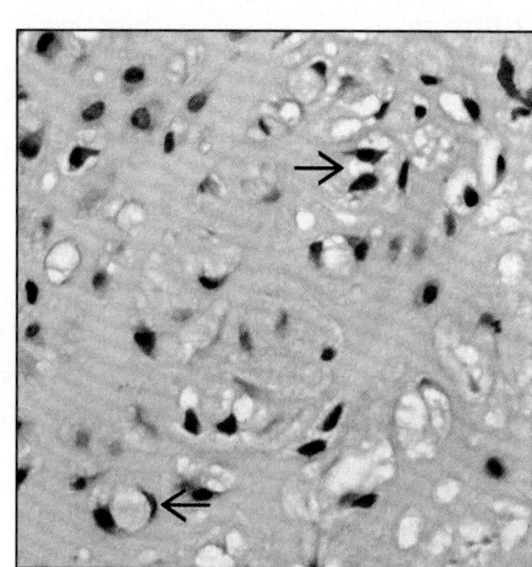

__(Left)__ Medium-power view shows the kind of hypercellularity that may be expected in an enchondroma of the small bones of the hands or feet. __(Center)__ The chondrocytes in this enchondroma are mildly atypical. The nuclei are large and round with cleared chromatin and conspicuous nucleoli ➢. Radiographs would help with a benign diagnosis. __(Right)__ Sometimes more than 1 chondrocyte can be seen within a single lacunar space ➔.

CHONDROBLASTOMA

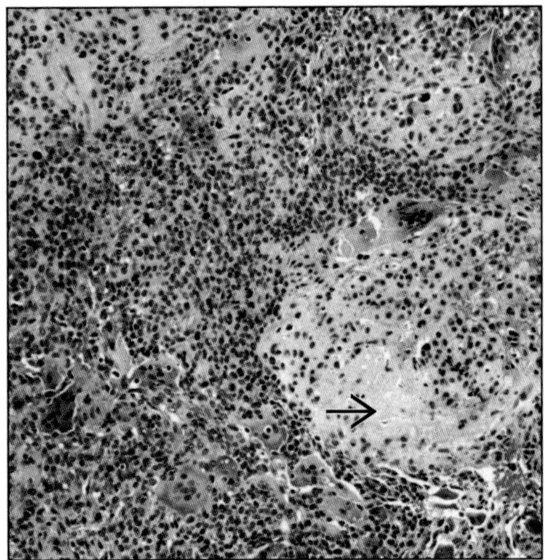

Hematoxylin & eosin shows sheets of small, round to oval cells with islands of chondroid ⇒. Scattered giant cells are present.

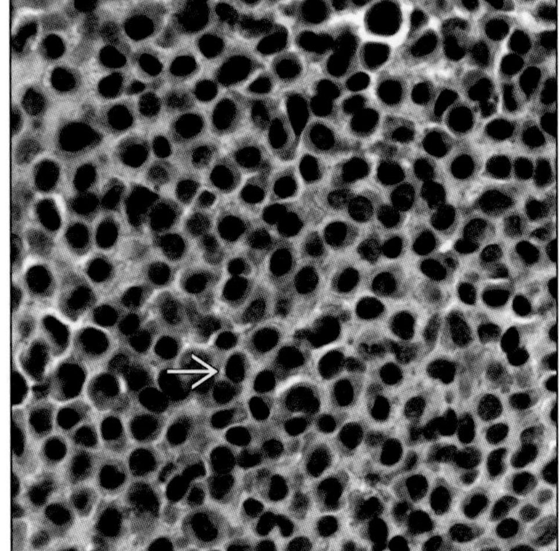

Hematoxylin & eosin shows sheets of lesional cells with distinct borders and eosinophilic cytoplasm. The nuclei are uniform with longitudinal grooves ⇒.

TERMINOLOGY

Synonyms

- Calcifying giant cell tumor
- Epiphyseal chondromatous giant cell tumor

Definitions

- Benign cartilaginous neoplasm most often arising in epiphysis of skeletally immature patients

ETIOLOGY/PATHOGENESIS

Neoplastic

- Structural anomalies of chromosomes 5 and 8 reported

CLINICAL ISSUES

Epidemiology

- Age
  - Wide age range but most frequent in 2nd decade

Site

- Long bones in 75% of cases
  - Proximal or distal femur, proximal tibia, proximal humerus
  - Epiphyseal location most common, followed by epimetaphyseal region
- Other sites: Acetabulum, ilium, talus, calcaneus, patella, temporal bone

Presentation

- Localized pain
  - Duration of months to years reported
  - Soft tissue swelling with rare joint effusion
  - Temporal bone cases associated with hearing loss, tinnitus, and vertigo

Treatment

- Surgical approaches
  - Simple curettage with bone grafting curative in 80-90% of cases

Prognosis

- Local recurrence risk 14-20%
  - Temporal bone recurrence is higher (up to 50%)
  - Cytologic atypia in recurrence does not indicate malignant transformation
- Rare metastasis in histologically benign chondroblastoma
  - Usually occurs after surgical manipulation
  - Pulmonary metastasis most frequent
  - Metastatic disease usually cured by surgical resection
- Malignant chondroblastoma reported
  - No reliable histologic features to predict aggressive behavior
  - Molecular markers: Rearrangement of *8q21*, *TP53* mutation, increased proliferative activity
  - May represent misclassification of sarcoma

IMAGE FINDINGS

General Features

- Central or eccentric, epiphyseal-based lytic lesion with sharp borders
  - May cross open physis to involve metaphysis
  - Typically 3-6 cm
- Sclerotic rim ± expansion of bone
  - Periosteal reaction more common in flat or small tubular bones
- Matrix calcification identified in 25-30% of cases
- MR may show edema

MACROSCOPIC FEATURES

General Features

- Tan to pink, focally calcified tissue
- Hemorrhagic or cystic component possible when associated with aneurysmal bone cyst

CHONDROBLASTOMA

Key Facts

Terminology

- Benign, cartilaginous neoplasm most often arising in epiphysis of skeletally immature patients

Clinical Issues

- Localized pain
- Long bones in 75% of cases
- Proximal or distal femur, proximal tibia, proximal humerus
- Simple curettage with bone grafting curative in 80-90% of cases
- Rare metastasis in histologically benign chondroblastoma

Image Findings

- Central or eccentric, epiphyseal-based lytic lesion with sharp borders
- Thin sclerotic border in some cases
- May cross open physis to involve metaphysis

Microscopic Pathology

- Uniform, round to polygonal cell with well-defined cytoplasmic border
- Round to oval nucleus with clefts or longitudinal grooves, "coffee bean"
- Variable nodules of amorphous eosinophilic chondroid present
- Network of pericellular calcification: "Chicken wire" calcification (~ 30%)
- S100 and vimentin positive
- Secondary aneurysmal bone cyst in > 1/3 of cases

MICROSCOPIC PATHOLOGY

Histologic Features

- Sheets of uniform, round to polygonal cells with well-defined cytoplasmic borders
  - Clear to eosinophilic cytoplasm
  - Round to oval nucleus with clefts or longitudinal grooves, "coffee bean"
  - Mitotic activity allowed but no atypical mitoses
  - Focal, cytologically atypical cells do not change prognosis
- Scattered, osteoclast-type giant cells identified
- Variable nodules of amorphous basophilic to eosinophilic chondroid present (75%)
  - Mature hyaline cartilage rare
- Network of pericellular calcification: "Chicken wire" calcification (~ 30%)
- Special stains
  - S100 and vimentin positive
  - Reticulin outlines each individual cell
  - Focal positive staining with cytokeratin
- Secondary aneurysmal bone cyst in > 1/3 of cases

Predominant Pattern/Injury Type

- Sheets

Predominant Cell/Compartment Type

- Cartilaginous

DIFFERENTIAL DIAGNOSIS

Chondromyxoid Fibroma

- Involves metaphysis not epiphysis

Giant Cell Tumor

- Radiographically lacks sclerotic border
- Lacks calcification and chondroid differentiation

Langerhans Cell Histiocytosis

- CD1a positive
- Associated, mixed, inflammatory infiltrate

Chondrosarcoma

- Cellular pleomorphism with prominent nucleoli
- Lacks sheets of uniform cells

Chondroblastic Osteosarcoma

- CT imaging shows bony expansion with periosteal reaction
- Cellular pleomorphism with atypical mitotic figures
- Malignant osteoid production

DIAGNOSTIC CHECKLIST

Pathologic Interpretation Pearls

- Uniform, small, oval cells with longitudinal groove
- Foci of eosinophilic chondroid in majority of cases
- "Chicken wire" calcification in 30%
- S100 immunostain positive

SELECTED REFERENCES

1. de Silva MV et al: Chondroblastoma: varied histologic appearance, potential diagnostic pitfalls, and clinicopathologic features associated with local recurrence. Ann Diagn Pathol. 7(4):205-13, 2003
2. Jain M et al: Cytological features of chondroblastoma: a case report with review of the literature. Diagn Cytopathol. 23(5):348-50, 2000
3. Kilpatrick SE et al: Chondroblastoma of bone: use of fine-needle aspiration biopsy and potential diagnostic pitfalls. Diagn Cytopathol. 16(1):65-71, 1997
4. Turcotte RE et al: Chondroblastoma. Hum Pathol. 24(9):944-9, 1993
5. Edel G et al: Chondroblastoma of bone. A clinical, radiological, light and immunohistochemical study. Virchows Arch A Pathol Anat Histopathol. 421(4):355-66, 1992
6. Kurt AM et al: Chondroblastoma of bone. Hum Pathol. 20(10):965-76, 1989
7. Kunze E et al: Histology and biology of metastatic chondroblastoma. Report of a case with a review of the literature. Pathol Res Pract. 182(1):113-23, 1987

CHONDROBLASTOMA

Radiologic and Microscopic Features

(Left) *Radiograph shows a well-defined, lytic lesion in the femoral epiphysis with a sclerotic rim.* ***(Right)*** *Hematoxylin & eosin shows sheets of uniform lesional cells with giant cells ➙ and islands of eosinophilic chondroid matrix ➙.*

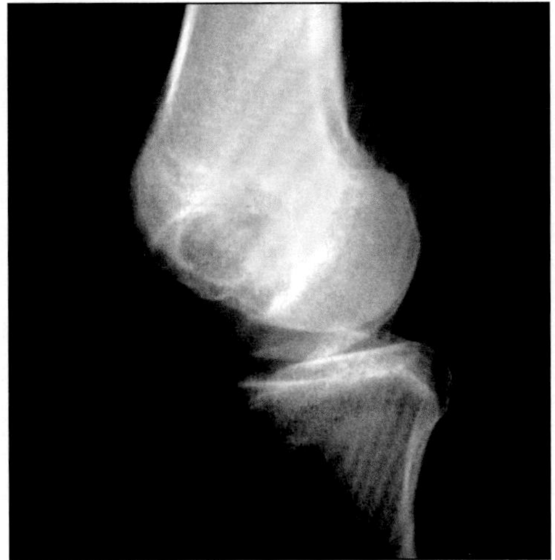

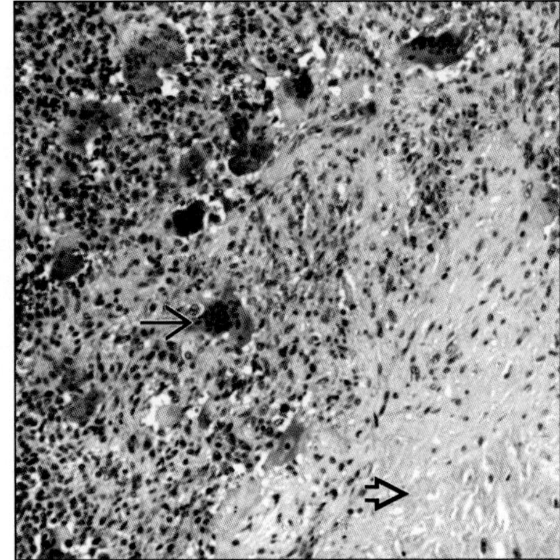

(Left) *Hematoxylin & eosin shows sheets of lesional cells separated by a fine network of "chicken wire" calcification ➙. Prominent nuclear grooves ➙ are present.* ***(Right)*** *Lesional cells have discrete cell borders. A reticulin stain can be used to outline each individual tumor cell.*

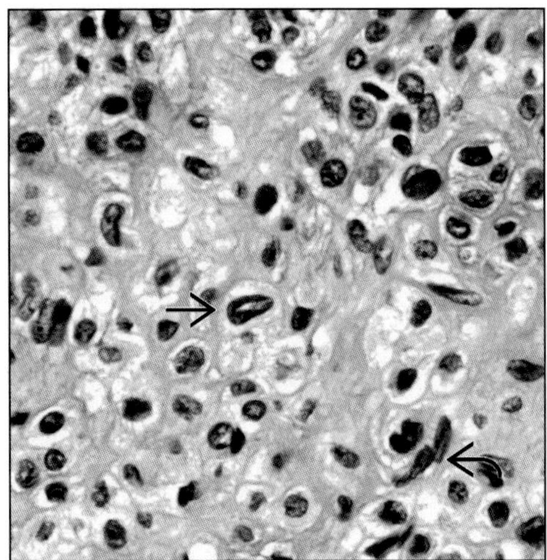

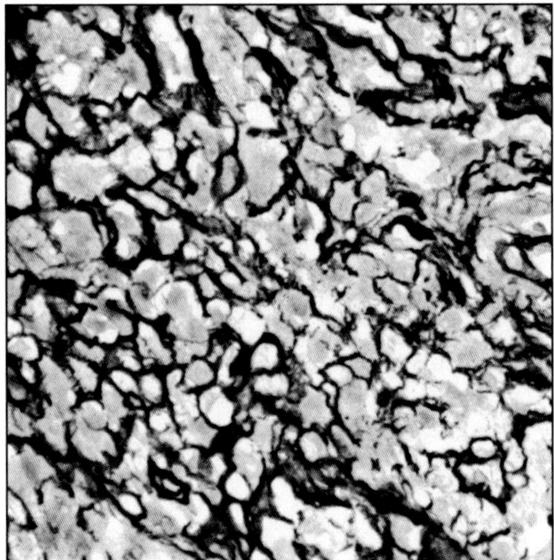

(Left) *Hematoxylin & eosin shows islands of metaplastic osteoid ➙. Unlike osteosarcoma, the surrounding cells in a chondroblastoma are uniform and lack significant cytologic atypia.* ***(Right)*** *Hematoxylin & eosin shows a chondroblastoma with a secondary aneurysmal bone cyst, which is characterized by large, blood-filled spaces ➙ adjacent to sheets of lesional chondroblasts.*

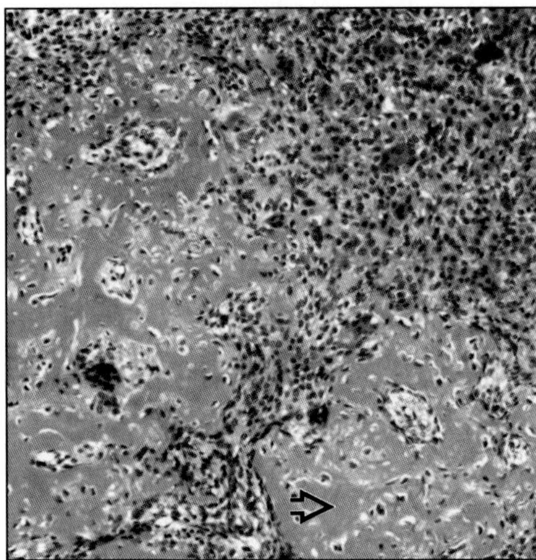

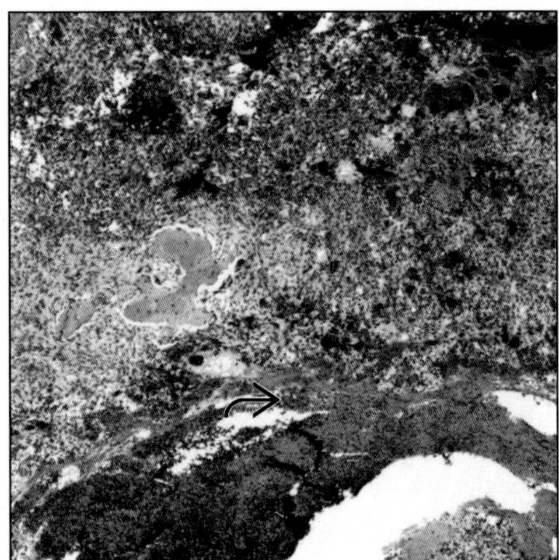

Differential Diagnosis

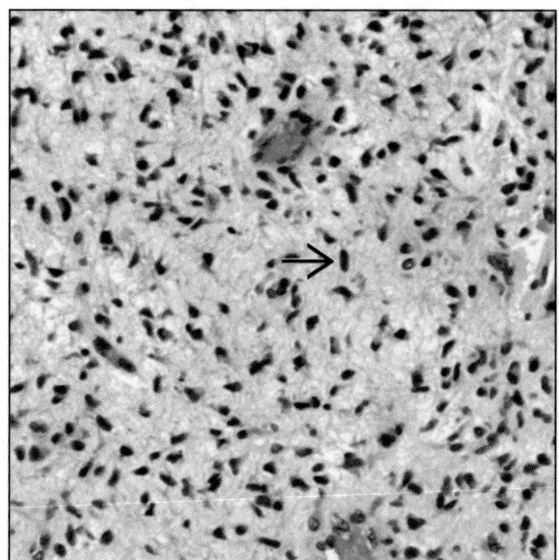

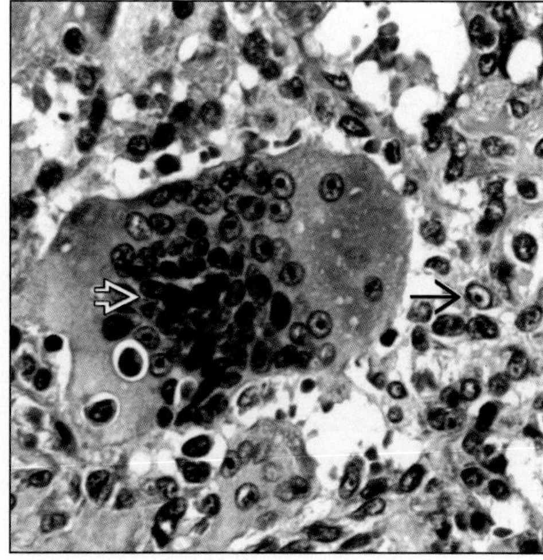

(Left) *Hematoxylin & eosin of chondromyxoid fibroma shows oval to spindled cells ➙ scattered within a myxoid stroma.* ***(Right)*** *Hematoxylin & eosin of a giant cell tumor shows scattered lesional cells with distinct nucleoli ➙ rather than grooves. Lesional cells have variable cytoplasm and irregular borders. Giant cells with numerous nuclei ➙, which are identical to those in the single cells, are prominent.*

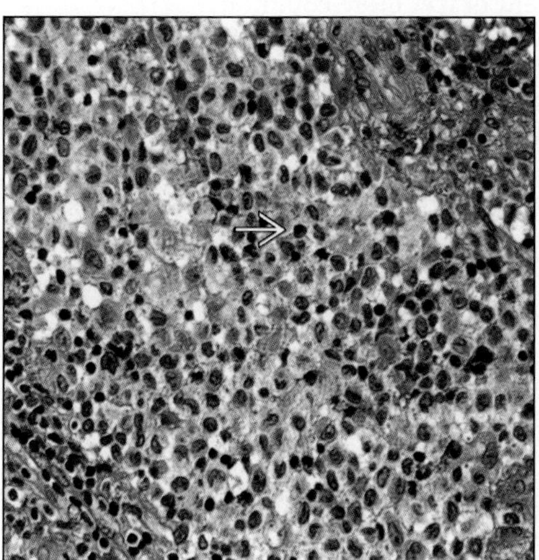

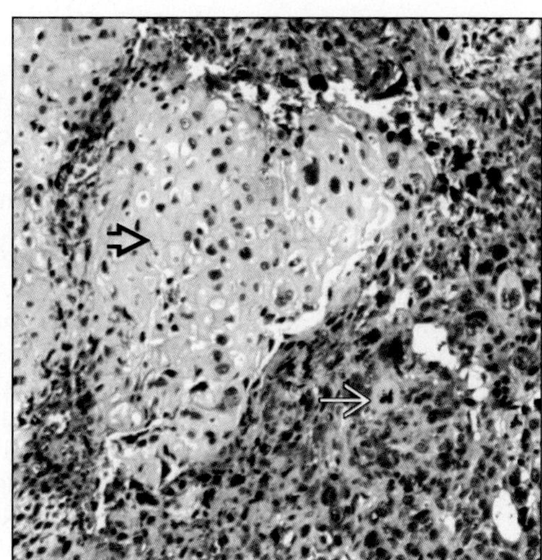

(Left) *Hematoxylin & eosin of Langerhans cell histiocytosis shows sheets of cells with longitudinal grooves. A mixed inflammatory infiltrate with eosinophils ➙ is present. Calcification and chondroid matrix are absent.* ***(Right)*** *Hematoxylin & eosin of an osteosarcoma shows markedly pleomorphic cells, loose and embedded in a chondroid matrix ➙. Prominent atypical mitoses ➙ are present. A malignant osteoid, though not seen, must be present.*

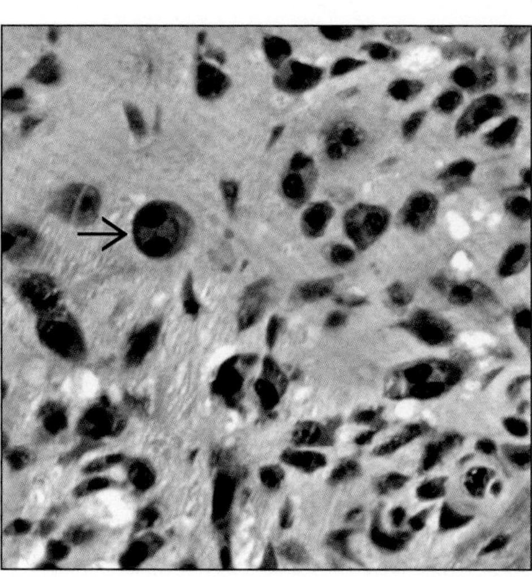

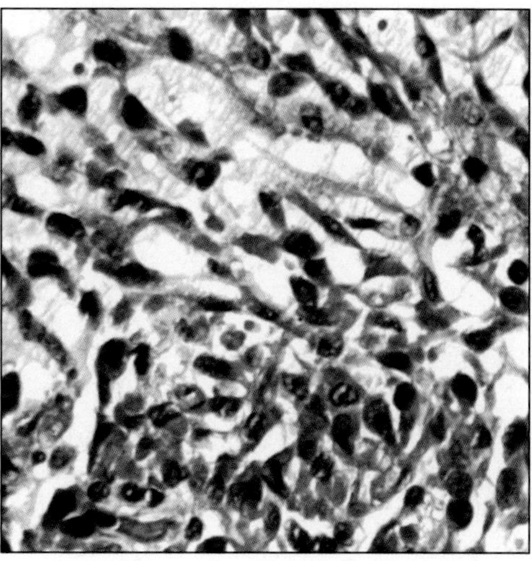

(Left) *Hematoxylin & eosin of a chondrosarcoma shows lesional cells with atypical nuclear features, including binucleation ➙ embedded in a chondroid matrix.* ***(Right)*** *Hematoxylin & eosin of a chondrosarcoma shows pleomorphic chondrocytes with prominent nucleoli streaming through a chondromyxoid background. Chondrosarcomas lack sheets of uniform cells with distinct borders and nuclear grooves.*

CHONDROMYXOID FIBROMA

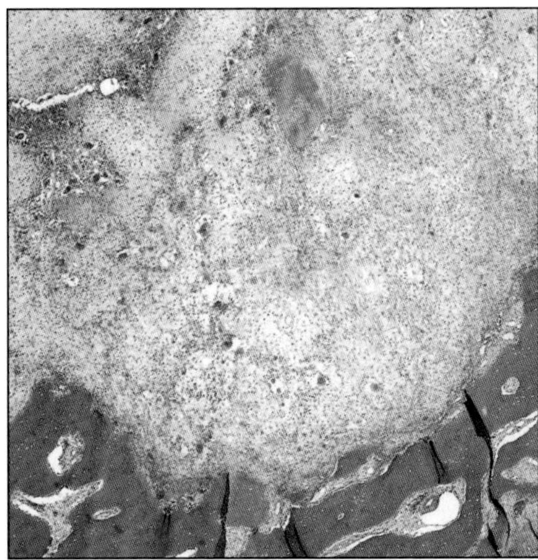

H&E stained section shows a lobulated growth pattern of chondromyxoid fibroma at low power, with central areas of loose myxoid stroma and scattered osteoclastic giant cells.

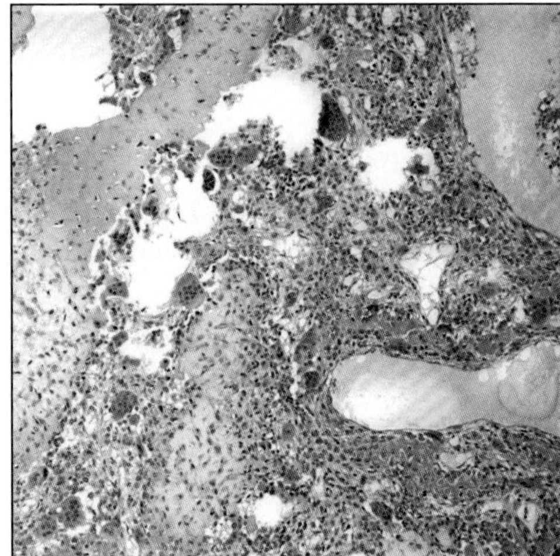

H&E stained section shows increased cellularity at the periphery of a chondromyxoid fibroma, including scattered giant cells and cells with long processes arranged in a reticular pattern.

TERMINOLOGY

Abbreviations

- Chondromyxoid fibroma (CMF)

Synonyms

- Fibromyxoid chondroma, myxofibrous chondroma

Definitions

- Rare, benign intramedullary tumor composed of immature myxoid mesenchymal tissue with features of primitive cartilaginous differentiation

ETIOLOGY/PATHOGENESIS

Pathogenesis

- Originates from cartilage-forming connective tissue

CLINICAL ISSUES

Epidemiology

- Incidence
  - Rare, < 1% of bone tumors
- Age
  - Wide age range with peak in 2nd and 3rd decades
    - 75% occur in patients younger than 30 years
- Gender
  - Male predominance (M:F = 2:1)
- Ethnicity
  - No racial predilection

Site

- Lower extremities more common than upper extremities
- 60% occur in long bones
  - Around knee (50%)
    - Distal femur common location
  - Proximal tibia (30%)
- Short tubular bones of hands and feet (25%)
  - Involvement of feet more common
- Pelvis (8%)
- Almost always metaphyseal (95%)
- Distribution can be widespread, however, with involvement of cranium and bones of hands
  - Lesions that occur in spine and sacrum, although uncommon, tend to be more aggressive

Presentation

- Pain
  - Most common complaint at presentation
  - Tends to be mild and chronic
  - Regional tenderness is typically only finding on physical examination
- Local swelling is often present when tumor involves small bone
  - Tumefaction may be found when tumor involves bones of hands or feet
- Occasionally lesion is asymptomatic and incidental radiologic finding

Natural History

- Benign tumor
- Can cause damage by continued growth and extension into soft tissues
- Malignant degeneration is rare
  - Reported in association with radiation therapy
- Recurrence can occur
  - Likely due to incomplete curettage
    - Less likely with implantation of allograft bone chips or polymethylmethacrylate
    - Tumors treated by excision do not recur
  - More common in young patients (< 20 years of age)

Treatment

- Surgical approaches
  - Curettage and bone grafting for stage 2 lesions
  - En bloc resection with marginal margin for stage 3 lesions
    - Ideal in cases of aggressive lesions where removal of tumor will not cause significant loss of function

CHONDROMYXOID FIBROMA

Key Facts

Terminology
- Rare, benign intramedullary tumor composed of immature myxoid mesenchymal tissue with features of primitive cartilaginous differentiation

Clinical Issues
- Rare, < 1% of bone tumors
- 75% occur in patients younger than 30 years of age
- Most common sites: Proximal tibia, distal femur, pelvis, and bones of feet
- Almost always metaphyseal
- Pain is most common complaint at presentation
- Curettage and bone grafting for stage 2 lesions
- En bloc resection with marginal margin for stage 3 lesions

Image Findings
- Eccentric, metaphyseal location
- Lucent with sharp, sclerotic, and scalloped margins
- Only rarely see matrix calcification

Macroscopic Features
- Resection specimens are lobulated with distinct margins
- Surrounding bone is sclerotic

Microscopic Pathology
- Lobulated pattern of growth
- Periphery of lobules are hypercellular
- Bland spindled and stellate-shaped cells

- Radiation therapy contraindicated due to risk of malignant transformation

Prognosis
- Recurrence is rare

IMAGE FINDINGS

Radiographic Findings
- Round to ovoid eccentric lytic lesion within metaphysis
- Geographic pattern of bone destruction
- Lucent with sharp, sclerotic, and scalloped margins
  - In small tubular bones, soft tissue extension may be present, but periosteum is intact
- Occasionally see septa within lesion
- Only rarely see matrix calcification
- No visible periosteal reaction (unless fractured)
- Can break through cortex and infiltrate into surrounding soft tissues (rare)

MR Findings
- Useful for determining soft tissue extension

CT Findings
- NECT
  - Well-defined lytic lesion, ± matrix calcification
  - Cortical expansion and soft tissue extension covered by thin layer of periosteal new bone
  - Most sensitive modality for visualizing presence of chondroid matrix calcification
- CECT: Enhancement

MACROSCOPIC FEATURES

General Features
- Translucent and blue-gray, sometimes resembling hyaline cartilage
  - Cartilage is softer than typical hyaline cartilage but is not viscous or liquid, as typically seen with myxoid areas of chondrosarcoma
- Resection specimens are lobulated with distinct margins
  - Surrounding bone is sclerotic

Size
- 1-10 cm; mean: 3-4 cm

MICROSCOPIC PATHOLOGY

Histologic Features
- Lobulated pattern of growth
  - Micro- or macrolobular
  - Periphery of lobules are hypercellular
    - May see giant cells
  - Well circumscribed
- Benign giant cells are present between lobules
- Myxoid stroma
  - Rarely see well-formed hyaline cartilage
- Solid cellular areas may contain ovoid cells resembling those seen in chondroblastoma
- Secondary changes, such as aneurysmal bone cyst, may be seen
- Necrosis and mitoses are not typical findings

Cytologic Features
- Bland spindled and stellate-shaped cells
  - Rare nuclei appear atypical
    - Larger cells with hyperchromatic nuclei but preserved nuclear to cytoplasmic ratio (pseudomalignant or pseudoanaplastic cells)
  - Tumor cells have long processes which form reticular pattern

ANCILLARY TESTS

Cytology
- Hypercellular chondromyxoid fragments always present
  - Stellate to spindle-shaped cells embedded in metachromatic chondromyxoid stroma
- Low smear cellularity

CHONDROMYXOID FIBROMA

- May see mild nuclear atypia
- High-power view of stellate and spindled cells may show foamy cytoplasm
- Giant cells are common

Immunohistochemistry

- Spindle cells at rim of myxoid or chondroid matrix of CMF are myofibroblastic cells
  - Immunoreactive for smooth muscle actin, muscle-specific actin, desmin, H-caldesmon, and calponin
- Myxoid and chondroid matrix
  - Matrix cells are immunoreactive for SOX9, S100, and collagen type II
    - Collagen staining can be quite variable

Cytogenetics

- Abnormalities of chromosome 6 are common
  - Rearrangement of long arm of chromosome 6 at bands q13 and q25
  - Pericentric inversions
    - Inv(6)(p25;q13)
    - Inv(6)(p25;q23)
  - Rearrangements in 3 distinct breakpoint cluster regions
    - 6p23-p25, 6q12-q15, and 6q23-q27
- Clonal translocation t(1;5)(p13;p13)
- Aberrations in chromosomes 2 and 5
- Gain of 13q and losses of 1p, 12q, 16p, 17p, 19p, 19q, 20q, and 22q

DIFFERENTIAL DIAGNOSIS

Benign Lesions

- **Chondroblastoma**
  - Epiphyseal lesion
  - Not characterized by lobular growth pattern with peripheral hypercellularity
  - Calcified matrix in 50%
  - Most common complaint is history of several months to years of pain involving joint
    - May be accompanied by swelling, decreased mobility, or gait abnormality
  - Most occur in long bones
    - Temporal bone and calcaneus are also common sites
- **Enchondroma**
  - Contains true hyaline cartilage
  - Tumor cells are round
  - Painless, often discovered incidentally
  - Associated with Maffucci and Ollier syndromes
  - Centrally located
    - Intramedullary lesion with rarification and variable amounts of mineralization
    - Ring calcifications
- **Fibrous dysplasia with myxoid change**
  - Absence of lobular architecture
  - Associated with trabeculae of immature woven bone that lack osteoblastic rimming
  - Central location
  - Internal septations rare
  - No periosteal reaction

Malignant Lesions

- **Chondrosarcoma**
  - Associated with hyaline cartilage and pools of viscous liquid myxoid matrix
  - Permeates surrounding bone, both microscopically and radiographically
    - Cortical destruction
    - Soft tissue extension
  - Majority of patients in 4th through 6th decades of life
- **Chondroblastic osteosarcoma**
  - Contains hyaline cartilage, may be focal
  - Atypical spindle cells
    - Dense and sheet-like and associated with osteoid
  - Absence of lobular architecture
  - Malignant radiographic appearance

DIAGNOSTIC CHECKLIST

Pathologic Interpretation Pearls

- Benign neoplasm composed of nodules with myxoid matrix and spindled to stellate spindle cells
- Always have benign appearance
- Lobular pattern of growth

STAGING

Surgical Staging for Benign Musculoskeletal Tumors

- Stage 1: Latent
- Stage 2: Active
- Stage 3: Aggressive

SELECTED REFERENCES

1. Konishi E et al: Immunohistochemical analysis for Sox9 reveals the cartilaginous character of chondroblastoma and chondromyxoid fibroma of the bone. Hum Pathol. 41(2):208-13, 2010
2. Bergman S et al: Fine-needle aspiration biopsy of chondromyxoid fibroma: an investigation of four cases. Am J Clin Pathol. 132(5):740-5, 2009
3. Lersundi A et al: Chondromyxoid fibroma: a rarely encountered and puzzling tumor. Clin Orthop Relat Res. 439:171-5, 2005
4. Tallini G et al: Correlation between clinicopathological features and karyotype in 100 cartilaginous and chordoid tumours. A report from the Chromosomes and Morphology (CHAMP) Collaborative Study Group. J Pathol. 196(2):194-203, 2002
5. Dürr HR et al: Chondromyxoid fibroma of bone. Arch Orthop Trauma Surg. 120(1-2):42-7, 2000
6. Wu CT et al: Chondromyxoid fibroma of bone: a clinicopathologic review of 278 cases. Hum Pathol. 29(5):438-46, 1998

Diagrammatic and Other Features

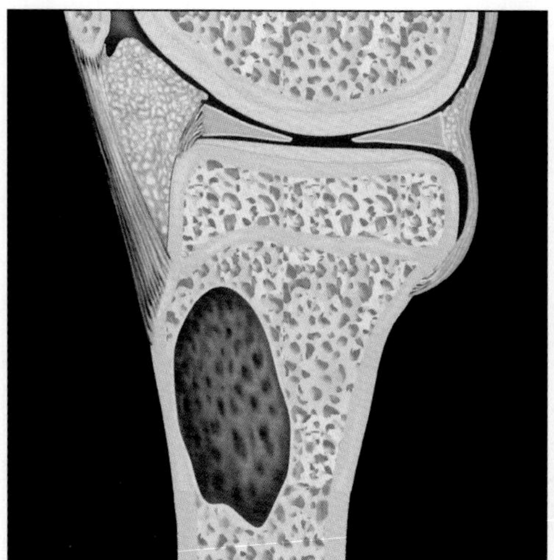

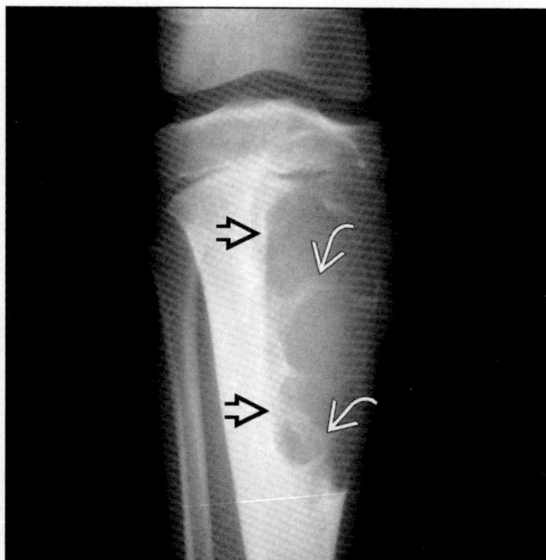

*(**Left**) Sagittal graphic of chondromyxoid fibroma shows a lytic, slightly lobulated lesion with thin sclerotic margin involving the tibial metaphysis. (**Right**) Anteroposterior radiograph of the knee shows a radiolucent lobulated lesion in tibial metadiaphysis, exhibiting a geographic type of bone destruction, sclerotic scalloped borders ➩, and internal septa ➦.*

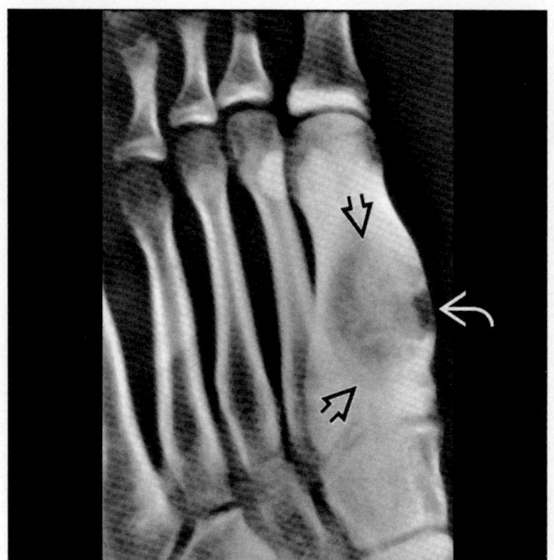

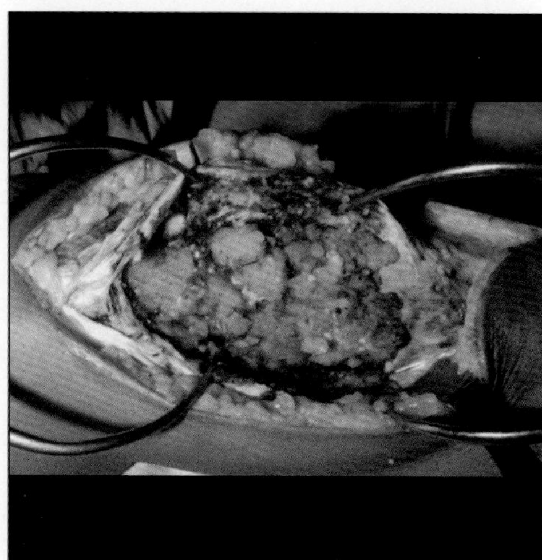

*(**Left**) Anteroposterior radiograph of the left foot shows a radiolucent slightly lobulated lesion with thin sclerotic margins ➩ in the 1st metatarsal bone. Note the focal cortical disruption ➦, which led to pain and local swelling. (**Right**) Intraoperative photograph of a chondromyxoid fibroma shows a cartilaginous, lobulated, well-marginated mass.*

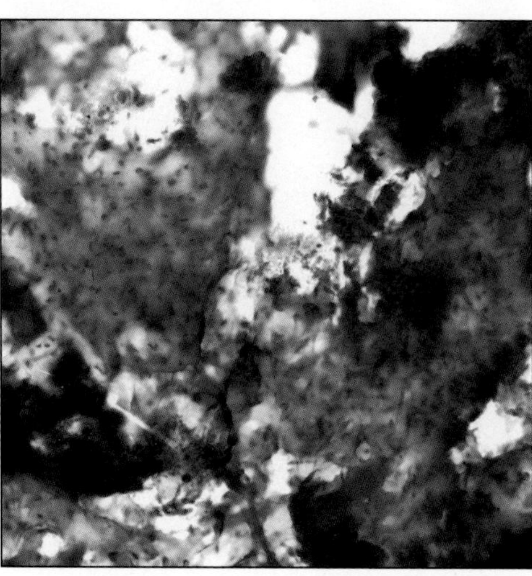

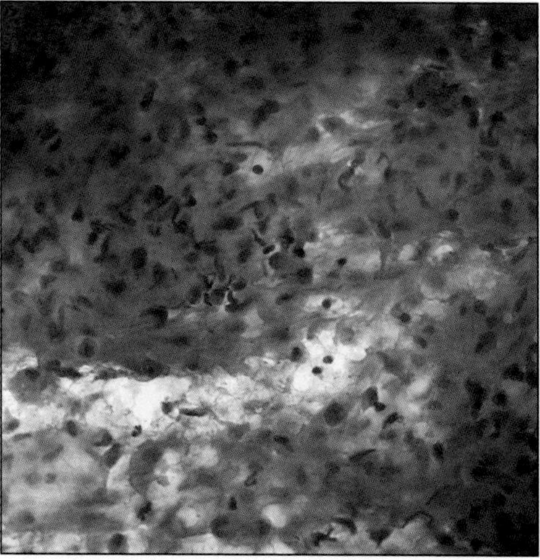

*(**Left**) Smear preparation shows hypercellular chondromyxoid fragments consisting of bland stellate- to spindle-shaped cells embedded in a chondromyxoid stroma. (**Right**) High-power view of smear preparation highlights the bland nature of spindled and stellate cells in a myxoid background. The nuclear to cytoplasmic ratio should not be increased and typically no cellular atypia or pleomorphism are present.*

CHONDROMYXOID FIBROMA

Microscopic Features

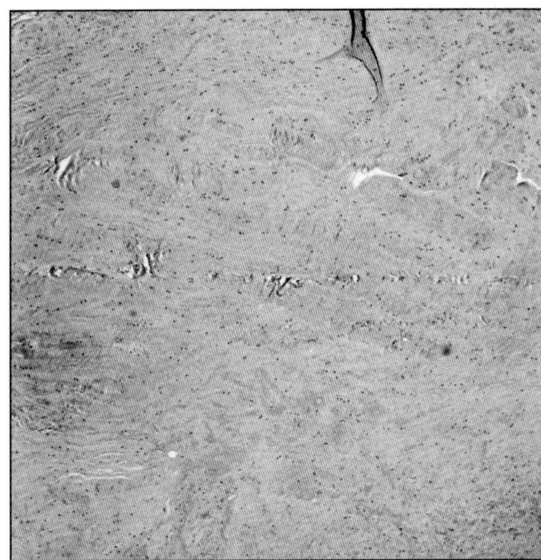
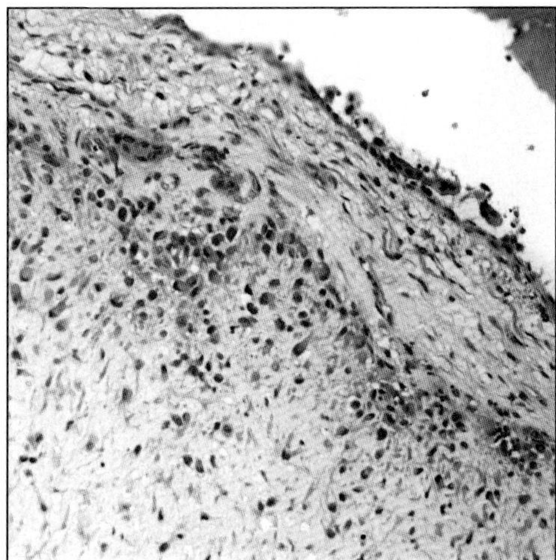

(Left) *Low-power view of a chondromyxoid fibroma shows a bland lesion composed of inconspicuous, bland stellate and spindled cells scattered throughout a myxoid background.* ***(Right)*** *Section of chondromyxoid fibroma shows more cellularity at the periphery of the lesion with collections of spindled to stellate cells with polygonal nuclei, fine chromatin, and eosinophilic cytoplasmic extensions.*

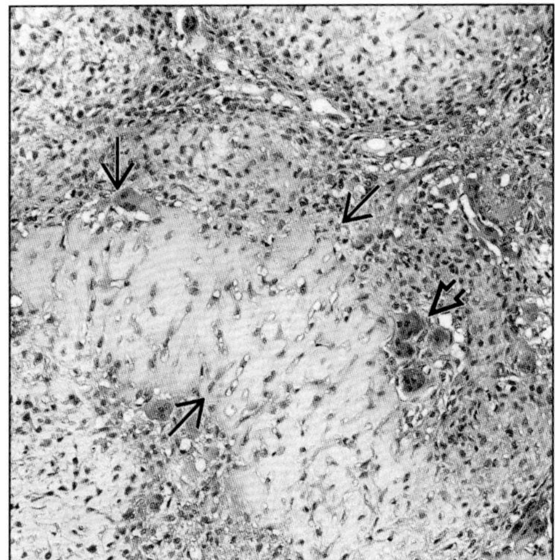
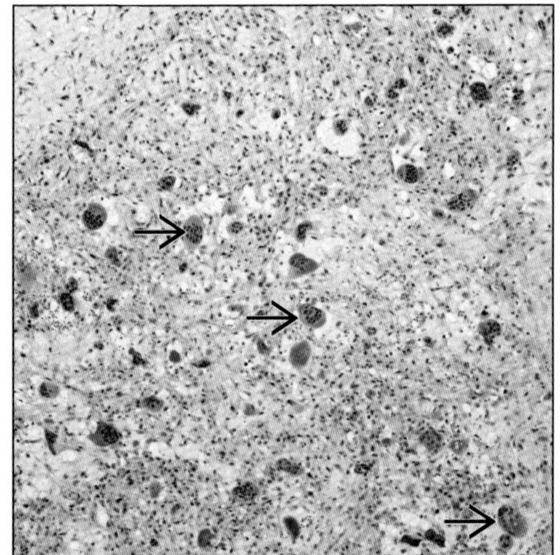

(Left) *This section shows a central area of ill-defined cartilage ⇒ surrounded by lobules of loose myxoid stroma. Note the clusters of osteoclastic giant cells ⇨.* ***(Right)*** *Chondromyxoid fibroma with larger numbers of scattered osteoclastic giant cells ⇒ is shown here.*

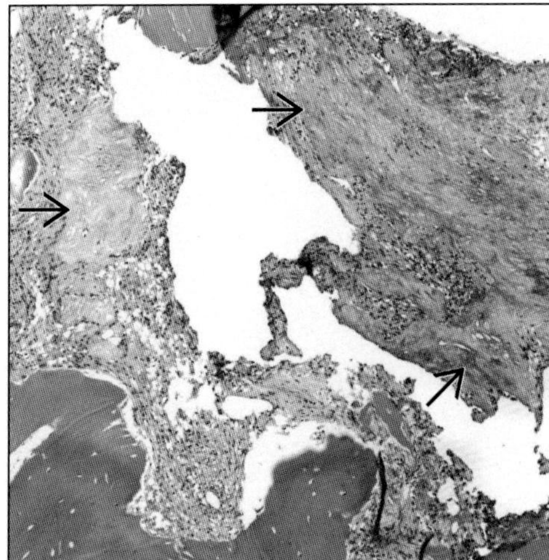
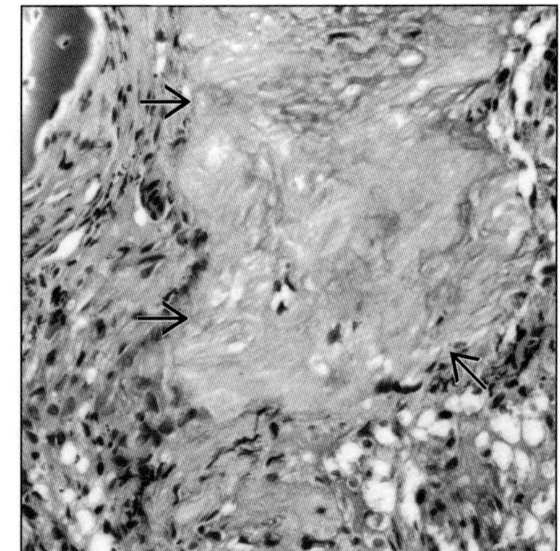

(Left) *At higher magnification, chondromyxoid fibroma has a chondroid appearance in the central portion of the tumor lobules ⇒.* ***(Right)*** *High-power view shows an island of myxoid matrix ⇒ surrounded by bland spindled cells.*

Differential Diagnosis

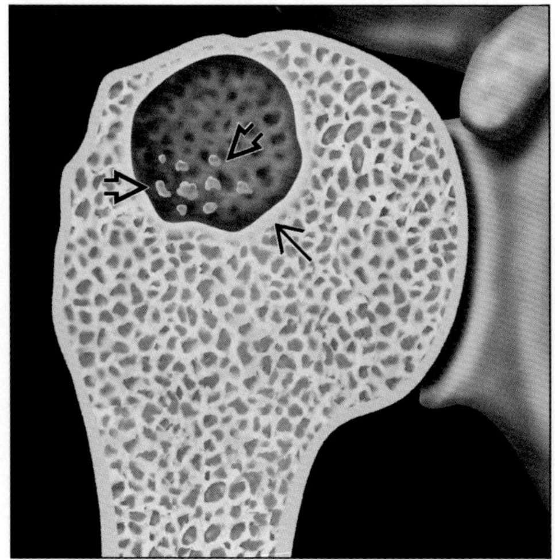

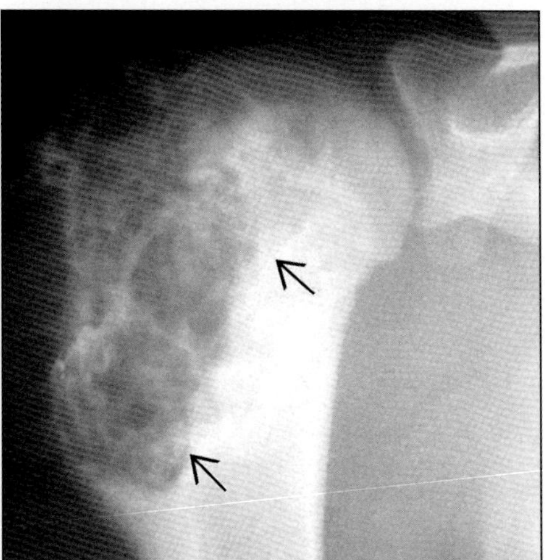

***(Left)** Coronal graphic of a chondroblastoma shows lytic epiphyseal lesion with chondroid matrix ⇨ involving the humeral head. Well-defined sclerotic margin is shown →. **(Right)** Anteroposterior radiograph of a chondroblastoma in the humeral epiphysis shows a multilobulated, lytic, expansile lesion → with a chondroid matrix (complex-appearing, stippled internal calcifications). Such matrix calcification is rare in chondromyxoid fibromas and helps distinguish the 2 lesions.*

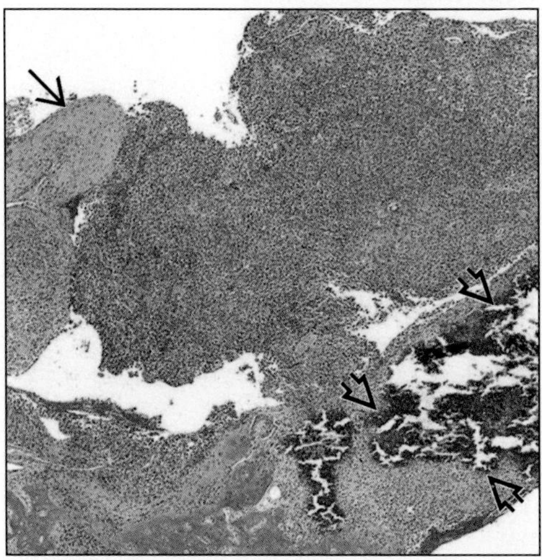

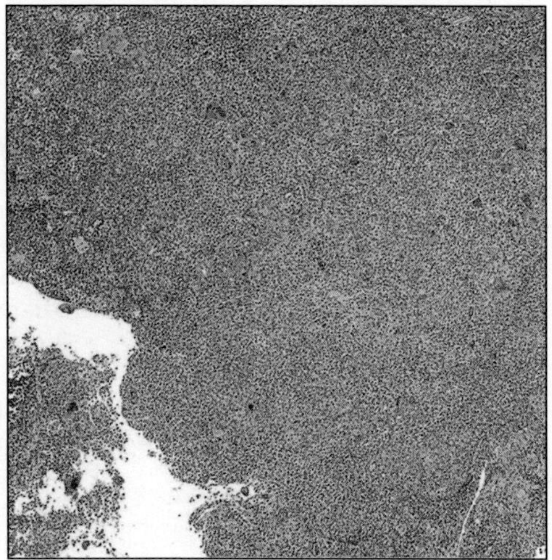

***(Left)** Low-power view of chondroblastoma shows a highly cellular lesion with peripheral zones of amphophilic fibrochondroid matrix → and areas of delicate pericellular or "chicken-wire" calcification ⇨. **(Right)** Low-power view shows a solid area of a chondroblastoma composed of sheets of round to ovoid cells admixed with osteoclast-like giant cells.*

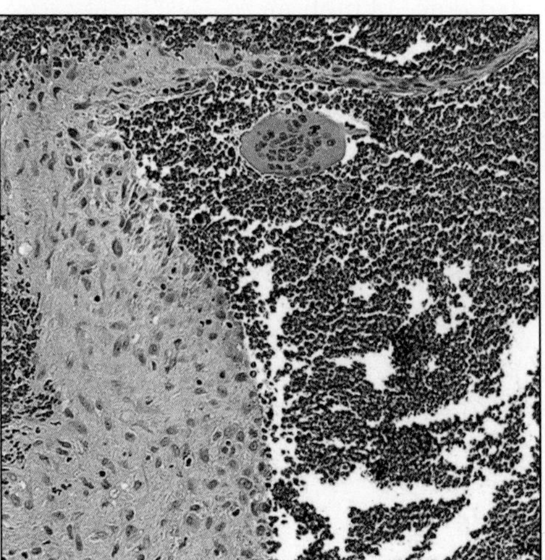

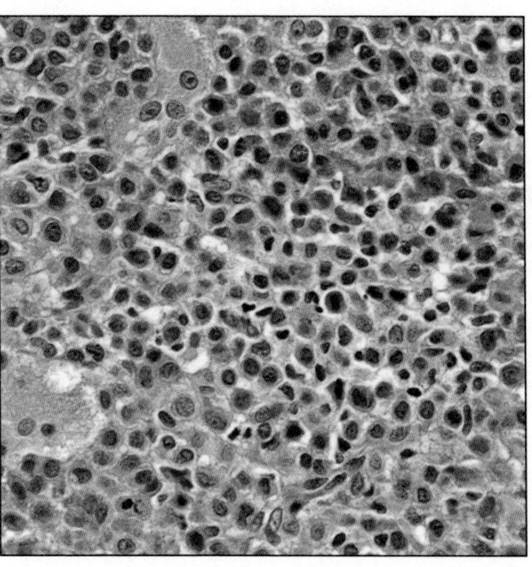

***(Left)** This photomicrograph shows a secondary aneurysmal bone cyst complicating a chondroblastoma. **(Right)** High-power view highlights the mononuclear cells of chondroblastoma. Some cells contain eccentric nuclei with abundant eosinophilic cytoplasm.*

OSTEOID OSTEOMA

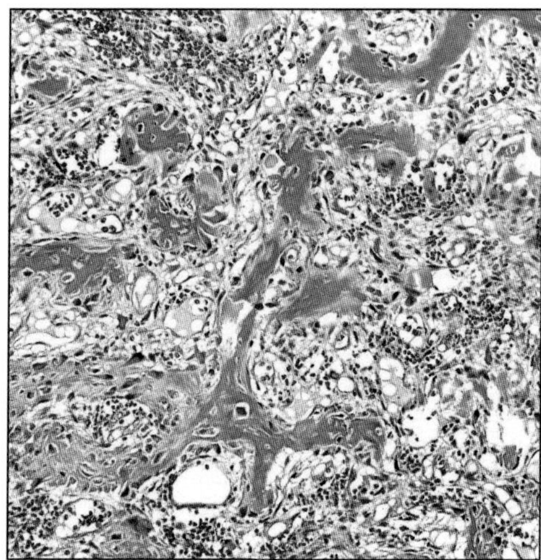

Nidus shows an interlacing network of osteoid and bony trabeculae with variable mineralization.

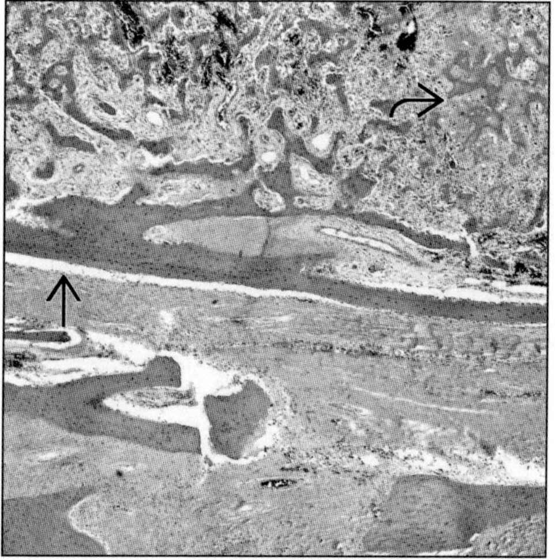

Low-power magnification shows a well-circumscribed nidus surrounded by reactive sclerosis ➡. Varying degrees of osteoid mineralization can be visualized within the nidus ➡.

TERMINOLOGY

Abbreviations

- Osteoid osteoma (OO)

Definitions

- Benign bone-forming neoplasm
- Characterized by limited growth potential
- Usually less than 1 cm in dimension

CLINICAL ISSUES

Epidemiology

- Incidence
  - 2-3% of all bone tumors
  - 10-20% of benign bone tumors
- Age
  - Predominates between ages of 5-20 years
- Gender
  - More common in males
    - M:F ratio = 2-3:1
- Ethnicity
  - Rare in African-American population

Site

- 65-80% of lesions occur in metaphysis or diaphysis of long bones (cortical)
  - Femur/tibia: 53-60%
  - Rare localizations
    - Intramedullary
    - Subperiosteal
    - Epiphyseal
    - Apophyseal
- 20% occur in short bones of hands and feet
  - Phalanges are most common sites, followed by carpal bones
- Approximately 10% occur in spine
  - Posterior elements: 90%
  - Vertebral body: 10%
- Extremely rare in skull and facial bones

Presentation

- Pain
  - Nocturnal
  - Localized and continuous
  - Relieved by aspirin or other nonsteroidal anti-inflammatory drugs (NSAIDs)
    - Pain relief usually occurs within 30 minutes
  - Exacerbated by alcohol intake
  - Mediated by 2 major factors
    - Presence of nerve endings in tumor
    - High levels of prostaglandins within nidus, which produce inflammatory reaction
- Symptoms in specific locations
  - Proximal femoral shaft
    - Pain may be referred to knee joint
  - Intraarticular
    - Present with 1 or more symptoms of arthritis, including pain, soft tissue swelling, joint effusion, or decreased range of motion
  - Lesions adjacent to growth plates
    - Over time leads to growth disturbances with subsequent limb length inequality or axial deviation
  - Spinal lesions
    - May present as stiff scoliosis or lordosis
    - Pain often mimics radiculopathy of disc herniation secondary to paravertebral muscle spasm
- Tenderness over site of involvement
- May be localized swelling
  - Especially when lesion involves superficially located bone such as tibia
- Involved extremity may show disuse atrophy

Laboratory Tests

- Elevated urinary excretion of major prostacyclin metabolite (2,3-dinor-6-keto-PGF1α)
  - Returns to normal after removal of nidus

OSTEOID OSTEOMA

Key Facts

Terminology
- Benign bone-forming neoplasm
- Usually less than 1 cm in dimension
- Characterized by limited growth potential

Clinical Issues
- Accounts for 2-3% of all bone tumors
- Predominates between ages of 5-20 years
- More common in males
- Typically associated with nocturnal pain that is often relieved by aspirin or other NSAIDs
- More than 50% occur in long bones of lower extremity, particularly femur and tibia
- Lesion is typically cortico-diaphyseal or metaphyseal
- Not associated with malignant transformation
- Lesions may spontaneously regress

Image Findings
- Area of cortical thickening and sclerosis containing lucent nidus of less than 1 cm

Macroscopic Features
- Nidus consists of sharply demarcated, round, red granular area
- Surrounding sclerotic bone has appearance of ivory

Microscopic Pathology
- Interlacing network of osteoid and bony trabeculae, with variable mineralization
- Sharply demarcated from surrounding sclerotic bone

- Normal CBC
  - White blood count elevated with infectious process
- Normal erythrocyte sedimentation rate (ESR)
  - Typically elevated with infectious process
  - May be elevated with malignant lesions

Natural History
- Many cases have been reported in which injury precedes onset of lesion
- No growth progression
- Not associated with malignant transformation
- Lesions may spontaneously regress
  - Average time to regression is 6 years

Treatment
- Surgical approaches
  - En-bloc surgical excision of lesion
    - Can be difficult to localize nidus because of surrounding reactive bone
    - Large portion of bone must be excised to ensure complete removal of nidus
  - Curettage
    - Removes less bone than en bloc excision
    - Nidus can be visualized, curetted, and treated with a high-speed burr to ensure complete removal
    - Intraoperative use of tetracycline fluorescence or bone scintigraphy can often aid in locating lesion
  - CT-guided techniques: Simple and effective ways to treat OOs, especially in small children
    - Radiofrequency ablation
    - Laser ablation
- Drugs
  - Primary goal of treatment is pain control
    - NSAIDs are effective in approximately 50% of patients

Prognosis
- Complete removal of nidus results in cure
  - Associated with immediate resolution of pain
- Incomplete nidus removal has been associated with recurrence
- To date, there have not been any documented reports of an OO undergoing malignant change

IMAGE FINDINGS

Radiographic Findings
- Cortical lesion
  - Radiolucent central nidus
    - Less than 1.0 cm
    - Surrounding dense sclerosis
  - Periosteal reaction may be present
- Cancellous/intraarticular lesion
  - Mild reactive sclerosis
  - Joint effusion, synovitis
- Subperiosteal lesion
  - Round soft tissue mass adjacent to cortex
  - Absence of surrounding reactive changes is common
- Lesions near growth plate may be associated with limb overgrowth
- Children mount more of sclerotic response than adults

Ultrasonographic Findings
- Color Doppler
  - Increased vascularity of nidus
  - Can be used to localize lesion for biopsy

MR Findings
- May show extensive bone marrow edema, which can obscure nidus
- Can show synovitis and joint effusion with intraarticular lesion

CT Findings
- Nonenhanced CT
  - Small, well-defined, round/oval nidus surrounded by sclerosis
  - Use thin sections, 1-2 mm
- Contrast-enhanced CT
  - Can be valuable in differentiation of OO from chronic osteomyelitis (Brodie abscess)
    - Osteoid osteoma: Dramatically enhancing central nidus
    - Chronic osteomyelitis: Relatively avascular

OSTEOID OSTEOMA

MACROSCOPIC FEATURES

General Features

- Nidus consists of sharply demarcated, round, red granular area
- Cortical lesions
  - Surrounding sclerotic bone has appearance of ivory
    - Thickened cortex
- Intramedullary lesions
  - Usually no associated sclerosis

MICROSCOPIC PATHOLOGY

Histologic Features

- Nidus
  - Interlacing network of osteoid and bony trabeculae
  - Variable mineralization
  - Central portion tends to be more mineralized than periphery
  - Sharply demarcated from surrounding sclerotic bone
- 2 histologic patterns associated with bony trabeculae associated with nidus
  - Thin and arranged in random tangle of anastomoses
  - Thickened
    - Shows cement lines that are suggestive of pagetoid bone
- Single layer of osteoblasts rim bony trabeculae
  - Small
  - Polygonal
  - Not cytologically atypical
- Intratrabecular spaces
  - Proliferation of capillaries
  - Scattered spindled fibroblasts
- Cartilaginous differentiation may be present
  - Unusual within nidus
- Adjacent synovium
  - Proliferation of lymphocytes and plasma cells

Cytologic Features

- Osteoblasts are small and polygonal
  - No cytological atypia

Predominant Pattern/Injury Type

- Not applicable

Predominant Cell/Compartment Type

- Osteogenic cell
- Bony trabeculae
- Fibroblast

ANCILLARY TESTS

Cytology

- Fine-needle aspiration diagnosis not commonly done for these lesions
  - Technically difficult in presence of sclerotic bone
  - If sample is obtained, it is composed of small osteoblasts and scattered fibroblasts

Cytogenetics

- Reported in only a handful of cases
  - Partial deletion of long arm of chromosome 22 [del(22)(q31.1)]
  - Loss of distal long arm of chromosome 17

DIFFERENTIAL DIAGNOSIS

Osteoblastoma

- Most common sites of involvement
  - Vertebral column
  - Long tubular bones
  - Jaw
- Always larger than 2 cm
- Rarely associated with nidus radiographically

Chronic Osteomyelitis (Brodie Abscess)

- Considered in radiographic differential diagnosis of OO
  - Presence of cortical destruction correlates with chronic osteomyelitis
- Classically present with pain and systemic symptoms, such as chills and fever
- Inflammatory infiltrate is composed mostly of plasma cells
- Bone marrow fibrosis consists of loose fibrous tissue, not spindle cell proliferation

Stress Fractures

- May simulate OO clinically and radiographically
- Show reactive new bone formation in form of fracture callus
- Lack rounded nidus-like characteristics of OO

DIAGNOSTIC CHECKLIST

Clinically Relevant Pathologic Features

- History of nocturnal pain relieved by NSAIDs

Pathologic Interpretation Pearls

- Nidus with interlacing network of osteoid and bony trabeculae

SELECTED REFERENCES

1. Aschero A et al: Percutaneous treatment of osteoid osteoma by laser thermocoagulation under computed tomography guidance in pediatric patients. Eur Radiol. 19(3):679-86, 2009
2. Malik AA et al: New techniques for localisation and excision of osteoid osteoma. J Hand Surg Eur Vol. 33(3):389-91, 2008
3. Ghanem I: The management of osteoid osteoma: updates and controversies. Curr Opin Pediatr. 18(1):36-41, 2006
4. Lee EH et al: Osteoid osteoma: a current review. J Pediatr Orthop. 26(5):695-700, 2006
5. Gebhardt MC et al: Case records of the Massachusetts General Hospital. Case 8-2005. A 10-year-old boy with pain in the right thigh. N Engl J Med. 352(11):1122-9, 2005

Diagrammatic and Radiologic Features

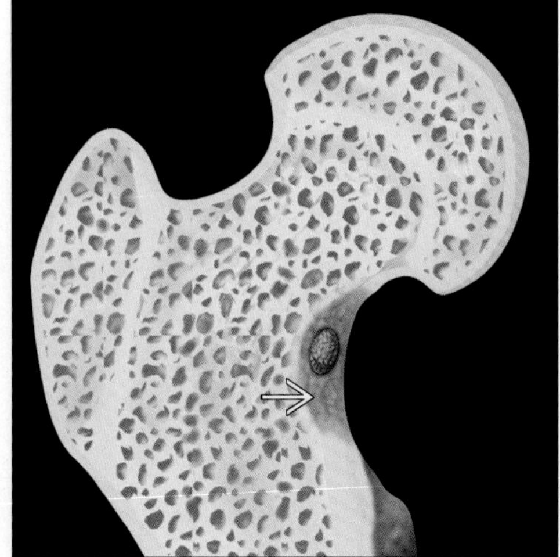

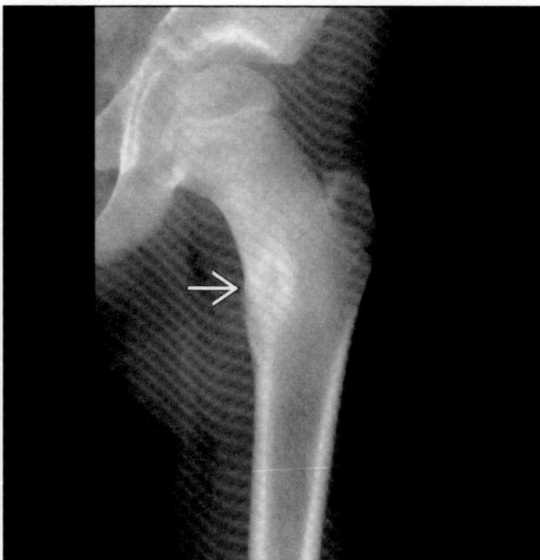

*(**Left**) Coronal graphic shows intracortical osteoid osteoma in the femoral neck. Nidus (in red) and surrounding sclerosis are shown ➡. (**Right**) Anteroposterior radiograph shows radiolucent nidus with surrounding sclerosis in the right femoral intertrochanteric region ➡.*

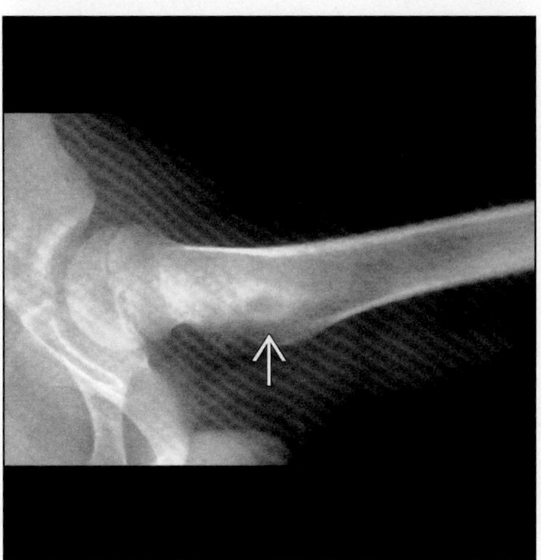

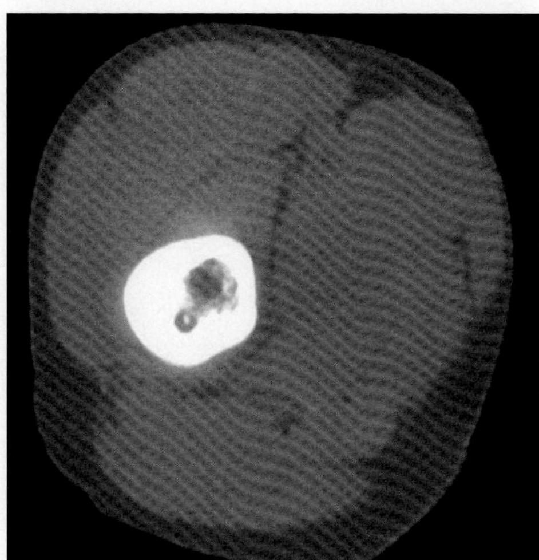

*(**Left**) Lateral radiograph shows radiolucent nidus with surrounding periosteal reaction in the proximal femoral metaphysis ➡. (**Right**) Axial CT scan shows radiolucent nidus with central sclerosis and surrounding periosteal reaction in the femoral cortex.*

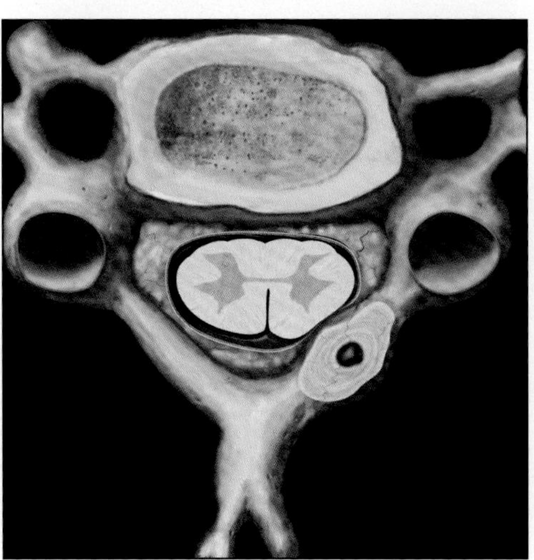

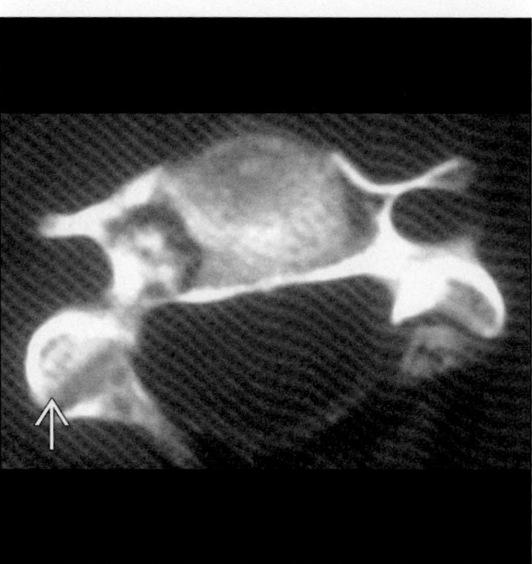

*(**Left**) Axial graphic shows a small, highly vascular tumor nidus of osteoid osteoma in the left lamina, surrounded by dense reactive bone. (**Right**) Axial NECT shows a low-attenuation nidus with central calcifications in the right pedicle of C4 extending into the lamina ➡.*

OSTEOID OSTEOMA

Gross and Microscopic Features

*(**Left**) Gross photograph shows round, sharply demarcated, reddish nidus, surrounded by sclerotic bone. (**Right**) Low-power magnification typically shows a well-circumscribed nidus surrounded by reactive sclerosis.*

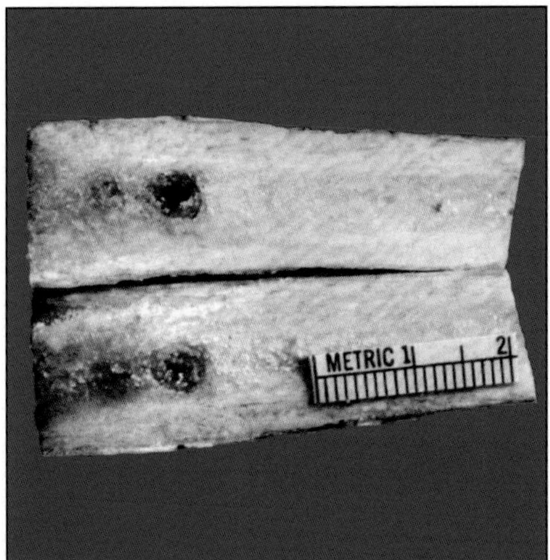

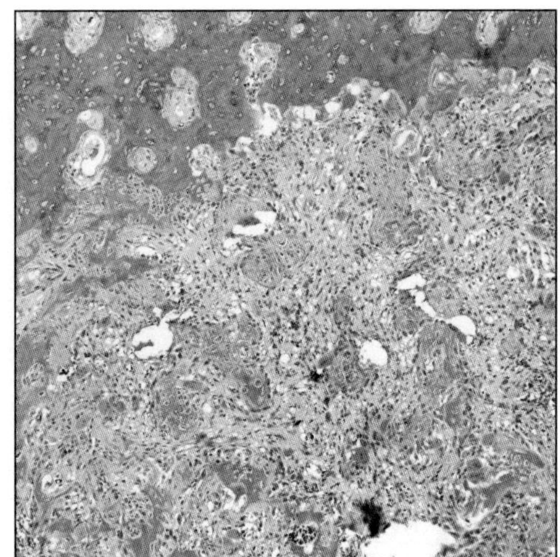

*(**Left**) Low-power magnification shows abrupt transition ⇒ from an area of reactive sclerosis to nidus characterized by an interlacing network of osteoid and bony trabeculae. (**Right**) This nidus contains numerous irregular bony trabeculae separated by intratrabecular spaces containing a proliferation of capillaries and scattered spindled fibroblasts.*

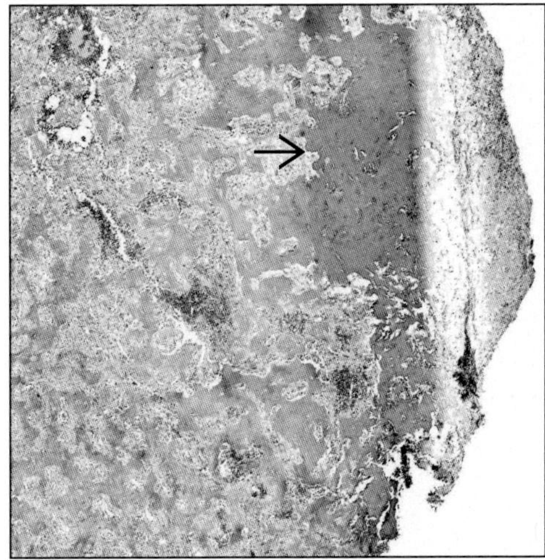

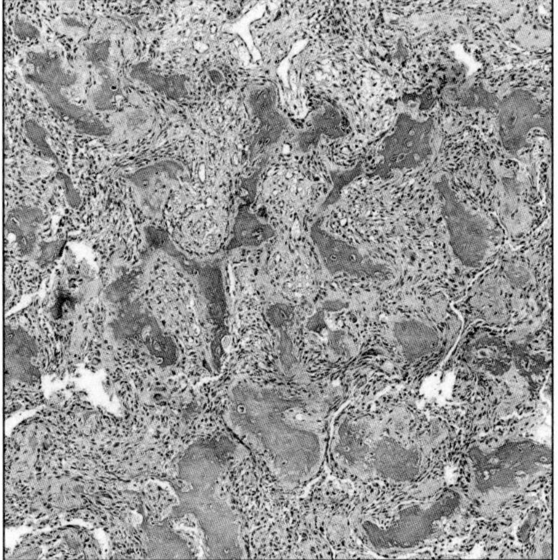

*(**Left**) Higher power magnification shows intratrabecular space filled with dilated capillaries ⇗ and scattered spindled fibroblasts. Bony trabecula is rimmed by single layer of small, polygonal osteoblasts ⇒. (**Right**) High-power magnification highlights the vascular nature of the nidus with numerous dilated capillaries ⇒.*

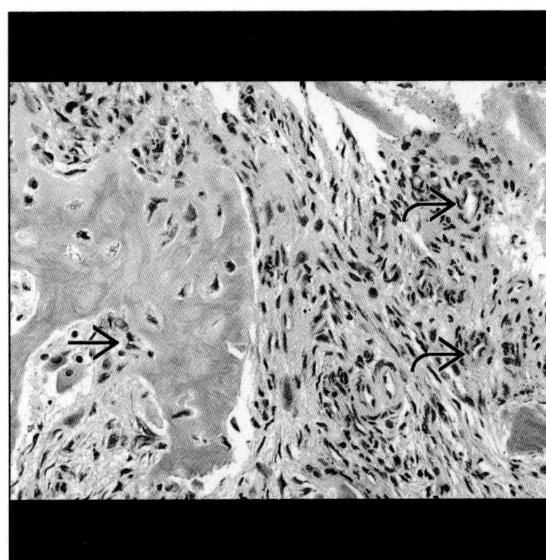

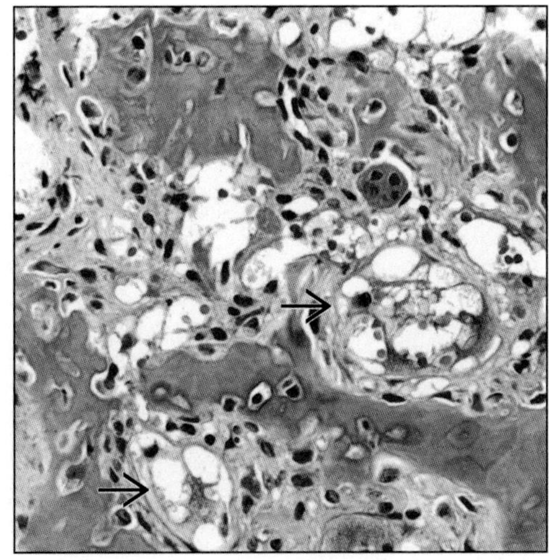

Differential Diagnosis

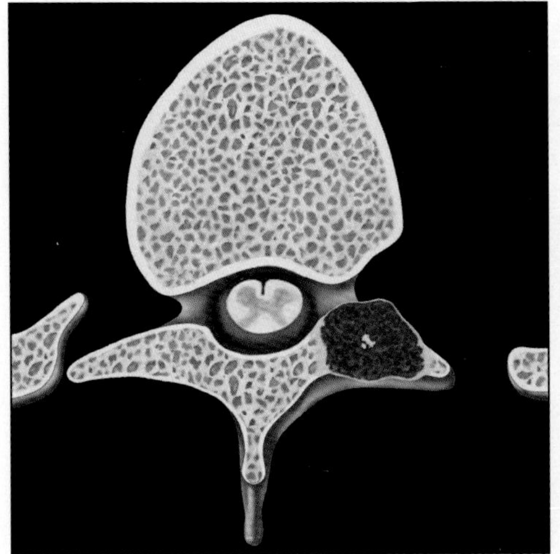

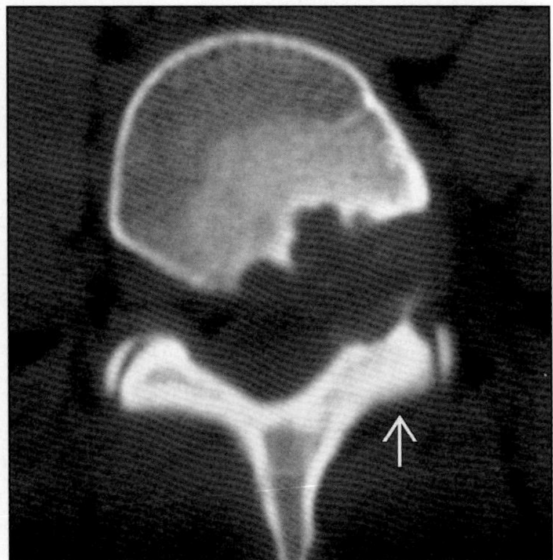

(Left) *Axial graphic shows an osteoblastoma (in red) involving the posterior elements. Central calcifications are shown in white.* ***(Right)*** *Axial NECT shows an expansile circumscribed lytic lesion with scalloped margins involving the vertebral body and posterior elements* ➔.

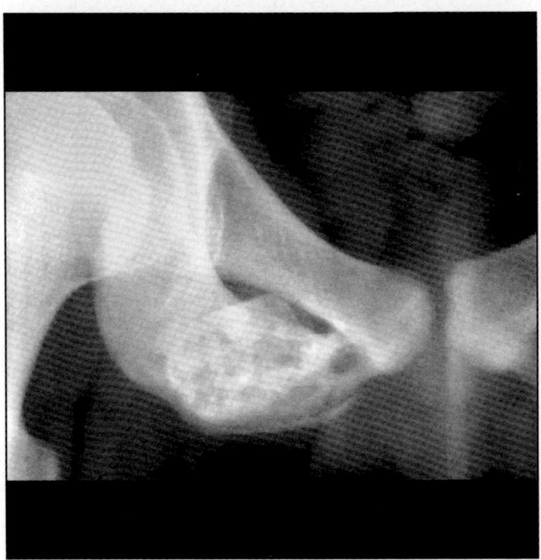

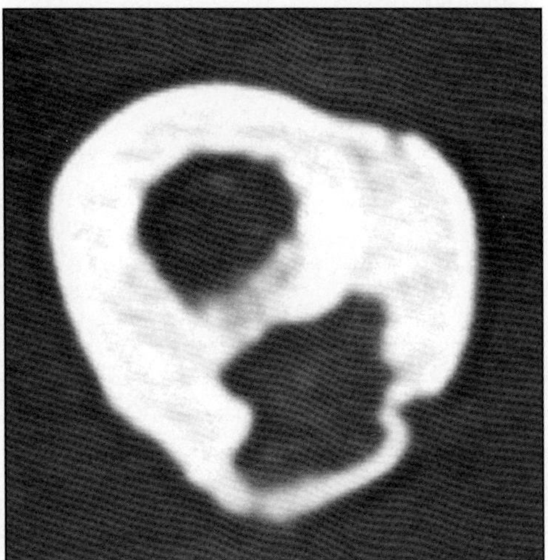

(Left) *Anteroposterior radiography shows a circumscribed lesion with central ossifications involving the inferior pubic ramus.* ***(Right)*** *Axial NECT shows a well-defined lytic lesion with surrounding sclerosis involving the femoral diaphysis.*

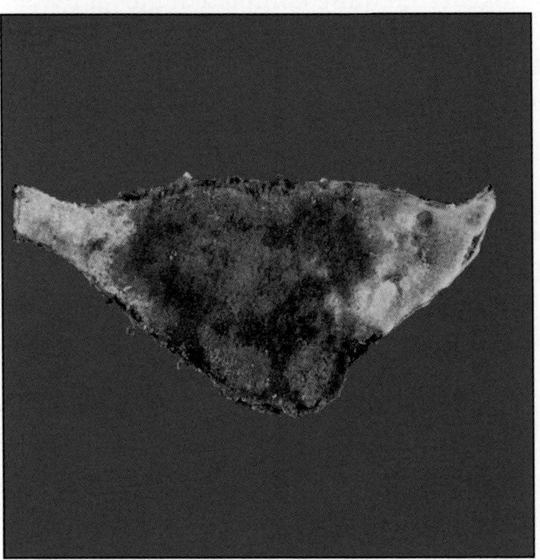

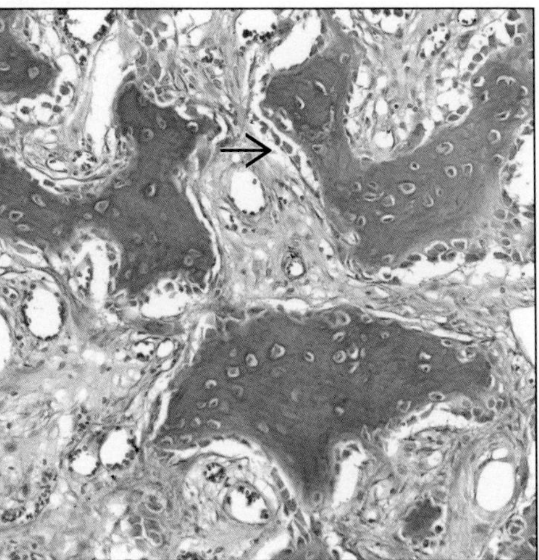

(Left) *The tissue of this osteoblastoma involving the right occipital bone of a 13-year-old boy shows a well-demarcated lytic lesion with areas of hemorrhage.* ***(Right)*** *The typical appearance of an osteoblastoma shows anastomosing bony trabeculae surrounded by a loose fibrovascular stroma. The bony trabeculae are rimmed by a single layer of small, polygonal osteoblasts* ➔.

OSTEOBLASTOMA

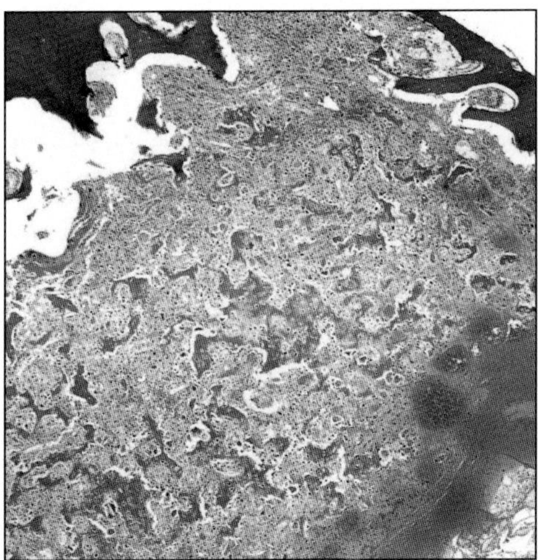

Low-power view demonstrates an osteoblastoma arising in the pedicle of L5 in a 16-year-old male showing a well-circumscribed lesion with prominent demarcation from the surrounding bone.

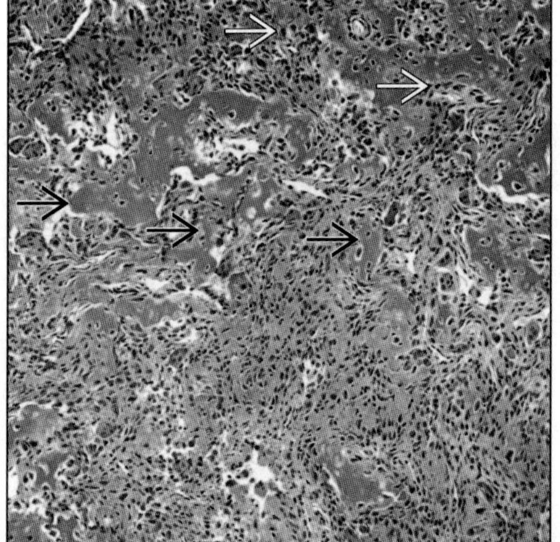

High-power view of vertebral osteoblastoma highlights the interanastomosing trabeculae ⇨ rimmed by osteoblasts ➡.

TERMINOLOGY

Abbreviations

- Osteoblastoma (OB)

Synonyms

- Giant osteoid osteoma

Definitions

- Benign tumor-forming osteoid

ETIOLOGY/PATHOGENESIS

Etiology

- Unknown

CLINICAL ISSUES

Epidemiology

- Incidence
  - < 1% of all primary bone tumors and 3% of all benign bone tumors
- Age
  - 90% occur in 2nd to 3rd decades of life
- Gender
  - M:F = 2-2.5:1

Site

- 40% occur in spine and 30% in long bones
- > 50% occur in diaphysis
- Approximately 1/2 are located eccentrically while the other 1/2 are intracortical
- Periosteal reactions are extremely rare

Presentation

- Most common signs/symptoms
  - Localized pain of long duration is usually presenting complaint, and physical examination often reveals tender mass lesion
    - Prostaglandins released by tumor cause severe peritumoral edema
  - Vertebral tumors can cause compression of spinal cord or peripheral nerve roots with associated neurological deficit such as scoliosis, neurologic symptoms, and gait disturbance
  - Not uncommon to see atrophy of muscle groups in region of tumor
  - Patients younger than 10 years may rarely present with weight loss, fever, anemia, and osteomalacia that resolve with removal of tumor

Natural History

- Grows slowly

Treatment

- Surgical approaches
  - Curettage with bone graft or methylmethacrylate placement
  - Marginal en bloc resection of symptomatic lesions
  - Spinal lesions often require complete removal by curettage or excision and may require bone grafting to stabilize vertebral column

Prognosis

- 10-15% recurrence for typical OB
- 50% recurrence for aggressive OB

Classification Criteria

- Classical OB
- Aggressive OB, sometimes called pseudomalignant OB
  - Concept is controversial

IMAGE FINDINGS

General Features

- Best diagnostic clue
  - Expansile, circumscribed, lytic lesion involving extremities and posterior elements of spine

OSTEOBLASTOMA

Key Facts

Etiology/Pathogenesis

- Histologically similar to osteoid osteomas, producing osteoid and primitive woven bone

Clinical Issues

- < 1% of all primary bone tumors and 3% of all benign bone tumors
- 90% occur in 2nd to 3rd decades of life
- M:F = 2-2.5:1
- 40% occur in spine and 30% in long bones
- Not uncommon to see scoliosis or atrophy of muscle groups in region of tumor

Image Findings

- Expansile, circumscribed, lytic lesion involving extremities and posterior elements of spine

Macroscopic Features

- Highly vascular tumor composed of granular and friable hemorrhagic, red lesional tissue
- > 1.5-2 cm; average size is 3 cm in diameter
- Circumscribed mass, often surrounded by shell of cortical bone or periosteum

Microscopic Pathology

- Haphazardly arranged irregular osteoid admixed with loose fibrovascular connective tissue and vascular channels
- Prominent osteoblastic rimming of osteoid
- Osteoid merges with adjacent normal bone at periphery

Radiographic Findings

- Expansile, circumscribed, lytic lesion that may be associated with reactive sclerosis and variable central calcification and matrix
- > 75% are associated with cortical expansion, and 20% are associated with cortical destruction
- Approximately 15% may be associated with aneurysmal bone cyst

CT Findings

- Expansile lytic lesion with or without matrix mineralization
  - Adjacent periosteal reaction, sclerosis, and cortical erosions
  - Aggressive OB may disrupt cortex and has soft tissue component

MACROSCOPIC FEATURES

General Features

- Gross findings
  - Circumscribed red, granular mass, often surrounded by shell of cortical bone or periosteum
  - Presence of secondary aneurysmal bone cyst often indicated by prominent cystic spaces
  - Epithelioid morphology correlates strongly with multifocal lesions, typically as multiple nidi in same bone

Size

- > 1.5-2 cm; average size is 3 cm in diameter

MICROSCOPIC PATHOLOGY

Histologic Features

- Histologically similar to osteoid osteomas, producing osteoid and primitive woven bone
- Haphazardly arranged irregular osteoid admixed with loose fibrovascular connective tissue and vascular channels
- Osteoid merges with adjacent normal bone at periphery
- Prominent osteoblastic rimming of osteoid, which is often arranged as interanastomosing trabeculae

ANCILLARY TESTS

Cytogenetics

- Involvement of chromosomes 1 and 14 appears to be recurrent in osteoblastoma

DIFFERENTIAL DIAGNOSIS

Osteoid Osteoma

- Smaller, < 2 cm, with predilection for axial skeleton
- Can regress spontaneously

Aneurysmal Bone Cyst

- Radiographically see fluid-fluid levels
- No matrix calcification
- Secondary aneurysmal bone cysts are common in OB

Osteosarcoma

- Sarcoma containing bone matrix
  - More aggressive appearance on radiographs and CT scan with cortical breakthrough and permeative growth pattern at periphery
- Wider zone of transition and soft tissue component

SELECTED REFERENCES

1. Berry M et al: Osteoblastoma: a 30-year study of 99 cases. J Surg Oncol. 98(3):179-83, 2008

OSTEOBLASTOMA

Radiologic and Other Features

(Left) Axial graphic shows an osteoblastoma ➪ involving the posterior elements of a vertebra. Central calcifications are shown in white. *(Right)* Axial NECT of an osteoblastoma shows an expansile circumscribed lytic lesion with scalloped margins involving the vertebral body and posterior elements ➔.

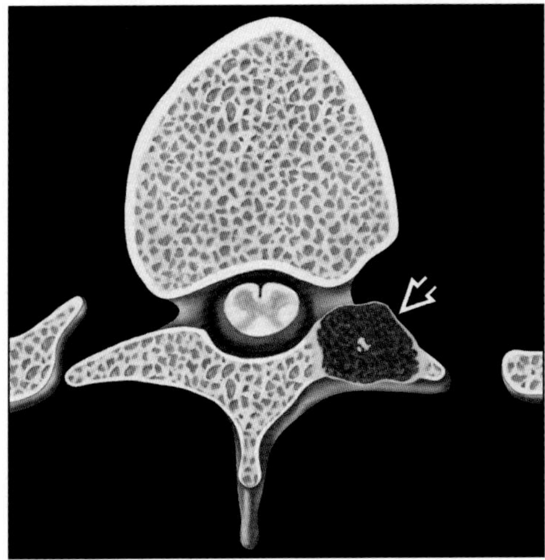

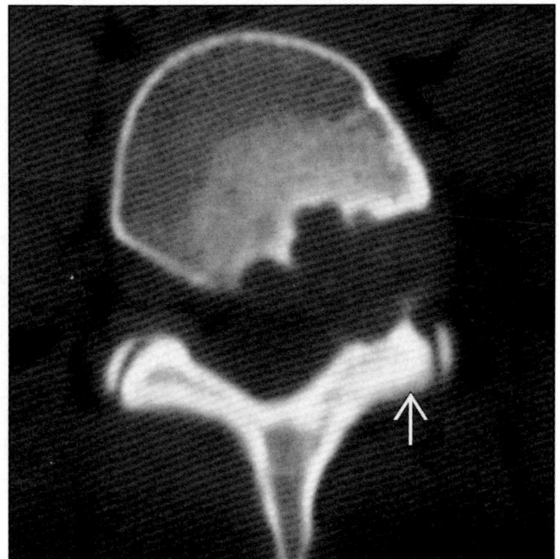

(Left) Anteroposterior radiography of an osteoblastoma shows a circumscribed lesion with central ossifications involving the inferior pubic ramus. *(Right)* Axial NECT of an osteoblastoma shows a well-defined lytic lesion with surrounding sclerosis involving the femoral diaphysis.

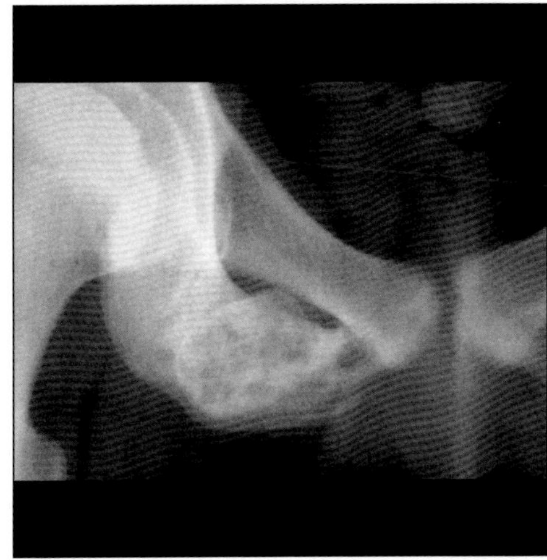

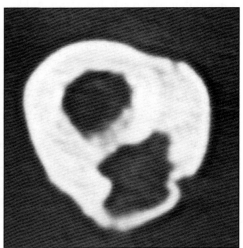

(Left) The tissue of this osteoblastoma involving the right occipital bone of a 13-year-old boy shows a well-demarcated lytic lesion with areas of hemorrhage. *(Right)* Section of osteoblastoma shows expansion of a central lesion with a rim of reactive bone and associated cortical expansion.

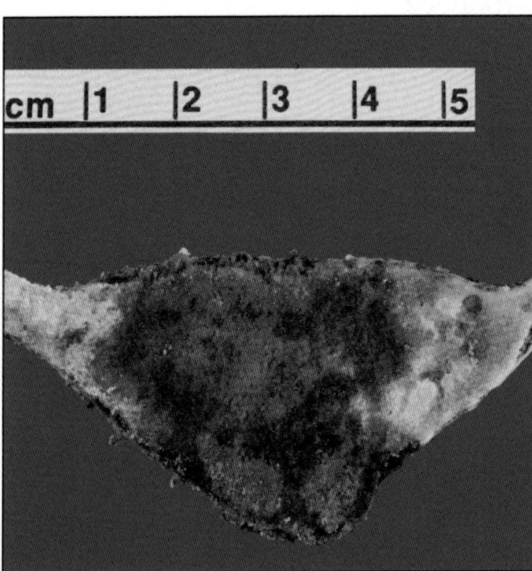

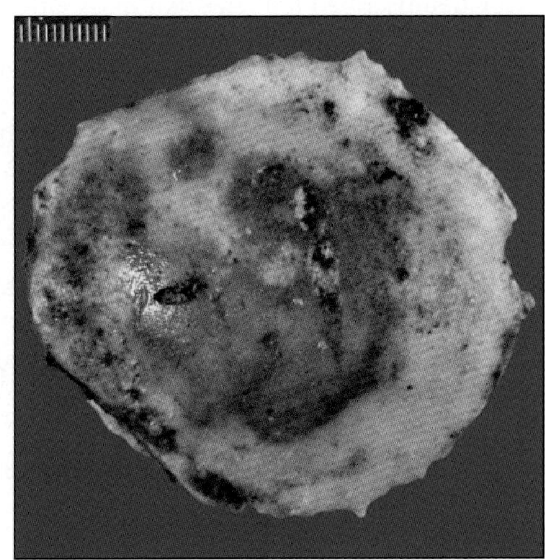

OSTEOBLASTOMA

Microscopic Features

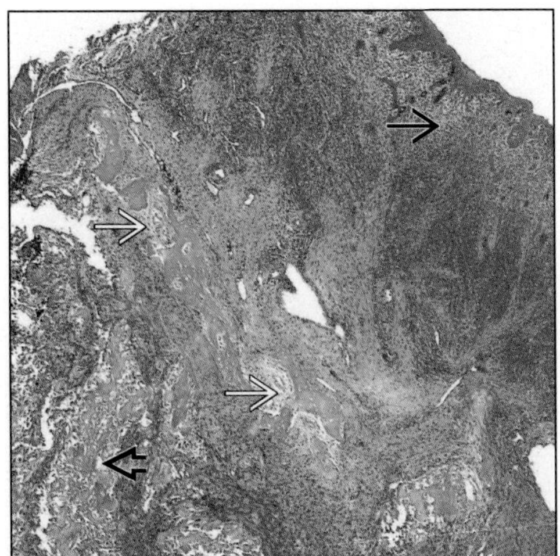

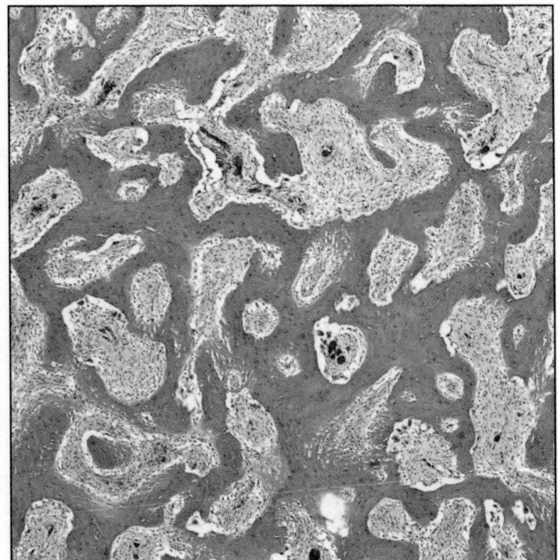

(Left) *Low-power view of a mandibular osteoblastoma shows ulcerated oral mucosa ➔ present on top of the lesion. The osteoblastoma is well circumscribed and surrounded by a rim of sclerotic bone ➔. Note the trabecular anastomosing network in the center of the lesion ➔.* ***(Right)*** *Central portion of an osteoid osteoma highlights the anastomosing trabecular network. The trabeculae are lined by an inconspicuous layer of small osteoblasts.*

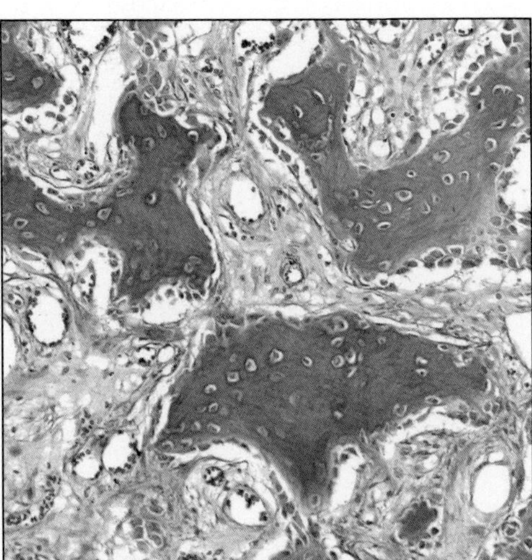

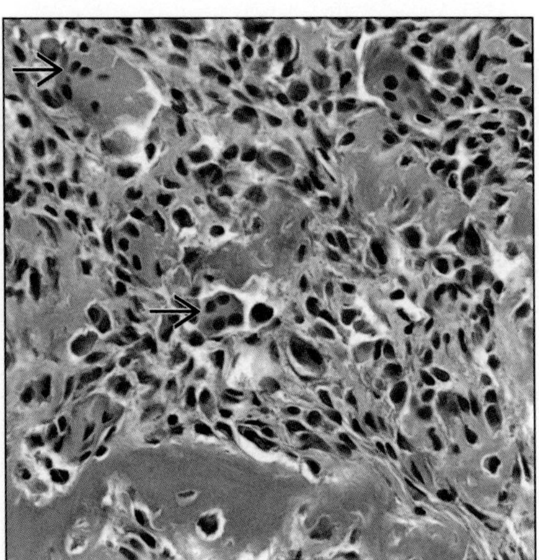

(Left) *The typical appearance of an osteoblastoma shows anastomosing bony trabeculae surrounded by a loose fibrovascular stroma. The bony trabeculae are rimmed by a single layer of small, polygonal osteoblasts.* ***(Right)*** *Skull osteoblastoma in a 14-year-old girl shows collections of epithelioid osteoblasts aggregating between the anastomosing trabeculae. Only mild atypia and pleomorphism are appreciated. A few osteoclastic giant cells ➔ are also present.*

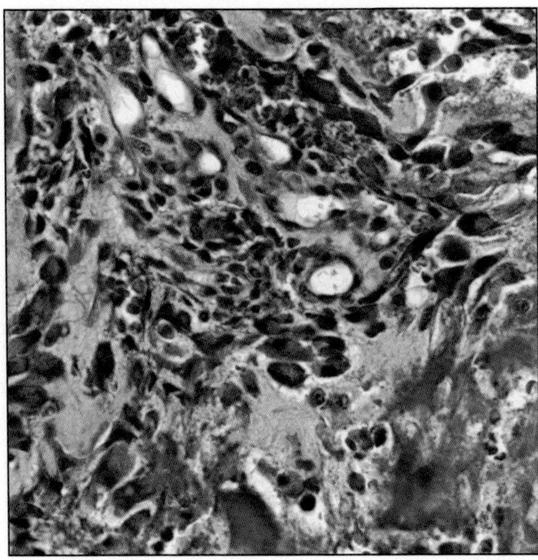

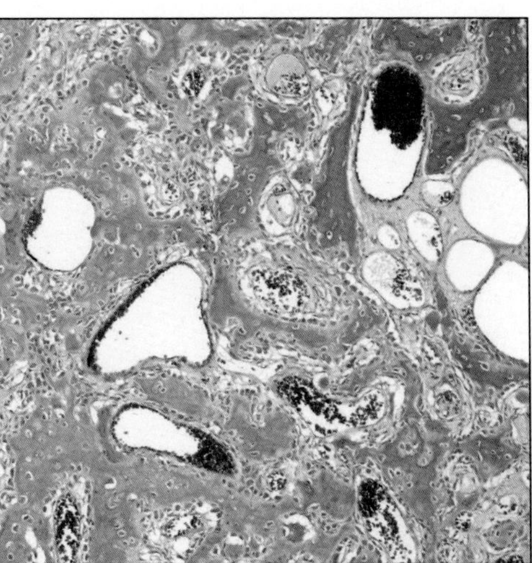

(Left) *This recurrent aggressive maxillary osteoblastoma in a 10-year-old girl contains large pleomorphic epithelioid osteoblasts with abundant eosinophilic cytoplasm and large vesicular nuclei with prominent nucleoli.* ***(Right)*** *A secondary aneurysmal bone cyst characterized by small cystic spaces filled with erythrocytes and surrounded by loose fibrous stroma can be seen in the background of this osteoblastoma.*

Differential Diagnosis

*(**Left**) Axial graphic shows a highly vascular tumor nidus of osteoid osteoma in the left lamina, surrounded by dense reactive bone. (**Right**) Axial NECT shows a low-attenuation nidus with central calcifications in the right pedicle of C4 extending into the lamina.*

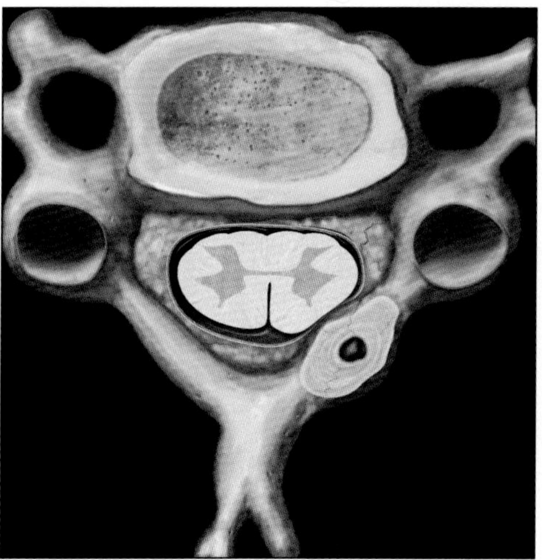

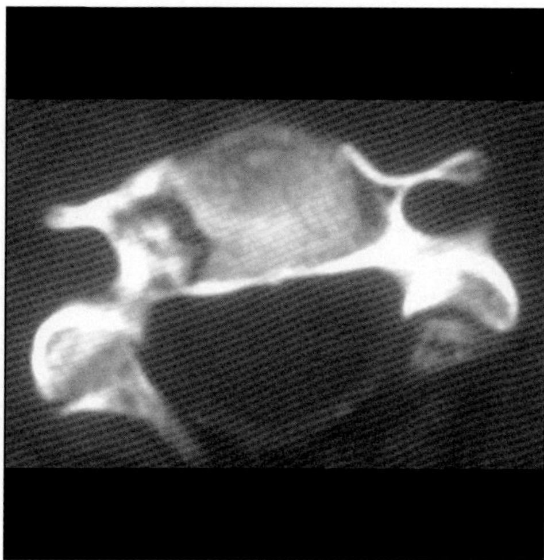

*(**Left**) Gross photograph of an osteoid osteoma shows a round, sharply demarcated, reddish nidus surrounded by sclerotic bone. (**Right**) Low-power magnification of an osteoid osteoma shows a well-circumscribed nidus surrounded by reactive sclerosis ⇾.*

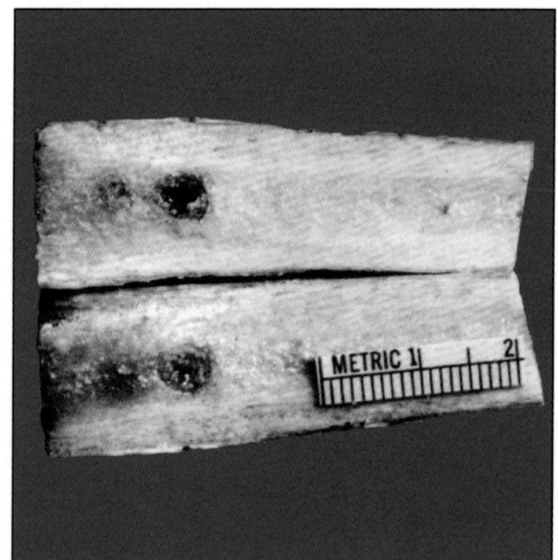

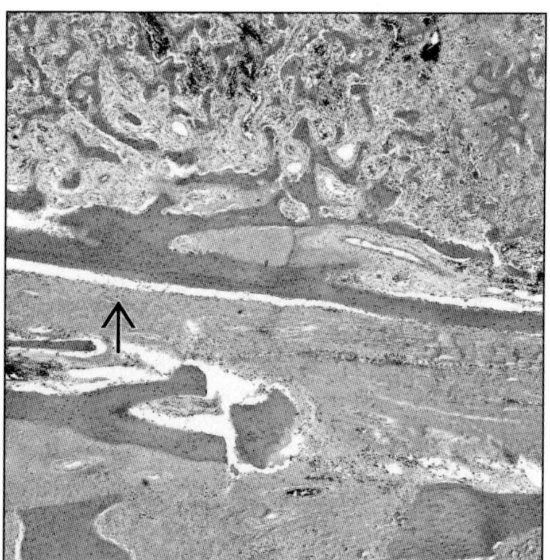

*(**Left**) Nidus of an osteoid osteoma shows an interlacing network of osteoid and bony trabeculae with variable mineralization. (**Right**) High-power magnification of an osteoid osteoma highlights the vascular nature of the nidus with numerous dilated capillaries ➔.*

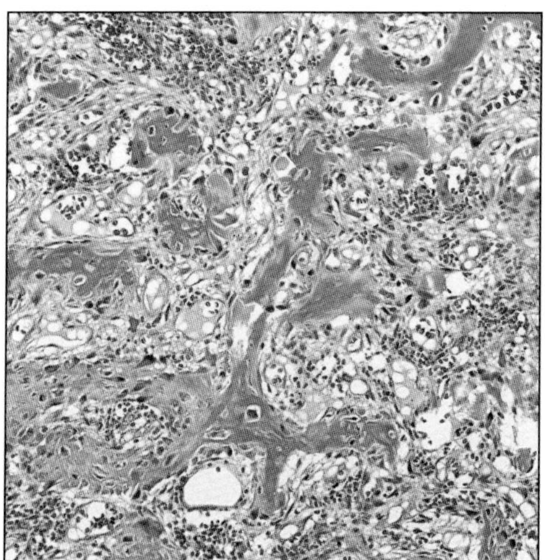

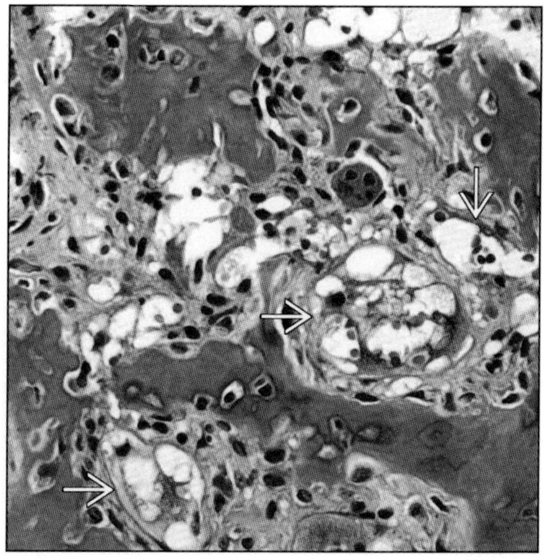

Diagrammatic and Microscopic Features

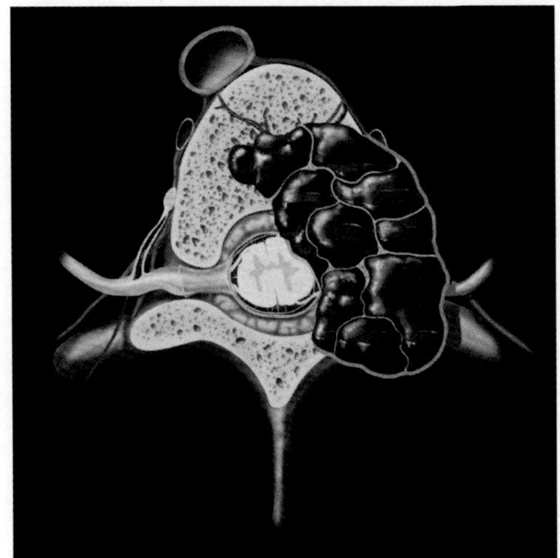

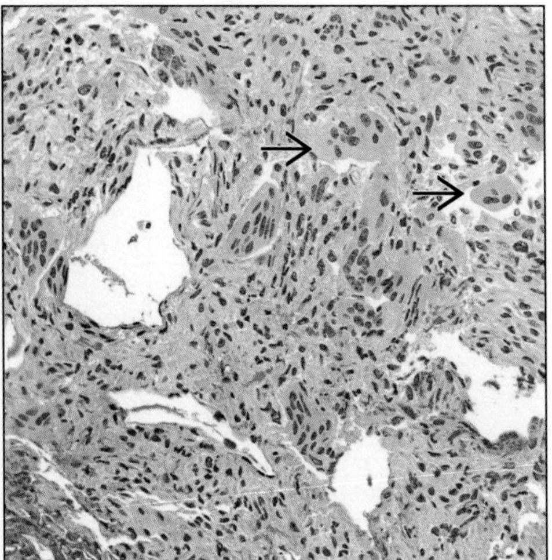

(Left) *Axial graphic shows an aneurysmal bone cyst characterized by an expansile, multicystic mass located in the posterior vertebral body and pedicle extending into the epidural space. Fluid-fluid levels are characteristic.* ***(Right)*** *A high-power view of an aneurysmal bone cyst shows cystic spaces surrounded by a fibrohistiocytic stroma. Note the osteoclastic giant cells floating within the cystic spaces ⇨, a common finding in aneurysmal bone cysts.*

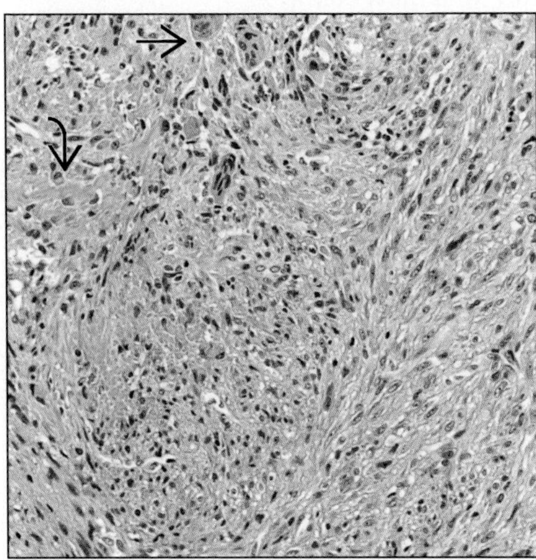

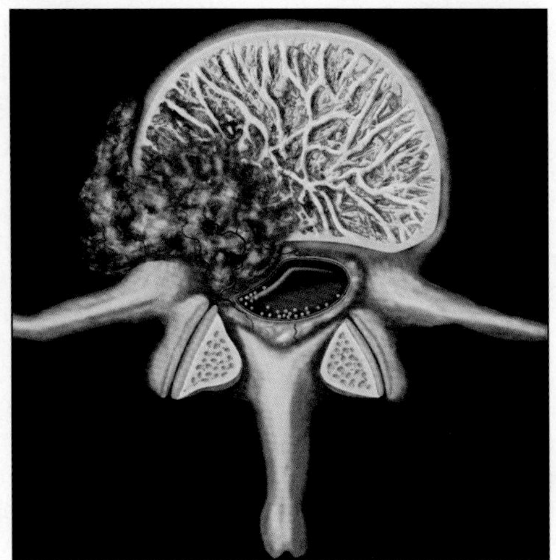

(Left) *Solid aneurysmal bone cyst shows clusters of osteoclastic giant cells ⇨ and immature osteoid ⮫ within a fibrohistiocytic stroma. Note the absence of interanastomosing trabeculae and osteoblasts associated with osteoblastoma.* ***(Right)*** *Axial graphic shows an osteosarcoma arising in the background of Paget disease, destroying the cortex and invading adjacent soft tissues. The tumor has a wide zone of transition.*

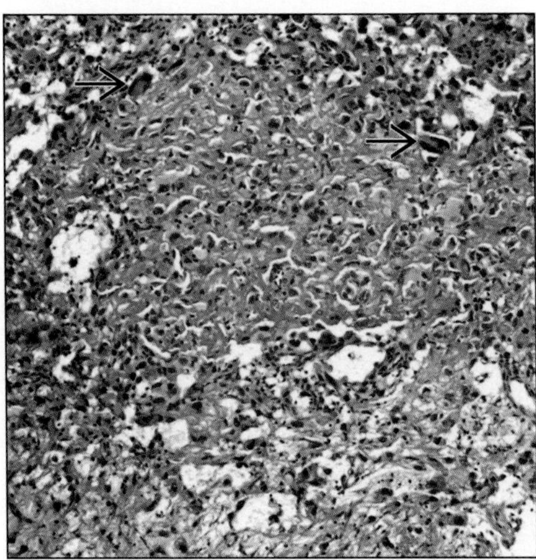

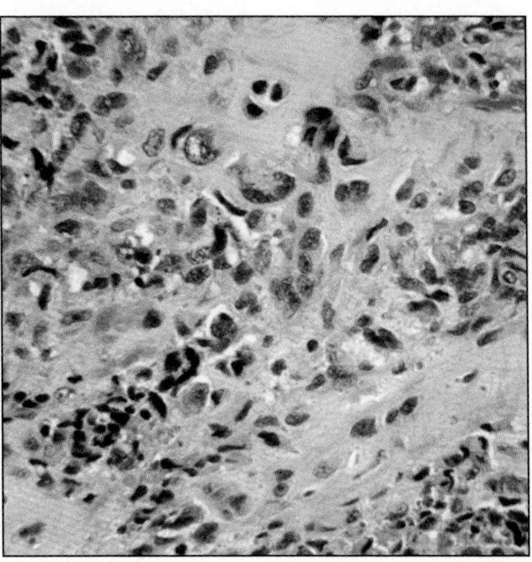

(Left) *High-grade osteosarcoma shows small interanastomosing trabeculae surrounded by malignant cells. Note the mitoses ⇨ at the periphery of the lesion, a finding absent in osteoblastoma.* ***(Right)*** *High-power view of high-grade osteosarcoma shows large atypical, pleomorphic tumor cells with abundant eosinophilic cytoplasm and centrally or eccentrically located nuclei. Note the osteoid matrix intimately associated with the tumor cells.*

OSTEOMA

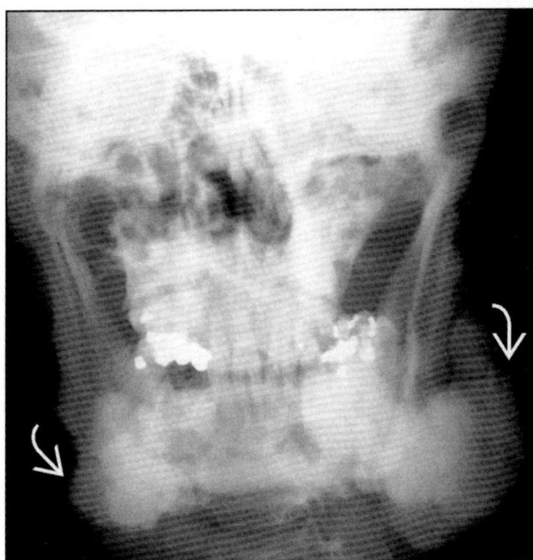

AP radiograph shows gnathic bones in a patient with Gardner syndrome. Large lobulated osteomas arise from surface of mandible bilaterally ➡. Radiodense masses are well circumscribed from surrounding soft tissues.

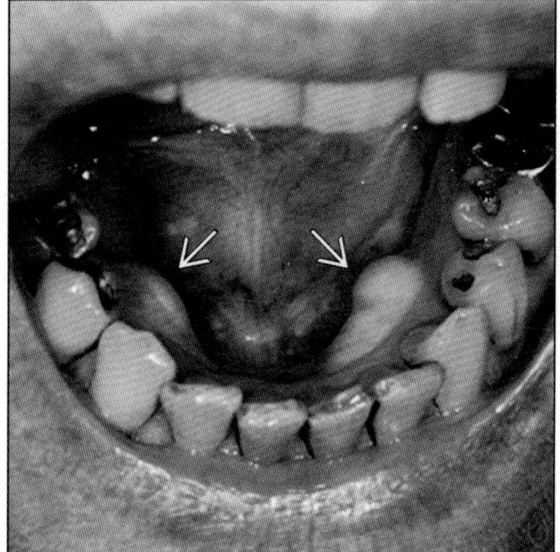

Clinical photograph of torus mandibularis shows bilateral tan-white masses that bulge into the oral cavity from inner surface of mandible ➡. The tumors are oblong, with long axis parallel to mandible. (Courtesy T. Dodson, MD.)

TERMINOLOGY

Abbreviations

- Osteoma (OS)

Synonyms

- Button osteoma
- Ivory exostosis
- Torus palatinus (when arising on palate)
- Torus mandibularis (when arising on mandible)

Definitions

- Benign surface bone-forming tumor usually composed of cortical type bone
  - Minority are composed of trabecular bone: Trabecular/cancellous osteoma

CLINICAL ISSUES

Epidemiology

- Incidence
  - Paranasal sinus osteoma: 3-4%
  - Cranial osteoma at autopsy: 4-5%
  - Accounts for 0.03% of biopsied primary bone tumors
- Age
  - Most common in 4th to 6th decade of life
  - Approximately 5% are diagnosed before age of 20
- Gender
  - Male:female ratio is 1:1

Site

- Craniofacial skeleton most common
  - Often located in frontal and ethmoid sinuses (75%)
    - Incidence of paranasal sinus osteoma: 3-4%
  - Sphenoid sinus
  - Inner and outer surfaces of cranium
  - Gnathic bones especially palate and mandible
- Appendicular skeleton rare
  - Long tubular bones
    - Femur and tibia most common
  - Multiple lesions should raise possibility of Gardner syndrome

Presentation

- Slow-growing small lesions that are usually incidental finding
- Large lesions produce symptoms related to anatomic location
  - Paranasal and sinus tumors cause obstruction and secondary mucocele
  - Orbital tumors cause exophthalmos; double, blurred, or loss of vision
  - Appendicular tumors can manifest as hard palpable mass
  - Oral tumors can interfere with mastication
- Usually solitary
- Extremity tumors may form firm palpable mass
- May be initial presentation of Gardner syndrome
  - Patients commonly have multiple osteomas

Treatment

- Observation
- Simple excision

Prognosis

- Excellent
  - No recurrence

IMAGE FINDINGS

General Features

- Uniformly radiodense surface lesion
- Ovoid to mushroom-shaped and well demarcated from soft tissue
- Broad base of attachment to underlying cortex with which it merges
- Well-formed periosteal reaction along margin of attachment may be present

OSTEOMA

Key Facts

Terminology
- Benign surface bone-forming tumor usually composed of cortical type bone

Clinical Issues
- Usually small and solitary
- Commonly asymptomatic and incidental finding
- Most frequently develop in craniofacial skeleton
- Appendicular tumors are very uncommon
- Multiple lesions raise possibility of Gardner syndrome
- Asymptomatic lesions can be observed
- Symptomatic lesions can be conservatively excised

Image Findings
- Small and uniformly radiodense
- Sharply marginated with well-formed periosteal reaction
- Oval to dome-shaped with broad attachment to cortical surface
- Underlying cortex is not involved

Macroscopic Features
- Generally < 2 cm in diameter; round, tan-white, and hard
- Resembles cortical bone with which it merges

Microscopic Pathology
- Consists mainly of lamellar bone admixed with some woven bone
- Bone has cortical-type architecture
- Minority of osteomas composed of trabecular type bone
- Lesional osteoblasts and osteocytes usually inconspicuous

  - Periosteal reaction appears as very well-formed Codman triangle
- No cortical involvement

MR Findings
- Mass has low signal intensity on T1- and T2-weighted images
  - Lesion does not enhance with contrast

CT Findings
- Oval well-delineated surface mass composed of bone with cortical appearance

Bone Scan
- May show increased or no radiotracer uptake

MACROSCOPIC FEATURES

General Features
- Generally < 2 cm in diameter
- Oval, round, or hemispheric
- Hard
- Tan to white
- Resembles cortical bone with which it merges
- Well-formed triangular-shaped subperiosteal reactive bone may surround attachment site to cortex

MICROSCOPIC PATHOLOGY

Histologic Features
- Consist of admixture of lamellar and woven bone with Haversian-like systems
- Infrequently consist of interconnecting trabeculae of bone
- May contain fibrous component, mimicking fibroosseous lesion
- Osteoblasts rimming bone are inconspicuous, small, and flat
  - Actively growing lesions contain plump, metabolically active osteoblasts
    - Metabolically active osteoblasts have abundant eosinophilic cytoplasm and nuclei polarized away from bone-forming surface
- Surface osteoblasts and osteocytes have nuclei containing condensed chromatin and very small or no visible nucleoli

DIFFERENTIAL DIAGNOSIS

Bone-Forming Lesions
- Parosteal osteosarcoma
  - Contains spindle cell component
- Juxtacortical myositis ossificans
  - Composed of cancellous bone
- Melorheostosis
  - "Dripping candle wax" configuration on imaging
- Osteochondroma
  - Has cartilage cap

DIAGNOSTIC CHECKLIST

Pathologic Interpretation Pearls
- Well-formed bone and banal cytology helps distinguish osteoma from osteosarcoma
- Intact cortex and absence of cartilage excludes osteochondroma
- Hypocellularity of lesion is evidence against myositis ossificans
- Melorheostosis and osteoma are similar histologically

SELECTED REFERENCES

1. Alexander AA et al: Paranasal sinus osteomas and Gardner's syndrome. Ann Otol Rhinol Laryngol. 116(9):658-62, 2007
2. Eppley BL et al: Large osteomas of the cranial vault. J Craniofac Surg. 14(1):97-100, 2003
3. Greenspan A. Benign bone-forming lesions: osteoma et al: Clinical, imaging, pathologic, and differential considerations. Skeletal Radiol. 22(7):485-500, 1993
4. O'Connell JX et al: Solitary osteoma of a long bone. A case report. J Bone Joint Surg Am. 75(12):1830-4, 1993

OSTEOMA

Radiologic and Clinical Features

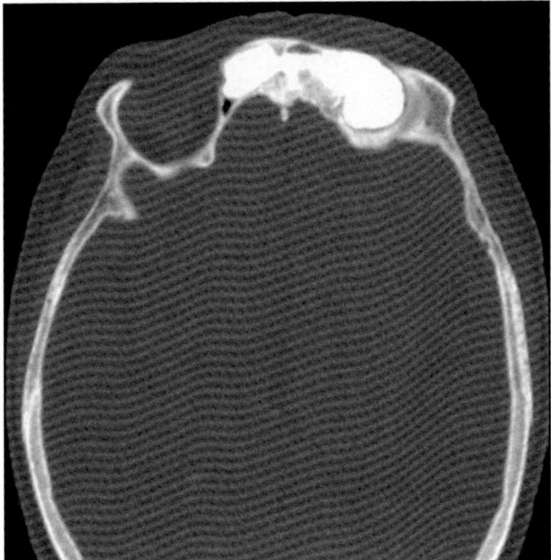

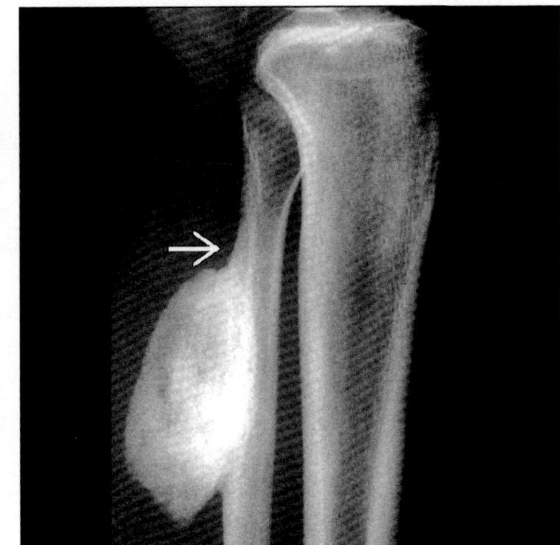

*(**Left**) CT scan shows a homogeneously dense lesion occupying the entire frontal sinus, a typical location for sinus osteoma. The tumor has a broad site of attachment to the surface of the cortex that forms the wall of the sinus. (**Right**) Radiograph of proximal lower leg shows a dense, well-defined ossific mass on the surface of the proximal fibula. There is thick, periosteal bone apposition proximally that is triangular in shape ➔.*

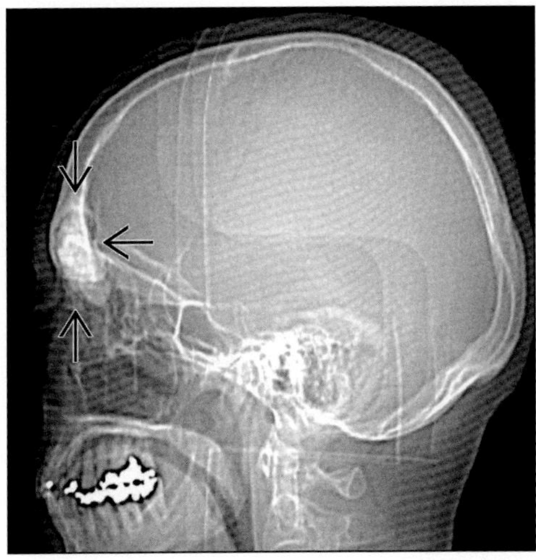

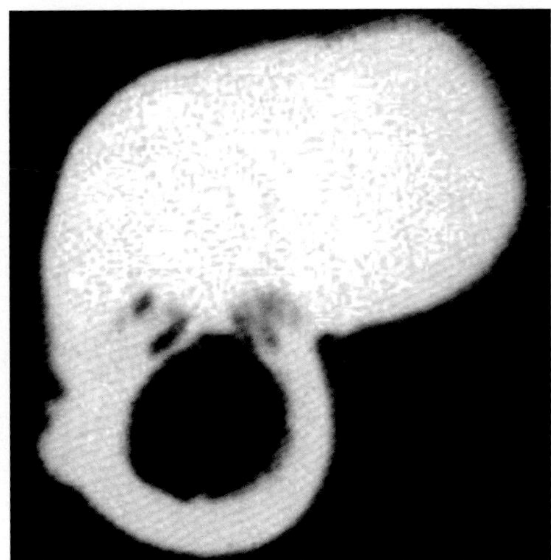

*(**Left**) Radiograph of lateral view of the skull shows a dense, sclerotic osteoma in the frontal sinus ➔. The well-circumscribed mass arises from the cortex delineating the sinus and fills much of the cavity. (**Right**) CT shows a well-defined, homogeneously sclerotic mass, contiguous with the outer cortex of the femur and extending into the soft tissues. The underlying cortex contains cylindrical lucencies, which contain feeding blood vessels that branch into the tumor.*

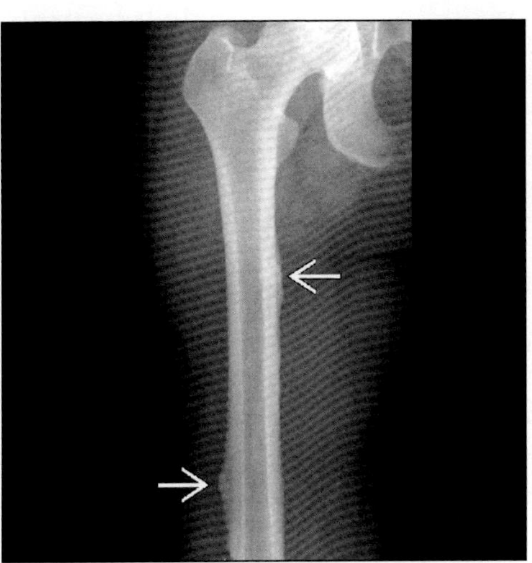

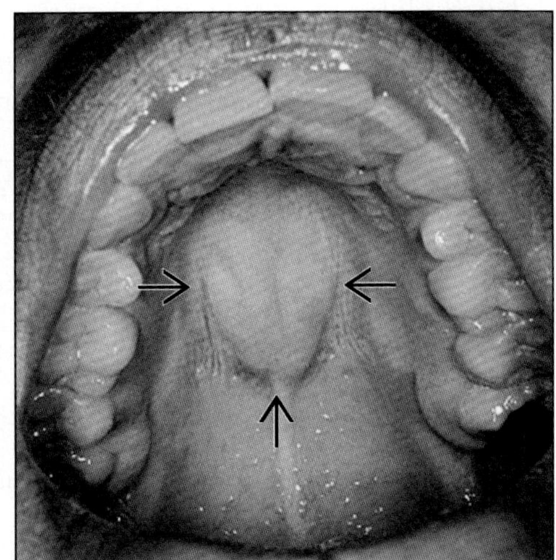

*(**Left**) AP radiograph of the femur in a patient with Gardner syndrome shows 2 elongate sessile osteomas. The masses protrude from the medial and lateral surfaces of the cortex ➔ and merge with the underlying bone. (**Right**) In this clinical photograph of torus palatinus, the mass appears as a midline oval tan-white lesion ➔ beneath the oral mucosa lining. The mucosa is intact and translucent. (Courtesy T. Dodson, MD.)*

OSTEOMA

Gross and Microscopic Features

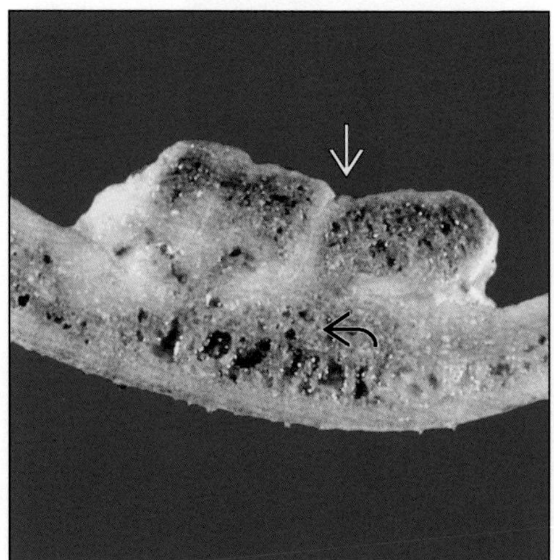

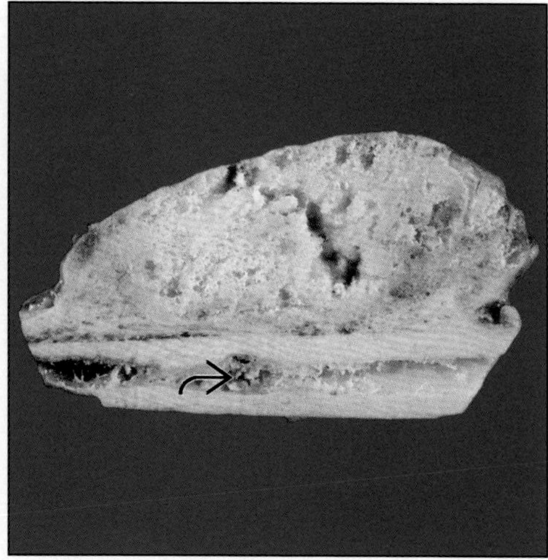

(Left) *Gross photograph shows cancellous osteoma that arises from the inner table of the skull ⮫. The bilobed tumor ➡ has a cancellous appearance with the intertrabecular spaces filled with marrow.* ***(Right)*** *Gross photograph shows large osteoma of long bone. The tan-white mass is composed of an admixture of cortical and cancellous bone. The underlying cortex is intact, and the medullary cavity is filled with fat ⮫.*

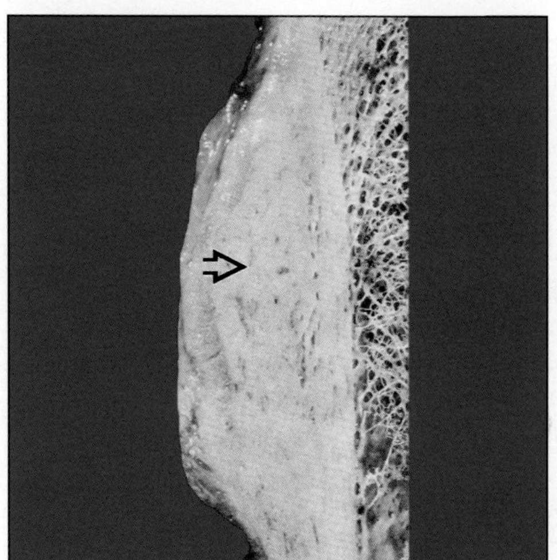

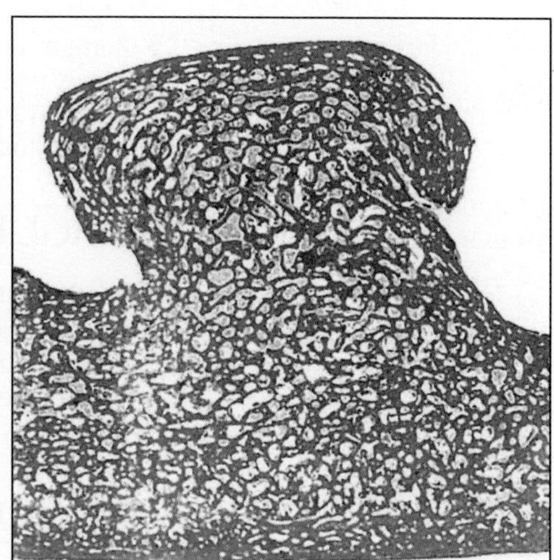

(Left) *Osteoma is composed of hard, dense, compact bone ⇨ with a broad attachment to the underlying cortex. A triangular-shaped zone of subperiosteal bone is present proximal and distal to the osteoma.* ***(Right)*** *Hematoxylin & eosin stain shows a cancellous osteoma of skull. The tumor merges with the underlying inner table. The surface of the lesion is composed of a thin plate of cortical-type bone, and the central component consists of interconnecting trabeculae of mainly lamellar bone.*

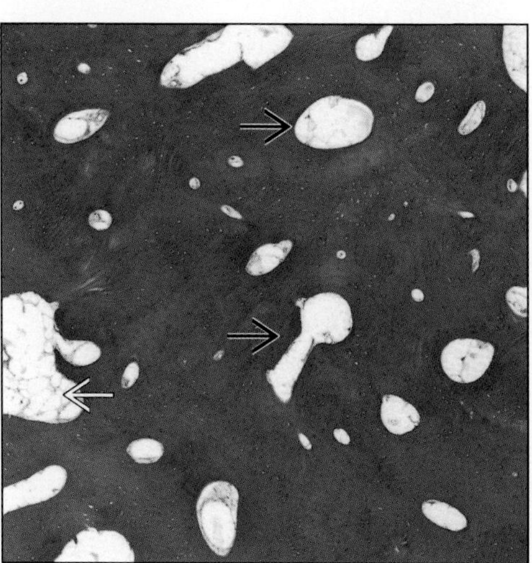

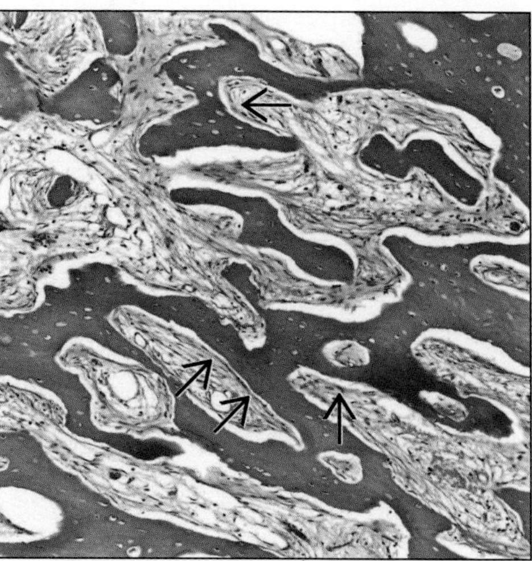

(Left) *Hematoxylin & eosin of osteoma shows haversian-like canals → that are prominent and vary in size and shape. The lining osteoblasts are small, and osteocytes are numerous. Some of the spaces are filled with fatty marrow ➡.* ***(Right)*** *Hematoxylin & eosin section of cancellous osteoma shows that the interconnecting trabeculae are covered by prominent osteoblasts →. The bone is surrounded by loose connective tissue.*

GIANT CELL TUMOR

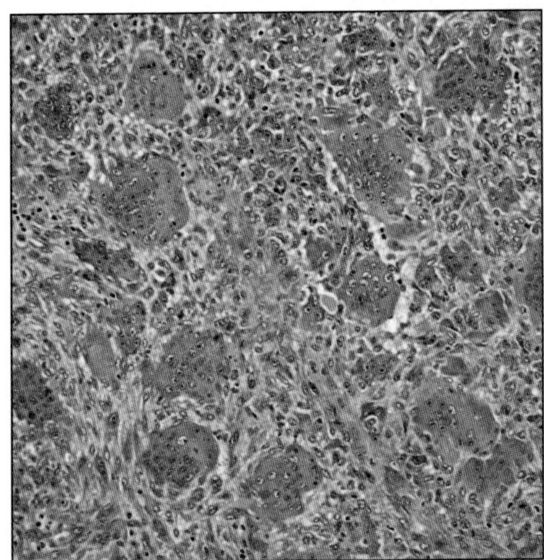

This example of a giant cell tumor shows typical giant cells with numerous nuclei evenly spaced among mononuclear cells that have similar nuclei.

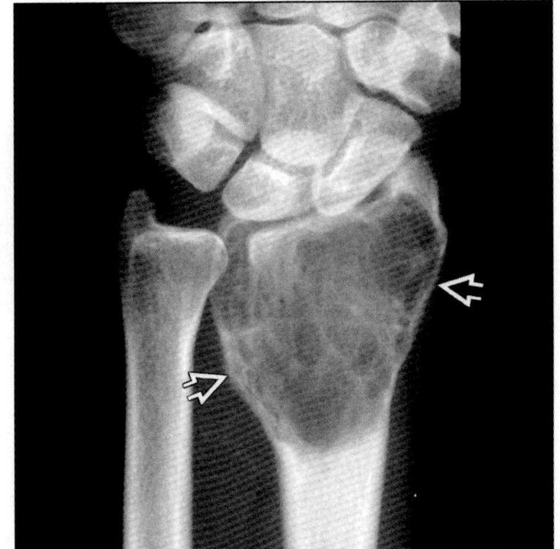

Radiograph of the wrist shows a large, lytic, expansile lesion ➡ involving the distal radius. Giant cell tumors are typically located in the epiphyses of long bones, with the distal radius being a common site.

TERMINOLOGY

Abbreviations

- Giant cell tumor (GCT)

Definitions

- Benign, giant cell-containing tumor of bone with predilection for skeletally mature women

CLINICAL ISSUES

Epidemiology

- Age
  - Usually in 3rd to 4th decade of life
  - After skeletal maturity
- Gender
  - Much more common in females
- Ethnicity
  - More common in people of Chinese descent

Site

- Epiphyses of long bones most common
  - Distal femur
  - Proximal tibia
  - Distal radius
- Sacrum
- Any portion of skeleton may be involved
- GCTs in small bones of hands tend to be more aggressive

Presentation

- Pain
- Localized swelling
- Pathologic fracture
- Rare complication of Paget disease of bone

Treatment

- Surgical approaches
  - Excision preferred over curettage
    - High recurrence rate after curettage

Prognosis

- Benign, but locally aggressive
- Rarely can metastasize to lung or lymph nodes
  - Survival not affected if met is surgically resected
- Malignancy is extremely uncommon

IMAGE FINDINGS

Radiographic Findings

- Purely lytic destructive lesion
  - Mineralization is unusual
- Often extends to articular cartilage
- In soft tissue, can have eggshell type of ossification

MACROSCOPIC FEATURES

General Features

- Usually soft and dark brown
- Can be fleshy white or pink
- Large collections of foam cells cause yellow color
- Often cystic

MICROSCOPIC PATHOLOGY

Histologic Features

- Multinucleated giant cells
  - Uniform distribution
  - Can have up to 50 or more nuclei
  - Nuclei are large with inconspicuous nucleoli
- Mononuclear cells
  - Round to oval
  - Nuclei resemble those of giant cells
- Can have brisk mitoses
  - No atypical mitoses
- Variant features common
  - Secondary aneurysmal bone cyst changes
    - Hemorrhage
    - Hemosiderin deposits

GIANT CELL TUMOR

Key Facts

Clinical Issues

- Usually in 3rd to 4th decade of life
- Skeletally mature women
- Epiphyses of long bones most common
  - Distal femur, proximal tibia, distal radius, sacrum
- Benign, but locally aggressive
- Excision preferred over curettage
  - High recurrence rate after curettage

Image Findings

- Purely lytic destructive lesion

Microscopic Pathology

- Multinucleated giant cells
  - Can have up to 50 or more nuclei
- Mononuclear cells
  - Nuclei resemble those of giant cells
- Variant features common
  - Secondary aneurysmal bone cyst changes
  - Collections of foam cells
  - Spindled mononuclear cells with storiform pattern can dominate
- **Giant cell tumor of tendon sheath**
  - Nodular tenosynovitis (localized form)
  - Pigmented villonodular synovitis (diffuse form)

Top Differential Diagnoses

- Solid aneurysmal bone cyst (reparative granuloma)
- Osteosarcoma
- Hyperparathyroidism
- Chondroblastoma

  - Collections of foam cells
    - May indicate involution
    - Mononuclear cells tend to spindle in areas with foam cells
  - Spindled mononuclear cells with storiform pattern can dominate
- Foci of reactive bone can be present, especially at periphery
- Rarely can find new bone within substance of tumor
- **Giant cell tumor of tendon sheath**
  - Nodular tenosynovitis (localized form)
    - Usually in hands or nonarticular areas of arm/leg
    - Cellular with evenly distributed giant cells
    - Hemosiderin
  - Pigmented villonodular synovitis (diffuse form)
    - Knee or ankle joints
    - Not encapsulated, grows around joint cavity
    - More aggressive with extension into soft tissue and joint erosion
    - Similar histology as nodular localized form
- **Malignant giant cell tumor**
  - Extremely uncommon
  - Benign giant cell tumor with juxtaposed spindle cell sarcoma **or** previous documentation of prior benign giant cell tumor in same location

DIFFERENTIAL DIAGNOSIS

Solid Aneurysmal Bone Cyst (Reparative Granuloma)

- Most common in mandible or maxilla
- Giant cells cluster in areas of hemorrhage
  - Giant cell tumor is more homogeneous
- May have new bone or osteoid formation

Osteosarcoma

- More frequent in adolescent boys
- Malignant osteoid with highly atypical cells

Hyperparathyroidism

- Diaphysis of long bones, jaw, skull
- Giant cells cluster in cellular, fibrous stroma
- Laboratory findings of hypocalcemia, hypophosphatemia

Chondroblastoma

- Calcification or chondroid differentiation

SELECTED REFERENCES

1. Alberghini M et al: Morphological and immunophenotypic features of primary and metastatic giant cell tumour of bone. Virchows Arch. 456(1):97-103, 2010
2. Arroud M et al: Giant-cell tumor of the fourth metacarpal bone in children: case report. J Pediatr Orthop B. 19(1):86-9, 2010
3. Errani C et al: Giant cell tumor of the extremity: A review of 349 cases from a single institution. Cancer Treat Rev. 36(1):1-7, 2010
4. Jakowski JD et al: Fine-needle aspiration biopsy of the distal extremities: a study of 141 cases. Am J Clin Pathol. 133(2):224-31, 2010
5. Moskovszky L et al: Centrosome abnormalities in giant cell tumour of bone: possible association with chromosomal instability. Mod Pathol. 23(3):359-66, 2010
6. Ulu MO et al: Giant cell tumor of the frontal bone in an 18-month-old girl: a case report. Cen Eur Neurosurg. 71(2):104-7, 2010
7. Abdel-Motaal MM et al: Soft-tissue recurrence of giant cell tumor of bone associated with pulmonary metastases. Gulf J Oncolog. (5):49-53, 2009
8. Cho HS et al: Giant cell tumor of the femoral head and neck: result of intralesional curettage. Arch Orthop Trauma Surg. Epub ahead of print, 2009
9. Sulzbacher I et al: Expression of platelet-derived growth factor-alpha receptor and c-kit in giant cell tumours of bone. Pathology. 41(7):630-3, 2009

GIANT CELL TUMOR

Microscopic and Other Features

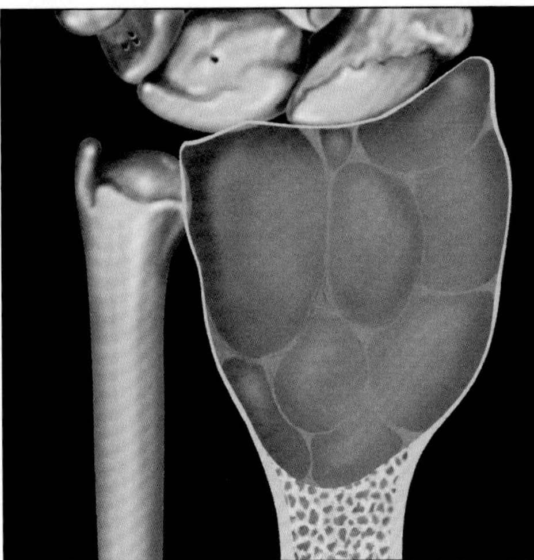

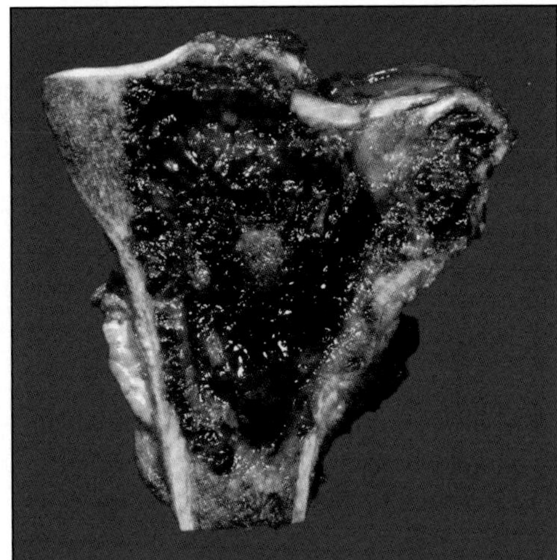

(Left) *Coronal graphic shows expansile lytic lesion with trabeculations extending to subchondral bone. Thinned but intact cortex is shown.* ***(Right)*** *Coronal gross pathology shows brown-reddish tumor involving the proximal tibia with extension to subchondral bone and through the cortex. Areas of hemorrhage and cyst formation are noted.*

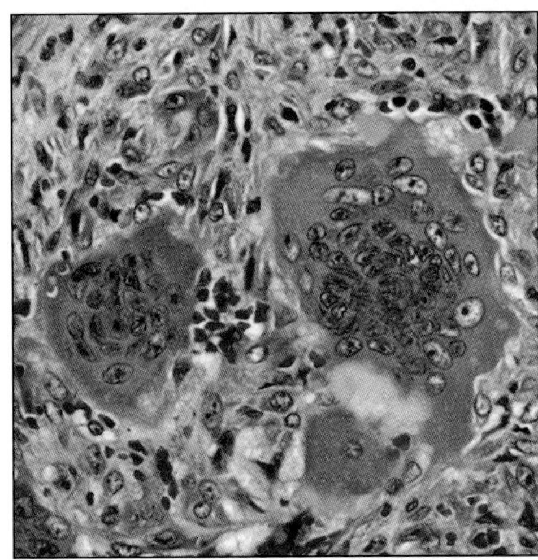

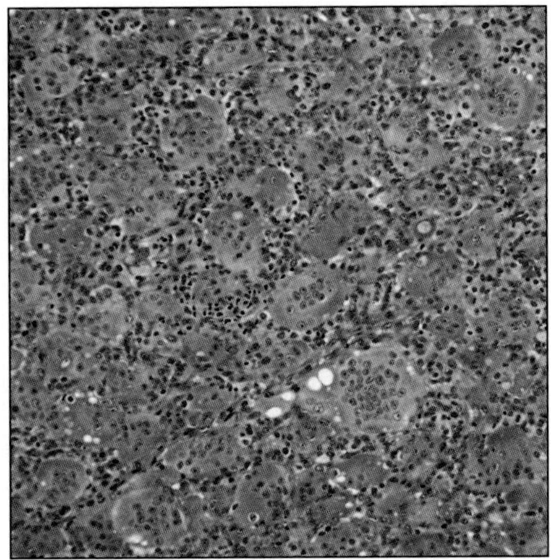

(Left) *H&E shows 2 giant cells typical of giant cell tumor. Individual nuclei are large with mostly inconspicuous nucleoli, and resemble the nuclei of the background mononuclear cells. The number of nuclei in a giant cell can reach well over 50.* ***(Right)*** *This giant cell tumor shows the giant cells to be back-to-back. The giant cells of giant cell tumor are usually evenly distributed, although their density varies from case to case.*

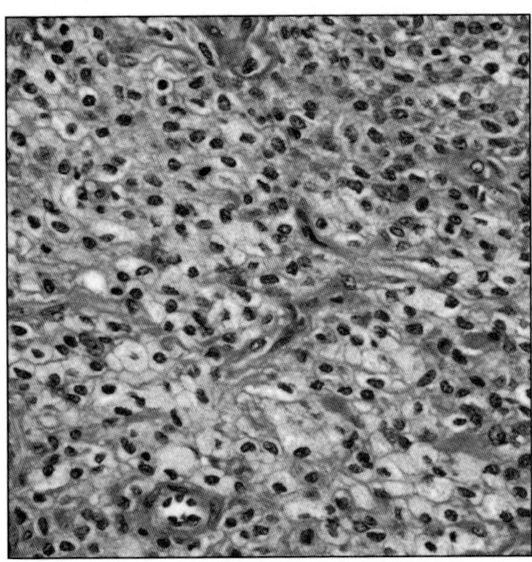

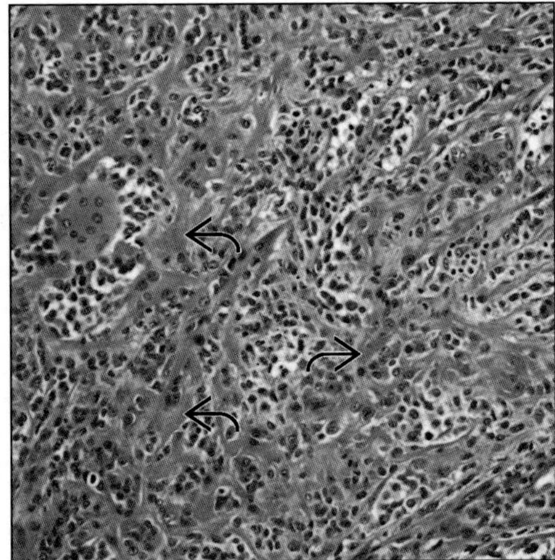

(Left) *Clusters of foam cells like this can be seen in giant cell tumors as a sign of involution. While these clusters are usually small and scattered throughout the lesion, they can be dominant and may obscure the correct diagnosis.* ***(Right)*** *This giant cell tumor of tendon sheath shows characteristic giant cells and mononuclear cells dissecting among dense collagen fibers* ➔.

Variant Microscopic Features

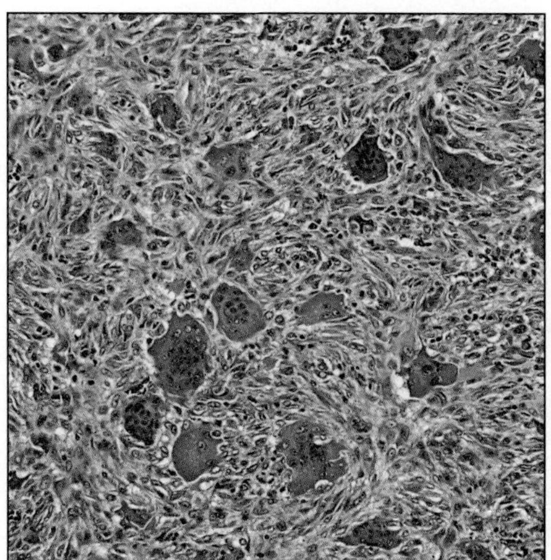

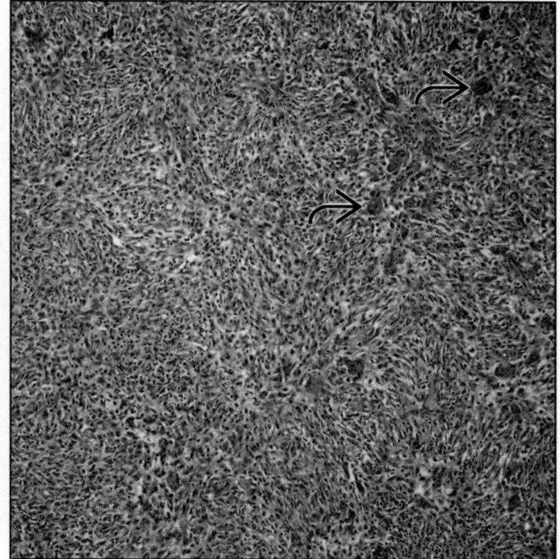

(Left) *The background mononuclear cells in this GCT are spindled, a common variation. Sometimes the spindle cells can be present in a storiform pattern with only a few giant cells, mimicking a spindle cell neoplasm.* ***(Right)*** *This GCT has a large area of spindled mononuclear cells with only a few scattered giant cells ⮫. Areas like this may raise the possibility of benign histiocytoma or nonossifying fibroma. Careful examination of all the tissue can make the correct diagnosis.*

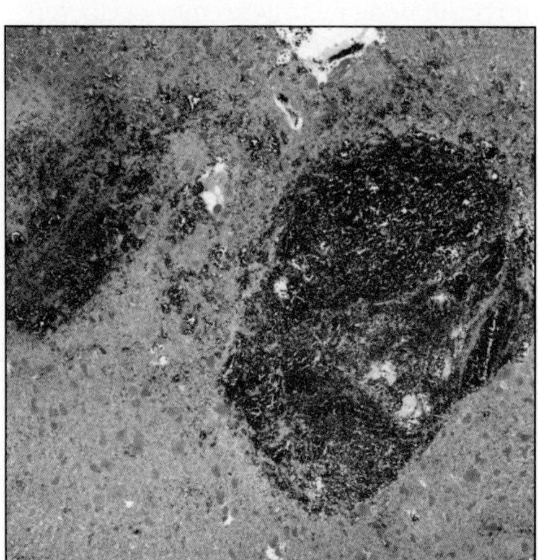

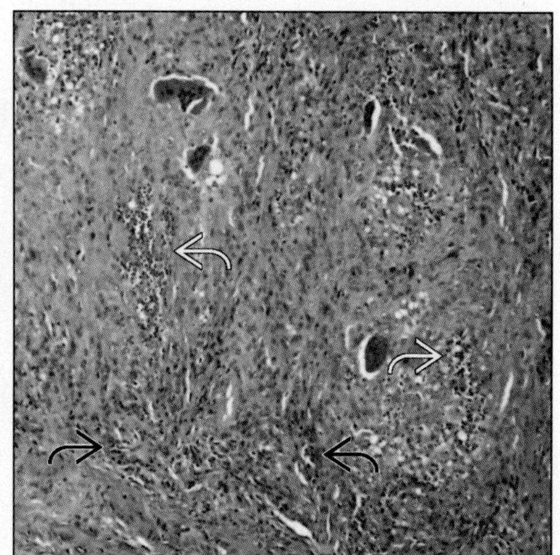

(Left) *This giant cell tumor has large collections of red blood cells. This is a common finding in giant cell tumors that have undergone secondary aneurysmal bone cyst change.* ***(Right)*** *This giant cell tumor shows scattered red blood cells ➡ and hemosiderin pigment ⮫. This is another common change in giant cell tumors that have undergone secondary aneurysmal bone cyst change.*

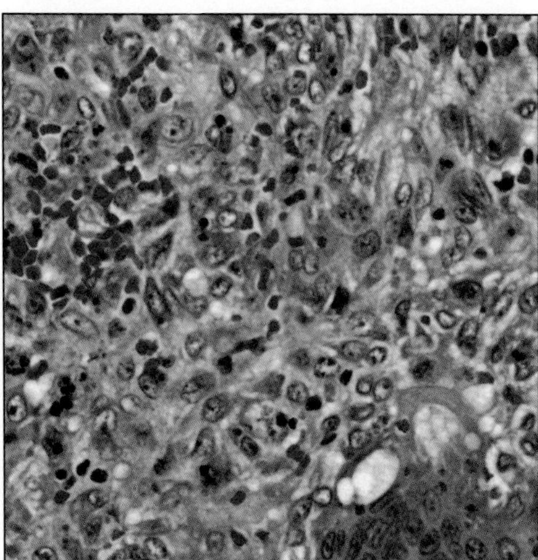

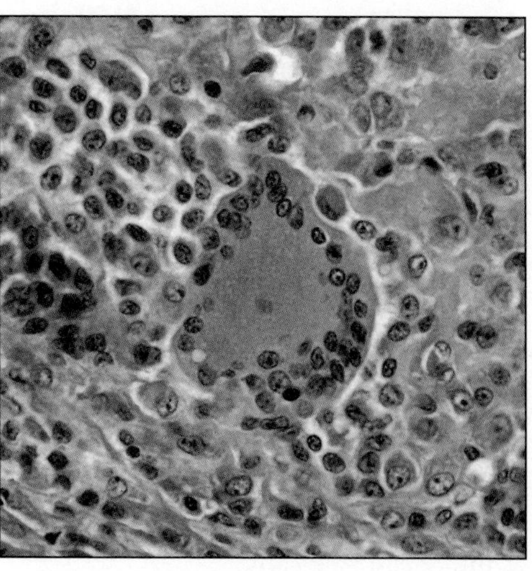

(Left) *Scattered red blood cells and hemosiderin are seen in a giant cell tumor with secondary aneurysmal bone cyst change.* ***(Right)*** *This giant cell in a giant cell tumor looks like a Touton giant cell seen in juvenile xanthogranuloma. Examination of the entire specimen should lead to the correct diagnosis.*

ADAMANTINOMA

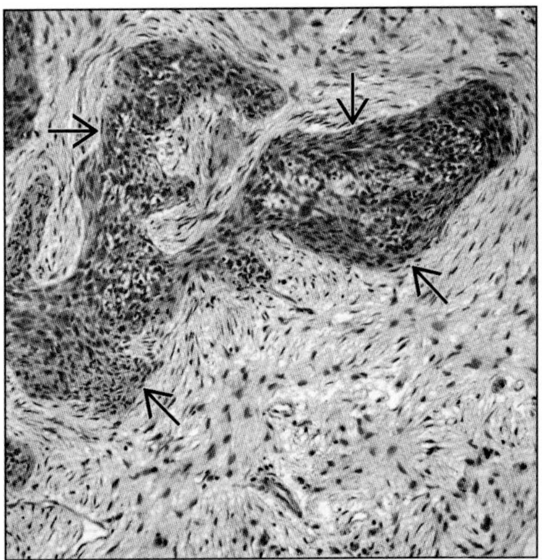

The biphasic nature of adamantinoma is easily seen here, with an irregular island of epithelial cells ⇒ within a loose, spindled stroma.

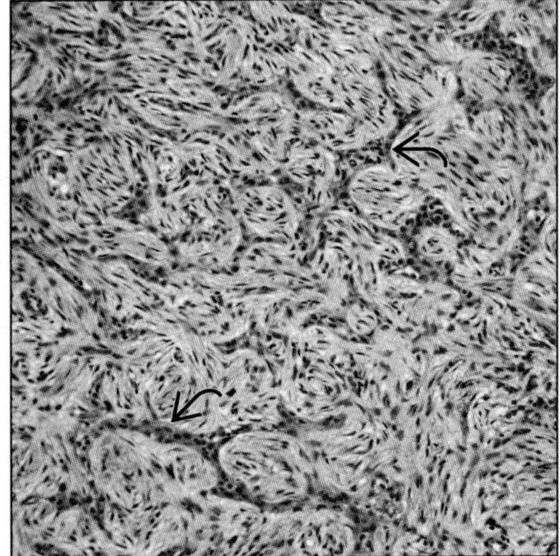

In this adamantinoma, cords of epithelial cells ⇒ infiltrate spindled stroma. The relative proportions of epithelial to spindled cells vary widely from case to case.

TERMINOLOGY

Definitions

- Rare, low-grade malignancy of bone with likely epithelial origin

CLINICAL ISSUES

Epidemiology

- Incidence
  - Extremely rare
- Age
  - Young adults
- Gender
  - Males slightly more common than females

Site

- > 90% in diaphysis of tibia
- Most of remainder in fibula, radius, or ulna

Presentation

- Pain
- Swelling
- Long duration of symptoms before diagnosis
  - Slow-growing tumor

Treatment

- Surgical approaches
  - Resection gives best outcomes
- Drugs
  - Chemotherapy has not been shown to be effective
- Radiation
  - Not useful, adamantinoma is highly radioresistant

Prognosis

- Low-grade malignancy
- Excellent prognosis if resected
  - Resection can be difficult as tumor can be locally aggressive
- Pulmonary or lymph node metastases may occur very late

IMAGE FINDINGS

Radiographic Findings

- Large lesion involving shaft of bone
- Involves cortex and medullary cavity
- Large areas of sclerosis mixed with lucent areas
- May have satellite lesions

MACROSCOPIC FEATURES

General Features

- Firm, fibrous
- Generally well circumscribed
- May have areas of cystic change, hemorrhage, or necrosis

Size

- 3-15 cm

MICROSCOPIC PATHOLOGY

Histologic Features

- Biphasic
- Epithelial islands in fibrous stroma
  - Amounts of epithelium and fibrous stroma vary
- Epithelial cells arranged in cords or nests
  - Central loose area
  - Peripheral palisading
  - May have squamous differentiation and rarely keratinization
  - Moderate cytologic atypia at most
  - Few mitoses
- Fibrous areas look like osteofibrous dysplasia
- Some have purely spindled pattern

ADAMANTINOMA

Key Facts

Clinical Issues
- Young adults
- > 90% in diaphysis of tibia
- Long duration of symptoms before diagnosis
- Excellent prognosis if resected
- Pulmonary or lymph node metastases may occur very late

Microscopic Pathology
- Epithelial islands in fibrous stroma

Ancillary Tests
- Epithelial cells strongly positive for keratin

Top Differential Diagnoses
- Osteofibrous dysplasia (ossifying fibroma)
  - May be related to adamantinoma
- Fibrous dysplasia
- Metastatic carcinoma

  - Spindled cells will cluster and merge into less cellular areas
  - Spindle cell tumor in cortex of tibia is nearly diagnostic for adamantinoma

Cytologic Features
- Biphasic nature can be seen on fine needle aspiration

ANCILLARY TESTS

Immunohistochemistry
- Epithelial cells strongly positive for keratin

Cytogenetics
- Complex chromosomal abnormalities, including trisomies

DIFFERENTIAL DIAGNOSIS

Osteofibrous Dysplasia (Ossifying Fibroma)
- Spindled cells with woven bone with osteoblastic rimming
- Single cells and rare clusters of keratin-positive cells can be seen
  - May be related to adamantinoma
- Occurs in young children
- Painless and rapidly growing

Fibrous Dysplasia
- Spindle cells produce woven bone without osteoblastic rimming
- Common in jawbones, skull, ribs, femur
- Asymptomatic except for pathologic fracture or mass deformity

Metastatic Carcinoma
- Rare below knee
- Older patients

SELECTED REFERENCES

1. Bishop JA et al: Primary tibial adamantinoma diagnosed by fine needle aspiration. Diagn Cytopathol. 38(3):198-201, 2010
2. Szendroi M et al: Adamantinoma of long bones: a long-term follow-up study of 11 cases. Pathol Oncol Res. 15(2):209-16, 2009
3. Gleason BC et al: Osteofibrous dysplasia and adamantinoma in children and adolescents: a clinicopathologic reappraisal. Am J Surg Pathol. 32(3):363-76, 2008
4. Jain D et al: Adamantinoma: A clinicopathological review and update. Diagn Pathol. 3:8, 2008
5. Khanna M et al: Osteofibrous dysplasia, osteofibrous dysplasia-like adamantinoma and adamantinoma: correlation of radiological imaging features with surgical histology and assessment of the use of radiology in contributing to needle biopsy diagnosis. Skeletal Radiol. 37(12):1077-84, 2008
6. Piña-Oviedo S et al: Primary adamantinoma of the rib. Unusual presentation for a bone neoplasm of uncertain origin. Pathol Oncol Res. 14(4):497-502, 2008

IMAGE GALLERY

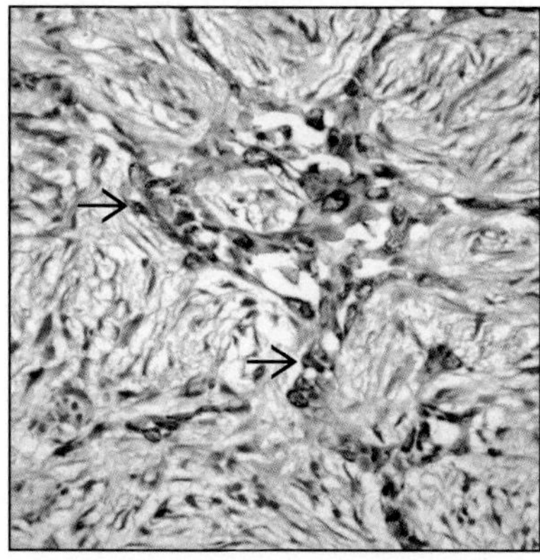

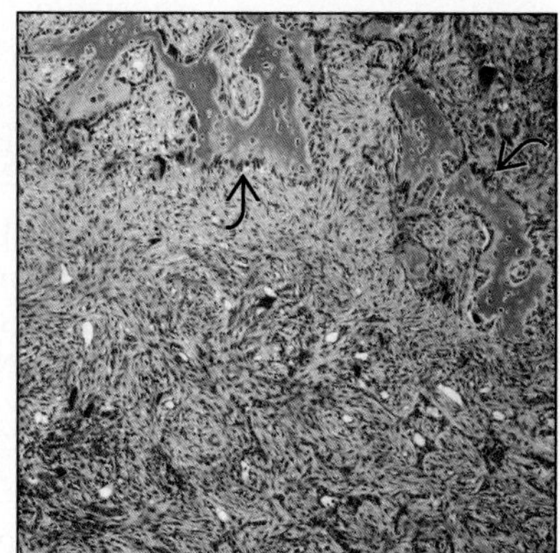

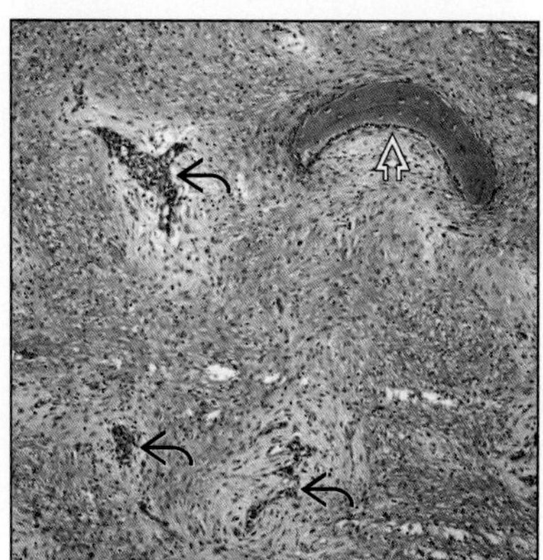

(Left) *The epithelial cells in adamantinoma are keratin positive ⇨.* ***(Center)*** *Low-power view of this adamantinoma shows reactive bony trabeculae rimmed by osteoclasts ⇨. In a small biopsy, the differential would include osteofibrous dysplasia.* ***(Right)*** *This adamantinoma shows small islands of epithelial cells ⇨ within a collagenous fibrous stroma. Also present is a reactive bony trabecula rimmed by osteoblasts ➡.*

ANEURYSMAL BONE CYST

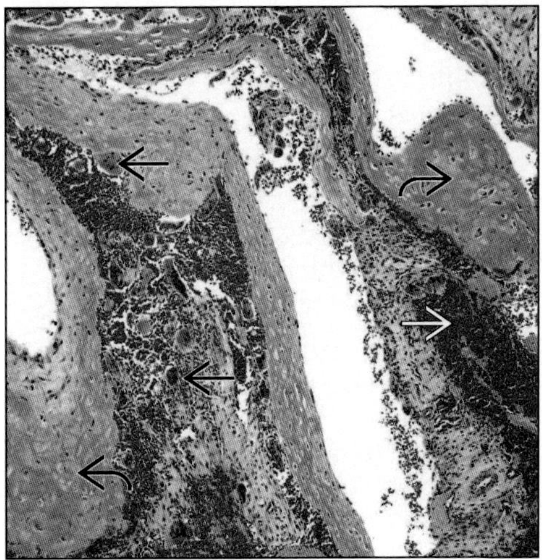

The characteristic features of aneurysmal bone cyst include hemorrhage ➡, giant cells ➡, and thin osteoid ➡.

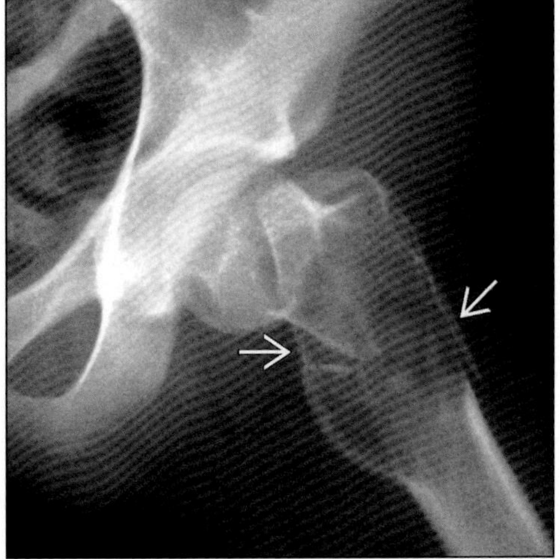

Anteroposterior radiograph shows a lytic expansile lesion in the proximal femoral metaphysis with pathologic fracture ➡.

TERMINOLOGY

Abbreviations

- Aneurysmal bone cyst (ABC)

Definitions

- Solitary expansile lesion, most commonly involving long bones or spine

ETIOLOGY/PATHOGENESIS

Developmental Anomaly

- Proposed etiology for secondary ABCs implicates venous obstruction or arteriovenous fistula formation after bone trauma
- Chromosomal abnormalities in primary ABCs indicate clonal tumor

CLINICAL ISSUES

Epidemiology

- Age
  - 1st and 2nd decade of life
  - Usually before skeletal maturity
- Gender
  - Slightly more common in females

Site

- Metaphysis of long bones
  - Eccentric
- Dorsal elements of spine
  - Not seen in coccyx
  - Can affect multiple vertebrae
  - Cord compression is common

Presentation

- Pain, tenderness
- Swelling

Natural History

- ABC is secondary reactive lesion in many cases
- Can coexist with many tumors, such as
  - Osteoblastoma
  - Chondroblastoma
  - Nonossifying fibroma
  - Fibrous dysplasia

Treatment

- Surgical approaches
  - Curettage

Prognosis

- Benign but locally aggressive
- Commonly recurs after curettage

IMAGE FINDINGS

Radiographic Findings

- Lytic destructive lesion
- Soft tissue extension surrounded by reactive new bone (eggshell)
- Can look malignant

MR Findings

- Loculated pattern
- Fluid levels

MACROSCOPIC FEATURES

General Features

- Wall is soft and fibrous
- Spaces contain fresh blood and blood clot
- Very rare to get intact ABC in gross room

MICROSCOPIC PATHOLOGY

Histologic Features

- **Always look for secondary tumors**

ANEURYSMAL BONE CYST

Key Facts

Terminology
- Solitary expansile lesion, most commonly involving long bones or spine

Clinical Issues
- 1st and 2nd decade of life
- Secondary reactive lesion in many cases
- Can coexist with many tumors
- Benign but locally aggressive

Image Findings
- Can look malignant

Microscopic Pathology
- **Always look for secondary tumors**
- Blood-filled cystic spaces
- Fibrous septa separate cystic spaces
  - Septae contain spindle cells, giant cells, hemosiderin, osteoid
- Most ABCs have some solid areas
- **Solid ABC/giant cell reparative granuloma**
  - Most common in mandible, maxilla, and small bones of hands and feet
  - 2nd to 3rd decade of life
  - No cystic cavities grossly or microscopically

Ancillary Tests
- 17p13 rearrangement is characteristic

Top Differential Diagnoses
- Giant cell tumor
- Telangiectatic osteosarcoma
- Simple bone cyst
- Low-grade osteosarcoma

- Blood-filled cystic spaces
  - Spaces are **not** lined by endothelium
- Fibrous septa separate cystic spaces
  - Septa composed of loose spindled cells and giant cells
  - Septa also contain
    - Immature bone or unmineralized osteoid
    - Hemosiderin
    - Foam cells
    - Chronic inflammation
- Most ABCs have some solid areas
  - Loose spindled areas
  - Fine or trabecular osteoid
- **Solid ABC/giant cell reparative granuloma**
  - Most common in mandible, maxilla, and small bones of hands and feet
  - 2nd to 3rd decade of life
  - No cystic cavities grossly or microscopically
  - Giant cells, hemorrhage, hemosiderin, osteoid, and new bone formation

ANCILLARY TESTS

Cytogenetics
- 17p13 rearrangement is characteristic
  - Present in primary but not secondary ABCs
- t(16;17)(q22;p13) most common translocation
  - *CDH11-USP6* fusion gene, upregulates *USP6* oncogene
- Other *USP6* fusions also reported

DIFFERENTIAL DIAGNOSIS

Giant Cell Tumor
- Epiphyses of long bones in young adults
- Background cells resemble giant cells

Telangiectatic Osteosarcoma
- Resembles ABC on low power
- Marked cytologic atypia
  - Atypical cells can be few in number, making distinction from ABC difficult in some cases

Simple Bone Cyst
- Frequently has secondary ABC changes
- Has cementum

Low-Grade Osteosarcoma
- Hypocellular spindle cell lesion
- No giant cells

SELECTED REFERENCES

1. Chan G et al: Case report: primary aneurysmal bone cyst of the epiphysis. Clin Orthop Relat Res. 468(4):1168-72, 2010
2. Docquier PL et al: Histology can be predictive of the clinical course of a primary aneurysmal bone cyst. Arch Orthop Trauma Surg. 130(4):481-7, 2010
3. Subach BR et al: An unusual occurrence of chondromyxoid fibroma with secondary aneurysmal bone cyst in the cervical spine. Spine J. 10(2):e5-9, 2010
4. Gopalakrishnan CV et al: Intracranial intradural aneurysmal bone cyst: a unique case. Pediatr Neurosurg. 45(4):317-20, 2009
5. van de Luijtgaarden AC et al: Metastatic potential of an aneurysmal bone cyst. Virchows Arch. 455(5):455-9, 2009
6. Lin PP et al: Aneurysmal bone cysts recur at juxtaphyseal locations in skeletally immature patients. Clin Orthop Relat Res. 466(3):722-8, 2008
7. Panagopoulos I et al: Fusion of the COL1A1 and USP6 genes in a benign bone tumor. Cancer Genet Cytogenet. 180(1):70-3, 2008
8. Oliveira AM et al: Aneurysmal bone cyst variant translocations upregulate USP6 transcription by promoter swapping with the ZNF9, COL1A1, TRAP150, and OMD genes. Oncogene. 24(21):3419-26, 2005
9. Oliveira AM et al: USP6 (Tre2) fusion oncogenes in aneurysmal bone cyst. Cancer Res. 64(6):1920-3, 2004
10. Oliveira AM et al: USP6 and CDH11 oncogenes identify the neoplastic cell in primary aneurysmal bone cysts and are absent in so-called secondary aneurysmal bone cysts. Am J Pathol. 165(5):1773-80, 2004

ANEURYSMAL BONE CYST

Gross and Microscopic Features

(Left) Gross pathology shows hemorrhagic and cystic lesion with multiple septations ("blood-filled sponge"). **(Right)** The giant cells in aneurysmal bone cyst can be quite large with very many nuclei, reminiscent of giant cell tumor. However, in aneurysmal bone cyst, the giant cells do not resemble the background mononuclear cells. Many ABCs have solid areas such as this; if the entire specimen has no blood-filled spaces, the diagnosis of solid ABC can be made.

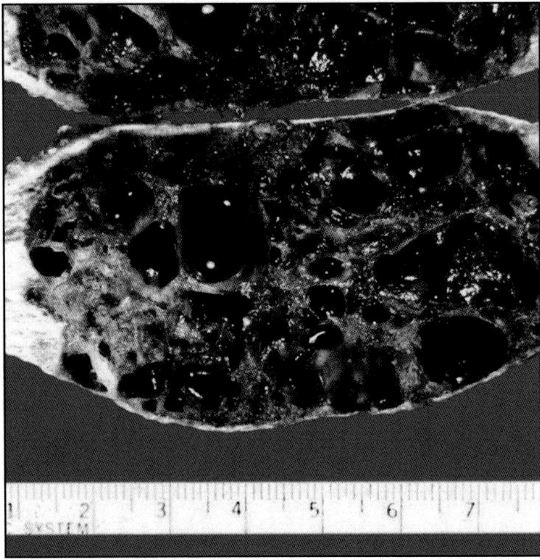

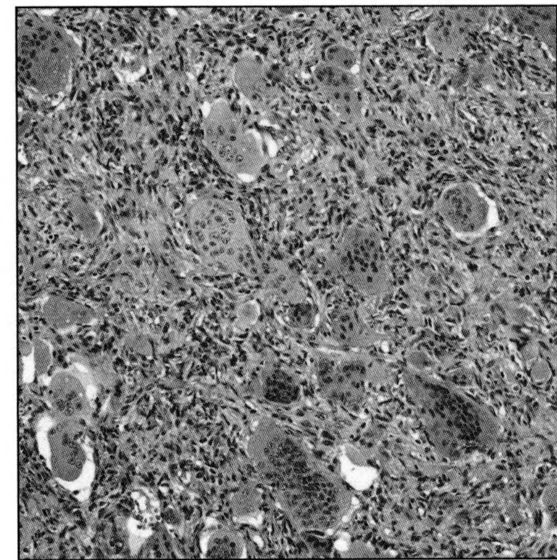

(Left) Aneurysmal bone cyst often has a loose spindled stroma that resembles granulation tissue →. An island of immature osteoid is also present ➔. **(Right)** The blood-filled spaces of aneurysmal bone cyst do not have an endothelial lining ➔. Instead, the "lining" is composed of giant cells and loose fibrous stroma.

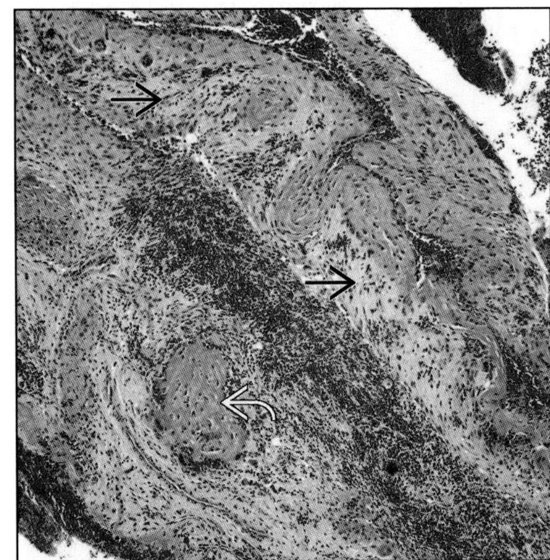

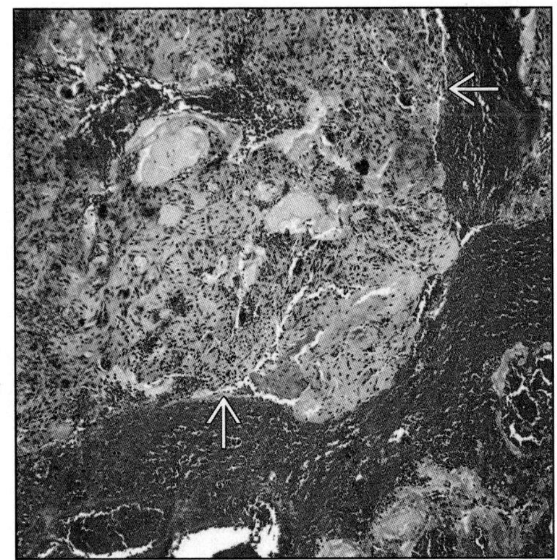

(Left) Hemosiderin pigment ➔ is nearly always seen in aneurysmal bone cyst. Combined with the surrounding hemorrhage and giant cells, these are classic findings of aneurysmal bone cyst. However, ABC-like changes can be seen along with many bone tumors, and it is important to look for evidence of other tumors. **(Right)** Sometimes the blood-filled spaces in ABC are small. Even still, the septae contain giant cells and hemosiderin pigment.

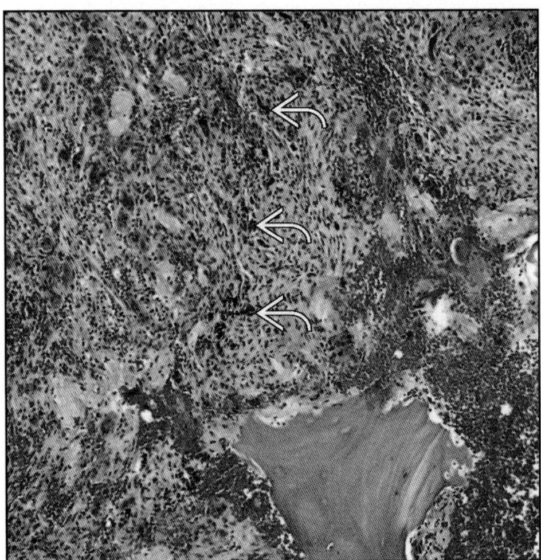

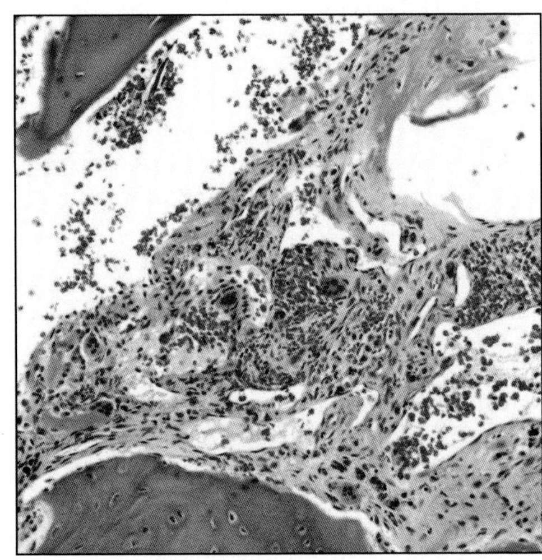

Differential Diagnosis

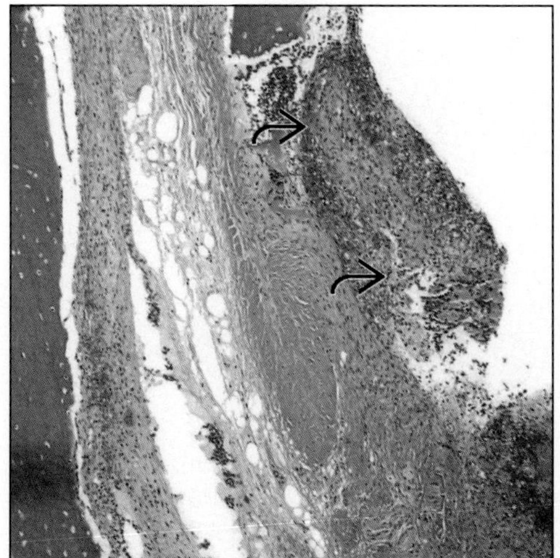

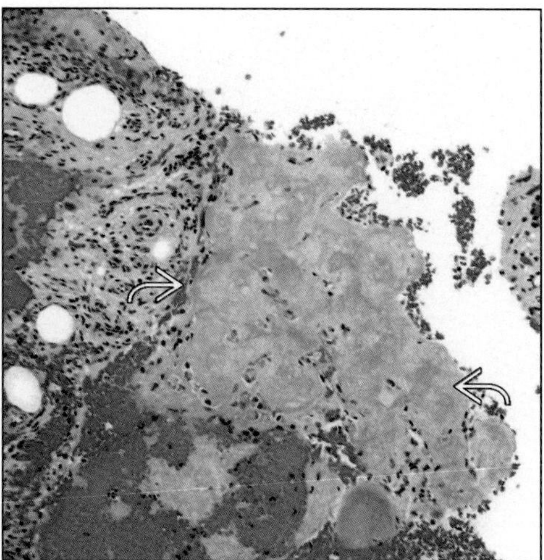

(Left) *This simple/unicameral bone cyst has secondary ABC changes ➢, with hemorrhage, giant cells, and hemosiderin pigment. This is common in simple bone cysts. The correct diagnosis can be made by finding cementum and with the help of the surgeon's gross impression and the radiology report.* ***(Right)*** *Finding cementum ➢ in a simple bone cyst helps make the correct diagnosis when there are ABC-like changes.*

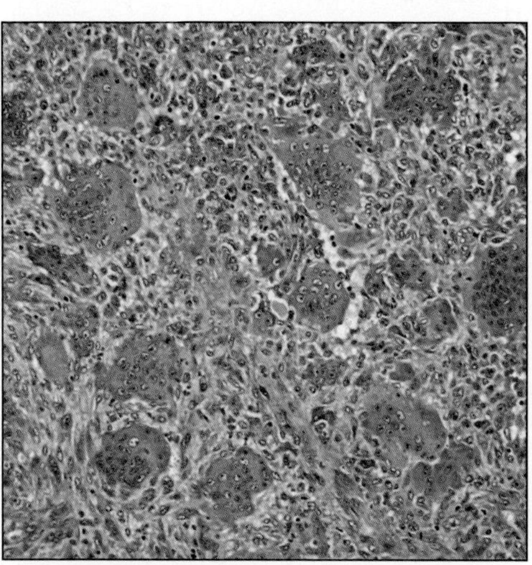

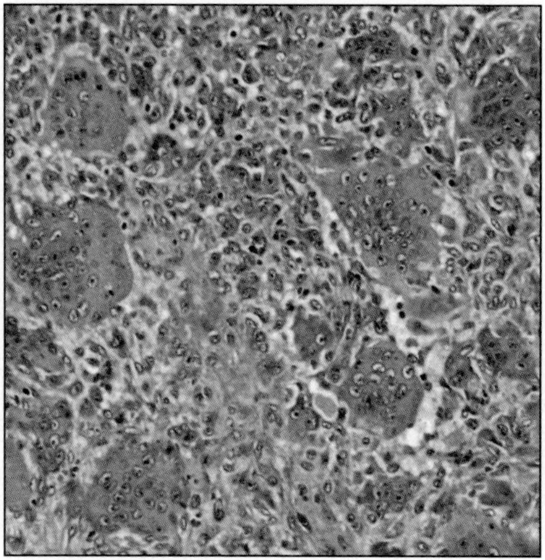

(Left) *The histologic differential diagnosis between ABC and giant cell tumor (seen here) can be difficult. The clinical history is the best help. Giant cell tumors are commonly seen in the epiphyses of skeletally mature women, whereas ABCs are seen in the metaphyses of older children.* ***(Right)*** *In giant cell tumor (seen here), the giant cell nuclei are similar to those of the background mononuclear cells. This is a helpful feature in differentiating from aneurysmal bone cyst.*

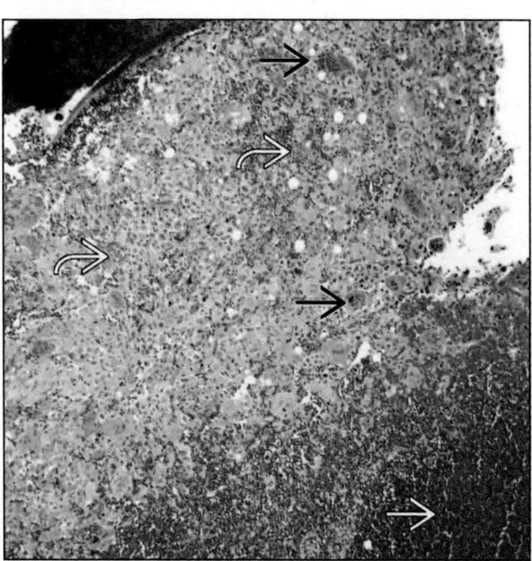

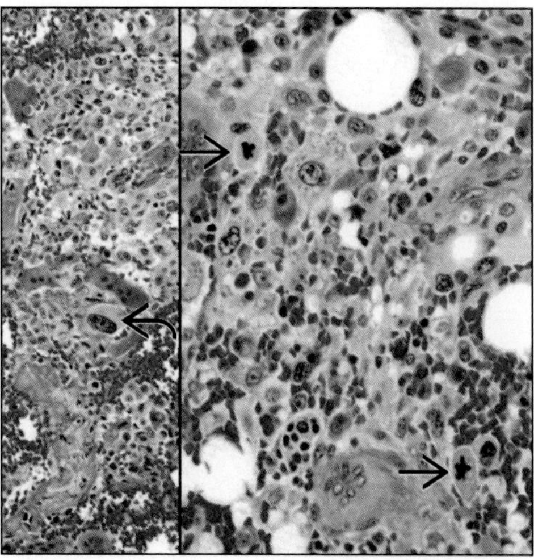

(Left) *This telangiectatic osteosarcoma can easily be mistaken for an aneurysmal bone cyst at low power. Note hemorrhage ➡, giant cells ➡, and hemosiderin pigment ➢.* ***(Right)*** *While the low-power view of telangiectatic osteosarcoma can mimic aneurysmal bone cyst, high-power view of the osteosarcoma reveals large malignant cells ➢ and atypical mitoses ➡.*

SIMPLE BONE CYST

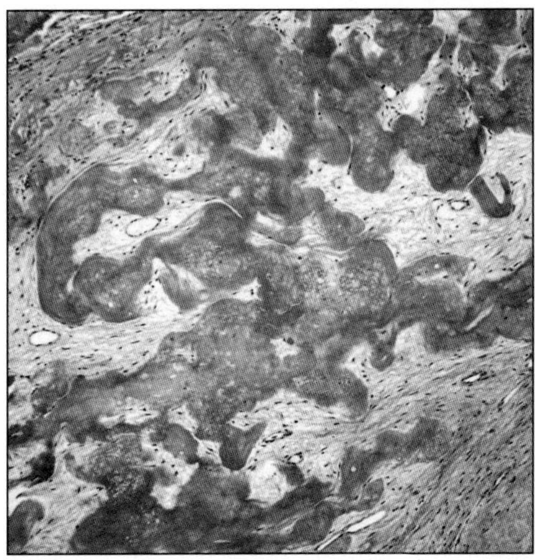

This eosinophilic, somewhat fibrillar, amorphous material is cementum, a diagnostic (though sometimes hard to find) feature of simple/unicameral bone cyst.

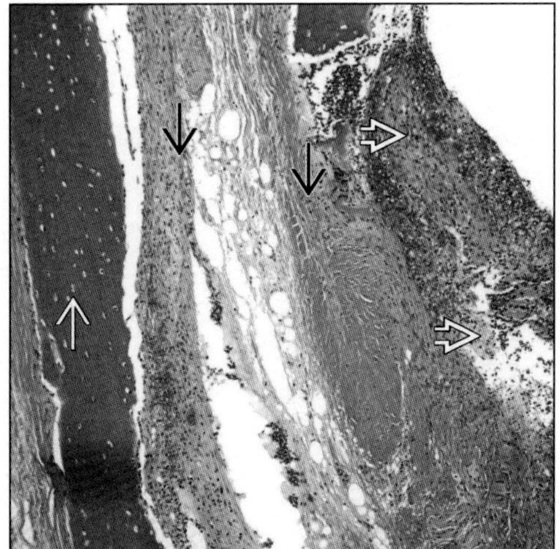

Features of simple/unicameral bone cyst include benign bone ➔ with a fibrous or spindle cell lining ⇒. Secondary changes of hemorrhage and giant cells ➔ are common.

TERMINOLOGY

Abbreviations

- Simple bone cyst (SBC)

Synonyms

- Unicameral bone cyst
- Solitary bone cyst

Definitions

- Benign, solitary cyst in metaphysis of long bones

ETIOLOGY/PATHOGENESIS

Developmental Anomaly

- Proposed theories include blockage of interstitial fluid drainage or venous obstruction

CLINICAL ISSUES

Epidemiology

- Age
  - 1st and 2nd decades of life
- Gender
  - Much more common in males

Site

- Most common
  - Proximal humerus
  - Proximal femur
- Less common
  - Tibia
  - Fibula
  - Radius
  - Ulna
- Older patients (> 20 years)
  - Ilium
  - Calcaneus

Presentation

- Asymptomatic unless pathologic fracture

Treatment

- Watch and wait
- Steroid injection
- Burr holes
- Curettage with bone grafting if above conservative measures do not work

Prognosis

- Benign
- Those that do not fracture likely regress since these are uncommon in adults
- Recurrence common after curettage
  - Especially in younger children with lesions near growth plate

IMAGE FINDINGS

Radiographic Findings

- Well-defined lucent lesion with thin sclerotic rim
- May have pseudoloculated appearance
- Generally does not expand bone
- Over time SBC appears to migrate away from epiphyseal plate

MACROSCOPIC FEATURES

General Features

- Unilocular cyst with thin lining and filled with clear fluid
- Secondary changes can cause multiloculation or bloody fluid
- Extremely rare to receive intact SBC in gross room

SIMPLE BONE CYST

Key Facts

Terminology
- Unicameral bone cyst
- Solitary bone cyst
- Benign, solitary cyst in metaphysis of long bones

Clinical Issues
- 1st and 2nd decades of life
- Much more common in males
- Proximal humerus
- Proximal femur

Microscopic Pathology
- Cementum
- Fragments of fibrous lining
- Secondary changes very common

Top Differential Diagnoses
- Aneurysmal bone cyst

MICROSCOPIC PATHOLOGY

Histologic Features
- Cementum
  - Amorphous, somewhat fibrillar, eosinophilic material
  - May represent calcified fibrin
  - Considered by many to be diagnostic finding
- Benign bony fragments
- Fragments of fibrous lining
  - Spindled cells and giant cells
- Secondary changes very common
  - Hemorrhage
  - Hemosiderin deposits
  - Granulation tissue
  - Cholesterol clefts
  - Fibrin
  - Calcification
  - Reactive bone

DIFFERENTIAL DIAGNOSIS

Aneurysmal Bone Cyst
- When in long bones, most often in diaphysis
- More abundant blood, hemosiderin, and giant cells
- No cementum
- Can be very difficult to differentiate ABC from SBC with ABC-like changes

Giant Cell Tumor
- Solid with even distribution of giant cells
- More common in women

Fibrous Dysplasia
- Not cystic
- Fibrosis with woven bone

Hemangioma
- Very rare in long bones
- Blood-filled cavernous spaces are endothelial-lined

SELECTED REFERENCES

1. Jordanov MI: The "rising bubble" sign: a new aid in the diagnosis of unicameral bone cysts. Skeletal Radiol. 38(6):597-600, 2009
2. Cho HS et al: Unicameral bone cysts: a comparison of injection of steroid and grafting with autologous bone marrow. J Bone Joint Surg Br. 89(2):222-6, 2007
3. Hammoud S et al: Unicameral bone cysts of the pelvis: a study of 16 cases. Iowa Orthop J. 25:69-74, 2005
4. Singh S et al: Unusually large solitary unicameral bone cyst: case report. J Orthop Sci. 8(4):599-601, 2003
5. Tsirikos AI et al: Unicameral bone cyst in the spinous process of a thoracic vertebra. J Spinal Disord Tech. 15(5):440-3, 2002
6. Wilkins RM: Unicameral bone cysts. J Am Acad Orthop Surg. 8(4):217-24, 2000

IMAGE GALLERY

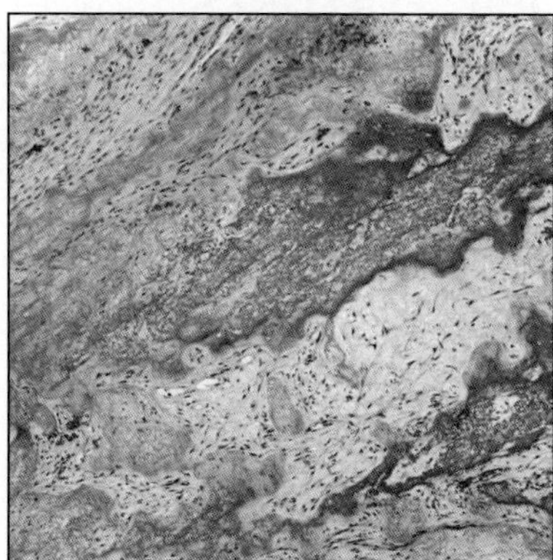

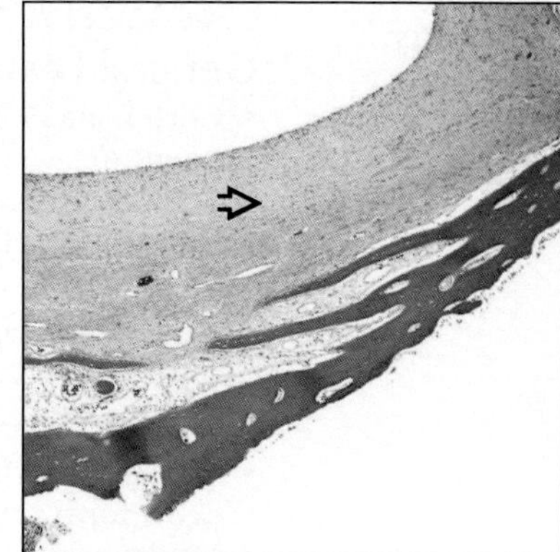

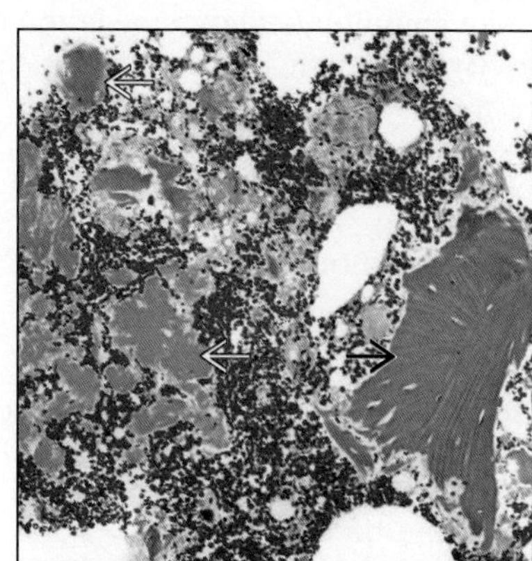

(Left) *The cementum in this simple/unicameral bone cyst has a blue hue typical of calcification or mineralization.* ***(Center)*** *Simple/unicameral bone cysts are frequently received in fragments. A lucky fragment may show a nice fibrous lining ⇨.* ***(Right)*** *This field shows the contrast between a normal bony fragment ⇨ and the amorphous fibrillar cementum ➡ in a simple/unicameral bone cyst.*

NONOSSIFYING FIBROMA

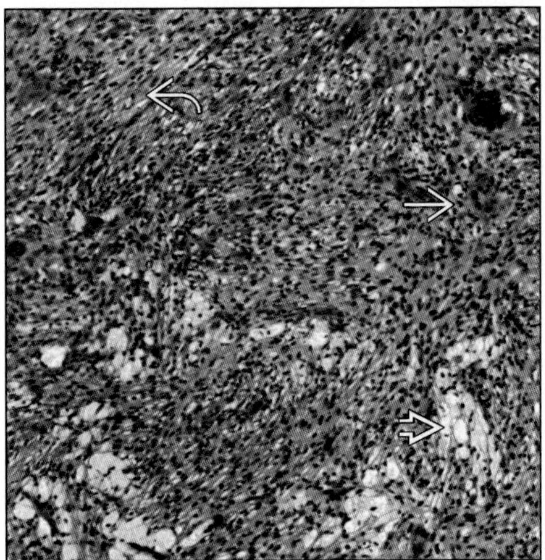

Hematoxylin & eosin stain shows sheets of spindled lesional cells ➡ with admixed foam cells ➡ and giant cells ➡. Cells are uniform and without cellular pleomorphism.

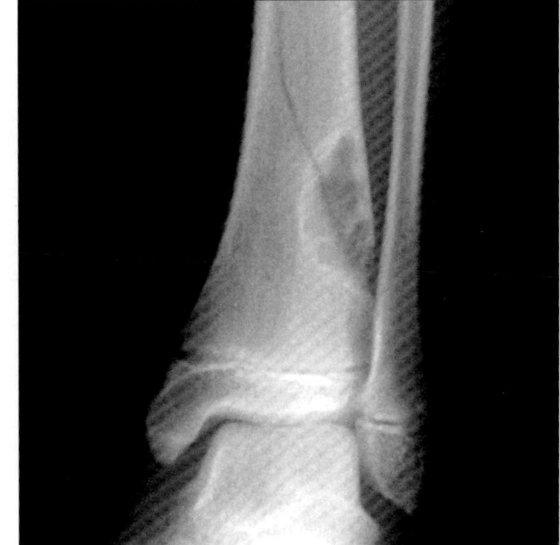

Anteroposterior radiography shows a lytic lesion with well-defined sclerotic, scalloped borders and an associated pathologic fracture involving the distal femoral metaphysis.

TERMINOLOGY

Abbreviations

- Nonossifying fibroma (NOF)

Synonyms

- Metaphyseal fibrous defect
- Nonosteogenic fibroma
- Fibrous cortical defect
  - Limited only to bony cortex

Definitions

- Proliferation of spindle cells involving cortex and medullary cavity of long bones

ETIOLOGY/PATHOGENESIS

Developmental Anomaly

- May be defect in ossification

CLINICAL ISSUES

Epidemiology

- Incidence
  - Most common benign bone lesion of skeleton
    - Asymptomatic lesions in up to 35% of children ages 4-8 years
- Age
  - Most common in 1st 2 decades
- Gender
  - More common in males

Site

- Long bone involvement
  - Adjacent to knee most common location
  - Rare flat bone involvement
- Metaphyseal location
- May be multifocal

Presentation

- Usually asymptomatic, incidental radiographic findings
- May present as pathologic fracture
- Local pain or swelling reported

Treatment

- Options, risks, complications
  - Observation if classic radiographic presentation and bone not at risk of fracture
    - If > 50% of bone involved, at risk of fracture
- Surgical approaches
  - Curettage and bone grafting curative

Prognosis

- No risk of malignant transformation

IMAGE FINDINGS

General Features

- Expansile, lytic lesion with scalloped, sclerotic borders
  - Lesional long axis parallels long axis of affected bone

MACROSCOPIC FEATURES

General Features

- Cortex may be thinned but is intact (unless pathologic fracture)
  - Lesional tissue well demarcated
- Curettings yellow to brown fibrous tissue

MICROSCOPIC PATHOLOGY

Histologic Features

- Sheets of storiform spindled cells
  - Uniform nuclei
- Multinucleated giant cells

NONOSSIFYING FIBROMA

Key Facts

Clinical Issues

- Usually asymptomatic and are incidental radiographic findings
  - May present with pathologic fracture
- Most common in 1st 2 decades
- Long bone involvement
  - Metaphyseal location
  - Adjacent to knee most common location
- No risk of malignant transformation

Image Findings

- Expansile, lytic lesion with scalloped, sclerotic border

Microscopic Pathology

- Sheets of storiform spindled cells
  - Foam cells, giant cells, and hemosiderin
- Mitotic figures identified
- Associated pathologic fracture
  - Associated reactive bone formation and necrosis

- Histiocytic foam cells
- Hemosiderin
- Mitotic figures identified
- Associated pathologic fracture
  - New reactive bone formation
  - Necrosis

Predominant Pattern/Injury Type

- Sheets
- Spindled
- Storiform

Predominant Cell/Compartment Type

- Mesenchymal, fibroblast
- Histiocyte/macrophage
- Multinucleated giant cell

DIFFERENTIAL DIAGNOSIS

Giant Cell Tumor

- Lack storiform pattern
- Nonmetaphyseal
- Giant cells more numerous
  - Higher numbers of nuclei per giant cell

Benign Fibrous Histiocytoma

- Adult presentation
- Unusual location

Malignant Fibrous Histiocytoma

- Cellular pleomorphism

Osteosarcoma

- In setting of pathologic fracture with reactive bone formation
  - Diagnosis of osteosarcoma requires malignant osteoid
  - Cellular pleomorphism with osteosarcoma

DIAGNOSTIC CHECKLIST

Pathologic Interpretation Pearls

- Sheets of spindled cells
  - Admixed foam cells, giant cells, hemosiderin

SELECTED REFERENCES

1. Betsy M et al: Metaphyseal fibrous defects. J Am Acad Orthop Surg. 12(2):89-95, 2004
2. Biermann JS: Common benign lesions of bone in children and adolescents. J Pediatr Orthop. 22(2):268-73, 2002
3. Jee WH et al: Nonossifying fibroma: characteristics at MR imaging with pathologic correlation. Radiology. 209(1):197-202, 1998
4. Moser RP Jr et al: Multiple skeletal fibroxanthomas: radiologic-pathologic correlation of 72 cases. Skeletal Radiol. 16(5):353-9, 1987
5. Mandell GA et al: Fibrous lesions in the lower extremities in neurofibromatosis. AJR Am J Roentgenol. 133(6):1135-8, 1979
6. Steiner GC: Fibrous cortical defect and nonossifying fibroma of bone. A study of the ultrastructure. Arch Pathol. 97(4):205-10, 1974

IMAGE GALLERY

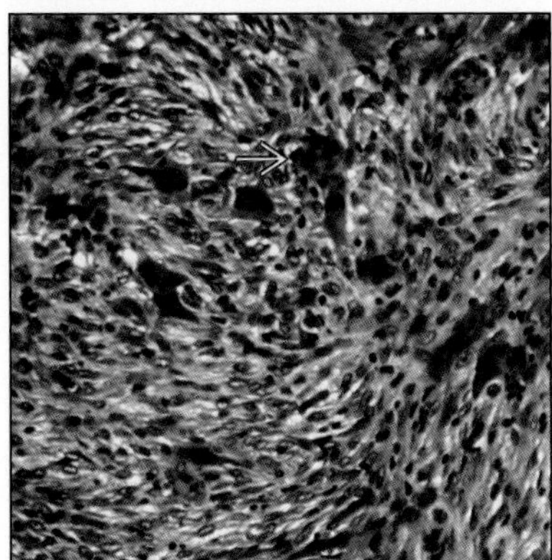

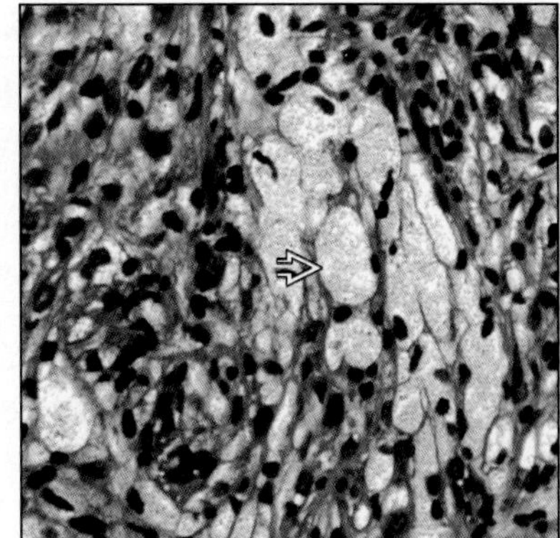

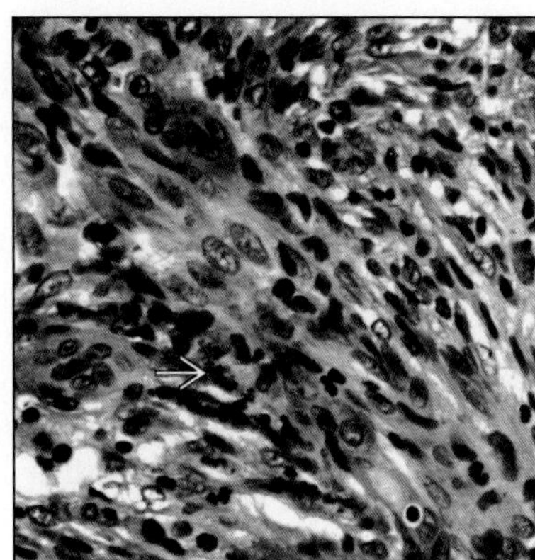

*(**Left**) Hematoxylin & eosin shows a storiform pattern of spindled cells with admixed multinucleated giant cells. Giant cells ➡ have a smaller number of nuclei than typically seen in giant cell tumor. (**Center**) Hematoxylin & eosin shows clusters of lipid-laden macrophages or foam cells ➡. These cells give gross tissue a yellow-brown color. (**Right**) Hematoxylin & eosin shows deposits of hemosiderin ➡, which can be confirmed with iron stain. Hemosiderin can be free or in macrophages.*

FIBROUS DYSPLASIA

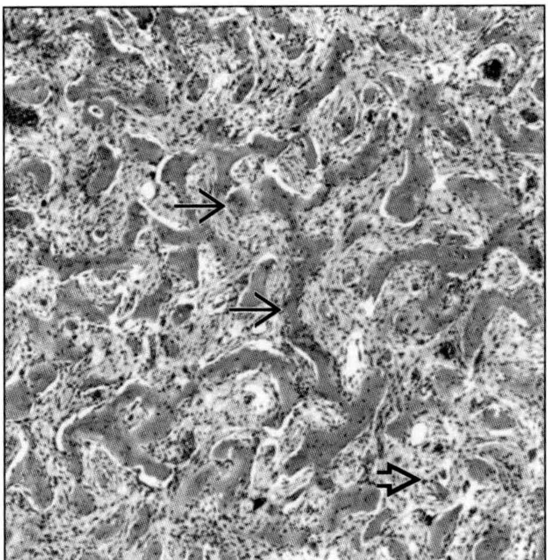

Hematoxylin & eosin stain shows irregular spicules of bone ➔ arranged in a haphazard manner in a background of bland fibrous tissue ➲. Fibroblasts produce variably cellular collagenous matrix.

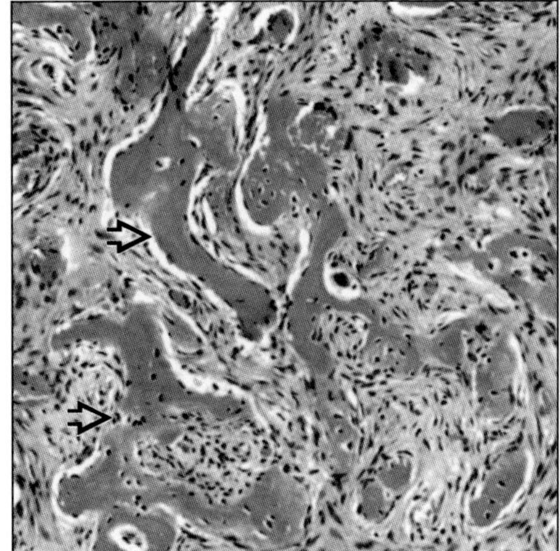

Hematoxylin & eosin shows bony spicules or so-called Chinese characters ➲. Spicules are irregularly arranged without functional architecture. Cytologic atypia and cellular pleomorphism are absent.

TERMINOLOGY

Abbreviations

- Fibrous dysplasia (FD)

Synonyms

- Fibrocartilaginous dysplasia

Definitions

- Defect in ossification with fibrous proliferation and spicules of disorganized bone in medullary cavity

ETIOLOGY/PATHOGENESIS

Neoplastic

- 12p13, trisomy 2, activating mutations of G proteins

CLINICAL ISSUES

Epidemiology

- Age
  - Can occur any age; most frequent at 20-30 years
- Gender
  - Equal sex distribution

Site

- Monostotic: 6x more common than polyostotic form
  - Craniofacial bones, femur, tibia, and ribs
    - Occurs more often in long bones of women and ribs and skull bones of men
- Polyostotic: Seen in younger age group
  - Femur, pelvis, and tibia

Presentation

- Asymptomatic, incidental imaging finding
- Localized swelling, pain, pathologic fracture, bony deformity, or exophthalmos with skull involvement
- Associations
  - McCune-Albright syndrome: Polyostotic FD, skin pigmentation, endocrine hyperactivity, precocious puberty
  - Mazabraud syndrome: FD and intramuscular or soft tissue myxoma

Treatment

- Surgical approaches
  - Curettage and bone grafting or observation if asymptomatic with classic imaging

Prognosis

- Rare malignant transformation
  - Most frequently fibrosarcoma
  - Chondrosarcoma also reported
  - Not associated with history of radiation

IMAGE FINDINGS

General Features

- Metaphyseal or diaphyseal lesion with ground-glass matrix
- Bony expansion with sharp borders
- Soft tissue involvement and periosteal reaction absent

MACROSCOPIC FEATURES

General Features

- Tan-gray, firm-fibrous to gritty tissue
  - Cystic component with clear fluid
  - Cartilaginous component

MICROSCOPIC PATHOLOGY

Histologic Features

- Mixed fibrous and osseous lesion
- Cytologically bland spindled fibroblasts with collagenous matrix
- Scattered, irregular, curvilinear spicules of woven bone

FIBROUS DYSPLASIA

Key Facts

Terminology

- Benign intramedullary fibroosseous lesion which may be multifocal

Clinical Issues

- Monoostotic form: Head (35%), femur and tibia (30%), ribs (20%)
- Polyostotic form: Femur, pelvis, and tibia

Image Findings

- Metaphyseal or diaphyseal expansion with sharp borders

Microscopic Pathology

- Spindle cells with irregular, curvilinear trabeculae of woven bone
- Focal cartilage, degenerative change, ABC

  - Round, psammomatous or cementum-like bone possible
  - Lacks osteoblastic rimming
- Secondary features
  - Foci of hyaline cartilage, usually small component, common in femoral neck region
  - Degenerating cystic areas with foam cells, multinucleated giant cells, myxoid change
  - Aneurysmal bone cyst

Predominant Cell/Compartment Type

- Mesenchymal, osteocyte

DIFFERENTIAL DIAGNOSIS

Paget Disease

- Bony trabeculae are lined by plump osteoblasts and osteoclasts

Giant Cell Reparative Granuloma

- Predominantly fibrous background
- Mature bony trabeculae are lined by osteoblasts

Osteosarcoma

- Greater degree of cellularity and pleomorphism
- Atypical mitoses
- Permeates surrounding soft tissues; correlate with imaging

Osteofibrous Dysplasia

- Bony trabeculae are lined by osteoblasts

DIAGNOSTIC CHECKLIST

Pathologic Interpretation Pearls

- Irregular bony spicules
  - "Chinese characters"
  - Lacks osteoblastic rimming
- Bland spindle cell proliferation lacking cytologic atypia

SELECTED REFERENCES

1. Huening MA et al: Fine-needle aspiration of fibrous dysplasia of bone: a worthwhile endeavor or not? Diagn Cytopathol. 36(5):325-30, 2008
2. Riminucci M et al: The pathology of fibrous dysplasia and the McCune-Albright syndrome. Pediatr Endocrinol Rev. 4 Suppl 4:401-11, 2007
3. Hoshi M et al: Malignant change secondary to fibrous dysplasia. Int J Clin Oncol. 11(3):229-35, 2006
4. Fitzpatrick KA et al: Imaging findings of fibrous dysplasia with histopathologic and intraoperative correlation. AJR Am J Roentgenol. 182(6):1389-98, 2004
5. Ippolito E et al: Natural history and treatment of fibrous dysplasia of bone: a multicenter clinicopathologic study promoted by the European Pediatric Orthopaedic Society. J Pediatr Orthop B. 12(3):155-77, 2003
6. Cohen MM Jr: Fibrous dysplasia is a neoplasm. Am J Med Genet. 98(4):290-3, 2001

IMAGE GALLERY

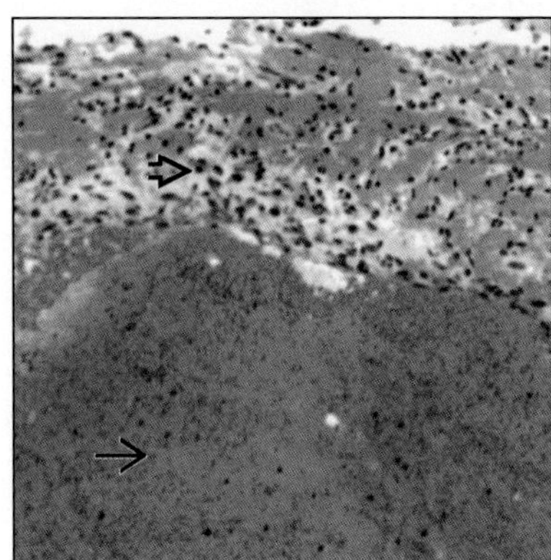

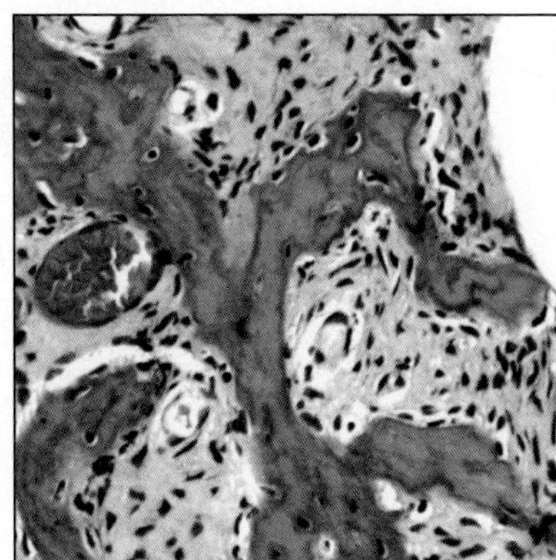

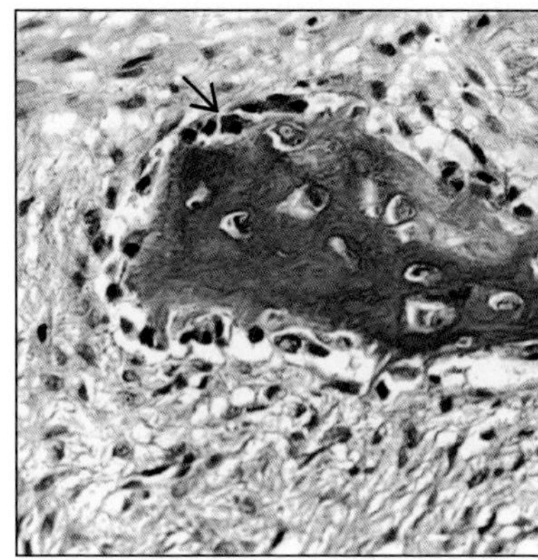

(Left) *Hematoxylin & eosin shows a secondary aneurysmal bone cyst, a frequent finding in cases of FD. A thin organizing rim of fibrous tissue ⇨ lines a cystic space, which lacks a true endothelial lining & is filled with blood ⇨.* ***(Center)*** *Hematoxylin & eosin shows a higher power view of the bony spicules. Note the absence of osteoblastic rimming. Bony spicules show changes of remodeling.* ***(Right)*** *Hematoxylin & eosin shows a case of osteofibrous dysplasia, which is characterized by the presence of ⇨ osteoblastic rimming. This feature is absent in FD.*

CHORDOMA

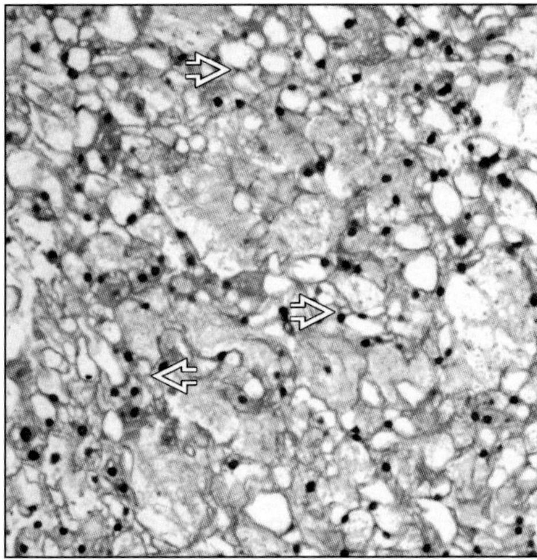

The defining cell of chordoma is the physaliferous cell, a vacuolated cell that sometimes has a "soap bubble" appearance. Many physaliferous cells are seen here ⇨ within a myxoid background.

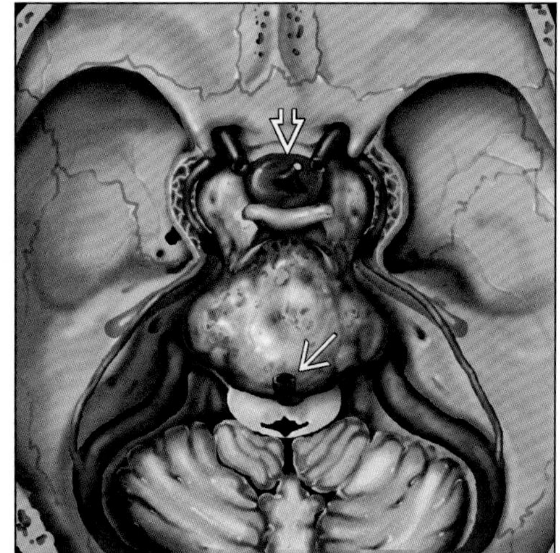

Graphic of the skull base viewed from above shows a large clival chordoma pushing posteriorly to indent the pons and basilar artery ➡. Basi-sphenoid invasion is also seen lifting the pituitary gland ⇨.

TERMINOLOGY

Definitions

- Malignant tumor arising from notochordal elements

ETIOLOGY/PATHOGENESIS

Developmental Anomaly

- Embryonic notochord is midline structure in embryo
- Notochord remnants can persist in axial skeleton

CLINICAL ISSUES

Epidemiology

- Age
  - Uncommon in patients under 20 years old
  - < 5% occur in children
- Gender
  - More common in females

Site

- Always midline
  - Base of skull, clivus (45%)
  - Sacrum (40%)
  - Spine
    - Cervical (10%)
    - Thoracic (2%)
    - Lumbar (2%)

Presentation

- Pain
- Neurological abnormality

Treatment

- Surgical approaches
  - En bloc resection for best outcome
  - Recurrence common

Prognosis

- Slow growing, but can be very aggressive
  - ~ 40% 10-year survival
- Dedifferentiation has been reported

IMAGE FINDINGS

Radiographic Findings

- Irregular areas of destruction
- Intratumoral calcifications
- When in sacrum, often extends to presacral space
  - Sacral lesions can be difficult to identify on x-ray

MACROSCOPIC FEATURES

General Features

- Soft, lobulated, gray-brown, somewhat mucoid

Size

- Usually several centimeters

MICROSCOPIC PATHOLOGY

Histologic Features

- Lobulated
  - May not be apparent on small biopsy
- Cords of small cells
  - Epithelioid or spindled
  - Many cells have vacuolated cytoplasm
    - Physaliferous cells
    - Vacuoles contain mucin and glycogen
- Myxoid stroma
- **Chondroid chordoma**
  - Chordoma at base of skull with extensive chondroid differentiation
  - Much better prognosis

CHORDOMA

Key Facts

Terminology

- Malignant tumor arising from notochordal elements

Clinical Issues

- < 5% occur in children
- Always midline
- Recurrence common

Microscopic Pathology

- Physaliferous cells

Top Differential Diagnoses

- Chondrosarcoma
- Metastatic carcinoma
- Myxopapillary ependymoma
- Chordoid meningioma
- Myxoid liposarcoma

ANCILLARY TESTS

Immunohistochemistry

- Tumor cells are positive for
  - S100
  - Keratin
  - Epithelial membrane antigen (EMA)
  - Vimentin

Electron Microscopy

- Multilayered structures composed of rough endoplasmic reticulum and mitochondria

DIFFERENTIAL DIAGNOSIS

Chondrosarcoma

- Keratin(-)
- Lack fibrous septa

Metastatic Carcinoma

- S100(-)
- Usually no lobulated pattern

Myxopapillary Ependymoma

- Keratin(-)

Chordoid Meningioma

- Often intermixed with typical meningioma
- Usually S100(-)

Myxoid Liposarcoma

- Has lipoblasts
- Usually found in extremities
- Characteristic chromosomal translocation; t(12;16)

SELECTED REFERENCES

1. Choi GH et al: Pediatric cervical chordoma: report of two cases and a review of the current literature. Childs Nerv Syst. Epub ahead of print, 2010
2. Ferraresi V et al: Chordoma: clinical characteristics, management and prognosis of a case series of 25 patients. BMC Cancer. 10:22, 2010
3. Nishiguchi T et al: Lumbar vertebral chordoma arising from an intraosseous benign notochordal cell tumour: radiological findings and histopathological description with a good clinical outcome. Br J Radiol. 83(987):e49-54, 2010
4. Strano S et al: Primary chordoma of the lung. Ann Thorac Surg. 89(1):302-3, 2010
5. Tena-Suck ML et al: Chordoid meningioma: a report of ten cases. J Neurooncol. Epub ahead of print, 2010
6. Kumar P et al: Chordoma with increased prolactin levels (pseudoprolactinoma) mimicking pituitary adenoma: a case report with review of the literature. J Cancer Res Ther. 5(4):309-11, 2009
7. Larizza L et al: Update on the cytogenetics and molecular genetics of chordoma. Hered Cancer Clin Pract. 3(1):29-41, 2005

IMAGE GALLERY

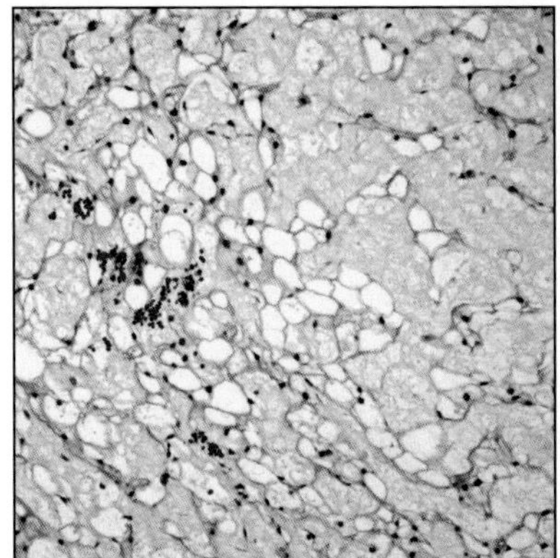

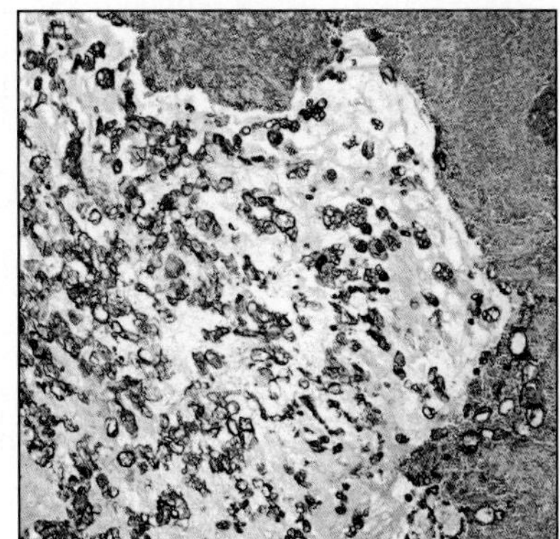

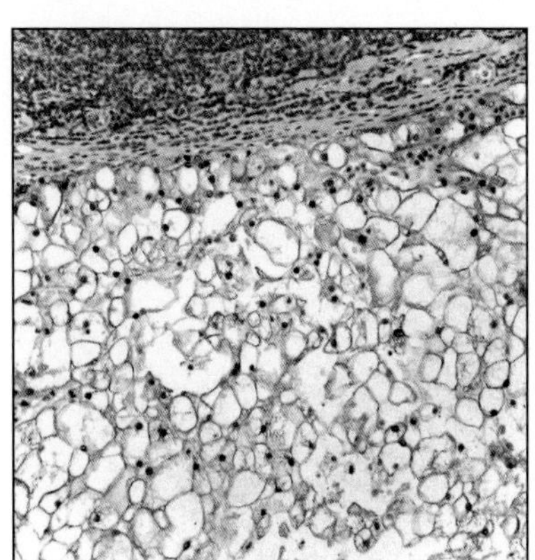

(Left) *Chordoma has a myxoid background, which can vary in amount. Some areas, like this, can look like myxoid liposarcoma; however, lipoblasts are not found.* ***(Center)*** *Chordoma is positive for cytokeratin. This is useful in differentiating from chondrosarcoma, myxopapillary ependymoma, and myxoid liposarcoma (these are CK negative).* ***(Right)*** *Chordoma is positive for S100. This is useful in the differential from metastatic carcinoma, which would be S100 negative.*

CHONDROSARCOMA

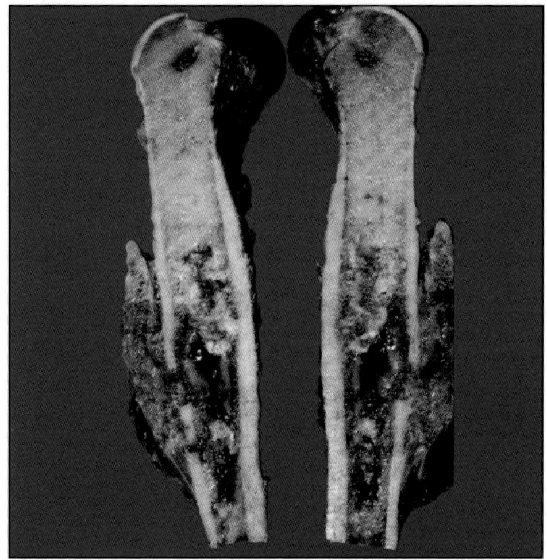

Gross photograph shows a lobulated, cartilaginous tumor with ill-defined margins and soft tissue extension.

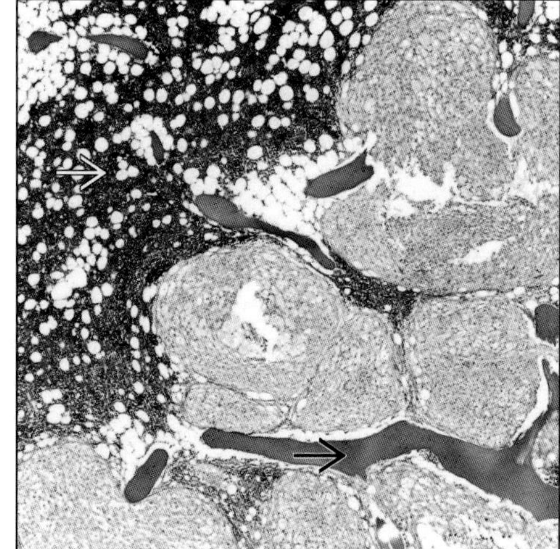

This chondrosarcoma shows the usual lobular architecture. The tumor surrounds normal bony trabeculae ⇨ and is seen pushing into marrow space ➡.

TERMINOLOGY

Synonyms

- Conventional chondrosarcoma

Definitions

- Malignant neoplasm of cartilage-producing cells

ETIOLOGY/PATHOGENESIS

Primary vs. Secondary Chondrosarcoma

- ~ 14% of chondrosarcomas arise secondary to a preexisting condition
  - Multiple hereditary exostosis (Ollier disease)
  - Chondrodysplasia

CLINICAL ISSUES

Epidemiology

- Age
  - Adults in their 40s to 50s
  - Unusual in patients under 16 years
- Gender
  - M:F = 2:1

Site

- Pelvis: 25%
- Ribs and sternum: 12%
- Femur: 15%
- Humerus: 10%
- Tibia: 5%
- Spine and sacrum: 5%
- Craniofacial bones: 2%
- Soft tissue (extraskeletal chondrosarcoma)

Presentation

- Dull aching pain at rest
  - Can be severe at night
  - May be present several months to years
- Soft tissue swelling
- Pathologic fracture is rare

Treatment

- Complete surgical excision
- Chemotherapy and radiation used only for grade 3 tumors

Prognosis

- Lesion of axial skeleton and proximal limbs tend to be more malignant
- Grade I
  - Rarely metastasize, can recur locally
  - 90% 5-year survival
- Grade II
  - 10-15% metastasize
  - 81% 5-year survival
- Grade III
  - Frequently metastasize, especially to lung
  - 29% 5-year survival

IMAGE FINDINGS

Radiographic Findings

- Fusiform, lucent defect with scalloped inner cortex
- Thickened cortex
- Punctate calcifications
- May have soft tissue extension

MACROSCOPIC FEATURES

General Features

- Lobulated
- Gray-white to bluish
- Calcification may be seen grossly
- Mucoid degeneration or necrosis

Size

- 1-40 cm (mean = 10 cm)

CHONDROSARCOMA

Key Facts

Terminology
- Malignant neoplasm of cartilage-producing cells

Etiology/Pathogenesis
- About 14% of chondrosarcomas arise secondary to preexisting condition

Clinical Issues
- Adults in their 40s to 50s
- M:F = 2:1
- Common sites
  - Pelvis: 25%
  - Femur: 15%
  - Ribs and sternum: 12%
  - Humerus: 10%

Microscopic Pathology
- Grade I
  - Must rely on radiology and clinical presentation for accurate diagnosis
- Grade II
- Grade III
- Trabeculae of normal bone may be found embedded in tumor
- Subtypes include
  - Clear cell chondrosarcoma
  - Dedifferentiated chondrosarcoma
  - Mesenchymal chondrosarcoma

Top Differential Diagnoses
- Chondroblastic osteosarcoma
- Small round cell tumors
  - In differential of mesenchymal chondrosarcoma

MICROSCOPIC PATHOLOGY

Histologic Features
- Grade I
  - Histologically similar to benign enchondromas
  - Any myxoid change suggests malignancy
  - Must rely on radiology and clinical presentation for accurate diagnosis
- Grade II
  - Increased cellularity
  - Increased nuclear size and binucleation
  - Nucleoli often present
- Grade III
  - Marked cellular atypia
- Trabeculae of normal bone may be found embedded in tumor
- Mitoses are rare
- **Clear cell chondrosarcoma**
  - Epiphysis of long bones
  - Radiology may look benign
  - Cells with well-defined cytoplasmic membranes and clear cytoplasm
  - Cells arranged in lobules, often with central bony trabeculae
  - Areas of conventional low-grade chondrosarcoma often seen
- **Dedifferentiated chondrosarcoma**
  - Low-grade chondrosarcoma abruptly juxtaposed with high-grade spindle cell sarcoma
    - Sarcoma may be fibrosarcoma, osteosarcoma, or malignant fibrous histiocytoma (MFH)
  - Very poor prognosis
- **Mesenchymal chondrosarcoma**
  - Young adults
  - More common in females
  - More common in jaws, ribs
  - Islands of well-differentiated chondrosarcoma within a small round cell tumor
    - Chondroid islands may calcify or ossify
  - Hemangiopericytomatous pattern
  - Unpredictable prognosis

ANCILLARY TESTS

Immunohistochemistry
- Vimentin and S100 positive

DIFFERENTIAL DIAGNOSIS

Chondroblastic Osteosarcoma
- Gradual transition from high-grade cartilaginous neoplasm to spindle cell neoplasm

Small Round Cell Tumors
- In differential of mesenchymal chondrosarcoma
- Chondroid lobules or well-differentiated cartilage not seen in small round cell tumors

SELECTED REFERENCES

1. Küpeli S et al: Sacral mesenchymal chondrosarcoma in childhood: a case report and review of the literature. Pediatr Hematol Oncol. 27(7):564-73, 2010
2. De Cecio R et al: Congenital intracranial mesenchymal chondrosarcoma: case report and review of the literature in pediatric patients. Pediatr Dev Pathol. 11(4):309-13, 2008
3. Weinberg J et al: Periosteal chondrosarcoma in a 9-year-old girl with osteochondromatosis. Skeletal Radiol. 34(9):539-42, 2005
4. Pierz KA et al: Pediatric bone tumors: osteosarcoma ewing's sarcoma, and chondrosarcoma associated with multiple hereditary osteochondromatosis. J Pediatr Orthop. 21(3):412-8, 2001
5. Chou P et al: Chondrosarcoma of the head in children. Pediatr Pathol. 10(6):945-58, 1990
6. Fletcher JA et al: Complex cytogenetic aberrations in a well-differentiated chondrosarcoma. Cancer Genet Cytogenet. 41(1):115-21, 1989
7. Aprin H et al: Chondrosarcoma in children and adolescents. Clin Orthop Relat Res. (166):226-32, 1982

CHONDROSARCOMA

Radiologic and Microscopic Features

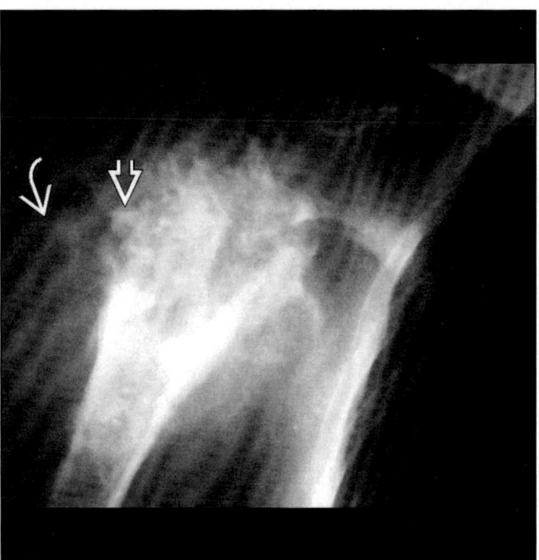

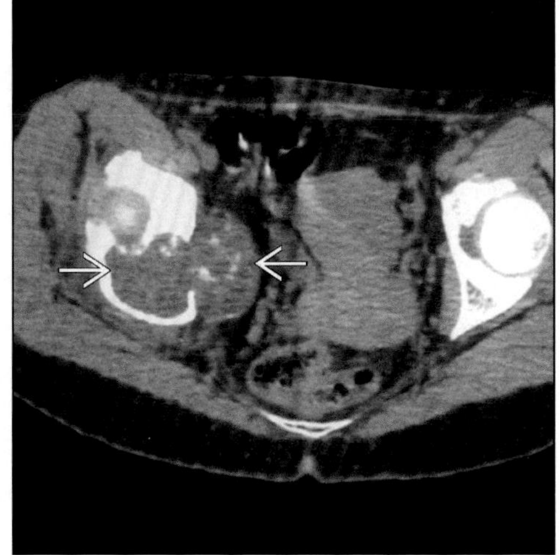

(Left) *Anteroposterior radiograph shows a destructive lesion in the proximal humerus with the areas of ring and arc-like calcifications ➡, cortical destruction, and associated soft tissue extension ➡.* ***(Right)*** *Nonenhanced CT shows a destructive lesion in the right acetabulum with cortical destruction and associated soft tissue mass ➡. Note the calcified matrix.*

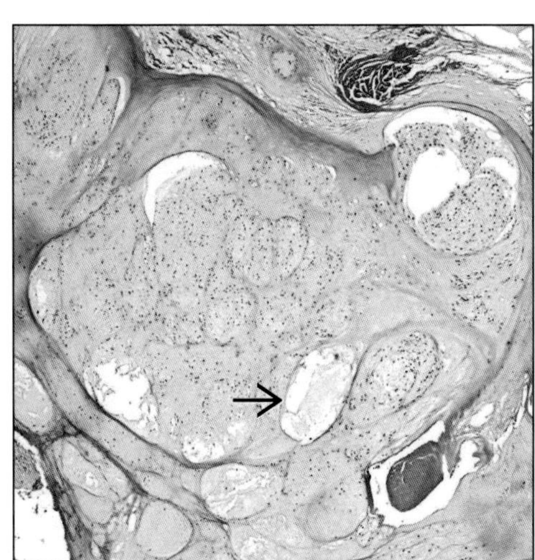

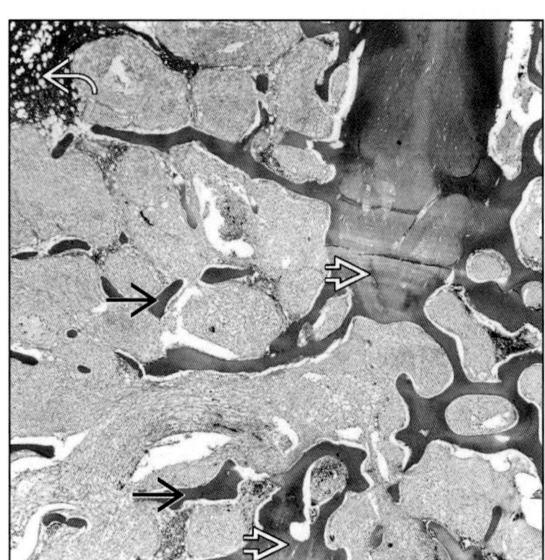

(Left) *This grade 2 chondrosarcoma shows the usual lobular architecture. Areas of myxoid degeneration ➡ are present. Myxoid areas in cartilaginous tumors are indications of malignancy.* ***(Right)*** *This grade 2 chondrosarcoma has the usual lobular architecture and surrounds normal bony trabeculae ➡. The tumor is also seen breaking through the epiphyseal plate ➡ and pushing into normal bone marrow ➡.*

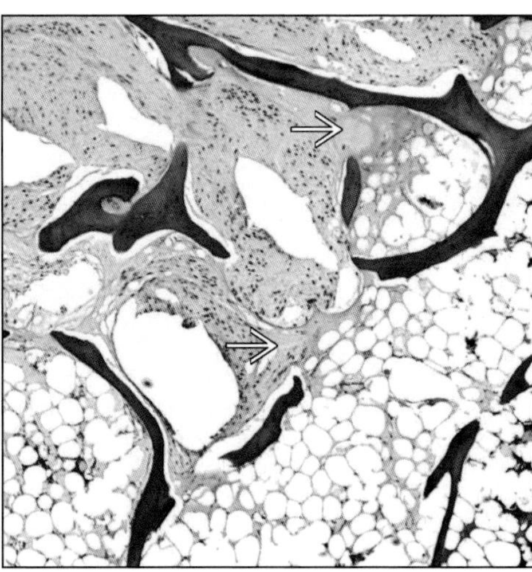

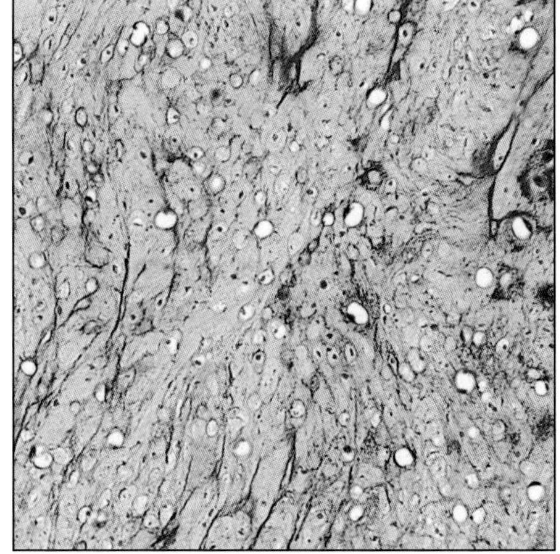

(Left) *This grade 2 chondrosarcoma has small myxoid areas ➡ and is seen infiltrating into the marrow space. The usual lobular architecture is not as prominent here.* ***(Right)*** *This section from a chondrosarcoma shows extensive myxoid change, which is indicative of malignancy. On histology alone, this area could be mistaken for a myxoid liposarcoma. Radiology and clinical information is very important when diagnosing chondrosarcoma.*

Microscopic Features

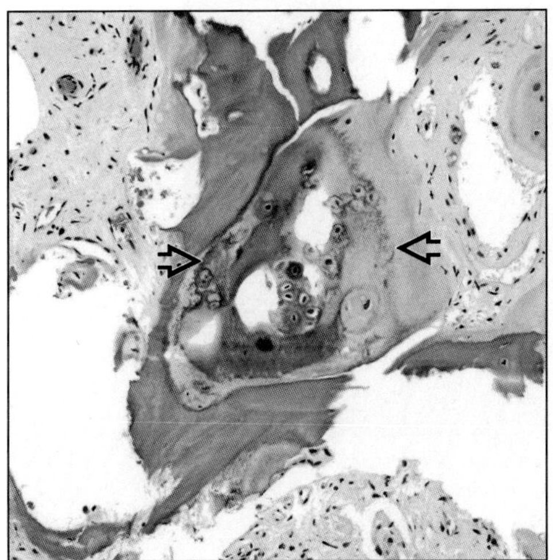

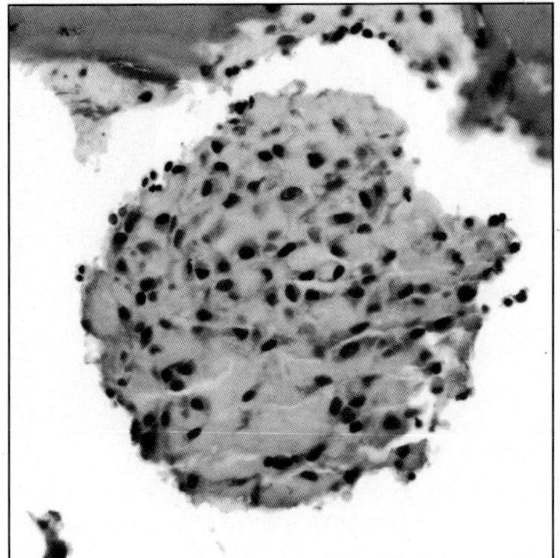

(Left) *Biopsy or curettage is often low yield. In this case, this small fragment of malignant cartilage ⇨ was the only diagnostic area. Here, the chondrocytes are large with prominent nucleoli.* ***(Right)*** *This is another example of a low-yield sample. This fragment was the only diagnostic tissue present. In some cases, immunohistochemistry may be helpful; chondrosarcoma is positive for vimentin and S100.*

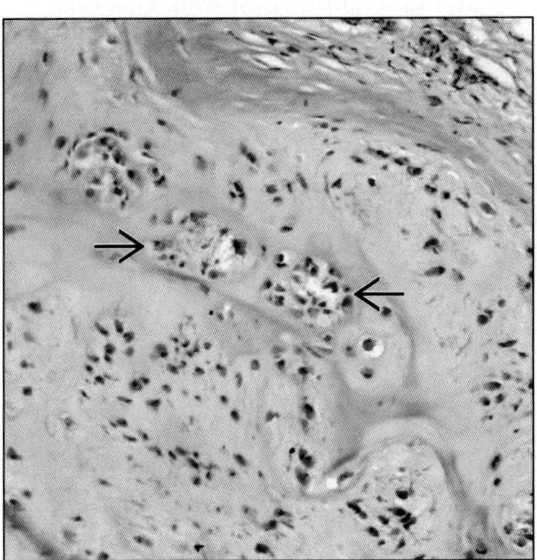

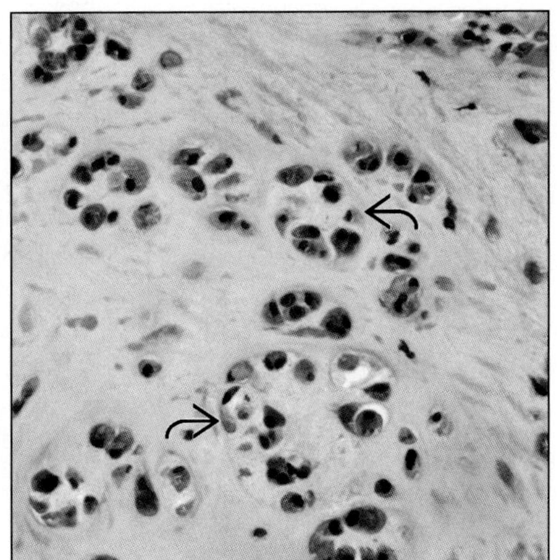

(Left) *In chondrosarcoma, lacunae often contain more than 1 chondrocyte →. The chondrocytes are large and atypical.* ***(Right)*** *In this grade 2 chondrosarcoma, multiple chondrocytes are seen in a single lacunar space ↷. The chondrocytes have large, hyperchromatic nuclei, and prominent nucleoli are also often seen.*

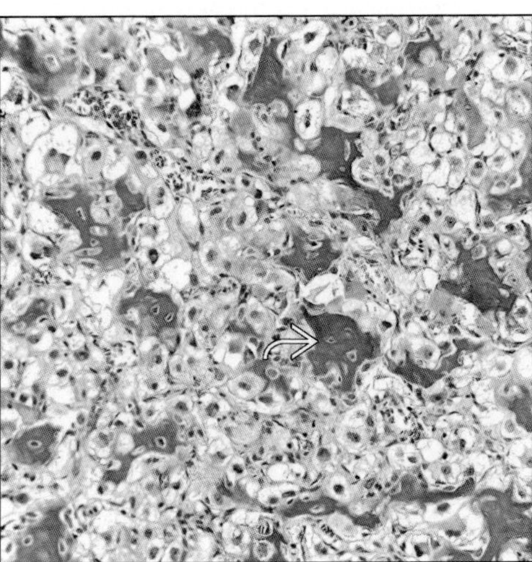

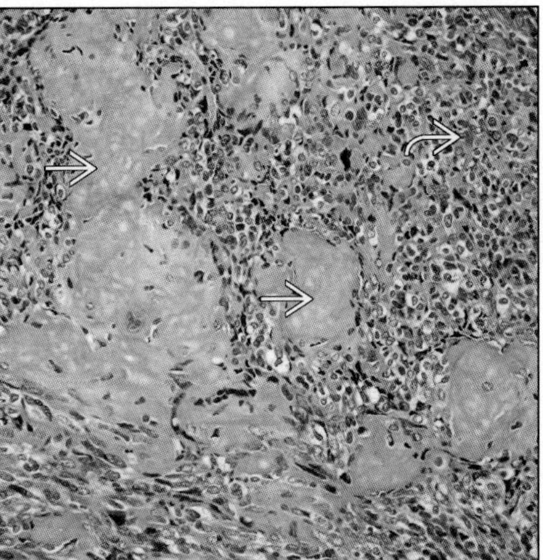

(Left) *This is an example of clear cell chondrosarcoma (grade 3). The cytoplasm is clear, and the cell membranes are distinct. Fragments of woven bone are present* ↷*.* ***(Right)*** *This is an example of mesenchymal chondrosarcoma. There are sheets of small round cells* ↷ *with interspersed cartilaginous islands* →*.*

EWING SARCOMA

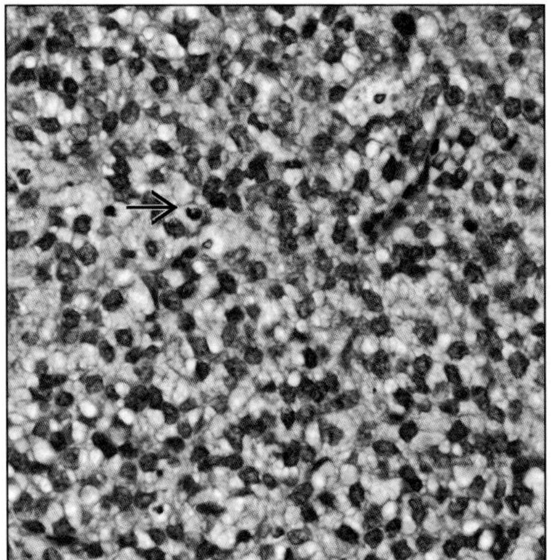

Monotonous proliferation of round blue cells with vacuolated cytoplasm secondary to the deposition of glycogen. Mitoses may be infrequent, but scattered pyknotic nuclei are easily identified ⇒.

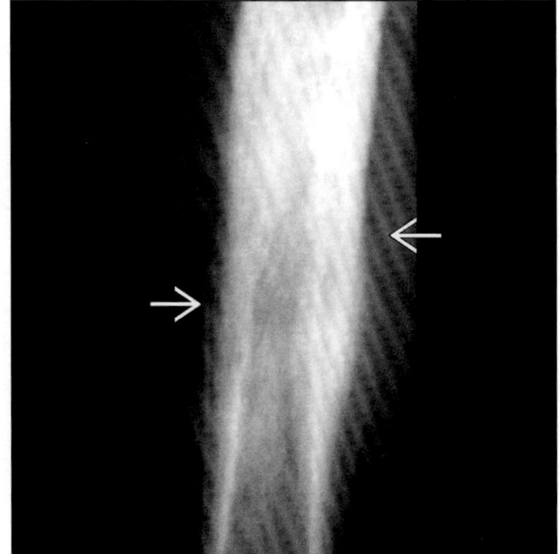

AP radiograph shows a poorly defined diaphyseal lesion with permeative bone destruction and aggressive periosteal reaction ⇒, typical of Ewing sarcoma.

TERMINOLOGY

Abbreviations

- Ewing sarcoma (EWS)

Definitions

- "Small round blue cell" malignant neoplasm of bone and soft tissue
- Ewing sarcoma/primitive neuroectodermal tumor family
  - Primitive neuroectodermal tumors (PNETs) have overlapping histologic and immunohistochemical features with EWS
  - t(11;22) is seen in PNETs
  - Many support that EWS and PNETs are histogenetically related and represent a spectrum of disease
- Askin tumor
  - Malignant small blue cell tumor of thoracopulmonary region
  - Histologically similar to EWS/PNETs

CLINICAL ISSUES

Epidemiology

- Age
  - Most patients with EWS/PNETs or extraskeletal EWS are adolescents or young adults
  - Rarely seen in children < 5 years of age
- Ethnicity
  - Rarely seen in African-Americans

Site

- Develops in diaphysis or metaphysis of long bones
  - Most often femur, tibia, and humerus
  - Also seen in scapulae, ribs, and pelvic bones
- PNETs
  - Commonly arise in the extremities
- Extraskeletal EWS
  - Seen in paravertebral region, chest wall, and soft tissue of lower extremities

Presentation

- Pain and tenderness of affected bone for weeks or months
- Systemic symptoms such as fever and weight loss
- Swelling and tenderness
- Pathologic fracture

Prognosis

- High incidence of early metastatic spread
  - Lungs or other bones
- Adjuvant chemotherapy with radiation and surgical resection has dramatically improved prognosis
  - 50-60% 5-year survival
- Favorable prognostic factors include
  - Age < 10 years
  - Tumor < 8 cm in greatest dimension
  - Tumor of extremity rather than pelvis

IMAGE FINDINGS

Radiographic Findings

- Lytic, "moth-eaten" mottled appearance
- Laminated periosteal reactive bone giving "onion peel" or "hair on end" appearance
  - This pattern is seen secondary to prominent periosteal new bone formation
  - This appearance is not diagnostic of EWS
- Cortex overlying tumor can be irregularly thinned or thickened

MACROSCOPIC FEATURES

General Features

- Bone destruction
- Intramedullary and soft tissue involvement is often greater than suggested on plain films

Key Facts

Terminology
- Many support that EWS and PNETs are histogenetically related and represent spectrum of disease

Clinical Issues
- Favorable prognostic factors include
  - Age < 10 years
  - Tumor < 8 cm in greatest dimension
  - Tumor of extremity rather than pelvis

Image Findings
- Laminated periosteal reactive bone giving an "onion peel" or "hair on end" appearance

Microscopic Pathology
- Uniform population of "small round blue cells"
- Cells borders are indistinct
- Glycogen staining is seen with periodic acid-Schiff staining in majority of cases
- Areas of hemorrhage and necrosis are typical

Ancillary Tests
- CD99 (O13) shows classic membranous pattern
- CD99 (O13) positivity should be considered supportive for, but not diagnostic of, EWS
- t(11;22)(q24;q12)
- t(21;22)(q22;q12)
- *EWS* gene on chromosome 22 is fused with either *FLI1* gene on chromosome 11 or *ERG* gene on chromosome 21
- These hybrid transcripts can be detected by reverse transcriptase-polymerase chain reaction

- Gray, tan, or white poorly demarcated fleshy lesion
- Hemorrhage, cystic degeneration, and necrosis

MICROSCOPIC PATHOLOGY

Histologic Features
- Uniform population of "small round blue cells"
- Finely granular nuclear chromatin
- Several small nucleoli may be seen
- Mitoses are typically sparse
- Scattered apoptotic cells are easily identified
- Cells borders are indistinct
- Cytoplasm may contain vacuoles
  - Glycogen staining is seen with periodic acid-Schiff staining in majority of cases
- Areas of hemorrhage and necrosis are typical
- In areas of necrosis, viable cells are perivascular in distribution
- Areas of neuroectodermal differentiation (Homer Wright rosettes) may be seen
- Extraskeletal EWS may rarely have spindle cell morphology
- "Atypical EWS"
  - Small subset (5%) of tumors with larger, pleomorphic nuclei and more noticeable mitotic figures
  - Also known as "large cell EWS"
  - Prognosis is similar to that of classic EWS

ANCILLARY TESTS

Immunohistochemistry
- CD99 (O13) shows classic membranous pattern
  - This marker is sensitive but not specific
  - CD99 (O13) positivity should be considered supportive for, but not diagnostic of, EWS
- Cells also commonly express vimentin and FLI-1

Cytogenetics
- t(11;22)(q24;q12)
- *EWS* gene on chromosome 22 is fused with the *FLI1* gene on chromosome 11
  - 90-95% of cases have reciprocal translocation between chromosomes 11 and 22
- Multiple types of *EWS-FLI1* fusions exist
  - Patients with type 1 fusions may have better prognosis than those with other fusion types
    - Type 1 fusion: *EWS* exons 1-7 fuse to *FLI1* exons 6-9
- t(21;22)(q22;q12)
- *EWS* gene on chromosome 22 is fused with *ERG* gene on chromosome 21
  - Less common translocation seen in approximately 10% of EWS
  - At least 4 *EWS-ERG* fusions types have been documented
- These hybrid transcripts can be detected by reverse transcriptase-polymerase chain reaction
- Other tumor defining translocations include
  - t(7;22)(p22;q12) *EWS-ETV1*
  - t(17;22)(q12;q12) *EWS-E1AF*
  - t(2;22)(q33;q12) *EWS-FEV*
  - t(1;22)(p36;q12) *EWS-ZSG*
- These translocation are rare, accounting for < 5% of EWS cases
- Break-apart FISH probes for EWS locus can be used for these rare translocations
- FISH can be performed on touch preparations made from fresh tissue or formalin-fixed paraffin-embedded tissue

Molecular Genetics
- Translocations can also be detected by RT-PCR on frozen or formalin-fixed paraffin-embedded tissue

DIFFERENTIAL DIAGNOSIS

Osteomyelitis
- Also presents with fever, anemia, leukocytosis, and elevated sedimentation rate
- Acute osteomyelitis can simulate EWS and lymphomas on imaging

EWING SARCOMA

Immunohistochemistry

Antibody	Reactivity	Staining Pattern	Comment
CD99	Positive	Cell membrane	Sensitive but not specific
FLI-1	Positive	Nuclear	Sensitive but not specific
Vimentin	Positive		Useful as control marker
Synaptophysin	Positive		Variable reactivity
NSE	Positive		Variable reactivity
CD45	Negative		Lymphoid marker
CD79-α	Negative		Lymphoid marker
Desmin	Negative		Muscle marker
Myogenin	Negative		Muscle marker
S100	Negative		Schwannian, melanocytic, chondrocytic
EMA	Negative		Epithelial marker

  - Capillary proliferation and reactive new bone formation is seen in association with acute inflammation
- Plasma cells and lymphocytes predominate in chronic osteomyelitis

Osteosarcoma
- Usually occurs in metaphysis
- Malignant tumor cells produce osteoid matrix

Rhabdomyosarcoma
- Tumor cells are positive for immunohistochemical markers desmin and myogenin
- In embryonal rhabdomyosarcoma, nucleus is eccentrically placed, and cytoplasm appears more eosinophilic and granular in contrast to EWS
- t(2;13)(q35;q14) and t(1;13)(p36;q14) are seen in alveolar rhabdomyosarcoma

Metastatic Neuroblastoma
- Catecholamine levels are elevated
- Patients usually present within 1st 2 years of life
- Presence of neurofibrils, unless poorly differentiated

Lymphoma/Leukemia
- Polymorphic cellular infiltrate in contrast to more uniform EWS cells
- Cells tend to have more dyscohesive appearance
- CD45(+)

REPORTING CONSIDERATIONS

Key Elements to Report
- Distance of tumor from bone and soft tissue margins
- Presence or absence of lymph-vascular invasion
- Percent tumor necrosis in post-treatment resections

SELECTED REFERENCES

1. Indelicato DJ et al: Chest wall Ewing sarcoma family of tumors: long-term outcomes. Int J Radiat Oncol Biol Phys. 81(1):158-66, 2011
2. Ban SP et al: Congenital paraspinal Ewing sarcoma family of tumors with an epidural extension. J Clin Neurosci. 17(12):1599-601, 2010
3. Charbord P: Bone marrow mesenchymal stem cells: historical overview and concepts. Hum Gene Ther. 21(9):1045-56, 2010
4. Dirksen U et al: Approaching Ewing sarcoma. Future Oncol. 6(7):1155-62, 2010
5. Gangwal K et al: Emergent properties of EWS/FLI regulation via GGAA microsatellites in Ewing's sarcoma. Genes Cancer. 1(2):177-187, 2010
6. Ginsberg JP et al: Long-term survivors of childhood Ewing sarcoma: report from the childhood cancer survivor study. J Natl Cancer Inst. 102(16):1272-83, 2010
7. Jinawath N et al: Complex rearrangement of chromosomes 1, 7, 21, 22 in Ewing sarcoma. Cancer Genet Cytogenet. 201(1):42-47, 2010
8. Kumagai A et al: Detection of SYT and EWS gene rearrangements by dual-color break-apart CISH in liquid-based cytology samples of synovial sarcoma and Ewing sarcoma/primitive neuroectodermal tumor. Am J Clin Pathol. 134(2):323-31, 2010
9. Le Deley MC et al: Impact of EWS-ETS fusion type on disease progression in Ewing's sarcoma/peripheral primitive neuroectodermal tumor: prospective results from the cooperative Euro-E.W.I.N.G. 99 trial. J Clin Oncol. 28(12):1982-8, 2010
10. Mitchell BD et al: Ewing sarcoma mimicking a peripheral nerve sheath tumor. J Clin Neurosci. Epub ahead of print, 2010
11. Morris CD: Pelvic bone sarcomas: controversies and treatment options. J Natl Compr Canc Netw. 8(6):731-7, 2010
12. van Doorninck JA et al: Current treatment protocols have eliminated the prognostic advantage of type 1 fusions in Ewing sarcoma: a report from the Children's Oncology Group. J Clin Oncol. 28(12):1989-94, 2010
13. Herrero-Martín D et al: Stable interference of EWS-FLI1 in an Ewing sarcoma cell line impairs IGF-1/IGF-1R signalling and reveals TOPK as a new target. Br J Cancer. 101(1):80-90, 2009
14. Saito Y et al: Congenital Ewing sarcoma in retroperitoneum with multiple metastases. Pediatr Blood Cancer. 51(5):698-701, 2008
15. González I et al: EWS/FLI-1 oncoprotein subtypes impose different requirements for transformation and metastatic activity in a murine model. J Mol Med. 85(9):1015-29, 2007
16. Lewis TB et al: Differentiating Ewing's sarcoma from other round blue cell tumors using a RT-PCR translocation panel on formalin-fixed paraffin-embedded tissues. Mod Pathol. 20(3):397-404, 2007

Radiologic and Gross Features

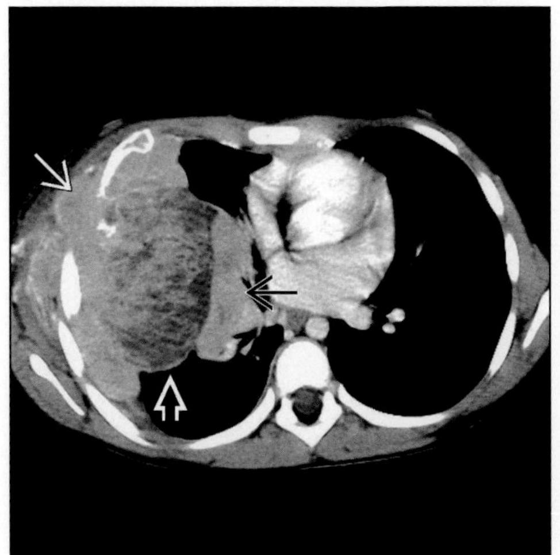

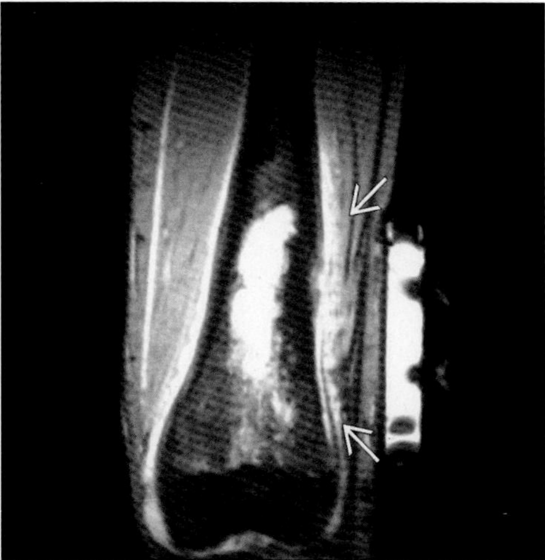

(Left) *Axial CECT shows a large Askin tumor with compression atelectasis of the right lung. The tumor involves the pleura, multiple ribs, and chest wall.* ***(Right)*** *Coronal T2WI FS MR shows abnormal high signal in the distal femoral diaphysis, consistent with tumor involvement. Note the associated soft tissue mass and cortical destruction.*

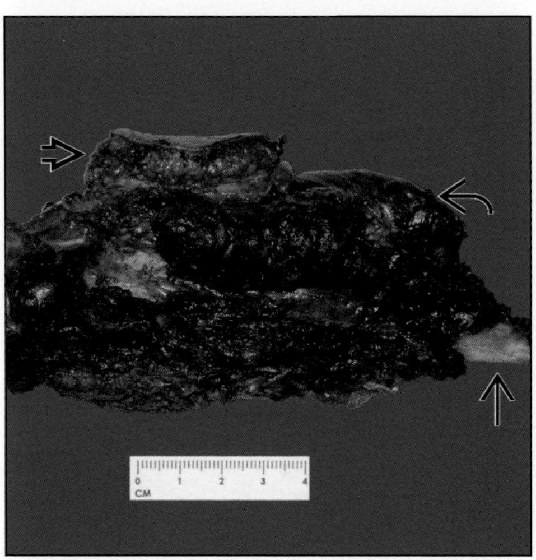

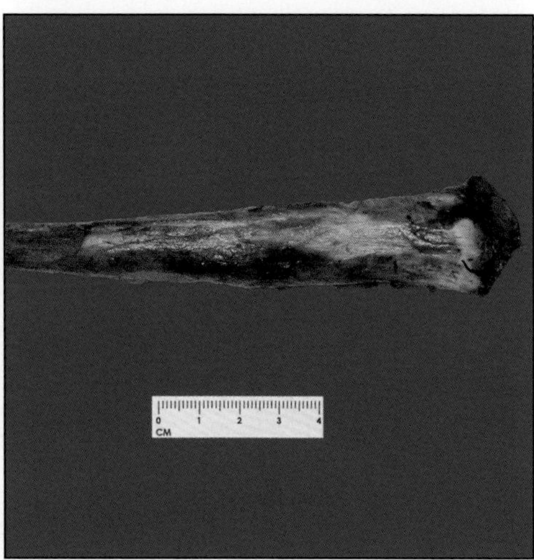

(Left) *Post-treatment resection of EWS involving the fibula shows adjacent soft tissue. Skeletal muscle and biopsy tract is also excised. Sections of the biopsy tract and soft tissue margins closest to tumor should be submitted for microscopic examination. (Courtesy L. Erickson, PA.)* ***(Right)*** *Post-treatment resection for EWS shows that the soft tissue and skeletal muscle have been removed from the fibula. (Courtesy L. Erickson, PA.)*

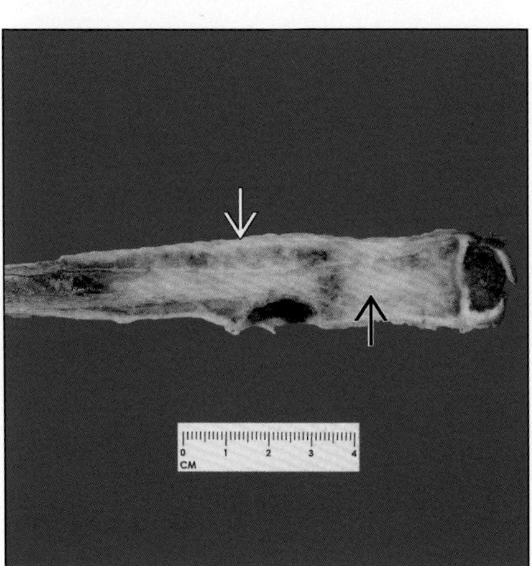

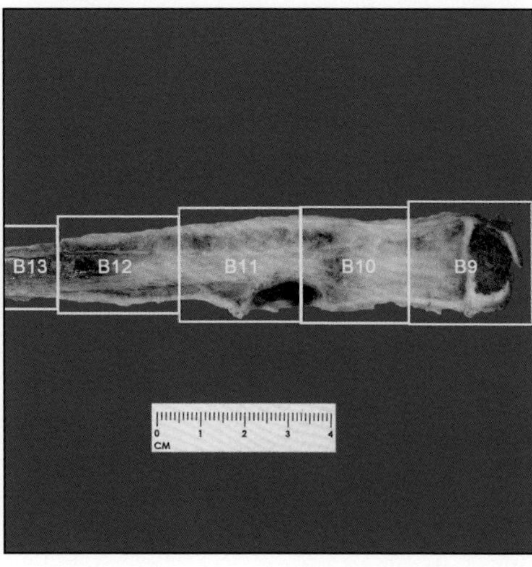

(Left) *Gross specimen of EWS involving the fibula. Treated osseous EWS shows a tan-gray lesion with widening of the bone, hemorrhage, and necrosis. Cystic degeneration may also be seen. (Courtesy L. Erickson, PA.)* ***(Right)*** *Section mapping is a useful tool for identifying the location of viable tumor and percentage of viable tumor. (Courtesy L. Erickson, PA.)*

EWING SARCOMA

Microscopic Features

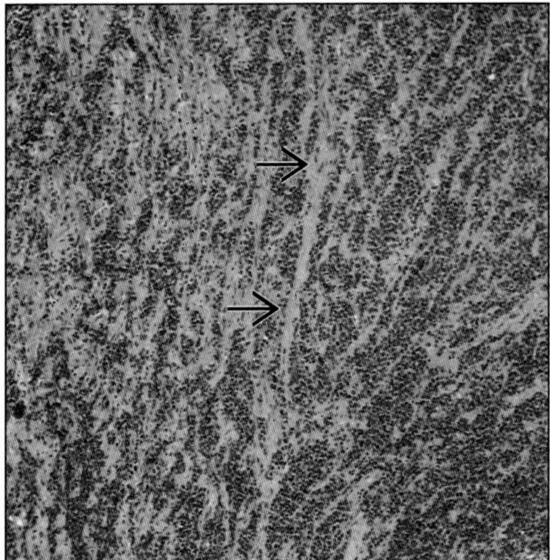

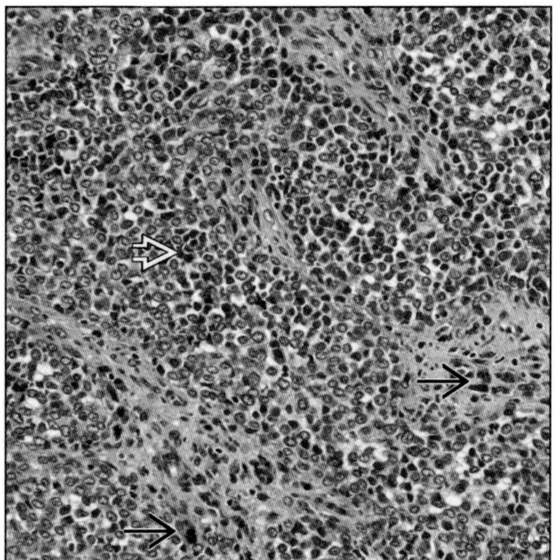

(Left) *Monotonous sheets of tumor cells are separated by thick fibrous septa →, a feature one would not encounter in lymphoma.* ***(Right)*** *Fibrous septa separate EWS tumor cells. The sheets of cells have a bubbly appearance secondary to cytoplasmic glycogen. Note areas of hemorrhage ➡ and scattered hemosiderin-laden macrophages →.*

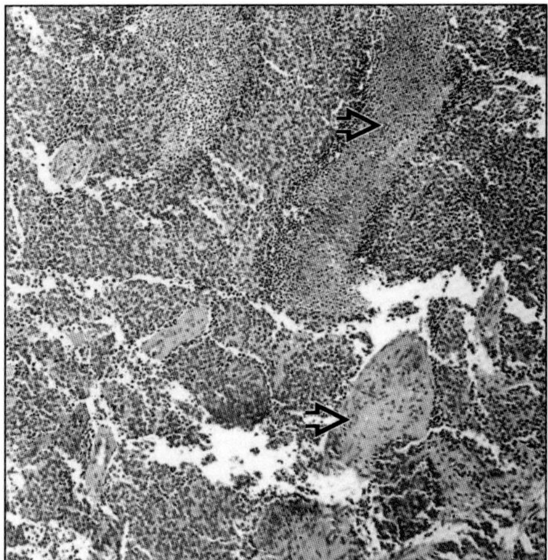

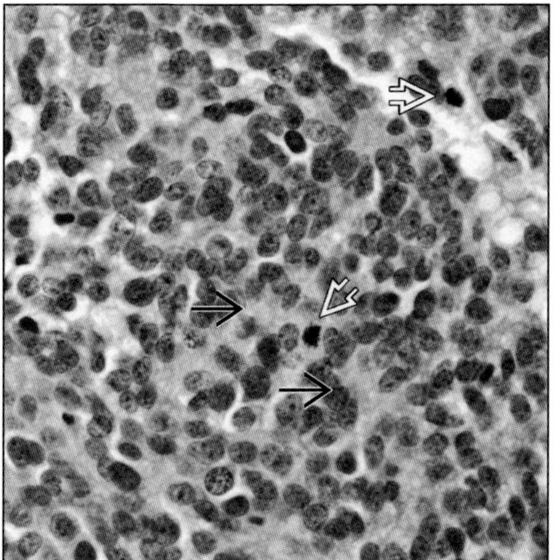

(Left) *Thick fibrous septa ➡ separate lobules of monotonous tumor cells.* ***(Right)*** *Mitotic activity is usually not prominent in EWS; however, several mitotic figures are seen here ➡. Cytoplasmic borders are indistinct, and there is some suggestion of rosette formation →.*

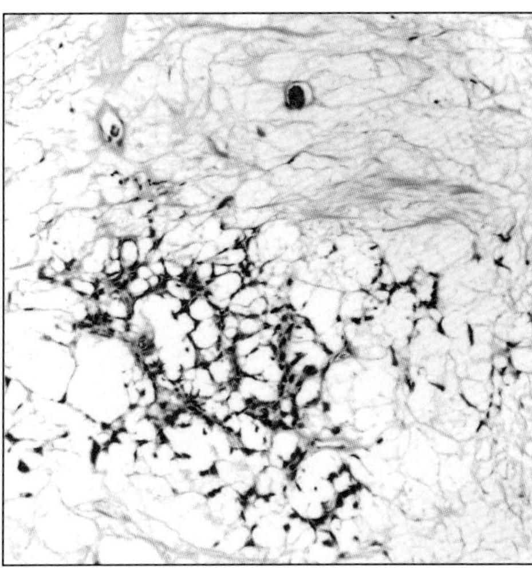

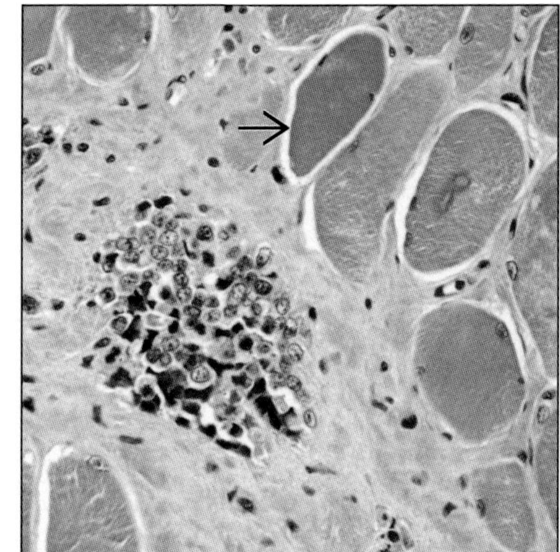

(Left) *Viable EWS tumor cells are seen in a post-treatment resection specimen.* ***(Right)*** *A small nest of viable EWS tumor cells in a post-treatment soft tissue section is shown. Note the skeletal muscle fibers →. The distance to the nearest soft tissue margin should be noted in the pathology report.*

Microscopic Features

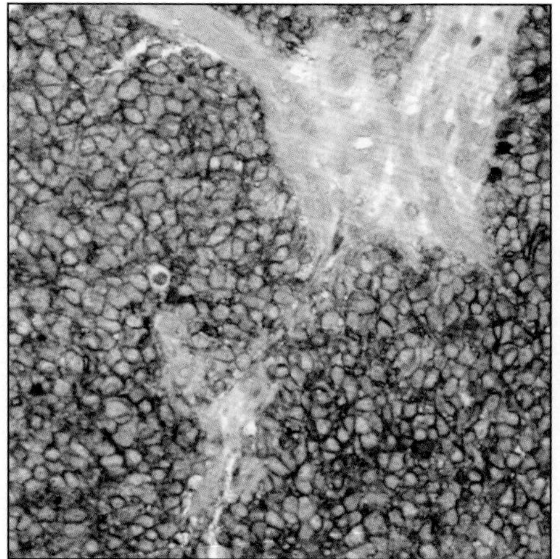

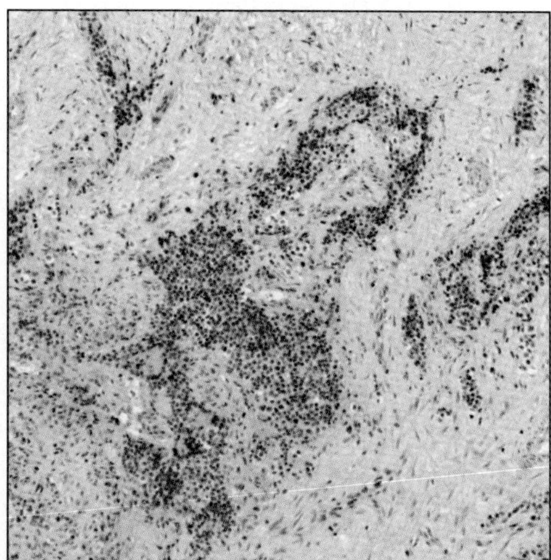

(Left) *Immunohistochemical staining with antibody to CD99 antigen shows a membranous staining pattern. Positive CD99 staining in itself is not diagnostic of EWS and should be performed as part of an immunohistochemical panel.* ***(Right)*** *FLI-1 shows a nuclear staining pattern. Endothelial cell nuclei should also stain, serving as a good internal control.*

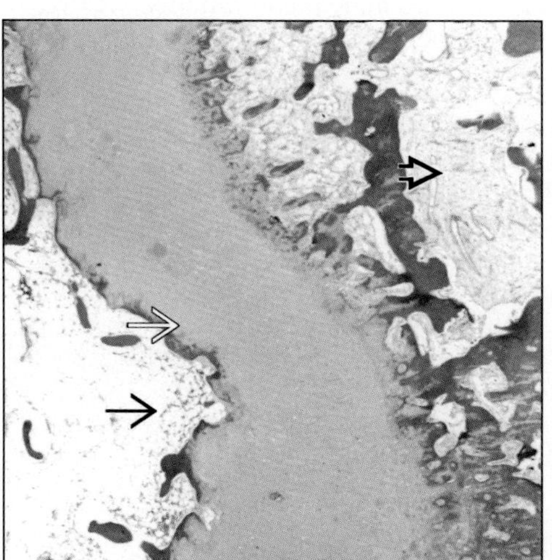

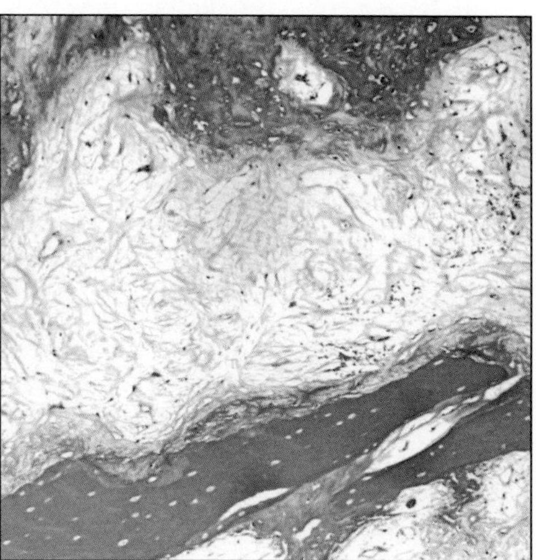

(Left) *Treated EWS ⇨ is seen in the upper right. Note the epiphyseal plate ➡ and uninvolved marrow → to the left.* ***(Right)*** *Histologic findings in treated EWS include necrosis, myxoid stromal change, and decreased cellularity as observed in this image.*

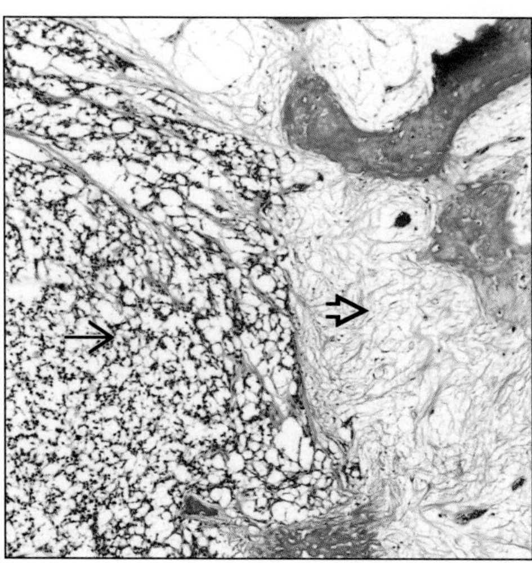

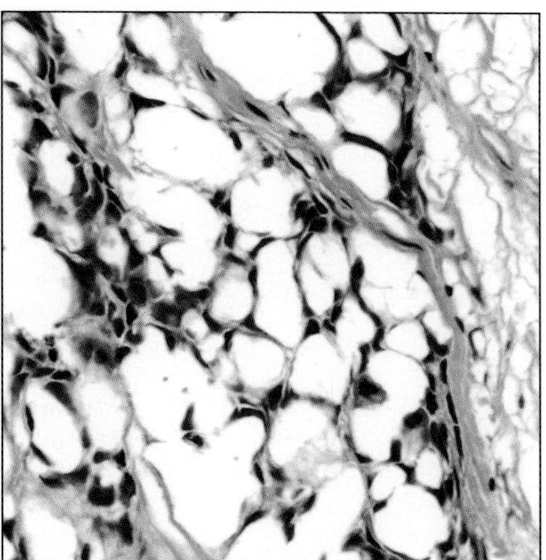

(Left) *Treated EWS shows areas of viable tumor → and necrosis with myxoid stromal change ⇨.* ***(Right)*** *Viable tumor cells in a post-treatment EWS resection specimen is shown. The nuclei are hyperchromatic and angulated. In some cases, residual tumor can mimic alveolar rhabdomyosarcoma by taking on a pseudoalveolar architecture.*

OSTEOSARCOMA

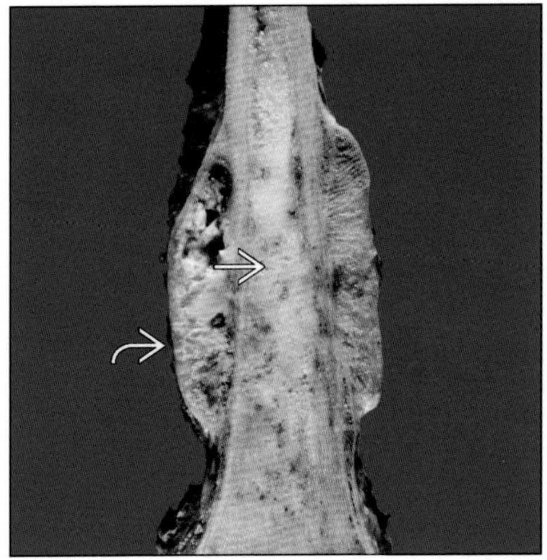

Gross specimen of a conventional osteosarcoma. From the typical metaphyseal origin, the tumor can spread along the marrow cavity ➔ and lift and perforate the cortex ➔.

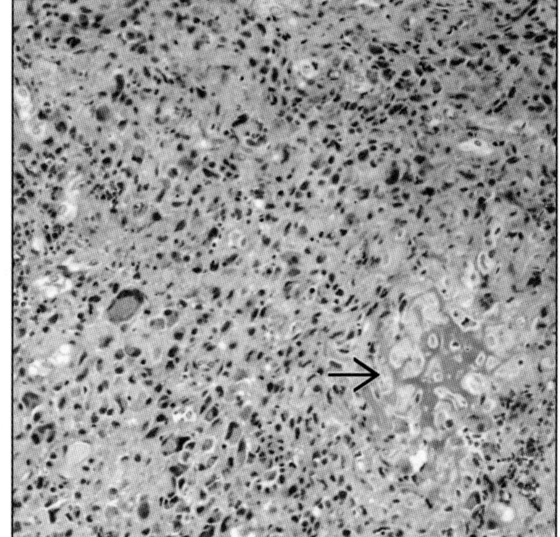

The key feature for diagnosis of osteosarcoma is the identification of osteoid ➔ that is produced directly by the tumor cells. Osteosarcomas are highly malignant tumors with marked pleomorphism.

TERMINOLOGY

Abbreviations

- Osteosarcoma (OS)

Definitions

- Malignant tumor (of mesenchymal origin) in which a bony matrix or osteoid is produced by tumor cells
- Several histologic subtypes exist (WHO Classification)
  - Conventional OS
    - Chondroblastic
    - Fibroblastic
    - Osteoblastic
  - Telangiectatic OS
  - Small cell OS
  - Low-grade central OS
  - Secondary (post-irradiation) OS
  - Parosteal OS
  - Periosteal OS
  - High-grade surface OS
- All are considered high-grade malignancies except
  - Parosteal OS: Considered a grade I lesion
  - Periosteal OS: Considered a grade II or grade III lesion
  - Low-grade intraosseous variants: Considered grade I lesions

CLINICAL ISSUES

Epidemiology

- Incidence
  - Most common nonhematopoietic bone malignancy
- Age
  - Occurs most often in 2nd decade of life
    - 60% of patients are < 25 years of age
    - Extremely rare in children < 5 years of age
  - Patients with low-grade central OS and parosteal OS tend to be older
- Gender
  - Conventional OS has male predominance
  - Parosteal OS and periosteal OS have female predominance

Site

- Metaphyses of long bones
  - At sites of peak mitotic activity for bone cells
    - Distal femur
    - Proximal tibia
    - Proximal humerus
  - However, OS can arise in any bone
  - Parosteal OS occurs most often on posterior aspect of distal femur
    - Patients present with inability to flex knee joint
  - Periosteal OS most often involves diaphysis of femur or tibia

Presentation

- Nonspecific clinical symptoms such as pain and swelling

Treatment

- Biopsy followed by neoadjuvant chemotherapy
- Tumor response is assessed by radiologic imaging
- Surgical resection of treated primary tumor
- If histologic response to treatment is poor, additional chemotherapy may be used

Prognosis

- Significant indicator of prognosis is histologic response to preoperative chemotherapy
  - Osteoblastic and chondroblastic OS tend to be less responsive to chemotherapy than fibroblastic and telangiectatic variants
- Several grading systems for tumor response exist
- The Children's Oncology Group uses system developed by L.E. Wold
  - I: No treatment effect present
  - II: Some treatment effect
    - A: > 50% viable tumor remaining post treatment
    - B: 5-50% viable tumor remaining post treatment

OSTEOSARCOMA

Key Facts

Terminology

- Malignant tumor in which a bony matrix or osteoid is produced by tumor cells
- All osteosarcoma variants are considered high-grade malignancies except
  - Parosteal osteosarcoma: Considered a grade I lesion
  - Periosteal osteosarcoma: Considered a grade II or grade III lesion
  - Low-grade intraosseous variants: Considered grade I lesions

Clinical Issues

- Most common nonhematopoietic bone malignancy
- 60% of patients are younger than 25 years of age
- Extremely rare in children < 5 years of age
- Occurs in metaphyses of long bones
- Significant indicator of prognosis is histologic response to preoperative chemotherapy

Macroscopic Features

- Heavily mineralized tumors that are hard, gritty, or hemorrhagic
- Spreads throughout medullary cavity
- Soft tissue involvement has fish-flesh appearance that surrounds bone

Microscopic Pathology

- Malignant tumor cells produce osteoid matrix
- Homogeneous and eosinophilic with lace-like irregular contours and osteoblastic rimming
- Thin basophilic trabeculae
- Can resemble fungal hyphae

  - III: < 5% viable tumor remaining post treatment
  - IV: No viable tumor remaining
- > 90% chemotherapy-induced necrosis is associated with a 90% disease-free survival rate
- Conventional OS
  - 60-80% disease-free survival with surgery and chemotherapy
  - Tends to metastasize to lungs
    - 20-80% of patients have lung metastases at time of diagnosis
    - Excision of lung metastases is thought to prolong survival
  - Less frequently metastasizes to other bones, pleura, and heart
  - Rarely metastasizes to lymph nodes, brain, and gastrointestinal tract
  - Presentation with pathologic fracture has been associated with poorer overall survival
  - Involvement of craniofacial bone (excluding jaw) and vertebral bodies is associated with poor prognosis
  - Loss of heterozygosity of *RB* gene is associated with poor prognosis
  - Tumor involving jaw bones is associated with good prognosis
  - Subclassification of conventional osteosarcoma has no prognostic significance
- Telangiectatic OS
  - Prognosis is similar to conventional OS
  - Highly chemosensitive
- Small cell OS
  - Extremely rare tumor with poor prognosis
- Low-grade central OS
  - Prognosis is excellent
    - However, 15% of patients develop a high-grade osteosarcoma
  - May locally recur
  - Limited potential for metastatic disease
- Secondary (post-irradiation) OS
  - Prognosis is similar to conventional OS
  - Typically, long latent period (10-15 years) between irradiation and development of sarcoma
  - Amount of radiation received also varies from 12-240 Gy
- Parosteal OS
  - Excellent prognosis
  - Local recurrence with inadequate excision
  - Rarely metastasizes
- Periosteal OS
  - Excellent prognosis
- High-grade surface OS
  - Prognosis is similar to conventional OS

IMAGE FINDINGS

Radiographic Findings

- Can be variable
- Destruction of bone with extension into soft tissue
- Codman triangle
  - As tumor destroys cortex, periosteum is lifted
  - Reactive new bone formation is seen between cortex and lifted periosteum
- Amount of mineralization depends on histologic subtype
- Parosteal OS shows heavily ossified mass with broad base attached to cortex
- Periosteal OS creates saucer-like defect of cortex
  - Sunburst appearance; parallel arrays of mineralization in soft tissue

MACROSCOPIC FEATURES

General Features

- Heavily mineralized tumors that are hard, gritty, or hemorrhagic
  - Grittiness depends on amount of osteoid production
- Spreads throughout medullary cavity
  - Skip lesions or satellite nodules may be seen
- Usually does not extend through epiphyseal plates
- Destroys cortical bone
- Elevates periosteum
- Soft tissue involvement has fish-flesh appearance that surrounds bone

OSTEOSARCOMA

- Conventional OS
  - Chondroblastic subtype may have areas of cartilage
- Telangiectatic OS
  - Resembles cavity containing a blood clot or hemorrhagic cavity separated by septa
- Low-grade central OS
  - Firm, fibrous appearance
- Parosteal OS
  - Occurs on bone surface
  - Encircles involved bone
  - Firm, hard mass
  - Invades surrounding skeletal muscle
  - May have areas that appear to be cartilaginous cap or plate
- Periosteal OS
  - Chondroid appearance
- High-grade surface OS
  - Occurs on bone surface
  - May have some medullary involvement

Sections to Be Submitted

- Soft tissue margins nearest tumor
- Areas of soft tissue extension and interface with tumor
- Bony margins
- Pretreatment surgical biopsy site with skin and soft tissue
- Joint and synovial surfaces should be submitted if suspicious for involvement by tumor
- Entire longitudinal bone slab with section map

Important Grossing Points

- After external soft tissue surfaces are examined and inked, bone can be cut longitudinally
  - This cut should include 2 greatest dimensions of the tumor mass
- The following should be documented
  - Tumor extent and appearance
  - Tumor size in 3 dimensions
  - Distance of tumor from resection margins
  - Presence of cortical breakthrough
  - Soft tissue extension
  - Medullary extension
  - Involvement of epiphyseal plate or joint
  - Skip areas of tumor away from main mass

MICROSCOPIC PATHOLOGY

Histologic Features

- Malignant tumor cells produce osteoid matrix
  - Homogeneous and eosinophilic with lace-like irregular contours and osteoblastic rimming
  - Thin basophilic trabeculae
    - Can resemble fungal hyphae
- Vascular invasion and areas of necrosis are common
- Conventional OS can be divided into 3 subtypes, based on predominant matrix
  - Chondroblastic
    - Lobules of malignant cartilage are seen in addition to osteoid production
    - Osteoid matrix can be seen within chondroid lobules
    - Cells within lacunae are markedly anaplastic
    - Cellularity and spindling increases at periphery of lobules
    - Approximately 1/4 of all OS are chondroblastic
  - Fibroblastic
    - Predominant spindle cell pattern with little osteoid matrix
    - Approximately 1/4 of all OS are fibroblastic
  - Osteoblastic
    - Unmineralized osteoid or mineralized trabeculae
    - At least 1/2 of all OS are osteoblastic
  - Some lesions may contain giant cells
    - When numerous, consider diagnosis of giant cell-rich osteosarcoma
- Telangiectatic OS
  - Resembles aneurysmal bone cysts; however, the stromal cells are pleomorphic
- Small cell OS
  - Resembles Ewing sarcoma or malignant lymphoma
  - Must see osteoid or bony matrix
- Low-grade central OS
  - Hypocellular spindle cell population with minimal cytologic atypia
  - Sparse mitotic figures
  - Spindle cell component surrounds bony trabeculae and permeates marrow space
  - Amount of osteoid production varies
  - Bone production is evident as well-formed bony trabeculae
    - Can mimic fibrous dysplasia
- Secondary (post-irradiation) OS
  - Histologically indistinguishable from conventional OS
- Parosteal OS
  - Hypocellular spindle cell population without cytologic atypia
  - Abundant collagen
  - Well-formed bony trabeculae
  - Lace-like osteoid is not present
  - Rare mitotic figures
  - Variable amounts of cartilage, sometimes forming cap over lesion
  - Entrapment of skeletal muscles in spindle cell population at edge of lesion
- Periosteal OS
  - Moderately well-differentiated chondroblastic osteosarcoma
  - Lobular pattern with atypical chondrocytes
    - Bone formation may be seen in center of lobule
  - Spindle cells are seen at periphery
    - These cells produce matrix
- High-grade surface OS
  - Histologically resembles conventional OS but is on the bone surface
  - Typically anaplastic and may be osteoblastic, fibroblastic, or chondroblastic

Post-Treatment Changes

- Post-treatment viable tumor cells are atypical cells with hyperchromatic smudged chromatin and vacuolated cytoplasm
- Percent viable tumor is a qualitative assessment
- Ghost cells with loss of cellular detail
- Granulation tissue formation

Osteosarcomas Categorized by Location*	
Arising within the Bone	**Arising from the Bone Surface**
Conventional osteosarcoma	Parosteal osteosarcoma
Secondary (post-irradiation) osteosarcoma	Periosteal osteosarcoma
Telangiectatic osteosarcoma	High-grade surface osteosarcoma
Low-grade central osteosarcoma	
Small cell osteosarcoma	

**Osteosarcomas can be divided broadly into 2 groups: Those that occur within the bone and constitute the majority of osteosarcomas and those that occur on the bone surface.*

- Hemosiderin deposition
- Inflammation
- Fibrosis

ANCILLARY TESTS

Cytogenetics

- High-grade OS shows complex karyotypes with numerous structural and numerical alterations
- Low-grade OS can show ring chromosomes

DIFFERENTIAL DIAGNOSIS

Exuberant Fracture Callous

- Resembles sarcoma but without atypia or atypical mitotic figures

Myositis Ossificans

- Benign fibro-osseous lesion with zonation, cellular stroma, and new bone
- Early lesions are highly cellular with immature fibroblasts centrally, brisk mitotic activity, and focal hemorrhage

Giant Cell Tumor

- Regular and uniform distribution of stromal cells and giant cells
- 1/3 have focal deposition of osteoid or bone
- No cellular atypia or atypical mitotic figures

Osteochondroma

- May resemble parosteal OS because of cartilaginous cap
- Intertrabecular spaces are filled by fatty marrow and not spindle cell proliferation as in OS
- Imaging shows continuity of marrow space between bone and osteochondroma

DIAGNOSTIC CHECKLIST

Clinically Relevant Pathologic Features

- Pathology report should note percent of remaining viable tumor in post-treatment resection specimens

SELECTED REFERENCES

1. Benjamin RS et al: Pediatric and adult osteosarcoma: comparisons and contrasts in presentation and therapy. Cancer Treat Res. 152:355-63, 2010
2. Blattmann C et al: Enhancement of radiation response in osteosarcoma and rhabdomyosarcoma cell lines by histone deacetylase inhibition. Int J Radiat Oncol Biol Phys. 78(1):237-45, 2010
3. Du LQ et al: Knockdown of Rad51 expression induces radiation- and chemo-sensitivity in osteosarcoma cells. Med Oncol. Epub ahead of print, 2010
4. Eftekhari F: Imaging assessment of osteosarcoma in childhood and adolescence: diagnosis, staging, and evaluating response to chemotherapy. Cancer Treat Res. 152:33-62, 2010
5. Ferguson PC et al: Clinical and functional outcomes of patients with a pathologic fracture in high-grade osteosarcoma. J Surg Oncol. 102(2):120-4, 2010
6. Koob M et al: Intercostal myositis ossificans misdiagnosed as osteosarcoma in a 10-year-old child. Pediatr Radiol. 40 Suppl 1:S34-7, 2010
7. Leithner A et al: Wikipedia and osteosarcoma: a trustworthy patients' information? J Am Med Inform Assoc. 17(4):373-4, 2010
8. Li J et al: Limb salvage surgery for calcaneal malignancy. J Surg Oncol. 102(1):48-53, 2010
9. Mayerson JL: Limb salvage: An acceptable option in select patients with pathologic fracture in high grade osteosarcoma. J Surg Oncol. 102(2):119, 2010
10. Moon A et al: Expression of heat shock proteins in osteosarcomas. Pathology. 42(5):421-5, 2010
11. Morris CD: Pelvic bone sarcomas: controversies and treatment options. J Natl Compr Canc Netw. 8(6):731-7, 2010
12. Smida J et al: Genomic alterations and allelic imbalances are strong prognostic predictors in osteosarcoma. Clin Cancer Res. 16(16):4256-67, 2010
13. Wittig JC et al: Osteosarcoma of the proximal tibia: limb-sparing resection and reconstruction with a modular segmental proximal tibia tumor prosthesis. Ann Surg Oncol. 17(11):3021, 2010
14. Worch J et al: Osteosarcoma in children 5 years of age or younger at initial diagnosis. Pediatr Blood Cancer. 55(2):285-9, 2010
15. Yoshida A et al: Immunohistochemical analysis of MDM2 and CDK4 distinguishes low-grade osteosarcoma from benign mimics. Mod Pathol. 23(9):1279-88, 2010
16. Coffin CM et al: Treatment effects in pediatric soft tissue and bone tumors: practical considerations for the pathologist. Am J Clin Pathol. 123(1):75-90, 2005

OSTEOSARCOMA

Radiologic Features

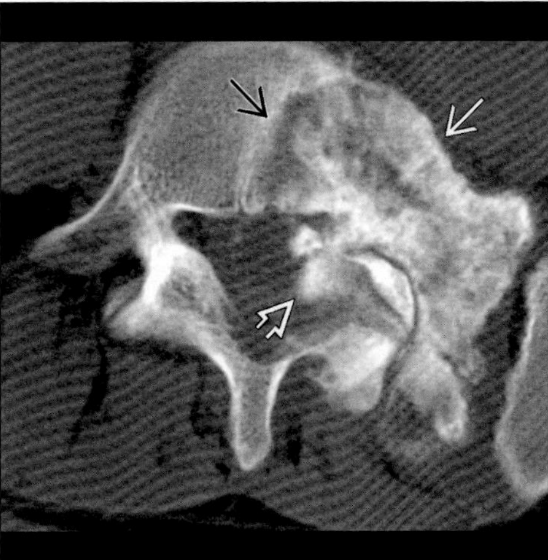

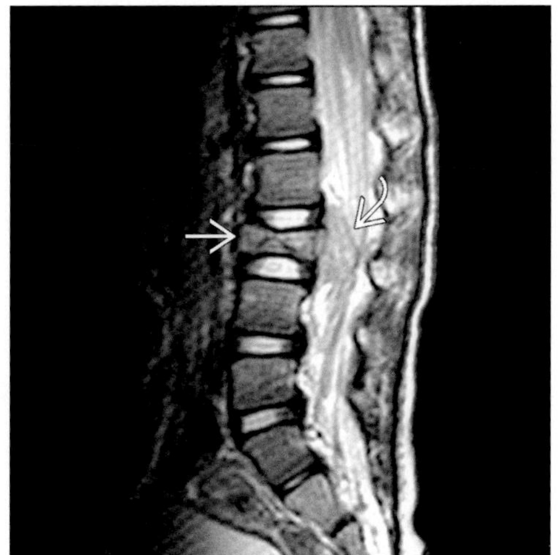

(Left) *Axial bone CT shows an osteoid containing tumor in the left side of L5, expanding the vertebral body ➔ and extending into the spinal canal ➔. Note the moth-eaten bone destruction and wide zone of transition ➔.* ***(Right)*** *Sagittal STIR MR shows a compression fracture of the 3rd lumbar vertebral body ➔. The bone marrow is replaced with tumor, which permeates through the cortex and into the spinal canal ➔, indicating an aggressive process.*

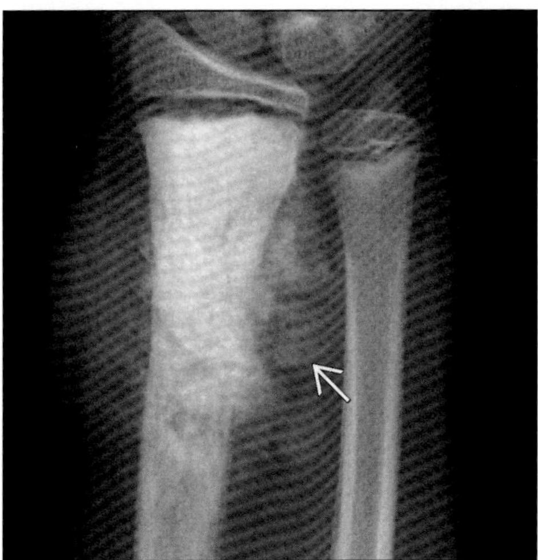

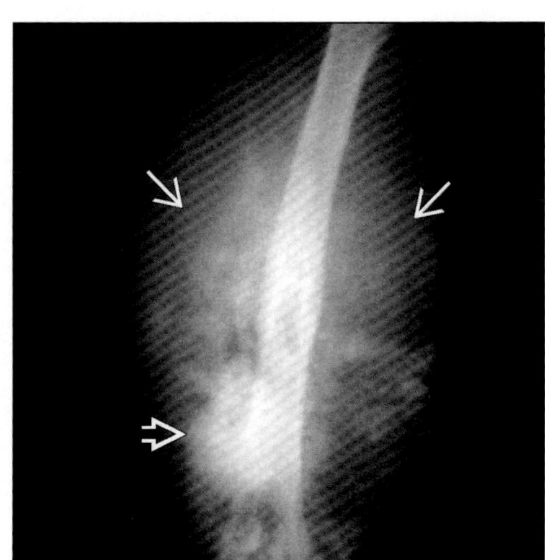

(Left) *Radiograph of the forearm shows diffuse medullary and cortical bone destruction with associated aggressive periosteal reaction. Cloud-like osteoid matrix is seen within the soft tissue mass ➔.* ***(Right)*** *Lateral radiograph of the femur shows medullary and cortical bone destruction with associated periosteal reaction of the sunburst type ➔. Soft tissue extension with new bone formation is present ➔.*

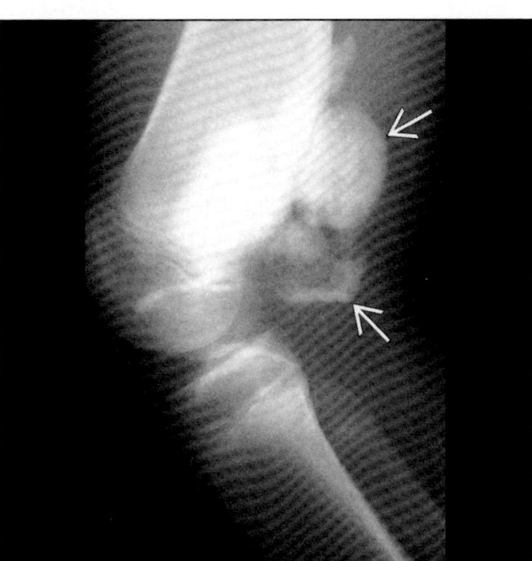

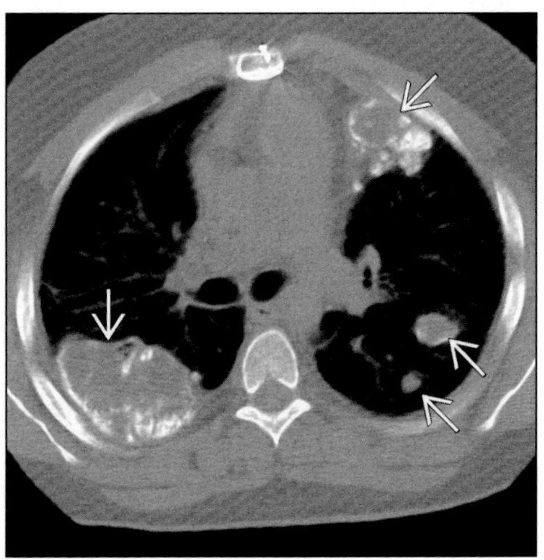

(Left) *Lateral radiograph shows a lobulated sclerotic mass ➔ arising from the metaphyseal surface of the posterior distal femur, consistent with parosteal osteosarcoma.* ***(Right)*** *Axial CT shows pleural and parenchymal lung metastases ➔ in this patient with a large pelvic osteogenic sarcoma. Note areas of ossification within the metastases.*

Radiologic and Gross Features

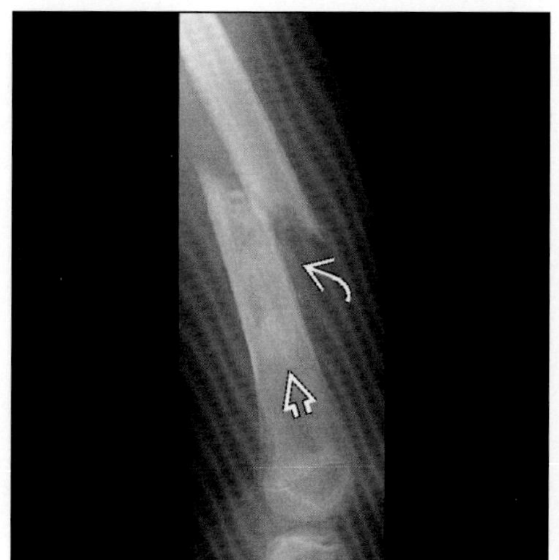

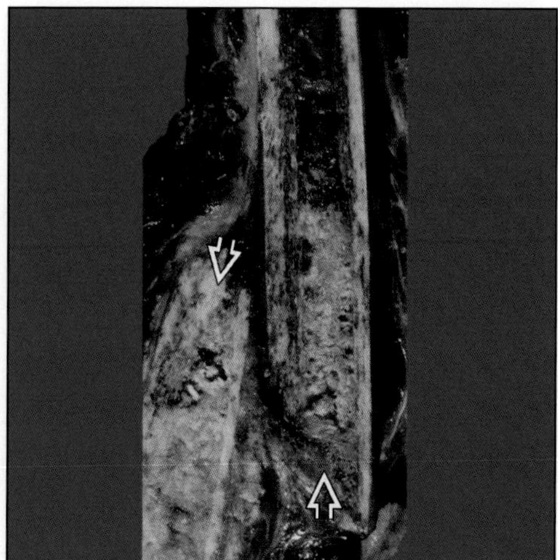

(Left) *Lateral radiograph of the femur shows a pathologic fracture secondary to weakening from an osteosarcoma. The tumor extends distally with abnormal medullary bone* ➡ *and periosteal reaction* ➡*.* ***(Right)*** *Gross specimen shows abnormal bone marrow* ➡ *at the site of the fracture. Presentation with a pathologic fracture has been associated with a poorer overall survival.*

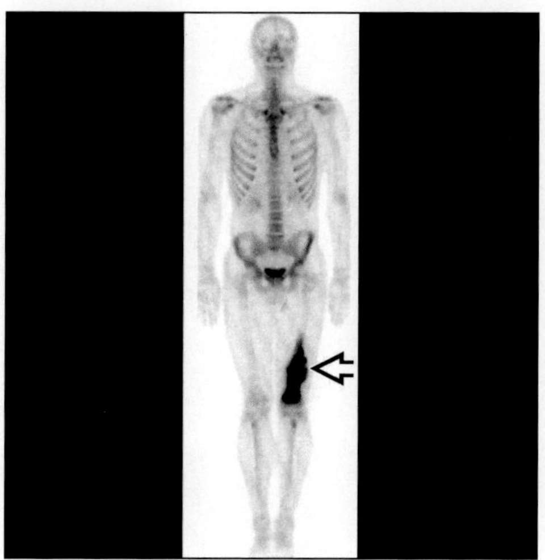

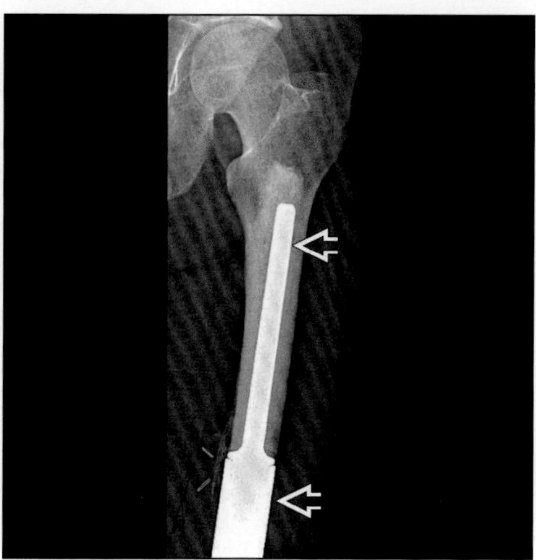

(Left) *A technetium (Tc-99m) bone scan shows intense uptake by an osteosarcoma in the left distal femur* ➡*. An MR would need to be performed to detail the exact extent of involvement that is essential for treatment planning.* ***(Right)*** *A wide resection of the tumor was performed and a long stem modular prosthesis* ➡ *put in its place.*

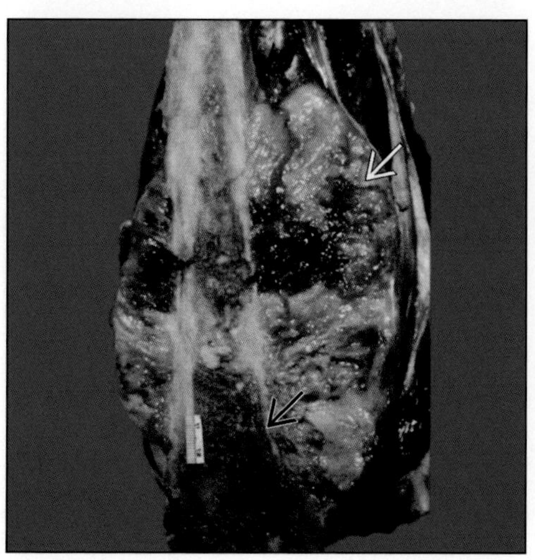

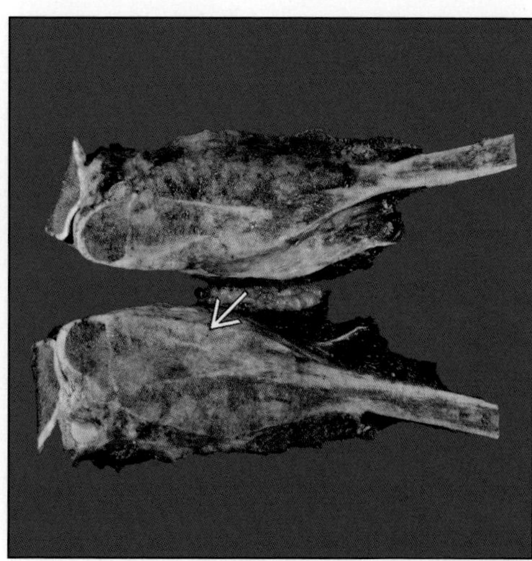

(Left) *Coronal gross pathology section shows a yellow-brown tumor with hemorrhagic areas* ➡ *in the femoral metadiaphysis with cortical destruction and extraosseous extension* ➡*.* ***(Right)*** *Osteosarcoma with extensive soft tissue involvement. The tumor has a fish-flesh appearance* ➡*. The gross appearance can vary a great deal, from firm and gritty to hemorrhagic depending on the amounts of bone, cartilage, cellular stroma, and vessels.*

OSTEOSARCOMA

Gross and Microscopic Features

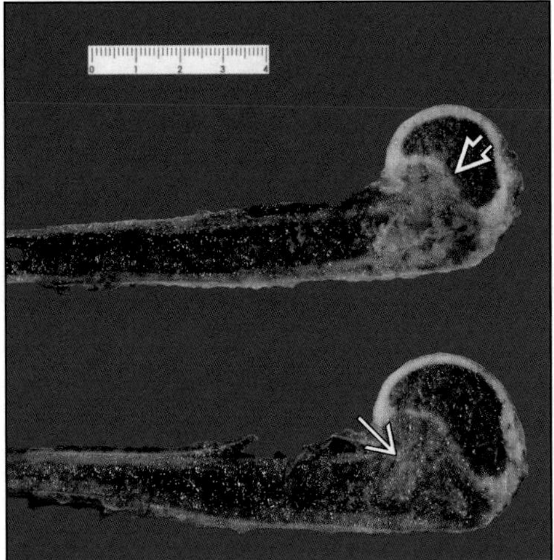

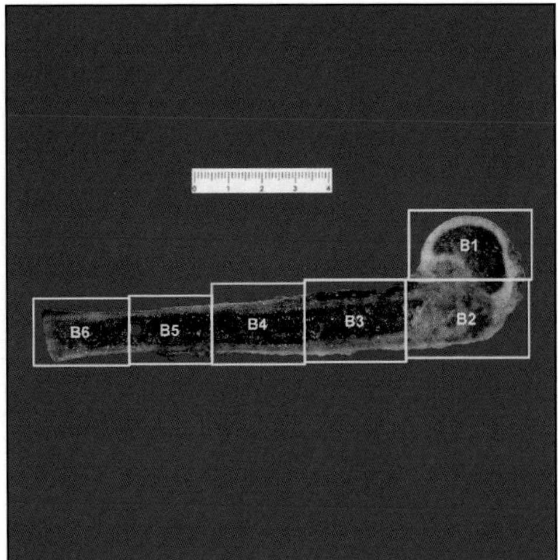

(Left) *Proximal humerus is shown. Note the classic metaphyseal origin ➡ and how the tumor respects the epiphyseal line ➡. (Courtesy L. Erickson, PA.)* ***(Right)*** *An entire longitudinal cross section should be submitted for histologic evaluation. This is an example of section mapping to document the sites of microscopic sections. (Courtesy L. Erickson, PA.)*

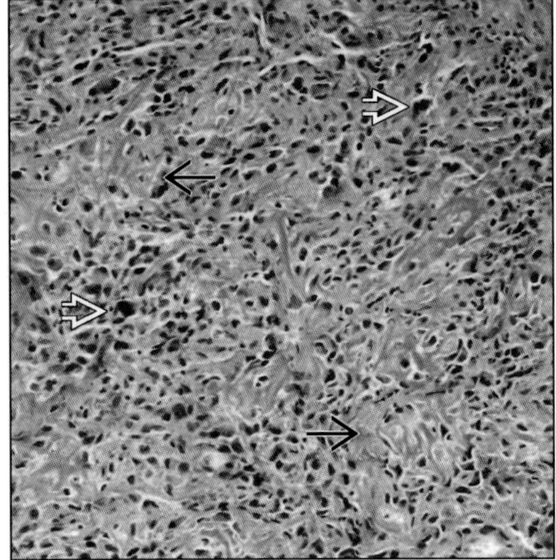

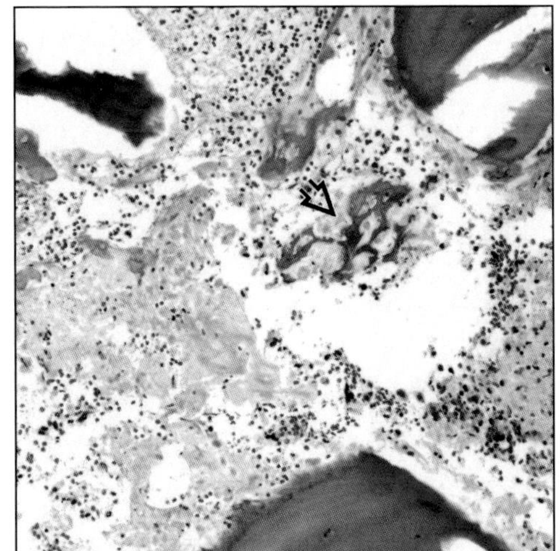

(Left) *H&E shows conventional osteosarcoma with fine, eosinophilic osteoid ➡ and pleomorphic, malignant stromal cells ➡.* ***(Right)*** *Thin, basophilic trabeculae of neoplastic bone can mimic fungal hyphae ➡.*

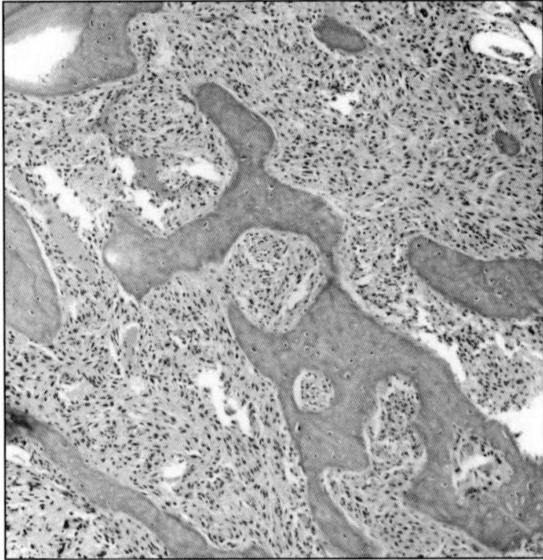

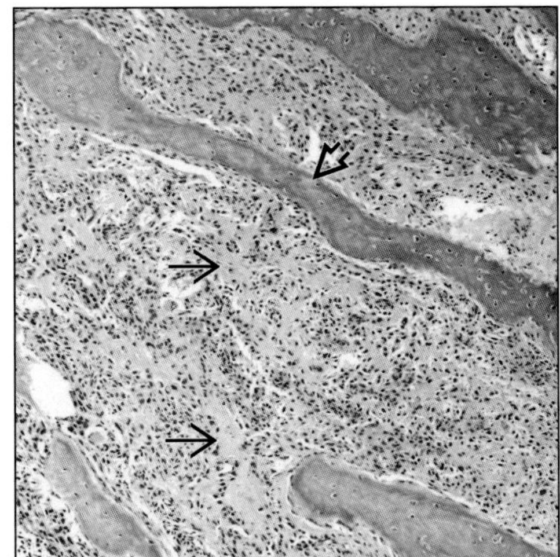

(Left) *H&E shows conventional osteosarcoma permeating between bony trabeculae.* ***(Right)*** *Note the light eosinophilic osteoid ➡, produced by the malignant stromal cells, in contrast to preexisting benign bony trabeculae ➡. Osteosarcoma may destroy the preexisting trabeculae or simply grow around them.*

Microscopic Features

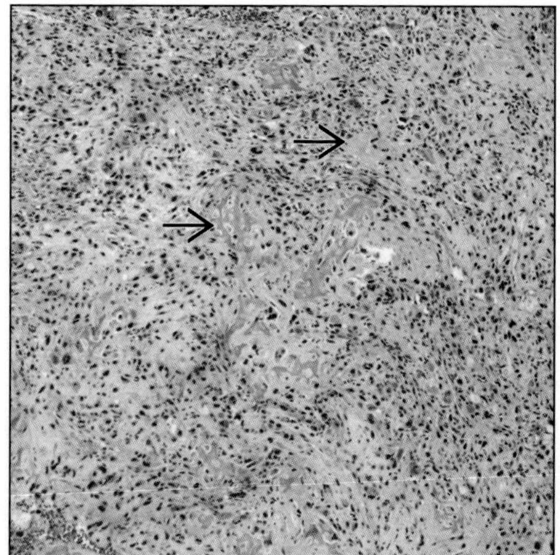

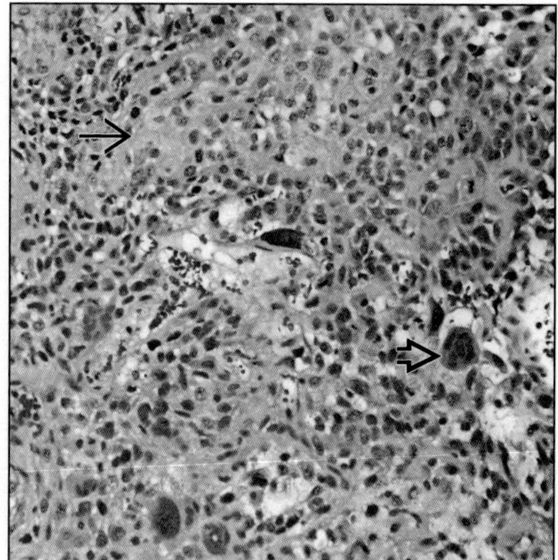

(Left) *H&E shows conventional osteosarcoma with a pleomorphic, bizarre, spindle cell stroma/matrix and osteoid production ➔.* ***(Right)*** *Approximately 1/4 of osteosarcomas may have scattered giant cells ➔ throughout the stroma. It is important not to mistake this lesion for a giant cell tumor. The presence of osteoid ➔ is diagnostic of osteosarcoma.*

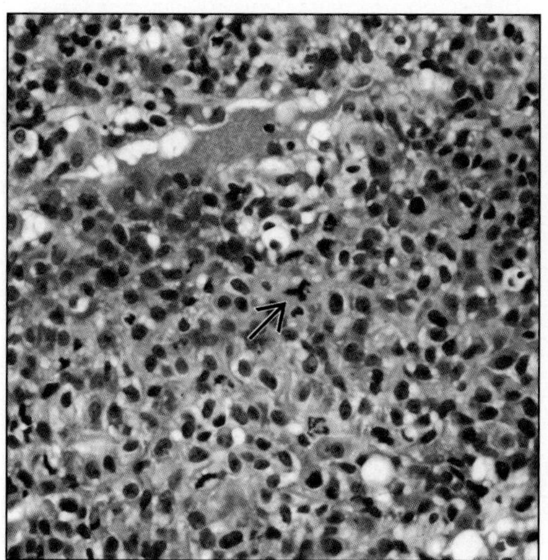

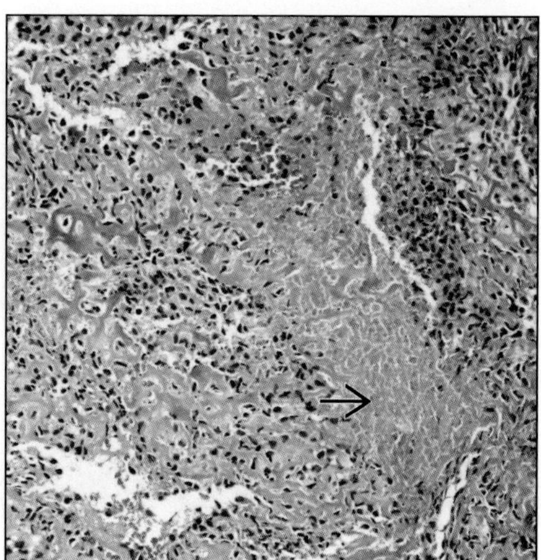

(Left) *H&E shows osteosarcoma with numerous mitotic figures. Note the atypical tripolar mitotic figure ➔.* ***(Right)*** *Areas of hemorrhage and necrosis ➔ may be present. In this example of osteosarcoma prominent areas of necrosis are highlighted.*

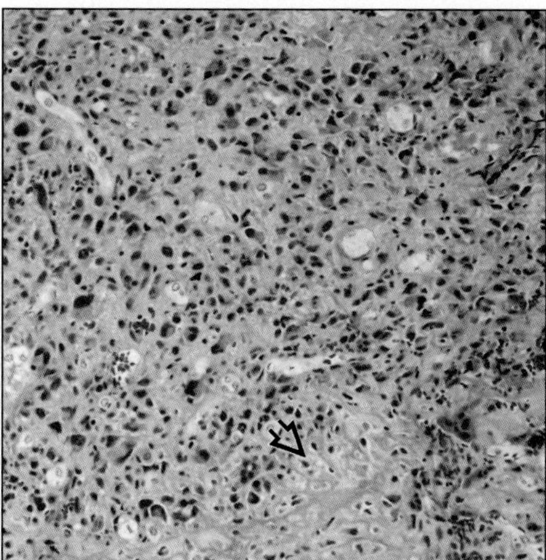

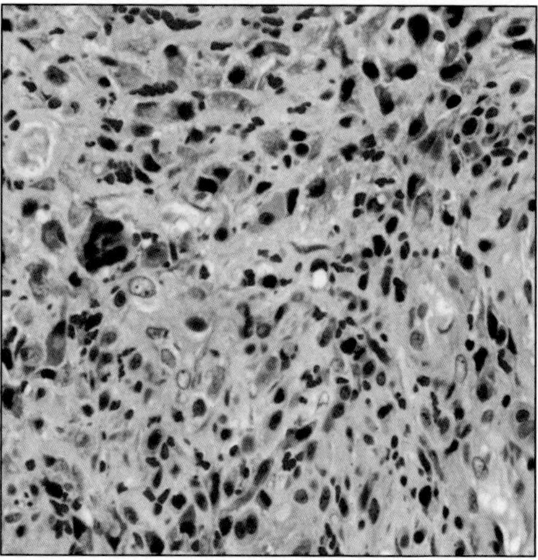

(Left) *Malignant bone (calcified osteoid) or osteoid ➔ is formed directly by tumor cells.* ***(Right)*** *H&E shows conventional osteosarcoma with pleomorphic, bizarre stromal cells. Tumor cells can vary greatly in size and shape and may be spindle, oval, or round.*

OSTEOSARCOMA

Microscopic Features

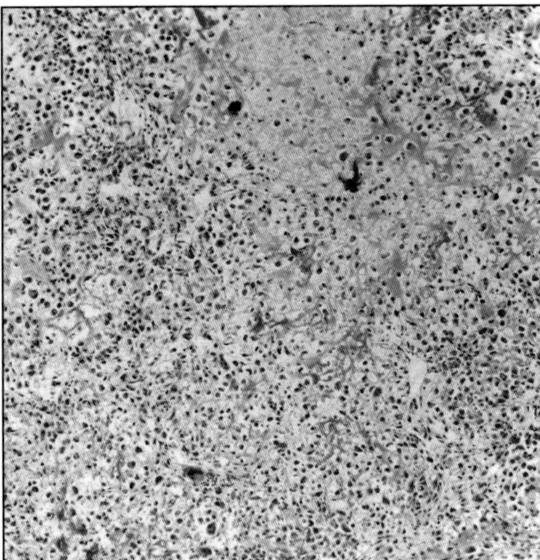

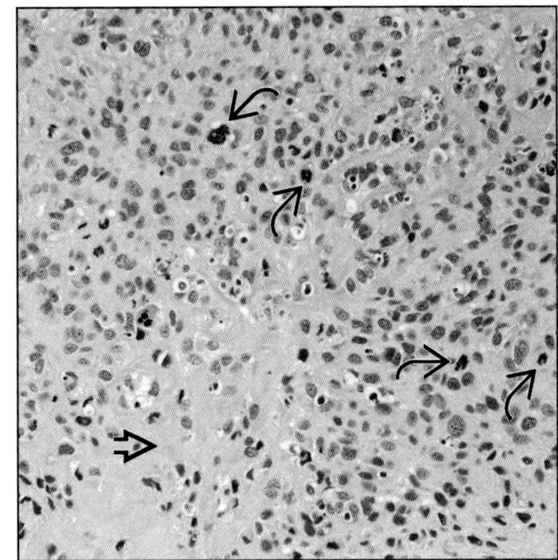

(Left) *Conventional osteosarcoma is shown. Osteoid can take on a lace-like appearance.* ***(Right)*** *Hematoxylin & eosin shows conventional osteosarcoma. Osteoid ⇨ may resemble hyalinized collagen; however, it is more homogeneous or glassy rather than fibrillary in appearance. Note the pleomorphism and numerous mitotic figures ↷.*

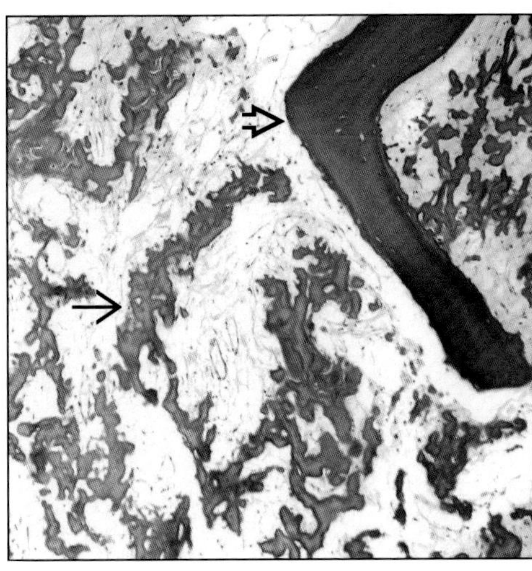

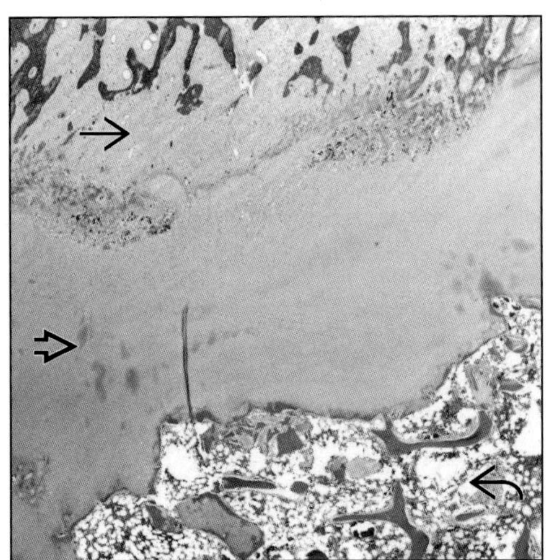

(Left) *Treated osteosarcoma contains blue spiculated bone →. Note the trabecular bone to the right ⇨. Malignant bone is more basophilic and has irregular borders when compared to benign trabecular bone.* ***(Right)*** *Hematoxylin & eosin shows conventional osteosarcoma, post-treatment specimen. OS rarely crosses the epiphyseal plate ⇨. Conventional OS with treatment effect is seen above →, while uninvolved marrow is below ↷.*

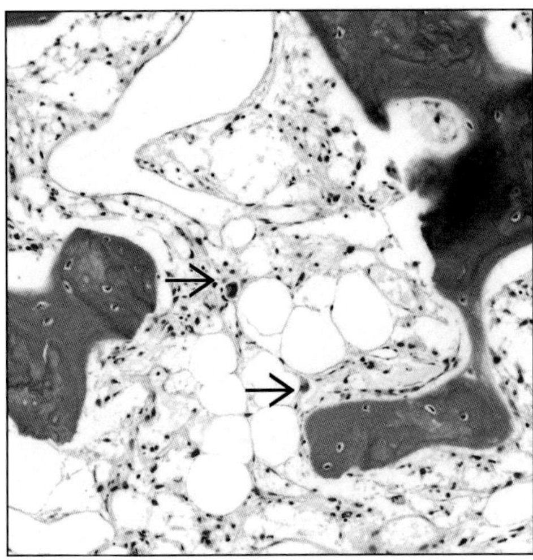

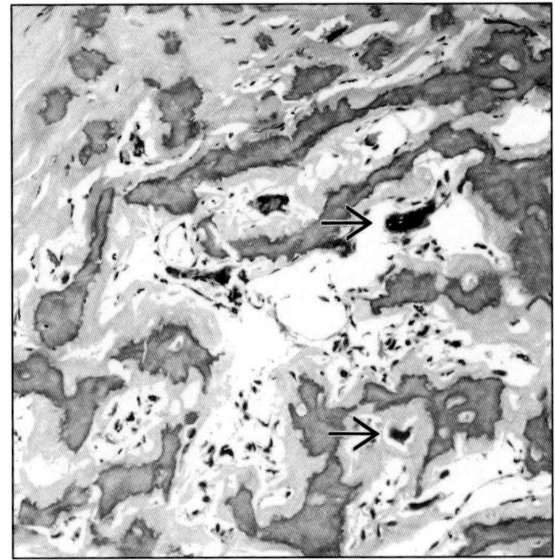

(Left) *Conventional OS, post treatment is shown. Note the scattered viable tumor cells →. Areas of necrosis, fibrosis, and calcification (not shown in image) are typically seen in the background of post-treatment specimens.* ***(Right)*** *Post-treatment viable tumor cells are atypical cells with hyperchromatic nuclei, smudged chromatin, and vacuolated cytoplasm →. These cells are typically sparse.*

Microscopic Features

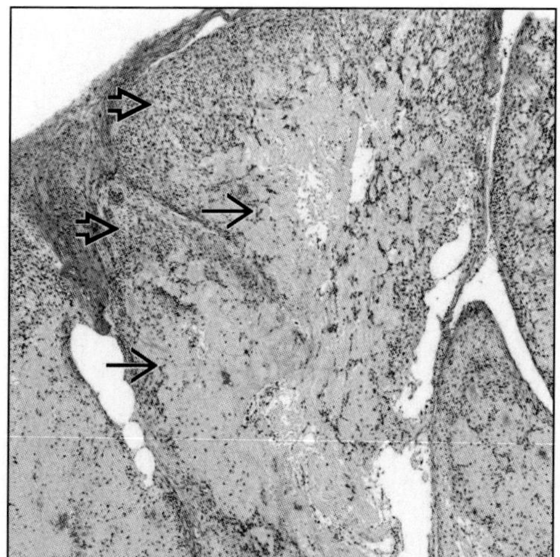

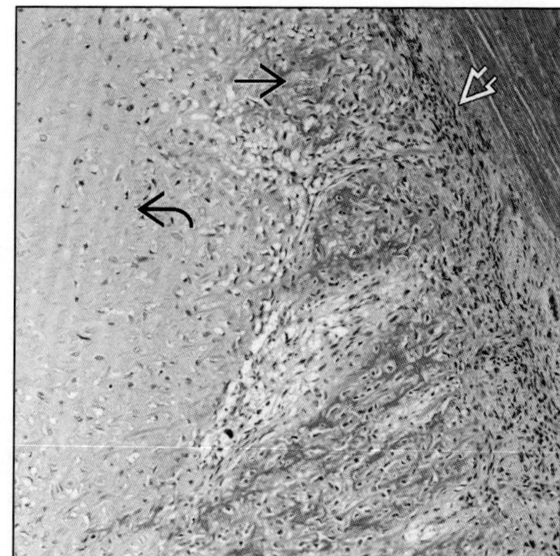

(Left) *H&E shows chondroblastic osteosarcoma with lobules of cartilage that are more cellular at their periphery.* ***(Right)*** *Chondroblastic osteosarcoma is shown. A lobule of malignant cartilage is rimmed by osteoid. Note the increased cellularity and spindle cell population at the periphery.*

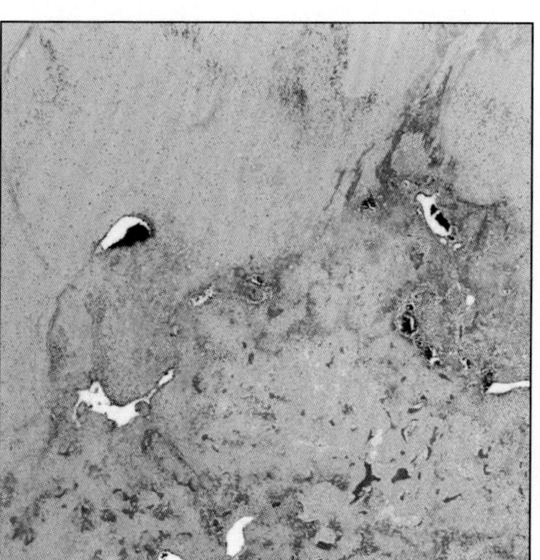

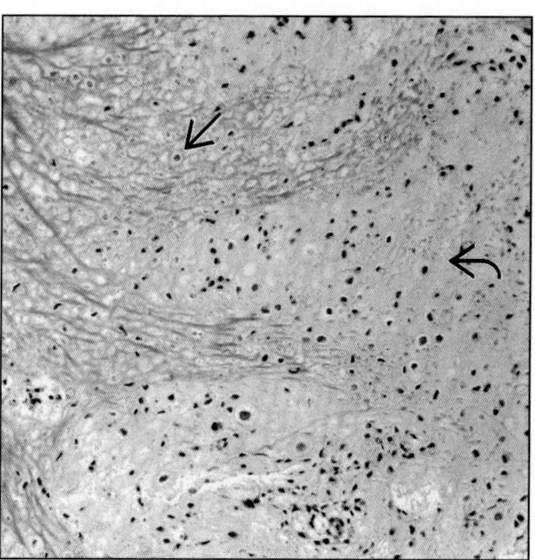

(Left) *Low-power view of chondroblastic osteosarcoma shows lobular architecture.* ***(Right)*** *A malignant bone tumor should be diagnosed as osteosarcoma when osteoid is identified, regardless of the amount of cartilage formation. The cells within the lacunae of the cartilaginous component show marked anaplasia.*

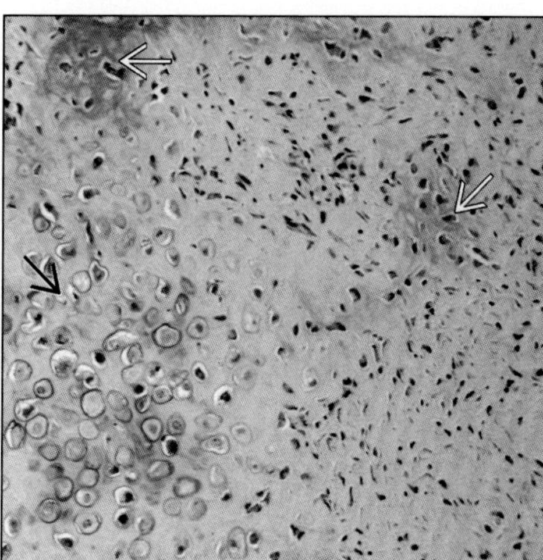

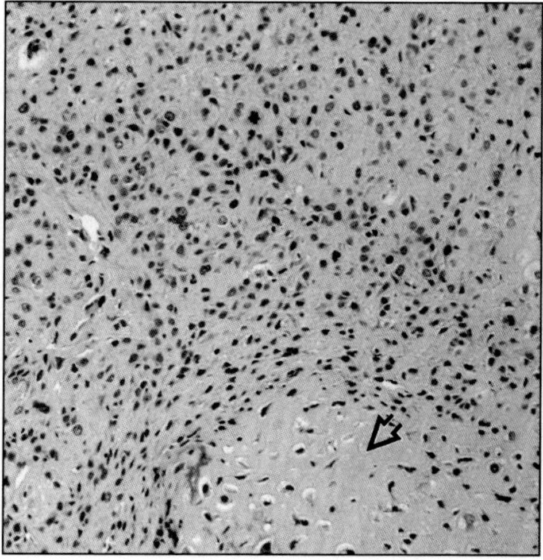

(Left) *Cartilage may be immature, myxoid, or mineralized. Note the osteoid production. In some cases, osteoid can be found in the center of the chondroid lobules.* ***(Right)*** *Marked pleomorphism is seen in both the stromal cells and the cells within the lacunae of the chondroid lobule.*

OSTEOSARCOMA

Gross and Microscopic Features

*(**Left**) Telangiectatic osteosarcoma is shown. The tumor can resemble a blood clot or a "bag of blood." (**Right**) This telangiectatic osteosarcoma has a hemorrhagic red-brown gross appearance similar to that of an aneurysmal bone cyst.*

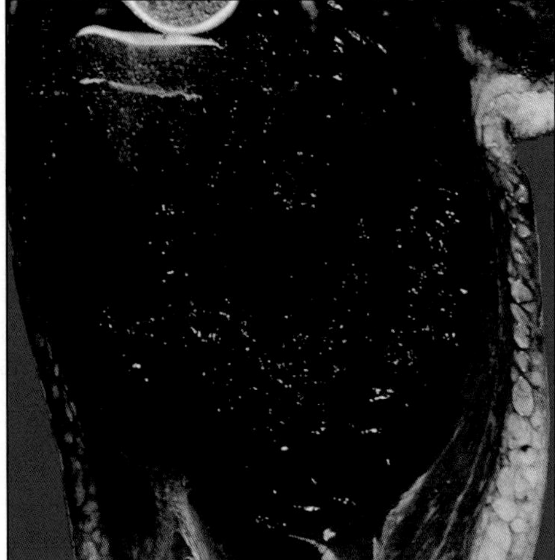

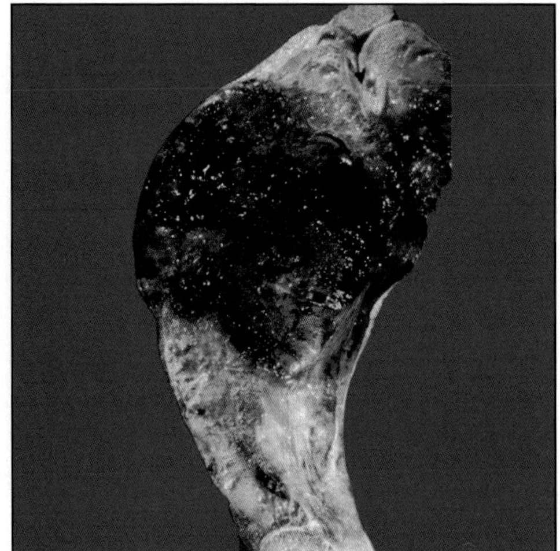

*(**Left**) Telangiectatic osteosarcoma and aneurysmal bone cyst can resemble each other at low power. Atypical cells in the septa are diagnostic of telangiectatic osteosarcoma. (**Right**) In this case of telangiectatic osteosarcoma, spaces filled with blood are separated by septae. Note the scattered giant cells ➔.*

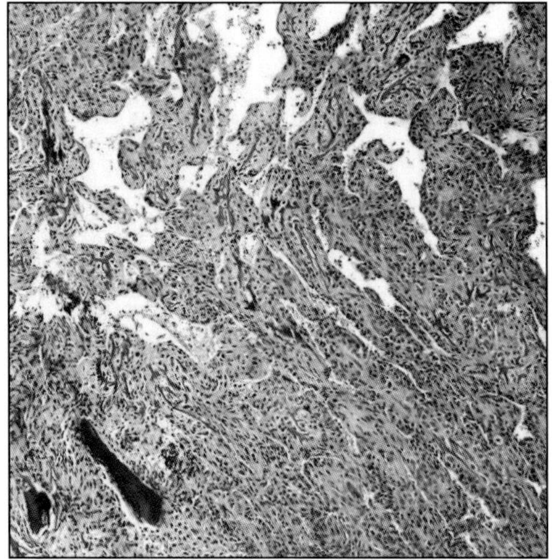

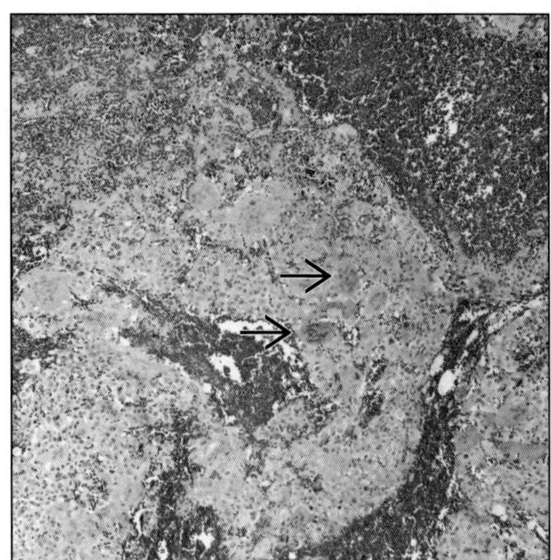

*(**Left**) Malignant stromal cells ➔ and the presence of osteoid ➔ distinguishes telangiectatic osteosarcoma from aneurysmal bone cyst. (**Right**) Telangiectatic osteosarcoma shows atypical mitotic figures ➔ and hemosiderin-laden macrophages ➔.*

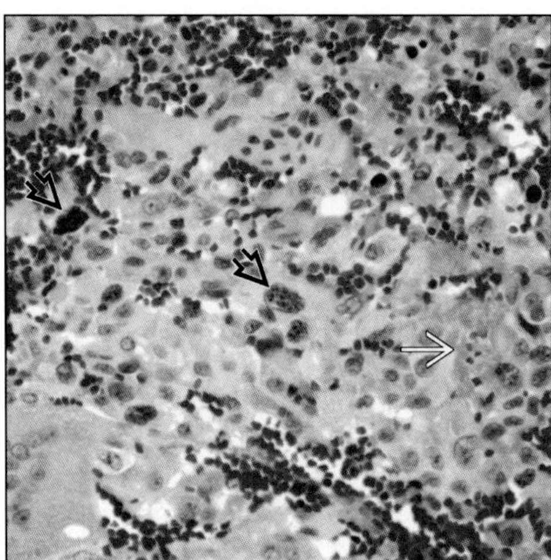

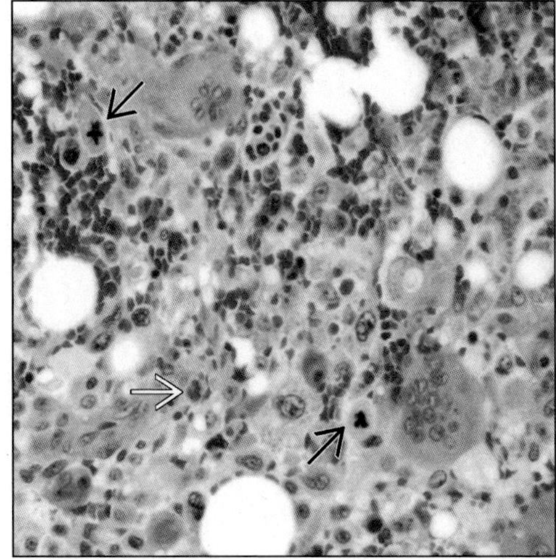

Gross and Microscopic Features

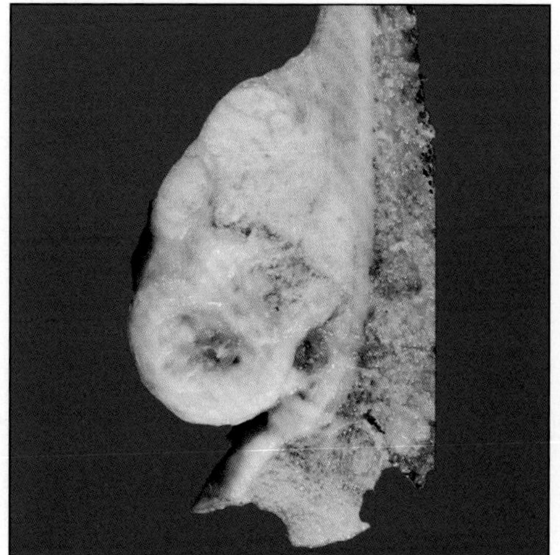

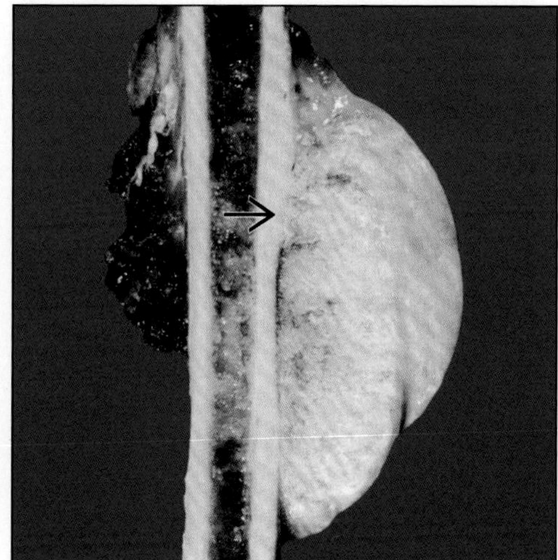

(Left) *Parosteal osteosarcoma, also known as juxtacortical osteosarcoma, frequently arises along the posterior aspect of the lower femoral shaft.* ***(Right)*** *Parosteal osteosarcoma forms a large, lobulated mass. Sometimes a cartilaginous cap or plate is present. This type of osteosarcoma tends to encircle the bone, and there is minimal involvement of the cortex* →.

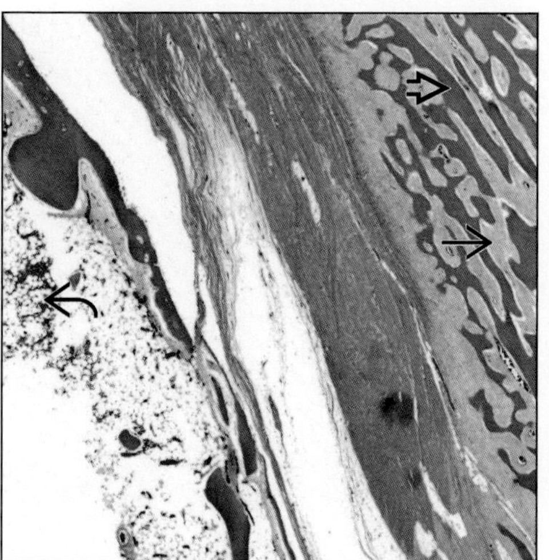

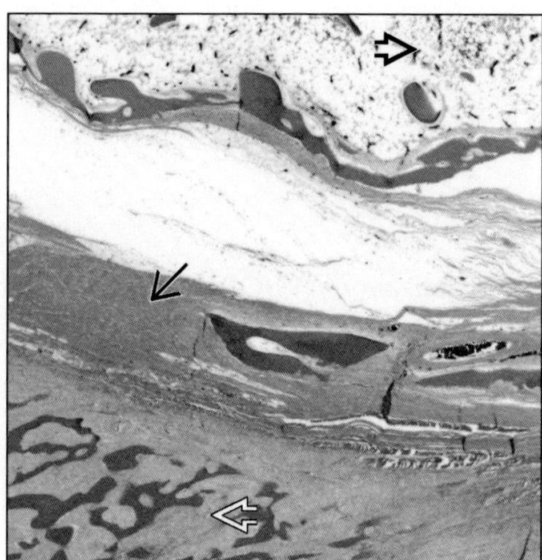

(Left) *Parosteal osteosarcoma is shown. This is a low-grade lesion composed of hypocellular spindle cell stroma* → *and bone formation is the form of trabeculae* ⇨. *Normal cortical bone and marrow elements* ↗ *are present on the left.* ***(Right)*** *In this case of parosteal osteosarcoma, there is minimal involvement of the cortex* →. *Tumor* ➡ *is seen along the bottom of the photomicrograph, and normal marrow is present at the top* ⇨.

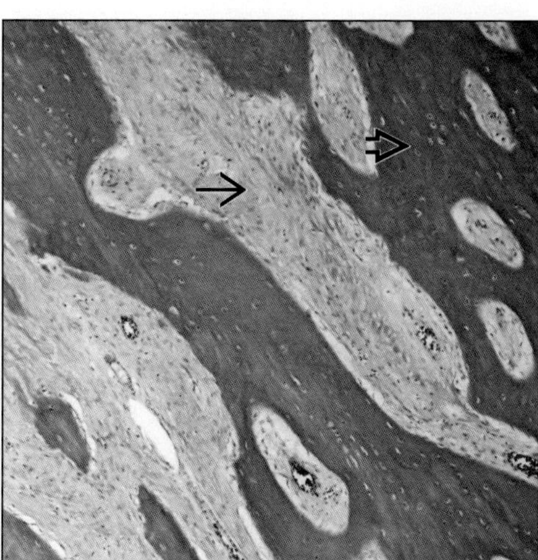

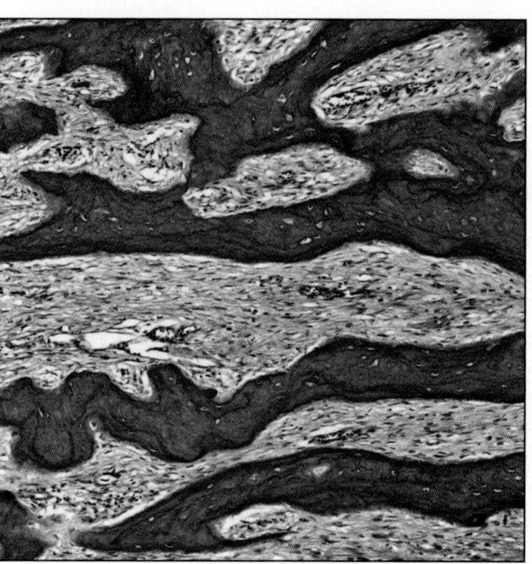

(Left) *Microscopically, there is well-formed bone* ⇨ *with a fibrous, spindle cell stroma* →. *Evidence of malignancy, such as cytologic atypia, is subtle, which can lead to a misdiagnosis. Mitotic figures are rare.* ***(Right)*** *In this case of parosteal osteosarcoma, the bone appears to arise directly from the moderately cellular spindle cell stroma.*

PROTOCOL FOR BONE TUMOR SPECIMENS

Bone: Biopsy

Surgical Pathology Cancer Case Summary (Checklist)

Specimen

Specify bone involved (if known): ___________________________

___ Not specified

Procedure

___ Core needle biopsy

___ Curettage

___ Excisional biopsy

___ Other (specify): ___________________________

___ Not specified

Tumor Site (select all that apply)

___ Epiphysis or apophysis

___ Metaphysis

___ Diaphysis

___ Cortex

___ Medullary cavity

___ Surface

___ Tumor involves joint

___ Tumor extension into soft tissue

___ Cannot be determined

Tumor Size

Greatest dimension: _________ cm

*Additional dimensions: _________ x _________ cm

___ Cannot be determined

Histologic Type (World Health Organization [WHO] classification of bone tumors)

Specify: ___________________________

___ Cannot be determined

****Mitotic Rate***

*Specify: _________ /10 high-power fields (HPF)

(1 HPF x 400 = 0.1734 mm²; X40 objective; most proliferative area)

Necrosis

___ Not identified

___ Present

Extent: _________ %

___ Cannot be determined

Histologic Grade

Specify: _________

___ Cannot be determined

****Lymph-Vascular Invasion***

*___ Not identified

*___ Present

*___ Indeterminate

****Additional Pathologic Findings***

*Specify: ___________________________

Ancillary Studies

Immunohistochemistry

Specify: ___________________________

___ Not performed

Cytogenetics

Specify: ____________________________

___ Not performed

Molecular pathology

Specify: ____________________________

___ Not performed

Radiographic Findings (if available)

Specify: ____________________________

___ Not available

Data elements with asterisks are not required. These elements may be clinically important but are not yet validated or regularly used in patient management. Adapted with permission from College of American Pathologists, "Protocol for the Examination of Specimens from Patients with Tumors of Bone." Web posting date February 2011, www.cap.org.

Bone: Resection

Surgical Pathology Cancer Case Summary (Checklist)

Specimen

Specify bone involved (if known): ____________________________

___ Not specified

Procedure

___ Intralesional resection

___ Marginal resection

___ Segmental/wide resection

___ Radical resection

___ Other (specify): ____________________________

___ Not specified

Tumor Site (select all that apply)

___ Epiphysis or apophysis

___ Metaphysis

___ Diaphysis

___ Cortical

___ Medullary cavity

___ Surface

___ Tumor involves joint

___ Tumor extension into soft tissue

___ Cannot be determined

Tumor Size

Greatest dimension: ________ cm

*Additional dimensions: ________ x ________ cm

___ Cannot be determined

___ Multifocal tumor/discontinuous tumor at primary site (skip metastasis)

Histologic Type (World Health Organization [WHO] classification of bone tumors)

Specify: ____________________________

___ Cannot be determined

**Mitotic Rate*

*Specify: ________ /10 high-power fields

(1 HPF x 400 = 0.1734 mm^2; X40 objective; most proliferative area)

Necrosis (macroscopic or microscopic)

___ Not identified

___ Present

Extent: ________ %

Histologic Grade

Specify: ____________________________

___ Not applicable

___ Cannot be determined

PROTOCOL FOR BONE TUMOR SPECIMENS

Margins

___ Cannot be assessed

___ Margins uninvolved by sarcoma

Distance of sarcoma from closest margin: ________ cm

Specify margin (if known): ___________________________

___ Margin(s) involved by sarcoma

Specify margin(s) if known: ___________________________

**Lymph-Vascular Invasion*

*___ Not identified

*___ Present

*___ Indeterminate

Pathologic Staging (pTNM)

TNM descriptors (required only if applicable) (select all that apply)

___ m (multiple)

___ r (recurrent)

___ y (post-treatment)

Primary tumor (pT)

___ pTX: Primary tumor cannot be assessed

___ pT0: No evidence of primary tumor

___ pT1: Tumor ≤ 8 cm in greatest dimension

___ pT2: Tumor > 8 cm in greatest dimension

___ pT3: Discontinuous tumors in the primary bone site (not including skip metastasis)

Regional lymph nodes (pN)

___ pNX: Regional lymph nodes cannot be assessed

___ pN0: No regional lymph node metastasis

___ pN1: Regional lymph node metastasis

Specify: Number examined: ________

Number involved: ________

Distant metastasis (pM)

___ Not applicable

___ pM1a: Lung

___ pM1b: Metastasis involving distant sites other than lung (including skip metastases)

*Specify site(s), if known: ___________________________

**Additional Pathologic Findings*

Specify: ___________________________

Ancillary Studies

Immunohistochemistry

Specify: ___________________________

___ Not performed

Cytogenetics

Specify: ___________________________

___ Not performed

Molecular pathology

Specify: ___________________________

___ Not performed

Radiographic Findings (if available)

Specify: ___________________________

___ Not available

Pre-resection Treatment (select all that apply)

___ No therapy

___ Chemotherapy performed

___ Radiation therapy performed

___ Therapy performed, type not specified

___ Unknown

Treatment Effect (select all that apply)

___ Not identified

___ Present

*Specify percentage of necrotic tumor: ________ %

___ Cannot be determined

**Data elements with asterisks are not required. These elements may be clinically important but are not yet validated or regularly used in patient management. Adapted with permission from College of American Pathologists, "Protocol for the Examination of Specimens from Patients with Tumors of Bone." Web posting date February 2011, www.cap.org.*

PROTOCOL FOR PNET/EWING SARCOMA SPECIMENS

Ewing Sarcoma/Primitive Neuroectodermal Tumor: Biopsy

Surgical Pathology Cancer Case Summary Checklist

Procedure

___ Core needle biopsy
___ Incisional biopsy
___ Excisional biopsy
___ Other (specify): ____________________________
___ Not specified

Tumor Site

Specify site (if known): ____________________________
___ Not specified

Tumor Size

Greatest dimension: _________ cm
*Additional dimensions: _________ x _________ cm
___ Cannot be determined

****Extent of Osseous Tumors (select all that apply)***

*___ Diaphysis
*___ Metaphysis
*___ Medullary cavity
*___ Tumor extension into soft tissue
*___ Other (specify): ____________________________
*___ Not specified
*___ Cannot be determined

****Extent of Primary Extraosseous Tumors (select all that apply)***

*___ Dermal
*___ Subcutaneous/suprafascial
*___ Subfascial
*___ Intramuscular
*___ Intraabdominal/pelvic
*___ Retroperitoneal
*___ Other (specify): ____________________________
*___ Not specified
*___ Cannot be determined

Margins (for excisional biopsy only)

___ Cannot be assessed
___ Margins negative for tumor
Distance of tumor from closest bone margin: _________ cm
Distance of tumor from closest soft tissue margin: _________ cm
___ Margin(s) positive for sarcoma
Specify margin(s): ____________________________

****Lymph-Vascular Invasion***

*___ Not identified
*___ Present
*___ Indeterminate

Pre-biopsy Treatment (select all that apply)

___ No therapy
___ Chemotherapy performed
___ Radiation therapy performed
___ Therapy performed, type not specified
___ Unknown

PROTOCOL FOR PNET/EWING SARCOMA SPECIMENS

Necrosis Post Chemotherapy

___ Necrosis not identified

___ Necrosis present

*Specify extent of total specimen: ________ %

___ Cannot be determined

___ Not applicable

****Additional Pathologic Findings***

*Specify: ____________________

****Ancillary Studies***

***Cytogenetics**

*Specify: ____________________

*___ Not performed

***Molecular pathology**

*Specify: ____________________

*___ Not performed

*Protocol applies to pediatric and adult patients with osseous and extraosseous Ewing sarcoma family of tumors, including peripheral ES/PNET. *Data elements with asterisks are not required. These elements may be clinically important but are not yet validated or regularly used in patient management. Adapted with permission from College of American Pathologists, "Protocol for the Examination of Specimens from Patients with Primitive Neuroectodermal Tumor (PNET)/Ewing Sarcoma (ES)." Web posting date: February 2011, www.cap.org.*

Ewing Sarcoma/Primitive Neuroectodermal Tumor: Resection

Surgical Pathology Cancer Case Summary (Checklist)

Procedure

___ Resection

___ Amputation (specify type): ____________________

___ Other (specify): ____________________

___ Not specified

Tumor Site

Specify site(s): ____________________

___ Not specified

Tumor Size

Greatest dimension: ________ cm

*Additional dimensions: ________ x ________ cm

___ Cannot be determined

****Extent of Tumor (primary osseous tumors) (select all that apply)***

*___ Diaphysis

*___ Metaphysis

*___ Medullary cavity

*___ Tumor extension into soft tissue

*___ Other (specify): ____________________

*___ Not specified

*___ Cannot be determined

****Extent of Tumor (primary extraosseous tumors) (select all that apply)***

*___ Dermal

*___ Subcutaneous

*___ Subfascial

*___ Intramuscular

*___ Intraabdominal/pelvic

*___ Retroperitoneal

*___ Other (specify): ____________________

*___ Not specified

*___ Cannot be determined

Margins

___ Cannot be assessed

PROTOCOL FOR PNET/EWING SARCOMA SPECIMENS

___ Margins negative for tumor

Distance of tumor from closest bone margin: ________ cm

Distance of tumor from closest soft tissue margin: ________ cm

___ Margin(s) positive for sarcoma

Specify margin(s): ________________________

*Lymph-Vascular Invasion

*___ Not identified

*___ Present

*___ Indeterminate

Pre-resection Treatment (select all that apply)

___ No therapy

___ Chemotherapy performed

___ Radiation therapy performed

___ Therapy performed, type not specified

___ Unknown

Necrosis Post Chemotherapy

___ Necrosis not identified

___ Necrosis present

*Specify extent of total mass: ________ %

___ Cannot be determined

___ Not applicable

*Ancillary Studies

***Cytogenetics**

*Specify: ________________________

*___ Not performed

***Molecular pathology**

*Specify: ________________________

*___ Not performed

Pathologic Staging (pTNM)

TNM descriptors (required only if applicable) (select all that apply)

___ m (multiple primary tumors)

___ r (recurrent)

___ y (post-treatment)

Primary tumor (pT)

For primary osseous tumors

___ pTX: Primary tumor cannot be assessed

___ pT0: No evidence of primary tumor

___ pT1: Tumor ≤ 8 cm in greatest dimension

___ pT2: Tumor > 8 cm in greatest dimension

___ pT3: Discontinuous tumors in the primary bone site (not including skip metastases)

For primary extraosseous tumors

___ pTX: Primary tumor cannot be assessed

___ pT0: No evidence of primary tumor

___ pT1a: Tumor ≤ 5 cm in greatest dimension, superficial tumor

___ pT1b: Tumor ≤ 5 cm in greatest dimension, deep tumor

___ pT2a: Tumor > 5 cm in greatest dimension, superficial tumor

___ pT2b: Tumor > 5 cm in greatest dimension, deep tumor

Lymph nodes

Regional lymph nodes (pN)

___ pNX: Cannot be assessed

___ pN0: No regional lymph node metastasis

___ pN1: Regional lymph node metastasis

___ No regional lymph nodes submitted or found

Number of regional lymph nodes examined

Specify: _________

___ Number cannot be determined (explain): ____________________________

Number of regional lymph nodes involved

Specify: _________

___ Number cannot be determined (explain): ____________________________

Nonregional lymph nodes

___ Cannot be assessed

___ No nonregional lymph node metastasis

___ Nonregional lymph node metastasis

___ No nonregional lymph nodes submitted or found

Number of nonregional lymph nodes examined

Specify: _________

___ Number cannot be determined (explain): ____________________________

Number of nonregional lymph nodes involved

Specify: _________

___ Number cannot be determined (explain): ____________________________

Distant metastasis

For primary osseous tumors

___ Not applicable

___ pM1a: Lung

___ pM1b: Metastasis involving distant sites other than lung (including skip metastases)

*Specify site(s), if known: ____________________________

For primary extraosseous tumors

___ Not applicable

___ pM1: Distant metastasis

*Specify site(s), if known: ____________________________

***Additional Pathologic Findings**

*Specify: ____________________________

**Data elements with asterisks are not required. These elements may be clinically important but are not yet validated or regularly used in patient management.*

Breast

Neoplasm, Benign

Neoplasm, Borderline

Neoplasm, Malignant Primary

JUVENILE HYPERTROPHY

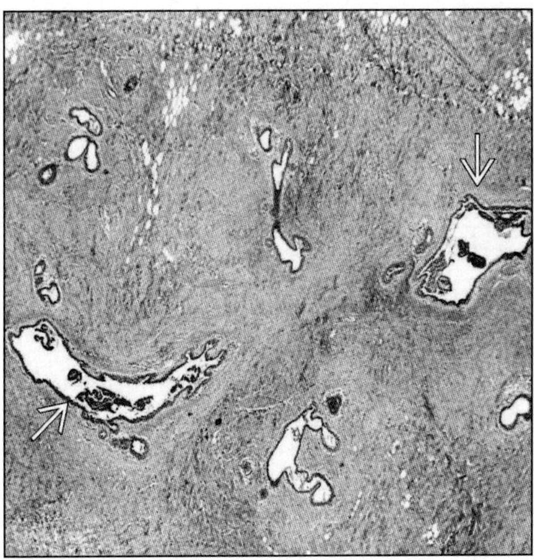

High-power view of JH shows large dilated ducts ➔ in a background of abundant hypocellular fibrous tissue. Note the absence of lobules.

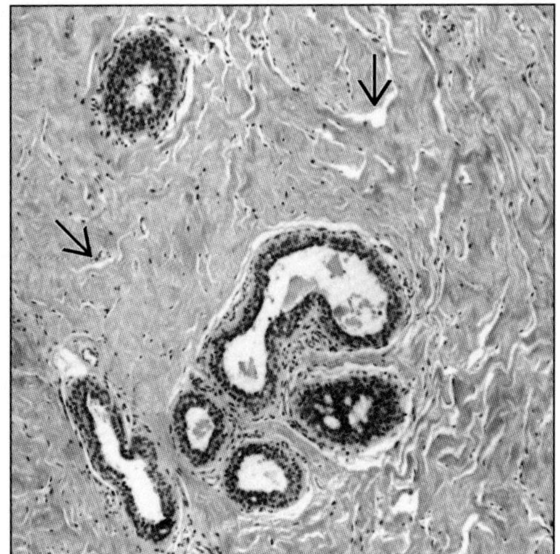

Classic features of JH, which include large dilated ducts in a background of fibrous stroma, are shown. Note the slit-like vascular spaces, which resemble pseudoangiomatous stromal hyperplasia ➔.

TERMINOLOGY

Abbreviations

- Juvenile hypertrophy (JH)

Synonyms

- Juvenile hyperplasia
- Juvenile gigantomastia
- Macromastia
- Virginal hypertrophy

Definitions

- Excessive unilateral or bilateral breast enlargement that occurs over relatively short period of weeks to months in peripubertal females

ETIOLOGY/PATHOGENESIS

Developmental Anomaly

- Thought to be related to local estrogen hypersensitivity of estrogen receptors
- Various studies have shown normal levels of estradiol, prolactin, luteinizing hormone, and follicle-stimulating hormone

CLINICAL ISSUES

Epidemiology

- Incidence
  - True incidence remains unknown

Presentation

- Rapid unilateral or bilateral breast enlargement
  - Usually symmetrically and diffusely enlarged
  - Mastalgia
  - Skin hyperemia
  - Dilated subcutaneous veins
  - Skin necrosis and ulceration may also be present
- Typically occurs shortly after menarche
- Familial pattern of JH reported
  - Associated with nail dysplasia
- Pathology limited to breast with otherwise normal growth and development

Natural History

- Most patients experience a period of brisk growth over 6 months followed by a period of sustained growth over several years
- Does not spontaneously resolve/involute

Treatment

- Surgical approaches
  - Surgical options often pursued at presentation or following breast growth
  - Reduction mammoplasty
    - Associated with frequent recurrences
  - Subcutaneous mastectomy with areola-nipple complex preservation
    - Often pursued following recurrences
- Pharmacologic approaches
  - Anti-estrogen agents
    - Tamoxifen: Effective in arresting recurrent breast enlargement following reduction
    - Useful adjunct that may allow stable results when combined with reduction mammaplasty
    - Must address elevated risk of endometrial cancer
  - Oral contraceptives
    - Variable results
    - Not proven to be effective

Prognosis

- Benign condition
- Profound impact on social and psychological well-being
- Frequent recurrences
  - More commonly recur with early onset of hypertrophy

JUVENILE HYPERTROPHY

Key Facts

Terminology

- Excessive unilateral or bilateral breast enlargement that occurs over a relatively short period of weeks to months in peripubertal females

Etiology/Pathogenesis

- Thought to be related to local estrogen hypersensitivity of estrogen receptors

Clinical Issues

- Usually symmetrically and diffusely enlarged
- Benign condition with frequent recurrences

Microscopic Pathology

- Proliferation of breast connective tissue and ducts
- Overall appearance similar to gynecomastia

MACROSCOPIC FEATURES

General Features

- Homogeneous gray-tan to yellow cut surface

MICROSCOPIC PATHOLOGY

Microscopic Features

- Proliferation of breast connective tissue and ducts
  - Dense hypocellular stroma
  - Ducts show varying degrees of cystic dilatation and intraductal hyperplasia
  - Absence of lobular units in areas of hypertrophy
- Overall appearance similar to gynecomastia
- Fibrous stroma may show pseudoangiomatous appearance
- Collagenous fibrosis and cellular myxoid hyperplasia can be seen

DIFFERENTIAL DIAGNOSIS

Juvenile Fibroadenoma

- Greater degree of stromal cellularity and epithelial hyperplasia
- Most often unilateral

Phyllodes Tumor

- Greater degree of stromal cellularity
- Stromal overgrowth
- More commonly unilateral

Breast Malignancy

- Exceedingly rare
- More relevant to differential with unilateral breast enlargement
- More likely to encounter extramammary metastatic disease

SELECTED REFERENCES

1. Chung EM et al: From the archives of the AFIP: breast masses in children and adolescents: radiologic-pathologic correlation. Radiographics. 29(3):907-31, 2009
2. Dancey A et al: Gigantomastia--a classification and review of the literature. J Plast Reconstr Aesthet Surg. 61(5):493-502, 2008
3. Govrin-Yehudain J et al: Familial juvenile hypertrophy of the breast. J Adolesc Health. 35(2):151-5, 2004
4. Baker SB et al: Juvenile gigantomastia: presentation of four cases and review of the literature. Ann Plast Surg. 46(5):517-25; discussion 525-6, 2001
5. Kupfer D et al: Juvenile breast hypertrophy: report of a familial pattern and review of the literature. Plast Reconstr Surg. 90(2):303-9, 1992

IMAGE GALLERY

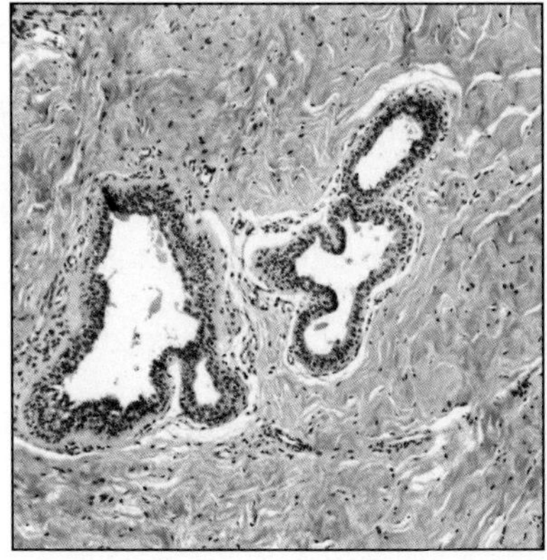

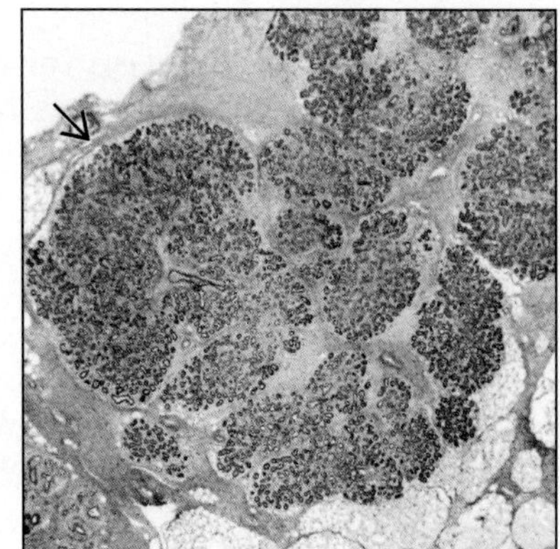

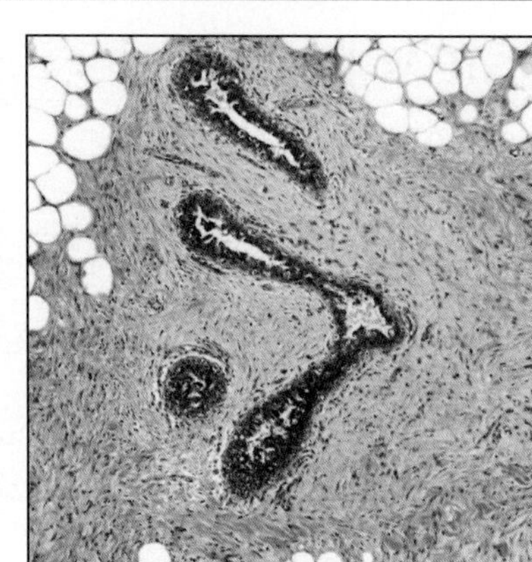

(Left) *High-power view of JH highlights many of the classic features, which include large ducts set in a hypocellular stroma that may show pseudoangiomatous stromal hyperplasia-like features.* ***(Center)*** *This example of JH taken from an excisional biopsy in a 16-year-old female shows very distinct lobule formation ⇒. Other areas showed more classic features.* ***(Right)*** *Juvenile hypertrophy commonly shows overlapping features with gynecomastia as illustrated here.*

PSEUDOANGIOMATOUS STROMAL HYPERPLASIA

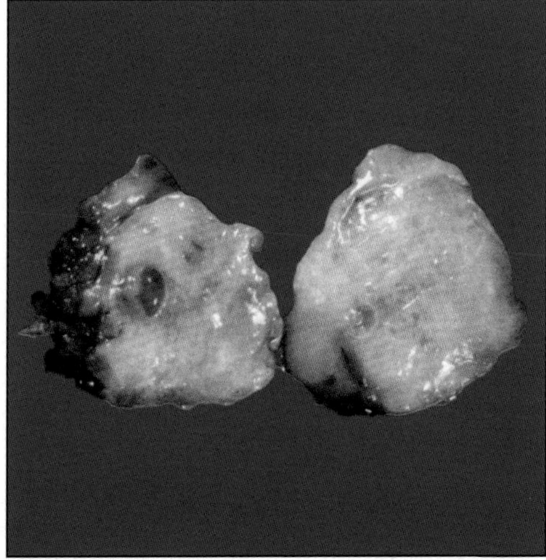

This case of PASH shows a well-circumscribed, firm, rubbery mass with a white cut surface. (Courtesy R. Flinner, MD.)

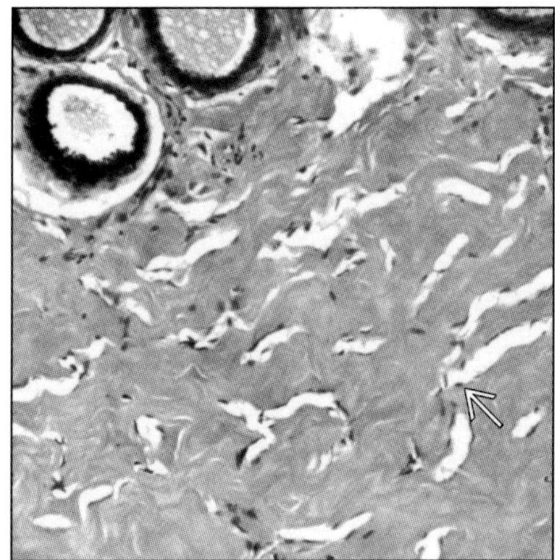

Thin slit-like channels lined by attenuated myofibroblasts ➔ and devoid of red blood cells are set in a hyalinized collagenous stroma. (Courtesy R. Flinner, MD.)

TERMINOLOGY

Abbreviations

- Pseudoangiomatous stromal hyperplasia (PASH)

Synonyms

- Pseudoangiomatous hyperplasia of mammary stroma

Definitions

- Benign, hormonally stimulated myofibroblastic proliferation associated with stromal clefting (i.e., forming pseudovascular spaces)

ETIOLOGY/PATHOGENESIS

Hormonal

- Myofibroblastic proliferation likely due to hormonal stimulation or hormonal imbalance
- Similar stromal changes are seen in gynecomastia and juvenile hyperplasia
- Some carcinomas invade with pattern suggesting that they involve clefts seen in PASH
- Has been suggested that clefts are prelymphatic channels that drain into true lymphatics

CLINICAL ISSUES

Epidemiology

- Age
  - Described in patients in 2nd decade of life
  - Occurs most frequently in women of childbearing age
  - Postmenopausal women receiving hormonal therapy may also be affected

Presentation

- Incidental finding in approximately 23% of biopsies
- Palpable mass or radiographic density
  - Circumscribed or ill defined
- PASH frequently grows in size
  - Rapid growth can occur during pregnancy and may be associated with peau d'orange and skin necrosis
  - Rapid growth also seen during adolescence
- Young patients typically present with
  - Painless, firm, rubbery, movable mass
    - Can mimic fibroadenoma clinically and radiographically

Treatment

- Mass-forming PASH should be biopsied to exclude malignancy
- If malignancy excluded, no other treatment necessary
- Surgical excision recommended for symptomatic or growing masses

Prognosis

- Benign lesion
- Recurrence rate of up to 18%
- Spontaneous regression described

IMAGE FINDINGS

Mammographic Findings

- Circumscribed or ill-defined mass
- Calcifications are not characteristic

Ultrasonographic Findings

- Borders may be well defined, or ill-defined mass may be present

MR Findings

- Smooth-bordered mass with enhancement is characteristic
  - May be clumped enhancement or an irregular mass

MACROSCOPIC FEATURES

General Features

- Mass-forming PASH

PSEUDOANGIOMATOUS STROMAL HYPERPLASIA

Key Facts

Terminology
- Pseudoangiomatous stromal hyperplasia (PASH)
- Benign hormonally stimulated myofibroblastic proliferation associated with stromal clefting (i.e., forming pseudovascular spaces)

Etiology/Pathogenesis
- Majority of affected persons are women of childbearing age
- Postmenopausal women taking hormonal therapy may also be affected
- Similar stromal changes are seen in gynecomastia and juvenile hyperplasia

Clinical Issues
- Incidental finding in approximately 23% of biopsies
- May form palpable mass or radiographic density
  - Circumscribed or ill defined
  - Frequently grow in size

Microscopic Pathology
- Prominent slit-like stromal clefts set in hyalinized collagenous stroma
- Slits are lined by bland stromal myofibroblasts
- IHC will confirm that cells are myofibroblasts

Top Differential Diagnoses
- Vascular lesions
- Myofibroblastoma
- Fibrous tumors

Diagnostic Checklist
- Most important lesion in differential diagnosis is angiosarcoma

  - Can appear as firm, rubbery, circumscribed white nodule
  - Size can range from 1-11 cm in diameter
- Large clefts seen grossly in some fibroadenomas and phyllodes tumors are not present

MICROSCOPIC PATHOLOGY

Histologic Features
- Prominent slit-like stromal clefts set in hyalinized collagenous stroma
- Slits are lined by bland stromal myofibroblasts
- Clefts can involve both inter- and intralobular stroma and appear to invade into lobules
- Spaces are devoid of red blood cells

ANCILLARY TESTS

Immunohistochemistry
- Spindle cells immunoreactive for desmin, vimentin, SMA (variable), SMHC, CD34, estrogen receptor(+/-), progesterone receptor(+/-), and Bcl-2(+/-)
- Spindle cells negative for FVIII-related antigen and CD31

DIFFERENTIAL DIAGNOSIS

Vascular Lesions
- Anastomosing slit-like spaces involving lobules of PASH can mimic angiosarcoma
- In most angiosarcomas, there will be nuclear pleomorphism, mitoses, and solid areas or tufting
- In vascular lesions, spaces will be filled with blood
- Immunoperoxidase studies will distinguish endothelial cells of vascular lesions from myofibroblasts of PASH

Myofibroblastoma
- Well-circumscribed myofibroblastic lesion
- Short fascicles of bland spindle cells admixed with collagenous bands
- Tumors form solid masses of spindle cells and do not proliferate around ducts and lobules
- Generally more cellular than PASH
  - Fascicular PASH can mimic myofibroblastoma, particularly on core needle biopsy

Fibrous Tumors
- Proliferations of interlobular fibroblasts that surround ducts and lobules
- Lack characteristic stromal clefting
- Epithelial elements are usually scant and atrophic in appearance

DIAGNOSTIC CHECKLIST

Pathologic Interpretation Pearls
- Histologic findings are not specific for mass-forming lesion on core needle biopsy
  - Confirm that biopsies are representative of circumscribed or ill-defined mass
- Differentiate from angiosarcoma
  - PASH will lack cytologic atypia and may be circumscribed
  - Immunohistochemical studies (if necessary)

SELECTED REFERENCES

1. Damiani S et al: Malignant neoplasms infiltrating pseudoangiomatous' stromal hyperplasia of the breast: an unrecognized pathway of tumour spread. Histopathology. 41(3):208-15, 2002
2. Powell CM et al: Pseudoangiomatous stromal hyperplasia (PASH). A mammary stromal tumor with myofibroblastic differentiation. Am J Surg Pathol. 19(3):270-7, 1995
3. Anderson C et al: Immunocytochemical analysis of estrogen and progesterone receptors in benign stromal lesions of the breast. Evidence for hormonal etiology in pseudoangiomatous hyperplasia of mammary stroma. Am J Surg Pathol. 15(2):145-9, 1991
4. Ibrahim RE et al: Pseudoangiomatous hyperplasia of mammary stroma. Some observations regarding its clinicopathologic spectrum. Cancer. 63(6):1154-60, 1989

PSEUDOANGIOMATOUS STROMAL HYPERPLASIA

Radiologic, Gross, and Microscopic Features

*(**Left**) MLO mammography of the right breast in a patient with biopsy-proven PASH shows a circumscribed mass with a prominent lucent halo ➔. (**Right**) Ultrasound shows a smooth, oval, solid mass with a hyperechoic rim ➔, heterogeneous internal echoes, and posterior enhancement ➔ in this case of biopsy-proven PASH.*

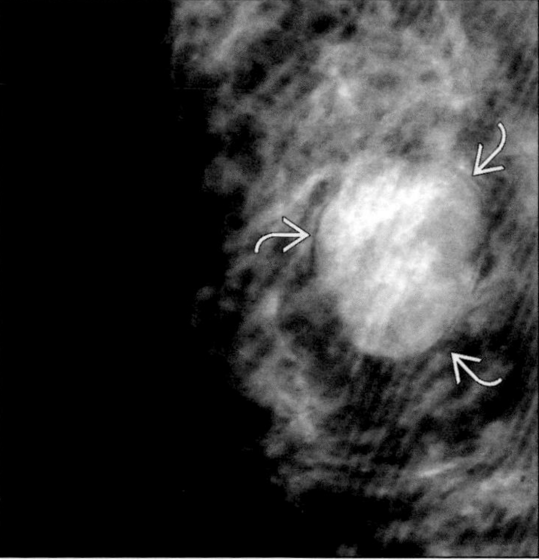

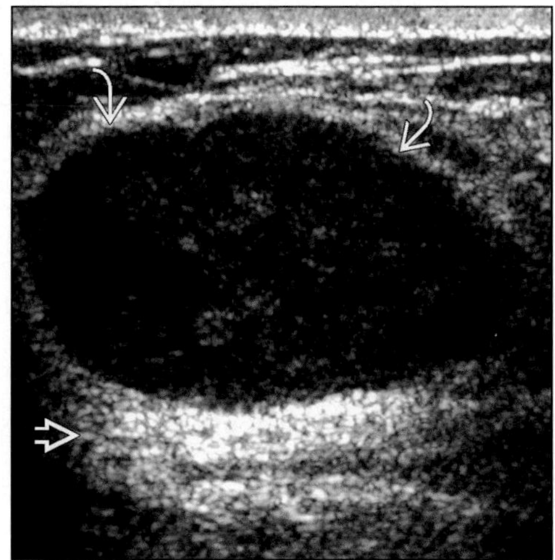

*(**Left**) Some cases of PASH form firm, rubbery, circumscribed masses. This lesion has been bisected to show the white whorled surface of the tumor ➔ within an area of yellow adipose tissue. (**Right**) The small slit-like spaces ➔ characteristic of PASH are present in and around normal ducts and lobules. In this case, the cells form a discrete mass with a circumscribed border ➔.*

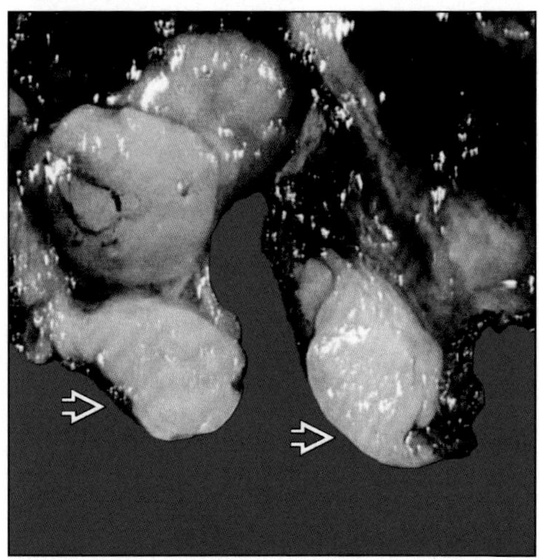

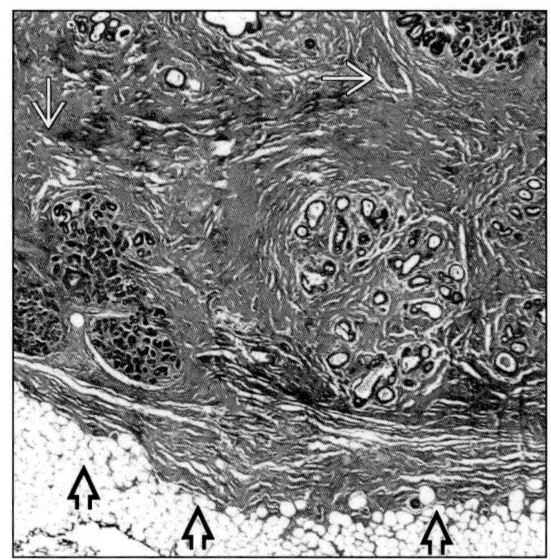

*(**Left**) Low-power view of PASH shows the numerous slit-like spaces set in a collagenous stroma adjacent to and surrounding a small breast lobule. (**Right**) High-power view of PASH shows the slit-like pseudovascular spaces that are lined by more plump myofibroblastic cells ➔.*

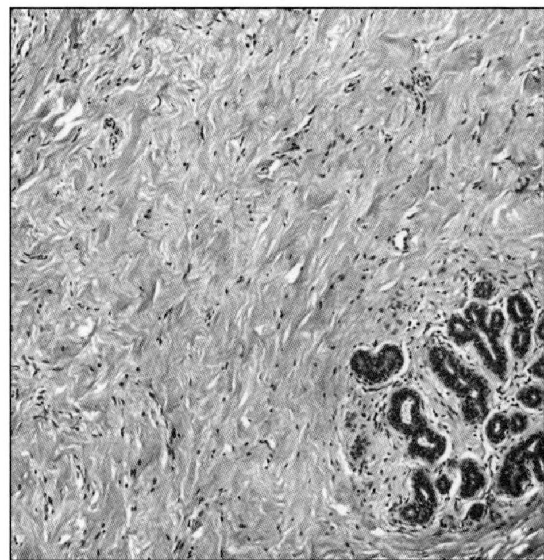

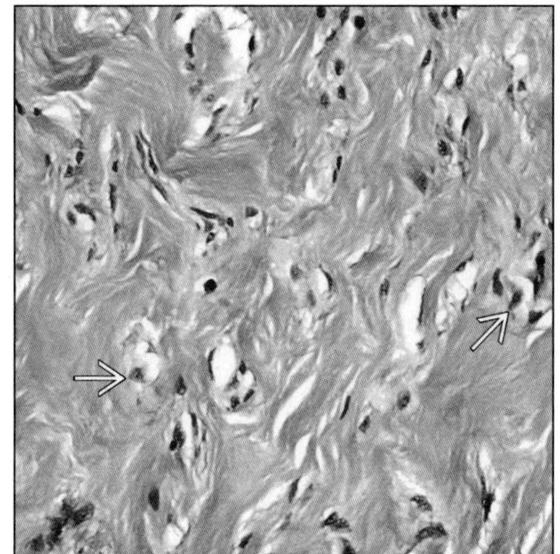

Ancillary Techniques and Differential Diagnosis

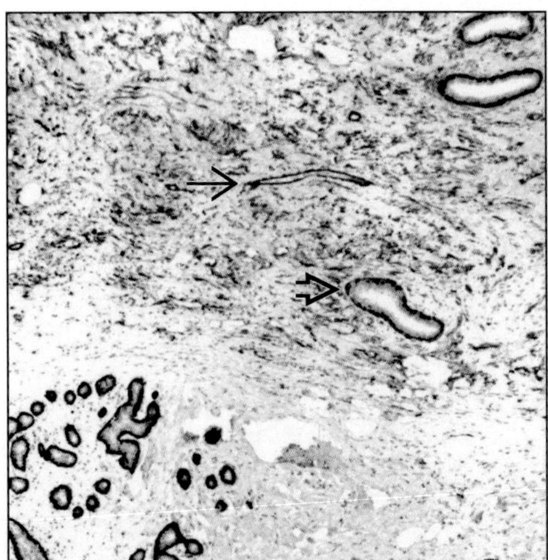

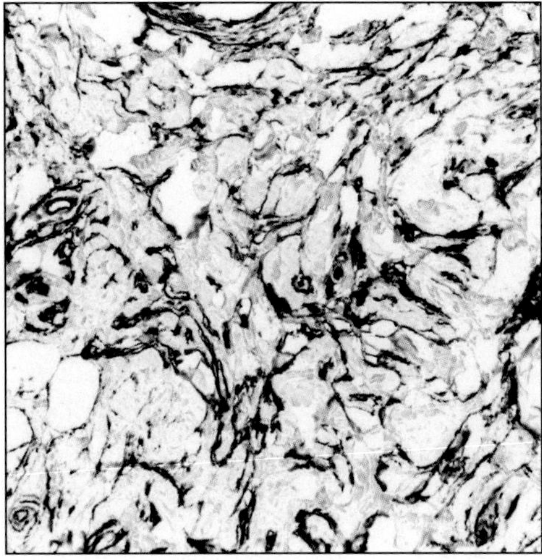

(Left) *The myofibroblasts forming PASH are immunoreactive for smooth muscle myosin heavy chain and are more abundant in the area of PASH (top) than in normal stroma (bottom). Myoepithelial cells ⇨ and endothelial cells → are also positive for this marker.* ***(Right)*** *The myofibroblasts of PASH are positive for CD34, as are almost all stromal lesions of the breast. The 2 exceptions are fibromatosis and nodular fasciitis.*

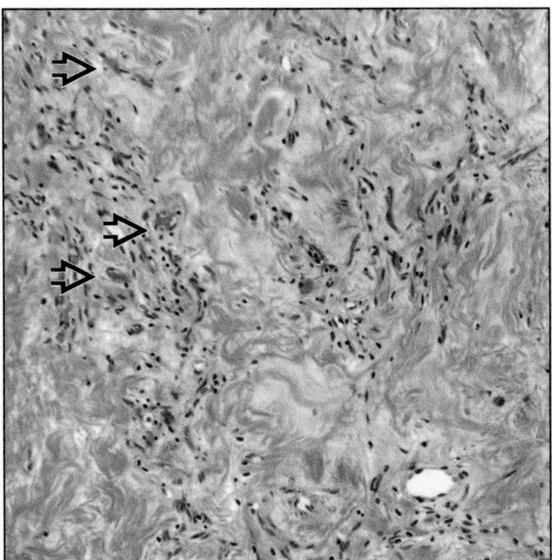

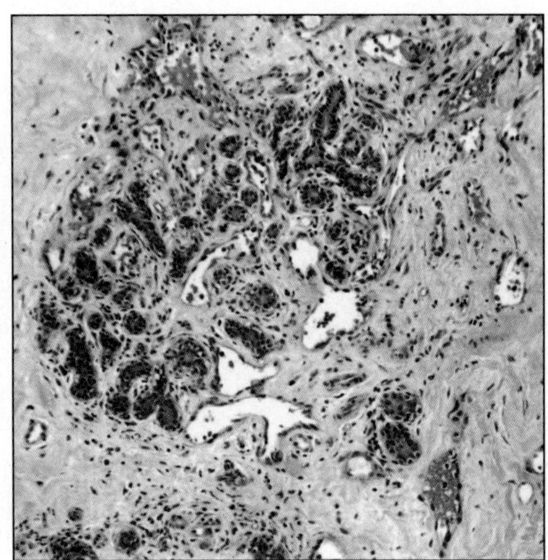

(Left) *PASH can mimic the appearance of a low-grade angiosarcoma due to the clefting that simulates anastomosing blood vessels. However, angiosarcomas will have red blood cells in the lumens of the vessels ⇨, as shown here. In other areas of this angiosarcoma, nuclear atypia was more apparent.* ***(Right)*** *Angiosarcomas are seen invading into lobules. The stromal clefting of PASH may also involve intralobular stroma. However, the other diagnostic features of angiosarcoma will not be present.*

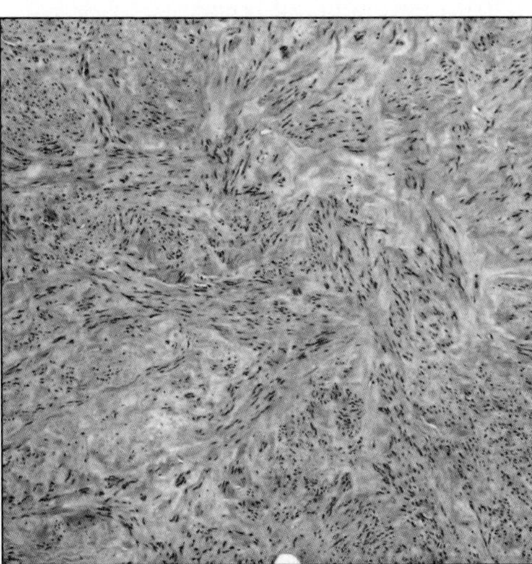

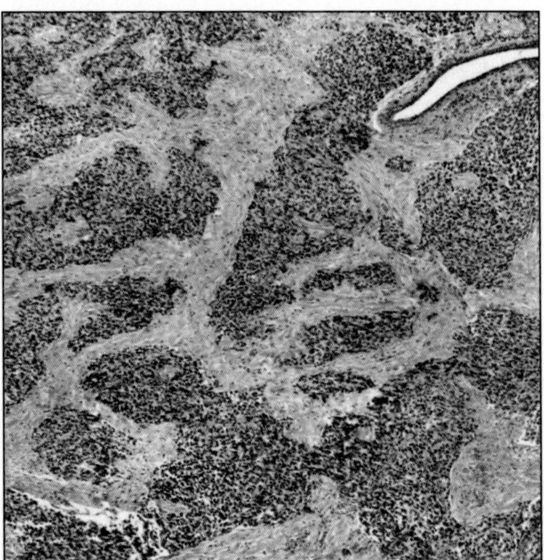

(Left) *Myofibroblastomas consist of short fascicles of cytologically bland spindle cells admixed with bands of hyalinized collagen. Epithelial elements will not be present within the lesion. Fascicular PASH may have a similar appearance, but it surrounds ducts and lobules.* ***(Right)*** *It has been suggested that the clefts of PASH are prelymphatic spaces in the stroma. Some carcinomas, such as this one, appear to involve similar anastomosing spaces in the stroma.*

GYNECOMASTIA

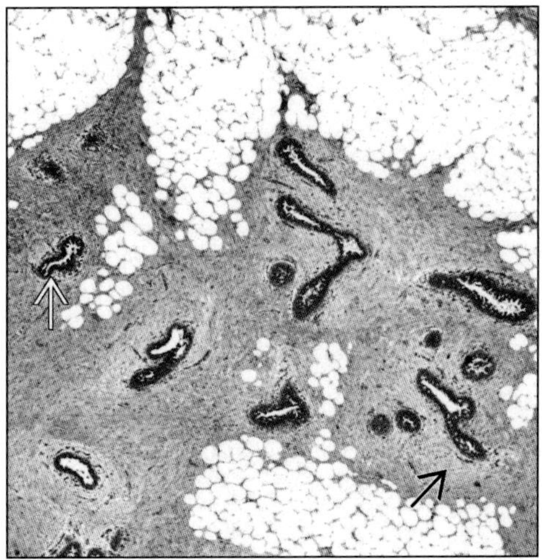

Low-power view shows early stage gynecomastia characterized by increased numbers of ducts ➡ surrounded by a loose, pale-appearing periductal stroma ➡.

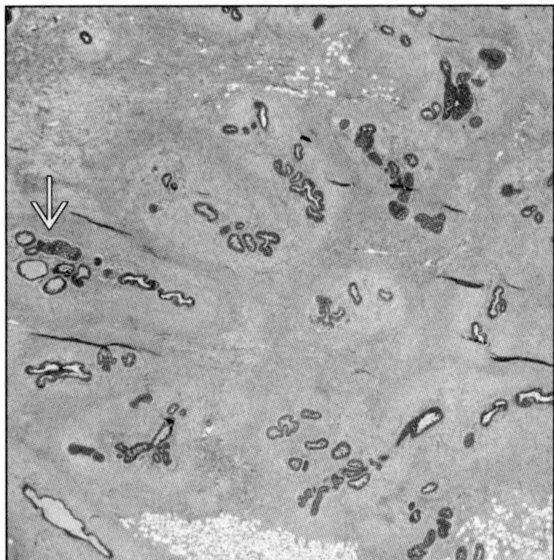

Low-power view highlights increased numbers of ducts with abortive lobule formation ➡ that are surrounded by loose periductal stroma.

TERMINOLOGY

Abbreviations

- Sex hormone binding globulin (SHBG)
- Human chorionic gonadotropin (HCG)
- Atypical ductal hyperplasia (ADH)
- Ductal carcinoma in situ (DCIS)

Definitions

- Pubertal gynecomastia
  - Benign enlargement of glandular and stromal tissue in male breast not associated with underlying pathology

ETIOLOGY/PATHOGENESIS

Absolute Excess of Estrogens

- Exogenous estrogens
- Endogenous estrogen production
  - Tumors
    - Leydig cell tumors
    - HCG secreting tumors (Leydig cell stimulation)
    - Adrenocortical tumors
  - Other causes
    - Aromatase excess syndrome, drugs, alcoholic cirrhosis, aging, obesity, hyperthyroidism, elevated leptin levels

Absolute Deficiency of Androgens

- Primary hypogonadism
  - Klinefelter syndrome
    - Gynecomastia is associated with increased risk of developing breast cancer
- Secondary hypogonadism
  - Pituitary/hypothalamic disease, surgery, radiation

Altered Androgen/Estrogen Ratio

- Puberty, elevated SHBG levels, aging, refeeding gynecomastia, renal failure and dialysis, cirrhosis, hyperthyroidism, drugs

Decreased Androgen Activity

- Androgen receptor defects
- Drugs

CLINICAL ISSUES

Epidemiology

- Age
  - Trimodal age distribution
    - Neonates, pubertal boys, and elderly men
- Ethnicity
  - Prevalence similar among white and black adolescents

Presentation

- Enlargement of breast
  - Bilateral in 2/3
  - Can be asymmetric
  - May be tender
- Common, 50-70% of all pubertal boys
- Family history reported in 1/2 of patients

Laboratory Tests

- Not recommended with normal history and physical exam

Natural History

- Pubertal gynecomastia
  - Typically appears at least 6 months after onset of male secondary sex characteristics
  - Regresses within 1-2 years
  - Persistence beyond age 17 is uncommon

Treatment

- Drugs
  - Medical therapy most effective in early stages
    - Antiestrogens, aromatase inhibitors, androgens
- Surgical excision
  - May be necessary in later stages
- Reassurance and observation in most cases

GYNECOMASTIA

Key Facts

Terminology

- Benign enlargement of glandular and stromal tissue in male breast not associated with underlying pathology

Clinical Issues

- Typically appears at least 6 months after onset of male secondary sex characteristics
- Regresses within 1-2 years

Microscopic Pathology

- Proliferation of mammary ductules in fibroconnective tissue stroma
- Ductal hyperplasia
- Loose and edematous periductal stroma

Top Differential Diagnoses

- Pseudogynecomastia (lipomastia)
- Breast carcinoma

Prognosis

- Clinical gynecomastia not shown to be risk factor for development of breast carcinoma

MACROSCOPIC FEATURES

General Features

- Well-circumscribed oval or disc-shaped mass
- Elastic consistency

MICROSCOPIC PATHOLOGY

Microscopic Features

- Proliferation of mammary ductules in fibroconnective tissue stroma
  - Ductal hyperplasia
    - Cell tufting with protrusion into duct lumens is characteristic
    - Florid ductal hyperplasia seen in early lesions
    - Solid, cribriform, or papillary growth patterns
    - ± apocrine metaplasia
    - Architectural and cytological features may warrant diagnosis of ADH in some cases
    - Associated cancer risk for ADH in gynecomastia is unknown
    - Threshold for diagnosis of DCIS should be high
  - Lobule formation may be seen
  - Loose and edematous periductal stroma
  - Varying numbers of lymphocytes and plasma cells
  - Component of pseudoangiomatous stromal hyperplasia can be seen
  - Stromal fibrosis and hyalinization become prominent with time

DIFFERENTIAL DIAGNOSIS

Pseudogynecomastia (Lipomastia)

- Enlargement of adipose tissue
- Often associated with obesity
- No enlargement of glandular tissue

Breast Carcinoma

- Rare in males
- Hard, eccentric, asymmetric mass
- Axillary lymphadenopathy
- Bloody nipple discharge

Other Clinical Considerations

- Hemangiomas, lipomas, neurofibromas, and dermoid cysts

SELECTED REFERENCES

1. Nordt CA et al: Gynecomastia in adolescents. Curr Opin Pediatr. 20(4):375-82, 2008
2. Cakan N et al: Gynecomastia: evaluation and treatment recommendations for primary care providers. Clin Pediatr (Phila). 46(6):487-90, 2007
3. Narula HS et al: Gynecomastia. Endocrinol Metab Clin North Am. 36(2):497-519, 2007

IMAGE GALLERY

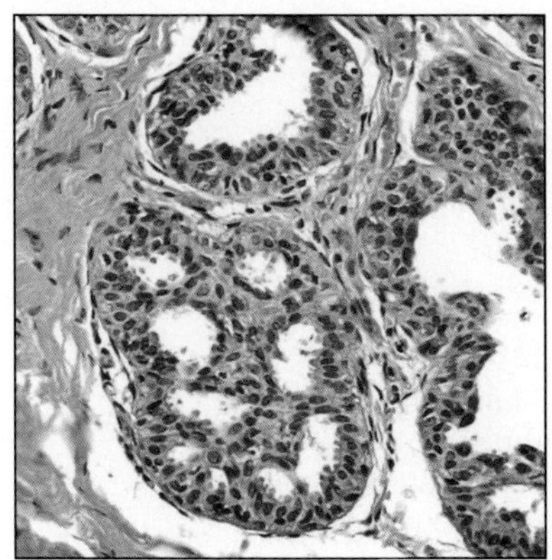

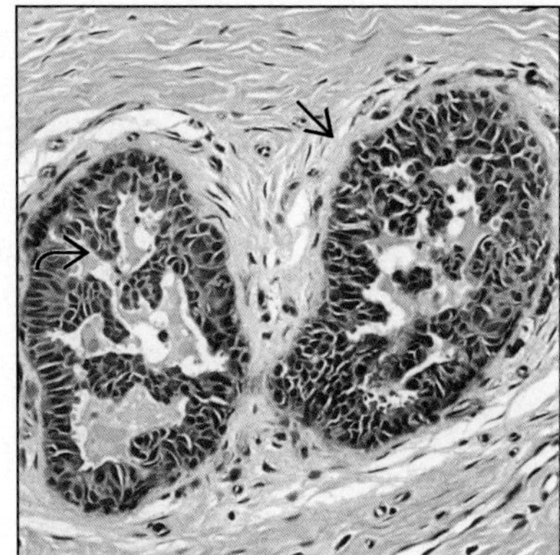

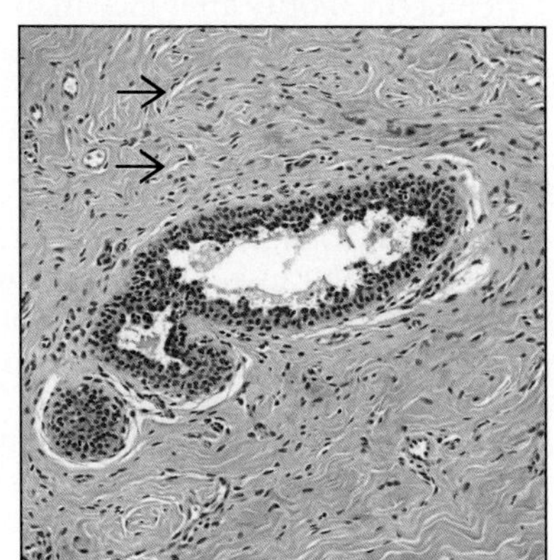

(Left) *High-power view shows ductal hyperplasia with a cribriform pattern of growth. Note the lack of loose periductal stroma indicative of a later, fibrous stage of gynecomastia.* ***(Center)*** *Characteristic features of gynecomastia are shown, including loose periductal stroma ⇒ and ductal hyperplasia with tapering tufts of epithelium ⇒ that protrude into the lumen.* ***(Right)*** *The pseudoangiomatous stromal hyperplasia component ⇒ of gynecomastia is shown.*

JUVENILE FIBROADENOMA

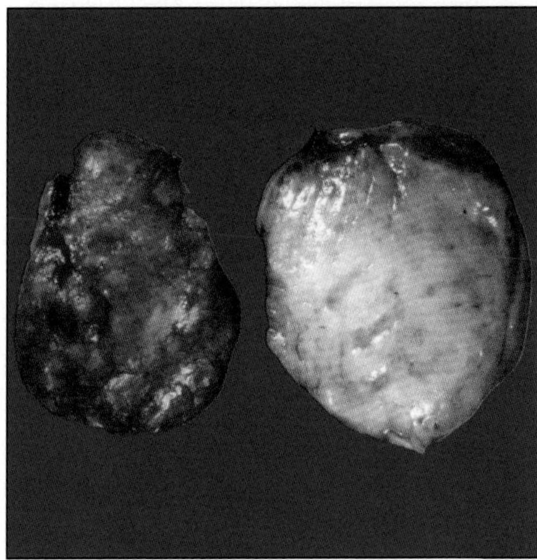

Gross photograph of a "giant" juvenile fibroadenoma demonstrates a fairly uniform gray-white soft cut surface. (Courtesy R. Flinner, MD.)

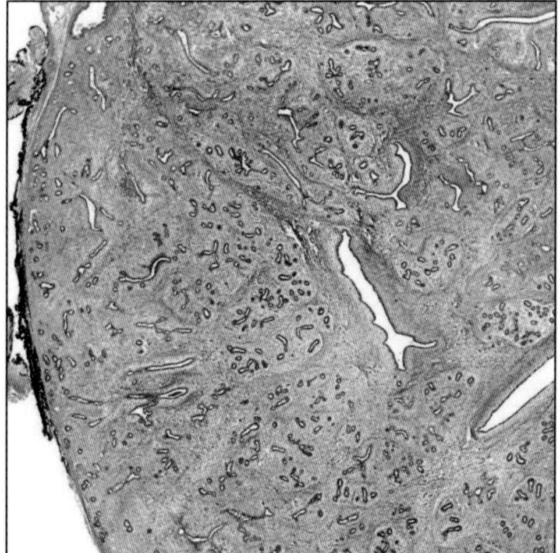

Low-power view of a juvenile fibroadenoma shows a proliferation of glandular and stromal elements. Note the lack of stromal overgrowth and uniform stromal cellularity.

TERMINOLOGY

Synonyms

- Cellular fibroadenoma/adenofibroma
- Hypercellular fibroadenoma
- Giant fibroadenoma
- Juvenile adenofibroma
- Fetal fibroadenoma

Definitions

- Rare variant of fibroadenoma that occurs predominantly in adolescents
- Characterized by rapid growth, large size, increased stromal cellularity, and greater degree of epithelial hyperplasia

CLINICAL ISSUES

Epidemiology

- Incidence
  - Peaks in late adolescence
  - Accounts for < 4% of all fibroadenomas
- Age
  - Tumor of adolescence (11-19 years of age)
  - Often occur shortly after menarche
  - Reported in middle-aged females
- Ethnicity
  - More frequent in African-American patients

Presentation

- Unilateral macromastia
  - Most common cause of unilateral macromastia and breast asymmetry in adolescent women
- Solitary mass
- Rapid growth
  - May double in size over period of months
  - Distortion of overlying skin may be present
  - Compression of adjacent breast tissue
- Venous distension
- Simulates juvenile (virginal) hypertrophy

Treatment

- Local excision with reconstruction
- Preservation of normal breast tissue should be emphasized

Prognosis

- Excellent
- Recurrences
  - Extremely rare in solitary lesions
  - More common with multiple and bilateral tumors
  - May show features of adult fibroadenoma

MACROSCOPIC FEATURES

General Features

- Large circumscribed mass
- Softer in consistency than typical fibroadenoma

Size

- By definition > 5 cm in diameter
- Often > 10 cm in diameter

MICROSCOPIC PATHOLOGY

Predominant Pattern/Injury Type

- Biphasic
- Pericanalicular pattern of growth

Predominant Cell/Compartment Type

- Epithelial, glandular
- Mesenchymal

Microscopic Features

- Biphasic epithelial and stromal lesion
- Stromal hypercellularity
  - Uniformly hypercellular stroma
    - Lacks periductal concentration
    - Lacks stromal overgrowth

JUVENILE FIBROADENOMA

Key Facts

Terminology

- Characterized by rapid growth, large size, increased stromal cellularity, and greater degree of epithelial hyperplasia

Clinical Issues

- Tumor of adolescence (11-19 years of age)
- Often occur shortly after menarche
- More frequent in African-American patients
- Unilateral macromastia

Macroscopic Features

- By definition > 5 cm in diameter

Microscopic Pathology

- Biphasic epithelial and stromal lesion
  - Uniformly hypercellular stroma
  - Intraductal epithelial hyperplasia
- Lacks leaf-like growth pattern of benign phyllodes tumor

    - Lacks cytologic atypia
    - Variable mitotic activity (1-5 mitoses/10 HPF)
- Intraductal epithelial hyperplasia
  - Cytologic atypia may be present
- Lacks leaf-like growth pattern of benign phyllodes tumor
- Lacks stromal myxoid and or mucinous changes of adult-type fibroadenoma

DIFFERENTIAL DIAGNOSIS

Fibroadenoma, Adult-Type

- More firm rubbery consistency
- Smaller in size (2-3 cm in diameter)
- Grow slowly
- Less cellular stroma
- Stromal myxoid &/or mucinous changes

Benign Phyllodes Tumor

- Periductal concentration of stromal cellularity
- Stromal overgrowth
- Leaf-like pattern of growth
- Typically lack prominent intraductal epithelial hyperplasia
- Rare in children

Juvenile (Virginal) Hypertrophy

- Rapid and symmetric breast enlargement
- Unilateral enlargement can occur
- Histologic features similar to those of gynecomastia

Mammary Hamartoma

- Detected mammographically as demarcated density with radiolucent halo
- Composed of mammary ducts, lobules, collagenous stroma, and adipose tissue

Lipoma

- Composed of mature adipose tissue surrounded by capsule
- Lacks glandular and stromal elements

Fibrocystic Change

- Cord-like nodularity
- Cyclic premenstrual mastalgia
- Characteristic morphologic changes include
  - Cyst formation, fibrosis, epithelial hyperplasia, apocrine metaplasia, and chronic inflammation

SELECTED REFERENCES

1. Jayasinghe Y et al: Fibroadenomas in adolescence. Curr Opin Obstet Gynecol. 21(5):402-6, 2009
2. Greydanus DE et al: Breast disorders in children and adolescents. Prim Care. 33(2):455-502, 2006
3. Kuijper A et al: Histopathology of fibroadenoma of the breast. Am J Clin Pathol. 115(5):736-42, 2001
4. Pike AM et al: Juvenile (cellular) adenofibromas. A clinicopathologic study. Am J Surg Pathol. 9(10):730-6, 1985

IMAGE GALLERY

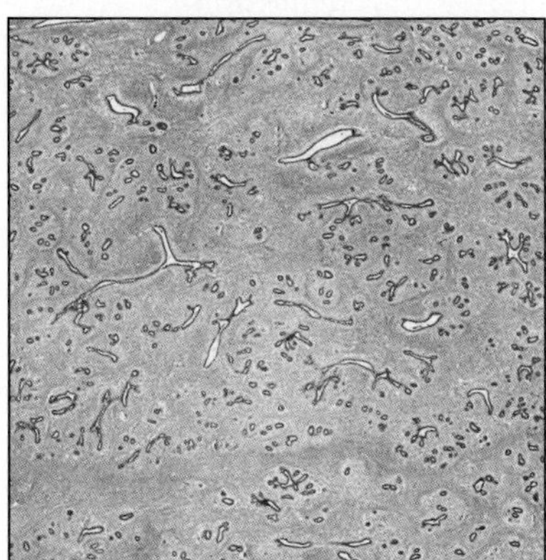

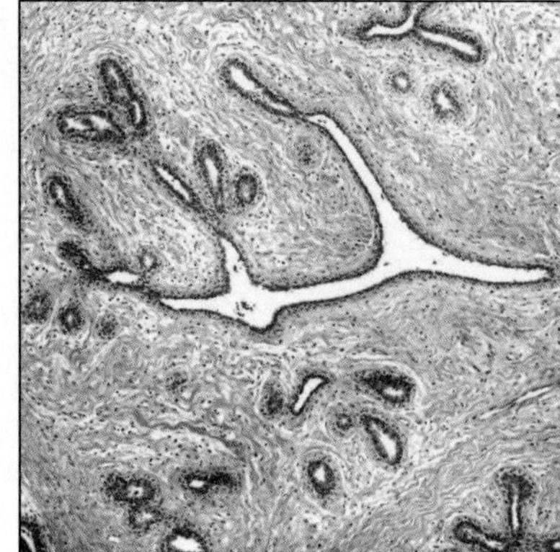

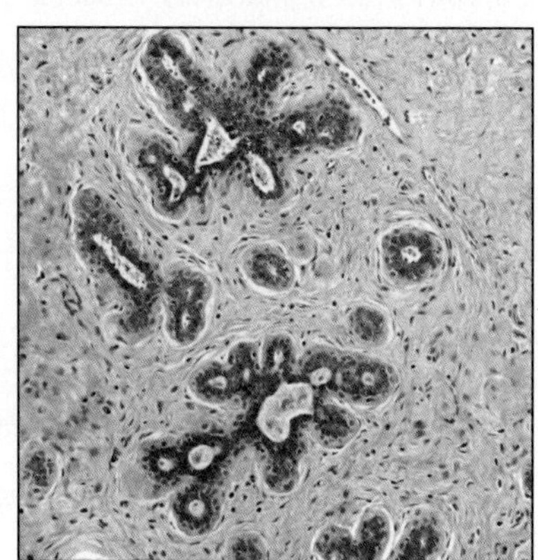

(Left) *The proliferation of glandular and stromal elements without stromal overgrowth and concentrated periductal cellularity help distinguish this tumor from a benign phyllodes tumor.* ***(Center)*** *Medium-power view of this juvenile fibroadenoma highlights a pericanalicular pattern of growth and a moderately hypercellular stroma.* ***(Right)*** *High-power view of a juvenile fibroadenoma highlights the uniform increase in stromal cellularity.*

FIBROADENOMA

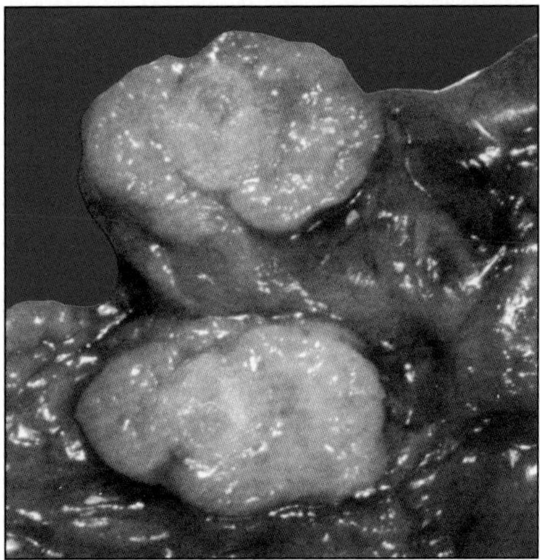

A well-circumscribed and bisected fibroadenoma shows the typical bulging, tan-white cut surface. (Courtesy R. Flinner, MD.)

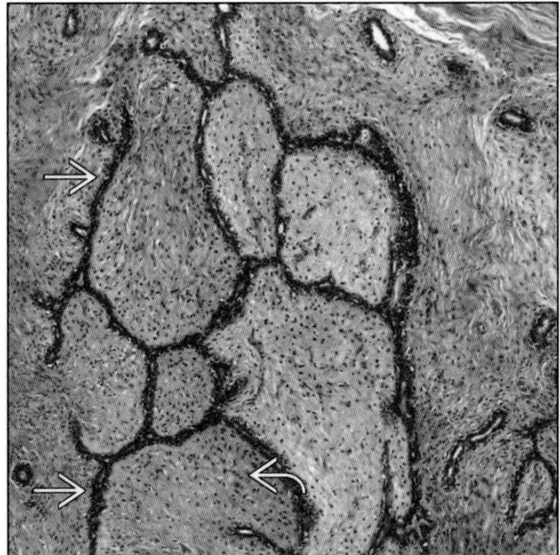

Medium-power view shows a typical fibroadenoma. Note the glandular component ➡ that is compressed and distorted by the stromal proliferation ↪ that shows a uniformly even cellularity.

TERMINOLOGY

Abbreviations

- Fibroadenoma (FA)

Synonyms

- Fibroepithelial lesion
- Adenofibroma

Definitions

- Benign proliferation of glandular and stromal elements
- Variants
  - Complex FA: Include cysts > 3 mm, sclerosing adenosis, epithelial calcifications, or papillary apocrine change
  - Cellular FA: Hypercellular stroma
  - Juvenile FA: Cellular stroma or of large size
  - Giant FA: Large size (> 500 g or > 5-10 cm in diameter)

ETIOLOGY/PATHOGENESIS

Etiology/Pathogenesis

- Proliferation of intralobular stromal cells stimulates growth of lobular epithelial cells
- Most are polyclonal hyperplasias of lobular stroma
- Expression of steroid receptors thought to play a role

CLINICAL ISSUES

Epidemiology

- Incidence
  - Most common benign tumor of female breast
  - Most common cause of breast masses in adolescent girls
  - Population prevalence reported between 2.2-13%
- Age
  - Can occur at any age
  - Peak incidence in 2nd and 3rd decades
- Ethnicity
  - More common in African-American young women

Site

- Upper outer quadrant
- May occur anywhere
- Bilateral in 10-15%

Presentation

- Self-detected breast mass
- Rubbery, smooth, mobile mass
- Well circumscribed

Natural History

- Slow growth
- 10-40% of FA in adolescents will regress

Treatment

- Surgical approaches
  - Most can be diagnosed by core needle biopsy and followed radiographically for signs of regression
  - Indications for surgical excision include
    - Rapid growth and > 5 cm in diameter
    - Distortion of breast architecture with overlying skin changes
    - Persistent mass without regression
    - Multiple &/or bilateral masses
    - Stromal hypercellularity
    - Cystic changes seen by ultrasound
    - Signs or symptoms concerning for malignancy
    - History of malignancy or prior chest radiation
    - Presence of high-risk genetic mutation or syndrome
    - Histologically complex fibroadenoma

Prognosis

- Excellent
- Malignant transformation of epithelial component is extremely rare

FIBROADENOMA

Key Facts

Terminology
- Benign proliferation of glandular and stromal elements

Clinical Issues
- Most common benign tumor of female breast
- Most common cause of breast masses in adolescent girls
- Can occur at any age
- Peak incidence in 2nd and 3rd decades
- Associated with slightly increased risk of breast carcinoma (1.5-2x)
- Rare cancer syndromes associated with development of multiple FA
  - Mafucci syndrome, Cowden syndrome, and Carney complex

Macroscopic Features
- Well circumscribed and unencapsulated

Microscopic Pathology
- Proliferation of both stromal and glandular elements

Top Differential Diagnoses
- Phyllodes tumor
  - Greater degree of stromal cellularity and overgrowth
- Fibroadenomatoid changes
  - Lacks circumscription
- Tubular adenoma
  - May resemble pericanalicular growth pattern of FA
  - Intracanalicular pattern is often present in FA

- FAs are included in "proliferative breast disease without atypia"
  - Associated with slightly increased risk of breast carcinoma (1.5-2x)
  - Increased risk is to both breasts
  - Risk may only apply to women with complex FAs

Syndrome Associations
- Rare cancer syndromes associated with the development of multiple FA
  - Mafucci syndrome, Cowden syndrome, and Carney complex

MACROSCOPIC FEATURES

General Features
- Well circumscribed and unencapsulated
- Smooth multinodular surface
- Pale tan-pink or white fibrous appearance

MICROSCOPIC PATHOLOGY

Cytologic Features
- Aggregates of cells with papillary configuration (antler-like resemblance)
- Clusters of spindle cells

Microscopic Features
- Proliferation of both stromal and glandular elements
- Glandular component
  - Contains inner epithelial and outer myoepithelial layers
  - May show
    - Metaplastic changes (most commonly apocrine), cystic changes, and sclerosing adenosis
    - Proliferative changes
  - Component of atypical ductal hyperplasia and carcinoma in situ is rare
- Stromal component
  - Bland and relatively uniform cellularity
  - Myxoid stromal change may be seen
  - Hyalinized stroma and calcifications more common in older patients
  - Multinucleated giant cells and heterologous elements are rarely seen
- 2 growth patterns
  - Intracanalicular
    - Distortion, stretching, and compression of glands by stromal proliferation
  - Pericanalicular
    - Glands with open lumina surrounded by stroma
- Patterns often coexist

DIFFERENTIAL DIAGNOSIS

Phyllodes Tumor
- Greater degree of stromal cellularity and overgrowth
- May represent FA that has undergone somatic mutation
- May be confused with intracanalicular pattern of FA

Fibroadenomatoid Changes
- Lacks circumscription
- Smaller in size

Tubular Adenoma
- May resemble the pericanalicular growth pattern of FA
- Intracanalicular pattern is often present in FA

SELECTED REFERENCES

1. Chung EM et al: From the archives of the AFIP: breast masses in children and adolescents: radiologic-pathologic correlation. Radiographics. 29(3):907-31, 2009
2. Jayasinghe Y et al: Fibroadenomas in adolescence. Curr Opin Obstet Gynecol. 21(5):402-6, 2009
3. Dehner LP et al: Pathology of the breast in children, adolescents, and young adults. Semin Diagn Pathol. 16(3):235-47, 1999
4. Greenberg R et al: Management of breast fibroadenomas. J Gen Intern Med. 13(9):640-5, 1998

FIBROADENOMA

Radiologic, Gross, and Microscopic Features

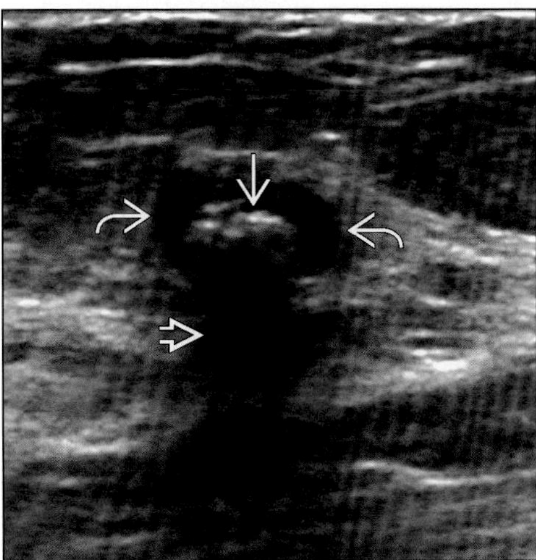

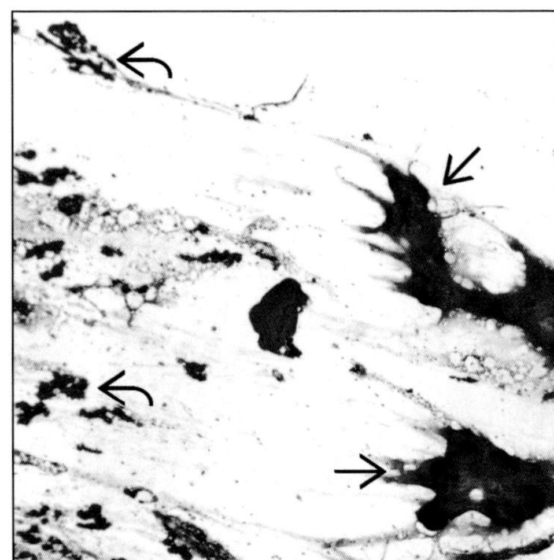

(Left) *Radial ultrasound of a fibroadenoma shows an oval circumscribed hypoechoic mass ➡. Coarse, echogenic macrocalcifications ➡ cause posterior shadowing ➡.* ***(Right)*** *Fine needle aspiration of a FA from low power shows several large fragments of fibrous tissue ➡ and numerous small fragments of glandular tissue ➡, many of which show a delicate branching pattern.*

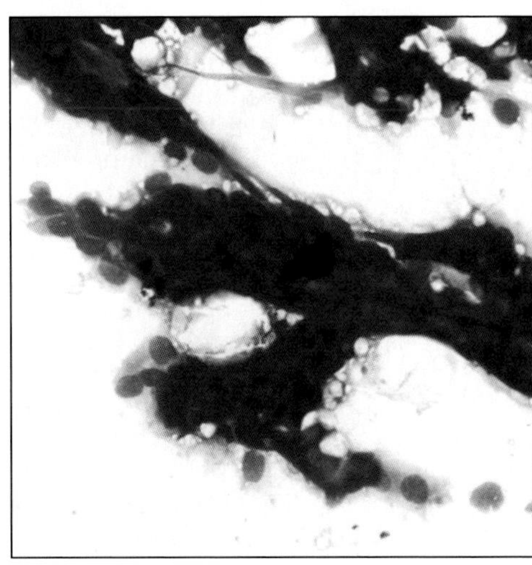

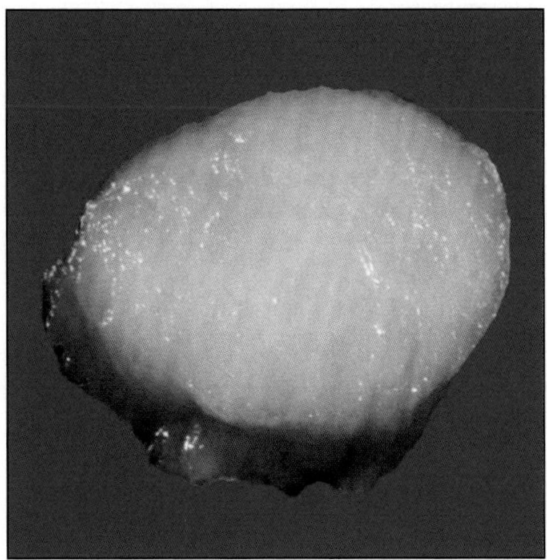

(Left) *Fine needle aspiration of a FA at high power illustrates the delicate antler-like branching pattern of the epithelial cells that is characteristic of this tumor.* ***(Right)*** *A gross photograph of a myxoid FA is shown. Myxoid FAs have been reported in patients with Carney syndrome; however, it is important to note that most patients with myxoid FAs or FAs with prominent myxoid change do not have this syndrome. (Courtesy R. Flinner, MD.)*

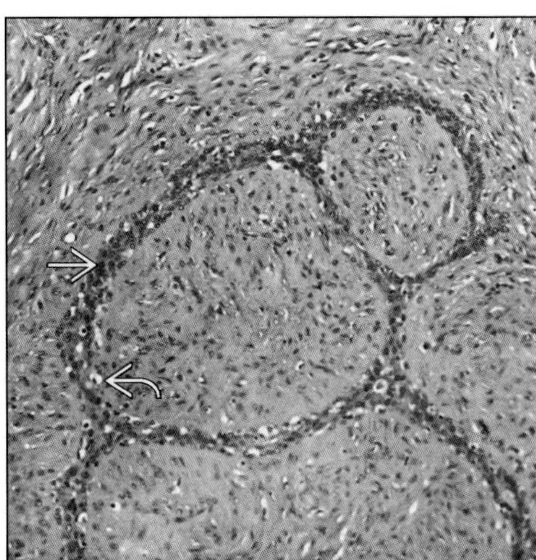

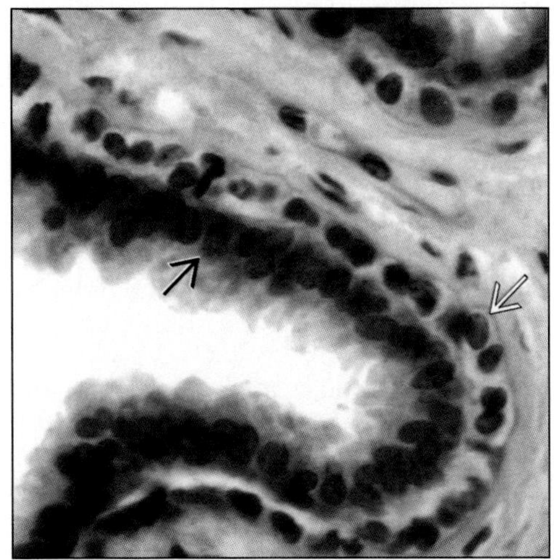

(Left) *High-power view of an FA, intracanalicular pattern, highlights the compressed and distorted glands. Occasional myoepithelial cells ➡ with clear cytoplasm are seen underlying the epithelial cells ➡.* ***(Right)*** *High-power view of the glandular component of a FA highlights a distinct myoepithelial cell layer ➡ and an overlying layer of bland epithelial cells ➡. Immunostains, such a smooth muscle actin, calponin, and p63 can be used to highlight the myoepithelial cells.*

Microscopic Features

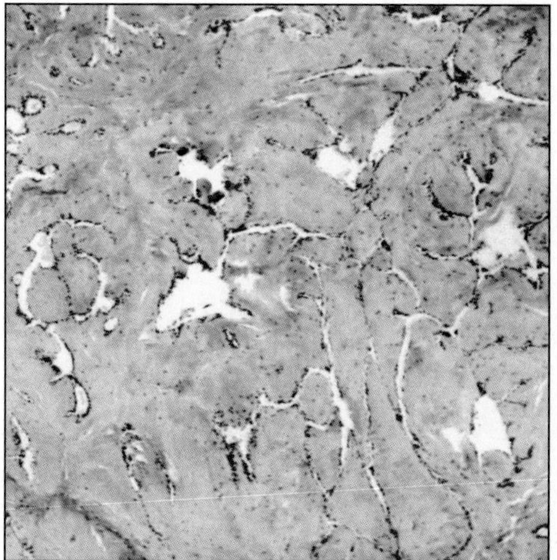

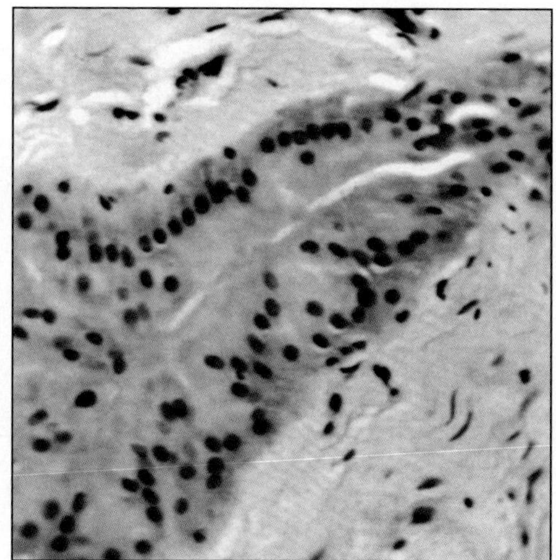

(Left) *An FA with prominent stromal hyalinization is shown. Calcifications can often be seen in cases that have undergone stromal hyalinization. These features are more common in older women. (Courtesy R. Flinner, MD.)* ***(Right)*** *High-power view shows an FA with apocrine metaplasia, as noted by the small bland nuclei and abundant eosinophilic cytoplasm. Squamous metaplasia, although less frequent, may also be seen. (Courtesy R. Flinner, MD.)*

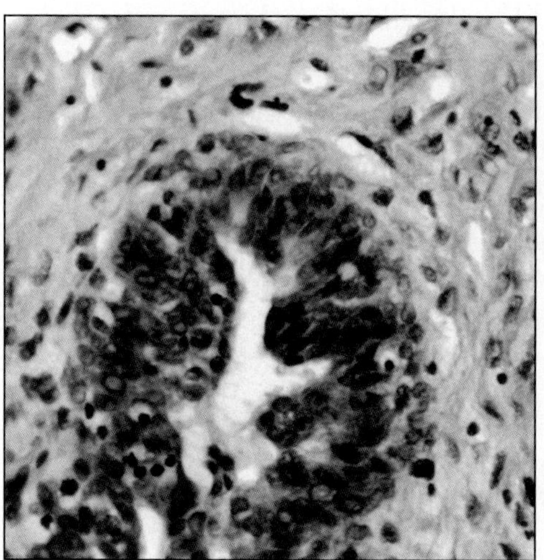

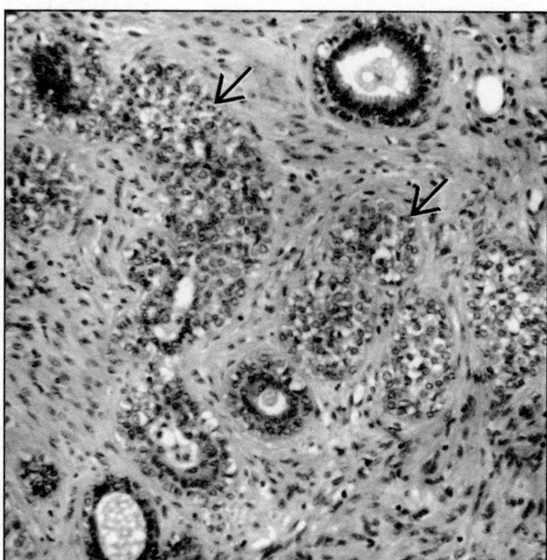

(Left) *High-power view of a FA with a component of usual ductal hyperplasia (UDH). Note the crowded, bland, overlapping and streaming nuclei that are characteristic of UDH. (Courtesy R. Flinner, MD.)* ***(Right)*** *Shown here is an FA with a component of lobular carcinoma in situ (LCIS). Note the small, round, and dyscohesive cells that fill and distend the glands ⇒. (Courtesy R. Flinner, MD.)*

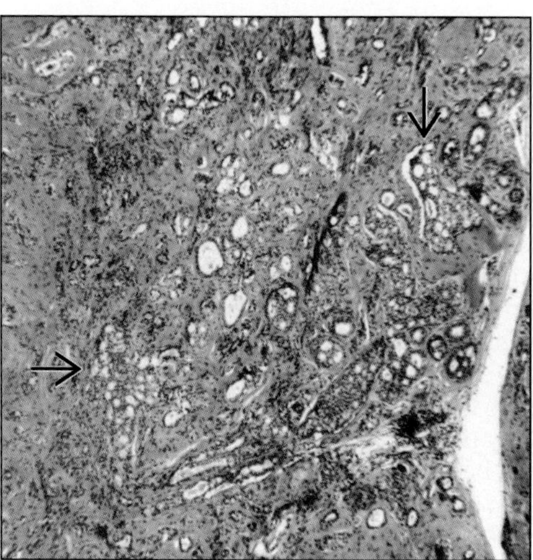

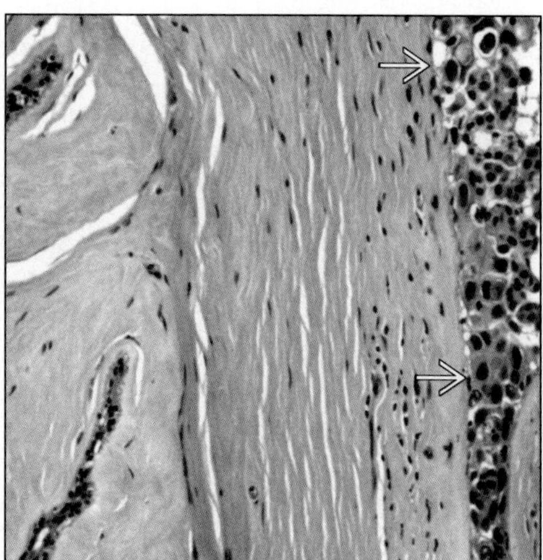

(Left) *Shown here is an FA with a distinct component of ductal carcinoma in situ (DCIS) ⇒. Although very rare, epithelial proliferative changes, such as LCIS and DCIS, can occur. (Courtesy R. Flinner, MD.)* ***(Right)*** *Shown at high power is an FA (left) adjacent to a component of high-grade DCIS ➡. (Courtesy R. Flinner, MD.)*

FIBROCYSTIC CHANGE

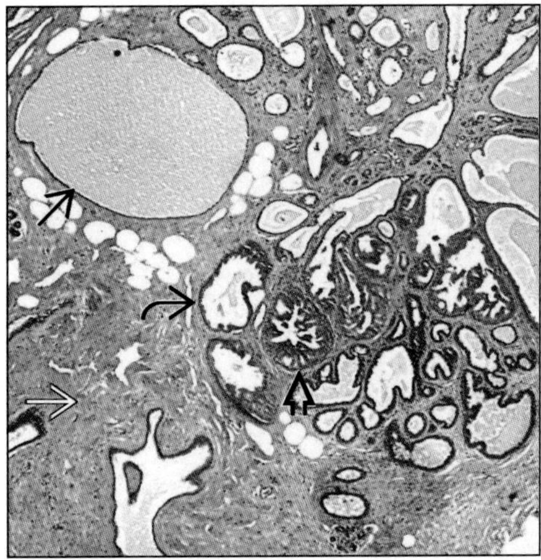

Low-power view shows many of the characteristic features of fibrocystic change, including cysts ➔, fibrosis ➔, and apocrine metaplasia ➔ with proliferative changes seen in many of the ducts ➔.

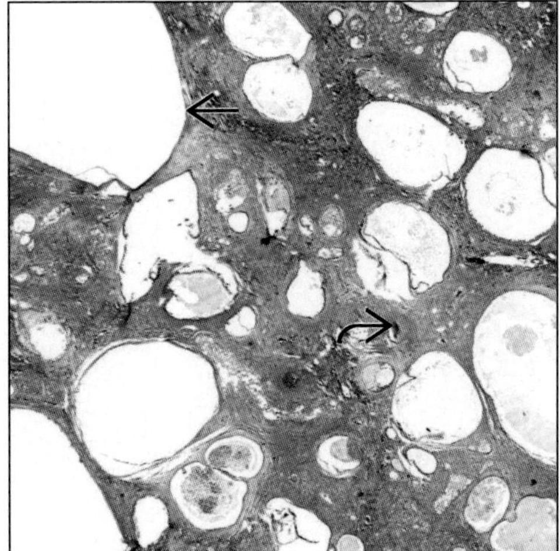

A predominance of cysts ➔ separated by stromal fibrosis ➔ is illustrated in this example of fibrocystic change of the breast.

TERMINOLOGY

Abbreviations

- Fibrocystic change (FCC)

Synonyms

- Fibrocystic disease
- Cystic disease
- Cystic mastopathy

Definitions

- Hormonal-induced proliferative and cystic changes that occur in adolescent and adult female breast
- Changes considered more physiologic in nature than overt disease
- Encompasses constellation of conditions

ETIOLOGY/PATHOGENESIS

Unclear

- Linked to estrogen and progesterone imbalances

CLINICAL ISSUES

Epidemiology

- Incidence
  - Frequency increases with age
    - 10% of women younger than 21 years
    - 25% of women during menstruating years
    - 50% of women during perimenopausal period
- Age
  - More common in premenopausal women
  - Changes usually lessen in postmenopausal women
  - Most common between 25-45 years
- Ethnicity
  - Proliferative components more common in Caucasians

Presentation

- Breast tenderness
- Breast nodules and lumps
- Cord-like thickenings
- Symptoms develop over time and fluctuate over course of menstrual cycle
- Symptoms most often bilateral
- Bloody nipple discharge may be seen
- Frequent family history of breast carcinoma

Natural History

- Not considered to be precancerous in most instances; however
  - Proliferative changes seen as component of FCC may carry ↑ risk of developing breast cancer in either breast
    - Proliferative changes: Lobular and ductal hyperplasia, sclerosing adenosis, papillomas, etc.
    - Nonproliferative: Cysts, apocrine metaplasia

Treatment

- Dependent on severity of condition
  - Most often supportive
- Drugs
  - Analgesics
  - Oral contraceptives
    - Beneficial in as many as 90% of patients
    - Statistical data indicate lower frequency of fibrocystic change among long-term users
  - Danazol, bromocriptine, and tamoxifen have been used in adult women
    - No proven value in adolescent girls
    - Possible adverse affects include teratogenicity and masculinization
- Reassurance of benign nature

Prognosis

- Excellent
- Proliferative changes may carry ↑ risk of developing breast cancer in either breast

FIBROCYSTIC CHANGE

Key Facts

Terminology
- Hormonal-induced proliferative and cystic changes that occur in adolescent and adult female breast
- Changes considered more physiologic in nature than overt disease

Clinical Issues
- Frequency increases with age
- More common in premenopausal women, between 25-45 years
- Typically presents with
  - Breast tenderness
  - Breast nodules and lumps
  - Cord-like thickenings
- Proliferative changes seen as a component of FCC may carry ↑ risk of developing breast cancer in either breast

Microscopic Pathology
- Basic morphologic changes include
  - Cysts
  - Apocrine metaplasia
  - Fibrosis
  - Calcifications
  - Chronic inflammation
  - Epithelial hyperplasia
  - Fibroadenomatoid change (less frequent)

Top Differential Diagnoses
- Benign breast cysts
- Juvenile papillomatosis
  - Microscopic features can overlap
- Mammary duct ectasia
  - May coexist with FCC of breast

IMAGE FINDINGS

General Features
- Best diagnostic clue
  - Mammographically dense breasts
  - Scattered punctate calcifications and fluctuating cysts
  - Findings can be focal, regional, or diffuse

Mammographic Findings
- Changing pattern of bilateral, partially circumscribed, partially obscured masses due to cysts developing and regressing

Ultrasonographic Findings
- Scattered echogenic foci due to calcifications
  - May occasionally be seen in cysts
- Simple cysts
- Complicated cysts
- Clustered microcysts
- Complex cystic and solid masses
  - Mixture of fibrosis and cystic changes
  - Ruptured or inflamed cysts
  - Often difficult to distinguish from malignancy and require biopsy
- Echogenic tissue due to ↑ fibrosis
  - Heterogeneous echotexture when mixed with residual fat
- Discrete masses due to fibrosis
  - Mixed hyper- and hypoechoic ovoid mass
  - Uniformly echogenic mass
  - Can appear irregular with shadowing, often requiring biopsy

MACROSCOPIC FEATURES

General Features
- Fibrocystic appearance
- Larger cysts may have bluish cast
  - "Blue dome cysts" of Bloodgood
- Cysts contain cloudy to clear fluid

MICROSCOPIC PATHOLOGY

Predominant Pattern/Injury Type
- Fibrous
- Cystic
  - Macro- and microcysts

Microscopic Features
- Changes primarily affect terminal duct lobular unit (TDLU)
- Basic morphologic changes include
  - Cysts
    - Micro- and macroscopic cyst formation (ductal dilatation)
    - Small cysts may surround larger cysts
    - Epithelial lining, columnar or cuboidal
    - Ruptured cysts often associated with stromal inflammatory response, foamy macrophages, and cholesterol clefts
  - Apocrine metaplasia
    - Observed in normal tubules as well as dilated and cystic structures
    - Lining cells indistinguishable from those lining apocrine sweat glands
    - Cells have abundant granular eosinophilic cytoplasm
    - Metaplasia may be partial or complete
    - Apical "apocrine snouts" are frequently seen
  - Fibrosis
    - Variable degrees are frequently present
    - Thought to be secondary to cyst rupture
  - Calcifications
    - Calcium phosphate or calcium oxalate
    - Infrequent feature
    - More common component of duct ectasia
  - Chronic inflammation
    - Common feature secondary to cyst rupture
    - Composed of lymphocytes, plasma cells, and histiocytes
  - Epithelial hyperplasia
    - Most show only minimal degree without atypia
    - Possible relationship to carcinoma

- Fibroadenomatoid change
  - Infrequent finding
  - Histologically resembles fibroadenoma
  - Lacks circumscription observed in classic fibroadenoma
- Duct ectasia
  - Not considered component of fibrocystic change but often coexists
  - Calcifications are more common
  - Lack epithelial hyperplasia and apocrine metaplasia
  - Often associated with chronic inflammatory reaction secondary to luminal material escaping from duct into surrounding stroma
- Other features may include
  - Adenosis
  - Papillomatosis

DIFFERENTIAL DIAGNOSIS

Benign Breast Cysts

- Common nonproliferative lesions noted in adolescents but more frequently seen in adults
- Typically lack the combination of findings of fibrocystic change
- Ovoid to round structures lined by epithelium
- Contain sterile clear to brown to blood-tinged fluid
- Typically not fixed to breast tissue
- May include
  - Solitary large "blue-domed" cysts
    - Contain fluid of various colors (green, yellow, black)
    - May be confused with fibroadenoma or breast cancer
  - Simple single cysts
  - Galactoceles
    - Develop from overdistension of lactiferous ducts
    - Subareolar mass with yellow discharge
  - Cysts occurring secondary to traumatic fat necrosis
- Evaluate by fine needle aspiration ± ultrasound

Juvenile Papillomatosis

- More commonly presents as unilateral breast mass
- Well circumscribed
- Microscopic features can overlap
- Displays a combination of cysts and ectatic ducts of variable size
- Cysts impart Swiss cheese-like appearance from low power

Mammary Duct Ectasia

- May coexist with FCC of breast
- More likely to contain calcifications and to be associated with chronic inflammation
- More likely to present with bloody nipple discharge than FCC
- Commonly seen in premenopausal parous women
- Microscopic appearance shows dilatation of large ducts with accumulation of luminal fatty detritus and fibrous thickening of duct wall
- Typically lacks epithelial hyperplasia and apocrine metaplasia

Breast Carcinoma

- Exceedingly rare in adolescents
- Rule out with careful evaluation of hyperplastic epithelial components and fibrous components for possible invasive carcinoma
- Retention of normal breast architecture and circumscription helps distinguish benign vs. malignant breast lesions

DIAGNOSTIC CHECKLIST

Pathologic Interpretation Pearls

- Most common morphologic changes include
  - Cyst formation
  - Fibrosis
  - Apocrine metaplasia
- Careful evaluation of proliferative components necessary for accurate risk assessment

Considerations

- FCC is within a spectrum of normal breast physiology
  - Not an indication for diagnostic mammography per se in absence of focal symptoms or abnormalities on screening
- Focal pain not a sign of malignancy, though US can be performed for reassurance
- Calcifications are frequently (~ 16%) present in both benign and malignant processes
- Assure adequate sampling of suspicious calcifications
- Random sampling of benign dense breast tissue will often yield fibrosis
- Assure correlation of imaging and histopathologic findings: Discordant result should be rebiopsied

Fine Needle Aspiration/Needle Biopsy

- Should be performed in patients with macrocysts and whenever clinical, ultrasonic, &/or mammographic examinations are suspicious for carcinoma

SELECTED REFERENCES

1. Chung EM et al: From the archives of the AFIP: breast masses in children and adolescents: radiologic-pathologic correlation. Radiographics. 29(3):907-31, 2009
2. Greydanus DE et al: Breast disorders in children and adolescents. Prim Care. 33(2):455-502, 2006
3. Imamoglu M et al: Bloody nipple discharge in children: possible etiologies and selection of appropriate therapy. Pediatr Surg Int. 22(2):158-63, 2006
4. Dehner LP et al: Pathology of the breast in children, adolescents, and young adults. Semin Diagn Pathol. 16(3):235-47, 1999
5. Drukker BH: Fibrocystic change of the breast. Clin Obstet Gynecol. 37(4):903-15, 1994
6. Fiorica JV: Fibrocystic changes. Obstet Gynecol Clin North Am. 21(3):445-52, 1994

Radiologic and Microscopic Features

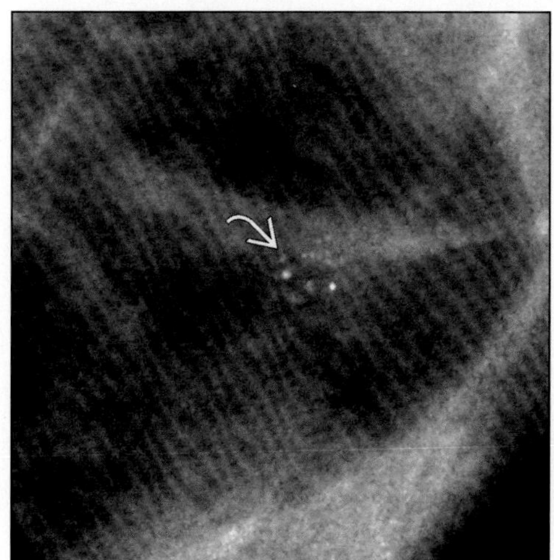

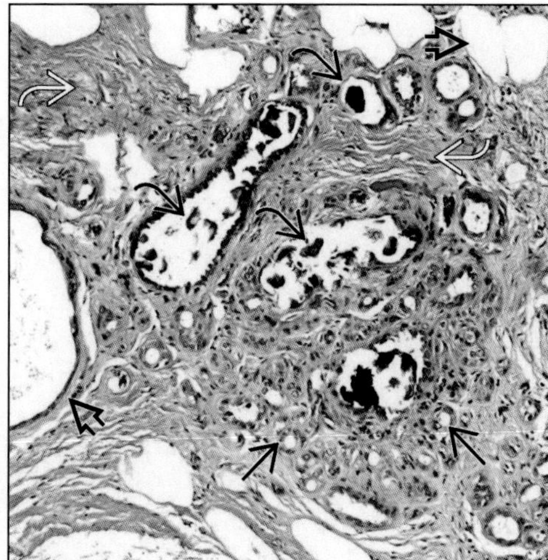

(Left) *Lateral mammography magnification shows clustered pleomorphic calcification ➦ identified on baseline screening. Stereotactic 11-g biopsy showed FCC with ductal hyperplasia and sclerosing adenosis.* ***(Right)*** *H&E from an 11-g stereotactic biopsy shows typical FCC with cysts ⇨, fibrosis ➦, and adenosis →. Numerous calcifications are evident in microcysts ➦.*

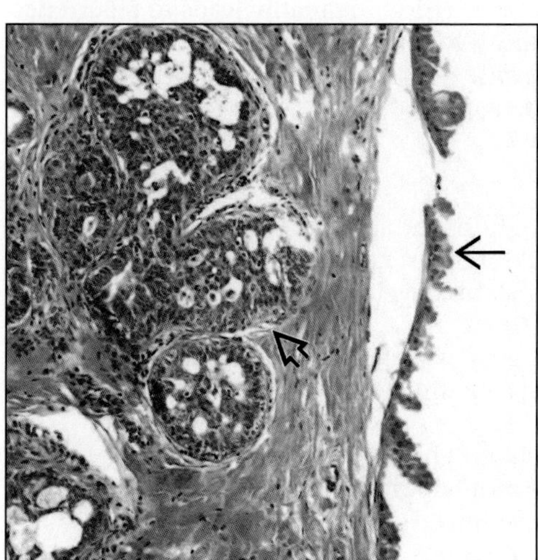

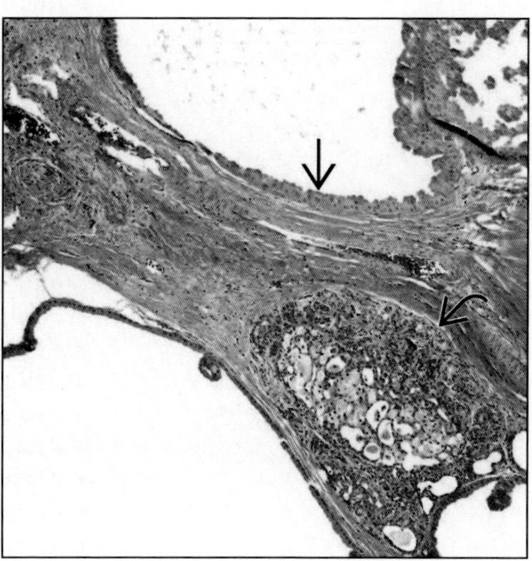

(Left) *High-power view of FCC illustrates a large cystic duct with apocrine metaplasia → and several neighboring ducts that show features of usual ductal hyperplasia ⇨. Note the small round nuclei, abundant eosinophilic cytoplasm, and apical snouts that are characteristic of apocrine metaplasia in FCC.* ***(Right)*** *Medium-power view of of FCC illustrates prominent apocrine metaplasia → within the cysts with some areas showing focal adenosis ➦.*

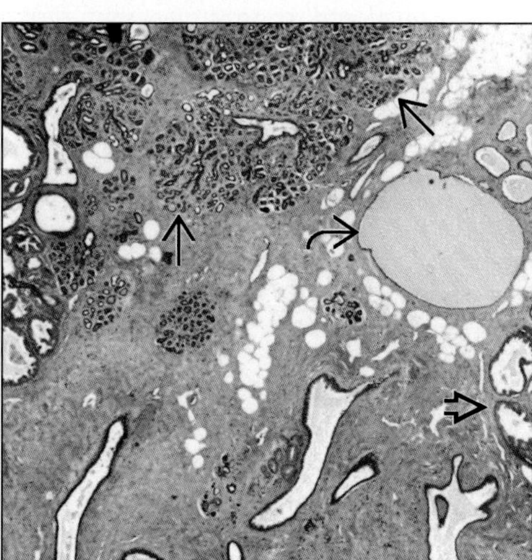

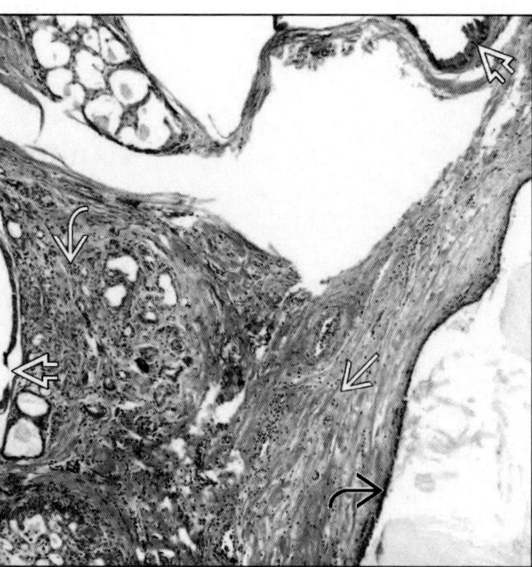

(Left) *Low-power view shows areas of normal breast tissue/ lobules → and adjacent FCC characterized by cysts ➦, stromal fibrosis, and apocrine metaplasia ⇨.* ***(Right)*** *Large cysts ➦ lie adjacent to areas of fibrosis →, adenosis ➦, and apocrine metaplasia ⇨ in this example of FCC of the breast.*

JUVENILE PAPILLOMATOSIS

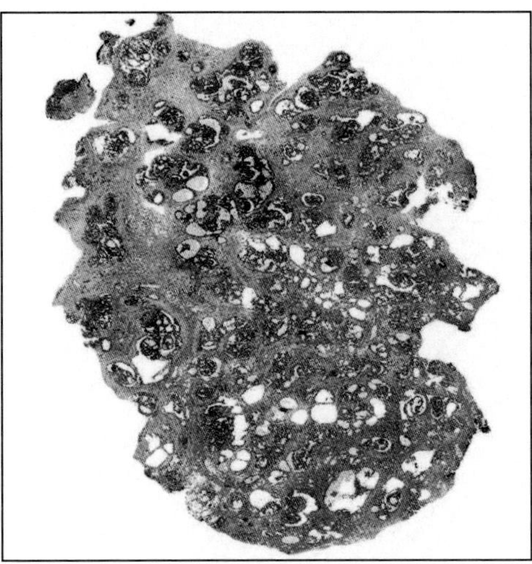

Whole mount scanned slide illustrates the well-circumscribed nature and low-power resemblance of "Swiss cheese" imparted by the numerous cysts in this example of juvenile papillomatosis.

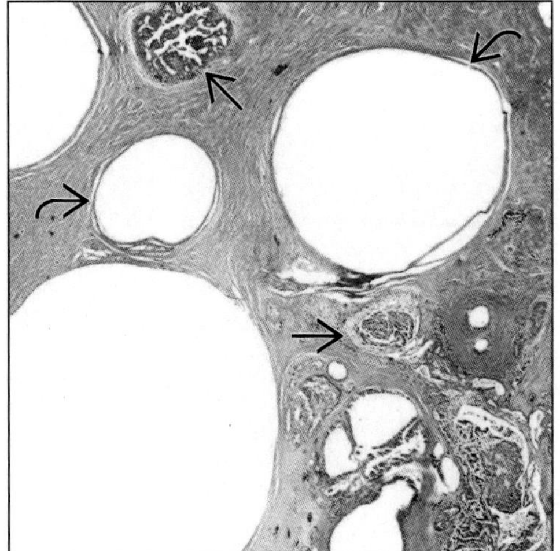

Low-power view illustrates a combination of cysts ⮫ and papillomatosis ➔ that are characteristic of juvenile papillomatosis.

TERMINOLOGY

Abbreviations

- Juvenile papillomatosis (JP)

Synonyms

- Swiss cheese disease

Definitions

- Benign breast tumor of young women featuring numerous cysts and ectatic ducts with epithelial hyperplasia, papillomatosis, and apocrine metaplasia

CLINICAL ISSUES

Epidemiology

- Age
  - Mean age at diagnosis 23 years (range: 12-48 years)
  - Majority of patients are < 26 years of age
- Gender
  - Female predominance
  - Very rare cases of JP occurring in males reported

Presentation

- Unilateral breast mass
  - Localized and discrete
  - Rare presentations of bilateral and multifocal disease
- Nipple discharge and pain
- Often thought clinically to represent fibroadenoma, cystic disease, mastitis, and carcinoma
- Frequent maternal family history of breast cancer
  - Up to 50-60% of cases may report family history of breast cancer
  - Approximately 10% of these patients subsequently develop breast cancer
- Reported association with neurofibromatosis type 1

Treatment

- Surgical approaches
  - Complete excision
    - Incomplete excision invariably leads to recurrence
  - Careful clinical follow-up for patient and family is recommended
  - No current evidence to justify prophylactic mastectomy

Prognosis

- Excellent prognosis for unilateral lesions without family history of breast carcinoma
- Subsequent risk for developing carcinoma has not been well defined
  - Patients at greatest risk of having associated or developing subsequent carcinoma have 1 or more of the following
    - Positive family history of breast cancer
    - Atypical proliferative lesions
    - Bilateral lesions
    - Multifocal lesions
    - Recurrent lesions
  - Risk appears greatest in patients with positive family history of breast cancer and recurrent lesions

IMAGE FINDINGS

Mammographic Findings

- Similar to those observed in fibroadenomas &/or cysts

MACROSCOPIC FEATURES

General Features

- Cystic breast mass
  - Cysts impart Swiss cheese-like appearance
- Interspersed dense stroma
- Calcifications may be present
- Well-circumscribed

Size

- Range from 1-8 cm in diameter

JUVENILE PAPILLOMATOSIS

Key Facts

Terminology
- Benign breast tumor of young women featuring numerous cysts and ectatic ducts with epithelial hyperplasia, papillomatosis, and apocrine metaplasia

Clinical Issues
- Mean age at diagnosis 23 years (range: 12-48 years)
- Often thought clinically to represent fibroadenoma, cystic disease, mastitis, and carcinoma
- Frequent maternal family history of breast cancer
- Excellent prognosis for unilateral lesions without family history of breast carcinoma
- Risk for developing carcinoma not well defined

Microscopic Pathology
- Combination of cysts and ectatic ducts

Top Differential Diagnoses
- Fibroadenoma
- Fibrocystic change

MICROSCOPIC PATHOLOGY

Microscopic Features
- Combination of cysts and ectatic ducts of variable size
  - Cysts and ducts may display
    - Flat epithelium
    - Apocrine metaplasia
    - Epithelial hyperplasia (usual and atypical)
    - Papillary hyperplasia (papillomatosis)
    - Intraluminal secretions with foamy histiocytes
- Other described features
  - Sclerosing adenosis
  - Lobular hyperplasia
  - Fibroadenomatous change
  - Focal necrosis
    - Often associated with epithelial atypia
  - Concurrent breast carcinoma (rare)
    - More frequently associated with family history of breast cancer
    - Patients tend to be slightly older (mean age of 27 years)

DIFFERENTIAL DIAGNOSIS

Fibrocystic Change
- Presents as breast tenderness with nodules, lumps, and cord-like thickenings
- More often bilateral
- Symptoms may fluctuate over course of menstrual cycle
- Microscopic features may overlap
- Papillomatosis is less frequent feature

Fibroadenoma
- Most common benign tumor of female breast
- Solitary, palpable, firm, mobile mass
- Typically < 3 cm in size
- Biphasic proliferation of glandular and stromal elements
- Typically lack cystic component

Fibroadenomatoid Changes
- Same features as fibroadenoma but does not form discrete mass
- May be component of JP

Breast Carcinoma
- Exceedingly rare in adolescents
- Rule out with careful evaluation of hyperplastic epithelial component

SELECTED REFERENCES

1. Rosen PP et al: Juvenile papillomatosis of the breast. A follow-up study of 41 patients having biopsies before 1979. Am J Clin Pathol. 93(5):599-603, 1990
2. Rosen PP et al: Juvenile papillomatosis and breast carcinoma. Cancer. 55(6):1345-52, 1985
3. Rosen PP et al: Juvenile papillomatosis (Swiss cheese disease) of the breast. Am J Surg Pathol. 4(1):3-12, 1980

IMAGE GALLERY

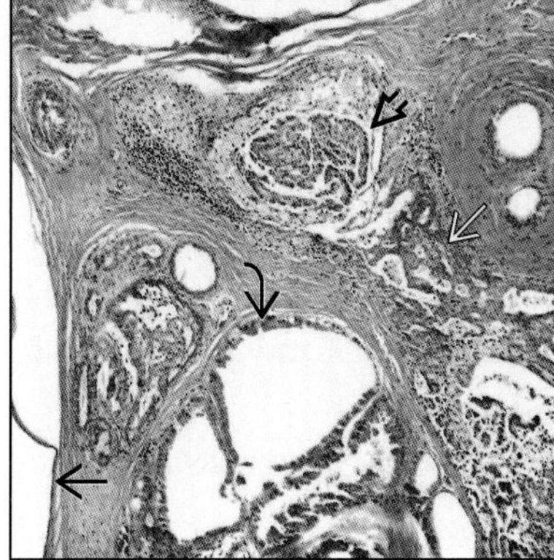

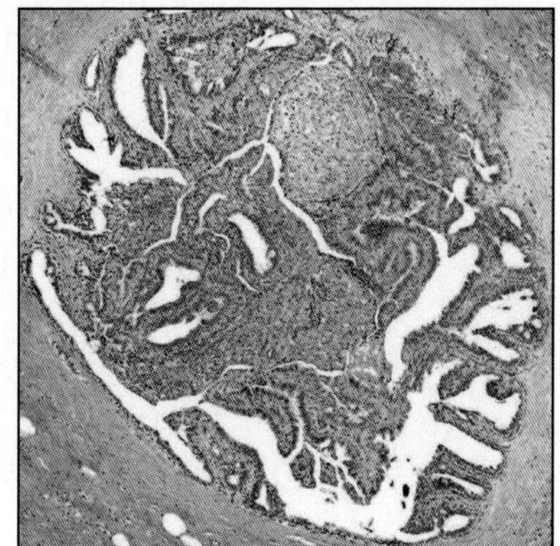

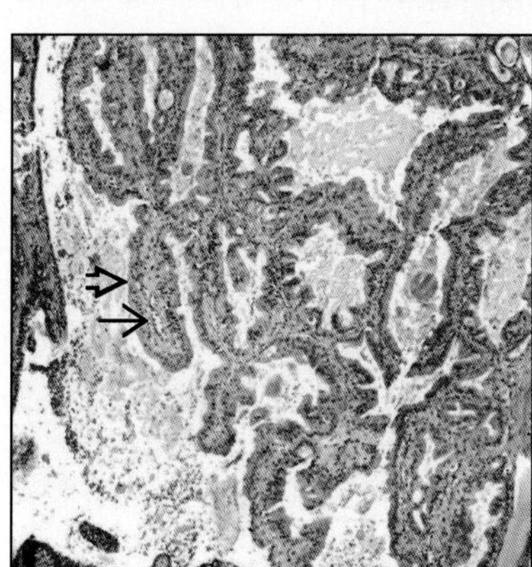

(Left) *A combination of cysts ➔, apocrine metaplasia ➔, usual ductal hyperplasia ➔, and papillomatosis ➔ is shown in this example of juvenile papillomatosis.* ***(Center)*** *The presence of papillomatosis in conjunction with numerous cysts in a well-defined mass is characteristic of JP.* ***(Right)*** *High-power view illustrates the benign nature of the papillomas, which show fibrovascular cores ➔, lined by both epithelial and myoepithelial cells ➔.*

TUBULAR ADENOMA

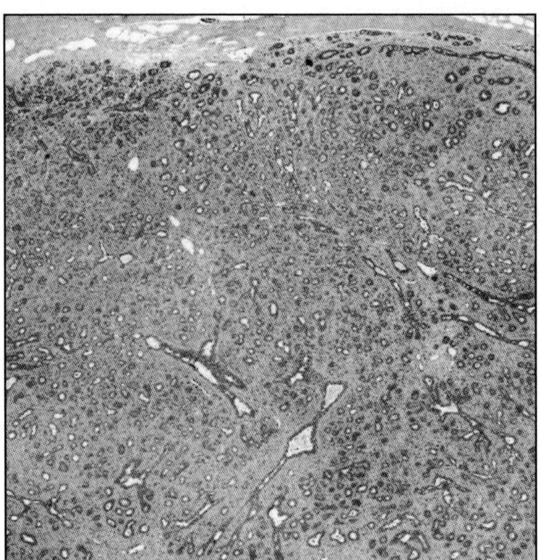

Low-power view shows a sharply circumscribed nodule composed of tightly packed tubular/acinar structures with little intervening stroma, characteristic of a tubular adenoma.

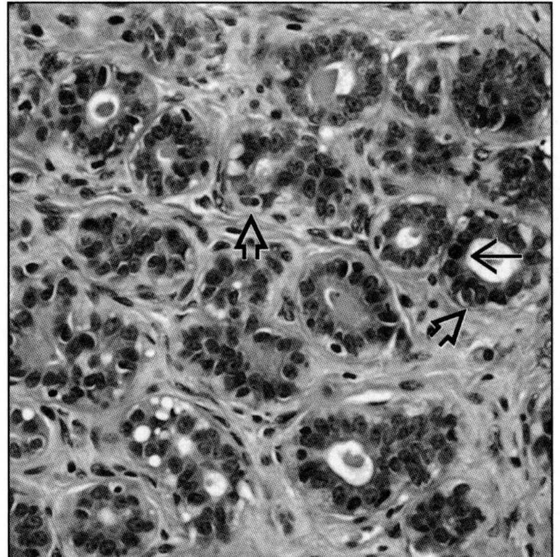

High-power view of this tubular adenoma highlights the tightly packed acini composed of a layer of epithelial cells ➔ and an inconspicuous layer of myoepithelial cells ➢.

TERMINOLOGY

Synonyms

- Pure adenoma

Definitions

- Rare, well-demarcated benign tumor of breast that usually occurs in young women
- Some consider it a variant of fibroadenoma with predominance of epithelial elements

CLINICAL ISSUES

Presentation

- Solitary, well-circumscribed mass
- Most common signs/symptoms
  - Painless, mobile mass
- Typically women of reproductive age; 90% < age 40
- No association with exogenous hormones or pregnancy

Treatment

- Options, risks, complications
  - Percutaneous core biopsy may provide definitive diagnosis

Prognosis

- Excellent; no reported increased breast cancer risk

IMAGE FINDINGS

General Features

- Best diagnostic clue
  - Circumscribed mass

Mammographic Findings

- Characteristics similar to those of fibroadenoma (FA)
  - Circumscribed mass: Oval, lobulated, round
  - May be partially indistinctly marginated
- Microcalcifications may be present
  - Tightly packed punctate and amorphous microcalcifications
  - Unlike FA, no "popcorn" calcifications reported

Ultrasonographic Findings

- Grayscale ultrasound
  - Characteristics similar to FA
  - Circumscribed mass: Oval, lobulated, round
  - May be partially indistinctly marginated
  - Homogeneously hypoechoic
  - May have echogenic rim

MACROSCOPIC FEATURES

General Features

- Circumscribed, well-defined mass
- Soft
- Tan-brown cut surface

MICROSCOPIC PATHOLOGY

Cytologic Features

- Benign ductal cells
- 3-dimensional cohesive balls and tubular structures
- Highly cellular smears
- Scant to absent stroma
- Myoepithelial cells often seen with sheets of ductal cells
- Often confused with fibroadenoma

Predominant Cell/Compartment Type

- Acini
  - Composed of both epithelial and myoepithelial cells

Microscopic Features

- Homogeneously tightly packed tubular/acinar structures

TUBULAR ADENOMA

Key Facts

Terminology
- Well-demarcated benign tumor of breast

Clinical Issues
- Solitary, painless, mobile mass
- Excellent prognosis

Microscopic Pathology
- Homogeneously tightly packed tubular/acinar structures
- Scant intervening connective tissue

Top Differential Diagnoses
- Fibroadenoma
  - Proliferation of both glandular and fibrous components
- Lactating adenoma
  - Pregnant and lactating women
- Apocrine adenoma
  - Composed exclusively of apocrine cells

  - Lined by double cell layer of epithelial and myoepithelial cells
    - Myoepithelial cells are often inconspicuous
  - Typically lack large ducts
  - Calcifications may be present and are often located in dilated acini
    - Thought to result from calcification of inspissated secretions
    - More common in older individuals
- Scant intervening connective tissue

DIFFERENTIAL DIAGNOSIS

Fibroadenoma
- Proliferation of both glandular and fibrous components
- More abundant stroma
- Epithelial component consists of large ducts
- Some lesions may show mixed features
  - When mixed features are present, diagnosis of fibroadenoma is typically made
  - Diagnosis of tubular adenoma is reserved for lesions with purely acinar units and scant stroma

Lactating Adenoma
- Pregnant and lactating women
- May represent tubular adenoma or fibroadenoma with lactational change
- Prominent tubular and lobular elements with secretory activity

Apocrine Adenoma
- Form of adenoma composed exclusively of apocrine cells
- Exceptionally rare

Phyllodes Tumor
- Less than 1% of all breast tumors
- More common among older females
- Well-defined lesion
- Biphasic proliferation of both stromal and epithelial cells
- Typically show dominance of stromal over glandular component, "stromal overgrowth"

SELECTED REFERENCES

1. Soo MS et al: Tubular adenomas of the breast: imaging findings with histologic correlation. AJR Am J Roentgenol. 174(3):757-61, 2000
2. Kumar N et al: Characterization of tubular adenoma of breast--diagnostic problem in fine needle aspirates (FNAs). Cytopathology. 9(5):301-7, 1998
3. Liu K et al: Cytologic features of a combined tubular adenoma and fibroadenoma of the breast. Diagn Cytopathol. 16(2):184-6, 1997
4. Maiorano E et al: Tubular adenoma of the breast: an immunohistochemical study of ten cases. Pathol Res Pract. 191(12):1222-30, 1995
5. Moross T et al: Tubular adenoma of breast. Arch Pathol Lab Med. 107(2):84-6, 1983

IMAGE GALLERY

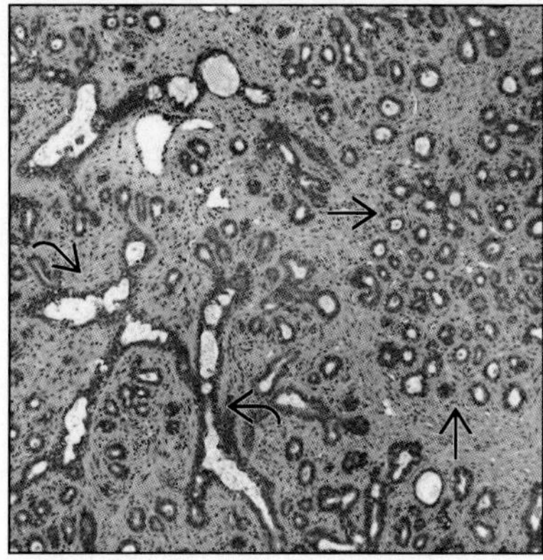

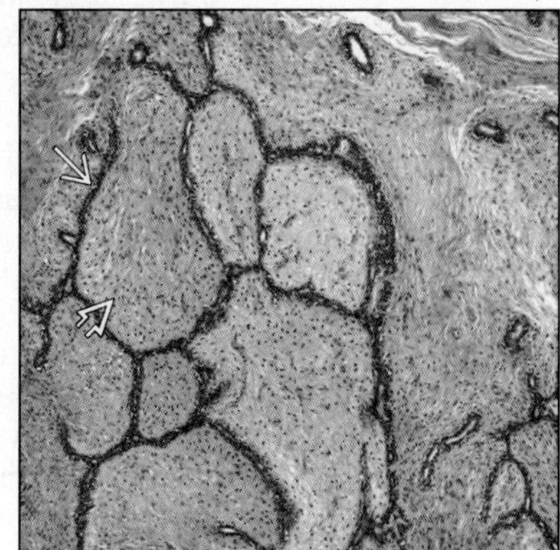

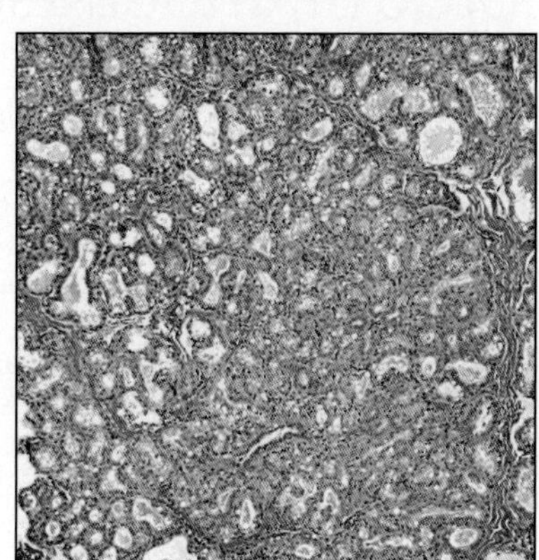

(Left) *Medium-power view illustrates a tubular adenoma with some features suggestive of fibroadenoma, pericanalicular pattern ⇗, and other areas of classic tubular adenoma →.* ***(Center)*** *Low-power view of a classic fibroadenoma is shown. Note the proliferation of both epithelial ➡ and stromal elements ⇨.* ***(Right)*** *Low-power view of a lactational adenoma is shown. Note the hyperplastic lobules with abundant glandular secretions.*

PHYLLODES TUMOR

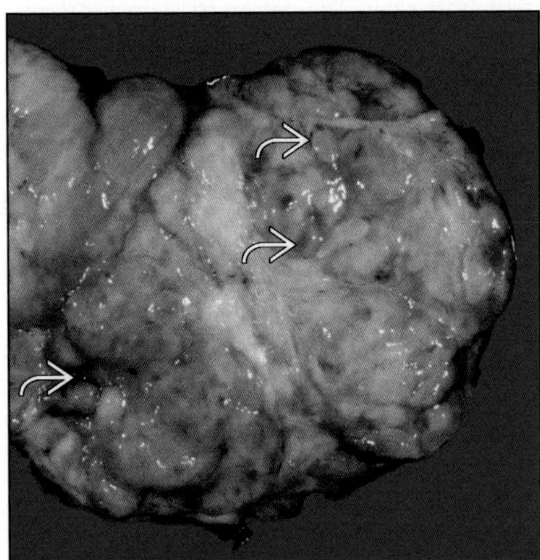

Gross photograph of PT shows circumscribed borders and a bulging mucoid-appearing cut surface. The characteristic whorled pattern with cleft-like spaces resembling leaf buds ➡ is seen here.

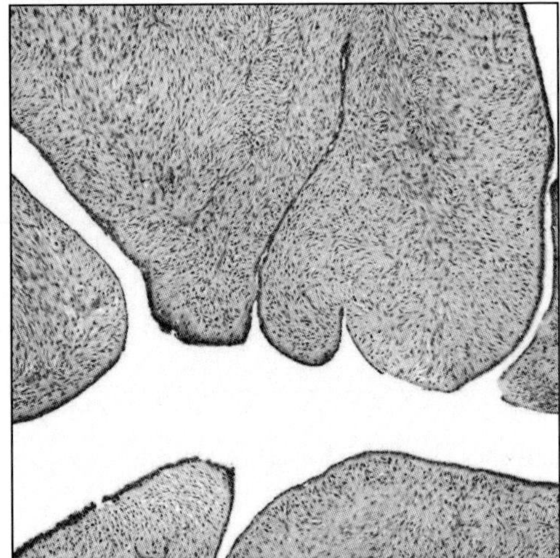

The leaf-like projections of mildly hypercellular stroma are covered by epithelium in this example of a benign PT. Minimal atypia and mitotic activity was present within the stroma.

TERMINOLOGY

Abbreviations

- Phyllodes tumor (PT)

Synonyms

- Cystosarcoma phyllodes
- Periductal stromal tumor
  - Probable origin from specialized periductal stromal elements
  - Term "phyllodes tumor" favored

Definitions

- Term derived from Greek word "phyllos" (leaf)
- Uncommon biphasic lesion of breast characterized by
  - Proliferating foci of hypercellular stroma lined by epithelium, forming variably sized cystic spaces
  - Growth pattern resulting in clefts and leaf-like fronds of tissue within lesion
- Broad spectrum of biologic and clinical behavior
  - Classified into 3 groups based on their morphologic features
    - Benign, borderline, and malignant

ETIOLOGY/PATHOGENESIS

Fibroepithelial Proliferation

- Stromal cells likely arise from fibroblasts of specialized intralobular stroma
- Epithelial cells are benign and not clonal; stimulated to proliferate by stromal cells
  - Tumor is formed by clonal proliferation of neoplastic spindle cells
  - Potential for independent and invasive growth
  - Ability to metastasize in some cases
- Some PT may arise from a preexisting fibroadenoma
  - May represent clonal progression

CLINICAL ISSUES

Epidemiology

- Incidence
  - Uncommon
    - Comprise < 1% of all breast tumors
- Age
  - Can occur at any age
    - Most common in middle-aged or elderly women
- Ethnicity
  - May be more commonly seen in younger women from the Far East

Presentation

- Painless, firm, palpable mass
  - Typically well defined clinically and by imaging
  - Most common presentation
- Clinical history of increasing size favors diagnosis of PT
- Malignant lesions tend to be larger than benign lesions
  - Relationship can be inconsistent

Treatment

- Surgical approaches
  - Vast majority follow benign clinical course
  - Complete local excision is recommended
    - Incompletely excised lesions at risk for local recurrence
    - Recurrence rates tend to increase from benign to malignant subtypes
    - May be related to infiltrative border of malignant lesions

Prognosis

- Difficult to predict prognosis
- All PT can recur
  - Depends on adequacy of surgical excision
- Classified into benign, borderline, and malignant categories based on combination of histologic features

PHYLLODES TUMOR

Key Facts

Terminology

- Uncommon biphasic lesion of breast characterized by
  - Proliferating foci of hypercellular stroma lined by epithelium, forming variably sized cystic spaces

Clinical Issues

- < 1% of all breast tumors
- Can occur at any age
- Vast majority follow benign clinical course
- Classified into benign, borderline, and malignant categories based on combination of histologic features
  - Stromal cellularity and pleomorphism
  - Stromal mitotic activity
  - Presence or absence of stromal overgrowth
  - Invasion of surrounding breast parenchyma at interface of lesion
  - Malignant heterologous elements (e.g., rhabdomyosarcoma or liposarcoma)

Macroscopic Features

- Well-defined lobulated lesion

Microscopic Pathology

- Biphasic proliferation of spindle cells and epithelial elements
- Epithelial proliferation creates cleft-like spaces lined by a bilayer of epithelial and myoepithelial cells
- Stromal cells often show condensation (hypercellularity) adjacent to epithelium

Top Differential Diagnoses

- Fibroadenoma with cellular stroma
- Metaplastic carcinoma with spindle cell elements
- Primary sarcoma of the breast

  - Stromal cellularity and pleomorphism
  - Stromal mitotic activity
  - Presence or absence of stromal overgrowth
  - Invasion of surrounding breast parenchyma at interface of lesion
  - Malignant heterologous elements (e.g., rhabdomyosarcoma or liposarcoma)

- Proliferation markers and other molecular markers have been studied
  - Correlate with conventional histologic classification
    - Do not provide additional prediction for recurrence or metastases beyond morphology
    - Not routinely used in clinical practice
- PT rarely can metastasize (10-20% in most series)
  - Most distant metastases develop from tumors classified as malignant

IMAGE FINDINGS

General Features

- Circumscribed mass lesion
  - May have history of slow or rapid growth
  - Calcifications are not a characteristic feature

Mammographic Findings

- Well-defined circumscribed mass
- Partially indistinct margins favor more aggressive lesion

Ultrasonographic Findings

- Typically a hypoechoic lesion
  - Internal hyperechoic striations
  - May demonstrate intramural cystic spaces
    - This feature favors more aggressive lesion

MACROSCOPIC FEATURES

General Features

- Well-defined lobulated lesions with bosselated borders
- May be multinodular
- Cut surface shows
  - Bulging tan-gray tissue
  - Whorled appearance
  - Clefts and cystic spaces (cauliflower-like appearance)
  - Hemorrhage and necrosis may be present (suggests malignancy)
- Higher grade lesions may show tongues of tumor protruding into adjacent breast parenchyma

MICROSCOPIC PATHOLOGY

Histologic Features

- Biphasic proliferation of spindle cells and epithelial elements
  - Epithelial proliferation creates cleft-like spaces lined by a bilayer of epithelial and myoepithelial cells
    - Benign in most cases
    - Usual ductal hyperplasia can be seen in some lesions
    - Lobular carcinoma in situ (LCIS) or ductal carcinoma in situ (DCIS) can be seen (rare)
  - Stromal component
    - Stromal cells often show condensation (hypercellularity) adjacent to epithelium
    - Evaluation of stromal component is used to classify and assess biologic potential
    - Most malignant PT show overgrowth of overtly sarcomatous element within stroma
    - Malignant component may be present in only a portion of lesion; therefore, adequate sampling is important
- Histologic features used to classify as malignant PT
  - Marked stromal hypercellularity
  - Marked stromal cell atypia/nuclear pleomorphism
  - Stromal pattern
    - Marked stromal overgrowth
    - Full high-power field (HPF) of stroma devoid of glandular elements
    - Feature most frequently associated with recurrence &/or metastasis in majority of studies
  - Stromal mitotic activity
    - > 10 mitoses/10 HPF

PHYLLODES TUMOR

Morphologic Classification of Phyllodes Tumors			
Morphologic Criterion	**Benign**	**Borderline**	**Malignant**
Tumor borders	Pushing/circumscribed borders	± infiltrative borders	Infiltrative border
Stromal cellularity	Low	Intermediate	High
Mitotic figures (per 10 HPFs)	< 5	5-10	> 10
Stromal pleomorphism	Mild	Moderate	Marked
Stromal overgrowth	Absent or very focal	Usually focal	May be extensive
Heterologous stromal elements	Absent	Absent	May be present
Incidence of metastases	< 1%	< 10%	10-20%

- Margins
  - Invasion into surrounding breast parenchyma
- Some authors include necrosis and heterologous elements as criteria for malignant PT
- No single feature consistently defines PT as malignant
- Benign PT can be difficult to distinguish from cellular fibroadenomas

Margins

- Assessment of tumor/parenchymal interface is important
  - Circumscribed borders are typical of benign PT
  - Infiltrative borders characteristic of borderline and malignant PT
- Infiltration of tumor cells into adjacent breast tissue may be responsible for local recurrence
  - Assessment of margins in re-excision specimens can be difficult
  - Reactive fibroblasts from prior surgery can be difficult to distinguish from tumor cells

DIFFERENTIAL DIAGNOSIS

Fibroadenoma with Cellular Stroma

- Uniform distribution of glandular and stromal elements with no stromal overgrowth
  - PT typically show dominance of stromal over glandular component
- Minimal cytologic atypia
- Mitotic figures are virtually absent

Metaplastic Carcinoma with Spindle Cell Elements

- Cytokeratin stains helpful
  - Highlight malignant spindle cells
- Neoplastic epithelioid nests of cells merging with spindle cell elements often seen

Primary Sarcoma of the Breast

- Extremely rare event
- Diagnosis should be made only after thorough sampling of lesion
  - Exclude malignant PT with prominent stromal overgrowth (look for biphasic pattern)
  - Exclude high-grade metaplastic carcinoma (look for epithelioid nests and cytokeratin expression)

Metastatic Spindle Cell Tumors

- Clinical history for prior malignancies
  - Exclude metastatic spindle cell carcinoma, melanoma of soft tissue sarcoma in some cases

DIAGNOSTIC CHECKLIST

Pathologic Interpretation Pearls

- Distinctive characteristics for PT
  - Heterogeneous mass with regional variation and disorganization of glandular and stromal components
  - Stromal > glandular components
  - Malignant PT requires at least focally overt sarcomatous overgrowth of stroma
- Assessment of margins is important
  - Infiltrative borders (tumor/parenchymal interface) may indicate potential for local recurrence

SELECTED REFERENCES

1. Lv S et al: Chromosomal aberrations and genetic relations in benign, borderline and malignant phyllodes tumors of the breast: a comparative genomic hybridization study. Breast Cancer Res Treat. 112(3):411-8, 2008
2. Barrio AV et al: Clinicopathologic features and long-term outcomes of 293 phyllodes tumors of the breast. Ann Surg Oncol. 14(10):2961-70, 2007
3. Grabowski J et al: Malignant phyllodes tumors: a review of 752 cases. Am Surg. 73(10):967-9, 2007
4. Lee AH et al: Histological features useful in the distinction of phyllodes tumour and fibroadenoma on needle core biopsy of the breast. Histopathology. 51(3):336-44, 2007
5. Taira N et al: Phyllodes tumor of the breast: stromal overgrowth and histological classification are useful prognosis-predictive factors for local recurrence in patients with a positive surgical margin. Jpn J Clin Oncol. 37(10):730-6, 2007
6. Tan PH et al: Phyllodes tumors of the breast: the role of pathologic parameters. Am J Clin Pathol. 123(4):529-40, 2005
7. Tomita T et al: Phyllodes tumor of borderline malignancy: seven year follow up with immunohistochemical study. Pathol Int. 55(9):585-9, 2005

Radiologic and Microscopic Features

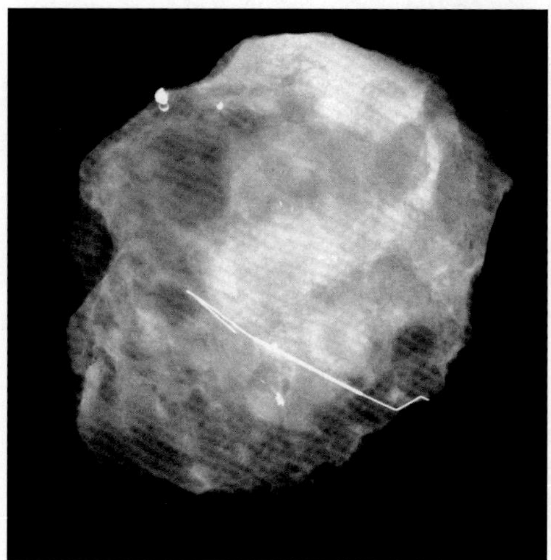

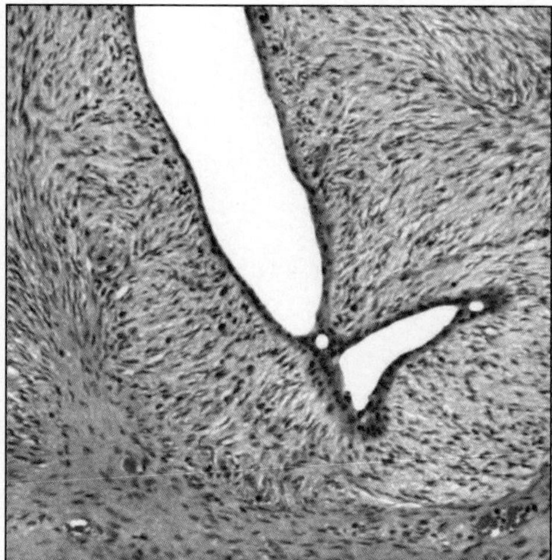

(Left) *The typical imaging finding associated with a PT is that of a circumscribed or lobulated mass as seen here. The radiographic appearance may overlap with fibroadenoma and other benign lesions.* ***(Right)*** *The stromal cells in this example of a benign PT show condensation/ hypercellularity adjacent to the epithelium. (Courtesy R. Flinner, MD.)*

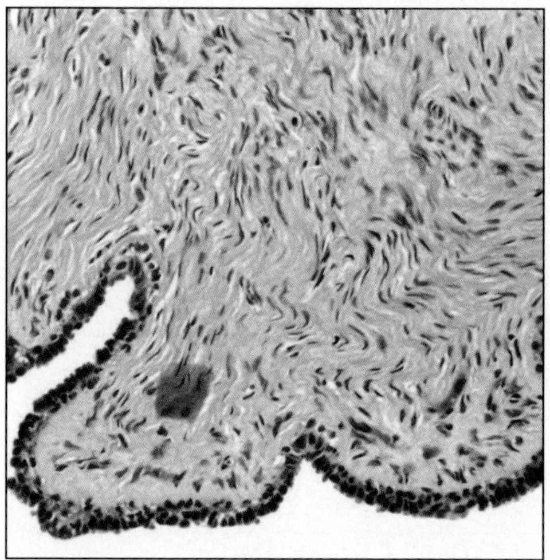

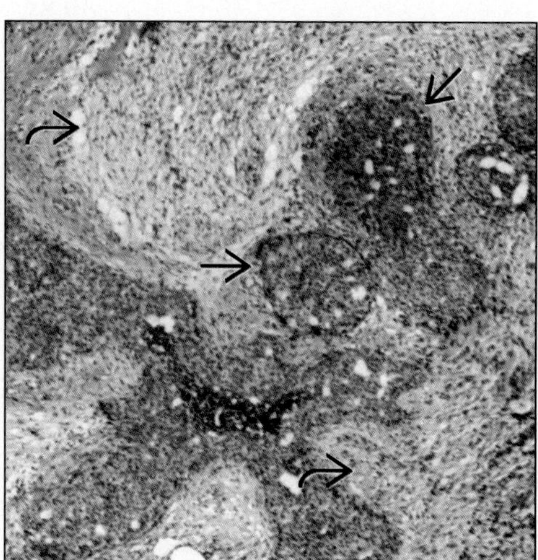

(Left) *High-power image shows the mildly hypercellular stroma covered by epithelium in this benign PT. Note the bland spindle-shaped nuclei and rare mitotic figures.* ***(Right)*** *This borderline PT shows DCIS ⇒ within the epithelial component. The surrounding stroma ⇒ showed modest stromal hypercellularity and nuclear atypia. The occurrence of DCIS and LCIS within the epithelial component is a rare occurrence. (Courtesy R. Flinner, MD.)*

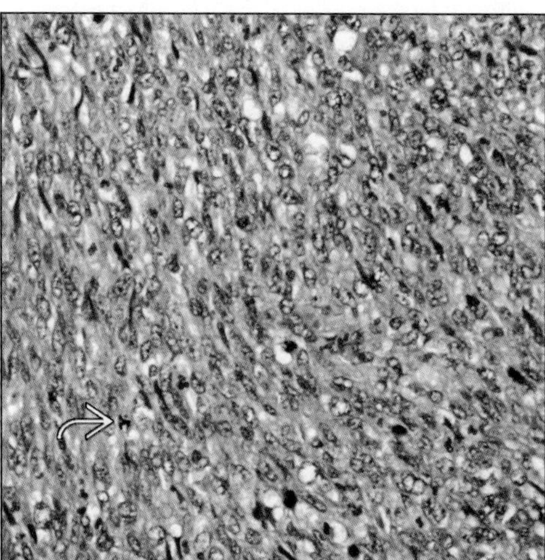

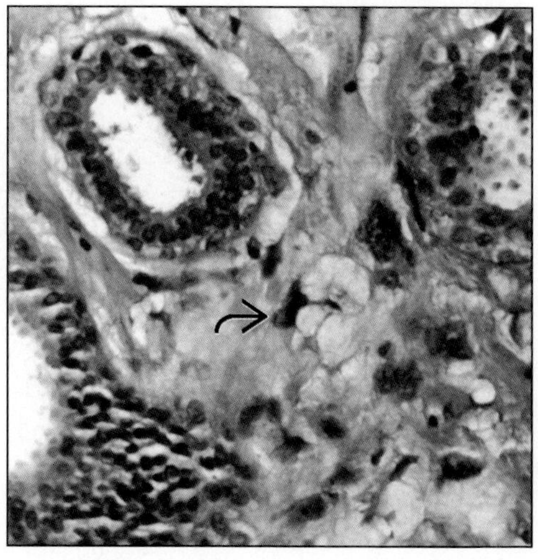

(Left) *High-power image of stroma from a malignant PT shows marked nuclear atypia and frequent mitotic figures ⇒.* ***(Right)*** *This malignant PT shows scattered lipoblasts ⇒ indicative of liposarcomatous differentiation. Although the stroma in malignant PT most commonly resembles fibrosarcoma, heterologous differentiation may be seen. Other examples include osteosarcoma, rhabdomyosarcoma, and chondrosarcoma. (Courtesy R. Flinner, MD.)*

SECRETORY CARCINOMA

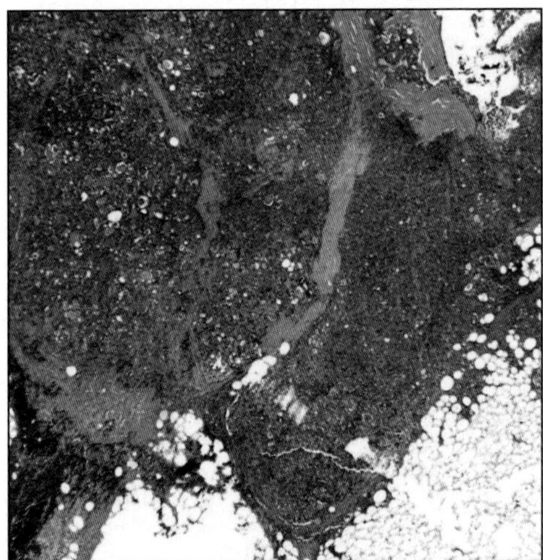

Nests of tumor cells separated by hyalinized bands of fibrous connective tissue are seen in this example of a secretory carcinoma. Central areas of hyalinization are also commonly seen features.

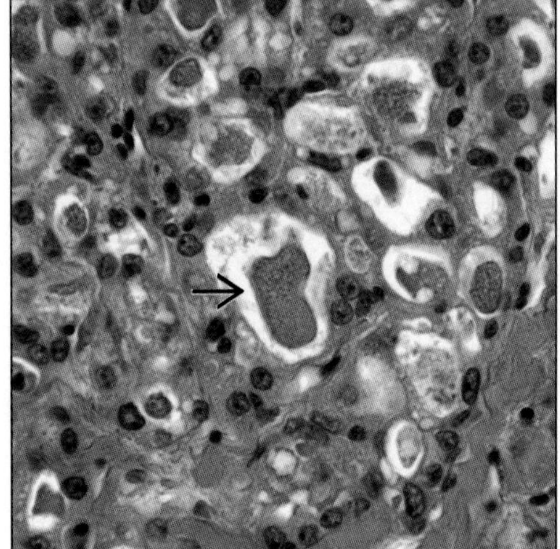

The small uniform glands are filled with dense eosinophilic secretory material ➔. This feature is characteristic of this tumor. The material is positive for PAS and Alcian blue.

TERMINOLOGY

Synonyms

- Juvenile breast carcinoma (this name is discouraged as majority of cases occur in older patients)

Definitions

- Very rare type of breast cancer characterized by specific translocation and occurring over wide age range from children to adults

CLINICAL ISSUES

Epidemiology

- Incidence
  - Very rare type of invasive breast carcinoma (< 0.2% of breast carcinomas)
- Age
  - Occurs over wide range: < 5 years to > 80 years (median: 25 years)

Presentation

- In young women and men, carcinoma is generally in subareolar location due to presence of breast tissue at this site
- Not associated with pregnancy or lactation, although histologic appearance mimics lactating breast tissue

Treatment

- Majority of patients have been treated surgically with excision of breast and lymph nodes
- Too few patients to determine benefit of chemotherapy and radiation
  - Rare patients with metastatic secretory carcinoma who received chemotherapy progressed during treatment

Prognosis

- Majority of patients remain free of disease after surgical excision
  - About 30% of patients have axillary lymph node metastases
- Local recurrences can occur in residual breast tissue or in chest wall many years after initial surgery
- In rare cases, systemic metastases have resulted in death of patient
  - Only 5 cases with distant metastases have been reported

IMAGE FINDINGS

Mammographic Findings

- May appear as circumscribed or irregular densities
  - Calcifications may be present
- No specific imaging features

MACROSCOPIC FEATURES

General Features

- Gross tumors are firm and lobulated or circumscribed
  - No gross features that are specific for secretory carcinoma

MICROSCOPIC PATHOLOGY

Histologic Features

- Generally grows as nests of cells
  - Separated by thick fibrous bands giving lobulated appearance
    - Less frequently, carcinoma has irregular invasive pattern into adjacent stroma
- 3 main growth patterns are recognized
  - Solid
  - Microcystic ("honeycomb")
  - Tubular
- Cells typically have uniform round nuclei with minimal pleomorphism and small nucleoli
- Mitoses are absent or infrequent

SECRETORY CARCINOMA

Key Facts

Clinical Issues

- Very rare type of invasive breast carcinoma (< 0.2% of breast carcinomas)
- Occurs over wide age range: < 5 years to > 80 years (median: 25 years)
- Majority of patients have been treated surgically with excision of breast tumor and lymph nodes

Microscopic Pathology

- Characterized by proliferation of tubules containing characteristic eosinophilic secretory material
- Cells have typical bubbly or granular cytoplasm and are strongly positive for S100
- These carcinomas have characteristic balanced translocation, t(12;15)(p13;q25), resulting in *ETV6-NTRK3* gene fusion product
  - Same translocation occurs in pediatric mesenchymal cancers (congenital fibrosarcoma and congenital cellular mesoblastic nephroma) and adult acute myeloid leukemia
- Majority of secretory carcinomas are negative for ER, PR, and HER2
- Although secretory carcinomas have immunohistochemical similarities to basal-like carcinomas, genetic/molecular relationship with this group is unclear

Top Differential Diagnoses

- Invasive ductal carcinoma of other types
- Lactational changes in normal breast tissue
- Granular cell tumor
- Microglandular adenosis (MGA)
- Cystic hypersecretory carcinoma (CHC)

- Cytoplasm has typical bubbly (vacuolated) or granular cytoplasm due to secretory material
  - Cells are positive for periodic acid-Schiff and Alcian blue
  - Signet ring cells may be present
  - Some carcinomas have apocrine appearance
- Tumor cell lumens contain characteristic dense eosinophilic secretory material
  - Also positive for periodic acid-Schiff and Alcian blue
- May be associated with DCIS
  - Papillary and cribriform types of DCIS are most common
  - Same gene translocation found in secretory carcinomas is also present in associated DCIS
  - Central comedo-like necrosis is uncommon but may occur
  - Associated DCIS is histologically similar to invasive carcinoma
  - IHC for myoepithelial cells may be necessary to distinguish circumscribed nests of invasive carcinoma from DCIS

ANCILLARY TESTS

Immunohistochemistry

- Majority of secretory carcinomas are negative for ER
  - About 1/2 of cases are reported to be positive for PR
- Majority of secretory carcinomas are negative for HER2
- Secretory carcinomas are strongly positive for S100 (nuclear and cytoplasmic)
  - Also positive for CEA and smooth muscle actin (~ 80%)
- Negative for GCDFP-15 and nuclear p63
  - Cytoplasmic p63 positivity may be present
- Secretory carcinomas express some markers typical of "luminal" carcinomas
  - Cytokeratin 8/18 positive in ~ 100% (but may be weak and focal)
  - E-cadherin positive in ~ 100%
- Secretory carcinomas express markers typical of basal-like carcinomas
  - Basal cytokeratin 5/6 positive in ~ 80%
  - Basal cytokeratin 14 positive in ~ 30%
  - EGFR (HER1) positive in ~ 50%
  - CD117 (C-Kit) positive in ~ 70% (but may be weak and focal)
- Although secretory carcinomas have immunohistochemical similarities to basal-like carcinomas, genetic/molecular relationship with this group is unclear

Molecular Studies

- Secretory carcinomas have characteristic balanced translocation: t(12;15)(p13;q25), which results in a *ETV6-NTRK3* gene fusion product
  - *ETV6* (TEL) encodes *E26* transformation-specific (ETS) transcription factor active in hematopoiesis and angiogenesis
  - *NTRK3* encodes neurotrophic tyrosine receptor kinase 3, which is predominantly expressed in central nervous system
- Same translocation occurs in pediatric mesenchymal cancers
  - Congenital fibrosarcoma and congenital cellular mesoblastic nephroma
  - Translocation may be seen in adult acute myeloid leukemia
  - This translocation has not been reported in other types of breast cancer
- Loss of heterozygosity (LOH) is not seen at 17p13 (the *P53* gene locus); LOH is present at this site in 47% of breast carcinomas of no special type
- Comparative genomic hybridization shows 2.0 alterations per carcinoma including gains of 8q or 1q and losses of 22q
- Results of molecular profiling tests (such as Oncotype DX [Genomic Health; Redwood City, CA]) should be interpreted with caution
  - Validity of results has not been determined in rare tumor types such as secretory carcinoma

SECRETORY CARCINOMA

DIFFERENTIAL DIAGNOSIS

Invasive Ductal Carcinoma of Other Types

- Other types of breast carcinomas can have granular eosinophilic &/or vacuolated cytoplasm
  - Apocrine carcinomas, acinic cell carcinomas
- Immunohistochemical pattern of negativity for ER, PR, HER2, and GCDFP-15 and positivity for S100
  - Helpful to support the diagnosis of secretory carcinoma
- In some cases, it may be helpful to confirm diagnosis of secretory carcinoma with molecular studies for translocation

Lactational Changes in Normal Breast Tissue

- Occur in breast tissue with normal underlying architecture
  - Occasionally, these changes are pronounced and form circumscribed masses ("lactational adenomas")
- Solid, cribriform, and infiltrative patterns are not present
- During pregnancy and lactation, lumens appear empty as secretory products are water soluble and dissolve during processing
- Luminal eosinophilic secretions seen in secretory carcinoma are not present

Granular Cell Tumor

- Solid variant of secretory carcinoma can resemble granular cell tumor
- In most cases, tubule formation with intratubular secretions will exclude diagnosis of granular cell tumor
- Immunohistochemical studies can be used to confirm cytokeratin expression in secretory carcinomas
- Both granular cell tumors and secretory carcinomas are strongly positive for S100

Microglandular Adenosis (MGA)

- MGA and secretory carcinomas have several features in common
  - Characterized by tubules containing dense eosinophilic material
  - Typically negative for ER, PR, and HER2 and strongly positive for S100
  - Have invasive pattern but do not (MGA) or rarely (secretory carcinoma) metastasize or cause death of patient
- MGA is usually not confused with secretory carcinoma due to absence of solid and cribriform growth patterns
- In 1 reported case of MGA, t(12;15) translocation characteristic of secretory carcinoma was not found

Cystic Hypersecretory Carcinoma (CHC)

- Consists of grossly evident cystic spaces filled with densely eosinophilic secretory material
  - Spaces are lined by cells with pleomorphic hyperchromatic nuclei and scant cytoplasm
  - Bland nuclei and abundant foamy cytoplasm of secretory carcinomas are not typical
- Majority of cases of CHC are in situ carcinomas
  - Rare associated invasive carcinomas are poorly differentiated and have solid growth pattern
  - Invasive carcinoma lacks secretory features of in situ carcinoma
  - Nuclei may be centrally clear (similar to papillary thyroid carcinoma)

DIAGNOSTIC CHECKLIST

Clinically Relevant Pathologic Features

- Very rare variant of invasive breast cancer
  - Very wide age range for presentation
  - May occur in adolescents or in young children

Pathologic Interpretation Pearls

- Secretory carcinoma will have characteristic morphologic appearance, immunophenotype, and molecular alterations
  - Bubbly or granular cytoplasm
  - Negativity for ER, PR, HER2, and GCDFP-15; positivity for S100
  - Balanced translocation, t(12;15)(p13;q25), that results in *ETV6-NTRK3* gene fusion product
- Immunohistochemistry and molecular studies may be helpful to confirm diagnosis

SELECTED REFERENCES

1. Geyer FC et al: Microglandular adenosis or microglandular adenoma? A molecular genetic analysis of a case associated with atypia and invasive carcinoma. Histopathology. 55(6):732-43, 2009
2. Lambros MB et al: Genomic profile of a secretory breast cancer with an ETV6-NTRK3 duplication. J Clin Pathol. 62(7):604-12, 2009
3. Laé M et al: Secretory breast carcinomas with ETV6-NTRK3 fusion gene belong to the basal-like carcinoma spectrum. Mod Pathol. 22(2):291-8, 2009
4. Arce C et al: Secretory carcinoma of the breast containing the ETV6-NTRK3 fusion gene in a male: case report and review of the literature. World J Surg Oncol. 3:35, 2005
5. Bratthauer GL et al: Antibodies targeting p63 react specifically in the cytoplasm of breast epithelial cells exhibiting secretory differentiation. Histopathology. 47(6):611-6, 2005
6. Ozguroglu M et al: Secretory carcinoma of the breast. Case report and review of the literature. Oncology. 68(2-3):263-8, 2005
7. Diallo R et al: Secretory carcinoma of the breast: a distinct variant of invasive ductal carcinoma assessed by comparative genomic hybridization and immunohistochemistry. Hum Pathol. 34(12):1299-305, 2003
8. Rivera-Hueto F et al: Long-term prognosis of teenagers with breast cancer. Int J Surg Pathol. 10(4):273-9, 2002
9. Herz H et al: Metastatic secretory breast cancer. Non-responsiveness to chemotherapy: case report and review of the literature. Ann Oncol. 11(10):1343-7, 2000
10. Maitra A et al: Molecular abnormalities associated with secretory carcinomas of the breast. Hum Pathol. 30(12):1435-40, 1999

Microscopic Features

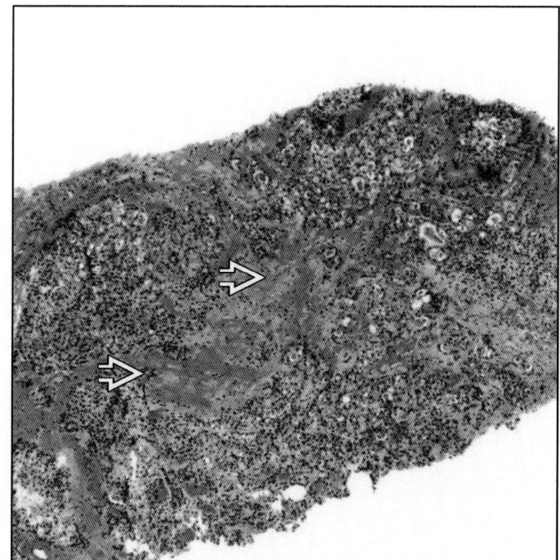

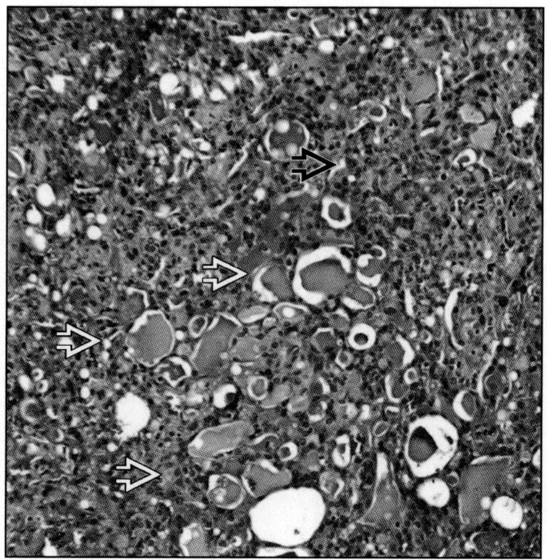

(Left) *This core needle biopsy shows irregular nests of tumor cells in a dense stroma. Note the thick bands of dense fibrosis ⇨ separating nests of tumor cells, a characteristic feature of secretory carcinoma.* ***(Right)*** *This carcinoma has both microcystic ⇨ and solid ⇨ patterns. The lumens are filled with characteristic eosinophilic secretory material. Some cases mimic lactating breast, but true lactation has empty spaces as milk is water soluble and does not survive processing.*

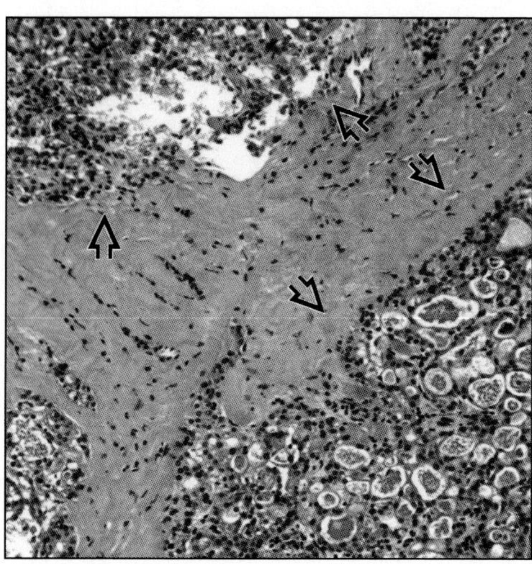

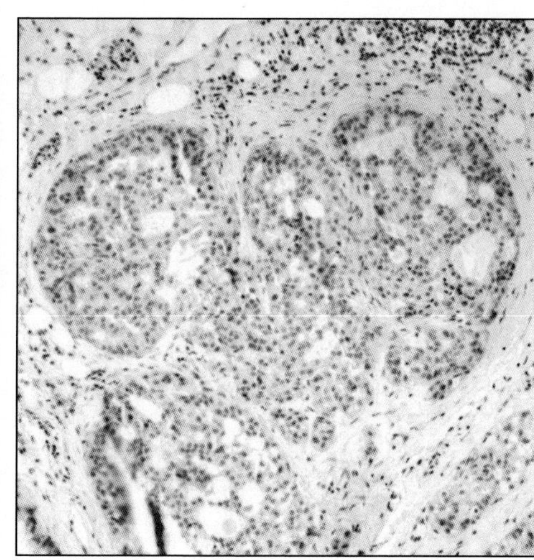

(Left) *The nests of tumor cells can appear well circumscribed ⇨ and surrounded by dense tissue. IHC studies for myoepithelial cells may be necessary to distinguish invasive carcinoma from DCIS.* ***(Right)*** *Secretory carcinomas are typically negative for ER (as seen here), PR, and HER2. Nevertheless, these carcinomas have a favorable prognosis. The results of some prognostic tests, such as Oncotype DX, are likely to be inaccurate for this rare tumor type.*

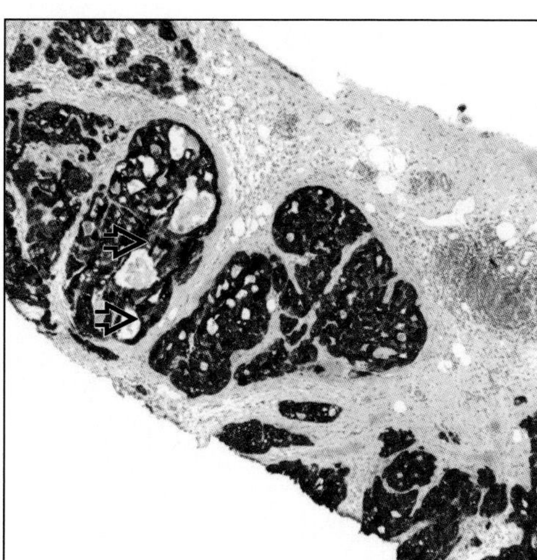

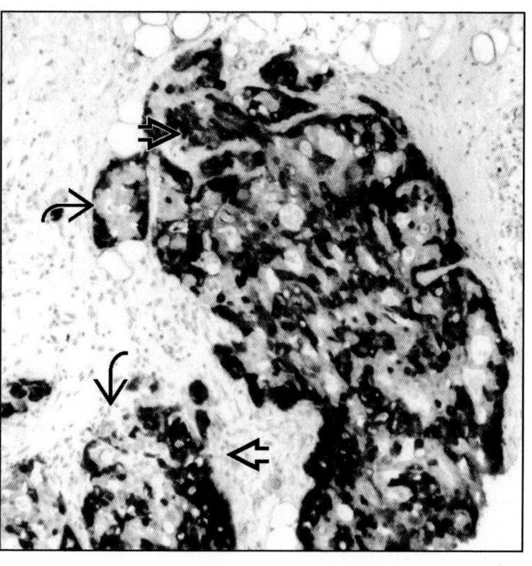

(Left) *Tumor cells are positive for cytokeratin (AE1/AE3; red cytoplasm). No myoepithelial cells are identified using p63 (brown nuclei), showing that the circumscribed nests of cells are invasive carcinoma. Focal cytoplasmic positivity for p63 is present ⇨. This finding has been reported in cells with a secretory phenotype.* ***(Right)*** *Secretory carcinomas are strongly positive for S100. This carcinoma shows marked heterogeneity with both positive ⇨ and negative ↗ cells.*

Central Nervous System

Neoplasm, Benign

Neoplasm, Malignant Primary

Protocol for the Examination of Specimens from Patients with Tumors of the Brain/Spinal Cord

GANGLION CELL TUMORS

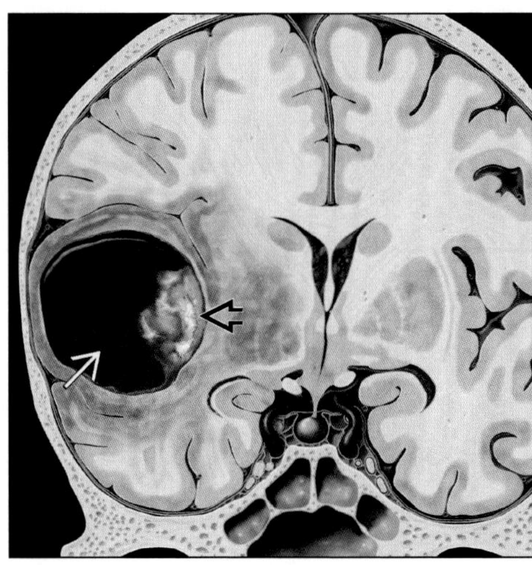

Coronal graphic shows the classic appearance of a GCT: Superficial mass centered in the cortex or subarachnoid space, composed of a cyst ➔ with mural nodule ⊳.

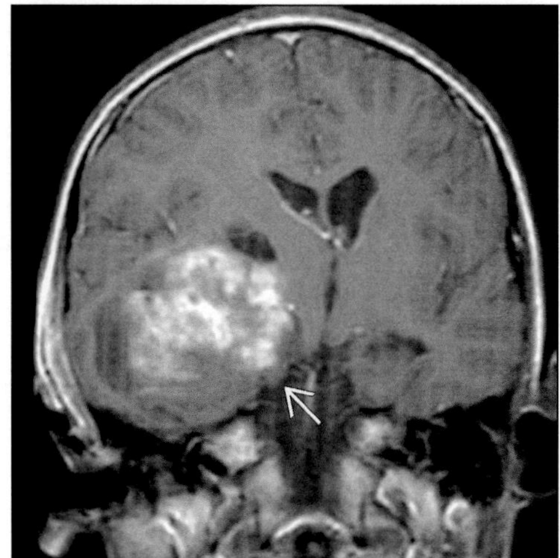

Coronal T1WI C+ MR shows a large, heterogeneous right temporal mass with cystic and enhancing solid components ➔. Note no significant surrounding edema.

TERMINOLOGY

Abbreviations

- Ganglion cell tumors (GCT)

Definitions

- Benign, well-differentiated, slow-growing neuroepithelial tumors
- Composed predominantly of large, mature, dysmorphic neoplastic cells resembling pyramidal neurons or well-developed ganglion cells
- Either exclusively (gangliocytoma) or admixed with neoplastic glial cells (ganglioglioma)

ETIOLOGY/PATHOGENESIS

Histogenesis of GCTs

- Gangliocytomas may be malformative (hamartomas)
  - Cortical dysplasia seen adjacent to some GCTs
- Gangliogliomas associated with developmental lesions
  - Particularly neuronal migration disorders
  - Lesional glia cells: Neoplastic vs. reactive
  - Monoclonal origin in some cases: *TSC2* gene
- Alternatively, from pluripotential progenitor cells
  - Divergent differentiation: Glial and neuronal lines
- Presence of less mature neurons ("ganglioid cells")
  - Stepwise neoplastic transformation to larger cells
- Possibly differentiated remnants of embryonal tumors
  - Neuroblastoma, primitive neuroectodermal tumor

CLINICAL ISSUES

Epidemiology

- Incidence
  - Gangliogliomas: 0.4-1.3% of all brain tumors
    - Up to 9% in some pediatric populations
- Age
  - Children, young adults (1st and 2nd decades of life)

Site

- Mostly supratentorial, especially temporal lobe
- Also reported in cerebellum, optic nerve, brainstem, pineal, pituitary, spinal cord

Presentation

- Cerebral location: History of seizures, headache
- Mass: ↑ intracranial pressure (ICP), hydrocephalus
- Symptoms precede diagnosis by mean of 3-4 years

Natural History

- Slow-growing, indolent lesion: Long history of seizures
- May extend to subarachnoid space but not aggressive

Treatment

- Surgical approaches
  - Simple, even partial resection may relieve symptoms

Prognosis

- Excellent long-term prognosis, almost never fatal
- Infrequent recurrence (< 10 % of cases)
  - After incomplete removal → less favorable prognosis
- Rare malignant transformation (< 5 % of cases)
  - Mostly limited to glial component
  - Histologic anaplasia does not predict outcome

IMAGE FINDINGS

MR Findings

- Hypointense on T1WI, hyperintense on T2WI
- Solid, nodular, or rim-like enhancement

CT Findings

- Cyst with contrast-enhancing mural nodule
  - Or circumscribed, solid mass
- Iso- or hypodense, heterogeneous
- Typically contrast enhancing, calcified
- Superficial cerebral tumors: Scalloped calvarium
  - Erode inner skull table → bone remodeling
    - Result of chronic compression

Key Facts

Terminology
- Benign, well-differentiated tumors with dysplastic ganglion cells, either alone (gangliocytoma) or with neoplastic glial cells (ganglioglioma)

Clinical Issues
- Slow-growing, indolent lesions: History of seizures
- Cyst with contrast-enhancing mural nodule
- Resectable, excellent prognosis, almost never fatal

Macroscopic Features
- Mostly supratentorial (cortical), temporal lobe
- Often calcified (gritty), rare hemorrhage or necrosis

Microscopic Pathology
- Compact (not infiltrative) with dysplastic neurons
  - Large pleomorphic vesicular hyperchromatic nuclei
  - Irregular apical dendrites, coarse peripheral Nissl
- Eosinophilic granular bodies, lymphocytes
- Ganglioglioma: Additional neoplastic glial cells
  - Pleomorphic, GFAP-positive cells, mostly astrocytic
- Anaplastic ganglioglioma (WHO grade III)
  - Anaplastic component usually glial (GFAP positive)
  - Frequent mitoses, necrosis, resembles glioblastoma

Ancillary Tests
- Neoplastic neurons: Positive, granular synaptophysin
- S100, GFAP stain glial component, intermediate cells
- CD34(+), MAP2(-) (recent studies)
- MIB-1 labeling: Low (< 3%) in glial component

Top Differential Diagnoses
- Infiltrating glioma: Diffuse, not contrast enhancing
- Trapped normal neurons: Uniform, differentiated
  - Polar cytoplasm, apical dendrites, no atypia

MACROSCOPIC FEATURES

General Features
- Superficial, centered in cortex or subarachnoid space
- Solid or cystic tumors, with little mass effect
- Well-circumscribed nodule, frequently in cyst wall
- Often calcified (gritty), rare hemorrhage or necrosis

Sections to Be Submitted
- Mural nodule entirely (if small), portion of cyst wall

MICROSCOPIC PATHOLOGY

Gangliocytoma
- Compact growth pattern (not infiltrative)
  - Cellularity similar to or less than normal gray matter
  - Architecturally disorganized (hamartomatous)
  - Lack small neurons or specialized glia (perineuronal oligodendrocytes, reactive astrocytes)
- Neuropil-rich fibrillar background (neuritic processes)
  - Reticulin fibers (often perivascular)
  - Nonneoplastic astrocytes; rarely pigmented cells
- Microvascular proliferation may occur
  - Usually capillary proliferation in cyst wall
  - May be more glomeruloid in parenchyma
  - Not of clinical significance
- Cytologically abnormal, dysplastic multipolar neurons
  - Poorly formed, irregularly arranged apical dendrites
    - Uncoordinated, not "oriented" toward pia
  - Large pleomorphic vesicular hyperchromatic nuclei
    - Bi- or multinucleated, with prominent nucleoli
    - Intranuclear cytoplasmic inclusions
  - Coarse, irregular, peripherally misplaced Nissl
  - Granulovacuolar degeneration
    - Cytoplasmic vacuoles with basophilic granules
  - Neurofibrillary cytoplasmic tangles
    - Basophilic; silver, tau protein, ubiquitin positive
- "Ganglioid cells": Less mature, intermediate neurons
- By definition: Lack mitotically active "neuroblasts"
- Eosinophilic granular bodies (EGBs)
  - Aggregates of small round droplets
  - Eosinophilic, hyaline, PAS positive
  - In astrocyte cytoplasm or interstitium
- Perivascular lymphocytes common
- Microcalcifications (calcospherites) common

Ganglioglioma
- As in gangliocytoma, but more complex
- Prominent neoplastic glial cell component
  - Pleomorphic, GFAP-positive cells
  - Most often astrocytic, fibrillar type
    - Glassy cytoplasm, short processes, Rosenthal fibers
  - May be piloid (pilocytic) or oligodendroglioma-like
  - Glial component may infiltrate brain parenchyma
- Neuronal elements
  - Vesicular, often multiple nuclei, prominent nucleoli
  - Variable Nissl substance, discrete cell borders
- Neuronal, glial components: Admixed or distinct
  - Often with lobular architecture
    - Nests of neoplastic cells, trapped or encircled
    - Reticulin-, collagen-rich interlobular stroma
  - Microcyst-rich pattern
    - Smaller ganglion cells and piloid glia
  - Mixed ganglion cells, astrocytes in fibrillar stroma
- Desmoplasia common in classic gangliogliomas
  - Especially those involving subarachnoid space
  - Trichrome-positive, reticulin-rich matrix
  - May be focal in other lesions
- Rare GCTs may have melanotic features

Histologic Variants
- **Anaplastic ganglioglioma (WHO grade III)**
  - Anaplastic component usually glial (GFAP[+])
    - Rarely anaplastic neuronal component or both
  - Frequent mitoses, necrosis, resembles glioblastoma
  - Aggressive like malignant gliomas, tend to recur
  - Diagnose only when clear GCT component present
- **Dysplastic cerebellar gangliocytoma (WHO grade I)**
  - Rare, benign, mass-forming nonneoplastic lesion (a.k.a. Lhermitte-Duclos disease)
  - In young adults: Sporadic or in Cowden disease
    - *PTEN* mutation: Phosphorylated AKT in neurons
  - Cerebellar dysfunction, ↑ ICP, CSF obstruction

GANGLION CELL TUMORS

- Slow-growing, treated by surgical excision
- T2WI MR: Characteristic striped cerebellar mass
- Enlarged folia, but gyriform/laminar architecture
- ↑ thickness of internal granule cell layer
  - Massive enlargement, hypertrophic neurons
  - Haphazardly oriented, apolar, may be bizarre
  - Superficial (near Purkinje cell layer) > deeper
- Molecular layer: ↑ myelinated axons, vacuolated

- **Desmoplastic infantile ganglioglioma (WHO grade I)**
  - Rare tumor in infants (< 1 year old)
  - Massive, supratentorial, superficial, dura attached
    - Fills and expands subarachnoid space
    - Reaches cortex along perivascular spaces
  - Macrocephaly, ↑ ICP, neurologic deficits
  - Resection is difficult, but long survival is common
  - Discrete, contrast-enhancing, solid-cystic mass
  - Mostly acellular, reticulin-rich collagenous matrix
    - Spindled and storiform, merges with glioneuronal
    - Dark on T2WI MR, "woody" texture grossly
  - Small, GFAP(+) astrocytes
    - Oval nuclei, glassy cytoplasm, gemistocytic
  - Neuronal component difficult to identify
    - Ganglion cells are sparse, may have EGBs
    - Synaptophysin, chromogranin positive
  - May have highly cellular, mitotically active areas
    - Resembling embryonal tumors, high-grade glioma
    - Microvascular proliferation, palisading necrosis
    - Unclear prognostic significance, may be aggressive
  - No ganglia → Desmoplastic infantile **astrocytoma**
- **Ganglioneurocytoma**
  - Central neurocytoma variant ("differentiated")
    - Fibrillary neuropil background (synaptophysin[+])
    - Variable numbers of ganglion and "ganglioid" cells
  - "Ganglioid" cells: Small neurons, less prominent nucleoli, inconspicuous Nissl substance
  - Often parenchymal; may be papillary or lipomatous
- **Ganglioglioneurocytoma**
  - Central neurocytoma with ganglion cells and glia
  - Benign, well circumscribed, resectable
  - Cystic, calcified, focally contrast enhancing
  - Fibrillar background may be more prominent
  - GFAP(+) neoplastic cells (glial component)
- **Papillary glioneuronal tumor**
  - Paraventricular deep white matter, often temporal
  - Contrast enhancing, cystic, pseudopapillary
  - Hyalinized vessels, perivascular GFAP(+) cells
  - Single layer of small, pseudostratified, cuboidal cells
  - Collections of neurocytes, intermixed ganglion cells

ANCILLARY TESTS

Cytology

- Ganglion cells better preserved than in frozen sections
  - Ample cytoplasm, open chromatin, visible nucleoli
  - Larger, rounder than normal ganglion cells
- Fibrillar background of glial cell processes, EGBs

Frozen Sections

- Ganglion cells undergo freezing artifact
  - Smudgy, disfigured nuclei, may be hyperchromatic
  - May be misdiagnosed as malignant astrocytes
- Consider clinical, radiologic context
  - Solid, discrete, contrast-enhancing lesion
  - Little mass effect, cystic with mural nodule
  - In young patient: Suggests GCT
- Histologic support for GCT
  - Nodular, calcified, EGBs, perivascular lymphocytes

Immunohistochemistry

- Synaptophysin in neoplastic neurons
  - Fine granular surface positivity
  - Not specific: Normal neurons may be similar
- Chromogranin mirrors presence of dense core granules
  - Punctate cytoplasmic staining in neuronal cells
- NeuN stains nucleus, cytoplasm of large ganglion cells
- S100, GFAP stain glial component, intermediate cells
  - But will also stain nonneoplastic astrocytes
- Some tumor cells stain with neuronal & glial markers
- Collagen type IV, laminin stain stroma
  - Especially in longstanding nodular tumors
- GCTs: CD34(+), MAP2(-) (recent studies)
- MIB-1 labeling: Low (< 3%) in glial component
  - Almost absent in neuronal component
  - ↑ MIB-1, p53: Aggressive behavior, recurrence

Cytogenetics

- Various abnormal karyotypes described in GCTs
  - Involving chromosomes 5, 6, and 7

Electron Microscopy

- Abundant dense core granules in ganglion cells
  - If present, raise suspicion for GCT
  - Inconspicuous in normal CNS neurons
- Microtubule-containing cell processes (axons)
- Synaptic junctions, neurosecretory vesicles seen
- Neurofibrillary tangles: Paired helical filaments
- Astrocytes: Intermediate filaments, basal lamina

DIFFERENTIAL DIAGNOSIS

Normal Brain Tissue

- Ordered, organized complexity
- Cytologically normal neurons, no binucleate forms
- Generally lacks calcifications

Cortical Dysplasia and Tubers

- Abnormal neurons in cortex, subcortical white matter
  - Large, glassy, astrocyte-like cells
- Not a discrete, compact mass; lacks lymphocytes

Infiltrating Glioma

- Especially oligodendroglioma (gray matter)
- Infiltrating, diffuse tumor; no contrast enhancement
- "Perineuronal satellitosis" (tumor cells around ganglia)

Trapped Normal Neurons

- Uniform, differentiated; lacks atypia, pleomorphism
- No association with smaller "ganglioid" forms
- Polar cytoplasm, apical dendrites oriented toward pia
- Generally lack granular surface synaptophysin staining

Dysembryoplastic Neuroepithelial Tumor

- Cortical lesion, nodules of oligodendroglia-like cells
- Large neurons, "floating" in small mucin pools
  - Little dysmorphism or atypia

Pleomorphic Xanthoastrocytoma
- May contain large, neuron-like astrocytes
- Infiltrating cortical component
  - May overrun normal ganglion cells

Pilocytic Astrocytoma
- Large, amphophilic multinucleated cells
  - Not ganglion cells
- CD34(-), MAP2(+)

Meningioangiomatosis
- Enlarged vessels entrap islands of cortex
- Crowded ganglion cells resemble gangliocytoma
- Plaque-like intracortical lesion, not a round mass

Extraventricular Neurocytoma
- Usually overrun by oligodendroglioma-like neurocytes
- May contain ganglion cells

Ganglion Cell "Metaplasia"
- In hypothalamic hamartoma, pituitary adenoma

DIAGNOSTIC CHECKLIST

Clinically Relevant Pathologic Features
- Slow-growing, WHO grade I or II neoplasms
  - Characteristic common clinical, radiologic features
  - Well-differentiated, circumscribed lesions
  - "Cyst with mural nodule" appearance
    - Radiologically or grossly
  - Local extension into subarachnoid, leptomeninges
    - Do not misinterpret as aggressive behavior
    - Little infiltration into brain parenchyma
  - Histologically EGBs are common
  - Differential diagnosis
    - Gangliocytoma, ganglioglioma (GCTs)
    - Pilocytic astrocytoma
    - Pleomorphic xanthoastrocytoma
    - Extraventricular neurocytoma
- Ganglioglioma: Most common tumor (40%) associated with chronic temporal lobe epilepsy
- GCTs tend to be overdiagnosed
  - Normal neurons trapped in a glioma
    - Misinterpreted as dysplastic

Pathologic Interpretation Pearls
- Distinction between ganglioglioma, gangliocytoma
  - May be difficult, transitional entities exist
  - Large pleomorphic cells may resemble both astrocytes and ganglion cells
  - Uncertain neoplastic nature of glial component
    - Generally, neoplastic astrocytes lack prominent symmetric process of reactive glia
  - Best called "GCTs" in this situation
- Mitotic figures and diagnosis of GCT
  - Occasional mitoses compatible with GCT
  - Significant numbers of mitoses raise differential
    - Infiltrating glioma with trapped neurons
    - Less likely: Anaplastic change in glial component
- Neurofibrillary change, granulovacuolar degeneration
  - In cytoplasm of neoplastic ganglion cells
  - Similar to change of Alzheimer disease
  - No diagnostic significance
    - Neoplastic neurons can undergo degeneration
    - Neurofibrillary change can occur without amyloid
- Perivascular lymphocytes in GCTs
  - Characteristic, but not diagnostic
- EGBs common in many low-grade tumors
  - Most numerous in GCTs, particularly gangliogliomas

GRADING

Gangliocytoma
- By definition WHO grade I

Ganglioglioma (WHO Grade I or II)
- Grade II: Atypical features, ↑ cellularity
  - ↑ proliferation activity: MIB-1 labeling > 5%

Anaplastic Ganglioglioma (WHO Grade III)
- Substantial mitotic activity, MIB-1 labeling > 10%
- Microvascular proliferation, necrosis

Ganglioglioma with Glioblastoma Changes
- In the glial component (WHO grade IV)
- No set criteria for distinction from grade III

SELECTED REFERENCES

1. Karremann M et al: Anaplastic ganglioglioma in children. J Neurooncol. 92(2):157-63, 2009
2. Yam B et al: Radiology-pathology conference: incidental posterior mediastinal ganglioneuroma. Clin Imaging. 33(5):390-4, 2009
3. Luyken C et al: Supratentorial gangliogliomas: histopathologic grading and tumor recurrence in 184 patients with a median follow-up of 8 years. Cancer. 101(1):146-55, 2004
4. Blümcke I et al: Gangliogliomas: an intriguing tumor entity associated with focal epilepsies. J Neuropathol Exp Neurol. 61(7):575-84, 2002
5. De Munnynck K et al: Desmoplastic infantile ganglioglioma: a potentially malignant tumor? Am J Surg Pathol. 26(11):1515-22, 2002
6. Nowak DA et al: Lhermitte-Duclos disease (dysplastic cerebellar gangliocytoma): a malformation, hamartoma or neoplasm? Acta Neurol Scand. 105(3):137-45, 2002
7. Hirose T et al: Ganglioglioma: an ultrastructural and immunohistochemical study. Cancer. 79(5):989-1003, 1997
8. Prayson RA et al: Cortical architectural abnormalities and MIB1 immunoreactivity in gangliogliomas: a study of 60 patients with intracranial tumors. J Neuropathol Exp Neurol. 54(4):513-20, 1995
9. Wolf HK et al: Ganglioglioma: a detailed histopathological and immunohistochemical analysis of 61 cases. Acta Neuropathol. 88(2):166-73, 1994
10. Zentner J et al: Gangliogliomas: clinical, radiological, and histopathological findings in 51 patients. J Neurol Neurosurg Psychiatry. 57(12):1497-502, 1994
11. Miller DC et al: Central nervous system gangliogliomas. Part 1: Pathology. J Neurosurg. 79(6):859-66, 1993
12. VandenBerg SR: Desmoplastic infantile ganglioglioma and desmoplastic cerebral astrocytoma of infancy. Brain Pathol. 3(3):275-81, 1993
13. Diepholder HM et al: A clinicopathologic and immunomorphologic study of 13 cases of ganglioglioma. Cancer. 68(10):2192-201, 1991

GANGLION CELL TUMORS

Microscopic Features

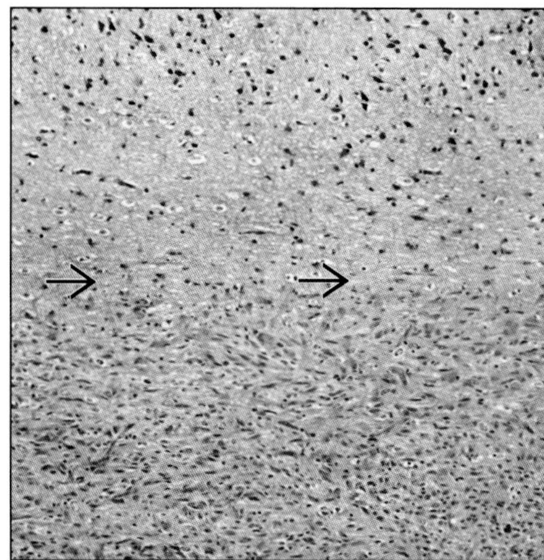

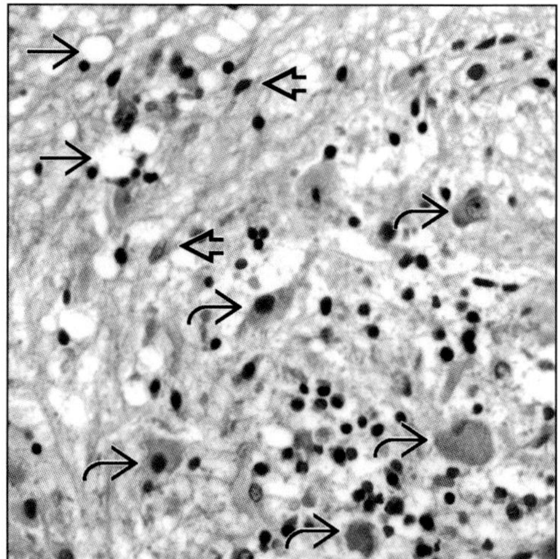

(Left) *Hematoxylin & eosin shows low-power view of a well-circumscribed ganglioglioma having compact growth pattern, without infiltration into adjacent brain parenchyma →.* ***(Right)*** *Hematoxylin & eosin shows high-power view of ganglioglioma with a microcystic appearance → and piloid glial cells ⇨ that resembles, and needs to be differentiated from, pilocytic astrocytoma. Numerous and crowded ganglion cells ↷ suggest a neoplastic lesion and a diagnosis of GCT should be considered.*

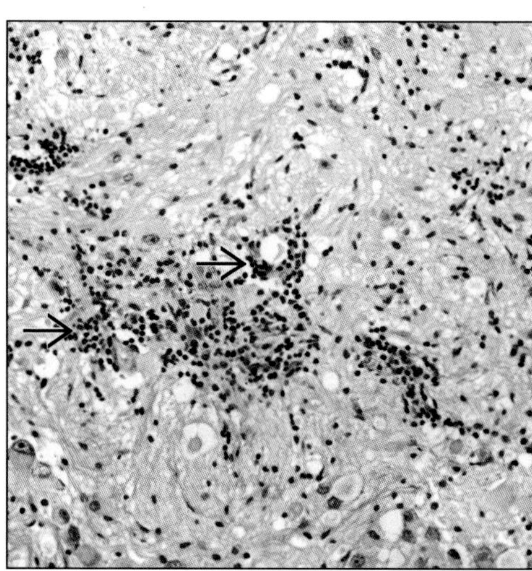

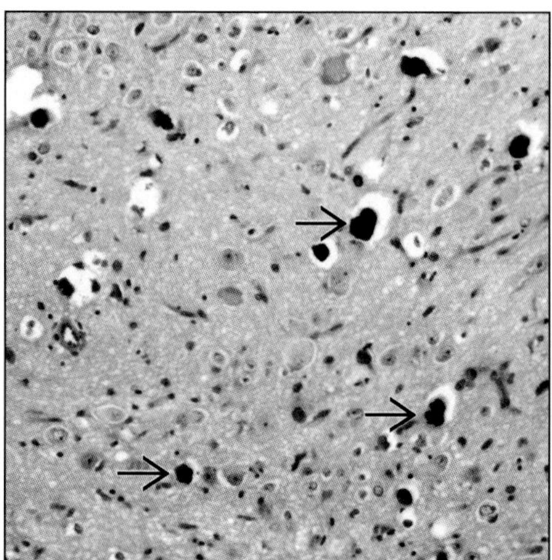

(Left) *Hematoxylin & eosin shows medium-power view of a ganglioglioma with prominent lymphoid aggregates, most of which are perivascular →. Perivascular lymphocytes are characteristic of, but not exclusive to, GCTs and should prompt consideration of the diagnosis.* ***(Right)*** *Hematoxylin & eosin shows high-power view of a ganglioglioma with abundant microcalcifications (calcospherites) →, which are commonly found in GCTs.*

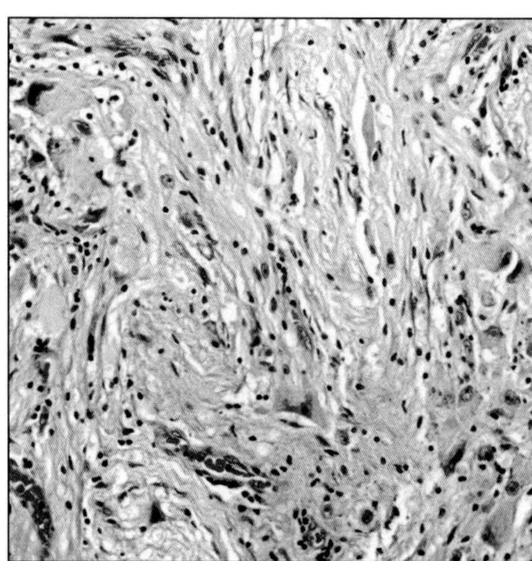

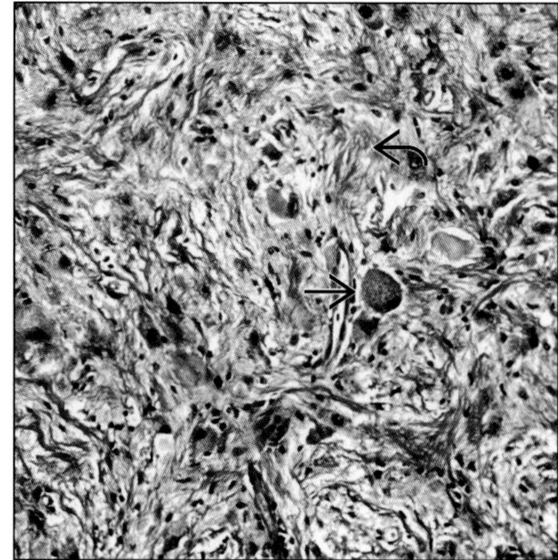

(Left) *Hematoxylin & eosin shows medium-power view of desmoplastic background, which is common in gangliogliomas, especially those that involve the subarachnoid space.* ***(Right)*** *Trichrome stain highlights the collagen-rich connective tissue (desmoplastic) stroma ↷ in a ganglioglioma. Note the ganglion cells that stand out →.*

Microscopic Features

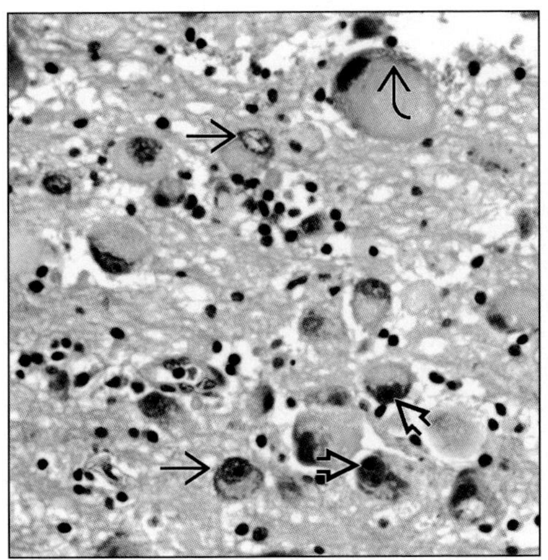
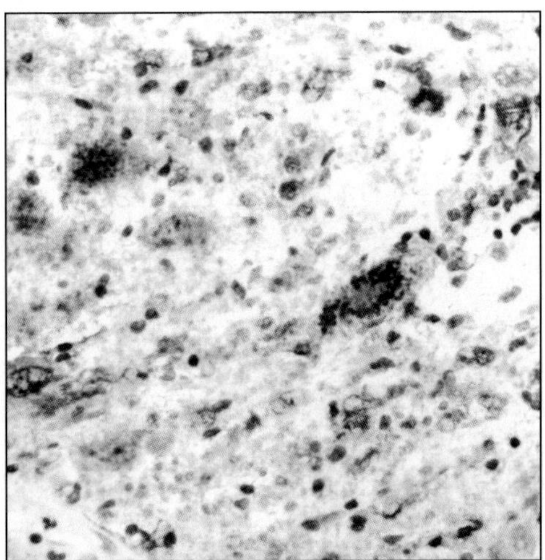

(Left) *Hematoxylin & eosin shows high-power view of a GCT with large, cytologically abnormal, dysplastic ganglion cells (neurons) having large, pleomorphic and vesicular nuclei ➔, prominent nucleoli ➔, and irregular, coarse, peripheral Nissl substance ➔.* ***(Right)*** *Synaptophysin immunohistochemical stain shows high-power view of ganglioglioma with neoplastic neuronal (ganglion) cells having a distinctive pattern of fine granular surface positivity.*

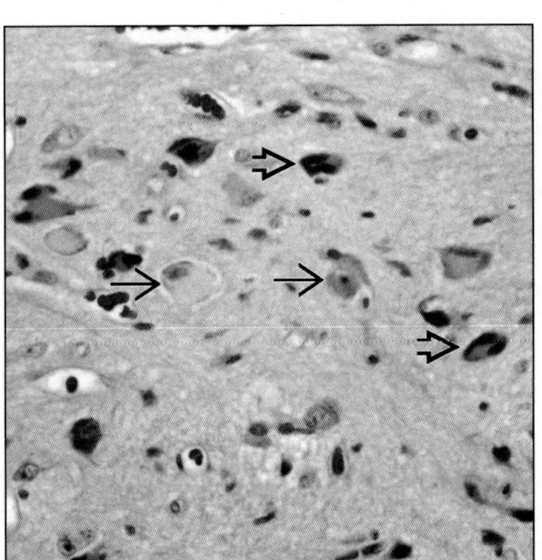
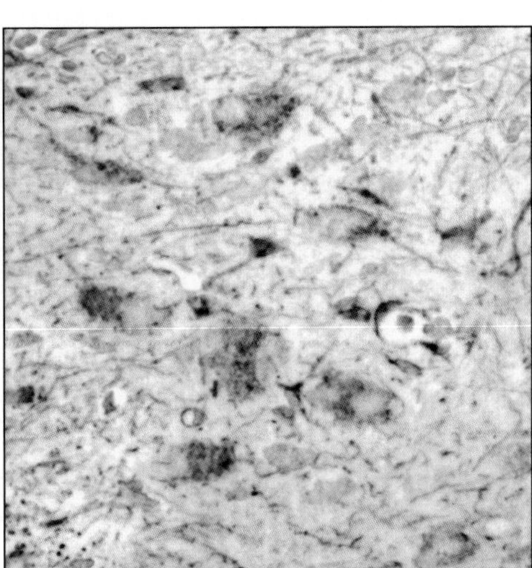

(Left) *H&E shows a ganglioglioma with admixed glial and neuronal components, which may be difficult to distinguish. Cells with prominent nucleoli and peripherally misplaced Nissl ➔ are probably ganglion cells. Cells with glassy eosinophilic cytoplasm and hyperchromatic nuclei ➔ are probably glial, with the phenotype of gemistocytic astrocytes.* ***(Right)*** *GFAP immunostain shows some cells in this ganglioglioma staining positive, highlighting their glial (mostly astrocytic) differentiation.*

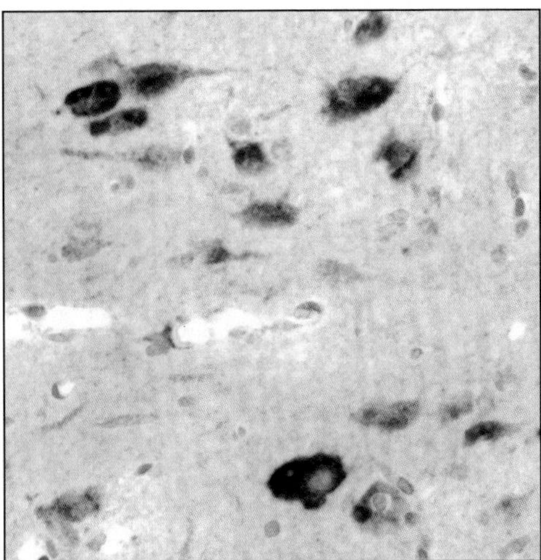
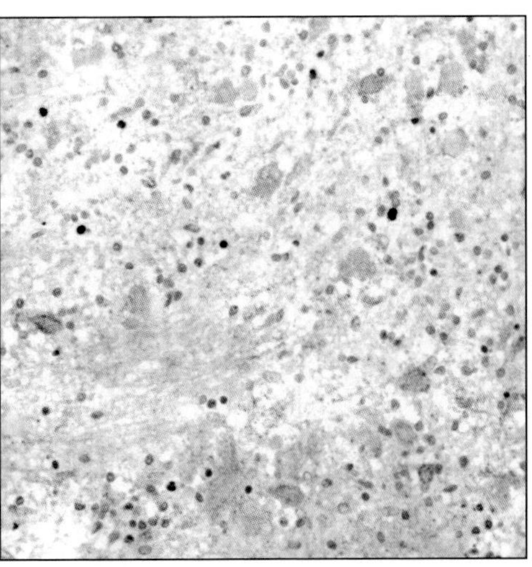

(Left) *NeuN immunohistochemical stain shows high-power view of ganglioglioma with some neoplastic cells having positive staining in their nuclei and cytoplasm, confirming their neuronal phenotype.* ***(Right)*** *Ki-67 immunohistochemical stain in a ganglioglioma shows the low (< 3%) MIB-1 labeling index.*

SUBEPENDYMAL GIANT CELL TUMOR

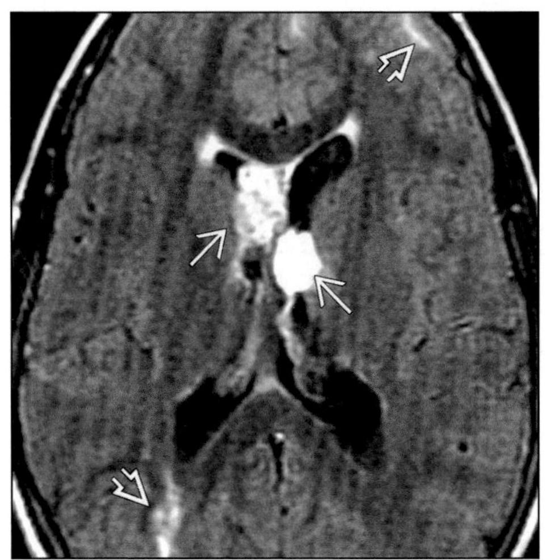

Axial FLAIR shows hyperintense bilateral subependymal giant cell tumors ➡. Hyperintense parenchymal tubers ⇨ are also common in patients with tuberous sclerosis.

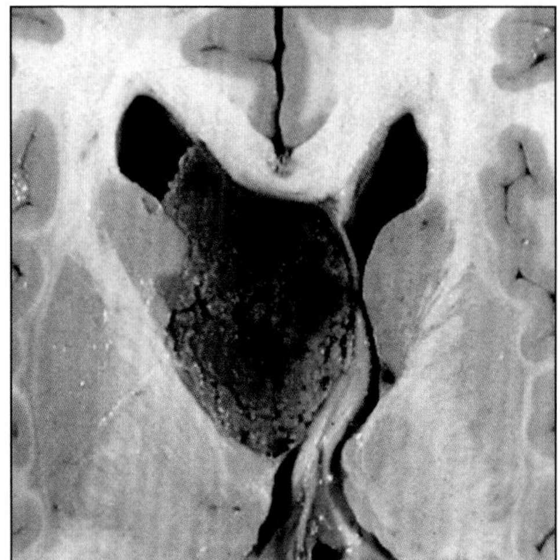

Gross photograph shows a SEGT at the wall of the lateral ventricle, near the foramen of Monro, in a patient with tuberous sclerosis complex. (Courtesy R. Hewlitt, MD.)

TERMINOLOGY

Abbreviations

- Tuberous sclerosis (complex) (TSC)
- Subependymal giant cell tumor (SEGT)

Synonyms

- Subependymal giant cell astrocytoma (SEGA) synonymous with SEGT
- Bourneville or Bourneville-Pringle disease synonymous with TSC

Definitions

- Histologically benign (WHO grade I), slow-growing, discrete, periventricular tumor with glioneuronal features, seen almost exclusively in TSC

ETIOLOGY/PATHOGENESIS

Tuberous Sclerosis (Complex) (TSC)

- Phakomatosis (neurocutaneous genetic syndrome)
- Autosomal dominant in ~ 50% of patients
  - High penetrance, but phenotypic variability
- De novo mutations in substantial number of patients
  - 50-66% thought to be sporadic
- Germline mutations: Tumor suppressor genes
  - *TSC1* gene (chromosome 9q) hamartin protein
  - *TSC2* gene (chromosome 16p) tuberin protein
  - Mutation incidence: *TSC2* > *TSC1* (5:1)
  - Similar phenotypes → unknown if part of same pathway

Manifestations of TSC

- Widespread hamartomatous lesions
- CNS: Cortical tubers, subcortical glioneuronal hamartomas (white matter heterotopias), subependymal hamartomas, intraocular hamartomas
- Skin: Cutaneous facial angiofibromas ("sebaceous adenomas"), hypomelanotic macules, shagreen patches ("peau chagrin"), subungual fibromas
- Angiomyolipoma (kidney), rhabdomyoma (heart), lymphangioleiomyomatosis (lung), hamartomatous intestinal polyps, visceral cysts, liver hamartomas

Histogenesis of SEGT

- Considered distinct, circumscribed astrocytoma
  - Usually has mixed glioneuronal phenotype
    - Glial (astrocytic, ependymal) differentiation
    - Neuronal/neuroendocrine differentiation
- Evolves from enlarging subependymal hamartomas
- Regional localization, ependymal phenotypic features
  - Questionable origin from ependyma of circumventricular organs

TSC Gene Defect

- Dysgenetic event early in development
  - Possibly along astrocytic lineage
  - Disruption of neuronal migration
  - Abortive differentiation, abnormal migration
- Results in tubers, subependymal nodules
  - Questionable neoplastic transformation to SEGT
  - Capable of glioneuronal differentiation

CLINICAL ISSUES

Epidemiology

- Incidence
  - SEGT: In 3-19% of patients with confirmed TSC
  - TSC incidence: 0.01-0.02%
- Age
  - Typically presents during childhood, adolescence
    - Average age at diagnosis: ~ 13 years
  - Congenital examples in premature infants
  - TSC manifestations usually present by 10 years old
- Gender
  - No sex predilection reported

Site

- Wall of lateral ventricle, at level of basal ganglia
  - Classically near foramen of Monro

SUBEPENDYMAL GIANT CELL TUMOR

Key Facts

Terminology
- Benign (WHO grade I), slow-growing, discrete, periventricular glioneuronal tumor in TSC

Etiology/Pathogenesis
- TSC: Autosomal dominant phakomatosis
  - High penetrance, phenotypic variability
  - Tumor suppressor genes *TSC1*, *TSC2*
  - Widespread hamartomas: CNS, skin, organs

Clinical Issues
- SEGT: In 3-19% of patients with confirmed TSC
- Typically presents during childhood, adolescence
- Wall of lateral ventricle, near foramen of Monro
- CSF obstruction, ↑ intracranial pressure (ICP)
- Longstanding history of seizures, epilepsy
- Nodules, SEGTs enlarge on serial imaging

Macroscopic Features
- Solitary or bilateral, discrete intraventricular mass
- Calcified (gritty), cystic, vascular, hemorrhagic

Microscopic Pathology
- Epithelioid eosinophilic cells, eccentric nuclei
- Pyramidal cells with vesicular nuclei, nucleoli
- Nuclear pleomorphism, atypia: Not malignant
- Vascular stroma, hemorrhage, calcification
- Rare mitoses, necrosis, vascular proliferation

Ancillary Tests
- GFAP, S100, neuronal markers: Variably positive

Diagnostic Checklist
- Subependymal nodule, SEGT: Histologically identical
- SEGT: Diagnostic of TSC, may be 1st manifestation

- Subependymal hamartomas often coexist anteriorly
- Rarely: 3rd ventricle, paraventricular (in parenchyma)
  - Possible origin in paramedian channels
    - Between lateral and 3rd ventricles

Presentation
- CSF obstruction, ↑ intracranial pressure (ICP)
  - Headache, papilledema, hydrocephalus
  - Acute (spontaneous) hemorrhage may occur
- Longstanding history of seizures, epilepsy
  - TSC-related cortical tubers, white matter heterotopia
- Other TSC-related symptoms
  - Autistic withdrawal, mental retardation, behavioral abnormalities, infantile spasms

Natural History
- Subependymal hamartomas, SEGTs
  - Can show progressive growth
  - Enlargement on serial imaging studies
- Often extends into foramen of Monro, 3rd ventricle
  - Causing CSF obstruction
- Malignant transformation, metastasis
  - Exceptionally rare: Only single cases reported

Treatment
- Surgical approaches
  - Principal treatment, large lesions can be debulked
  - Favorable postoperative course

Prognosis
- Good prognosis, long survival after (sub)total resection
  - May recur after resection → re-excise
- SEGT may be cause of death in TSC
  - Due to ↑ ICP (herniation), seizures, hemorrhage

IMAGE FINDINGS

General Features
- Location
  - Intraventricular, demarcated from caudate nucleus
    - Adjacent to and obstructing foramen of Monro
- Morphology
  - Nodular, multicystic, vascular, variably calcified

MR Findings
- Other features of TSC often present
  - Calcified subependymal nodules in lateral ventricles
    - "Candle drippings" or "gutterings"
  - Cortical tubers with rarefaction or cyst formation
    - Hyperintense on T2-weighted MR
  - Linear abnormalities, white matter hypomyelination

CT Findings
- Contrast-enhancing, solid, discrete, bulky mass
- Heterogeneous mixed hypo- and isodense regions

MACROSCOPIC FEATURES

General Features
- Solitary or bilateral, discrete intraventricular mass
- Dome-shaped, broadly based, smooth-surfaced
- Soft to firm, gray or pink (well perfused)
- May be calcified (gritty) or have cystic degeneration
- Obvious vascular elements, variable hemorrhage

MICROSCOPIC PATHOLOGY

Histologic Features
- Sharp demarcation from brain parenchyma
  - May be only minimally infiltrative
  - Growth in solid pattern or clusters
- Coarse, astroglial fibrillar background
  - May form vaguely rosette-like structures
  - Larger, irregular (vs. ependymal pseudorosettes)
- Prominent microvascular stroma
  - Dilated channels, thin hyalinized walls
  - Old and recent hemorrhage may be present
- Calcospherites, perivascular calcification

Cytologic Features
- Large, plump, polygonal epithelioid cells
  - Glassy eosinophilic or dark red cytoplasm
  - Phenotypically astrocytic, resemble gemistocytes
  - Bipolar or multipolar, with eccentric nuclei

SUBEPENDYMAL GIANT CELL TUMOR

- Giant pyramidal cells, may be multinucleated
  - Round vesicular nuclei, distinct nucleoli
  - Fine granular chromatin, resemble ganglion cells
  - Intranuclear inclusions of cytoplasm
- Smaller, spindle or fusiform cells also seen
  - Long processes, loose growth in fascicles
- Occasional nuclear pleomorphism, atypia
  - Rare mitoses, necrosis, vascular proliferation
  - Do not signify malignancy
- Mast cells commonly present, T cells sometimes

Subependymal Hamartoma

- Elevated, calcified nodules, smaller than SEGT
- Anteriorly in lateral ventricles, near foramen of Monro
  - May enlarge sufficiently to obstruct CSF
- Large cells with abundant eosinophilic cytoplasm
  - Histologically indistinguishable from SEGT

Cortical Tuber

- Firm, nodular lesion in cerebral or cerebellar cortex
- Abnormal cortical lamination, dysmorphic neurons
- Variable numbers of large eosinophilic cells
  - Histologically identical to those in SEGT

ANCILLARY TESTS

Cytology

- Glassy cytoplasm, eccentric nuclei
- Fibrillar cell processes (1 pole, opposite nucleus)

Immunohistochemistry

- Astrocytic differentiation (large, spindle cells)
  - GFAP: May be focal or weak, in cell processes
  - S100: Usually strong and widespread
- Neuronal differentiation (ganglioid cells)
  - Class III β-tubulin (TUJ1), neuropeptides
  - Synaptophysin, neurofilament, chromogranin, NSE
- MIB-1 labeling index generally low (mean: ~ 1%)
- Tuberin: Positive in cortical tubers, not SEGT
- HMB-45: Positive in systemic lesions of TSC
  - Not present in SEGT or other CNS hamartomas

Cytogenetics

- Loss of heterozygosity in *TSC1*, *TSC2* (some SEGTs)
- Chromosomal imbalances are rare

Electron Microscopy

- Aggregates of intermediate filaments, microtubules
  - In cytoplasm, cytoplasmic processes
- Junctions to pial membrane, capillary basal lamina
- Electron-dense lysosomes, secretory granules
- Nissl-like stacks of rough endoplasmic reticulum
- Ependymal differentiation: Blepharoplasts, 9+2 cilia

DIFFERENTIAL DIAGNOSIS

Gemistocytic Astrocytoma

- Infiltrative, intraparenchymal lesion in older adults
- Uniform processes around entire cell circumference

Giant Cell Glioblastoma

- Intraparenchymal tumor, poor prognosis
- Giant, histologically malignant cells

Ependymoma

- Perivascular pseudorosettes, true ependymal rosettes
- Smaller, less astrocytic cells, lack vesicular nuclei

DIAGNOSTIC CHECKLIST

Clinically Relevant Pathologic Features

- Subependymal nodule, SEGT: Histologically identical
  - Criteria to distinguish the 2 are inconsistent
  - Currently, lesion considered tumor (i.e., SEGT)
    - Clinically: Large enough to cause symptoms (e.g., hydrocephalus), usually > 1-1.2 cm
    - Radiologically: Growth on serial imaging or contrast enhancing
- SEGT: Virtually diagnostic of TSC
  - May be 1st manifestation of TSC
    - Subclinical (forme fruste): 30-40% of TSC cases
  - Follow-up MR may identify tubers, hamartomas
  - Should probably also undergo genetic counseling
- Large symptomatic lesion in foramen of Monro
  - Probably SEGT until proven otherwise
- Slow-growing asymptomatic SEGTs in TSC
  - Discovered during routine radiologic screening
- Anaplastic features in SEGT do not affect outcome

Pathologic Interpretation Pearls

- Other CNS neoplasms with mast cells
  - Meningioma, hemangioblastoma
- Large cells of SEGT differ from gemistocytic astrocytes
  - More cytoplasm
  - Less hyperchromatic vesicular nuclei
  - Asymmetric fibrillar cell processes
    - Only on cell surface opposite nucleus

SELECTED REFERENCES

1. Buccoliero AM et al: Subependymal giant cell astrocytoma (SEGA): Is it an astrocytoma? Morphological, immunohistochemical and ultrastructural study. Neuropathology. 29(1):25-30, 2009
2. Goh S et al: Subependymal giant cell tumors in tuberous sclerosis complex. Neurology. 63(8):1457-61, 2004
3. Sharma MC et al: Subependymal giant cell astrocytoma--a clinicopathological study of 23 cases with special emphasis on histogenesis. Pathol Oncol Res. 10(4):219-24, 2004
4. Lopes MB et al: Immunohistochemical characterization of subependymal giant cell astrocytomas. Acta Neuropathol. 91(4):368-75, 1996
5. Hirose T et al: Tuber and subependymal giant cell astrocytoma associated with tuberous sclerosis: an immunohistochemical, ultrastructural, and immunoelectron and microscopic study. Acta Neuropathol. 90(4):387-99, 1995
6. Sinson G et al: Subependymal giant cell astrocytomas in children. Pediatr Neurosurg. 20(4):233-9, 1994
7. Shepherd CW et al: Subependymal giant cell astrocytoma: a clinical, pathological, and flow cytometric study. Neurosurgery. 28(6):864-8, 1991
8. Bonnin JM et al: Subependymal giant cell astrocytoma. Significance and possible cytogenetic implications of an immunohistochemical study. Acta Neuropathol. 62(3):185-93, 1984

Microscopic Features

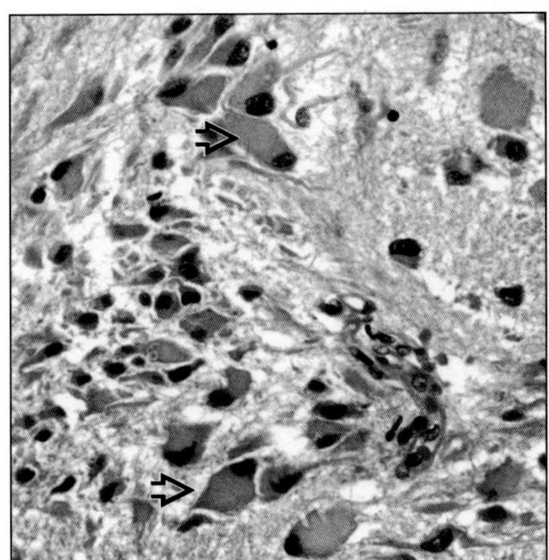

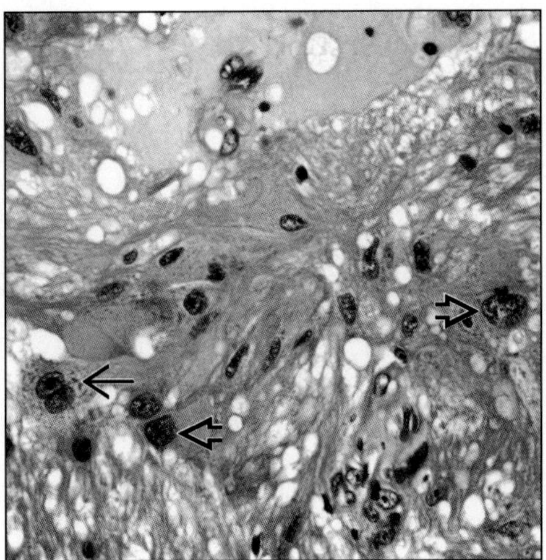

(Left) Hematoxylin & eosin shows a high-power view of the classic large cells in SEGT with glassy eosinophilic cytoplasm and eccentric nuclei ➡, distinctively resembling gemistocytic astrocytes. **(Right)** Hematoxylin & eosin shows a high-power view of tumor cells in SEGT with a more characteristically neuronal appearance. These cells may be binucleated →, and have large, round, and vesicular nuclei ➡ with fine granular chromatin and prominent nucleoli.

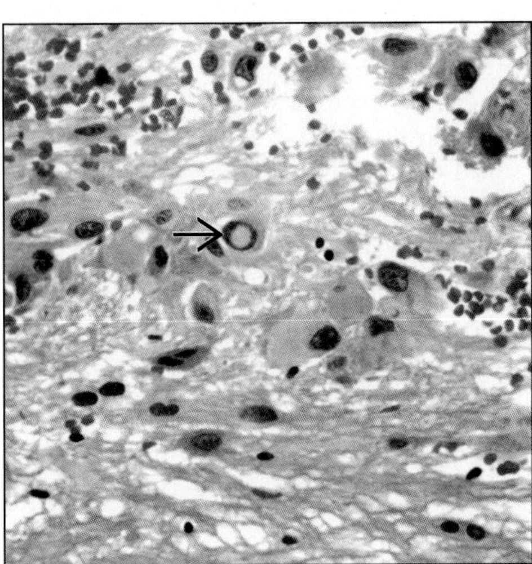

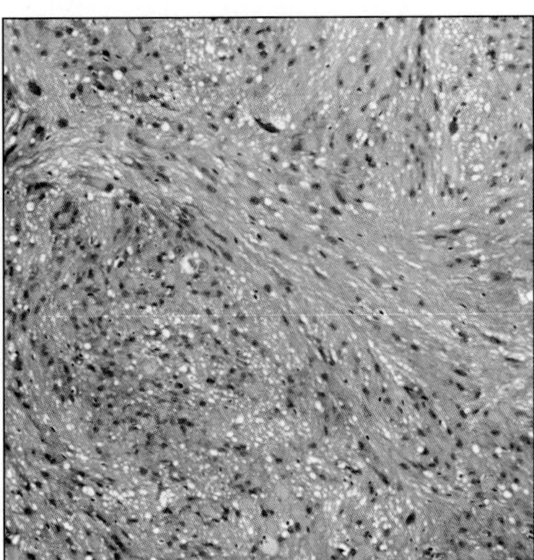

(Left) Hematoxylin & eosin shows a high-power view of the tumor cells in SEGT that resemble neuronal or ganglion cells, and which may have intranuclear inclusions of cytoplasm →. **(Right)** Hematoxylin & eosin shows a low-power view of SEGT with relatively coarse, fibrillary astroglial background where some tumor cells are smaller with a more fusiform or spindle appearance, long processes, and growth in loose fascicles.

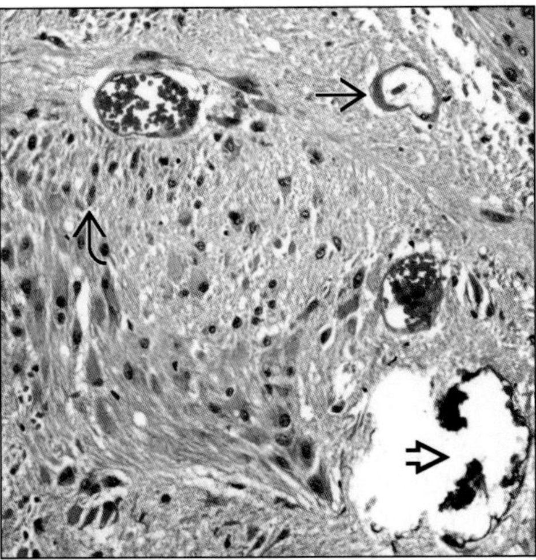

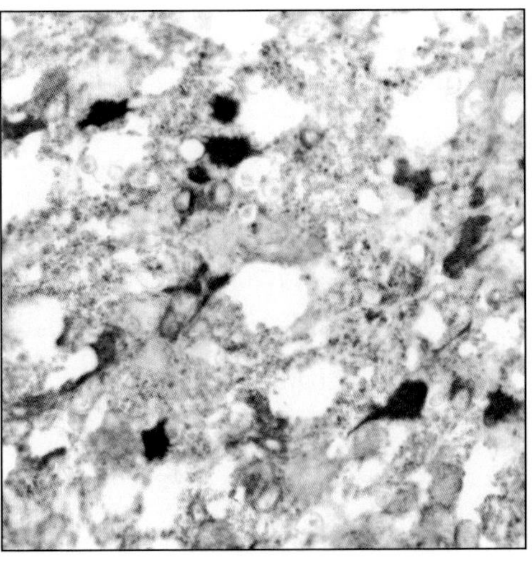

(Left) Hematoxylin & eosin shows a medium-power view of SEGT with dilated vascular channels having hyalinized walls →, prominent calcospherites and calcifications ➡, and vaguely rosette-like ↗ perivascular arrangement of tumor cells. **(Right)** GFAP immunostain shows a high-power view of SEGT where most cells stain positive, supporting the astrocytic differentiation of the tumor.

CRANIOPHARYNGIOMA

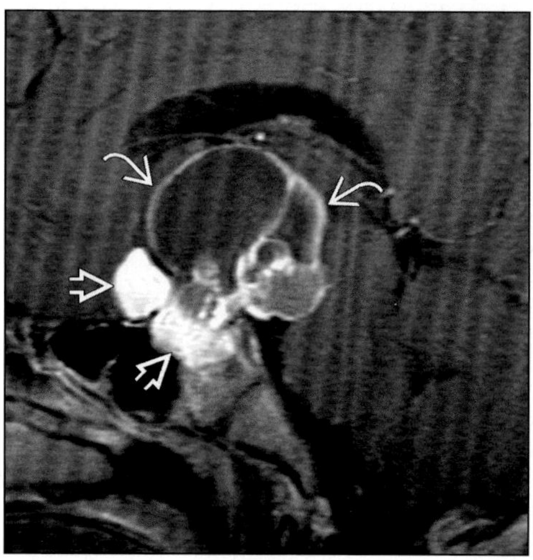

Sagittal MR shows a complex, partially cystic suprasellar mass with enhancing rim ➔ and solid components ➔. This is the classic appearance of craniopharyngioma.

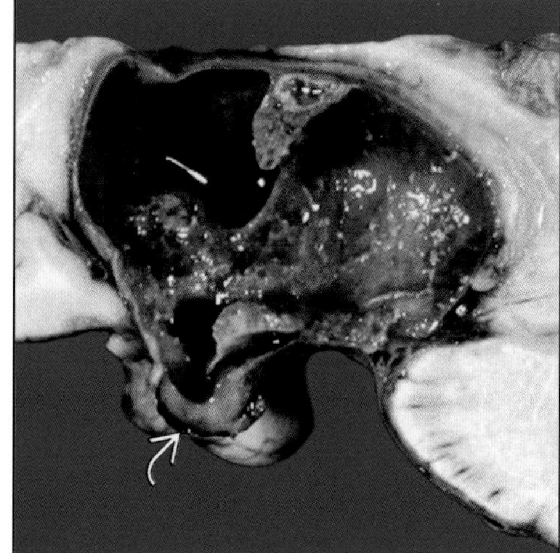

Gross photograph shows a classic ACP with mixed solid and cystic components. Note the intrasellar extension ➔, which is a common finding. (Courtesy R. Hewlett, MD.)

TERMINOLOGY

Abbreviations

- Adamantinomatous craniopharyngioma (ACP)
- (Squamous) papillary craniopharyngioma (PCP)

Synonyms

- Suprasellar papillary squamous epithelioma = PCP

Definitions

- Slow-growing, partially cystic, relatively rare epithelial neoplasms of sellar region
- Histologically benign (WHO grade I) but with location-related adverse sequelae
- 2 clinicopathologically distinct variants
  - Adamantinomatous craniopharyngioma
    - Sellar epithelial neoplasm of childhood with similarity to odontogenic tumors
  - Papillary craniopharyngioma
    - Well-differentiated, squamous pseudopapillary neoplasm in 3rd ventricle of adults

ETIOLOGY/PATHOGENESIS

Theories of Histogenesis/Derivation

- Embryogenetic hypothesis
  - Neoplastic transformation of ectodermal epithelium
    - Rathke pouch (cleft)
    - Hypophyseal-pharyngeal (craniopharyngeal) duct
  - Fails to develop into adenohypophysis
  - Differentiates into tooth primordia → ACP
    - ACP express pituitary hormones, chromogranin, human chorionic gonadotropin (hCG)
  - Differentiates into oral mucosa → PCP
    - PCP have focal cilia, goblet cells
  - Similar cytokeratin expression profiles
- Developmental aberration (variant of embryogenetic)
  - "Misplaced odontogenic epithelium"
  - Embryonic rests with enamel organ potential
  - ACP resembles jaw ameloblastoma (adamantinoma) or keratinizing and calcifying odontogenic cyst
  - Occasional ACP have erupted teeth
- Metaplasia of adenohypophyseal cells
  - Squamous metaplastic cells/nests
    - In anterior pituitary stalk (pars tuberalis)
    - Frequency of metaplasia ↑ with age
    - May better explain PCP derivation
    - Metaplastic nests occurrence peaks with ↑ age, but ACP incidence ↓ with age
- Rare examples exist with mixed ACP and PCP features
  - Possible histologic transition between 2 variants
- Subset of craniopharyngiomas shown to be monoclonal

CLINICAL ISSUES

Epidemiology

- Incidence
  - 2-5% of primary intracranial tumors
    - 5-15% of non-neuroepithelial childhood intracranial tumors
  - ACP:PCP ratio = 10:1
- Age
  - ACP
    - Peak in 1st and 2nd decades of life (5-14 years old)
    - Rare congenital examples, or in elderly
  - PCP
    - Almost exclusively in adults (peak: 50-75 years old)

Site

- ACP
  - Typically suprasellar or intrasellar
    - ~ 20-25% restricted to sellar region
  - 50-70% extend anteriorly, to retroclival area, or middle fossa
  - Rare ectopic sites

CRANIOPHARYNGIOMA

Key Facts

Etiology/Pathogenesis
- ACP resembles jaw ameloblastoma (adamantinoma) or keratinizing and calcifying odontogenic cyst
- Neoplastic ectodermal epithelium, Rathke pouch

Clinical Issues
- 5-15% of non-neuroepithelial childhood intracranial tumors, ACP:PCP ratio = 10:1
- ACP: Peak 5-14 years old, suprasellar or intrasellar
  - 50-70% extend anteriorly (retroclival, middle fossa)
- Hypothalamic-pituitary axis dysfunction
- CSF obstruction, ↑ intracranial pressure
- Mass effect: Visual disturbances, headache
- Cognitive impairment, chemical meningitis (spillage)
- Gross total resection, avoid operative damage nearby
  - Irregular margins: Difficult resection
- 60-95% recurrence-free and overall 10-year survival

Macroscopic Features
- Cystic, necrotic debris, fibrous tissue, calcification
- Characteristic fluid contents ("machine oil")

Microscopic Pathology
- "Clover leaf": Broad and anastomosing trabeculae
- Peripherally palisaded columnar-appearing cells
  - With "wet keratin," practically diagnostic of ACP
- Internal, loose squamous cells ("stellate reticulum")
- Compact, nodular "wet keratin" whorls
- Inflammatory, foreign body-type giant cell reaction
- Nuclear β-catenin staining (only seen in ACP)

Diagnostic Checklist
- PCP: Pseudopapillary tumor in 3rd ventricle of adults
  - Simple, well-differentiated squamous epithelium
  - Fibrovascular cores, focal cilia, goblet cells

    - Sphenoid bone, nasopharynx, posterior fossa (cerebellopontine angle), optic chiasm, pineal
- PCP
  - Usually suprasellar, tends to involve 3rd ventricle

Presentation
- Often insidious
  - Delay between disease onset and actual diagnosis
- Hypothalamic-pituitary axis dysfunction
  - Hypopituitarism
    - Growth retardation, diabetes insipidus, amenorrhea, precocious or delayed puberty
- Cerebrospinal fluid (CSF) obstruction
  - ↑ intracranial pressure
    - Mostly in pediatric patients
  - Hydrocephalus, headache, nausea, vomiting
- Mass effect (proximity to optic chiasm)
  - Visual disturbance or loss, headache
- Cognitive impairment
  - Diminished mental acuity, personality changes
- Chemical meningitis
  - Spillage of irritant cholesterol-rich cyst contents into CSF

Natural History
- Histologically benign and slow growing
  - But behavior is unpredictable
  - Delicate structures involved
  - High morbidity, mortality
    - Surgery may be difficult
- May recur after incomplete resection
  - Especially without adjuvant radiotherapy (58%)
- Meningeal/CSF seeding and spread: Exceptionally rare

Treatment
- Options, risks, complications
  - Operative damage to nearby structures
    - Hypothalamus, optic nerve
    - Benefit of total resection controversial
  - Uncommon ectopic recurrence
    - Due to CSF dissemination or intraoperative implantation
- Surgical approaches
  - Gross total resection
    - Reduces recurrence to 10-20%
    - May be more successful in PCP (better defined borders)
    - Irregular margins in ACP pose difficulty in achieving good surgical planes
- Adjuvant therapy
  - Radiotherapy
    - For incomplete resections, recurrence
    - Reduces recurrence after subtotal resection to 30%
  - Newer approaches: Brachytherapy, chemotherapy
    - No clear consensus as to best treatment
- Preoperative assessment
  - Ophthalmologic examination
  - Testing for endocrine deficiencies
    - Growth hormone (GH), luteinizing hormone (LH), follicle-stimulating hormone (FSH), adrenocorticotrophic hormone (ACTH), thyroid-stimulating hormone (TSH)

Prognosis
- 60-95% recurrence-free and overall 10-year survival
  - Lesions > 5 cm diameter
    - Markedly worse prognosis
- Recurrences often adhere to local structures
  - May become unresectable as a result
  - May have higher Ki-67 labeling index
    - ~ 13% in lesions that recurred in 1 study
    - Vs. ~ 3% in nonrecurring lesions
    - Prognostic significance unclear
- Single reports of malignant transformation
  - To squamous cell carcinoma
  - After local radiation therapy
- Good prognostic factors (lower risk of recurrence)
  - Small size (< 4 cm)
  - Favorable site
  - Complete (gross total) surgical resection
  - Age > 5 years
  - Absence of severe hypothalamic involvement
  - Ki-67 labeling index < 7%

CRANIOPHARYNGIOMA

IMAGE FINDINGS

General Features

- ACP
  - Lobulated, intra- or suprasellar mass
  - Partly calcified, especially peripherally
    - May be seen in plain radiographs
- PCP
  - More solid, generally lack calcification

MR Findings

- ACP
  - Bright cystic areas in pre-contrast T1WI
    - Due to protein-rich contents

CT Findings

- ACP
  - Contrast enhancing, cystic

MACROSCOPIC FEATURES

General Features

- ACP
  - Fill suprasellar region, adhere to vessel/nerves at brain base
  - Irregular interference with adjacent brain
    - Especially pituitary stalk, after recurrence
  - Cystic with necrotic debris, fibrous tissue, calcification
  - Characteristic fluid contents ("machine oil")
    - a.k.a. "machinery oil"
    - Opaque, thick, yellow-brown fluid
    - Contains shiny cholesterol crystals
    - Orthogonal, notched (under polarized light)
- PCP
  - Mostly solid, less cystic, with conspicuous papillations
  - Well-circumscribed, smooth interface with brain parenchyma
    - May be encapsulated
  - Lacks calcifications, "machine oil"

Size

- Most (60-80%) of craniopharyngiomas are 2-4 cm
  - Rare giant lesions (up to 12 cm) described

MICROSCOPIC PATHOLOGY

Predominant Pattern/Injury Type

- Neoplastic
- Cystic

Predominant Cell/Compartment Type

- Epithelial, squamous

Histologic Features, ACP

- Characteristic architectural appearance
  - Resembles "clover leaf"
  - Broad and anastomosing trabeculae
  - Sheets, nodules, whorls, lobules, cords of cells
- Orderly arranged squamous epithelium
  - Peripherally palisaded columnar-appearing cells
    - Resting on basement membrane
  - Intervening layer of polygonal cells
  - Internal, loosely aggregated stellate squamous cells
    - So-called "stellate reticulum"
  - Final layer of of flat, plate-like squamous cells
    - May keratinize and merge with keratin whorls
- Compact, nodular "wet keratin" whorls
  - Plump, eosinophilic, keratinized cells
  - Necrotic cells with ghost nuclei
  - Often undergo dystrophic calcification or even ossification
- Cystic degeneration common
  - Epithelium becomes flattened, attenuated, fibrotic
- Inflammatory and foreign body-type giant cell reaction
  - Often caused by necrotic keratinous debris
  - Chronic histiocytic reaction (xanthoma cells)
  - Cholesterol clefts
- Rarely, melanosomal pigment may be present

Histologic Features, PCP

- Simple, well-differentiated squamous epithelium
  - Resembles oropharyngeal mucosa
  - Generally in solid sheets
  - Separate (dehisce), forming "crack" artifacts
    - Result in arborizing pseudopapillary appearance
- Prominent anastomosing fibrovascular stroma cores
- Small epithelial or collagenous whorls
- Focal cilia, mucin-producing columnar (goblet) cells
- Small numbers of chronic inflammatory cells may be seen

ANCILLARY TESTS

Cytology

- Sheets of cohesive monomorphous epithelium
- Nodules of "wet keratin" in ACP

Immunohistochemistry

- Nuclear β-catenin staining
  - Only seen in ACP
- Often EMA/MUC1(+)
- May also be ERP, PRP, IGF-1 receptor, and somatostatin positive
  - Uncertain biologic significance
  - Treating craniopharyngioma cell cultures with progesterone and IGF-1 receptor inhibitors may result in growth arrest
- Usually cytokeratin positive
  - Especially CK7
  - Reported negative for CK8, CK20

Cytogenetics

- Few chromosomal abnormalities reported
  - Translocations, deletions, increased DNA copies
- Mutations in exon 3 of β-catenin (tumor suppressor gene)
  - Resulting in nuclear accumulation
  - Transcriptional activation of Wnt pathway
  - Found exclusively in ACP

Electron Microscopy

- Evidence of squamous differentiation

- Intermediate filament bundles
- Well-formed desmosomes
- Basal lamina on cells abutting stroma

DIFFERENTIAL DIAGNOSIS

Dermoid or Epidermoid Cyst

- Uniloculated, with fibrous capsule
- Contain dry, flaky, lamellar keratin
- Lined by attenuated stratified squamous epithelium
- Cells uniformly mature toward surface
  - Keratinization (thin anucleate squamous), keratohyaline granules
- Lack palisaded cells, calcification, histiocytes, debris, or "machine oil"

Xanthogranuloma of Sellar Region

- Intrasellar cyst with degenerative changes
- Cholesterol clefts, macrophages, debris, hemosiderin
- Mostly seen in adolescents, young adults
- Smaller size: Better resectability, outcome

Rathke Cleft Cyst

- Especially with squamous metaplasia vs. PCP
- Lack solid growth component
- Extensive ciliation, mucin production (goblet cells)
- May have epithelial atrophy, xanthogranulomatous change
- CK8 and CK20 positive

Pilocytic Astrocytoma

- Gliotic parenchyma near infiltrative ACP margins
- More cellular; have microcysts, granular bodies

DIAGNOSTIC CHECKLIST

Clinically Relevant Pathologic Features

- Gross appearance
- ACP
  - Cyst fluid or CSF may contain ↑ HCG levels
  - May be rarely complicated by abscess
    - Abundant neutrophils seen
- ACP after radiation or recurrence
  - Mostly degenerative, fibrotic, with amorphous debris
    - Xanthogranulomatous reaction
  - Diagnostic epithelium difficult to identify
  - Look for diagnostic features
- PCP
  - Generally more indolent behavior
  - Smaller size, less extension into surroundings
  - More respectable, lower recurrence rate

Pathologic Interpretation Pearls

- Practically diagnostic of ACP
  - Adamantinomatous epithelium
    - Palisading peripherally
    - Stellate reticulum
  - "Wet keratin"
    - Often calcified
- Highly suggestive of ACP but not pathognomonic
  - Calcification
  - Necrotic debris
  - Cholesterol clefts
  - Fibrohistiocytic reaction (xanthoma cells)
  - "Machine oil"
- Features lacking in PCP
  - Peripherally palisading epithelium
  - "Wet keratin"
  - "Machine oil"
  - Calcification
  - Cholesterol clefts
- ACP margins may infiltrate surrounding brain parenchyma
  - Resulting in dense reactive piloid gliosis
  - Rosenthal fibers may be seen
  - Resembles pilocytic astrocytoma
    - Do not misdiagnose

SELECTED REFERENCES

1. Gleeson H et al: 'Do no harm': management of craniopharyngioma. Eur J Endocrinol. 159 Suppl 1:S95-9, 2008
2. Karavitaki N et al: Craniopharyngiomas. Endocrinol Metab Clin North Am. 37(1):173-93, ix-x, 2008
3. Muller HL: Childhood craniopharyngioma. Recent advances in diagnosis, treatment and follow-up. Horm Res. 69(4):193-202, 2008
4. Garnett MR et al: Craniopharyngioma. Orphanet J Rare Dis. 2:18, 2007
5. Garrè ML et al: Craniopharyngioma: modern concepts in pathogenesis and treatment. Curr Opin Pediatr. 19(4):471-9, 2007
6. Ohmori K et al: Craniopharyngiomas in children. Pediatr Neurosurg. 43(4):265-78, 2007
7. Rodriguez FJ et al: The spectrum of malignancy in craniopharyngioma. Am J Surg Pathol. 31(7):1020-8, 2007
8. Jane JA Jr et al: Craniopharyngioma. Pituitary. 9(4):323-6, 2006
9. May JA et al: Craniopharyngioma in childhood. Adv Pediatr. 53:183-209, 2006
10. Karavitaki N et al: Craniopharyngiomas in children and adults: systematic analysis of 121 cases with long-term follow-up. Clin Endocrinol (Oxf). 62(4):397-409, 2005
11. Tavangar SM et al: Craniopharyngioma: a clinicopathological study of 141 cases. Endocr Pathol. 15(4):339-44, 2004
12. Burger PC et al: Surgical pathology of the nervous system and its coverings. Philadelphia: Churchill Livingstone. 475-83, 2002
13. Janzer RC et al: Craniopharyngioma. In Kleihues P et al: Pathology and Genetics: Tumors of the Nervous System. Lyon: IARC Press. 244-6, 2000
14. Miller DC: Pathology of craniopharyngiomas: clinical import of pathological findings. Pediatr Neurosurg. 21 Suppl 1:11-7, 1994

CRANIOPHARYNGIOMA

Microscopic Features of ACP

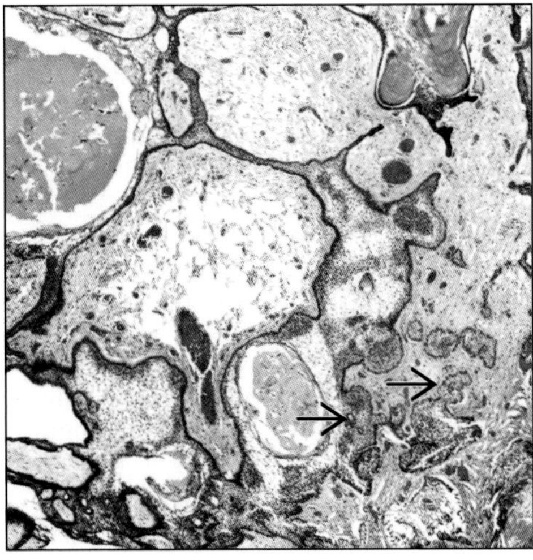
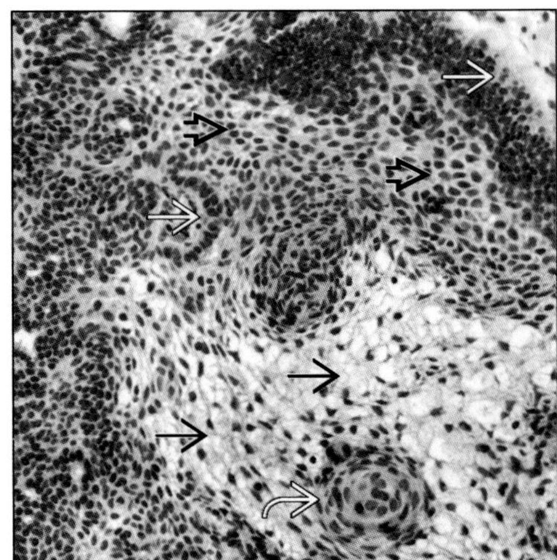

(Left) *Hematoxylin & eosin shows low-power view of ACP with cystic change and broad anastomosing trabeculae of epithelium that resemble clover leaves →.* ***(Right)*** *H&E shows a high-power view of ACP with characteristic, orderly arranged layers: Outer, peripherally palisading columnar-type cells →, intervening polygonal cells →, & internal loose aggregates of stellate squamous cells → ("stellate reticulum"). A final layer of flat, plate-like squames → merges with whorls, which will eventually become "wet keratin."*

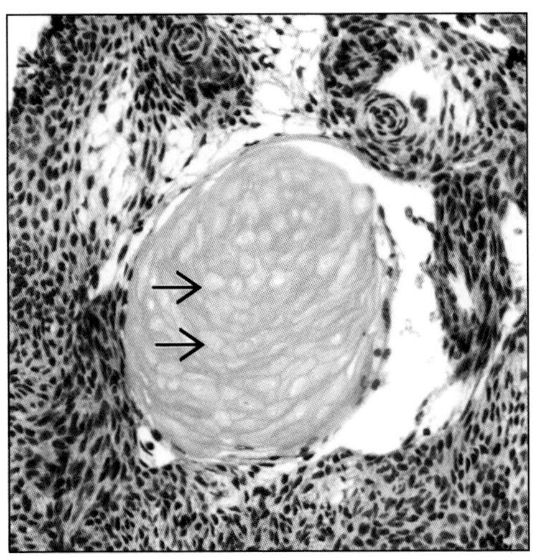
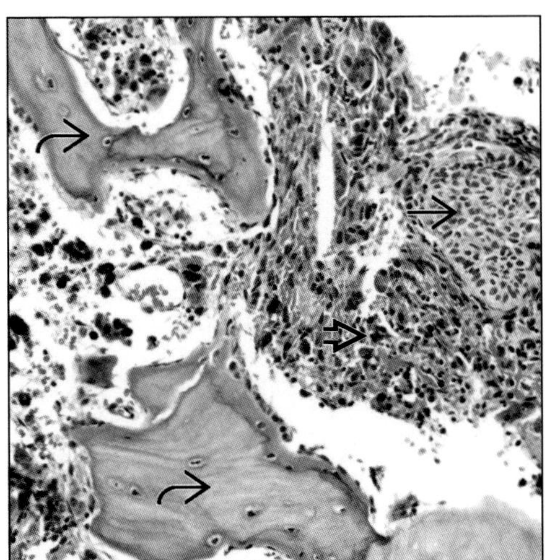

(Left) *Hematoxylin & eosin shows a high-power view of ACP with a classic "wet keratin" whorl: A compact nodule of plump, eosinophilic, and necrotic keratinized cells with ghost nuclei →. Practically diagnostic of ACP, these can often undergo calcification.* ***(Right)*** *Hematoxylin & eosin shows a medium-power view of ACP with adamantinomatous epithelium →, old hemorrhage →, and ossification →, which can be seen as the result of longstanding, extensive dystrophic calcification.*

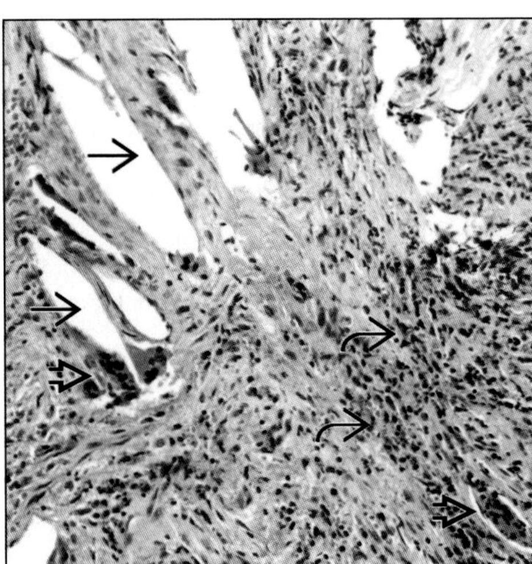
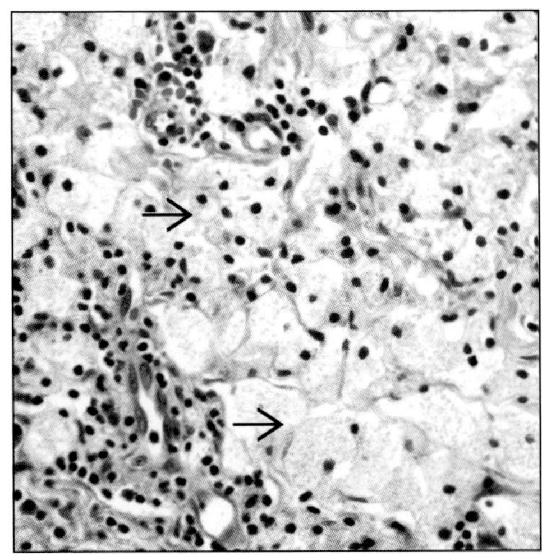

(Left) *Hematoxylin & eosin shows a medium-power view of ACP with foreign body reaction characterized by cholesterol clefts →, multinucleated giant cells →, and old hemorrhage composed of hemosiderin-laden macrophages →.* ***(Right)*** *Hematoxylin & eosin shows a high-power view of foamy histiocytes → (xanthoma cells), part of the chronic inflammatory reaction that is commonly seen in ACP.*

Microscopic Features of PCP

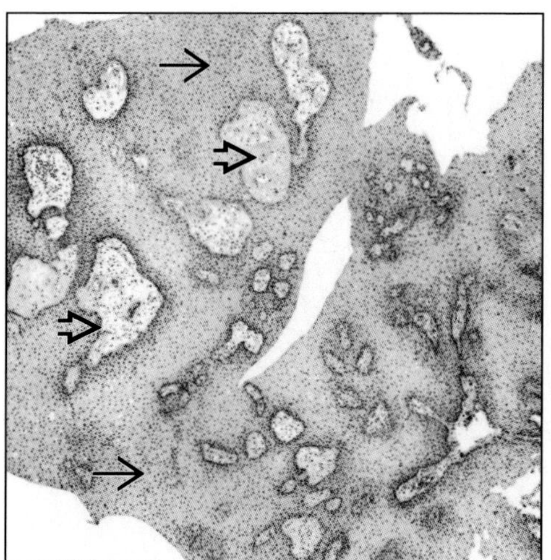

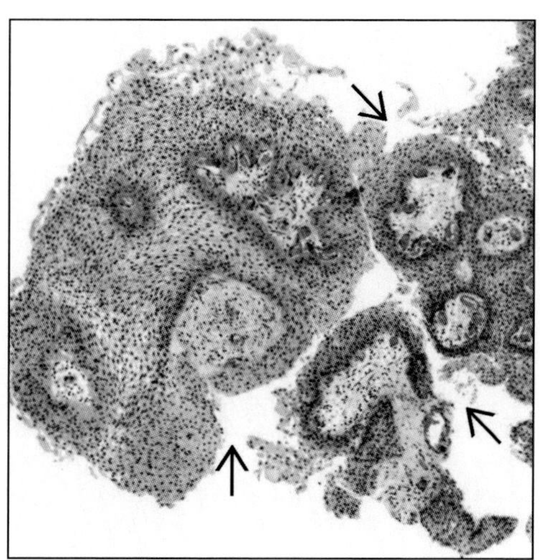

(Left) Hematoxylin & eosin shows a low-power view of a suprasellar mass composed of solid sheets of well-differentiated squamous epithelium ➔ overlying prominent anastomosing cores of fibrovascular stroma ➲. This appearance, which resembles oropharyngeal mucosa, is classic for PCP. **(Right)** Hematoxylin & eosin shows a medium-power view of PCP where fragments of tissue separate (dehisce), resulting in "cracks" ➔ that give the appearance of arborizing papillae (pseudopapillary).

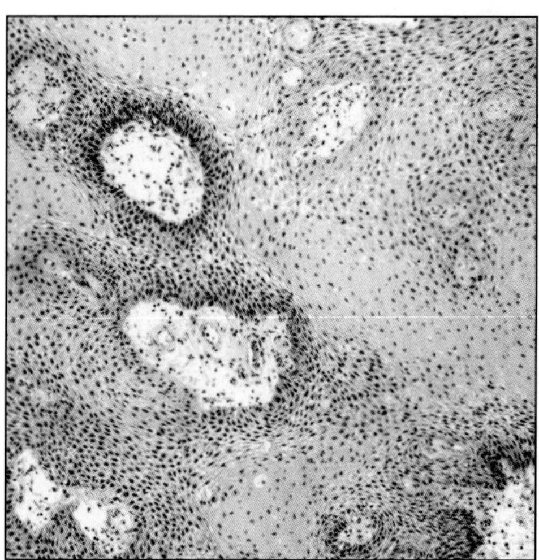

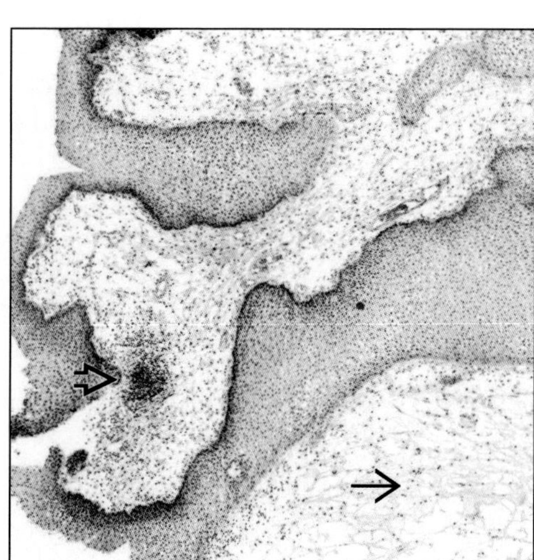

(Left) Hematoxylin & eosin shows a high-power view of PCP characterized by mature squamous epithelium without the peripheral palisading, "wet keratin," or "stellate reticulum" features seen in classic ACP. **(Right)** Hematoxylin & eosin shows a medium-power view of PCP with edematous change ➔ and focal chronic inflammation ➲, features that are commonly seen in the fibrovascular stroma.

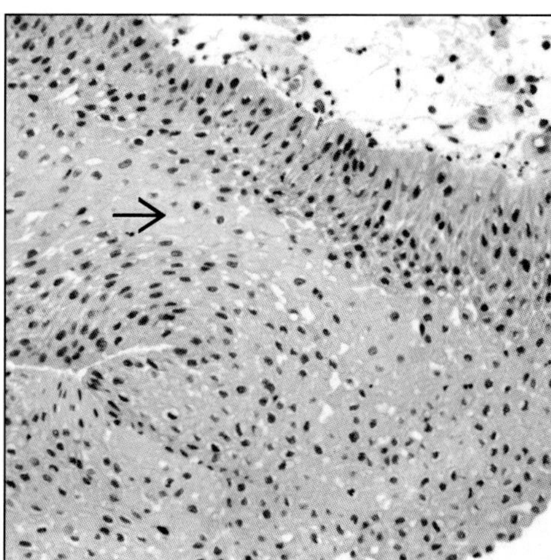

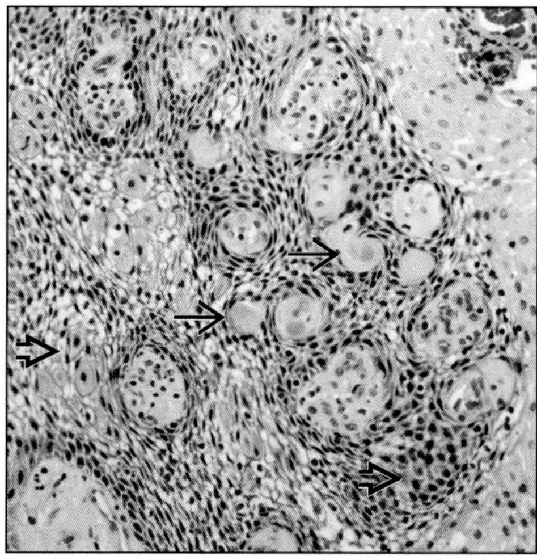

(Left) Hematoxylin & eosin shows a high-power view of a PCP with well-differentiated squamous epithelium showing the graded maturation ➔ commonly seen in all squamous mucosal surfaces, such as in the oropharyngeal cavity. **(Right)** Hematoxylin & eosin shows a high-power view of PCP where small epithelial ➲ or collagenous ➔ whorls can be seen but not to the extent of the "wet keratin" whorls of ACP.

MENINGIOANGIOMATOSIS

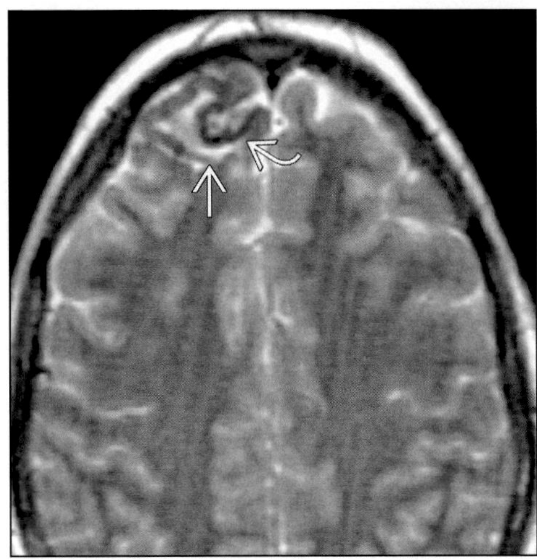

Axial T2WI MR shows focal curvilinear cortical hypointensity ➡ that corresponded to calcification and underlying edema ➡ in the subcortical white matter.

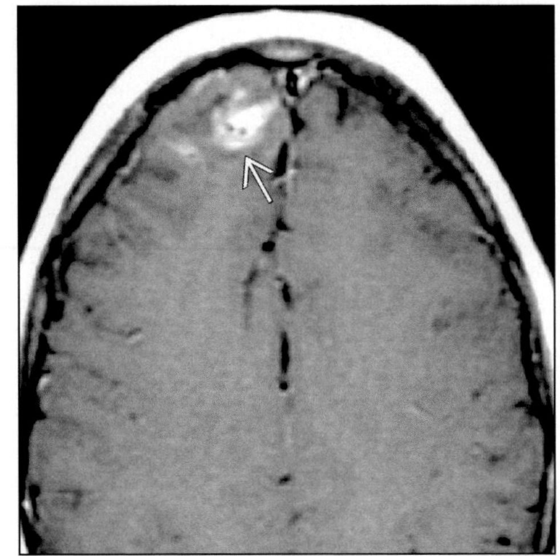

Axial T1WI MR with contrast shows leptomeningeal and gyriform cortical enhancement ➡ in the right superior frontal gyrus, likely due to proliferation of blood vessels and meningothelial cells.

TERMINOLOGY

Abbreviations

- Meningioangiomatosis (MA)
- Neurofibromatosis type 2 (NF2)

Synonyms

- (Meningeal) meningiomatosis

Definitions

- Rare, benign, most likely nonneoplastic lesion
- Focal, plaque-like, and mostly intracortical, involving leptomeninges and subarachnoid space with perivascular ingrowth into cerebral cortex
- Proliferation of meningothelial and fibroblast-like cells with leptomeningeal calcification
- Originally described in association with NF2

ETIOLOGY/PATHOGENESIS

Histogenesis

- Meningothelial cell origin favored
  - Meningothelial features of proliferating cells
    - Histologic, immunohistochemical, ultrastructural
    - Psammoma bodies, epithelioid appearance
  - Rare concurrence of MA with meningioma
    - Both meningioma and MA occur in NF2
- Alternatively from perivascular mesenchymal cells
  - Fibroblasts, pericytes

Neoplastic vs. Nonneoplastic Process

- Most cases (~ 75%) are sporadic
  - ~ 25% arise in NF2
  - Sporadic MA may be forme fruste of NF2
    - *NF2* gene deletion found in only rare sporadic cases
- Appears more reactive or hamartomatous
  - Developmental, malformative lesion
  - Vascular-type malformations often accompany phakomatoses (NF2)

CLINICAL ISSUES

Epidemiology

- Incidence
  - Rare, ~ 100 cases reported in literature
- Age
  - Children, young adults
  - Only 10% are > 40 years old
- Gender
  - M > F (2:1) in sporadic MA

Site

- Intracortical (90%)
  - Most (70%) are located in frontotemporal region
  - Right > left hemisphere (2:1)
- Rare extracortical lesions have been described
  - 3rd ventricle, thalamus, brainstem
  - More likely to occur in NF2
- Usually single when sporadic
  - May be multifocal in NF2

Presentation

- Long history of intractable partial seizures/epilepsy
- Persistent headaches, nausea
- May be asymptomatic in NF2
  - Discovered incidentally at autopsy

Natural History

- Slow-growing lesion

Treatment

- Surgical approaches
  - Complete surgical removal

Prognosis

- Excellent
  - Generally cured by surgical excision
  - Recurrences have not been reported
- Variable postoperative resolution of seizures
  - Up to 70% of patients need to continue on anti-epileptics

MENINGIOANGIOMATOSIS

Key Facts

Terminology
- Rare, benign, probably nonneoplastic lesion
- Originally described in association with NF2

Etiology/Pathogenesis
- Most (~ 75%) are sporadic, ~ 25% arise in NF2

Clinical Issues
- Children, young adults, male > female
- Intracortical (90%), mostly in frontotemporal region
  - Right > left hemisphere (2:1)
- Long history of intractable partial seizures/epilepsy
  - May be asymptomatic in NF2
- Generally cured by surgical excision
  - Variable postoperative resolution of seizures

Image Findings
- Cortical mass with enhancement, calcification

Macroscopic Features
- Firm, discrete, vascular, plaque-like superficial mass
- Intracortical ingrowth from overlying subarachnoid

Microscopic Pathology
- Perivascular sheaths of proliferating cells
  - Elongated, spindle, or fusiform, fibroblast-like
  - May be meningothelial, forming nodules or lobules
- Serpentine vessels, often with hyalinized walls
- Scattered psammoma bodies or calcospherites
- Trapped neurons, may show neurodegeneration

Ancillary Tests
- Some perivascular cells are EMA(+)
- MIB-1 labeling index low (< 1-2%)

IMAGE FINDINGS

General Features
- Best diagnostic clue
  - Cortical mass with enhancement
  - Calcification but generally little mass effect

MR Findings
- Superficial, hypointense (dark) mass on T2WI
  - Due to fibrous tissue and calcium content
- Mild hyperintense vasogenic edema
  - In underlying white matter

CT Findings
- Leptomeningeal and cortical mass
  - White (calcified), may be enhancing
- Rare hemorrhage, cysts
- Surrounding low-density edema

MACROSCOPIC FEATURES

General Features
- Firm, dense, discrete, vascular, plaque-like superficial mass
  - Psammomatous calcification or osteoid formation
- Intracortical ingrowth from overlying subarachnoid space
  - Follows, thickens, and obscures contours of cortex
- Serpentine vessels often seen overlying lesion

Size
- Generally small, < 5 cm

MICROSCOPIC PATHOLOGY

Histologic Features
- Cortex largely replaced by nodular fibrous tissue
  - Leptomeningeal meningothelial and meningovascular proliferation
  - Small islands of intervening gliotic parenchyma
  - Trapped cortical neurons, may show neurodegenerative changes
    - Neurofibrillary tangles (NFT), granulovacuolar degeneration, Pick bodies
- Scattered psammoma bodies or calcospherites common
  - Osseous metaplasia (osteoid) in advanced cases
- Serpentine vessels, often with hyalinized walls
  - In tumor and in overlying subarachnoid/ leptomeninges
  - Resemble vascular malformation
    - But usually of similar caliber, evenly spaced

Cytologic Features
- Perivascular sheaths of proliferating cells
  - Elongated, spindle or fusiform, fibroblast-like
  - May be meningothelial, forming nodules or lobules
  - Occasional palisading, mimic schwannoma
  - Can have relatively high nuclear to cytoplasmic ratio
    - But generally lack atypia, mitoses, or necrosis

Predominant Pattern/Injury Type
- Perivascular
- Serpentine
- Calcification
- Ossification

Predominant Cell/Compartment Type
- Mesenchymal, spindle
- Fibroblast
- Meningothelial

ANCILLARY TESTS

Immunohistochemistry
- Some perivascular cells are EMA positive
  - More spindled, fibroblastic areas are negative
- MIB-1 labeling index low (< 1-2%)
- TAU(+) NFT in trapped neurons

Electron Microscopy

- Meningothelial features
  - Cellular plasma membrane interdigitations
  - Scattered cytoplasmic intermediate filaments
  - Well-formed desmosomes, gap junctions
- Paired helical filaments (NFT) in trapped neurons

DIFFERENTIAL DIAGNOSIS

Invasive Meningioma

- Extraaxial with ragged, tongue-like invasion into parenchyma
- Less fibroblastic appearing
- Malignant cases have atypia, mitoses, necrosis
- EMA(+), high MIB-1 labeling

Vascular Malformation

- Less organized, unevenly spaced vessels
- Usually hemorrhagic
- Lacks intervening islands of gliotic cortex

Ganglion Cell Tumor

- Less collagen, no intracortical meningothelial cells
- Clearly cytologically abnormal neurons
- Perivascular lymphocytes

Calcifying Pseudotumor (Pseudoneoplasm)

- Usually extraaxial, or in craniospinal meninges
- Bosselated calcific mass
- Amorphous granular or fibrillar material

Intracranial Schwannoma

- Spindle cells with obvious palisading
- Encapsulated
- Strong positivity for S100

DIAGNOSTIC CHECKLIST

Clinically Relevant Pathologic Features

- Tissue distribution
- Gross appearance
- Age distribution
- Raises possibility that patient has NF2
  - Sporadic MA generally lack *NF2* gene mutations
- Meningioma-associated MA is probably neoplastic
  - Perivascular spread along Virchow-Robin spaces
- Relatively little mass effect, symptoms
  - Given size/location

Pathologic Interpretation Pearls

- Consider clinical and radiologic context
  - Intracortical, superficial mass, dark on T2WI MR
- Characteristic histomorphologic features
  - Perivascular proliferation of spindle cells
  - Small, uniform blood vessels with hyalinized walls
  - Intervening gliotic parenchyma with neurodegeneration
  - Calcification/ossification, psammoma bodies
- Meningeal sarcomatosis
  - Not to be confused with MA
  - Refers to diffuse leptomeningeal sarcoma
    - Not a circumscribed mass
  - Most are poorly differentiated "spindle cell" sarcomas
    - Many end up being carcinomas, lymphomas, or gliomas
    - Based on immunohistochemistry results

SELECTED REFERENCES

1. Deb P et al: Meningioangiomatosis with meningioma: an uncommon association of a rare entity--report of a case and review of the literature. Childs Nerv Syst. 22(1):78-83, 2006
2. Omeis I et al: Meningioangiomatosis associated with neurofibromatosis: report of 2 cases in a single family and review of the literature. Surg Neurol. 65(6):595-603, 2006
3. Wang Y et al: Histopathological study of five cases with sporadic meningioangiomatosis. Neuropathology. 26(3):249-56, 2006
4. Perry A et al: Insights into meningioangiomatosis with and without meningioma: a clinicopathologic and genetic series of 24 cases with review of the literature. Brain Pathol. 15(1):55-65, 2005
5. Koutsopoulos AV et al: Meningioangiomatosis with predominantly cellular pattern. Neuropathology. 23(2):141-5, 2003
6. Savargaonkar P et al: Meningioangiomatosis: report of three cases and review of the literature. Ann Clin Lab Sci. 33(1):115-8, 2003
7. Kim NR et al: Childhood meningiomas associated with meningioangiomatosis: report of five cases and literature review. Neuropathol Appl Neurobiol. 28(1):48-56, 2002
8. Takeshima Y et al: Meningioangiomatosis occurring in a young male without neurofibromatosis: with special reference to its histogenesis and loss of heterozygosity in the NF2 gene region. Am J Surg Pathol. 26(1):125-9, 2002
9. Chakrabarty A et al: Meningioangiomatosis: a case report and review of the literature. Br J Neurosurg. 13(2):167-73, 1999
10. Giangaspero F et al: Meningioma with meningioangiomatosis: a condition mimicking invasive meningiomas in children and young adults: report of two cases and review of the literature. Am J Surg Pathol. 23(8):872-5, 1999
11. Wiebe S et al: Meningioangiomatosis. A comprehensive analysis of clinical and laboratory features. Brain. 122 (Pt 4):709-26, 1999

Microscopic Features

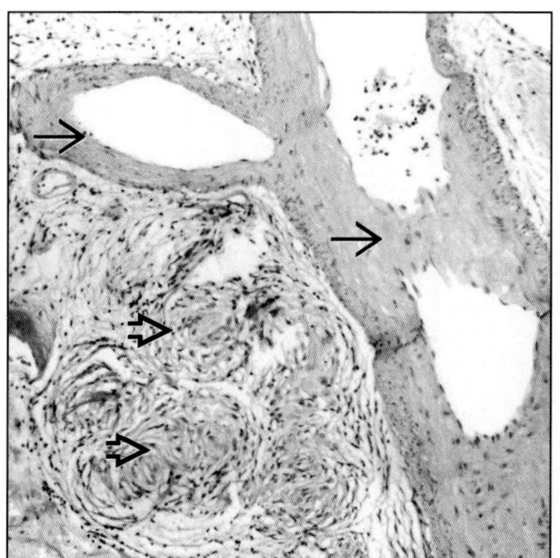

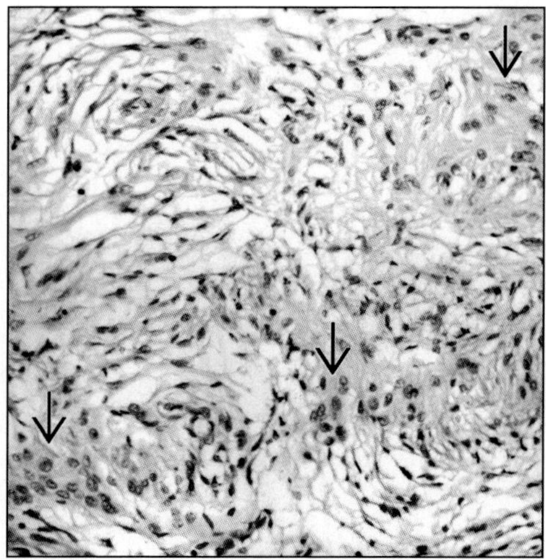

(Left) *H&E stained paraffin section shows medium-power magnification of MA with large vessels* → *in the subarachnoid space resembling a vascular malformation and surrounded by perivascular proliferation of tissue with a meningothelial appearance* ⇒. ***(Right)*** *H&E section at a high-power magnification shows perivascular proliferation of spindle cells* →.

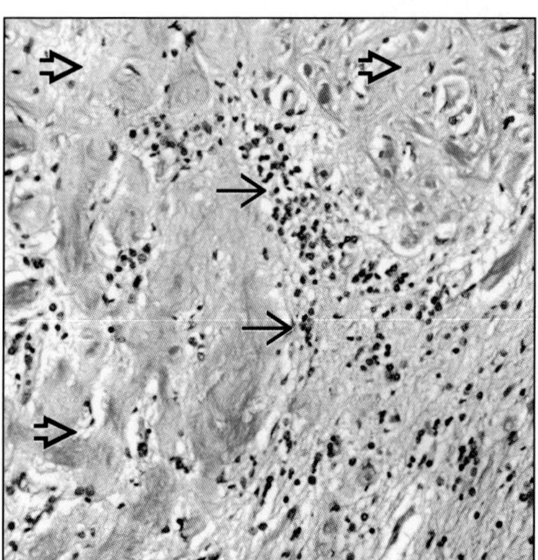

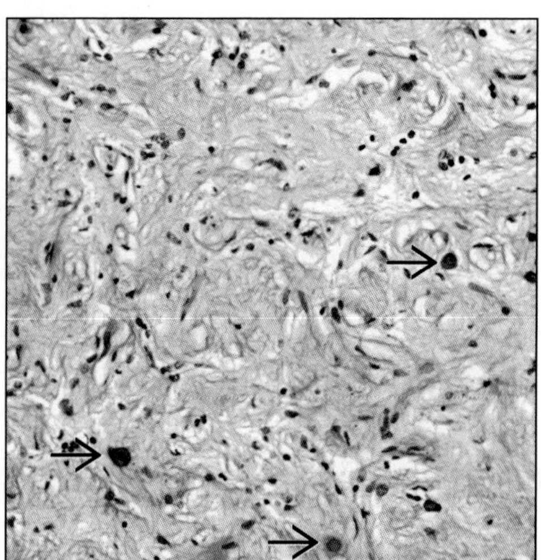

(Left) *High-power magnification of H&E section shows gliotic brain parenchyma* → *trapped in between tongues of MA* ⇒ *that are growing intracortically.* ***(Right)*** *High magnification of H&E section shows area of MA with more nodular fibrous appearance and prominent calcospherites* →.

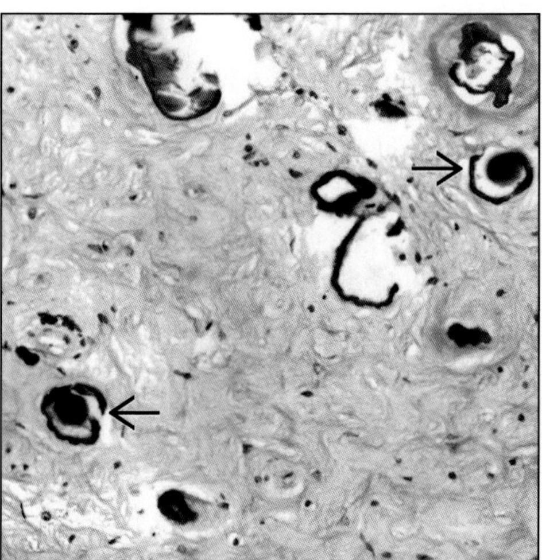

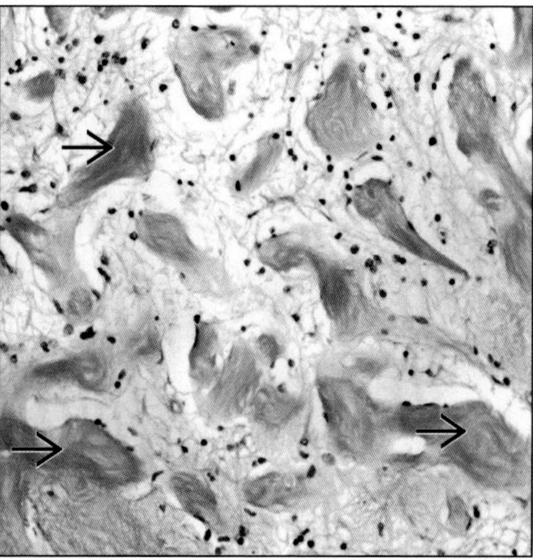

(Left) *High magnification of H&E section shows largely fibrous tissue of MA with psammoma bodies* →. ***(Right)*** *Medium-power magnification of H&E section shows more advanced lesion of MA where osseous metaplasia (osteoid* →*) has largely replaced calcifications in the fibrous tissue.*

CHOROID PLEXUS TUMORS

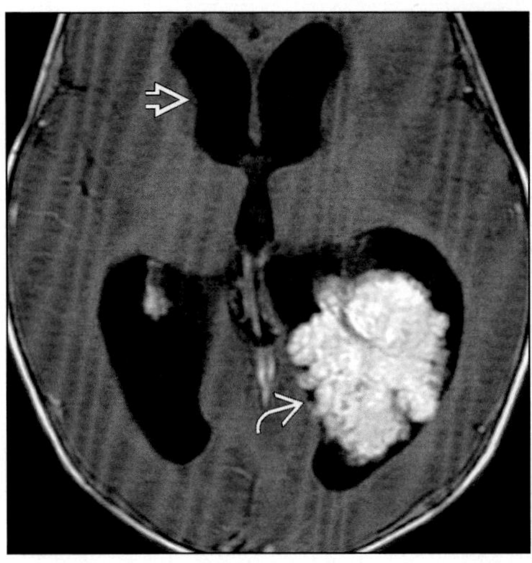

Axial contrast-enhanced MR shows a choroid plexus papilloma ➔ in the lateral ventricle. Ventriculomegaly ➢ is due to CSF overproduction by the tumor.

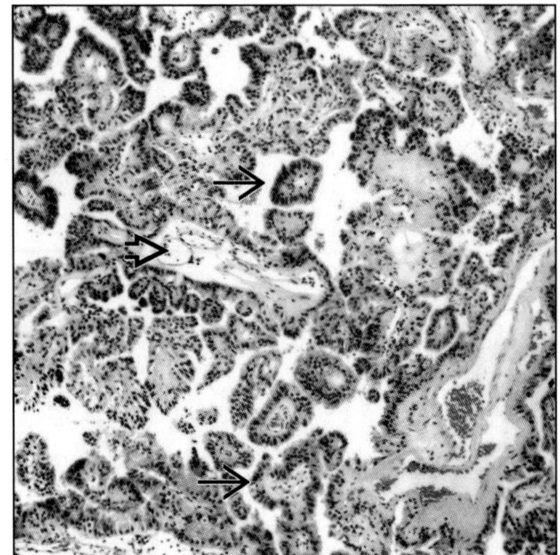

Hematoxylin & eosin shows medium-power view of well-differentiated CPP with delicate papillary fronds ➔ and underlying fibrovascular connective tissue stroma ➢.

TERMINOLOGY

Abbreviations

- Choroid plexus papilloma (CPP)
- Choroid plexus carcinoma (CPC)

Definitions

- Uncommon papillary epithelial neoplasms occurring mostly in children, derived from and closely resembling choroid plexus of cerebral ventricles
- CPP (WHO grade I): Slow growing, benign, resectable
- Atypical CPP (WHO grade II): Intermediate lesions
- CPC (WHO grade III): Malignant, invasive, seeds CSF

ETIOLOGY/PATHOGENESIS

Histogenesis and Differentiation

- Neuroepithelial derivation → glial differentiation
- Histogenesis of "ectopic" (extraventricular) lesions
  - Arise from primitive ectopic choroid plexus
  - Normal choroid tufts outside foramen of Luschka

Molecular Abnormalities

- Loss of chromosome 22: *hSNF5/INI1* gene implicated
  - Preserved protein expression in majority of CPC
  - May represent atypical teratoid/rhabdoid tumors
- SV40 polyomaviruses implicated
  - Tumor induction in SV40 T-antigen transgenic mice
  - SV40 genomic sequences found in choroid tumors

Familial Syndromes

- Mostly sporadic; some occur in genetic syndromes
- Aicardi syndrome: X-linked dominant syndrome
  - Psychomotor retardation, infantile spasms/seizures, corpus callosum agenesis, lacunar chorioretinopathy
- Li-Fraumeni syndrome: Germline *TP53* mutations
- von Hippel-Lindau disease: Chromosome 3 allele loss
  - Rare tumor sites, e.g., cerebellopontine angle (CPA)

CLINICAL ISSUES

Epidemiology

- Incidence
  - 0.4-0.6% of intracranial tumors
    - 2-5% in infants/children
  - CPP:CPC = 3-5:1
- Age
  - Most frequent brain tumor in 1st year of life (15%)
    - Rarely congenital: Diagnosed in utero or at birth
    - Smaller peak in adults: Incidental autopsy finding
  - CPC presents by 3 years old (median: 24-26 months)

Site

- Ventricles: Lateral (50%) > 4th (30-40%) > 3rd (5-15%)
  - Children/infants: Lateral ventricles most common
  - Adults: 4th ventricle most common
- Bilateral or multifocal tumors reported (5%)
- Rare extraventricular sites
  - CPA, suprasellar, spinal epidural space, middle ear

Presentation

- CSF outflow obstruction or overproduction/secretion
  - ↑ intracranial pressure: Headache, nausea, vomiting, strabismus/diplopia, ataxia, lethargy
  - Hydrocephalus, macrocephaly (in infants < 2 years)
- CSF seeding: Symptoms throughout neuraxis
- Extension into parenchyma: Focal neurologic deficits
- Spontaneous intraventricular or subarachnoid bleed

Natural History

- Progression from CPP to CPC: Unusual
- May fill, expand, and obliterate ventricle lumen
- May extend toward cerebral cortex or temporal horn
- May cause pressure to bone, pseudocystic destruction

Treatment

- Options, risks, complications
  - Intraoperative hemorrhage → incomplete resection
  - Persistent subdural fluid (ventricular dilation)

CHOROID PLEXUS TUMORS

Key Facts

Terminology
- Papillary epithelial neoplasms of choroid plexus
- CPP (WHO grade I): Slow growing, benign, resectable
- CPC (WHO grade III): Malignant, invasive, seeds CSF

Clinical Issues
- 0.4-0.6% of intracranial tumors (2-5% in children)
  - CPP:CPC = 3-5:1
- Lateral (50%, children) > 4th ventricle (30%, adults)
- CSF outflow obstruction or overproduction/secretion
  - ↑ intracranial pressure, hydrocephalus
- Gross resection: Most important prognostic factor
- CPC rare in adults → favor metastatic carcinoma

Image Findings
- Discrete, iso- to hyper-dense, intraventricular mass
- Intensely and homogeneously contrast enhancing

Macroscopic Features
- Cauliflower-like, cystic, calcified, hemorrhagic
- CPC: Invasive, destructive, hemorrhagic, necrotic

Microscopic Pathology
- CPP: Well-differentiated, delicate papillary fronds
  - Single cell layer, cuboidal/columnar epithelium
  - Maintained polarity: Basal monomorphic nuclei
- Atypical CPP: No clear diagnostic criteria
  - ↑ mitotic figures (generally ≥ 2/10 HPF)
- CPC: Marked architectural complexity, solid areas
  - Atypia, necrosis, brain invasion, > 5 mitoses/10 HPF

Ancillary Tests
- S100, CAM5.2, vimentin, prealbumin: Positive
- GFAP(+) epithelial cells and fibrillar processes
- CPC: > 10-15% Ki-67 staining (CPP < 5-10%)

- Surgical approaches
  - Simple excision almost always curative in CPP
  - May be difficult in highly vascular, invasive CPC
  - Recurrent CPC: Re-excise, adjuvant therapy
- Adjuvant therapy
  - Effectiveness is controversial in CPC
  - Chemotherapy debatable for low-grade CPC
  - Radiotherapy withheld (young age of patients)

Prognosis
- Gross total resection: Most important prognostic factor
- CPP: 5-year survival after resection near 100%
  - Occasional mitoses, infiltration, cytologic atypia
    - Not prognostically significant
  - CSF seeding may rarely occur
    - Usually clinically asymptomatic and undetectable
- Atypical CPP: Usually follow benign course (like CPP)
  - Uncertain prognostic significance
  - Local recurrence may become more malignant
- CPC: 5-year survival around 30-50%
  - More rapid growth, less favorable outcome
  - CSF seeding common (> 60%)
  - Systemic metastases exceedingly rare

IMAGE FINDINGS

CT Findings
- Discrete, iso- to hyperdense, intraventricular mass
- Intensely and homogeneously contrast enhancing
- Lobular or papillary, often calcified, cystic
- CPC: Peritumoral edema, parenchymal invasion

MACROSCOPIC FEATURES

General Features
- Generally well circumscribed, globular, soft
- May extend into cerebral tissue with broad tumor edge
- Lobular or papillary (cauliflower-like), gray/brown-red
- Cystic, calcified (gritty), highly vascular (hemorrhagic)
- CPC: Invasive, destructive, hemorrhagic, necrotic

MICROSCOPIC PATHOLOGY

Choroid Plexus Papilloma
- Well differentiated, lacks significant atypia
  - Distinctive papillary architecture, delicate fronds
  - Underlying fibrovascular connective tissue stroma
- Uniform epithelium resting on basement membrane
  - Single cell layer, cuboidal to columnar
  - More crowded, columnar (elongated), pleomorphic than "hobnail," "cobblestone" normal choroid
  - May have acinar, tubular, or "adenomatous" patterns
  - Maintained polarity: Apical eosinophilic cytoplasm
    - Round/oval, basally located monomorphic nuclei
- Metaplastic/regressive/degenerative changes
  - Concretions, calcification, even psammoma bodies
  - Hyalinization, sclerosis of stroma (may be extensive)
  - Osseous, cartilaginous (chondroid) metaplasia
  - Oncocytic, mucinous or xanthomatous change
  - Brown melanin pigment (lipofuscin-derived)

Atypical Choroid Plexus Papilloma
- No clear diagnostic criteria
  - Some loss of papillary architecture
- Difficult to grade, only few malignant features
  - ↑ cellularity, crowding, ↑ nuclear to cytoplasmic ratio
  - Some cytologic atypia, nuclear pleomorphism
  - ↑ mitotic figures (generally ≥ 2/10 HPF)

Choroid Plexus Carcinoma
- Marked architectural complexity
  - Partially solid, nonpapillary growth pattern
  - Disarray, complex glands, cribriform structures
- Diffuse, destructive invasion of brain parenchyma
- Marked cytologic atypia (malignant)
  - Nuclear pleomorphism, ↑ nuclear to cytoplasmic ratio
  - Obvious necrosis
  - ↑ and atypical mitoses (> 5/10 HPF)
- Most CPCs retain epithelial phenotype
  - Papillation, cell nests with defined borders
- High-grade or anaplastic carcinomas

CHOROID PLEXUS TUMORS

- Sheets of small tumor cells (resemble embryonal)
- Perinuclear halos appear oligodendroglioma-like
- Undifferentiated, pleomorphic or giant cells
  - Resembling atypical teratoid/rhabdoid tumors
- May contain better differentiated areas
  - Poorly formed papillae, uniform plump cells
  - Allow diagnosis as CPC
- Eosinophilic hyaline droplets seen in CPC of infancy
  - α-1-antitrypsin: PAS(+), diastase resistant
    - CSF level predicts recurrence, progression

ANCILLARY TESTS

Cytology

- Papillary fragments in well-differentiated tumors
- CPP: Nuclear uniformity, cohesiveness
- CPC: High cellularity, mitoses, necrosis
  - Cytologic atypia: Nuclear pleomorphism, nucleoli

Immunohistochemistry

- **CPP**: S100, CAM 5.2, Vimentin: Positive
  - CEA, EMA/MUC1: Generally negative
  - Transthyretin (pre-albumin): Positive, patchy
  - GFAP(+) epithelial cells and fibrillar processes
    - In areas with ependymal differentiation
  - Laminin(+) basement membrane
- **CPC**: Less likely S100, GFAP, transthyretin positive
  - Higher proportion of p53 nuclear staining
  - ↑ MIB-1 proliferation index (Ki-67 immunostaining)
    - CPC: > 10-15% nuclear staining (CPP < 5-10%)

Cytogenetics

- Multiple chromosomal imbalances, both CPP and CPC
  - Especially gains of chromosomes 5, 7, 9, and 12

Electron Microscopy

- Maintained apical-basal polarity of normal choroid
- Apical microvilli, few cilia, tight junction complexes
  - Abnormal cilia (9+0 microtubule configuration)
- Lateral desmosomes, interdigitating cell membranes
- Subluminal basal lamina (basement membrane)
- Intermediate filaments suggest glial differentiation
- Fenestrated capillaries, mitochondria-rich oncocytes

DIFFERENTIAL DIAGNOSIS

Choroid Plexus with Villous Hypertrophy

- Regular, uncrowded cells with cobblestone appearance
- Lack of contrast-enhancing intraventricular mass
- Usually GFAP negative; very low Ki-67 labeling

Papillary Ependymoma

- Ependymal epithelial surface and fibrillary glial stroma
- True ependymal rosettes, perivascular pseudorosettes
- Lack prominent PAS/laminin-positive basal lamina
- Vimentin/GFAP(+); CK8/18/CAM5.2(-)

Metastatic Carcinoma

- Intraparenchymal lesions in adults, vs. CPC
- CEA-M, EMA/MUC1, EpCAM/BER-EP4/CD326 positive
- S100, GFAP, synaptophysin, prealbumin negative

Atypical Teratoid/Rhabdoid Tumor (AT/RT)

- In posterior fossa of infants, vs. CPC
- EMA/MUC1 positive rhabdoid cells: Eccentric pleomorphic nuclei, abundant eosinophilic cytoplasm
- Abnormalities in *INI1* gene (FISH) or loss of nuclear staining (IHC)

Small Cell Embryonal Tumors

- Usually less pleomorphic and papillary than CPC
- Medulloepithelioma may appear papillary

Papillary Endolymphatic Sac Tumor

- Extraaxial, in CPA vs. CPP/well-differentiated CPC
- Less papillary, simpler epithelium

Germ Cell Tumors

- Embryonal carcinoma, endodermal sinus tumor, etc.
- Usually α-fetoprotein, CD117, or PLAP positive

DIAGNOSTIC CHECKLIST

Clinically Relevant Pathologic Features

- Histologic features of poor prognosis
  - Correlate with recurrence, fatal outcome
    - Frequent/atypical mitoses, necrosis, brain invasion
    - Absence of marked stromal edema
    - Absence of prealbumin staining
    - < 50% cells with strong positivity for S100

Pathologic Interpretation Pearls

- Rosenthal fibers, piloid gliosis suggest chronicity
- CPC rare in adults → favor metastatic carcinoma
- Distinction between CPP and low-grade CPC
  - Somewhat arbitrary, subjective
  - Most consistent criteria: ↑ mitoses, cytologic atypia
- Invasion of brain parenchyma may be seen in CPP
  - More common in CPC, but not diagnostic

GRADING

Criteria for Malignancy (CPC)

- Marked cytologic atypia, nuclear pleomorphism
- Hypercellularity, loss of polarity, brain infiltration
- Frequent and atypical mitoses, necrosis
- Vascular proliferation, hemorrhage

SELECTED REFERENCES

1. Wrede B et al: Atypical choroid plexus papilloma: clinical experience in the CPT-SIOP-2000 study. J Neurooncol. 95(3):383-92, 2009
2. Gopal P et al: Choroid plexus carcinoma. Arch Pathol Lab Med. 132(8):1350-4, 2008
3. Kamaly-Asl ID et al: Genetics of choroid plexus tumors. Neurosurg Focus. 20(1):E10, 2006
4. Gupta N: Choroid plexus tumors in children. Neurosurg Clin N Am. 14(4):621-31, 2003
5. Rickert CH et al: Tumors of the choroid plexus. Microsc Res Tech. 52(1):104-11, 2001
6. Berger C et al: Choroid plexus carcinomas in childhood: clinical features and prognostic factors. Neurosurgery. 42(3):470-5, 1998

Microscopic Features of CPP

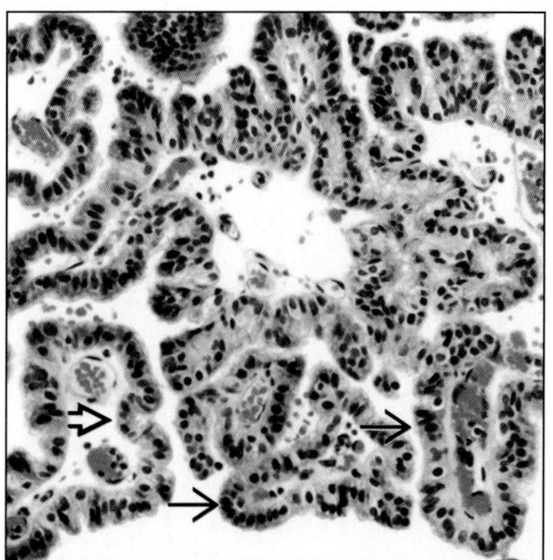

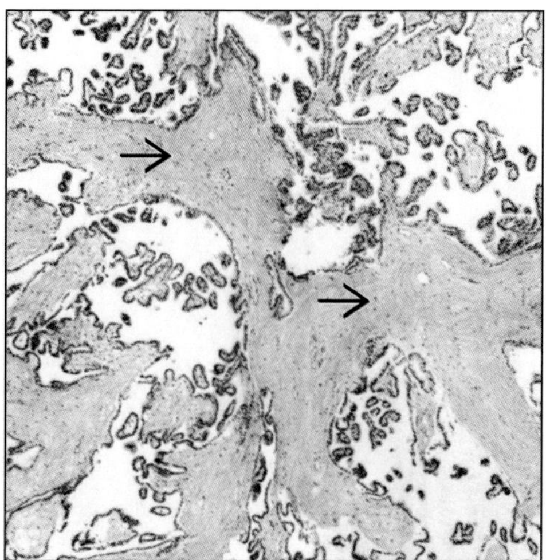

(Left) *Hematoxylin & eosin shows high-power view of CPP with single cell layer of well-differentiated cuboidal to columnar epithelium* ➙ *resting on a basement membrane* ➙. *CPP epithelium is more crowded than normal choroid plexus, but cells maintain their polarity with basal monomorphic round nuclei and apical eosinophilic cytoplasm.* ***(Right)*** *Hematoxylin & eosin shows low-power view of CPP with extensive hyalinization and sclerosis* ➙ *of connective stroma.*

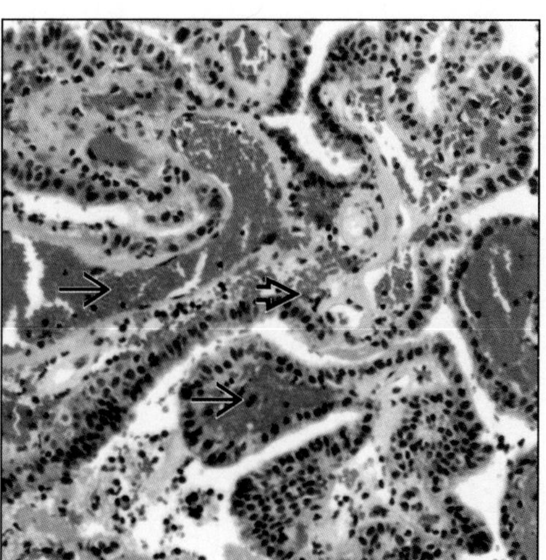

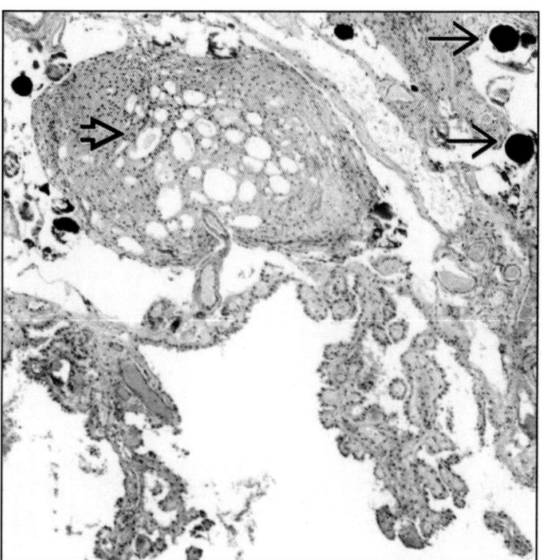

(Left) *Hematoxylin & eosin shows a high-power view of very vascular CPP with congested stromal capillaries* ➙ *that can lead to intraoperative hemorrhage. Hemosiderin-laden macrophages can also be seen* ➙. ***(Right)*** *Hematoxylin & eosin shows a low-power view of CPP with microcystic change* ➙ *and many calcified concretions* ➙ *that often exhibit concentric laminations (psammoma bodies).*

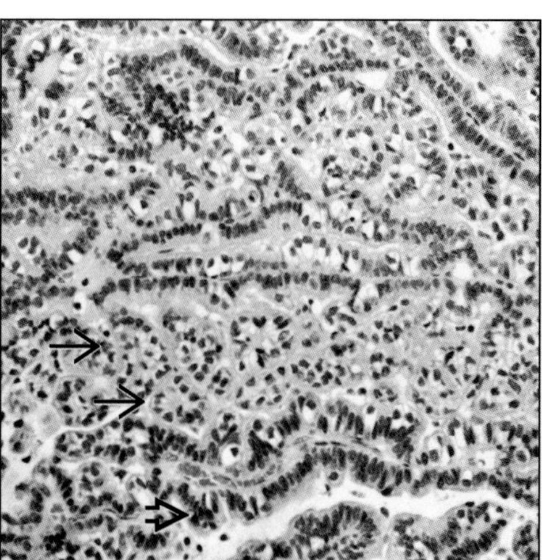

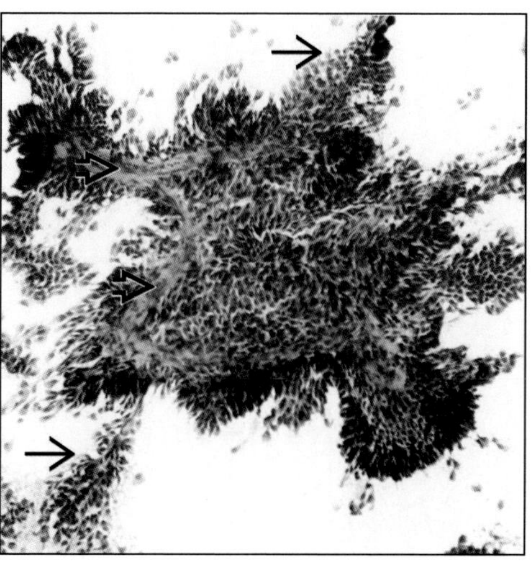

(Left) *Hematoxylin & eosin shows a high-power view of CPP with acinar or tubular architecture* ➙ *in between the more classic papillary formations* ➙. *In some instances, this has been described as "adenomatous change" or choroid plexus adenoma.* ***(Right)*** *Hematoxylin & eosin shows a high-power view of a cytologic smear preparation from a CPP with evident papillary architecture* ➙ *and fibrovascular cores* ➙.

CHOROID PLEXUS TUMORS

Atypical CPP and CPC

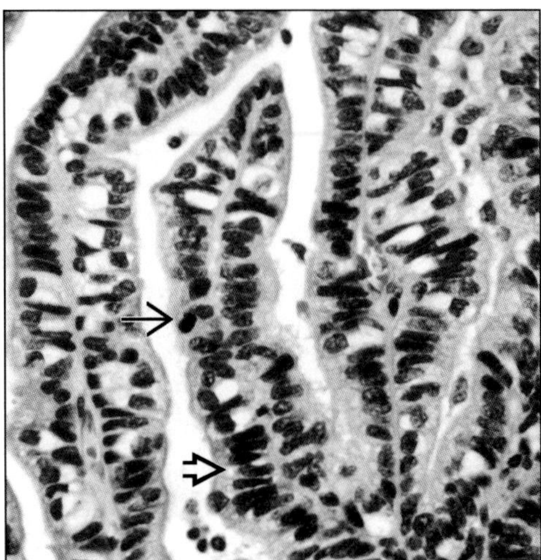

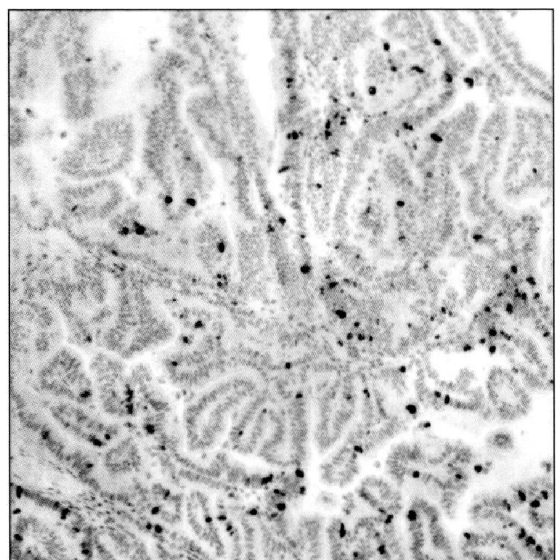

(Left) *High-power view shows atypical CPP with high cellularity, nuclear crowding, and increased nuclear to cytoplasm ratio. Cytologic atypia, nuclear pleomorphism ⇨, and occasional mitoses → are present. While subjective, these features warrant the diagnosis of atypical CPP in this case.* ***(Right)*** *Ki-67 immunostain in an atypical CPP shows a Ki-67 labeling index as high as 5-10%, which is characteristic in these lesions, but less than what would be seen in a CPC.*

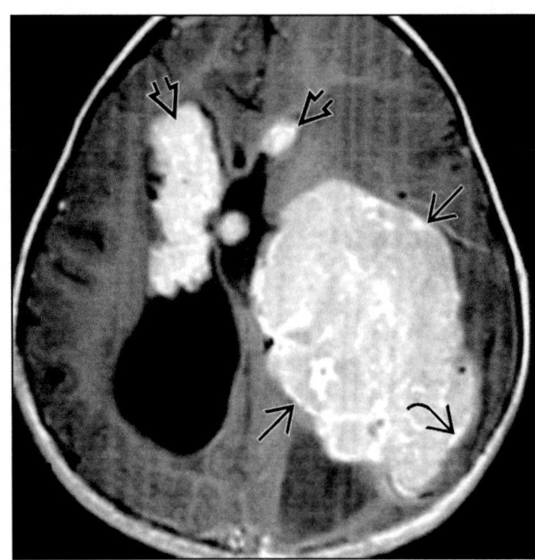

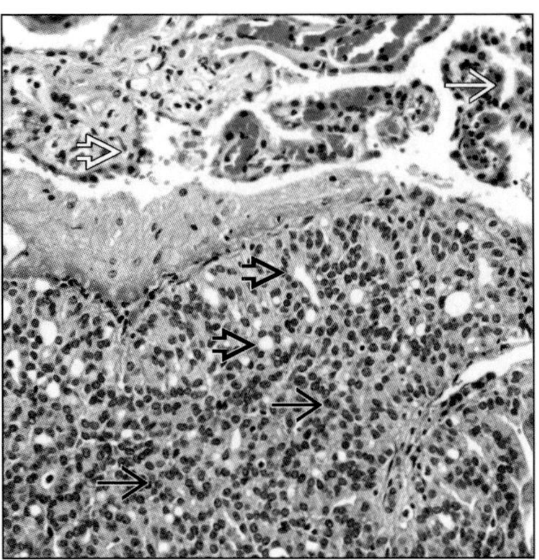

(Left) *Axial contrast-enhanced MR shows a large robustly enhancing left trigonal choroid plexus carcinoma →. There is ependymal invasion ↗ and intraventricular tumor seeding ⇨.* ***(Right)*** *High-power view of hypercellular CPC shows areas of solid growth → and cribriform architecture ⇨. In contrast, normal choroid plexus consists of a single cell layer of papillary epithelium with "hobnail" ⇨ or "cobblestone" → appearance.*

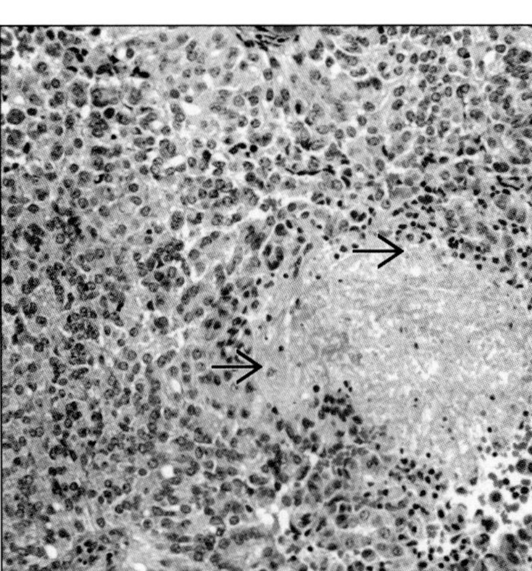

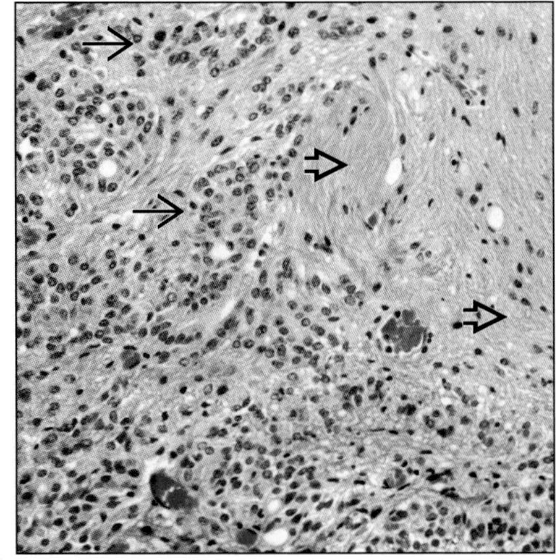

(Left) *High-power view of CPC shows an area of necrosis having a rim of cellular debris condensation around the periphery → ("geographic necrosis"). Together with hypercellularity, mitoses, cytologic atypia, and solid growth with loss of polarity, these features warrant the diagnosis of CPC.* ***(Right)*** *Hematoxylin & eosin shows high-power view of CPC with tumor nests → infiltrating into brain parenchyma ⇨. While not diagnostic, brain invasion is more commonly seen in CPC than CPP.*

Immunohistochemical Features and Differential Diagnosis

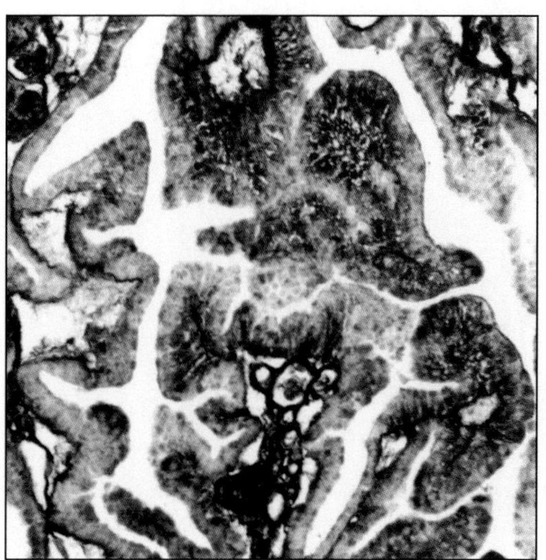

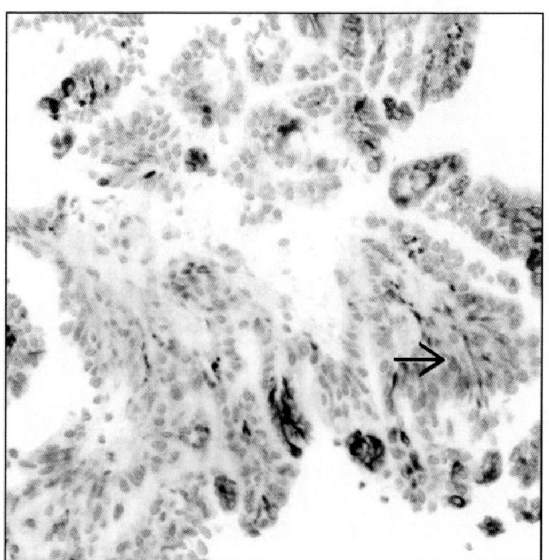

(Left) *Prealbumin (transthyretin) immunostain is strongly and diffusely positive in CPP, but less so in CPC. In some studies, this stain was useful in discriminating CPP/CPC from other entities in the differential.* ***(Right)*** *GFAP immunostain in CPP is weakly and focally positive in areas of ependymal differentiation ➔, being useful in differentiating CPP from papillary ependymoma (where GFAP is strongly positive) and CPC from metastatic adenocarcinoma (where GFAP is negative).*

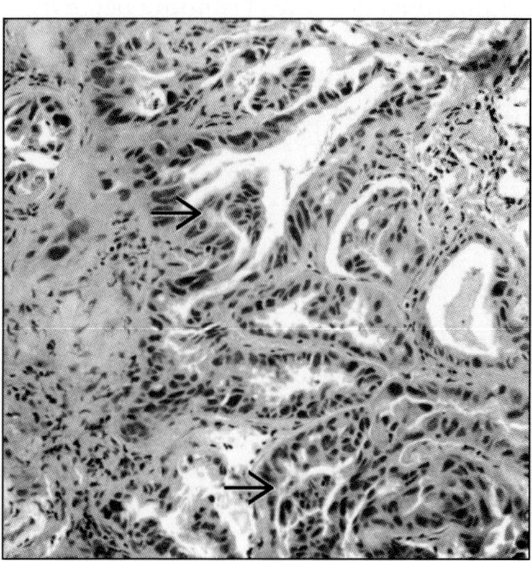

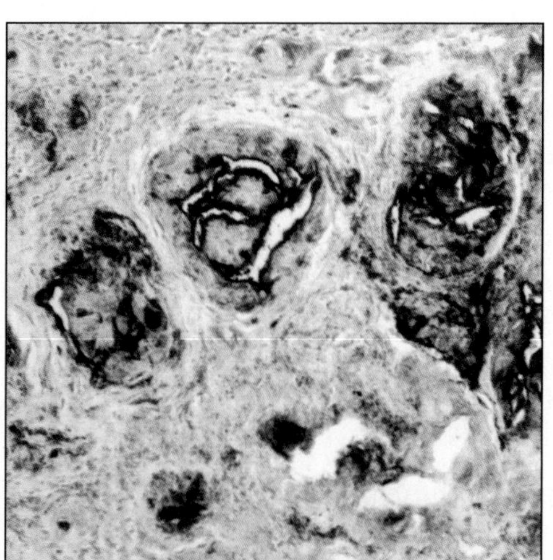

(Left) *Hematoxylin & eosin shows a high-power view of metastatic adenocarcinoma in the brain with glandular structures that can focally assume papillary architecture ➔ and be confused with CPC.* ***(Right)*** *EMA/MUC1 immunostain is strongly and diffusely positive in metastatic adenocarcinoma in the brain. CEA and other epithelial markers would also be positive, in contrast to CPP/CPC where EMA and CEA are generally negative. However, some cytokeratins, such as CAM5.2, can be positive in CPP/CPC.*

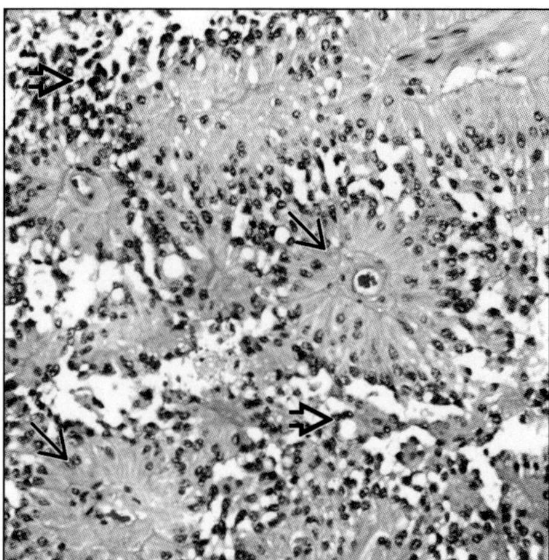

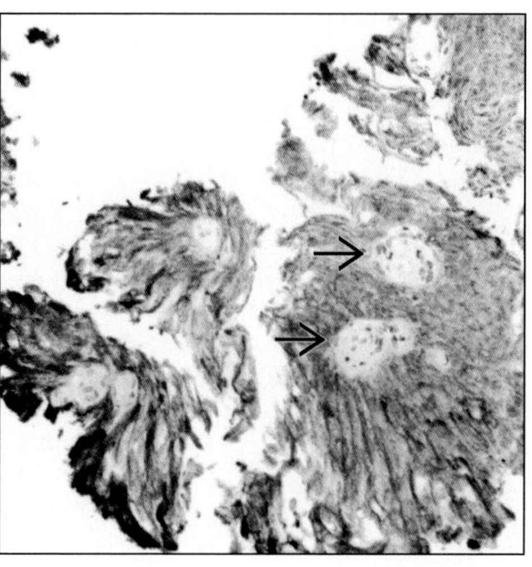

(Left) *Hematoxylin & eosin shows a high-power view of a papillary ependymoma with vaguely papillary architecture of the ependymal surface ➢, but characteristic perivascular pseudorosettes ➔ formed by fibrillary glial processes.* ***(Right)*** *GFAP immunostain shows strong and diffuse positivity in a papillary ependymoma (in contrast to CPP), highlighting the glial fibrillary processes that are radially oriented around vessels ➔, forming perivascular pseudorosettes.*

PINEAL PARENCHYMAL TUMORS

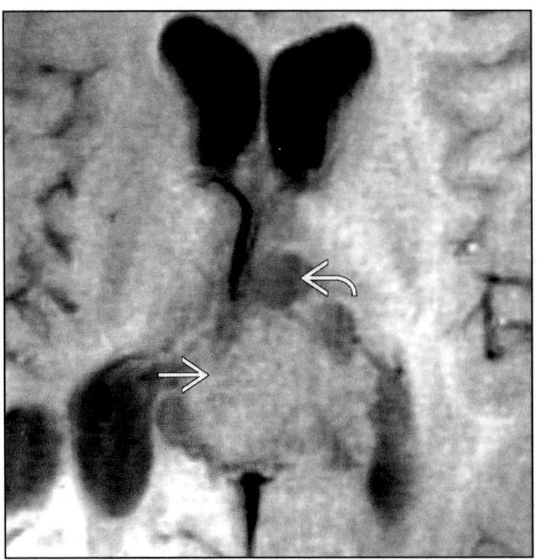

Axial T1WI MR shows a large, heterogeneous pineal mass with solid ➡ and cystic ➡ components in a 32 year old with headache and Parinaud ophthalmoplegia, compatible with pineocytoma.

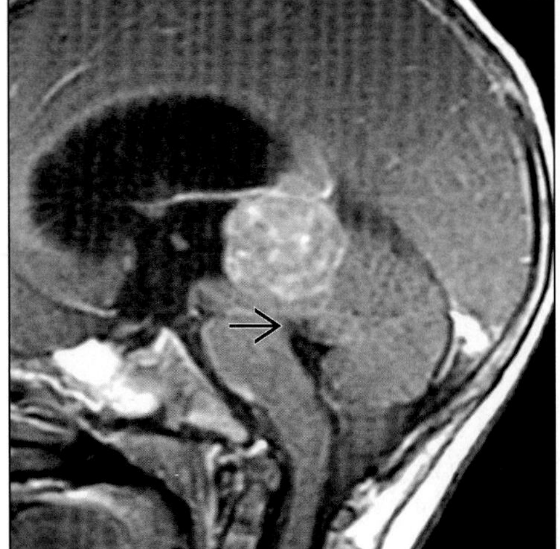

Sagittal T1WI C+ MR shows a heterogeneously enhancing pineal mass consistent with pineoblastoma. Proximity of the lesion to a cerebral aqueduct ➡ causes hydrocephalus.

TERMINOLOGY

Abbreviations

- Pineal parenchymal tumor (PPT)
- PPT of intermediate differentiation (PPTID)

Synonyms

- "True pinealomas"

Definitions

- Neuroepithelial tumors of the pineal gland, derived from pineocytes or their embryonal precursors
- Pineocytoma (WHO grade I)
  - Well-differentiated, histologically benign, slow-growing tumor of young adults
  - Pineocytomatous rosettes, divergent phenotypes
  - Unlikely local invasion or CSF spread
  - Cured by excision, relatively favorable prognosis
- PPTID (WHO grade II or III)
  - Intermediate histologic features (vs. grades I & IV)
  - Unpredictable growth rate, clinical behavior
    - In between pineocytoma and pineoblastoma
- Pineoblastoma (WHO grade IV)
  - Highly malignant, poorly differentiated, primitive (embryonal) neuroectodermal tumor of children
  - Rapid growth, local infiltration, CSF dissemination
  - Resistant to radiochemotherapy, fatal outcome

ETIOLOGY/PATHOGENESIS

Histogenesis

- Pineal gland
  - Derivative of epithalamic roof plate of diencephalon
  - Pineocytes: Specially modified neurons
    - Photosensory and neuroendocrine functions
- PPTs share morphology
  - With cells of developing pineal gland and retina
    - Melanin pigment, cilia (9+0 microtubule pattern)
    - Photoreceptor differentiation
  - Common immunohistochemical staining patterns
    - Interphotoreceptor retinoid-binding protein
    - Retinal S-antigen, rhodopsin

Differentiation

- Pineocytomas
  - Well differentiated, mature
  - Clearly neuronal tumors with features of pineocytes
- PPTIDs
  - In middle of differentiation spectrum
- Pineoblastomas
  - Poorly differentiated, primitive

Genetic Associations

- Familial adenomatous polyposis (FAP)
- With (familial) bilateral retinoblastoma
  - Termed "trilateral retinoblastoma" syndrome
  - Dismal prognosis: < 1 year survival after diagnosis

CLINICAL ISSUES

Epidemiology

- Incidence
  - Pineal region tumors
    - < 1% of all intracranial neoplasms
    - 5-10% of pediatric brain tumors
  - ~ 50% are germ cell tumors
  - 15-30% are PPTs
    - Pineoblastoma, pineocytoma: 35-50% each
    - PPTID: 10-20%
- Age
  - Pineocytomas
    - Mostly in young to middle-aged adults
    - 3rd to 6th decades (mean age 38-45 years old)
  - Pineoblastomas
    - Occur mostly in childhood
    - 1st 2 decades of life
- Gender
  - Pineoblastoma
    - 2:1 male preponderance, reported in 1 study

PINEAL PARENCHYMAL TUMORS

Key Facts

Terminology

- Pineocytoma (WHO grade I)
  - Well-differentiated, histologically benign, slow-growing tumor of young adults
  - Pineocytomatous rosettes, divergent phenotypes
  - Cured by excision, relatively favorable prognosis
- PPTID (WHO grade II or III)
  - Intermediate histologic features (vs. grades I & IV)
  - Unpredictable growth rate, clinical behavior
  - In between pineocytoma and pineoblastoma
  - Lack pineocytomatous rosettes, overt small cells
- Pineoblastoma (WHO grade IV)
  - Highly malignant, poorly differentiated, primitive (embryonal) neuroectodermal tumor of children
  - Rapid growth, local infiltration, CSF dissemination
  - Resistant to radiochemotherapy, fatal outcome

Clinical Issues

- Pineal tumors: 5-10% of pediatric brain tumors
  - ~ 50% are germ cell tumors, 15-30% are PPTs
- CSF obstruction, intracranial pressure, hydrocephalus
- Mass effect on adjacent structures: Gait ataxia
  - Upward gaze paresis (Parinaud ophthalmoplegia)
- Hypothalamic/endocrine abnormalities
- Rarely intratumoral hemorrhage (pineal apoplexy)
- Gross total resection, chemotherapy for high grade

Diagnostic Checklist

- Histologically biphasic, "mixed" tumors
  - If small cell areas: Considered pineoblastoma
- Grading: Correlates with clinical variables, outcome
  - Cellularity, mitoses per HPF, necrosis
  - Immunostaining for neuronal markers

Site

- Pineal gland and adjacent region

Presentation

- Aqueduct (CSF) obstruction, ↑ intracranial pressure
  - Hydrocephalus, headache
  - Change in mental status
- Mass effect on adjacent structures
  - Neuro-ophthalmologic dysfunction (brainstem)
    - Upward gaze paresis (Parinaud ophthalmoplegia)
  - Gait ataxia (compressive cerebellar dysfunction)
- Hypothalamic/endocrine abnormalities
  - Endocrinopathy; e.g., precocious puberty
- Rarely intratumoral hemorrhage (pineal apoplexy)
- Interval between initial symptoms and diagnosis
  - Median of 4 years for pineocytoma
  - As little as 1 month in pineoblastoma

Natural History

- Pineocytomas
  - Typically remain localized in pineal region
    - May indent or extend into posterior 3rd ventricle
  - May compress adjacent structures
    - Cerebral aqueduct, brainstem, cerebellum
  - Rarely transform to malignant pineoblastoma
    - May explain histogenesis of "mixed" tumors
- Pineoblastomas
  - Local invasion, CSF/leptomeningeal seeding
  - CNS, vertebral column metastases
    - Most common cause of death
  - Rare extracranial metastases

Treatment

- Surgical approaches
  - Goal is gross total resection
- Adjuvant therapy
  - Chemotherapy for pineoblastoma, PPTID
- Radiation
  - When margins are close
  - Unclear value, avoided in infants

Prognosis

- Grading correlates with survival
- Pineocytoma
  - Essentially benign
    - No metastases reported (when strictly defined)
  - 86% 5-year survival in 1 study
  - Cure often achieved
    - Only occasional examples of recurrences
- PPTID
  - Intermediate between pineocytoma/pineoblastoma
  - ~ 75% 5-year survival for grade II tumors
  - ~ 40% 5-year survival for grade III tumors
- Pineoblastoma
  - Carry poor prognosis
  - Few patients survive more than 2 years
    - Median postsurgical survival: 24-30 months
  - Best prognostic features (affect survival)
    - Completeness of tumor resection
    - Extent of disease (CSF examination, spine MR)

IMAGE FINDINGS

MR Findings

- Homogeneously contrast enhancing
- Hypointense on T1W, hyperintense on T2W images

CT Findings

- Pineocytoma
  - Well-circumscribed, discrete round mass in midline
  - Isodense with homogeneous contrast enhancing
  - Occasional cystic change, peripheral calcification
  - Accompanying mild hydrocephalus
- Pineoblastoma
  - Large, poorly demarcated, homogeneous mass
  - Infiltration of surrounding tissues depends on grade
  - Hyperdense, heterogeneous contrast enhancement
  - Infrequent calcification, common hydrocephalus

MACROSCOPIC FEATURES

General Features

- Pineocytoma
  - Well-circumscribed, relatively discrete mass

    - Displace rather than invade adjacent structures
  - Gray-tan, soft, granular, homogeneous cut surfaces
  - May have small cysts, scant hemorrhage
  - Necrosis generally absent
    - Unless vascular compromise in large tumors
- Pineoblastoma
  - Soft, friable, gelatinous, poorly demarcated
  - Hemorrhagic, focally necrotic, rarely calcified

Size

- Pineocytomas are generally < 3 cm

MICROSCOPIC PATHOLOGY

Pineocytoma

- Well-differentiated neoplasm, moderate cell density
  - Sheets, clusters, or ill-defined lobular pattern
- Small to moderately sized, uniform, mature cells
  - Resemble pineocytes, larger than pineoblastoma
  - Round to oval nuclei
    - Fine dispersed chromatin, inconspicuous nucleoli
  - Moderate, homogeneous, eosinophilic cytoplasm
- Short cytoplasmic processes with club-shaped endings
  - Often perivascular terminal expansions
  - Highlighted by silver, neurofilament stains
- Uncommon nuclear pleomorphism, hyperchromasia
  - If present, considered "degenerative atypia"
  - Rare mitoses, occasional necrosis (no palisading)
  - Occasional multinucleated giant cells, bizarre nuclei
- "Pineocytomatous rosettes"
  - Peripheral, cytologically bland, mature cells
  - Delicate fibrillar processes form nuclear-free zones
  - Eosinophilic, circular or stellate neuropil-like foci
  - Larger, more irregular, lack lumens of other rosettes
- Stroma
  - Delicate network of vascular channels
    - Lined by single layer of endothelial cells
  - Scant reticulin fibers, some microcalcifications
- Often exhibits divergent differentiation
  - Neuronal differentiation: Ganglion cells
    - Single cells or large islands of neuropil
  - Glial (astrocytic) or neuroglial
  - Melanocytic, photoreceptor, or mesenchymal

PPTID

- Intermediate features (not a precise definition)
- Compared to pineocytoma
  - ↑ cellularity, anaplasia, mitotic activity, no necrosis
  - ↓ size of nuclei, cytoplasm, neurofilament staining
  - But not as much as pineoblastoma
- Absence of large pineocytomatous rosettes

Pineoblastoma

- Poorly differentiated
  - Very cellular, resemble other embryonal tumors
  - Patternless sheets of densely packed "small blue cells"
  - Rarely papillary pattern may be present
- Round to irregular hyperchromatic nuclei
  - Indistinct cell borders, scant cytoplasm
  - High nuclear:cytoplasmic ratio, occasional nucleoli
- Very mitotically active
  - Prominent apoptosis, necrosis
  - Large cell/anaplastic features may be present
  - Microcalcifications, vascular proliferation seen
- Frequently present rosettes
  - Neuroblastic (Homer Wright)
    - Delicate, radially arranged silver-positive processes
  - Retinoblastic/neurosensory (Flexner-Wintersteiner)
    - Small lumen with radially arranged tumor cells
  - More rarely "fleurettes" may be present
    - Rare form of photoreceptor differentiation
    - Small lumens surrounded by 2 layers of cells
    - Inner and outer "visual receptor layers"
    - Cytoplasmic extensions project into rosette center
  - Pineocytomatous rosettes generally absent
- May be biphasic
  - Areas of intermediate grade or pineocytoma-like

Pineal Anlage Tumor

- Pineoblastoma with additional differentiation
  - Retinal/ciliary epithelium differentiation
    - Pigmented (melanin-containing) tubules
  - Cartilaginous or rhabdomyoblastic differentiation

ANCILLARY TESTS

Immunohistochemistry

- Tumor cells/fibrillar areas: Positive neuronal markers
  - Synaptophysin, neurofilament, chromogranin, NSE
- Variable immunostaining
  - S100, TAU protein, PGP9.5, class III β-tubulin
- Evidence of photoreceptor/sensory differentiation
  - Immunopositivity for retinal S-antigen, rhodopsin
- GFAP(+) cell processes may be present
  - Suggest glial differentiation (glassy cytoplasm)
  - Should not be considered evidence of glioma
- MIB-1 labeling index (Ki-67 immunostain)
  - Pineoblastomas: > 8%
  - PPTIDs: 3-10%
  - Pineocytomas: < 1-3%

Cytogenetics

- Few studies, some chromosomal imbalances described
- Monosomy/deletions in chromosomes 11, 12, 22
  - May be related to tumor progression

Electron Microscopy

- Ultrastructural features of pineocytic differentiation
- Microtubules, intermediate or helical filaments
  - In fibrillar centers of pineocytomatous rosettes
- Membrane-bound, (electron) dense-core granules
- Club-shaped termini of cells with clear vesicles
  - Synapse-like junctions ("vesicle-crowned rods")
- Neurosensory (photoreceptor) cilia
  - With 9+0 configuration of microtubules
- Retinoblastic differentiation
  - Flexner-Wintersteiner rosettes
- Correlate with level of differentiation
  - Most abundant in pineocytomas
  - Least abundant in pineoblastomas

DIFFERENTIAL DIAGNOSIS

Normal Pineal Gland Parenchyma

- Compact, small, well-defined lobular tissue
- Little cytoplasm, large pale nuclei
- Absent MIB-1 labeling, pineocytomatous rosettes
- Neurofilament/GFAP highlight processes, lobularity

Pineal Cyst

- Largely macrocystic, especially with fluid level
- External delicate connective tissue
- Attenuated layer of lobular pineal parenchyma
- Internal dense fibrillar gliosis
  - Granular bodies, Rosenthal fibers

Medulloblastoma

- By definition, in cerebellum (pineoblastoma in pineal)
- Pale islands, desmoplastic reticulin-rich stroma
- Rarely contain Flexner-Wintersteiner rosettes

Germ Cell Tumors

- Most common tumors of pineal region (50-65%)
- Germinoma
  - PLAP(+), clear cytoplasm, lymphocytes
- Embryonal carcinoma
  - Often AFP or HCG positive
- Typical or atypical teratoma

Gliomas

- Astrocytic or ependymal type
- Synaptophysin(-), GFAP(+)
- Biphasic architecture of pilocytic astrocytoma

Papillary Tumor of the Pineal Region

- Rare neuroepithelial tumor
- Most often located in posterior 3rd ventricle
- Papillary and compact, solid, sheet-like architecture
- Strong immunopositivity for cytokeratins
- Features suggesting ependymal differentiation
  - Membranous dot-like immunopositivity for EMA
  - Ultrastructurally junctions, lumens with microvilli

DIAGNOSTIC CHECKLIST

Clinically Relevant Pathologic Features

- Divergent differentiation in pineocytomas
  - Does not influence prognosis (still excellent)

Pathologic Interpretation Pearls

- Glial differentiation in PPTs is rare
  - Cells with ample cytoplasm
  - GFAP(+) processes, fibrillar background
- Nuclear pleomorphism in PPT
  - With well-formed, large pineocytomatous rosettes
  - Not evidence of malignancy
  - Pineocytoma with degenerative changes
- Diagnosis of PPTID
  - In absence of pineocytomatous rosettes
  - No overtly small cell appearance (pineoblastoma)
  - Not biphasic tumors with both components
- Histologically biphasic tumors
  - Recognizable pineoblastoma
  - Additional areas of intermediate differentiation
  - a.k.a. "mixed pineocytoma/pineoblastoma"
    - Although term "mixed" also applied to PPTID
  - Should be considered to be pineoblastoma

GRADING

Criteria

- Partly based on personal, anecdotal experience
  - ↑ cellularity, mitoses per high-power field (HPF)
  - Presence of necrosis portends worse prognosis
  - Immunostaining for neuronal markers
    - Corresponds to neuropil-like fibrillar areas
- 4 grades correlate with clinical variables, outcome
  - Largely equivalent to WHO classification categories
  - PPTs have continuous spectrum of differentiation

Grade I (Pineocytoma)

- Pineocytomatous rosettes, no mitoses or necrosis
- Strong immunopositivity for neuronal markers
  - Neurofilament, synaptophysin, chromogranin

Grade II (PPTID)

- < 6 mitoses/10 HPF, strong neurofilament staining

Grade III (PPTID)

- < 6 mitoses/10 HPF, no/weak neurofilament staining
- > 6 mitoses/10 HPF, strong neurofilament staining
- May be considered pineoblastoma by WHO criteria

Grade IV (Pineoblastoma)

- Small cell tumor with aggressive clinical behavior
- > 6 mitoses/10 HPF, no/weak neurofilament staining

SELECTED REFERENCES

1. Sato K et al: Pathology of pineal parenchymal tumors. Prog Neurol Surg. 23:12-25, 2009
2. De Girolami U et al: Pathology of tumors of the pineal region. Rev Neurol (Paris). 164(11):882-95, 2008
3. Pusztaszeri M et al: Pineal parenchymal tumors of intermediate differentiation in adults: case report and literature review. Neuropathology. 26(2):153-7, 2006
4. Hirato J et al: Pathology of pineal region tumors. J Neurooncol. 54(3):239-49, 2001
5. Fauchon F et al: Parenchymal pineal tumors: a clinicopathological study of 76 cases. Int J Radiat Oncol Biol Phys. 46(4):959-68, 2000
6. Jouvet A et al: Pineal parenchymal tumors: a correlation of histological features with prognosis in 66 cases. Brain Pathol. 10(1):49-60, 2000
7. Scheithauer BW: Pathobiology of the pineal gland with emphasis on parenchymal tumors. Brain Tumor Pathol. 16(1):1-9, 1999
8. Tsumanuma I et al: Clinicopathological study of pineal parenchymal tumors: correlation between histopathological features, proliferative potential, and prognosis. Brain Tumor Pathol. 16(2):61-8, 1999
9. Schild SE et al: Pineal parenchymal tumors. Clinical, pathologic, and therapeutic aspects. Cancer. 72(3):870-80, 1993
10. Scheithauer BW: Neuropathology of pineal region tumors. Clin Neurosurg. 32:351-83, 1985

PINEAL PARENCHYMAL TUMORS

Microscopic Features of Pineocytoma

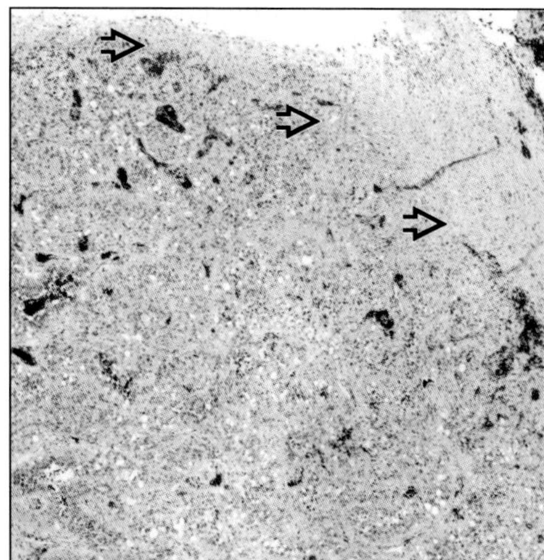

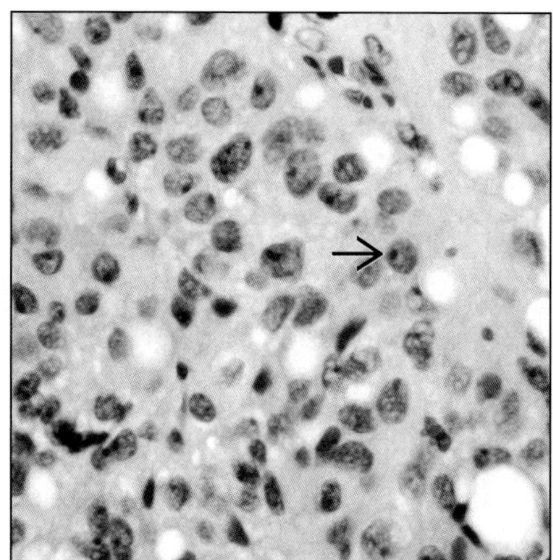

(Left) *Hematoxylin & eosin shows a low-power view of pineocytoma having moderate cellularity, a vaguely lobular growth pattern and a well-demarcated border ⇨ from adjacent normal brain parenchyma.* ***(Right)*** *Hematoxylin & eosin shows a high-power view of pineocytoma composed of mature-appearing cells resembling pineocytes with round to oval nuclei, finely dispersed open chromatin, and inconspicuous nucleoli →.*

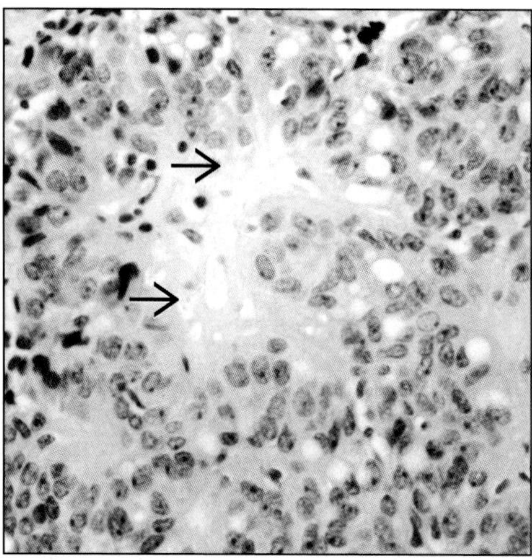

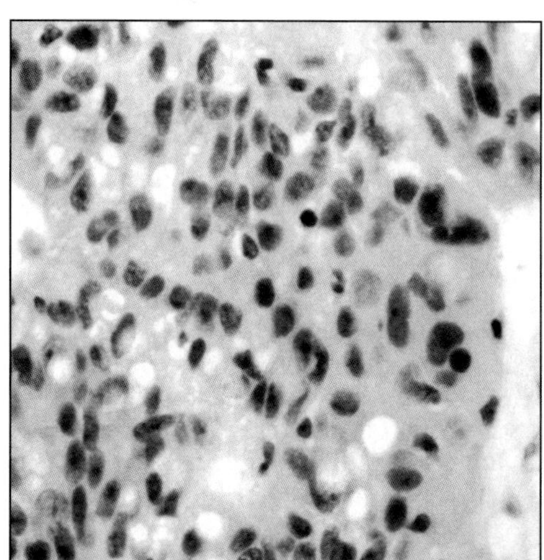

(Left) *Hematoxylin & eosin shows a high-power view of pineocytoma with "pineocytomatous rosettes" consisting of delicate, fibrillar cell processes forming stellate nuclear-free zones →. These are larger and more irregularly shaped foci of eosinophilic neuropil than neuroblastic rosettes and lack the lumen of retinoblastic rosettes.* ***(Right)*** *H&E shows a high-power view of pineocytoma with nuclear pleomorphism and hyperchromasia, considered "degenerative atypia" and not by itself diagnostic of a higher grade lesion.*

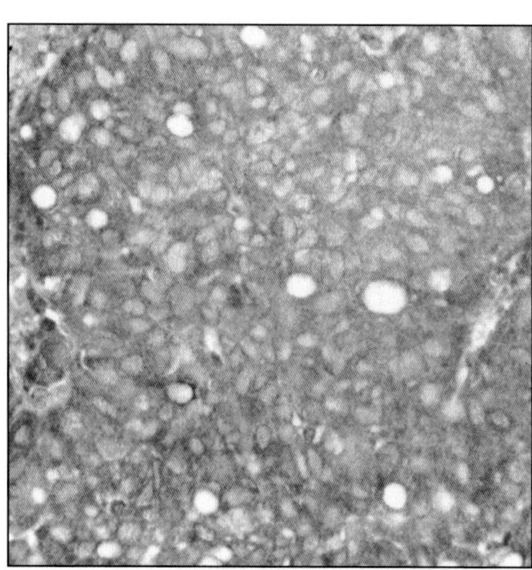

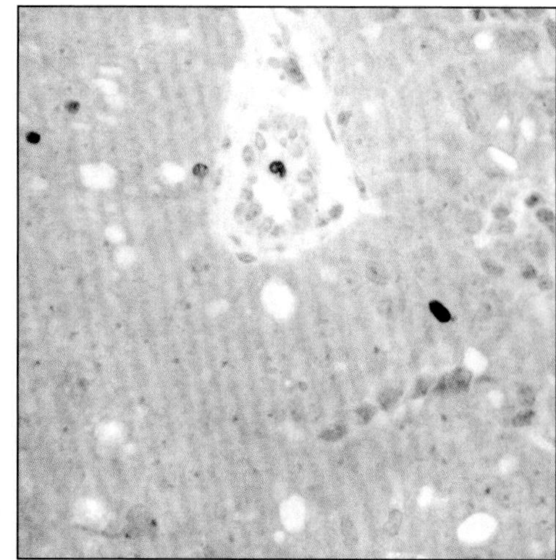

(Left) *Synaptophysin immunohistochemical stain shows a high-power view of pineocytoma with strong and diffuse positive staining in tumor cells and processes. Along with other neuronal markers, this is considered evidence of differentiation and a characteristic of low-grade pineal parenchymal lesions.* ***(Right)*** *Ki-67 immunohistochemical stain shows a high-power view of pineocytoma with a very low MIB-1 labeling index, consistent with a low-grade lesion.*

Microscopic Features of Pineoblastoma

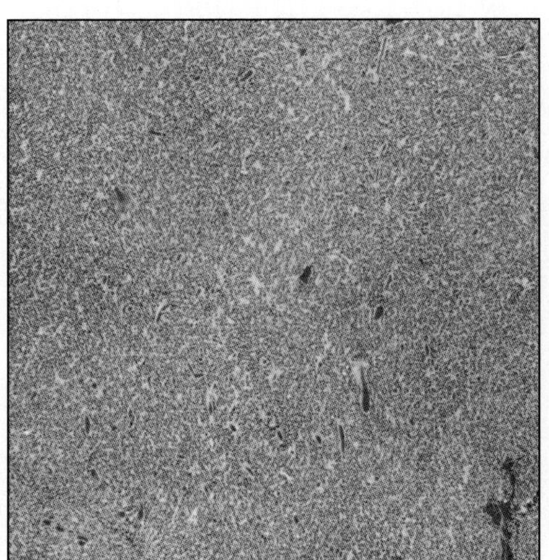

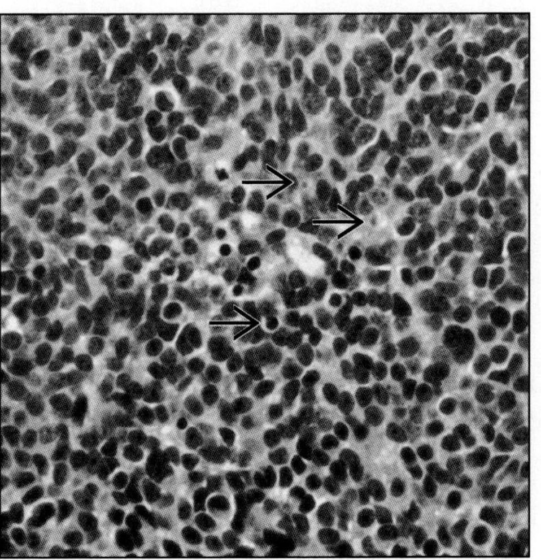

(Left) *Hematoxylin & eosin shows a low-power view of pineoblastoma, composed of very cellular, patternless sheets of densely packed "small blue cells." A tumor this hypercellular is unlikely to be low grade.* ***(Right)*** *Hematoxylin & eosin shows a high-power view of pineoblastoma with crowded small cells having little cytoplasm, high nuclear to cytoplasmic ratio, indistinct cell borders, and round hyperchromatic nuclei. Apoptotic figures ⇨ and mitoses are usually prominent.*

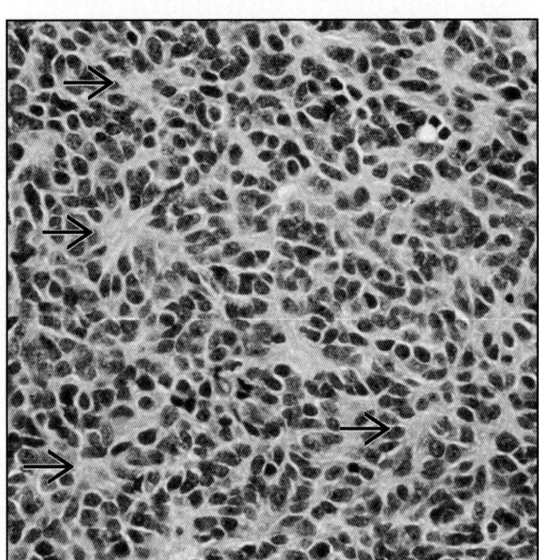

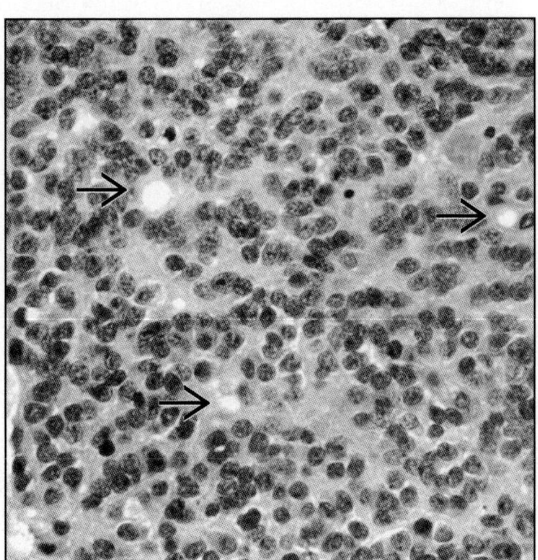

(Left) *Hematoxylin & eosin shows a high-power view of pineoblastoma with numerous small neuroblastic (Homer Wright) rosettes ⇨ composed of delicate, radially arranged cell processes, resulting in nuclear-free areas.* ***(Right)*** *H&E shows a high-power view of pineoblastoma with retinoblastic (Flexner-Wintersteiner) rosettes ⇨ composed of small lumens radially surrounded by tumor cells. These are considered evidence of neurosensory/photoreceptor differentiation.*

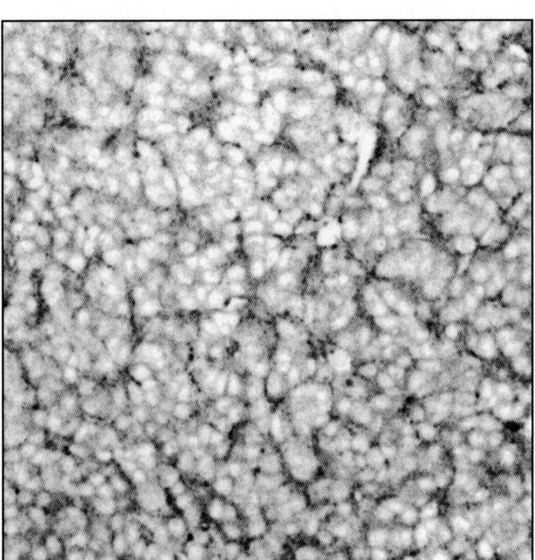

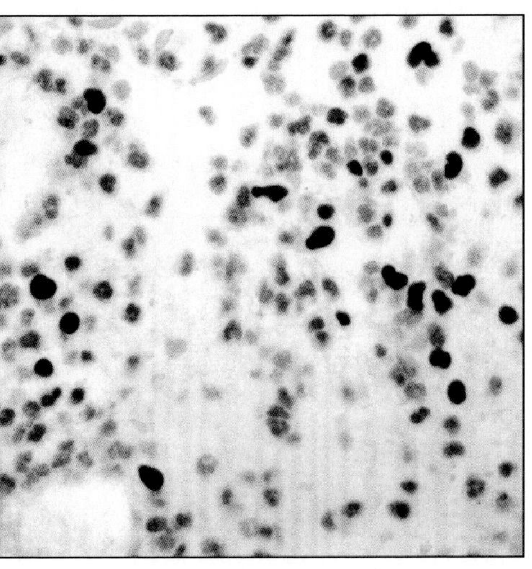

(Left) *Synaptophysin immunohistochemical stain shows a high-power view of pineoblastoma where the nuclear-free central zones of neuroblastic rosettes are strongly positive, corresponding to tumor cell processes. Scattered individual tumor cells may also be positive.* ***(Right)*** *Ki-67 immunohistochemical stains shows a high-power view of pineoblastoma with a relatively high labeling index, something that distinguishes these tumors from more low-grade lesions.*

PILOCYTIC ASTROCYTOMA

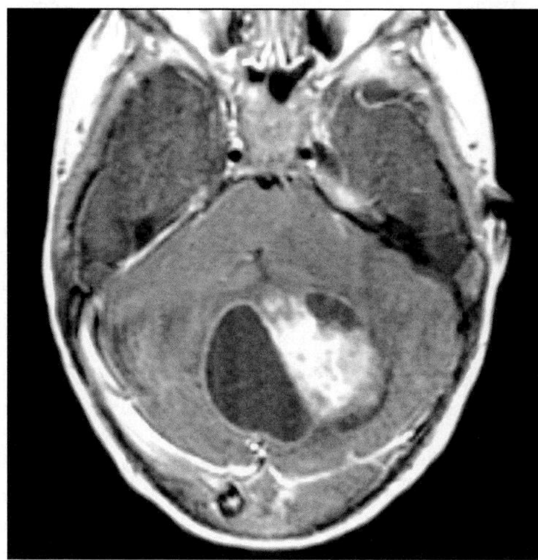

Axial T1 MR shows a heterogeneously contrast-enhancing cerebellar mass with cystic components compressing the 4th ventricle.

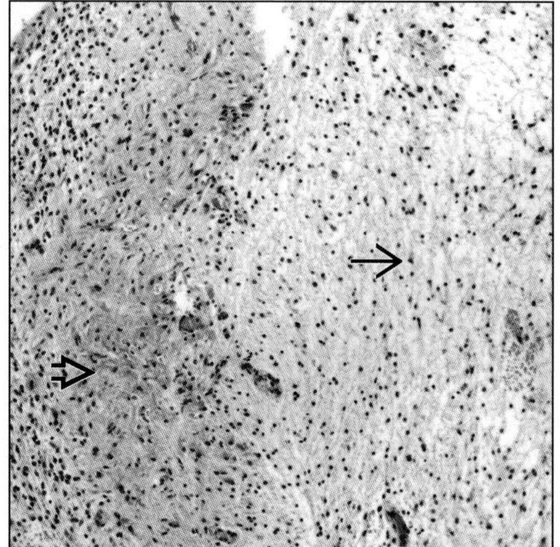

H&E section shows a medium-power view of classic biphasic histology in pilocytic astrocytoma with dense fibrillar piloid areas ⇨ and loose microcystic areas →.

TERMINOLOGY

Synonyms

- Juvenile pilocytic astrocytoma
- Piloid, "cystic" or "childhood" astrocytoma
- Spongioblastoma (original Bailey and Cushing term)

Definitions

- Slow-growing, benign (WHO grade I) astrocytic tumor
- Well-circumscribed, midline CNS lesion in children
- Grossly cystic with mural nodule, biphasic histology

ETIOLOGY/PATHOGENESIS

Histogenesis

- Unresolved cell of origin, various possibilities
  - Bipolar astrocyte, prone to forming Rosenthal fibers
  - Distinct immature glial precursor cell
    - "Spongioblast" or tanycyte (ependymoglial cell)
- Distinct genetic abnormalities acquired
  - Frequently occur in neurofibromatosis type 1 (NF1) (especially in optic nerve)
  - Sporadic lesions show 17q LOH (location of *NF1*)

CLINICAL ISSUES

Epidemiology

- Incidence
  - 6% of intracranial tumors (< 1 per 100,000 per year)
  - Most common pediatric primary brain tumor (30%)
    - 2nd after embryonal tumors in infants
- Age
  - Peak incidence 8-13 years old; > 70% in < 20 years old
  - Cerebral/spinal lesions tend to manifest at older age

Site

- Mostly axial (ventricles, midline), throughout neuraxis
  - 12-18% in cerebellum ("cerebellar astrocytoma")
    - Secondary invasion of brainstem in up to 30%
  - 8-20% in cerebral hemispheres
    - Especially in medial temporal lobe
  - 3-5% in optic nerve ("optic nerve glioma"), chiasm
    - Often extends into hypothalamus, 3rd ventricle
  - 3-6% in brainstem ("brainstem glioma")
    - Often dorsal/exophytic, in medulla/midbrain
  - Spinal cord, thalamus, basal ganglia, infundibulum

Presentation

- Long symptom history prior to presentation/diagnosis
- Neurological symptoms depend on tumor site
  - Cerebellum: ↑ ICP, CSF obstruction, hydrocephalus
    - Papilledema, headache, ataxia, nausea, vomiting
  - Optic nerve: Visual acuity/field defects, proptosis
  - Hypothalamus: Endocrine, electrolyte imbalance
    - Diabetes insipidus, precocious puberty
  - Brainstem: Cranial nerve deficits, CSF obstruction
  - Supratentorial: Mass effect, ↑ ICP, seizures/epilepsy
  - Thalamus/basal ganglia: ↑ ICP, weakness/paresis

Natural History

- Slow growth: Symptoms may long precede diagnosis
  - May be constant in size or regress, especially in NF1
- Tends to extend/invade meninges, subarachnoid space
  - Especially in optic nerve, cerebellar lesions, in NF1
    - **Not** criterion of malignancy, rare CSF seeding
- May have multiple synchronous/metachronous lesions
  - Mostly in NF1; if NF1 excluded, cause is CSF spread
- Malignant progression uncommon, rarely reported
- Clinical "recurrence" may instead be post-op cyst
- "Progressive": Rapidly enlarging/developing symptoms
  - Not necessarily indicative of malignant progression
  - May be due to expansion of tumor cyst

Treatment

- Surgical approaches
  - Complete surgical resection is the goal
    - May be difficult due to lesion location
- Adjuvant therapy

PILOCYTIC ASTROCYTOMA

Key Facts

Terminology
- Slow-growing, benign (grade I) astrocytic tumor
- Well-circumscribed, midline CNS lesion in children
- Grossly cystic with mural nodule, biphasic histology

Clinical Issues
- Most common pediatric primary brain tumor (30%)
- Peak incidence 8-13 years old; > 70% in < 20 years old
- Axial (ventricles, midline), throughout neuraxis
- Long symptom history before presentation/diagnosis
- Tends to extend into meninges, subarachnoid space
- 5- and 10-year survival > 80%, regardless of location
- No histopathologic criteria predict clinical outcome

Image Findings
- Discrete, iso- to hypodense, contrast-enhancing mass
- Cystic, round-oval lesions with mural nodule(s)

Macroscopic Features
- Well delineated, expansive rather than infiltrative
- Gray-pink, soft, with cysts/mucoid degeneration

Microscopic Pathology
- Biphasic pattern, but not always present/identifiable
- Mature, trapped ganglion cells often present
- Degenerative hyalinized vessels, hemosiderin
  - Necrosis, calcifications are uncommon
- Nuclear pleomorphism may be extensive
  - But mitoses, proliferation rare (MIB-1 ~ 1%)
- Anaplastic pilocytic astrocytoma (grade III)
  - Overt anaplasia, necrosis, vascular proliferation
- Pilomyxoid astrocytoma (grade II)
  - Mucoid with monotonous, small angiocentric cells

  - No evidence for benefit of radiation on survival
    - Avoided due to long-term sequelae in children
    - Usually reserved for 1st or 2nd recurrence
  - Chemotherapy for progressing, unresectable lesions

Prognosis
- Long recurrence-free intervals (> 20 years) are typical
  - Depends on completeness of surgical resection
- 5- and 10-year survival > 80%, regardless of location
  - Approaches 100% after complete surgical resection
- No histopathologic criteria to predict clinical outcome
- Pilomyxoid variant might have worse prognosis

IMAGE FINDINGS

MR Findings
- Hypo- to isointense on T1, hyperintense on T2

CT Findings
- Discrete, iso- to hypodense, contrast-enhancing mass
- Lack of peritumoral edema, uncommon calcifications
- Cystic, round-oval lesions with mural nodule(s)
  - Especially cerebellar, supratentorial lesions
- Fusiform enlargement ("pencil-shaped glioma")
  - Longitudinal growth within spinal cord, optic nerve

MACROSCOPIC FEATURES

General Features
- Well delineated, expansive rather than infiltrative
- Gray-pink, soft, with cysts/mucoid degeneration
- Optic: Infiltrate/expand nerve underneath sheath
- Spinal cord: Multi-segment ("holocord astrocytoma")

MICROSCOPIC PATHOLOGY

Histologic Features
- Relatively solid, but may permeate brain parenchyma
- Biphasic pattern of intermingled components
- Ratio of each varies widely, not always identifiable
- Highly fibrillar, dense "piloid" areas
  - Sheets or islands of compact, elongated, bipolar cells
  - Marked, long, hair-like processes; Rosenthal fibers
  - Tend to be more "lobular" in tumor periphery
  - Infiltrative pilocytic areas dominate in optic glioma
- Loosely structured, microcystic, "wet" areas
  - May predominate over fibrillar areas in cerebellum
  - Small vacuoles, often coalesce into larger cavities
    - Filled with amorphous eosinophilic fluid
  - Stellate, multipolar cells with round-oval nuclei
    - Short, afibrillar cytoplasmic processes
- Glomeruloid microvascular proliferation
  - May be extensive, especially along tumor cyst wall
  - Secondary to VEGF secretion by tumor cells
  - Presence does **not** signify malignancy
- Reticulin fibers and desmoplasia
  - Especially in areas of subarachnoid space invasion
  - Silver stain highlights extensive reticulin deposits
  - Fibrocollagenous septa in peritumoral sulci
- Degenerative/regressive changes
  - Longstanding lesions of cerebellum, cerebral cortex
  - Extensively hyalinized vessels, often telangiectatic
    - Similar to vascular malformation, hemangioma
  - Hemosiderin deposits, perivascular lymphocytes
  - Necrosis or calcifications are uncommon

Cytologic Features
- Relatively hypocellular, highly fibrillar dense matrix
- Classic elongated, uni- or bipolar neoplastic astrocytes
  - Form parallel or interdigitating bundles or whorls
  - Uniform oval nuclei, open chromatin, small nucleoli
  - Thin, hair-like processes with intermediate filaments
- Round/stellate cells, resemble protoplasmic astrocytes
  - Especially in areas of cystic/mucoid degeneration
  - Lose processes; weakly GFAP positive or negative
- Oligodendroglia-like intracellular mucin accumulation
- Nuclear pleomorphism may be present, even extensive
  - Hyperchromasia, degenerative atypia
  - Multinucleated giant cells
    - "Pennies on a plate" nuclear arrangement
  - But mitoses rare, cell proliferation not increased
    - 30% of tumors may have a solitary mitosis
- Mature ganglion cells present, especially in cerebellum

PILOCYTIC ASTROCYTOMA

- Mostly trapped normal neurons (Purkinje cells)
- If dysmorphic, neoplastic: Pilocytic ganglioglioma
  - Especially in temporal lobe

Cytoplasmic Accumulations (Inclusions)

- Rosenthal fibers (RFs)
  - Bright eosinophilic, beaded cytoplasmic bodies
  - Corkscrew-shaped, 1 blunt and 1 tapered end
  - Red on Mason trichrome, blue on Luxol fast blue
  - Restricted to compact pilocytic/fibrillar areas
- Eosinophilic granular bodies (EGBs)
  - Bright eosinophilic PAS(+) protein droplets
  - More frequent in less fibrillar, microcystic areas

Pilomyxoid Astrocytoma (WHO Grade II)

- "Infantile" form, mostly in hypothalamus, cerebellum
- More likely to recur locally, seed CSF
- Monotonous, small, elongated GFAP-positive cells
  - Radially oriented around vessels ("angiocentric")
    - Similar to perivascular pseudorosettes
- Mucoid, but usually lacks microcysts, RFs, EGBs
- Mitoses, necrosis may be present

Anaplastic Pilocytic Astrocytoma (WHO Grade III)

- Malignant astrocytoma within pilocytic astrocytoma
  - Overt anaplasia, necrosis, vascular proliferation
  - Increased proliferation: ↑ MIB-1 index, ↑ mitoses
- Rare, < 3-5% of all pilocytic astrocytomas
  - Often in setting of prior irradiation

ANCILLARY TESTS

Frozen Sections

- Biphasic pattern often obscured
- Helpful: Microcysts, hyalinized vessels, RFs, EGBs

Immunohistochemistry

- GFAP(+) piloid cells, especially in fibrillar areas
- RFs, EGBs: Ubiquitin, αB-crystallin positive
- MIB-1 index: Mean 1%, focally up to 5-10%

Cytogenetics

- Frequent trisomy 7 or 8; LOH at 17q
- Significant aneuploidy, but *P53* mutations rare

Electron Microscopy

- Intermediate filaments in elongated piloid cells
- RFs: Well-delineated, amorphous, electron dense
- EGBs: Membrane-bound, electron dense, up to 20 μm

Smear Preparation

- Uniform bland nuclei, RFs, EGBs
- Elongated, bipolar cells with long, fine processes

DIFFERENTIAL DIAGNOSIS

Piloid Gliosis

- Dense fibrillar tissue, often with many RFs
- Usually lacks microcystic component
- Little vessel hyalinization, no cytologic atypia

Diffuse Astrocytoma

- Not circumscribed, cystic, or contrast enhancing
- Usually lacks RFs, EGBs, hyalinized vessels

Pleomorphic Xanthoastrocytoma

- Superficial, leptomeningeal location
- More cellular, pleomorphic, and fascicular
- Perivascular lymphocytes, reticulin, foamy cytoplasm
- Lacks RFs or spongy microcystic areas

Ganglioglioma

- Solid, noninfiltrative, microcystic, with RFs and EGBs
- Perivascular lymphocytes, reticulin-rich stroma
- Contains dysmorphic, neoplastic neurons

DIAGNOSTIC CHECKLIST

Clinically Relevant Pathologic Features

- Often grossly cystic with mural nodule
  - Nodule is neoplastic, needs to be biopsied/excised
- Extensive nuclear pleomorphism may be present
  - No associated anaplasia or unfavorable prognosis
- 15-20% of NF1 patients develop pilocytic astrocytomas
  - Especially of optic nerve, can be bilateral
  - 30% of patients with optic nerve lesions have NF1

Pathologic Interpretation Pearls

- Biphasic histology not always present or required
- RFs: Characteristic, but not specific, finding
  - Be cautious of diagnosis in absence of RFs
  - Also seen in piloid gliosis, other tumors
- EGBs: Not specific, seen in slow-growing CNS lesions

GRADING

"Atypical" Lesions

- Increased cellularity &/or vascular proliferation

"Malignant" Lesions

- Brisk mitotic activity, vascular proliferation, necrosis
- However, still little association with survival rates

SELECTED REFERENCES

1. Scarabino T et al: Supratentorial low-grade gliomas. Neuroradiology. J Neurosurg Sci. 49(3):73-6, 2005
2. Koeller KK et al: From the archives of the AFIP: pilocytic astrocytoma: radiologic-pathologic correlation. Radiographics. 24(6):1693-708, 2004
3. Komotar RJ et al: Pilomyxoid astrocytoma: a review. MedGenMed. 6(4):42, 2004
4. Giannini C et al: Classification and grading of low-grade astrocytic tumors in children. Brain Pathol. 7(2):785-98, 1997
5. Krieger MD et al: Recurrence patterns and anaplastic change in a long-term study of pilocytic astrocytomas. Pediatr Neurosurg. 27(1):1-11, 1997
6. Kleihues P et al: Histopathology, classification, and grading of gliomas. Glia. 15(3):211-21, 1995
7. Tomlinson FH et al: The significance of atypia and histologic malignancy in pilocytic astrocytoma of the cerebellum: a clinicopathologic and flow cytometric study. J Child Neurol. 9(3):301-10, 1994

Microscopic Features

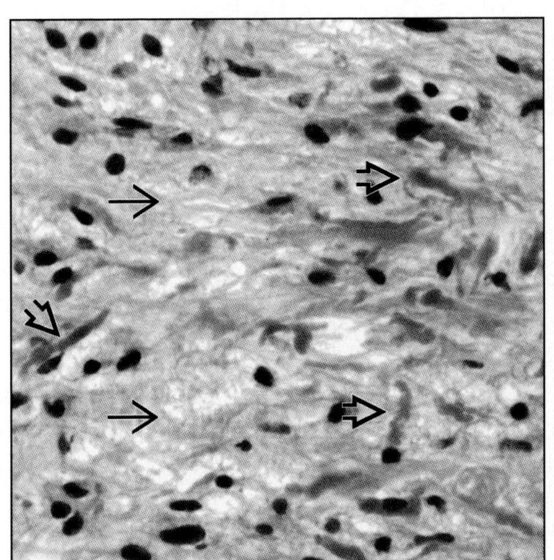

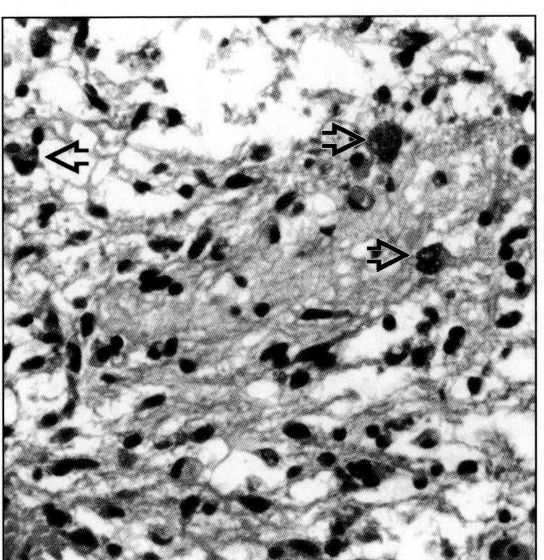

(Left) Rosenthal fibers ⇨ are bright eosinophilic cytoplasmic inclusions with a beaded, cork-screw shape, often with 1 blunt and 1 tapered end. While not specific for pilocytic astrocytomas, they are highly characteristic and mostly found in the more compact, fibrillar parts → of the tumor. ***(Right)*** Occasional nuclear hyperchromasia and pleomorphism ⇨ is common in pilocytic astrocytomas, but without accompanying mitotic activity or increased cell proliferation.

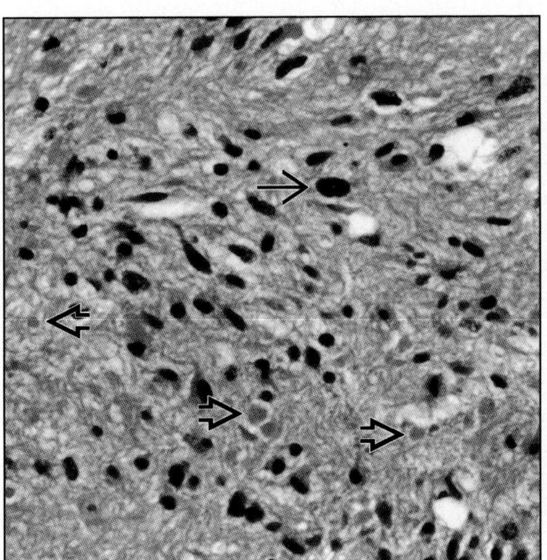

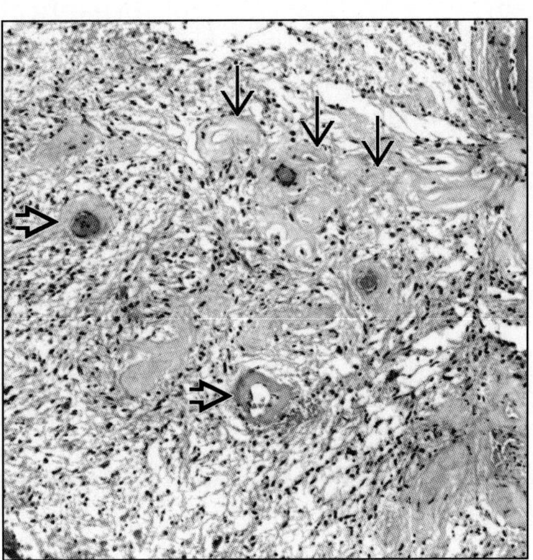

(Left) H&E section shows a high-power view of eosinophilic granular bodies ⇨, which are cytoplasmic, round protein droplets found in pilocytic astrocytomas and other slow-growing CNS tumors. Occasional giant cells → with multiple nuclei appearing like "pennies on a plate" can be present in pilocytic astrocytomas. ***(Right)*** H&E section shows a medium-power view of pilocytic astrocytoma with hyalinized vessels ⇨ which, when aggregated →, can resemble vascular malformation or angioma.

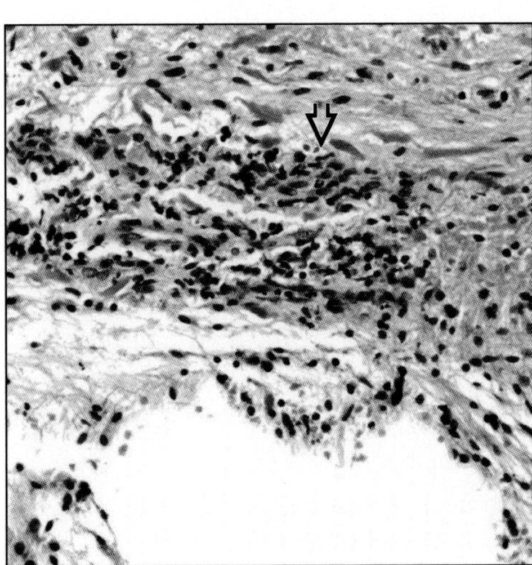

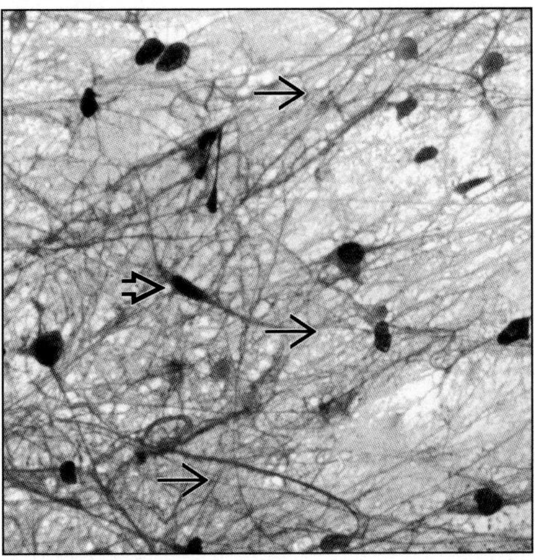

(Left) H&E section shows a medium-power view of glomeruloid microvascular proliferation ⇨, which can be present in pilocytic astrocytoma, especially along the cyst wall, and does not signify a high-grade glioma. ***(Right)*** H&E stained smear preparation shows a high-power view of the uniform, bland nuclei of pilocytic astrocytoma and elongated, bipolar cells ⇨ with long, fine, hair-like processes →, creating a meshwork.

PLEOMORPHIC XANTHOASTROCYTOMA

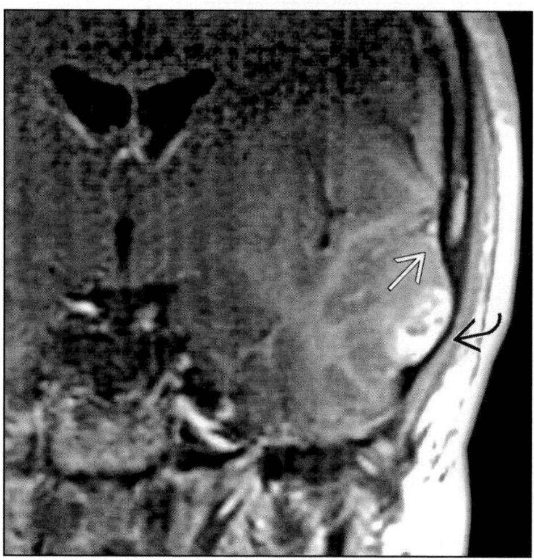

Coronal T1 MR shows a contrast-enhancing, superficial cortical mass with thickening of adjacent meninges ➡ and skull remodeling ⇨, but little peritumoral edema.

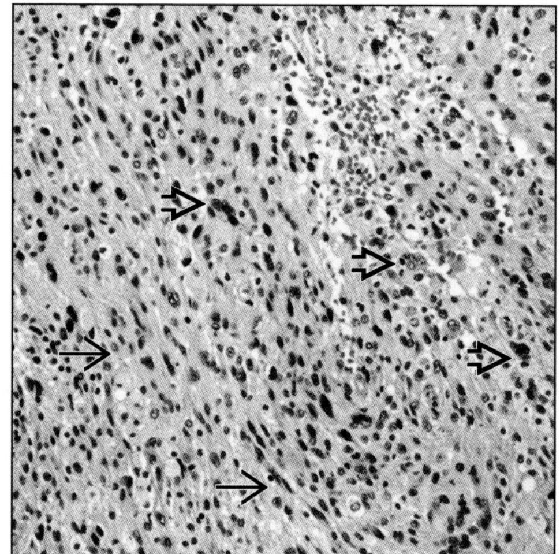

H&E shows high-power view of PXA with characteristic pleomorphic, bizarre tumor cells, including giant cells ⇨, and a focal fascicular growth pattern →.

TERMINOLOGY

Abbreviations

- Pleomorphic xanthoastrocytoma (PXA)

Definitions

- Superficial, circumscribed, meningocerebral, WHO grade II astrocytic tumor of children/young adults
- Cytologic pleomorphism, giant cells, xanthomatous change, reticulin-rich stroma, GFAP immunoreactivity

ETIOLOGY/PATHOGENESIS

Histogenesis

- Possible origin from subpial astrocytes
  - Produce basal lamina that envelops them
- Neuronal differentiation seen in most PXAs
  - Possible multipotential precursor cell

Genetics

- PXAs may be more common in malformative states
  - Associations: Cortical dysplasia, ganglionic lesions
- Rare reports of PXA in neurofibromatosis type 1
  - No familial clustering or other genetic associations

CLINICAL ISSUES

Epidemiology

- Incidence
  - < 1% of all astrocytic gliomas, pediatric CNS tumors
- Age
  - 1st 2 decades of life; 65% are < 18 years old
  - Occasional reports of cases in older patients

Site

- Involves meninges, cerebral cortex (meningocerebral)
  - But dura usually unaffected
- 98% are supratentorial, 50% involve temporal lobe
- Rare reported cases in cerebellum, spinal cord, retina

Presentation

- Long history of seizures (superficial cerebral location)
  - But may remain subclinical

Natural History

- Slow-growing tumor with long symptom-free periods
- May rarely cause abrupt hemorrhage
- Can be multicentric, especially in post-op recurrence
- 15-20% recur (mean of 6 years after surgical removal)
- Diffuse leptomeningeal/CSF spread uncommon

Treatment

- Surgical approaches
  - Complete surgical resection considered curative
    - Difficult if poor interface with brain parenchyma
    - Follow-up: Clinical/radiologic observation
  - Re-excise or debulk lesions after recurrence
- Radiation
  - Considered for higher grade lesions, unclear benefit

Prognosis

- Generally favorable, despite pleomorphic histology
  - Overall 5- and 10-year survival: > 80% and > 70%
    - Recurrence-free: > 70% and > 60%, respectively
  - Median postoperative survival: 18 years
- Related to extent of resection, mitotic activity, necrosis
  - > 5 mitoses/10 HPF: Higher recurrence rate
  - Malignant transformation: Less favorable outcome

IMAGE FINDINGS

MR Findings

- Isointense on T1, hyperintense on T2-weighted images

CT Findings

- Superficial, discrete, contrast-enhancing mass
- About 50% appear as nodule in wall of cyst
- Little mass effect/peritumoral edema (slow growth)
- Inner skull table often remodeled, "scalloped"
  - Due to chronic pressure from tumor

PLEOMORPHIC XANTHOASTROCYTOMA

Key Facts

Terminology
- Pleomorphic xanthoastrocytoma (PXA)
- Superficial, circumscribed, meningocerebral, WHO grade II astrocytic tumor of children/young adults

Clinical Issues
- < 1% of all astrocytic gliomas, pediatric CNS tumors
- 1st 2 decades of life; 65% are < 18 years old
- 98% are supratentorial, 50% involve temporal lobe
- Long history of seizures, but may remain subclinical
- Complete surgical resection considered curative
- Overall 5- and 10-year survival: > 80% and > 70%

Image Findings
- Superficial, discrete, contrast-enhancing mass
- About 50% appear as nodule in wall of cyst
- Little mass effect/peritumoral edema (slow growth)

Microscopic Pathology
- Compact, expansile, noninfiltrating, in subarachnoid
- Tongues into cerebral cortex along perivascular spaces
- Large, hyalinized vessels; dense reticulin-rich stroma
- Loose, perivascular chronic inflammatory infiltrate
- Pleomorphic, cytologically bizarre neoplastic cells
- Glassy, variably fibrillar, GFAP(+) cytoplasm
- Xanthomatous (lipidized, foamy) cell vacuolization
- Often contains EGBs; mitoses/necrosis mostly absent
- Large atypical ganglionic cells occasionally present
- PXA with anaplastic features
  - > 5 mitoses/10 HPF, vascular proliferation, necrosis
  - Higher recurrence rate, less favorable outcome
- Reconsider PXA diagnosis in the absence of
  - Reticulin-rich stroma
  - Discrete, superficial, contrast-enhancing cystic mass

MACROSCOPIC FEATURES

General Features
- Firm, well-circumscribed, superficial nodule or plaque
- Often cystic, with dark yellow clear/serous fluid
- Yellow-orange mural nodule, vascular/hemorrhagic
- Contiguously attached/extending to leptomeninges
  - Sharp interface with underlying brain grossly

MICROSCOPIC PATHOLOGY

Histologic Features
- Compact or lobulated, expansile, noninfiltrating
  - Often expands within subarachnoid space
  - May invade brain, despite gross circumscription
- Extends tongues into underlying cerebral cortex
  - Along perivascular Virchow-Robin spaces
- Fascicular growth pattern, especially in periphery
  - May be storiform, akin to fibrohistiocytic lesions
  - Or more closely packed and "epithelioid"
- Large muscular arteries within tumor substance
  - Of size normally seen in subarachnoid
  - Hyalinized vessels, especially superficially
  - Some have been termed "angiomatous" PXAs
- Abundant, dense, reticulin-rich intercellular stroma
  - Mostly around vessels, solid areas of pleomorphism
  - Around individual or groups of tumor cells
- Loose, perivascular chronic inflammatory infiltrate
  - T lymphocytes and occasionally plasma cells
  - May infiltrate diffusely into surrounding tumor
- May have infiltrating component at brain interface
  - Resembles diffuse astrocytoma, but not prognostic
- Calcifications in adjacent cortex, but rare in tumor

Cytologic Features
- Pleomorphic, cytologically bizarre neoplastic cells
  - Vary in number, size, shape, density
  - Round, irregular, elongated or spindle; may be giant
    - Resemble large polar cells of sarcomatous tumors
  - Large, multiple or multilobed hyperchromatic nuclei
  - Glassy, variably fibrillar, GFAP(+) cytoplasm
- Xanthomatous (lipidized, foamy) vacuolization of cells
  - Intracellular lipid droplets, oil red O positive
- Eosinophilic granular bodies (EGBs)
  - Small cytoplasmic aggregates of protein droplets
  - Eosinophilic, hyaline, PAS(+) material
- Large atypical ganglionic cells occasionally present
  - Trapped nonneoplastic neuronal cells, or
  - Binucleated neoplastic lesional neuronal cells
- Mitoses and necrosis generally absent
  - Unless anaplastic

ANCILLARY TESTS

Frozen Sections
- Pleomorphism does not always signify high grade
  - Especially if circumscribed, enhancing, or superficial
  - If no brisk mitoses, vascular proliferation, necrosis
- EGBs, xanthomatous change are helpful, reassuring

Immunohistochemistry
- GFAP immunoreactivity may be weak or focal
  - Confirms astrocytic nature of tumor cells
- S100 positivity, often widespread
- Abundant CD68(+) macrophages, microglial cells
- Ganglionic cells: Synaptophysin &/or NF positive
- MIB-1 index: Mean 2%; ~ 10-20% in anaplastic areas

Cytogenetics
- Complex karyotypes, subtelomeric gains/losses seen
  - Especially chromosome 9 loss (in up to 50%)
- Low incidence of *TP53* or other gene mutations
  - May be more prevalent in PXAs with anaplasia

Electron Microscopy
- Intermediate filaments in glial cell processes
- Basal lamina envelops cell bodies, processes
  - Corresponds to silver stain-positive reticulin
- Ganglion cells: ER, microtubules, dense-core granules

Smear Preparation
- Glial cells with varying nuclear pleomorphism
  - May find EGBs in astrocytic processes

PLEOMORPHIC XANTHOASTROCYTOMA

DIFFERENTIAL DIAGNOSIS

Glioblastoma Multiforme

- Especially giant cell type
- Rarely superficial, cystic, or solidly enhancing
- Highly infiltrative, widely pleomorphic, ↑ mitoses
- Generally lacks EGBs, has little reticulin

Pilocytic Astrocytoma

- Also compact, noninfiltrating, and solidly enhancing
- More biphasic and microcystic, with Rosenthal fibers
- Less compact, less cellular, less pleomorphic

Ganglioglioma

- Also cyst forming, in temporal lobe of young patients
- Generally much less pleomorphic

DIAGNOSTIC CHECKLIST

Clinically Relevant Pathologic Features

- Age distribution
- Symptom complex
- Tissue distribution
- Cytoplasmic features
- "Anaplastic" PXAs less aggressive than glioblastomas
  - Most cases survive > 3 years
- Growth patterns within PXA may vary
  - Wide sampling important, especially mural nodule

Pathologic Interpretation Pearls

- EGBs are not entirely sensitive or specific
  - Seen in many CNS tumors, not only PXAs
  - Indicate chronicity, characteristic of low-grade, slow-growing, discrete glioneuronal tumors
    - Pilocytic astrocytoma
    - Ganglion cell tumors
  - Avoid diagnosis of malignancy in their presence
  - Hyalinized vessels also seen in slow-growing tumors
  - EGBs can be absent in as many as 20% of PXAs
- Reconsider PXA diagnosis in absence of
  - Reticulin-rich stroma
  - Discrete, superficial, contrast-enhancing cystic mass
- Xanthomatous change is often difficult to identify
  - Not necessary for diagnosis
- Rosenthal fibers generally not present in PXA
  - Except in peritumoral gliotic brain parenchyma
- PXAs with neoplastic neuronal (ganglion) component
  - Best thought as PXA with ganglionic differentiation
  - Rather than ganglioglioma (WHO grade I)
- Necrosis generally absent in PXAs
  - If present: Search for mitoses, anaplastic features

GRADING

PXA with Anaplastic Features

- Preferred WHO term
- Either de novo or in preexisting PXAs
  - But most cases lack history of irradiation therapy
- Higher grade, anaplastic histology in 15-20% of PXAs
  - High mitotic activity (> 5 per 10 HPF)
  - Endothelial microvascular proliferation, necrosis
- More monomorphically atypical than pleomorphic
  - Small cell, epithelioid appearance
- Higher recurrence rate
  - Unclear if aggressive adjuvant therapy is needed
    - Especially if completely excised
  - Unclear whether these are true grade III lesions

SELECTED REFERENCES

1. Fu YJ et al: Intraventricular pleomorphic xanthoastrocytoma with anaplastic features. Neuropathology. 30(4):443-8, 2010
2. Grau E et al: Subtelomeric analysis of pediatric astrocytoma: subchromosomal instability is a distinctive feature of pleomorphic xanthoastrocytoma. J Neurooncol. 93(2):175-82, 2009
3. Okazaki T et al: Primary anaplastic pleomorphic xanthoastrocytoma with widespread neuroaxis dissemination at diagnosis--a pediatric case report and review of the literature. J Neurooncol. 94(3):431-7, 2009
4. Zakrzewska M et al: Prevalence of mutated TP53 on cDNA (but not on DNA template) in pleomorphic xanthoastrocytoma with positive TP53 immunohistochemistry. Cancer Genet Cytogenet. 193(2):93-7, 2009
5. Hirose T et al: Pleomorphic xanthoastrocytoma: a comparative pathological study between conventional and anaplastic types. Histopathology. 52(2):183-93, 2008
6. Hamlat A et al: Cerebellar pleomorphic xanthoastrocytoma: case report and literature review. Surg Neurol. 68(1):89-94; discussion 94-5, 2007
7. Marton E et al: Malignant progression in pleomorphic xanthoastrocytoma: personal experience and review of the literature. J Neurol Sci. 252(2):144-53, 2007
8. Weber RG et al: Frequent loss of chromosome 9, homozygous CDKN2A/p14(ARF)/CDKN2B deletion and low TSC1 mRNA expression in pleomorphic xanthoastrocytomas. Oncogene. 26(7):1088-97, 2007
9. Gil-Gouveia R et al: Pleomorphic xanthoastrocytoma of the cerebellum: illustrated review. Acta Neurochir (Wien). 146(11):1241-4, 2004
10. Yin XL et al: Genetic imbalances in pleomorphic xanthoastrocytoma detected by comparative genomic hybridization and literature review. Cancer Genet Cytogenet. 132(1):14-9, 2002
11. Sharma MC et al: Pigmented pleomorphic xanthoastrocytoma: report of a rare case with review of the literature. Arch Pathol Lab Med. 125(6):808-11, 2001
12. Giannini C et al: Classification and grading of low-grade astrocytic tumors in children. Brain Pathol. 7(2):785-98, 1997
13. Tonn JC et al: Pleomorphic xanthoastrocytoma: report of six cases with special consideration of diagnostic and therapeutic pitfalls. Surg Neurol. 47(2):162-9, 1997
14. Pahapill PA et al: Pleomorphic xanthoastrocytoma: case report and analysis of the literature concerning the efficacy of resection and the significance of necrosis. Neurosurgery. 38(4):822-8; discussion 828-9, 1996
15. van Roost D et al: Clinical, radiological, and therapeutic features of pleomorphic xanthoastrocytoma: report of three patients and review of the literature. J Neurol Neurosurg Psychiatry. 60(6):690-2, 1996
16. Davies KG et al: Pleomorphic xanthoastrocytoma--report of four cases, with MRI scan appearances and literature review. Br J Neurosurg. 8(6):681-9, 1994
17. Whittle IR et al: Pleomorphic xanthoastrocytoma. Report of four cases. J Neurosurg. 70(3):463-8, 1989

Microscopic Features

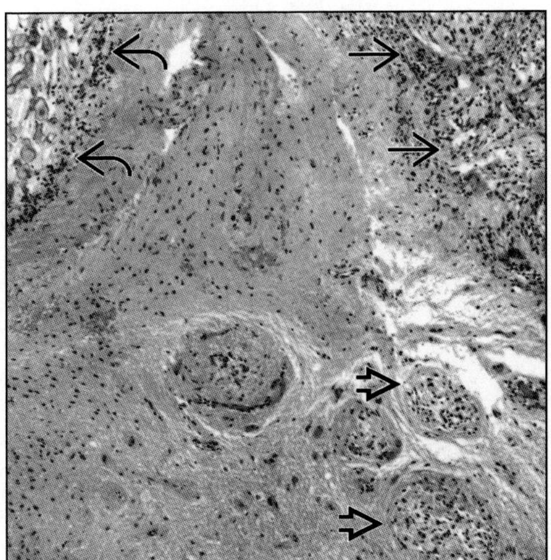

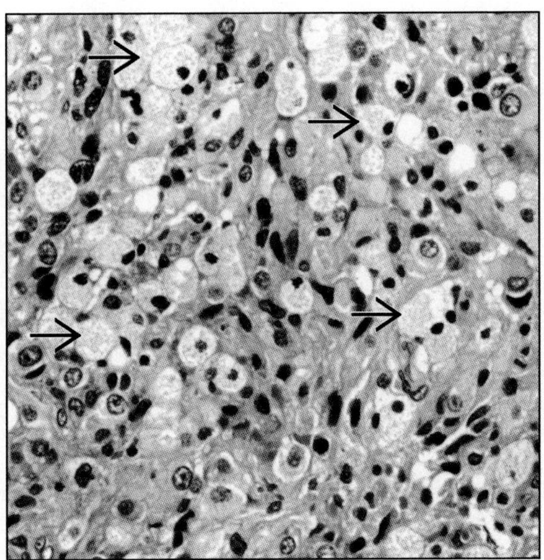

(Left) *H&E section shows low-power view of PXA, characteristically growing within subarachnoid space* → *and extending along perivascular Virchow-Robin spaces* ⇨. *In this case, there is sharp interface with the underlying brain parenchyma, which has calcifications* ↷. ***(Right)*** *H&E shows high-power view of xanthomatous change* →, *foamy vacuolization in tumor cells due to intracellular lipid droplets. Often difficult to identify, it is not required for the diagnosis of PXA.*

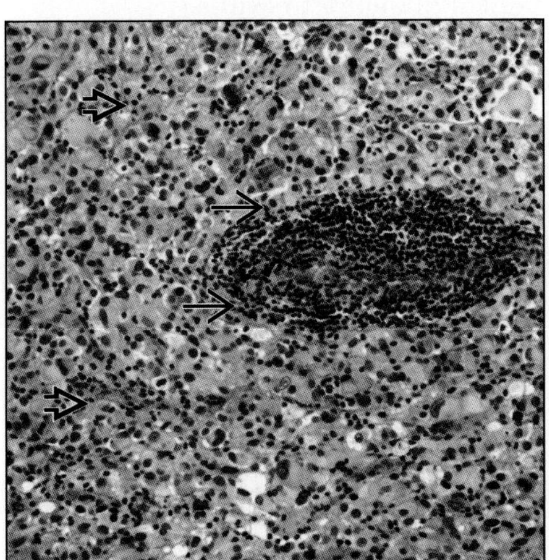

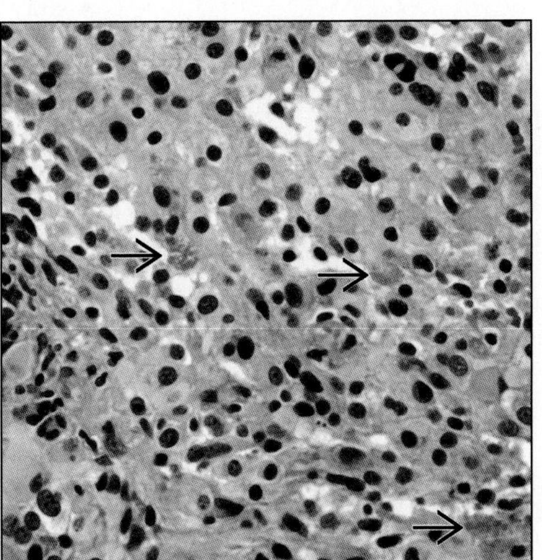

(Left) *H&E shows a high-power view of PXA with prominent perivascular chronic inflammation* →, *mostly composed of T cells and occasional plasma cells. Some inflammatory cells infiltrate between the surrounding tumor cells* ⇨. ***(Right)*** *H&E shows a high-power view of EGBs* →, *round cytoplasmic aggregates of hyaline protein droplets, commonly found in PXA as well as in other well-differentiated, slow-growing, discrete glioneuronal neoplasms.*

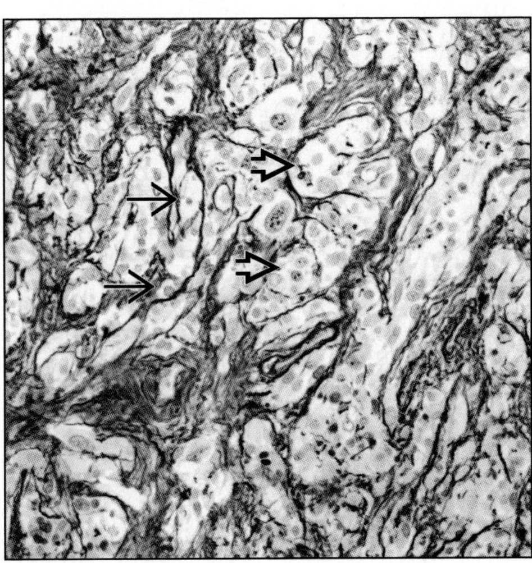

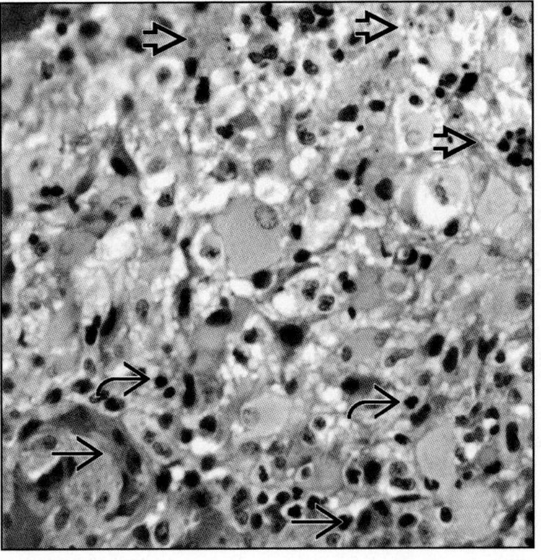

(Left) *Reticulin stain shows a high-power view of PXA with abundant, dense reticulin-rich stroma that envelops individual* → *or clusters* ⇨ *of tumor cells. This finding is highly characteristic of PXA, the diagnosis being suspect in its absence.* ***(Right)*** *H&E shows a high-power view of PXA with histologic anaplasia, including microvascular proliferation* →, *necrosis* ⇨, *and increased mitotic figures* ↷, *features associated with increased recurrence rate and a less favorable outcome.*

OLIGODENDROGLIOMA

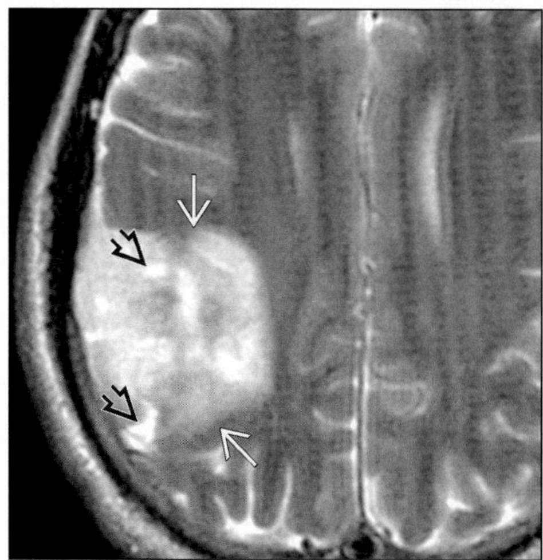

Axial T2WI MR shows a heterogeneous cortical/subcortical mass ➔ with cystic change ⊳. Despite a circumscribed appearance, oligodendrogliomas have infiltrating margins.

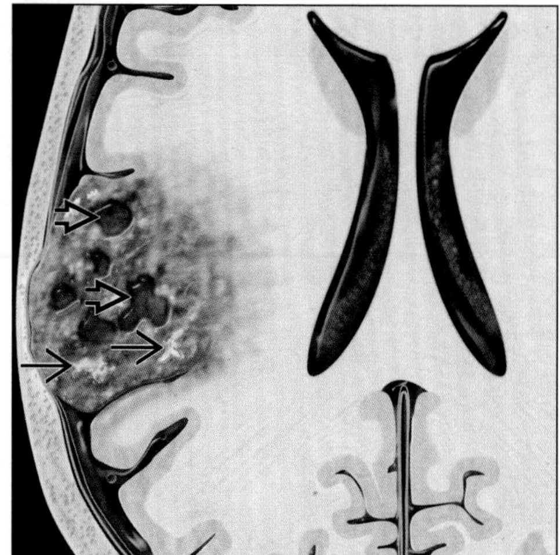

Graphic shows the gross appearance of an oligodendroglioma superficially expanding the cerebral cortex and containing chalky calcifications ➔ and cystic degeneration ⊳.

TERMINOLOGY

Synonyms

- Malignant = anaplastic oligodendroglioma

Definitions

- Diffusely infiltrating glioma, mostly in subcortical white matter of cerebral hemispheres, composed of neoplastic cells resembling oligodendrocytes
- WHO grades: II (well differentiated), III (anaplastic)
- Chromosome 1p/19q deletion portends better response to chemotherapy and improved prognosis
- Mixed glioma (oligoastrocytoma): Phenotypic features of both oligodendroglioma and astrocytoma

ETIOLOGY/PATHOGENESIS

Environmental Exposure

- In rats, induced experimentally with nitrosoureas
- Human cases reported after prior irradiation
- Viral sequences (SV40, JC, BK) identified in some cases

Histogenesis

- Morphologic characteristics suggest transformation of oligodendrocytes, but evidence is circumstantial
- Originating cell may be immature glial precursor
  - Dedifferentiation of putative bipotential stem cell
    - Oligodendrocyte type 2 astrocyte progenitor
  - May explain occasional immunoreactivity for GFAP
  - Possible common precursor in oligoastrocytoma
- Oligodendrocytes may be related to neurons
  - Some tumors have neurosecretory-like granules
  - Some staining for Hu protein, NMDA receptor 1
  - Ultrastructural findings suggest distinct neoplasm

Genetics

- Translocation between chromosomes 1 and 19
  - Results in 1p/19q codeletion
  - Incidence varies (40-90%)
    - Not entirely sensitive or specific
    - May be present in some astrocytomas
  - Corresponding gene mutations not yet identified
    - Several gene candidates exist
- As yet, undetected point mutations may also exist
  - Occasional reports of familial clustering
- *TP53* mutation generally rare in oligodendrogliomas
  - LOH seen in < 10-15% of cases
  - Virtually mutually exclusive with 1p/19q deletions
- Mixed glioma histogenesis is unclear
  - In 1 study both components had 1p/19q deletion

CLINICAL ISSUES

Epidemiology

- Incidence
  - 0.2-0.3 per 100,000 population annually
  - Approximately 2-5% of all primary brain tumors
    - 5-25% of all intracranial gliomas
- Age
  - Most occur in adults
    - Peak in 4th-6th decade; mean age: 40-45 years
    - Infratentorial lesions tend to occur slightly earlier
  - 5-7% arise in infancy/childhood
- Gender
  - Variable, slight male preponderance (3:2 to 2:1)

Site

- Throughout neuraxis, mostly in cerebral hemispheres
  - 90% in supratentorial white matter
  - 50-65% involve frontal lobe
  - Remaining lobes: Temporal > parietal > occipital
  - 50% involve multiple lobes, 20% bilateral
- Rare lesions in cerebellum, brainstem
- Unusual spinal/leptomeningeal lesions in children

Presentation

- Long symptomatic period (1-5 years) before diagnosis
- Seizures (epileptic), may also be focal/localizing
  - Due to diffuse involvement of cerebral cortex
- Focal neurologic deficits

OLIGODENDROGLIOMA

Key Facts

Clinical Issues

- 2-5% of all primary brain tumors, 5-25% of gliomas
- Most occur in adults, 5-7% arise in infancy/childhood
- 90% in supratentorial white matter (50-65% frontal)
- Long symptomatic period (seizures) before diagnosis
- Slow growing, indolent, but often recur locally
- Common leptomeningeal or CSF spread
- Gross total resection, adjuvant chemoradiation
  - 1p/19q deletion: Favorable response, prognosis
- Resected, well-differentiated lesions: Good prognosis

Image Findings

- Well circumscribed, heterogeneous, may enhance
  - Hemorrhagic, cystic, calcified

Macroscopic Features

- Soft, gelatinous, gray-pink, calcified (gritty)

Microscopic Pathology

- Diffusely infiltrating glioma of cerebral cortex
- Monomorphic: Round nuclei, small nucleoli
- Clear perinuclear vacuolization ("halo")
  - Processing artifact, absent in frozen sections
- Arborizing microvascular pattern ("chicken wire")
- Microcalcifications, microcysts, extracellular mucin
- Perineuronal satellitosis, subpial aggregates
- Circumscribed "clones" within tumor
- Focal "minigemistocytes": Astrocytic appearing
  - Prominent, eccentric pink cytoplasm
- Anaplastic oligodendroglioma (WHO grade III)
  - Hypercellularity, atypia, nuclear pleomorphism
  - Increased mitoses, necrosis, vascular proliferation
- Mixed glioma (oligoastrocytoma)
  - Both astrocytoma, oligodendroglioma components

- Increased intracranial pressure, headache
  - Larger posterior fossa lesions (obstruction)

Natural History

- Most are generally slow growing, indolent
- Local recurrence is most common cause of death
  - Relapse less likely in lesions with 1p/19q deletion
- Malignant progression (dedifferentiation) may occur
  - Less commonly than in astrocytomas
- Leptomeningeal or CSF spread is common (1-14%)
- Extracranial metastases: Bone, lung, liver
  - More common than in other gliomas
    - Especially in higher grade lesions
- Oligodendrogliomatosis
  - Diffuse leptomeningeal spread
  - May be component of gliomatosis cerebri

Treatment

- Surgical approaches
  - Generally thought unresectable (infiltrating glioma)
    - But surgery is mainstay of treatment
    - For diagnosis, reduction of mass effect
  - Attempt at gross total resection
    - At least of radiologic abnormality
- Adjuvant therapy
  - In unresected or higher grade lesions
    - Radiation &/or chemotherapy (PCV, thiotepa)
    - Favorable response in 1p/19q deleted lesions
  - Not in largely excised well-differentiated lesions
    - Unless neoplasm recurs

Prognosis

- Well-differentiated lesions carry good prognosis
  - Survival rates: 5-year (~ 75%), 10-year (~ 60%)
    - After gross total resection
  - Rates are 1/2 if subtotal resection or higher grade
  - Better than astrocytomas of comparable grade
- Prognosis still guarded: Recurrence after > decade
- 1p/19q deletion significantly improves prognosis
  - Median postoperative survival ~ 10-15 years
    - (vs. ~ 2-5 years without codeletion)
  - Survival advantage also in anaplastic lesions
    - But may not apply to pediatric lesions

IMAGE FINDINGS

MR Findings

- Hypointense on T1WI, hyperintense on T2WI
- Variable mass effect, little peritumoral edema
- Well-circumscribed margin with brain parenchyma
- Heterogeneous: Hemorrhage, cystic degeneration

CT Findings

- Superficially seated, usually large intracortical lesion
  - Rare, deep-seated lesions may cross corpus callosum
- Hypo- or isodense, well demarcated
- Absent or minimal contrast enhancement
- Higher grade (anaplastic) lesions may enhance
  - But lack rim or ring pattern of glioblastoma
- Calcification common (30-90%) but not diagnostic
  - Usually intracortical and curvilinear, gyriform

MACROSCOPIC FEATURES

General Features

- Soft, gelatinous, gray-pink
  - May be densely calcified (gritty)
- Thickened and expanded cerebral cortex
  - But relatively well circumscribed overall
- Often superficial, may infiltrate leptomeninges
  - May create marked desmoplastic reaction
- Cystic degeneration, intratumoral hemorrhage
- Higher grade lesions are more cellular, "fleshy"
  - But lack central necrosis of glioblastoma

Size

- Mean size at presentation: 3.5 cm

MICROSCOPIC PATHOLOGY

Histologic Features

- Generally diffusely infiltrating glioma
  - Obscures normal architecture, gray-white junction
    - Despite relatively sharp macroscopic interface
- Prominent, circumscribed "clones" within tumor

OLIGODENDROGLIOMA

- Nodules of ↑ cellularity, atypia, mitotic activity
- MIB-1 labeling index is higher
- Less common growth patterns
  - Cohesive ribbons, nests, or clusters of cells
  - Parallel palisades of tumor cells with long nuclei
  - Sarcoma-like areas, especially in higher grade lesions
- "Secondary structures" often form
  - Perineuronal satellitosis
    - Atypical tumor cells orbit large cortical neurons
    - In larger numbers than normal oligodendroglia
  - Perivascular collections, rare focal pseudorosettes
  - Subpial aggregates
- Microcalcifications very common (90% of tumors)
  - Perivascular or stromal laminated calcospherites
  - In tumor and surrounding cortex
  - Bone may form in highly calcified lesions
  - However, not specific for oligodendrogliomas
- Characteristic microvascular pattern
  - Interconnected delicate blood vessels
  - Geometric branching: Short arcs, angular segments
    - May arborize, likened to "chicken wire"
  - Separate out lobules of tumor cells
  - Glomeruloid microvascular proliferations absent
- Extracellular mucin or microcysts are common
  - Protein-rich, amphophilic, PAS(+) fluid
  - Peripheral vacuolization
    - Resembles dysembryoblastic neuroepithelial tumor
  - Not true cysts (not lined by epithelium)

Cytologic Features

- Very monomorphic/monotonous appearance
  - Uniform cell density, moderate cellularity
    - Distributed in delicate eosinophilic matrix
  - Scant rim of cytoplasm
  - Round nuclei of similar size and shape
    - Delicate, open, and bland chromatin
    - Small prominent nucleoli
- Artifactual swelling due to fixation/preparation
  - Clear perinuclear vacuolization ("halo")
    - Likened to "fried eggs" or "honeycomb"
  - Absent in cytology smears and frozen sections
- Focally, cells may resemble astrocytes
  - Faintly gliofibrillar appearance
    - But rarely have cell processes
  - Prominent, eccentric pink cytoplasm
    - Often GFAP(+)
    - May have hyaline, brightly eosinophilic fibrils, and cell bodies that resemble Rosenthal fibers
  - Termed "minigemistocytes," "gliofibrillary oligodendrocytes," or "transitional cells"
    - Retain oligodendroglial nuclear appearance
    - More common in higher grade lesions
- Neurocytic differentiation occasionally seen
  - Neurocytic rosettes or fibrillar neuropil islands
  - Synaptophysin(+)
  - Especially among tumors with 1p/19q deletions
- Reactive astrocytes often seen within tumor
  - Evenly distributed GFAP(+) stellate cells
  - Long, uniform, symmetric processes
  - Do not diagnose as mixed glioma

Predominant Pattern/Injury Type

- Neoplastic

Predominant Cell/Compartment Type

- Nervous, glial

Anaplastic Oligodendroglioma (Grade III)

- Estimated 20-55% of all oligodendrogliomas
- Evolve from well-differentiated lesion or arise de novo
- Preferentially in adults, slight male predominance
- Focal or diffuse histologic features of malignancy
  - Markedly increased cellularity and cytologic atypia
  - Nuclear pleomorphism, hyperchromasia, coarseness
  - Increased mitotic activity, prominent apoptoses
- Retain some "oligodendroglial" cytologic features
  - Round nuclei, perinuclear halos, few processes
- Gliofibrillary oligodendrocytes, minigemistocytes
- Necrosis, usually without geographic pseudopalisading
- Microvascular hypertrophy (glomeruloid proliferation)

Mixed Glioma (Oligoastrocytoma)

- Incidence varies: 2-10% of all intracranial gliomas
- 2 histologic subtypes
  - Biphasic ("compact"): Distinct populations of cells
    - Astrocytic areas: Frankly fibrillar or gemistocytic
  - Other variants may be more hybrid ("diffuse")
    - Intermixed astrocytic/oligodendroglial areas
- Generally > 20-50% astroglial component required
  - Distinction may make little sense clinically
    - Treated like similar grade oligodendroglioma
    - Respond favorably to PCV chemotherapy
    - Especially when harboring 1p/19q deletions
  - Clinical, radiologic, macroscopic similarities
    - Common molecular alterations in 2 components
    - Monoclonal neoplasms from single precursor cell
- Anaplastic oligoastrocytoma (WHO grade III)
  - Histologic features of anaplasia
    - In either or both glial components

ANCILLARY TESTS

Frozen Sections

- Nuclei: Absent halos, ↑ hyperchromasia and angularity
  - More difficult to distinguish from astrocytoma
- Intraoperative distinction not crucial
  - Diagnose as "low-grade infiltrating glioma"
    - Unless anaplastic
- Helpful findings suggesting oligodendroglioma
  - Cortical involvement, perineuronal satellitosis
  - Nuclear roundness, obvious nucleoli
  - Mucin-filled microcysts, calcifications

Immunohistochemistry

- No specific oligodendroglial marker exists to date
- Generally express S100 protein, LEU-7 (CD56)
- Usually negative for GFAP, vimentin
  - Reactive astrocytes, "transitional cells" may stain
- Anaplastic lesions may be GFAP, vimentin positive
  - Distinction from glioblastoma difficult
- Neuronal markers negative (synaptophysin, NeuN)
  - Trapped axons and neuropil may be positive
- MIB-1 proliferation index may be prognostically useful

- Correlates with cellularity, degree of atypia, survival
- p53 staining absent in classic oligodendrogliomas
  - Especially those with 1p/19q deletion

Cytogenetics

- Chromosome 1p and 19q loss (entire arm of both)
  - Common in strictly defined oligodendrogliomas
  - Retained arms (1q, 19p): Derivative chromosome
  - May be less common in pediatric tumors
- Predicts treatment response, better survival
  - Tumor suppressor genes not yet identified
- *P53* mutation lacking in lesions with 1p/19q deletion
- Anaplastic lesions accumulate genetic abnormalities

Electron Microscopy

- Rare pericellular spiral lamination (membrane whorls)
  - Reminiscent of normal myelin sheath formation
- May have microtubule-containing short processes
  - Distinguish from astrocytoma (glial filaments)
- Neurosecretory-like granules may be seen
  - Probably represent small lysosomes
- Intermediate filaments in astrocyte-like cells
  - Amorphous, electron-dense cytoplasmic structures
  - Resemble eosinophilic Rosenthal fibers

Cytology (Smear Preparation)

- Round "naked" nuclei, open chromatin, small nucleoli
- Paucity of cell processes, little fibrillarity
  - May see "glassy" cytoplasm of minigemistocytes

DIFFERENTIAL DIAGNOSIS

Normal or Increased Oligodendrocytes

- Cluster around neurons (satellitosis)
- Preferentially around arteriovenous malformations
- Usually in deeper white matter
- Neoplastic cells: Numerous, in higher cortex levels
  - Nuclei are larger with coarser chromatin

Reactive Gliosis

- Lacks cytologic atypia; nuclei are normal
- Contains reactive, GFAP-positive astrocytes

Demyelinating Disease

- Lipid-laden macrophages with granular cytoplasm
  - Oligodendrocytes have more clear cytoplasm
- Active phase of disease is contrast enhancing
- PAS, Luxol fast blue, KP-1 (CD68) positive

Cerebral Infarct

- Distinct clinical presentation
- Macrophage-rich, contains dying "red" neurons

Progressive Multifocal Leukoencephalopathy

- Clinical setting of immunosuppression
- No cortical involvement on imaging
- Inclusion-baring oligodendrocytes
- Reactive astrocytes, many macrophages

Diffuse Astrocytoma

- Distinctively fibrillar background
- More abundant cytoplasm, mitoses
- Usually more irregular, pleomorphic nuclei
  - Elongated, angulated, hyperchromatic
- Generally lacks prominent nucleoli, halos
- Lacks calcification, "chicken wire" vasculature

Clear Cell Ependymoma

- Sharply circumscribed, contrast enhancing
  - Pushing (displacing) rather than infiltrating border
- GFAP and vimentin positive
- Perivascular pseudorosettes of tapering processes
- True rosettes (canals): Cellular polarity, microlumina
- EM features: Microvilli, cilia, junctional complexes
- Dot-like intracytoplasmic EMA staining

Central Neurocytoma

- Intraventricular, discrete, contrast-enhancing mass
- Positive for neuronal markers (synaptophysin)
- Microtubule processes, clear vesicles, granules

Dysembryoplastic Neuroepithelial Tumor

- Multinodular intracortical lesion
  - Surrounded by disorganized cortical "dysplasia"
- Loosely textured "specific glioneuronal element"
  - Intercellular mucin, floating dysmorphic neurons
- Long history of partial complex seizures in children
- Lacks perineuronal satellitosis, 1p/19q deletions

Pilocytic Astrocytoma

- Contrast-enhancing cyst with mural nodule

Clear Cell Meningioma

- Whorls, thick-walled vessels, collagenous stroma
- EMA positive, PAS (diastase sensitive) positive

Ganglioglioma

- Discrete contrast-enhancing mass
- Gliofibrillary stroma, neoplastic ganglion cells
- Mesenchymal elements, chronic inflammatory cells

Metastatic Clear Cell Carcinoma

- Especially vs. anaplastic oligodendroglioma
- Solid with sharply defined (pushing) borders
- Positive for EMA, cytokeratin (low molecular weight)

Primary CNS Lymphoma

- Macrophage-rich, especially after steroid treatment
- Positive for lymphoid markers (CD45, CD20)

DIAGNOSTIC CHECKLIST

Clinically Relevant Pathologic Features

- Nuclear features
- Invasive pattern
- Symptom complex
- Symptom time frame
- Oligodendrogliomas may be underdiagnosed
  - Expanded molecular criteria (1p/19q deletion)
  - Incidence may be up to 20-30% of all gliomas
- Prognostically **unfavorable** features
  - Focal neurologic deficits, ↑ intracranial pressure
  - Hypercellularity, increased mitoses, necrosis
  - Higher nuclear/cytoplasm ratio, pleomorphism
  - Endothelial (microvascular) proliferation
  - ↑ proliferative activity
    - ≥ 6 mitoses/10 HPF
    - MIB-1 index > 3-5%

OLIGODENDROGLIOMA

- Presence of radiologic contrast enhancement
- Blood group A patients (in 1 study)
- Prognostically **favorable** characteristics
  - Age younger than 40 years old at presentation
  - Presentation: Seizures or normal neurologic exam
  - Low tumor grade (WHO grade II)
  - Microcysts, calcifications on CT scan
  - 1p/19q codeletion
  - Frontal lobe (or other hemispheric) location
  - Macroscopically complete resection
  - Higher performance status
- "Mixed gliomas" tend to be genetically divisible
  - Have either *P53* mutation or 1p/19q deletion
- "Aggressive" oligodendrogliomas
  - Lack histologic atypia, but behave aggressively
    - Clinically &/or radiologically
    - Symptomatic, enlarging, enhancing on CT/MR

Pathologic Interpretation Pearls

- 2 most important histopathologic features
  - Monomorphic, infiltrating appearance
  - Regular round nuclei, perinuclear halos
- Useful mnemonics
  - "Chicken wire" vasculature and "fried egg" nuclei
- Trapped normal ganglion cells a common feature
  - Since oligodendrogliomas infiltrate cortex
  - Do not misinterpret as ganglioglioma
- Identification of "oligodendroglial features"
  - Helpful to include in report
    - In any mixed glioma or glioblastoma
  - Should be examined for presence of 1p/19q deletion
    - Ultimately determines prognosis, treatment

GRADING

Well-Differentiated Oligodendroglioma

- WHO grade II
- Low to moderate cellularity, mild atypia
- Infrequent mitoses
- Absent microvascular proliferation or necrosis
- "Clonal" nodules of increased atypia can be present

Anaplastic Oligodendroglioma

- WHO grade III
- Diagnosis based on presence of unequivocal anaplasia
  - Hypercellularity, increased nuclear to cytoplasm ratio
  - Readily evident (prominent, increased) mitoses
  - Nuclear pleomorphism: Coarser, prominent nucleoli
  - Vascular (endothelial) proliferation, necrosis
- Prognostic significance of each feature not clear
  - Conflicting results
- But retain histologic features of oligodendrogliomas
  - Cell uniformity and nuclear "roundness"
  - May need better differentiated areas to diagnose

Grade IV Oligodendroglioma vs. Glioblastoma (Grade IV Astrocytoma)

- Microvascular (endothelial) proliferation
- Geographic, pseudopalisading necrosis
- Most authors would diagnose as glioblastoma, unless clear cut oligodendroglial differentiation is present
  - Nuclear uniformity, roundness, perinuclear halos
- Grade IV is controversial in oligodendrogliomas
  - Glioblastoma is by definition astrocytic
- Consensus term for this entity
  - "Glioblastoma with oligodendroglial features"
- Molecular analysis for 1p/19q deletion
  - Helps with diagnosis, prognosis, treatment

SELECTED REFERENCES

1. Cairncross G et al: Gliomas with 1p/19q codeletion: a.k.a. oligodendroglioma. Cancer J. 14(6):352-7, 2008
2. Van den Bent MJ et al: Oligodendroglioma. Crit Rev Oncol Hematol. 66(3):262-72, 2008
3. Aldape K et al: Clinicopathologic aspects of 1p/19q loss and the diagnosis of oligodendroglioma. Arch Pathol Lab Med. 131(2):242-51, 2007
4. van den Bent MJ: Anaplastic oligodendroglioma and oligoastrocytoma. Neurol Clin. 25(4):1089-109, ix-x, 2007
5. Koeller KK et al: From the archives of the AFIP: Oligodendroglioma and its variants: radiologic-pathologic correlation. Radiographics. 25(6):1669-88, 2005
6. Ueki K: Oligodendroglioma: impact of molecular biology on its definition, diagnosis and management. Neuropathology. 25(3):247-53, 2005
7. van den Bent MJ: Diagnosis and management of oligodendroglioma. Semin Oncol. 31(5):645-52, 2004
8. Ellis TL et al: Oligodendroglioma. Curr Treat Options Oncol. 4(6):479-90, 2003
9. Engelhard HH et al: Oligodendroglioma and anaplastic oligodendroglioma: clinical features, treatment, and prognosis. Surg Neurol. 60(5):443-56, 2003
10. Reifenberger G et al: Oligodendroglioma: toward molecular definitions in diagnostic neuro-oncology. J Neuropathol Exp Neurol. 62(2):111-26, 2003
11. Engelhard HH et al: Oligodendroglioma: pathology and molecular biology. Surg Neurol. 58(2):111-7; discussion 117, 2002
12. Engelhard HH: Current diagnosis and treatment of oligodendroglioma. Neurosurg Focus. 12(2):E2, 2002
13. Hussein MR et al: Advances in diagnosis and management of oligodendroglioma. Expert Rev Anticancer Ther. 2(5):520-8, 2002
14. van den Bent MJ: New perspectives for the diagnosis and treatment of oligodendroglioma. Expert Rev Anticancer Ther. 1(3):348-56, 2001
15. Reifenberger G et al: Anaplastic oligoastrocytoma. In Kleihues P et al: Pathology and Genetics: Tumors of the Nervous System. Lyon: IARC Press. 68-9, 2000
16. Reifenberger G et al: Anaplastic oligodendroglioma. In Kleihues P et al: Pathology and Genetics: Tumors of the Nervous System. Lyon: IARC Press. 62-4, 2000
17. Reifenberger G et al: Oligoastrocytoma. In Kleihues P et al: Pathology and Genetics: Tumors of the Nervous System. Lyon: IARC Press. 65-7, 2000
18. Reifenberger G et al: Oligodendroglioma. In Kleihues P et al: Pathology and Genetics: Tumors of the Nervous System. Lyon: IARC Press. 56-61, 2000
19. Fortin D et al: Oligodendroglioma: an appraisal of recent data pertaining to diagnosis and treatment. Neurosurgery. 45(6):1279-91; discussion 191, 1999
20. Brandes AA et al: Clinical, pathological and therapeutic aspects of oligodendroglioma. Cancer Treat Rev. 24(2):101-11, 1998
21. Peterson K et al: Oligodendroglioma. Cancer Invest. 14(3):243-51, 1996

OLIGODENDROGLIOMA

Microscopic Features

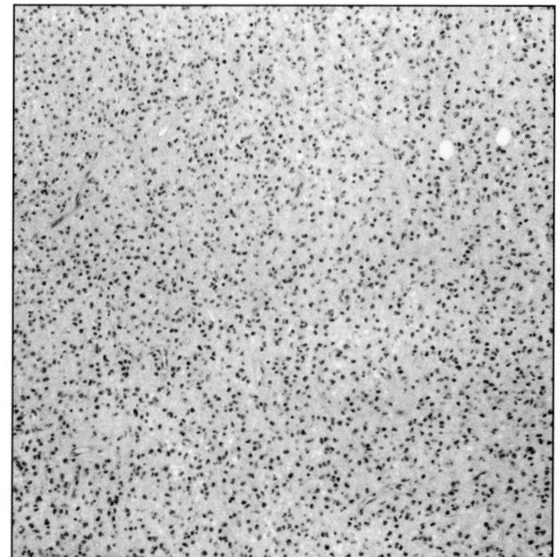

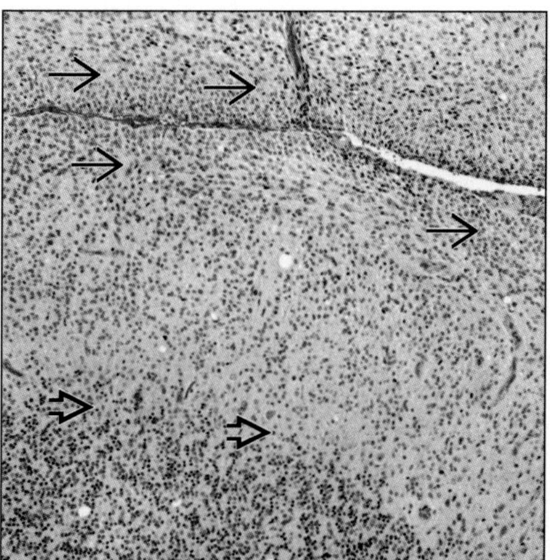

(Left) *H&E shows a low-power view of oligodendroglioma with a very monotonous and monomorphic appearance, having uniform cell density, and moderate cellularity in an eosinophilic background matrix.* ***(Right)*** *H&E shows a medium-power view of a diffusely infiltrating oligodendroglioma that, even though circumscribed grossly, obscures the normal cerebral cortex architecture, blurs the gray-white matter junction ⇨, and forms secondary structures, such as subpial aggregates →.*

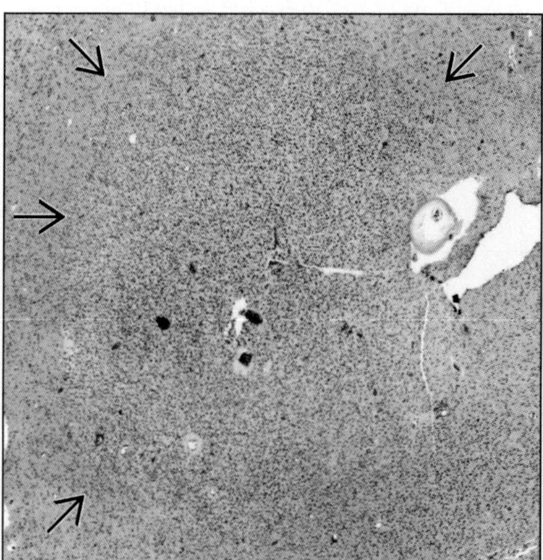

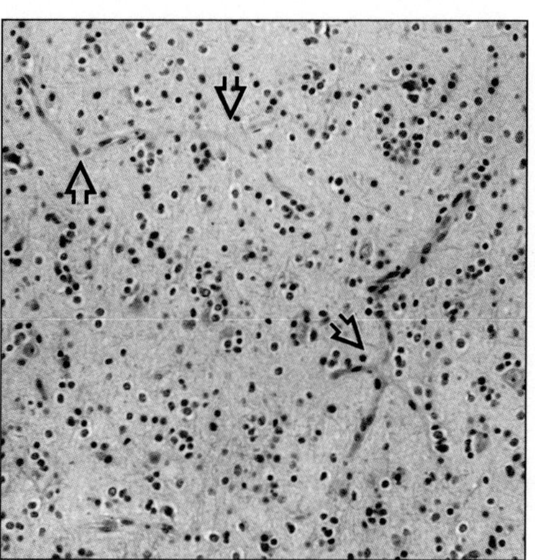

(Left) *H&E shows a low-power view of a prominent circumscribed "clone" → within an oligodendroglioma. Such nodules commonly have increased cellularity and mitoses.* ***(Right)*** *H&E shows a high-power view of characteristic vascular pattern in oligodendroglioma. Delicate interconnected capillaries often exhibit geometric branching ⇨ with arcuate or angular segments that appear to arborize, akin to "chicken wire."*

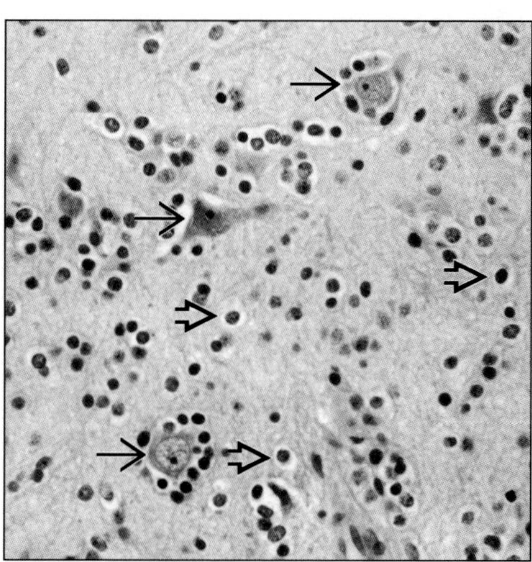

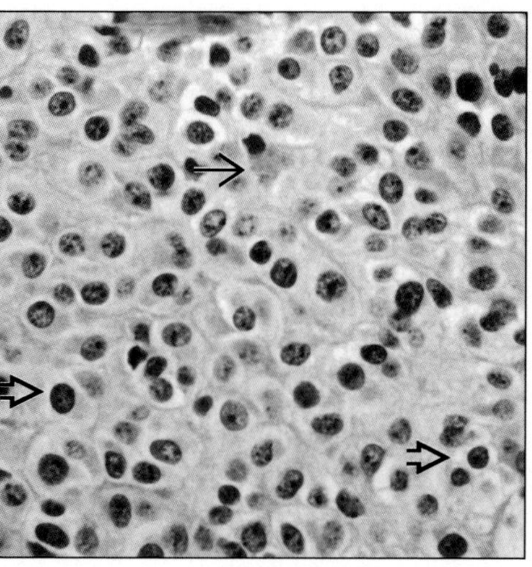

(Left) *H&E shows a high-power view of perineuronal satellitosis in oligodendroglioma in which neoplastic cells orbit large cortical neurons →. Clear perinuclear vacuolizations ⇨ ("halos"), an artifact of fixation and processing, are also present in most tumor cells.* ***(Right)*** *H&E shows a high-power view of oligodendroglioma with "minigemistocytes" → that resemble astrocytes due to their prominent eosinophilic cytoplasm. Perinuclear halos ⇨ are also present.*

OLIGODENDROGLIOMA

Microscopic and Other Features

*(Left) H&E shows medium-power view of microcalcifications ⇨, mostly in the form of laminated calcospherites. A very common but not specific finding in oligodendrogliomas, microcalcifications can be present in perivascular or stromal locations in the tumor or in surrounding cortex. **(Right)** Low-power view shows microcysts → filled with protein-rich amphophilic fluid. A common finding in oligodendroglioma, these microcysts are not true cysts since they are not lined by epithelium.*

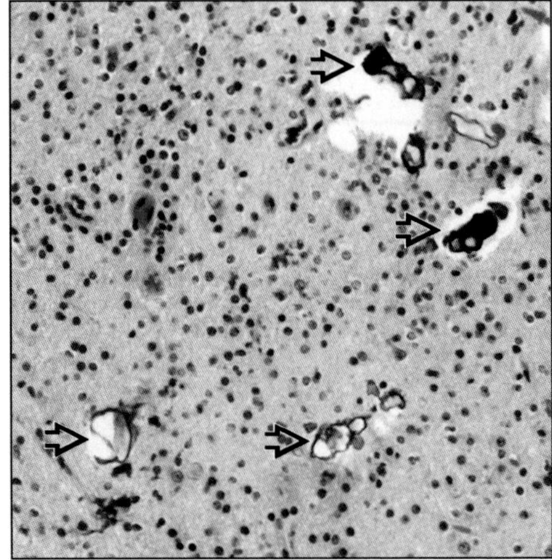

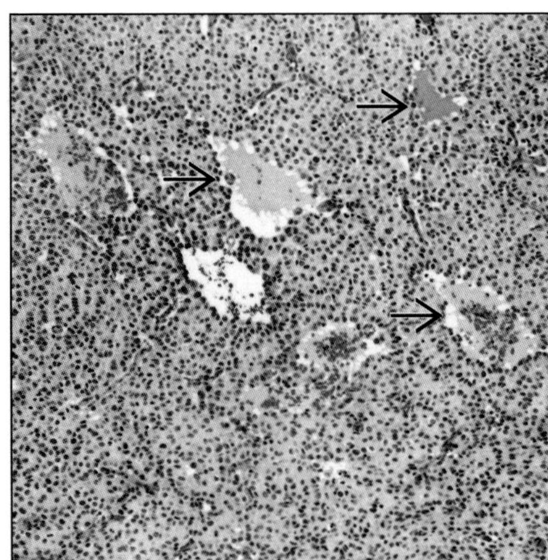

*(Left) Axial gadolinium-enhanced MR shows intense heterogeneous enhancement with ependymal extension ➡. This newly present enhancement represents malignant progression in a previously treated oligodendroglioma. **(Right)** Smear H&E preparation shows a high-power view of oligodendroglioma cells with round, often "naked" nuclei → that have open chromatin and small nucleoli. Overall, there is little fibrillarity and few cell processes. Perinuclear halos are not present since they represent fixation artifact.*

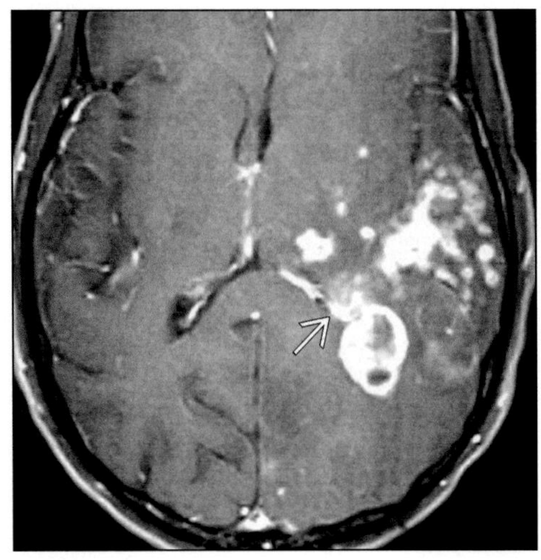

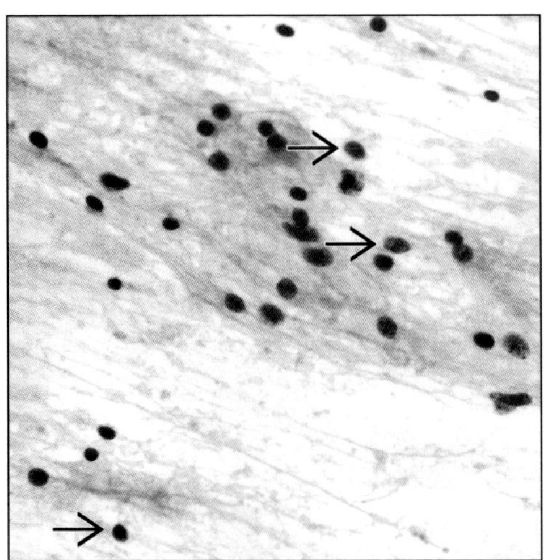

*(Left) Immunohistochemistry for GFAP shows a high-power view of an oligodendroglioma with trapped reactive astrocytes that have GFAP-positive cell processes →. Most tumor cells are negative for GFAP ⇨. **(Right)** Immunohistochemistry for Ki-67 shows a very high MIB-1 proliferation index, approaching 60-70%. Combined with unequivocal anaplasia present on H&E sections, this is an unfavorable prognostic feature in this anaplastic oligodendroglioma.*

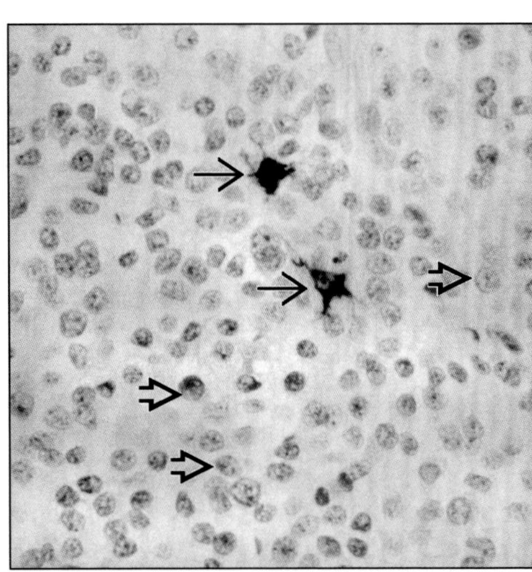

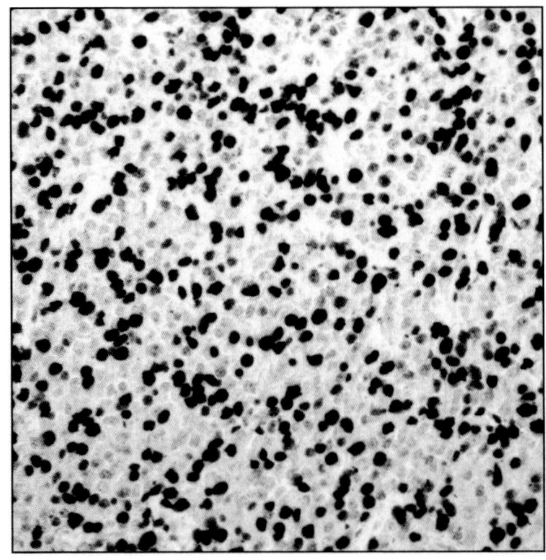

Variant Microscopic Features

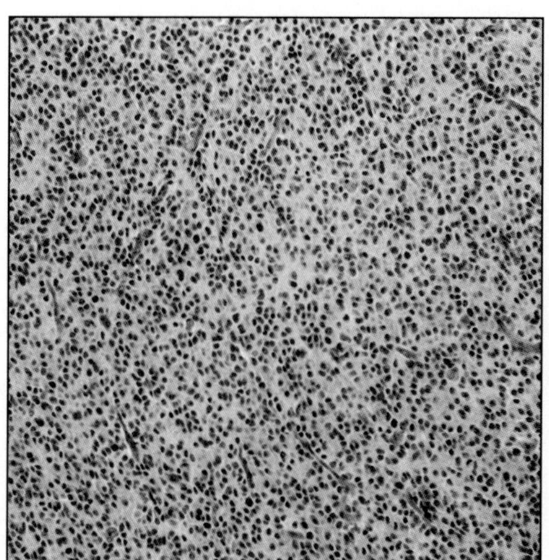

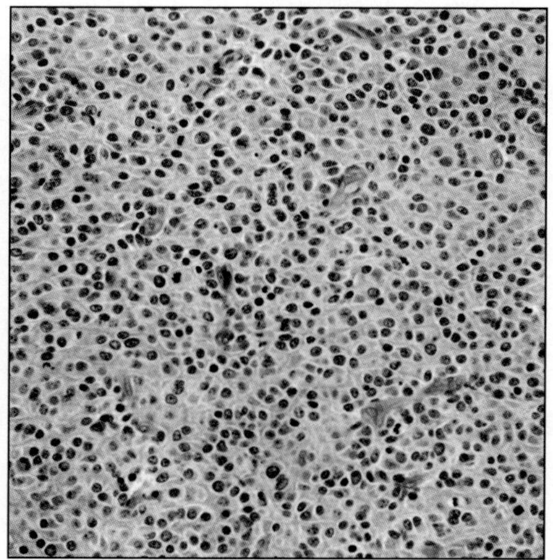

(Left) *H&E shows a medium-power view of an anaplastic oligodendroglioma that has markedly increased cellularity and nuclear pleomorphism evident even at this magnification.* ***(Right)*** *H&E shows a high-power view of anaplastic oligodendroglioma with features of malignancy (cytologic atypia, nuclear pleomorphism, and hyperchromasia). Overall, it retains features of oligodendroglioma, such as cell uniformity and monomorphism, with round nuclei and perinuclear halos.*

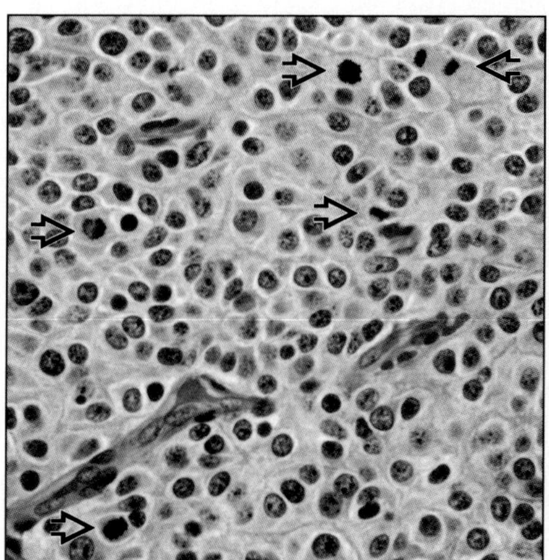

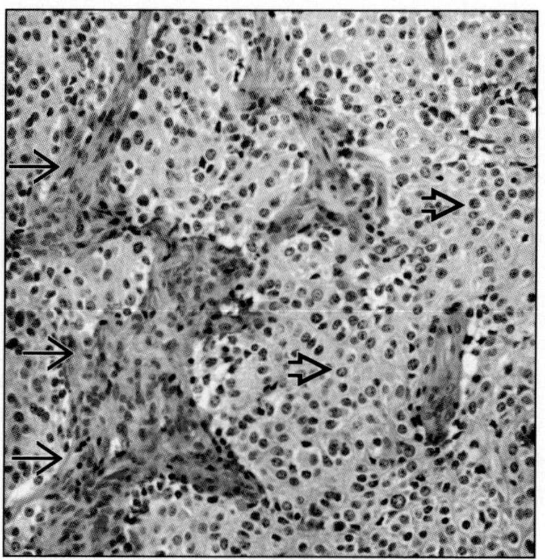

(Left) *H&E shows a high-power view of anaplastic oligodendroglioma with increased mitoses ⇨, an unfavorable prognostic feature.* ***(Right)*** *H&E shows a medium-power view of "glomeruloid" microvascular hypertrophy. These vascular channels, lined by multiple rows of proliferating endothelial cells →, are almost pathognomonic of a malignant glioma (in this case, an anaplastic oligodendroglioma composed of monotonous cells with round nuclei and perinuclear halos ⇨).*

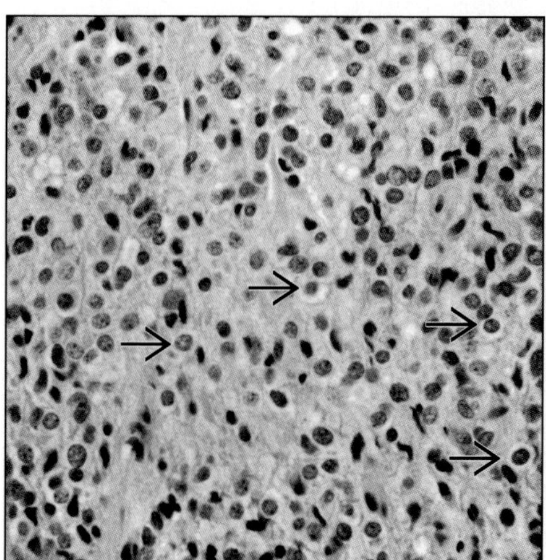

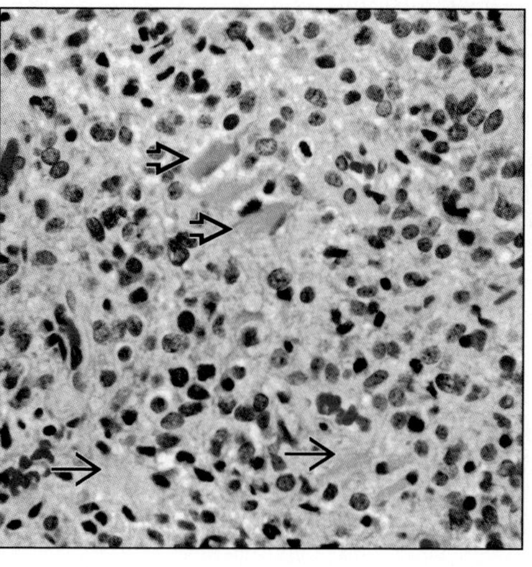

(Left) *H&E shows high-power view of a mixed glioma with 2 distinct populations of neoplastic cells. In this field, a classic oligodendroglioma appearance is evidenced by monomorphic cells with round nuclei and perinuclear halos →.* ***(Right)*** *H&E shows high-power view of a mixed glioma with a more astrocytic gliofibrillar appearance → and frankly gemistocytic cells ⇨. This degree of nuclear pleomorphism and atypia is more in keeping with an astrocytic differentiation.*

EPENDYMOMA

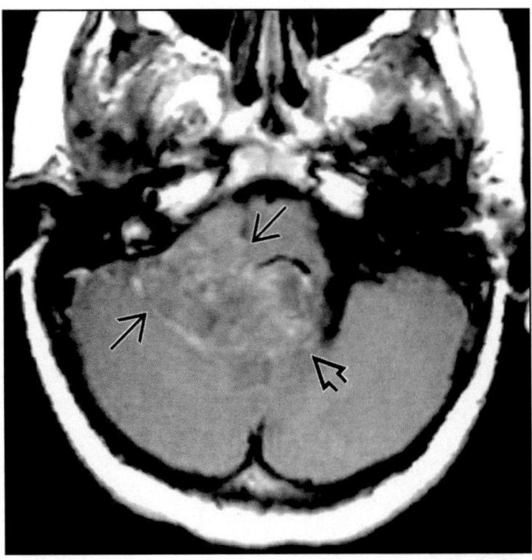

Axial T1WI MR shows heterogeneous enhancement in an ependymoma, extending from the 4th ventricle ⇨ through the foramen of Luschka into the CPA cistern →.

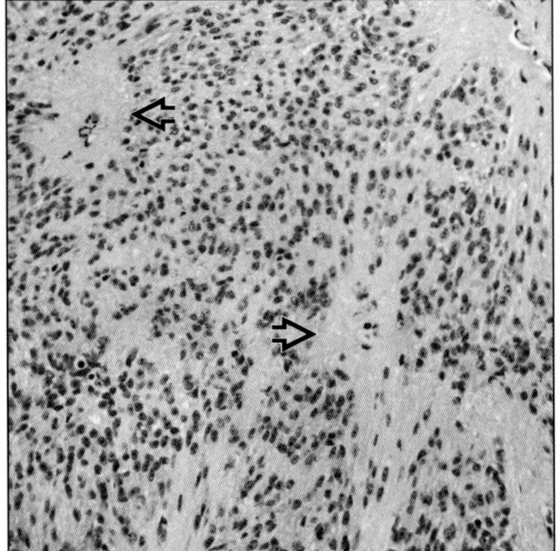

Hematoxylin & eosin shows the classic low-power appearance of ependymoma with monomorphic cellular areas interrupted by perivascular nuclear-free zones ⇨.

TERMINOLOGY

Definitions

- Slow-growing (WHO grade II) neuroectodermal tumor of neoplastic ependymal cells with mixed gliofibrillary and neuroepithelial appearance
- Mostly arising from wall of cerebral ventricles or spinal canal in children and young adults

ETIOLOGY/PATHOGENESIS

Infectious Agents

- SV40 polyoma virus Tag (large T antigen)-related DNA
  - Identified in some ependymomas, not confirmed
  - SV40-contaminated polio vaccine implicated

Genetic Syndromes

- ↑ incidence (2-5%) in neurofibromatosis type 2 (NF2)
  - May be multifocal in these patients
  - *NF2* tumor suppressor gene (chromosome 22)
- Case reports of other hereditary forms of ependymoma
  - Turcot syndrome, MEN1, *TP53* germline mutation

Histogenesis

- From neuroepithelial lining of ventricles, central canal
- Outside ventricles (intraparenchymal, extraneural)
  - From fetal/embryonic ependymal remnants (rests)

CLINICAL ISSUES

Epidemiology

- Incidence
  - Annual incidence: ~ 2 per million
  - 6-12% of intracranial tumors in children
    - 30% in < 3 years old
  - Most common neuroectodermal tumor of spinal cord (50-60%)
- Age
  - Infratentorial: 2 months to 16 years old
    - Mean age: ~ 6 years old
  - 2nd peak for spinal ependymomas in 4th decade
  - Supratentorial: Adult > pediatric patients
- Gender
  - M = F

Site

- Infratentorial > supratentorial (2:1)
- Posterior fossa (4th ventricle) > spinal cord (cervical, cervicothoracic) > lateral (rarely 3rd) ventricle
- May occur outside ventricular system
  - Cerebral cortex, subarachnoid space
- Rare extraneural sites
  - Ovary, pre-/post-sacral soft tissue, mediastinum/lung

Presentation

- Symptoms begin insidiously, improve during the day
  - Generally depend on tumor size and location
- Infratentorial (4th ventricle, posterior fossa)
  - Symptoms due to CSF flow obstruction
    - Hydrocephalus, ↑ intracranial pressure (ICP)
    - Headache, nausea, vomiting, dizziness
  - Obstructive hydrocephalus, sudden death may occur
  - Ataxia, nystagmus, paresis
- Supratentorial
  - Focal neurologic deficits, local mass effect, seizures
  - Less likely: ↑ ICP, head enlargement (< 2 years old)
- Spinal cord: Motor and sensory deficits, back pain

Natural History

- Generally indolent tumors
  - May undergo transformation, be locally destructive
- Posterior fossa tumors
  - In floor or roof of 4th ventricle
  - May extend to cervical canal, cerebellopontine angle, cisterna magna
- Infrequent (5-10%) spread via CSF, subarachnoid space
  - Mostly in infratentorial anaplastic ependymomas
- Rare extraneural metastases (lung)
  - In pre- or post-sacral soft tissue ependymomas

EPENDYMOMA

Key Facts

Terminology

- Slow-growing (grade II) ependymal tumor with glio-fibrillary/neuroepithelial appearance, arising in ventricles or spinal canal of children, young adults

Clinical Issues

- 6-12% childhood intracranial tumors (30% < 3 years)
- Posterior fossa > spinal cord > lateral/3rd ventricles
- Less often: Cortex, subarachnoid space, extraneural
- Symptoms: CSF obstruction (hydrocephalus, ↑ ICP)
- Total resection (50% cases), possibly chemoradiation
- Poor outcome: Posterior fossa, CSF spread, incomplete resection, anaplastic histology, young age

Image Findings

- Contrast enhancing, heterogeneous, circumscribed
- Intratumoral hemorrhage, calcification, cystic change

Microscopic Pathology

- Well circumscribed, uniform cells, round nuclei
- True rosettes: Columnar cells around central lumen
  - Diagnostic of ependymoma but not always present
- Perivascular pseudorosettes (nuclear-free zones)
  - GFAP-positive cell processes radially around vessels
- Variants: Cellular, papillary, clear cell (grade III), tanycytic, myxopapillary (grade I), giant cell
- Anaplastic (grade III): Unfavorable prognosis
  - Mitotic activity (> 5-10 mitoses per 10 HPF)
  - Vascular proliferation, pseudopalisading necrosis

Ancillary Tests

- 22q deletions/translocations; NF2 association
- EM: Cilia, blepharoplasts, microvilli, cell junctions

Treatment

- Surgical approaches
  - Complete (gross total) resection
    - Possible in ~ 50% of cases
    - Most important prognostic variable
- Adjuvant therapy
  - Chemoradiation role remains limited, controversial
  - "High-risk" patients (especially intracranial tumors)
    - < 3 years old, preoperative metastases, anaplastic histology, residual disease

Prognosis

- Survival: ~ 60% at 5 years, 45-50% at 10 years
- Poor correlation between histology and outcome
  - Variation in grading, subjective interpretation
- Reported indicators of poor outcome
  - Posterior fossa, supratentorial/intraparenchymal
    - Spinal ependymomas: More favorable outcome
  - Cerebrospinal (CSF), leptomeningeal dissemination
  - Incomplete tumor resection
  - Anaplastic histologic features
    - ↑ mitoses, proliferation (> 4% MIB-1 label index)
    - Hypercellular, less differentiated foci
    - Reduce 10-year survival by 1/2 (25%)
  - Young age (< 3 years; especially dismal < 2 years)
    - More common anaplasia, posterior fossa location
- Recurrence usually locally, within 2-3 years of surgery
  - May occur in up to 40-50% of cases
  - More difficult to excise, resistant to chemoradiation
- Collins law
  - Time interval from surgery to symptomatic recurrence < time interval from conception to initial presentation/diagnosis (i.e., age + 9 months)
    - Little postoperative recurrence risk after this time
  - Assumes similar pre- and postoperative growth rates
    - But anaplastic progression can be seen

IMAGE FINDINGS

MR Findings

- Low intensity on T1WI, high intensity on T2WI
- Well circumscribed, variably gadolinium enhancing
- Ventricular or brainstem displacement
- Hydrocephalus or syrinx (spinal cord) present
- Intratumoral hemorrhage, calcification, cystic change
- Infrequent edema, brain invasion

CT Findings

- Hyper-/isodense, contrast enhancing, heterogeneous

MACROSCOPIC FEATURES

General Features

- Soft, gray-red, fleshy solid mass
- Focal necrosis, hemorrhage, or cystic change
- May be gritty, chalky due to calcification

MICROSCOPIC PATHOLOGY

Histologic Features

- Well circumscribed, expansile, lobulated
  - Sharp transition with surrounding parenchyma
  - May be more infiltrative in spinal cord
  - In ventricles, surfaced by residual ependyma
- Glial/fibrillar elements generally dominate
  - Background fibrillary meshwork (cell processes)
- Moderately cellular, monomorphic, patternless
  - Uniform cells, round nuclei, clumped chromatin
  - Absent or rare mitoses
  - Occasional, focal, nonpalisading necrosis
- Characteristic neuroepithelial elements
  - Closely arranged cells, epithelioid groups (rosettes)
- True ependymal rosettes/canals
  - Columnar epithelial cells around central lumen
  - PTAH-positive blepharoplasts in apical surface
- Perivascular pseudorosettes
  - Tumor cells radially arranged around blood vessels
  - Fibrillary "cuffs" of cytoplasmic processes
  - Result in perivascular "nuclear-free zones"
- Degenerative/regressive changes
  - Myxoid change, intratumoral hemorrhage
  - Hemosiderin, especially in intramedullary tumors

EPENDYMOMA

- Small eosinophilic granules, vacuoles, melanin
- Foam cells, sometimes prominent ("lipidized")
- Hyalinization of vessel walls, calcification
- Rare cartilaginous/osseous metaplasia

Predominant Pattern/Injury Type

- Neoplastic

Predominant Cell/Compartment Type

- Nervous, glial

Histologic Variants

- Cellular ependymoma
  - Classic type, increased cellularity, densely packed
  - Fewer true rosettes or pseudorosettes formed
  - May have mitoses, but only focally
  - Epithelioid variant: Prominent cell clusters
- Papillary ependymoma
  - Rare; well-formed pseudopapillary structures
  - Columnar cells resting on glial fibrillary stroma
- Clear cell ependymoma
  - Oligodendroglial-like perinuclear clearing (halo)
  - Calcospherites may also be present
  - Often supratentorial, in young children
  - Usually WHO grade III
    - Atypia, ↑ mitotic activity, vascular proliferation
- Tanycytic ependymoma
  - Hypocellular, fibrillar; true rosettes typically absent
  - Spindle, bipolar tumor cells in bundles or fascicles
    - Akin to paraventricular ependymoglia (tanycytes)
  - Predilection for spinal cord
- Myxopapillary ependymoma (WHO grade I)
  - Lumbar spinal cord location; may erode bone
    - Cauda equina, filum terminale, conus medullaris
  - Cauda equina syndrome
    - Compressed nerve roots → pain, lower extremity weakness, sphincter dysfunction
  - Lobulated, highly vascular, gelatinous
  - Papillary architecture of epithelial/glial tumor cells
  - Microcystic connective tissue, perivascular mucin
- Giant cell ependymoma
  - Term used in 2 different instances
  - Low-grade spinal cord lesions (filum terminale)
    - With degenerative nuclear atypia, low mitoses
  - Intracranial anaplastic ependymoma
    - Unusually high nuclear pleomorphism

Anaplastic Ependymoma (WHO Grade III)

- Constitutes about 30% of ependymal tumors
  - Often intracranial: Posterior fossa, intraparenchymal
  - Unfavorable outcome, especially in children
  - Typically develop/grow rapidly, cause ↑ ICP
  - Diffusely invade, destroy surrounding parenchyma
  - Contrast enhancement on MR imaging
- Defining histologic features not consistent/universal
  - Hypercellular, poorly differentiated
  - Cytologic atypia and nuclear pleomorphism
  - Brisk mitotic activity (> 5-10 mitoses per 10 HPF)
  - "Glomeruloid" microvascular proliferation
  - Pseudopalisading ("geographic") necrosis
  - Absence of embryonal (PNET) components or ependymoblastic rosettes
- EM may be needed to prove ependymal differentiation
- High MIB-1 index (mean: ~ 30%); may be p53(+)

Subependymoma (WHO Grade I)

- Clinically indolent tumors, rare in children
  - Usually in 4th or lateral ventricle
- Microscopic features
  - Clusters of small, uniform, bland nuclei
  - Amidst dense gliofibrillary background
  - Microcystic change, calcification, hemosiderin
  - Degenerative nuclear atypia, occasional mitoses
  - Coagulative, nonpalisading necrosis
- May also have ependymal rosettes
  - "Mixed ependymoma/subependymoma"
    - WHO grade II
  - Ependymoma component determines prognosis

ANCILLARY TESTS

Immunohistochemistry

- GFAP(+) cell processes around vessels
  - Normal, mature ependymal cells are GFAP negative
- S100, vimentin, nestin: Diffusely positive
- EMA(+) and CD99(+) luminal (apical) surfaces
  - Dot-like perinuclear cytoplasmic EMA expression in well-differentiated tumors
- Only focal cytokeratin positivity
- Negative for neuronal antigens (synaptophysin)

Cytogenetics

- Monosomy 22 or deletions/translocations of 22q
  - 30% of cases
  - Especially in spinal cord ependymomas
- Less frequent abnormalities: Chromosomes 6, 9, 11, 17
- Amplification of *MDM2* implicated in ~ 35% of cases

Electron Microscopy

- Maintain characteristic structures of ependymal cells
  - Preserved polarity, luminal surface structures
    - Cilia (9+2), blepharoplasts, microvilli
  - Complex lateral junctions (zonulae adherentes)
  - Glial processes with 10 nm intermediate filaments
- Lack neurosecretory granules
- No basement membrane on internal surface
- Intracellular lumina ("microrosettes") may be seen
  - With "abortive" cilia and microvilli

DIFFERENTIAL DIAGNOSIS

Medulloblastoma

- In posterior fossa vs. anaplastic ependymoma
- ↑ ↑ cellularity, mitotic activity; Homer Wright rosettes
- May have perivascular fibrillar zones
- Synaptophysin positive

Pilocytic Astrocytoma

- Especially in spinal cord, 4th ventricle
- Less cellular, more piloid, microcystic
- Rosenthal fibers can also be seen in ependymomas

(Diffuse) Astrocytoma

- Especially in posterior fossa, 4th ventricle
- Infiltrating, more fibrillary, cytologically atypical
- Lacks true rosettes, perivascular pseudorosettes

Oligodendroglioma
- In cerebral hemispheres vs. clear cell ependymoma
- Infiltrates surrounding brain parenchyma
- Lacks true rosettes, perivascular pseudorosettes

Choroid Plexus Papilloma
- In ventricles vs. papillary ependymoma
- Frond-like epithelial papillae with fibrovascular cores
- Smooth basement membrane, collagen stroma
- GFAP/vimentin(-), cytokeratin(+)

Pituitary Adenoma
- In sella turcica
  - Primary ependymomas do not occur in sella turcica
- Synaptophysin(+), GFAP(-)

Pilomyxoid Glioma
- In suprasellar region, 3rd ventricle
- More myxoid and microcystic, less cellular

Central Neurocytoma
- In foramen of Monro, 3rd ventricle
- Highly cellular, very monomorphic
- Synaptophysin/chromogranin(+), GFAP(-)

Glioblastoma Multiforme (Small Cell Type)
- Intraparenchymal vs. malignant ependymoma
- Infiltrative, diffuse growth pattern
- High mitotic rate, pseudopalisading necrosis
- Mostly astrocytic histologic features
- May have vague perivascular fibrillar areas

Schwannoma
- In spinal cord vs. tanycytic ependymoma
- Strongly diffusely S100(+), GFAP(-)
- Characteristically biphasic: Antoni A and B areas

Meningioma
- In extraventricular sites vs. tanycytic ependymoma
- Papillary meningioma vs. papillary ependymoma
- Usually will have recognizable meningothelial areas
- EMA(+), GFAP(-)

Paraganglioma
- In filum terminale vs. myxopapillary ependymoma
- Nested, reticulin-rich, epithelioid; ganglion cells
- Chromogranin, synaptophysin positive

Metastatic Carcinoma
- Differentiate from cellular or papillary ependymoma
- Diffusely strongly cytokeratin positive
- S100/GFAP(-)

Ependymoblastoma
- Supratentorial vs. anaplastic ependymoma
- Distinct primitive neuroectodermal tumor (PNET)
- Characteristic "ependymoblastic" rosettes
- Background sheets of undifferentiated cells
- Perivascular pseudorosettes absent

DIAGNOSTIC CHECKLIST

Clinically Relevant Pathologic Features
- Focal atypia, mitotic activity, hypercellularity
  - Generally not sufficient to grade as anaplastic
    - Unless these features predominate
  - May portend a less favorable prognosis
- Nonpalisading necrosis common in posterior fossa
  - Do not overdiagnose as anaplastic ependymoma
- Proliferation markers may help with prognosis
  - MIB-1 labeling index (Ki-67 immunostain)
  - > 20-25% positive (nuclear) staining associated with decreased survival (in some studies)
- Clear cell ependymomas
  - Worse prognosis, early recurrence, rare metastases
- Past inclusion of ependymoblastomas in ependymoma
  - May have overestimated metastases, poor outcome

Pathologic Interpretation Pearls
- True ependymal rosettes
  - Diagnostic of ependymomas but not always seen
  - Usually in more differentiated neoplasms
- Hypocellular, fibrillar lesions, often with gemistocytes
  - Not a mixed glioma ("ependymoastrocytoma")
  - These are ependymomas clinically, radiologically
- Frozen section diagnosis
  - Guides surgical decision for complete resection
  - Cytologic features resemble astrocytes
  - Perivascular pseudorosettes helpful
- Smear preparation diagnosis
  - Cellular aggregates retain cohesion
  - Cytoplasmic processes around vessels
  - Round/oval uniform nuclei, small nucleoli

SELECTED REFERENCES

1. Mridha AR et al: Anaplastic ependymoma with cartilaginous and osseous metaplasia: report of a rare case and review of literature. J Neurooncol. 82(1):75-80, 2007
2. Reni M et al: Ependymoma. Crit Rev Oncol Hematol. 63(1):81-9, 2007
3. Krieger MD et al: Effects of surgical resection and adjuvant therapy on pediatric intracranial ependymomas. Expert Rev Neurother. 5(4):465-71, 2005
4. Boccardo M et al: Tanycytic ependymoma of the spinal cord. Case report and review of the literature. Neurochirurgie. 49(6):605-10, 2003
5. Chamberlain MC: Ependymomas. Curr Neurol Neurosci Rep. 3(3):193-9, 2003
6. Grill J et al: Childhood ependymoma: a systematic review of treatment options and strategies. Paediatr Drugs. 5(8):533-43, 2003
7. Teo C et al: Ependymoma. Childs Nerv Syst. 19(5-6):270-85, 2003
8. Maksoud YA et al: Intracranial ependymoma. Neurosurg Focus. 13(3):e4, 2002
9. Wiestler OD et al: Ependymoma. In Kleihues P et al: Pathology and Genetics: Tumors of the Nervous System. Lyon: IARC Press. 72-81, 2000
10. Bouffet E et al: Intracranial ependymomas in children: a critical review of prognostic factors and a plea for cooperation. Med Pediatr Oncol. 30(6):319-29; discussion 329-31, 1998
11. Schiffer D et al: Prognosis of ependymoma. Childs Nerv Syst. 14(8):357-61, 1998
12. Min KW et al: Clear cell ependymoma: a mimic of oligodendroglioma: clinicopathologic and ultrastructural considerations. Am J Surg Pathol. 21(7):820-6, 1997

EPENDYMOMA

Microscopic Features

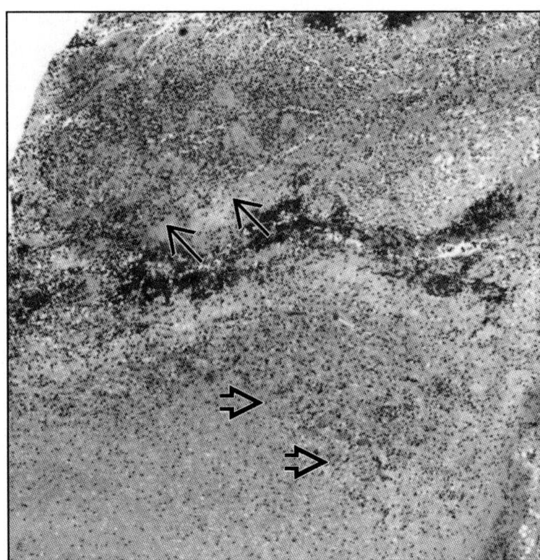

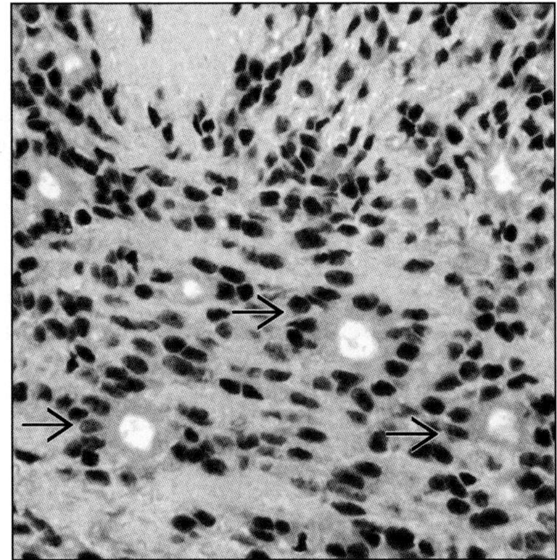

(Left) *Hematoxylin & eosin shows a low-power view of an ependymoma with a relatively well-circumscribed border ➙. Hemorrhage separates the tumor from adjacent parenchyma with reactive gliosis ➲. Anaplastic or spinal cord tumors may diffusely infiltrate normal nervous tissue.* ***(Right)*** *Hematoxylin & eosin shows a high-power view of true ependymal rosettes ➙ with more epithelial-appearing tumor cells forming a central lumen, defined by their apical surface.*

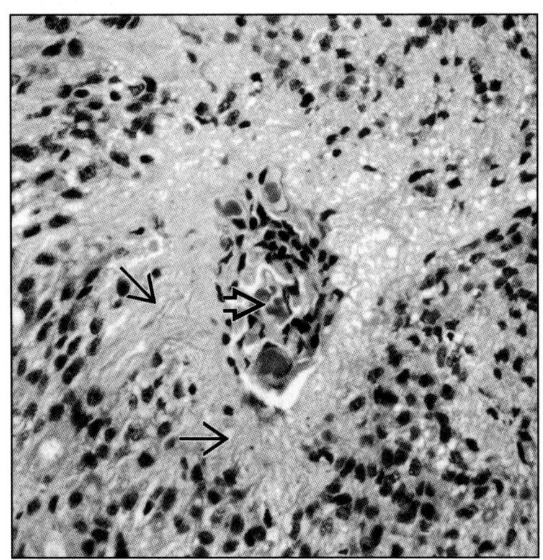

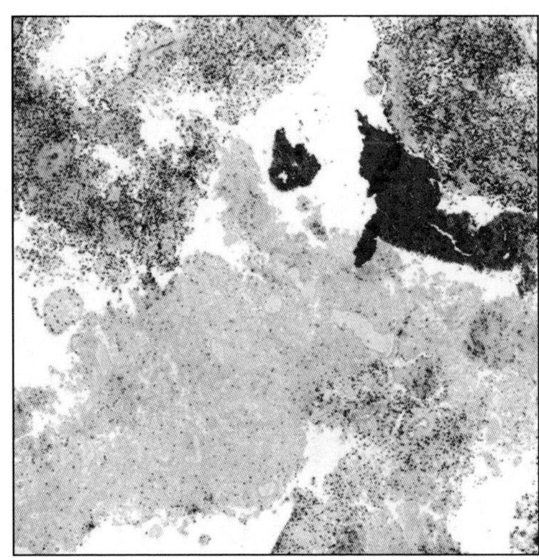

(Left) *Hematoxylin & eosin shows a medium-power view of a pseudorosette formed by more glial-appearing tumor cells. Their processes ➙, radially arranged around a central vessel ➲, result in a perivascular nuclear-free zone.* ***(Right)*** *Hematoxylin & eosin shows a low-power view of a 4th ventricle ependymoma with nonpalisading, coagulative necrosis. This type of necrosis (as opposed to the geographic kind) is common in this location and does not qualify this tumor as anaplastic.*

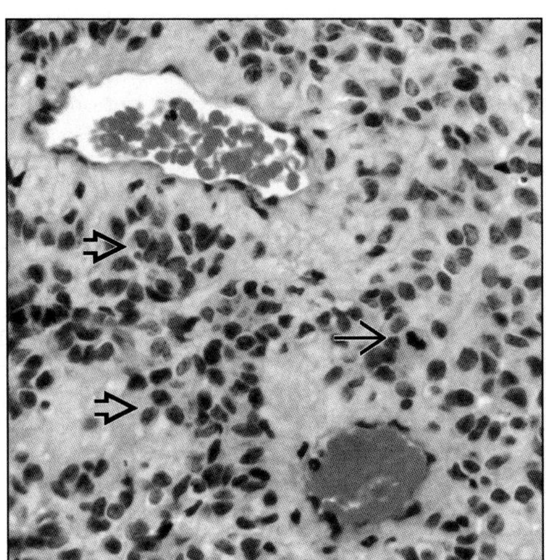

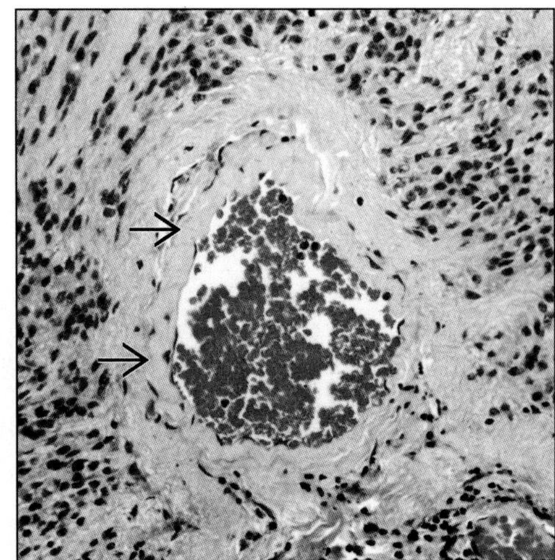

(Left) *Hematoxylin & eosin shows a high-power view of an ependymoma with focally increased cellularity, high nuclear to cytoplasmic ratio ➲, mild cytologic atypia, and occasional mitosis ➙. These features, unless predominant, do not suffice for the diagnosis of anaplastic ependymoma.* ***(Right)*** *Hematoxylin & eosin shows a medium-power view of a perivascular pseudorosette with hyalinization ➙ of the vessel wall, a characteristic example of degenerative change in ependymomas.*

Variant Microscopic Features

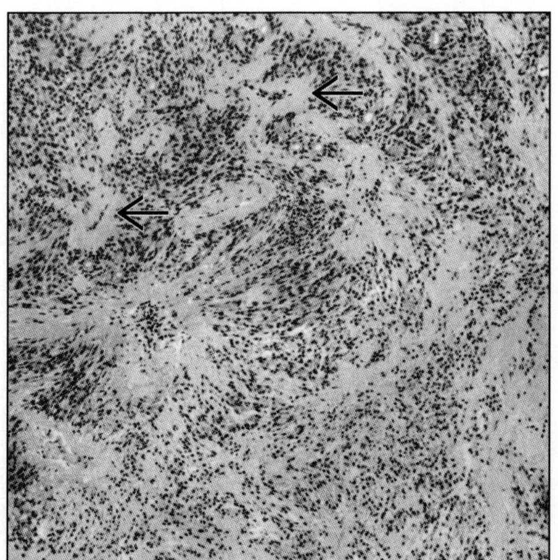

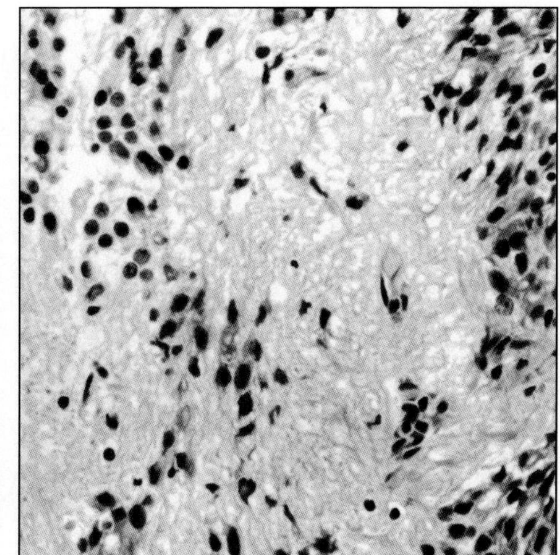

(Left) *Hematoxylin & eosin shows a low-power view of a cellular ependymoma, the most classic variant, where areas of densely packed tumor cells alternate with nuclear-free zones of perivascular pseudorosettes ➔.* ***(Right)*** *H&E shows a high-power view of a hypocellular, fibrillar area where rosettes are inconspicuous. These tumors should not be diagnosed as mixed glioma (or "ependymoastrocytoma") if the area is occurring in an otherwise convincing ependymoma.*

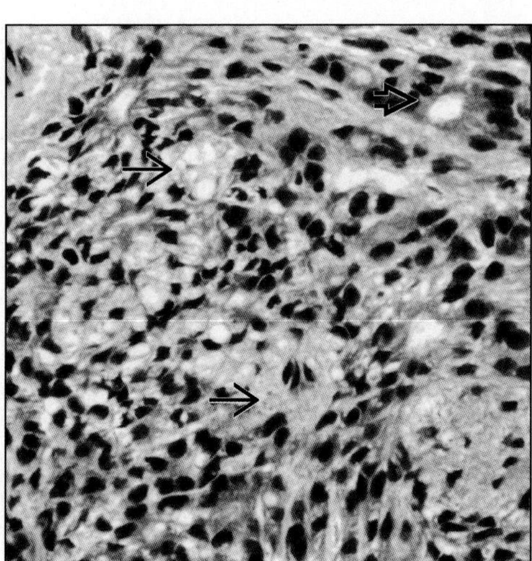

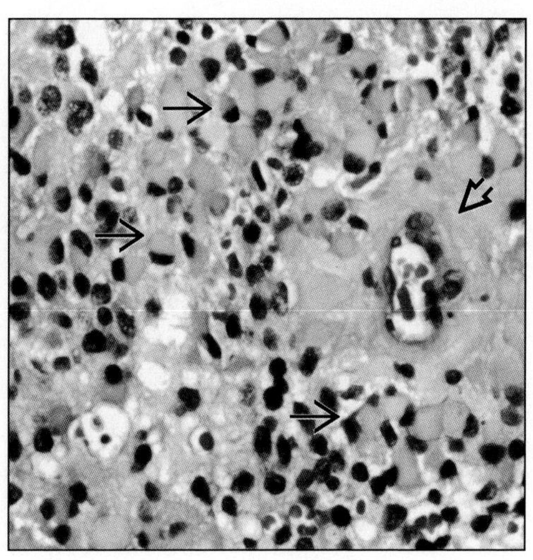

(Left) *Hematoxylin & eosin shows a high-power view of an ependymoma with foam cells ➔, a commonly seen degenerative change. When areas like this are very prominent, the tumor can be referred to as a "lipidized" ependymoma. True ependymal rosettes ➔ are also present.* ***(Right)*** *Hematoxylin & eosin shows a high-power view of an ependymoma with a perivascular pseudorosette ➔ and numerous cells ➔ that resemble gemistocytic astrocytes.*

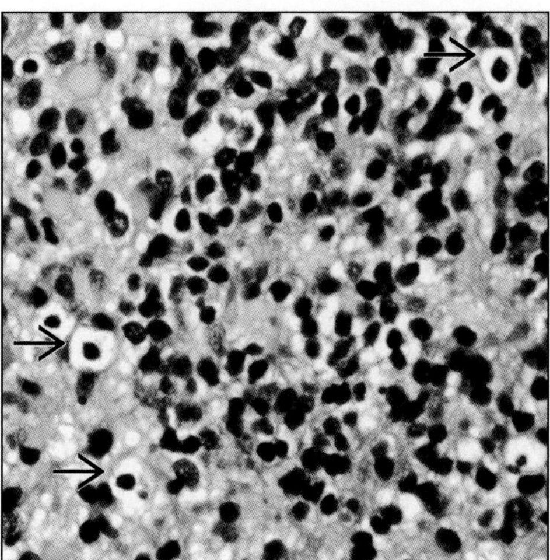

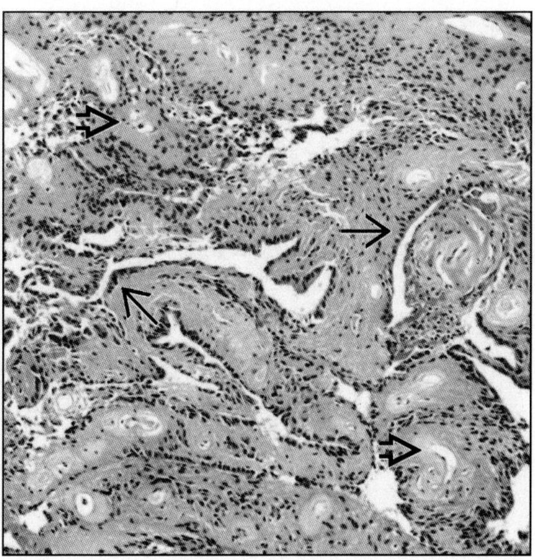

(Left) *Hematoxylin & eosin shows a high-power view of a frontal lobe clear cell ependymoma with tumor cells having perinuclear halos ➔, resembling oligodendroglioma. These generally have anaplastic features and behave like grade III neoplasms.* ***(Right)*** *Hematoxylin & eosin shows a medium-power view of a papillary ependymoma with columnar cell-lined ➔ fronds of gliofibrillary stroma containing perivascular pseudorosettes ➔.*

EPENDYMOMA

Ancillary Techniques

*(**Left**) Hematoxylin & eosin shows a frozen section slide where ependymomas can look deceptively fibrillar and "astrocytic." However, the presence of perivascular pseudorosettes ⇨ can be very helpful in arriving at the correct diagnosis. (**Right**) Hematoxylin & eosin shows an intraoperative smear preparation slide where aggregates of tumor cells retain their cohesiveness, have round uniform nuclei →, and cytoplasmic processes ⇨ are distinctly oriented around blood vessels ↩.*

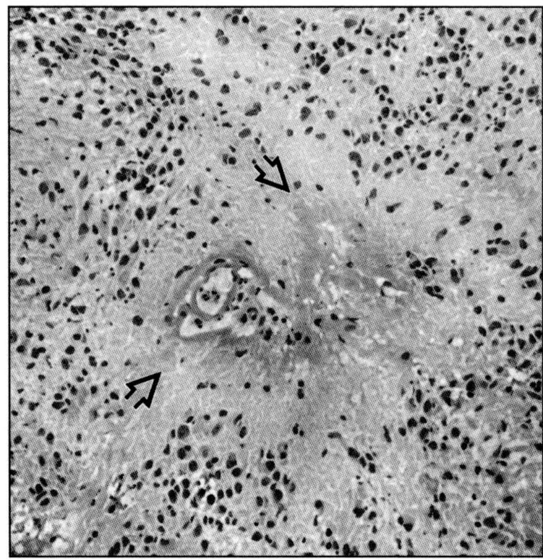

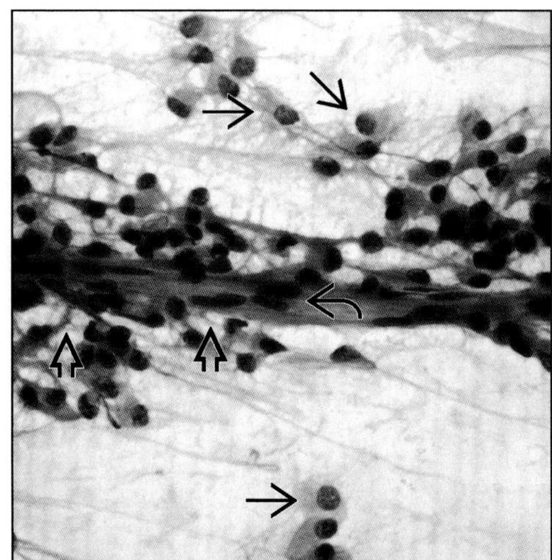

*(**Left**) Immunohistochemical stain with an antibody against glial fibrillary acidic protein (GFAP) highlights tumor cell processes → forming perivascular pseudorosettes ⇨. (**Right**) Immunohistochemical stain with an antibody against vimentin shows diffuse cytoplasmic positivity in ependymoma tumor cells.*

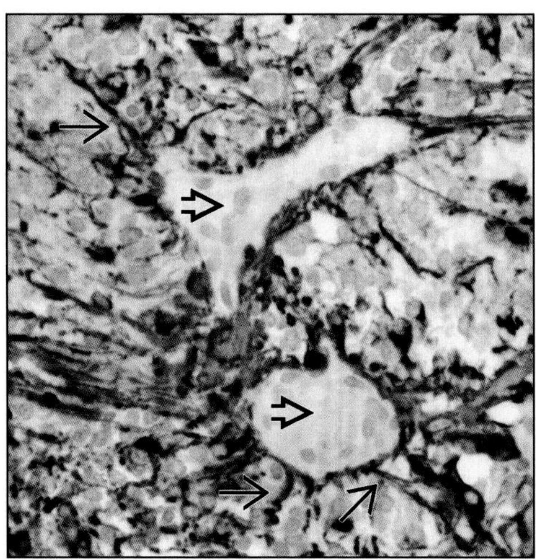

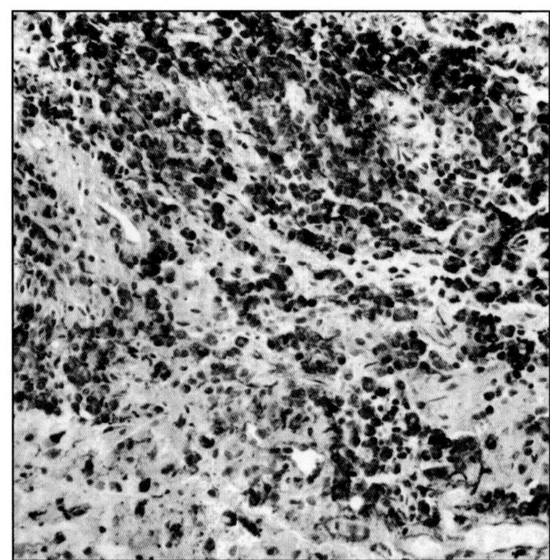

*(**Left**) Immunohistochemical stain with an antibody against S100 protein shows diffuse positivity in ependymomas, especially in areas with more cellular, epithelioid features. (**Right**) Immunohistochemical stain with an antibody against epithelial membrane antigen (EMA) shows characteristic dot-like perinuclear positivity →, thought to represent the luminal surface of intracytoplasmic microrosettes.*

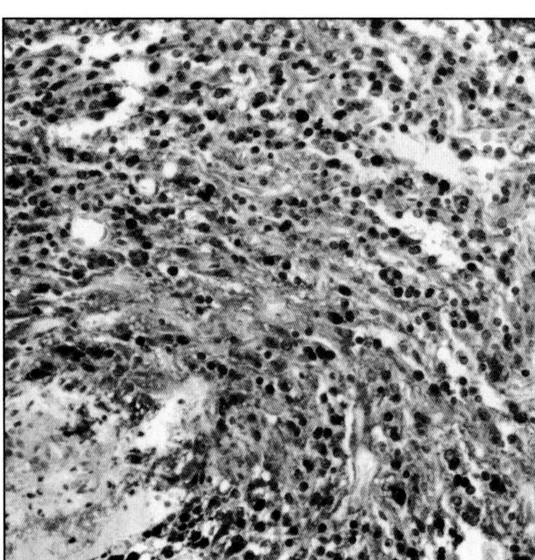

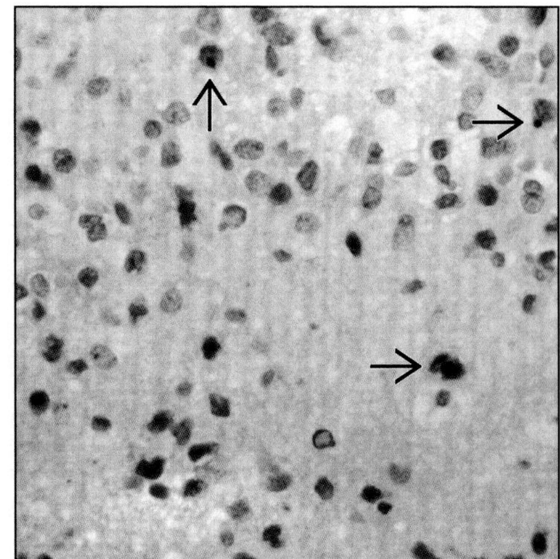

Microscopic Features of Anaplastic Ependymoma

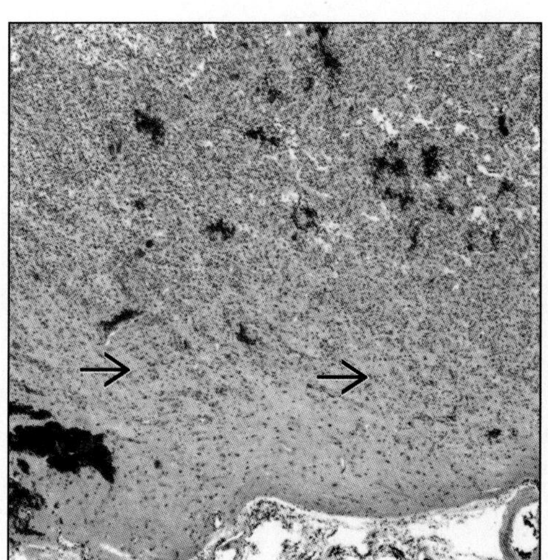

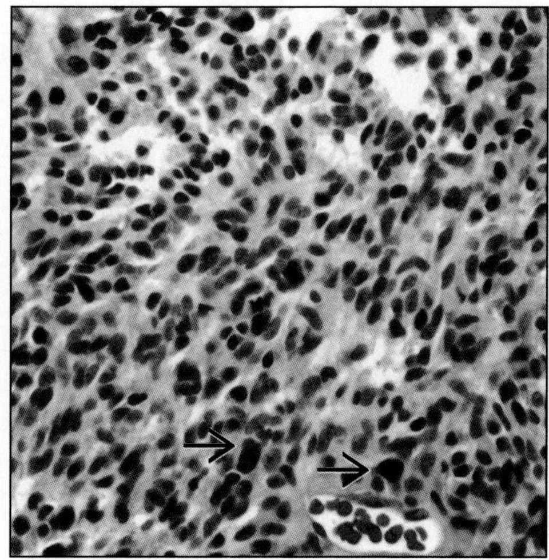

(Left) *Hematoxylin & eosin shows a low-power view of anaplastic ependymoma (grade III), having a more infiltrative border* ⇒ *with adjacent brain tissue than grade II lesions.* ***(Right)*** *Hematoxylin & eosin shows a high-power view of anaplastic ependymoma (grade III). These tumors are hypercellular and poorly differentiated with cytologic atypia and nuclear pleomorphism* ⇒.

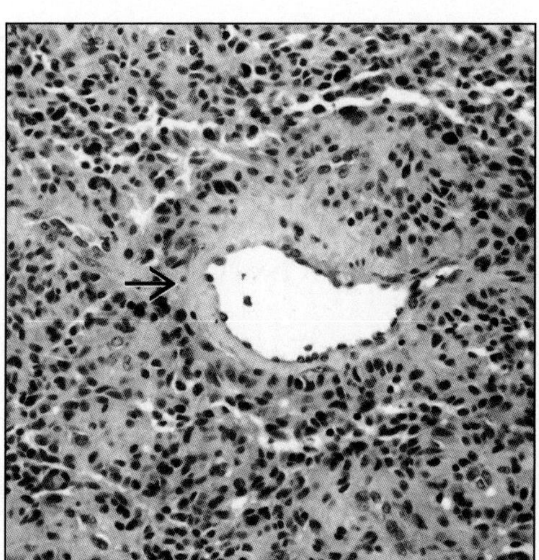

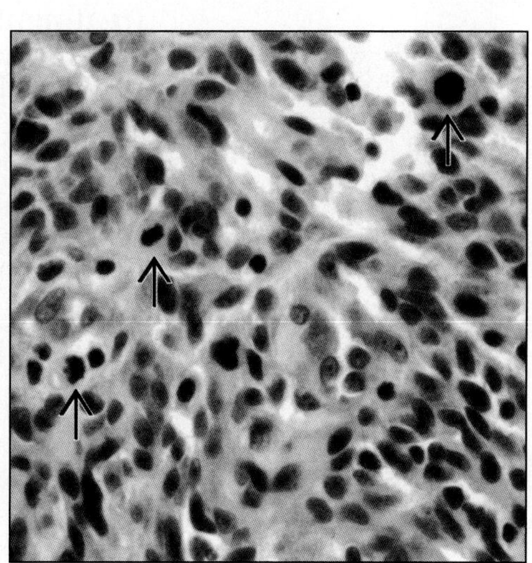

(Left) *Hematoxylin & eosin shows a high-power view of anaplastic ependymoma (grade III), where despite the increased cellularity, perivascular pseudorosettes* ⇒ *are still identifiable. In their absence, electron microscopy may be needed to correctly identify the histogenesis of the tumor.* ***(Right)*** *Hematoxylin & eosin shows a high-power view of anaplastic ependymoma (grade III) with high mitotic activity. Generally more than 5-10 mitoses* ⇒ *are found per 10 HPF.*

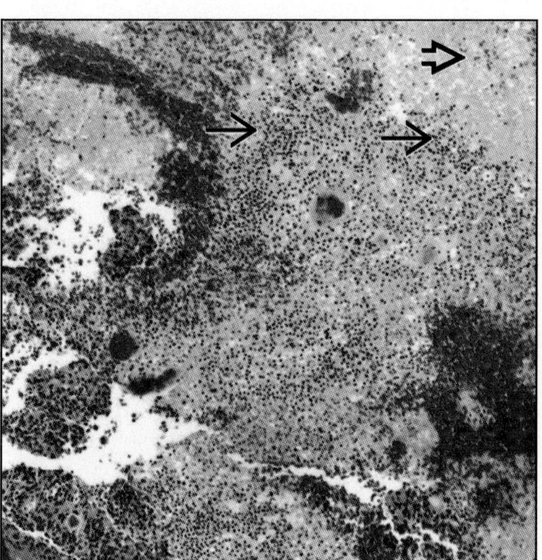

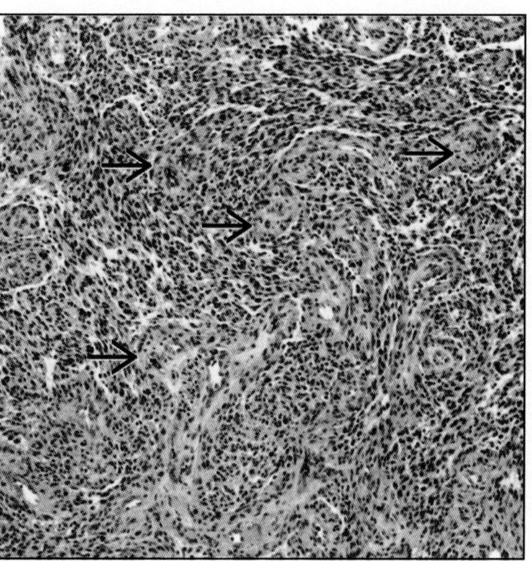

(Left) *Hematoxylin & eosin shows a low-power view of an anaplastic ependymoma (grade III) with pseudopalisading ("geographic") necrosis, where areas of nuclear condensation* ⇒ *can be seen adjacent to areas of necrotic tumor* ⇨. ***(Right)*** *Hematoxylin & eosin shows a high-power view of an ependymoma with "glomeruloid" endothelial cell (microvascular) proliferation* ⇒, *a histologic feature generally associated with anaplastic (grade III) ependymomas.*

EPENDYMOBLASTOMA

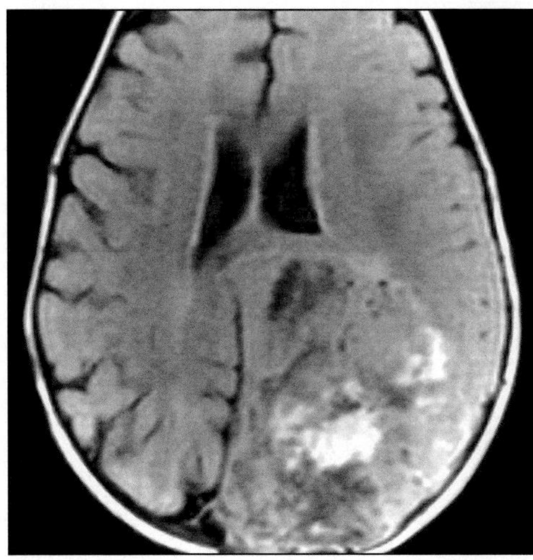

Axial FLAIR MR shows large, inhomogeneous mass in the left occipital lobe with elevation of the ventricle and corpus callosum. Histology showed ependymoblastic rosettes.

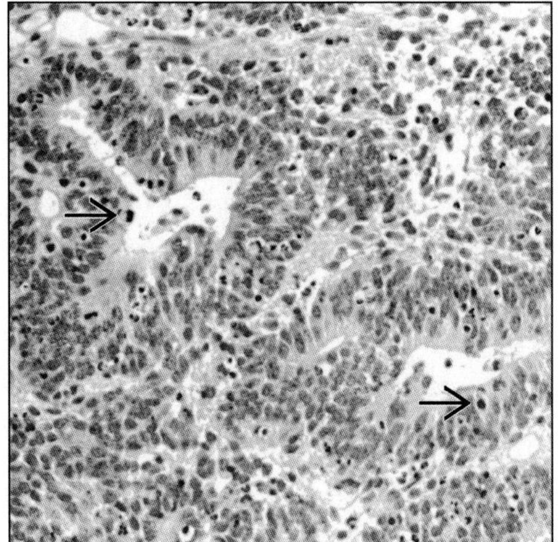

H&E shows ependymoblastoma with small cells having a high nuclear to cytoplasmic ratio and ependymoblastomatous rosettes with abluminal mitotic figures ➔. (Courtesy P. Burger, MD.)

TERMINOLOGY

Definitions

- Rare, highly malignant (WHO grade IV) embryonal brain tumor of infants and young children with ependymoblastic rosettes in primitive cell background
- For some authors, not specific diagnostic entity, but histologic feature in other malignant CNS tumors

ETIOLOGY/PATHOGENESIS

Histogenesis

- WHO (2007): Considered a variant of supratentorial CNS primitive neuroectodermal tumors (PNET)
- Arises from periventricular neuroepithelial precursors
  - Incompletely differentiated, immature ependyma

CLINICAL ISSUES

Epidemiology

- Incidence
  - Very rare; < 100 cases reported in literature
- Age
  - Neonates, young children (congenital to 5 years old)

Site

- Supratentorial; frontoparietal location most common
  - Usually associated with lateral or 4th ventricles
- Sacrococcygeal, 1° leptomeningeal cases reported

Presentation

- Rapid onset of clinical manifestations over weeks
- Young children: ↑ intracranial pressure, hydrocephalus
- Older children: Focal neurologic deficits
- May have elevated serum α-fetoprotein

Natural History

- Rapid growth, CSF dissemination, extraneural mets

Treatment

- Attempt at gross total surgical resection
- Postoperative radiation may prolong survival

Prognosis

- Mean survival time after presentation or diagnosis
  - 1-2 years (aggressive therapy); 2 months (without)
  - Overall 5-year survival: ~ 15%
- Completeness of resection may predict outcome

IMAGE FINDINGS

MR Findings

- Contrast-enhancing, large, discrete, deeply seated mass
- Surrounded by extensive peritumoral edema

MACROSCOPIC FEATURES

General Features

- Soft, fleshy, friable, gray-white mass
- Highly vascular, hemorrhagic, partially cystic

MICROSCOPIC PATHOLOGY

Histologic Features

- Relatively well demarcated from adjacent brain
  - But often infiltrates parenchyma, leptomeninges
- Distinctive, multilayered, concentric rosettes
  - "Ependymoblastic" or "ependymoblastomatous"
  - Pseudostratified, ependymal-type tubules
- Inner true rosette around slit-like or round lumen
  - Polarized cells with defined apical surface
  - Internal limiting membrane (terminal bar)
  - Faint stippling (blepharoplasts; PTAH[+])
  - Abluminal mitoses, coarse chromatin, nucleoli
- Outer layer merges with densely cellular background
  - Compact, undifferentiated neuroectodermal cells
  - Small cells with delicate cytoplasmic processes

EPENDYMOBLASTOMA

Key Facts

Terminology
- Rare, highly malignant (WHO grade IV) embryonal brain tumor (PNET) with ependymoblastic rosettes

Clinical Issues
- Neonates, young children (congenital to 5 years old)
- Supratentorial, usually associated with ventricles
  - ↑ intracranial pressure, hydrocephalus
- Rapid, aggressive growth; 15% 5-year survival
- Gross total resection; postoperative radiation

Microscopic Pathology
- Well demarcated, but invasive into parenchyma
- Distinctive, multilayered "ependymoblastic" rosettes
  - Inner true rosette of polarized cells around lumen
  - Outer layer merges with primitive cell background

Top Differential Diagnoses
- Anaplastic ependymoma
  - Perivascular pseudorosettes, true 1-layer rosettes
  - Vascular proliferation, pseudopalisading necrosis

  - Round/oval nuclei, high nuclear to cytoplasmic ratio
- Microvascular proliferation generally absent
- Variable, focal, nongeographic necrosis

ANCILLARY TESTS

Immunohistochemistry
- S100, cytokeratin, vimentin, nestin: Variably positive

Electron Microscopy
- Occasional, glial-like cytoplasmic filaments
- Cells constituting rosettes may contain
  - Short, lateral, or apical junctional complexes
  - "Abortive" cilia (some with 9+2 configuration)
  - Microvilli, basal bodies oriented toward lumen

DIFFERENTIAL DIAGNOSIS

Anaplastic Ependymoma
- Perivascular pseudorosettes, true single-layer rosettes
- Microvascular proliferation, pseudopalisading necrosis
- Lacks background of small primitive embryonal cells

Medulloblastoma
- Cerebellar location; Homer Wright rosettes (no lumen)

Embryonal Tumor with Abundant Neuropil and True Rosettes (ETANTR)
- Biphasic pattern: Abundant, finely fibrillar neuropil
  - Admixed, densely cellular areas with true rosettes

Medulloepithelioma
- Tubular, cannalicular, or papillary neuroepithelium
- Neuroectodermal differentiation: Glial, neuronal, etc.

DIAGNOSTIC CHECKLIST

Pathologic Interpretation Pearls
- "Ependymoblastomatous" rosettes
  - Characteristic apical (juxtaluminal) mitoses
  - Similar to Flexner-Wintersteiner rosettes
    - Often larger, more elliptical, with slit-like lumens
  - May also be seen in other primitive tumors
    - ETANTR, PNET, medulloepithelioma
    - Divergent differentiation in primitive tumors
    - Some favor abolishing term "ependymoblastoma"
- Do not use "ependymoblastoma" for anaplastic ependymoma (histologically distinct neoplasms)

SELECTED REFERENCES

1. Judkins AR et al: Ependymoblastoma: dear, damned, distracting diagnosis, farewell!*. Brain Pathol. 20(1):133-9, 2010
2. Becker LE et al: Ependymoblastoma. In Kleihues P et al: Pathology and Genetics: Tumors of the Nervous System. Lyon: IARC Press. 127-8, 2000
3. Cruz-Sanchez FF et al: Ependymoblastoma: a histological, immunohistological and ultrastructural study of five cases. Histopathology. 12(1):17-27, 1988
4. Mørk SJ et al: Ependymoblastoma. A reappraisal of a rare embryonal tumor. Cancer. 55(7):1536-42, 1985

IMAGE GALLERY

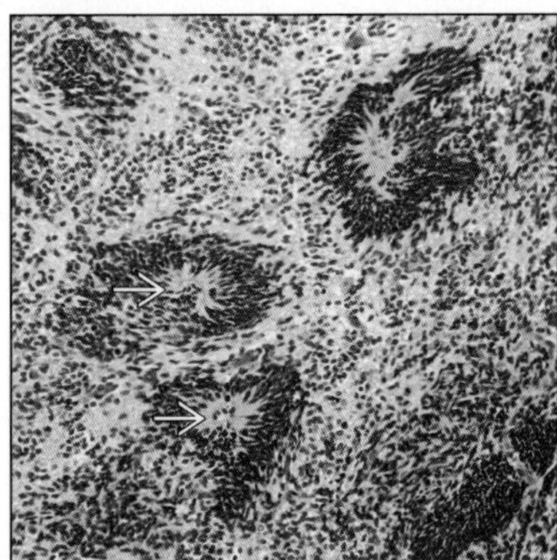
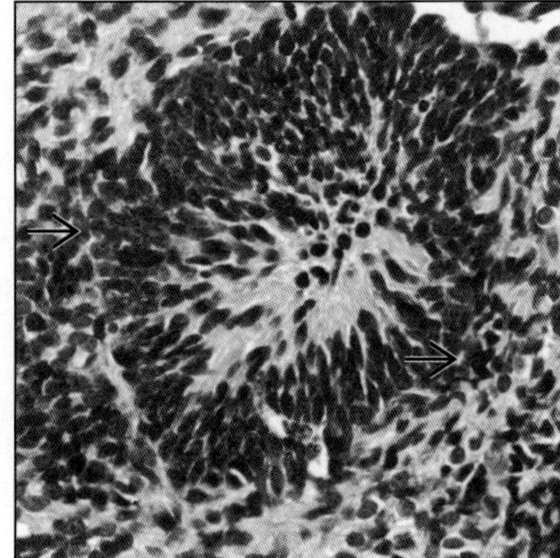
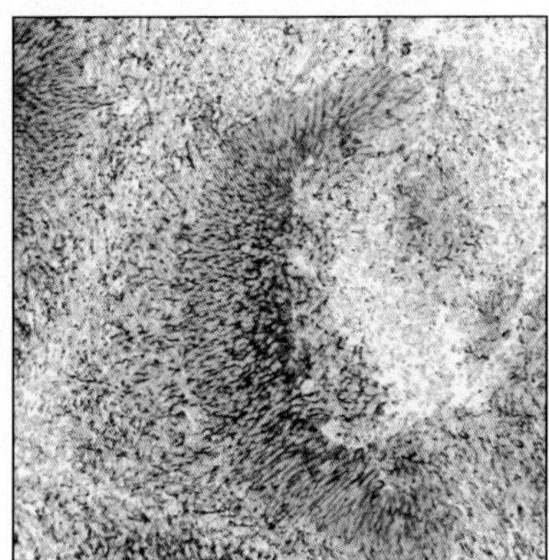

(Left) *Hematoxylin & eosin shows ependymoblastoma with concentric, multilayered ependymoblastomatous rosettes with inner true rosettes centered around slit-like or round lumens ➡. (Courtesy E. Rushing, MD.)* ***(Center)*** *Higher magnification shows an ependymoblastomatous rosette with pseudostratified, ependymal-type tubules lined by polarized cells and an outer layer that merges with the cellular background ➡. (Courtesy E. Rushing, MD.)* ***(Right)*** *Nestin-positive cells of ependymoblastomatous rosettes are shown. (Courtesy E. Rushing, MD.)*

DIFFUSE ASTROCYTOMA (LOW GRADE)

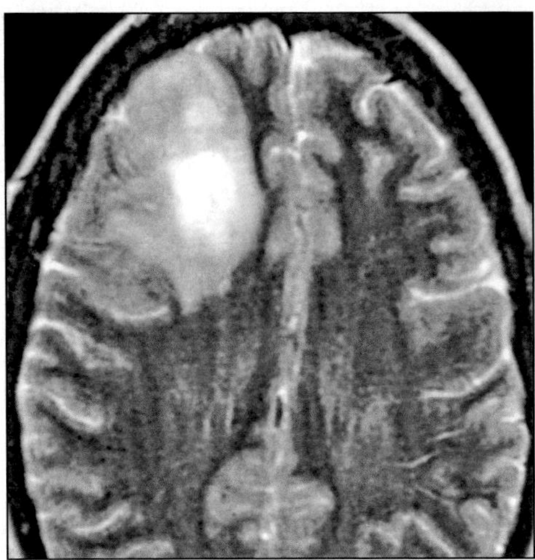

Axial T2W MRI shows a hyperintense, diffuse mass in the frontal lobe white matter with central hyperintensity, suggesting cystic change. Note the infiltrative margins.

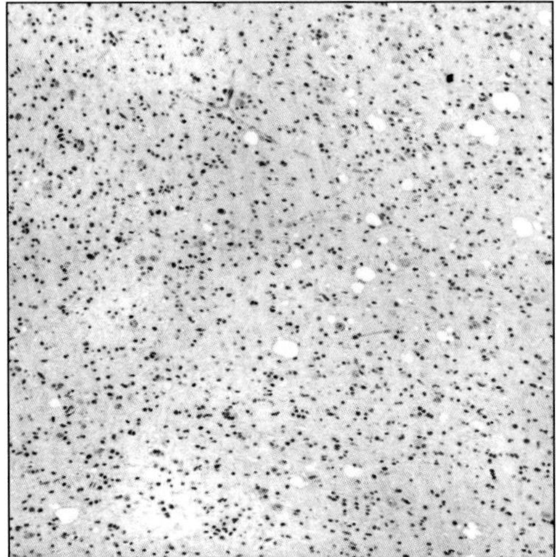

H&E shows low-power view of mildly hypercellular, well-differentiated neoplastic astrocytes diffusely infiltrating white matter with ill-defined borders.

TERMINOLOGY

Synonyms

- Well-differentiated (WHO grade II) astrocytoma
- Fibrillary astrocytoma

Definitions

- Well-differentiated (grade II), slow-growing, diffusely infiltrating intraparenchymal astrocytic neoplasm
- Mostly involves cerebral white matter of young adults, with intrinsic tendency for malignant progression/ degeneration to anaplastic astrocytoma, glioblastoma

ETIOLOGY/PATHOGENESIS

TP53 Mutation

- Astrocytomas in patients with germline mutations
  - Especially higher grade lesions
- Mutations present in most lesions that progress
  - Especially in gemistocytic astrocytomas
- Clonal expansion seen with higher grade or recurrence

Familial/Genetic Syndrome Associations

- Li-Fraumeni syndrome
- Multiple enchondromatosis type 1 (Ollier disease)
- Neurofibromatosis type 1

CLINICAL ISSUES

Epidemiology

- Incidence
  - 5-15% of all astrocytomas
- Age
  - Young adults: 20-45 years old (mean age: 34 years)
- Gender
  - Slight male predominance (1.2:1)

Site

- Supratentorial: Mostly in cerebral hemispheres
  - Frontal, temporal lobes (30% of cases each)
  - Less often in brainstem, spinal cord, cerebellum
- Children: More often in brainstem, thalamus
- "Tectal glioma": Unclear relation
  - Slow-growing, periaqueductal, nonpilocytic

Presentation

- Cerebral lesions
  - Seizures, mass effect, ↑ intracranial pressure
  - Subtle changes in speech, vision, sensation, behavior
    - May be present earlier (months before diagnosis)
- Brainstem lesions
  - "Long tract" signs, 6th cranial nerve dysfunction

Natural History

- Can remain well differentiated for years
  - Good long-term survival
- May undergo anaplastic transformation
  - Causes neurologic deficits, leads to death
  - Mean time of progression to grade IV: 3-5 years
  - More likely in gemistocytic astrocytomas, adults

Treatment

- Surgical approaches
  - Attempt at gross total resection
- Adjuvant therapy
  - Value of radiation therapy remains debatable
    - Depends on symptoms, volume of residual tumor
    - Improves survival after subtotal resection

Prognosis

- Mean survival 4-12 years (most: 5-8 years after surgery)
  - 10-year survival < 20% in adults
- Main prognostic factors
  - Extent of surgical resection
  - Neurologic status at presentation (Karnofsky score)
- Less favorable prognosis
  - MIB-1 labeling index > 5%, *P53* mutation
  - Thalamus/pons lesions
    - Tend to be unresectable, unresponsive to radiation
- Presence of microcysts: Better prognosis

DIFFUSE ASTROCYTOMA (LOW GRADE)

Key Facts

Terminology
- Well-differentiated (grade II), slow-growing, diffusely infiltrating intraparenchymal astrocytic neoplasm
- Mostly in cerebral white matter of young adults, with intrinsic tendency for malignant progression

Clinical Issues
- 5-15% of all astrocytomas
- Young adults: 20-45 years old (mean age: 34 years)
- Cerebral hemispheres (frontal, temporal lobes)
- Children: More often in brainstem, thalamus
- Seizures, mass effect, ↑ intracranial pressure
- May undergo anaplastic transformation in 3-5 years
- Surgical treatment: Attempt at gross total resection
- Mean survival: 4-12 years, 5-8 years after surgery
- Less favorable prognosis: MIB-1 > 2%, *p53* mutation

Image Findings
- Hypointense on T1; hyperintense on T2, FLAIR
- Enhancement: Prior radiotherapy or transformation

Macroscopic Features
- Infiltrative, diffuse, ill-defined; distorts white matter
- Gray-yellow, soft-gelatinous to firm, gritty or calcified
- ↑ discrete, hemorrhagic, necrotic: Suggests high grade

Microscopic Pathology
- Hypercellular astrocytes, moderate atypia, no mitoses
- Loose fibrillar, often microcystic background matrix
- GFAP(+) processes, MIB-1 < 2%, p53(+)

Diagnostic Checklist
- Focal necrosis in low-grade lesions may be ischemic
- Astrocytoma with single mitosis: Probably grade II

- Pediatric grade II astrocytomas more favorable
  - 10-year survival rate reported as high as 82%
  - Malignant transformation less likely (< 20%)
  - Control may be achieved by surgery alone

IMAGE FINDINGS

MR Findings
- Hypointense on T1; hyperintense on T2, FLAIR
- Mostly diffuse, ill-defined, confined to white matter
- Generally little edema or vasogenic effect
- Low-grade (II) lesions lack gadolinium enhancement
  - If enhancement is present, it suggests
    - Prior radiotherapy or malignant transformation
    - Possible diagnosis of pilocytic astrocytoma
- Thalamic lesions tend to be symmetric or bilateral
- Brainstem lesions: Diffusely enlarge, no distinct mass
  - "Hypertrophy" with radiographic "whiteout"
  - Centered in the pons, engulfing basilar artery
- Spinal cord lesions: Ill-defined fusiform enlargement
  - May span many segments, associated with syrinx

CT Findings
- Ill-defined, homogeneous mass of low density
- Lack contrast enhancement; may be calcified, cystic

MACROSCOPIC FEATURES

General Features
- Infiltrative, diffuse, ill-defined borders
  - Enlarge/distort but do not destroy white matter
  - Expand gyri, obscure gray-white matter junction
- Gray-yellow, soft-gelatinous to firm, gritty or calcified
  - Focal spongy, clear fluid-filled microcysts
- ↑ discrete, hemorrhagic, necrotic: Suggests high grade

MICROSCOPIC PATHOLOGY

Histologic Features
- Diffusely infiltrating, well-differentiated astrocytes
  - May appear well circumscribed at low magnification
  - Irregularly distributed, mostly in white matter
    - Between myelinated axons of entrapped neurons
  - Loose fibrillar, often microcystic background matrix
- Increased cellularity, density of astrocytes
  - 2-3x more than normal
  - Some lesions are only barely hypercellular
    - Diagnosis depends on recognizing cytologic atypia
- "Secondary structures" often present
  - Neuronal satellitosis
    - Neoplastic cells cluster around cortical neurons
  - Subpial aggregates of neoplastic astrocytes
    - More typical in oligodendrogliomas
- Amorphous/lamellar calcifications (< 10% of lesions)

Cytologic Features
- Moderate atypia, hyperchromasia, and pleomorphism
  - Larger, more irregular/coarse nuclei than normal
- Eosinophilic cytoplasm with short fibrillar processes
  - Cytoplasm may be inconspicuous ("naked" nuclei)
  - Perinuclear halos may be present

"Gemistocytic" Astrocytoma
- Variant with > 20% gemistocytic neoplastic astrocytes
  - Common in astrocytomas, rarely occur in pure form
- Plump, angular cells; abundant "glassy" cytoplasm
- Eccentrically placed asymmetric nuclei; small nucleoli
- "Corona" of short, random, coarse fibrillary processes
- Eosinophilic bodies of fibril-rich cytoplasm
  - Resemble Rosenthal fibers
- Perivascular lymphocytic infiltrates, germinal centers
- Areas of small cells with scattered mitoses common
  - Higher MIB-1 labeling index
  - May explain tendency for anaplastic progression
  - Considered equivalent to WHO grade III by some

Protoplasmic Astrocytoma
- Rare hypocellular variant with scant GFAP expression
- Small cell bodies, few processes, low fibrillarity
- Mucoid degeneration, microcyst formation
- Absent mitotic activity, low MIB-1 index

DIFFUSE ASTROCYTOMA (LOW GRADE)

Meningeal Gliomatosis
- Leptomeningeal glioma, no parenchymal component
- From small heterotopic glial nodules or protrusions
- Mostly near foramen of Luschka, or caudal spinal cord
- Enhancing, thickening, and opacifying leptomeninges
- Histologically, most are diffuse grade II astrocytomas

ANCILLARY TESTS

Frozen Sections
- Artifact causes ice crystals misinterpreted as microcysts
  - Also conceals degree of hypercellularity
- Helpful findings that suggest astrocytoma
  - Perineuronal satellitosis
  - Nuclear hyperchromasia and angulation

Immunohistochemistry
- GFAP(+) prominent processes, perinuclear rim
  - Also accentuates coexisting reactive astrocytes
- Neurofilament protein stains trapped normal axons
- May be positive for p53, especially gemistocytic lesions
- Vimentin(+) cell bodies and cytoplasmic/nuclear S100 positivity maybe present
- MIB-1 index generally 1-2%

Cytogenetics
- Gains of chromosome 7q, *P53* mutations seen
  - Both thought to confer worse prognosis

Electron Microscopy
- Intermediate filaments in cell body and processes
  - Of limited diagnostic significance
    - Does not distinguish neoplastic from reactive

Smear Preparation
- Nuclear atypia and pleomorphism
- Finely fibrillar background of cell processes
  - Fewer, shorter, more asymmetric than normal

DIFFERENTIAL DIAGNOSIS

Normal Brain Parenchyma
- Lacks hypercellularity, nuclear atypia, pleomorphism

Reactive Piloid Gliosis
- Chronic process around longstanding lesions/tumors
- Mostly in hypothalamus, cerebellum, spinal cord
- Densely fibrillar, paucicellular, rich in Rosenthal fibers

Subacute ("Fibrillary") Gliosis
- Uniformly spaced, hypertrophic reactive astrocytes
- But only minimally increased in number, lack atypia

Demyelinating Disease
- Widely separated reactive astrocytes, no clustering
  - Abundant, radiating cytoplasmic processes
- Rich in foamy macrophages, perivascular lymphocytes

Progressive Multifocal Leukoencephalopathy
- JC virus infection, in immunosuppressed (e.g., AIDS)
- Pleomorphic astrocytes, bizarre hyperchromatic nuclei
- Foamy macrophages, oligodendrocytic inclusions

Pilocytic Astrocytoma
- Discrete contrast-enhancing cystic mass, mural nodule
- Biphasic histologic pattern, hyalinized blood vessels
- Rosenthal fibers, eosinophilic granular bodies

Oligodendroglioma
- Monotonous cells, round nuclei, clear cytoplasm, halo
- Calcifications, "chicken wire" vasculature

DIAGNOSTIC CHECKLIST

Clinically Relevant Pathologic Features
- Some propose 1.5% MIB-1 cutoff between grades II/III
  - Shorter survival seen with MIB-1 index > 4-5%

Pathologic Interpretation Pearls
- Focal necrosis in low-grade lesions maybe ischemic
  - Do not overdiagnose as grade IV (glioblastoma)
  - In absence of aggressive histology/radiology
- Single mitosis theoretically qualifies for grade III
  - Reluctantly accepted, may be due to tumor sampling
    - Carries more weight if in small biopsy tissue
  - "Astrocytoma with single mitosis": Grade II by some
    - If well sampled and well scanned microscopically
- "Minigemistocytes"
  - Eccentric, spherical, GFAP(+) cytoplasmic mass
  - Hyaline, faint fibrillar appearance akin to inclusion
  - Common in oligodendroglioma, also in astrocytoma
- If ambiguity between astrocytoma-oligodendroglioma
  - Diagnose as "well-differentiated, infiltrating glioma"
    - Especially on frozen section
  - Consider diagnosis of "mixed oligoastrocytoma"
    - If significant, convincing oligodendroglial features
- Microcysts of varying size/shape helpful for diagnosis
  - Uncommon in gliosis
  - Differ from linear clefts of freezing artifact

GRADING

WHO/St. Anne-Mayo System
- Features in grading of infiltrating astrocytic neoplasms
  - Atypia, mitoses, vascular proliferation, necrosis
- Grade II: Only 1 feature present, usually nuclear atypia
- Grade III (anaplastic or malignant astrocytoma)
  - 2 features present, typically atypia and mitoses
- Grade IV (glioblastoma): 3-4 features present
  - Often exhibit necrosis, microvascular proliferation
  - Should also have hypercellularity, atypia, ↑ mitoses

SELECTED REFERENCES

1. Perry A: Pathology of low-grade gliomas: an update of emerging concepts. Neuro Oncol. 5(3):168-78, 2003
2. Cohen KJ et al: Pediatric glial tumors. Curr Treat Options Oncol. 2(6):529-36, 2001
3. Stieber VW: Low-grade gliomas. Curr Treat Options Oncol. 2(6):495-506, 2001
4. Giannini C et al: Classification and grading of low-grade astrocytic tumors in children. Brain Pathol. 7(2):785-98, 1997
5. Kleihues P et al: Histopathology, classification, and grading of gliomas. Glia. 15(3):211-21, 1995

Microscopic Features

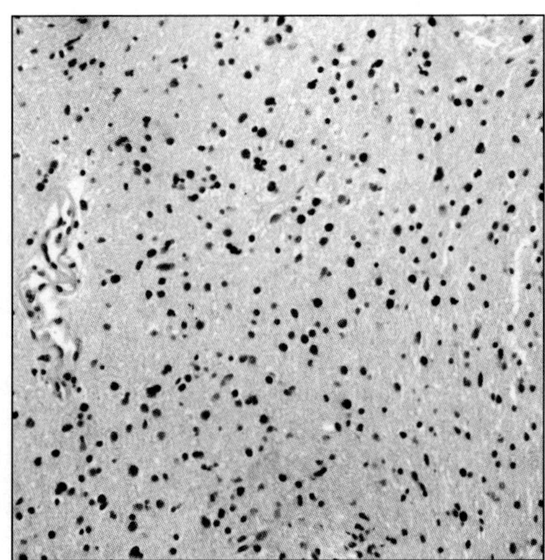

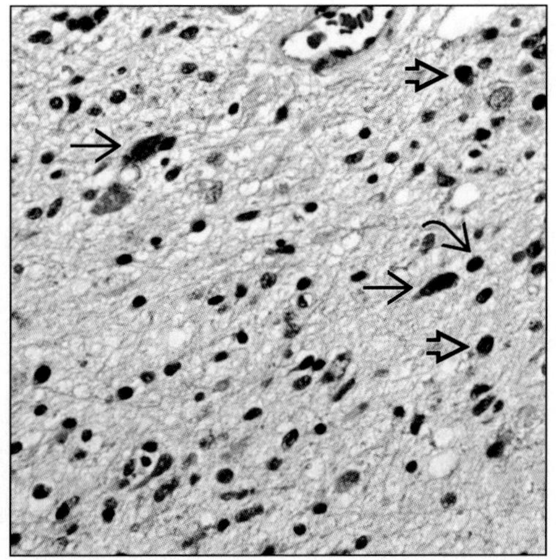

(Left) *H&E shows medium-power view of low-grade diffuse astrocytoma with 2-3x increased cellularity vs. normal white matter. Neoplastic cells are irregularly distributed in a loosely fibrillar background.* ***(Right)*** *High-power view shows cytologically atypical, but well-differentiated astrocytes ⇒ with nuclear enlargement, hyperchromasia, and pleomorphism. Cytoplasm varies from inconspicuous ("naked" nuclei ↗) to slightly eosinophilic with short fibrillar processes ⇨.*

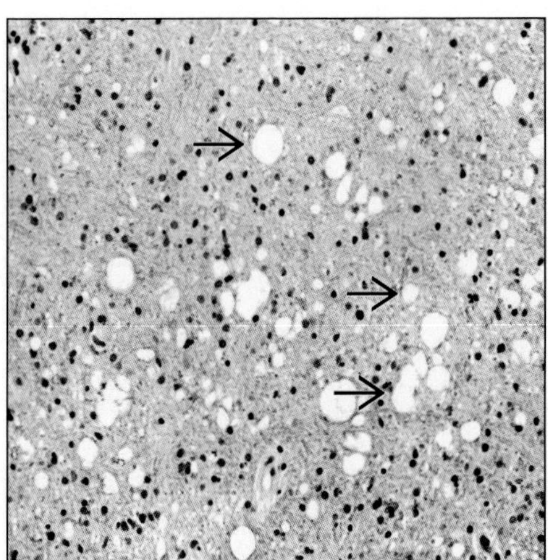

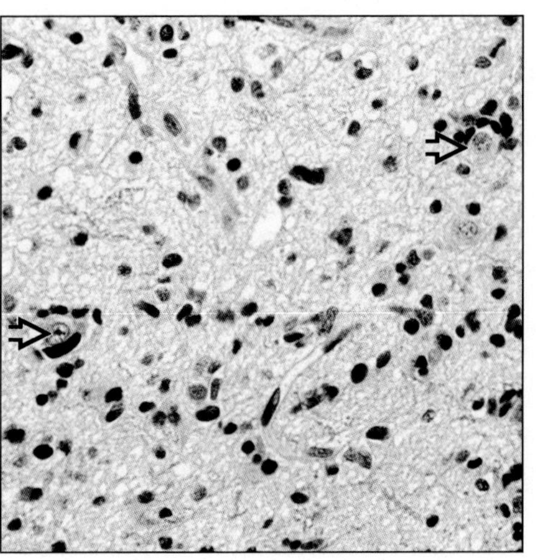

(Left) *H&E shows medium-power view of low-grade diffuse astrocytoma with background microcysts ⇒ of varying size and shape, a helpful finding; they are uncommon in reactive gliosis and differ from the linear clefts of freezing artifact.* ***(Right)*** *High-power view shows perineuronal satellitosis, where neoplastic cells cluster around cortical neurons ⇨, a "secondary structure" that suggests astrocytoma. Background cellularity is only mildly increased and mitoses are absent.*

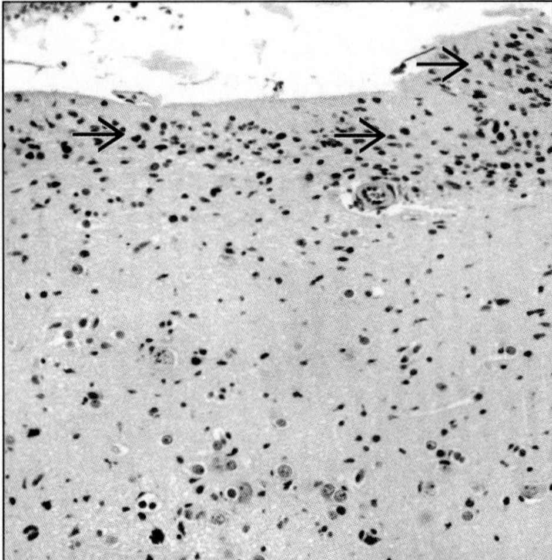

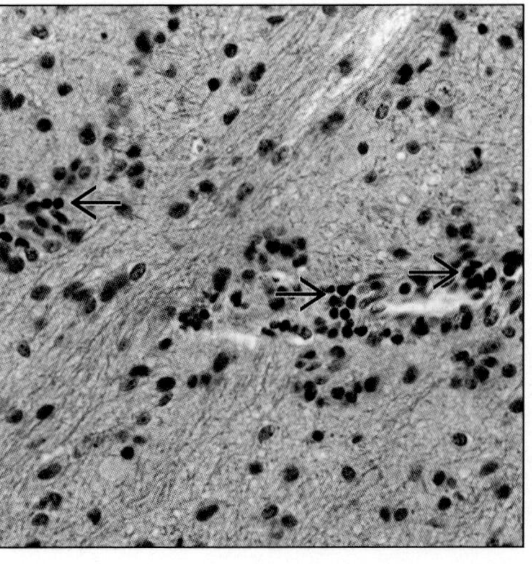

(Left) *H&E shows medium-power view of low-grade diffuse astrocytoma with subpial aggregates of neoplastic cells ⇒. Even though more common in oligodendrogliomas, this "secondary structure" is suggestive of a glioma.* ***(Right)*** *High-power view shows perivascular infiltrates of mature lymphocytes ⇒. These are more often seen in gemistocytic astrocytoma, where they can even develop germinal centers.*

DIFFUSE ASTROCYTOMA (LOW GRADE)

Ancillary Techniques

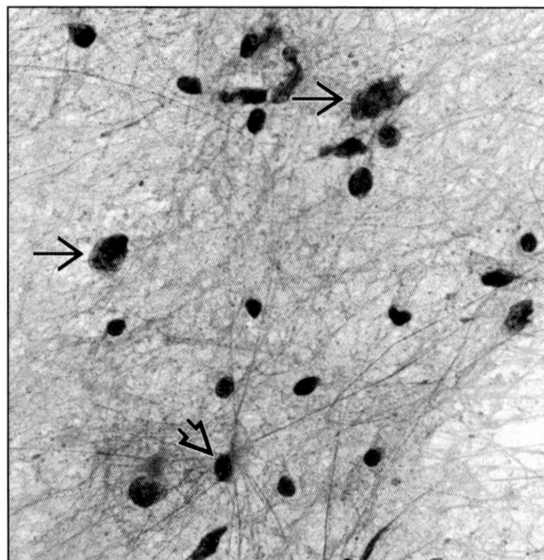

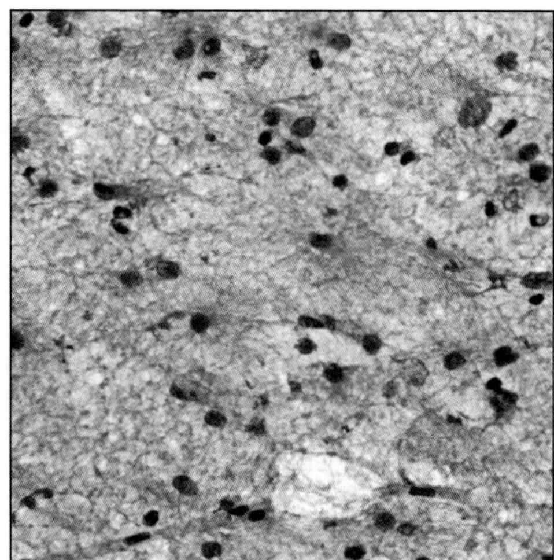

(Left) *High-power view of smear preparation (H&E stain) shows astrocytes with nuclear atypia and pleomorphism ⇨ between finely fibrillar processes, which are generally fewer, shorter, and more asymmetric than normal reactive astrocytes ⇨.* ***(Right)*** *High-power view of frozen section (H&E stain) shows ice crystal artifact that may be misinterpreted as microcysts. The degree of hypercellularity is also hidden. However, the presence of nuclear hyperchromasia and angulation suggests astrocytoma.*

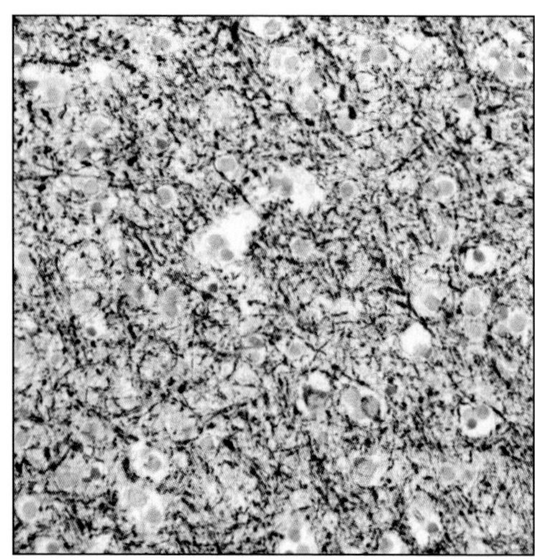

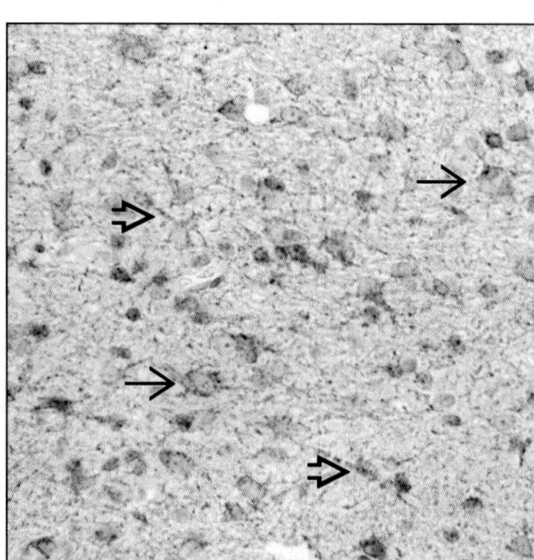

(Left) *High-power view of immunohistochemical stain for neurofilament protein highlights the myelinated axons of normal neurons "trapped" between irregularly distributed neoplastic astrocytes.* ***(Right)*** *High-power view of immunohistochemical stain for GFAP shows prominent positive astrocytic processes ⇨. Staining can also be seen in a perinuclear rim ⇨ distribution around neoplastic cells. Note that GFAP immunostain also accentuates coexisting reactive astrocytes.*

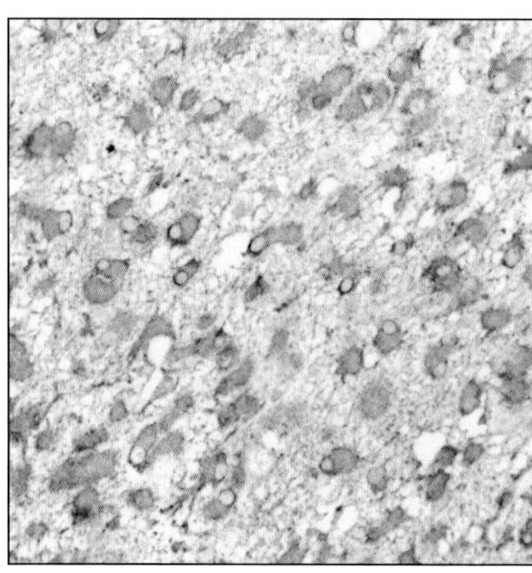

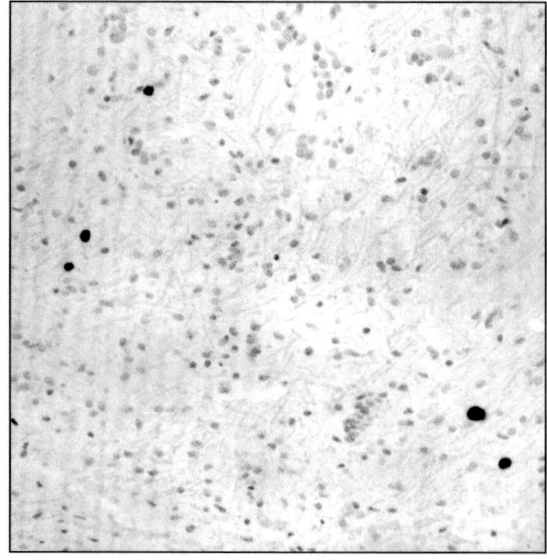

(Left) *High-power view of immunohistochemical stain for GFAP in a gemistocytic astrocytoma demonstrates positive staining of abundant cytoplasm in angular and plump neoplastic cells with eccentric, asymmetric nuclei.* ***(Right)*** *High-power view of immunohistochemical stain for Ki-67 (MIB-1 proliferation index) shows staining in approximately 1-2% of cells, compatible with low-grade astrocytoma. Even though a cutoff in the MIB-1 index is not universally applied, lesions with levels higher than 5% behave more aggressively.*

Differential Diagnosis

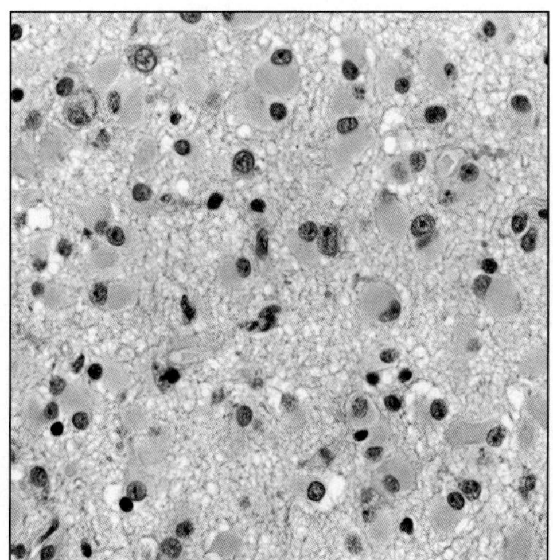

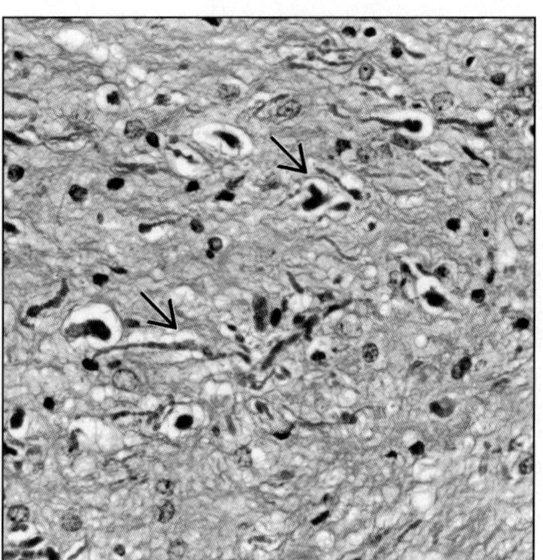

(Left) *H&E shows high-power view of gemistocytic astrocytoma, a variant with prominent gemistocytic astrocytes having abundant "glassy" eosinophilic cytoplasm, eccentrically placed asymmetric nuclei, and small nucleoli.* ***(Right)*** *H&E shows high-power view of piloid gliosis, a reactive chronic process near longstanding lesions (in this case, a craniopharyngioma). Note the paucicellular appearance with densely fibrillar matrix and plenty of Rosenthal fibers ➙.*

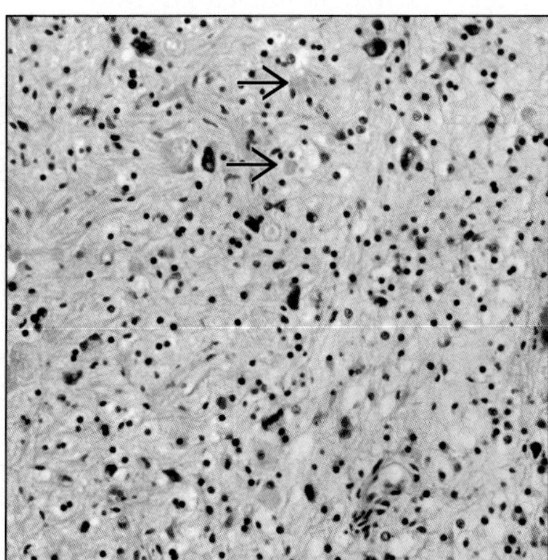

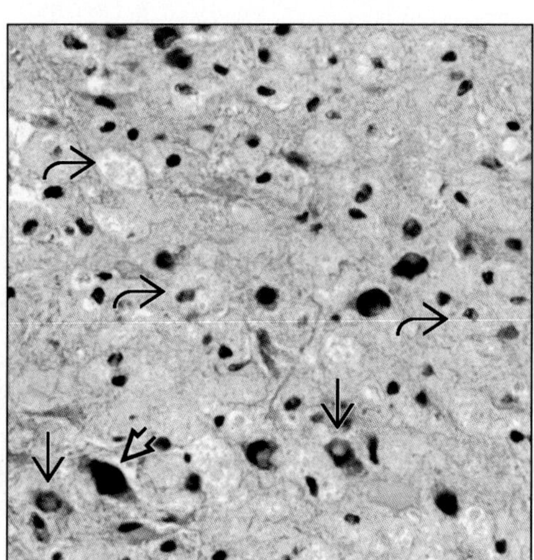

(Left) *H&E shows high-power view of pilocytic astrocytoma with characteristic biphasic histology (loose cystic areas on the right, more densely cellular areas on the left) and eosinophilic granular bodies ➙.* ***(Right)*** *H&E shows high-power view of progressive multifocal leukoencephalopathy with pleomorphic astrocytes ➙ and characteristic oligodendrocytic nuclear inclusions ➙. Note the foamy macrophages ➙ seen in this and other demyelinating diseases.*

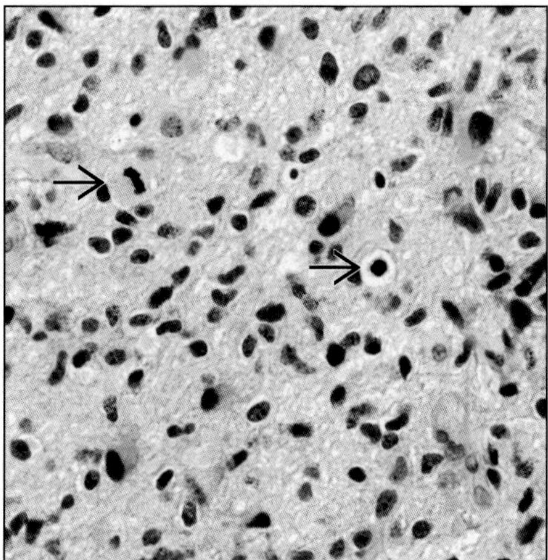

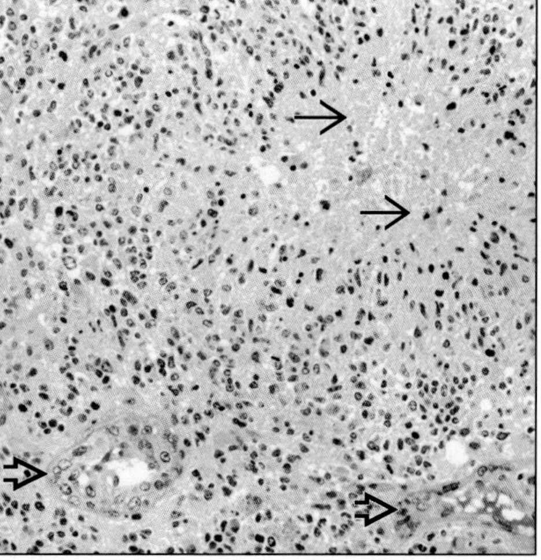

(Left) *H&E shows high-power view of anaplastic astrocytoma. While astrocytoma with a "solitary mitosis" may behave more favorably, the presence of easily identifiable mitoses ➙ (2 in this field) with this degree of accompanying hypercellularity is compatible with a grade III lesion.* ***(Right)*** *H&E shows high-power view of glioblastoma. The presence of tumor necrosis ➙ with peripheral pseudopalisading nuclei &/or microvascular proliferation ➙ is typical of glioblastoma multiforme.*

ANAPLASTIC ASTROCYTOMA

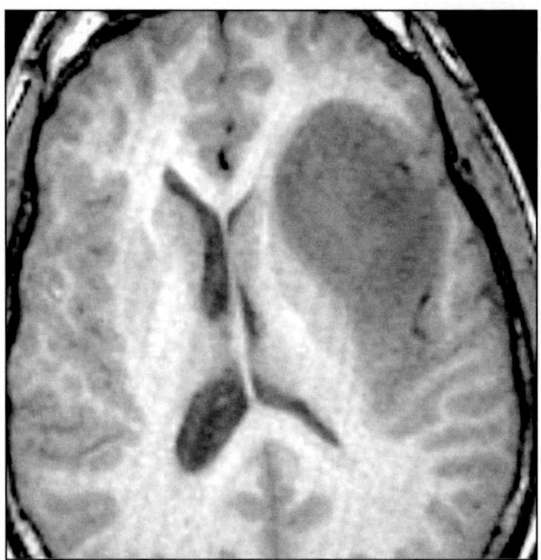

Axial T1WI MR shows an infiltrative, hypointense left temporal lesion with mild mass effect. No enhancement was seen after contrast, which is typical of an anaplastic astrocytoma.

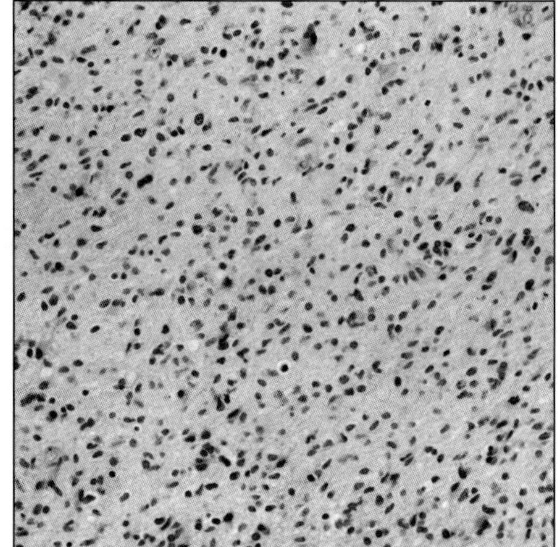

This H&E section shows an anaplastic astrocytoma with increased cellularity and pleomorphism. Note the lack of pseudopalisading necrosis and microvascular proliferation.

TERMINOLOGY

Synonyms

- Malignant (high-grade) astrocytoma (WHO grade III)

Definitions

- Biologically aggressive, diffusely infiltrating high-grade astrocytoma with focal or scattered anaplasia, mitoses

ETIOLOGY/PATHOGENESIS

Evolves From Low-Grade Astrocytoma (75%)

- *TP53* mutation present in > 90% of cases
- Suggests role in neoplastic progression/transformation
- Some lesions may arise de novo, but difficult to prove

CLINICAL ISSUES

Epidemiology

- Age
  - Peak: 4th-5th decades (mean diagnosis: 41 years)
  - Decade later than grade II, decade earlier than IV
- Gender
  - Male predominance (1.8:1)

Site

- Proclivity for cerebral hemispheres (white matter)
- Rarely: Optic nerve/chiasm, cerebellum, spinal cord
- Children: Pons/thalamus additionally involved

Presentation

- Neurologic deficits, seizures, ↑ intracranial pressure

Natural History

- Clinical deterioration/recurrence in low-grade lesion
  - Suggests progression/transformation to grade III/IV
- Transformation to glioblastoma within 2 years

Prognosis

- Survival usually not beyond 2-4 years after therapy
- Favorable prognostic factors (improved survival)
  - Presentation at young age and complete gross resection
  - High preoperative performance (Karnofsky score)
  - Presence of oligodendroglial component and MIB-1 < 5%
- Well-differentiated astrocytoma with solitary mitosis
  - Behaves well, prognosis similar to grade II
- Chromosome 10, EGFR, PTEN abnormalities
  - Portend poorer prognosis, akin to glioblastoma

IMAGE FINDINGS

CT/MR Findings

- Ill-defined, infiltrating mass of low density
- Often has partial/focal/patchy enhancement
  - But not ring/rim enhancement of glioblastoma

MACROSCOPIC FEATURES

General Features

- Often shows cortical/gyral expansion, pallor
  - Large degree of mass effect, but no tissue destruction
- May appear discrete, but border is often infiltrating
- Peritumoral edema, mass shifts, increased pressure
  - Associated with rapid tumor growth

MICROSCOPIC PATHOLOGY

Histologic Features

- ↑ cellular, pleomorphic, hyperchromatic (vs. grade II)
- Broad histologic spectrum, variable appearance
  - Well-differentiated astrocytoma (as in grade II)
    - But with increased mitoses or MIB-1 > 3-4%
  - Atypia (anaplasia), hypercellularity (as in grade IV)
    - But lacking necrosis, microvascular proliferation
- Clusters of gemistocytes or giant cells may be seen

ANAPLASTIC ASTROCYTOMA

Key Facts

Terminology
- Aggressive, diffusely infiltrating high-grade astrocytoma, + focal/scattered anaplasia, mitoses

Clinical Issues
- 4th-5th decades; cerebral hemispheres (white matter)
- Clinical deterioration/recurrence in low-grade lesion
- Survival/transformation to glioblastoma: 2-4 years
- Favorable prognosis: Young, gross resection, single mitosis, MIB-1 < 5%, oligodendroglial component

Image Findings
- Infiltrating, patchy (but no ring) enhancement

Macroscopic Features
- Mass effect, cortical/gyral expansion, pallor

Microscopic Pathology
- ↑ cellularity, pleomorphism, hyperchromasia, mitoses
- Lack pseudopalisading necrosis, vascular proliferation
- GFAP(+), MIB-1 typically 5-10%

Granular Cell Astrocytoma
- Rare infiltrating astrocytoma; between 5th-8th decades
- Radiology: Mass effect, contrast enhancement, edema
- Granular cytoplasm eccentrically displaces nucleus
  - Autophagic lysosomal, PAS(+) vacuoles
- Mitotically active, even necrotic (mostly grade III, IV)
- Poor prognosis: Death in 2 years, despite radiotherapy

Gliomatosis Cerebri
- Infiltrating glioma involving ≥ 2 contiguous sites
  - Often bilateral or spanning corpus callosum
- Extensive T2 and FLAIR hyperintensity
- Little parenchymal destruction, more effacing
- Typically grade III, some are bland (grade II), indolent
- May have elongated rod-like nuclei (microgliomatosis)

ANCILLARY TESTS

Frozen Sections
- Freezing artifact: Nuclear angulation, hyperchromasia
  - Care needed not to overgrade or misdiagnose
- Mitoses may be difficult to find, but aid in diagnosis
- Necrosis, vascular proliferation suggest glioblastoma

Immunohistochemistry
- GFAP and vimentin positive
- MIB-1 index typically 5-10%, almost always > 3%

DIFFERENTIAL DIAGNOSIS

Reactive Gliosis
- Much less cellular, pleomorphic, or mitotically active

Demyelinating Disease
- Macrophage-rich, multinucleated cells

Oligodendroglioma
- Round uniform nuclei, perinuclear clearing (halo)
- More cortical, neuronal satellitosis, subpial aggregates

Pilocytic Astrocytoma
- Discrete contrast-enhancing cyst with mural nodule
- Biphasic; Rosenthal fibers/eosinophilic granular bodies

DIAGNOSTIC CHECKLIST

Pathologic Interpretation Pearls
- Characteristics that suggest glioblastoma (grade IV)
  - Rim/ring enhancement around central necrosis
  - Pseudopalisading necrosis, vascular proliferation
  - Adequate sampling crucial for correct diagnosis
- Sufficient oligodendroglial histologic component
  - Suggests oligoastrocytoma; 1p/19q testing indicated

SELECTED REFERENCES

1. Reddy AT et al: Pediatric high-grade gliomas. Cancer J. 9(2):107-12, 2003

IMAGE GALLERY

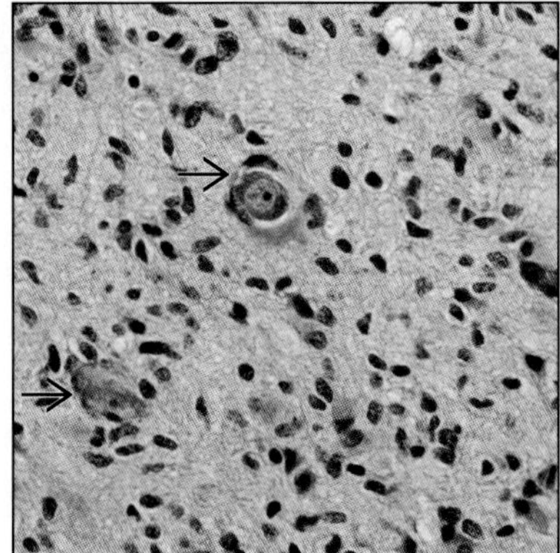

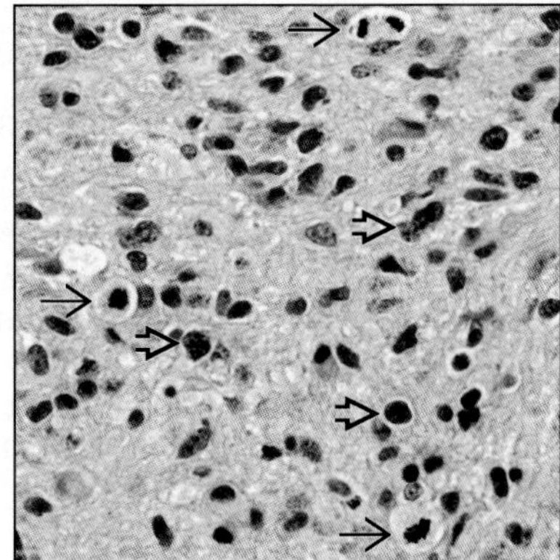

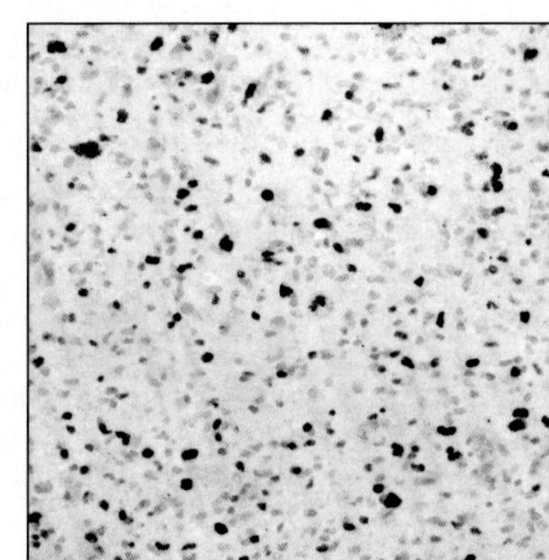

*(**Left**) This high-power view of an anaplastic astrocytoma shows neoplastic astrocytes surrounding cortical neurons ⇒ (perineuronal satellitosis). This is typical of infiltrating astrocytomas. (**Center**) Note the cytologic atypia ⇨ and mitoses ⇒ in this anaplastic astrocytoma. Even if anaplasia was absent, this amount of mitotic activity is not compatible with a low-grade diffuse astrocytoma. (**Right**) Immunohistochemical staining with MIB-1 shows an increased proliferation index (around 15-20%), typical of high-grade astrocytoma.*

GLIOBLASTOMA

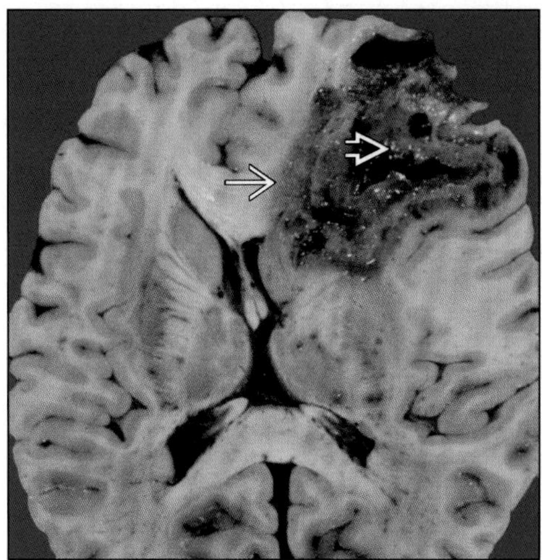

Characteristic heterogeneous gross appearance of GBM: Central necrosis ⇨ surrounded by hemorrhage, edema, and infiltrating tumor →. (Courtesy R. Hewlett, MD.)

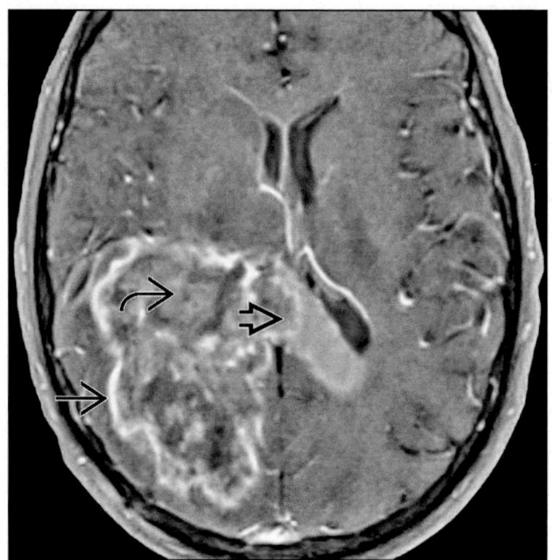

Axial T1 C+ MRI shows peripheral ring enhancement →, central necrosis ↷, and extension across the splenium of the corpus callosum ⇨, all characteristic of GBM.

TERMINOLOGY

Synonyms

- Glioblastoma (spongioblastoma) multiforme (GBM)
- High-grade (malignant) astrocytoma (WHO grade IV)

Definitions

- Highly malignant (WHO grade IV) astrocytic neoplasm mostly of cerebral hemispheres, typically in adults
- Fast-growing, poorly differentiated hypercellular tumor with mitoses, microvascular proliferation, and necrosis

ETIOLOGY/PATHOGENESIS

Secondary GBM (Type I or "Progressive")

- Evolves/progresses from lower grade astrocytoma
  - Diffuse (grade II) or anaplastic (grade III)
    - Mean interval of 4-5 years
  - Temporal/spatial association
    - Lower grade areas coexist, often multiple
  - Oligodendroglioma may also progress to GBM
- Sequential accumulation of genetic alterations
  - Early and frequent *TP53* mutation (> 70%)
  - Rare *EGFR* amplification/overexpression (< 10%)
  - *PDGFR* overexpression; LOH 10, 17p, 19q
- More common in women, younger patients, children

Primary GBM (Type II or "De Novo")

- No evidence of less malignant precursor lesion
  - Shorter clinical history (< 3 months)
  - Densely cellular, homogeneously anaplastic
  - Lower grade lesion possibly overrun/obscured
- Distinctly different genetic mutations
  - *EGFR* amplification or overexpression (> 50%)
  - Less common *P53* mutation (10%)
  - *PTEN* mutation, *CDNK2A* (*p16*) deletion
- Older patients; represents most GBMs (90%)

Pediatric High-Grade Astrocytomas

- Common *TP53* mutation, rare *EGFR* amplification
  - Especially brainstem lesions
- Some evidence of DNA mismatch repair
  - Resulting microsatellite instability (MSI)

Genetic Predisposition/Familial Syndromes

- Turcot syndrome, Maffucci syndrome, NF1
- Multiple enchondromatosis type I (Ollier disease)
- Germline *TP53* mutations (Li-Fraumeni syndrome)

Prior Ionizing Radiation

- Only known environmental risk for high-grade glioma
  - Considered a contributing factor in < 1% of patients
- Site of GBM needs to be within prior irradiation field
- Average latency period: 10-15 years

Rare Unproven Associations

- Meningioma, AIDS, demyelinating diseases

Multifocal Glioblastoma

- Independent, polyclonal lesions proven in 3-5% cases
  - Usually limited to inherited predisposing syndromes
- True multicentricity/multifocality difficult to measure
  - May be from widespread extension (satellite lesions)

CLINICAL ISSUES

Epidemiology

- Incidence
  - 2-3 cases per 100,000 people per year
  - Most common intracranial neoplasm (12-15%)
    - 5-10% of childhood intracranial neoplasms
  - Most common astrocytic tumor (50-70%)
- Age
  - Any age; peak: 45-70 years (70%)
  - ~ 9% in children, rare congenital cases
- Gender
  - Slight male predominance (3:2)

GLIOBLASTOMA

Key Facts

Terminology
- Highly malignant (grade IV) astrocytic neoplasm

Etiology/Pathogenesis
- Secondary GBM: From lower grade astrocytoma
  - In 4-5 years; women, children; *TP53* mutation
- Primary GBM (90%): No evidence of precursor lesion
  - Short history; older patients; *EGFR* amplification

Clinical Issues
- Most common intracranial neoplasm (12-15%)
- Peak: 45-70 years old (70%); ~ 9% in children
- Cerebral hemispheres: Frontal, temporal, parietal
- Abrupt onset, rapid/relentless symptom progression
- Expansile neoplasm; poor prognosis (3-9 months)
- Rapid infiltration of CNS along white matter fibers
- Debulking/palliative surgery, chemoradiation

Image Findings
- Irregular ring enhancement around central necrosis
- Broad, ill-defined peripheral edema/infiltrating tumor

Macroscopic Features
- Poorly demarcated; irregular infiltration of cortex
- Red-brown hemorrhage, central yellow necrosis

Microscopic Pathology
- Poorly differentiated, highly anaplastic astrocytes
  - Nuclear pleomorphism, brisk mitotic activity
- Subpial, subependymal, perineuronal aggregates
- Vascular proliferation, pseudopalisading necrosis
  - 1 or both generally required for diagnosis
- Perivascular lymphocytes, metaplastic areas seen
- Variants: Small cell, giant cell, gliosarcoma
- GFAP(+) cells; MIB-1 index > 10%

Site
- Mostly cerebral hemispheres (subcortical white matter)
  - Frontal, temporal, parietal > occipital lobes
- Brainstem ("malignant brainstem glioma"), thalamus
  - Mostly in children
- May be bilaterally symmetrical or multifocal (20%)
- Rare: Cerebellum, optic nerve, spinal cord, ventricles

Presentation
- Abrupt onset, rapid/relentless symptom progression
- Increased intracranial pressure (life-threatening)
- Epileptic seizures, acute intracranial hemorrhage
- Nonspecific neurologic symptoms, but may be focal
- Mental status/personality changes, headache, nausea
- Pons lesions: Long tract/cranial nerve signs, ataxia

Natural History
- Aggressive, expansile neoplasm with poor prognosis
  - Due to lack of localization, late detection
- Rapid infiltration/invasion/spread within CNS
  - Adjacent cortex, basal ganglia, subependymal
- Along compact white matter (myelinated) fibers
  - Corpus callosum to contralateral hemisphere
    - "Butterfly glioma" (bilateral, symmetric lesion)
  - Fornix, internal capsule, optic radiation, anterior commissure, perivascular (Virchow-Robin) spaces
  - May lead to multifocality at presentation
  - Provide pathway for post-treatment recurrence
- Subarachnoid space/CSF seeding in ~ 10%
  - Especially after long postoperative period
  - More common in brain stem, spinal cord lesions
- Cranial (dural/skull) extension: Less common
- Rare distant systemic spread (hematogenous)
  - Bone, lymph nodes, liver, lung
  - Usually after surgical intervention
- Multifactorial cause of death
  - Local effects, progressive deficits, radionecrosis
  - Pulmonary embolism a common complication

Treatment
- Surgical approaches
  - More successful with better demarcated lesions
  - Often for debulking or supportive/palliative reasons
- Adjuvant therapy
  - Radiation, chemotherapy are standard treatment
    - Fail to improve outcome or prevent recurrence

Prognosis
- Mean postoperative survival time: 3-9 months
  - 5-year survival rates < 20% in most studies
- Reduced survival correlated with
  - *EGFR* amplification/overexpression
  - Loss of chromosome 10; lack of *TP53* mutation
  - MIB-1 index (Ki-67 immunostain) > 7.5%
  - Brainstem, spinal cord location
  - Extent of necrosis
- Favorable prognostic factors
  - Young patient age (< 45 years old)
  - Secondary GBM (vs. primary/de novo)
  - Larger extent (gross total) resection
  - High performance status (Karnofsky scale)
  - Long duration of preoperative symptoms
  - Presence of better differentiated component
  - Giant cell GBM, oligodendroglial component

IMAGE FINDINGS

General Features
- Best diagnostic clue
  - Irregular ring enhancement around central necrosis
- Location
  - Usually solitary but may form satellite lesions
    - Primary lesion: Deep seated; satellites: Superficial

MR Findings
- T1WI: Isointense to hypointense, necrotic, cystic mass
  - Irregular, thick rim of contrast enhancement
    - Corresponds to highly cellular, vascular neoplasm
  - Infiltrating glioma extends beyond enhancing rim
- T2WI/FLAIR: Heterogeneous, hyperintense mass
  - Broad, ill-defined peripheral area of low attenuation
    - Corresponds to edema and infiltrating tumor

GLIOBLASTOMA

CT Findings
- Irregularly shaped, iso-/hypodense, expansile mass
- Peripheral ring-like contrast enhancement
- Dark, hypodense central area of necrosis
- Marked mass effect, surrounding edema

PET
- Malignant tumors: ↑ cellularity, ↑ glucose metabolism
- GBM: ↑ FDG uptake; also correlates with ↓ survival

Imaging Findings for Giant Cell GBM
- Discrete, subcortical solid mass; lacks central necrosis
- Homogeneous enhancement: Resembles metastasis

MACROSCOPIC FEATURES

General Features
- Generally ill defined, poorly demarcated
  - Irregular infiltration of cortex, expansion of gyri
  - Appears better demarcated than WHO grade II/III
- Discrete extension into subarachnoid, meninges
  - Desmoplastic, collagen-rich reaction
  - May resemble extraaxial meningioma or metastasis
- Red-brown areas of recent and remote hemorrhage
  - Usually small, multiple, and diffuse
  - May form large thrombosed hypervascular mass
- Central yellow necrotic areas with myelin breakdown
  - May involve up to 80-90% of tumor mass
  - Liquefactive necrosis can lead to macroscopic cysts

Sections to Be Submitted
- Generously sample tumor, including
  - Nonnecrotic, gray, fleshy, viable areas
    - To achieve diagnostic histology
  - Less dense-appearing peripheral areas
    - To identify precursor glioma, if present
  - Necrotic, hemorrhagic areas
    - To find pseudopalisading, vascular proliferation

Size
- Often very large, occupying much of lobe

Giant Cell GBM and Gliosarcoma
- May be well demarcated, firm, resemble metastasis

MICROSCOPIC PATHOLOGY

Histologic Features
- Variable histologic appearance ("multiforme")
  - Loose aggregates or cellular sheets of neoplastic cells
  - Prominent intersecting bundles or fascicles
- More heterogeneity seen in secondary GBM
  - In terms of size, fibrillarity, process formation
  - Lower grade areas (WHO II, III) may coexist
    - Abrupt or continuous transition to GBM
- Architectural organization of tumor in zones
  - Central regions of coagulative necrosis
    - Corresponds to radiologic dark hypodense area
  - Surrounded by rims of densely cellular tissue
    - Correspond to radiologic contrast enhancement
  - Peripheral tumor cells infiltrating brain parenchyma
    - Correspond to surrounding radiologic edema
- Prominent "secondary structures" (of Scherer)
  - Perivascular/subpial/subependymal aggregates
  - Perineuronal satellitosis
  - Fusiform tumor cells within myelinated pathways
  - Especially in areas of infiltration into cortex
    - Interaction of neoplastic cells with native brain
- Microvascular (endothelial) proliferation
  - Glomeruloid capillary tufts (microvascular)
    - Multilayered, proliferating endothelial cells
    - May also include smooth muscle cells, pericytes
    - Usually along edge of necrotic, ischemic tumor
    - Glioma-secreted angiogenic substances (VEGF)
    - Vascular thrombosis often present
  - 2nd form of vascular hyperplasia
    - Medium-sized vessels (not truly "microvascular")
    - Intraluminal endothelial cell proliferation
    - Less common, poorer prognosis
- Geographic tumor necrosis
  - Small, irregular, band-like, or serpiginous areas
  - Outlined by "pseudopalisading" pattern
    - Radially oriented, small, fusiform tumor cells
  - Central area of necrotic fibrillary network
  - Probably secondary to hypoxia-induced apoptosis
  - Coalesce into larger necrotic areas
    - Necrotic tumor cells, vessels
    - Eventually lack pseudopalisading
    - Often in primary GBM, indicate poorer prognosis
    - Correspond to radiologic nonenhancing areas
    - Ischemic, due to insufficient blood supply
    - Macrophages not prominent
- Perivascular lymphocyte collections
  - Mostly CD8(+) T cells, fewer CD4(+) T cells
  - Some B cells, rare plasma cells
  - Especially in gemistocytic or giant cell areas
  - May be associated with better prognosis
- Infiltration into meninges, dura, vascular adventitia
  - Mesenchymal fibrosis, desmoplasia
  - Reticulin and collagen-rich matrix
- Metaplastic areas common
  - Gland-like ribbons of epithelioid cells
    - "Adenoid glioblastoma"
    - Myxoid or mucinous, microcystic background
  - Squamous epithelial whorls, keratin pearls
  - Cartilaginous/osseous metaplasia

Cytologic Features
- Severe nuclear atypia, pleomorphism, hyperchromasia
- Poorly differentiated, highly anaplastic astrocytic cells
  - Bipolar, fusiform, round, or rhabdoid
  - Small cells to giant "grotesque" forms
  - Multinucleated (up to 20 nuclei) cells common
- Variable amounts of "glassy" eosinophilic cytoplasm
  - Betrays astrocytic nature of neoplasm
  - Gemistocytes with eccentrically displaced nucleus
- Brisk mitotic activity, apoptosis often seen
- Epithelioid cells often present
  - Prominent plump cytoplasm, distinct cell borders
  - Round-oval nuclei with prominent nucleoli
- Granular cells with PAS(+) cytoplasm
- Lipidized cells with foamy cytoplasm

Predominant Pattern/Injury Type
- Neoplastic

GLIOBLASTOMA

- Hypercellular
- Infiltrative
- Necrosis, coagulative

Predominant Cell/Compartment Type

- Nervous, glial

Small Cell Astrocytoma (Small Cell GBM)

- Distinct histologic variant, especially in 1° GBM
  - Monomorphic, undifferentiated cells, bland nuclei
  - Fibrillar/fascicular background, little cytoplasm
- May resemble anaplastic oligodendroglioma, but
  - Has nuclear pleomorphism, prominent mitoses
  - Frequent *EGFR* amplification, *PTEN* deletion
  - Lacks chromosome 1p/19q deletions

Giant Cell GBM

- ~ 5% of GBM; younger age; similar presentation
- ↑ *P53* and *PTEN* mutations, ↓ *EGFR* amplification
- Very large, pleomorphic cells, often multinucleated
  - More angulated, often with prominent nucleoli
  - > 20% multinucleated cells required for diagnosis
- Reticulin/collagen-rich stroma, tends to be firm
- Tend to be better circumscribed, more subcortical
  - May have slightly better prognosis as a result
- Contains scattered lymphocytes, often perivascular

Gliosarcoma

- ~ 2% of GBM; same prognosis/presentation/behavior
- GBM with mesenchymal (sarcomatous) component
  - Clonal cytogenetic abnormalities, *P53* mutations
    - Suggests phenotypic variance of same lesion
    - Not separate, additional neoplasm (i.e., collision)
- Firm, well-circumscribed, often temporal lobe mass
- Hyperdense, homogeneous enhancement
  - Mimics meningioma
- Mesenchymal component resembles fibrosarcoma
  - Fascicles of spindle cells, herringbone pattern
- May be more pleomorphic, undifferentiated
  - Akin to so-called malignant fibrous histiocytoma
- Malignant cartilage, bone, and muscle areas described
- Characteristic, prominent intercellular reticulin matrix
- Occasional spindle cells, desmoplasia in GBM
  - Not sufficient for diagnosis of gliosarcoma
  - Need unequivocally malignant mesenchymal tissue
    - Nuclear atypia, mitotic activity, necrosis
- Rule out malignant meningioma, fibrosarcoma
  - GFAP immunoreactivity in glial areas

ANCILLARY TESTS

Frozen Sections

- Fibrillary background betrays astrocytic nature
- Freezing artifact may underestimate hypercellularity
- Vascular proliferation, mitoses, necrosis: Malignant
- Normal gray matter may appear oligocellular, necrotic
  - Would lack pseudopalisading peripheral nuclei

Immunohistochemistry

- GFAP(+) spindle cells and gemistocytes
  - Establish neoplasm as glial in origin
  - Small undifferentiated cells usually lack staining
  - Reactive, polar astrocytes also positive
- Often vimentin and S100 positive
- MIB-1 labeling index almost always >10%
  - Especially in small cell areas around necrotic foci
- *EGFR* usually amplified, p53 usually positive
- May also be cytokeratin (AE1/AE3), EMA positive
  - Especially in epithelioid/adenoid areas

Molecular Genetics

- *EGFR* amplification/overexpression or *P53* mutation
  - Tend to be mutually exclusive events
- LOH on chromosomes 10, 17p, 19q
- *PTEN* mutations, *p16* deletions, *PDGFR* amplification

Electron Microscopy

- Contains cytoplasmic intermediate filaments
  - Suggestive, but not diagnostic, of glioma
  - Presence depends on degree of differentiation
- Lacks well-formed desmosomes, tonofilaments
- Basement membrane at stromal interface

Smear Preparation

- Evidences hypercellularity, nuclear pleomorphism
- Mitotic activity helps establish malignancy
- Cells may be small, bipolar, with scant cytoplasm
- Fine fibrillar processes exclude lymphoma, carcinoma

DIFFERENTIAL DIAGNOSIS

Evolving Infarct

- Macrophage rich, usually spares large vessels
- Liquefactive rather than coagulative necrosis

Demyelinating Disease ("Tumefactive")

- Macrophages, evenly distributed reactive astrocytes
- Generally lacks geographic necrosis

Radionecrosis

- After radiation therapy for head/neck neoplasms
- Subcortical white matter, with microcalcifications
- Confluent, nonpalisading, coagulative necrosis
- Less cellular/atypical than GBM, but may be gliotic
- Fibrinoid necrosis, hyaline thickening of vessels

Pleomorphic Xanthoastrocytoma

- Solid, enhancing, superficial, cystic mass
- Cellular pleomorphism, nuclear atypia
- Only occasional mitoses, infrequent necrosis
- Contains eosinophilic granular bodies

Pilocytic Astrocytoma

- Discrete mass, enhancing cyst with mural nodule
- May contain glomeruloid vascular tufts
  - Lacks proliferating endothelium in large vessels
- Rosenthal fibers, eosinophilic granular bodies

Anaplastic Oligodendroglioma

- Obvious and unequivocal oligodendroglial features
  - Nuclear uniformity, halos, chicken-wire vasculature
- Exhibits chromosome 1p/19q deletions
- Generally lacks significant pseudopalisading necrosis
  - Unclear whether necrosis should upgrade diagnosis
    - No change in survival observed vs. WHO grade III

GLIOBLASTOMA

Anaplastic Oligoastrocytoma

- Separate, distinct astrocytic and oligodendroglial areas
- Chromosome 1p/19q deletions in approximately 20%
- If necrosis present, designate as grade IV
  - Malignant oligoastrocytoma (WHO grade IV), or
  - Glioblastoma with oligodendroglial component
    - Prognosis is slightly better than regular GBM

Malignant Ependymoma

- Solid, well circumscribed, not infiltrating
- True rosettes, perivascular pseudorosettes

Metastatic Carcinoma

- Discrete, not infiltrating, typically multiple lesions
- Collagenous stroma, lacks glial fibrillarity
- Larger, cohesive, more epithelioid cells
  - Discrete borders, prominent nucleoli
- Nonpalisading necrosis spares perivascular cuffs
- Microvascular proliferation in surrounding tissue only
- AE1/AE3, membranous EMA positive; GFAP(-)

Primary (CNS) or Secondary Lymphoma

- May be infiltrative, but homogeneously enhancing
- Lacks cohesion or reactive astrocytes within tumor
- Perivascular, intravascular lymphoma cells
- Frequent apoptosis, macrophages (histiocytes)
- Large, vesicular, indented nuclei, prominent nucleoli
- Immunoreactive for LCA (CD45), lymphoid markers

DIAGNOSTIC CHECKLIST

Clinically Relevant Pathologic Features

- Age distribution
- Symptom time frame
- Gross appearance
- Tissue distribution
- Cytoplasmic features
- Nuclear features
- Mitotic rate
- Mutually exclusive genetic pathways of pathogenesis
  - Primary GBM (*EGFR*) vs. secondary GBM (*P53*)
    - GBM is common phenotypic endpoint
- Vascular proliferation suggests malignancy
  - Also in anaplastic oligodendroglioma/ependymoma
  - Nonglomeruloid neovascularization seen in infarcts
    - Endothelial hypertrophy rather than hyperplasia
  - Glomeruloid-type microvascular proliferation
    - Also in low-grade gliomas (pilocytic astrocytoma)
    - But lack intraluminal large vessel proliferation
- Radiotherapy effect (tumoral radionecrosis)
  - Often eradicates small, undifferentiated cells
  - Reactive astrocytes with radiation-induced atypia
  - Foci of parenchymal necrosis
    - Patchy, discrete or ill-defined, often calcified
    - Without pseudopalisading nuclei in periphery
  - Thickened, hyalinized vessels with fibrinoid necrosis
- Previously irradiated vs. recurrent GBM
  - Reoperation for debulking, decompression
  - Expanding, contrast-enhancing mass with edema
  - Distinction guides adjuvant chemotherapy
  - Recurrent "active" tumor cells
    - Undifferentiated, small cells with little cytoplasm
    - Spontaneous pseudopalisading tumor necrosis
    - Proliferating, mitotically active, high MIB-1 index
  - Residual persistent or quiescent tumor
    - Generally paucicellular
    - Large pleomorphic cells with abundant cytoplasm
    - Actively proliferating, hypercellular tumor absent

Pathologic Interpretation Pearls

- GBM usually exhibits great histologic heterogeneity
  - May cause diagnostic problems/difficulties
    - Especially with little tissue (needle biopsy)
  - Some lesions are histologically monomorphic
    - WHO has dropped term "multiforme" from GBM
- Evidence required for diagnosis of GBM
  - Infiltrative, hypercellular, pleomorphic astrocytes
  - Mitotic activity, microvascular proliferation, necrosis
    - Peripheral pseudopalisading not always present
  - Absent GFAP staining does not exclude diagnosis
  - Acute inflammation may be prominent
    - Need to differentiate from abscess

Diagnosis on Stereotactic Needle Biopsy

- Small size, fragmentation, sampling: Hinder diagnosis
- Anaplasia, hypercellularity, mitoses suggest high grade
- Presence of coagulative necrosis strongly favors GBM
  - As opposed to infarct (macrophage-rich)
- Sampling of better differentiated astrocytoma area
  - Especially from noncontrast-enhancing area
  - May lead to undergrading in secondary GBM

GRADING

High Grade

- Glioblastoma corresponds to WHO grade IV
  - All variants (gliosarcoma, giant cell GBM)
- Equivalent to St. Anne/Mayo grade 4
  - Diagnosis requires 3 of 4 histologic criteria
    - Atypia, mitoses, necrosis, vascular proliferation
    - Usually all 4 features are present

SELECTED REFERENCES

1. Hargrave D: Paediatric high and low grade glioma: the impact of tumour biology on current and future therapy. Br J Neurosurg. 23(4):351-63, 2009
2. Karremann M et al: Pediatric giant cell glioblastoma: New insights into a rare tumor entity. Neuro Oncol. 11(3):323-9, 2009
3. Brat DJ et al: Surgical neuropathology update: a review of changes introduced by the WHO classification of tumours of the central nervous system, 4th edition. Arch Pathol Lab Med. 132(6):993-1007, 2008
4. Arslantas A et al: Genomic alterations in low-grade, anaplastic astrocytomas and glioblastomas. Pathol Oncol Res. 13(1):39-46, 2007
5. Miller CR et al: Glioblastoma. Arch Pathol Lab Med. 131(3):397-406, 2007
6. Sathornsumetee S et al: Diagnosis and treatment of high-grade astrocytoma. Neurol Clin. 25(4):1111-39, x, 2007
7. Reddy AT et al: Pediatric high-grade gliomas. Cancer J. 9(2):107-12, 2003
8. Cohen KJ et al: Pediatric glial tumors. Curr Treat Options Oncol. 2(6):529-36, 2001

Gross and Microscopic Features

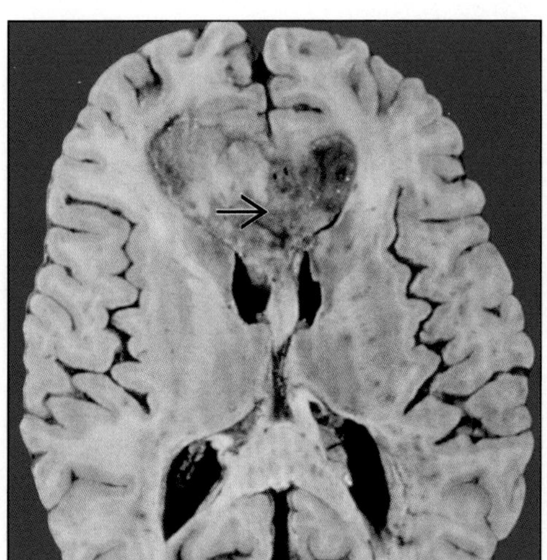

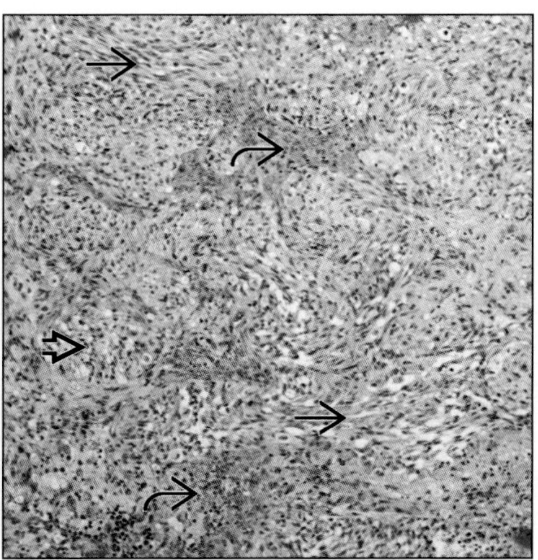

(Left) *Extension of GBM along white matter fibers of the corpus callosum ➔ often leads to a bilateral, symmetric lesion ("butterfly glioma"). (Courtesy R. Hewlett, MD.)* ***(Right)*** *H&E shows medium-power view of the variable histologic features often present in GBM, hence the name ("multiforme"). Intersecting bundles or fascicles of fusiform or spindle cells ➔ alternate with more loose aggregates of epithelioid cells ➔ and are separated by areas of microvascular proliferation ➔.*

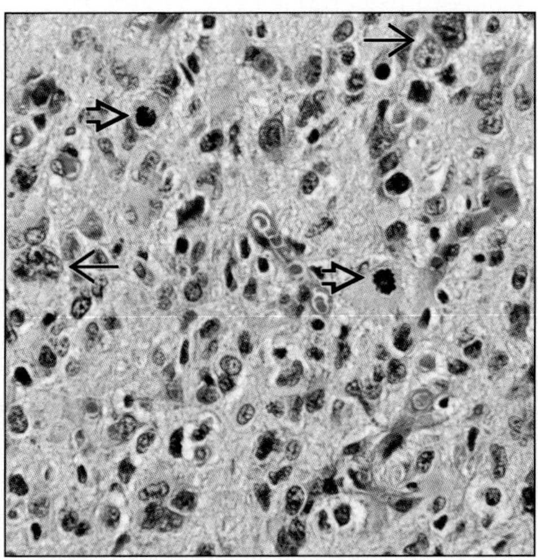

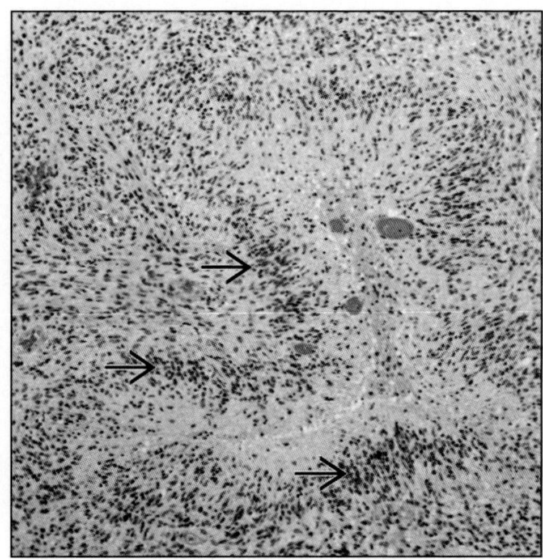

(Left) *High-power view shows hypercellularity, pleomorphic nuclei ➔, and prominent mitoses ➔. The background fibrillarity and "glassy" eosinophilic cytoplasm betray the astrocytic nature of this neoplasm, which, even in the absence of necrosis or vascular proliferation, should prompt consideration of a GBM.* ***(Right)*** *Medium-power view of classic pattern of geographic, serpiginous necrosis in GBM is outlined by radially arranged, "pseudopalisading" tumor cells ➔.*

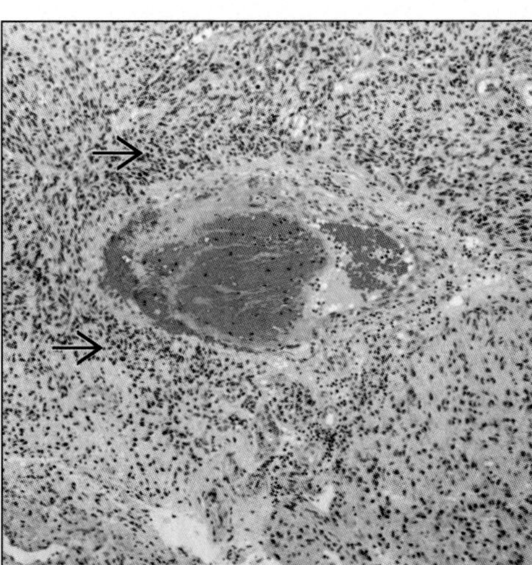

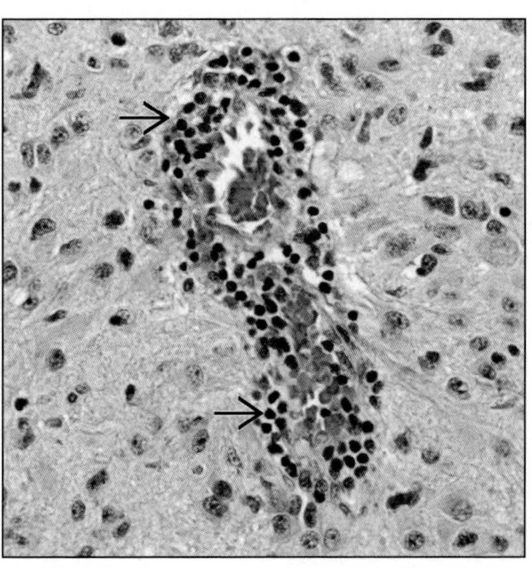

(Left) *Medium-power view shows perivascular aggregates of tumor cells ➔, one of the "secondary" structures (of Scherer) prominent in all astrocytic neoplasms and especially common in GBM.* ***(Right)*** *High-power view shows perivascular collections of lymphocytes ➔ (mostly T cells), which are common in gemistocytic or giant cell areas of GBM and may be associated with a better prognosis.*

GLIOBLASTOMA

Microscopic Features

(Left) H&E shows high-power view of "glomeruloid" tufts ⇒ of multilayered, proliferating endothelial cells signifying (micro)vascular proliferation, one of the cardinal features of GBM seen mostly around necrotic, ischemic tumor areas. ***(Right)*** High-power view shows the 2nd, less common form of vascular proliferation where endothelial cells in medium-size vessels proliferate intraluminally ⇒. This finding is more restricted to higher grade gliomas and signifies a poorer prognosis.

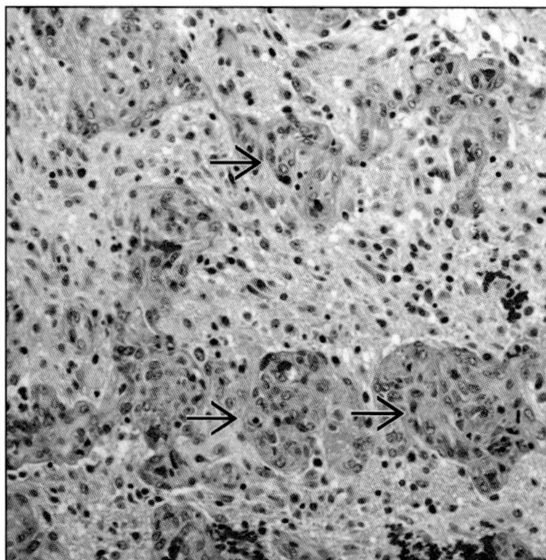

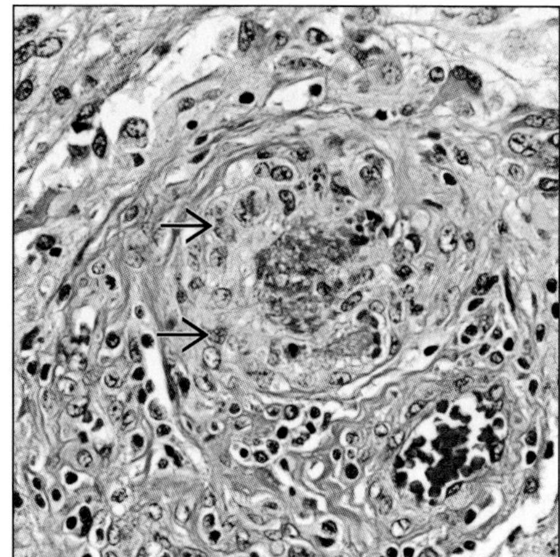

(Left) In this high-power view of an oligodendroglioma-like area in a GBM, cells have more round and uniform nuclei ⇒ and exhibit perinuclear clearing ("halo"). Whether designated as a GBM with oligodendroglial component or a grade IV oligoastrocytoma, evaluation of chromosome 1p/19q deletions is important for further clinical management. ***(Right)*** On high-power view, epithelioid cells ⇒ in a GBM have prominent plump cytoplasm, distinct cell borders, and round-oval nuclei, often with nucleoli.

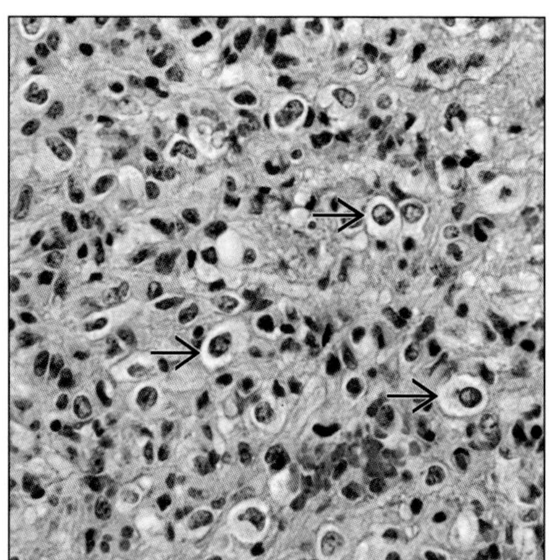

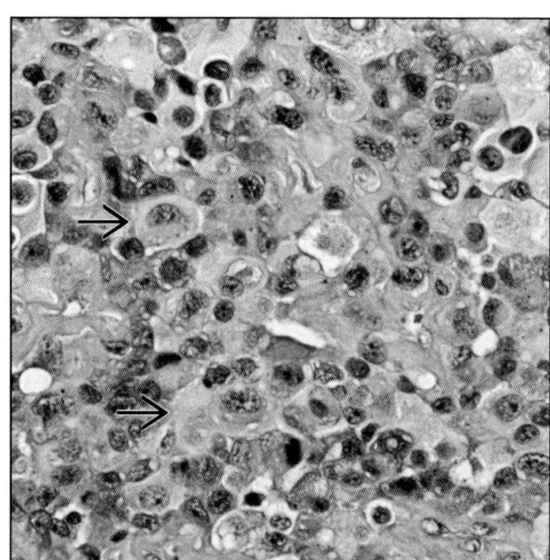

(Left) Medium-power view shows GBM with cell nests amidst a myxoid background, rendering a more mesenchymal appearance. Metaplastic areas such as this (e.g., cartilagenous, squamous metaplasia, etc.) are common in GBM. ***(Right)*** On medium-power view, GBM is seen with giant pleomorphic cells ⇨ and bubbly secretions within many microcysts ⇒ of varying size. The overall appearance of this tumor with hemorrhage and an almost clear cell pattern is reminiscent of renal cell carcinoma, an important differential diagnosis.

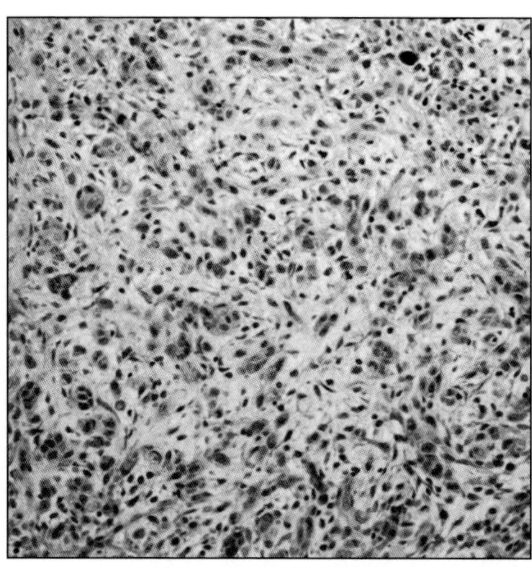

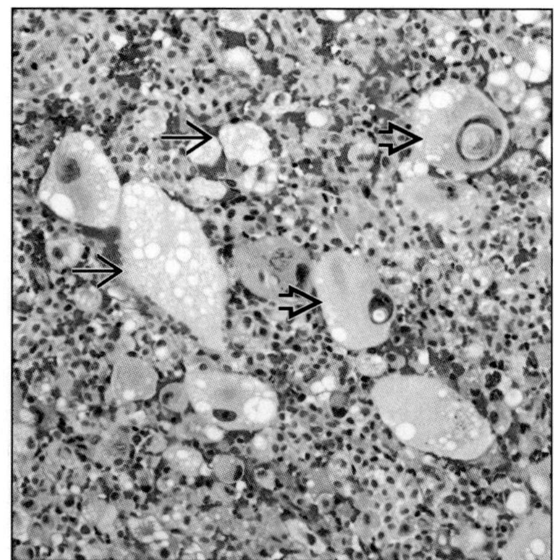

Ancillary Techniques

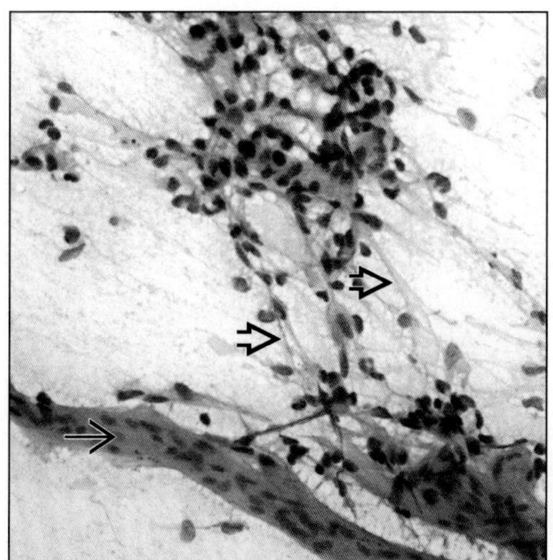

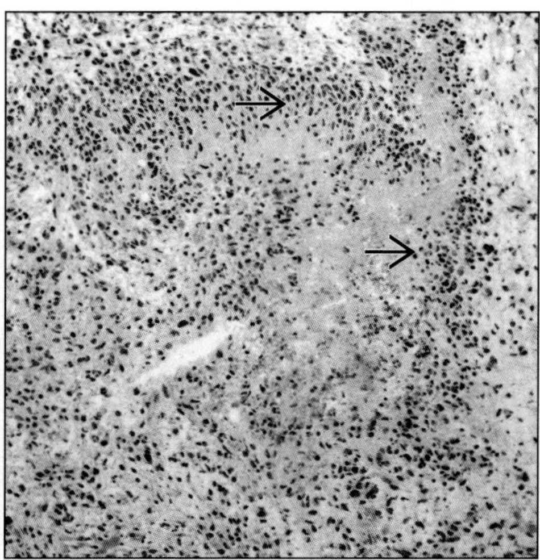

(Left) *High-power view of an H&E stained smear preparation from a GBM provides evidence of background fibrillarity* ⇨ *and helps establish the astrocytic nature of the tumor while excluding a metastasis. The prominent vessels* → *signify vascular proliferation.* ***(Right)*** *Medium-power view shows H&E stained frozen section from a GBM. While freezing artifact may underestimate the cellularity, the presence of pseudopalisading necrosis* → *establishes this lesion as malignant.*

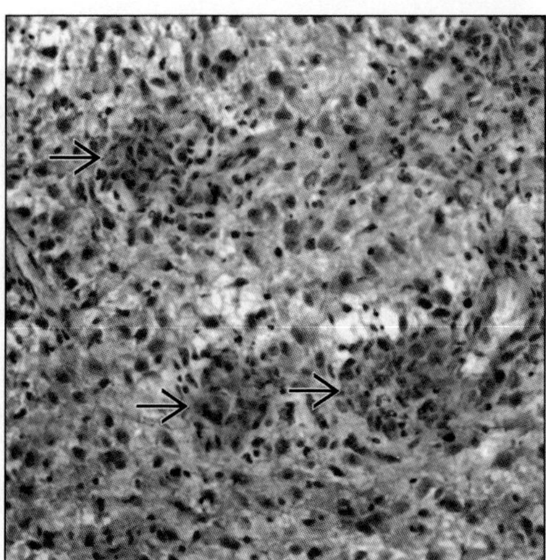

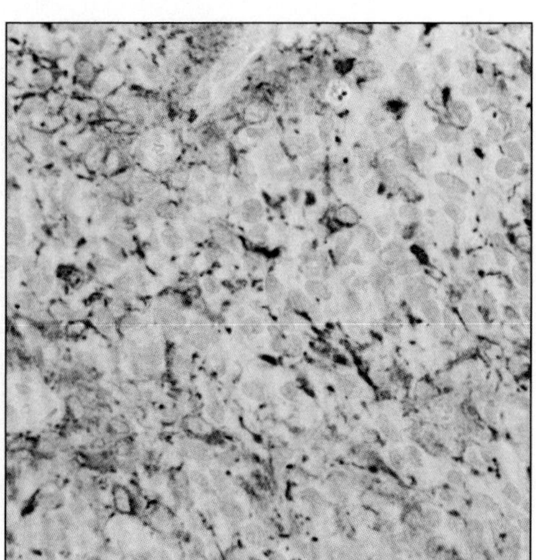

(Left) *In this high-power view of an H&E stained frozen section from a GBM, vascular proliferation is evident as small glomeruloid capillary tufts* → *of proliferating endothelial cells. Harder to recognize than in permanent sections, vascular proliferation is highly suggestive of a high-grade glioma.* ***(Right)*** *High-power view of a GFAP immunohistochemical stain shows diffuse positivity in the cytoplasm and processes of most cells in this GBM, establishing its glial nature.*

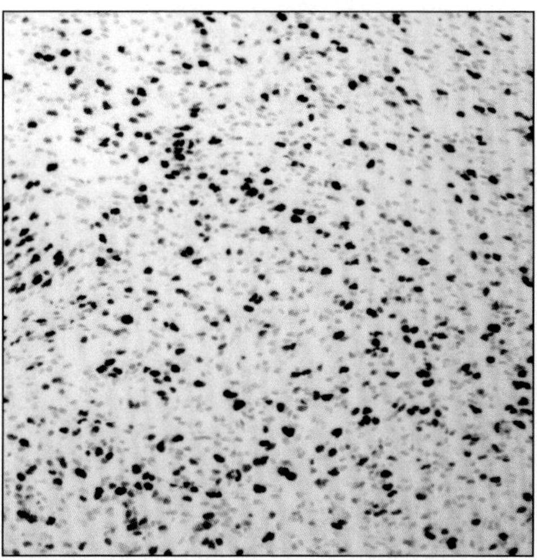

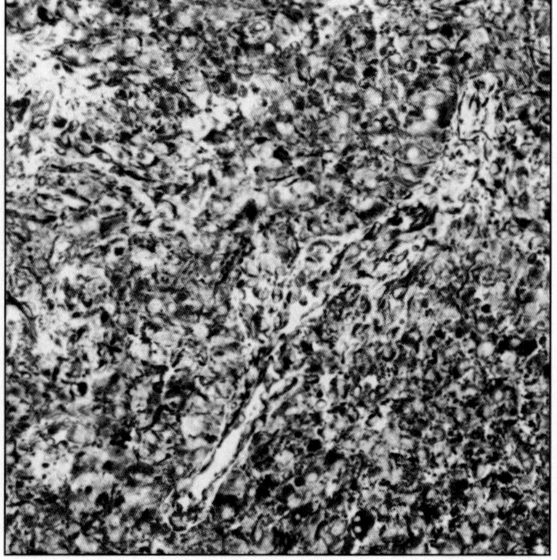

(Left) *Medium-power view of a Ki-67 immunohistochemical stain shows GBM with MIB-1 proliferation index estimated at approximately 30-40%. MIB-1 index is almost always > 10% in GBM.* ***(Right)*** *Medium-power view of a vimentin immunohistochemical stain is almost always strongly and diffusely positive in GBM. This serves as a useful internal control that the lesion is still immunoreactive.*

GLIOBLASTOMA

Variant Microscopic Features

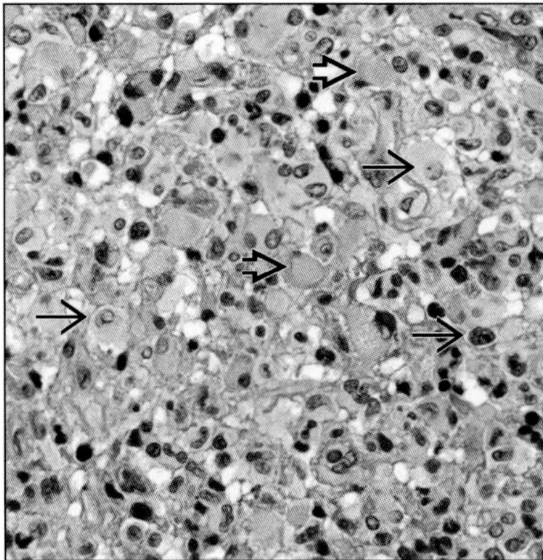

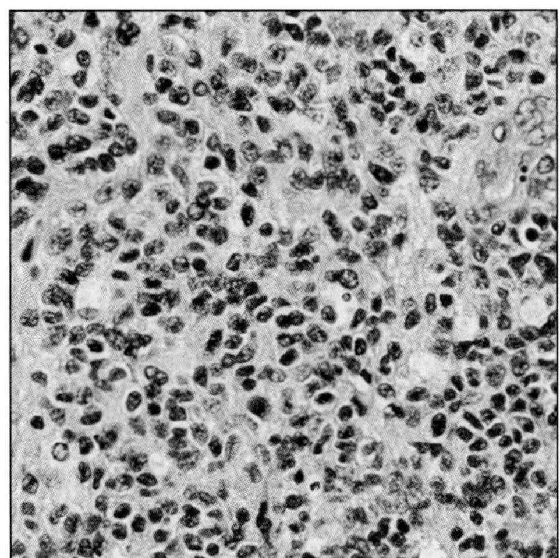

(Left) *H&E shows high-power view of GBM with prominent gemistocytes ⇨ having bright pink eosinophilic cytoplasm and eccentrically displaced nuclei. More epithelioid cells → with plump cytoplasm, round nuclei, and nucleoli are also present.* ***(Right)*** *High-power view shows small cell GBM with monomorphic small cells lacking differentiation and having little cytoplasm and relatively bland nuclei. These lesions may resemble anaplastic oligodendroglioma.*

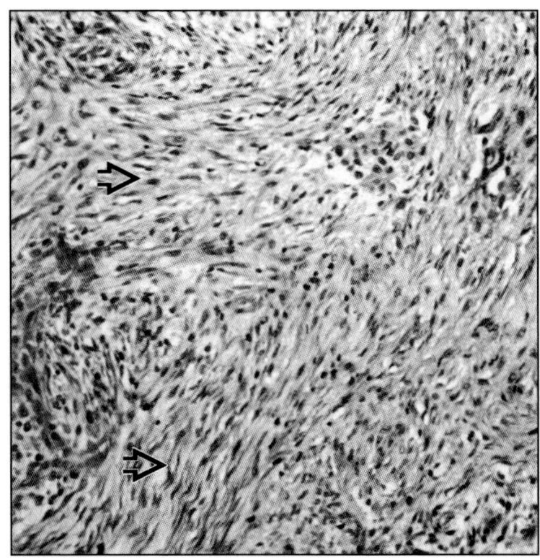

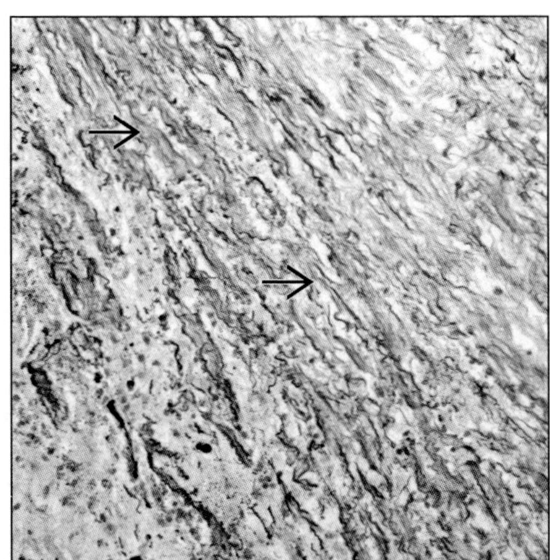

(Left) *Medium-power view shows the mesenchymal component in a gliosarcoma. Often resembling fibrosarcoma, gliosarcoma consists of intersecting fascicles ⇨ of spindle cells in a herringbone pattern. Elsewhere in the lesion, areas of convincing astrocytic differentiation were present.* ***(Right)*** *Reticulin stain shows a medium-power view of gliosarcoma where the intercellular matrix → demonstrates prominent reticulin positivity.*

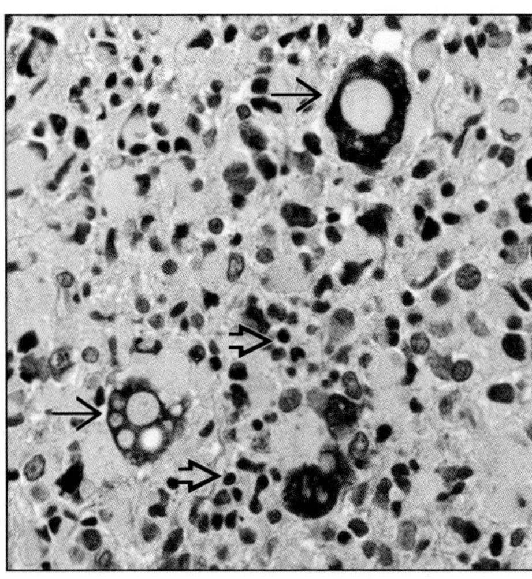

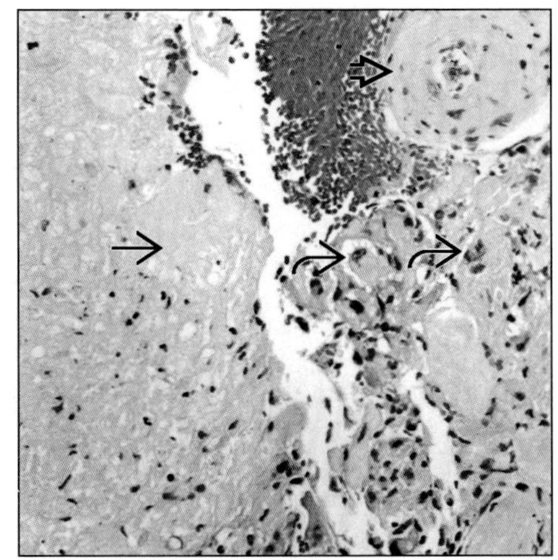

(Left) *High-power view shows GBM with very large, pleomorphic ("grotesque") cells → that are often multinucleated. Lesions with a prominent component of such cells are termed "giant cell GBM" and often contain scattered lymphocytes ⇨.* ***(Right)*** *Medium-power view shows irradiated GBM with areas of nonpalisading, coagulative necrosis → and a residual paucicellular tumor ↷ with cells having abundant cytoplasm. Note the hyalinized vessel ⇨ and absence of a proliferating, recurrent tumor.*

Differential Diagnosis

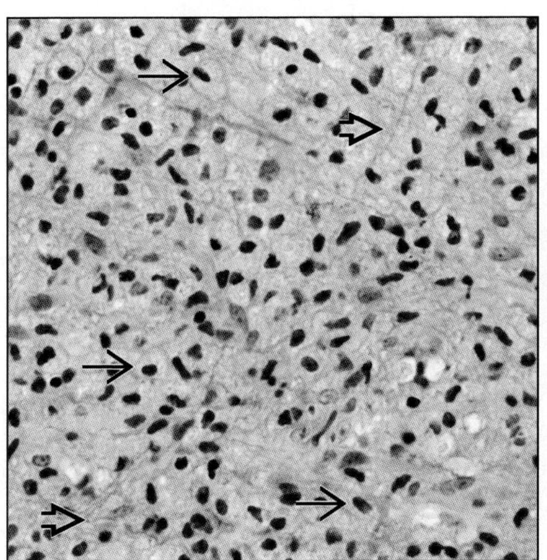

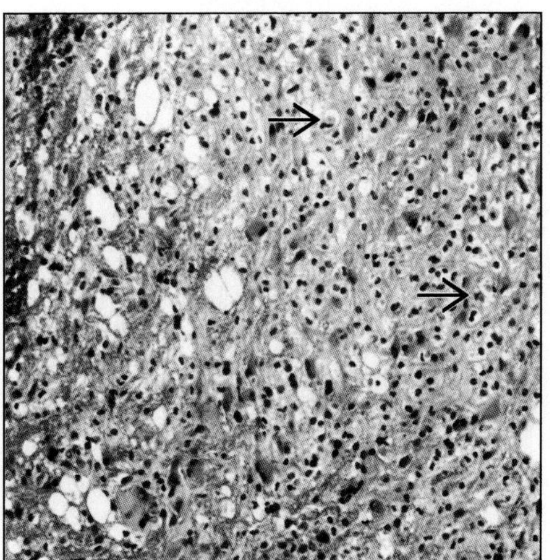

(Left) *H&E shows high-power view of a mass-forming ("tumefactive") demyelinating lesion. Macrophages* → *are diffusely infiltrating between reactive astrocytes whose processes* ⇨ *provide the background fibrillarity.* ***(Right)*** *Luxol fast blue/ H&E shows medium-power view of a demyelinating lesion where clumps of phagocytosed myelin (stained blue) can be seen within the macrophages* → *infiltrating the lesion. Still myelinated areas are present on the left part of the image.*

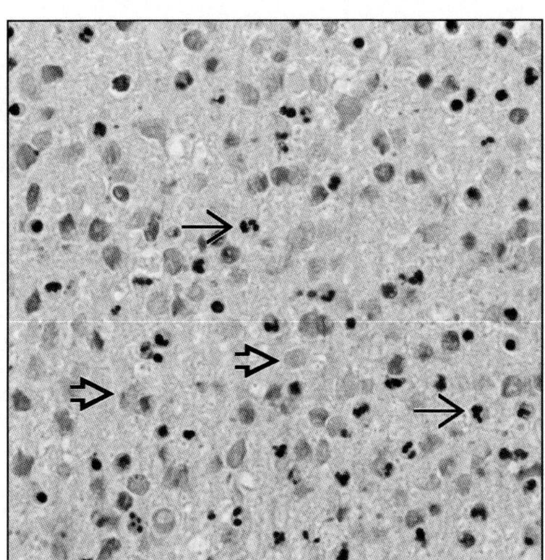

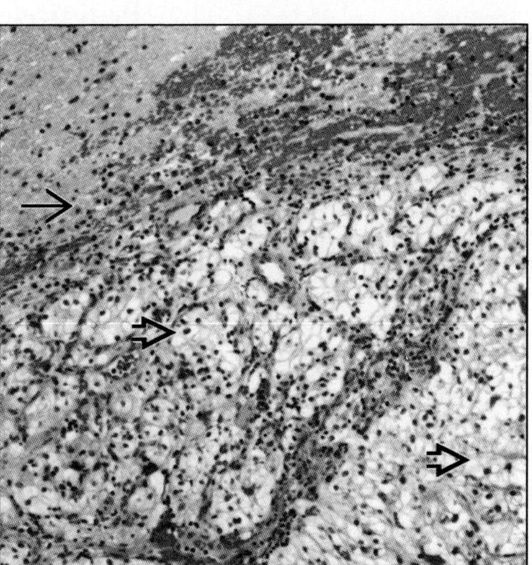

(Left) *H&E shows a high-power view of a relatively new, evolving infarct. Neutrophils* → *are diffusely infiltrating between dying neurons &/or glia* ⇨ *whose nuclei are starting to disappear.* ***(Right)*** *Medium-power view of renal cell carcinoma metastatic to the brain shows the tumor as characteristically composed of clear cells* ⇨*. The lesion is discrete and has a noninfiltrating border with the surrounding brain* →*.*

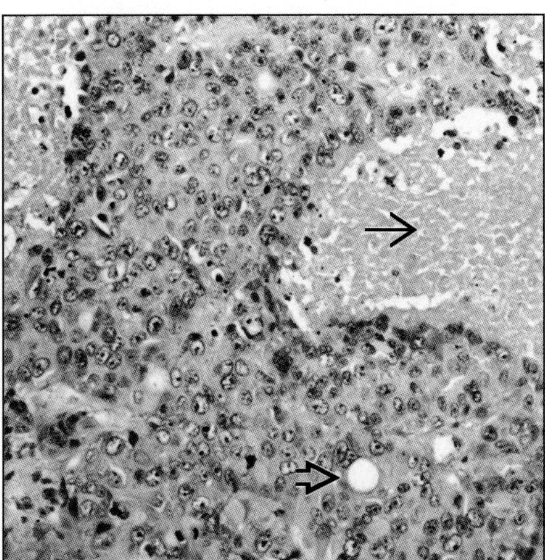

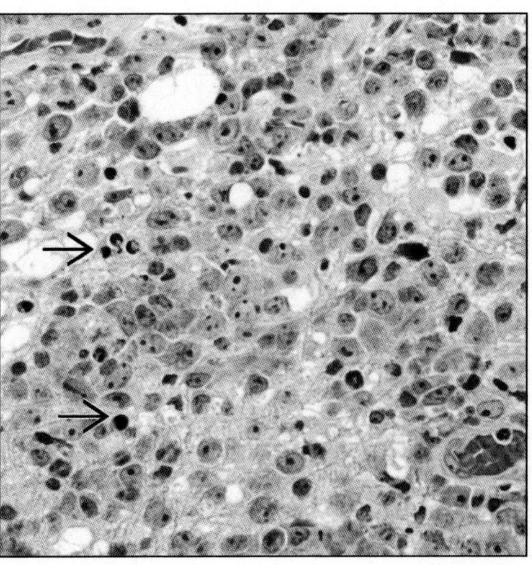

(Left) *High-power view of breast carcinoma metastatic to the brain shows malignant cells that are cohesive and epithelioid and form structures resembling glandular lumens* ⇨*. Necrotic areas* →*, when present, tend to be nonpalisading.* ***(Right)*** *High-power view shows primary CNS lymphoma with sheets of malignant cells that lack cohesion and have large vesicular nuclei and prominent nucleoli. Apoptotic bodies* → *and macrophages are common.*

MEDULLOEPITHELIOMA

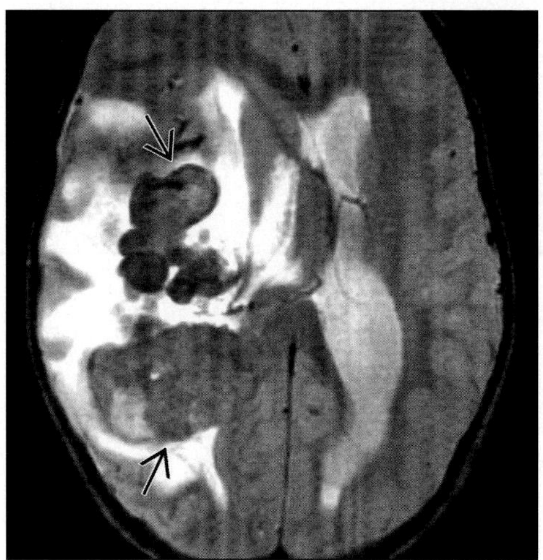

Axial T2WI MR shows a large inhomogeneous hypointense mass ⇒ in periventricular right cerebral hemisphere with marked edema in the white matter and internal capsule.

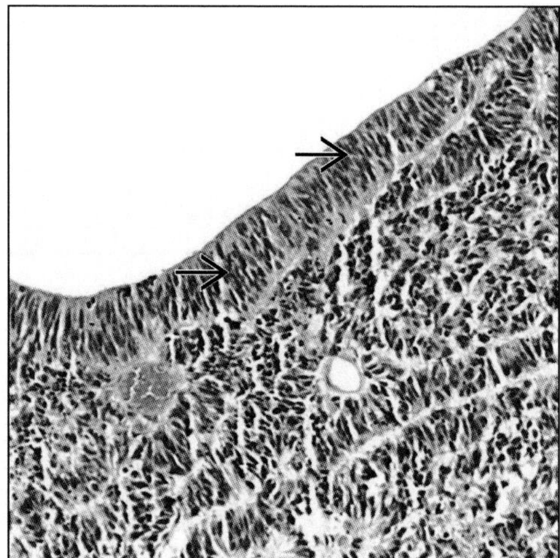

H&E shows a high-power view of medulloepithelioma with glandular structures composed of pseudostratified ⇒, columnar-cuboidal epithelium. (Courtesy P. Burger, MD.)

TERMINOLOGY

Definitions

- Rare, malignant (WHO grade IV), embryonal brain tumor affecting young children, composed of neuroepithelial structures mimicking primitive neural tube

ETIOLOGY/PATHOGENESIS

Histogenesis

- May be derived from primitive subependymal cell
  - Neoplastic transformation in early development vs. abnormal re-expression of early neural tube genes
- Recapitulates medullary epithelium of germinal matrix
- Embryonal tumor: Conceptually related to teratoma

CLINICAL ISSUES

Epidemiology

- Age
  - 6 months to 5 years old (mean age: 29 months)
  - Rare adult and congenital cases described

Site

- Mostly in CNS (supratentorial and infratentorial)
  - Cerebral hemispheres (periventricular location)
  - Also in cerebellum, brainstem, distal spinal cord
- Reported in cauda equina, presacral area, sciatic nerve
- Variant ocular group: Ciliary body, retina, optic nerve
  - Behave well; enucleation is curative

Presentation

- Symptoms related to increased intracranial pressure
  - Headache, nausea, vomiting, lethargy
- Seizure, neuropathy, hemiparesis, tremor

Treatment

- Gross total resection, but local recurrence common
- Optimal approach unknown; chemoradiation used

Prognosis

- Rapid growth, diffuse CSF dissemination
- Death within 1 year of diagnosis (mean: 5-9 months)
  - Occasional long-term survivors reported
- Systemic metastases (beyond neuraxis) rare

IMAGE FINDINGS

MR Findings

- T1-weighted: Hypointense or isotense
- Gadolinium enhancement variable; ↑ with progression

CT Findings

- Circumscribed, heterogeneous, cystic, calcified mass
- Isodense to hypodense with peritumoral edema
- Little or no enhancement with intravenous contrast

MACROSCOPIC FEATURES

General Features

- Large, well-circumscribed, soft, and friable mass
- Areas of cystic change, hemorrhage, and necrosis
- Fibrosis, calcification, and ossification reported

MICROSCOPIC PATHOLOGY

Histologic Features

- Glandular structures (tubular, trabecular, papillary)
  - Pseudostratified columnar to cuboidal epithelium
  - Resembles canal-like structure of neural tube
  - Vimentin, bFGF, IGF-1, and MAP5 positive
  - Nestin positive in basal aspect, EMA on surface
- Inner luminal surface
  - Amorphous, may have small membranous blebs
  - No cilia, microvilli, or blepharoplasts
- External limiting membrane (outer surface)
  - Continuous basement membrane
  - PAS(+), collagen type IV positive

Key Facts

Terminology
- Rare, malignant (WHO grade IV), embryonal brain tumor affecting young children, composed of neuroepithelial structures mimicking primitive neural tube

Clinical Issues
- Cerebral hemispheres (periventricular location)
- Variant ocular group: Behave well after enucleation
- Symptoms related to increased intracranial pressure
- Poor prognosis: Recurrence, CSF dissemination

Macroscopic Features
- Cystic, hemorrhagic, necrotic, calcified, fibrotic

Microscopic Pathology
- Glandular structures (tubular, trabecular, papillary)
  - Amorphous inner luminal surface with blebs
  - External PAS(+) basement membrane
  - Abundant mitotic figures, near luminal surface
- Sheets of immature, cytologically malignant cells
  - Divergent differentiation: Neuroglial, mesenchymal

- Immature, cytologically malignant cells
  - Large nuclei, coarse chromatin, visible nucleoli
  - Abundant mitotic figures, near luminal surface
- Divergent differentiation
  - Distinct patternless sheets of primitive cells
  - Neuronal/neuroblastic: Homer Wright rosettes, ganglion cells, NSE/NF/synaptophysin(+)
  - Astrocytic: Maturity spectrum, GFAP(+)
  - Oligodendroglial: Round nuclei, perinuclear halos
  - Ependymoblastomatous and ependymal rosettes
  - Mesenchymal: Bone, cartilage, fat, striated muscle
- Pigmented medulloepithelioma variant
  - Tubular epithelium with melanin (melanosomes)

ANCILLARY TESTS

Electron Microscopy
- Primitive lateral junctions (zonulae adherentes)

DIFFERENTIAL DIAGNOSIS

Medulloblastoma
- Generally lacks neural tube-like epithelium
- Hyperdense, enhancing on CT
- Responds to treatment

Choroid Plexus Carcinoma
- Papillary architecture
- Lacks neuroectodermal differentiation
- S100, cytokeratin positive

Ependymoblastoma
- Cilia, microvilli by EM
- Generally lacks divergent differentiation

Immature Teratoma
- Contains fetal-appearing tissue from all 3 germ layers
- PLAP, AFP, CEA positive

DIAGNOSTIC CHECKLIST

Clinically Relevant Pathologic Features
- Location, characteristic histomorphology distinguishes from other primitive neuroectodermal tumors (PNETs)

Pathologic Interpretation Pearls
- Characteristic gland-like appearance of epithelium
- Abundant mitotic figures, mostly near luminal surface
- Nestin preferentially stains basal neuroepithelium

SELECTED REFERENCES

1. Moftakhar P et al: Long-term survival in a child with a central nervous system medulloepithelioma. J Neurosurg Pediatr. 2(5):339-45, 2008
2. Donner LR et al: Peripheral medulloepithelioma: an immunohistochemical, ultrastructural, and cytogenetic study of a rare, chemotherapy-sensitive, pediatric tumor. Am J Surg Pathol. 27(7):1008-12, 2003
3. Molloy PT et al: Central nervous system medulloepithelioma: a series of eight cases including two arising in the pons. J Neurosurg. 84(3):430-6, 1996

IMAGE GALLERY

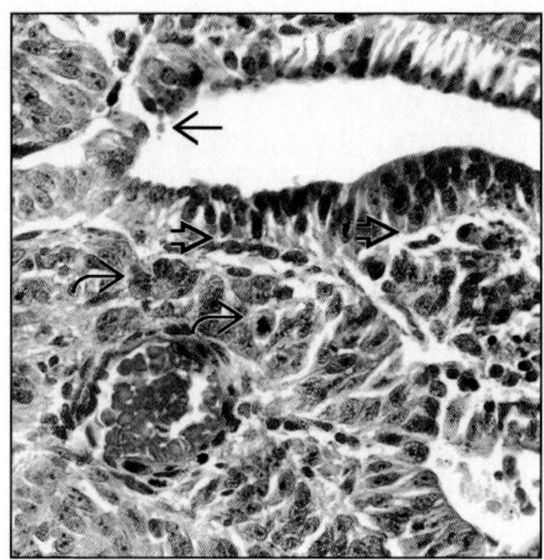

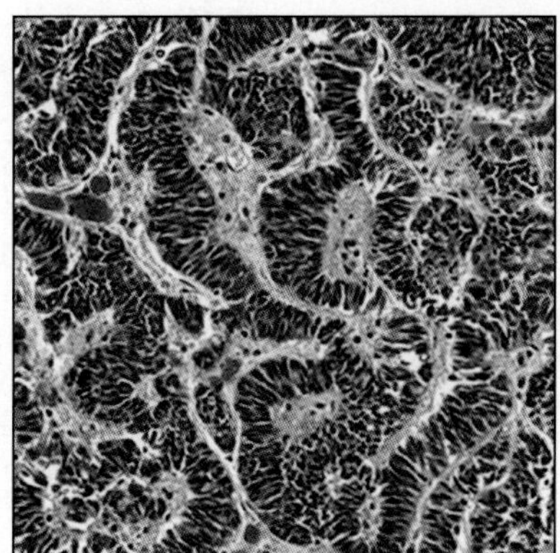

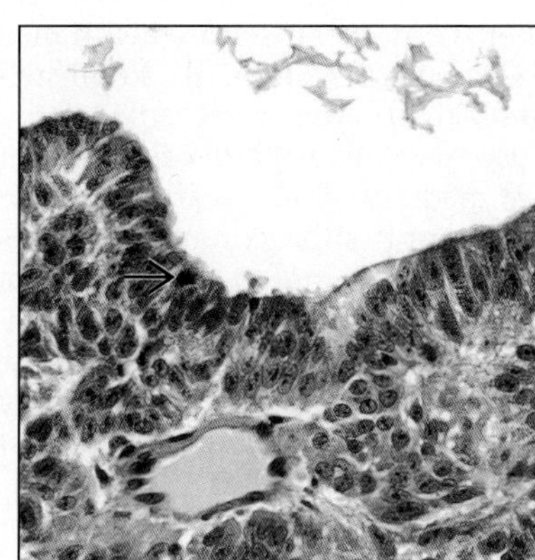

(Left) *H&E shows a high-power view of glandular structures resembling neural tube, having an inner luminal surface with small membranous blebs ➔, an external basement membrane ⮕, & merging with patternless sheets of primitive cells ↗. (Courtesy P. Burger, MD.)* ***(Center)*** *H&E shows a high-power view of tubular/trabecular glandular structures. (Courtesy P. Burger, MD.)* ***(Right)*** *H&E shows a high-power view of malignant cells with large nuclei, coarse chromatin, prominent nucleoli, & mitotic figures ➔ near the luminal surface. (Courtesy P. Burger, MD.)*

MEDULLOBLASTOMA

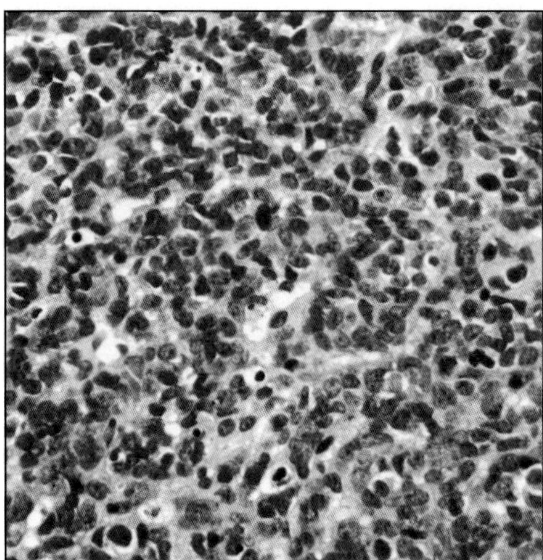

H&E shows a high-power view of medulloblastoma with classic appearance of hypercellular patternless sheets of monotonous, undifferentiated "small round blue cells."

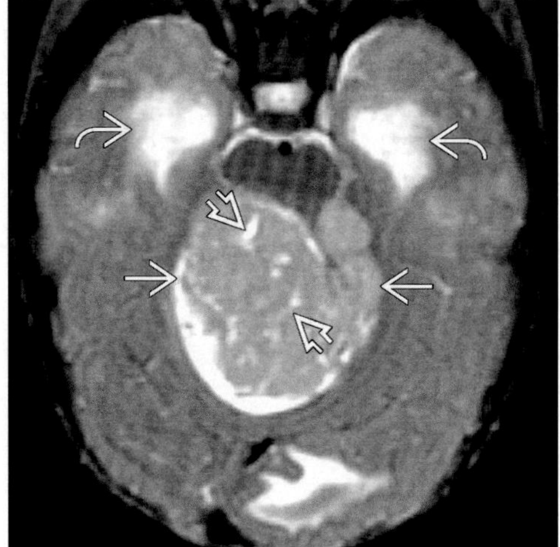

Axial T2-weighted MR shows a large mass filling and expanding the 4th ventricle, causing hydrocephalus. It appears mildly heterogeneous due to small cysts and clefts in the tumor.

TERMINOLOGY

Synonyms

- Cerebellar/posterior fossa primitive neuroectodermal tumor (PNET)

Definitions

- Malignant (WHO grade IV), poorly differentiated, embryonal neuroepithelial tumor of "small blue cells"
- In cerebellum/4th ventricle, mostly of children, with tendency for leptomeningeal and CSF spread

ETIOLOGY/PATHOGENESIS

Infectious Agents

- JC, SV40 (large T antigen) viruses implicated
  - In experimental animal models

Genetics

- 1-2% arise in setting of Gorlin syndrome
  - Autosomal dominant, multiple lesions
  - *PTCH1* mutations (activation of *shh* pathway)
- Some arise in setting of Turcot syndrome (type 2)
  - Colorectal polyposis (adenomas) and carcinoma
  - *APC*, *β-catenin* mutations (*Wnt* signaling pathway)
- Other syndromes associated with medulloblastoma
  - Li-Fraumeni, Coffin-Siris, Rubinstein-Taybi
- Familial cases, yet undefined genetic abnormalities
  - Also have increased risk for leukemia/lymphoma
- Most medulloblastomas arise sporadically
  - Commonly show chromosome 17p LOH (30-50%)
  - Same genetic mutations as syndromic lesions
    - *APC*, *β-catenin*, *PTCH1*, *p53* (each at 5-15% rate)
  - Other abnormalities in signaling pathways described
    - *EGFR/TrkC* (tyrosine receptor kinases)
    - *Notch/CXCR4*, *survivin* (apoptosis)

Histogenesis

- Proliferating (mitotically active) precursor stem cells
  - External granular cell layer of cerebellum
    - Regulated by *shh/PTCH1*, neuronal differentiation
    - Possible origin of nodular/desmoplastic variant
  - Subventricular (subependymal) germinal matrix cells
    - Possible common histogenesis of all PNETs
  - More than 1 cell of origin also possible
- Dysplastic foci: Medullary velum or cerebellar vermis
  - Migration of undifferentiated cells with age
    - May explain more lateral tumor location in adults

CLINICAL ISSUES

Epidemiology

- Incidence
  - 0.5-0.7 per 100,000 children annually
  - 2nd most common pediatric CNS tumor (15-25%)
    - 40% of pediatric cerebellar tumors
  - Most common malignant brain tumor of childhood
- Age
  - Usually in 1st 2 decades of life (mean: 6-8 years)
    - 10-15% occur in infants; 70% occur < 16 years old
  - Some occur in adults (nodular/desmoplastic variant)
  - Rare congenital: Prenatal malignant transformation
- Gender
  - Slight male predominance (1.5-2:1)

Site

- Posterior fossa (cerebellum/4th ventricle) by definition
  - Children: 75% originate in vermis (median)
    - Often project into and obstruct the 4th ventricle
  - Adults: Involve cerebellar hemispheres (lateral)

Presentation

- Brief (< 3 month) symptom duration before diagnosis
- Cerebellar symptoms: Nystagmus, diplopia
  - Midline lesions: Truncal ataxia, unsteady gait
  - Hemispheric lesions: Appendicular ataxia, dysmetria
- Signs and symptoms of increased intracranial pressure
  - Due to 4th ventricle (CSF outflow) obstruction
  - Hydrocephalus, lethargy, irritability, papilledema
  - Headache, AM vomiting, nausea, "sun-setting" sign

MEDULLOBLASTOMA

Key Facts

Terminology
- Malignant embryonal neuroepithelial tumor (PNET)
- Posterior fossa, children, leptomeningeal/CSF spread

Etiology/Pathogenesis
- Some arise in genetic syndromes (Gorlin, Turcot)
- Most arise sporadically (but similar mutations)

Clinical Issues
- 2nd most common pediatric CNS tumor (15-25%)
- Usually in 1st 2 decades of life (mean: 6-8 years)
- Nystagmus, diplopia, ataxia, unsteady gait, dysmetria
- ↑ intracranial pressure (obstruction), hydrocephalus
- Surgery, craniospinal radiation, chemotherapy
- 50-80% have > 5 years disease-free survival
- Poor prognosis: Age < 3, incomplete resection, CSF/ metastases at presentation, histologic anaplasia

Image Findings
- Discrete, homogeneous mass with peritumoral edema
- Infrequent cysts, calcification, hemorrhage (10%)

Microscopic Pathology
- Hypercellular, monotonous, small round blue cells
- Round, hyperchromatic nuclei; scant cytoplasm
- Neuroblastic differentiation: Rosettes, ganglion cells
- Glial differentiation: GFAP(+) fibrillar processes
- Nodular/desmoplastic: 7-15%, pale islands, reticulin
  - Better prognosis, cerebellar hemispheres of adults
- Extensive nodularity: < 2-5%, infants, best prognosis
- Large cell areas in 2-5%, anaplasia in up to 20-25%
- Myogenic &/or melanotic/epithelial differentiation
- Synaptophysin, NFP, NSE positive (fibrillar areas)
- MIB-1 (> 20%), i17q, *c-Myc/N-Myc* amplification

- Referred deficits due to craniospinal dissemination

Natural History
- Extension into leptomeninges, subarachnoid (CSF)
  - Common, up to 30-50% of patients at presentation
  - Brainstem infiltration, "drop mets" to spinal cord
  - Lateral spread along pia, perivascular penetration
    - Particularly in nodular/desmoplastic lesions
- Collin law: Embryonal tumors arise prenatally
  - Assumes steady growth rate of neoplasm
  - Postoperative period of risk for recurrence
    - Time interval from inception to presentation
    - i.e., 9 months + patient's age at diagnosis
  - Considered cured if disease-free beyond this interval
- Relapse seen within 2 years (75%), but often > 10 years
  - Local (cerebellum); neuraxis dissemination occurs
  - Late, systemic (extraneural) metastases (in 5%)
    - Bone, lymph nodes, liver, lung, peritoneum
- Large cell/anaplastic lesions: Aggressive behavior
  - Prone to recurrence and CSF/extraneural spread
- Differentiation to mature neurons rare
  - During local growth or at metastatic sites
  - Usually seen in very nodular lesions
- Patients may succumb to malignant glioma
  - Radiation induced or emergence of glial component

Treatment
- Options, risks, complications
  - Combination of surgery, radiation, chemotherapy
  - Radiation complications (especially in very young)
    - Affects child's physical, intellectual development
    - 2° malignant glioma, schwannoma, meningioma
  - Surgery (postoperative) complications
    - Posterior fossa (cerebellar) mutism (in 5-10%)
- Surgical approaches
  - Tissue diagnosis, tumor reduction, achieve CSF flow
- Adjuvant therapy
  - Highly responsive to radiation/chemotherapy
- Radiation
  - Craniospinal radiotherapy throughout neuraxis
    - Reduces chance of recurrence, CSF spread
  - Avoid radiation in infants (chemotherapy alone)

Prognosis
- Has improved dramatically with combined modalities
- 50-80% have > 5 years disease-free survival
  - 80-90% in average-risk, 25% in high-risk patients
- Unfavorable prognostic factors
  - Clinical/radiologic (any one classifies as high risk)
    - Age < 3 years old
    - Incomplete or partial surgical resection
    - CSF dissemination or metastases at presentation
  - Histologic features of malignancy (anaplasia)
    - Necrosis, increased mitoses, pleomorphism
    - Large cell areas: Large vesicular nuclei, nucleoli
  - Immunohistochemical/cytogenetic features
    - Overexpression of *GFAP, P53, c-Myc, N-Myc*
    - 17p LOH or isochromosome 17q (i17q)
- Favorable prognostic factors
  - Excessive nodularity, neuronal differentiation
  - Older age (> 10 years) and adults
  - Hemispheric location (more amenable to resection)
  - High apoptosis rate may be prognostically favorable
  - Evidence of nuclear β-catenin accumulation

IMAGE FINDINGS

MR Findings
- Iso- or hypointense; heterogeneously enhancing
- Leptomeningeal disease: Nodular enhancement
- Lesions with extensive nodularity: Botryoid

CT Findings
- Hyper- to isodense; moderate, solid enhancement
- Discrete, homogeneous mass with peritumoral edema
- Hemispheric lesions in adults may appear extraaxial
- Infrequent cysts, calcification, hemorrhage (10%)

PET Findings
- Metabolic activity evaluates treatment response

MEDULLOBLASTOMA

MACROSCOPIC FEATURES

General Features

- Relatively discrete, delineated, expansive mass
- Soft, gray-pink, granular; occasionally hemorrhagic
- May have strips of necrosis, but not extensive
- Firmness with subarachnoid invasion (desmoplasia)
  - White, porcelain-like thickening of meninges

MICROSCOPIC PATHOLOGY

Histologic Features

- Various architectural patterns, often in same lesion
- Usually solid/circumscribed, may invade parenchyma
  - Ribbon-like palisading cells within molecular layer
- Common apoptoses, especially in high-grade lesions
- Rare extensive, geographic, pseudopalisading necrosis
- Absent collagen (except in nodular/desmoplastic)
- Rare calcifications (except necrotic/apoptotic areas)
- Rare hemorrhage, microvascular proliferation

Cytologic Features

- Hypercellular with monotonous small, round cells
  - Round, oval, or elongated hyperchromatic nuclei
- Vary considerably in degree of cytologic atypia
  - Small, dark, bland uniform nuclei, scarce mitoses
  - Overtly atypical (anaplastic), mitotically active

"Classic" (Undifferentiated) Medulloblastoma

- Patternless sheets of densely packed small round blue cells with scant cytoplasm
- Neuronal/neuroblastic differentiation in most cases
  - Immunohistochemical (synaptophysin) or by EM
- Significant variation: Cytologic atypia, mitotic activity

Neuroblastic or Neuronal Differentiation

- Most consistent lineage of differentiation in all PNETs
  - Not recognized as variant/subtype by all (e.g., WHO)
- Well-formed Homer Wright rosettes usually present
  - Most common neuroblastic element (in up to 40%)
  - Cells surrounding small, circular, fibrillar zone
    - Delicate, synaptophysin-positive processes
    - Microtubule/neurofilament-containing neurites
- May manifest as large neoplastic mature ganglion cells
  - Lack uniformity of normal cerebellar neurons
  - Nuclear (binucleation), architectural abnormalities
  - Less mature, ganglioid cells: Smaller nuclei, nucleoli
- Irregular fibrillar zones, akin to neoplastic neuropil
  - When perivascular, resemble pseudorosettes
    - But synaptophysin(+), GFAP(-)
- Some lesions have extensive neuronal differentiation
  - Termed "cerebellar ganglioneuroblastoma"

Glial or Glioneuronal Differentiation

- True incidence of this variant difficult to estimate
  - Identification of glial elements difficult on H&E
  - Not recognized as variant/subtype by all (e.g., WHO)
- GFAP(+), coarse gliofibrillary processes
  - In nodule periphery (nodular/desmoplastic lesions)
  - Extranodular small cells with scant cytoplasm
- Exclude reactive astrocytes (in periphery, near vessels)

Nodular/Desmoplastic Medulloblastoma

- Approximately 7-15% of all medulloblastomas
- Tends to occur in cerebellar hemispheres of adults
- More common in patients with Gorlin syndrome
- ↓ cellularity, mitoses than classic medulloblastoma
- Thought to have more favorable prognosis
- Prominent, hypocellular nodules ("pale islands")
  - Cytologically uniform, monotonous, bland cells
  - Neurocytic/neuroblastic differentiation
    - Synaptophysin positive, microtubule processes
    - Ganglioid cells or large neurons are rare
    - May have oligodendroglia-like perinuclear halos
  - Mature cells with more cytoplasm, ↓ mitotic rate
  - Apoptoses may be more prominent in these areas
  - Larger, more ganglioid cells with prominent nucleoli
    - At nodule edge, within fibrillar anuclear areas
- Collagen-rich ("desmoplastic") internodular areas
  - Extranodular tissue is rich in reticulin fibers
    - May occasionally compress nodules into columns
  - ↑ cellularity, cytologic atypia, mitoses, MIB-1 index

Medulloblastoma with Extensive Nodularity

- Also termed "with advanced neuronal differentiation"
- Rare (< 2-5%), mostly in infants, distinct radiology
- May mature to more differentiated ganglion cell tumor
  - Also termed "cerebellar neuroblastoma"
- Almost exclusively nodular, little internodular stroma
- Large areas of finely fibrillar background, focal Ca++
- Streaming small uniform neurocyte-like ganglioid cells
  - Usually mitotically inactive; best prognosis

Large Cell/Anaplastic Medulloblastoma

- Anaplasia in up to 20-25%; Large cell areas in 2-5%
- Markedly atypical and pleomorphic ("anaplastic") cells
  - ↑ mitoses, necrosis, very high proliferation index
  - Nuclear irregularity, hyperchromasia, molding
  - Many apoptoses, often confluent
    - Debris engulfed by tumor cells wrapping around it
- Sheets and lobules of large round cells
  - More abundant cytoplasm, prominent nucleoli
  - Often arise in background of histologic anaplasia
  - Probably represent tumor progression

Medullomyoblastoma

- Mostly in males; almost exclusively < 7 years old
- At least focal myogenic differentiation
  - Globular eosinophilic cytoplasm (rhabdomyoblastic)
  - Occasionally visible cross striations (strap cells)
  - Positive for myogenin, desmin, muscle-specific actin
  - EM: Primitive sarcomeres, Z bands
- Considered a histologic variant of medulloblastoma
  - Similar genetic changes and clinical behavior
  - More broadly: PNET with myogenic differentiation

Melanotic Medulloblastoma

- Few reported cases; shows aggressive behavior
- At least focal pigmented epithelial differentiation
  - Small tubulopapillary formations
    - Finely granular cytoplasmic melanin pigment
  - Cytokeratin, S100, HMB-45 positive
  - EM: Melanosomes, premelanosomes
- Distinct entity from intracranial melanotic neuroectodermal tumor of infancy ("progonoma")

Large Cell Melanotic Medullomyoblastoma

- Large cell/anaplastic medulloblastoma with areas of additional myogenic and melanotic differentiation
- Presence of isochromosome 17q, *c-Myc* amplification
  - Supports histologic variant of medulloblastoma
  - Not a variant of teratoma or progonoma

ANCILLARY TESTS

Immunohistochemistry

- Synaptophysin(+), especially in fibrillar areas
  - Homer Wright rosettes, pseudorosettes, pale islands
- Neurofilament, microtubule associated protein (MAP)
  - In areas neuronal differentiation, large ganglion cells
- NSE, vimentin, nestin immunoreactivity
- Retinal S antigen, rhodopsin immunoreactivity
  - In areas of photoreceptor differentiation (up to 50%)
- Significance of GFAP immunoreactivity controversial
  - Reactive astrocytes: Perivascular, evenly spaced
  - Glial differentiation in medulloblastoma
    - Focal: In fibrillar areas, stellate cells in pale islands
    - Small atypical extranodular cells (scant cytoplasm)
- MIB-1 proliferation index (Ki-67 immunostain)
  - Often > 20%, as high as 50%; less in pale islands

Cytogenetics

- Duplication/translocation resulting in i(17q)
  - Most common abnormality (in 30-50%)
- Amplification of *c-Myc* (chr. 2p), *N-Myc* (chr. 8q)
  - 20-40% of tumors, especially large cell/anaplastic

Electron Microscopy

- Evidence of neuroblastic differentiation
  - Processes containing aligned microtubules
  - Neurosecretory granules, clear vesicles, synapses
- Glial differentiation: Intermediate filament processes

Smear Preparation

- Hyperchromatic, pleomorphic nuclei; varying atypia
- Homer Wright rosettes; cell wrapping/engulfment

DIFFERENTIAL DIAGNOSIS

Normal Internal Granular Cell Layer

- Densely packed, little cytoplasm, but small cells
- No atypia, pleomorphism, or proliferative activity

Ependymoma

- More fibrillar, less cellular, more likely calcified
- More and better developed perivascular pseudorosettes
- GFAP(+); synaptophysin(-)

High-Grade Infiltrating Astrocytoma

- More fibrillar, pleomorphic; diffusely invasive
- GFAP(+); synaptophysin(-)

Pilocytic Astrocytoma

- Less cellular, more cystic (biphasic); GFAP(+)

Metastatic Small Cell Carcinoma

- Rare in children
- CK, EMA positive; synaptophysin, GFAP negative

Atypical Teratoid/Rhabdoid Tumor

- Children < 2 years; large areas of hemorrhage, necrosis
- Large cells with eccentric cytoplasmic filaments
- *INI1* (chr. 22q) deleted; synaptophysin negative

Cerebellar Liponeurocytoma

- Also termed lipomatous (lipidized) medulloblastoma
- Low-grade neuronal tumor; mostly in adults
- Foci of lipidized (foamy) cells in neurocytoma

DIAGNOSTIC CHECKLIST

Clinically Relevant Pathologic Features

- Chang staging system
  - Extent of local growth/tumor size (T): T1-T4
    - 3 cm size cutoff
    - Invasion into ventricles, canal, adjacent structures
  - Extent of metastatic tumor spread (M): M0-M4
    - Cytologic, gross, or radiologic CSF involvement
    - Neuraxis seeding, extraneural metastatic spread
- Terminology: PNET vs. medulloblastoma
  - Some authors consider all such tumors PNETs
    - Subdivide by location: Peripheral, supratentorial
    - Medulloblastoma = "cerebellar PNET"
  - Others argue that medulloblastoma is distinct
    - Biologically, clinically, histopathologically

SELECTED REFERENCES

1. Dhall G: Medulloblastoma. J Child Neurol. 24(11):1418-30, 2009
2. Entz-Werle N et al: Medulloblastoma: what is the role of molecular genetics? Expert Rev Anticancer Ther. 8(7):1169-81, 2008
3. Gilbertson RJ et al: The origins of medulloblastoma subtypes. Annu Rev Pathol. 3:341-65, 2008
4. Gulino A et al: Pathological and molecular heterogeneity of medulloblastoma. Curr Opin Oncol. 20(6):668-75, 2008
5. Polydorides AD et al: Large cell medulloblastoma with myogenic and melanotic differentiation: a case report with molecular analysis. J Neurooncol. 88(2):193-7, 2008
6. Rossi A et al: Medulloblastoma: from molecular pathology to therapy. Clin Cancer Res. 14(4):971-6, 2008
7. Crawford JR et al: Medulloblastoma in childhood: new biological advances. Lancet Neurol. 6(12):1073-85, 2007
8. Polkinghorn WR et al: Medulloblastoma: tumorigenesis, current clinical paradigm, and efforts to improve risk stratification. Nat Clin Pract Oncol. 4(5):295-304, 2007
9. Ellison D: Classifying the medulloblastoma: insights from morphology and molecular genetics. Neuropathol Appl Neurobiol. 28(4):257-82, 2002
10. Weil MD: Primitive neuroectodermal tumors/ medulloblastoma. Curr Neurol Neurosci Rep. 2(3):205-9, 2002
11. Packer RJ et al: Medulloblastoma: clinical and biologic aspects. Neuro Oncol. 1(3):232-50, 1999
12. Reddy AT et al: Medulloblastoma. Curr Opin Neurol. 12(6):681-5, 1999
13. Giordana MT et al: Prognostic factors in medulloblastoma. Childs Nerv Syst. 14(6):256-62, 1998
14. Tomlinson FH et al: Medulloblastoma: I. Clinical, diagnostic, and therapeutic overview. J Child Neurol. 7(2):142-55, 1992
15. Tomlinson FH et al: Medulloblastoma: II. A pathobiologic overview. J Child Neurol. 7(3):240-52, 1992

MEDULLOBLASTOMA

Microscopic Features

(Left) H&E shows a high-power view of classic (undifferentiated) subtype of medulloblastoma with densely packed small round blue cells having little cytoplasm. While there is some degree of variation in nuclear size, there is not enough atypia or pleomorphism for this lesion to be considered anaplastic. ***(Right)*** H&E shows high-power view of neuroblastic differentiation in medulloblastoma, seen as Homer Wright rosettes ⇒ with tumor cells radially arranged around small fibrillar areas.

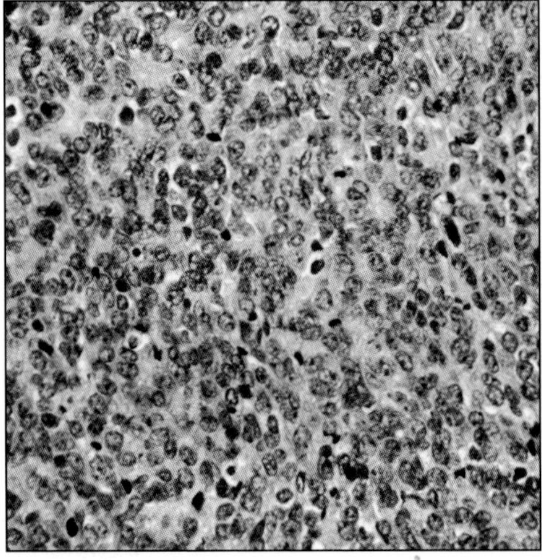

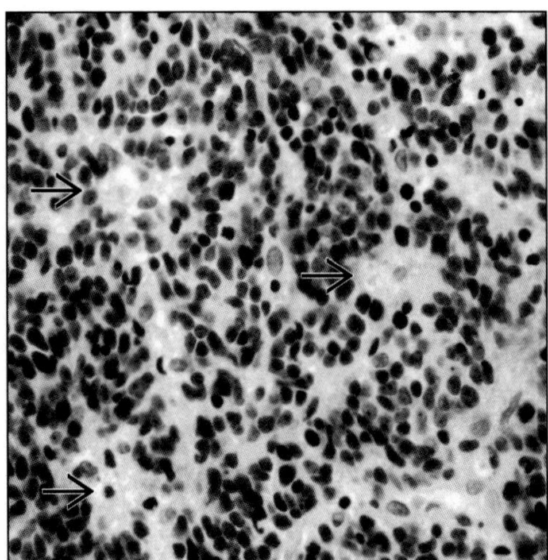

(Left) H&E shows high-power view of medulloblastoma with prominent nuclear molding ⇒ and cell wrapping ➲, often around engulfed apoptotic debris. These features are commonly seen in areas of anaplasia, witnessed here by large irregular nuclei with increased atypia and pleomorphism. ***(Right)*** H&E section shows high-power view of classic medulloblastoma with increased mitoses ⇒, the rate of which can vary significantly. However, in this case, most nuclei are small, uniform, and not very hyperchromatic.

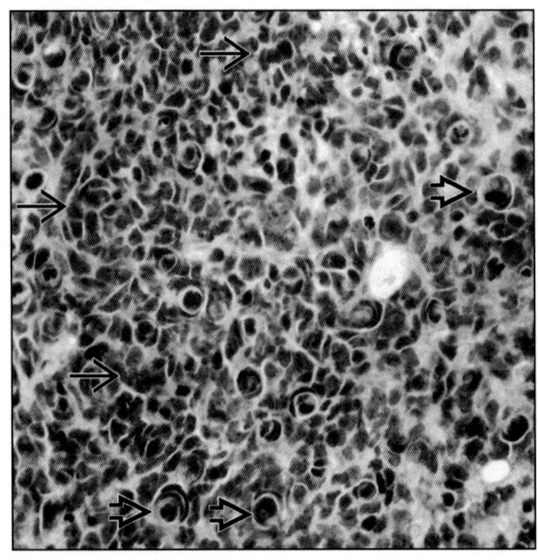

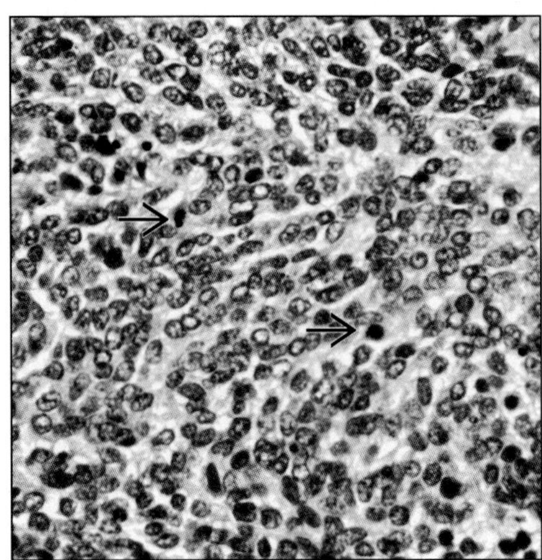

(Left) H&E shows a medium-power view of medulloblastoma with areas of necrosis ⇒. This is often focal and usually does not show the pseudopalisading, "geographic" quality of the type of necrosis commonly associated with high-grade gliomas. ***(Right)*** H&E shows a medium-power view of medulloblastoma with cystic areas ⇒, which are not very common, but contribute to the heterogeneous radiologic appearance of the tumor.

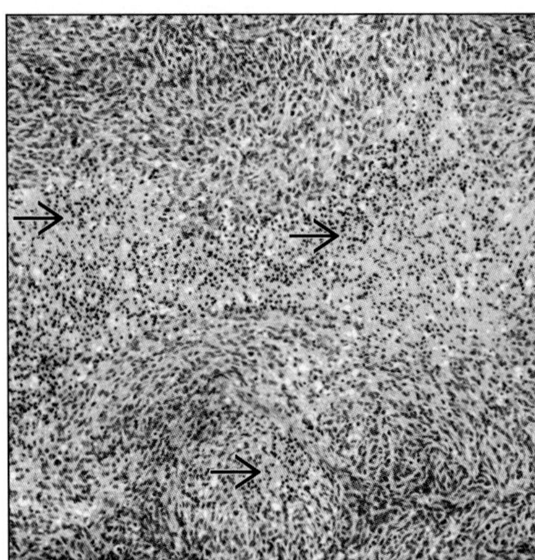

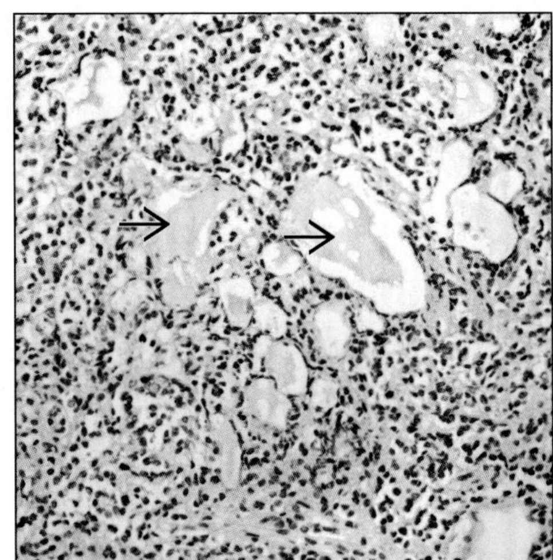

Nodular/Desmoplastic Medulloblastoma

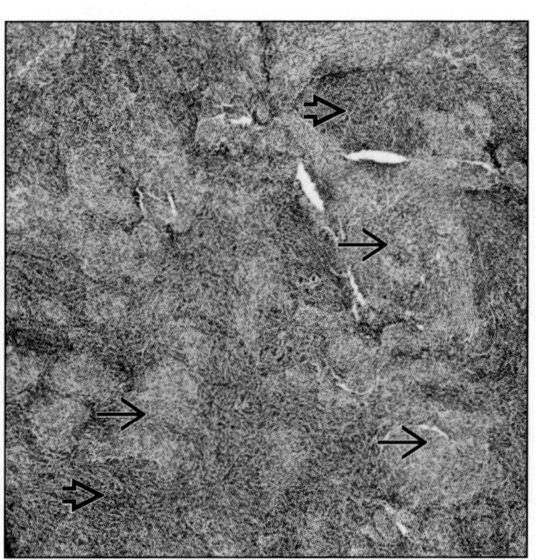

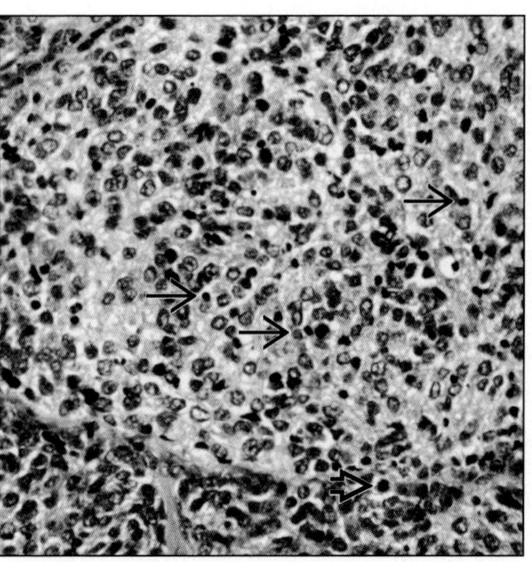

(Left) *H&E shows a low-power view of nodular/desmoplastic medulloblastoma with hypocellular nodules ⇒ juxtaposed against an internodular background of increased cellularity ⇨, giving the appearance of "pale islands."* ***(Right)*** *H&E shows a high-power view of nodular/desmoplastic medulloblastoma where apoptoses ⇒ are more prominent within nodules, but mitoses ⇨ and occasionally cytologic atypia are more evident in extranodular areas.*

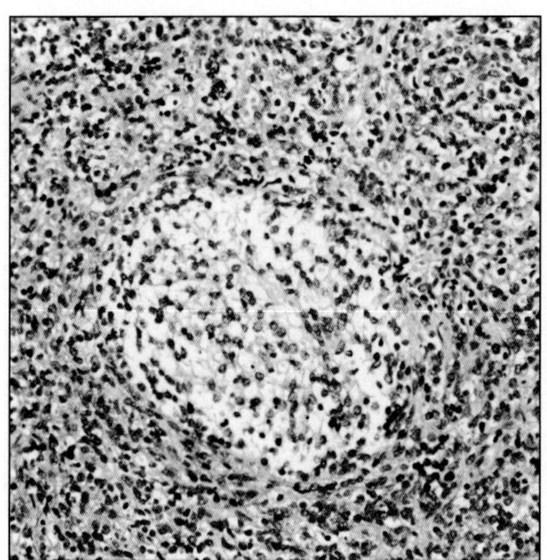

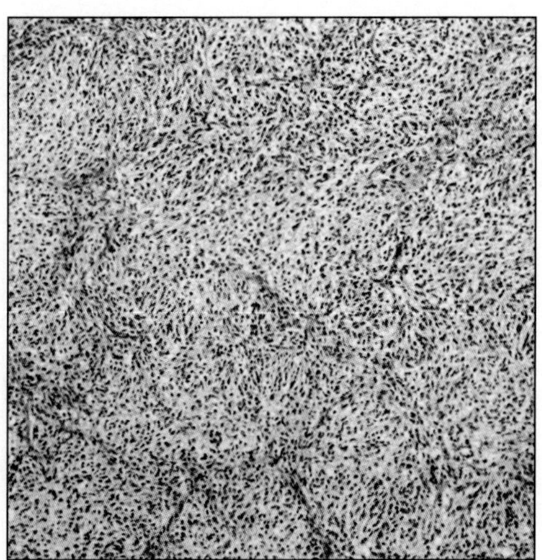

(Left) *Medium-power view shows medulloblastoma at 1 extreme of the nodular/desmoplastic spectrum where the rare nodule is small and poorly formed. Neuroblastic/neurocytic differentiation is evident in these nodules with cell processes resulting in fine fibrillarity, giving the nodule its pale look.* ***(Right)*** *Medium-power view shows medulloblastoma with extensive nodularity, the opposite end of the spectrum, composed almost entirely of nodules with very little extranodular tissue.*

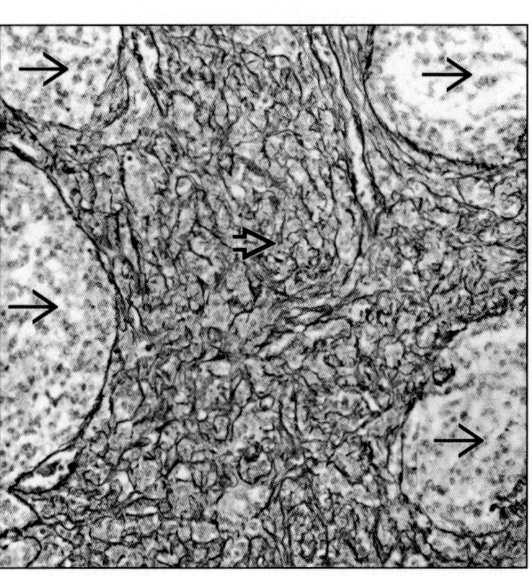

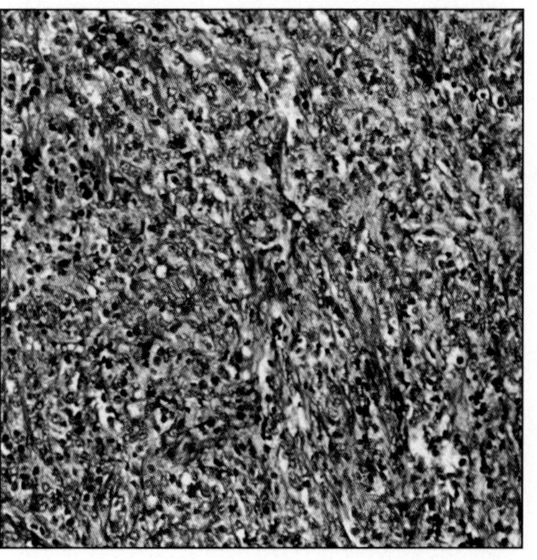

(Left) *Reticulin stain shows a medium-power view of nodular/desmoplastic medulloblastoma with abundant fibers ⇨ surrounding individual tumor cells and small clusters in the hypercellular internodular region, but absent staining in the nodules ⇒, reinforcing the "pale island" appearance.* ***(Right)*** *Trichrome stain shows a medium-power view of a desmoplastic area in medulloblastoma. Collagen deposition (here stained blue) can compress tumor cells into thin columns.*

MEDULLOBLASTOMA

Variant Microscopic Features

(Left) **H&E section shows a high-power view of large cell medulloblastoma where larger cells have more abundant cytoplasm and round nuclei with prominent nucleoli ➔. *(Right)* H&E section shows a high-power view of melanotic differentiation in medulloblastoma, seen as tubulopapillary epithelial formations ➔ with cells containing finely granular, cytoplasmic melanin pigment.**

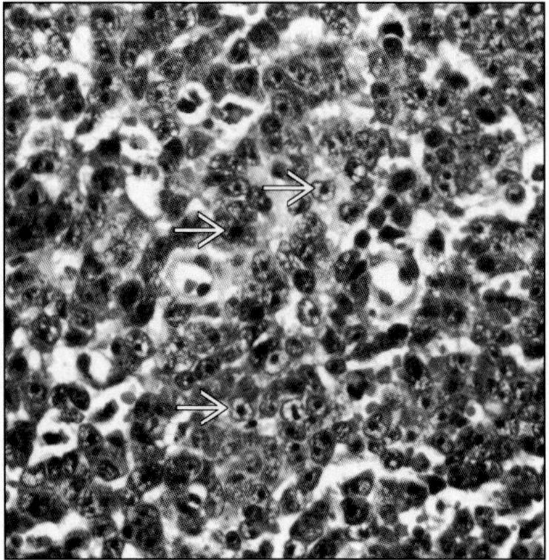

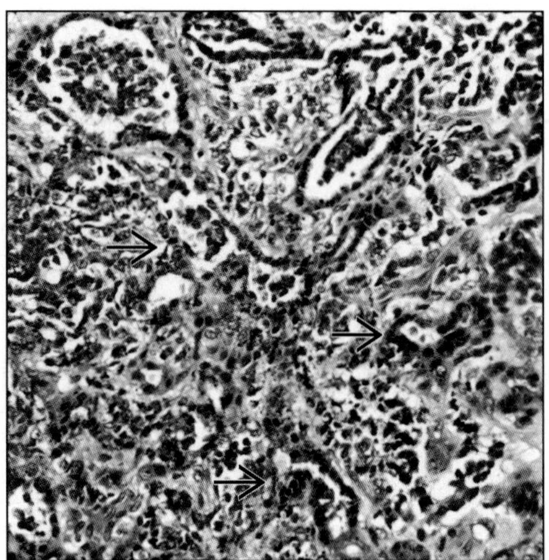

(Left) *Immunohistochemical stain for cytokeratin AE1/AE3 shows a high-power view of melanotic medulloblastoma where the areas of melanotic/epithelial differentiation in the tumor are immunoreactive.* ***(Right)*** *Immunohistochemical stain for HMB-45 shows a high-power view of melanotic medulloblastoma where the pigmented cells in the tubular areas of the tumor are immunoreactive.*

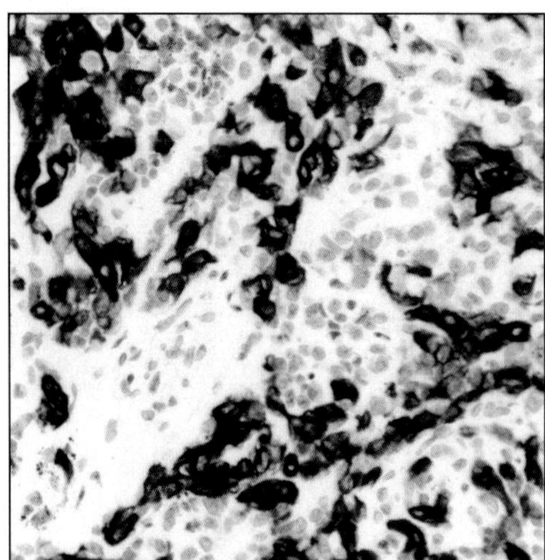

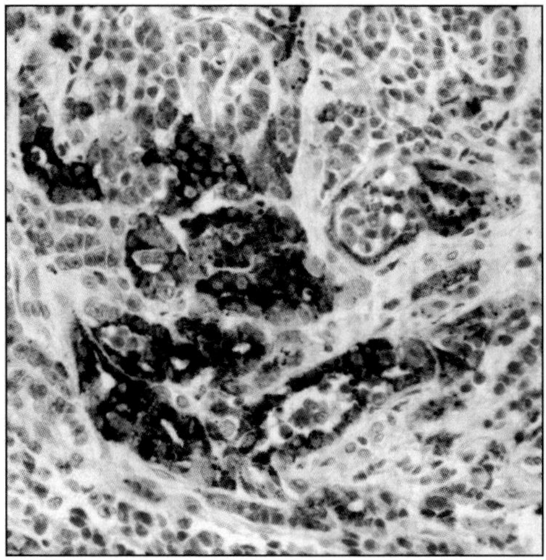

(Left) *H&E section shows a high-power view of rhabdomyoblastic differentiation in medulloblastoma with myoblasts ➔ having eccentric nuclei and prominent, globular and eosinophilic cytoplasm.* ***(Right)*** *Immunohistochemical stain for Desmin shows a high-power view of medullomyoblastoma where tumor cells with rhabdomyoblastic differentiation are immunoreactive. (Courtesy A. Perry, MD.)*

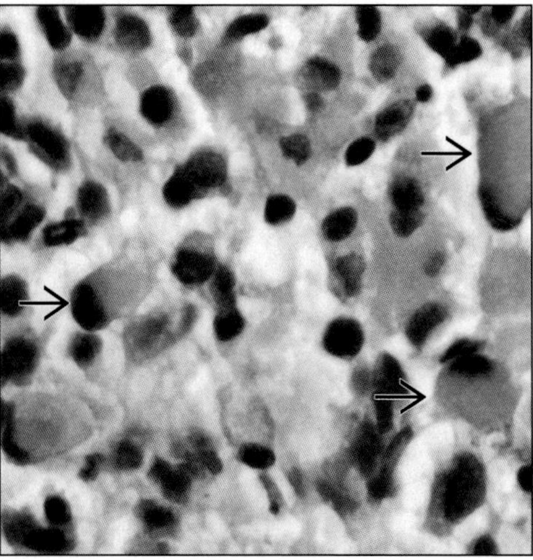

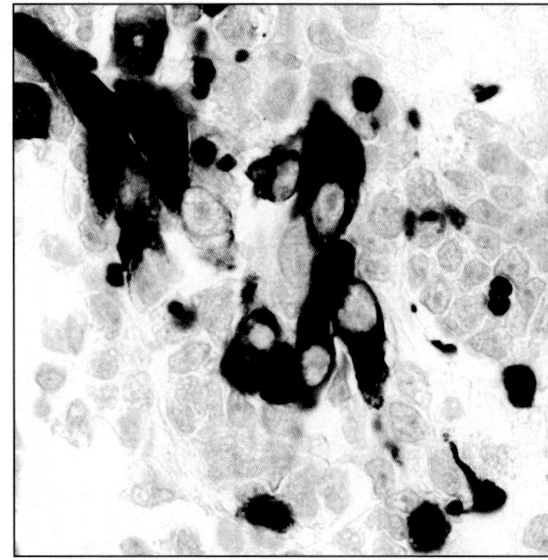

Ancillary Techniques

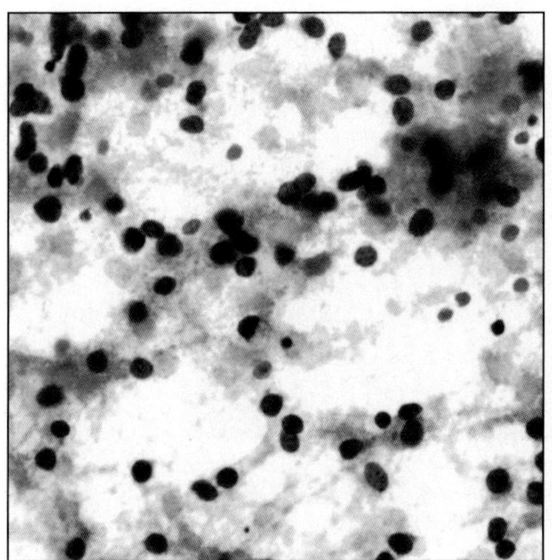

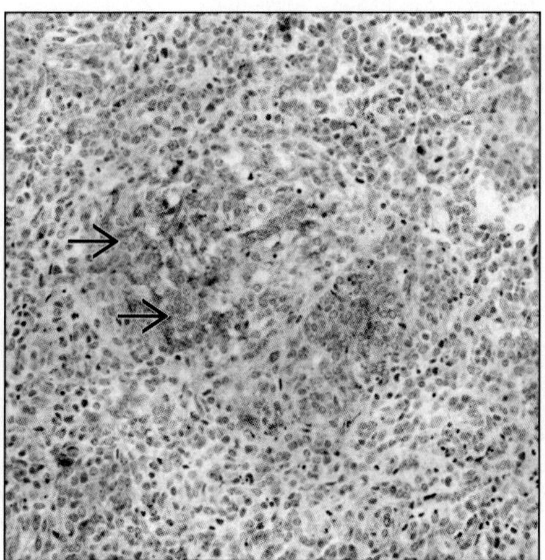

(Left) *H&E stain of smear preparation shows a high-power view of classic medulloblastoma composed of small, uniform, dark cells with little variation in size and shape and scant cytoplasm.* ***(Right)*** *Immunohistochemical stain for synaptophysin shows a medium-power view of nodular/desmoplastic medulloblastoma where the pale islands of nodular regions are now dark ➔ because the neurocytic fibrillar areas are immunoreactive.*

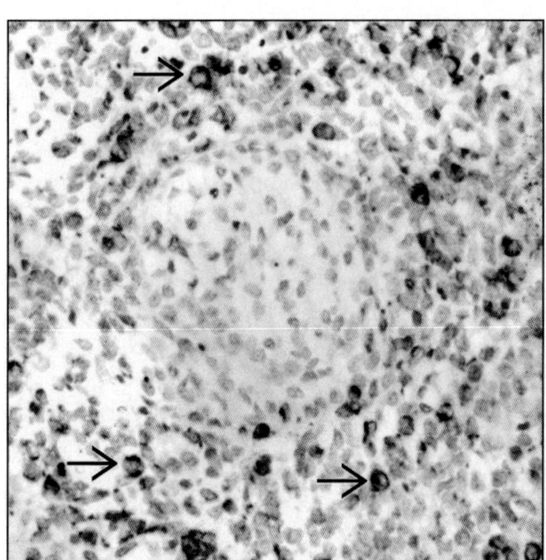

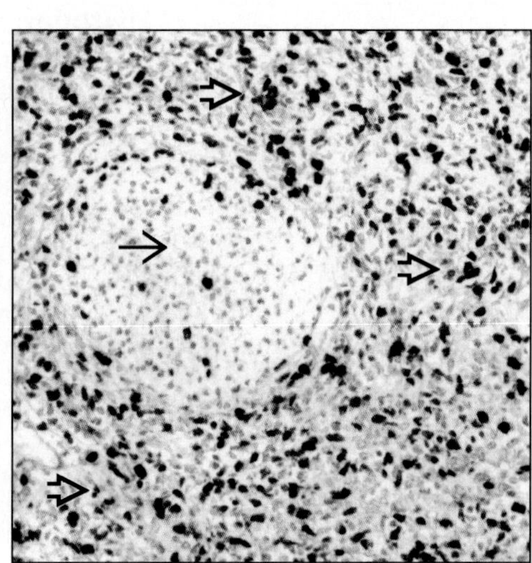

(Left) *Immunostain for GFAP in nodular/desmoplastic medulloblastoma shows small atypical tumor cells with little cytoplasm and few processes ➔ in the extranodular areas to be positive, indicative of glial differentiation.* ***(Right)*** *Immunostain for Ki-67 in nodular/desmoplastic medulloblastoma shows the percentage of immunoreactivity (MIB-1 proliferation index) to be higher in the extranodular regions ➔ as opposed to the pale islands ➔.*

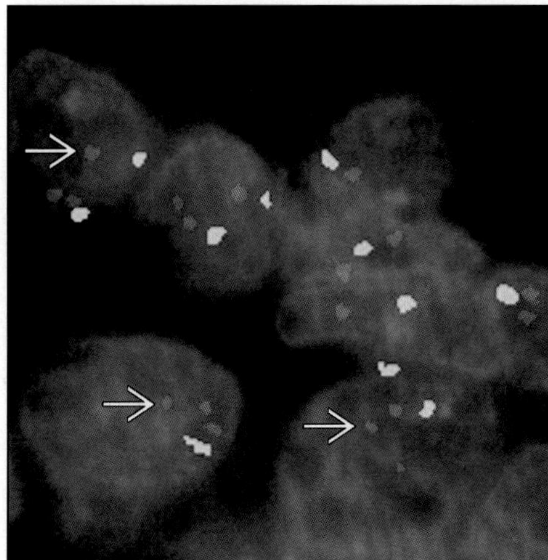

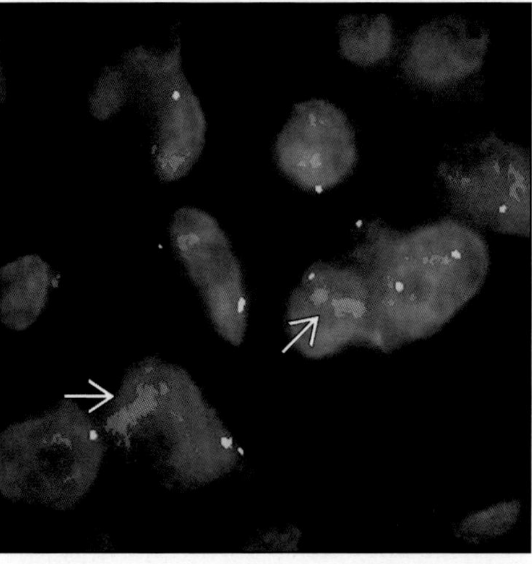

(Left) *FISH in a medulloblastoma shows an extra copy of chromosome 17q ➔ in each tumor cell, consistent with isochromosome 17q. Red signal is the NF1 gene on 17q11.2; green signal is the centromere of chromosome 17. (Courtesy A. Perry, MD.)* ***(Right)*** *FISH in a medulloblastoma shows a high-level amplification of the c-Myc gene ➔ in tumor cells. Red signal is the c-Myc gene; green signal is the centromere of chromosome 8. (Courtesy A. Perry, MD.)*

PRIMITIVE NEUROECTODERMAL TUMOR

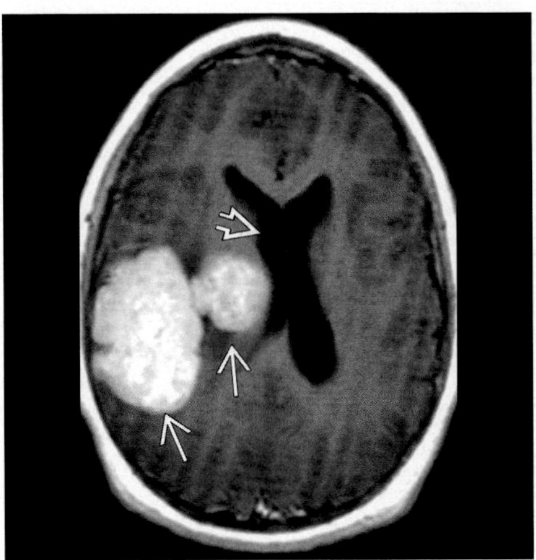

Axial T1 contrast-enhanced brain MR shows a bilobed, right hemispheric PNET with sharply defined borders ➡ and mass effect with compression of the ventricle ⇨.

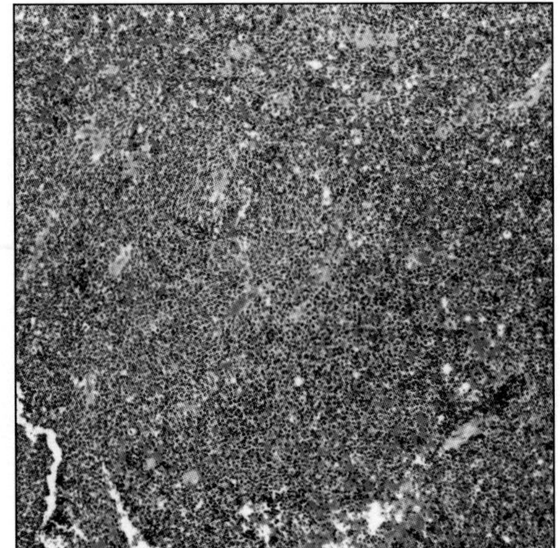

H&E shows a medium-power view of PNET with the classic appearance of patternless, hypercellular sheets of undifferentiated, "small round blue cells."

TERMINOLOGY

Abbreviations

- Primitive neuroectodermal tumor (PNET)

Synonyms

- Embryonal neuroepithelial tumor
- Medulloblastoma = PNET of cerebellum
- "Cerebral medulloblastoma" = supratentorial PNET
- Pineoblastoma = PNET of pineal region
- Askin tumor = chest wall/thoracopulmonary PNET
- Peripheral neuroepithelioma = peripheral nerve PNET
- Cerebral neuroblastoma = PNET with distinct neuronal differentiation
- Cerebral ganglioneuroblastoma = PNET with advanced neuronal differentiation (ganglion cells)

Definitions

- Malignant (WHO grade IV), poorly differentiated, embryonal, "small round blue cell" neuroepithelial tumor of nervous system, with predilection for children and capacity for divergent differentiation

ETIOLOGY/PATHOGENESIS

Environmental Exposure

- Complication after prophylactic skull irradiation
  - Within 7-9 years after treatment for leukemia (ALL)
  - Transformation of persisting progenitor cells, vs. acceleration of already initiated neoplastic process

Genetics

- Peripheral neuroblastoma: Chromosome 1p deletion
- Retinoblastoma: *Rb* gene mutations (13q14)
- Peripheral neuroepithelioma, Askin tumor: t(11;22)
- Central PNETs: Rare chromosome 17 abnormalities
- von Hippel-Lindau: Divergent differentiation in PNET
  - Adipose tissue, smooth muscle
- Germline *P53* mutations rarely described

Histogenesis

- PNET: Term initially used to describe embryonal tumors akin to medulloblastoma but outside the cerebellum
  - Expanded to include other embryonal CNS tumors
    - Olfactory/adrenal neuroblastoma, retinoblastoma
    - Medulloepithelioma, ependymoblastoma
    - Peripheral neuroepithelioma, Askin tumor
  - Subdivided: Central (CNS), peripheral (PNS) PNETs
- Morphologic similarities: Medulloblastoma and PNETs
  - Assumed to share common histogenetic origins
  - Pluripotential progenitor cells
    - Subependymal germinal matrix (lateral ventricles)
    - Neoplastic transformation at various CNS sites
  - Different molecular characteristics, gene expression
    - Suggests divergent histogenesis pathways instead
- Alternatively: PNET from primitive neuroepithelial cell
  - Retains capacity for divergent differentiation
    - Neuronal, glial, ependymal features

CLINICAL ISSUES

Epidemiology

- Incidence
  - PNETs overall: 15-25% of pediatric CNS tumors
    - Supratentorial PNETs less common (2.5%)
    - Medulloblastoma:supratentorial PNET ratio varies from 5:1 to 25:1
- Age
  - Most (80%) occur in 1st decade of life
  - Peak in 1st 3 years; mean: 5.5 years
- Gender
  - Slight male predominance (1.5-2:1)

Site

- Supratentorial (cerebral hemispheres, suprasellar)
  - Mostly in frontoparietal region
  - Arise in cortex or deep periventricular white matter
- Intrapontine, spinal cord examples rare, but described

Key Facts

Terminology
- Malignant (grade IV) poorly differentiated embryonal neuroepithelial tumor of nervous system
- PNET term initially used for embryonal tumors akin to medulloblastoma but outside cerebellum

Clinical Issues
- PNETs overall: 15-25% of pediatric CNS tumors
  - Supratentorial PNETs less common (2.5%)
- Peak in 1st 3 years, mean age: 5.5 years
- Site: Supratentorial (cerebral hemispheres, suprasellar)
  - Rare intrapontine, spinal cord examples
  - Pineoblastoma, medulloblastoma, retinoblastoma
  - Peripheral nerve PNET (related to Ewing sarcoma)
- Locally aggressive, recurrence, CSF/meningeal spread
  - Distant mets: Bone, liver, lung, nodes, peritoneum
- 5-year survival: 30-40% for extracerebellar PNET
- Treatment: Complete surgical resection, if possible
  - Radiation of entire neuraxis if patient age allows
- Poor prognosis (high risk): Age < 3 years, incomplete resection, or extensive/CSF disease at presentation

Image Findings
- Well defined, contrast enhancing; little/no edema

Macroscopic Features
- Pink-red, well demarcated, soft or firm (desmoplastic)
- Cysts, necrosis, hemorrhage, calcification (in 50-70%)

Microscopic Pathology
- Sheets/lobules of monotonous, dense hypercellularity
- Small nuclei, scant cytoplasm, inconspicuous nucleoli
- Neuronal, astroglial, or mesenchymal differentiation
- Usually NSE, NFP, or synaptophysin positive
- Prominent mitoses; MIB-1 index generally high

  - Need to exclude "drop mets" from medulloblastoma
- Certain specific locations termed accordingly
  - Pineoblastoma (pineal gland), medulloblastoma
  - Olfactory/adrenal neuroblastoma, retinoblastoma
- Peripheral neuroepithelioma (peripheral nerve PNET)
  - In adrenal gland, sympathetic ganglia
  - More often in adults

Presentation
- Symptoms related to site of tumor, local mass effect
- Cerebral lesions
  - Seizures, disturbed consciousness
  - Focal neurologic deficits (e.g., motor, visual)
  - ↑ intracranial pressure, macrocephaly (infants)
- Suprasellar lesions
  - Visual disturbance, endocrine (pituitary) problems
- Peripheral PNETs
  - Weakness, pain, sensory disturbance

Natural History
- Locally aggressive behavior, tendency to recur
- Prone to extensive CSF spread or meningeal invasion
  - ~ 20% of infants at presentation
  - Primary tumor often not found
- Distant (extracranial) metastases
  - Bone, liver, lung, lymph nodes, peritoneum
  - More common than in other brain tumors

Treatment
- Options, risks, complications
  - At risk for long-term neurocognitive sequelae
- Surgical approaches
  - Complete resection, if possible
- Adjuvant therapy
  - High-dose chemotherapy role unclear, still debated
    - Probably beneficial, at least in high-risk groups
  - Radiation of entire neuraxis when patient age allows

Prognosis
- Extracerebellar PNET: Poor prognosis in children
  - 5-year survival: 30-40%, but improving
    - With more aggressive (adjuvant) treatment
    - Compared with 75-85% for medulloblastoma
- Pineoblastoma: More favorable outcome
- Poor prognosis (high-risk group): Any of the following
  - Age < 2-3 years old (infants)
  - Subtotal or incomplete resection
  - Disseminated or locally extensive at presentation

IMAGE FINDINGS

MR Findings
- Hypointense; contrast enhancing with gadolinium
- Cystic or necrotic areas hyperintense on T2WI
- Intratumoral hemorrhage hypointense on T2WI

CT Findings
- Bulky, well-defined tumor mass, contrast enhancing
- Iso- to hyperdense; solid or cystic; necrotic areas
- Calcification (in 50-70%); little peritumoral edema

MACROSCOPIC FEATURES

General Features
- Pink-red, soft, usually well-demarcated mass
  - Tan and firm, if desmoplastic
- Common intratumoral cystic degeneration, necrosis, hemorrhage, and calcification

Size
- Variable size; may be massive if parenchymal
  - Cerebral lesions usually larger than suprasellar

MICROSCOPIC PATHOLOGY

Histologic Features
- Sheets or lobules with diffuse, dense cellularity
  - May be linearly arranged, streaming
  - Less prominent, inconspicuous stroma
- Neuronal/neuroblastic differentiation commonly seen
  - Homer Wright rosettes: Cells radially arranged around fibrillar, nuclear-free zones
  - Rare true ependymal, Flexner-Wintersteiner rosettes
  - Focal ganglioid cells or even mature neurons

- Diffuse, eosinophilic, fibrillar background matrix
- May also exhibit astroglial differentiation
  - Abundant, eccentric, eosinophilic cytoplasm
  - Occasional oligodendroglial, ependymal features
- Mesenchymal differentiation
  - Rhabdomyoblastic, adipocytic, smooth muscle
  - Variable fibrocollagenous (desmoplastic) component
- Melanotic (pigmented) epithelial cells
- Calcification, single-cell necrosis present
  - More frequent than in medulloblastomas
- Hemorrhage and focal necrosis may be present
  - But microvascular proliferation, pseudopalisading ("geographic") necrosis usually absent

Cytologic Features

- Monotonous, poorly differentiated, small round cells
- Small, round to elongated, hyperchromatic nuclei
  - May be larger, more pleomorphic, angular
- Scant cytoplasm, usually inconspicuous nucleoli
- Variable but usually prominent mitotic activity

ANCILLARY TESTS

Immunohistochemistry

- Usually NSE, NFP, synaptophysin positive
  - Especially in areas of neuronal differentiation
- Nestin immunoreactivity
  - Intermediate filament of neuroepithelial cells
- Desmin immunoreactivity
  - In areas of rhabdomyoblastic differentiation
- Retinal S antigen, rhodopsin immunoreactivity
  - In areas of photoreceptor differentiation
- May be immunoreactive for CD99 (*MIC2* product)
  - Characteristic of peripheral PNET/Ewing sarcoma
- Focal GFAP immunoreactivity often seen
  - In stellate, reactive, perivascular astrocytes
  - Rarely as positive rim of cytoplasm in tumor cells
    - Evidence of glial differentiation in the tumor
- MIB-1 proliferation index (Ki-67 immunostain)
  - Generally high but varies widely (0-85%)

Cytogenetics

- Translocation t(11;22)(q24;q12)
  - Olfactory neuroblastoma, peripheral PNET, Askin
  - Not in central PNET (suggests different histogenesis)
- Isochromosome 17q: 2 long arms, loss of short arm
  - 30-50% of cases (less than in medulloblastomas)
- *N-Myc* amplification (neuroblastoma), *TP53* mutation
- Double minutes (DM) in 10-20% of central PNETs

Electron Microscopy

- Round cells with scant cytoplasm, few organelles
- Occasional short, neuritic-type, microtubule processes
- Rare dense core, neurosecretory granules

DIFFERENTIAL DIAGNOSIS

Neuroblastoma

- Young children, less aggressive, better survival
- Shows adrenergic expression, metabolic excretion
- Neuronal differentiation (neurites, granules by EM)
  - Neurofilament(+); generally vimentin(-)

Malignant Glioma

- Especially small cell glioblastoma
- Generally larger, more pleomorphic cells and nuclei
- More widespread fibrillarity, GFAP immunoreactivity
- Microvascular proliferation, pseudopalisading necrosis

Atypical Teratoid/Rhabdoid tumor

- Especially in infants < 2 years old
- Large areas of hemorrhage, necrosis
- Large cells with eccentric cytoplasmic filaments
- *INI1* (22q) deletion/mutation; synaptophysin(-)

Metastatic Small Cell Carcinoma

- Rare in children
- CK, EMA positive; synaptophysin, GFAP negative

DIAGNOSTIC CHECKLIST

Clinically Relevant Pathologic Features

- Ewing sarcoma may be considered peripheral PNET
  - In bone/soft tissue but lacks neural differentiation
  - Common chromosomal translocation t(11;22)
  - But different clinical presentation, behavior

SELECTED REFERENCES

1. Brat DJ et al: Surgical neuropathology update: a review of changes introduced by the WHO classification of tumours of the central nervous system, 4th edition. Arch Pathol Lab Med. 132(6):993-1007, 2008
2. MacDonald TJ: Aggressive infantile embryonal tumors. J Child Neurol. 23(10):1195-204, 2008
3. Jakacki RI: Treatment strategies for high-risk medulloblastoma and supratentorial primitive neuroectodermal tumors. Review of the literature. J Neurosurg. 102(1 Suppl):44-52, 2005
4. Sarkar C et al: Recent advances in embryonal tumours of the central nervous system. Childs Nerv Syst. 21(4):272-93, 2005
5. McLean TW: Medulloblastomas and central nervous system primitive neuroectodermal tumors. Curr Treat Options Oncol. 4(6):499-508, 2003
6. Vogel H et al: Primitive neuroectodermal tumors, embryonal tumors, and other small cell and poorly differentiated malignant neoplasms of the central and peripheral nervous systems. Ann Diagn Pathol. 7(6):387-98, 2003
7. Bouffet E: Embryonal tumours of the central nervous system. Eur J Cancer. 38(8):1112-20, 2002
8. Dedeurwaerdere F et al: Primary peripheral PNET/Ewing's sarcoma of the dura: a clinicopathologic entity distinct from central PNET. Mod Pathol. 15(6):673-8, 2002
9. Taylor MD et al: Molecular insight into medulloblastoma and central nervous system primitive neuroectodermal tumor biology from hereditary syndromes: a review. Neurosurgery. 47(4):888-901, 2000
10. Jürgens HF: Ewing's sarcoma and peripheral primitive neuroectodermal tumor. Curr Opin Oncol. 6(4):391-6, 1994
11. Molenaar WM et al: Primitive neuroectodermal tumors of the central nervous system in childhood: tumor biological aspects. Crit Rev Oncol Hematol. 17(1):1-25, 1994
12. Dehner LP: Primitive neuroectodermal tumor and Ewing's sarcoma. Am J Surg Pathol. 17(1):1-13, 1993

Microscopic Features

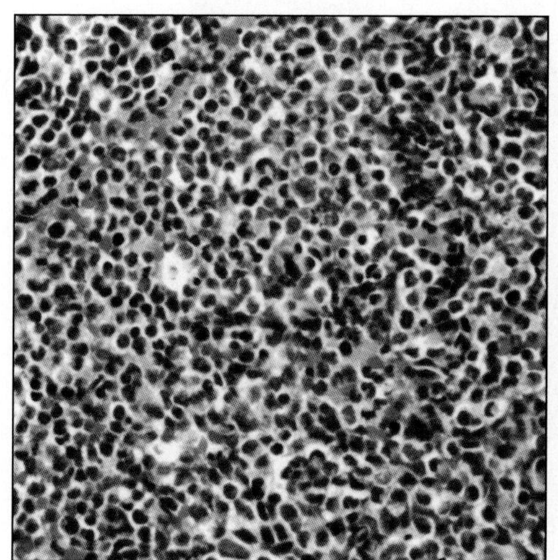

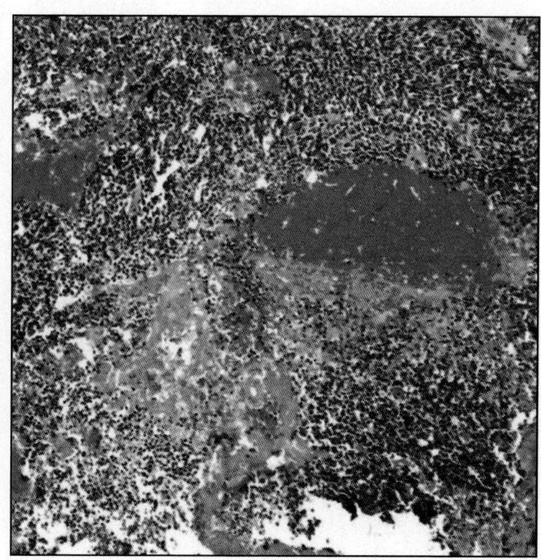

(Left) *H&E shows a high-power view of supratentorial PNET with patternless dense cellularity and inconspicuous stroma. Tumor cells are poorly differentiated but monomorphic due to their small round shape, scant cytoplasm, and inconspicuous nucleoli. Mitoses are usually numerous.* ***(Right)*** *H&E shows a medium-power view of supratentorial PNET with areas of hemorrhage and necrosis (which is usually not geographic or pseudopalisading).*

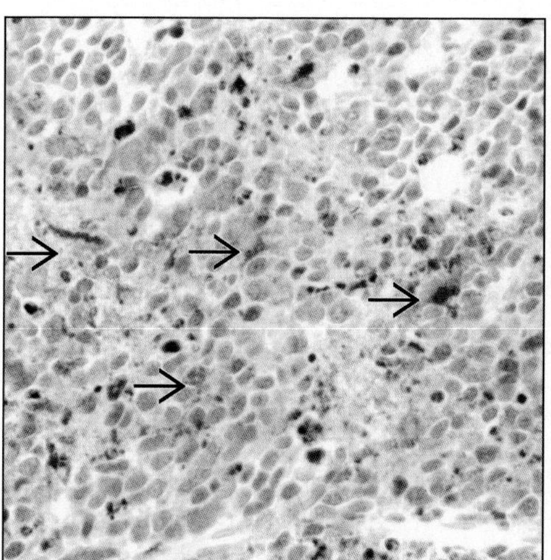

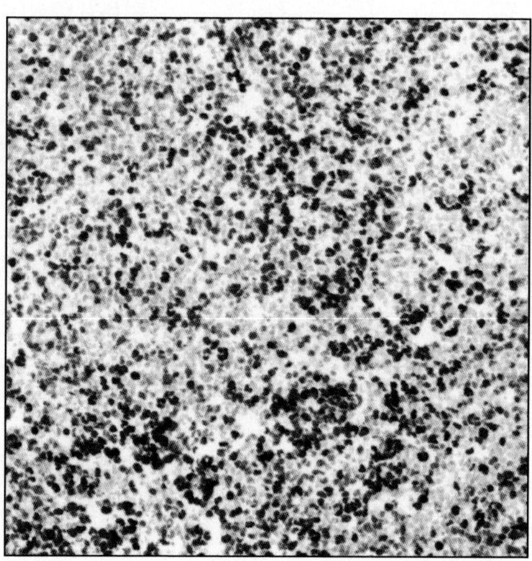

(Left) *Immunohistochemical stain for synaptophysin shows a high-power view of PNET, with highlighted areas of neuronal differentiation ⇒ characterized by nuclear-free fibrillar zones with tumor cells radially arranged around them, akin to neuroblastic Homer Wright rosettes.* ***(Right)*** *Immunohistochemical stain for Ki-67 shows a medium-power view of PNET with a very high MIB-1 proliferation index approaching 80-90%.*

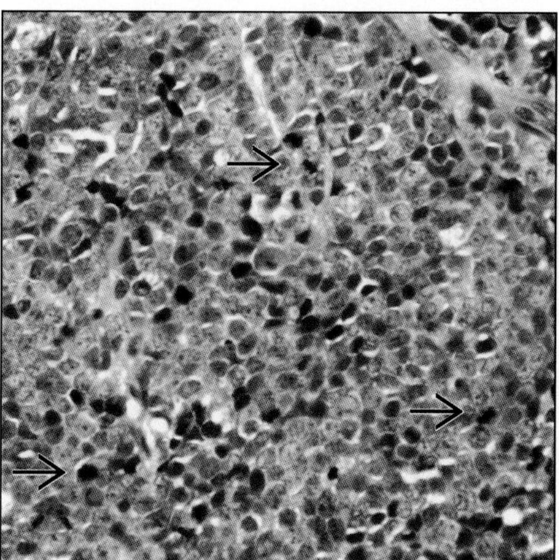

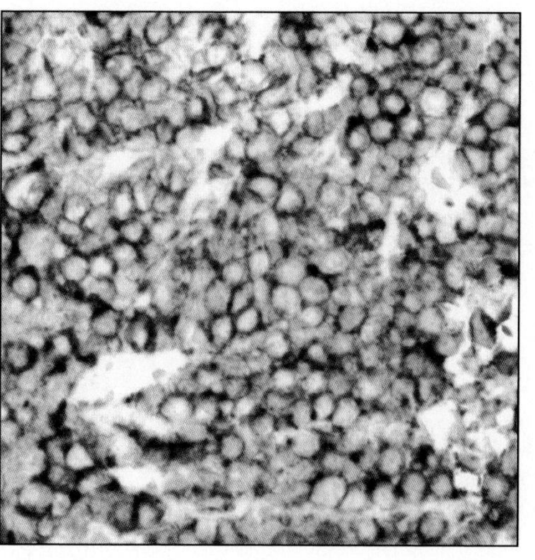

(Left) *H&E shows a high-power view of peripheral PNET from the area of the sciatic nerve with lobulated areas of dense cellularity composed of monotonous, poorly differentiated tumor cells with little cytoplasm and prominent mitoses ⇒.* ***(Right)*** *Immunohistochemical stain for CD99 shows a high-power view of peripheral PNET with strong membranous immunoreactivity in the tumor cells.*

ATYPICAL TERATOID/RHABDOID TUMOR

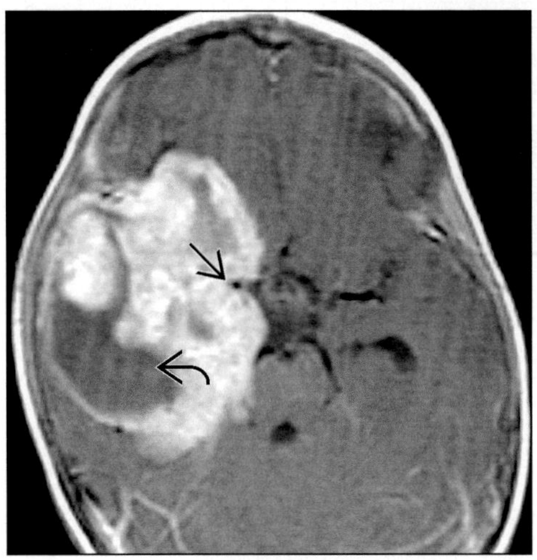

Axial T1WI MR with contrast shows a large enhancing mass centered in the right middle fossa with large lateral cystic component ⇨, encasing the right carotid terminus at the origin of the middle cerebral artery →.

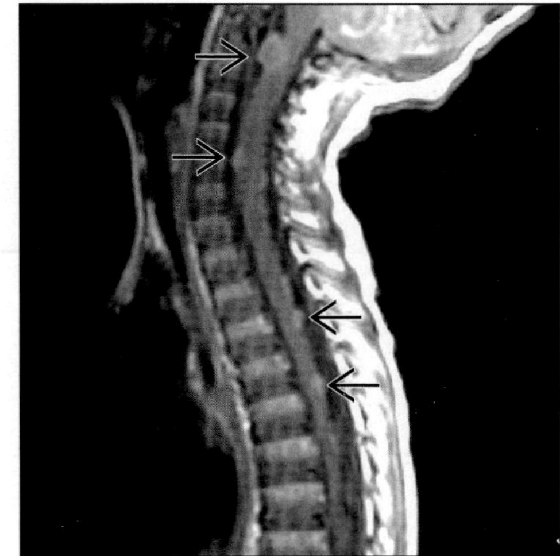

Sagittal T1WI MR with contrast shows multiple enhancing "drop mets" → along the ventral and dorsal surfaces of the cervical and thoracic cord from a posterior fossa AT/RT.

TERMINOLOGY

Abbreviations

- Atypical teratoid/rhabdoid tumor (AT/RT)

Synonyms

- Atypical teratoid tumor
- Rhabdoid tumor of CNS

Definitions

- Highly malignant CNS neoplasm (WHO grade IV)
  - Occurring in infants and young children
  - Similar to renal and extrarenal rhabdoid tumors
- Composed of distinctive large, often rhabdoid cells
  - Round eccentric nuclei
  - Eosinophilic cytoplasm of intermediate filaments
  - Prominent nucleoli
- Histologically divergent differentiation
  - Small cell/embryonal (PNET-like)
  - Epithelial
  - Mesenchymal
- Immunohistochemically polyphenotypic
  - Representing all germ layers

ETIOLOGY/PATHOGENESIS

Genetics

- Genetic abnormalities that define AT/RT
  - Deletions or monosomy of chromosome 22
  - Mutations in *hSNF5/INI1* gene (22q11.2)
  - Shared with other renal/extrarenal rhabdoid tumors
- 10-15% of AT/RT may not have detectable genetic abnormalities
- Germline *INI1* mutations have been described in patients with AT/RT or renal rhabdoid tumors
- Tumors reported occurring synchronously in monozygous twin infants

Histogenesis

- Histologically resembles malignant rhabdoid tumor of kidney of infancy or extrarenal rhabdoid tumors
  - Synchronous occurrence of renal rhabdoid tumor with intracranial tumors has been reported
    - May be medulloblastoma/PNET or AT/RT
- Disparate combination of histologic components
  - Suggests teratoma
    - However, AT/RT is consistently negative for germ cell markers
    - AT/RT does not exhibit as varied histologic differentiation patterns

CLINICAL ISSUES

Epidemiology

- Incidence
  - 1-2% of pediatric primary CNS tumors
    - 7-10% in infants (< 2 years old)
- Age
  - Generally present in 1st 2 years of life
    - > 90% younger than 5 years old
    - Median age at diagnosis: 16.5 months
  - Only rare examples reported in adults
- Gender
  - Males > females (3:2)

Site

- Most are intracranial
  - 50-60% infratentorial/posterior fossa
    - Cerebellum
    - Brainstem
    - Characteristically in cerebellopontine angle (CPA), invade adjacent structures
  - 30-40% supratentorial
    - Cerebral, suprasellar
- Rare intraspinal (~ 2%) examples reported
- ~ 2% may be multifocal

ATYPICAL TERATOID/RHABDOID TUMOR

Key Facts

Terminology
- Highly malignant CNS neoplasm (WHO grade IV)
- Defined by genetic abnormalities
  - Chromosome 22 deletion, *hSNF5/INI1* mutation

Clinical Issues
- Mostly (> 90%) in infants, young children
- 50-60% infratentorial, 30-40% supratentorial
- Nonspecific lethargy, vomiting, failure to thrive
- Gross total resection often not possible
  - Adjuvant chemotherapy/radiation have little effect
- Poor prognosis: Most die within 1 year of diagnosis
- Common CSF spread (drop mets), local recurrence

Image Findings
- Large, hyperdense, contrast-enhancing mass
- Commonly cystic and hemorrhagic

Macroscopic Features
- May surround cranial nerves and vessels
- Large, bulky, soft, and fleshy lesions

Microscopic Pathology
- Loose, disordered, complex architecture
- Divergent histologic patterns of differentiation
  - Rhabdoid, large cell, small cell/PNET-like, epithelial, and mesenchymal
- Variability in cell size/shape (rhabdoid to small cell)
  - Rhabdoid cells: Large and polygonal with round nuclei, prominent nucleoli, eosinophilic cytoplasm
- Necrosis and mitoses are common
- Polyphenotypic by immunohistochemistry
  - EMA/MUC1, GFAP, cytokeratins, vimentin positive
  - Loss of nuclear INI1; Ki-67 index: 30-80%

Presentation
- Variable
  - Depending on age, size, and location of tumor
- Infants
  - Nonspecific symptoms
  - Lethargy, vomiting, failure to thrive
    - Related to hydrocephalus
- More specific symptoms due to location
  - Cerebellar tumors
    - Head tilt, gait ataxia
  - CPA tumors
    - Cranial nerve (6th, 7th) palsy
  - Cerebral tumors
    - Seizures, visual changes
- Older children
  - Headache, hemiplegia

Natural History
- Large and rapidly enlarging
  - Can be massive
- 15-35% of patients present with CSF &/or leptomeningeal spread

Treatment
- Surgical approaches
  - Gross total resection often not possible
    - Large size
    - Attachment to surrounding structures
    - < 1/3 of tumors are amenable to surgery
  - Aim should be maximal safe resection
- Adjuvant therapy
  - Chemotherapy is mainstay of postsurgical adjuvant treatment
    - Usually has little impact
    - Slight prolongation of life
  - Some response to intrathecal chemotherapy
    - Usually not durable
  - Aggressive chemotherapy has little impact
- Radiation
  - Usually withheld initially
    - Due to young age of patients
  - May slightly prolong survival

Prognosis
- Highly malignant
  - Brief survival
    - 6 months to 1 year after diagnosis
- Early local recurrence
- Common CSF dissemination
- Systemic spread is rare

IMAGE FINDINGS

General Features
- More commonly necrotic than other malignant CNS tumors
- CSF metastases are often contrast enhancing

MR Findings
- T1-weighted imaging
  - Isointense
  - Hyperintense foci due to hemorrhage
- T2-weighted imaging
  - Heterogeneous mix of intensity
- Enhancement with gadolinium

CT Findings
- Large, hyperdense mass
- Intense, but nonhomogeneous contrast enhancement
- Cysts and hemorrhage are common

MACROSCOPIC FEATURES

General Features
- Large, bulky lesions
  - May be focally demarcated from adjacent parenchyma
- Soft, pink, and fleshy
  - Firm and white where more mesenchymal tissue is present
- Hemorrhagic, often necrotic
- May surround cranial nerves and vessels
  - Can invade parenchyma this way
- Deposits along CSF pathways are common

ATYPICAL TERATOID/RHABDOID TUMOR

- "Drop mets"

MICROSCOPIC PATHOLOGY

Histologic Features

- Loose, disordered, complex architecture
  - No clear structures present
- Distinctive large, often rhabdoid cells
  - Round eccentric nuclei
  - Eosinophilic cytoplasm of intermediate filaments
  - Prominent nucleoli
- Cells may be present in cords
  - Amidst a basophilic mucoid matrix
  - Resemble chordoma or trabecular pattern of renal rhabdoid tumors
- Other patterns of differentiation
  - Flexner-Wintersteiner or Homer Wright rosettes
    - Ependymal canals or neural tube-like structures rarely present
  - Epithelial patterns
    - Few small, gland-like spaces or nests
    - Rarely primitive squamous differentiation
- Necrosis is common
  - Often with dystrophic calcification
- Collagenous stroma may be present
- Broad, edematous fibrovascular septae
- In cerebellum, trapped choroid plexus may be present

Cytologic Features

- Wide spectrum of appearance
  - Variability in cell size and shape
  - From exclusively rhabdoid to predominantly small cell
    - 10-15% are exclusively composed of rhabdoid cells
- "Rhabdoid" phenotype
  - Large, plump, round or polygonal cells
  - Kidney-shaped (reniform) or round nuclei
    - Eccentric, vesicular, with prominent nucleoli
  - Ample eosinophilic cytoplasm
    - Finely granular and homogeneous
    - Often vacuolated (artifact)
  - Prominent spherical cytoplasmic inclusions
    - "Pink body"
  - Distinct cellular borders
- Large cells may not always be rhabdoid
  - Often medium-sized, with pale or clear cytoplasm
- Compact small cell areas resemble embryonal tumors
  - Primitive neuroectodermal tumor (PNET)-like
    - Sparse cytoplasm, dense nuclei
    - Nested pattern, within delicate fibrovascular stroma
  - Small spindle cells may have fascicular arrangement
    - Appears mesenchymal, sarcoma-like
- Abundant mitotic figures, often abnormal

Predominant Pattern/Injury Type

- Neoplastic

Predominant Cell/Compartment Type

- Rhabdoid

ANCILLARY TESTS

Cytology

- Smear preparations highlight hypercellularity, cytologic polymorphism
  - Rhabdoid cells, large pale cells, small primitive cells
  - Numerous apoptoses, mitoses

Immunohistochemistry

- Commonly positive but can be patchy
  - EMA/MUC1 (surface), GFAP, cytokeratins, vimentin
- Neuronal markers, occasionally positive
  - Neurofilament protein, chromogranin, synaptophysin
- Less frequently positive
  - Smooth muscle actin, S100
- Occasionally described
  - Insulin-like growth factor II and receptor type 1, cathepsin
  - Uncommon staining for desmin
    - Strap cells absent
  - Generally do not express germ cell markers
- Loss of nuclear reactivity for SNF5 (INI1)
  - Diagnostic of AT/RT
- High Ki-67 index
  - 30-80% in different studies

Cytogenetics

- Vast majority of AT/RT (90%)
  - Loss of all (monosomy) or part (deletion) of chromosome 22 by FISH
- Deletions, mutations in *hSNF5/INI1* gene
  - Maps to chromosome band 22q11.2
  - Loss of heterozygosity in cases where disomy is still present
    - Mutational analysis necessary for confirmation
    - Hot spots: Exons 1 and 9

Electron Microscopy

- Rhabdoid cell cytoplasm
  - Cytoplasmic inclusions
    - Tight, compact, whorled intermediate filaments
  - Occasionally, neurosecretory granules

DIFFERENTIAL DIAGNOSIS

Medulloblastoma/PNET

- Especially anaplastic/large cell variant
- More mitoses, apoptoses, cell wrapping
- More coarse, atypical, hyperchromatic nuclei
- EMA/MUC1 and cytokeratin negative
- Lack *INI1* gene or chromosome 22 abnormalities

Gemistocytic Astrocytoma

- Especially vs. overtly rhabdoid AT/RT
- Usually highly infiltrative
- GFAP(+), but EMA/MUC1(-)

Choroid Plexus Carcinoma

- Especially if high-grade cytology
- Usually supratentorial
- Cytokeratin(+), but EMA/MUC1(-)

Rhabdoid Meningioma

- Not as anaplastic as AT/RT
- EMA/MUC1(+), but GFAP(-)

DIAGNOSTIC CHECKLIST

Clinically Relevant Pathologic Features

- Age distribution
  - AT/RT tends to occur in younger infants/children than PNET
- Cytoplasmic features
- Metastatic distribution
- Mitotic rate
  - Typically do not respond to treatment
  - Worse prognosis than PNET

Pathologic Interpretation Pearls

- AT/RT characterized by histologic heterogeneity
  - Rhabdoid, PNET-like, epithelial, and mesenchymal features
  - But do not resemble teratomas in any other way
    - Lack midline location, germ cell markers
- Large pale cells with rhabdoid appearance
  - Virtually diagnostic of AT/RT
  - Confirmatory immunohistochemistry is important
    - EMA/MUC1 and GFAP positivity is critical
- Chromosome 22 or *INI1* abnormalities are important for diagnosis
  - Not essential if histology/immunohistochemistry is classic
  - Tumor with PNET-like histology and *INI1* mutation is AT/RT
  - Retained nuclear staining for SNF5 protein rules out AT/RT

SELECTED REFERENCES

1. Athale UH et al: Childhood atypical teratoid rhabdoid tumor of the central nervous system: a meta-analysis of observational studies. J Pediatr Hematol Oncol. 31(9):651-63, 2009
2. Biswas A et al: Atypical teratoid rhabdoid tumor of the brain: case series and review of literature. Childs Nerv Syst. 25(11):1495-500, 2009
3. de León-Bojorge B et al: Atypical teratoid/rhabdoid tumor of the central nervous system. Childs Nerv Syst. 25(11):1387; author reply 1389, 2009
4. Ertan Y et al: Atypical teratoid/rhabdoid tumor of the central nervous system: clinicopathologic and immunohistochemical features of four cases. Childs Nerv Syst. 25(6):707-11, 2009
5. Edgar MA et al: The differential diagnosis of central nervous system tumors: a critical examination of some recent immunohistochemical applications. Arch Pathol Lab Med. 132(3):500-9, 2008
6. Seno T et al: An immunohistochemical and electron microscopic study of atypical teratoid/rhabdoid tumor. Brain Tumor Pathol. 25(2):79-83, 2008
7. Warmuth-Metz M et al: CT and MR imaging in atypical teratoid/rhabdoid tumors of the central nervous system. Neuroradiology. 50(5):447-52, 2008
8. Biegel JA: Molecular genetics of atypical teratoid/rhabdoid tumor. Neurosurg Focus. 20(1):E11, 2006
9. Haberler C et al: Immunohistochemical analysis of INI1 protein in malignant pediatric CNS tumors: Lack of INI1 in atypical teratoid/rhabdoid tumors and in a fraction of primitive neuroectodermal tumors without rhabdoid phenotype. Am J Surg Pathol. 30(11):1462-8, 2006
10. Chen ML et al: Atypical teratoid/rhabdoid tumors of the central nervous system: management and outcomes. Neurosurg Focus. 18(6A):E8, 2005
11. Parwani AV et al: Atypical teratoid/rhabdoid tumor of the brain: cytopathologic characteristics and differential diagnosis. Cancer. 105(2):65-70, 2005
12. Reddy AT: Atypical teratoid/rhabdoid tumors of the central nervous system. J Neurooncol. 75(3):309-13, 2005
13. Strother D: Atypical teratoid rhabdoid tumors of childhood: diagnosis, treatment and challenges. Expert Rev Anticancer Ther. 5(5):907-15, 2005
14. Judkins AR et al: Immunohistochemical analysis of hSNF5/INI1 in pediatric CNS neoplasms. Am J Surg Pathol. 28(5):644-50, 2004
15. Dang T et al: Atypical teratoid/rhabdoid tumors. Childs Nerv Syst. 19(4):244-8, 2003
16. Bambakidis NC et al: Atypical teratoid/rhabdoid tumors of the central nervous system: clinical, radiographic and pathologic features. Pediatr Neurosurg. 37(2):64-70, 2002
17. Biegel JA et al: Alterations of the hSNF5/INI1 gene in central nervous system atypical teratoid/rhabdoid tumors and renal and extrarenal rhabdoid tumors. Clin Cancer Res. 8(11):3461-7, 2002
18. Biegel JA et al: The role of INI1 and the SWI/SNF complex in the development of rhabdoid tumors: meeting summary from the workshop on childhood atypical teratoid/rhabdoid tumors. Cancer Res. 62(1):323-8, 2002
19. Kleihues P et al: The WHO classification of tumors of the nervous system. J Neuropathol Exp Neurol. 61(3):215-25; discussion 226-9, 2002
20. Lee MC et al: Atypical teratoid/rhabdoid tumor of the central nervous system: clinico-pathological study. Neuropathology. 22(4):252-60, 2002
21. Packer RJ et al: Atypical teratoid/rhabdoid tumor of the central nervous system: report on workshop. J Pediatr Hematol Oncol. 24(5):337-42, 2002
22. Oka H et al: Clinicopathological characteristics of atypical teratoid/rhabdoid tumor. Neurol Med Chir (Tokyo). 39(7):510-7; discussion 517-8, 1999
23. Burger PC et al: Atypical teratoid/rhabdoid tumor of the central nervous system: a highly malignant tumor of infancy and childhood frequently mistaken for medulloblastoma: a Pediatric Oncology Group study. Am J Surg Pathol. 22(9):1083-92, 1998
24. Rorke LB et al: Central nervous system atypical teratoid/rhabdoid tumors of infancy and childhood: definition of an entity. J Neurosurg. 85(1):56-65, 1996

ATYPICAL TERATOID/RHABDOID TUMOR

Microscopic Features

*(**Left**) H&E section at high magnification shows occasional rhabdoid cells ⇨ in an AT/RT with eccentric round nuclei, prominent nucleoli, and eosinophilic cytoplasm. A rhabdoid phenotype is not always dominant in AT/RT and can be manifested with only focal rhabdoid features as in this case. (**Right**) H&E section at high magnification shows the disordered architecture of AT/RT and many medium to large cells with prominent nucleoli and pale or clear cytoplasm but not overt rhabdoid features.*

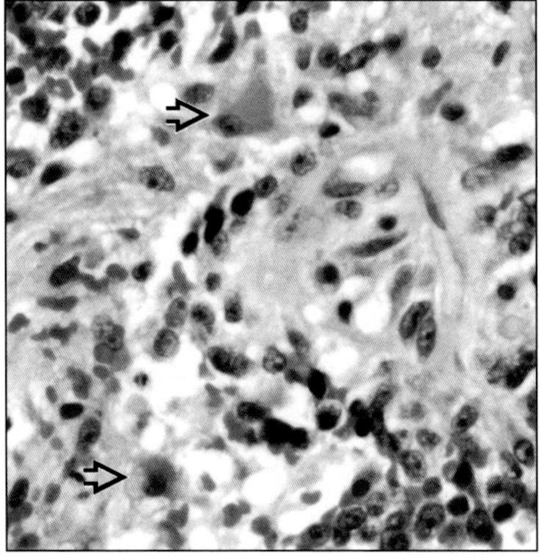

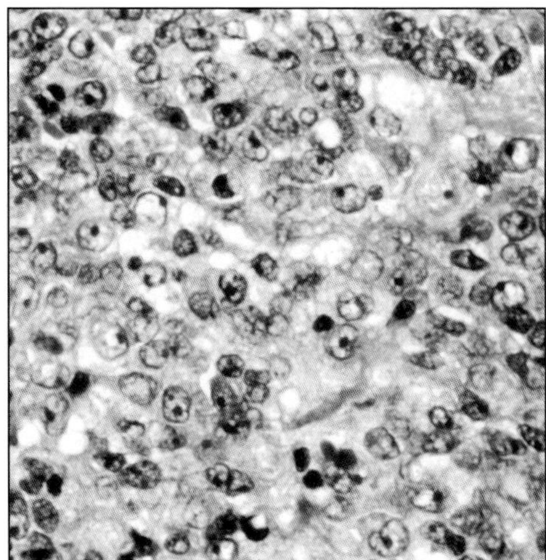

*(**Left**) H&E section at high magnification shows an area of an AT/RT that has small cell/embryonal features with sparse cytoplasm and small dense nuclei, resembling a PNET. (**Right**) H&E section at medium magnification shows the prominent fascicular and sarcoma-like arrangement of spindle cells that can be seen in components of AT/RT with mesenchymal differentiation.*

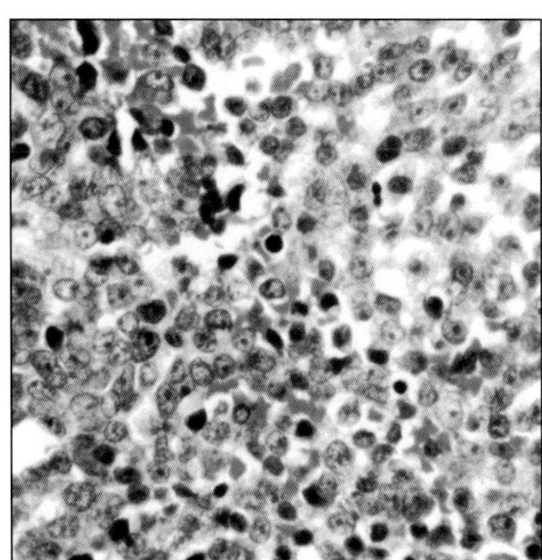

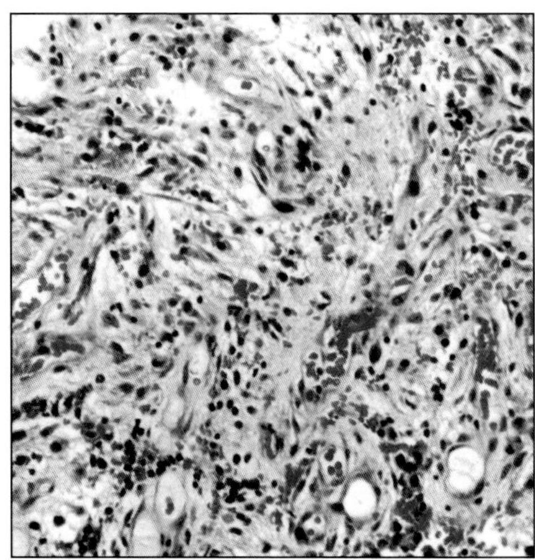

*(**Left**) H&E section at high magnification shows numerous and prominent mitotic figures →, often seen in AT/RT. (**Right**) H&E section at low magnification shows AT/RT with hemorrhage and necrosis, a common finding.*

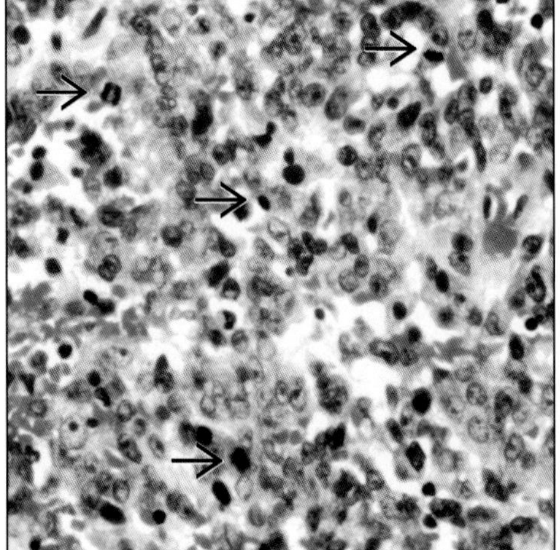

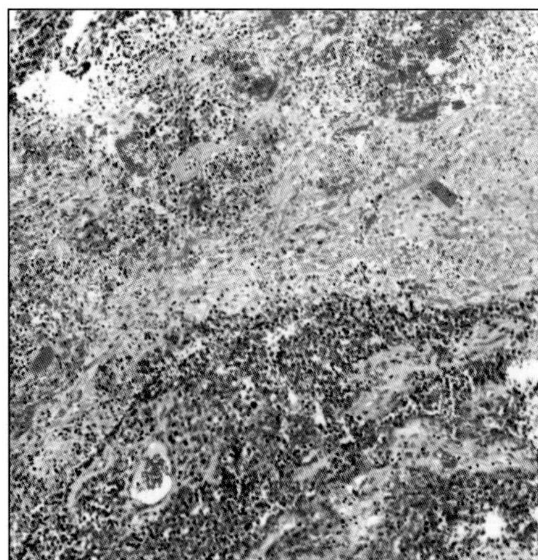

Immunohistochemical Features

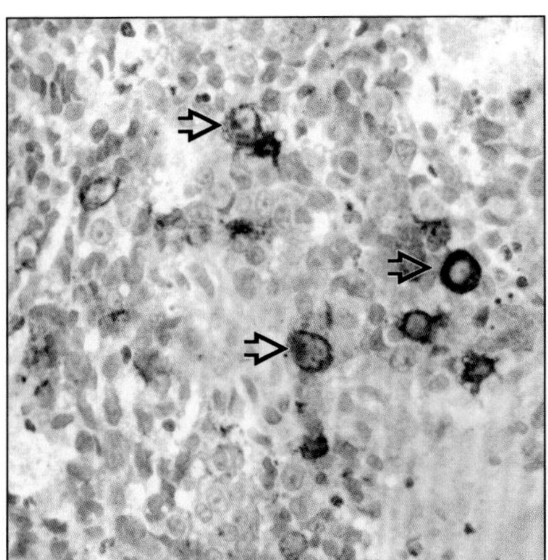
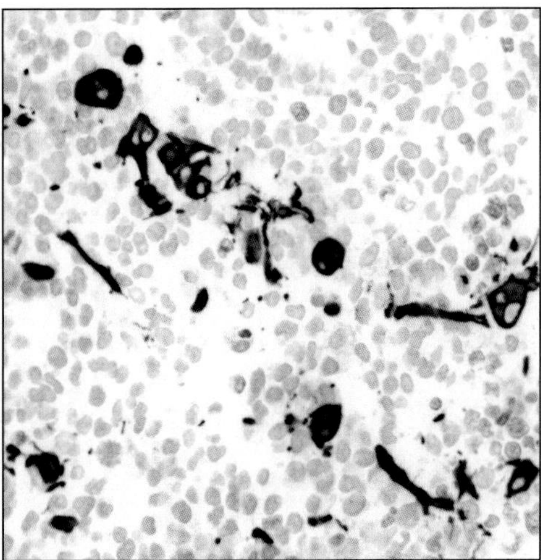

***(Left)** Immunohistochemical staining for EMA/MUC1 shows focal surface staining ➩, a characteristic of AT/RT observed most often in areas with large or rhabdoid cells. **(Right)** Immunohistochemical staining for GFAP shows patchy positive staining, which can be seen in both the large/rhabdoid cell and small cell/PNET-like areas.*

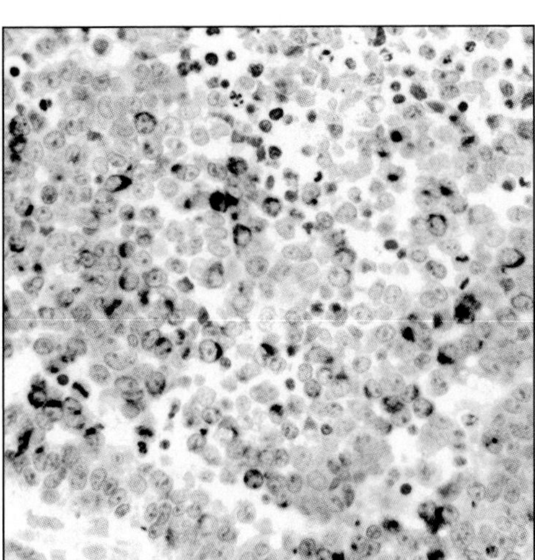
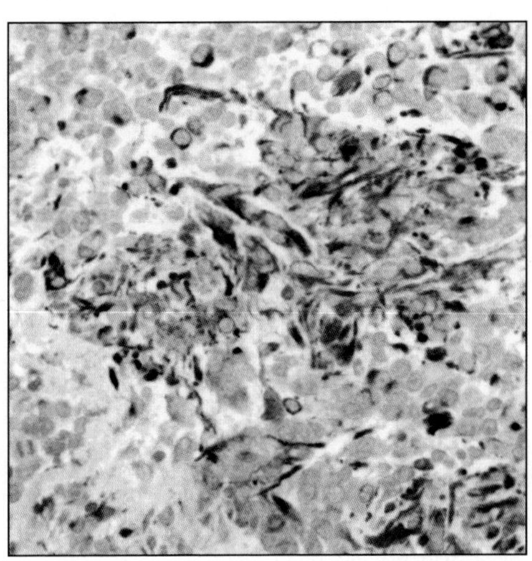

***(Left)** Immunohistochemical staining for neurofilament protein can be positive in some AT/RTs along with other markers of neuronal differentiation. **(Right)** Immunohistochemical staining for vimentin is often diffusely and strongly positive in AT/RT.*

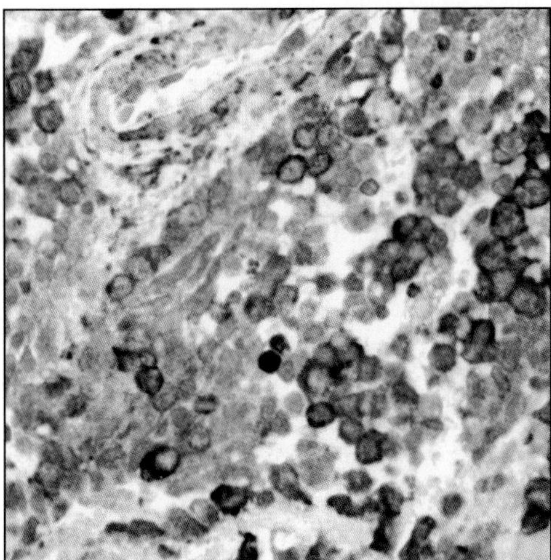
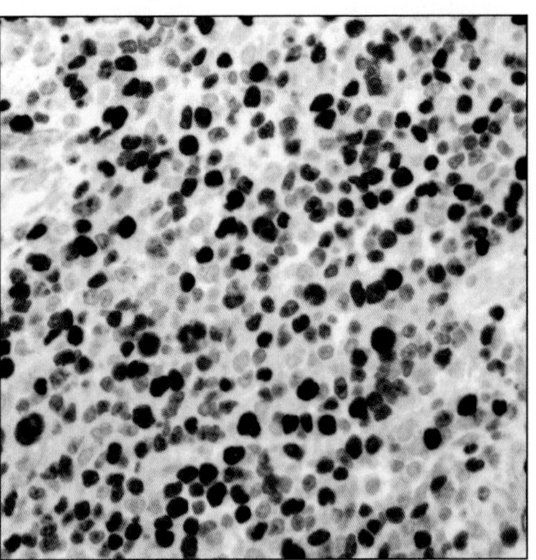

***(Left)** Immunohistochemical staining for smooth muscle actin can be positive in some areas. **(Right)** Immunohistochemical staining for Ki-67 shows a MIB-1 proliferation index that is characteristically very high, often more than 50%.*

PROTOCOL FOR BRAIN/SPINAL CORD TUMOR SPECIMENS

Brain/Spinal Cord

Biopsy/Resection

*History of Previous Tumor/Familial Syndrome

*___ None known

*___ Known (specify, if known: ___________________________)

*___ Not specified

Specimen Type/Procedure

___ Open biopsy

___ Resection

___ Stereotactic biopsy

___ Other (specify): ___________________________

___ Not specified

Specimen Handling (check all that apply)

___ Squash/smear/touch preparation

___ Frozen section

___ Tissue for electron microscopy

___ Frozen tissue

___ Unfrozen for routine permanent paraffin sections

___ Other (specify): ___________________________

___ Not specified

*Specimen Size

*___ Greatest dimension: _________ cm

*___ Additional dimensions: _________ x _________ cm (for fragmented tissue, aggregate size may be given)

*___ Cannot be determined

Laterality

___ Right

___ Left

___ Bilateral

___ Not specified

___ Not applicable

Tumor Site (check all that apply)

___ Skull

*Specify further (e.g., frontal, parietal, temporal, occipital), if known: ___________________________

___ Dura

*Specify further (e.g., cerebral [convexity/lobe, falx, tentorium, sphenoid wing, skull base, other], spinal, or other), if known: ___________________________

___ Leptomeninges

*Specify further (e.g., cerebral [convexity/lobe], spinal, or other), if known: ___________________________

___ Brain/cerebrum

*Specify lobe(s) (e.g., frontal, temporal, parietal, occipital), if known: ___________________________

___ Brain, other

___ Basal ganglia

___ Thalamus

___ Hypothalamus

___ Pineal

___ Cerebellum

___ Cerebellopontine angle

___ Suprasellar

___ Sella

___ Other (specify, if known: ___________________________)

___ Cranial nerve

*Specify I-XII, if known: _________

___ Ventricle
*Specify lateral, 3rd, 4th, cerebral aqueduct, if known: ___________________________
___ Brainstem
*Specify midbrain, pons, or medulla, if known: ___________________________
___ Spine (vertebral column)
*Specify bony level (e.g., C5, T2, L3), if known: ___________________________
___ Spinal cord
*Specify bony level (e.g., C5, T2, L3), if known: ___________________________
*Specify spinal location (e.g., extradural, intradural-extramedullary, intramedullary, conus medullaris filum terminale), if known: ___________________________
___ Spinal nerve root(s)
*Specify bony level (e.g., C5, T2, L3), if known: ___________________________
*Specify location (e.g., intradural, foramen), if known: ___________________________
___ Cranial or peripheral nerve
*Specify site, if known: ___________________________
___ Ganglion
*Specify site, if known: ___________________________
___ Other (specify): ___________________________
___ Not specified

Histologic Type and Grade (Applicable World Health Organization [WHO] Classification and Grade) (check all that apply)

Astrocytic tumors
___ Pilocytic astrocytoma (WHO grade I)
___ Pilomyxoid astrocytoma (WHO grade II)
___ Subependymal giant cell astrocytoma (WHO grade II)
___ Pleomorphic xanthoastrocytoma (WHO grade II)
___ Pleomorphic xanthoastrocytoma with anaplastic features (WHO grade not assigned)
___ Diffuse astrocytoma (WHO grade II)
  ___ Fibrillary astrocytoma (WHO grade II)
  ___ Protoplasmic astrocytoma (WHO grade II)
  ___ Gemistocytic astrocytoma (WHO grade II)
___ Anaplastic astrocytoma (WHO grade III)
___ Glioblastoma (WHO grade IV)
  ___ Giant cell glioblastoma (WHO grade IV)
  ___ Gliosarcoma (WHO grade IV)
___ Gliomatosis cerebri (usually WHO grade III; diagnosis requires clinical-pathological correlation)
___ Astrocytoma, not otherwise characterized (WHO grades I-IV)

Oligodendroglial tumors
___ Oligodendroglioma (WHO grade II)
___ Anaplastic oligodendroglioma (WHO grade III)

Oligoastrocytic tumors (mixed glioma)
___ Oligoastrocytoma (WHO grade II)
___ Anaplastic oligoastrocytoma (WHO grade III)

Ependymal tumors
___ Subependymoma (WHO grade I)
___ Myxopapillary ependymoma (WHO grade I)
___ Ependymoma (WHO grade II)
  ___ Cellular ependymoma (WHO grade II)
  ___ Papillary ependymoma (WHO grade II)
  ___ Clear cell ependymoma (WHO grade II)
  ___ Tanycytic ependymoma (WHO grade II)
___ Anaplastic ependymoma (WHO grade III)

Choroid plexus tumors
___ Choroid plexus papilloma (WHO grade I)

PROTOCOL FOR BRAIN/SPINAL CORD TUMOR SPECIMENS

____ Atypical choroid plexus papilloma (WHO grade II)
____ Choroid plexus carcinoma (WHO grade III)

Other neuroepithelial tumors

____ Astroblastoma (WHO grade not assigned)
____ Chordoid glioma of 3rd ventricle (WHO grade II)
____ Angiocentric glioma (WHO grade I)

Neuronal and mixed neuronal-glial tumors

____ Dysplastic gangliocytoma of cerebellum (Lhermitte-Duclos) (WHO grade I)
____ Desmoplastic infantile astrocytoma/ganglioglioma (WHO grade I)
____ Dysembryoplastic neuroepithelial tumor (WHO grade I)
____ Gangliocytoma (WHO grade I)
____ Ganglioglioma (WHO grade I)
____ Anaplastic ganglioglioma (WHO grade III)
____ Central neurocytoma (WHO grade II)
____ Extraventricular neurocytoma (WHO grade II)
____ Cerebellar liponeurocytoma (WHO grade II)
____ Papillary glioneuronal tumor (PGNT) (WHO grade I)
____ Rosette-forming glioneuronal tumor of 4th ventricle (RGNT) (WHO grade I)
____ Paraganglioma of spinal cord (WHO grade I)

Tumors of pineal region

Pineal parenchymal tumors
- ____ Pineocytoma (WHO grade I)
- ____ Pineal parenchymal tumor of intermediate differentiation (WHO II-III)
- ____ Pineoblastoma (WHO grade IV)

____ Papillary tumor of pineal region (WHO grade II-III)

Embryonal tumors

____ Medulloblastoma, not otherwise characterized (WHO grade IV)
- ____ Desmoplastic/nodular medulloblastoma (WHO grade IV)
- ____ Medulloblastoma with extensive nodularity (WHO grade IV)
- ____ Anaplastic medulloblastoma (WHO grade IV)
- ____ Large cell medulloblastoma (WHO grade IV)

____ Central nervous system (CNS) primitive neuroectodermal tumor (PNET) (WHO grade IV)
- ____ Medulloepithelioma (WHO grade IV)
- ____ Neuroblastoma (WHO grade IV)
- ____ Ganglioneuroblastoma (WHO grade IV)
- ____ Ependymoblastoma (WHO grade IV)

____ Atypical teratoid/rhabdoid tumor (WHO grade IV)

Tumors of cranial and paraspinal nerves

____ Schwannoma (WHO grade I)
- ____ Cellular (WHO grade I
- ____ Plexiform (WHO grade I)
- ____ Melanotic (WHO grade I)

____ Neurofibroma (WHO grade I)
- ____ Plexiform (WHO grade I)

____ Perineurioma (WHO grade I)
- ____ Intraneural perineurioma (WHO grade I)
- ____ Soft tissue perineurioma (WHO grade I)

____ Ganglioneuroma (WHO grade I)
____ Malignant peripheral nerve sheath tumor (MPNST) (WHO grade II-IV)
- ____ Epithelioid (WHO grade II-IV)
- ____ MPNST with divergent mesenchymal &/or epithelial differentiation (WHO grade II-IV)

Tumors of meninges/meningothelial cells

____ Meningioma (WHO grade I)
- ____ Meningothelial (WHO grade I)

____ Fibrous (fibroblastic) (WHO grade I)
____ Transitional (mixed) (WHO grade I)
____ Psammomatous (WHO grade I)
____ Angiomatous (WHO grade I)
____ Microcystic (WHO grade I)
____ Secretory (WHO grade I)
____ Lymphoplasmacyte-rich (lymphoplasmacytic) (WHO grade I)
____ Metaplastic (WHO grade I)
____ Atypical meningioma (WHO grade II)
____ Clear cell meningioma (WHO grade II)
____ Chordoid meningioma (WHO grade II)
____ Anaplastic meningioma (WHO grade III)
____ Papillary meningioma (WHO grade III)
____ Rhabdoid meningioma (WHO grade III)
____ Other (specify): __________________________

Mesenchymal (nonmeningothelial) tumors

____ Lipoma
____ Angiolipoma
____ Hibernoma
____ Liposarcoma (intracranial)
____ Solitary fibrous tumor
____ Fibrosarcoma
____ Malignant fibrous histiocytoma
____ Leiomyoma
____ Leiomyosarcoma
____ Rhabdomyoma
____ Rhabdomyosarcoma
____ Chondroma
____ Chondrosarcoma
____ Osteosarcoma
____ Osteochondroma
____ Hemangioma
____ Epithelioid hemangioendothelioma
____ Hemangiopericytoma
____ Angiosarcoma
____ Kaposi sarcoma
____ Chordoma
____ Mesenchymal, nonmeningothelial tumor, other (specify type): __________________________
____ Sarcoma, primary CNS (specify type, if possible): __________________________

Primary melanotic tumors

____ Diffuse melanocytosis
____ Melanocytoma
____ Malignant melanoma
____ Meningeal melanomatosis

Tumors of uncertain histogenesis

____ Hemangioblastoma (WHO grade I)

Lymphoma and hematopoietic tumors

____ Malignant lymphoma (specify type, if possible): __________________________
____ Plasmacytoma
____ Granulocytic sarcoma
____ Hematopoietic neoplasm, other (specify type, if possible): __________________________

Germ cell tumors

____ Germinoma
____ Embryonal carcinoma

PROTOCOL FOR BRAIN/SPINAL CORD TUMOR SPECIMENS

____ Yolk sac tumor
____ Choriocarcinoma
____ Teratoma, mature
____ Teratoma, immature
____ Teratoma with malignant transformation
____ Malignant mixed germ cell tumor
Specify components, e.g., germinoma, embryonal, yolk sac, choriocarcinoma, teratoma: ____________

Tumors of sellar region
____ Craniopharyngioma, adamantinomatous (WHO grade I)
____ Craniopharyngioma, papillary (WHO grade I)
____ Granular cell tumor (WHO grade I)
____ Pituicytoma (WHO grade I)
____ Spindle cell oncocytoma (WHO grade I)
____ Pituitary adenoma
Specify nonfunctional or hormone expression (if known): ____________
____ Pituitary carcinoma
____ Pituitary hyperplasia
____ Other (specify): ____________

Other/nonclassifiable
____ Other(s) (specify): ____________
____ Malignant neoplasm, type cannot be determined

Histologic Grade (WHO histologic grade)

____ Not applicable
____ Cannot be determined
____ WHO grade I
____ WHO grade II
____ WHO grade III
____ WHO grade IV
____ WHO grade not assigned
____ Other (specify): ____________

Margins (for resections of malignant peripheral nerve sheath tumors only)

____ Cannot be assessed
____ Margins not involved by tumor
____ Margins involved by tumor
*Specify, if possible: ____________

**Ancillary Studies (check all that apply)*

*____ None performed
*____ Immunohistochemistry (specify): ____________
*____ Electron microscopy
*____ Molecular genetic studies (specify): ____________
*____ 1p deletion identified
*____ 1p deletion not identified
*____ 19q deletion identified
*____ 19q deletion not identified
*____ Other (specify): ____________
*____ Other (specify): ____________

**Additional Pathologic Findings*

*Specify: ____________

**Data elements with asterisks are not required for accreditation purposes for the Commission on Cancer. These elements may be clinically important but are not yet validated or regularly used in patient management. Alternatively, the necessary data may not be available to the pathologist at the time of pathologic assessment of this specimen. Adapted with permission from College of American Pathologists, "Protocol for the Examination of Specimens from Patients with Tumors of the Brain/Spinal Cord." Web posting date June 2008; protocol effective date: February 2009, www.cap.org.*

Endocrine

Neoplasm, Benign

Neoplasm, Malignant Primary

Protocol for the Examination of Specimens from Patients with Tumors of the Thyroid Gland

Protocol for the Examination of Specimens from Patients with Carcinoma of the Adrenal Gland

Protocol for the Examination of Specimens from Patients with Neurobolastoma

GANGLIONEUROMA

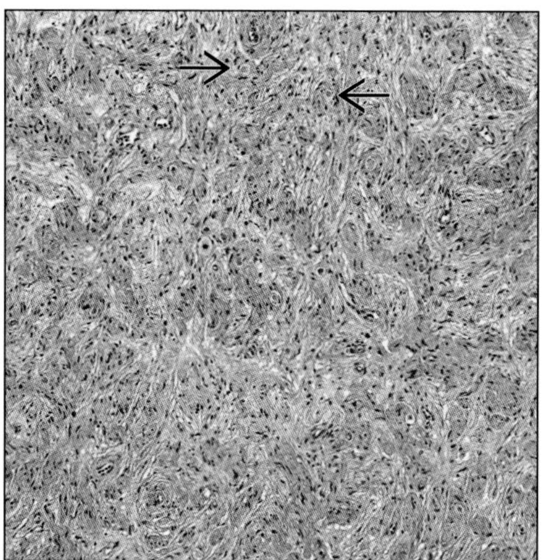

Low-power view of this ganglioneuroma (GN) shows a background of Schwann cells (spindled wavy cells in bundles) with scattered mature ganglion cells ⮕.

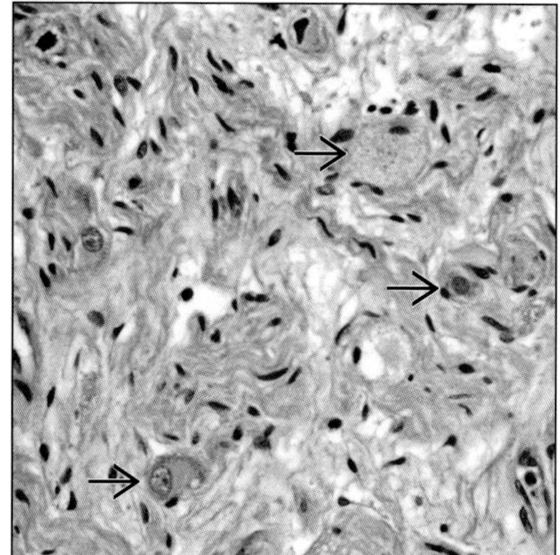

High-power view of a GN shows mature ganglion cells ⮕ with abundant eosinophilic to amphophilic cytoplasm, an eccentric nucleus, and prominent nucleolus; they are surrounded by Schwann cells.

TERMINOLOGY

Abbreviations

- Ganglioneuroma (GN)

Synonyms

- Schwannian stroma-dominant neuroblastic tumor

Definitions

- Most differentiated tumor on maturational spectrum of peripheral neuroblastic tumors

ETIOLOGY/PATHOGENESIS

Developmental Anomaly

- De novo tumor most common
- Therapy-induced maturation of preexisting neuroblastoma
  - Occurs in primary and metastatic sites

CLINICAL ISSUES

Epidemiology

- Age
  - Older than 10 years
- Gender
  - Male = female

Site

- Most common
  - Posterior mediastinum
  - Retroperitoneum
- Less common
  - Adrenal gland
  - Skin
  - GI tract

Presentation

- Commonly asymptomatic
- Rarely can present with
  - Hypertension
  - Watery diarrhea
  - Hypokalemia
  - Virilization
  - Sweating
- Associated syndromes/diseases include
  - Cowden syndrome
  - Tuberous sclerosis
  - Juvenile polyposis
  - Neurofibromatosis type 1
  - Multiple endocrine neoplasia type 2B

Laboratory Tests

- Urinary or serum catecholamines elevated in up to 40% of patients
  - More common if tumor is very large
  - Very high levels should prompt search for neuroblastomatous foci

Treatment

- Surgical approaches
  - Excision usually curative

Prognosis

- Generally benign
- Rarely can undergo malignant transformation
  - Usually resembles malignant peripheral nerve sheath tumor

MACROSCOPIC FEATURES

General Features

- Well circumscribed
- Fibrous capsule
- Gray to yellow cut surface

GANGLIONEUROMA

Key Facts

Terminology

- Most differentiated tumor on maturational spectrum of neuroblastic tumors

Clinical Issues

- Patients older than 10 years
- Posterior mediastinum most common site
- Surgical excision usually curative

Microscopic Pathology

- Maturing GN: Spectrum of maturation of ganglion cells
- Mature GN: Fully mature ganglion cells

Top Differential Diagnoses

- Ganglioneuroblastoma, intermixed
- Neurofibroma

MICROSCOPIC PATHOLOGY

Histologic Features

- No mitoses
- Rarely may have adipose tissue
- Ganglion cells may be pigmented

International Neuroblastoma Pathology Classification

- **Maturing GN**
  - Predominantly schwannian stroma
  - Scattered collections of differentiating neuroblasts, maturing ganglion cells, and fully mature ganglion cells
    - Neuroblastic elements do not form nests; they are individual cells
- **Mature GN**
  - Typical ganglioneuroma
  - Varying numbers of fully mature ganglion cells and Schwann cells in bundles
  - Variable amounts of collagen in bundles
  - Lymphocytic infiltrate common
    - May need immunohistochemistry to rule out neuroblastomatous component

ANCILLARY TESTS

Molecular Genetics

- GN does not show *N-Myc* amplification

DIFFERENTIAL DIAGNOSIS

Ganglioneuroblastoma, Intermixed

- Nests of neuroblastic elements
  - Whereas in maturing GN, neuroblastic elements are present as single cells

Neurofibroma

- Ganglion cells may be widely scattered and hard to find in small biopsies of GN

SELECTED REFERENCES

1. Bacci C et al: Multiple spinal ganglioneuromas in a patient harboring a pathogenic NF1 mutation. Clin Genet. 77(3):293-7, 2010
2. Dai X et al: Multiple ganglioneuromas: a report of a case and review of the ganglioneuromas. Clin Neuropathol. 28(3):193-6, 2009
3. Gershon TR et al: Enteric neural crest differentiation in ganglioneuromas implicates Hedgehog signaling in peripheral neuroblastic tumor pathogenesis. PLoS One. 4(10):e7491, 2009
4. Moon SB et al: Vasoactive intestinal polypeptide-producing ganglioneuromatosis involving the entire colon and rectum. J Pediatr Surg. 44(3):e19-21, 2009
5. Patterson AR et al: Ganglioneuroma of the mandible resulting from metastasis of neuroblastoma. Int J Oral Maxillofac Surg. 38(2):196-8, 2009
6. Zugor V et al: Retroperitoneal ganglioneuroma in childhood--a presentation of two cases. Pediatr Neonatol. 50(4):173-6, 2009

IMAGE GALLERY

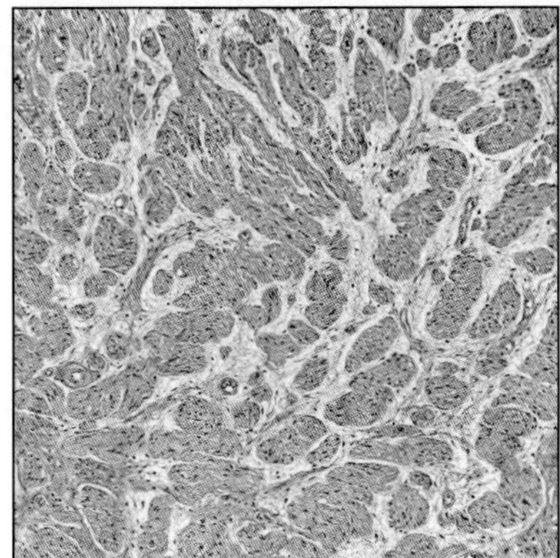

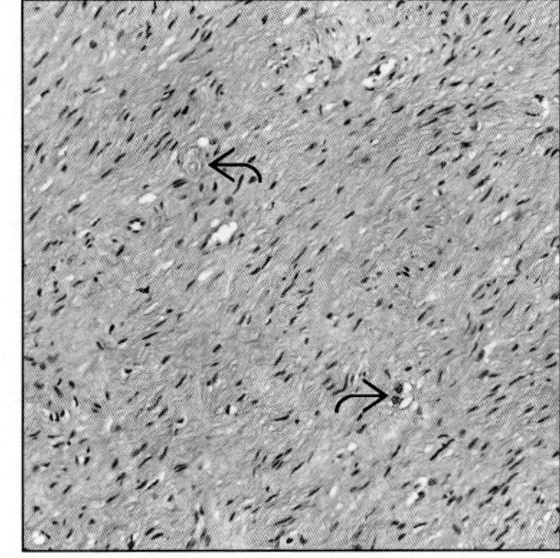

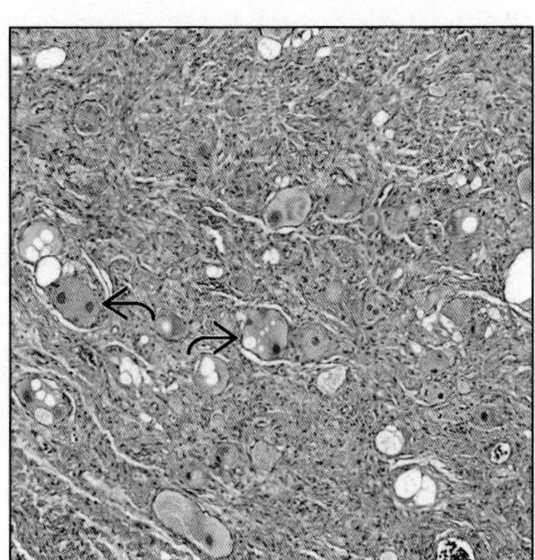

(Left) *This GN has neurofibroma-like features (spindled wavy cells within a myxoid type matrix). Careful examination will reveal ganglion cells.* ***(Center)*** *The schwannian stroma in GN may be dense and intermixed with collagen. Mature ganglion cells are still identified ➙.* ***(Right)*** *The mature ganglion cells in a GN may be quite large and may be binucleate ➙.*

ADRENAL CORTICAL ADENOMA

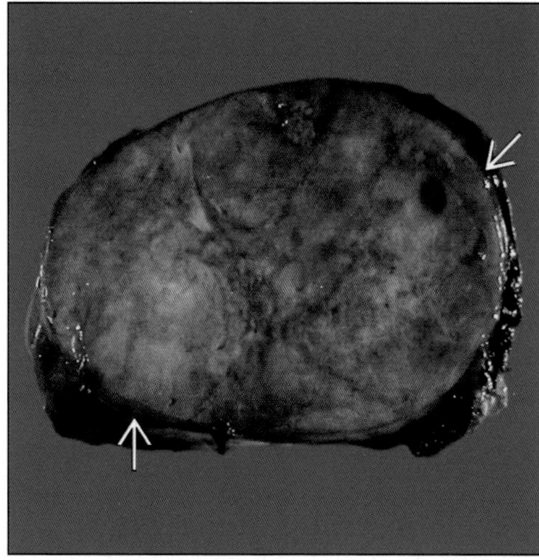

Gross photograph shows an encapsulated ➔, large adrenal cortical adenoma almost replacing the entire adrenal gland. The cut surface is marbled yellow-brown and free of necrosis and hemorrhage.

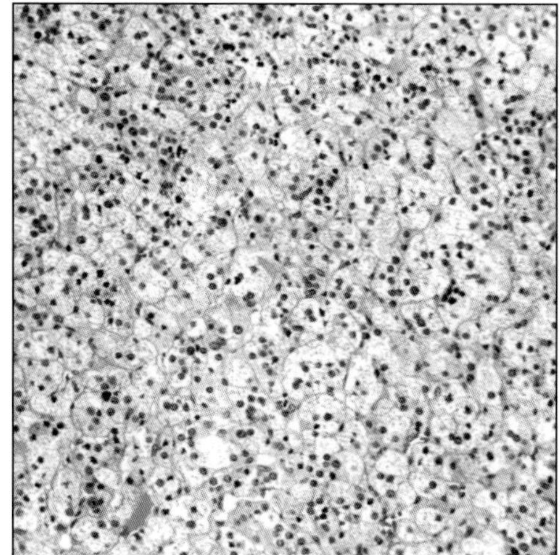

H&E stained section of adrenal gland adenoma shows sheets of bland cells with vacuolated, clear cytoplasm and uniform round nuclei.

TERMINOLOGY

Abbreviations

- Adrenal cortical adenoma (ACA)

Definitions

- Benign tumor of adrenal gland cell origin
- Cortical adenomas are functionally heterogeneous group of benign neoplasms that can differentiate toward any of the cortical layers
  - Most ACAs are nonfunctional in adults
  - In children, functional tumors are more common
  - Tumors can be associated with overproduction of glucocorticoids (Cushing syndrome), mineralocorticoids (Conn syndrome), or androgenic/estrogenic steroids (androgenital syndrome)
    - Tumors associated with Cushing syndrome and Conn syndrome are typically unilateral
    - Benign cortical tumors may be associated with syndromes of virilization or feminization, but presence of pure androgenital syndrome, particularly feminization, should raise possibility of malignancy
- Adrenal incidentaloma
  - Incidentally found structure in adrenal gland during abdominal examination with use of imaging methods
  - Autopsy series show 10-20% incidence

ETIOLOGY/PATHOGENESIS

Associated Abnormalities

- Multiple endocrine neoplasia syndromes (MEN)

CLINICAL ISSUES

Epidemiology

- Incidence
  - Most common adrenal tumor of all incidentalomas
    - Incidence increases in patients with diabetes or hypertension
    - Occurs in up to 9% of population (post-mortem data)
- Age
  - Prevalence of ACA increases with age
    - Peak at 60-69 years and decreasing thereafter
  - Adenomas associated with Cushing syndrome
    - 20% of cases occur before puberty
    - 80% of patients are female
  - Adenomas associated with Conn syndrome
  - Virilizing adenomas
    - 50% of cases occur before puberty
    - 80% of patients are female
- Gender
  - M = F

Presentation

- Most common signs/symptoms
  - Asymptomatic incidental CT imaging finding
    - More common in adult population
  - Cushing syndrome: Moon facies, truncal obesity, purple striae, and buffalo hump
  - Conn syndrome: Hypertension and weakness
  - Virilization in females or feminization in males

Laboratory Tests

- Tumors associated with overproduction of glucocorticoids (Cushing syndrome)
  - Low baseline secretion of ACTH (corticotropin)
  - Lack of suppressibility of cortisol secretion after 1 mg dexamethasone
    - Confirm with serum ACTH concentration and high-dose dexamethasone suppression test
  - Supranormal 24-hour urinary cortisol excretion

ADRENAL CORTICAL ADENOMA

Key Facts

Terminology

- Cortical adenomas are functionally heterogeneous group of benign neoplasms that can differentiate toward any of the cortical layers
- Tumors can be associated with overproduction of glucocorticoids (Cushing syndrome), mineralocorticoids (Conn syndrome), or androgenic/ estrogenic steroids (androgenital syndrome)

Clinical Issues

- Prevalence of ACA increases with age
- Surgical excision is primary treatment for hyperfunctioning ACAs
- No treatment is undertaken when patient is asymptomatic and adenoma is nonfunctional

Macroscopic Features

- Presents as sharply circumscribed or encapsulated masses

Microscopic Pathology

- Histologic appearance cannot reliably predict accompanying clinical presentation

Diagnostic Checklist

- Histologic appearance of adrenal cortical adenoma cannot be used to predict associated endocrine abnormality or syndrome
- Most frequent endocrine abnormality associated with adrenal cortical adenoma is primary hyperaldosteronism followed by Cushing syndrome

  - Disturbed cortisol circadian rhythm
  - Blunted plasma ACTH responses to corticotropin-releasing hormone
- Tumors associated with overproduction of mineralocorticoids (Conn syndrome)
  - Excessive amount of secreted aldosterone results in the following
    - Urinary loss of potassium
    - Retention of sodium
    - Suppressed renin levels
    - Hypertension
    - Muscle weakness
  - Diagnosis should be suspected when hypokalemia is found in patient with hypertension
    - Confirm by demonstrating nonsuppressible aldosterone excretion in conjunction with normal cortisol excretion
    - Elevated ratio of plasma aldosterone to plasma renin activity

Treatment

- Surgical approaches
  - Surgical excision is primary treatment for hyperfunctioning ACAs
- No treatment is undertaken when patient is asymptomatic and adenoma is nonfunctional

Prognosis

- Excellent with incidentaloma and when nonfunctioning
- Hypersecretory ACAs are cured by surgical removal of involved adrenal gland

IMAGE FINDINGS

General Features

- Best diagnostic clue
  - CT is study of choice to confirm diagnosis of ACA
  - If suspect ACA alone, NECT is sufficient to confirm diagnosis
    - Attenuation < 10 Hounsfield units (HU) is diagnostic

Ultrasonographic Findings

- Grayscale ultrasound
  - May show mass lesion in suprarenal area
    - Right suprarenal mass seen more clearly than left side due to acoustic window provided by liver

MR Findings

- T1WI and T2WI show varied signal intensity
- Lipid-rich ACA
  - T1WI out of phase: ↑ signal drop-out (lipid-rich)
  - T1WI in phase: Hyperintense
- T1WI C+
  - During early phase, ACA shows enhancement
  - Delayed phase: > 50% washout is seen

CT Findings

- Nonenhanced CT
  - Smooth, well defined, round or oval in shape
  - Homogeneous soft tissue mass of 0-20 HU
  - Lipid-rich ACA (70% of cases)
    - Low attenuation (< 10 HU)
    - Characteristic and diagnostic of adenoma
  - Lipid-poor adrenal adenoma (30% of cases)
    - Attenuation varies from 10-30 HU
    - Difficult to differentiate from metastases on NECT
  - Cushing syndrome due to ACA
    - Remainder of ipsilateral gland and contralateral adrenal gland are atrophic due to ↓ ACTH levels
    - ↑ cortisol levels: Feedback inhibition of pituitary ACTH
  - Conn syndrome due to ACA
    - Remainder of ipsilateral gland and contralateral adrenal gland appear normal
  - Large adenomas
    - More heterogeneous than small adenomas
    - ± cystic degeneration, calcifications, hemorrhage
- Contrast-enhanced CT
  - Enhancing adrenal mass that "de-enhances" rapidly
    - During enhanced phase, attenuation varies between 40-50 HU
    - At 10 minutes, during delayed phase, attenuation decreasing to 20-25 HU

- Washout of adenoma: 10 minutes post injection > 50%
- Washout pattern of enhancement is diagnostic for adenoma
  - No follow-up is required if seen
  - Similar washout pattern is seen in lipid-rich and lipid-poor adenomas

MACROSCOPIC FEATURES

General Features

- Tumors associated with Cushing syndrome
  - On cross section, these adenomas vary from yellow to brown
    - Occasional examples of heavily pigmented (black) adenomas have been reported
  - Present as sharply circumscribed or encapsulated masses
  - Adjacent cortex and contralateral adrenal gland are atrophic due to suppression of pituitary ACTH secretion by tumor hormone secretion
- Adenomas associated with Conn syndrome
  - Characteristically bright yellow
    - Rarely, black adenomas have been associated with Conn syndrome
  - Often poorly demarcated from adjacent cortex
    - Pseudocapsule may be identified
- Virilizing adenomas
  - Sharply circumscribed or encapsulated
  - Pale-tan to brown on cross section
- Oncocytic ACAs
  - Dark tan to mahogany brown cut surface
- Nonfunctional adenomas
  - Yellow to brown in color
  - May be multicentric
  - Not associated with atrophy of normal cortical tissue
- Necrosis is rare in all types of cortical adenomas
- Cystic degeneration often occurs in larger tumors

Size

- Tumors associated with Cushing syndrome usually weigh 10-50 grams and measure 3-4 cm in average diameter
  - Examine with particular care to rule out malignancy when > 100 grams
- Adenomas associated with hyperaldosteronism (Conn syndrome) measure < 2 cm in diameter
  - Round to ovoid in configuration
- Virilizing adenomas are usually large and often weigh ≥ 1,000 grams
- Nonfunctional adenomas are small (usually < 3 cm)

MICROSCOPIC PATHOLOGY

Histologic Features

- Adenomas associated with Cushing syndrome
  - Most often composed of small nests, cords, or alveolar arrangements of vacuolated clear cells that most closely resemble those of normal fasciculata
  - Generally, adenoma cells (lipid-laden) are somewhat larger than normal cortical cells
  - Variable numbers of compact-type (lipid-depleted) cells are also evident
  - Black adenomas may be composed exclusively of lipochrome-rich compact cells that contain eosinophilic cytoplasm with prominent granular yellow-brown pigment (lipofuscin)
  - Nuclear to cytoplasmic ratio is generally low and mitotic activity is rare
  - A few single cells and small groups of cells may have enlarged hyperchromatic nuclei
  - Typically, nuclei are vesicular with small, distinct (dot-like) nucleoli
  - Occasional adenomas may exhibit considerable fibrosis
  - Larger adenomas may show foci of myelolipomatous change or calcification
  - Cortex adjacent to functional adenoma and in contralateral adrenal gland is typically atrophic
- Adenomas associated with Conn syndrome
  - Tumor cells are generally arranged in small nests and cords
  - Can resemble cells of glomerulosa, fasciculata, or reticularis or combine features of both glomerulosa and fasciculata (hybrid cells)
  - Fasciculata adjacent to aldosterone-secreting adenomas is of normal thickness
  - Hyperplasia of zona glomerulosa may also be present
  - In patients treated with spironolactone, some cells within adenoma may contain lamellated eosinophilic inclusions (spironolactone bodies) measuring up to 10 μm in diameter
    - Often demarcated from adjacent cytoplasm by halo
- Virilizing/feminizing adenomas
  - Smaller tumors have alveolar pattern of growth
  - Larger tumors tend to have more solid or diffuse growth patterns
  - Most tumor cells have low nuclear to cytoplasmic ratio
  - Single cells and small groups may exhibit nuclear enlargement and hyperchromasia
  - Cytoplasm is usually eosinophilic and granular
  - Sex steroid-producing adenomas are not associated with atrophy of adjacent cortex or contralateral adrenal gland
- Oncocytic ACAs
  - Cells with abundant granular eosinophilic cytoplasm
  - Focal marked nuclear pleomorphism
  - Nuclear pseudoinclusions may be seen
- Histologic appearance cannot reliably predict accompanying clinical presentation

ANCILLARY TESTS

Cytology

- Fine-needle aspiration biopsy specimens show round to polyhedral cells with round nuclei and foamy cytoplasm
- Numerous naked nuclei in background of granular to foamy material may be present

Histochemistry

- Oil red O
  - Reactivity: Positive
  - Staining pattern
    - Intracellular neutral lipid is positive
  - Stain must be performed on fresh frozen tissue
    - Alcohol fixation removes lipids

Cytogenetics

- Clonality studies using X-chromosome inactivation analysis have shown that some adenomas are clonal while others are polyclonal
  - Monoclonal adenomas are larger than polyclonal lesions and have higher prevalence of nuclear pleomorphism

PCR

- Activating mutations of exon 3 of β-catenin gene are frequent in ACAs

Electron Microscopy

- Adenomas associated with Cushing syndrome
  - Contain cells that most closely resemble cells of normal fasciculata or reticularis
  - Cytoplasm typically contains abundant smooth endoplasmic reticulum and variable numbers of lipid droplets
  - Mitochondria are round to ovoid and show predominance of forms with tubulovesicular or exclusively vesicular cristae
    - Lamelliform cristae may also be present
- Tumors associated with Conn syndrome
  - Mitochondria manifest tubular or vesicular cristae typical of zona glomerulosa
  - Spironolactone bodies most closely resemble myelin figures
- Virilizing/feminizing adenomas
  - Mitochondria are of tubulolamellar type
- Oncocytic ACA
  - Numerous, closely packed mitochondria

DIFFERENTIAL DIAGNOSIS

Nodular or Macronodular Hyperplasia

- Usually multiple nodules rather than single dominant nodule
- Adjacent cortex and contralateral adrenal gland will commonly appear hypertrophic
- Almost always bilateral, except for rare pigmented nodules, which are more commonly unilateral
- Usually asymptomatic and found incidentally
  - Treatment is typically medical rather than surgical management when presenting symptom is endocrine syndrome

Adrenal Cortical Carcinoma

- Usually large mass with gross evidence of hemorrhage and necrosis
- Infiltrative borders typically invading into surrounding tissue
- Tumor cells show marked pleomorphism and frequent mitotic activity
- Vascular or capsular invasion are common

Pheochromocytoma

- Arises from adrenal medulla with normal adrenal cortex stretched out over its cortex
- Red-brown in color with areas of hemorrhage or cystic degeneration if large
- Organoid growth pattern with nests of cells ("zellballen") and delicate vascular septae
- Immunohistochemistry
  - Immunoreactive for neurofilament, chromogranin, synaptophysin, and S100 (in sustentacular cell pattern)
  - Vimentin: Negative
- Active tumors present with signs and symptoms of excess norepinephrine and epinephrine, including intermittent hypertensive episodes
  - Characteristically associated with secretion of norepinephrine
- Electron microscopy shows cells with neurosecretory granules

DIAGNOSTIC CHECKLIST

Pathologic Interpretation Pearls

- Histologic appearance of adrenal cortical adenoma cannot be used to predict associated endocrine abnormality or syndrome
- Most frequent endocrine abnormality associated with adrenal cortical adenoma is primary hyperaldosteronism followed by Cushing syndrome
- Treatment is typically resection of adrenal gland containing adenoma

SELECTED REFERENCES

1. Ctvrtlík F et al: Differential diagnosis of incidentally detected adrenal masses revealed on routine abdominal CT. Eur J Radiol. 69(2):243-52, 2009
2. Kuruba R et al: Current management of adrenal tumors. Curr Opin Oncol. 20(1):34-46, 2008
3. McNicol AM: A diagnostic approach to adrenal cortical lesions. Endocr Pathol. 19(4):241-51, 2008
4. Tahar GT et al: Adrenocortical oncocytoma: a case report and review of literature. J Pediatr Surg. 43(5):E1-3, 2008

ADRENAL CORTICAL ADENOMA

Diagrammatic, Gross, and Radiologic Features

*(**Left**) Graphic shows a small lipid-rich mass ➔ within the adrenal gland. (**Right**) Gross photograph shows adrenal gland with an ovoid well-circumscribed mass ➔ arising within the adrenal cortex. The uninvolved cortex is compressed to 1 side ⇨.*

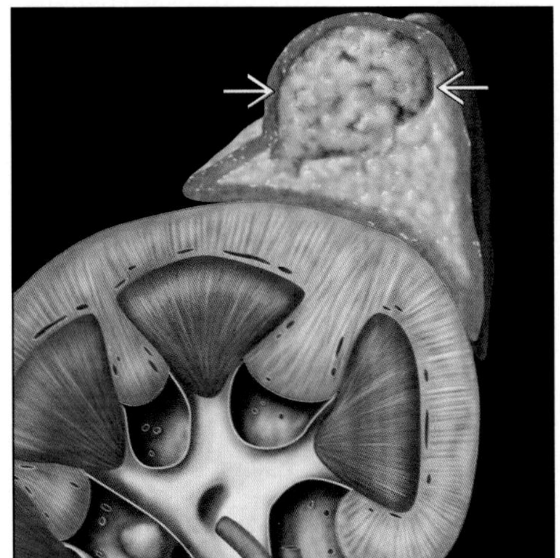

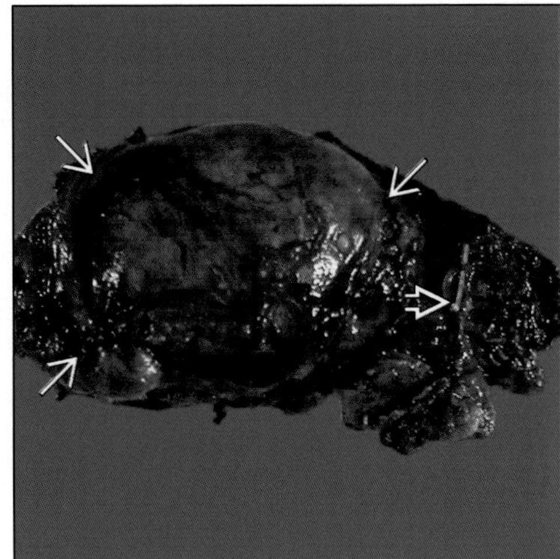

*(**Left**) Surgical photograph of a resected adenoma shows a 2 cm lipid-rich nodule ➔ within the adrenal gland. Note residual adrenal cortex beneath the nodule ⇨. (**Right**) Gross photograph shows an encapsulated adrenal cortical adenoma almost replacing the entire adrenal gland. The cut surface is yellow-brown and free of hemorrhage and necrosis. The residual adrenal gland is identified at the inferior portion of the specimen ➔.*

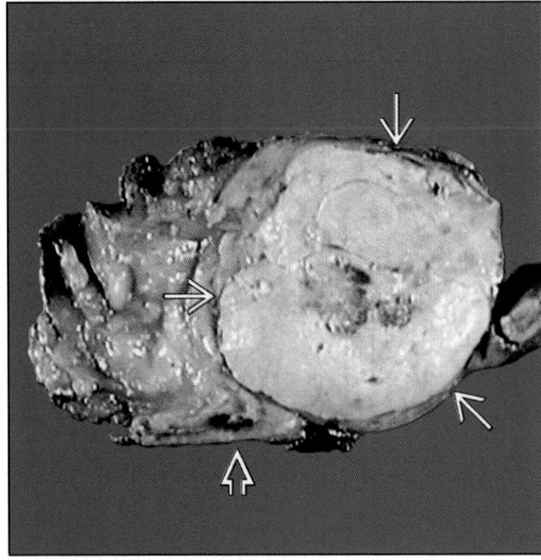

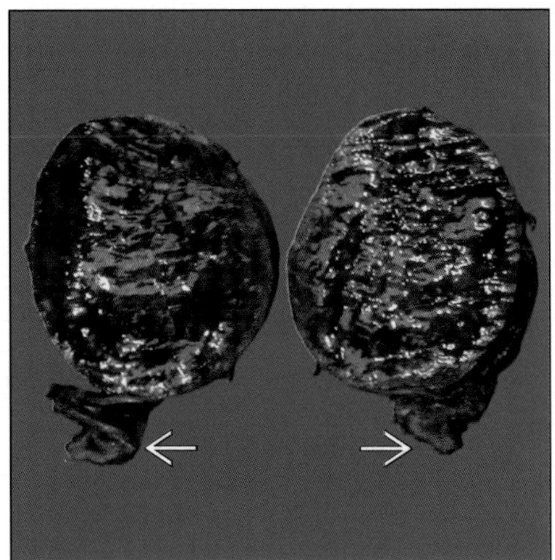

*(**Left**) Axial T1WI MR opposed phase GRE sequence shows bilateral, small adrenal masses ➔. (**Right**) Axial NECT shows a homogeneous low-density right adrenal adenoma ➔.*

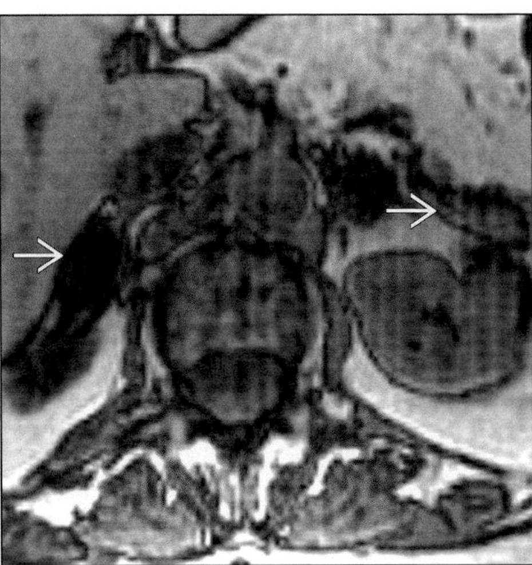

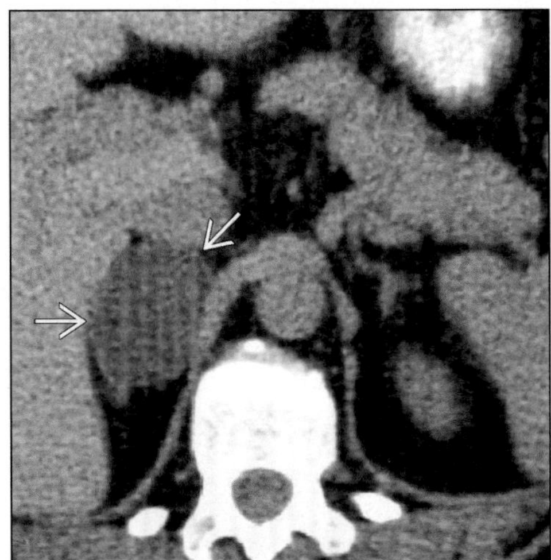

Microscopic Features

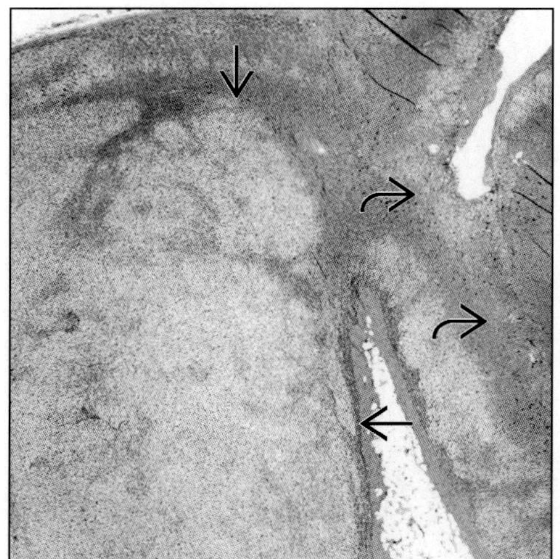

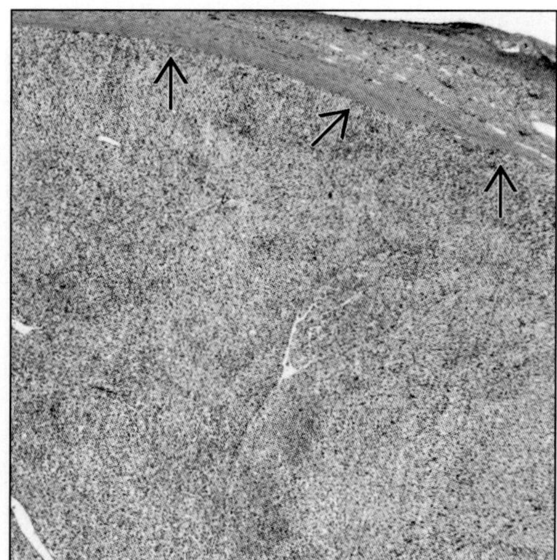

(Left) Low-power view shows a large nodule arising from the adrenal cortex ⇒. The uninvolved adrenal gland does not show significant compression ⇒. *(Right)* Low-power view of H&E stained section of adrenal cortical adenoma shows capsule ⇒.

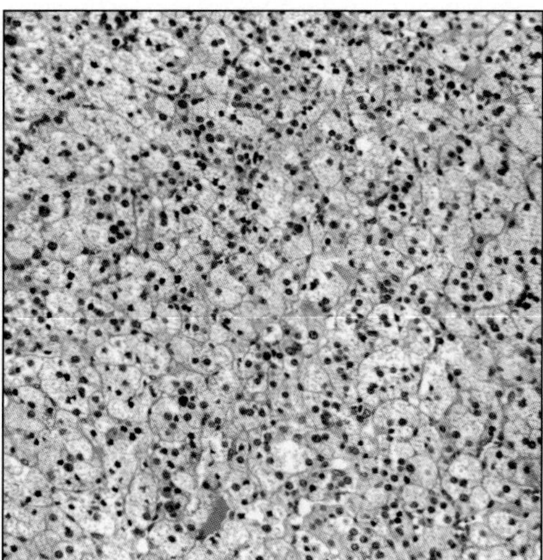

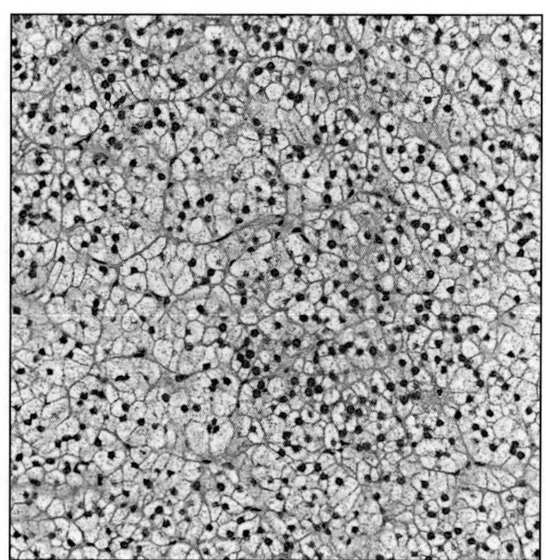

(Left) H&E stained section of adrenal cortical adenoma shows sheets of bland adrenal cortical-type cells with small, uniform nuclei and abundant vacuolated cytoplasm. Mitoses and necrosis are absent. *(Right)* H&E stained section shows an adrenal cortical adenoma from a patient with a clinical history of Cushing syndrome. Note the large population of vacuolated clear cells resembling the normal fasciculata of the adrenal cortex.

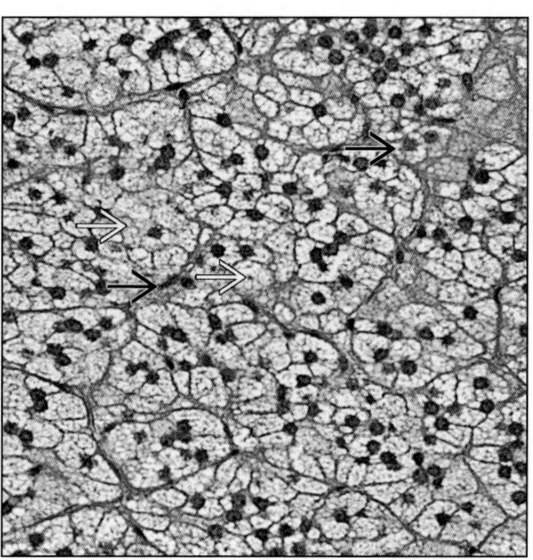

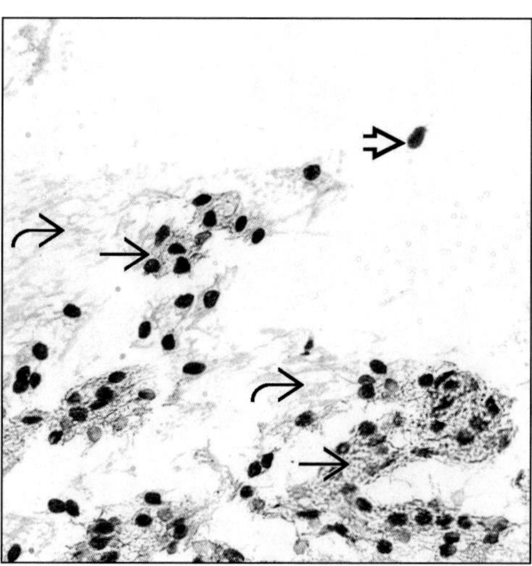

(Left) High-power view of H&E stained section shows vacuolated clear cells arranged in nests ⇒ and trabeculae. Note the lipid-depleted cells in the background ⇒. The nuclei are uniform in size and shape without significant pleomorphism. *(Right)* Touch prep of adrenal cortical adenoma shows polyhedral cells with round nuclei and foamy cytoplasm ⇒. Naked nuclei ⇒ are also present in a background of granular and foamy material ⇒.

ADRENAL CORTICAL ADENOMA

Differential Diagnosis

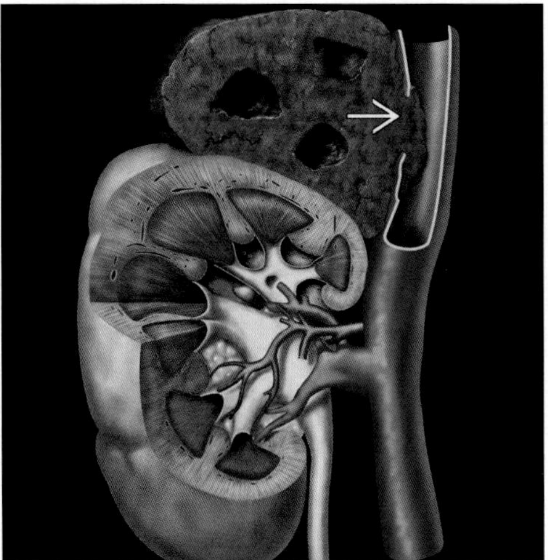

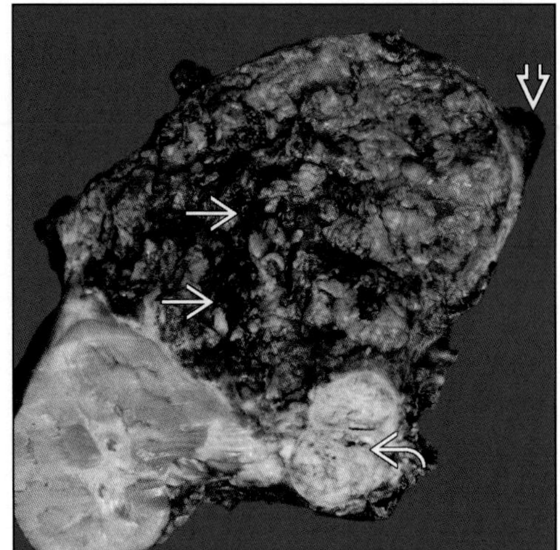

(Left) *Graphic shows large, hypervascular adrenal cortical carcinoma directly invading the inferior vena cava ➔.* ***(Right)*** *Gross photograph of adrenal cortical carcinoma shows almost complete replacement of the adrenal gland by a large tumor mass with areas of hemorrhage ➔ and necrosis ➔. Residual, compressed adrenal gland is identified ➔.*

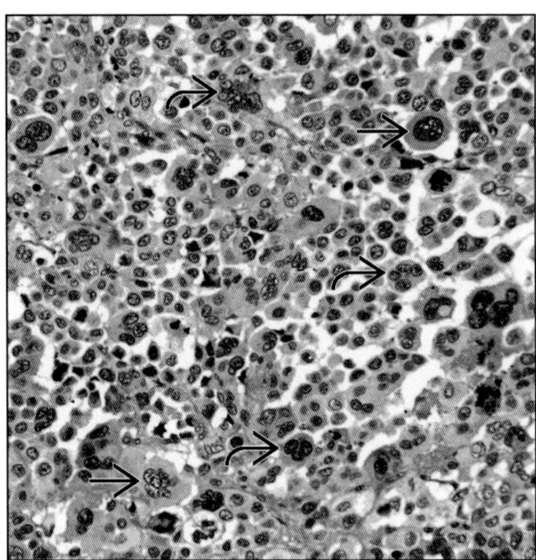

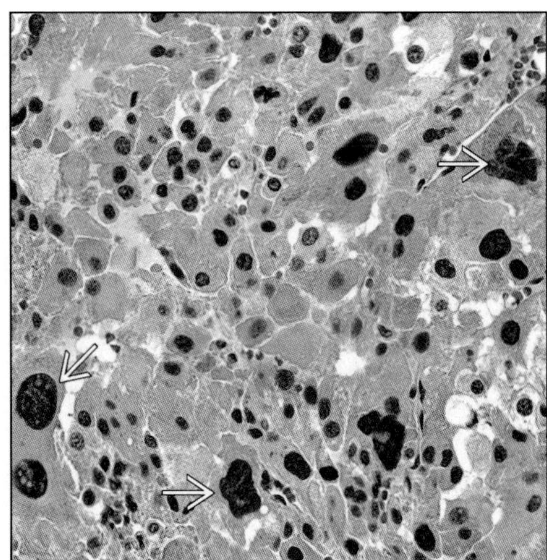

(Left) *H&E stained section of adrenal cortical carcinoma shows large pleomorphic ➔, some multinucleated ➔, tumor cells with eosinophilic cytoplasm and irregular cell borders. Prominent nucleoli are also readily identified.* ***(Right)*** *H&E stained section shows extreme nuclear pleomorphism on high power ➔ in this adrenal cortical carcinoma.*

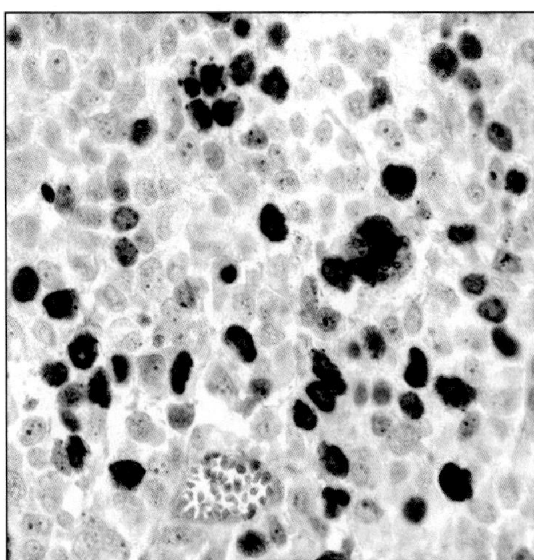

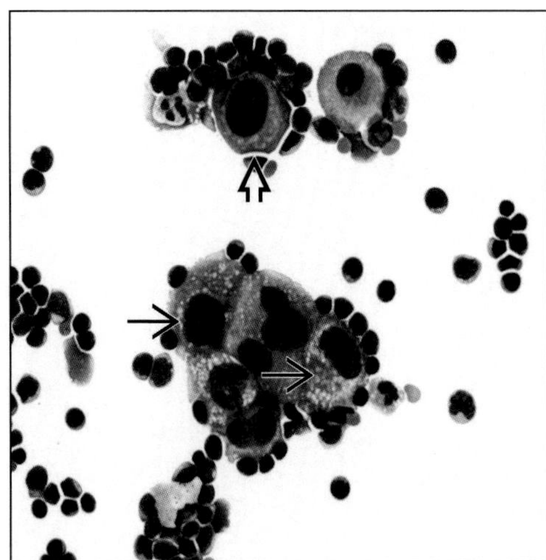

(Left) *Ki-67 (MIB-1) immunohistochemical stain shows nuclear staining in a number of cells, consistent with high mitotic index.* ***(Right)*** *Cytology of a fine needle aspiration from an adrenal cortical carcinoma shows large pleomorphic cells with large granular nuclei with irregular cell borders ➔ and vacuolated cytoplasm ➔.*

Differential Diagnosis

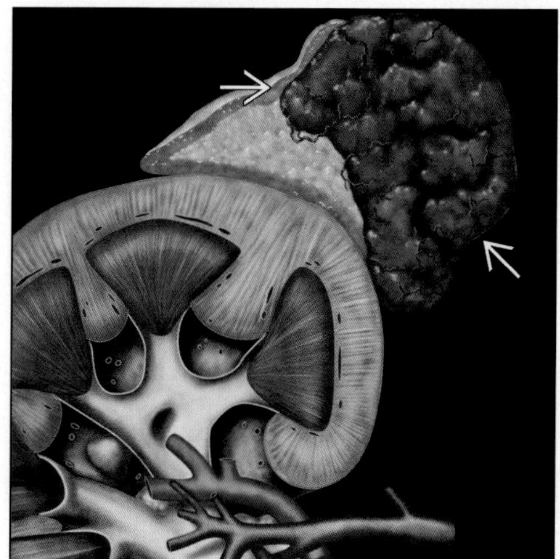

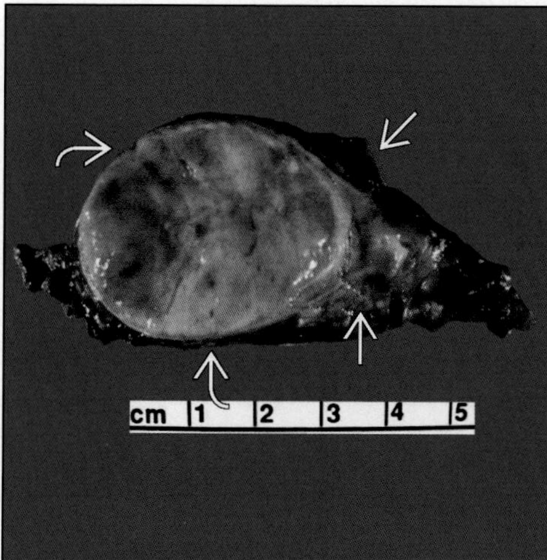

(Left) *Graphic shows a large, hypervascular, heterogeneous adrenal pheochromocytoma ➔.* ***(Right)*** *Gross photograph shows an ovoid, sharply circumscribed mass with a cut surface depicting a soft, variegated appearance with a tan-yellow to red-brown color ➔. Compressed adrenal cortex is present at 1 end of the specimen ➔.*

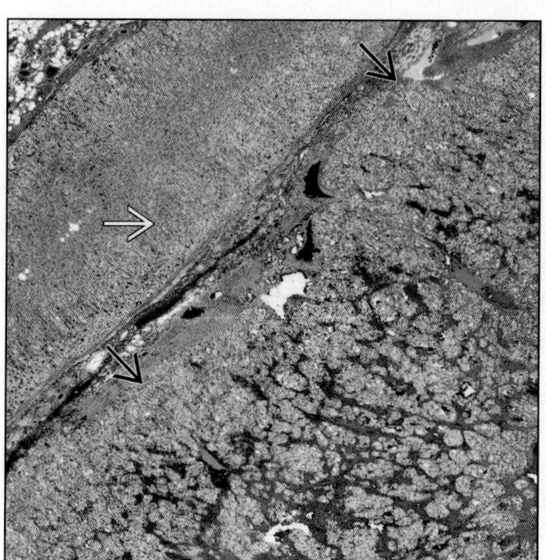

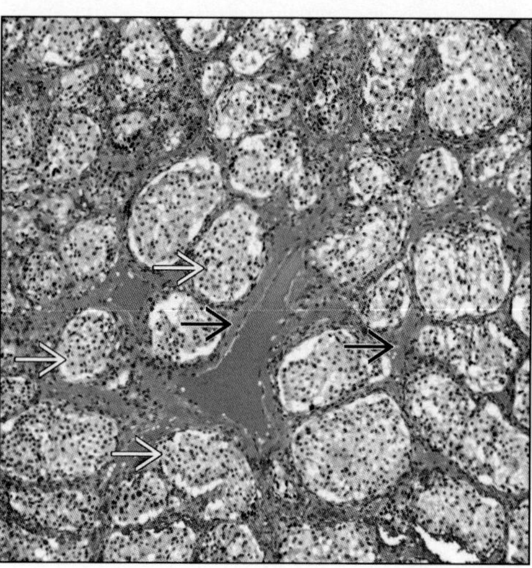

(Left) *H&E stained section shows nested tumor cells ➔ arising within the adrenal medulla adjacent to unremarkable adrenal cortex ➔.* ***(Right)*** *H&E stained section shows tumor cells arranged in well-defined nests ➔ called zellballen. The tumor nests are surrounded by thin strands of fibrovascular stroma ➔.*

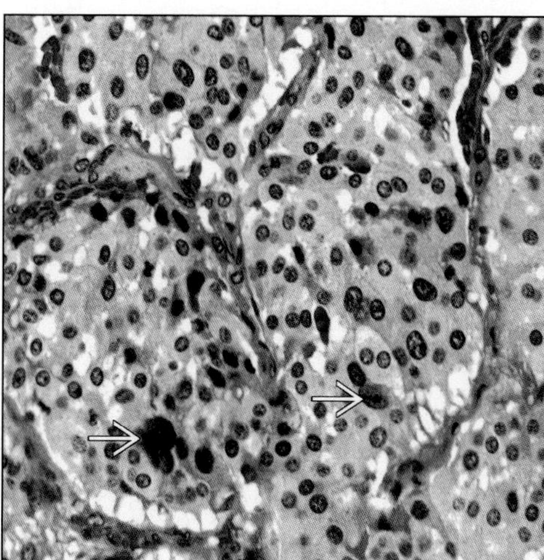

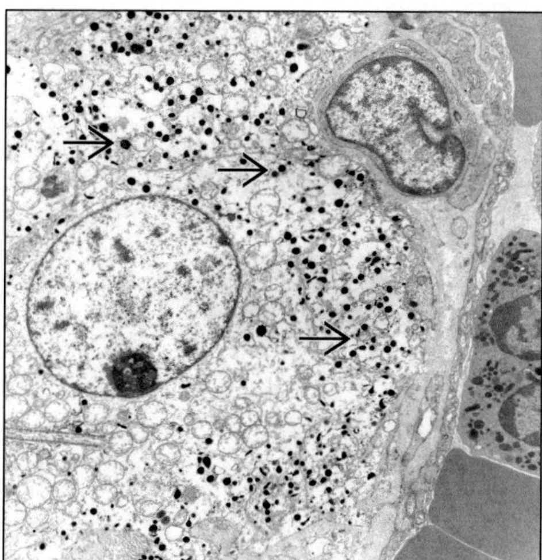

(Left) *High-power view of nested tumor cells shows a few cells with pleomorphic nuclei and irregular cell borders ➔.* ***(Right)*** *Electron micrograph shows numerous neurosecretory granules ➔ scattered throughout the cytoplasm of a pheochromocytoma tumor cell.*

FOLLICULAR ADENOMA

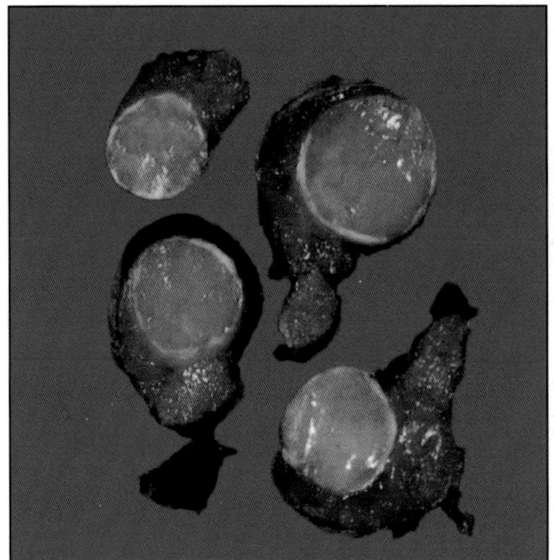

Cut surface of an encapsulated nodule shows lighter color than the background thyroid. A thick conspicuous capsule completely encircles the lesion as can be seen at several levels of dissection.

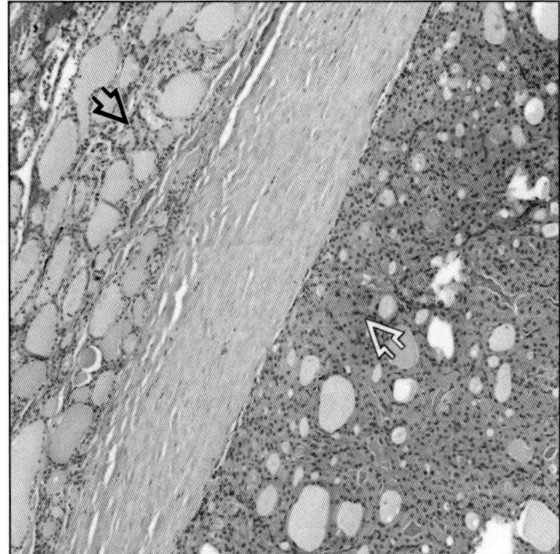

A thick fibrous capsule separates the normal thyroid tissue ➡ from the follicular adenoma ➡. Notice the distinct patterns and the sharp demarcation between the lesion and capsule.

TERMINOLOGY

Abbreviations

- Follicular adenoma (FA)

Synonyms

- Follicular thyroid adenoma (FTA)

Definitions

- Thyroid follicular cell-derived encapsulated benign neoplasm lacking diagnostic features of papillary thyroid carcinoma

ETIOLOGY/PATHOGENESIS

Environmental Exposure

- After radiation exposure
  - Gamma radiation during childhood
  - Follicular adenomas may arise < 10 years after exposure
  - May be associated with lymphocytic thyroiditis
  - Associated with other thyroid tumors
  - Age at diagnosis is usually 14 years younger than in patients with sporadic tumors
- In iodine-deficient areas
  - Patients in iodine-deficient areas are prone to have multiple adenomas
  - Follicular adenoma may be associated with follicular carcinoma
  - May be associated with nodular hyperplasia

As Part of Inherited Tumor Syndromes

- PTEN-hamartoma tumor syndrome (PHTS), Cowden disease, Bannayan-Riley-Ruvalcaba syndrome
  - Caused by germline mutation of *PTEN* gene in an autosomal dominant fashion
  - > 90% of individuals affected by PHTS manifest phenotype by age of 20 years
  - Affected individuals usually develop both benign and malignant tumors of breast, uterus, and thyroid
  - Affected individuals also develop multiple hamartomas of breast, colon, endometrium, and brain, and ganglioneuromatous proliferations
  - Thyroid tumors occur at younger age than sporadic tumors
  - May be associated with multiple follicular adenomas and follicular carcinomas
  - Often associated with multiple follicular adenomatous nodules
- Carney complex
  - Autosomal dominant disorder caused by mutations in *PRKAR1A* gene in 80% of affected families
  - < 750 cases have been identified as of 2010 (NIH Genetics Home Reference)
  - Carney complex (CNC) is defined as cardiac myxomas, multiple endocrine neoplasms, and spotty cutaneous pigmentation
  - Clinical manifestations can be numerous, and presentation is variable even within same kindred
  - Up to 75% of patients present with multiple thyroid nodules, most of which are FA
- Pendred syndrome
  - Autosomal recessive syndrome resulting from mutations in *SLC26A4 (PDS)* gene that codes for pendrin protein
  - Syndrome is characterized by bilateral sensorineural deafness, goiter, and hypothyroidism
  - > 100 mutations identified in *PDS* gene; most are family specific
  - Mutations in *PDS* gene lead to impaired iodine transport, which may cause subsequent goiter with possible hypothyroidism

CLINICAL ISSUES

Epidemiology

- Incidence
  - Incidence of thyroid nodules in children estimated at 1-1.5%

FOLLICULAR ADENOMA

Key Facts

Etiology/Pathogenesis

- Radiation exposure and iodine deficiency
- Inherited tumor syndromes: PTEN-hamartoma tumor syndrome (PHTS), Cowden disease, Bannayan-Riley-Ruvalcaba syndrome

Clinical Issues

- FA are common in areas of endemic goiter and iodine-deficient areas
- Occurs in all ages; mostly adults aged 20-50 years
- Most patients present with solitary nodule
- Multiple adenomas and association with adenomatous nodules are usually part of inherited tumor syndromes

Microscopic Pathology

- Histologic variants of FA
  - Microfollicular type
  - Macrofollicular type
  - Oncocytic type
  - Signet ring cell type
  - Adenoma with clear cells
  - Adenoma with bizarre nuclei
  - Atypical follicular adenoma

Top Differential Diagnoses

- Adenomatous nodules
- Follicular thyroid carcinoma
- Follicular variant of papillary thyroid carcinoma
- Parathyroid adenoma
- Medullary thyroid carcinoma
- Hyalinizing trabecular tumor

    - 50-70% of thyroid nodules in children are benign
  - FA is most common neoplasm of thyroid
  - FAs are common in areas of endemic goiter and iodine deficiency areas
- Age
  - Occurs in all ages; mostly adults aged 20-50 years
  - Occurs in younger age group when part of inherited nonmedullary thyroid tumor syndromes
- Gender
  - Female:male ratio of 6:1

Presentation

- Most patients present with solitary nodule
- Most adenomas lack uptake on iodine scans: Cold nodules
- Some adenomas can cause hyperthyroidism, so-called toxic adenomas, and take up iodine on scans
- Multiple adenomas and those associated with adenomatous nodules are usually part of inherited tumor syndromes

Treatment

- FAs are adequately treated by simple excision or lobectomy

Prognosis

- Behavior of these tumors is completely benign

IMAGE FINDINGS

Ultrasonographic Findings

- Ultrasound is best modality for initial evaluation of thyroid lesions
- Helpful in separation of single from multiple nodules (adenoma vs. adenomatoid nodules)
- Most FAs are single, solid, homogeneous masses with smooth borders and thin, well-defined, peripheral, echo-poor halo that represents the capsule
- Majority of FAs are isoechoic, but they can be hyper- or hypoechoic
- Pattern of peripheral blood vessels extending toward center of lesion is frequently present

MR Findings

- Often used in evaluation of recurrent tumors
- Nodule will appear as an iso- or hypointense lesion on T1WI and hyperintense on T2WI, with smooth regular margins
- Compression of adjacent normal gland can be seen

CT Findings

- Appears as solitary hypodense nodule
- Invasion and adenopathy can be evaluated
- Large FAs may show enhancement due to degeneration

MACROSCOPIC FEATURES

General Features

- Solitary nodule
- Can be multiple when part of a genetic syndrome
- Completely surrounded by thin sharp fibrous capsule
- Stands out from unaffected gland parenchyma
- Average size is 3 cm in diameter (range from 1-10 cm)
- Tan-gray to reddish brown cut surface, depending on cellularity and colloid content
- Secondary changes may occur in larger tumors
  - Hemorrhage
  - Degenerative changes
  - Cyst formation
  - Fibrosis and hyalinization

MICROSCOPIC PATHOLOGY

Histologic Features

- Encapsulated follicular-patterned neoplasm surrounded by well-defined fibrous capsule
- Variable architecture with different histologic patterns include
  - Normofollicular: Uniform-appearing follicles containing colloid
  - Macrofollicular: Large colloid-filled follicles
  - Microfollicular: Small follicles lined by flattened epithelial cells (a.k.a. fetal pattern)

FOLLICULAR ADENOMA

- Trabecular: Cells are grouped together forming trabeculae
- Solid: Cells in sheets
- Papillary: Papillary structures within large follicles or cystic spaces; may be confused with papillary thyroid carcinoma (PTC)

- Tumor architecture and cytologic appearance are very distinct from surrounding thyroid parenchyma
- Colloid is usually present within follicular lumen
- Cytoplasm is usually pale eosinophilic and can range from clear to oncocytic
- Nuclei are basal, evenly spaced, round to oval with homogeneously dark chromatin
- Nucleoli are rare, and when present, are small and eccentric
- Isolated bizarre nuclei are occasionally present
- Mitoses are very rare in follicular adenomas
- Can present with single or multiple combined morphological patterns with no difference in clinical behavior

Cytologic Features

- Cellularity is variable
- Rare variants have been reported, including clear cell, signet ring, and oncocytic follicular adenomas
- Cells are usually bland resembling normal follicular cells
- Pleomorphism, if present, does not indicate malignancy
- Nuclear to cytoplasmic ratio is variable, with clinically hot nodules tending to have more abundant cytoplasm

Histologic Variants

- Microfollicular type
- Macrofollicular type
- Oncocytic type
- Signet ring cell type
- Adenoma with clear cells
- Adenoma with bizarre nuclei
- Atypical follicular adenoma

ANCILLARY TESTS

Frozen Sections

- Should not be performed in follicular adenomas or other encapsulated follicular-patterned lesions
- Entire capsule should be evaluated to exclude invasion

Immunohistochemistry

- FA shows positive expression for keratins, TTF-1, and thyroglobulin
- Panel of markers that can assist in evaluation of encapsulated lesions with PTC features
  - CK19, HBME-1, galectin-3, and CITED-1 (often positive in PTC and negative in FA)
  - HBME-1 is most specific (up to 96%)
  - Strong expression of 2 or more of these markers (especially HBME-1) supports diagnosis of PTC
  - Lack of staining of 3 or 4 of the markers strongly supports diagnosis of FA

Cytogenetics

- Numerical chromosomal changes and translocation of 19p13 and 2p21 occur in minority of follicular adenomas

Molecular Genetics

- To date, no molecular test has been able to distinguish adenomatous nodules, follicular adenoma, and carcinoma with 100% sensitivity and specificity
- Activating point mutation of *NRAS* and *HRAS* is present in about 1/3 of follicular adenomas
- No *BRAF* mutation or *RET/PTC* rearrangement in follicular adenomas

DIFFERENTIAL DIAGNOSIS

Adenomatous Nodules

- Multiple nodules
- Variable-sized follicles
- No capsule

Follicular Thyroid Carcinoma

- Follicular-patterned neoplasm
- Characterized by vascular &/or capsular invasion if surrounded by fibrous capsule

Follicular Variant of Papillary Thyroid Carcinoma

- Follicular-patterned neoplasm with PTC nuclear features
  - Ground-glass nuclei (pale, clear, empty-appearing nuclei)
  - Intranuclear pseudoinclusions
  - Nuclear molding, grooves, & overlapping

Parathyroid Adenoma

- Smaller cells in a solid or microfollicular pattern

Medullary Thyroid Carcinoma

- Invasive growth
- "Salt and pepper" nuclear chromatin
- Cytoplasm is slightly granular

Hyalinizing Trabecular Tumor

- Trabecular growth pattern of medium-sized elongated cells with finely granular cytoplasm
- PAS positive basement membrane material

DIAGNOSTIC CHECKLIST

Pathologic Interpretation Pearls

- Pathologist's task is to differentiate malignant neoplasms, follicular carcinoma in particular, from numerous morphologic variants of follicular adenoma
  - Diagnosis of follicular carcinoma rests on demonstration of capsular or vascular invasion
  - Extensive sampling and histological examination of entire tumor capsule is essential
  - Topic of what constitutes capsular invasion (invasion into, all the way through, or presence of a few follicles within capsule) remains controversial among experts

Immunohistochemistry

Antibody	Reactivity	Staining Pattern	Comment
TTF-1	Positive	Nuclear	Strong nuclear staining
Thyroglobulin	Positive	Cytoplasmic	Strong in cytoplasm and luminal borders
CK-PAN	Positive	Cytoplasmic	
CK8/18/CAM5.2	Positive	Cytoplasmic	
CK19	Positive	Cytoplasmic	Present in ~ 1/2 of adenomas
Calcitonin	Negative		
Chromogranin-A	Negative		
CEA-M	Negative		
Galectin-3	Negative		Follicular adenomas may have scattered cells weakly positive in < 10% of cases
HBME-1	Negative		Distinguish from papillary carcinoma
Synaptophysin	Negative		

  - Deeper sectioning of suspicious tumor foci within capsule will often reveal invasion through entire capsule thickness
  - True invading tumor nests should be connected to main tumor mass, as free-standing foci may represent entrapment secondary to previous FNA biopsy
  - Isolated nodules outside capsule that are morphologically similar to tumor can only be considered invasion if a direct connection with main mass is seen histologically
- Atypical follicular adenoma
  - Term is reserved for encapsulated follicular lesions, which may show spontaneous necrosis, infarction, numerous mitoses, or increased cellularity
  - Atypical adenomas should have none of the features of papillary tumors and should lack capsular or vascular invasion
  - These tumors have benign clinical behavior

SELECTED REFERENCES

1. Laury AR et al: Thyroid pathology in PTEN-hamartoma tumor syndrome: characteristic findings of a distinct entity. Thyroid. 21(2):135-44, 2011
2. Nosé V: Thyroid cancer of follicular cell origin in inherited tumor syndromes. Adv Anat Pathol. 17(6):428-36, 2010
3. Westhoff CC et al: Clear cell follicular adenoma of the thyroid--a challenge in intra-operative diagnostics. Exp Clin Endocrinol Diabetes. 118(1):19-21, 2010
4. Osamura RY et al: Current practices in performing frozen sections for thyroid and parathyroid pathology. Virchows Arch. 453(5):433-40, 2008
5. Serra S et al: Controversies in thyroid pathology: the diagnosis of follicular neoplasms. Endocr Pathol. 19(3):156-65, 2008
6. Yeung MJ et al: Management of the solitary thyroid nodule. Oncologist. 13(2):105-12, 2008
7. Baloch ZW et al: Our approach to follicular-patterned lesions of the thyroid. J Clin Pathol. 60(3):244-50, 2007
8. Bertherat J: Carney complex (CNC). Orphanet J Rare Dis. 1:21, 2006
9. Marini F et al: Multiple endocrine neoplasia type 1. Orphanet J Rare Dis. 1:38, 2006
10. Rosai J et al: Pitfalls in thyroid tumour pathology. Histopathology. 49(2):107-20, 2006
11. Scognamiglio T et al: Diagnostic usefulness of HBME1, galectin-3, CK19, and CITED1 and evaluation of their expression in encapsulated lesions with questionable features of papillary thyroid carcinoma. Am J Clin Pathol. 126(5):700-8, 2006
12. LiVolsi VA et al: Use and abuse of frozen section in the diagnosis of follicular thyroid lesions. Endocr Pathol. 16(4):285-93, 2005
13. el-Sahrigy D et al: Signet-ring follicular adenoma of the thyroid diagnosed by fine needle aspiration. Report of a case with cytologic description. Acta Cytol. 48(1):87-90, 2004
14. Hirokawa M et al: Observer variation of encapsulated follicular lesions of the thyroid gland. Am J Surg Pathol. 26(11):1508-14, 2002

FOLLICULAR ADENOMA

Radiologic, Gross, and Microscopic Features

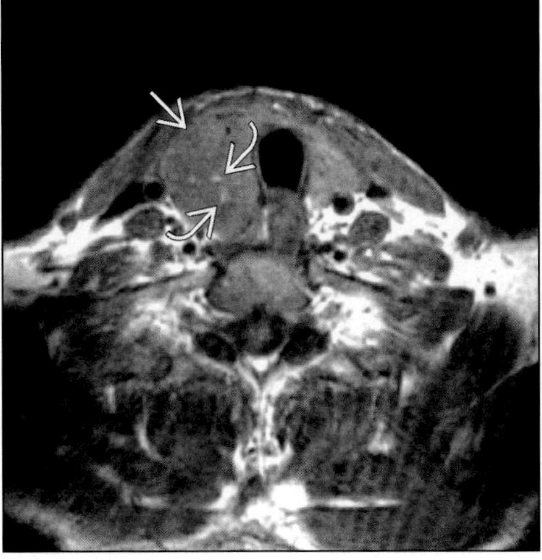

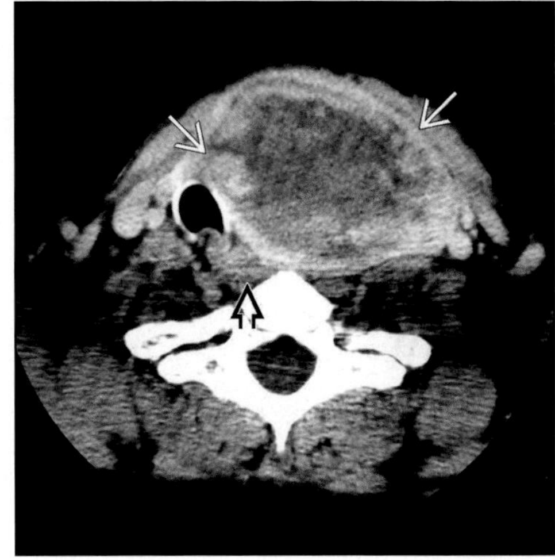

(Left) *Axial T1WI MR through the neck demonstrates the heterogeneous appearance of a right thyroid mass ➡. The mass is predominantly hypodense but has focal areas of T1 hyperintensity ➡.* ***(Right)*** *Axial contrast-enhanced CT through the neck demonstrates a large heterogeneous mass ➡ in the left thyroid lobe and extending into the superior mediastinum. There is significant mass effect on the larynx, trachea, and esophagus ➡, which are displaced laterally to the right.*

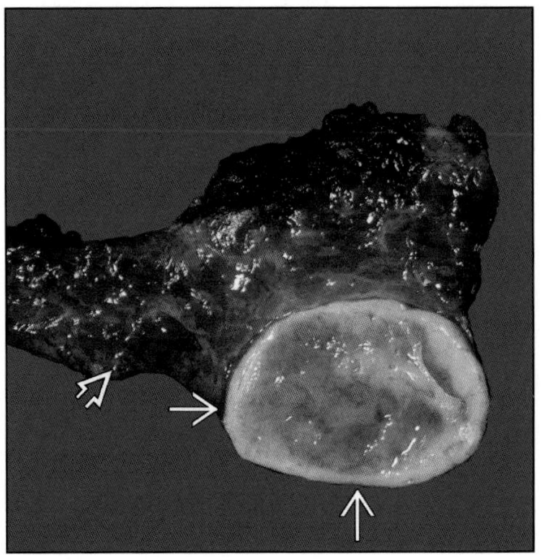

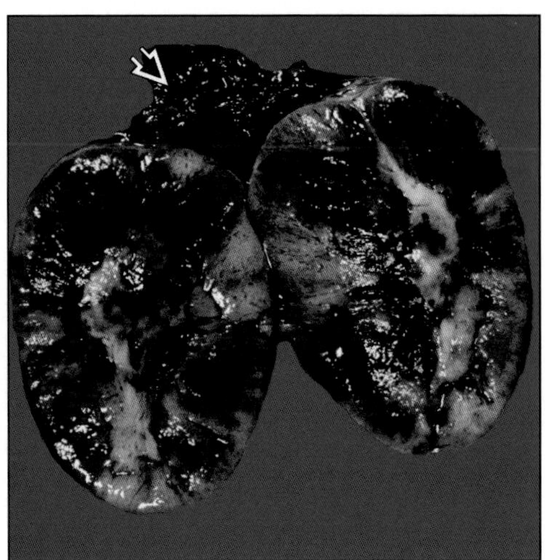

(Left) *Cross section shows a well-circumscribed, encapsulated lesion ➡ with a cut surface that is homogeneous and pale compared to normal thyroid tissue ➡. Extensive sampling of the tumor capsule throughout the lesion is critical to evaluate capsular &/or vascular invasion.* ***(Right)*** *There is a thin fibrous capsule separating this thyroid neoplasm from the surrounding compressed thyroid parenchyma ➡. This neoplasm has areas of hemorrhage and central degenerative changes.*

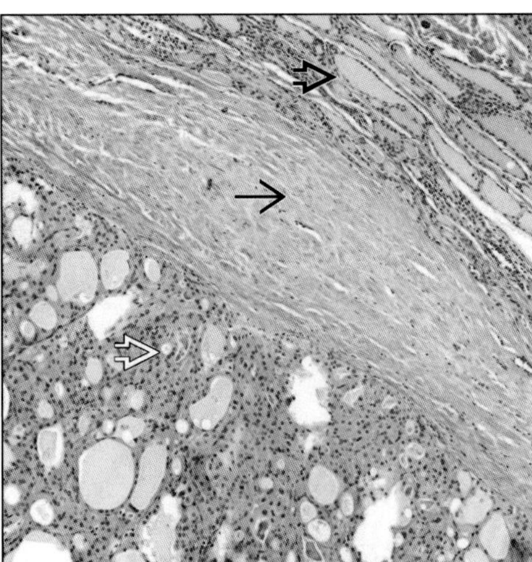

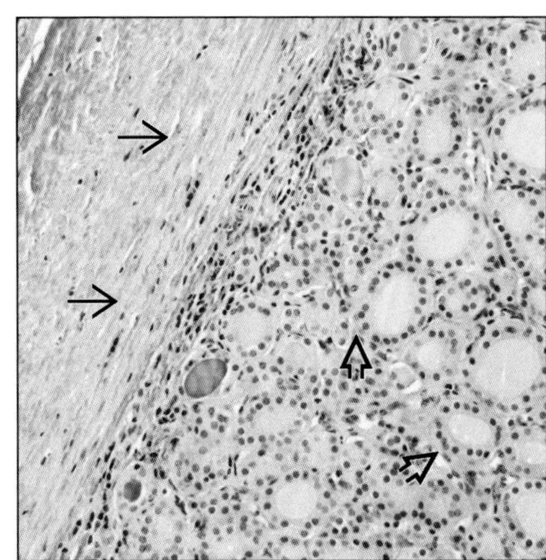

(Left) *This follicular adenoma ➡ is surrounded by a thick fibrous capsule ➡. The normal thyroid follicles ➡ surrounding the lesion are often elongated due to compression, and the follicular cells differ from the neoplastic cells.* ***(Right)*** *H&E shows a follicular neoplasm surrounded by a well-formed thick fibrous capsule, lacking invasion ➡. Follicles with colloid are surrounded by cuboidal cells with round regular nuclei and eosinophilic cytoplasm ➡.*

Microscopic Features

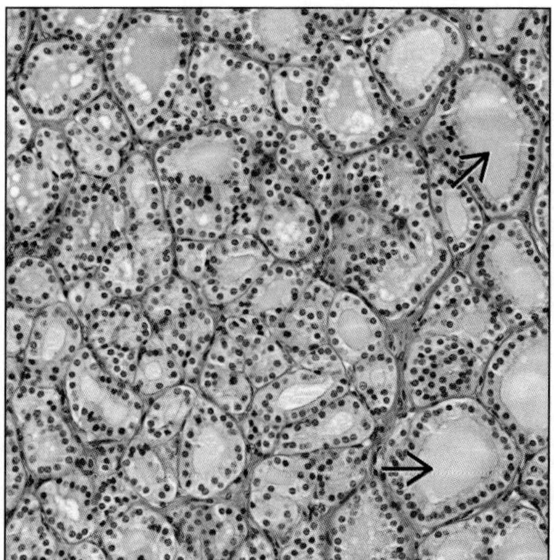
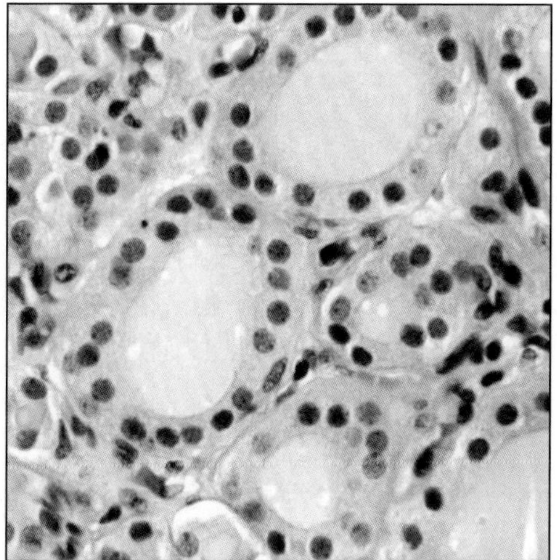

(Left) *This follicular adenoma shows typical follicular architecture with follicles of various sizes, lined by follicular cells with homogeneous regular nuclei, and with abundant colloid ⇒.* ***(Right)*** *High-power magnification shows bland follicular cells with regular, evenly spaced nuclei. Notice that the chromatin is homogeneous (unlike the nuclei of papillary carcinoma), and the cells respect each other's boundaries with minimal nuclear overlapping. Colloid is also present.*

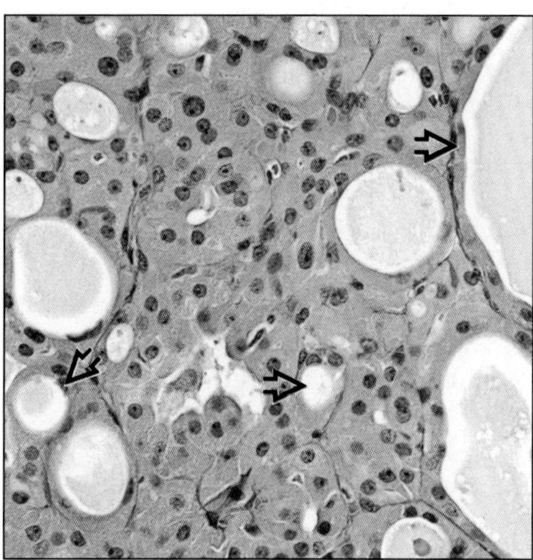
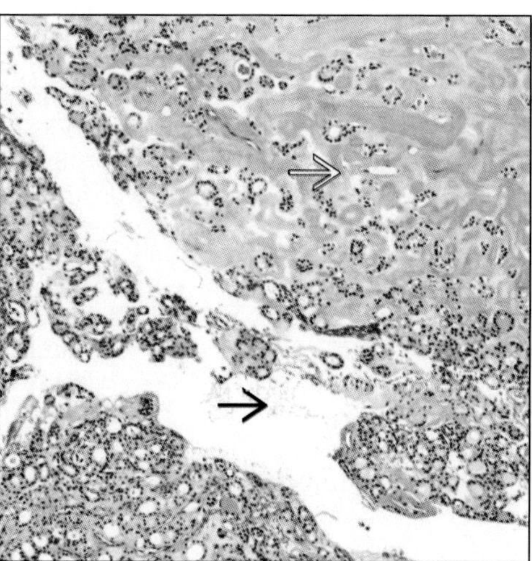

(Left) *This FA displays follicles formed by somewhat larger cells with abundant eosinophilic cytoplasm and homogeneous nuclei with conspicuous small nucleoli. The size of the follicles varies over a wide range. Colloid can be seen within most follicles ⇒.* ***(Right)*** *The follicular adenoma depicted here shows central degenerative changes. Edema is noted as empty spaces between the follicles ⇒. Prominent hyalinization with small residual follicles is usually present centrally ⇒.*

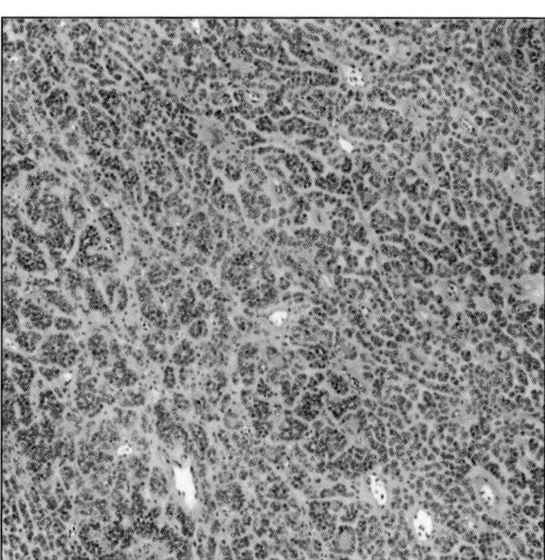
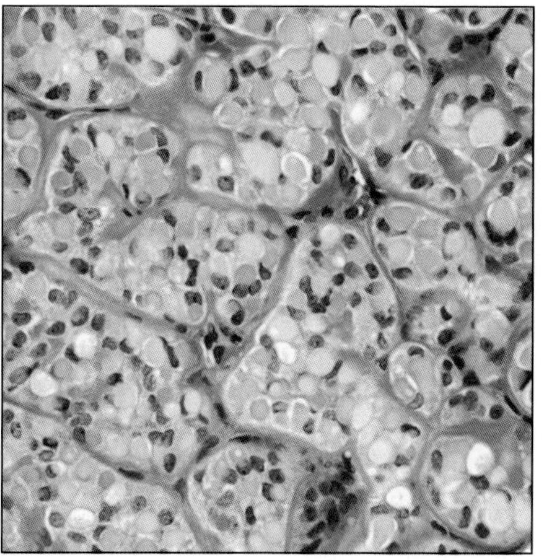

(Left) *Shown in this low-power photomicrograph is a follicular adenoma with small cell features displaying a mixed pattern of growth including solid nests, ribbons, and microfollicles. The transition of distinct patterns across the field is also illustrated.* ***(Right)*** *This follicular adenoma shows signet ring features in an alveolar pattern. The nests of signet ring cells are separated by thin fibrous trabeculae with rare follicle spaces showing colloid within the cytoplasm.*

NEUROBLASTOMA AND GANGLIONEUROBLASTOMA

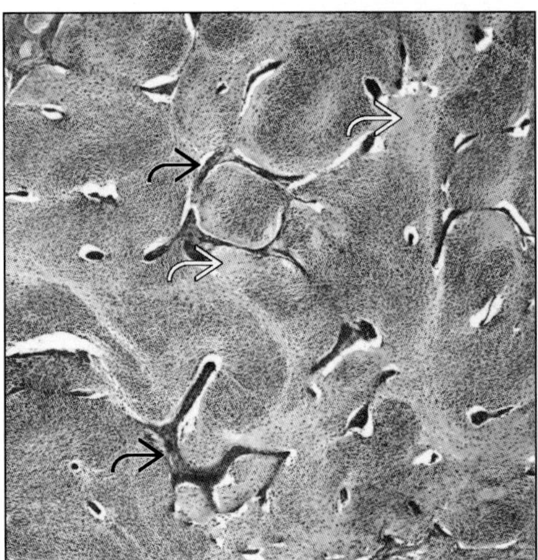

This low-power view of a poorly differentiated NB shows thin septae of schwannian stroma ➢. Pale, eosinophilic neuropil ➡ is seen between the nodules or nests of neuroblastoma cells.

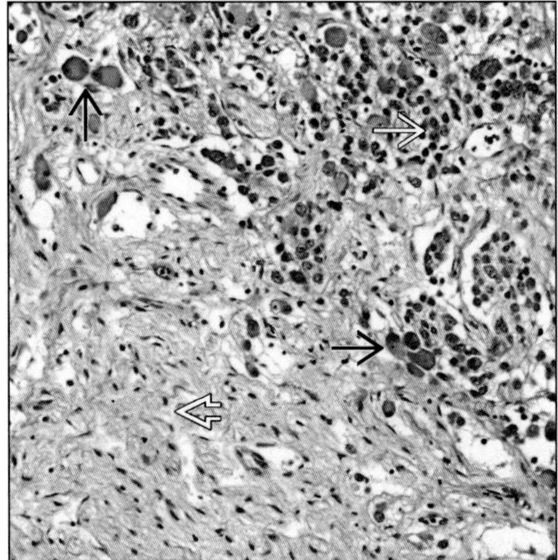

A typical intermixed GNB at medium power shows maturing ganglion cells ⇒, neuroblasts ➡, and abundant schwannian stroma ⇨.

TERMINOLOGY

Abbreviations

- Neuroblastoma (NB)
- Ganglioneuroblastoma (GNB)

Synonyms

- Schwannian stroma-poor neuroblastic tumor (neuroblastoma)
- Schwannian stroma-rich neuroblastic tumor (ganglioneuroblastoma)

Definitions

- Malignant tumor derived from primordial neural crest cells
- On maturational spectrum of neuroblastic tumors
  - NB is least differentiated
  - GNB is moderately differentiated

ETIOLOGY/PATHOGENESIS

Developmental Anomaly

- Derived from primordial neural crest cells
  - These cells migrate from spinal cord to adrenal medulla and sympathetic ganglia

CLINICAL ISSUES

Epidemiology

- Incidence
  - ~ 1 in 10,000 children
  - 3rd most common malignant tumor in children
    - Most common extracranial solid tumor in children
  - Usually sporadic
    - Some autosomal dominant familial cases have been seen
  - Screening not recommended
- Age
  - 1/2 diagnosed by age 2 years
  - 90% diagnosed by age 5 years
  - ~ 1/4 are congenital, with some detected prenatally on ultrasound
- Gender
  - Slight male predominance
- Ethnicity
  - Less common in African-Americans

Site

- Follows distribution of sympathetic ganglia
  - Paramidline from base of skull to pelvis
  - Most common in abdomen and retroperitoneum
- Adrenal medulla
- Dorsal root ganglia
- Metastases
  - Bone
  - Lymph nodes
  - Liver
  - Skin

Presentation

- Depends on age of patient, location of tumor, and associated clinical syndromes
- Most have nonspecific symptoms
  - Fever, weight loss, diarrhea, anemia, hypertension
- Fetuses may have hydrops
- Palpable mass in ~ 1/2
- ~ 2/3 have metastases on presentation
- "Blueberry muffin baby"
  - Blue-red cutaneous masses in infants
- Myoclonus-opsoclonus syndrome
  - Associated with good prognosis
  - Rapid, alternating eye movements and myoclonic movements of extremities
  - Resolves with tumor eradication
- Other associated syndromes include
  - Myasthenia gravis
  - Beckwith-Wiedemann syndrome
  - Cushing syndrome

NEUROBLASTOMA AND GANGLIONEUROBLASTOMA

Key Facts

Terminology

- Malignant tumor derived from primordial neural crest cells

Clinical Issues

- 3rd most common malignant tumor in children
- 90% diagnosed by age 5 years
- Common sites include adrenal medulla and sympathetic ganglia
- Presentation depends on age of patient, location of tumor, and associated clinical syndromes
- Urine catecholamines elevated in 95% of patients with NB

Microscopic Pathology

- International Neuroblastoma Pathology Committee Classification
  - Undifferentiated NB
  - Poorly differentiated NB
  - Differentiating NB
  - Nodular GNB
  - Intermixed GNB
- Mitotic-karyorrhectic index (MKI)

Ancillary Tests

- *N-Myc* amplification is associated with worse prognosis

Top Differential Diagnoses

- Alveolar rhabdomyosarcoma (ARMS)
- Ewing sarcoma/primitive neuroectodermal tumor (PNET)
- Lymphoma

  - Neurofibromatosis
  - Fetal hydantoin syndrome
  - Hirschsprung disease

Laboratory Tests

- Urine catecholamines (elevated in 95% of patients with NB)
  - Epinephrine
  - Norepinephrine
  - Homovanillic acid (HVA)
  - Vanillylmandelic acid (VMA)
    - VMA/HVA ratio > 1.5 associated with better prognosis
- Lactate dehydrogenase
  - > 1,500 IU/L associated with worse clinical outcome
- Ferritin
  - > 142 ng/mL associated with worse clinical outcome
- Neuron-specific enolase (NSE)
  - > 100 ng/mL associated with worse clinical outcome

Natural History

- 1-2% will spontaneously regress
  - Most in children under age 1 year
- NB can metastasize widely via lymphatics and vessels

Treatment

- Low risk
  - Surgery or observation alone
- Intermediate risk
  - Surgery and adjuvant chemotherapy
- High risk
  - Induction chemotherapy
  - Delayed tumor resection
  - Radiation of primary site
  - Myeloablative chemotherapy with stem cell recovery

Prognosis

- Favorable prognostic factors
  - Age < 1.5 years at diagnosis
  - Favorable histology
  - Stage 1, 2, or 4S
    - Related to location of tumor
  - No *N-Myc* amplification
  - Hyperdiploidy
  - No loss of 1p
  - High expression of TrKA
  - Normal serum ferritin, NSE, and LDH
  - Urinary VMA/HVA ratio > 1.5

IMAGE FINDINGS

General Features

- Extensive radiographic evaluation is required to determine extent of disease and identify metastatic foci
- Calcifications often seen in central portion of tumor

Bone Scan

- Radiolabeled metaiodobenzylguanidine (MIBG) incorporates into catecholamine-secreting cells and can detect neuroblastoma

MACROSCOPIC FEATURES

General Features

- **Neuroblastoma**
  - Fine membranous capsules
  - Cut surface is soft, fleshy, often with hemorrhage and necrosis
- **Ganglioneuroblastoma**
  - Cut surface is firm, gray-white
  - Nodular GNB must have grossly visible, usually hemorrhagic, nodules
  - Intermixed GNB can look like NB or ganglioneuroma (GN) depending on extent of differentiation

Size

- Average: 6-8 cm diameter

MICROSCOPIC PATHOLOGY

Histologic Features

- Neuroblasts

NEUROBLASTOMA AND GANGLIONEUROBLASTOMA

- Small round blue cells
- Very little cytoplasm
- Homer Wright pseudorosette
  - Neuroblasts forming ring around central core of cytoplasmic processes
- Ganglionic differentiation
  - Cells enlarge
  - Increased eosinophilic or amphophilic cytoplasm
  - Nuclear chromatin pattern becomes vesicular
  - Must have synchronous differentiation of cytoplasm and nucleus
- Neuropil
  - Fibrillar eosinophilic matrix
- Mitotic-karyorrhectic index (MKI)
  - Count of cells undergoing mitosis or karyorrhexis, per 5,000 cells
    - Can be estimated
  - Low: < 100 cells per 5,000
  - Intermediate: 100-200 cells per 5,000
  - High: > 200 cells per 5,000

International Neuroblastoma Pathology Committee Classification

- Shimada classification
  - **Undifferentiated NB**
    - No ganglionic differentiation
    - No neuropil
    - No or minimal Schwannian stroma
    - Often requires immunohistochemistry for accurate diagnosis
  - **Poorly differentiated NB**
    - < 5% of tumor cells show ganglionic differentiation
    - Neuropil background
    - No or minimal Schwannian stroma
  - **Differentiating NB**
    - > 5% of tumor cells show ganglionic differentiation
    - Usually more abundant neuropil
    - Usually more prominent Schwannian stroma (must be < 50%)
  - **Nodular GNB**
    - Grossly identifiable nodules will be neuroblastoma
    - Abrupt demarcation between stroma-poor neuroblastoma and stroma-rich component
    - Fibrous pseudocapsule often seen surrounding NB component
    - > 50% Schwannian stroma
  - **Intermixed GNB**
    - Microscopic nests of neuroblastoma within Schwannian stroma
    - > 50% Schwannian stroma
- Do not classify post-treatment resections
  - "Neuroblastoma with treatment effect" is sufficient
- May classify metastatic disease if resection/biopsy is pre treatment

ANCILLARY TESTS

Immunohistochemistry

- NSE
  - Most sensitive but least specific
  - Is found at least focally, even in very undifferentiated NBs
- S100
  - Positive in Schwannian stroma
- Other useful positive immunostains
  - Chromogranin
  - Synaptophysin
  - Protein gene product 9.5 (PGP9.5)
  - CD56

Cytogenetics

- *N-Myc*
  - Amplification is associated with worse prognosis
  - Usually seen in advanced disease
- DNA ploidy
  - Near-diploidy or tetraploidy is associated with worse prognosis
  - Hyperdiploidy is associated with better prognosis
- Loss of heterozygosity of 1p and 11q
  - Both associated with worse prognosis
- TrkA (high-affinity nerve growth factor receptor)
  - Increased expression associates with better prognosis

Electron Microscopy

- Wide range of cytologic differentiation
- Dense-core neurosecretory granules
  - Found in elongated cell processes
  - 100 nm in diameter
  - Dense core surrounded by clear halos and delicate outer membranes

DIFFERENTIAL DIAGNOSIS

Alveolar Rhabdomyosarcoma (ARMS)

- Clinical presentations may be similar
- ARMS shows more pleomorphic tumor cells than NB
- ARMS has more abundant cytoplasm than NB
- Immunohistochemistry shows ARMS positive for myogenic markers
- ARMS has characteristic t(1;13) or t(2;13)

Ewing Sarcoma (EWS)/Primitive Neuroectodermal Tumor (PNET)

- Patients with EWS/PNET usually older
- EWS/PNET has finely stippled chromatin and glycogen-filled cytoplasm
- EWS/PNET is usually CD99 positive whereas NB is negative

Lymphoma

- Will not be positive for NSE, synaptophysin, or chromogranin

Maturing Ganglioneuroma

- Differentiated from intermixed GNB in that GN has single cells instead of nests of cells within Schwannian stroma

Favorable vs. Unfavorable Histology in Neuroblastic Tumors

Tumor	Differentiation	MKI	Age	Histologic Classification
Neuroblastoma	Undifferentiated	Any MKI	Any age	Unfavorable histology
	Poorly differentiated	High MKI	Any age	Unfavorable histology
		Low or intermediate MKI	> 1.5 years	Unfavorable histology
			< 1.5 years	Favorable histology
	Differentiating	High MKI	Any age	Unfavorable histology
		Intermediate MKI	> 1.5 years	Unfavorable histology
			< 1.5 years	Favorable histology
		Low MKI	> 5 years	Unfavorable histology
			< 5 years	Favorable histology
Ganglioneuroblastoma	Nodular	**	**	Unfavorable or favorable
	Intermixed	N/A	Any age	Favorable histology
Ganglioneuroma	Mature or maturing	N/A	Any age	Favorable histology

***The determination of favorable vs. unfavorable histology in nodular GNB is based on the NB component.*

Prognosis Based on N-Myc Amplification and Histology

	Favorable Histology	Unfavorable Histology
N-Myc nonamplified	Excellent prognosis	Poor prognosis
N-Myc amplified	Rare	Extremely poor prognosis

Neuroblastoma Staging System

Stage	Definition
1	Localized tumor; complete gross resection; ipsilateral nodes negative
2A	Localized tumor; incomplete gross resection; nonadherent ipsilateral nodes negative
2B	Localized tumor ± complete gross resection; nonadherent ipsilateral nodes positive
3	Unresectable tumor that crosses midline ± positive nodes; or localized tumor with positive contralateral nodes
4	Distant metastases to nodes, bone, bone marrow, liver, skin, &/or other organs not stage 4S
4S	Localized primary tumor (stage 1 or 2) with metastases limited to skin, liver, &/or bone marrow

SELECTED REFERENCES

1. Ambros PF et al: International consensus for neuroblastoma molecular diagnostics: report from the International Neuroblastoma Risk Group (INRG) Biology Committee. Br J Cancer. 100(9):1471-82, 2009
2. Cohn SL et al: The International Neuroblastoma Risk Group (INRG) classification system: an INRG Task Force report. J Clin Oncol. 27(2):289-97, 2009
3. Chan EL et al: Favorable histology, MYCN-amplified 4S neonatal neuroblastoma. Pediatr Blood Cancer. 48(4):479-82, 2007
4. Tornóczky T et al: Pathology of peripheral neuroblastic tumors: significance of prominent nucleoli in undifferentiated/poorly differentiated neuroblastoma. Pathol Oncol Res. 13(4):269-75, 2007
5. Sano H et al: International neuroblastoma pathology classification adds independent prognostic information beyond the prognostic contribution of age. Eur J Cancer. 42(8):1113-9, 2006
6. Shimada H et al: TrkA expression in peripheral neuroblastic tumors: prognostic significance and biological relevance. Cancer. 101(8):1873-81, 2004
7. Tornóczky T et al: Large cell neuroblastoma: a distinct phenotype of neuroblastoma with aggressive clinical behavior. Cancer. 100(2):390-7, 2004
8. Peuchmaur M et al: Revision of the International Neuroblastoma Pathology Classification: confirmation of favorable and unfavorable prognostic subsets in ganglioneuroblastoma, nodular. Cancer. 98(10):2274-81, 2003
9. Shimada H: The International Neuroblastoma Pathology Classification. Pathologica. 95(5):240-1, 2003
10. Goto S et al: Histopathology (International Neuroblastoma Pathology Classification) and MYCN status in patients with peripheral neuroblastic tumors: a report from the Children's Cancer Group. Cancer. 92(10):2699-708, 2001
11. Shimada H et al: International neuroblastoma pathology classification for prognostic evaluation of patients with peripheral neuroblastic tumors: a report from the Children's Cancer Group. Cancer. 92(9):2451-61, 2001
12. Granata C et al: Features and outcome of neuroblastoma detected before birth. J Pediatr Surg. 35(1):88-91, 2000
13. Shimada H et al: Terminology and morphologic criteria of neuroblastic tumors: recommendations by the International Neuroblastoma Pathology Committee. Cancer. 86(2):349-63, 1999
14. Shimada H et al: The International Neuroblastoma Pathology Classification (the Shimada system). Cancer. 86(2):364-72, 1999

NEUROBLASTOMA AND GANGLIONEUROBLASTOMA

Radiologic and Gross Features

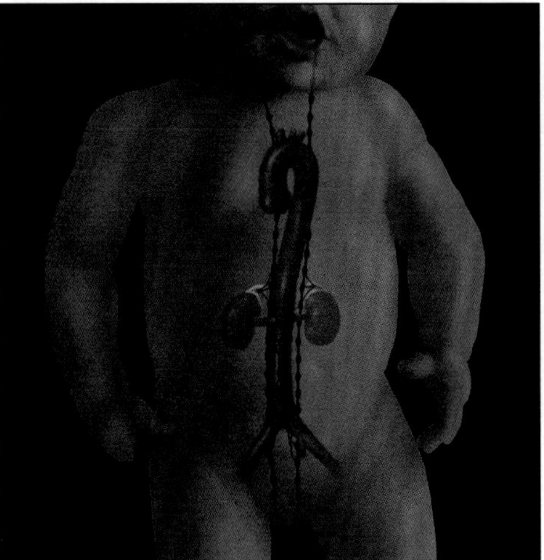

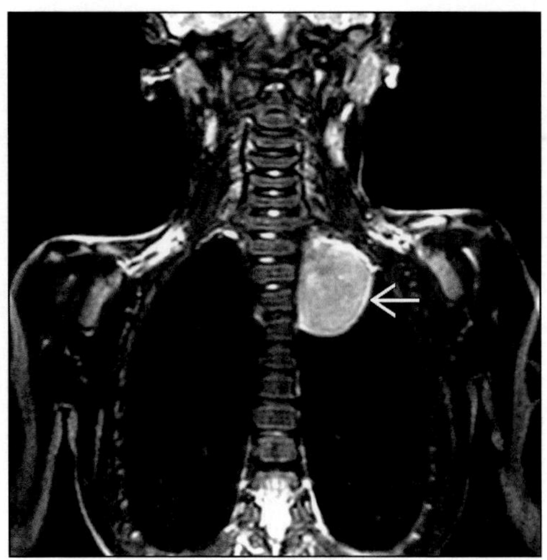

(Left) *Graphic shows the anatomic extent of the sympathetic chain (including adrenal gland) from cervical region to inferior pelvis. Neuroblastoma can arise anywhere along the sympathetic chain.* ***(Right)*** *Coronal T2-weighted MR in a case of ganglioneuroblastoma shows a mildly hyperintense posterior mediastinal mass ➔ with no adjacent osseous marrow signal abnormality.*

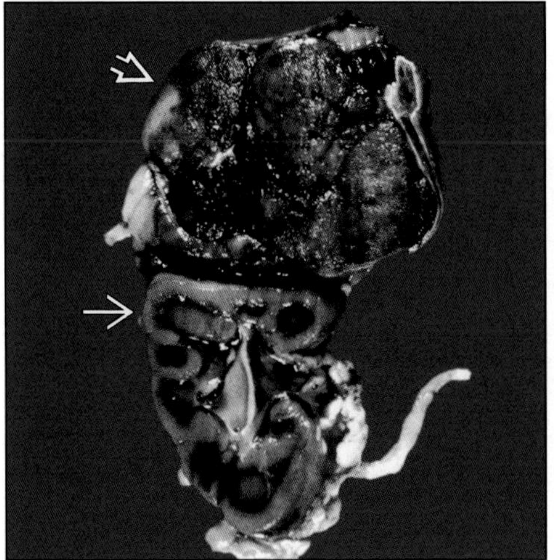

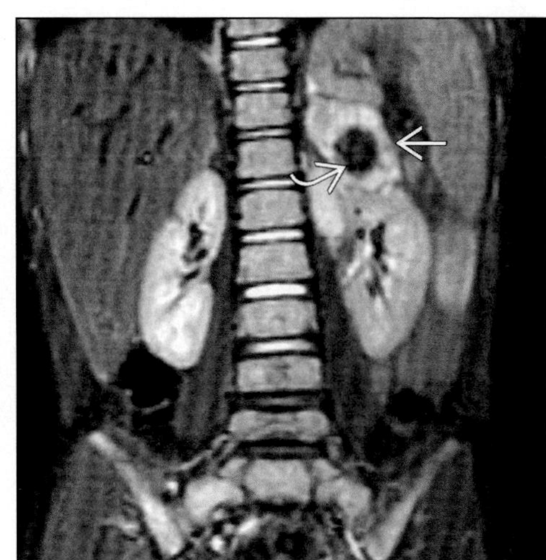

(Left) *Gross pathology shows an adrenal mass ⇨ compressing the upper pole of the kidney ➔. Neuroblastoma is often hemorrhagic with areas of necrosis and calcification.* ***(Right)*** *Coronal T2-weighted MR shows a left adrenal neuroblastoma ➔ with an area of central necrosis ↗.*

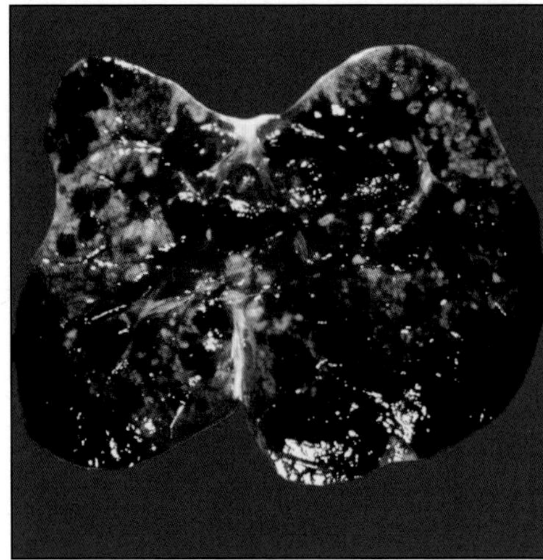

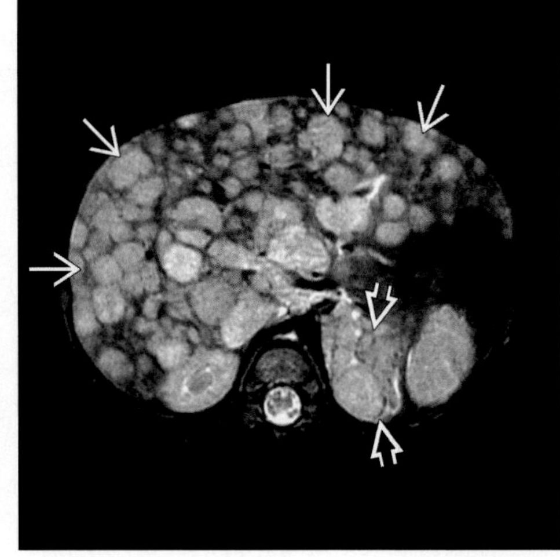

(Left) *Gross pathology of the liver shows diffusely metastatic neuroblastoma.* ***(Right)*** *Axial T2-weighted MR shows a left adrenal mass ⇨, which proved to be a neuroblastoma. It was widely metastatic with the liver filled with multiple high signal, nodular lesions ➔, with little normal remaining hepatic parenchyma.*

Microscopic Features of Neuroblastoma

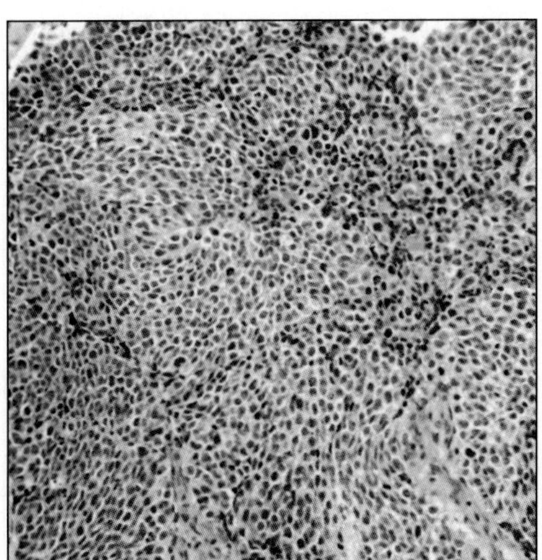

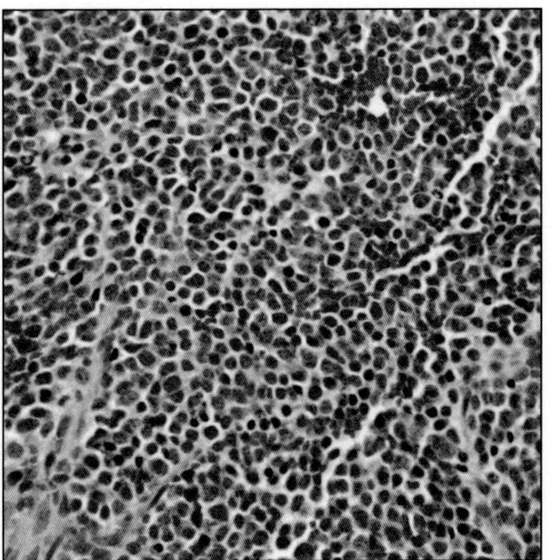

(Left) *This is the typical appearance of an undifferentiated NB. This is a small round cell tumor with no histologic evidence of differentiation. Immunohistochemical stains are required to make the diagnosis.* ***(Right)*** *This is an undifferentiated NB. The cells have scant cytoplasm and round to polygonal, deeply stained nuclei. On H&E this could be mistaken for Ewing sarcoma, alveolar rhabdomyosarcoma, or even lymphoma.*

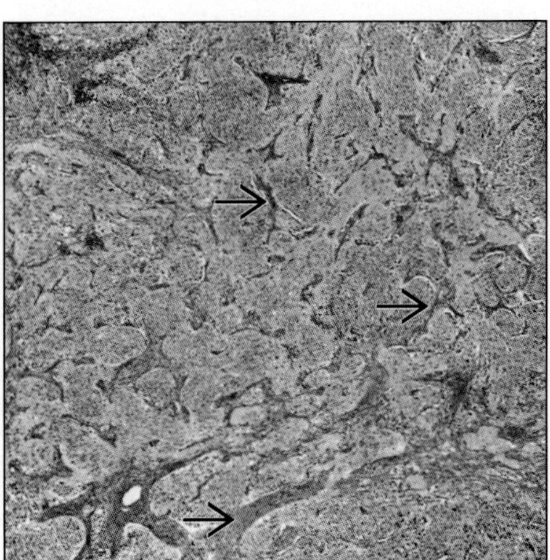

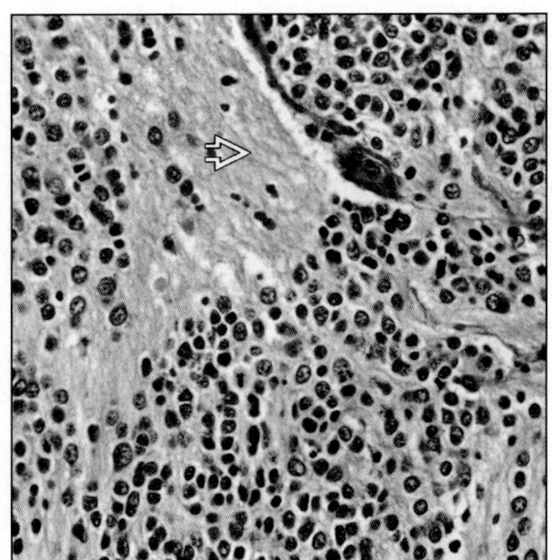

(Left) *This is a typical low-power view of a poorly differentiated NB. Small strips of schwannian stroma ⇒ separate the neuroblasts and neuropil into nests or nodules.* ***(Right)*** *This is a poorly differentiated NB. The small round cells are present within a background of neuropil ⇨. Neuropil is composed of tangled cell processes.*

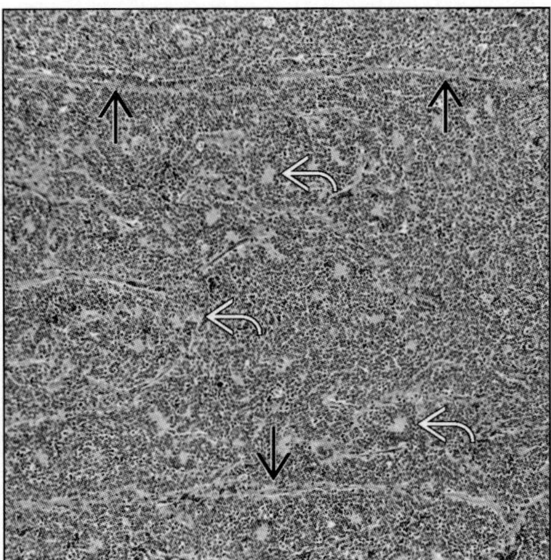

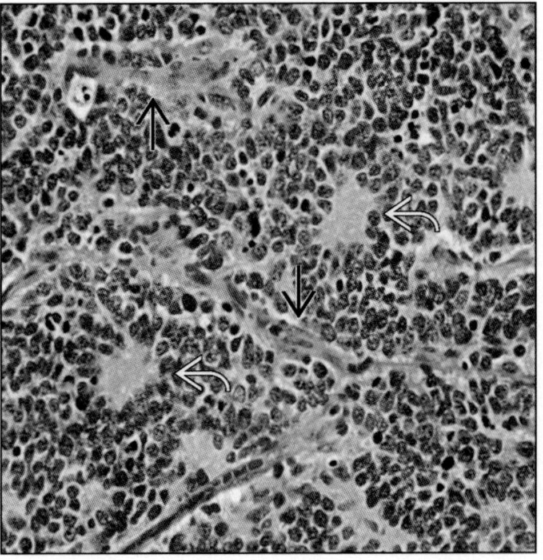

(Left) *This poorly differentiated NB shows scattered rosettes ↪, an early sign of differentiation. Also seen are thin bands of Schwannian stroma ⇒.* ***(Right)*** *Homer Wright rosettes ↪ are composed of neuroblasts surrounding a central core of neurites (cytoplasmic processes). These are seen in varying numbers in poorly differentiated NBs. Small bits of schwannian stroma ⇒ are also seen.*

NEUROBLASTOMA AND GANGLIONEUROBLASTOMA

Microscopic Features of Neuroblastoma

*(**Left**) Schwannian stroma in an NB is often present as thin septae composed of spindled, sometimes wavy, cells ⇒. (**Right**) Neuroblastomas are commonly hemorrhagic with areas of necrosis ⇒. These changes can also be seen after treatment. Neuroblastomas that have undergone treatment should not be classified in the International Neuroblastoma Pathology Classification system.*

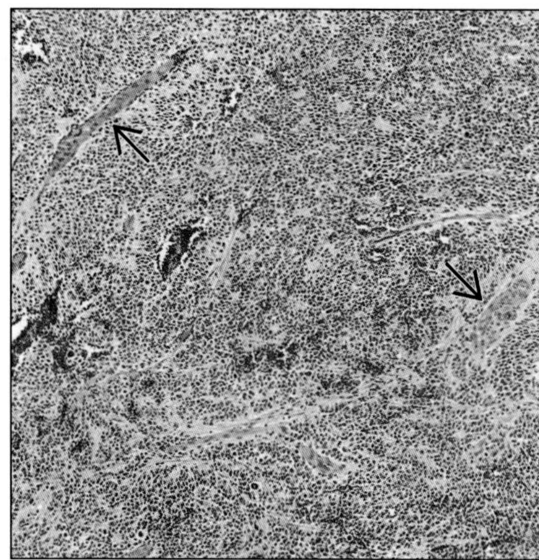

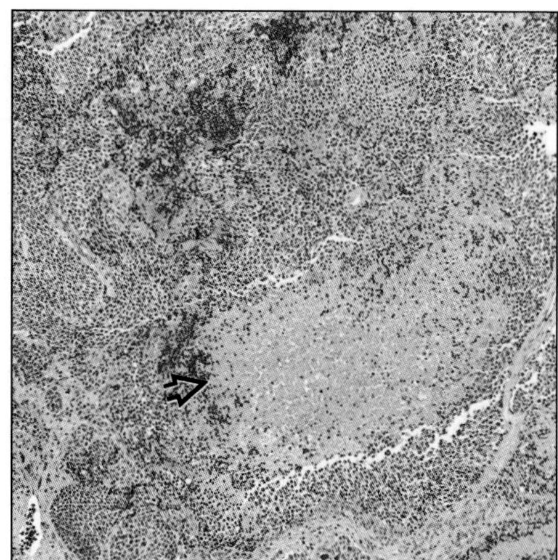

*(**Left**) This is a differentiating NB. More than 5% of the neuroblasts show differentiation with increased cytoplasm and vesicular nuclei. (**Right**) Differentiating neuroblasts ➡ are characterized by an increased amount of eosinophilic cytoplasm, an eccentrically placed nucleus, and vesicular chromatin.*

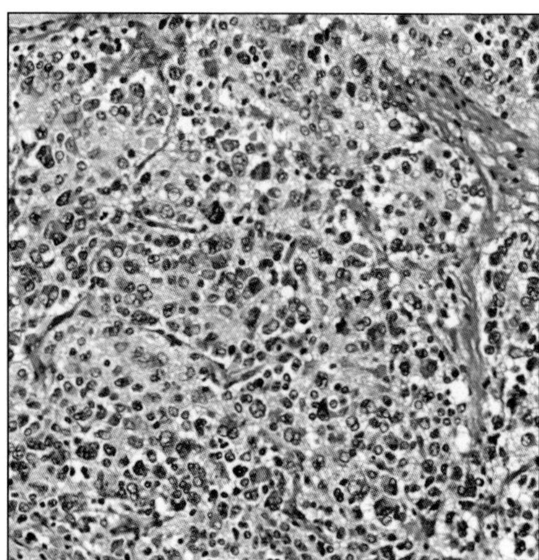

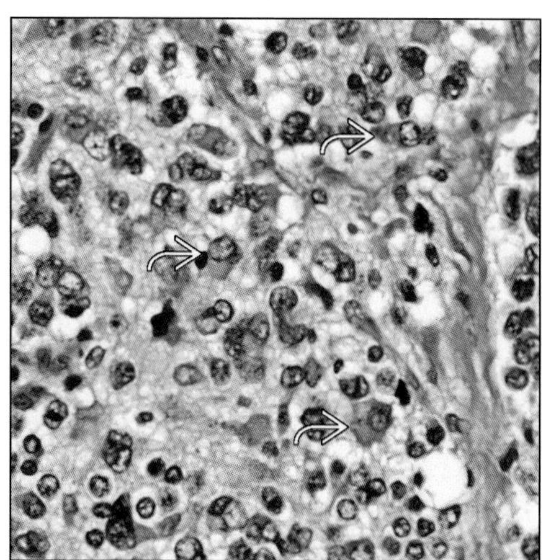

*(**Left**) The mitotic-karyorrhectic index (MKI) is determined by counting the number of mitoses ⇒ and karyorrhectic cells ➡ per 5,000 tumor cells. Estimating is acceptable, as counting 5,000 cells is tedious. MKI counts should be averaged over the entire tumor, and not just on the worst areas. (**Right**) This is an example of intermediate MKI in a poorly differentiated NB.*

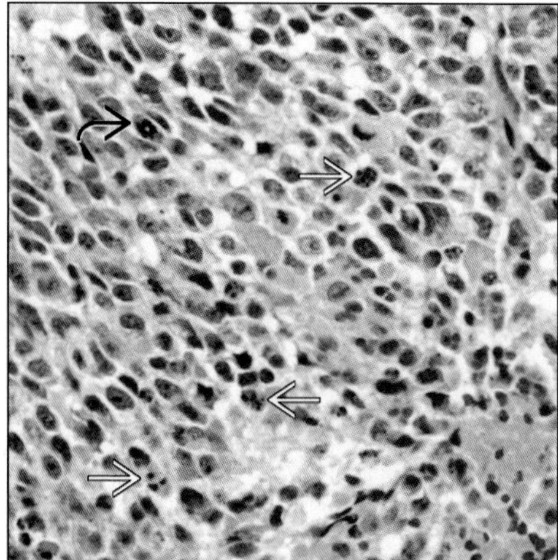

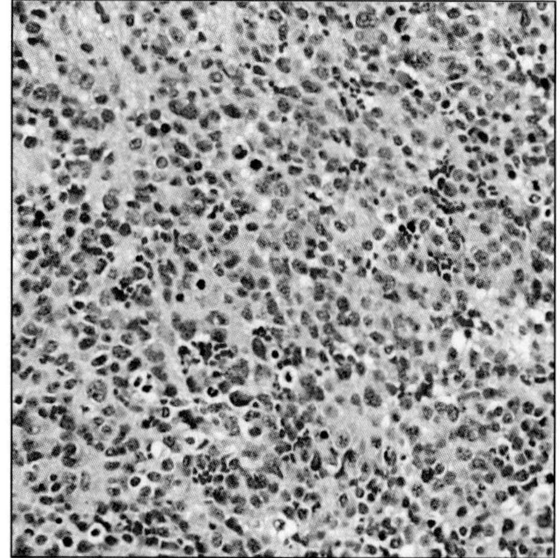

Additional Features of Neuroblastoma

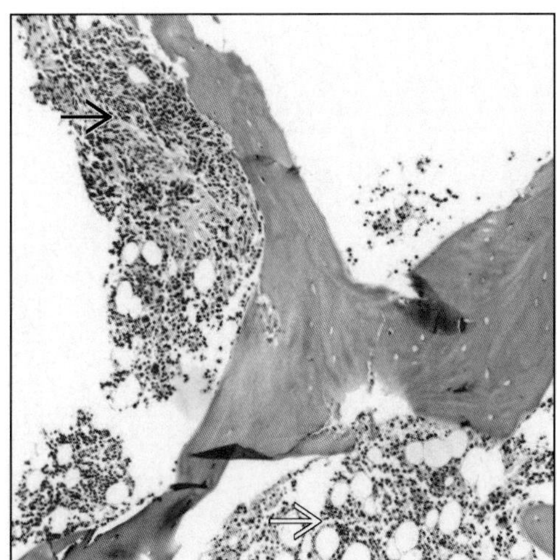

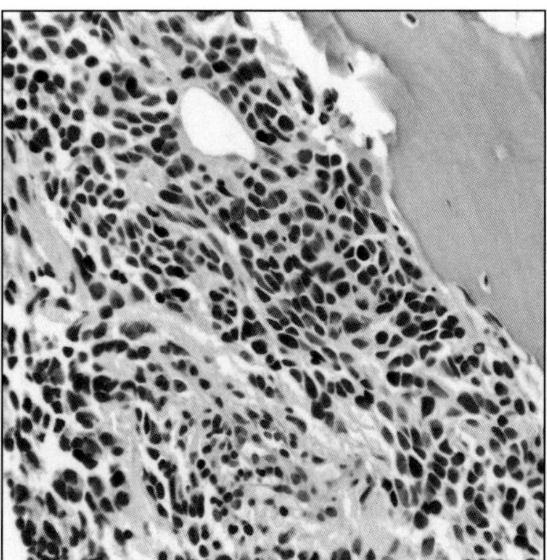

(Left) *This bone marrow core biopsy shows normal marrow at the bottom ➡ and a focus of metastatic NB at the top ➡. Notice how the architecture changes at the metastasis.* ***(Right)*** *This is a focus of metastatic NB in a bone marrow core biopsy. There is lack of normal trilineage hematopoiesis, which has been replaced by small round blue cells.*

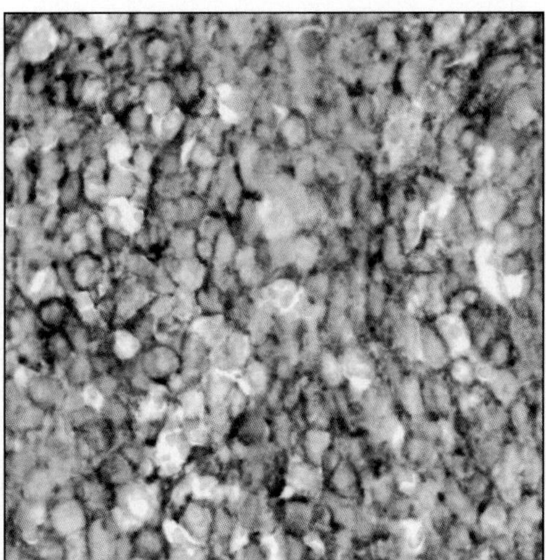

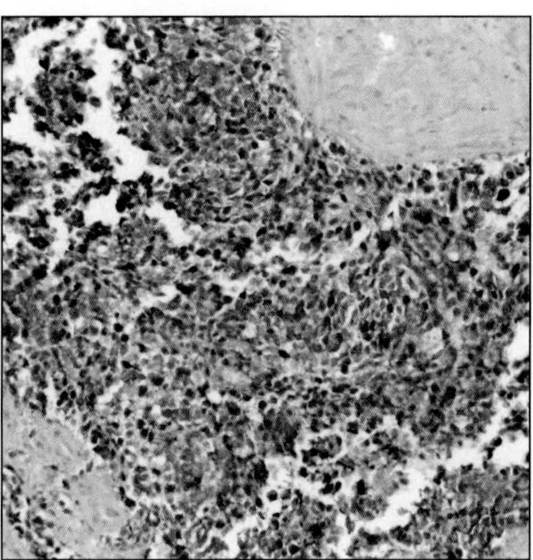

(Left) *Immunohistochemical staining for ALK1 in NB. There is strong membranous staining.* ***(Right)*** *Immunohistochemical staining for NSE in a NB shows strong cytoplasmic staining. NSE is a sensitive but not specific stain for NB, but is a useful member in a panel of stains when ruling out Ewing, alveolar rhabdomyosarcoma, or lymphoma.*

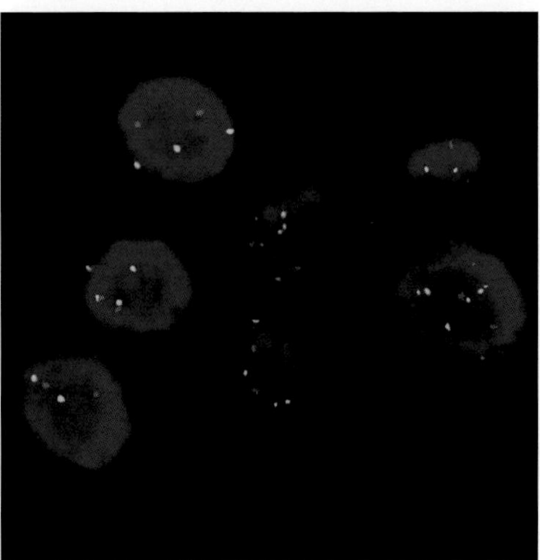

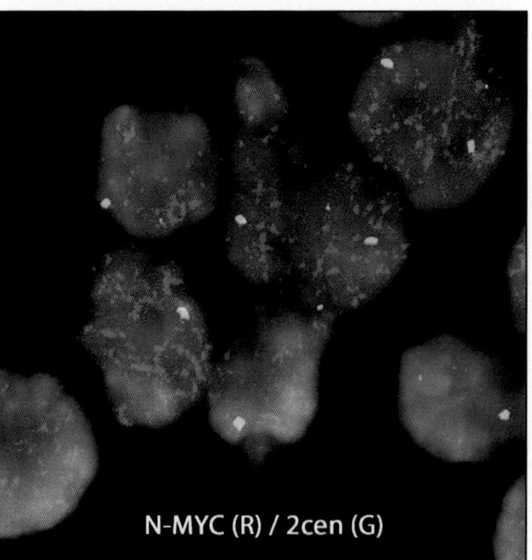

(Left) *Fluorescence in situ hybridization of this NB shows low-level N-Myc amplification (green). The degree of amplification is not important.* ***(Right)*** *Fluorescence in situ hybridization of this NB shows marked amplification of N-Myc (red), indicating poor prognosis. (Courtesy L. McGavran, PhD and K. Swisshelm, PhD.)*

NEUROBLASTOMA AND GANGLIONEUROBLASTOMA

Gross and Microscopic Features of Ganglioneuroblastoma

*(**Left**) This is a GNB from the mediastinum. While this image shows a tan, firm cut surface, the appearance of GNB depends on how much of the tumor is neuroblastic. (**Right**) This is the typical look of a nodular GNB on cut surface. The hemorrhagic nodule in the center ➡ is stroma-poor neuroblastoma, whereas the tan, fleshy rim ➡ is either ganglioneuroma or intermixed GNB. The diagnosis of nodular GNB requires grossly visible nodules.*

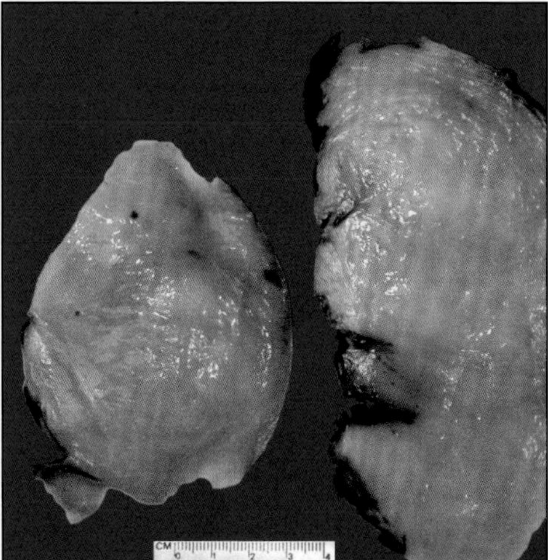

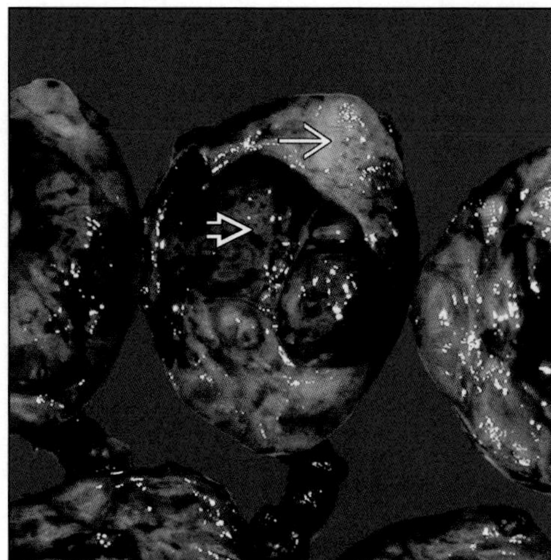

*(**Left**) This nodular GNB shows the pushing border between the stroma-poor neuroblastoma component ➡, and the ganglioneuroma component ➡. Often there will be a fibrous pseudocapsule between the 2 components. Even with this histologic picture, a grossly visible nodule is required to diagnose nodular GNB. (**Right**) In intermixed GNB, the nests of neuroblastoma can vary in size and maturation of neuroblasts. Here, a larger nest of immature neuroblasts is seen ➡.*

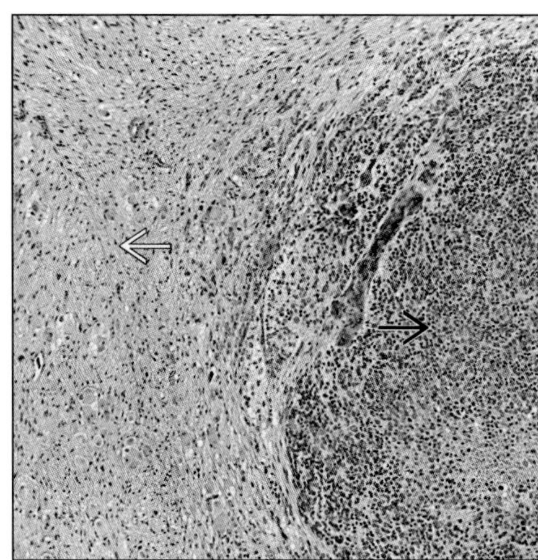

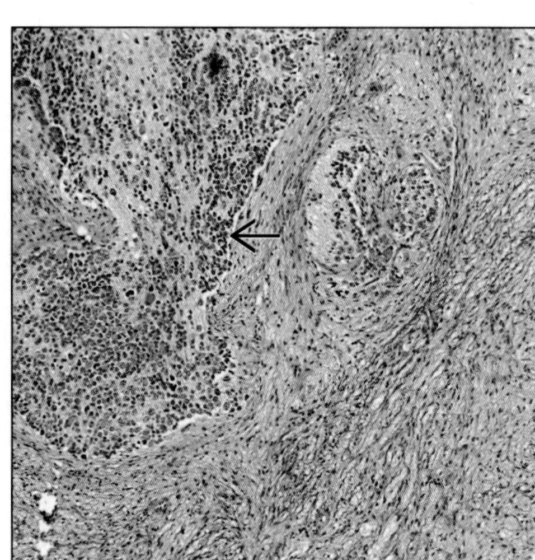

*(**Left**) To diagnose intermixed GNB, at least 50% of the tumor must be schwannian stroma. This is characterized by spindled, wavy cells in bundles of varying densities. (**Right**) This intermixed GNB shows nests ➡ of maturing neuroblasts, ganglion cells, and neuropil within a Schwannian stroma ➡.*

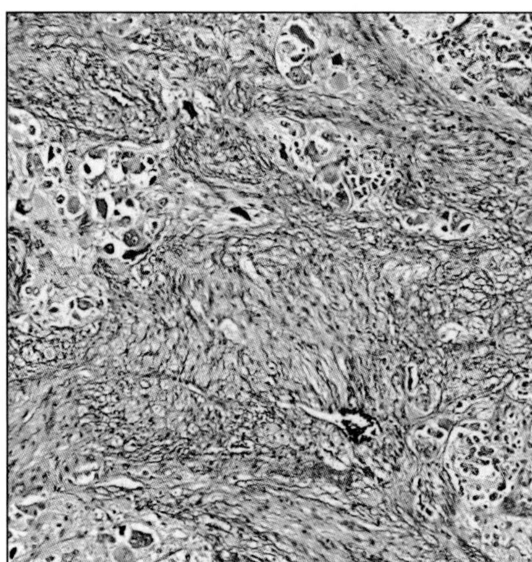

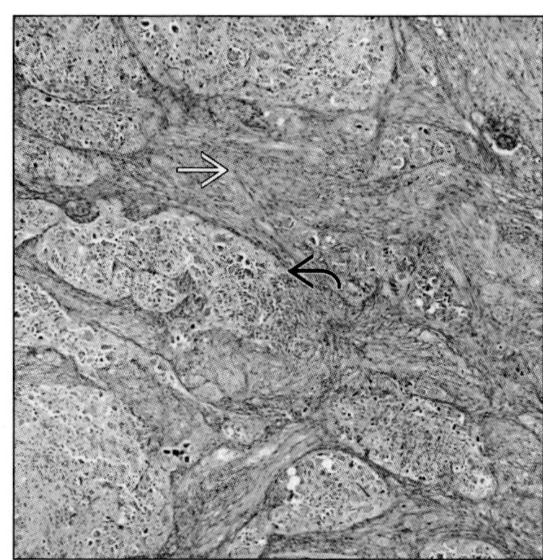

Microscopic Features of Ganglioneuroblastoma

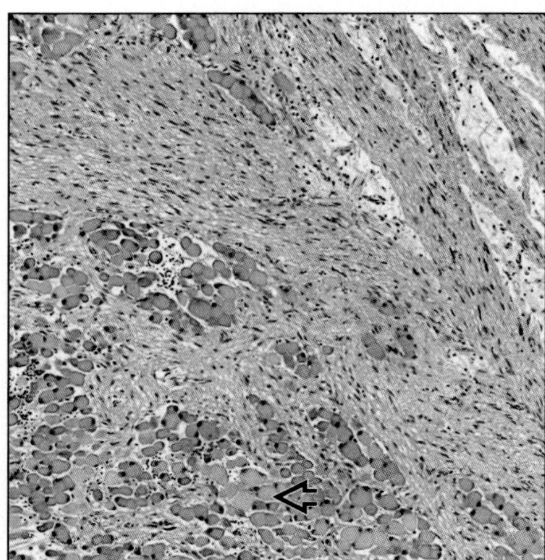

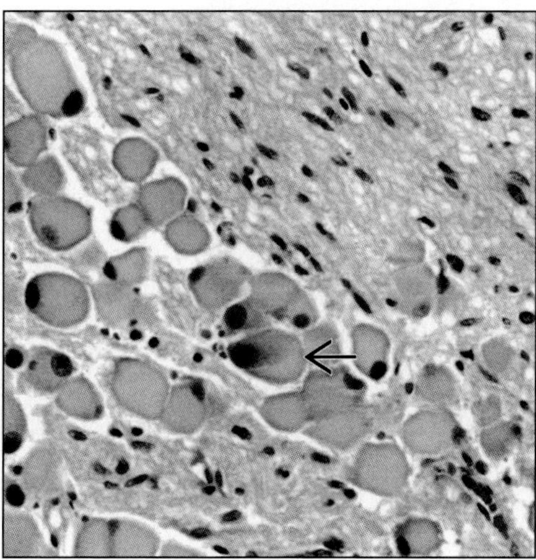

(Left) *The neuroblastomatous component of this intermixed GNB is predominantly (or nearly) mature ganglion cells ⇨. This is differentiated from a maturing ganglioneuroma (GN) by the ganglion cells present in clusters and not as single cells as in maturing GN.* ***(Right)*** *Mature ganglion cells → are characterized by abundant eosinophilic to amphophilic cytoplasm, eccentric nuclei, and prominent nucleoli. Nissl substance may or may not be present.*

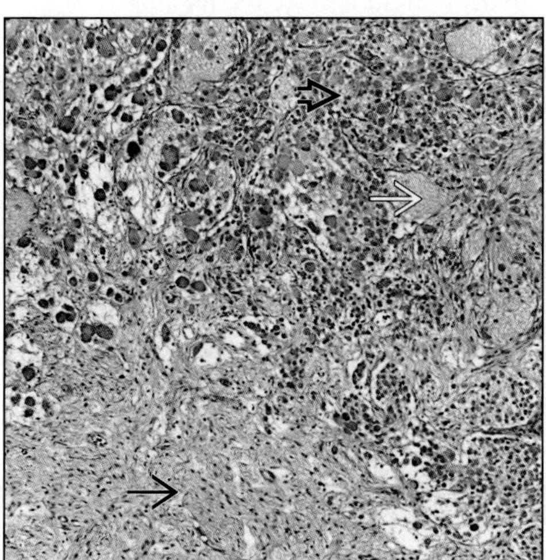

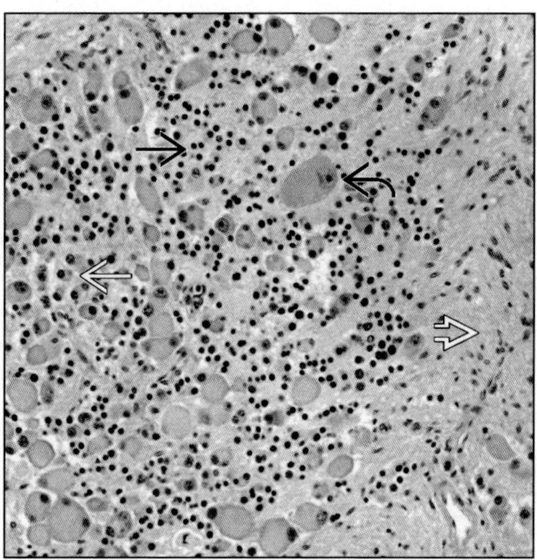

(Left) *Low-power view of this intermixed GNB shows maturing neuroblasts and ganglion cells ⇨, neuropil ➡, and schwannian stroma →.* ***(Right)*** *This intermixed GNB shows neuroblasts →, maturing neuroblasts ➡, and ganglion cells ↩ blending into schwannian stroma ⇨.*

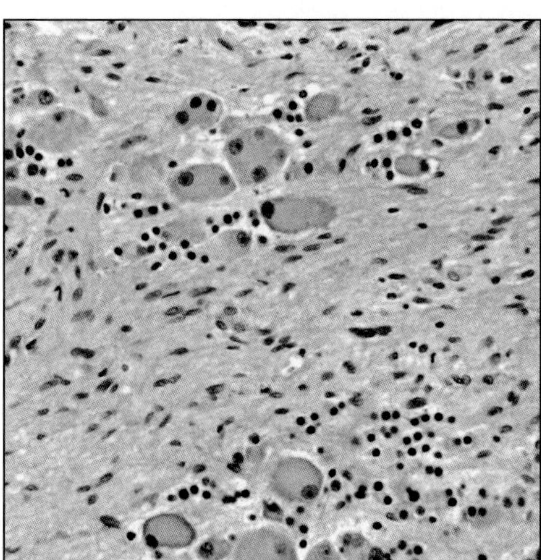

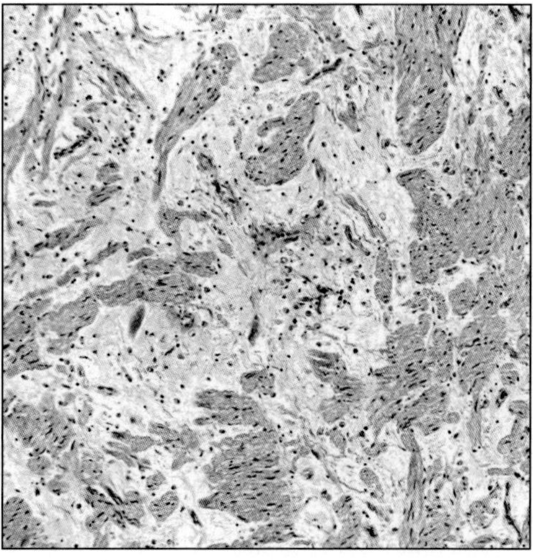

(Left) *This intermixed GNB could be mistaken for a maturing GN. In maturing GN, the tumor is predominantly composed of schwannian stroma, and individual neuroblastic cells merge into the schwannian stroma instead of forming distinct nests.* ***(Right)*** *This intermixed GNB could be mistaken for neurofibroma (spindled wavy cells in a myxoid background). Adequate sampling of the tumor specimen, generally 1 section per centimeter of tumor, is required to make an accurate diagnosis.*

ADRENAL CORTICAL CARCINOMA

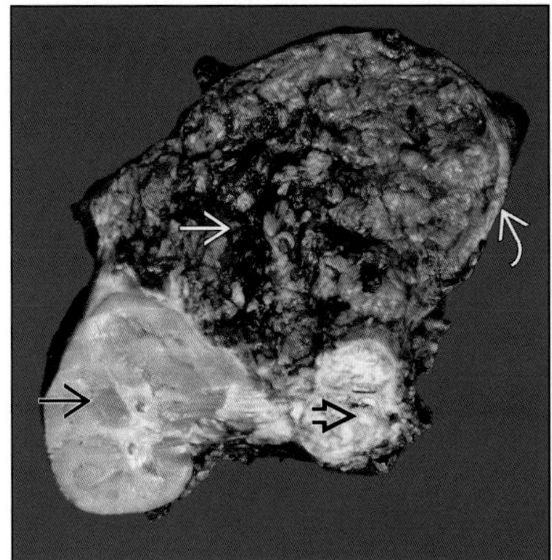

Gross image shows near complete replacement of adrenal gland by a large mass. Areas of hemorrhage ➔, necrosis ⇨, uninvolved kidney →, and residual adrenal gland ➔ are identified.

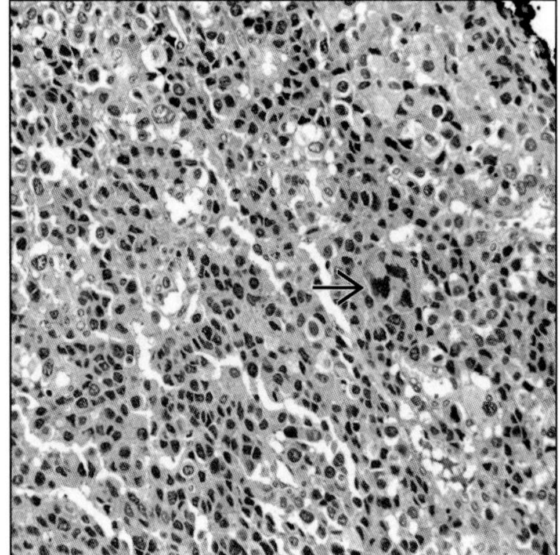

H&E stained section shows eosinophilic cells with marked nuclear pleomorphism →.

TERMINOLOGY

Abbreviations

- Adrenal cortical carcinoma (ACC)

Synonyms

- Adrenal carcinoma
- Adrenal cancer

ETIOLOGY/PATHOGENESIS

Associated with Multiple Hereditary Tumor Syndromes

- Li-Fraumeni syndrome
  - Frequency of ACC is up to 4% in Li-Fraumeni syndrome
- Beckwith-Wiedemann syndrome
  - Congenital overgrowth syndrome
  - Exophthalmos, macroglossia, gigantism
  - Development of childhood tumors
  - Mapped to 11p15.5 region
    - Genes located at 11p15 and implicated in pathogenesis of Beckwith-Wiedemann are *IGF-2*, *H19*, and *P57*
    - *IGF-2* is maternally imprinted
    - *H19* and *P57* are both paternally imprinted

Other Associations

- Somatic mutations in *P53* gene are often found in tumors of sporadic ACC
- 80-90% of sporadic ACCs are associated with rearrangement at 11p15 locus with overexpression of IGF-2
  - Overexpression of IGF-2 is associated with either duplications of paternal 11p15 allele or loss of maternal allele containing *H19* gene
- Loss of heterozygosity on chromosome 11q13 is also frequent occurrence
- In both benign and malignant ACCs, β-catenin accumulation has frequently been observed, indicating activation of Wnt-signaling pathway
  - Somatic mutations of β-catenin gene *CTNNB1* are seen in subset of these tumors
    - Thought to contribute to tumor progression

CLINICAL ISSUES

Epidemiology

- Incidence
  - 0.05-0.2% of all new cancers
  - 4% in general population
    - 1-2 per 1,000,000 population
  - 1/1,500 adrenal tumors are malignant
  - 20% have metastatic disease at presentation
- Age
  - Bimodal age distribution
    - Initial peak below age 5
    - Larger peak in 4th-5th decades
  - Surveillance epidemiology end results data
    - 14 new patient cases per year in individuals younger than 20 years
- Gender
  - F > M
    - Females account for 65-90% of all cases
    - Functioning tumors: More common in females
    - Nonfunctioning tumors: More common in males

Site

- Cortex of adrenal gland

Presentation

- Abnormal endocrine function
  - Hypersecretion of hormonal steroids in ACC is often presenting symptom but can also contribute to disease burden
    - Usually Cushing syndrome or sex steroid overproduction
  - Can severely affect quality of life

ADRENAL CORTICAL CARCINOMA

Key Facts

Clinical Issues

- Bimodal age distribution
- 1-2 per 1,000,000 population
- Stages I and II
  - Good prognosis after surgical removal
- Stages III and IV
  - Poor prognosis ± treatment
- Presentation
  - Abnormal endocrine function
  - Abdominal or flank tenderness

Image Findings

- Large, solid, unilateral adrenal mass with invasive margins (bilateral in 10%)

Macroscopic Features

- Average size: 14-15 cm

Microscopic Pathology

- Marked nuclear pleomorphism, hyperchromasia, and numerous mitotic figures are common findings
- Growth patterns may be alveolar, trabecular, or diffuse

Ancillary Tests

- Vimentin: Positive
- Inhibin-α: Positive
- Melan-A: Positive

Diagnostic Checklist

- Large size, vascular invasion, and high mitotic rates are features of more aggressive tumor
- Typical sites of metastasis include liver, lung, and lymph nodes

- Abdominal or flank tenderness
  - May present with palpable abdominal mass
  - Distant metastasis
    - Lungs, retroperitoneal nodes, and liver most common

Laboratory Tests

- Presentation with hormonally active malignancy
  - Cushing syndrome (30-40%): ↑ cortisol
    - Moon facies, truncal obesity, purple striae, and buffalo hump
  - Virilization in females (20-30%): ↑ androgens
    - 95% of children with functioning adrenal carcinoma present with virilization
  - Conn syndrome (primary hyperaldosteronism)
    - Hypertension and weakness
  - Feminization in males: ↑ androgens
- Other clinical syndromes at presentation
  - Hypoglycemia, polycythemia, and non-glucocorticoid-related insulin resistance

Natural History

- Rapid growth with local invasion and distant metastases
- Tumor thrombus: IVC and renal vein

Treatment

- Options, risks, complications
  - Due to high risk of recurrence, adjuvant therapy is recommended even after complete resection
  - Despite adjuvant measures, rate of recurrence after radical resection is still around 50%
- Surgical approaches
  - Radical surgery is standard therapy for patients with localized and regional ACC (stages I-III)
    - Small lesions: Laparoscopic adrenalectomy
    - Large lesions with extension: Radical resection of ipsilateral kidney, adrenal gland, and adjacent structures
    - Metastases also resected if possible
- Adjuvant therapy
  - Mitotane
    - Synthetic derivative of insecticide dichlorodiphenyltrichloroethane (DDT)
    - Proven to significantly reduce risk of recurrence and death
  - Mitotane in combination with cytotoxic drugs is used in patients with metastasized ACC
    - 2 most promising regimens are etoposide, doxorubicin, and cisplatin plus mitotane, or streptozotocin plus mitotane
  - VEGF is significantly elevated in tumor tissue and circulating blood in patients with ACC
    - VEGF and its receptor VEGF-R2 are strongly expressed in majority of ACCs, suggesting that vascular-targeted therapies may hold promise for patients with ACC
- Drugs
  - Radiolabeled metomidate
    - Specific tracer for molecular imaging of cytochrome p450 family 11B (Cyp11B) enzymes
    - Group of enzymes highly specific for adrenal cortex
    - Adrenocortical tissue shows high and specific tracer uptake in both primary tumor and ACC metastases
    - Preliminary experience has shown that high therapeutic doses can be achieved in patients with ACCs using iodine-labeled metomidate
- Radiation
  - Adjuvant tumor bed irradiation is often offered to patients with high risk for local recurrence

Prognosis

- Recent data from German ACC Registry demonstrated overall survival of 47% after 5 years and 41% after 10 years
- Stages I and II
  - Good prognosis after surgical removal
- Stages III and IV
  - Poor prognosis with or without treatment
  - 5-year survival for stage III disease is < 30%
  - In patients with metastases (stage IV), median survival is < 15 months and 5-year survival is 24%

ADRENAL CORTICAL CARCINOMA

- Children have better prognosis than adults

IMAGE FINDINGS

General Features

- Best diagnostic clue
  - Large, solid, unilateral adrenal mass with invasive margins (bilateral in 10%)
  - NECT + CECT: Study of choice to exclude adenoma
- Location
  - Suprarenal, usually unilateral (left > right)
- Size
  - Functioning tumors: Usually 5 cm at presentation
  - Nonfunctioning tumors: ≥ 10 cm
- Morphology
  - Large suprarenal invasive lesion
  - Usually contain hemorrhagic, cystic, and calcified areas

Ultrasonographic Findings

- Grayscale ultrasound
  - Variable appearance depending on size and contents
  - Small tumors
    - Echo pattern similar to renal cortex
  - Large tumors
    - Mixed heterogeneous echo pattern (due to areas of necrosis and hemorrhage)

MR Findings

- T1WI: Hypointense adrenal mass compared to liver
- T2WI: Hyperintense adrenal mass compared to liver
- T1WI C+: Heterogeneous enhancement (tumor necrosis)
- Multiplanar contrast-enhanced imaging
  - Renal vein, IVC, and adjacent renal parenchymal invasion well depicted on MR
  - Sagittal imaging helps to evaluate IVC invasion
  - Delineate tumor-liver interface if tumor is on right

CT Findings

- Solid, well-defined suprarenal mass with invasive margins
- Usually unilateral, may be bilateral (10% of cases)
- Typically associated with areas of hemorrhage, necrosis, fat, and calcification
  - 30% of tumors are associated with intratumoral calcification
- Variable enhancement secondary to necrosis and hemorrhage
- ± renal vein, IVC, and adjacent renal extension
- Metastases to lung bases, liver, or lymph nodes

MACROSCOPIC FEATURES

General Features

- Cut section pink to tan to yellow, depending on lipid content of tumor cells
- Commonly lobulated with areas of fibrosis, necrosis, hemorrhage, or calcification
- Invasion of adjacent structures is common

Size

- Large cortical masses
  - Usually > 100 g in adults and > 500 g in children
  - Usually > 6 cm and only rarely < 3 cm
    - Average: 14-15 cm

MICROSCOPIC PATHOLOGY

Histologic Features

- Varied cellular appearance depending on lipid content
  - Lipid-depleted cells appear as small cells with eosinophilic cytoplasm
  - Lipid-laden cells are large and vacuolated
- May be composed of cells resembling normal adrenal cortical cells
  - Marked nuclear pleomorphism, hyperchromasia, and numerous mitotic figures are common findings
  - Occasionally tumor cells are multinucleated and have single or multiple nucleoli
- Nuclear pseudoinclusions, representing invaginations of cytoplasm into nucleus, may be particularly striking
- Growth patterns may be alveolar, trabecular, or diffuse
  - Characteristic pattern shows broad trabeculae with anastomosing architecture
- Infiltrative growth pattern
- Irregularly shaped sinusoidal channels with flattened endothelial lining
- Vascular invasion is commonly identified
- Rarely intracytoplasmic eosinophilic hyaline globules may be seen
- Foci of myxoid change, pseudoglandular patterns, and spindle-cell growth may be prominent in some tumors
- Some ACCs may be composed of oncocytic cells
  - May be associated with Cushing syndrome or may be nonfunctional
  - Tend to have low mitotic activity (< 1/10 HPF)
  - Cytologic atypia is uncommon
- Features strongly suggestive of malignancy
  - Large tumor size
  - High-grade nuclear pleomorphism
  - Frequent mitoses (> 5/50 HPF), especially atypical mitoses
  - Broad fibrous bands
  - Necrosis (> 2 HPF in diameter)
  - Diffuse growth pattern (comprising > 30% of tumor)
  - Capsular or venous invasion
  - Predominantly lipid-depleted (nonclear) cells (< 25% of tumor composed of clear cells)
  - Metastasis

Predominant Pattern/Injury Type

- Heterogeneous

Predominant Cell/Compartment Type

- Epithelial

Two Histopathological Scoring Systems

- Weiss revisited index (WRI) score
  - Consists of the following parameters
    - Mitotic index
    - Clear cytoplasm < 25%
    - Abnormal mitoses

- Necrosis and capsular invasion
  - Each criterion is scored 0 when absent and 1 when present
    - Exceptions: Mitotic index and clear cytoplasm < 25%, which are scored 2 when present
  - Threshold for malignancy using WRI is ≥ 3
- van Slooten index (VSI)
  - Consists of 7 parameters, each with different weight (indicated between parentheses)
    - Regressive changes such as necrosis, hemorrhage, fibrosis, or calcification (5.7)
    - Structural changes (1.6)
    - Nuclear atypia (2.1)
    - Nuclear hyperchromasia (2.6)
    - Abnormal structure of nucleoli (4.1)
    - Mitotic activity > 2/10 HPFs (x 40 objective) (9)
    - Capsule &/or blood vessel invasion (3.3)
  - Total score is based on addition of parameters, if present, yielding score between 0 and 28.4
    - VSI threshold for malignancy is > 8
- Application of both scoring systems is recommended in case either one yields an equivocal result

ANCILLARY TESTS

Cytology

- ACCs generally contain single cells and poorly cohesive cell clusters in necrotic background
- Nuclear atypia and mitotic activity are common
  - However, some ACCs may contain very bland cells
- Cytoplasm varies from vacuolated to densely eosinophilic
- Rare spindle cells may be identified

Histochemistry

- Periodic acid-Schiff
  - Reactivity: Positive
  - Staining pattern
    - Hyaline globules

Immunohistochemistry

- Vimentin: Positive
- Inhibin-α: Positive
- Melan-A: Positive
- Ki-67 (MIB-1) should show strong nuclear reactivity in large proportion of cells, consistent with high mitotic activity
- p53: Positive if somatic mutations of *P53* gene are present
- May occasionally show immunoreactivity for neurofilament, S100, synaptophysin, and NSE
- Cytokeratin
  - Earlier studies indicated that ACCs were cytokeratin negative
  - More recent studies using microwave-induced antigen retrieval reveal positivity in substantial number of cases
  - CAM5.2 (for cytokeratins 8 and 18): Present focally in up to 60% of ACCs
  - Oncocytic ACCs are positive for cytokeratins using AE1/AE3 and CAM5.2 antibodies
- EMA: Negative

Cytogenetics

- Chromosomal instability has been described in ACCs
  - Abnormalities on chromosome 11, 13, or 17 are consistent findings
- Number of somatic aberrations in ACC predicts prognosis
- Cytotoxic drugs may further increase number of genomic alterations, thereby promoting tumor differentiation and resistance to current treatment modalities

Electron Microscopy

- Transmission
  - Prominent rough and smooth endoplasmic reticulum
  - Intracellular lipid droplets
  - Mitochondria are round, ovoid, or elongated
    - Contain tubular cristae

DIFFERENTIAL DIAGNOSIS

Adrenal Cortical Adenoma

- Smaller in size
  - Usually 3-6 cm in adults
- Well circumscribed, often encapsulated
- May show some nuclear pleomorphism
- Adult patients
  - No necrosis, increased mitoses, or invasion of capsule or vessels
- Pediatric patients
  - Commonly associated with high mitotic rate, necrosis, fibrous bands, and nuclear pleomorphism

Pheochromocytoma

- Arises from adrenal medulla with normal adrenal cortex stretched out over its surface
- Red-brown in color with areas of hemorrhage or cystic degeneration if large
- Organoid growth pattern with nests of cells ("zellballen") and delicate vascular septa
- Tumor > 3 cm in most cases
- Highly vascular tumor prone to hemorrhage and necrosis
- Immunohistochemistry
  - Immunoreactive for neurofilament, chromogranin, synaptophysin, and S100 (in sustentacular cell staining pattern)
  - Negative for vimentin
- Bilateral adrenal tumors in multiple endocrine neoplasia (MEN) 2A and 2B syndromes

Metastatic Renal Cell Carcinoma (RCC) (Clear Cell)

- Upper pole RCC mimics large ACC
- Often show very similar gross and microscopic features
- Cytokeratin and vimentin positive

ADRENAL CORTICAL CARCINOMA

Differential Diagnosis of Adrenal Cortical Carcinoma

Antibody	Cortical Carcinoma	Pheochromocytoma/ Chromocytoma	Renal Cell Carcinoma
Cytokeratin	±	-	+
Vimentin	+	±	+
Neurofilament	±	+	-
S100		+	±
EMA	-	-	+
Chromogranin	-	+	-
Synaptophysin	±	+	-
Calretinin	+	-	±
Inhibin	+	-	±

Criteria for Diagnosis of Adrenal Cortical Carcinoma

Criteria	van Slooten et al, 1985	Modified Weiss System, 2002
Common Histologic Features		
Venous invasion	+	
Pleomorphism/high-grade nuclei	+	
Necrosis	+	+
Mitoses	+	+
Capsular invasion	+	+
Other Histologic Features		
Atypical mitoses		+
Clear cells (< 25%)		+
Abnormal nucleoli	+	

DIAGNOSTIC CHECKLIST

Pathologic Interpretation Pearls

- Large size, vascular invasion, and high mitotic rates are features of more aggressive tumor
- Typical sites of metastasis include liver, lung, and lymph nodes

STAGING

TNM Stage I

- T1, N0, M0
  - T1: Tumor ≤ 5 cm, no local invasion
  - N0: No regional node
  - M0: No distant metastases

TNM Stage II

- T2, N0, M0
  - T2: Tumor ≥ 5 cm, no local invasion
  - N0: No regional node
  - M0: No distant metastases

TNM Stage III

- T1, N1, M0
  - N1: Positive regional nodes
- T2, N1, M0
- T3, N0, M0
  - T3: Tumors of any size with local invasion but without invasion of adjacent organs

TNM Stage IV

- Any T, any N, M1
  - M1: Distant metastases
- T3, N1, M0
- T4, N0, M0
  - T4: Tumor of any size with invasion of adjacent organs

SELECTED REFERENCES

1. Fassnacht M et al: New targets and therapeutic approaches for endocrine malignancies. Pharmacol Ther. 123(1):117-41, 2009
2. van Ditzhuijsen CI et al: Adrenocortical carcinoma. Neth J Med. 65(2):55-60, 2007
3. Michalkiewicz E et al: Clinical and outcome characteristics of children with adrenocortical tumors: a report from the International Pediatric Adrenocortical Tumor Registry. J Clin Oncol. 22(5):838-45, 2004
4. Aubert S et al: Weiss system revisited: a clinicopathologic and immunohistochemical study of 49 adrenocortical tumors. Am J Surg Pathol. 26(12):1612-9, 2002
5. van Slooten H et al: Morphologic characteristics of benign and malignant adrenocortical tumors. Cancer. 55(4):766-73, 1985

Diagrammatic and Gross Features

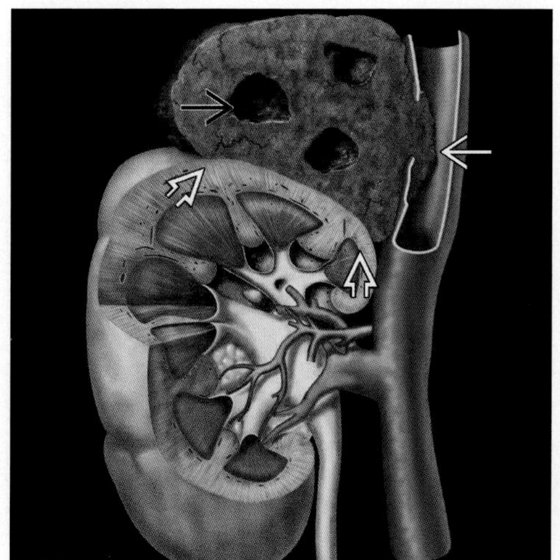

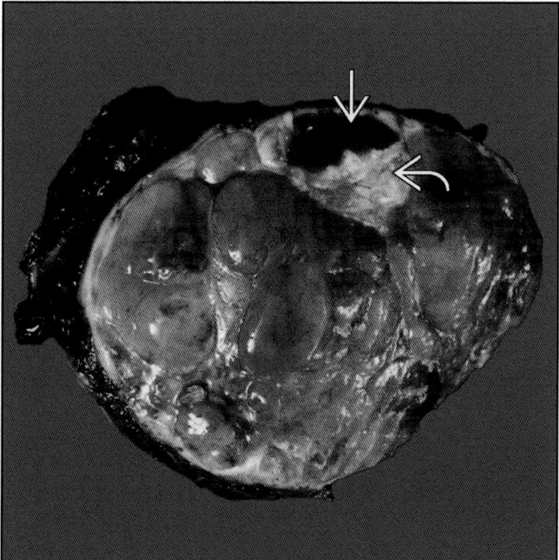

(Left) *Composite image shows a large right adrenal carcinoma with areas of necrosis ⇒, tumor invasion in the inferior vena cava ⇒, and compression of the right renal upper pole ⇒.* ***(Right)*** *Gross photograph shows nonencapsulated tumor within the adrenal gland with a focus of necrosis ⇒ and hemorrhage ⇒.*

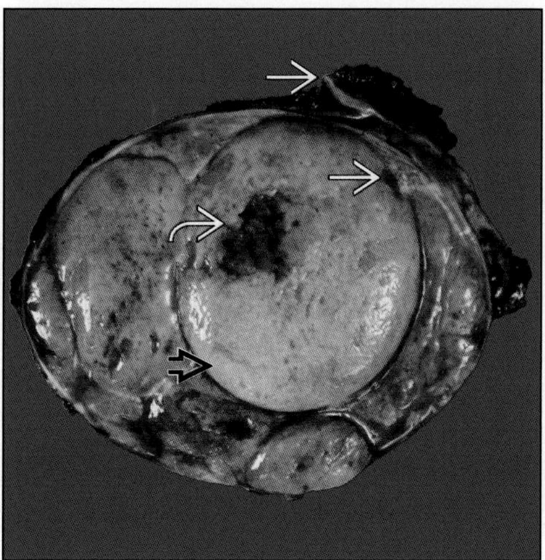

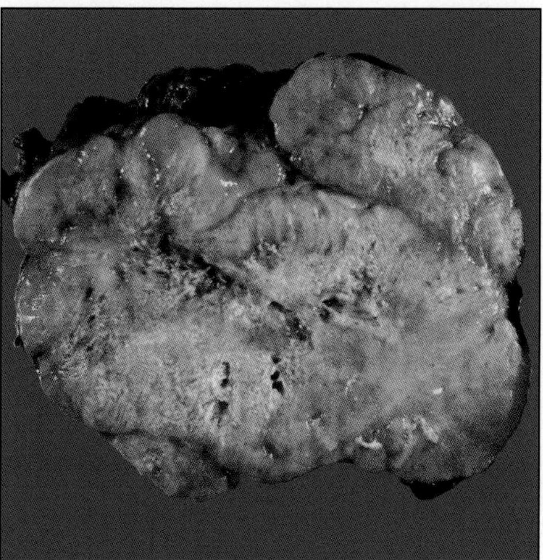

(Left) *Gross photograph of adrenal gland shows almost complete replacement by multiple red-brown tumor nodules ⇒ containing several areas of pinpoint hemorrhage ⇒. Residual adrenal gland ⇒ is seen at the superior edge of the picture.* ***(Right)*** *Gross photograph shows complete replacement of the adrenal gland by a pink-tan lobulated tumor.*

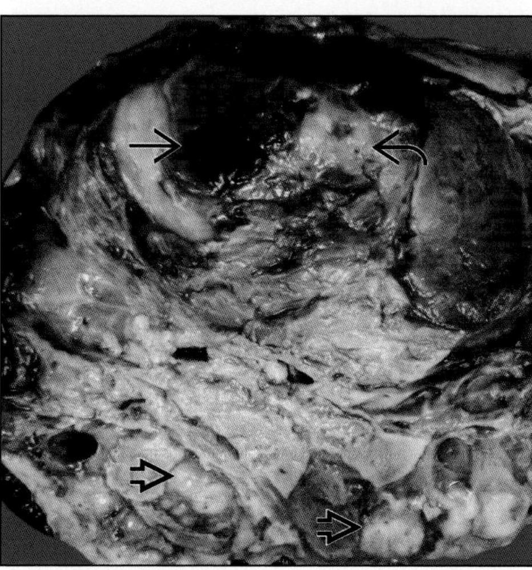

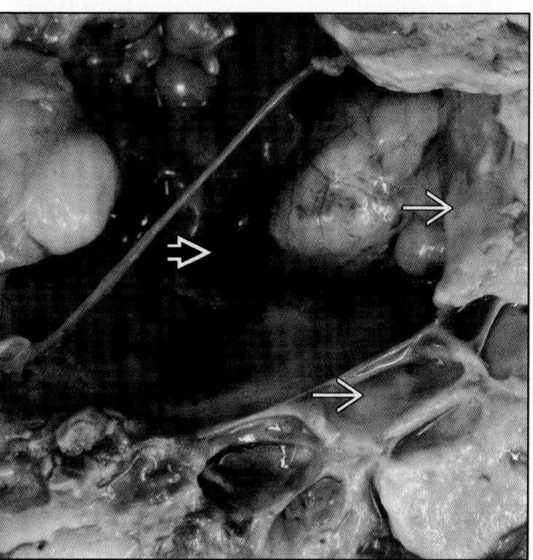

(Left) *Gross photograph of a large adrenal gland tumor shows extensive necrosis ⇒, hemorrhage ⇒, and multiple tumor nodules ⇒.* ***(Right)*** *Close-up shows an adrenal tumor composed of multiple tumor nodules with foci of hemorrhage ⇒ and lipid deposition ⇒.*

ADRENAL CORTICAL CARCINOMA

Microscopic Features

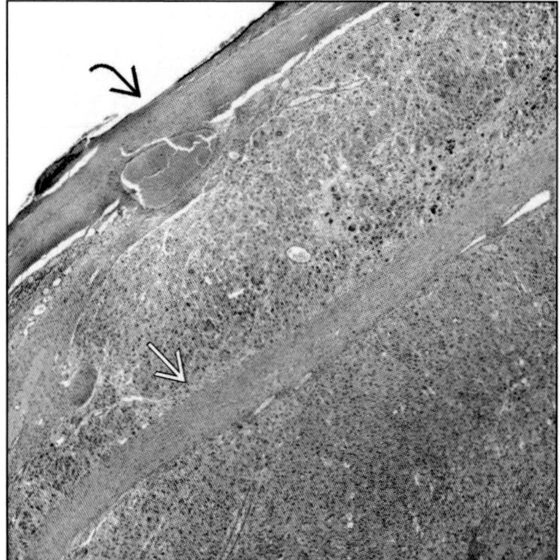

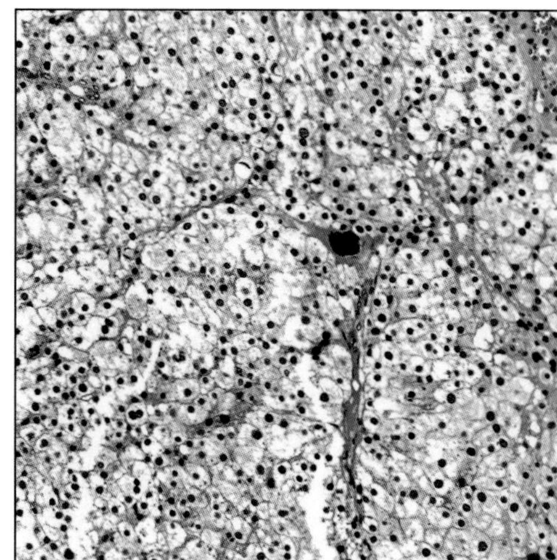

(Left) Low-power H&E stained section of ACC shows a thick capsule ➔ surrounding a tumor composed of eosinophilic cells. Large pleomorphic tumor cells with hyperchromatic chromatin can be seen scattered throughout the tumor. A large fibrous band ➔ runs down the middle of the tumor section. **(Right)** H&E stained section of ACC shows lobular pattern of growth.

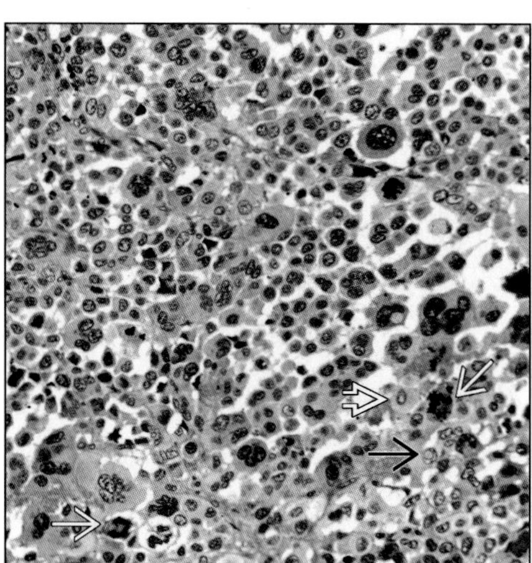

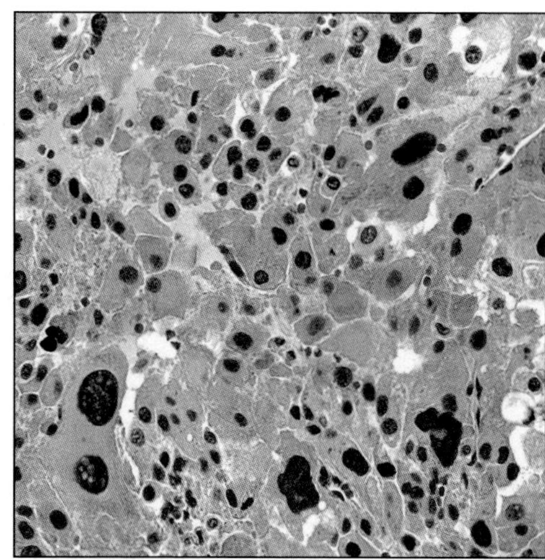

(Left) H&E stained section of ACC shows multiple large pleomorphic tumor cells with scattered atypical mitotic figures ➔ and focal incipient calcifications ➔. A few intranuclear "pseudoinclusions" are evident ➔. **(Right)** H&E stained section of ACC shows large pleomorphic tumor cells with hyperchromasia, lobulations, and irregular borders.

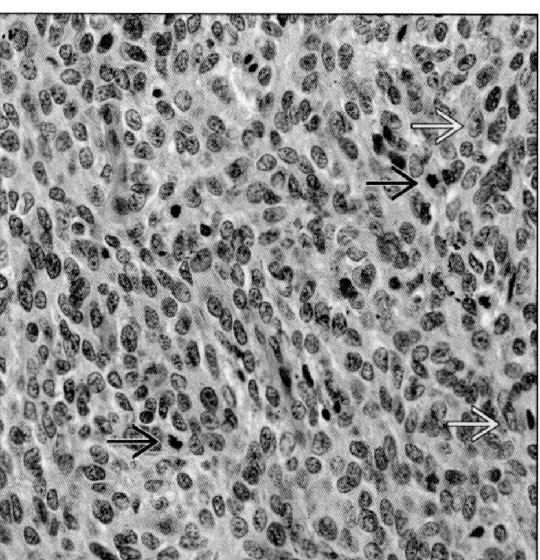

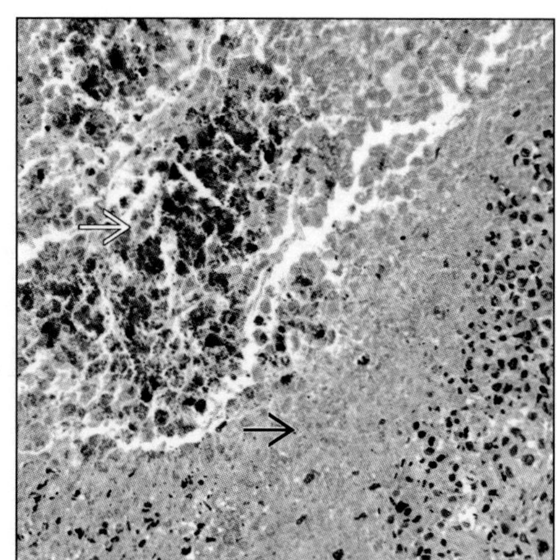

(Left) H&E stained section shows eosinophilic tumor cells with prominent nucleoli, scattered nuclear "pseudoinclusions" ➔, and numerous mitotic figures ➔. **(Right)** H&E stained section shows intratumoral necrosis ➔ and incipient calcification ➔.

Microscopic and Immunohistochemical Features

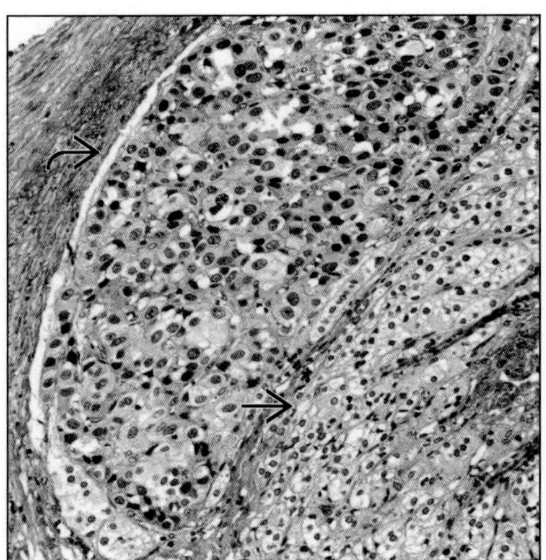

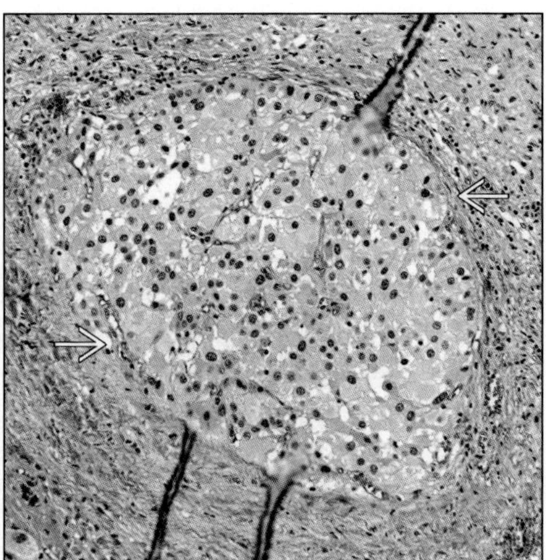

(Left) *H&E stained section shows intravascular tumor* ⮫ *adjacent to normal adrenal cortex* ⇨. *The tumor cells are large and pleomorphic when compared to the normal cortical cells, showing large nuclei with prominent nucleoli and abundant eosinophilic cytoplasm.* ***(Right)*** *An intravascular tumor* ➡ *completely fills the vessel lumen with compression of the endothelial lining. The surrounding fibrous tissue contains scattered lymphocytes.*

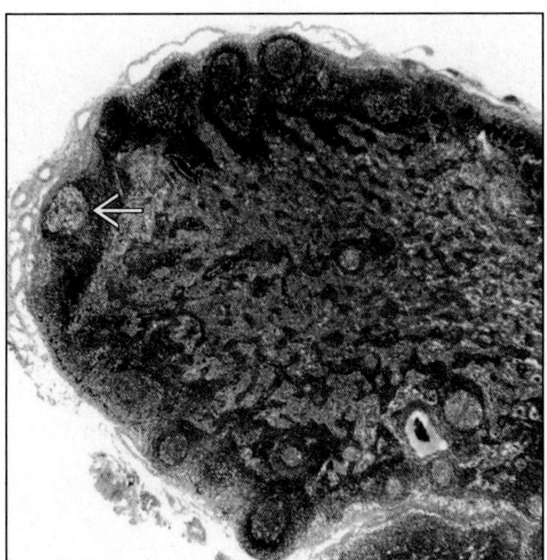

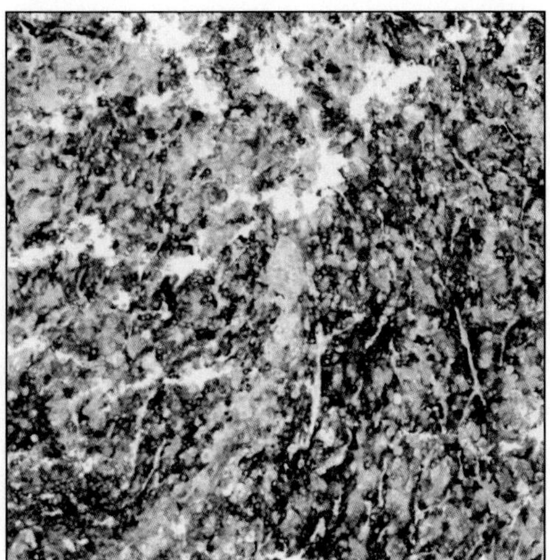

(Left) *H&E stained section of an abdominal lymph node shows a small focus of metastatic ACC* ➡ *just beneath the capsule. The lymph node shows preservation of follicular architecture at the periphery. The central portion of the lymph node shows dilated sinuses filled with clusters of histiocytes (sinus histiocytosis).* ***(Right)*** *Immunohistochemical stain for inhibin-α shows diffuse and strong cytoplasmic reactivity.*

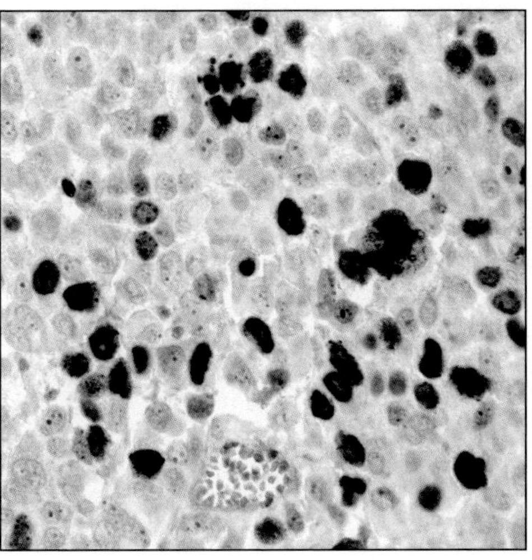

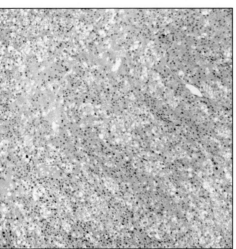

(Left) *Ki-67 (MIB-1) immunohistochemical stain shows > 20% of tumor cells with strong nuclear reactivity, consistent with a high mitotic index.* ***(Right)*** *Immunohistochemical stain shows tumor cells negative for p53. Positivity would support the presence of a somatic P53 mutation.*

Ancillary Techniques and Radiologic Features

(Left) *Fine needle aspiration shows large single cells and a cluster of poorly cohesive cells characterized by large, dense nuclei ➡, vacuolated cytoplasm ➡, and irregular cell borders ➡.* ***(Right)*** *Electron micrograph shows neoplastic cells with numerous lipid inclusions ➡, characteristic of steroid-producing tumors.*

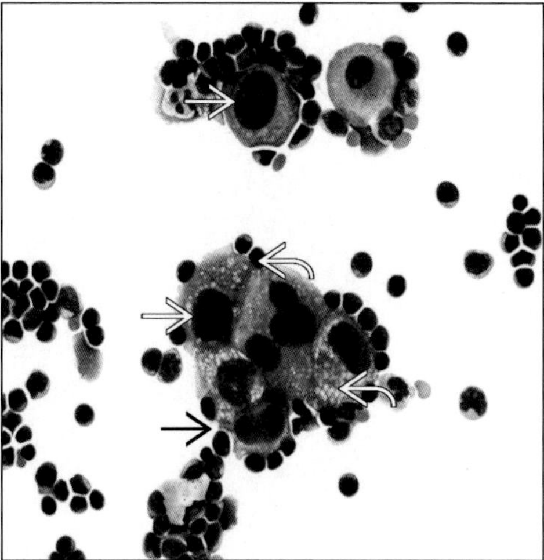

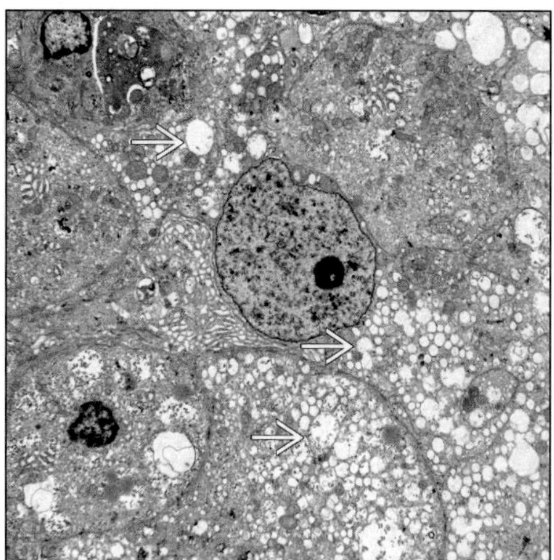

(Left) *Electron micrograph shows neoplastic cells with abundant smooth endoplasmic reticulum and mitochondria with tubular cristae ➡, characteristic of steroid-producing tumors.* ***(Right)*** *Transverse transabdominal ultrasound shows a huge, solid left adrenal cortical carcinoma ➡.*

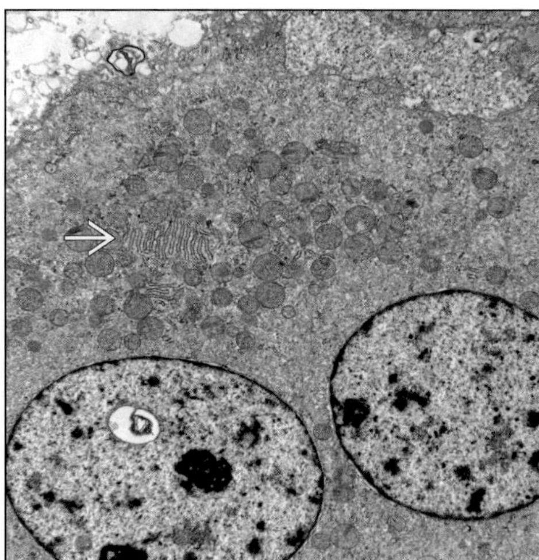

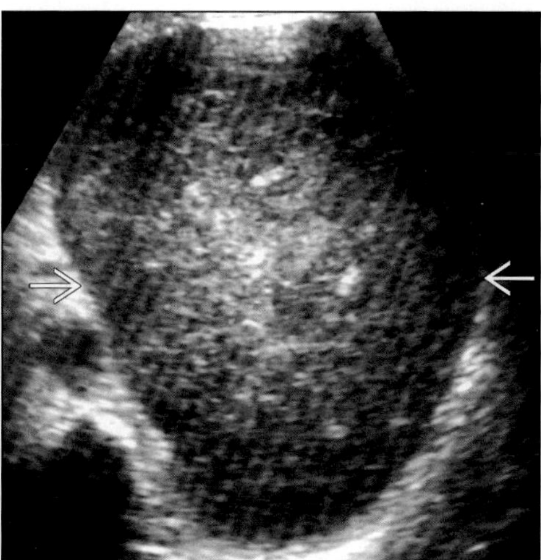

(Left) *Axial CECT shows a large, heterogeneous, partially calcified ➡ right adrenal cortical carcinoma ➡ with spontaneous retroperitoneal bleed.* ***(Right)*** *Axial T2WI MR shows a heterogeneous, large left adrenal cortical carcinoma ➡.*

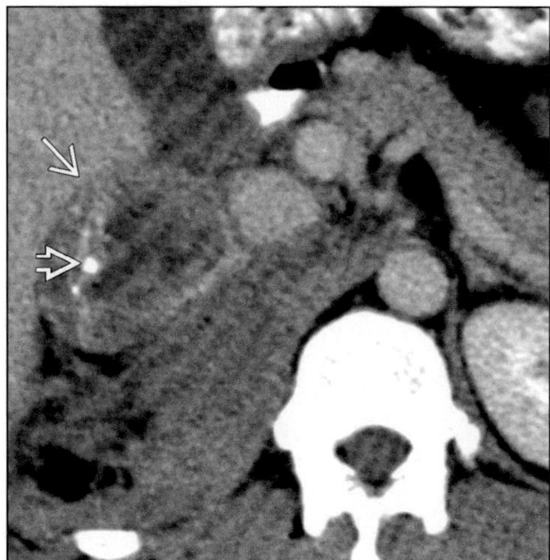

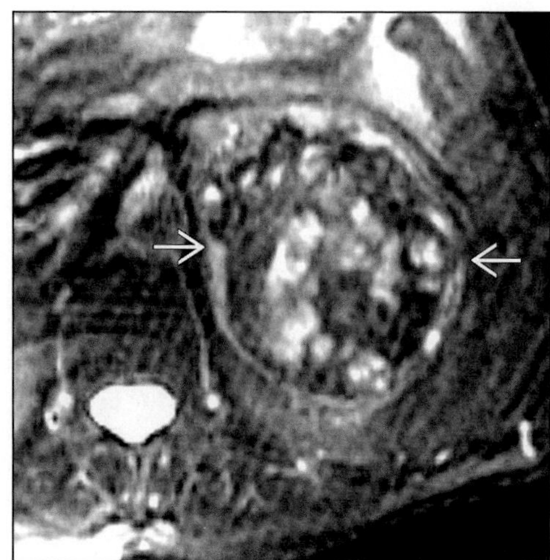

Differential Diagnosis

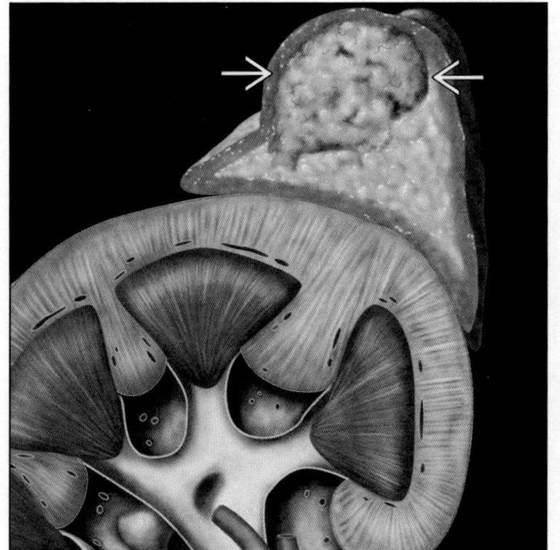

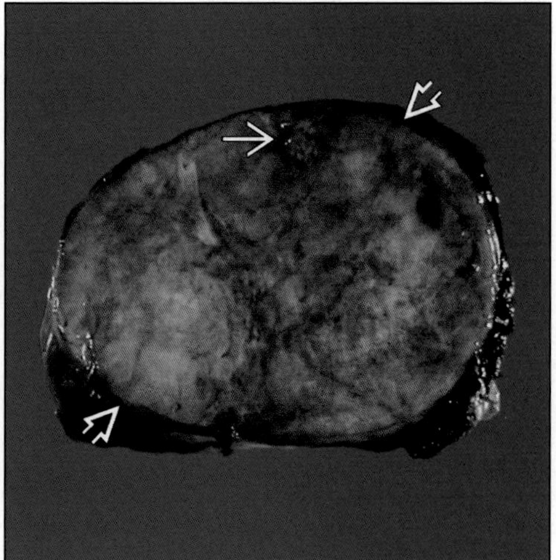

(Left) *Graphic of an adrenal cortical adenoma shows a small, lipid-rich mass ➡ within the adrenal gland.* ***(Right)*** *Gross photograph shows a well-circumscribed, encapsulated ➡ mass with residual small portion of adrenal cortex ➡. The cut surface of the adenoma is marbled yellow and brown and free of hemorrhage and necrosis.*

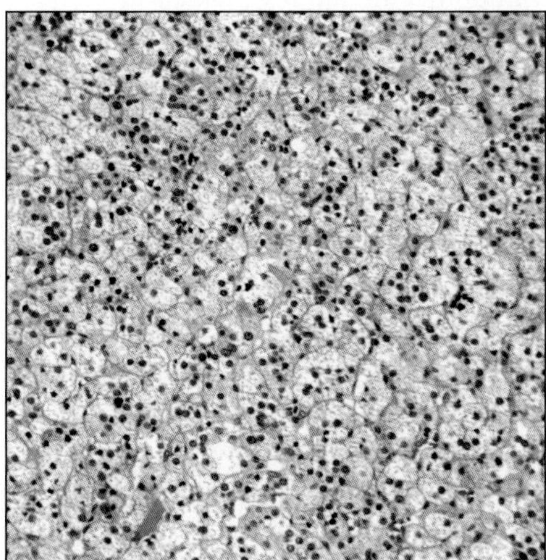

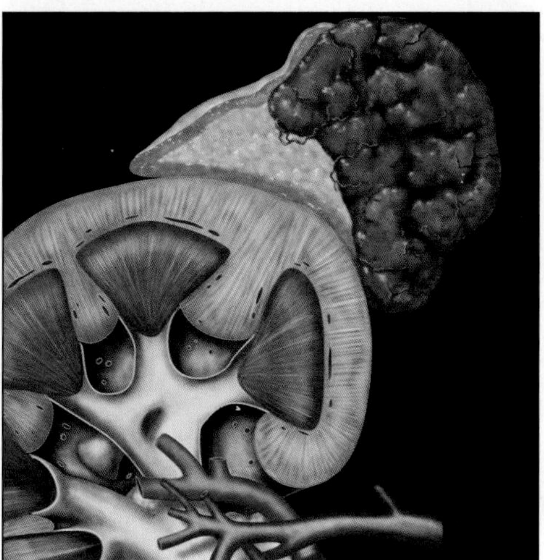

(Left) *H&E stained section of an adrenal adenoma shows cells with clear cytoplasm and small hyperchromatic nuclei lacking atypia, pleomorphism, and mitotic activity.* ***(Right)*** *Graphic shows heterogeneous, hypervascular adrenal pheochromocytoma.*

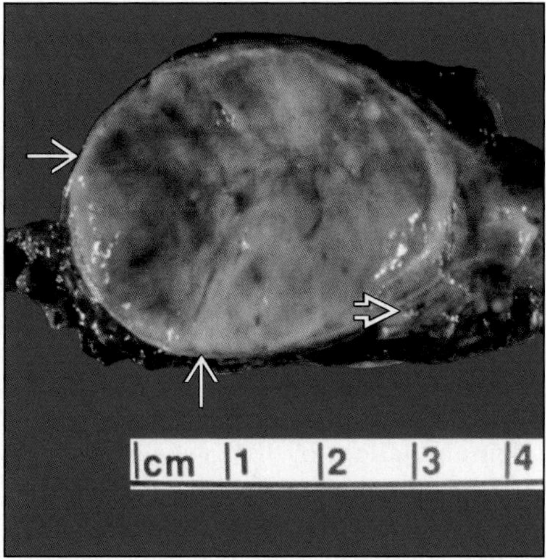

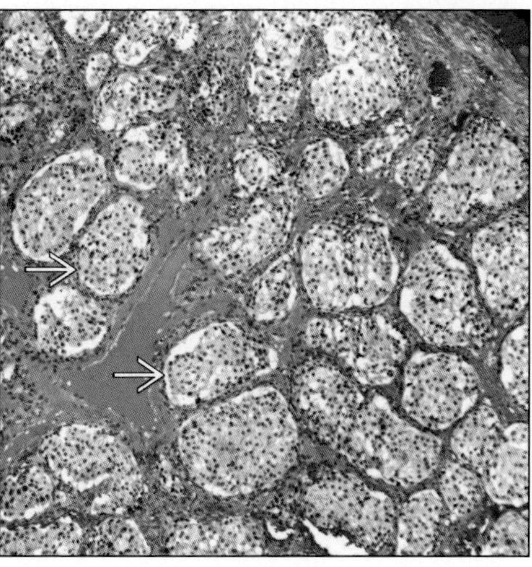

(Left) *Gross photograph shows a pheochromocytoma ➡ arising within the medulla of an adrenal gland. The mass is ovoid and sharply circumscribed from the adjacent uninvolved adrenal cortex ➡. Cut surface shows a soft, variegated appearance with an tan-yellow to a red-brown color.* ***(Right)*** *H&E stained section shows tumor cells of a pheochromocytoma arranged in well-defined nests called "zellballen" ➡.*

PAPILLARY THYROID CARCINOMA

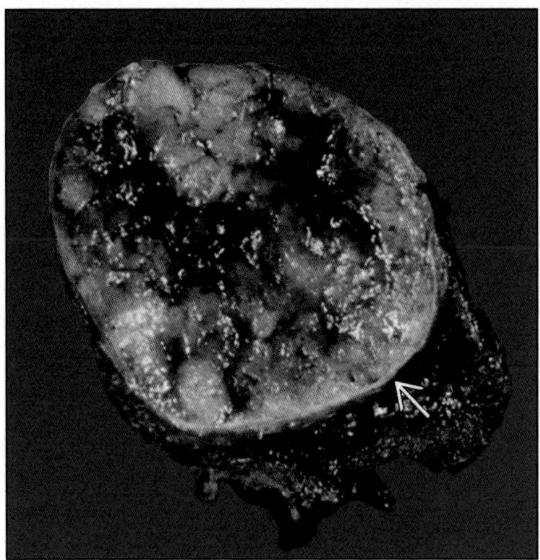

The cut surface of papillary thyroid carcinoma shows a granular appearance. The lesion is well circumscribed and has a thin capsule ➡ separating it from the adjacent normal parenchyma.

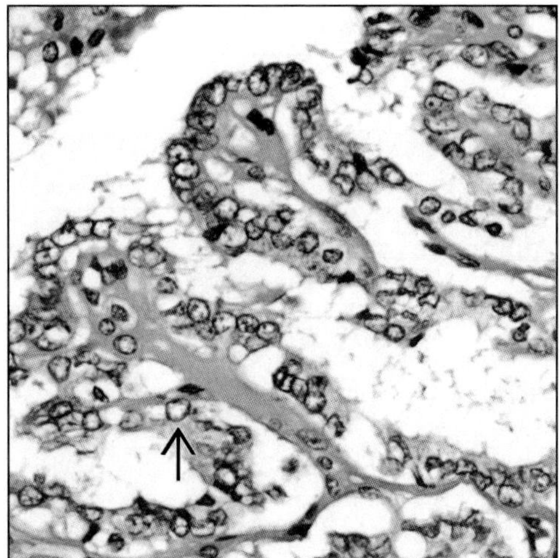

This photomicrograph demonstrates a papillary thyroid carcinoma with papillary architecture and fibrovascular cores. Note the irregularly shaped, clear nuclei ⇨ with irregular nuclear membranes.

TERMINOLOGY

Abbreviations

- Papillary thyroid carcinoma (PTC)

Synonyms

- Papillary carcinoma
- Thyroid papillary carcinoma (TPC)
- Papillary adenocarcinoma

Definitions

- Malignant epithelial neoplasm showing follicular cell differentiation characterized by distinctive nuclear features

ETIOLOGY/PATHOGENESIS

Environmental Exposure

- Radiation exposure
  - Only known predisposing factor in childhood development of papillary thyroid carcinoma
    - Children < 1 year of age who were exposed to Chernobyl fallout are at increased risk for thyroid cancer
    - Increased incidence in children who received head and neck radiation therapy for a prior head and neck neoplasm
    - Time from therapy to diagnosis of PTC is 9 years on average
- RET/PTC rearrangement
  - Most common chromosomal structural alteration in papillary thyroid carcinoma
  - Mutation leads to activation of RET proto-oncogene
  - Increased in children exposed to radiation (50-80%)
    - However, reported in children without radiation exposure (10-30%)
  - RET/PTC1
    - Associated with classic papillary histologic pattern
  - RET/PTC3
    - More common in children with radiation exposure
    - Associated with the follicular and solid histologic pattern of PTC
    - More aggressive tumors than those with the RET/PTC1 rearrangement

Tumor Predisposition Syndromes

- Carney complex
  - Autosomal dominant
  - Characterized by
    - Pigmented skin and mucosal lesions
    - Sertoli-Leydig cell tumors
    - Pituitary adenomas
    - Pigmented nodular adrenal disease
    - Thyroid tumors including PTC
- Familial adenomatous polyposis
  - Autosomal dominant syndrome caused by inherited germline mutations of *APC* gene (5q21)
  - FAP-associated PTC account for 2% of cases
  - FAP-associated PTC tend to be bilateral and multifocal
  - Histologically, majority are cribriform morular variant of PTC
    - Characteristic nuclear features are rarely identified
  - Prognosis is similar to conventional PTC
- Cowden syndrome
  - Part of the PTEN hamartomatous tumor syndrome
  - Patients are at increased risk for both benign and malignant tumors of the breast, thyroid, and endometrium

Somatic Mutations

- *BRAF* mutations
  - Activating point mutations of *BRAF* gene
  - Uncommon in children under 15 years of age with PTC
  - Uncommon in radiation-induced cases
  - *BRAF* mutations in PTC are associated with low expression of sodium iodide symporter genes,

PAPILLARY THYROID CARCINOMA

Key Facts

Etiology/Pathogenesis
- Most cases are sporadic
- Genetic alterations are common (*BRAF*, *RET/PTC*)
- Familial syndromes (Cowden, FAP, Carney complex)
- Increased incidence in children who received head and neck radiation therapy for a prior head and neck neoplasm
- RET/PTC rearrangement
  - ↑ in children exposed to radiation (50-80%)

Clinical Issues
- Most common histologic type of thyroid carcinoma in children
- Most are diagnosed in teen years
- Typically presents as palpable thyroid mass
- Regional lymph node metastasis is seen in up to 80% of children at presentation
- Children tend to present with more advanced disease than adults
- 10-year survival is nearly 100%

Microscopic Pathology
- Typically have branching papillae
- Follicles are often present
- Characteristic nuclear features must be present in majority of tumor cells
- Nuclei are crowded and frequently overlap
- Clear nucleoplasm with accentuated nuclear borders (margination of chromatin)
- Abundant nuclear grooves are present, resulting from infolding of nuclear membrane
- Psammoma bodies are found in approximately 1/2 of all cases
- Squamous metaplasia is common in pediatric cases

making these tumors refractory to radioactive iodine therapy
  - Associated with poor prognosis

CLINICAL ISSUES

Epidemiology
- Incidence
  - Most common histologic type of thyroid carcinoma in children
    - 80-90% of thyroid malignancies
    - Follicular variant of PTC accounts for 20% of cases
- Age
  - Most are diagnosed in teen years
  - Individual cases have been reported throughout childhood, including newborns
- Gender
  - Before puberty
    - Female:male = 1:1
  - During adolescence
    - Female:male = up to 6:1

Presentation
- Typically presents as a painless or tender palpable thyroid mass
- May present with enlarged cervical lymph nodes
  - Regional lymph node metastasis is seen in up to 80% of children at presentation

Treatment
- Surgical approaches
  - Surgical intervention is treatment of choice
    - PTC is found in contralateral lobe in 25% of cases
    - In this case a subtotal or total thyroidectomy is performed
  - Lymph node dissection if clinical or radiologic evidence of enlargement
- Radiation
  - Radioactive iodine ablation is instituted after thyroidectomy
    - Tumors must show radiolabel uptake in order to respond to radioablative therapies

Prognosis
- Children tend to present with more advanced disease than adults
  - Lymph node metastases
  - Pulmonary metastases
- Excellent prognosis; 10-year survival is nearly 100%
- Certain genetic mutations/rearrangements confer worse prognosis
  - *BRAF* mutation is seen in more aggressive tumors

MACROSCOPIC FEATURES

General Features
- Can be solitary nodule; however, multifocality is common (up to 65%)
- Various gross appearances
  - Can be solid or cystic
  - Typically firm, pale tan to white nodules (hemorrhagic area can also be present)
  - Appear granular or shaggy due to presence of papillae
- Cut surface may be gritty due to presence of psammoma bodies
- Areas of fibrosis may be present
- Lymph node metastasis usually solid whitish firm lesions, but cystic metastases do occur
- Well-circumscribed, encapsulated tumors tend to be classic papillary or follicular variant
- Poorly circumscribed lesions with fibrosis extending into perithyroidal soft tissue is likely sclerosing variant
  - Sclerosing variant is seen more often in children rather than adults

Size
- Varies widely, from microscopic up to 10 cm
- Mean: 1-3 cm

PAPILLARY THYROID CARCINOMA

MICROSCOPIC PATHOLOGY

Histologic Features

- Multiple different architectural patterns can be seen within same tumor (papillary, solid, cystic)
  - Typically have branching papillae
    - Delicate arborizing fronds with thin fibrovascular cores
    - Monolayer of neoplastic cells surround papillae, with haphazard nuclear arrangement
    - Stroma of papillae may be edematous, loose, myxoid, or hyalinized
  - Follicles are often present
    - Contain thick eosinophilic colloid within their lumens
    - Follicles may be enlarged, elongated, or irregularly shaped
- Characteristic nuclear features must be present in majority of tumor cells
  - In tumors without classical papillary architecture, diagnosis relies heavily on these characteristic nuclear features
  - Large ovoid nuclei with irregularly shaped nuclear membranes
    - Nuclei may be oval, elongated, crescent-shaped, asymmetric, angulated, or convoluted
  - Nuclei are crowded and frequently overlap
  - Powdery, ground glass ("Orphan Annie") nuclei
    - Clear nucleoplasm with accentuated nuclear borders (margination of chromatin)
    - May be an artifact of formalin fixation, as this feature is not seen with cytology preparations
  - Abundant nuclear grooves are present, resulting from infolding of nuclear membrane
    - Found in almost all cases
    - Discrete, longitudinal groove through long axis of nucleus, resembling coffee beans
  - Nuclear pseudoinclusions are usually present in a few tumor cells
    - Pale-staining, well-demarcated vacuoles resulting from nuclear herniations of cytoplasm
    - May not be present in some variants
    - 1 of the less frequently seen nuclear features
- Neoplastic cells can be polygonal, cuboidal, flattened, columnar, or hobnailed
- Cytoplasm is typically lightly eosinophilic but can also be oxyphilic or clear
- Neoplastic cells are 2-3x larger than normal follicular cells
  - Nuclear to cytoplasmic ratio is large
- Psammoma bodies are found in approximately 1/2 of all cases
  - Round, deep purple with concentric laminations
  - Seen within tumor, in association with tumor cells, or in lymphatic channels
  - May be only evidence of intrathyroid lymphatic spread or metastasis to lymph nodes
- Colloid is intensely eosinophilic when compared to surrounding nonneoplastic gland
  - Colloid is thicker and may even be scalloped along the edges
- Squamous metaplasia is common in pediatric cases
- Usually associated with patchy chronic inflammation and may be seen in background of lymphocytic thyroiditis
  - Lymphocytes, plasma cells, and histiocytes
  - Associated with improved prognosis

Cytologic Features

- Aspirates are obtained from fine needle aspiration biopsies and are diagnostic test of choice
  - Typically, aspirates are very cellular
    - Arranged in groups, sheets, and papillary tissue fragments
  - Cells are enlarged and may be irregularly shaped
    - Usually cuboidal but can be polygonal, columnar, spindled, or squamoid
  - Nuclei are enlarged and irregular in shape
    - Nuclear grooves are present
    - Chromatin is powdery
    - Small nucleoli may be present and are typically peripherally located
    - Nuclear pseudoinclusions are quite helpful when seen
  - Colloid is thick and ropy, resembling chewing gum
  - Psammoma bodies may also be present
  - Multinucleated giant cells are another helpful finding

Lymphatic/Vascular Invasion

- Seen in large number of cases
- Lymphatic invasion is most commonly seen

Margins

- Important to sample to determine completeness of excision and extrathyroid extension of tumor

Lymph Nodes

- Metastatic disease is common
- Metastatic deposits can be solid or cystic
- Psammoma bodies may be sole evidence of metastatic disease
- Benign inclusions in lymph nodes do not exist and should be considered metastases

Variants

- Many histopathological variants of papillary thyroid carcinoma exist, typically in combination with each other
- Tumor should be dominated by certain features to be categorized as a specific variant
- Variants seen in children include
  - Classic papillary type
  - Follicular variant
  - Solid type
  - Mixed papillary and follicular
  - Sclerosing variant
  - Cribriform morular variant (in FAP)
- **Follicular variant**
  - Common variant of papillary thyroid carcinoma
  - Composed of irregularly shaped follicles with few intrafollicular micropapillary structures
  - Eosinophilic colloid
  - Psammoma bodies rare
  - Intranuclear inclusions rare
  - May be completely encapsulated

 - HBME-1, galectin-3 and characteristic nuclear morphology of PTC are useful for differentiating from follicular carcinoma
- **Solid variant**
  - Solid sheets of tumor cells with characteristic nuclear morphology of PTC
  - More common in children
  - Should be distinguished from poorly differentiated/ insular carcinoma
- **Diffuse sclerosing variant**
  - Diffuse involvement of 1 or both thyroid lobes, often with extrathyroid extension of tumor
  - Most have *BRAF* mutation
  - Papillary and follicular architectures seen
  - Squamous metaplasia must be present and is often extensive
  - Lymphocytic infiltrate is seen
  - Psammoma bodies are abundant
  - Stromal fibrosis present
  - Regional and distant metastases are common
- **Cribriform morular variant**
  - Cribriform features, focal papillary architecture, squamoid morules, solid and spindled areas present
  - Most nuclei are hyperchromatic; however, some are clear and grooved
  - β-catenin nuclear positivity

ANCILLARY TESTS

Cytology

- Fine needle aspiration is typically initial diagnostic test for papillary thyroid carcinoma
  - Approximately 83% sensitivity and 92% specificity
- Typically performed with 27 to 25-g needle and guided by ultrasound
- Adequate samples must contain at least 6 groups of cells with 15-20 follicular cells per group
- Categorized as benign, suspicious, indeterminate, or malignant

Frozen Sections

- Often performed on suspicious ipsilateral or contralateral thyroid nodule
- Touch preps performed at time of frozen section are useful adjunct

Immunohistochemistry

- Rarely of value
  - Positive stains
    - Thyroglobulin, TTF-1, CK7, CK19, HBME-1, galectin-3, and CITED-1

DIFFERENTIAL DIAGNOSIS

Papillary Hyperplasia

- Papillary fronds extending into follicles
- Epithelium overlying papillae do **not** have features of papillary thyroid carcinoma
- Nuclei are hyperchromatic and basally oriented

Adenomatous Nodule

- Nodule composed of cells arranged in follicular pattern
- Cells are enlarged when compared to normal follicular cells
- Nuclei may be atypical but do not show characteristic papillary thyroid carcinoma features
  - Small number of cells may have nuclear clearing as fixation artifact, but they are few in number and usually centrally located

Follicular Thyroid Carcinoma

- Encapsulated lesions
- Neoplastic cells breach capsule
- Cells are arranged in follicular pattern
- Nuclei are round with granular chromatin
- Prominent nucleoli are seen
- Lack characteristic nuclear features of papillary carcinoma
  - Though cells with nuclear clearing may be seen in less well-preserved areas of tumor

Medullary Carcinoma

- Sheets or islands of irregular cells separated by thin fibrovascular septae
  - Other architectures may be seen (trabecular, papillary, cribriform, etc.)
- Cells are polygonal or spindly
- Nuclei are round to oval with fine chromatin
- Pleomorphism is not obvious
- Cytoplasm is granular, and mucin can be seen in about 1/2 of all tumor cells
- Amyloid stroma present in up to 80% of cases
- Calcitonin positive

Artifact/FNA Site Changes

- Areas of fibrosis, calcification, and hemorrhage seen following FNA biopsy
- Islands of follicular cells can be found within fibrotic areas
- Nuclei may be enlarged and pale staining
- Nuclei are round, not crowded, and lack nuclear grooves and inclusions or other features of papillary thyroid carcinoma

DIAGNOSTIC CHECKLIST

Pathologic Interpretation Pearls

- When classical papillary architecture is not present, nuclear features become extremely important
- Characteristic papillary thyroid carcinoma nuclear features must be present in majority of tumor cells
- Each variant has its own specific features required for diagnosis
- Age and extent of disease at diagnosis are main prognostic factors
  - Unfavorable histologic variants of PTC, such as tall cell, are uncommon in children

PAPILLARY THYROID CARCINOMA

Immunohistochemistry

Antibody	Reactivity	Staining Pattern	Comment
HBME-1	Positive	Cell membrane	More specific; also stains colloid
Galectin-3	Positive	Nuclear & cytoplasmic	Positive staining in nearly all papillary thyroid carcinomas
CK19	Positive	Cytoplasmic	Strong, can also be positive in reactive processes and chronic lymphocytic thyroiditis
MSG1	Positive	Nuclear & cytoplasmic	Equivalent to CITED-1; should be used with other immunohistochemical stains
FN1	Positive	Cell membrane	Luminal accentuation seen
TTF-1	Positive	Cytoplasmic	Strong, diffuse nuclear staining
Thyroglobulin	Positive	Cytoplasmic	Artifact can be a problem; staining may be lost in areas of squamous differentiation
Cyclin-D1	Positive	Nuclear	Positive metastatic disease and negative in nonmetastatic papillary carcinomas
CK7	Positive	Cytoplasmic	Stains almost all cells
AE1/AE3	Positive	Cytoplasmic	Stains almost all cells
Calcitonin	Negative		Useful for distinguishing from medullary thyroid carcinoma
CK20	Negative		

SELECTED REFERENCES

1. Barletta JA et al: Immunohistochemical staining of thyroidectomy specimens for PTEN can aid in the identification of patients with Cowden syndrome. Am J Surg Pathol. 35(10):1505-11, 2011
2. Biko J et al: Favourable course of disease after incomplete remission on (131)I therapy in children with pulmonary metastases of papillary thyroid carcinoma: 10 years follow-up. Eur J Nucl Med Mol Imaging. 38(4):651-5, 2011
3. Cochand-Priollet B et al: Immunocytochemistry with cytokeratin 19 and anti-human mesothelial cell antibody (HBME1) increases the diagnostic accuracy of thyroid fine-needle aspirations: preliminary report of 150 liquid-based fine-needle aspirations with histological control. Thyroid. 21(10):1067-73, 2011
4. Huang O et al: Sentinel lymph node biopsy is unsuitable for routine practice in younger female patients with unilateral low-risk papillary thyroid carcinoma. BMC Cancer. 11(1):386, 2011
5. Ito Y et al: Our experience of treatment of cribriform morular variant of papillary thyroid carcinoma; difference in clinicopathological features of FAP-associated and sporadic patients. Endocr J. 58(8):685-9, 2011
6. Moses W et al: Prevalence, clinicopathologic features, and somatic genetic mutation profile in familial versus sporadic nonmedullary thyroid cancer. Thyroid. 21(4):367-71, 2011
7. Nam JK et al: Is the BRAF(V600E) mutation useful as a predictor of preoperative risk in papillary thyroid cancer? Am J Surg. Epub ahead of print, 2011
8. Nosé V: Familial thyroid cancer: a review. Mod Pathol. 24 Suppl 2:S19-33, 2011
9. Torregrossa L et al: CXCR4 expression correlates with the degree of tumor infiltration and BRAF status in papillary thyroid carcinomas. Mod Pathol. Epub ahead of print, 2011
10. Dardas M et al: Thyroid cancer in Lebanese children and adolescents: a 15-year experience at a single institution. Pediatr Hematol Oncol. 26(6):439-47, 2009
11. González-González A et al: [Lung metastases in papillary thyroid carcinoma.] Med Clin (Barc). 133(20):807, 2009
12. Koo JS et al: Diffuse sclerosing variant is a major subtype of papillary thyroid carcinoma in the young. Thyroid. 19(11):1225-31, 2009
13. Massimino M et al: Conservative surgical approach for thyroid and lymph-node involvement in papillary thyroid carcinoma of childhood and adolescence. Pediatr Blood Cancer. 46(3):307-13, 2006
14. Powers PA et al: The MACIS score predicts the clinical course of papillary thyroid carcinoma in children and adolescents. J Pediatr Endocrinol Metab. 17(3):339-43, 2004
15. Eccles TG et al: Erythropoietin and the erythropoietin receptor are expressed by papillary thyroid carcinoma from children and adolescents. Expression of erythropoietin receptor might be a favorable prognostic indicator. Ann Clin Lab Sci. 33(4):411-22, 2003
16. Modi J et al: Papillary thyroid carcinomas from young adults and children contain a mixture of lymphocytes. J Clin Endocrinol Metab. 88(9):4418-25, 2003
17. Powers PA et al: Treatment of recurrent papillary thyroid carcinoma in children and adolescents. J Pediatr Endocrinol Metab. 16(7):1033-40, 2003
18. Powers PA et al: Tumor size and extent of disease at diagnosis predict the response to initial therapy for papillary thyroid carcinoma in children and adolescents. J Pediatr Endocrinol Metab. 16(5):693-702, 2003
19. Yagasaki H et al: [Development of severe aplastic anemia in a girl with Hashimoto's thyroiditis and papillary thyroid carcinoma.] Rinsho Ketsueki. 44(5):328-33, 2003
20. Harach HR et al: Occult papillary carcinoma of the thyroid. A "normal" finding in Finland. A systematic autopsy study. Cancer. 56(3):531-8, 1985

Gross and Microscopic Features

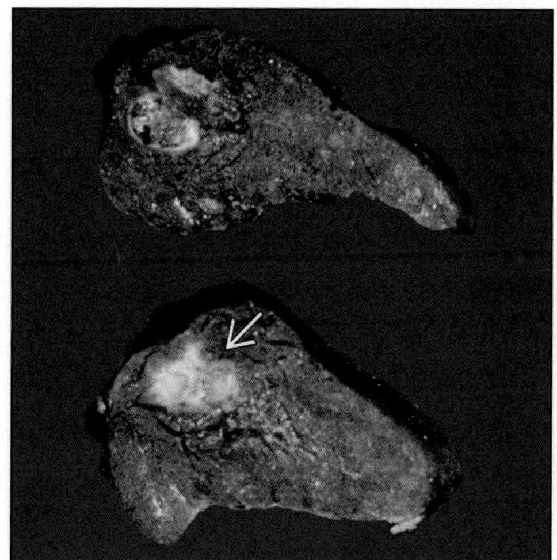

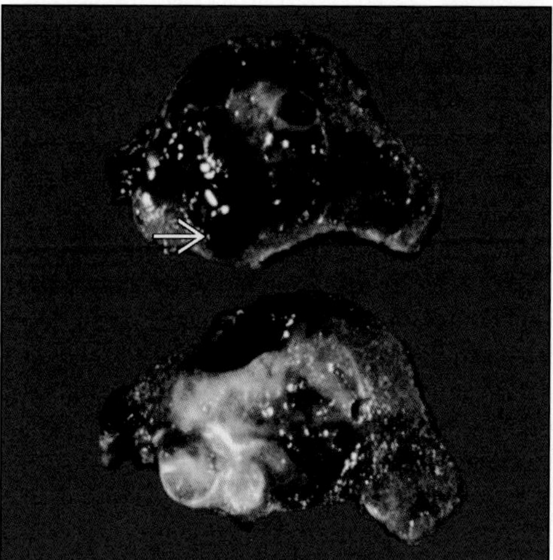

(Left) *This papillary thyroid carcinoma has an ill-defined border and an infiltrative appearance ➡. It is pale tan to whitish in color. The tumor is easily discernible from the adjacent normal thyroid parenchyma.* ***(Right)*** *This gross image of papillary thyroid carcinoma illustrates that some lesions may be partially cystic in nature. Hemorrhage ➡ is readily identified within the cystic spaces.*

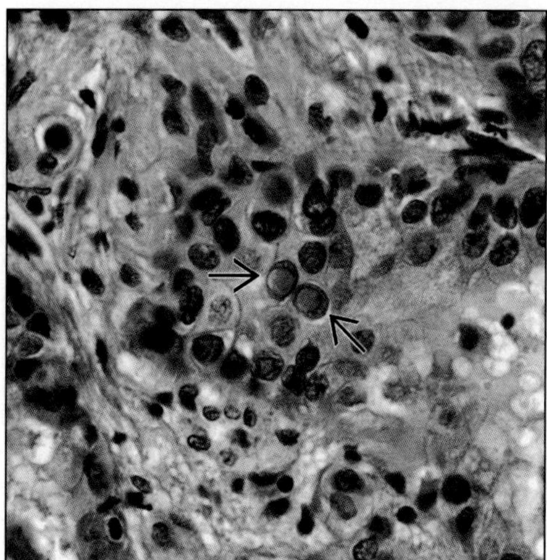

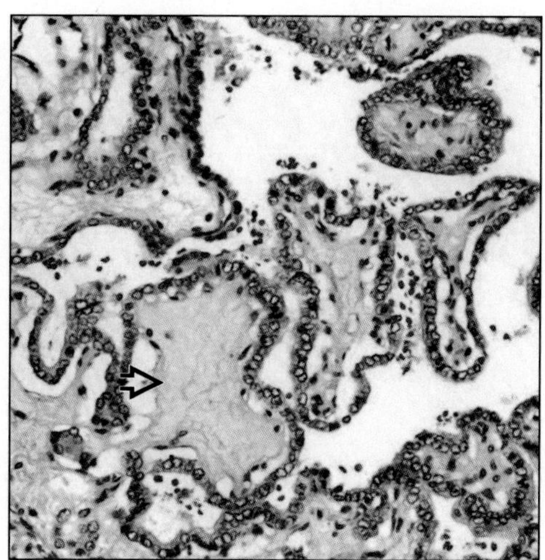

(Left) *Intranuclear inclusions ➡ are demonstrated in this photomicrograph. Note the crisp, punched-out border and eosinophilic color. Inclusions are typically round to oval in shape. They represent invaginations of the nuclear membrane.* ***(Right)*** *Papillary thyroid carcinoma, classical variant shows edematous papillae ⇨, which lack the thin delicate fibrovascular cores typically seen. Characteristic nuclear features are seen in the cells lining the papillae.*

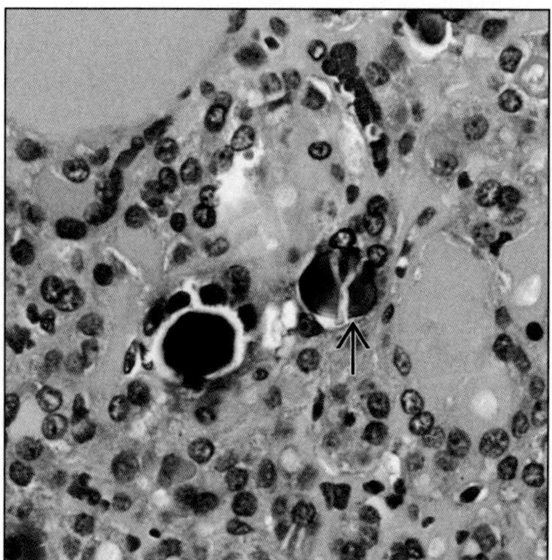

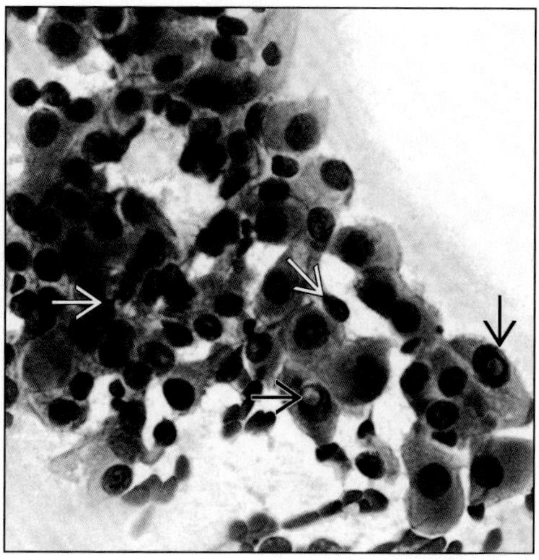

(Left) *2 psammoma bodies are seen in this photomicrograph. Note the concentric laminations ➡ demonstrated in this example. Due to processing, they typically fragment and cause artifacts and irregularities within paraffin sections.* ***(Right)*** *Characteristic cytological features of papillary thyroid carcinoma include enlarged tumor cells with abundant cytoplasm and nuclear inclusions ➡. Nuclear grooves ➡ can also be seen within the nuclei of some cells.*

PAPILLARY THYROID CARCINOMA

Microscopic Features

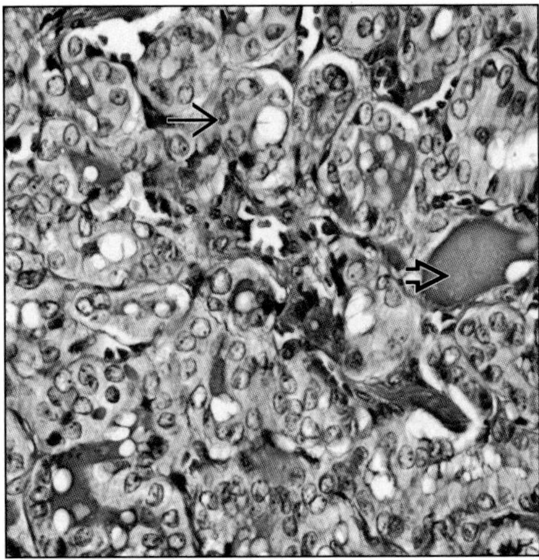

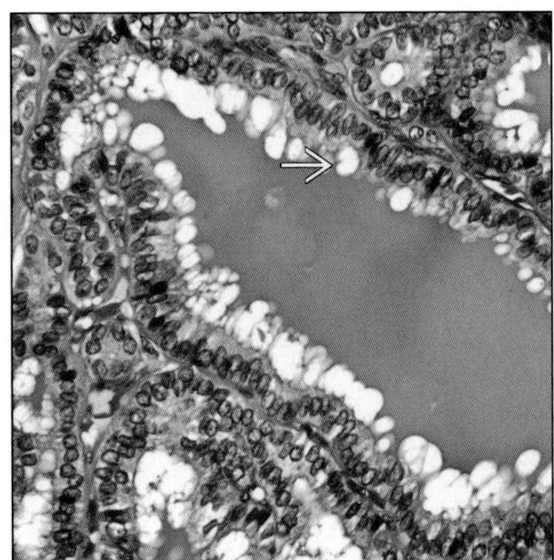

(Left) *Follicular variant, papillary thyroid carcinoma demonstrates a follicular architecture, increased nuclear to cytoplasmic ratio, and clear nuclei with irregular nuclear membranes. The follicles ➙ are small and have a thick eosinophilic colloid ➲.* ***(Right)*** *The tumor cells in the follicular variant of PTC are arranged in a follicular pattern. They demonstrate scalloping of colloid ➡, which is commonly seen in this variant.*

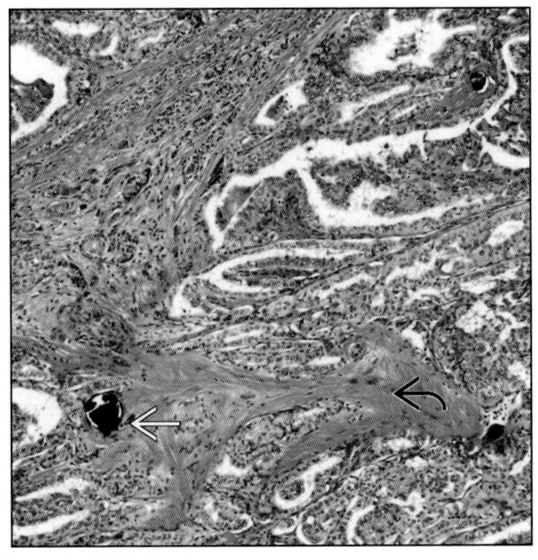

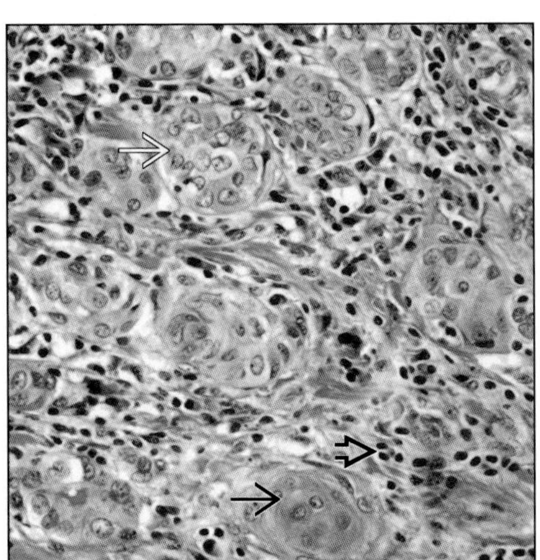

(Left) *Papillary thyroid carcinoma, diffuse sclerosing variant is characterized by thick fibrous bands ➦ associated with psammoma bodies ➡, a lymphocytic infiltrate, variable architecture, and squamous metaplasia.* ***(Right)*** *Diffuse sclerosing variant of papillary thyroid carcinoma demonstrates areas of squamous metaplasia ➙ adjacent to tumor cells with characteristic papillary carcinoma features ➡. A lymphoid infiltrate ➲ is present in association with tumor cells.*

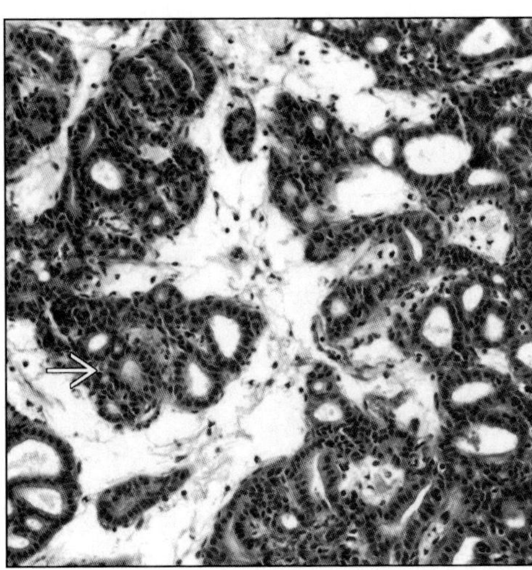

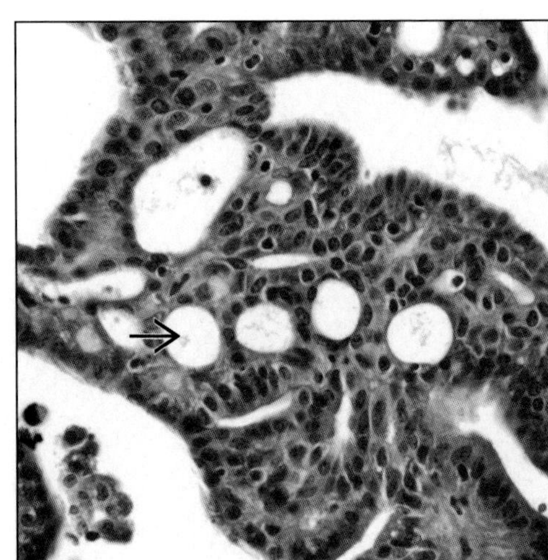

(Left) *This picture illustrates a cribriform morular variant of papillary carcinoma, with tumor cells arranged in a cribriform pattern, forming small gland-like structures ➡. These tumors are usually associated with morular component.* ***(Right)*** *Papillary thyroid carcinoma, cribriform morular variant demonstrates the characteristic "punched-out" cribriform pattern ➙, lacking colloid. The nuclei are enlarged and irregular, but are not as clear as other subtypes of papillary thyroid carcinoma.*

Microscopic and Immunohistochemical Features

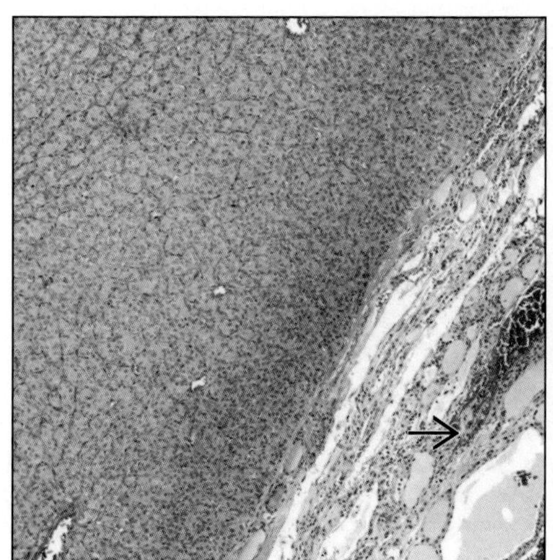

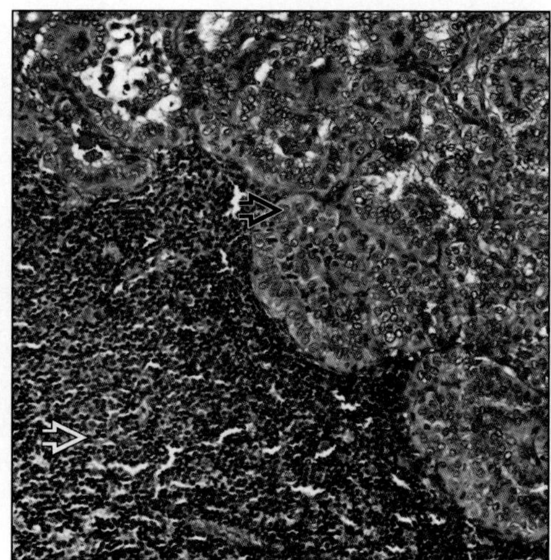

(Left) *Low magnification of the solid variant of papillary carcinoma shows solid architectural pattern, lacking colloid. Normal thyroid parenchyma is shown on right bottom corner* ➙. ***(Right)*** *This papillary thyroid carcinoma* ➙ *is metastatic to a lymph node* ➙. *Note the papillary architecture.*

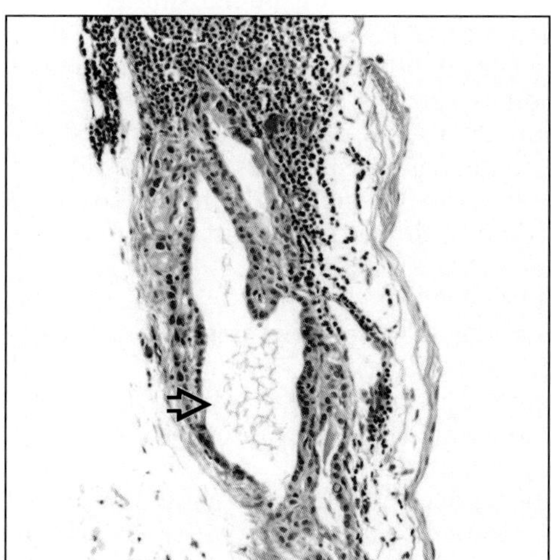

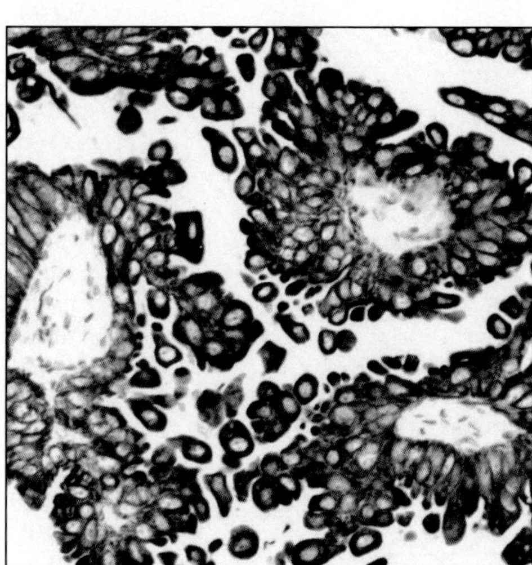

(Left) *Papillary thyroid carcinoma metastatic to a lymph node demonstrates cystic changes. Microscopically, this cystic structure* ➙ *is lined by cells with nuclear features characteristic of PTC.* ***(Right)*** *Immunostain for CK19 shows a pattern of staining typical of papillary thyroid carcinoma, with strong fibrillary cytoplasmic staining of neoplastic cells.*

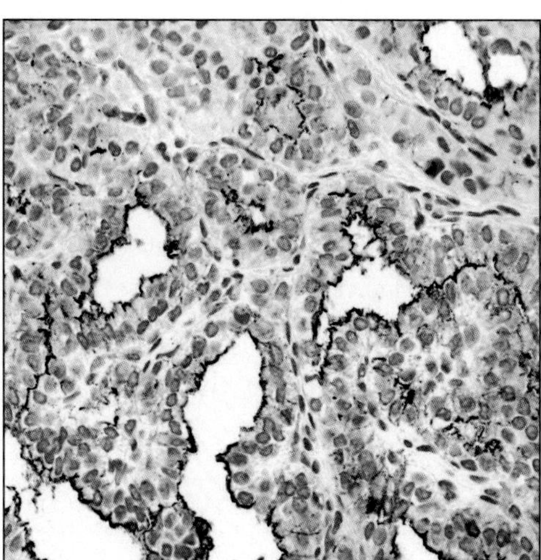

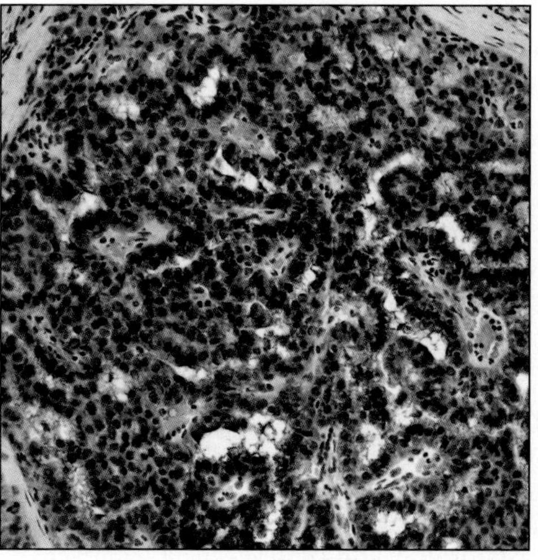

(Left) *HBME-1 immunostain demonstrates characteristic staining pattern with membranous and luminal borders in papillary thyroid carcinoma.* ***(Right)*** *Follicular variant of papillary thyroid carcinoma (PTC-FV) is usually characterized by an immunostain panel including HBME-1, galectin-3, and CK19. This panel has 87% sensitivity and 89% specificity for PTC-FV, while positive in only about 11% of follicular adenomas. In this photograph, galectin-3 immunostaining is strong and cytoplasmic.*

FOLLICULAR CARCINOMA

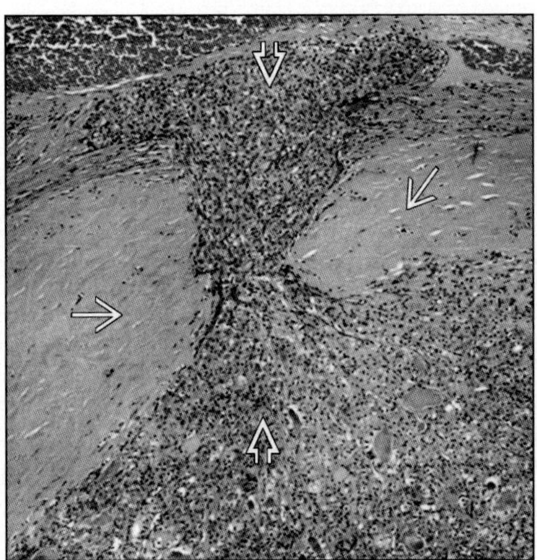

Photomicrograph depicts the classical "mushroom" sign of capsular invasion with tumor cells ⇨ invading across the entire thickness of the capsule ⇨.

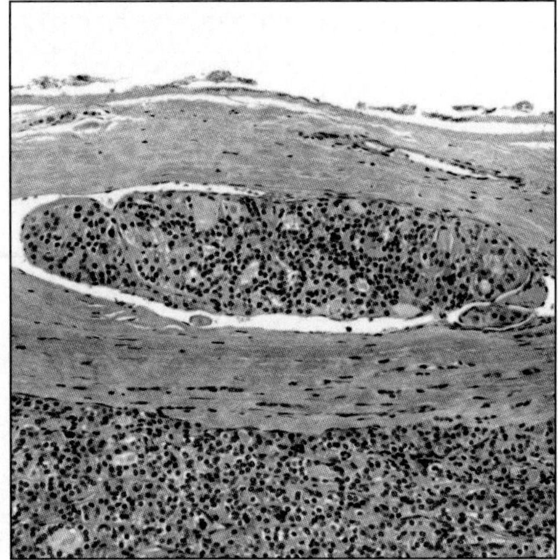

This image illustrates a hallmark in the diagnosis of follicular carcinoma. Vascular invasion is seen here as tumor cells present within a large capsular blood vessel.

TERMINOLOGY

Abbreviations

- Follicular carcinoma (FC)
- Follicular thyroid carcinoma (FTC)

Synonyms

- Follicular adenocarcinoma, oncocytic carcinoma, Hürthle cell carcinoma

Definitions

- Malignant epithelial tumor of thyroid
- Shows evidence of follicular cell differentiation
- Lacks diagnostic features of papillary thyroid carcinoma (PTC)

ETIOLOGY/PATHOGENESIS

Environmental Exposure

- Radiation exposure results in 5.2x relative risk for developing FTC
- Iodine deficiency is associated with higher risk for development of both adenomas and FTC

Preexisting Thyroid Disease

- Present in up to 15% of patients with FTC
- Dyshormonogenic goiter with chronic TSH stimulation may predispose to follicular neoplasms
- Associated with other thyroid tumors
- Lymphocytic thyroiditis and FTC may coexist
- Association between lymphocytic thyroiditis and FTC remains unclear

Inherited Tumor Syndromes

- Account for 4% of FTC in USA
- *PTEN*-hamartoma tumor syndrome
  - Cowden syndrome, Bannayan-Riley-Ruvalcaba syndrome (BRRS), proteus syndrome, and proteus-like syndrome
  - Germline mutation of *PTEN* gene transmitted in an autosomal dominant fashion
  - May be associated with multiple follicular adenomas and carcinomas
  - Affected individuals may develop benign and malignant tumors of breast, uterus, and thyroid
  - Individuals may also develop multiple hamartomas of breast, colon, endometrium, brain, and ganglioneuromatous proliferations
- Carney complex
  - Autosomal dominant disorder caused by mutations in *PRKAR1A* gene
  - Carney complex includes cardiac myxomas, multiple endocrine neoplasms, and spotty cutaneous pigmentation
  - 75% of patients develop multiple thyroid nodules
  - About 5% of patients may present with follicular or papillary carcinoma
- Werner syndrome
  - Autosomal recessive
  - Caused by mutations in *WRN* gene
  - Up to 3% of patients will have thyroid disease, usually FTC
- McCune-Albright syndrome
  - Triad of café au lait skin pigmentation, polyostotic fibrous dysplasia, and hyperfunctioning endocrinopathies
  - Associated with precocious puberty, hyperthyroidism, GH excess, and Cushing syndrome
  - Patients harbor postzygotic mutations in *GNAS1* gene as mosaics
  - Associated with FTC and papillary thyroid carcinomas

CLINICAL ISSUES

Epidemiology

- Incidence

FOLLICULAR CARCINOMA

Key Facts

Terminology

- Malignant epithelial tumor of thyroid that shows evidence of follicular cell differentiation

Clinical Issues

- Incidence of thyroid nodules in children estimated at 1-1.5%
  - 30-50% of thyroid nodules in children are malignant
- Differentiated thyroid cancers (e.g., FTC) account for 1-2% of all childhood malignancies
  - FTC accounts for up to 20% of all pediatric thyroid cancers
- Relatively good prognosis in pediatric age groups

Image Findings

- Scintigraphy scan shows cold nodule

Microscopic Pathology

- High cellularity with solid, trabecular, or microfollicular growth pattern
- Characterized by presence of invasion
- Commonly associated with a lymphocytic infiltration

Ancillary Tests

- *RAS* gene mutations found in 20-50%
- Up to 20% of FTC may show rearrangements of *PPARγ*

Top Differential Diagnoses

- Follicular adenoma
- Adenomatous nodule
- Papillary thyroid carcinoma, follicular variant

- Incidence of thyroid nodules in children estimated at 1-1.5%
  - 30-50% of thyroid nodules in children are malignant
  - 5-10% of thyroid nodules in adults are malignant
- Differentiated thyroid cancers (e.g., FTC) account for 1-2% of all childhood malignancies
- FTC accounts for up to 20% of all pediatric thyroid cancers
  - 2nd most common thyroid cancer in children after PTC

- Age
  - Affects children and adults
    - Most occur in 5th decade
    - Occur at earlier age when part of an inherited syndrome
- Gender
  - Female to male ratio of 5:1

Presentation

- Commonly present as asymptomatic thyroid mass/nodule
  - Nodule may be firm and fixed to surrounding tissue
- Widely disseminated disease at diagnosis more common in children than adults
  - More common with PTC
- At presentation patients are typically euthyroid

Laboratory Tests

- Thyrotropin (TSH), triiodothionine (T_3), free thyroxine (T_4), calcitonin, thyroglobulin, and thyroid antibody levels should be measured
  - Thyroid antibodies present in up to 25%

Treatment

- Management of thyroid carcinoma in children
  - Surgery
  - TSH suppression
    - Minimizes TSH-stimulated tumor growth
  - Radioiodine scanning and treatment
    - Routine radioactive iodine ablation of remaining normal thyroid is controversial in children
  - Monitoring of thyroglobulin levels
  - Thyroxine replacement
  - Total body scanning with ^{123}I recommended 6-8 weeks post surgery

Prognosis

- Relatively good prognosis in pediatric age groups
  - Children rarely die of disease
  - Mortality of 1-2% in most series
  - Low mortality even with distant metastases

IMAGE FINDINGS

Ultrasonographic Findings

- In minimally invasive disease, well-circumscribed nodule, usually > 1 cm is often present
- Indistinct margins, internal calcifications, and variable echodensity associated with malignant lesions
- Cannot distinguish follicular adenoma from FTC
- May be helpful in assessing lymph node involvement by thyroid carcinoma

Scintigraphy

- Scan shows cold nodule

MACROSCOPIC FEATURES

General Features

- Usually solitary
  - Round to ovoid encapsulated tumors
  - Tan to light brown
- Minimally invasive tumors
  - Thick irregular fibrous capsule
  - Grossly similar or indistinguishable from follicular adenoma
- Widely invasive carcinoma
  - Lack of capsule or extensive permeation of capsule
- Larger tumors may have areas of hemorrhage and necrosis

Sections to Be Submitted

- Weigh and record dimensions of thyroidectomy specimen

FOLLICULAR CARCINOMA

- Serially section through entire gland
- Identify nodule and note location, color, size, consistency, cystic changes, necrosis, and hemorrhage, if present
- Submit entire capsule, even in larger tumors, as invasion of capsule distinguishes follicular carcinomas from adenomas
- Evaluate extension of tumor into adjacent soft tissue and metastases to lymph nodes

Size

- Round to ovoid encapsulated tumors, 1-10 cm in diameter

Categories of Tumor

- Minimally invasive follicular carcinoma
- Widely invasive follicular carcinoma
- Oncocytic follicular carcinoma
  - Subtype formerly called oxyphil or Hürthle cell carcinoma

MICROSCOPIC PATHOLOGY

Histologic Features

- Thick fibrous capsule
- High cellularity with solid, trabecular, or microfollicular growth pattern
- Diffuse nuclear atypia
- Readily identified mitotic figures
- Commonly associated with a lymphocytic infiltrate
  - Inverse correlation with recurrence risk
- FTC characterized by the presence of invasion
- Spread is by vascular channels; does not invade lymphatics
- Oncocytic and clear cell variants are 2 main variants of FTC
  - Oncocytic variant may spread by lymphatic &/or vascular routes
- Criteria for capsular invasion
  - Tumor bud has invaded beyond outer contour of capsule
  - Tumor bud still clothed by thin capsule; however, it has extended through outer capsular surface
  - Presence of satellite nodule with cytoarchitectural and cellular features identical to those tumor cells
  - Classical mushroom-like bud that has totally transgressed fibrous capsule
- Criteria for vascular invasion
  - Blood vessels should be of larger caliber with an identifiable wall the size of a vein, and involved blood vessels must be located within or outside fibrous capsule (i.e., not within tumor)
  - Intravascular polypoid tumor growth must protrude into lumen, must be covered by endothelium, and it must be attached to wall of vessel and associated with a thrombus
  - Clusters of epithelial cells floating in vascular lumen, unattached to wall are **not** considered vascular invasion
- Extrathyroidal extension
  - Invasion into adipose tissue or skeletal muscle outside limits of thyroid

Cytologic Features

- Can vary from bland, resembling follicular cells, to pleomorphic atypical cells with bizarre nuclear features
- Hallmark of malignancy is vascular &/or capsular invasion irrespective of cytologic atypia, growth pattern or mitotic activity

ANCILLARY TESTS

Molecular Genetics

- Mutations in *RAS*, *PIK3CA*, and *PTEN* are found in FTC with higher frequency than in follicular adenomas
- *RAS* gene mutations found in 20-50%
- Accumulation of additional mutations, such as *TP53*, may be associated with progression to poorly differentiated carcinomas

Cytogenetics

- FTC may show rearrangements of peroxisome proliferator-activated receptor gamma (*PPARγ*)
- Translocation t(2,3)(q13;p25) leads to fusion of *PAX8* and *PPARγ* (*PAX8-PPARγ* rearrangement) detected by FISH
  - Rearrangements found in 25-50%

DIFFERENTIAL DIAGNOSIS

Follicular Adenoma

- Encapsulated benign neoplasm with variable architecture and histologic patterns
- Only features to reliably distinguish adenoma from FTC are capsular &/or vascular invasion

Adenomatous Nodule

- Frequently multiple, variable-sized follicles with no capsule or incomplete capsule
- May have abundant edematous or hyalinized stroma

Papillary Thyroid Carcinoma, Follicular Variant

- Follicular pattern of growth, can be encapsulated
- Usually show typical papillary carcinoma cytologic features
  - Ground-glass nuclei, intranuclear pseudo-inclusions, nuclear grooves, and nuclear overlapping
- Immunohistochemistry for HBME-1, galectin-3, and CK19 may help distinguish follicular variant of PTC from FTC

Hyperplastic Nodules in Hashimoto Thyroiditis

- Diffusely enlarged and firm thyroid
- Lymphocytic infiltration of stroma, formation of large lymphoid follicles
- Thyroid follicles are often small and atrophic, lined by Hürthle cells

Hyperplastic Nodules in Dyshormonogenetic Goiter
- Hypercellular nodules with varied appearances commonly solid and microfollicular
- Atypia with bizarre nuclei may be present
- Irregular areas of fibrosis at periphery of nodules may simulate capsular invasion

Medullary Thyroid Carcinoma
- Invasive growth pattern
- Slightly granular cytoplasm
- Salt and pepper nuclear chromatin
- Calcitonin, CEA, chromogranin, and synaptophysin positivity

Intrathyroid Parathyroid Tumor
- Solitary parathyroid adenomas within thyroid parenchyma may mimic thyroid carcinoma, as they appear as cold nodules on imaging studies
- Clinical picture of hyperparathyroidism should raise suspicion
- Histologic examination will confirm parathyroid tissue

Hyalinizing Trabecular Tumor
- Trabecular growth pattern with medium-sized elongated cells with granular cytoplasm
- No follicle formation and absent colloid
- PAS-positive basement membrane material
- Characteristic cytoplasmic and membranous Ki-67/ MIB-1 staining pattern

Congenital Abnormalities
- Thyroid hemiagenesis
  - May result in compensatory enlargement of single thyroid lobe

DIAGNOSTIC CHECKLIST

Clinically Relevant Pathologic Features
- Invasive pattern
- Metastatic distribution

Pathologic Interpretation Pearls
- Pathologist's most important task is differentiation between FTC and numerous variants of follicular adenoma and other benign neoplasms
- Diagnosis of FTC rests on demonstration of capsular or vascular invasion
- Determination of capsular invasion may be challenging, and to date there are no universally accepted criteria to define what constitutes capsular invasion
- Extensive sampling and histologic examination of entire capsule is essential in minimally invasive FTC
- Deeper sectioning of suspicious tumor foci within capsule will often reveal invasion through entire capsule
- Free-standing tumor foci within capsule may represent entrapment secondary to previous FNA biopsy
- Vascular invasion must be distinguished from artifactual impaction of tumor cells into vessels during processing

SELECTED REFERENCES

1. Paschke R et al: Thyroid nodule guidelines: agreement, disagreement and need for future research. Nat Rev Endocrinol. 7(6):354-61, 2011
2. Chia WK et al: Fluorescence in situ hybridization analysis using PAX8- and PPARG-specific probes reveals the presence of PAX8-PPARG translocation and 3p25 aneusomy in follicular thyroid neoplasms. Cancer Genet Cytogenet. 196(1):7-13, 2010
3. Mete O et al: Controversies in thyroid pathology: thyroid capsule invasion and extrathyroidal extension. Ann Surg Oncol. 17(2):386-91, 2010
4. Nosé V: Thyroid cancer of follicular cell origin in inherited tumor syndromes. Adv Anat Pathol. 17(6):428-36, 2010
5. Ohori NP et al: Contribution of molecular testing to thyroid fine-needle aspiration cytology of "follicular lesion of undetermined significance/atypia of undetermined significance". Cancer Cytopathol. 118(1):17-23, 2010
6. Ghossein R: Problems and controversies in the histopathology of thyroid carcinomas of follicular cell origin. Arch Pathol Lab Med. 133(5):683-91, 2009
7. Ghossein R: Update to the College of American Pathologists reporting on thyroid carcinomas. Head Neck Pathol. 3(1):86-93, 2009
8. Dinauer CA et al: Differentiated thyroid cancer in children: diagnosis and management. Curr Opin Oncol. 20(1):59-65, 2008
9. Dotto J et al: Familial thyroid carcinoma: a diagnostic algorithm. Adv Anat Pathol. 15(6):332-49, 2008
10. Josefson J et al: Thyroid nodules and cancers in children. Pediatr Endocrinol Rev. 6(1):14-23, 2008
11. Serra S et al: Controversies in thyroid pathology: the diagnosis of follicular neoplasms. Endocr Pathol. 19(3):156-65, 2008
12. Todd WU 4th et al: Thyroid follicular epithelial cell-derived carcinomas: an overview of the pathology of primary and recurrent disease. Otolaryngol Clin North Am. 41(6):1079-94, vii-viii, 2008
13. Baloch ZW et al: Our approach to follicular-patterned lesions of the thyroid. J Clin Pathol. 60(3):244-50, 2007
14. Dinauer C et al: Thyroid cancer in children. Endocrinol Metab Clin North Am. 36(3):779-806, vii, 2007
15. Rosai J et al: Pitfalls in thyroid tumour pathology. Histopathology. 49(2):107-20, 2006
16. Collins MT et al: Thyroid carcinoma in the McCune-Albright syndrome: contributory role of activating Gs alpha mutations. J Clin Endocrinol Metab. 88(9):4413-7, 2003

FOLLICULAR CARCINOMA

Radiologic and Other Features

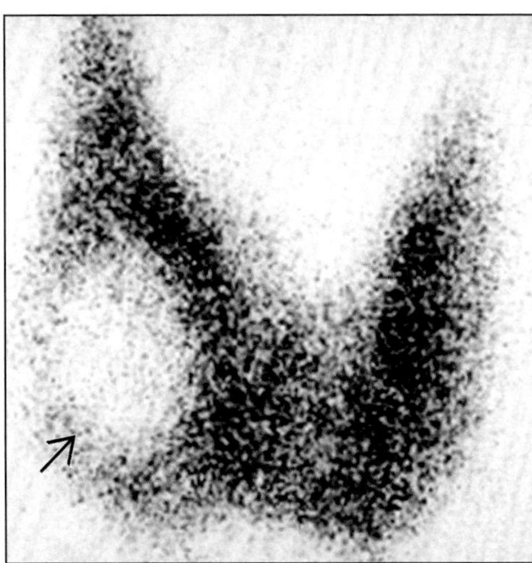

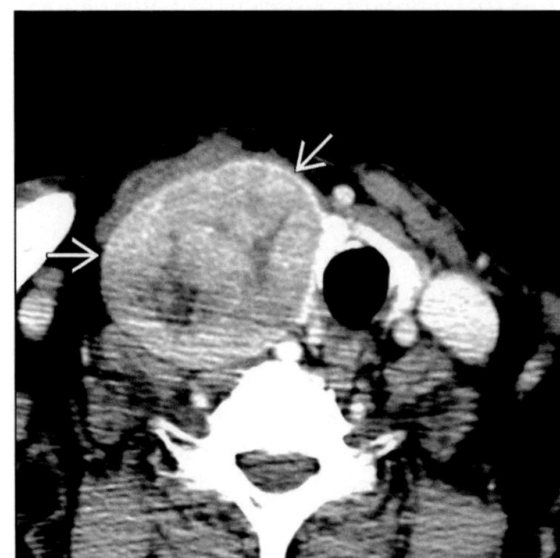

(Left) *Anterior planar ^{123}I nuclear medicine scan shows a cold nodule (differentiated thyroid carcinoma) in the right thyroid lobe ⇨. A cold nodule has an approximately 20% chance of being malignant.* ***(Right)*** *CT image shows a large, solid, well-circumscribed thyroid neoplasm ➡, lacking capsular invasion. This is a common but nonspecific finding in radiographic imaging of thyroid lesions, which may be seen with benign or malignant lesions.*

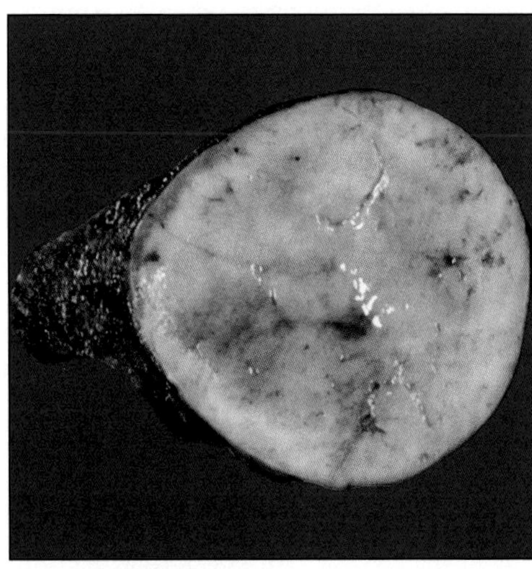

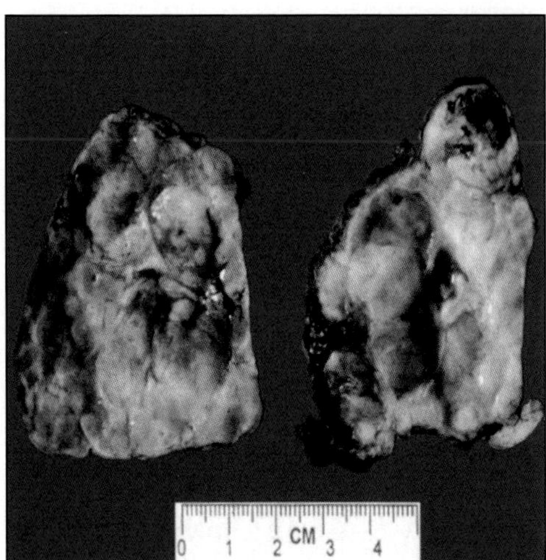

(Left) *A minimally invasive follicular carcinoma is shown presenting as an encapsulated, tan, fleshy nodule, indistinguishable from a follicular adenoma. Thorough examination of the capsule through extensive sampling is crucial to identify foci of capsular invasion.* ***(Right)*** *Unlike in minimally invasive FTC and follicular adenomas, the cut surface of widely invasive follicular carcinomas show an ill-defined diffuse tumoral mass with no discrete identifiable nodules or distinct sharp borders.*

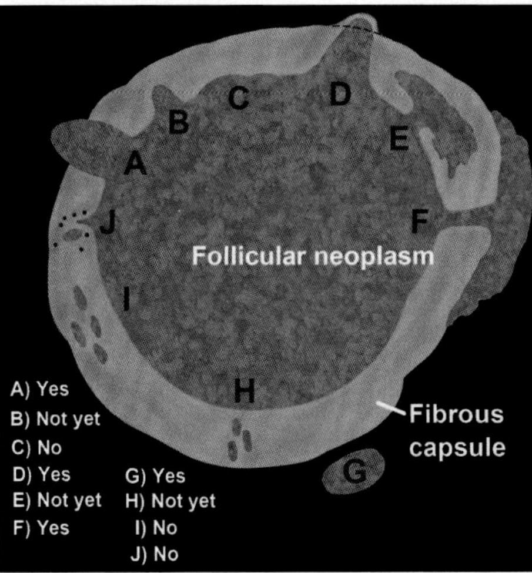

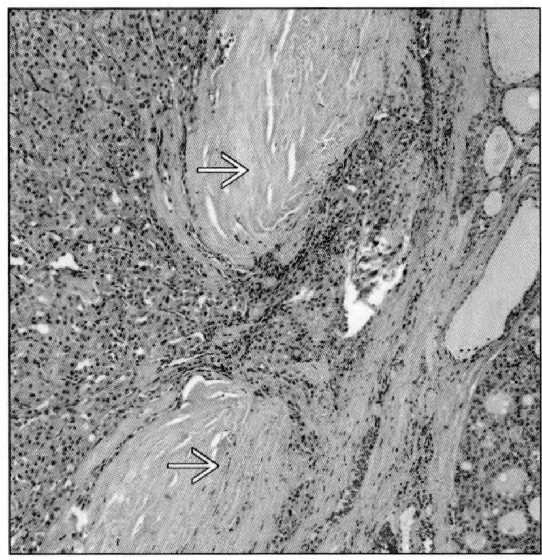

(Left) *A schematic drawing illustrates the criteria necessary to interpret and diagnose a follicular neoplasm based on capsular invasion. The follicular neoplasm is surrounded by a thick fibrous capsule with invasion on A, D, F, and G.* ***(Right)*** *Minimally invasive follicular carcinoma shows the point of invasion where the tumor capsule ➡ has been ruptured by malignant cells, which traverse across the entire capsule thickness and invade a large blood vessel along the way.*

Microscopic Features

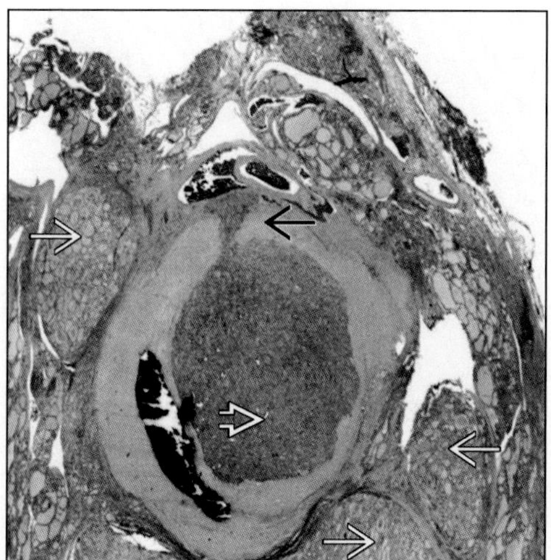

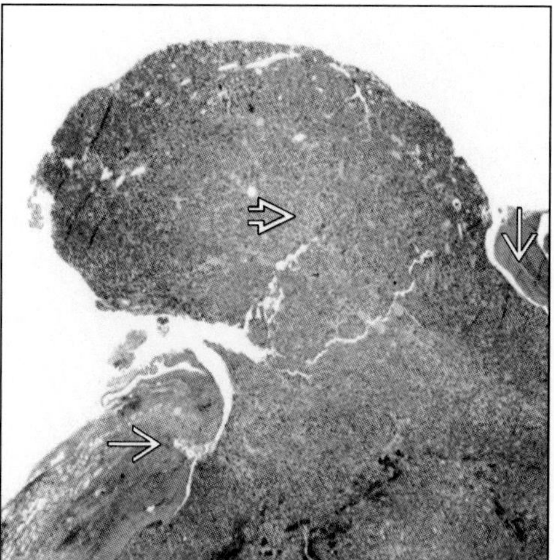

(Left) *Low-power photomicrograph shows multiple well-circumscribed adenomatous nodules ➔ and a single follicular carcinoma ➪. Full-thickness capsular invasion is easily recognizable ➙. This is a case in which the patient has PTEN-associated thyroid disease.* ***(Right)*** *A mass of neoplastic cells ➪ has breached the tumoral capsule in this microinvasive follicular carcinoma. The remaining portions of the ruptured capsule are shown ➔.*

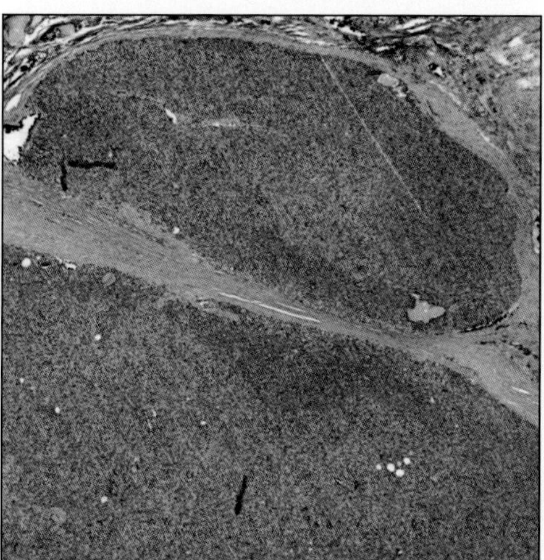

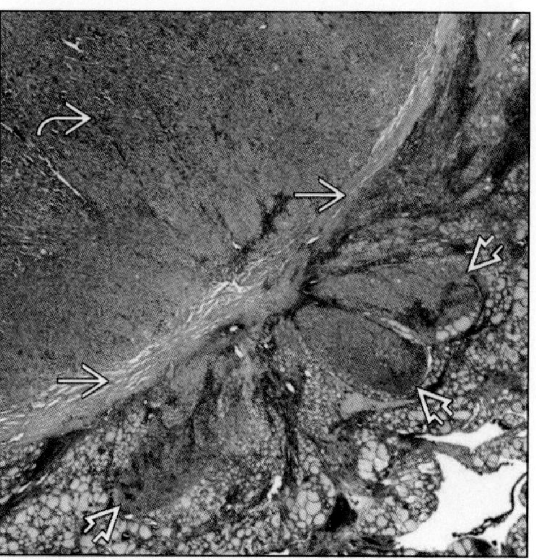

(Left) *Follicular carcinoma with cytologically identical satellite nodules indicates true capsular invasion, even without demonstration of the point of capsular penetration.* ***(Right)*** *Photomicrograph of a follicular carcinoma ➚ shows finger-like projections of the tumor ➪ protruding beyond the capsule ➔ into the surrounding thyroid parenchyma. Evaluation of deeper sections in such cases will often demonstrate the connection of the tumor on both sides of the capsule.*

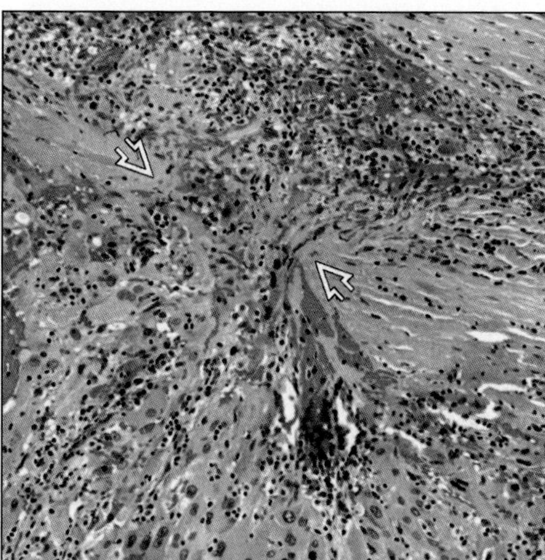

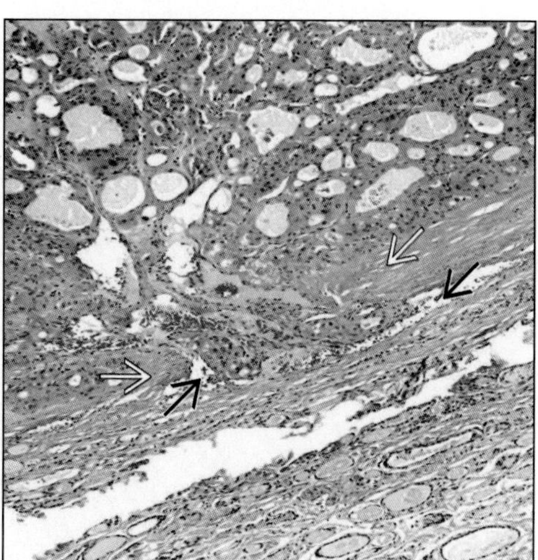

(Left) *H&E shows clear-cut capsular invasion where the tumor cells have ruptured the capsule and migrated into the adjacent parenchyma. A defect in the fibrous capsule is noted ➪.* ***(Right)*** *The neoplastic cells have penetrated halfway through the tumor capsule ➔ and reached a large vessel ➙. Even though the capsular invasion is only partial, vascular invasion in this case is sufficient to render a diagnosis of carcinoma.*

FOLLICULAR CARCINOMA

Microscopic Features

(Left) Tumor cells are present within a large capsular blood vessel ➞. The cells are attached to the vessel wall ➦. A rim of fibrous capsule is seen between the tumor thrombus and the remainder of the tumoral mass ➡. (Right) High-power micrograph shows 2 groups of tumor cells in a vessel within the tumor capsule ➡. The tumor cells are attached to the vessel wall ➦. Endothelial cells can be seen lining both tumor thrombi ➞.

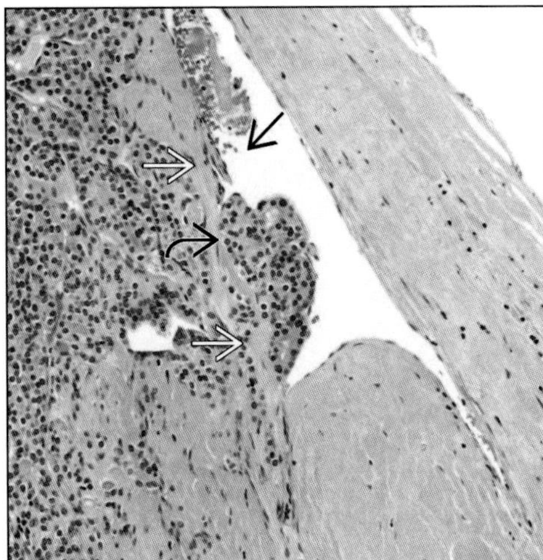

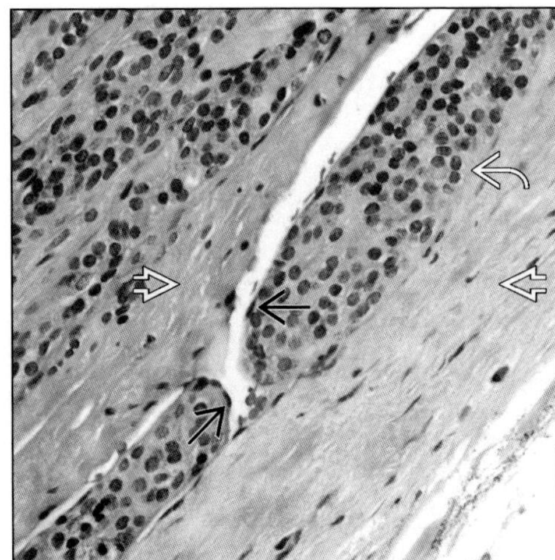

(Left) Microinvasive follicular carcinoma shows the point of invasion where tumor cells penetrate the capsule ➡ and reach a blood vessel ➦. (Right) In this example of vascular invasion, epithelial tumoral cells are present in the lumen of a vessel within the tumoral capsule. Note that the cluster of tumor cells is lined by endothelium ➡. The neoplastic cells are also associated with a thrombus, as evidenced by the fibrin and entrapped red blood cells ➡.

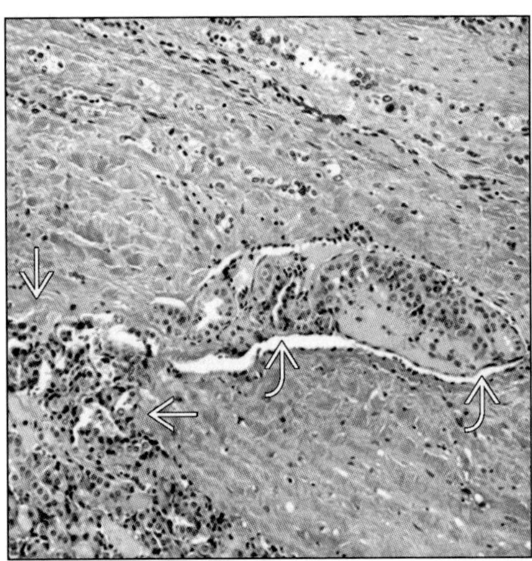

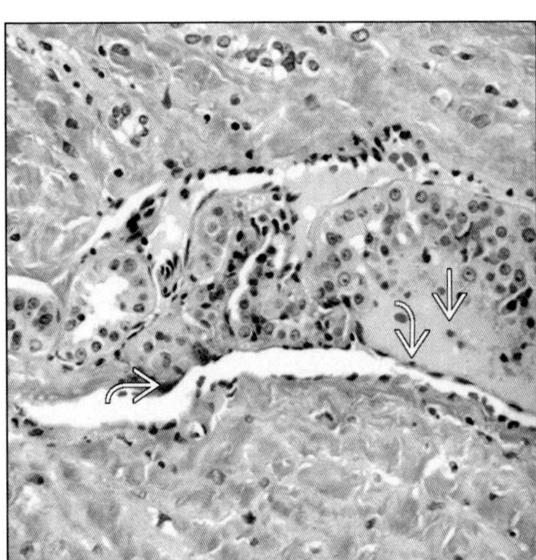

(Left) Low-power photomicrograph depicts a polypoid mass of tumor cells ➡ infiltrating the tumor capsule ➡ and invading a large vascular space ➞. The tumor mass is connected to the intravascular component. (Right) The neoplastic cells ➡ invading the capsular blood vessel ➦ have morphology identical to that of the underlying follicular carcinoma cells. They are small, with somewhat irregular nuclei. Numerous cells with hyperchromic nuclei are also present.

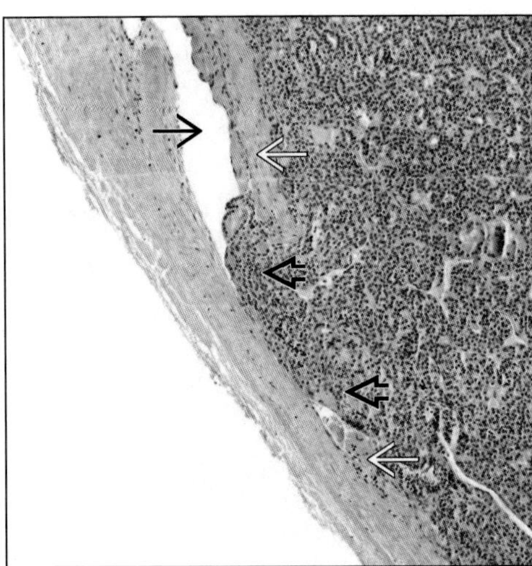

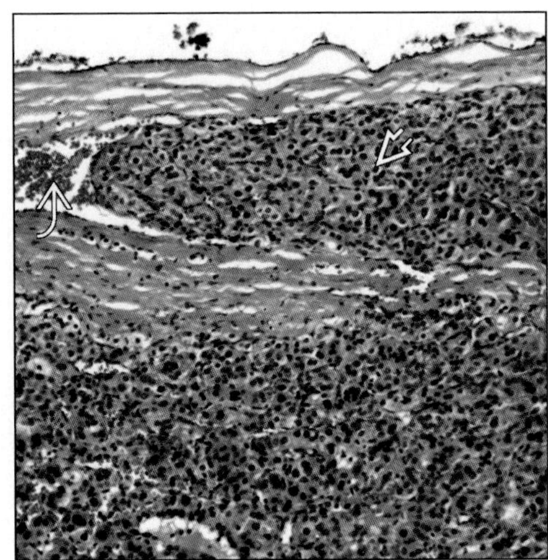

Microscopic and Cytologic Features

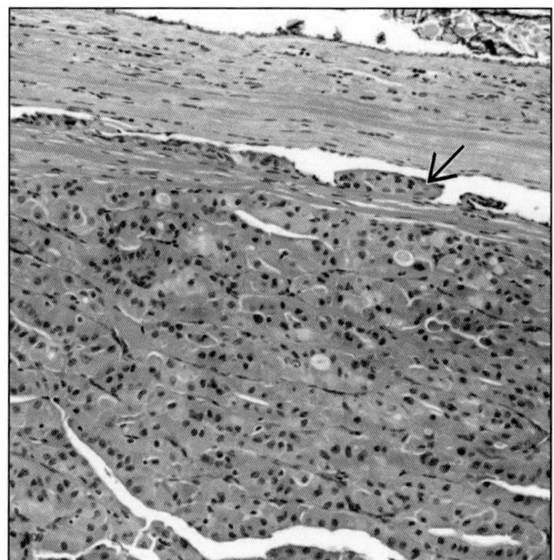

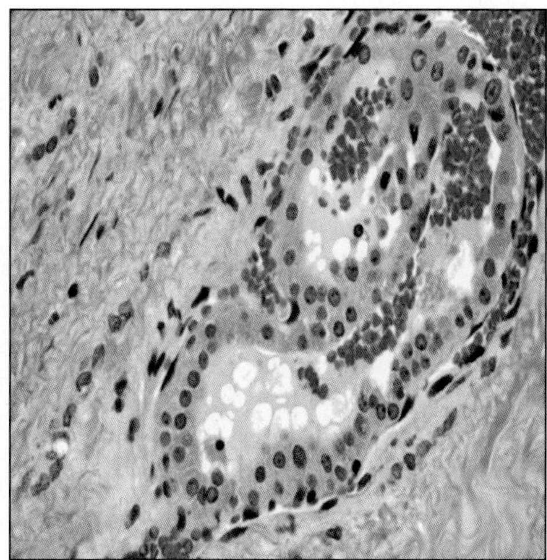

(Left) In follicular carcinomas with oncocytic features, the cells have a low nuclear to cytoplasmic ratio with uniform nuclei. The cytoplasm is abundant and pink. The tumor within the vascular space ➔ shares the same morphology. ***(Right)*** *High-power view shows a focus of vascular invasion in an oncocytic follicular carcinoma. The cells have monotonous, fairly regular nuclei and abundant eosinophilic cytoplasm. The tumor follicles are within vascular spaces.*

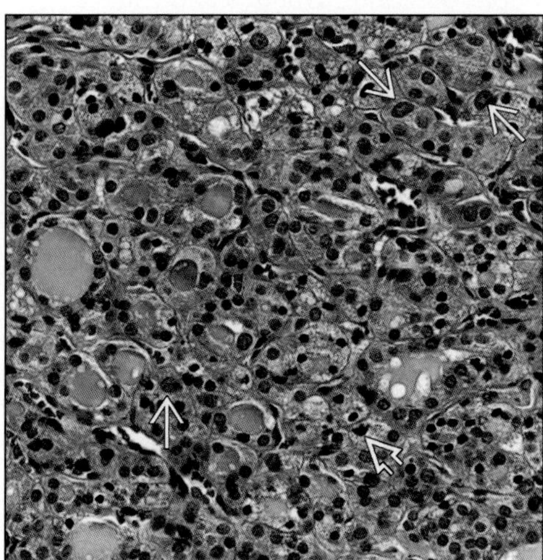

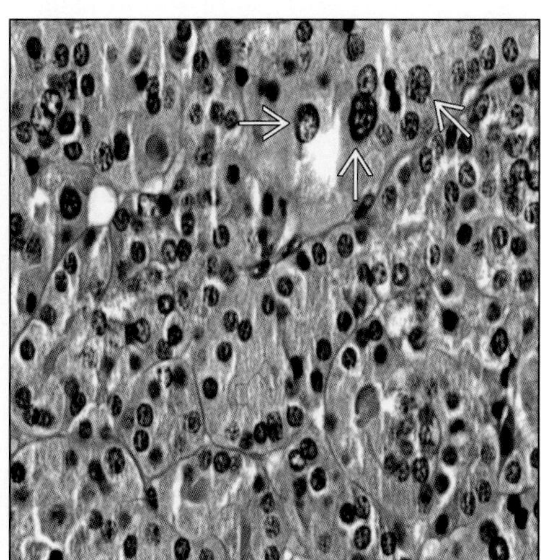

(Left) *Nuclear pleomorphism can be present to various degrees in follicular carcinoma. This case presents microfollicular architecture with few large irregular nuclei that may show nucleoli ➡. Colloid is present throughout the tumor. A mitotic figure is seen ⇨.* ***(Right)*** *High-power view of a FTC depicts pleomorphism and cellular atypia. The overall follicular architecture is preserved, but cells with pink granular cytoplasm and irregular large nuclei are present ➡.*

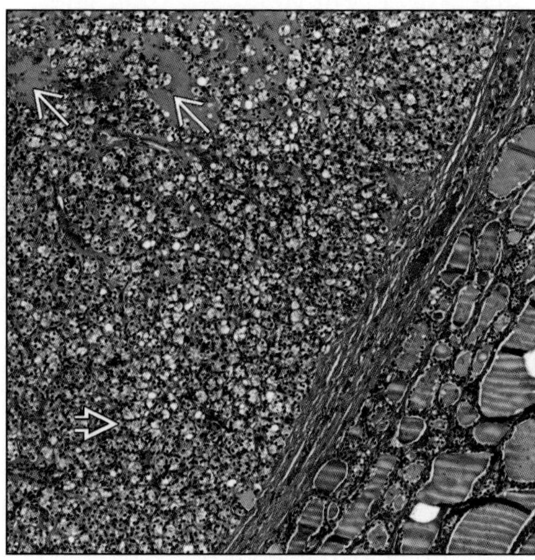

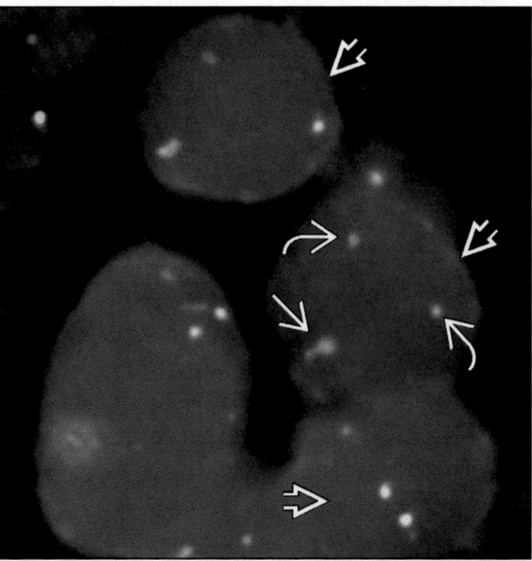

(Left) *Follicular carcinoma shows solid growth pattern with clear cells ⇨ and hyalinization ➡.* ***(Right)*** *Three cells ⇨ in this thyroid FNA specimen show typical rearrangements of PPARγ seen in FTC. A break-apart probe was used. Normal chromosomes should have green and red signal next to each other ➡. Rearrangement is shown as separate red and green signals ↪. Each of the affected cells shown here have 1 normal and 1 rearranged chromosome.*

MEDULLARY THYROID CARCINOMA

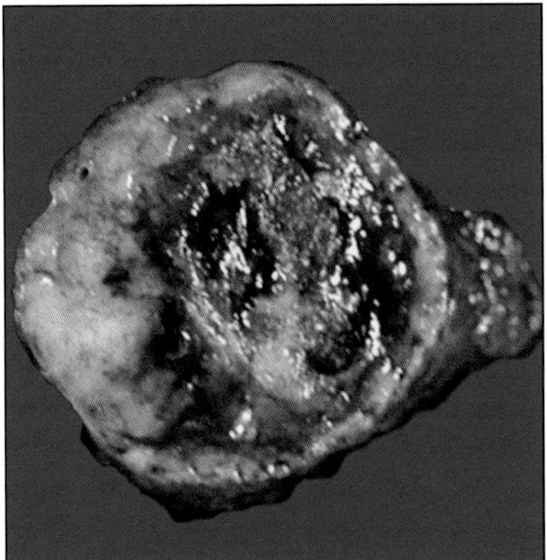

Gross cut surface of a thyroid lobe shows a well-circumscribed, white-gray-yellow thyroid tumor. Medullary thyroid carcinomas are usually firm and gritty. Areas of hemorrhage are present.

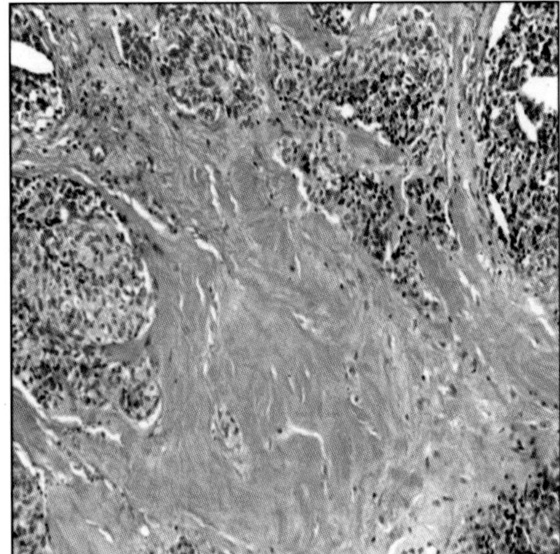

Medullary thyroid carcinoma shows a characteristic histological appearance with the presence of a highly cellular tumor with a variable amount of fibrosis and amyloid deposition.

TERMINOLOGY

Abbreviations

- Medullary thyroid carcinoma (MTC)

Synonyms

- Solid carcinoma
- Solid carcinoma with amyloid stroma
- C-cell carcinoma
- Medullary carcinoma (MC) of the thyroid
- Compact cell carcinoma
- Neuroendocrine carcinoma of the thyroid

Definitions

- Neuroendocrine tumor derived from C cells of the thyroid
- MTCs measuring < 1 cm in diameter are called medullary microcarcinomas (MMC)

ETIOLOGY/PATHOGENESIS

Associated Conditions

- Chronic hypercalcemia associated with increased incidence of sporadic MTC

Genetic Predisposition

- Hereditary forms of MTC are transmitted as autosomal dominant traits, usually with high penetrance
- MTC is seen in setting of MEN2 syndromes and familial MTC-only syndrome
  - **MEN2A:** MTC, parathyroid hyperplasia, pheochromocytoma, and pancreatic endocrine tumors
  - **MEN2B:** MTC, pheochromocytoma, and mucosal soft tissue tumors (notably neuromas)
  - **Familial MTC-only syndrome:** MTC not associated with other tumors
- MEN2 is caused by mutations in *RET* gene
  - Commonly activating point mutations
  - Exon 10 codons 609, 611, 618, 620 and exon 11 codon 634 responsible for 95% of MEN2A and 85% of FMTC
  - MEN2A: Up to 90% involve exon 11 codon 634
  - MEN2B: Up to 95% associated with exon 16 codon 918 mutation
  - Fusion genes with the tyrosine kinase domain of *RET* also occur
  - *RET* chromosomal rearrangements also associated with papillary carcinoma (*RET/PTC*)
  - Somatic *RET* mutations also present in 60% of sporadic MTCs

Precursor Lesions

- **Neoplastic C-cell hyperplasia**
  - NCCH is the precursor lesion in hereditary MTC
  - Clusters should have > 50 C cells
  - Also known as C-cell carcinoma in situ or medullary carcinoma in situ
  - These lesions harbor germline *RET* mutations
  - It is postulated that CCH progresses to MMC and eventually to MTC
  - C-cell clusters surrounding or invading follicles
  - Found in the vicinity of medullary carcinomas
  - Distinguishing CCH from MMC or intrathyroid spread of MTC may be difficult
- **Reactive C-cell hyperplasia**
  - Increase in the number of C-cells secondary to associated thyroid disorder (nodules, papillary or follicular carcinoma, inflammatory or autoimmune)
  - Cell groups contain < 50 cells
  - Lack pleomorphism, amyloid, fibrosis, or invasion of follicles
  - Difficult to visualize on H&E alone; requires calcitonin staining
- Role of CCH in sporadic MTC remains unknown
- Solid cell nests
  - Remnants of ultimobranchial body
  - Found in upper and middle regions of thyroid lobes

MEDULLARY THYROID CARCINOMA

Key Facts

Terminology
- Neuroendocrine tumor derived from C cells of thyroid
- MTCs measuring < 1 cm in diameter are called medullary microcarcinomas (MMC)

Etiology/Pathogenesis
- MTC is seen in setting of MEN2 and familial non-MEN MTC syndromes
- MEN2 is caused by mutations in *RET* gene
- Neoplastic C-cell hyperplasia (CCH) is the precursor lesion in hereditary MTC
- Role of CCH in sporadic MTC remains unknown

Clinical Issues
- 5-10% of all thyroid malignancies
- 75-80% are sporadic
- 20-25% are hereditary
- Increased serum calcitonin and CEA levels
- *RET* gene mutation analysis
- In patients with hereditary MTC, recommended age for prophylactic thyroidectomy is according to *RET* mutations
- 5- and 10-year survivals of 60-80% and 40-70%, respectively
- MMC (< 1 cm) 10-year survival of 74-100%

Ancillary Tests
- Positive for calcitonin and CEA

Diagnostic Checklist
- Desmoplasia and breach of the basement membrane helps differentiate CCH from MMC

- Clusters of flat epithelial cells lacking intercellular bridges
- Intimally associated with C cells

CLINICAL ISSUES

Epidemiology
- Incidence
  - 5-10% of all thyroid malignancies
    - 75-80% are sporadic
    - 20-25% are hereditary
  - Rising incidence due to calcitonin screening protocols and *RET* genetic testing
    - Increase in prophylactic thyroidectomies
    - Mostly MMC identified in familial cases
- Age
  - 50-60 years in sporadic cases
  - Familial cases can present from early childhood (mean age: 32 years)
- Gender
  - Slight female predominance in sporadic cases

Presentation
- Often presents as painless cold nodule
- Up to 50% have nodal metastases
- Up to 20% may present with distant metastases
- Symptoms of carcinoid and Cushing syndromes may be present
- Large tumors may lead to dysphagia and upper airway obstruction
- Nonthyroid findings: Mucosal neuromas; parathyroid, adrenal, pituitary, and pancreatic tumors
- MTC tends to metastasize early: Liver, lungs, bone, soft tissue outside the neck, brain, and bone marrow

Laboratory Tests
- Screening and monitoring tests are performed in patients at risk
  - History or presence of multiple endocrine neoplasias
  - Family history of MEN2 or familial MTC
  - Genetic counseling is recommended to assess patient-specific risk
- Increased serum calcitonin and CEA levels
- Abnormal pentagastrin-stimulated calcitonin response
- *RET* gene mutation analysis
  - Most commonly exons 10, 11, 13, 14, and 16 in hereditary forms
  - Mutations in codons 768, 790, 791, and 804 may predispose to a milder form of MTC with low penetrance, late onset, and without family history
  - Most common somatic mutation in sporadic MTC is M918T

Treatment
- Surgical approaches
  - Total thyroidectomy offers the best chance of cure
  - Associated neck dissections considered for tumors > 1 cm
  - Thyroidectomy recommendations for specific *RET* germline mutations
    - Codons 883, 918, or 922: Thyroidectomy by 1 year of age
    - Codons 611, 618, 620, or 634: Thyroidectomy before 5 years of age
    - Other mutations: Thyroidectomy once stimulated calcitonin screening turns abnormal
- Adjuvant therapy
  - Targeted tyrosine kinase, hormone therapy, chemotherapy, and anti-CEA treatments can be considered
- Radiation
  - For residual disease and palliation

Prognosis
- Considerable variation
- Overall 5- and 10-year survivals of 60-80% and 40-70%, respectively
- 10-year survival by tumor stage
  - Stage I: 100%, stage III: 65-85%, stage IV: 20-50%
- Better prognostic factors are tumor stage, young age, women, and familial forms
- Poor prognostic factors are necrosis, squamous metaplasia, < 50% calcitonin immunoreaction, CEA reactivity in the absence of calcitonin

MEDULLARY THYROID CARCINOMA

IMAGE FINDINGS

Scintigraphic Scan

- Cold nodule on iodine scan

MACROSCOPIC FEATURES

General Features

- Typically at junction of upper and middle 1/3 of the lobe
- Sporadic tumors tend to present as a solitary mass ± lymph node involvement
- Hereditary tumors are usually multicentric and bilateral
- Usually not encapsulated but well circumscribed
- Firm, yellow-white, gritty cut surface

Size

- Ranges from grossly undetectable to large, replacing entire gland
- Small tumors often seen in MEN2 patients after prophylactic thyroidectomy

Sections to Be Submitted

- In high-risk patients (MEN2 and familial MTC) who undergo prophylactic thyroidectomy, entire gland should be submitted to identify MMC and C-cell hyperplasia
- Specimen should be serially sectioned and submitted in toto from superior to inferior
- C cells are normally situated in upper and middle portions of the lobes
- In general, medullary carcinoma does not arise in isthmus

MICROSCOPIC PATHOLOGY

Histologic Features

- Histologic appearance is quite variable
- May mimic other thyroid carcinomas (follicular, papillary, insular, anaplastic)
- Most common morphology includes sheets, nests, trabeculae, or insular patterns
- Cells are round, polygonal, or spindle-shaped, separated by thin fibrovascular cores
- Cytoplasm can be clear, amphophilic or eosinophilic
- Nuclei are round to oval
- Chromatin is fine, granular and dispersed, typical of neuroendocrine tumors
- 80% show calcitonin positive amyloid in the stroma
- Variants: Follicular, papillary, clear cell, oncocytic, small cell, giant cell, melanotic, paraganglioma-like and squamous
- Vacuoles with mucin have been frequently described
- Psammoma-like concretions are occasionally seen

Cytologic Features

- Aspirates are hypercellular with loosely cohesive to noncohesive cells
- Spindle, polygonal, or bipolar cells often with excentric nuclei
- Hyperchromatic nuclei with coarse chromatin and moderate pleomorphism
- Amyloid may be seen in 50-70%
- Multinucleated giant tumor cells are common

Histologic Variants

- Variant patterns of medullary thyroid carcinoma may resemble a wide range of thyroid and extrathyroid tumors
- Staining for calcitonin is helpful in making distinction between MTC and the tumors it may mimic
  - Follicular carcinoma
  - Papillary or pseudopapillary carcinoma
  - Paraganglioma-like
  - Spindle cell
  - Clear cell
  - Oncocytic
  - Giant cell
  - Melanoma (with pigmentation)
  - Angiosarcoma

ANCILLARY TESTS

Histochemistry

- Congo red
  - Reactivity: Positive
  - Staining pattern
    - Amyloid shows light green birefringence with polarization

Immunohistochemistry

- Hallmark of MTC is positivity for calcitonin
- Tumor cells are also positive for neuroendocrine markers (chromogranin, synaptophysin) and CEA
- TTF-1 and low molecular weight keratins may be positive
- Progesterone receptor and S100 (in peripheral sustentacular cells) can be positive in MTC

Cytogenetics

- Identify rearrangements involving *RET* gene

Molecular Genetics

- *RET* gene sequencing is important to determine prognosis and timing of prophylactic thyroidectomy
  - Exons 10, 11, 13, 14, 15, and 16 cover 95% of cases

Electron Microscopy

- Transmission
  - Presence of neurosecretory granules confirms neuroendocrine origin of tumor
    - Electron-dense, membrane bound
  - Amyloid material is detected as fine fibrillary material within parenchymal space

DIFFERENTIAL DIAGNOSIS

Intrathyroid Tumor

- **Follicular carcinoma (FC)**
  - Thyroglobulin is positive
  - Nuclear features: Neuroendocrine chromatin in MTC compared to dark dense nuclei in FC
- **Undifferentiated carcinoma**

Differential Diagnosis of Medullary Thyroid Carcinoma by Immunohistochemistry

	MTC	PTC	PDC	ATC	PA/C	Para	Met C
Cytokeratin	+	+	+	+/-	+	-	+
Thyroglobulin	-	+	+	-	-	-	-
TTF-1	+	+	+	-	-	-	-/+
Chromogranin	+	-	-	-	+	+	+/-
Synaptophysin	+	-	-	-	+/-	+	+/-
Calcitonin	+	-	-	-	-	-	-
PTH	-	-	-	-	+	-	-
S100	-	-	-	-	-	+	-

MTC = medullary thyroid carcinoma; PTC = papillary thyroid carcinoma; PDC = poorly differentiated carcinoma; ATC = anaplastic thyroid carcinoma; PA/C = parathyroid adenoma/carcinoma; Para = paraganglioma; Met C = metastatic carcinoma.

  - Hemorrhage, necrosis, and high mitotic activity seen in undifferentiated carcinoma
  - Negative for calcitonin
- **Papillary thyroid carcinoma**
  - Intranuclear inclusions can be seen in both MTC and PTC
  - Nuclear features usually unique to PTC
  - PTC is calcitonin negative and thyroglobulin positive
- **Hyalinizing trabecular tumor**
  - Thyroglobulin positive, calcitonin negative
  - Hyalin material is not amyloid when stained by Congo red under polarized light
- **Paraganglioma**
  - Negative for calcitonin, zellballen with S100 positive sustentacular cells
- **Metastatic neuroendocrine tumors**
  - Can be positive for calcitonin and CEA in rare cases
  - Clinical and radiologic correlation may help in the differential
- **Intrathyroid parathyroid tumors**
  - PTH positive; calcitonin and thyroglobulin negative
  - Clear cytoplasm, defined cell border

Tumor in Lymph Nodes

- MTC metastatic to lymph nodes may be misdiagnosed as melanoma or metastatic neuroendocrine tumors
- Calcitonin and CEA immunostains should be performed in any suspicious case

Benign Conditions

- **Amyloid goiter**
  - May infiltrate fat, and Congo red is positive
  - Involves gland diffusely
  - Calcitonin stain is negative

DIAGNOSTIC CHECKLIST

Pathologic Interpretation Pearls

- Desmoplasia and break of follicular basement membrane helps differentiate C-cell hyperplasia from MMC
- Consider MTC and calcitonin staining in any suspicious thyroid tumor without colloid production

SELECTED REFERENCES

1. Marsh DJ et al: Multiple endocrine neoplasia: types 1 and 2. Adv Otorhinolaryngol. 70:84-90, 2011
2. Nosé V: Familial thyroid cancer: a review. Mod Pathol. 24 Suppl 2:S19-33, 2011
3. Eng C: Mendelian genetics of rare--and not so rare--cancers. Ann N Y Acad Sci. 1214:70-82, 2010
4. Pacini F et al: Medullary thyroid carcinoma. Clin Oncol (R Coll Radiol). 22(6):475-85, 2010
5. Phay JE et al: Targeting RET receptor tyrosine kinase activation in cancer. Clin Cancer Res. 16(24):5936-41, 2010
6. Richards ML: Familial syndromes associated with thyroid cancer in the era of personalized medicine. Thyroid. 20(7):707-13, 2010
7. Sadow PM et al: Mixed Medullary-follicular-derived carcinomas of the thyroid gland. Adv Anat Pathol. 17(4):282-5, 2010
8. Torino F et al: Medullary thyroid cancer: a promising model for targeted therapy. Curr Mol Med. 10(7):608-25, 2010
9. American Thyroid Association Guidelines Task Force et al: Medullary thyroid cancer: management guidelines of the American Thyroid Association. Thyroid. 19(6):565-612, 2009
10. Cakir M et al: Medullary thyroid cancer: molecular biology and novel molecular therapies. Neuroendocrinology. 90(4):323-48, 2009
11. Cerrato A et al: Molecular genetics of medullary thyroid carcinoma: the quest for novel therapeutic targets. J Mol Endocrinol. 43(4):143-55, 2009
12. Wells SA Jr et al: Targeting the RET pathway in thyroid cancer. Clin Cancer Res. 15(23):7119-23, 2009
13. Etit D et al: Histopathologic and clinical features of medullary microcarcinoma and C-cell hyperplasia in prophylactic thyroidectomies for medullary carcinoma: a study of 42 cases. Arch Pathol Lab Med. 132(11):1767-73, 2008
14. Tischler AS et al: Prophylactic thyroidectomy in multiple endocrine neoplasia type 2A. N Engl J Med. 353(26):2817-8; author reply 2817-8, 2005
15. Baloch ZW et al: Neuroendocrine tumors of the thyroid gland. Am J Clin Pathol. 115 Suppl:S56-67, 2001
16. Moline J, Eng C. Multiple endocrine neoplasia type 2. 1993-, 1999
17. DeLellis RA: Multiple endocrine neoplasia syndromes revisited. Clinical, morphologic, and molecular features. Lab Invest. 72(5):494-505, 1995

MEDULLARY THYROID CARCINOMA

Radiologic and Microscopic Features

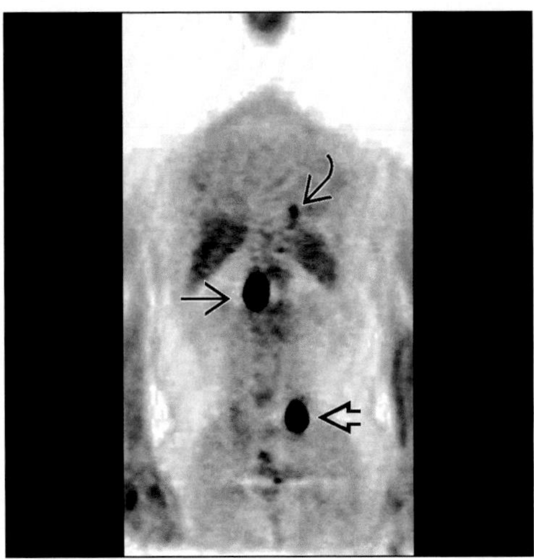
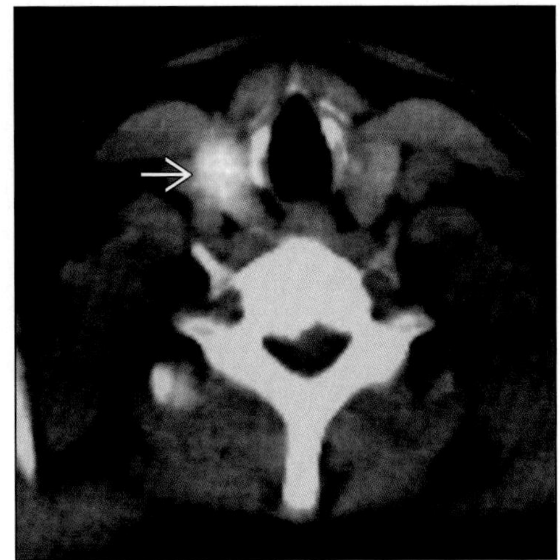

(Left) *Coronal FDG PET shows hypermetabolic foci in an upper lumbar vertebra ⇨, left sacroiliac region ⇨, and left lung ↷ in a patient with metastatic medullary thyroid cancer. Up to 20% of patients may have distant metastasis at the time of presentation.* ***(Right)*** *Fused transaxial fludeoxyglucose positron emission tomography/ computed tomography (FDG PET/CT) shows a focal hypermetabolic mass ➡ in the right thyroid lobe in a patient with medullary thyroid cancer.*

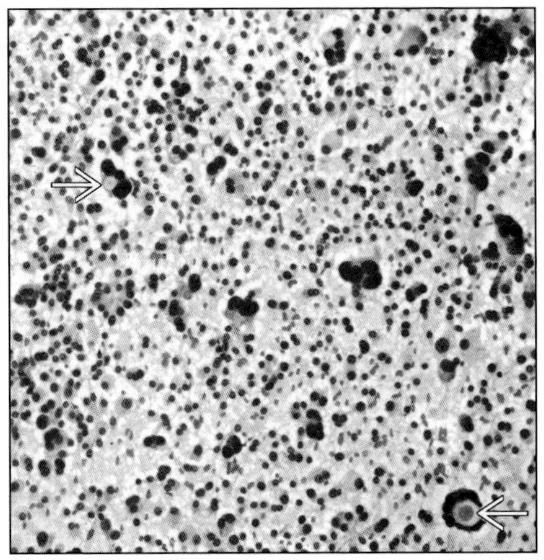
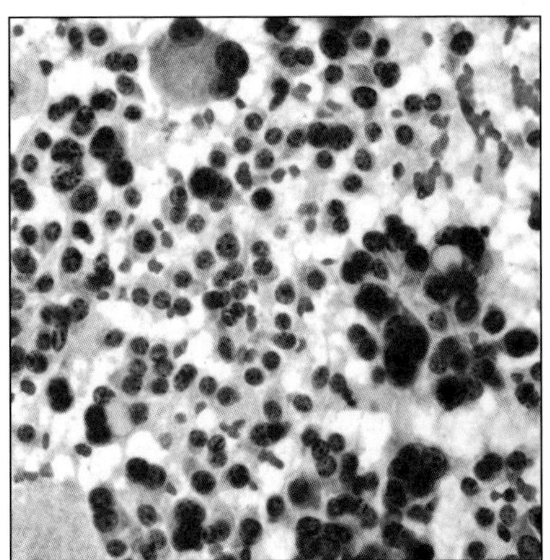

(Left) *FNA of a MTC shows a characteristic cellular specimen with clusters of loosely cohesive cells and small single cells in the background. Cells are round to oval and of variable sizes. Amyloid spheres ➡ can be seen in the background or associated with clusters of malignant cells. Colloid is notably absent.* ***(Right)*** *High magnification of a MTC FNA shows the "salt and pepper" quality of the nuclear chromatin. Many cells have have a plasmacytoid appearance with eccentric nuclei.*

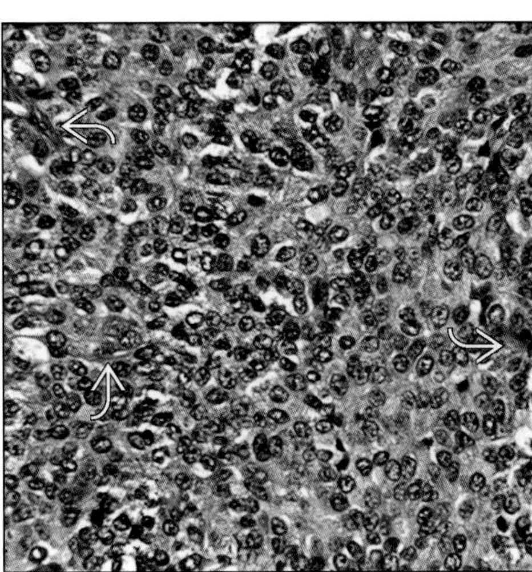
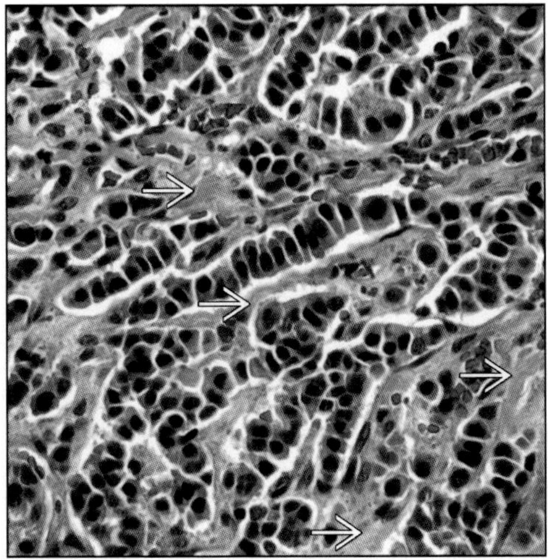

(Left) *Characteristic histopathological features of a MTC with solid growth pattern shown here include cohesive sheets and packets of round to polygonal tumor cells separated by thin fibrovascular cores ↷.* ***(Right)*** *MTC shows trabecular arrangement of anastomosing sheets of cells separated by dense hyalinized stroma ➡. Most cells have round to oval nuclei and polygonal cytoplasm and show mild to moderate pleomorphism. Amyloid deposits occur in over 70% of cases.*

MEDULLARY THYROID CARCINOMA

Gross and Microscopic Features

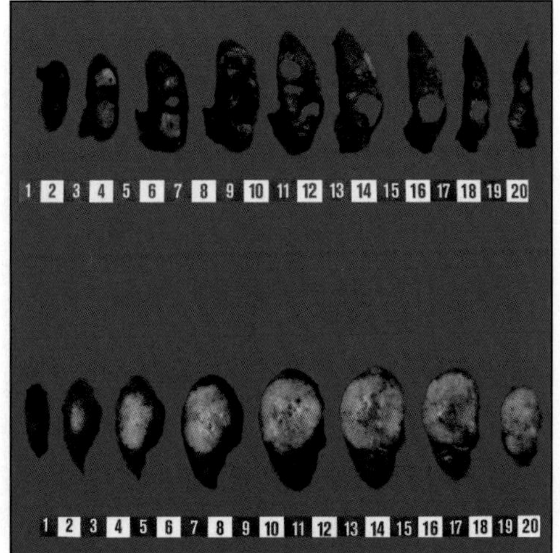

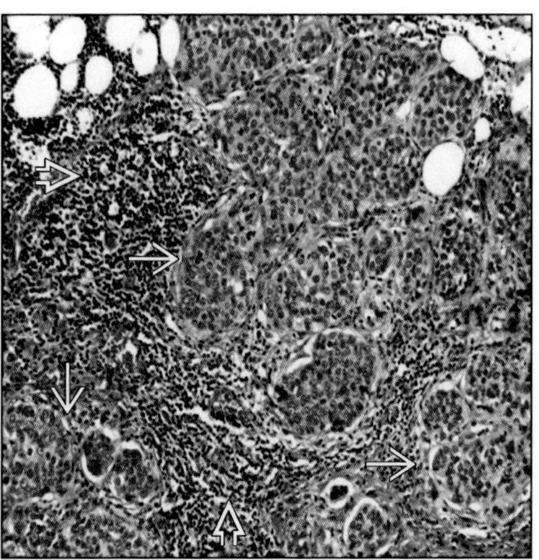

(Left) *Serial sections of both lobes of the thyroid gland show tumors. This is an example of familial medullary carcinoma, showing bilateral and multifocal tumors. Note the areas of cystic change in the upper series.* ***(Right)*** *MTC extending into extrathyroidal fibroadipose tissue shows multiple nests ➡ of small cells with scant cytoplasm and regular round nuclei, associated with marked inflammatory infiltrate ⇨.*

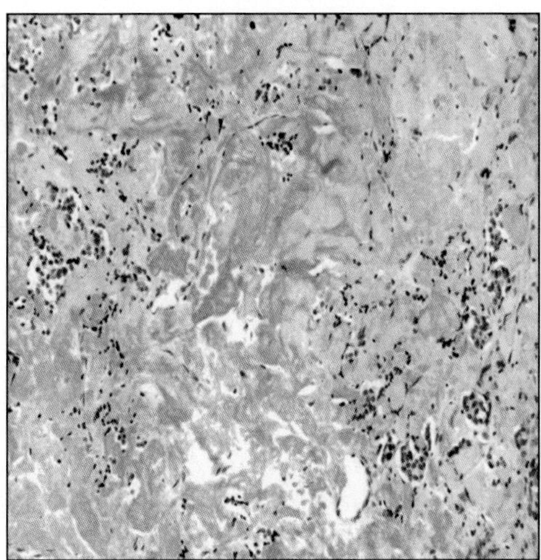

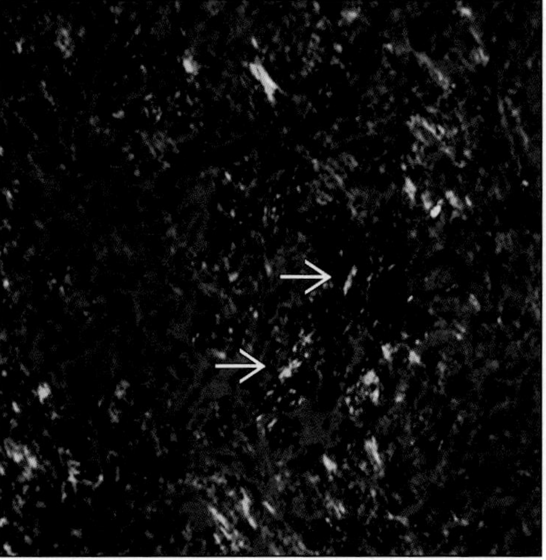

(Left) *This photomicrograph of a Congo red-stained tumor show extensive deposition of dense amorphous material suggestive of amyloid. Although not essential for the diagnosis of medullary thyroid carcinoma, variable amounts of amyloid are commonly seen in these tumors.* ***(Right)*** *Congo red-stained medullary thyroid carcinoma under polarized light reveals the characteristic apple-green birefringence ➡ confirming amyloid deposition.*

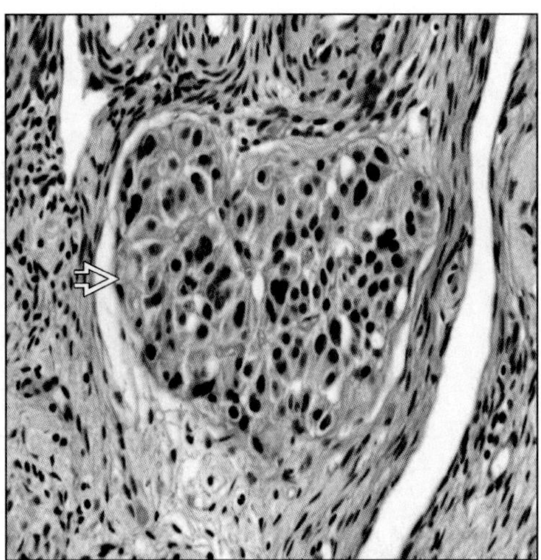

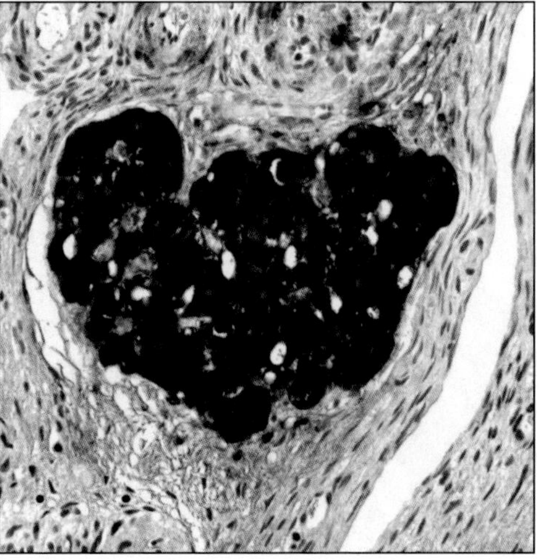

(Left) *A plug of malignant cells ⇨ is shown here invading a lymphatic space in a case of metastatic medullary thyroid carcinoma. The epithelioid cells have variable amounts of cytoplasm and moderate nuclear pleomorphism.* ***(Right)*** *Strong cytoplasmic calcitonin immunostaining highlights the C-cell nature of the tumor in the lymphovascular space and confirms the diagnosis of metastatic MTC to the ovary.*

MEDULLARY THYROID CARCINOMA

Microscopic and Immunohistochemical Features

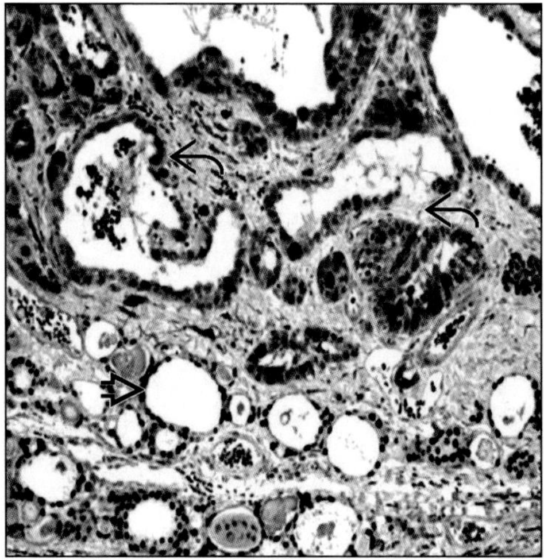

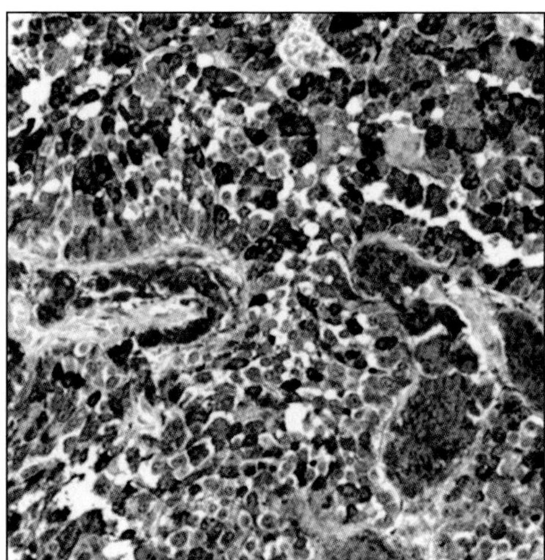

(Left) *Dual immunohistochemistry with chromogranin (red) and TTF-1 (brown) distinguishes the neuroendocrine-derived cells of a medullary thyroid carcinoma from the normal adjacent TTF-1 positive follicular cells. MTC cells have both TTF-1 and chromogranin positivity. The immunophenotypical distinction is especially important in cases with a follicular-patterned MTC morphology.* ***(Right)*** *Variable cytoplasmic calcitonin immunostaining is characteristic of MTC cells.*

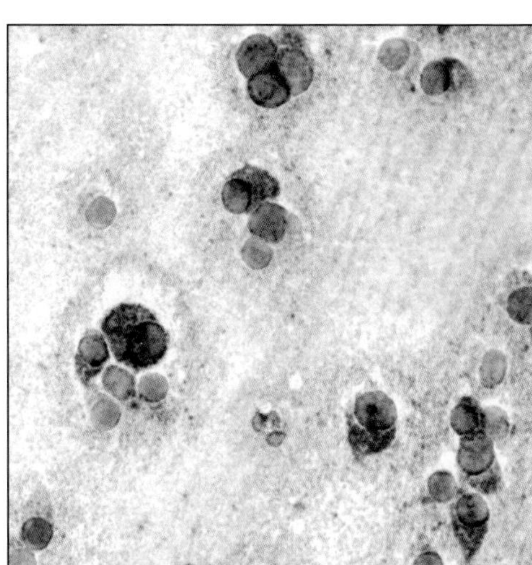

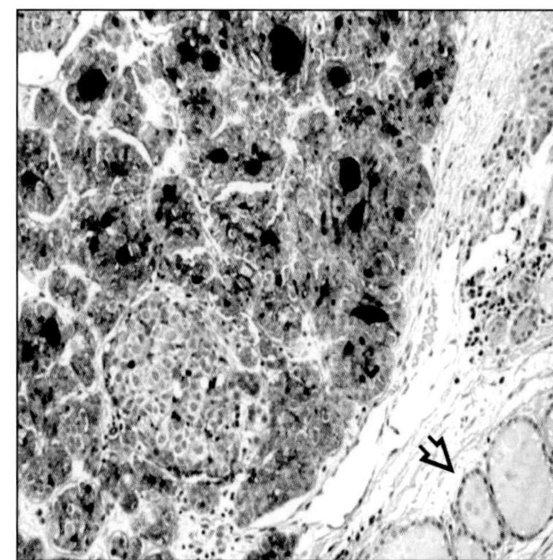

(Left) *Thyroid fine needle aspiration specimen immunocytological staining for calcitonin shows fine granular cytoplasmic pattern with variable intensity. The MTC cells in this case present the characteristic fine neuroendocrine-type nuclear chromatin.* ***(Right)*** *Carcinoembryonic antigen immunohistochemistry can be utilized for the confirmation of MTC. This stain typically gives a luminal and cytoplasmic staining pattern in MTC and is negative in normal thyroid.*

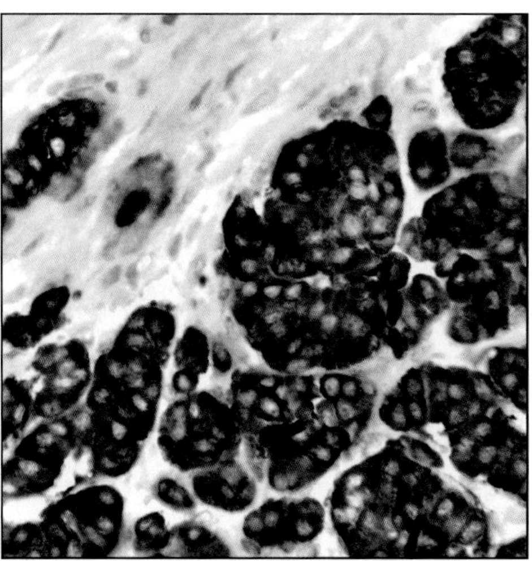

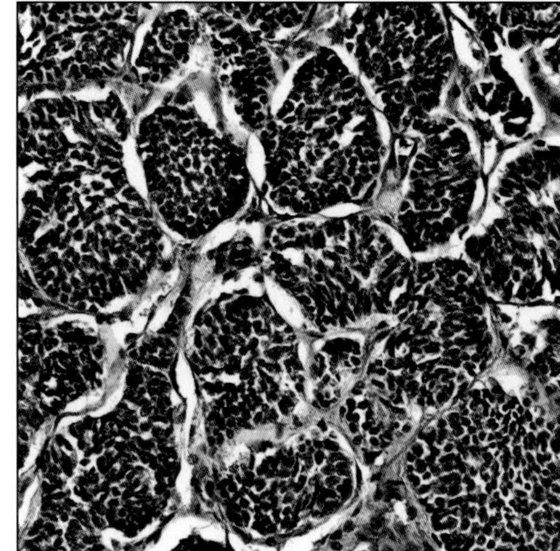

(Left) *Immunostaining for synaptophysin, as shown here, frequently gives strong diffuse cytoplasmic reactivity. Although calcitonin is the most specific stain for medullary thyroid carcinoma, other markers of neuroendocrine lineage can be helpful in establishing the diagnosis.* ***(Right)*** *The insular or organoid architecture is one of the more characteristic appearances for a medullary carcinoma. Note the delicate fibrovascular septations that surround the tumor nests.*

Metastatic Medullary Carcinoma

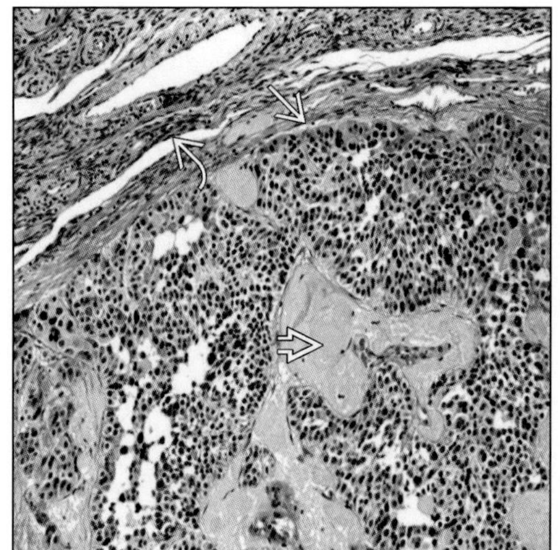

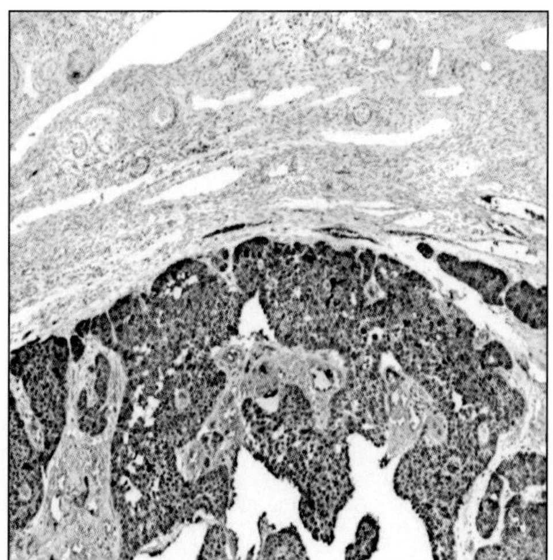

(Left) *This micrograph depicts an unusually aggressive case of medullary thyroid carcinoma metastatic to ovary. A well-defined nodule of tumors cells ➡ with interspersed areas of amyloid deposition ➡ can be seen. Compressed normal ovarian parenchyma ➡ is present surrounding the tumor.* ***(Right)*** *Section of ovary stained positive for calcitonin highlights the neoplasm and confirms medullary thyroid carcinoma as the origin for this metastatic lesion.*

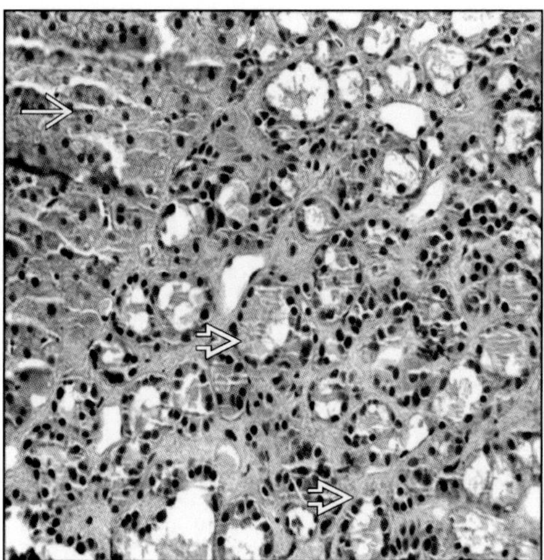

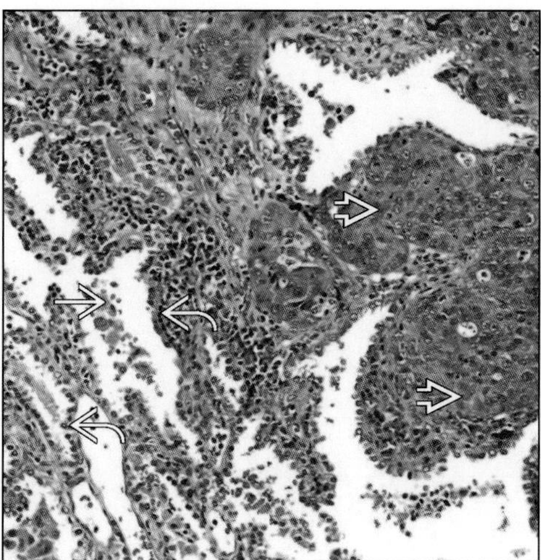

(Left) *A sharp border separates the liver metastasis of MTC ➡ from the surrounding hepatocytes ➡. Immunohistochemistry for calcitonin and thyroglobulin is helpful in establishing the diagnosis in challenging cases that mimic follicular carcinoma.* ***(Right)*** *An instance of medullary thyroid carcinoma metastatic to lung shows the lesion growing as a solid sheet of cells ➡ adjacent to alveoli lined by type II pneumocytes ➡ and filled with alveolar macrophages ➡.*

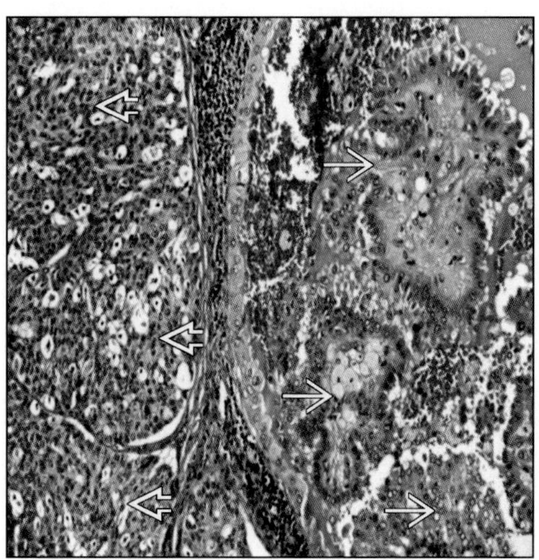

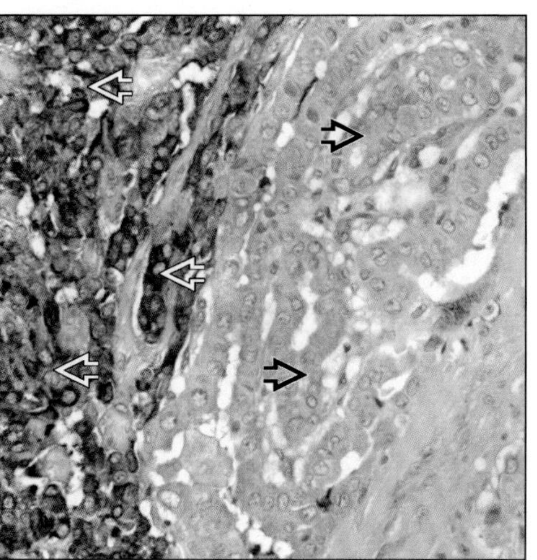

(Left) *Section of thyroid shows simultaneous medullary ➡ and papillary ➡ carcinomas of the thyroid. The distinct characteristic nuclear features of papillary thyroid carcinoma, such as large cleared nuclei and the papillary architecture, can be readily seen. The MTC nuclei are smaller and darker with neuroendocrine chromatin.* ***(Right)*** *Immunostain for calcitonin is strongly and diffusely positive in the cytoplasm of the MTC cells ➡ and negative in the adjacent PTC cells ➡.*

PROTOCOL FOR THYROID GLAND TUMOR SPECIMENS

Thyroid Gland: Resection

Pathology Cancer Case Summary (Checklist)

Procedure (select all that apply)

___ Thyroid lobectomy

 ___ Right

 ___ Left

___ Partial thyroidectomy (anything less than a lobectomy)

 ___ Right

 ___ Left

___ Hemithyroidectomy (lobe and part or all of isthmus)

 ___ Right

 ___ Left

___ Total thyroidectomy

___ Total thyroidectomy with central compartment dissection

___ Total thyroidectomy with right neck dissection

___ Total thyroidectomy with left neck dissection

___ Total thyroidectomy with bilateral neck dissection

___ Other (specify): ___________________________

___ Not specified

***Received**

*___ Fresh

*___ In formalin

*___ Other

Specimen Integrity

___ Intact

___ Fragmented

Specimen Size

Right lobe: _________ x _________ x _________ cm

Left lobe: _________ x _________ x _________ cm

Isthmus ± pyramidal lobe: _________ x _________ x _________ cm

Central compartment: _________ x _________ x _________ cm

Right neck dissection: _________ x _________ x _________ cm

Left neck dissection: _________ x _________ x _________ cm

*Additional dimensions (specify): _________ x _________ x _________ cm

***Specimen Weight**

*Specify: _________ g

Tumor Focality (select all that apply)

___ Unifocal

___ Multifocal (specify):

 ___ Ipsilateral

 ___ Bilateral

 ___ Midline (isthmus)

Dominant Tumor

Tumor laterality (select all that apply)

___ Right lobe

___ Left lobe

___ Isthmus

___ Not specified

Tumor size

Greatest dimension: _________ cm

*Additional dimensions: _________ x _________ cm

____ Cannot be determined

Histologic type (select all that apply)

____ Papillary carcinoma

Variant, specify:

____ Classical (usual)

____ Clear cell variant

____ Columnar cell variant

____ Cribriform-morular variant

____ Diffuse sclerosing variant

____ Follicular variant

____ Macrofollicular variant

____ Microcarcinoma (occult, latent, small, papillary microtumor)

____ Oncocytic or oxyphilic variant

____ Solid variant

____ Tall cell variant

____ Warthin-like variant

____ Other, specify: ____________________________

Architecture:

____ Classical (papillary)

____ Cribriform-morular

____ Diffuse sclerosing

____ Follicular

____ Macrofollicular

____ Solid

____ Other, specify: ____________________________

Cytomorphology:

____ Classical

____ Clear cell

____ Columnar cell

____ Oncocytic or oxyphilic

____ Tall cell

____ Follicular carcinoma

Variant, specify:

____ Clear cell

____ Oncocytic (Hürthle cell)

____ Other, specify: ____________________________

____ Poorly differentiated thyroid carcinomas, including insular carcinoma

____ Medullary carcinoma

____ Undifferentiated (anaplastic) carcinoma

____ Other (specify): ____________________________

____ Carcinoma, type cannot be determined

***Histologic grade**

*____ Not applicable

*____ GX: Cannot be assessed

*____ G1: Well differentiated

*____ G2: Moderately differentiated

*____ G3: Poorly differentiated

*____ G4: Undifferentiated

*____ Other (specify): ____________________________

Margins

____ Cannot be assessed

____ Margins uninvolved by carcinoma

*Distance of invasive carcinoma to closest margin: _________ mm

____ Margin(s) involved by carcinoma

PROTOCOL FOR THYROID GLAND TUMOR SPECIMENS

*Site(s) of involvement: ____________________________

Tumor capsule

____ Cannot be assessed
____ Totally encapsulated
____ Partially encapsulated
____ None

Tumor capsular invasion (select all that apply)

____ Cannot be assessed
____ Not identified
____ Present
Extent
____ Minimal
____ Widely invasive
____ Indeterminate

Lymph-vascular invasion (select all that apply)

____ Cannot be assessed
____ Not identified
____ Present
Extent
____ Focal (less than 4 vessels)
____ Extensive (4 or more vessels)
____ Indeterminate

***Perineural invasion**

*____ Not identified
*____ Present
*____ Indeterminate

Extrathyroidal extension (select all that apply)

____ Cannot be assessed
____ Not identified
____ Present:
Extent:
____ Minimal
____ Extensive

2nd Tumor (for multifocal tumors only)

Tumor laterality (select all that apply)

____ Right lobe
____ Left lobe
____ Isthmus
____ Not specified

Tumor size

Greatest dimension: _________ cm
*Additional dimensions: _________ x _________ cm
____ Cannot be determined

Histologic type (select all that apply)

____ Papillary carcinoma
Variant, specify:
____ Classical (usual)
____ Clear cell variant
____ Columnar cell variant
____ Cribriform-morular variant
____ Diffuse sclerosing variant
____ Follicular variant
____ Macrofollicular variant
____ Microcarcinoma (occult, latent, small, papillary microtumor)

___ Oncocytic or oxyphilic variant
___ Solid variant
___ Tall cell variant
___ Warthin-like variant
___ Other, specify: ___________________________

Architecture:

___ Classical (papillary)
___ Cribriform-morular
___ Diffuse sclerosing
___ Follicular
___ Macrofollicular
___ Solid
___ Other, specify: ___________________________

Cytomorphology:

___ Classical
___ Clear cell
___ Columnar cell
___ Oncocytic or oxyphilic
___ Tall cell

___ Follicular carcinoma

Variant, specify:

___ Clear cell
___ Oncocytic (Hürthle cell)
___ Other, specify: ___________________________

___ Poorly differentiated thyroid carcinomas, including insular carcinoma
___ Medullary carcinoma
___ Undifferentiated (anaplastic) carcinoma
___ Other (specify): ___________________________
___ Carcinoma, type cannot be determined

***Histologic grade**

*___ Not applicable
*___ GX: Cannot be assessed
*___ G1: Well differentiated
*___ G2: Moderately differentiated
*___ G3: Poorly differentiated
*___ G4: Undifferentiated
*___ Other (specify): ___________________________

Margins

___ Cannot be assessed
___ Margins uninvolved by carcinoma

*Distance of invasive carcinoma to closest margin: ________ mm

___ Margin(s) involved by carcinoma

*Site(s) of involvement: ___________________________

Tumor capsule

___ Cannot be assessed
___ Totally encapsulated
___ Partially encapsulated
___ None

Tumor capsular invasion (select all that apply)

___ Cannot be assessed
___ Not identified
___ Present

Extent

___ Minimal

PROTOCOL FOR THYROID GLAND TUMOR SPECIMENS

____ Widely invasive

____ Indeterminate

Lymph-vascular invasion (select all that apply)

____ Cannot be assessed

____ Not identified

____ Present

Extent

____ Focal (less than 4 vessels)

____ Extensive (4 or more vessels)

____ indeterminate

***Perineural invasion**

*____ Not identified

*____ Present

*____ Indeterminate

Extrathyroidal extension (select all that apply)

____ Cannot be assessed

____ Not identified

____ Present

Extent:

____ Minimal

____ Extensive

Pathologic Staging (pTNM)

TNM descriptors (required only if applicable) (select all that apply)

____ m (multiple primary tumors)

____ r (recurrent)

____ y (post-treatment)

Primary tumor (pT)**

____ pTX: Cannot be assessed

____ pT0: No evidence of primary tumor

____ pT1: Tumor size 2 cm or less, limited to thyroid

____ pT1a: Tumor 1 cm or less in greatest dimension limited to the thyroid

____ pT1b: Tumor > 1 cm but ≤ 2 cm in greatest dimension, limited to the thyroid

____ pT2: Tumor > 2 cm but ≤ 4 cm, limited to thyroid

____ pT3: Tumor > 4 cm limited to thyroid or any tumor with minimal extrathyroid extension (e.g., extension to sternothyroid muscle or perithyroid soft tissues)

____ pT4a: Moderately advanced disease. Tumor of any size extending beyond the thyroid capsule to invade subcutaneous soft tissues, larynx, trachea, esophagus, or recurrent laryngeal nerve

____ pT4b: Very advanced disease. Tumor invades prevertebral fascia or encases carotid artery or mediastinal vessels

Anaplastic carcinoma

____ pT4a: Intrathyroidal anaplastic carcinoma: Surgically resectable

____ pT4b: Extrathyroidal anaplastic carcinoma: Surgically unresectable

Regional lymph nodes (pN)***

____ pNX: Cannot be assessed

____ pN0: No regional lymph node metastasis

____ PN1a: Nodal metastases to level VI (pretracheal, paratracheal, and prelaryngeal/Delphian) lymph nodes

____ pN1b: Metastases to unilateral, bilateral, or contralateral cervical (levels I, II, III, IV, V) or retropharyngeal or superior mediastinal lymph nodes (level VII)

Specify: Number examined: ____

Number involved: ____

***Lymph node, extranodal extension**

*____ Not identified

*____ Present

*____ Indeterminate

Distant metastasis (pM)

____ Not applicable

____ pM1: Distant metastasis

*Specify site(s), if known: __________________________

*Source of pathologic metastatic specimen (specify): __________________________

Additional Pathologic Findings (select all that apply)

*____ Adenoma

*____ Adenomatoid nodule(s) or nodular follicular disease (e.g., nodular hyperplasia, goitrous thyroid)

*____ Diffuse hyperplasia (Graves disease)

*____ Thyroiditis:

- *____ Advanced
- *____ Focal (nonspecific)
- *____ Palpation
- *____ Other (specify): __________________________

*____ Parathyroid gland(s):

- *____ Within normal limits
- *____ Hypercellular
- *____ Other (specify): __________________________

*____ C-cell hyperplasia

*____ None identified

*____ Other (specify): __________________________

Ancillary Studies

*Specify type (e.g., histochemistry, immunohistochemistry, DNA analysis: __________________________

*Specify results: __________________________

Clinical History (select all that apply)

*____ Radiation exposure:

- *____ Yes (specify type): __________________________
- *____ No
- *____ Indeterminate

*____ Family history

*____ Other (specify): __________________________

**Data elements with asterisks are not required. These elements may be clinically important but are not yet validated or regularly used in patient management. **There is no category of carcinoma in situ (pTis) relative to carcinomas of thyroid gland. ***Superior mediastinal lymph nodes are considered regional lymph nodes (level VII). Midline nodes are considered ipsilateral nodes. Adapted with permission from College of American Pathologists, "Protocol for the Examination of Specimens from Patients with Carcinoma of the Thyroid Gland." Web posting date October 2009, www.cap.org.*

PROTOCOL FOR ADRENAL GLAND TUMOR SPECIMENS

Adrenal Gland

Biopsy (Core Needle, Incisional, Excisional); Resection

Specimen

Adrenal gland; received

___ Fresh

___ In formalin

___ Other (specify): ___________________________

Procedure

___ Needle biopsy (radiographically guided)

___ Adrenalectomy, total

___ Adrenalectomy, partial

___ Other (specify): ___________________________

___ Not specified

Specimen Integrity

___ Intact

___ Fragmented

Specimen Size

Greatest dimensions: _________ x _________ x _________ cm

*Additional dimensions (if more than 1 part): _________ x _________ x _________ cm

Specimen Laterality

___ Right

___ Left

___ Not specified

___ Other (specify): ___________________________

Tumor Size

Greatest dimension: _________ cm

*Additional dimensions: _________ x _________ cm

___ Cannot be determined (fragmented specimen)

Tumor Gland Weight

Specify: _________ g

**Tumor Description (select all that apply)*

*___Hemorrhagic

*___Necrotic

*___Invasion

*___ Capsule

*___ Vessels

*___ Extraadrenal (specify): ___________________________

*___Other (specify): ___________________________

Histologic Type

___ Adrenal cortical carcinoma

**Microscopic Tumor Extension*

*___Specify: ___________________________

Margins

___ Margins uninvolved by tumor

___ Margin(s) involved by tumor

Distance from closest margin: _________ mm or _________ cm

Specify margin(s) if possible: ___________________________

___ Cannot be determined

___ Not applicable

***Treatment Effect** (applicable to carcinomas treated with neoadjuvant therapy)*

*___ Not identified

*___ Present (specify): ____________________________

*___ Indeterminate

Lymph-Vascular Invasion (select all that apply)

___ Not identified

___ Present

  ___ Large vessel (venous)

  ___ Small vessel (capillary lymphatic)

___ Indeterminate

****Perineural Invasion***

*___ Not identified

*___ Present

*___ Indeterminate

****Lymph Nodes, Extranodal Extension***

*___ Not identified

*___ Present

*___ Indeterminate

Pathologic Staging (pTNM)

TNM descriptors (required only if applicable) (select all that apply)

___ m (multiple primary tumors)

___ r (recurrent)

___ y (post-treatment)

Primary tumor (pT)

___ pTX: Cannot be determined

___ pT0: No evidence of primary tumor

___ pT1: Tumor $\leq$ 5 cm in greatest dimension, no extraadrenal invasion

___ pT2: Tumor > 5 cm, no extraadrenal invasion

___ pT3: Tumor of any size with local invasion, but not invading adjacent organs#

___ pT4: Tumor of any size with invasion of adjacent organs#

Regional lymph nodes (pN)

___ pNX: Cannot be assessed

___ pN0: No regional lymph node metastasis

___ pN1: Regional lymph node metastasis

___ No nodes submitted or found

Number of lymph nodes examined

Specify: ________

___ Number cannot be determined (explain): ____________________________

Number of lymph nodes involved

Specify: ________

___ Number cannot be determined (explain): ____________________________

Distant metastasis (pM)

___ Not applicable

___ pM1: Distant metastasis

*Specify site(s), if known: ____________________________

****Additional Pathologic Findings (select all that apply)***

*___ None identified

*___ Tumor necrosis

*___ Degenerative changes

  *___ Calcifications

  *___ Hemorrhage

  *___ Cystic change

PROTOCOL FOR ADRENAL GLAND TUMOR SPECIMENS

*___Other (specify): ____________________________

Non-Pathology Findings (select all that apply)

*___Urinary 17-ketosteroids increased (10 mg/g creatinine/24 hours)

*___Hormone production

  *___ Cushing syndrome

  *___ Conn syndrome

  *___ Virilization/feminization

*___Weight loss

*___Other (specify): ____________________________

Ancillary Studies

  *Specify type(s): ____________________________

  *Specify result(s): ____________________________

Clinical History (select all that apply)

*___Neoadjuvant therapy

  *___ Yes (specify type): ____________________________

  *___ No

  *___ Indeterminate

*___Other (specify): ____________________________

**Data elements with asterisks are not required. These elements may be clinically important but are not yet validated or regularly used in patient management. #Adjacent organs include kidney, diaphragm, great vessels, pancreas, and liver. Note: There is no category of carcinoma in situ (pTis) relative to carcinomas of the adrenal gland. Adapted with permission from College of American Pathologists, "Protocol for the Examination of Specimens from Patients with Carcinoma of the Adrenal Gland." Web posting date February 2011, www.cap.org.*

Neuroblastoma

Resection, Biopsy

Specimen

___ Adrenal/periadrenal
___ Retroperitoneal, nonadrenal
___ Thoracic paraspinal
___ Cervical
___ Other (specify): ___________________________
___ Not specified

Procedure

___ Resection
___ Incisional biopsy
___ Other (specify): ___________________________
___ Not specified

****Specimen Size***

*Greatest dimension: _________ cm
*Additional dimensions: _________ x _________ cm

****Specimen Weight***

*Specify: _________ g

Specimen Laterality (select all that apply)

___ Right
___ Left
___ Midline
___ Other (specify): ___________________________
___ Not specified

Tumor Size

Greatest dimension: _________ cm
*Additional dimensions: _________ x _________ cm
___ Cannot be assessed

Tumor Weight (if separate from total specimen)

Specify: _________ g
___ Cannot be assessed

Patient Age

___ Not specified
___ < 18 months
___ ≥ 18 months and < 5 years
___ ≥ 5 years

Histologic Type (select all that apply)

___ Neuroblastoma
___ Ganglioneuroblastoma
    ___ Nodular subtype† (specify number of nodules: _________)
    ___ Intermixed subtype
___ Ganglioneuroma
___ Indeterminate
___ Cannot be assessed

Degree of Differentiation (neuroblastic component)

___ Undifferentiated
___ Poorly differentiated
___ Differentiating
___ Cannot be assessed

PROTOCOL FOR NEUROBLASTOMA TUMOR SPECIMENS

___ Not applicable

Mitotic-Karyorrhectic Index (MKI) (neuroblastic component)

___ Low (< 100 per 5,000 cells; < 2%)
___ Intermediate (100-200 per 5,000 cells; 2-4%)
___ High (> 200 per 5,000 cells; > 4%)
___ Indeterminate
___ Cannot be assessed
___ Not applicable

****Tumor Calcification***

*___ Present
*___ Not identified
*___ Cannot be assessed

Treatment History

___ No known presurgical chemotherapy
___ Presurgical chemotherapy given
___ Not specified

International Neuroblastoma Pathology Classification (INPC) (select all that apply)††

___ **Favorable histopathology**
  ___ Any age; ganglioneuroma (schwannian stroma-dominant); maturing or mature
  ___ Any age; ganglioneuroblastoma, intermixed (schwannian stroma-rich)
  ___ < 18 months old; neuroblastoma (schwannian stroma-poor) or nodular ganglioneuroblastoma;
    poorly differentiated or differentiating subtypes with low or intermediate mitosis-karyorrhexis index (MKI)
  ___ 18 months up to < 5 years old; neuroblastoma (schwannian stroma-poor)
    or nodular ganglioneuroblastoma; differentiating subtype and low MKI

___ **Unfavorable histopathology**
  ___ Any age; neuroblastoma (schwannian stroma-poor)
    or nodular ganglioneuroblastoma with undifferentiated histology and any MKI
  ___ < 18 months old; neuroblastoma (schwannian stroma poor)
    or nodular ganglioneuroblastoma with poorly differentiated or differentiating subtypes with high MKI
  ___ 18 months up to < 5 years old; neuroblastoma (schwannian stroma-poor or nodular ganglioneuroblastoma),
    poorly differentiated and any MKI, or differentiating and intermediate or high MKI
  ___ ≥ 5 years old; neuroblastoma (schwannian stroma-poor)
    or nodular ganglioneuroblastoma; any subtype and any MKI

___ Not applicable secondary to previous chemotherapy
___ Cannot be determined secondary to insufficient material
___ Indeterminate

Margins

___ Cannot be assessed
___ Margins uninvolved by tumor
___ Margin(s) involved by tumor
  Specify margin(s): ___________________________

****Lymph-Vascular Invasion***

*___ Not identified
*___ Present
*___ Indeterminate

Extent of Tumor

Primary tumor
  ___ Cannot be assessed
  ___ Encapsulated
  ___ Extracapsular extension without adjacent organ involvement
  ___ Extension into adjacent organs
  ___ Extension into spinal canal

Regional lymph nodes

____ Cannot be assessed

____ Regional lymph node metastasis not identified

____ Regional lymph node metastasis present

Specify site: ____________________________

Number of lymph nodes examined: _________

Number of lymph nodes involved by tumor: _________

Distant metastasis

____ Cannot be assessed

____ Distant metastasis

*Specify site(s), if known: ____________________________

International Neuroblastoma Staging System (INSS)#

____ Stage 1

Localized tumor with complete gross excision, ± microscopic residual disease

Representative ipsilateral nonadherent lymph nodes negative for tumor microscopically (nodes attached to and removed with primary tumor may be positive)

____ Stage 2A

Localized tumor with incomplete gross excision; representative ipsilateral nonadherent lymph nodes negative for tumor microscopically

____ Stage 2B

Localized tumor ± complete gross excision with ipsilateral nonadherent lymph nodes positive for tumor; enlarged contralateral lymph nodes must be negative microscopically

____ Stage 3

Unresectable unilateral tumor infiltrating across midline, ## ± regional lymph node involvement

Localized unilateral tumor with contralateral regional lymph node involvement

Midline tumor with bilateral extension by infiltration (unresectable) or by lymph node involvement

____ Stage 4

Any primary tumor with dissemination to distant lymph nodes, bone, bone marrow, liver, skin, &/or other organs (except as defined in stage 4S###)

____ Stage 4S

Localized primary tumor (as defined for stage 1, 2A, or 2B) with dissemination limited to skin, liver, &/or bone marrow### (limited to infants < 1 year old)

**Additional Pathologic Findings*

***MYCN amplification status †††**

*____ Not assessed

*____ Not amplified

*____ Amplified

*____ Gain

*____ Indeterminate

***Other**

*Specify: ____________________________

**Data elements with asterisks are not required. These elements may be clinically important but are not yet validated or regularly used in patient management. †For nodular (composite) ganglioneuroblastomas with > 1 nodule, degree of differentiation and mitotic-karyorrhectic index (MKI) must be given for each nodule. Please indicate differentiation and MKI for least favorable nodule in the checklist. ††INPC applies to untreated primary tumors and tumors in metastatic sites provided that there is sufficient material to classify histologically. Bone marrow biopsy is useful only for evaluation of degree of neuroblastic differentiation, but not eligible for MKI determination. #Multifocal primary tumors (e.g., bilateral adrenal primary tumors) should be staged according to greatest extent of disease, as defined above, and followed by a subscript "M." ##Midline is defined as vertebral column. Tumors originating on one side and crossing midline must infiltrate to or beyond opposite side of vertebral column. ###Marrow involvement in stage 4S should be minimal (i.e., < 10% of total nucleated cells identified as malignant on bone marrow biopsy or marrow aspirate). More extensive marrow involvement would be considered stage 4. Meta-iodobenzylguanidine (MIBG) scan (if performed) should be negative in bone marrow. †††Results of MYCN amplification information may not be available to the pathologist at the time of the report. Adapted with permission from College of American Pathologists, "Protocol for the Examination of Specimens from Patients with Neuroblastoma." Web posting date October 2009, www.cap.org.*

Head and Neck

Neoplasm, Benign

Neoplasm, Malignant Primary

Protocol for the Examination of Specimens from Patients with Retinoblastoma

Protocol for the Examination of Specimens from Patients with Carcinomas of the Salivary Glands

SALIVARY GLAND ANLAGE TUMOR

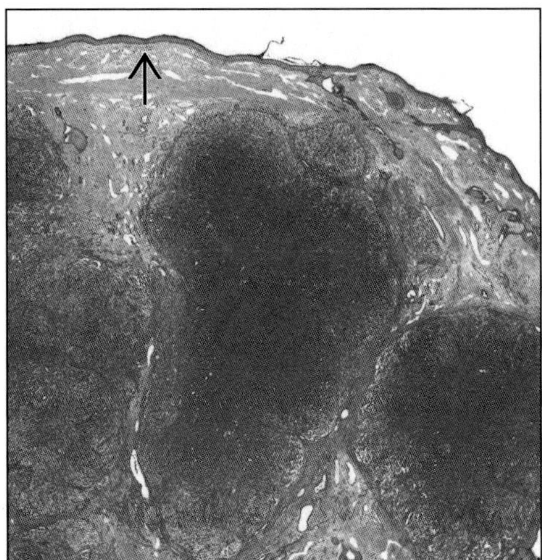

SGATs form a firm mass with a smooth or bosselated surface, covered by nonkeratinizing squamous epithelium ⇒. (Courtesy G. Ellis, DDS.)

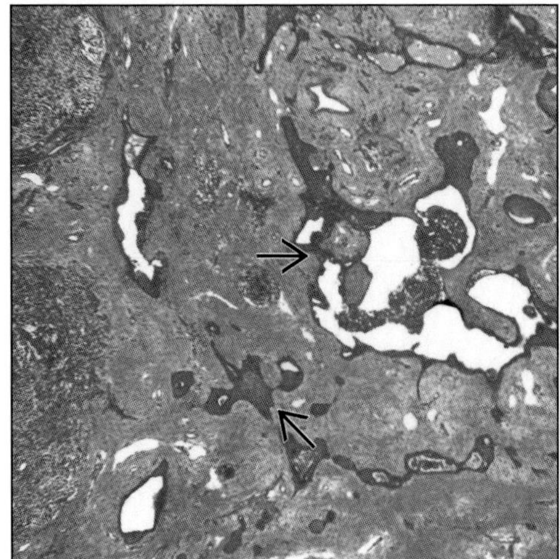

Solid and cystic nest ⇒ of squamous cells extend from the surface into a hypocellular stroma. (Courtesy G. Ellis, DDS.)

TERMINOLOGY

Abbreviations

- Salivary gland anlage tumor (SGAT)

Synonyms

- Congenital pleomorphic adenoma of nasopharynx

Definitions

- Extremely rare congenital lesion of midline nasopharynx
- Likely represents hamartoma of minor salivary gland origin

CLINICAL ISSUES

Site

- Posterior nasal septum
- Midline nasopharynx
  - Pedunculated mass attached by slender stalk to mucosa

Presentation

- Infants present in 1st days or weeks of life with
  - Respiratory distress
  - Feeding difficulties
  - Bleeding from nose and mouth
- Male predilection

Treatment

- Surgical approaches
  - Excision is curative

Prognosis

- No reported local recurrences

MACROSCOPIC FEATURES

General Features

- Firm mass
- Smooth surface
- Areas of hemorrhage and necrosis

Size

- Up to 4 centimeters

MICROSCOPIC PATHOLOGY

Histologic Features

- Peripheral biphasic pattern of squamous nests and duct-like structures
  - These structures extend from surface mucosa into deeper hypocellular stroma
- Cellular stromal nodules are present centrally
  - Composed of ovoid and spindled cells
  - Mesenchymal-appearing
- Tumor is covered by a nonkeratinizing squamous mucosa
- Mitotic figures may be present
- Histologic features are suggestive of pleomorphic adenoma, mucoepidermoid carcinoma, or synovial sarcoma
  - However, organoid pattern of SGAT is distinct

Predominant Pattern/Injury Type

- Organoid pattern resembles salivary gland embryogensis

ANCILLARY TESTS

Immunohistochemistry

- Epithelial structures are positive for cytokeratins
- Stromal nodules show variable positivity for cytokeratins and actin
  - Consistent with myoepithelial cells

Electron Microscopy

- Cells forming stromal nodules show ultrastructural evidence of myoepithelial differentiation

SALIVARY GLAND ANLAGE TUMOR

Key Facts

Terminology
- Extremely rare congenital lesion of midline nasopharynx
- Likely represents hamartoma of minor salivary gland origin

Clinical Issues
- Infants present in 1st days or weeks of life with respiratory or feeding difficulties
- Pedunculated mass attached by slender stalk to mucosa
- Male predilection
- Excision is curative

Microscopic Pathology
- Peripheral biphasic pattern of squamous nests and duct-like structures
- Cellular stromal nodules are present centrally

DIFFERENTIAL DIAGNOSIS

Dermoid Cyst
- Cystic lesion lined by keratinizing squamous epithelium
- Epithelium is associated with pilosebaceous structures

Teratoma
- Contains derivatives of all 3 germ layers

Encephalocele
- Contains brain and meningeal tissue

Nasal Glial Heterotopia
- Rare developmental abnormality
- Astrocytes and neuroglial fibers are intermixed with fibrovascular connective tissue stroma

Craniopharyngioma
- Adenomatous pattern characterized by nests and cords of squamoid cells
- Peripheral palisaded nuclei
- Calcification
- Keratin material
- Xanthogranulomatous inflammation

SELECTED REFERENCES

1. Tinsa F et al: Congenital salivary gland anlage tumor of the nasopharynx. Fetal Pediatr Pathol. 29(5):323-9, 2010
2. Lin L et al: [Congenital salivary gland anlage tumor: report of a case.] Zhonghua Bing Li Xue Za Zhi. 38(10):711-2, 2009
3. Mogensen MA et al: Salivary gland anlage tumor in a neonate presenting with respiratory distress: radiographic and pathologic correlation. AJNR Am J Neuroradiol. 30(5):1022-3, 2009
4. Vranic S et al: Hamartomas, teratomas and teratocarcinosarcomas of the head and neck: Report of 3 new cases with clinico-pathologic correlation, cytogenetic analysis, and review of the literature. BMC Ear Nose Throat Disord. 8:8, 2008
5. Herrmann BW et al: Congenital salivary gland anlage tumor: a case series and review of the literature. Int J Pediatr Otorhinolaryngol. 69(2):149-56, 2005
6. Cohen EG et al: Congenital salivary gland anlage tumor of the nasopharynx. Pediatrics. 112(1 Pt 1):e66-9, 2003
7. Boccon-Gibod LA et al: Salivary gland anlage tumor of the nasopharynx: a clinicopathologic and immunohistochemical study of three cases. Pediatr Pathol Lab Med. 16(6):973-83, 1996
8. Michal M et al: Salivary gland anlage tumor. A case with widespread necrosis and large cyst formation. Pathology. 28(2):128-30, 1996
9. Dehner LP et al: Salivary gland anlage tumor ("congenital pleomorphic adenoma"). A clinicopathologic, immunohistochemical and ultrastructural study of nine cases. Am J Surg Pathol. 18(1):25-36, 1994

IMAGE GALLERY

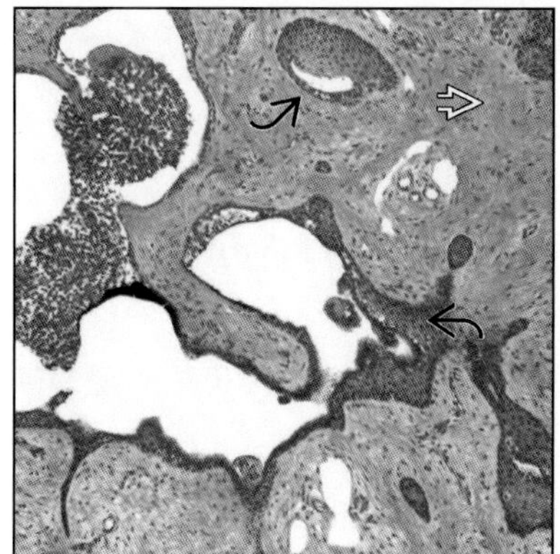

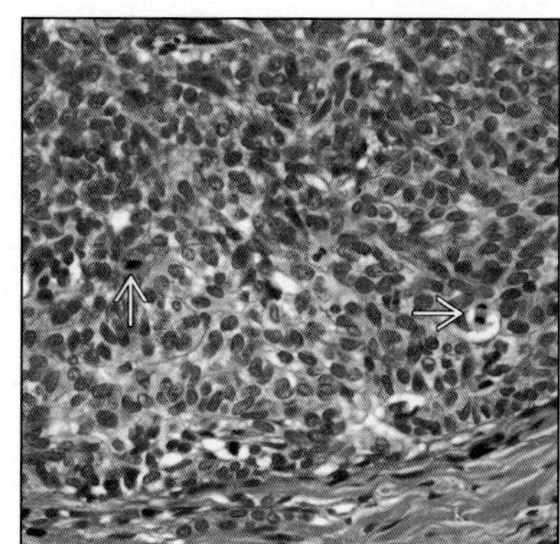

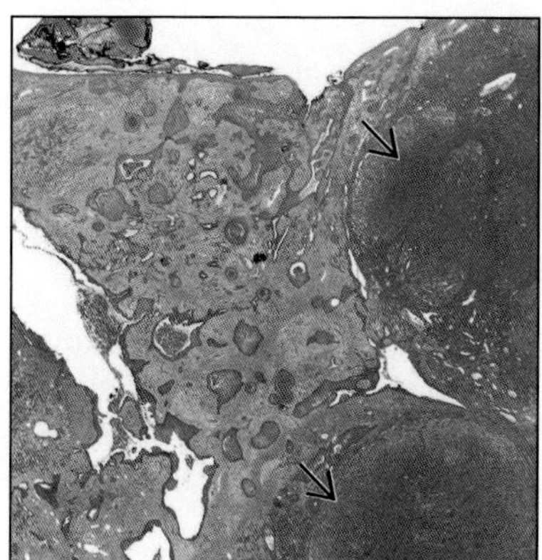

(Left) Epithelial structures ⇒ are surrounded by a hypocellular stroma ➡. (Courtesy G. Ellis, DDS.) *(Center)* The central stromal nodule consists of ovoid to spindled cells. Mitoses may be present ➡. (Courtesy G. Ellis, DDS.) *(Right)* Cellular stromal nodules are found centrally within the lesion ⇒. (Courtesy G. Ellis, DDS.)

SIALOBLASTOMA

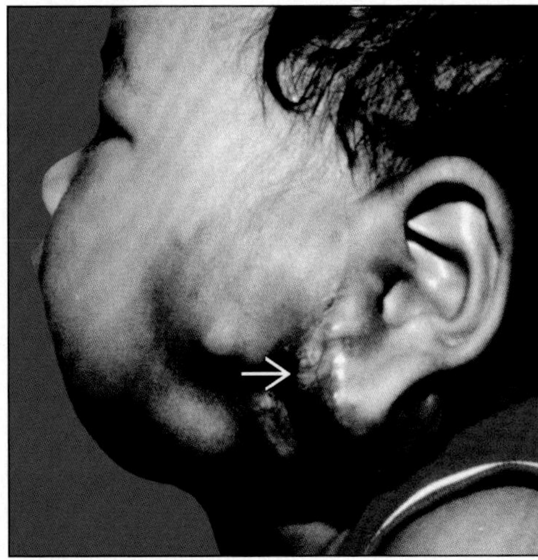

This parotid gland mass rapidly enlarged. Note the surface ulceration ➔ and involvement of the preauricular, retroauricular, and superior cervical regions.

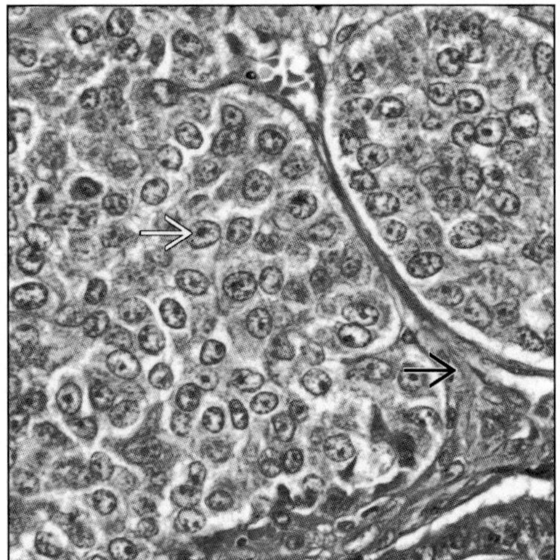

Nests of basaloid cells are separated by strands of fibrous connective tissue ⇒. The vesicular nuclei have single, prominent nucleoli ➔.

TERMINOLOGY

Synonyms

- Embryoma
- Congenital basal cell adenoma
- Congenital hybrid basal cell adenoma adenoid cystic carcinoma
- Monomorphic adenoma

Definitions

- Benign to low-grade malignant epithelial and myoepithelial neoplasm that resembles embryonic salivary gland

CLINICAL ISSUES

Presentation

- Mass most often seen in parotid gland, less frequently submandibular gland
- Growth may be rapid or slow
- Tumor may compromise airway
- Overlying skin may ulcerate
- Infrequently associated with nevus sebaceus and hepatoblastoma

Treatment

- Complete surgical excision
- Adjuvant therapy is avoided, if possible

Prognosis

- Biologic behavior is variable (benign, indolent, or aggressive)
- Surgery is curative in most cases
- Local recurrence seen in approximately 30% of cases
  - Usually within 4 years of diagnosis
- Regional metastasis can be seen in 10% of cases
  - Reported in cervical lymph nodes
- Distant metastasis is rare
  - Most commonly pulmonary metastasis

MACROSCOPIC FEATURES

General Features

- Gray, white, or yellow lobulated firm mass
- Areas of cystic change, hemorrhage, or necrosis can be seen
- Size ranges from 1-15 centimeters
- Satellite nodules may be present
- Typically freely mobile over deep structures but can be adherent to overlying skin

MICROSCOPIC PATHOLOGY

Histologic Features

- Resembles embryonic salivary gland at 3rd month of development
- Solid nests of basaloid cells are surrounded by strands of loose myxoid or loose fibrous connective tissue
  - Nest may show comedonecrosis (central necrosis)
- Predominately comprised of basaloid cells
  - Round to oval nuclei with fine chromatin pattern and small nucleoli
  - Can see significant nuclear pleomorphism
  - Scant, clear to pale cytoplasm, variable distinct cell borders
  - Peripheral palisading or cribriform architectural patterns
- Ductal structures may be present at periphery of basaloid epithelial nests
  - Cuboidal cells with eosinophilic cytoplasm
  - Spindle cells surround duct-like structures
- Loose myxoid or fibrous stroma
- Mitotic rate can be high
- Invasion into surrounding parenchyma, nerves, or blood vessels
- 2 major patterns of growth
  - Favorable histology
    - Partial encapsulation
    - Bland basaloid cells

Key Facts

Terminology
- Benign to low-grade malignant epithelial and myoepithelial neoplasm that resembles embryonic salivary gland

Clinical Issues
- Complete surgical excision
- Adjuvant therapy is avoided, if possible
- Local recurrence seen in approximately 30% of cases

Microscopic Pathology
- Solid nests of basaloid cells are surrounded by strands of loose myxoid or loose fibrous connective tissue
- Ductal structures may be present at periphery of basaloid epithelial nests

Ancillary Tests
- S100 protein positivity in basaloid cells; cytokeratin highlights ductal structures

- Unfavorable histology
  - Broad pushing infiltrative borders
  - Anaplastic basaloid cells with little cytoplasm
  - Associated with more aggressive clinical course

ANCILLARY TESTS

Immunohistochemistry
- Basaloid cells show positivity with S100 protein, actin, calponin, and p63
- Ductal structures show positivity with cytokeratin, epithelial membrane antigen, CK7, and CK19
- Spindle cells are variably positive for S100 and actin
  - Consistent with myoepithelial differentiation
- p53 expressed in tumors with more aggressive biologic behavior

DIFFERENTIAL DIAGNOSIS

Pleomorphic Adenoma
- Extremely rare in neonatal age group
- Chondroid matrix or stroma and oncocytic change
- No invasion

Basal Cell Adenoma
- Extremely rare in neonatal age group
- Lacks mitoses and pleomorphism
- May have excess basal lamina material

Adenoid Cystic Carcinoma
- Extremely rare in neonatal age group
- Palisading peg-/carrot-shaped cells
- Cribriform and sieve-like pattern is common
- Invasive lesion with perineural proclivity

Teratoma
- Tumors show elements from all 3 germinative layers
  - Endoderm
  - Ectoderm
  - Mesoderm

SELECTED REFERENCES

1. Williams SB et al: Sialoblastoma: a clinicopathologic and immunohistochemical study of 7 cases. Ann Diagn Pathol. 10(6):320-6, 2006
2. Mostafapour SP et al: Sialoblastoma of the submandibular gland: report of a case and review of the literature. Int J Pediatr Otorhinolaryngol. 53(2):157-61, 2000
3. Alvarez-Mendoza A et al: Diagnostic and therapeutic approach to sialoblastoma: report of a case. J Pediatr Surg. 34(12):1875-7, 1999
4. Brandwein M et al: Sialoblastoma: clinicopathological/immunohistochemical study. Am J Surg Pathol. 23(3):342-8, 1999
5. Luna MA: Sialoblastoma and epithelial tumors in children: their morphologic spectrum and distribution by age. Adv Anat Pathol. 6(5):287-92, 1999
6. Batsakis JG et al: Embryoma (sialoblastoma) of salivary glands. Ann Otol Rhinol Laryngol. 101(11):958-60, 1992

IMAGE GALLERY

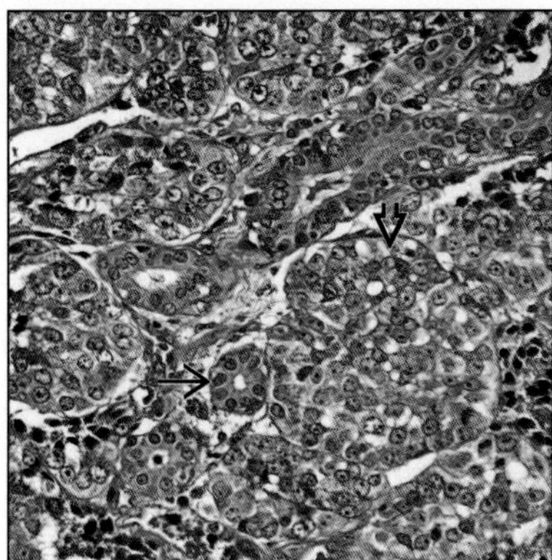

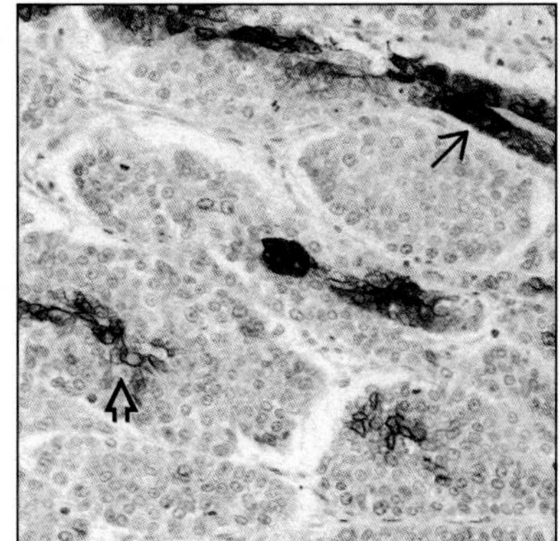

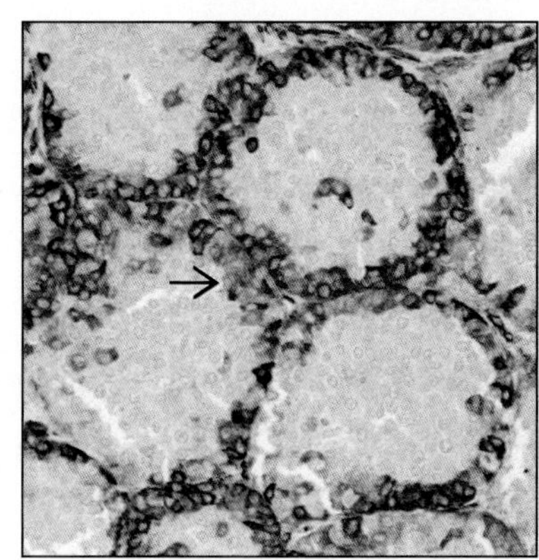

(Left) *This image highlights the biphasic appearance of the tumor. There are nests of basaloid cells ⇨ juxtaposed with ductules →.* ***(Center)*** *The ductal → and luminal ⇨ cells are highlighted with pan-cytokeratin immunohistochemistry. The biphasic appearance is accentuated with this stain. (Courtesy R. Foss, MD.)* ***(Right)*** *Smooth muscle actin shows a very strong decoration of the peripheral cells → in each of the lobules. (Courtesy R. Foss, MD.)*

PLEOMORPHIC ADENOMA

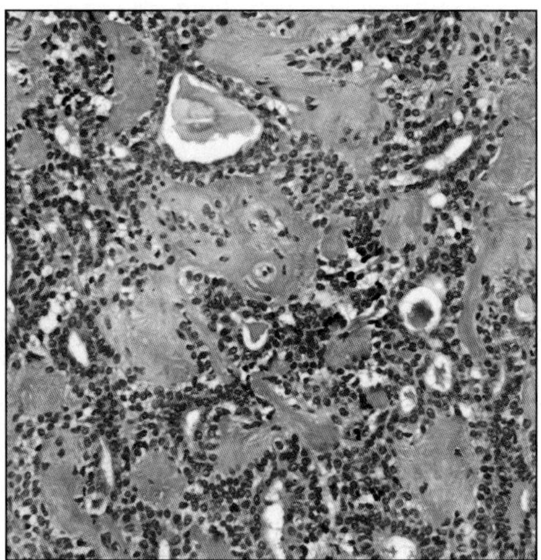

This tumor shows characteristic areas of tubular and ductal structures with a background of hyaline stroma. Pleomorphic adenomas, however, show amazing microscopic diversity.

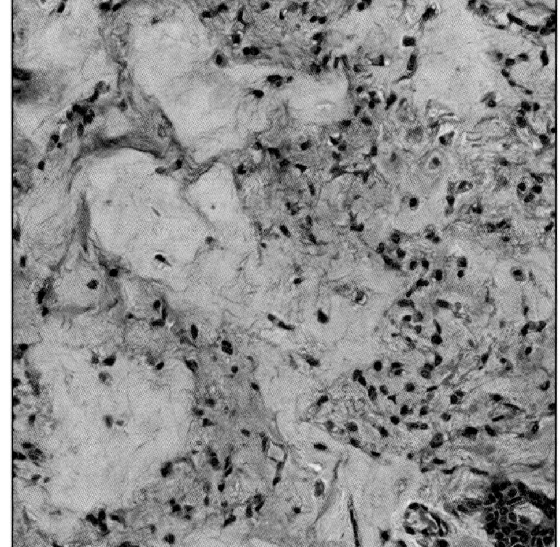

Hematoxylin & eosin shows a tumor with predominate myxoid stroma with focal epithelial structures. The ratio of epithelium and stroma can vary widely among tumors.

TERMINOLOGY

Abbreviations

- Pleomorphic adenoma (PA)

Synonyms

- Benign mixed tumor (BMT)
- Mixed tumor
- Chondroid syringoma
  - Only used if skin/dermis-based primary

Definitions

- Benign epithelial tumor that shows both epithelial and modified myoepithelial elements mixed with mesenchymal myxoid, mucoid, or chondroid-appearing material
  - Significant architectural diversity rather than cytologic pleomorphism

CLINICAL ISSUES

Epidemiology

- Incidence
  - Most common epithelial salivary tumor throughout childhood
  - Relatively uncommon in 1st 2 decades of life
- Age
  - Mean age at presentation in children is 12.4 years
- Gender
  - Males > females (in children; < 18 years old)

Site

- Parotid gland most common site
  - Superficial lobe most commonly
    - Inferior (lower pole) or "tail" of parotid gland
  - Deep lobe less frequently
    - Large lesions may compromise airway
- May involve minor salivary glands
  - Buccal mucosa
  - Upper lip
  - Palate
- Uncommon in submandibular and sublingual glands
- Can affect larynx, nasal cavity, ear, orbit, upper aerodigestive tract, gastrointestinal tract
- Rarely, may develop within ectopic salivary gland tissue

Presentation

- Usually a painless, slow-growing mass
- Single, smooth, mobile, firm nodule
- Paresthesia due to nerve compression is rare finding
- If pain is present, tumor is more likely to be infarcted

Natural History

- Slow growing
- Asymptomatic
- May reach enormous size if neglected
- Malignant transformation has not been reported in children

Treatment

- Surgical approaches
  - Parotid gland
    - Superficial parotidectomy
    - Extracapsular dissection (including rim of uninvolved tissue)
    - Facial nerve preservation when possible
  - Minor glands
    - Conservative, complete surgical excision
  - Submandibular gland
    - Complete excision
- Risks and complications
  - Surgical complications
    - Frey syndrome (gustatory sweating)
    - Decreased muscle control of face (if facial nerve is sacrificed)
    - Capsule disruption may result in "seeding" of tumor (increases likelihood of recurrence)
    - Enucleation only results in high recurrence rate (up to 50%)

Key Facts

Terminology
- Synonym: Benign mixed tumor
- Benign epithelial tumor that shows both epithelial and mesenchymal differentiation

Clinical Issues
- Most common epithelial salivary tumor throughout childhood
- Relatively uncommon in 1st 2 decades of life
- Parotid gland most common site
- Slow growing
- Minor salivary gland involvement is less common

Macroscopic Features
- Recurrent tumors are generally multinodular
- Irregular mass
- Parotid gland
  - Variably thick capsule
  - Rarely unencapsulated
- Minor glands
  - Poorly differentiated to absent capsule

Microscopic Pathology
- Innumerable cytologic and architectural patterns
- Epithelial tissue
- Mesenchymal-like tissue

Top Differential Diagnoses
- Myoepithelioma
- Basal cell adenoma
- Adenoid cystic

Prognosis
- Overall excellent long-term prognosis, although limited by recurrence of approximately 3.4% after 5 years and 6.8% after 10 years
  - Risk factors for recurrence
    - Histological subtype: Hypocellular (myxoid-rich stroma) variant
    - Other histological factors, such as the presence of pseudopods and multinodularity
    - Females
    - Young age at initial treatment
- No large series available in children

IMAGE FINDINGS

General Features
- Imaging provides information about exact anatomic site, extent of disease, and possible invasion or nodal metastases
- Ultrasound or CT are complementary and allow for image-guided fine needle aspiration
  - Excellent resolution and tissue characterization without radiation hazard, especially for superficial lobe lesions
- MR or CT is mandatory to evaluate tumor extent and exclude local invasion
  - Unilateral mass that shows post-contrast enhancement, has high T2 signal, and does not invade surrounding tissue planes is most likely PA
  - MR spectroscopy may separate Warthin from PA although not yet well accepted
- Ultrasonography is especially valuable in children since most tumors are benign and many are cystic or vascular (color Doppler for latter)
  - High-resolution sonography has nearly 100% sensitivity in detecting intraparotid tumors
  - Precisely outlines tumor borders
  - Can detect multiple or bilateral lesions
- Sialography delineates ductal system but is limited in tumor assessment

MACROSCOPIC FEATURES

General Features
- Irregular mass
- Fibrous capsule
  - Parotid gland
    - Variably thick incomplete capsule but rarely unencapsulated
  - Minor glands
    - Poorly developed to absent
- Cut surface homogeneous, white to white-tan
- Recurrent tumors are generally multinodular
- Hemorrhage and infarction
  - Secondary to FNA or previous surgical procedures

Size
- Majority from 2-5 cm
- Rarely, may be enormous

MICROSCOPIC PATHOLOGY

Histologic Features
- Innumerable architectural patterns
  - Solid
  - Tubular or trabecular
  - Cystic
- Epithelial tissue shows variable morphology
  - Spindle
  - Clear
  - Squamous
  - Basaloid
  - Plasmacytoid
- Mesenchymal-like tissue
  - Myxoid stroma
  - Myxochondroid
  - Hyaline stroma
  - Rarely lipomatous
- Duct structures
  - Lined by cuboidal &/or columnar epithelium
- Rarely, crystals are present

PLEOMORPHIC ADENOMA

  - Collagenous crystalloids: Eosinophilic needle shapes arranged radially
  - Tyrosine-rich crystalloids: Eosinophilic bunted shapes arranged tubularly
  - Crystalloids resembling oxalate crystals
- Occasionally, squamous metaplasia is identified
- Rarely, necrosis
- Rarely, sebaceous cells

ANCILLARY TESTS

Cytology

- Findings are variable
- Cellular smears with epithelial and mesenchymal cells and background stroma
- Clusters or cohesive groups of epithelial cells
  - Branching trabeculae of cells that drop off into stroma
  - Plasmacytoid or spindle cells
    - Bipolar myoepithelial cells with eccentric round nuclei
    - Spindled cells tend to embed within stroma
  - Round, ovoid to fusiform nuclei
  - Delicate nuclear chromatin distribution
  - Squamous and sebaceous cells may be seen
  - Atypia can be seen but tends to be single cell
- Fibrillar myxochondroid stroma
  - Feathered edge that blends and surrounds epithelial/myoepithelial cells
  - Cells may line up along edge of matrix, mimicking adenoid cystic carcinoma
  - Pale green with alcohol-fixed Papanicolaou stains
  - Deep purple to magenta with air-dried Romanowsky stains (Diff Quik®, Giemsa)
    - Striking metachromasia with Giemsa
  - Appears different from mucus, necrotic material, or inflammatory debris
- Presence of both epithelial and mesenchymal components required for diagnosis
- High cellularity with limited stroma should be diagnosed as "salivary gland neoplasm" to avoid misdiagnosis

Immunohistochemistry

- IHC is sensitive but not specific
- Cytokeratin panel, GFAP, S100, and SMA are recommended as all can show variable positivity

Cytogenetics

- 2 major cytogenetic abnormalities, with rearrangements involving
  - 8q12
    - Target gene is pleomorphic adenoma gene 1 (*PLAG1*), zinc finger transcription factor
    - Rearrangement and activation result in overexpression
  - 12q13-15
    - Target gene is high mobility group protein gene, *HMGA2* (or *HMGIC*), which is overexpressed
    - *HMGA2* encodes architectural transcription factor that promotes activation of gene expression
- Normal karyotype
- No large series available in children

Electron Microscopy

- Structurally modified myoepithelial cells show basal lamina, small microvilli, and well-developed desmosomes
- Cell arrangement and ultrastructure mimics normal salivary gland ducts
- Mesenchymal cells give modified myoepithelial cell appearance with tonofilaments, microfilaments, linear densities of plasma membrane, pinocytotic vesicles, and residua of basement membrane
- Elastic fibers are usually close to neoplastic myoepithelial-like cells

DIFFERENTIAL DIAGNOSIS

Myoepithelioma

- Essentially a cellular mixed tumor with no glandular differentiation and no myxochondroid matrix
- Perhaps part of spectrum of pleomorphic adenoma
- Very rare in pediatric population

Basal Cell Adenoma

- Uniform proliferation of basaloid cells
- Absence of myxochondroid stroma
- Prominent basal lamina encircles nests of cells
- Very rare in pediatric population

Adenoid Cystic Carcinoma

- Cells are predominately uniform in size with oval to angulated shape
- Variable patterns, but most have areas of amorphous eosinophilic hyalinized stroma
- Infiltrative margins
- Perineurial invasion
- Predominantly a tumor of adults

Mixed Tumor of Skin (Chondroid Syringoma)

- Essentially same histology but arising from skin

Polymorphous Low-Grade Adenocarcinoma

- Uniform oval cells
- Numerous growth patterns
- Unencapsulated
- Perineural invasion
- Almost exclusive to minor salivary glands
- **Almost exclusive to adults**

SELECTED REFERENCES

1. Bonet-Loscertales M et al: Multicentric recurrent parotid pleomorphic adenoma in a child. Med Oral Patol Oral Cir Bucal. 15(5):e743-5, 2010
2. Craver RD et al: Pediatric epithelial salivary gland tumors: spectrum of histologies and cytogenetics at a children's hospital. Pediatr Dev Pathol. 13(5):348-53, 2010
3. Köybaşı S et al: Submandibular gland pleomorphic adenoma in a seven-year-old child: a case report. Kulak Burun Bogaz Ihtis Derg. 20(4):210-3, 2010
4. Ito FA et al: Histopathological findings of pleomorphic adenomas of the salivary glands. Med Oral Patol Oral Cir Bucal. 14(2):E57-61, 2009

Immunohistochemistry

Antibody	Reactivity	Staining Pattern	Comment
CK-PAN	Positive	Cytoplasmic	Both ductal epithelial and spindle cells; variable positivity
S100	Positive	Nuclear & cytoplasmic	Myoepithelial cells
GFAP	Positive	Cytoplasmic	Myoepithelial cells and myxoid areas
Actin-sm	Positive	Cytoplasmic	Periductal and spindle cells; negative in plasmacytoid cells
Calponin	Positive	Cytoplasmic	Plasmacytoid cells
CK7	Positive	Cytoplasmic	Plasmacytoid cells
Vimentin	Positive	Cytoplasmic	Both epithelial and myoepithelial cells
p63	Positive	Nuclear	
SMHC	Positive	Cytoplasmic	Myoepithelial cells
CD10	Positive	Cytoplasmic	Myoepithelial cells
CD117	Negative		
CK20	Negative		

5. Redaelli de Zinis LO et al: Management and prognostic factors of recurrent pleomorphic adenoma of the parotid gland: personal experience and review of the literature. Eur Arch Otorhinolaryngol. 265(4):447-52, 2008
6. Shah SS et al: Glial fibrillary acidic protein and CD57 immunolocalization in cell block preparations is a useful adjunct in the diagnosis of pleomorphic adenoma. Arch Pathol Lab Med. 131(9):1373-7, 2007
7. da Cruz Perez DE et al: Salivary gland tumors in children and adolescents: a clinicopathologic and immunohistochemical study of fifty-three cases. Int J Pediatr Otorhinolaryngol. 68(7):895-902, 2004
8. Paris J et al: [Pleomorphic adenoma of the parotid: histopathological study.] Ann Otolaryngol Chir Cervicofac. 121(3):161-6, 2004
9. Stennert E et al: Recurrent pleomorphic adenoma of the parotid gland: a prospective histopathological and immunohistochemical study. Laryngoscope. 114(1):158-63, 2004
10. Alves FA et al: Pleomorphic adenoma of the submandibular gland: clinicopathological and immunohistochemical features of 60 cases in Brazil. Arch Otolaryngol Head Neck Surg. 128(12):1400-3, 2002
11. Hill AG: Major salivary gland tumours in a rural Kenyan hospital. East Afr Med J. 79(1):8-10, 2002
12. Verma K et al: Role of fine needle aspiration cytology in diagnosis of pleomorphic adenomas. Cytopathology. 13(2):121-7, 2002
13. Pinkston JA et al: Incidence rates of salivary gland tumors: results from a population-based study. Otolaryngol Head Neck Surg. 120(6):834-40, 1999
14. Yamamoto Y et al: DNA analysis at p53 locus in carcinomas arising from pleomorphic adenomas of salivary glands: comparison of molecular study and p53 immunostaining. Pathol Int. 48(4):265-72, 1998
15. Kilpatrick SE et al: Mixed tumors and myoepitheliomas of soft tissue: a clinicopathologic study of 19 cases with a unifying concept. Am J Surg Pathol. 21(1):13-22, 1997
16. Auclair PL et al: Atypical features in salivary gland mixed tumors: their relationship to malignant transformation. Mod Pathol. 9(6):652-7, 1996
17. Renehan A et al: An analysis of the treatment of 114 patients with recurrent pleomorphic adenomas of the parotid gland. Am J Surg. 172(6):710-4, 1996
18. Takai Y et al: Diagnostic criteria for neoplastic myoepithelial cells in pleomorphic adenomas and myoepitheliomas. Immunocytochemical detection of muscle-specific actin, cytokeratin 14, vimentin, and glial fibrillary acidic protein. Oral Surg Oral Med Oral Pathol Oral Radiol Endod. 79(3):330-41, 1995
19. Allen CM et al: Necrosis in benign salivary gland neoplasms. Not necessarily a sign of malignant transformation. Oral Surg Oral Med Oral Pathol. 78(4):455-61, 1994
20. Humphrey PA et al: Crystalloids in salivary gland pleomorphic adenomas. Arch Pathol Lab Med. 113(4):390-3, 1989
21. Campbell WG Jr et al: Characterization of two types of crystalloids in pleomorphic adenomas of minor salivary glands. A light-microscopic, electron-microscopic, and histochemical study. Am J Pathol. 118(2):194-202, 1985
22. Eveson JW et al: Salivary gland tumours. A review of 2410 cases with particular reference to histological types, site, age and sex distribution. J Pathol. 146(1):51-8, 1985

PLEOMORPHIC ADENOMA

Radiologic and Other Features

*(**Left**) Axial graphic shows the close relationship of the facial nerve ➔ to the parotid gland. Surgical excision requires the identification and preservation of the facial nerve when possible. (**Right**) T1 nonenhanced MR reveals a well-circumscribed hypointense tumor ➔ within the superficial lobe of the parotid gland. This tumor enhances with contrast and is commonly hyperintense on T2 MR sequences.*

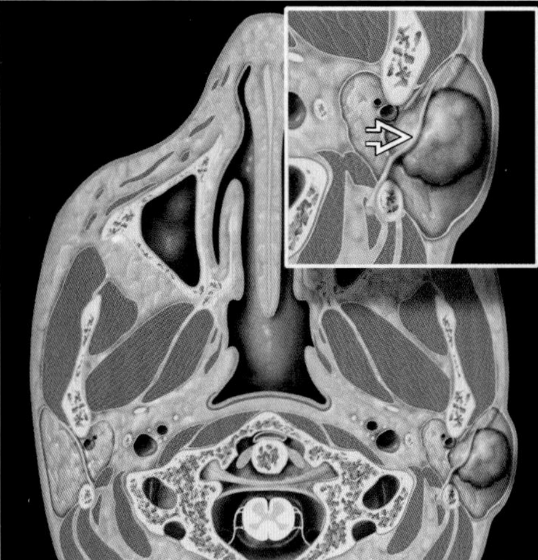

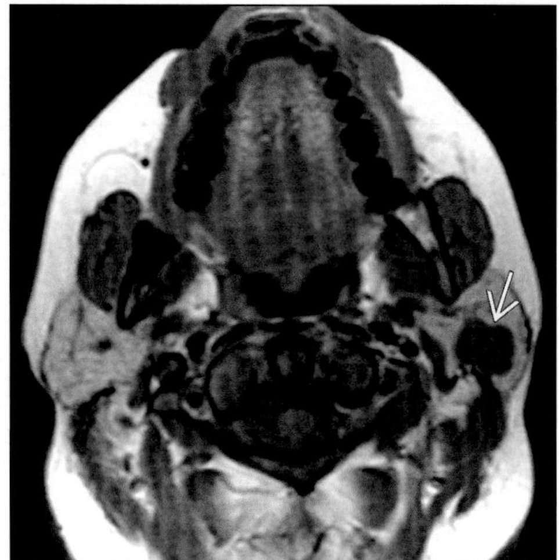

*(**Left**) CT with contrast shows a pleomorphic adenoma within the right submandibular gland ➔. The gland enhances more than the tumor, making identification on CT simple. About 50% of tumors of the submandibular gland are pleomorphic adenomas. (**Right**) This intraoperative photograph shows the removal of a pleomorphic adenoma, of minor salivary gland origin, via an intraoral approach. This patient had been aware of this tumor for more than 3 years prior to consenting to surgery.*

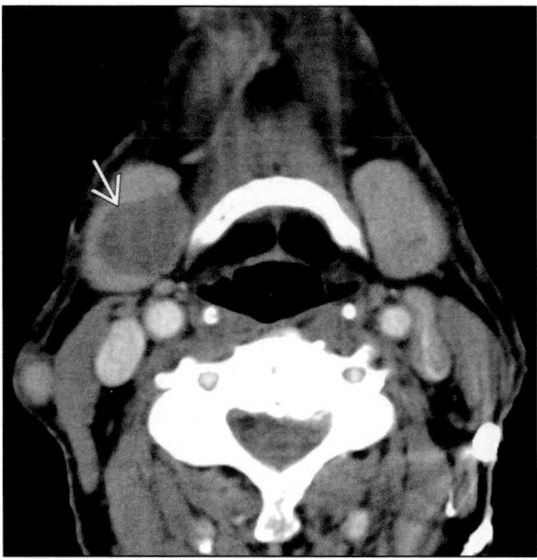

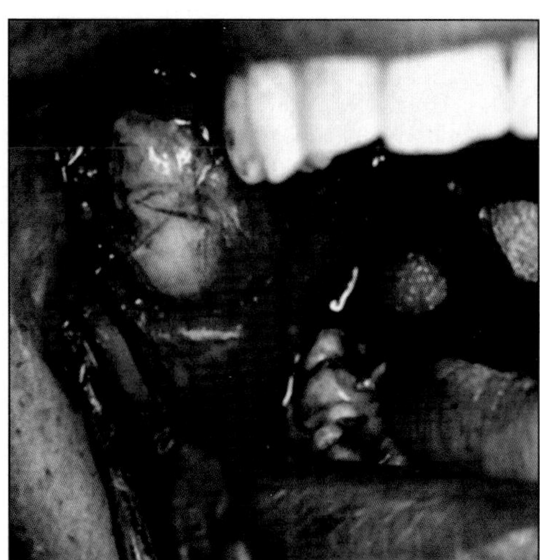

*(**Left**) Gross photograph shows a well-circumscribed, oval tumor. The cut surface is tan-pink to white. (**Right**) Gross photograph shows a formalin-fixed tumor with well-defined borders surrounded by normal gland and soft tissue. Note the focus of translucent tissue ➔, representing an area of myxochondroid tissue.*

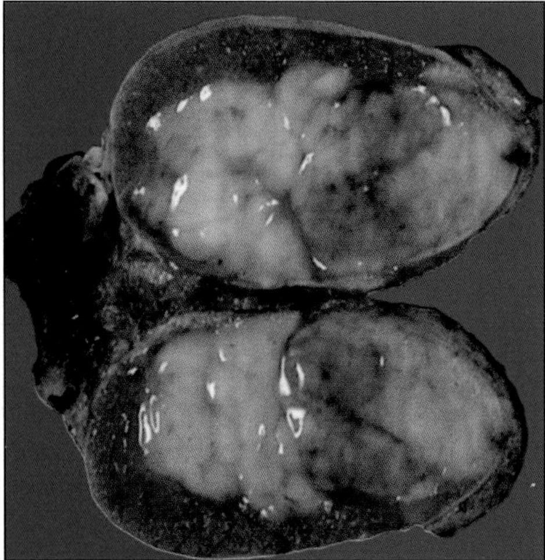

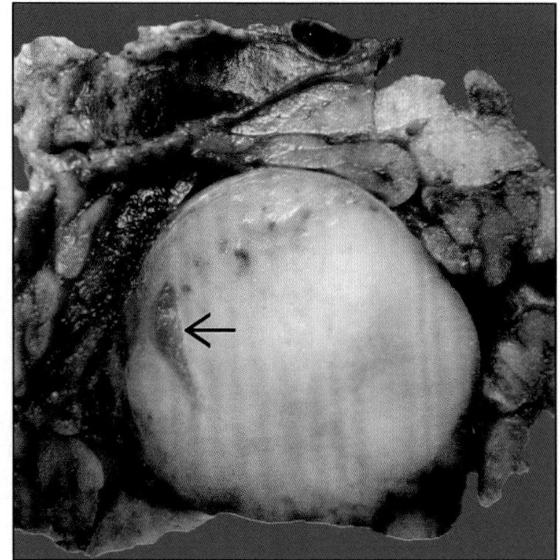

Microscopic Features

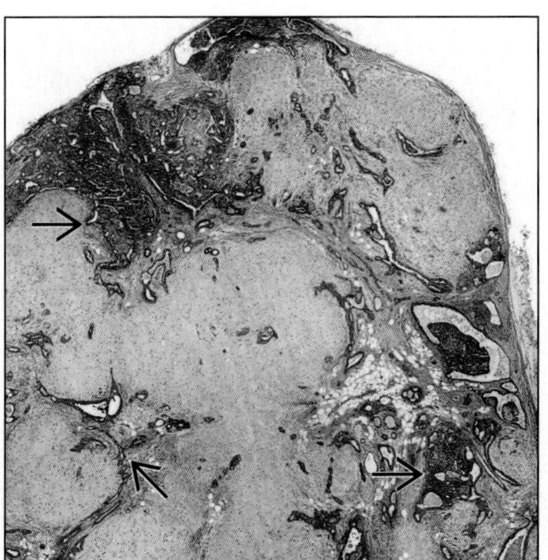

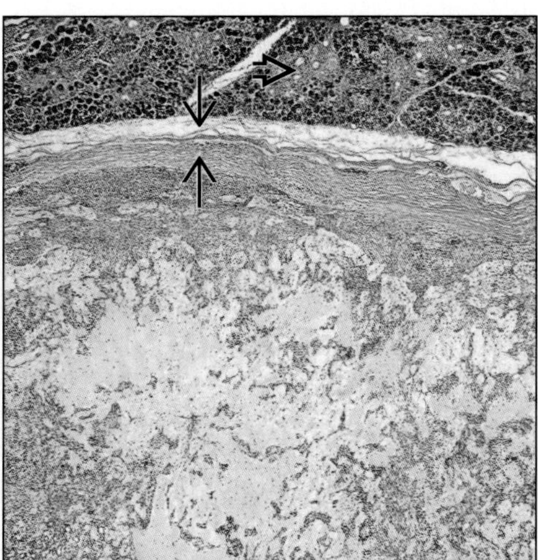

(Left) *Hematoxylin & eosin stained section shows a characteristic pleomorphic adenoma with varying patterns seen within a single section. Areas with ductal structures ⇒ are closely associated with a myxomatous stroma.* ***(Right)*** *This pleomorphic adenoma of a major gland shows a distinctive fibrous capsule ⇒ separating it from the associated salivary gland ⇒. Tumors of minor salivary glands may have an incomplete capsule; this is especially common in palatal tumors.*

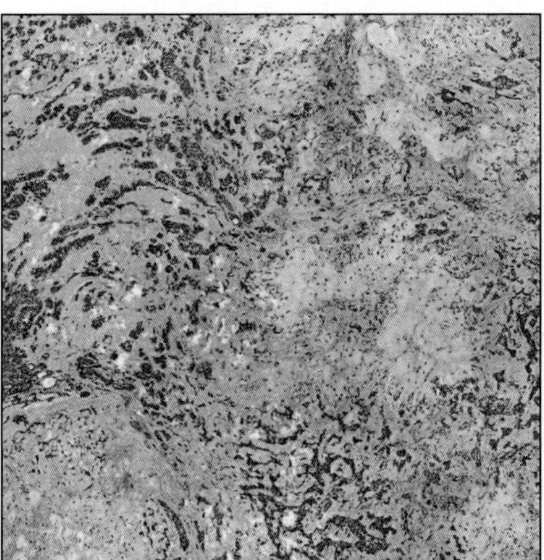

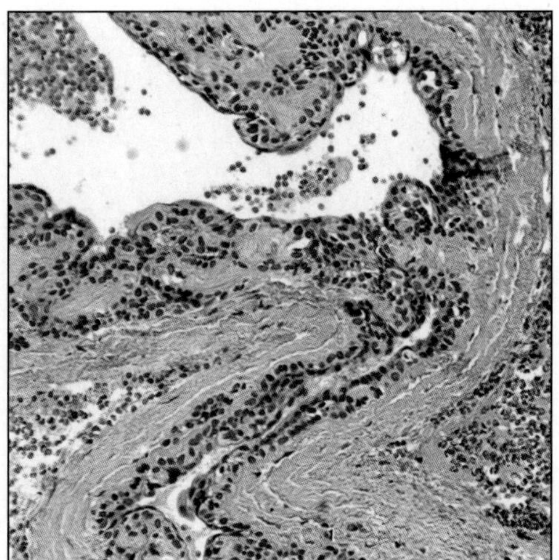

(Left) *Hematoxylin & eosin stained section of a pleomorphic adenoma shows a myxoid background with islands and anastomosing strands of epithelial cells.* ***(Right)*** *Medium-power view of a pleomorphic adenoma shows a cyst-like area. It is important to keep in mind the wide variety of architectural patterns seen in pleomorphic adenomas, which may include solid, tubular or trabecular, and cystic.*

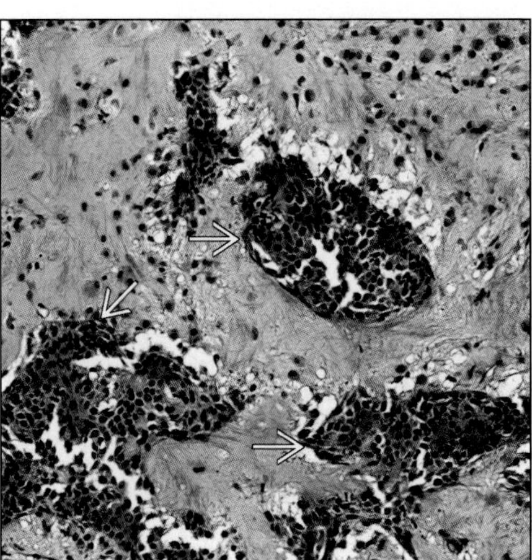

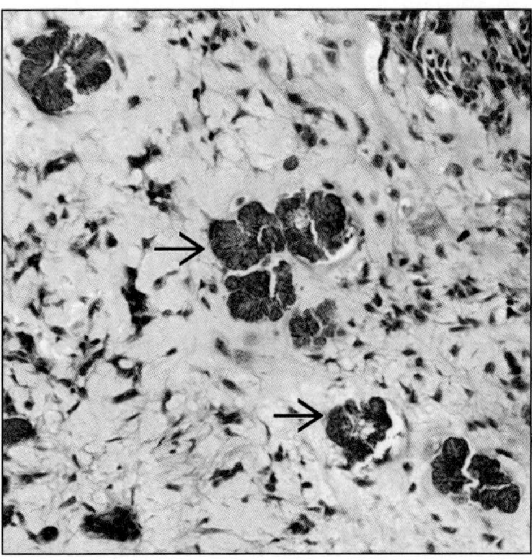

(Left) *Hematoxylin & eosin stained section of a pleomorphic adenoma shows focal solid areas composed of oval plasmacytoid cells ⇒.* ***(Right)*** *Hematoxylin & eosin stained section of this pleomorphic adenoma shows tyrosine-rich crystals ⇒ scattered in a myxoid stroma.*

PLEOMORPHIC ADENOMA

Microscopic and Cytologic Features

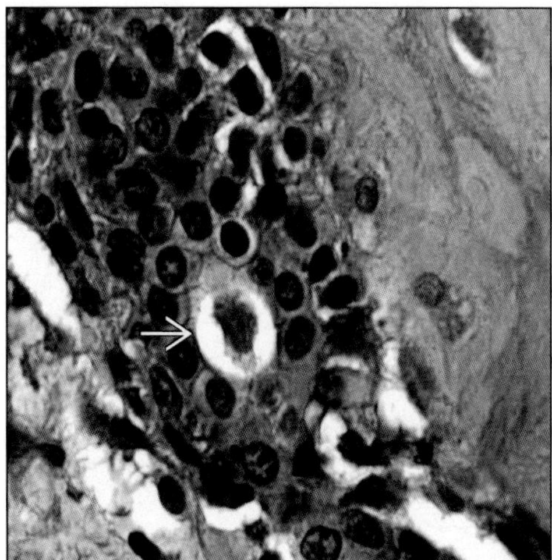
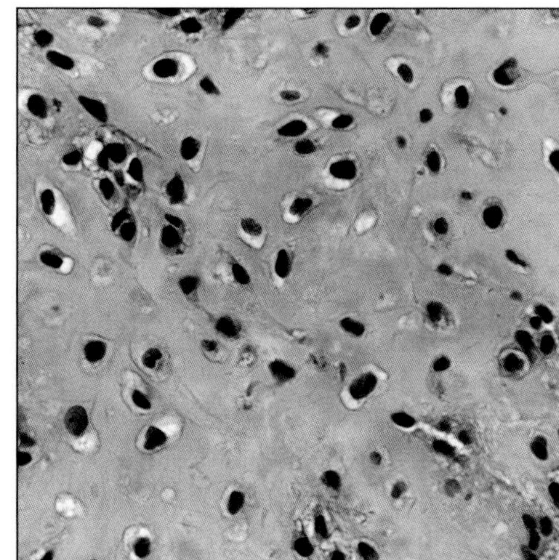

(Left) *High-power view of this pleomorphic adenoma highlights a duct ➡ lined by round to cuboidal luminal cells.* ***(Right)*** *A cartilaginous-like focus found in a pleomorphic adenoma is shown at high power.*

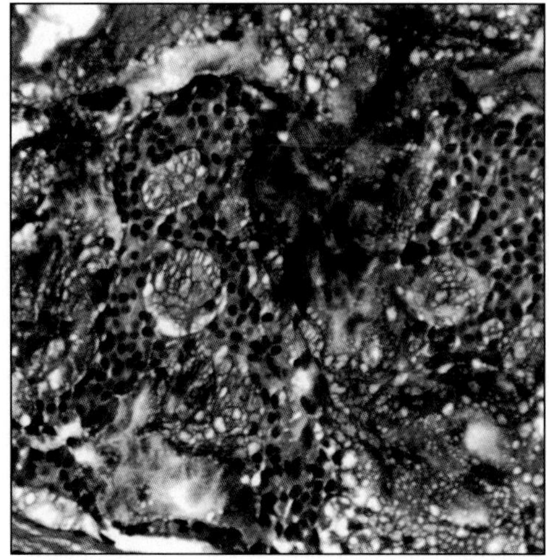
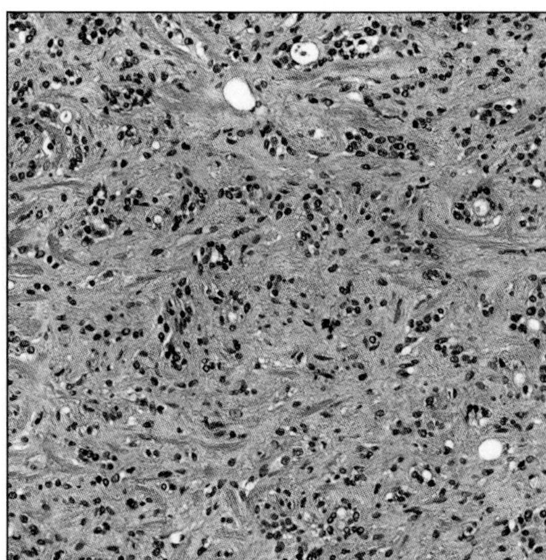

(Left) *Hematoxylin & eosin stained section highlights the blending of the epithelial cells with the mucinous-myxoid matrix material.* ***(Right)*** *Hematoxylin & eosin shows a very heavy, sclerotic fibrous connective tissue deposition in this pleomorphic adenoma. This heavy collagenized stroma is commonly seen in tumors that have undergone malignant transformation into a "carcinoma ex pleomorphic adenoma." Therefore, additional sections may be warranted when this feature is seen.*

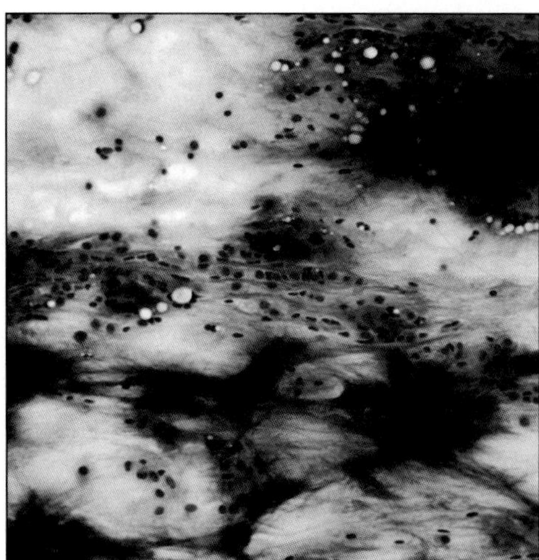
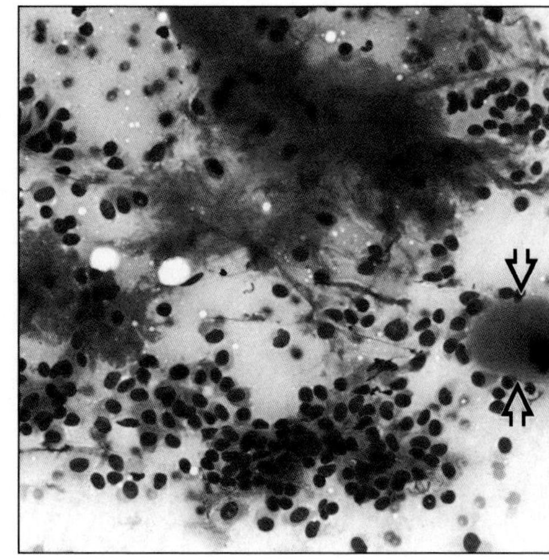

(Left) *Diff-Quik stained slide shows a fibrillar background stroma and a streaming of epithelial nuclei within the material. Small collections of epithelial cells are intermingled with the background myxoid-matrix material.* ***(Right)*** *Diff-Quik stained slide shows a bright magenta appearance to the fibrillar myxochondroid matrix material. Note how the epithelial-myoepithelial cells blend with the matrix, although only a single focus ⇨ shows a peripheral palisade of nuclei.*

Cytologic and Immunohistochemical Features

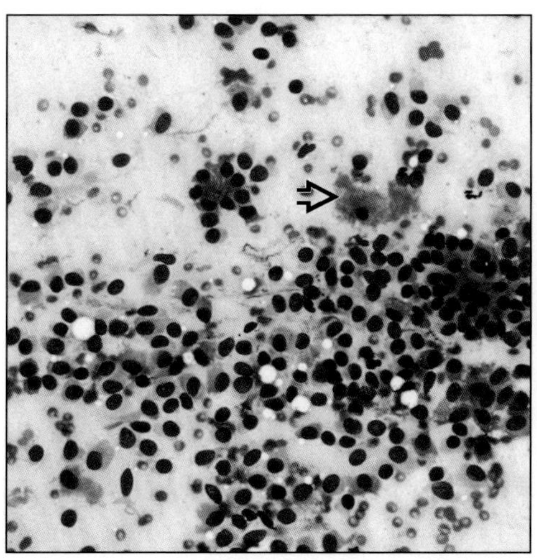

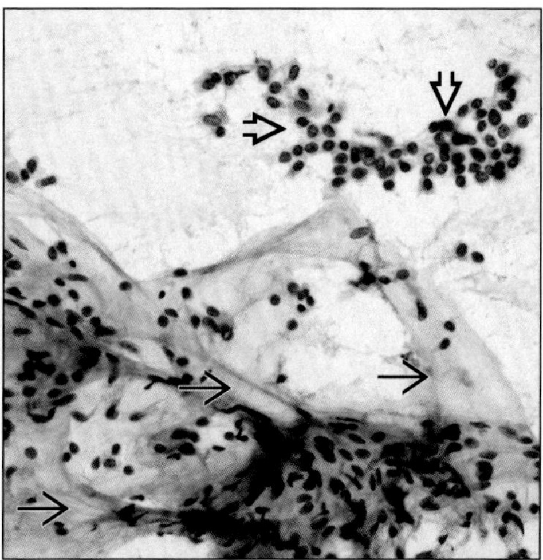

(Left) *Diff-Quik stained slide shows a much more cellular neoplastic proliferation with only a few foci of matrix material ➲ in this cellular pleomorphic adenoma. The cells have a plasmacytoid appearance, with eccentric nuclei that are round and regular.* ***(Right)*** *Papanicolaou stain shows the epithelial groups ➲ as well as the background stroma →, although the stroma is much less easy to definitively identify in comparison to the Diff-Quik preparations.*

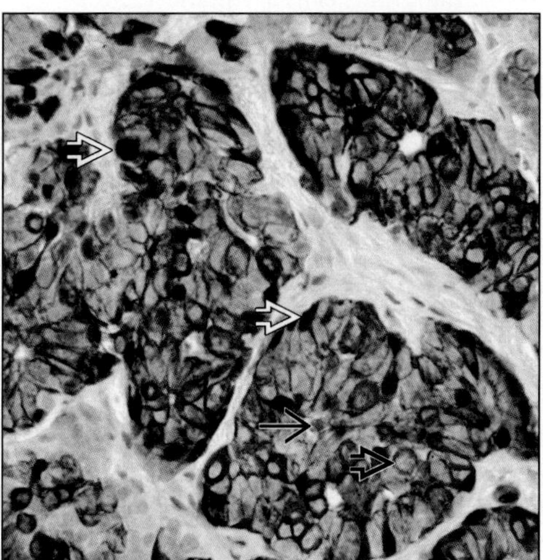

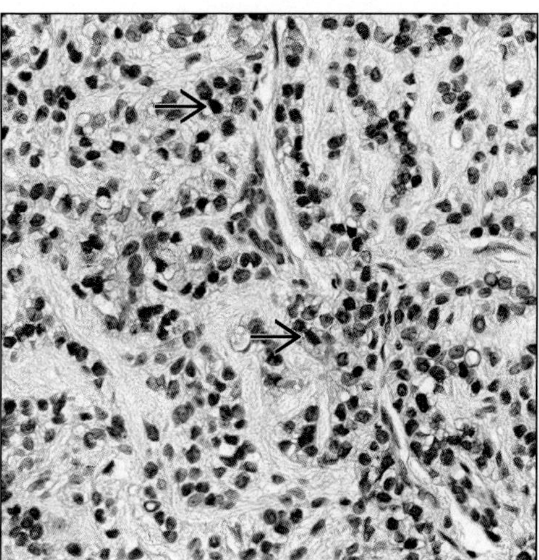

(Left) *This triple immunohistochemistry cocktail highlights the membrane of the epithelial cells (EMA) ➲, while the cytoplasm of the neoplastic cells is stained light brown (CK5/6) →, and the nuclei of the basal-myoepithelial cells are highlighted with p63 ➲.* ***(Right)*** *S100 staining shows nuclear and cytoplasmic reactivity for myoepithelial cells → but has variable reactivity for other cells in this example of a pleomorphic adenoma.*

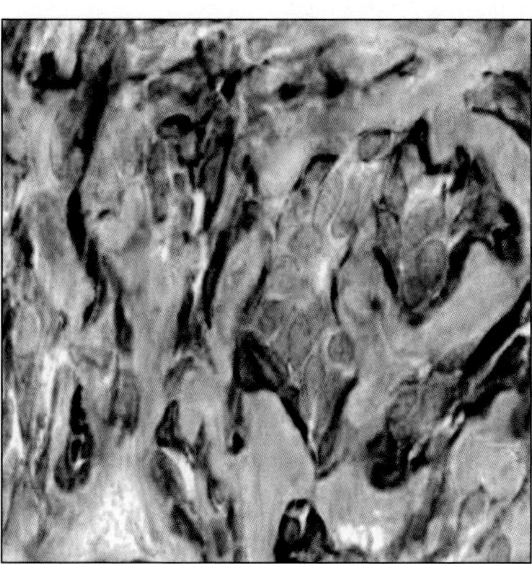

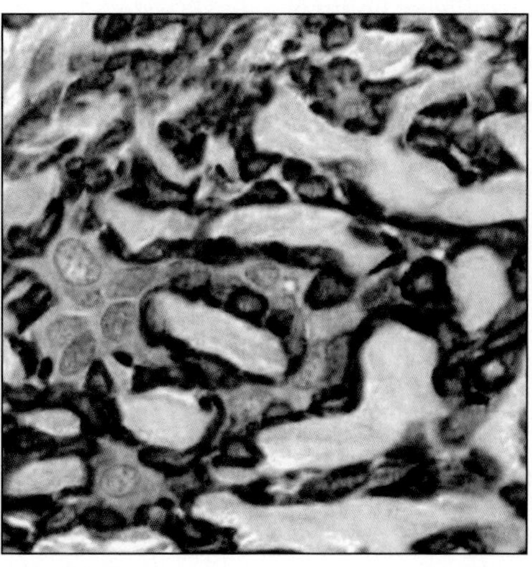

(Left) *Smooth muscle actin (SMA) shows cytoplasmic reactivity in spindle and polygonal myoepithelial cells.* ***(Right)*** *Glial fibrillary acidic protein (GFAP) shows dense reactivity for myoepithelial cells in the myxoid areas of the tumor.*

MUCOEPIDERMOID CARCINOMA

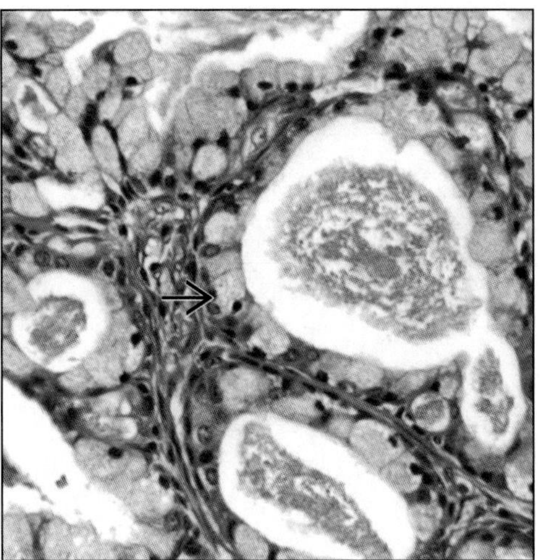

Hematoxylin & eosin shows small cystic spaces lined by mucous cells ⇒. These cells are large, ovoid, and have abundant foamy cytoplasm. The nuclei are frequently "squashed" toward the periphery.

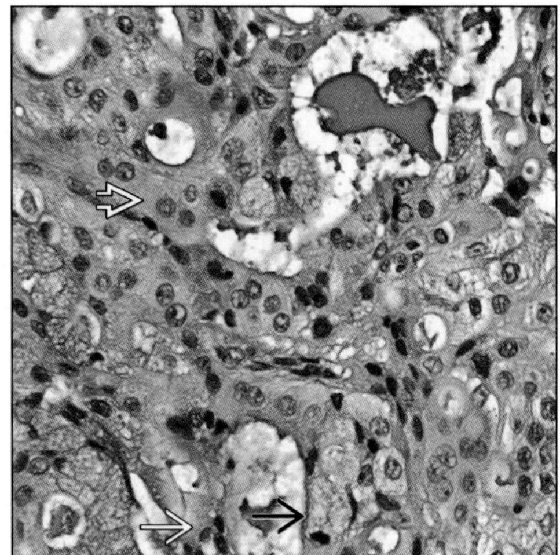

The presence of epithelial cells ➡, intermediate cells ➡, and mucocytes ⇒, although variable, is required for the diagnosis of mucoepidermoid carcinoma.

TERMINOLOGY

Abbreviations

- Mucoepidermoid carcinoma (MEC)

Definitions

- Malignant epithelial tumor with variable components of mucus, epidermoid, and intermediate cells

ETIOLOGY/PATHOGENESIS

Environmental Exposure

- Ionizing radiation
  - Latent period between irradiation and malignancy varies
    - Long-term follow-up is required

Pathogenesis of Primary Intraosseous Tumors

- Malignant transformation of epithelial lining of odontogenic cysts
  - Favored mechanism
- Malignant transformation of ectopic salivary gland tissue

CLINICAL ISSUES

Epidemiology

- Incidence
  - MEC accounts for 50% of malignant salivary gland tumors in children
  - Rare, comprising 0.08% of cancer in pediatric population
  - Only 5% of salivary gland MECs arise during childhood
- Age
  - Usually occurs in 5- to 15-year-old age group
  - Most common malignant salivary gland tumor in children
- Gender
  - Slight male predominance

Site

- Major glands
  - Parotid gland is most common location
- Minor glands
  - Palate or buccal mucosa
- Central (primary intraosseous)
  - Originates within jaws
    - Predilection for mandible

Presentation

- Painless, slow-growing mass
- Parotid gland
  - Usually asymptomatic solitary mass
  - Symptomatic
    - Pain, facial numbness, and paralysis
    - Drainage from ipsilateral ear
    - Dysphagia, trismus
- Minor glands
  - May be misdiagnosed clinically as reactive or inflammatory lesion
  - Swelling, fluctuant, red-blue mass
  - Secondary ulceration occasionally
  - Bleeding or drainage
  - Dysphagia, paresthesia
- Primary intraosseous
  - Radiolucent lesion on dental radiograph
  - Swelling, pain, facial asymmetry, trismus
- Rarely associated with other benign salivary gland tumors
  - Can be metachronous or synchronous
  - Pleomorphic adenoma, Warthin tumor, oncocytoma

Treatment

- Surgical approaches
  - Complete removal of tumor with adequate margins is treatment of choice

MUCOEPIDERMOID CARCINOMA

Key Facts

Terminology
- Malignant epithelial tumor with variable components of mucous, epidermoid, and intermediate cells

Clinical Issues
- Most common malignant salivary gland tumor
- Major glands most common, followed by minor salivary glands
- Low-grade tumors rarely metastasize
- Positive surgical margins are predictive of recurrence or residual tumor

Macroscopic Features
- Circumscribed, partially encapsulated, or poorly defined periphery

Microscopic Pathology
- Variably sized cystic spaces
- Contains intermediate cells, epidermoid cells, and mucocytes
  - Mucocytes are arranged in nests or are scattered
- Clear cells may be predominant
- Tumor-associated lymphoid proliferation (TALP)
- Tumor grading very helpful in predicting outcome and management

Ancillary Tests
- Mucicarmine(+) mucocytes

Top Differential Diagnoses
- Sialometaplasia
- Mucous extravasation reaction
- Squamous cell carcinoma
- Clear cell adenocarcinoma and epithelial-myoepithelial carcinoma

  - Major glands
    - Conservative excision for stage I and II parotid gland tumors
    - Preservation of facial nerve, if possible
    - Complete resection of submandibular gland
    - Neck dissection for metastatic disease, large tumors, or high-grade tumors
  - Minor glands
    - Excision with wide margin
    - Lesion infiltrating or closely abutting bone may require resection of bone
    - Neck dissection for metastatic disease, large tumors, or high-grade tumors
  - Primary intraosseous
    - Enucleation or curettage
    - Segmental resection
    - Neck dissection based on clinical findings
- Adjuvant therapy
  - Radiotherapy
    - Should be used with caution in children due to potential for long-term sequelae
    - Used when there are inoperable, positive margins
    - High-stage disease
  - Chemotherapy
    - May be useful for high-grade tumors

Prognosis
- Clinical stage and histologic grade are main prognostic factors
- MECs occurring in children have good prognosis
  - Majority of tumors are well differentiated
    - Rarely metastasize
- Positive surgical margins are predictive of recurrence
- Metastases
  - Predictive of poor prognosis
    - Lung, lymph node, bone, brain

IMAGE FINDINGS

General Features
- MR, CT, and radiographs used for major glands
  - Preoperative imaging studies to assess full extent of tumor and staging are recommended in children
- Minor gland tumors may show erosion of adjacent bone
- Primary intraosseous tumors are generally well-circumscribed radiolucencies

MACROSCOPIC FEATURES

General Features
- Circumscribed, partially encapsulated, or poorly defined periphery
- Cut surface
  - Pink, tan, or yellow
  - Cystic, sometimes with blood

Size
- Highly variable
  - From < 1 cm to large disfiguring masses

MICROSCOPIC PATHOLOGY

Histologic Features
- Variably sized cystic spaces
  - Often filled with mucin
  - Occasionally, papillary projections are present
- Epidermoid cells
  - Nests or scattered
  - Polygonal cells
- Intermediate cells
  - Large polygonal epidermoid cells
  - Small basal cells
  - Often found in nests or sheets
- Mucous cells
  - Intracytoplasmic mucin
  - Large or ovoid
  - Vacuolated or clear cytoplasm
  - In groups or individually scattered
- Clear cells
  - Usually < 10% of cells but can be dominant finding
  - Contain glycogen or mucin

MUCOEPIDERMOID CARCINOMA

- Spilled mucus
  - Incites inflammatory response
  - May be misinterpreted as mucous escape reaction
- Tumor-associated lymphoid proliferation (TALP)
  - Lymphoid cells with occasional germinal centers
  - May be confused with metastatic disease to a lymph node
- Necrosis, anaplasia, and mitoses variably present
- Perineural and vascular invasion can be seen
- Grading used for prognosis and management
- Sarcomatoid transformation may rarely be seen
- Sclerosing mucoepidermoid carcinoma
  - Fibrous stroma is plentiful and can be hyalinized
  - Inflammatory cells (eosinophils included) may be seen

ANCILLARY TESTS

Cytology

- Clusters of bland intermediate or epithelial cells
- Mucocytes within clusters
- Variable amounts of mucin in background
- May be hypocellular or acellular if cystic areas are sampled
- Papanicolaou stain: Epithelial cells with dense, green-blue cytoplasm
- Diff-Quik®: Mucocytes with intracellular, red-granular mucin droplet
  - Epithelial cells with light pink-purple cytoplasm

Frozen Sections

- Usually quite distinctive
- High-grade lesions may be misdiagnosed as squamous cell carcinoma

Immunohistochemistry

- p63
  - Strong, basal cell nuclear reaction
  - May highlight intermediate as well as epidermoid cells
  - Highly reactive lesions may indicate poor prognosis
- CK5/6
  - Highlights epidermoid-type cells but is often negative in transitional cells
- Ki-67
  - High expression seen with increased proliferation, usually indicative of high-grade tumor
  - Overexpression may serve as indicator of poor prognosis
- HER2
  - Tends to be strongly reactive in high-grade tumors
  - Overexpression may serve as indication for poor prognosis
  - Reactivity may guide future therapy with Herceptin®

Cytogenetics

- Not widely studied in pediatric MEC
- t(11;19)(q21-22;p13)
  - Fuses mucoepidermoid carcinoma translocated 1 (*MECT1*) (exon 1 of gene at 19p13) with mastermind-like gene family (*MAML2*) (exons 2-5 of gene at 11q21)

DIFFERENTIAL DIAGNOSIS

Sialometaplasia

- Usually in lobular pattern, lacking cystic growth, no intermediate cells
- Mucocytes are residual to salivary gland

Mucous Extravasation Reaction

- Lacks intermediate cells and epithelial cells
- Mucus found primarily in macrophages

Squamous Cell Carcinoma

- Extremely rare in children
- Usually has keratinization and well-developed intercellular bridges
- Lacks intermediate cells

Clear Cell Malignancies

- Rare in children
- Clear cell adenocarcinoma
  - Lacks intermediate cells or mucocyte differentiation
- Epithelial-myoepithelial carcinoma
  - Lacks intermediate cells, mucocyte differentiation
  - Shows distinct and characteristic biphasic glandular proliferation

Differential for Primary Intraosseous Tumors

- Glandular odontogenic tumor
- Reactive cyst with mucous metaplasia
- Clear cell odontogenic carcinoma

SELECTED REFERENCES

1. Cheuk W et al: Advances in salivary gland pathology. Histopathology. 51(1):1-20, 2007
2. do Prado RF et al: Calcifications in a clear cell mucoepidermoid carcinoma: a case report with histological and immunohistochemical findings. Oral Surg Oral Med Oral Pathol Oral Radiol Endod. 104(5):e40-4, 2007
3. Rahbar R et al: Mucoepidermoid carcinoma of the parotid gland in children: A 10-year experience. Arch Otolaryngol Head Neck Surg. 132(4):375-80, 2006
4. Triantafillidou K et al: Mucoepidermoid carcinoma of minor salivary glands: a clinical study of 16 cases and review of the literature. Oral Dis. 12(4):364-70, 2006
5. Haddad R et al: Herceptin in patients with advanced or metastatic salivary gland carcinomas. A phase II study. Oral Oncol. 39(7):724-7, 2003
6. Nguyen LH et al: HER2/neu and Ki-67 as prognostic indicators in mucoepidermoid carcinoma of salivary glands. J Otolaryngol. 32(5):328-31, 2003
7. Curry JL et al: Synchronous benign and malignant salivary gland tumors in ipsilateral glands: a report of two cases and a review of literature. Head Neck. 24(3):301-6, 2002
8. Foschini MP et al: Low-grade mucoepidermoid carcinoma of salivary glands: characteristic immunohistochemical profile and evidence of striated duct differentiation. Virchows Arch. 440(5):536-42, 2002
9. Guzzo M et al: Mucoepidermoid carcinoma of the salivary glands: clinicopathologic review of 108 patients treated at the National Cancer Institute of Milan. Ann Surg Oncol. 9(7):688-95, 2002

Immunohistochemistry

Antibody	Reactivity	Staining Pattern	Comment
CK-PAN	Positive	Cytoplasmic	Most cells, although only focally for mucocytes
CK5/6	Positive	Cytoplasmic	More common in epidermoid than in transitional cells
CK7	Positive	Cytoplasmic	More intense staining for intermediate/transitional cells
p63	Positive	Nuclear	Basal cell reaction; strong staining suggests worse prognosis
CK14	Positive	Cytoplasmic	
CK19	Positive	Cytoplasmic	
CK17	Positive	Cytoplasmic	
EpCAM/BER-EP4/ CD326	Positive	Cell membrane & cytoplasm	
HER2	Positive	Cell membrane	Greater degree of positivity, suggests higher grade tumor
Ki-67	Positive	Nuclear	The higher the proliferation index, the higher the grade of tumor and the worse the prognosis
CK20	Negative	Cytoplasmic	
S100	Negative	Nuclear & cytoplasmic	
GFAP	Negative	Cytoplasmic	
Actin-HHF-35	Equivocal	Cytoplasmic	5% positivity

Tumor Grading

Parameter	Point Value
Intracystic component < 20%	2
Neural invasion present	2
Necrosis present	3
4 or more mitoses per 10 high-power fields	3
Anaplasia	4
Grade	**Total point score**
Low	0-4
Intermediate	5-6
High	≥ 7

Modified from Auclair PL et al: Mucoepidermoid carcinoma of intraoral salivary glands. Evaluation and application of grading criteria in 143 cases. Cancer. 69(8):2021-30, 1992.

Histochemical Studies

Histochemical Stain	Reactivity	Staining Pattern	Comment
Mucicarmine	Positive	Cytoplasmic	Identifies mucocytes
Periodic acid-Schiff (PAS)	Positive	Cytoplasmic	Identifies glycogen
Alcian blue	Positive	Cytoplasmic	Identifies mucocytes
Periodic acid-Schiff with diastase	Negative		

10. Brandwein MS et al: Mucoepidermoid carcinoma: a clinicopathologic study of 80 patients with special reference to histological grading. Am J Surg Pathol. 25(7):835-45, 2001
11. Bentz BG et al: Masses of the salivary gland region in children. Arch Otolaryngol Head Neck Surg. 126(12):1435-9, 2000
12. Ellis GL: Clear cell neoplasms in salivary glands: clearly a diagnostic challenge. Ann Diagn Pathol. 2(1):61-78, 1998
13. Goode RK et al: Mucoepidermoid carcinoma of the major salivary glands: clinical and histopathologic analysis of 234 cases with evaluation of grading criteria. Cancer. 82(7):1217-24, 1998
14. Loyola AM et al: Study of minor salivary gland mucoepidermoid carcinoma differentiation based on immunohistochemical expression of cytokeratins, vimentin and muscle-specific actin. Oral Oncol. 34(2):112-8, 1998
15. Auclair PL: Tumor-associated lymphoid proliferation in the parotid gland. A potential diagnostic pitfall. Oral Surg Oral Med Oral Pathol. 77(1):19-26, 1994
16. Auclair PL et al: Mucoepidermoid carcinoma of intraoral salivary glands. Evaluation and application of grading criteria in 143 cases. Cancer. 69(8):2021-30, 1992
17. Callender DL et al: Salivary gland neoplasms in children. Arch Otolaryngol Head Neck Surg. 118(5):472-6, 1992
18. Gustafsson H et al: Mucoepidermoid carcinoma in a minor salivary gland in childhood. J Laryngol Otol. 101(12):1320-3, 1987

Radiologic and Other Features

*(**Left**) Axial contrast-enhanced computed tomography shows an invasive high-grade mucoepidermoid carcinoma involving the superficial lobe ➔ and deep lobe of the parotid gland ⇨. There is significant destruction of the parotid parenchyma by the tumor. Notice the single intraparotid lymph node ↷. (**Right**) Corresponding coronal T2-weighted magnetic resonance shows a well-defined, high signal tumor with cystic necrosis ➔. It could be easily mistaken for another tumor type.*

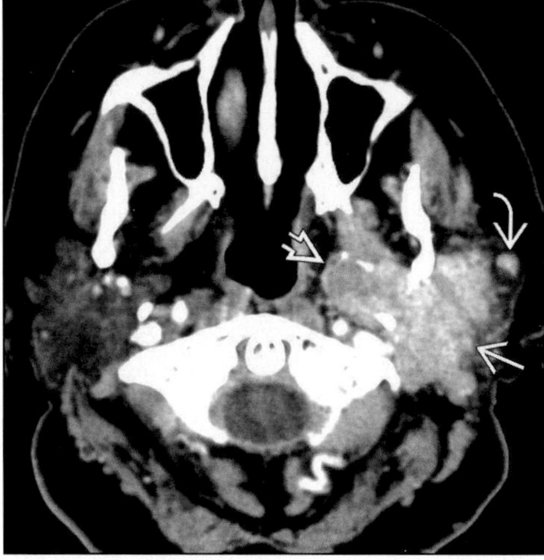

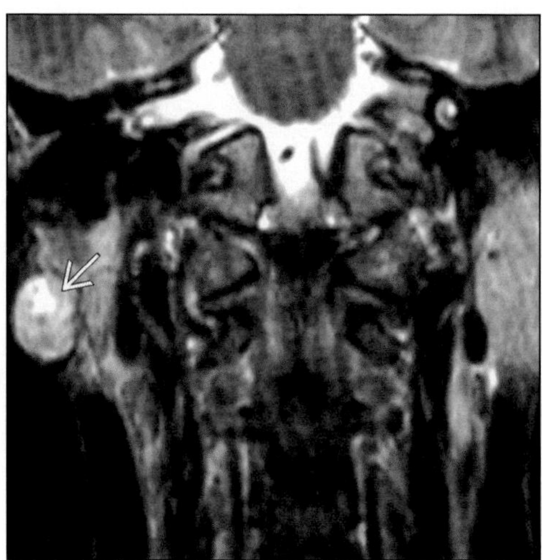

*(**Left**) Clinical photograph shows an ulcerated red mass of the posterior lateral hard palate ➔. Microscopic review confirmed a low-grade mucoepidermoid carcinoma arising from a minor salivary gland. Palate primaries usually do not have a capsule. (**Right**) Gross photograph shows a tumor with a tan-yellow cut surface. Mucoid material can be seen in the cystic spaces ➔. The remaining parenchyma is compressed toward the periphery.*

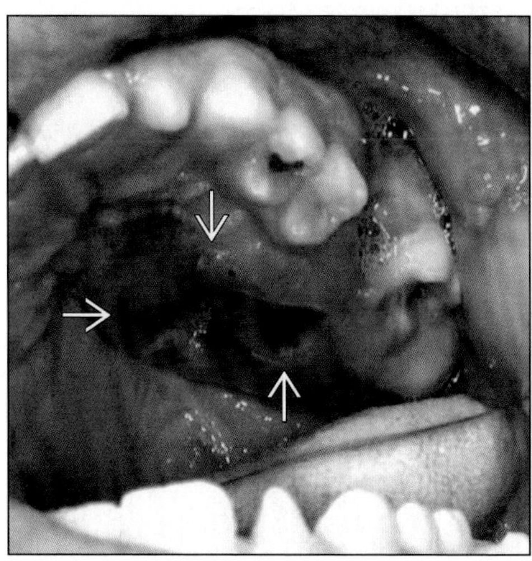

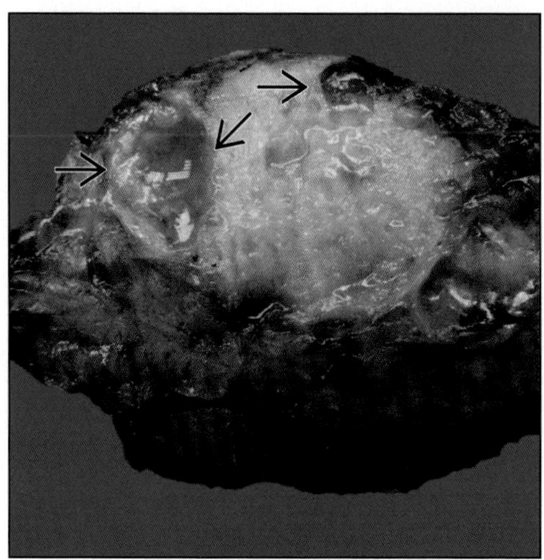

*(**Left**) Gross photograph shows a predominately unicystic mucoepidermoid carcinoma. The lumen was filled with thick, tenacious, mucoid material. This type of lesion can easily mimic a mucocele, clinically and macroscopically. (**Right**) Hematoxylin & eosin shows a neoplasm composed of numerous, variably sized cystic spaces lined by epithelium. Based on the greater than 20% cystic component, this pattern suggests a low-grade tumor.*

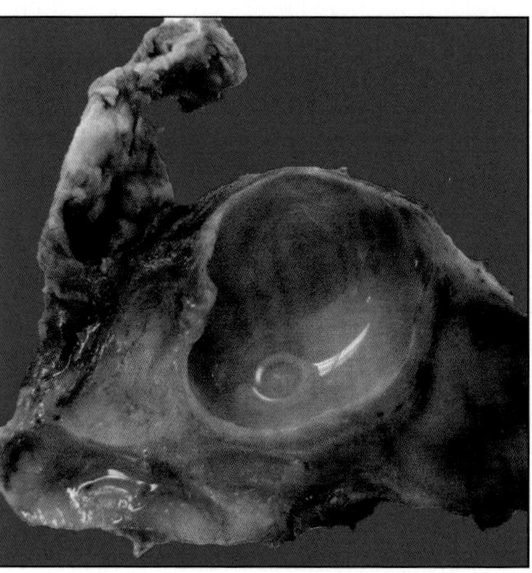

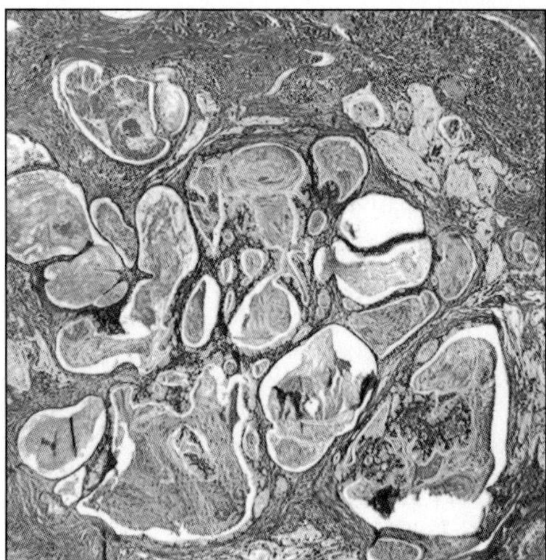

Microscopic Features

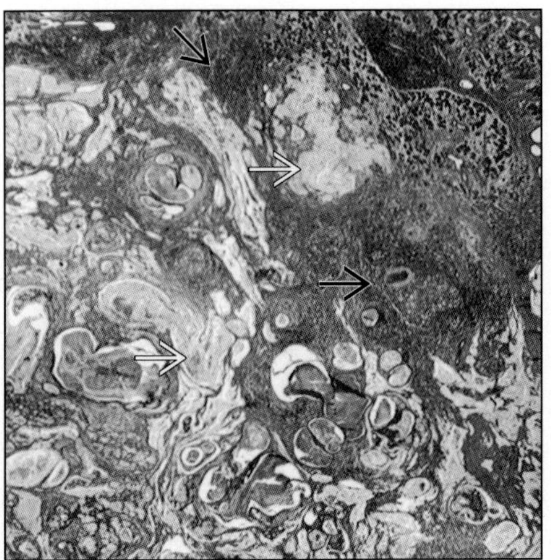

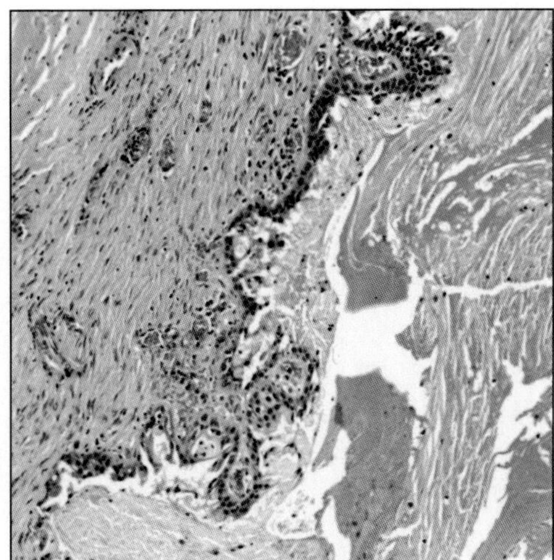

(Left) *Hematoxylin & eosin shows a cystic tumor with areas of spilled mucus ➡. It is not uncommon to have cysts of the tumor rupture, yielding free mucus, which incites an inflammatory response ➡. In small biopsies, these features may be misdiagnosed as a mucous escape reaction (mucocele).* ***(Right)*** *Shown here is a unicystic tumor in the parotid. Clinically it was thought to be a branchial cleft cyst.*

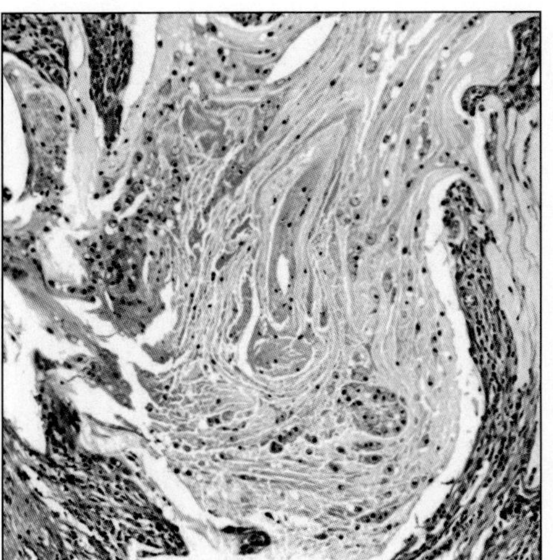

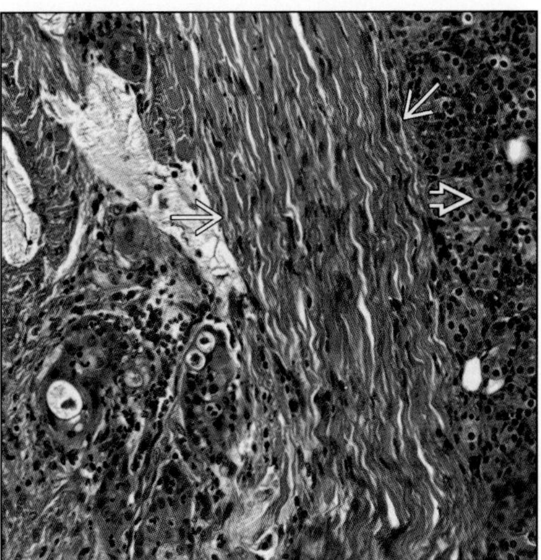

(Left) *Hematoxylin & eosin shows a pool of free mucus that has caused an inflammatory response. The mucinous material may contain inflammatory debris and histiocytes. These should not be mistaken for true "mucocytes," which should be sought in the lining epithelium.* ***(Right)*** *Hematoxylin & eosin shows an area of partial encapsulation ➡ separating the parotid gland ➡ from the tumor. Note the small cyst-gland spaces and extravasated mucus material within the tumor.*

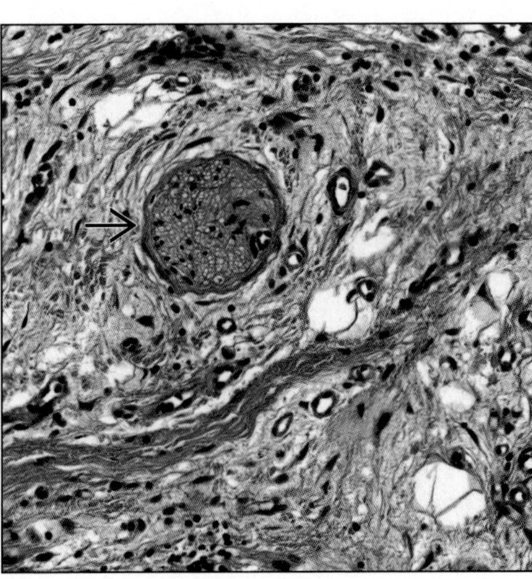

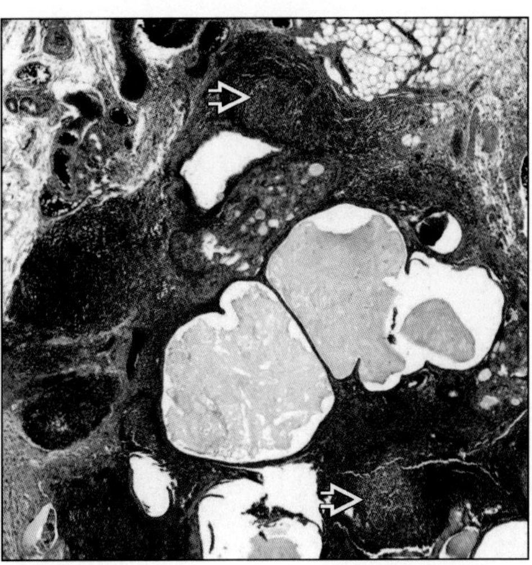

(Left) *The neoplastic cells invade beyond the contours of the tumor into the adjacent soft tissue. Sometimes, mucinous material will be present around nerves ➡. Isolated epithelial cells are frequently suspended in the mucus pools.* ***(Right)*** *This mucoepidermoid tumor has tumor-associated lymphoid proliferation (TALP). Well-formed germinal centers are easily identified ➡, but no capsule is seen, indicating that this in not metastatic disease to a lymph node.*

MUCOEPIDERMOID CARCINOMA

Microscopic Features

*(**Left**) The epidermoid and intermediate cell component of a mucoepidermoid carcinoma may undergo clear cell change. Sometimes, as in this case, it can be the dominant finding. The differential diagnosis expands when this is the case. (**Right**) Hematoxylin & eosin shows a tumor with a focus of clear cells. There are prominent intercellular borders with small hyperchromatic nuclei. Clear cells contain glycogen and, occasionally, mucin. A PAS or mucicarmine stain may be helpful.*

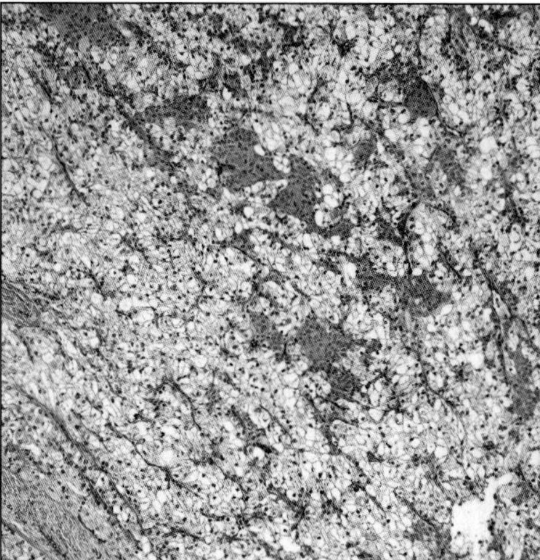

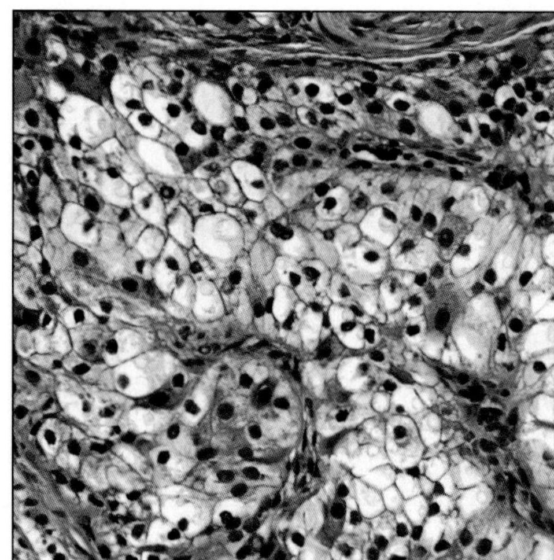

*(**Left**) The components of a mucoepidermoid carcinoma are frequently intermingled and blended. The mucocytes ⇒ are sometimes quite prominent but identified as single cells within the epidermoid/transitional cell component. There are no well-formed cystic spaces in this field. Inflammatory cells are frequently present. (**Right**) Hematoxylin & eosin shows cellular anaplasia and focal acute inflammation. Mucocytes can be seen ➡. These features are suggestive of a high-grade tumor.*

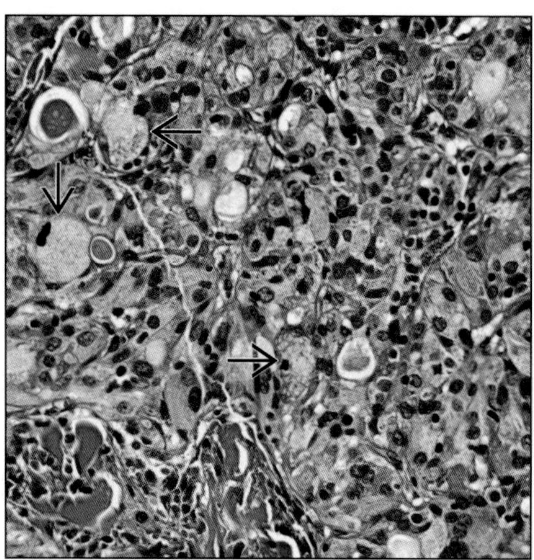

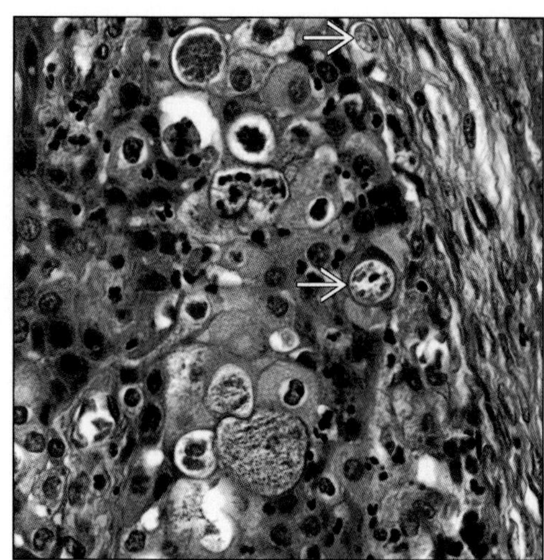

*(**Left**) Hematoxylin & eosin shows a high-power view of an atypical mitotic figure ⇒ within a pleomorphic high-grade tumor. There is a transitional epithelial proliferation immediately adjacent to this atypical mitotic figure. (**Right**) Hematoxylin & eosin shows a collection of mucous cells with foamy cytoplasm. The foamy cytoplasm can also be seen in histiocytes. It is for this reason that mucicarmine or other mucin stains need to be performed to confirm the diagnosis.*

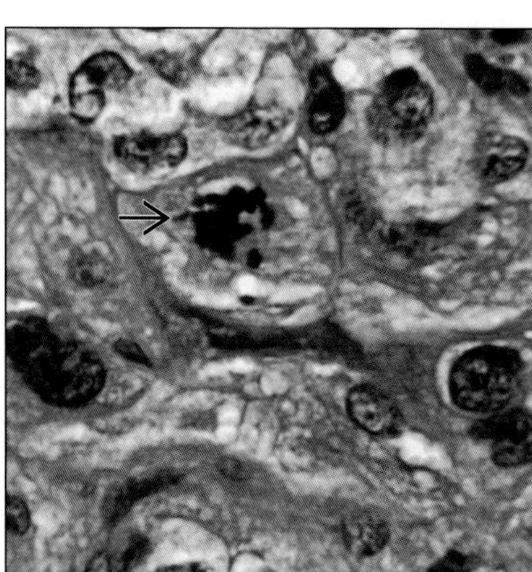

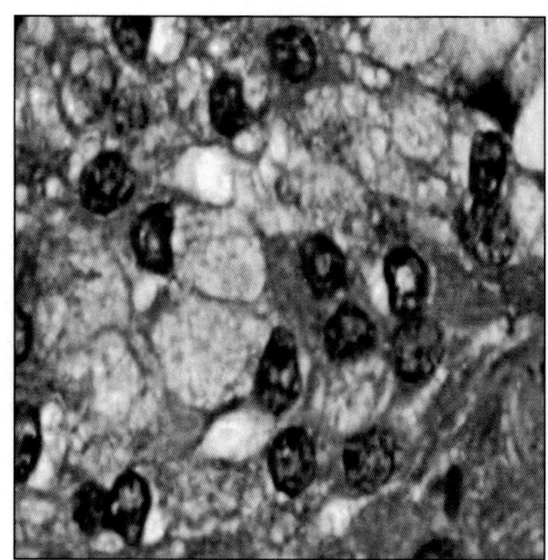

Ancillary Techniques

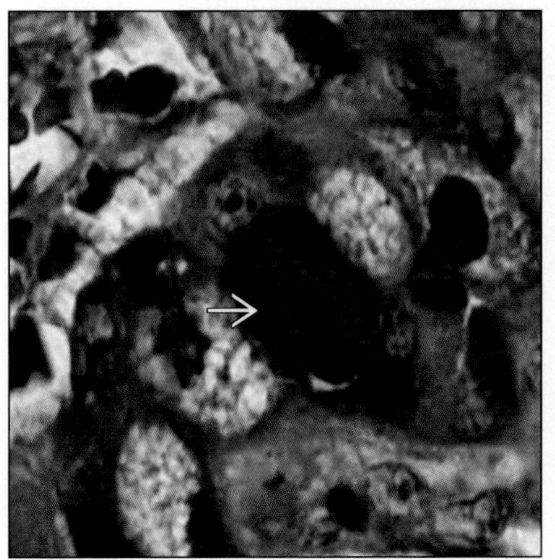

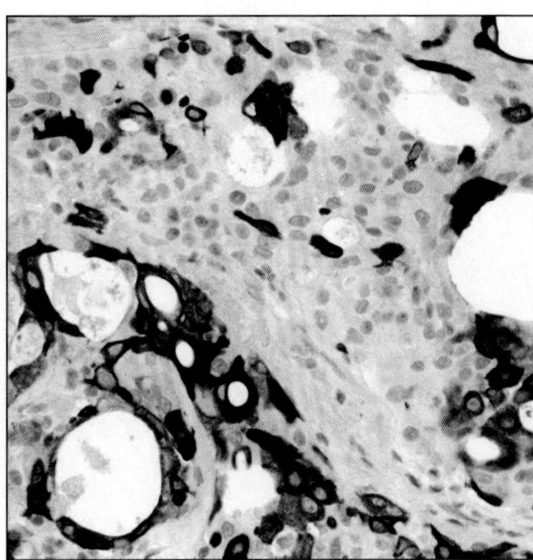

(Left) *Mucicarmine stain helps confirm intracytoplasmic mucin* ➔. *Oftentimes it is difficult to identify these cells with standard H&E staining. The surrounding cells appear to also have a "vacuolated" appearance but do not actually contain mucin. This finding highlights the need to perform histochemical stains to confirm the diagnosis.* ***(Right)*** *CK5/6 highlights the epithelial cells associated with the duct-like structures. There is a variable intensity to the staining.*

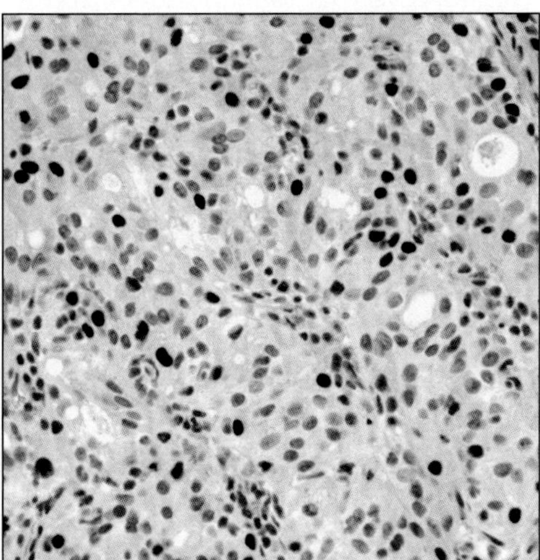

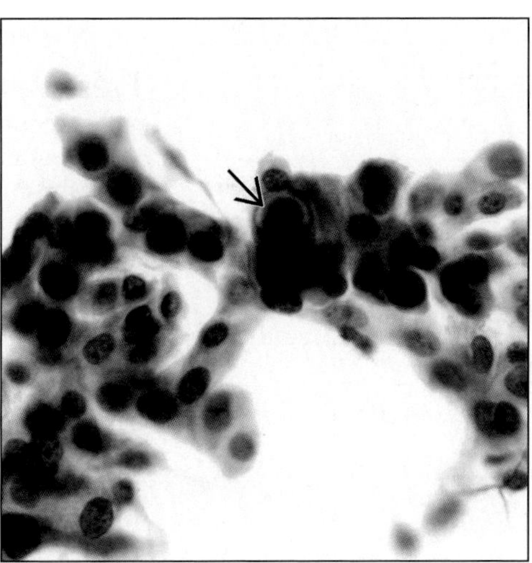

(Left) *p63 will highlight the nuclei of intermediate cells. There is not usually reactivity with mucocytes nor with the epidermoid cells.* ***(Right)*** *The cytology smear demonstrates sheets and clusters of epidermoid-transitional cells. The cytoplasm is opaque. There is a suggestion of a vacuole within the cytoplasm* ➔ *of 1 of the neoplastic cells.*

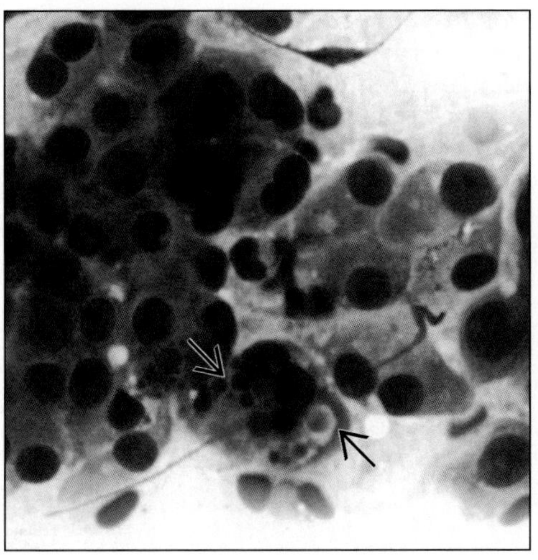

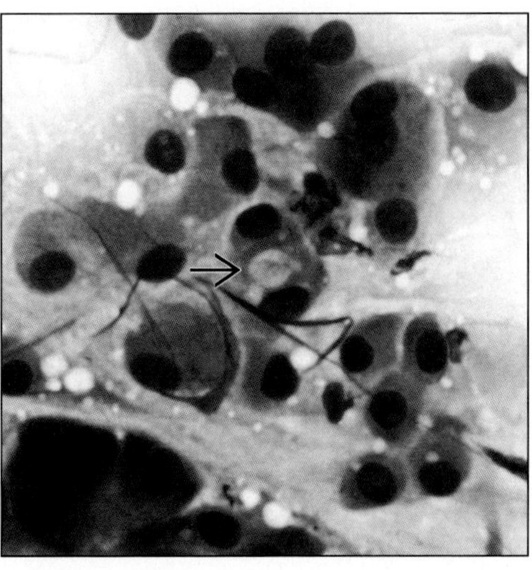

(Left) *There is a sheet-like distribution to these neoplastic epithelioid cells, making up the epidermoid component of this tumor. Note the mucin-filled cytoplasm* ➔ *highlighting a mucocyte in this smear. Mucin is usually a deep magenta. Often, it is present in the background.* ***(Right)*** *There is a well-formed mucocyte* ➔ *in the center of the field, surrounded by epidermoid or transitional cells. Note the "bluish" appearance to the cytoplasm, similar to squamous cells.*

RETINOBLASTOMA

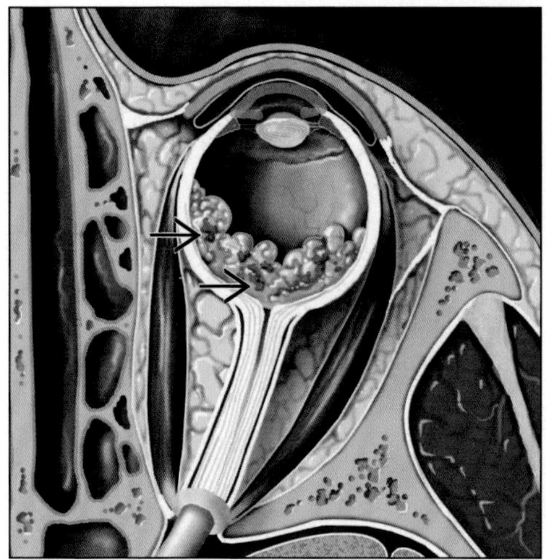

Axial graphic shows retinoblastoma with lobulated tumor extending through the limiting membrane into the vitreous. Punctate calcifications ⇒ are characteristic.

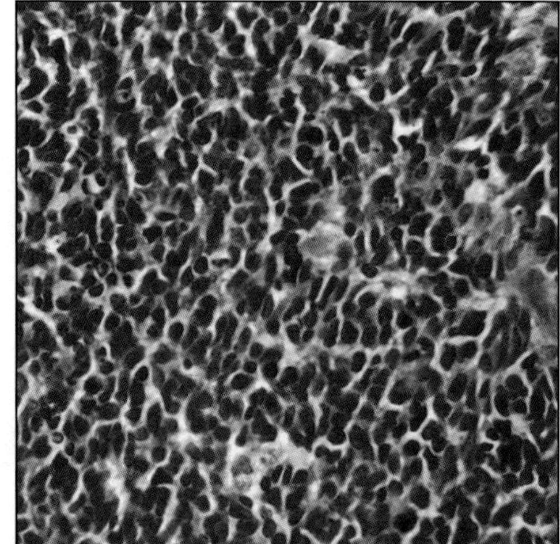

Retinoblastoma is a small round blue cell tumor. Tumor cells are present in sheets and have little cytoplasm. Calcifications and necrosis are common (though not seen here).

TERMINOLOGY

Abbreviations

- Retinoblastoma (RB)

Definitions

- Malignant retinal neoplasm arising from neuroectodermal cells

ETIOLOGY/PATHOGENESIS

Developmental Anomaly

- Loss or inactivation of both alleles of retinoblastoma gene (*RB* gene)
  - Located at 13q14
  - Tumor suppressor gene
- Knudson "2-hit" hypothesis
  - RB results from 2 independent mutations
  - 1st mutation may be either somatic (sporadic) or germinal (inherited)
  - 2nd mutation is sporadic

CLINICAL ISSUES

Epidemiology

- Incidence
  - Most common intraocular malignancy in children
- Age
  - Average age at diagnosis is 24 months
  - Younger in bilateral/familial cases
- Gender
  - No predilection
- Ethnicity
  - No predilection

Site

- Sporadic RB is usually unilateral
- Inherited RB is often bilateral
  - May include pineal tumor (so-called "trilateral" RB)
  - "Quadrilateral" RB is very rare and includes bilateral RB plus pineal and suprasellar tumors

Presentation

- Leukocoria (white pupil)
  - Frequently noticed in photographs
- Strabismus
- Decreased visual acuity
- Glaucoma
- Red, painful eye
- Up to 40% are familial
  - 5-10% have family history of RB
  - Remainder are new germline mutations

Treatment

- Depends on tumor size and intraocular location

Prognosis

- If treated within 1st year of life, additional tumor foci often develop
- If untreated, death within several years
- 2nd cancers common in patients with *RB* mutations
  - Incidence increases 1% per year of life
  - Incidence is higher in inherited RB
  - Osteosarcoma, sarcoma, melanoma, Hodgkin lymphoma, breast carcinoma
- Poor prognosis if direct scleral invasion or invasion of optic nerve
- 90% cure rate if noninvasive

IMAGE FINDINGS

General Features

- Calcified intraocular mass
- Diagnosis often made by imaging only

RETINOBLASTOMA

Key Facts

Etiology/Pathogenesis
- Loss or inactivation of both alleles of retinoblastoma gene (*RB* gene)
  - Knudson "2-hit" hypothesis

Clinical Issues
- Most common intraocular malignancy in children
- Average age at diagnosis: 24 months
- Up to 40% are familial
- 2nd cancers common in patients with *RB* mutations
  - Osteosarcoma, sarcoma, melanoma, Hodgkin lymphoma, breast carcinoma
- Leukocoria is most common clinical presentation

Image Findings
- Calcified intraocular mass
- Diagnosis often made by imaging only

Microscopic Pathology
- Small round blue cell tumor
- Variable appearance based on degree of differentiation
  - Flexner-Wintersteiner rosettes have central lumen
  - Fleurette shows photoreceptor differentiation
- Ischemic necrosis common
- Calcifications common

Top Differential Diagnoses
- Primitive neuroectodermal tumor (PNET)
- Leukemia/lymphoma
- Astrocytoma

MACROSCOPIC FEATURES

General Features
- Creamy white
- Calcifications
- Necrosis
- Growth patterns
  - Endophytic: Growth inward toward vitreous cavity
  - Exophytic: Growth outward toward subretinal space and choroid
    - Detaches retina; still may fill vitreous cavity
  - Diffuse infiltrating thickens retina

MICROSCOPIC PATHOLOGY

Histologic Features
- Small round blue cell tumor
- Variable appearance based on degree of differentiation
- Flexner-Wintersteiner rosettes
  - Tumor cells surround central lumen that contains acid mucopolysaccharide
  - Tumor nuclei are placed away from central lumen
- Homer Wright rosettes
  - Lack well-defined lumen
  - Less common in RB
- Fleurette
  - Photoreceptor differentiation (well-differentiated RB)
  - Pattern resembles a fleur-de-lis
- Ischemic necrosis common
  - Surrounds perivascular tumor cells
- Calcifications common
- May invade optic nerve and extend to brain or CSF

DIFFERENTIAL DIAGNOSIS

Primitive Neuroectodermal Tumor (PNET)
- If in eye, would be considered metastatic
- Calcifications and necrosis less common

Leukemia/Lymphoma
- Calcifications not seen, and necrosis much less common
- Immunohistochemical stains would help if needed
  - CD45 (LCA), Tdt

Astrocytoma
- Small round blue cell pattern generally not seen in astrocytoma
- GFAP immunohistochemistry would help if needed

SELECTED REFERENCES

1. Anand B et al: Prevalence of high-risk human papillomavirus genotypes in retinoblastoma. Br J Ophthalmol. 95(7):1014-8, 2011
2. Eagle RC Jr et al: Histopathologic observations after intra-arterial chemotherapy for retinoblastoma. Arch Ophthalmol. Epub ahead of print, 2011
3. Friedrich MJ: Retinoblastoma therapy delivers power of chemotherapy with surgical precision. JAMA. 305(22):2276-8, 2011
4. Gao YJ et al: Clinical characteristics and treatment outcome of children with intraocular retinoblastoma: a report from a Chinese cooperative group. Pediatr Blood Cancer. Epub ahead of print, 2011
5. Kashyap S et al: Clinical predictors of high risk histopathology in retinoblastoma. Pediatr Blood Cancer. Epub ahead of print, 2011
6. Palamar M et al: Evolution in regression patterns following chemoreduction for retinoblastoma. Arch Ophthalmol. 129(6):727-30, 2011
7. Serrano C et al: Low penetrance hereditary retinoblastoma in a family: what should we consider in the genetic counselling process and follow up? Fam Cancer. 10(3):617-21, 2011
8. Ghosh S et al: Diagnostic accuracy in retinoblastoma. J Indian Med Assoc. 108(8):509, 512-3, 2010

RETINOBLASTOMA

Clinical and Other Features

(Left) *Leukocoria, or white pupil, is a common presentation of retinoblastoma. This is frequently noticed in photographs. (Courtesy D. Shatzkes, MD.)* ***(Right)*** *This is a retinoblastoma as seen on funduscopic examination. The tumor ⇨ is white and fluffy. The optic nerve ➡ and macula ➪ are uninvolved. (Courtesy D. Dries, MD.)*

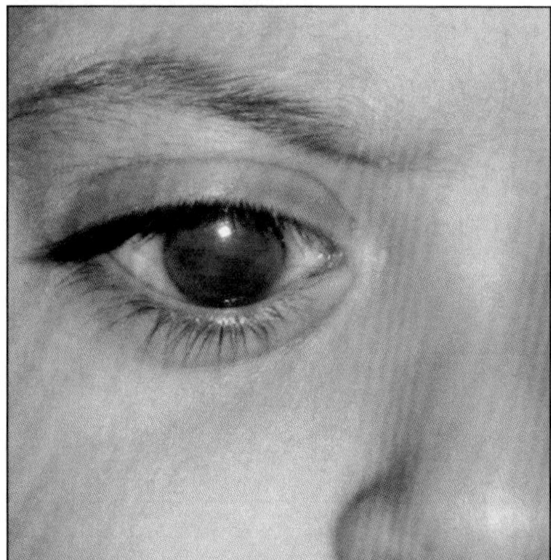

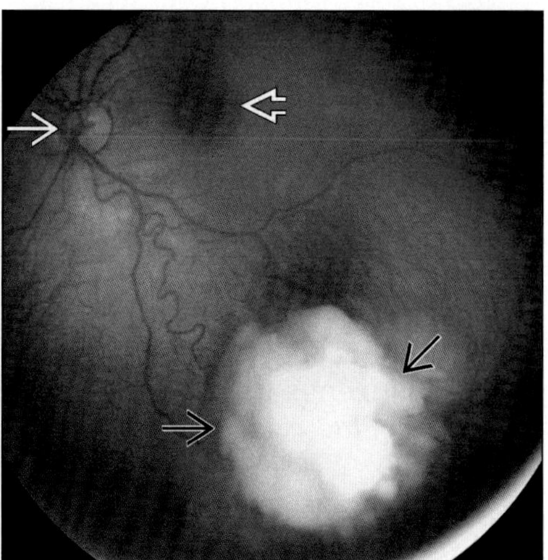

(Left) *Axial CT shows a large, lobulated, partially calcified left intraocular mass ➡, typical of retinoblastoma.* ***(Right)*** *Gross pathology shows the macroscopic appearance of the eye after exenteration. Retinoblastoma is a calcified mass that fills the vitreous cavity. (Courtesy B. Ey, MD.)*

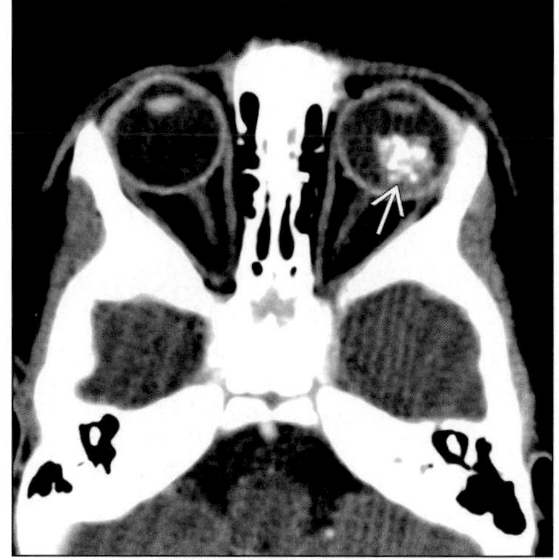

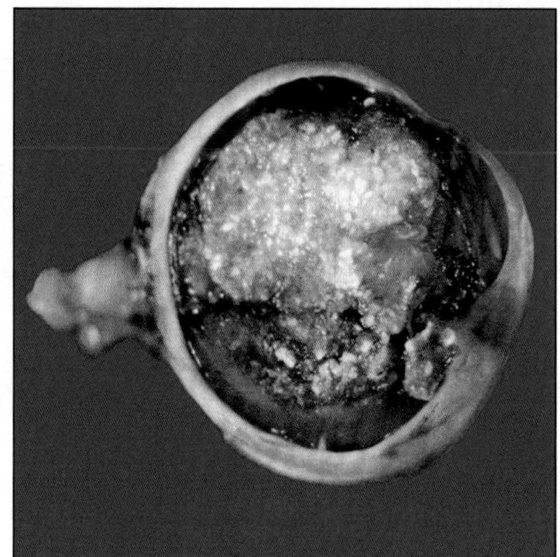

(Left) *Knudsen "2-hit" hypothesis is seen in which both copies of a tumor suppressor gene must be mutated in order for a tumor to develop. The 1st hit may be either inherited (somatic, germline) or sporadic. The 2nd hit is always sporadic.* ***(Right)*** *This whole mount of an eye exenteration specimen shows a subretinal (exophytic) retinoblastoma bulging into the vitreous space.*

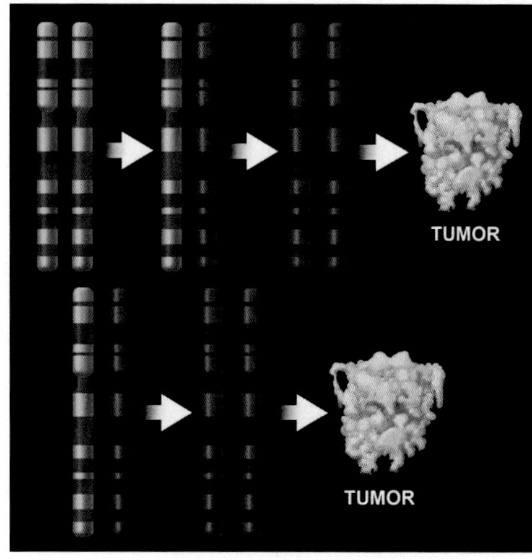

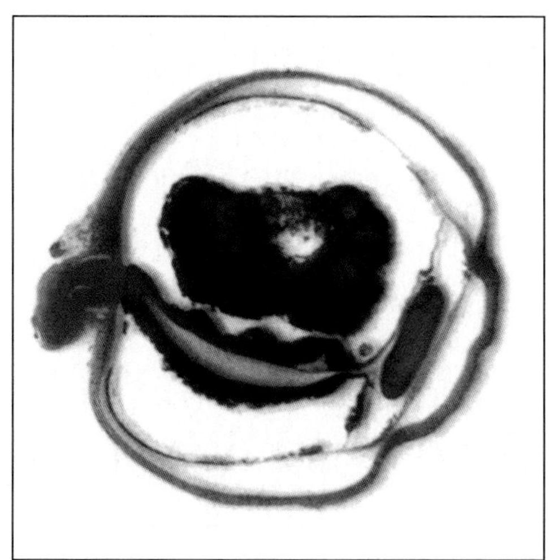

Microscopic Features

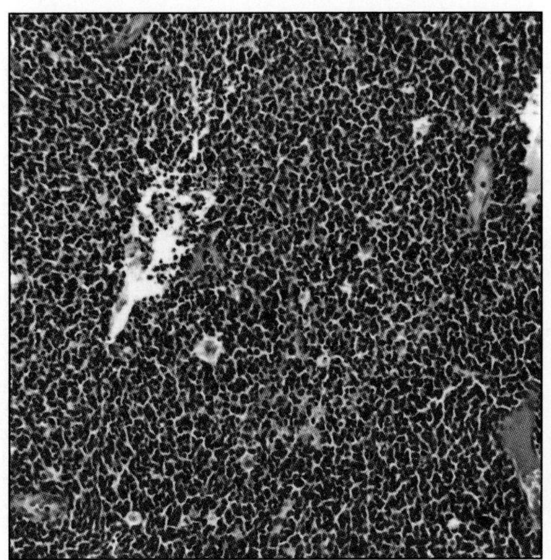

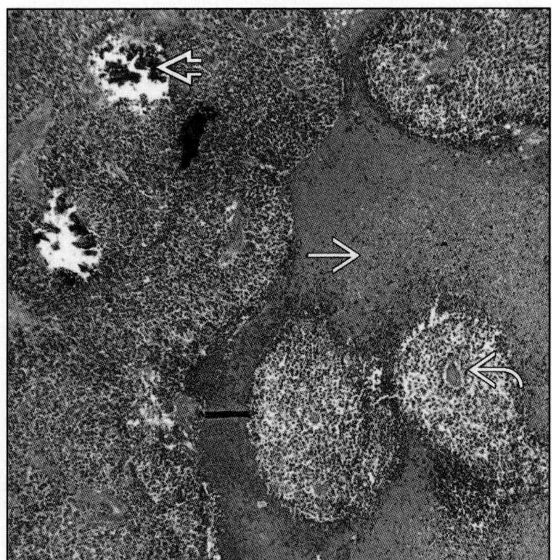

(Left) *Sheets of small round blue cells make up this poorly differentiated retinoblastoma. This field could be mistaken for PNET if the location was not known.* ***(Right)*** *Necrosis ➡ and calcifications ⇨ are very common in retinoblastoma. The necrosis is often seen around vascular spaces ↪, as the tumor outgrows its blood supply. Calcifications are an important marker in radiologic studies.*

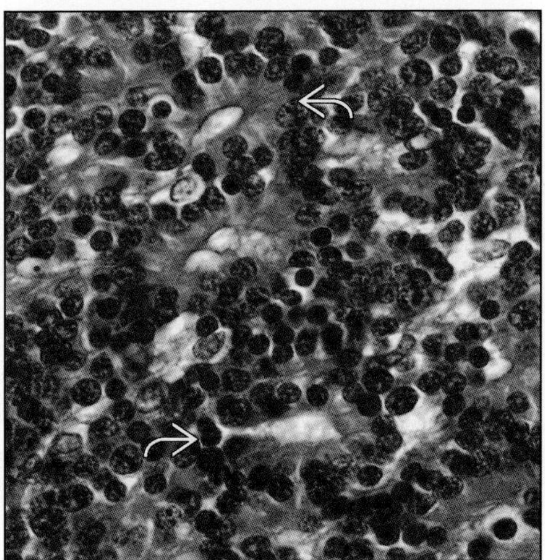

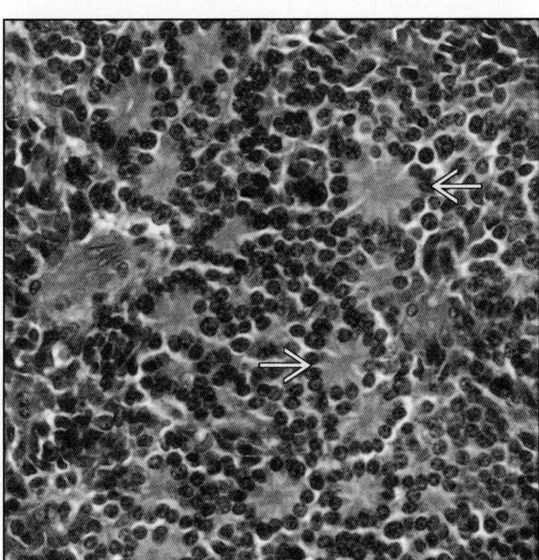

(Left) *Flexner-Wintersteiner rosettes ↪ are seen in moderately differentiated retinoblastomas. They have a central lumen filled with mucopolysaccharide, and the surrounding tumor cells have their nuclei located away from the lumen.* ***(Right)*** *Homer Wright rosettes ➡ can be seen in retinoblastoma but are much less common than Flexner-Wintersteiner rosettes. Homer Wright rosettes do not have central lumens.*

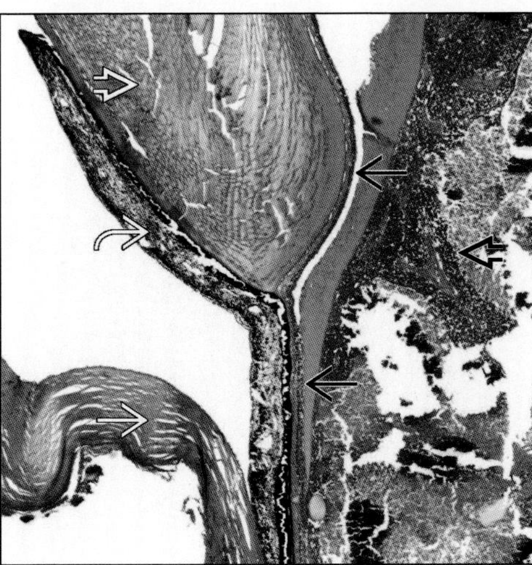

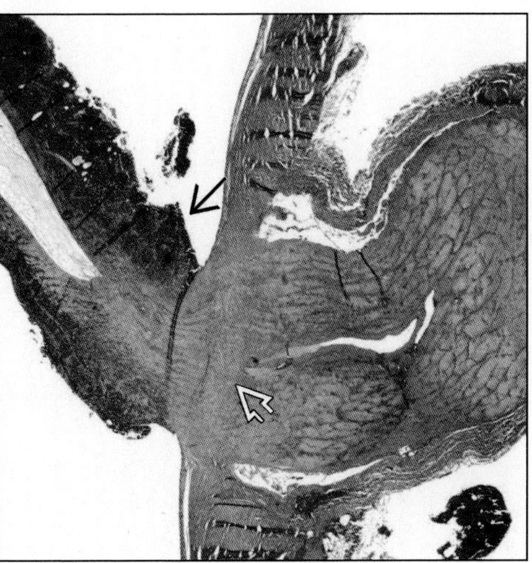

(Left) *While this retinoblastoma fills the vitreous cavity, it is exophytic since it is in the subretinal space. The cornea ➡, iris ↪, and lens ⇨ are anterior; the detached retina ➡ has been pushed up against the lens by the tumor ⇨.* ***(Right)*** *This retinoblastoma ➡ ends where the optic nerve ⇨ reaches the globe. Invasion of the optic nerve by retinoblastoma has a poor prognosis so careful examination is required.*

Retinoblastoma

Enucleation, Partial or Complete Exenteration

Procedure

___ Enucleation
___ Partial exenteration
___ Complete exenteration
___ Other (specify): ____________________________
___ Not specified

Specimen Size

For enucleation
Anteroposterior diameter: _________ mm
Horizontal diameter: _________ mm
Vertical diameter: _________ mm
Length of optic nerve: _________ mm
Diameter of optic nerve: _________ mm
___ Cannot be determined
For exenteration
Greatest dimension: _________ cm
*Additional dimensions: _________ x _________ cm
___ Cannot be determined

Specimen Laterality

___ Right
___ Left
___ Not specified

Tumor Site (macroscopic examination/transillumination) (select all that apply)

___ Cannot be determined
___ Supertemporal quadrant of globe
___ Superonasal quadrant of globe
___ Inferotemporal quadrant of globe
___ Inferonasal quadrant of globe
___ Other (specify): ____________________________

Tumor Basal Size on Transillumination

___ Cannot be determined
Anterior-posterior length: _________ x _________ mm
Transverse length: _________ x _________ mm

Tumor Size After Sectioning

___ Cannot be determined
Base at cut edge: _________ mm
Height at cut edge: _________ mm
Greatest height: _________ mm

Tumor Location After Sectioning

___ Cannot be determined
Distance from anterior edge of tumor to limbus at cut edge: _________ mm
Distance of posterior margin of tumor base from edge of optic disc: _________ mm

Tumor Involvement of Other Ocular Structures (select all that apply)

___ Cannot be determined
___ Cornea
___ Anterior chamber
___ Iris
___ Angle
___ Lens

___ Ciliary body
___ Vitreous
___ Retinal detachment
___ Optic disc
___ Choroid, minimal (solid tumor nest < 3 mm in maximum diameter [width or thickness])
___ Choroid, massive (solid tumor nest ≥ 3 mm in maximum diameter [width or thickness])
___ Sclera
___ Vortex vein
___ Orbit

Histologic Features (select all that apply)

___ Cannot be determined
___ Undifferentiated
___ Differentiated
    *___ Homer Wright rosettes
    *___ Flexner-Wintersteiner rosettes
    *___ Fleurettes
___ Necrotic

Growth Pattern

___ Cannot be determined
___ Endophytic
___ Exophytic
___ Combined endophytic/exophytic
___ Diffuse

Extent of Optic Nerve Invasion

___ Cannot be determined
___ None
___ Anterior to lamina cribrosa
___ At lamina cribrosa
___ Posterior to lamina cribrosa but not to end of nerve
___ To cut end of optic nerve

Histologic Grade

___ pGX: Grade cannot be assessed
___ pG1: Well differentiated
___ pG2: Moderately differentiated
___ pG3: Poorly differentiated
___ pG4: Undifferentiated

Margins (select all that apply)

___ Cannot be assessed
___ No tumor at margins
___ Tumor present at surgical margin of optic nerve
___ Extrascleral extension (for enucleation specimens)
___ Other margin(s) involved (specify): ____________________________

Pathologic Staging (pTNM)

TNM descriptors (required only if applicable) (select all that apply)
    ___ m (multiple primary tumors)
    ___ r (recurrent)
    ___ y (post-treatment)

Primary tumor (pT)
    ___ pTx: Primary tumor cannot be assessed
    ___ pT0: No evidence of primary tumor
    ___ pT1: Tumor confined to the eye with no optic nerve or choroidal invasion
    ___ pT2: Tumor with minimal optic nerve &/or choroidal invasion

PROTOCOL FOR RETINOBLASTOMA TUMOR SPECIMENS

____ pT2a: Tumor superficially invades optic nerve head but does not extend past lamina cribrosa **or** tumor exhibits focal choroidal invasion

____ pT2b: Tumor superficially invades optic nerve head but does not extend past lamina cribrosa **and** exhibits focal choroidal invasion

____ pT3: Tumor with significant optic nerve &/or choroidal invasion

____ pT3a: Tumor invades optic nerve past lamina cribrosa but not to surgical resection line **or** tumor exhibits massive choroidal invasion

____ pT3b: Tumor invades optic nerve past lamina cribrosa but not to surgical resection line **and** exhibits massive choroidal invasion

____ pT4: Tumor invades optic nerve to resection line or exhibits extraocular extension elsewhere

____ pT4a: Tumor invades optic nerve to resection line but no extraocular extension identified

____ pT4b: Tumor invades optic nerve to resection line and extraocular extension identified

Regional lymph nodes (pN)

____ pNX: Regional lymph nodes cannot be assessed

____ pN0: No regional lymph node involvement

____ pN1: Regional lymph node involvement (preauricular, cervical, submandibular)

____ pN2: Distant lymph node involvement

Distant metastasis (pM)

____ Not applicable

____ pM1: Metastasis to sites other than CNS

____ pM1a: Single lesion

____ pM1b: Multiple lesions

____ pM1c: CNS metastasis

____ pM1d: Discrete mass(es) without leptomeningeal &/or CSF involvement

____ pM1e: Leptomeningeal &/or CSF involvement

**Additional Pathologic Findings (select all that apply)*

*____None identified

*____Calcifications

*____Mitotic rate: Number of mitoses per 40x objective with a field area of 1.152 mm² (specify): _________

*____Apoptosis

*____Basophilic vascular deposits

*____Inflammatory cells

*____Hemorrhage

*____Neovascularization (specify site): ___________________________

*____Other (specify): ___________________________

Data elements with asterisks are not required. These elements may be clinically important but are not yet validated or regularly used in patient management. Adapted with permission from College of American Pathologists, "Protocol for the Examination of Specimens from Patients with Retinoblastoma." Web posting date February 2011, www.cap.org.

Major Salivary Glands

Incisional Biopsy, Excisional Biopsy, Resection

Specimen (select all that apply)

___ Parotid gland

  ___ Superficial lobe only

  ___ Deep lobe only

  ___ Total parotid gland

___ Submandibular gland

___ Sublingual gland

Received

___ Fresh

___ In formalin

___ Other (specify): ____________________________

Procedure (select all that apply)

___ Incisional biopsy

___ Excisional biopsy

___ Resection, parotid gland

  ___ Superficial parotidectomy

  ___ Total parotidectomy

___ Resection, submandibular gland

___ Resection, sublingual gland

___ Neck (lymph node) dissection (specify): ____________________________

___ Other (specify): ____________________________

___ Not specified

****Specimen Integrity***

*___ Intact

*___ Fragmented

Specimen Size

Greatest dimensions: _________ x _________ x ________ cm

*Additional dimensions (if more than 1 part): _________ x _________ x _________ cm

Specimen Laterality

___ Right

___ Left

___ Bilateral

___ Not specified

Tumor Site (select all that apply)

___ Parotid gland

  ___ Superficial lobe

  ___ Deep lobe

  ___ Entire parotid gland

___ Submandibular gland

___ Sublingual gland

___ Other (specify): ____________________________

___ Not specified

Tumor Focality

___ Single focus

___ Bilateral

___ Multifocal (specify): ____________________________

Tumor Size

Greatest dimension: _________ cm

*Additional dimensions: _________ x _________ cm

PROTOCOL FOR SALIVARY GLAND TUMOR SPECIMENS

___ Cannot be determined

Tumor Description (select all that apply)

*___ Encapsulated/circumscribed
*___ Invasive
*___ Solid
*___ Cystic
*___ Other (specify): ___________________________

Macroscopic Extent of Tumor (extent of invasion)

*Specify: ___________________________

Histologic Type (select all that apply)

___ Acinic cell carcinoma
___ Adenoid cystic carcinoma
___ Adenocarcinoma, not otherwise specified (NOS)
  ___ Low grade
  ___ Intermediate grade
  ___ High grade
___ Basal cell adenocarcinoma
___ Carcinoma ex pleomorphic adenoma (malignant mixed tumor)
  ___ Grade
    ___ Low grade
    ___ High grade
  ___ Invasion
    ___ Intracapsular (noninvasive)
    ___ Minimally invasive
    ___ Invasive
___ Carcinosarcoma (true malignant mixed tumor)
___ Clear cell adenocarcinoma
___ Cystadenocarcinoma
___ Epithelial-myoepithelial carcinoma
___ Large cell carcinoma
___ Low-grade cribriform cystadenocarcinoma
___ Lymphoepithelial carcinoma
___ Metastasizing pleomorphic adenoma
___ Mucoepidermoid carcinoma
  ___ Low grade
  ___ Intermediate grade
  ___ High grade
___ Mucinous adenocarcinoma (colloid carcinoma)
___ Myoepithelial carcinoma (malignant myoepithelioma)
___ Oncocytic carcinoma
___ Polymorphous low-grade adenocarcinoma
___ Salivary duct carcinoma
___ Sebaceous adenocarcinomas
  ___ Sebaceous adenocarcinoma
  ___ Sebaceous lymphadenocarcinoma
___ Sialoblastoma
___ Small cell (neuroendocrine) carcinoma
___ Squamous cell carcinoma, primary
___ Undifferentiated carcinoma, large cell type
___ Other (specify): ___________________________
___ Carcinoma, type cannot be determined

Histologic Grade

___ Not applicable

___ GX: Cannot be assessed
___ G1: Well differentiated
___ G2: Moderately differentiated
___ G3: Poorly differentiated
___ Other (specify): ___

*Microscopic Tumor Extension

*Specify: ___

Margins

___ Cannot be assessed
___ Margins uninvolved by carcinoma
Distance of tumor from closest margin: ___ mm or ___ cm
Specify margin, if possible: ___
___ Margin(s) involved by carcinoma
Specify margin(s), if possible: ___

*Treatment Effect (applicable to carcinomas treated with neoadjuvant therapy)

*___ Not identified
*___ Present (specify): ___
*___ Indeterminate

Lymph-Vascular Invasion

___ Not identified
___ Present
___ Indeterminate

Perineural Invasion

___ Not identified
___ Present
___ Indeterminate

Lymph Nodes, Extranodal Extension

___ Not identified
___ Present
___ Indeterminate

Pathologic Staging (pTNM)

TNM descriptors (required only if applicable) (select all that apply)
___ m (multiple primary tumors)
___ r (recurrent)
___ y (post-treatment)

Primary tumor (pT)†
___ pTX: Cannot be assessed
___ pT0: No evidence of primary disease
___ pT1: Tumor ≤ 2 cm in greatest dimension **without extraparenchymal extension**
___ pT2: Tumor > 2 cm but ≤ 4 cm in greatest dimension **without extraparenchymal extension**
___ pT3: Tumor > 4 cm &/or tumor **with extraparenchymal extension**
___ pT4a: Moderately advanced tumor
Tumor invades skin, mandible, ear canal, &/or facial nerve
___ pT4b: Very advanced local disease
Tumor invades skull base &/or pterygoid plates &/or encases carotid artery

Regional lymph nodes (pN)#
___ pNX: Cannot be assessed
___ pN0: No regional lymph node metastasis
___ pN1: Metastasis in single ipsilateral lymph node, ≤ 3 cm in greatest dimension
None > 6 cm in greatest dimension, or in bilateral or contralateral lymoph nodes, none > 6 cm in greatest dimension
___ pN2a: Metastasis in single ipsilateral lymph node, > 3 cm but ≤ 6 cm in greatest dimension
___ pN2b: Metastasis in multiple ipsilateral lymph nodes, none > 6 cm in greatest dimension

PROTOCOL FOR SALIVARY GLAND TUMOR SPECIMENS

____ pN2c: Metastasis in bilateral or contralateral lymph nodes, none > 6 cm in greatest dimension

____ pN3: Metastasis in lymph node, > 6 cm in greatest dimension

____ No nodes submitted or found

Number of lymph nodes examined

Specify: __________

____ Number cannot be determined (explain): ______________________________

Number of lymph nodes involved

Specify: __________

____ Number cannot be determined (explain): ______________________________

* Size (greatest dimension) of largest positive lymph node: __________

Distant metastasis (pM)

____ Not applicable

____ pM1: Distant metastasis

*Specify site(s), if known: ______________________________

**Additional Pathologic Findings (select all that apply)*

*____ Sialadenitis

*____ Tumor-associated lymphoid proliferation (TALP)

*____ Other (specify): ______________________________

**Ancillary Studies*

*Specify type(s): ______________________________

*Specify result(s): ______________________________

**Clinical History (select all that apply)*

*____ Neoadjuvant therapy

*____ Yes (specify type): ______________________________

*____ No

*____ Indeterminate

*____ Other (specify): ______________________________

**Data elements with asterisks are not required. These elements may be clinically important but are not yet validated or regularly used in patient management. †There is no category of carcinoma in situ (pTis) relative to carcinomas of salivary glands (major, minor). #Superior mediastinal lymph nodes are considered regional lymph nodes (level VII). Midline nodes are considered ipsilateral nodes. Adapted with permission from College of American Pathologists, "Protocol for the Examination of Specimens from Patients with Carcinomas of the Salivary Glands." Web posting date February 2011, www.cap.org.*

Respiratory

Neoplasm, Benign

PLEUROPULMONARY BLASTOMA

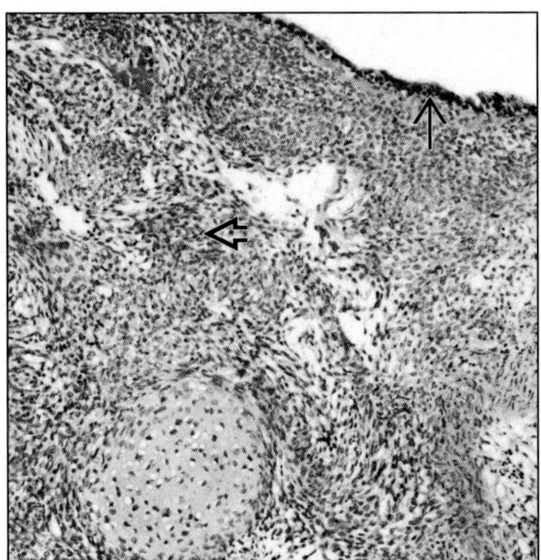

This low-power view of solid type III PPB shows benign epithelial component at upper right ⇒ overlying the malignant mesenchymal component ⇨.

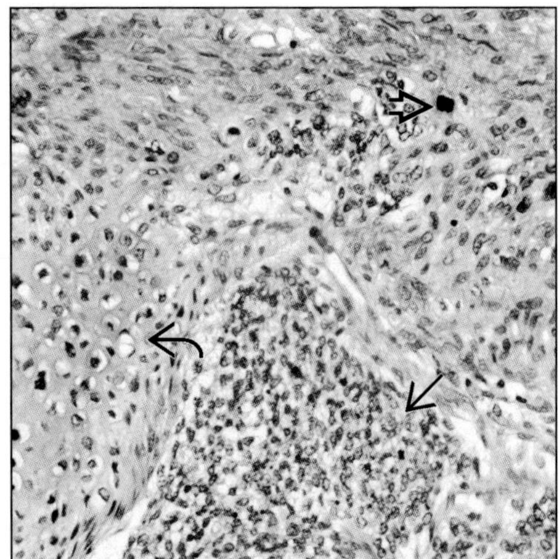

Solid component of PPB illustrated here consists of malignant cartilage ⇗, blastema ⇒, and spindle cell undifferentiated sarcoma with atypical mitotic figure ⇨.

TERMINOLOGY

Abbreviations

- Pleuropulmonary blastoma (PPB)

Synonyms

- Mesenchymal cystic hamartoma, malignant mesenchymoma, sarcoma arising in congenital cystic malformation

Definitions

- Embryonal tumor of lung and pleura with epithelial (benign) and mesenchymal (low- to high-grade malignant) components, presenting most often in early childhood

ETIOLOGY/PATHOGENESIS

Genetic Abnormality

- 20% are familial and associated with other extrapulmonary lesions in same patient or family members
- Extrapulmonary lesions include cystic nephroma (most common), rhabdomyosarcoma, and other embryonal tumors
- Variety of karyotypic abnormalities have been described; gain of chromosome 8, usually as trisomy 8, is very common
- Heterozygous germline mutations in *DICER1* have been identified in familial PPB
- Loss of DICER1 protein expression specifically in lung epithelium overlying mesenchymal component
- Loss of DICER1 in developing lung epithelium alters miRNA-dependent regulation of diffusible growth factors that promote mesenchymal cell proliferation
- Thus PPB may arise through a novel mechanism of non-cell-autonomous cancer initiation

CLINICAL ISSUES

Epidemiology

- Incidence
  - Extremely rare tumor, estimated incidence of 0.35-0.65 cases per 100,000 births
  - Most common malignancy of lung presenting in early childhood
- Age
  - Occurs almost exclusively in children, primarily in infants and toddlers, rare beyond 12 years of age
    - 94% present in children < 6 years old

Presentation

- Most common presentation is respiratory distress with or without pneumothorax
- May be detected incidentally in utero or postnatally
- May be solitary or multiple with additional lesions occurring synchronously or metachronously

Treatment

- Depends on type of PPB
- PPB I (cystic): Complete surgical resection; adjuvant chemotherapy if resection is incomplete
- PPB II (cystic and solid) and PPB III (solid): Complete surgical resection followed by adjuvant chemotherapy; radiation therapy for residual disease
- Close clinical follow-up for recurrence, metastasis, multifocal lesions, extrapulmonary lesions

Prognosis

- 5-year survival is 83% for type I and 42% for types II and III PPB
- Type I may recur as higher grade (II or III) lesions
- Metastases occur in 30% of types II and III lesions and may occur late
- Sites of metastases include central nervous system and bone

PLEUROPULMONARY BLASTOMA

Key Facts

Terminology

- Embryonal tumor of lung and pleura with epithelial (benign) and mesenchymal (low- to high-grade malignant) components, presenting most often in early childhood

Etiology/Pathogenesis

- 20% are familial and associated with other extrapulmonary lesions in same patient or family members
- Heterozygous germline mutations in *DICER1* have been identified in familial PPB

Macroscopic Features

- Type I: Peripheral- and pleural-based cysts, sometimes protruding from pleural surface, no solid nodules
- Type II: Both solid and cystic areas in varying proportions
- Type III: All solid, although areas of necrosis and cystic degeneration may be present

Microscopic Pathology

- PPB type I: Large cysts lined by single layer of cuboidal to flattened benign epithelium; within wall there are areas of hypercellularity composed of small blue to spindled cells, often forming cambium-like layer
- PPB types II and III have variable amount of solid areas composed of higher grade sarcomatous components (which may be undifferentiated), rhabdomyosarcomatous, or chondrosarcomatous

IMAGE FINDINGS

General Features

- Best diagnostic clue
  - Radiographically seen as unilocular or multilocular cyst, mixed cystic or solid lesion, or large solid mass often distorting contour of lung, located in periphery or protruding from pleura

MACROSCOPIC FEATURES

Subclassification

- Based on gross morphology
- Type I: Purely cystic
- Type II: Solid and cystic
- Type III: Purely solid

Gross Features

- Type I: Peripheral- and pleural-based cysts, sometimes protruding from pleural surface, no solid nodules
- Type II: Both solid and cystic areas in varying proportions
- Type III: All solid, although areas of necrosis and cystic degeneration may be present

MICROSCOPIC PATHOLOGY

Histologic Features

- PPB type I: Large cysts lined by single layer of cuboidal to flattened benign epithelium; within wall there are areas of hypercellularity composed of small blue to spindled cells, often forming cambium-like layer
- PPB types II and III have variable amount of solid areas composed of higher grade sarcomatous (which may be undifferentiated), rhabdomyosarcomatous, or chondrosarcomatous components
- Primitive/sarcomatous component is vimentin positive; may be focal myogenic differentiation on IHC staining

DIFFERENTIAL DIAGNOSIS

Congenital Pulmonary Airway Malformation Type 4 (CPAM 4)

- PPB type I has areas very similar to CPAM 4; however, latter has no immature/malignant component
- Cytogenetically, these are completely different lesions

Primary Sarcomas of Lung

- Synovial sarcoma can be distinguished by being focally keratin(+) and EMA(+) and diagnostic t(X;18) translocation
- Primary rhabdomyosarcoma of lung is very rare; many cases reported in the older literature are probably PPB type III

DIAGNOSTIC CHECKLIST

Pathologic Interpretation Pearls

- Cystic lesions need to be sampled extensively to differentiate benign CPAM 4 from low-grade malignant PPB I
- PPB I may recur as PPB II or III
- Margins of resection must be assessed

SELECTED REFERENCES

1. Hill DA et al: DICER1 mutations in familial pleuropulmonary blastoma. Science. 325(5943):965, 2009
2. Priest JR et al: Pulmonary cysts in early childhood and the risk of malignancy. Pediatr Pulmonol. 44(1):14-30, 2009
3. Dishop MK et al: Primary and metastatic lung tumors in the pediatric population: a review and 25-year experience at a large children's hospital. Arch Pathol Lab Med. 132(7):1079-103, 2008
4. Hill DA et al: Type I pleuropulmonary blastoma: pathology and biology study of 51 cases from the international pleuropulmonary blastoma registry. Am J Surg Pathol. 32(2):282-95, 2008
5. Taube JM et al: Pleuropulmonary blastoma: cytogenetic and spectral karyotype analysis. Pediatr Dev Pathol. 9(6):453-61, 2006

Types of Pleuropulmonary Blastoma

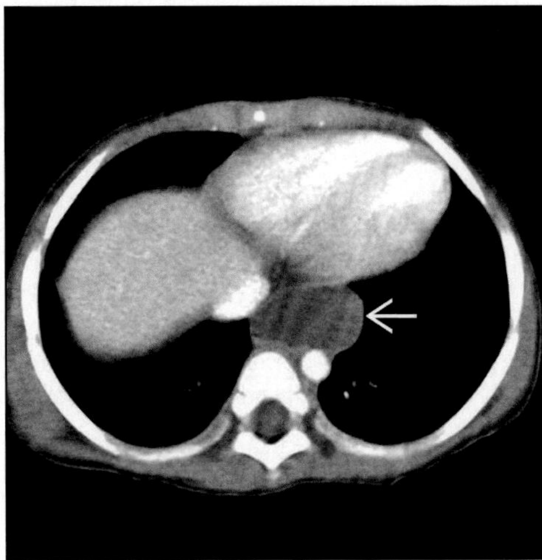

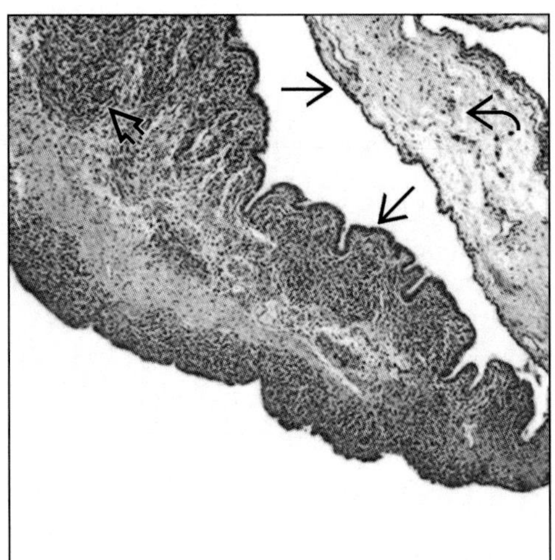

(Left) *Type I PPB: CT scan of chest shows a pleural-based cystic lesion with no solid component. (Courtesy B. Shehata, MD.)* ***(Right)*** *This histologic section from a type I PPB shows the diagnostic cystic spaces lined by a single layer of epithelium. The walls contain densely cellular (blastomatous) tumor as well as loose hypocellular tissue. (Courtesy B. Shehata, MD.)*

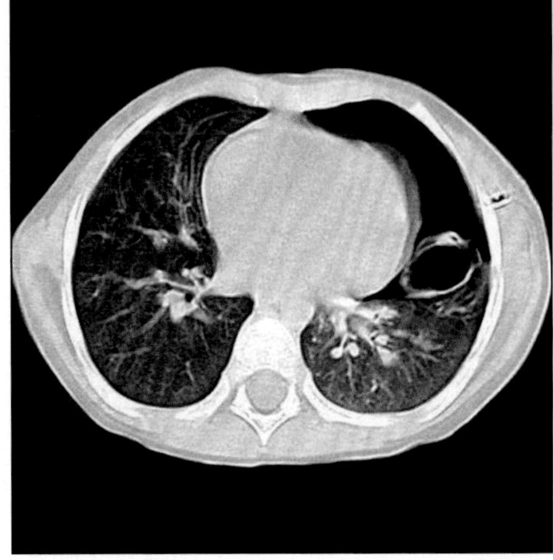

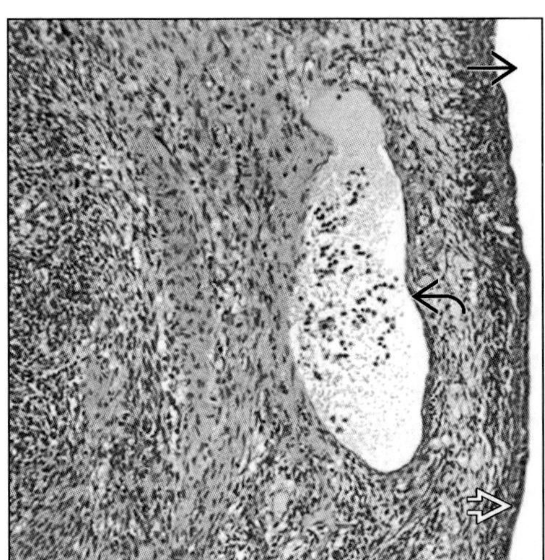

(Left) *CT scan of type II PPB shows a large cyst in the center of the left lung field, with some solid component in its wall. Part of the lung is collapsed. (Courtesy B. Shehata, MD.)* ***(Right)*** *This histologic section of a type II PPB has cystic space to the right, which is lined by a single layer of cuboidal cells, beneath which is the solid cellular component of the tumor composed of primitive cells. In addition, there is a smaller cyst. (Courtesy B. Shehata, MD.)*

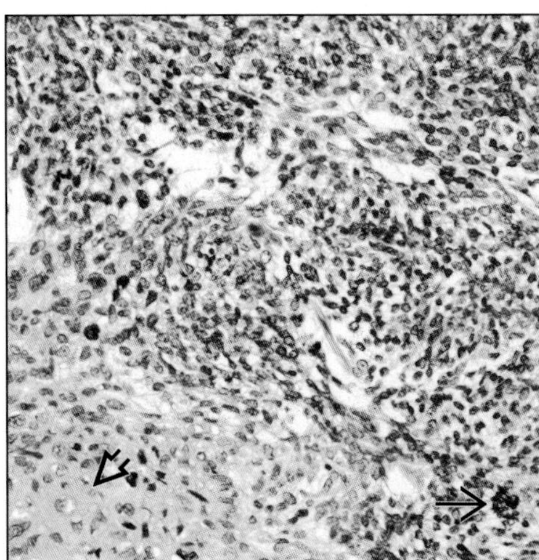

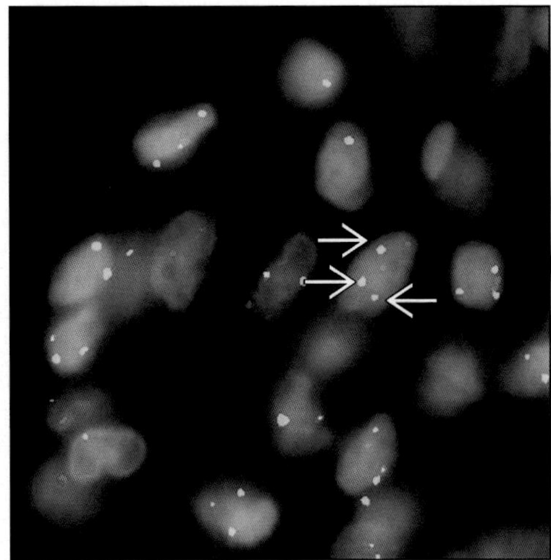

(Left) *High-power photomicrograph of a type III PPB shows a solid proliferation of malignant cells without any cyst formation. There is a blastomatous small cell component as well as focal cartilaginous differentiation. Note the atypical mitotic figure.* ***(Right)*** *FISH shows trisomy 8 (green dots) in many of the tumor cells of this pleuropulmonary blastoma. There is no evidence of trisomy 18 (red dots). (Courtesy B. Shehata, MD.)*

Differential Diagnosis

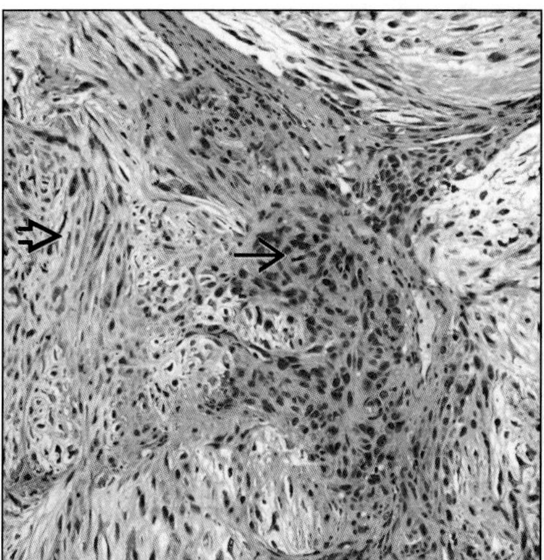

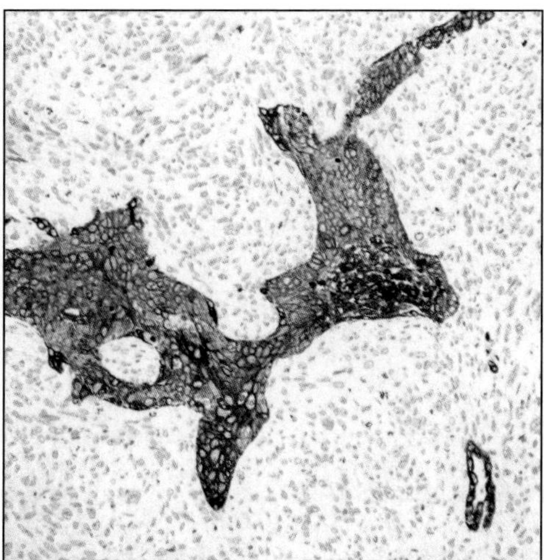

(Left) *This section of a carcinosarcoma, although extremely rare in children, shows the malignant epithelial ⇒ and sarcomatoid ⇨ components (in contrast to PPB, which shows only a malignant "sarcomatoid" component). The former forms irregular sheets of atypical cells while the latter is composed of spindles cells with myxoid stroma.* ***(Right)*** *This IHC stain with keratin AE1/AE3 shows strong staining of the epithelial component while the spindle cell component is negative.*

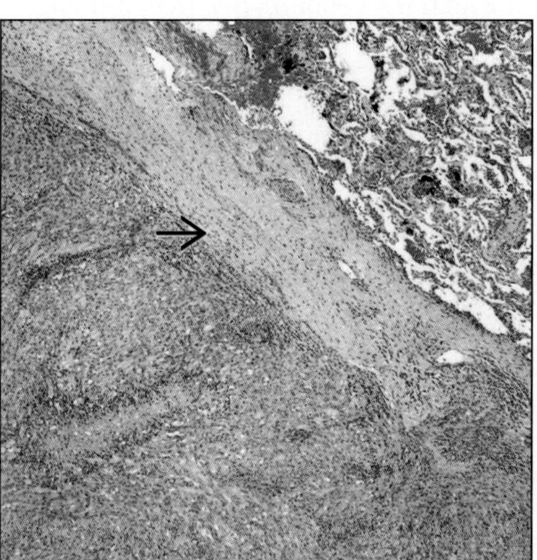

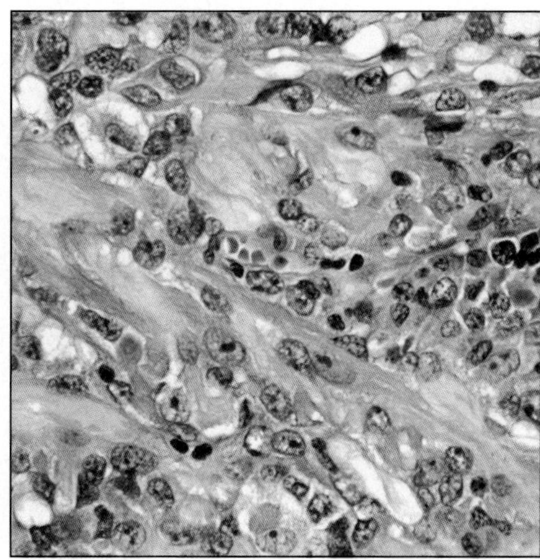

(Left) *This low-power view of rhabdomyosarcoma shows a cellular tumor involving the pulmonary artery (residual artery is seen in the middle ⇒) with uninvolved lung on the top right.* ***(Right)*** *This high-power view of rhabdomyosarcoma of the pulmonary artery shows a high-grade solid tumor, composed of dysplastic cells, some of which are spindled. The nuclei are vesicular and have prominent nucleoli.*

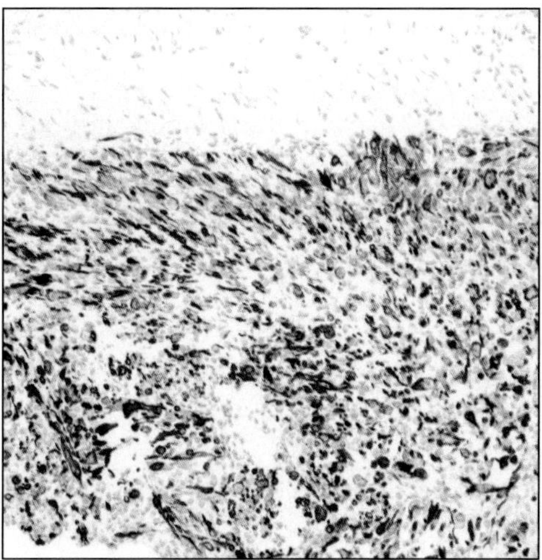

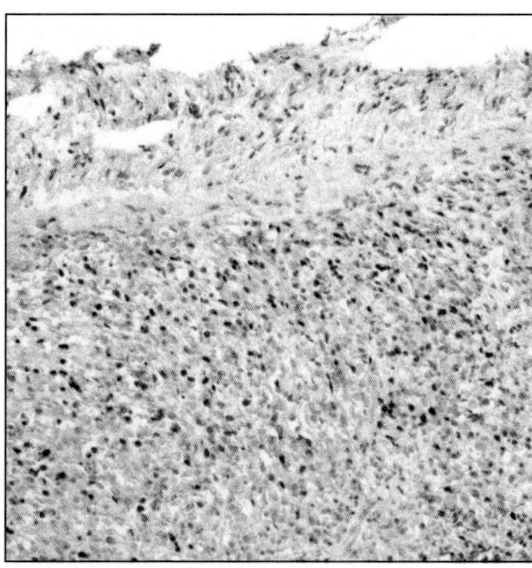

(Left) *IHC stain for desmin shows strong cytoplasmic staining of tumor cells in this rhabdomyosarcoma.* ***(Right)*** *IHC stain for myogenin in this rhabdomyosarcoma of pulmonary artery shows nuclear positivity in many of the tumor cells; thus, this is most consistent with embryonal rhabdomyosarcoma.*

LARYNGOTRACHEAL PAPILLOMATOSIS

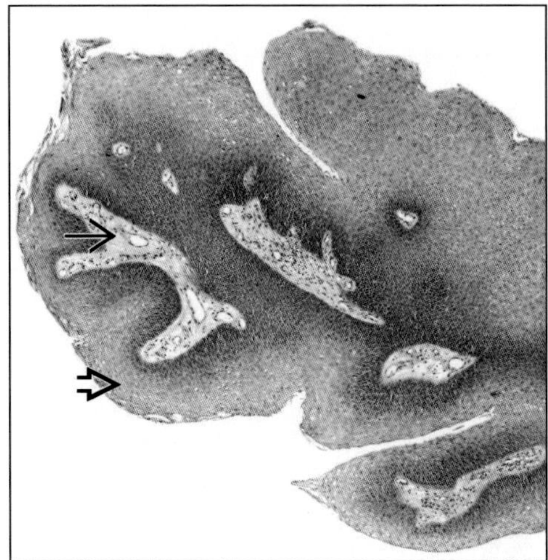

Low-power photomicrograph shows the typical appearance of a squamous papilloma removed through a laryngoscope. The fibrovascular core ➔ is covered by a multilayered squamous epithelium ➔.

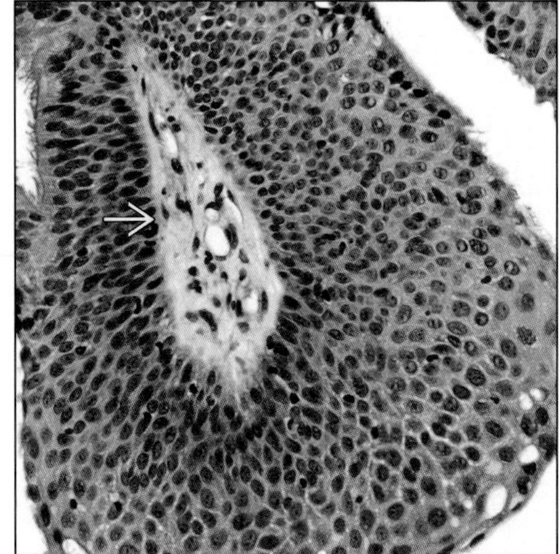

High-power view of a squamous papilloma shows the central slender fibrovascular core ➔ covered by multiple layers of squamous epithelium. Note the increasing maturation toward the surface.

TERMINOLOGY

Synonyms

- Laryngeal papillomatosis, recurrent respiratory papillomatosis

Definitions

- Multiple squamous papillomas, usually in larynx, occasionally extending into trachea and bronchi, caused by human papillomavirus (HPV) infection

ETIOLOGY/PATHOGENESIS

Infectious Agents

- Human papillomaviruses types 6 and 11 are associated with lesions
- HPV-11 infection is reported to be associated with more aggressive spread of lesions

CLINICAL ISSUES

Epidemiology

- Incidence
  - Most common benign epithelial tumors of larynx
- Age
  - Bimodal age distribution; 1st peak before 5 years (juvenile form), and 2nd peak at 20-40 years of age (adult form)
- Gender
  - Juvenile form has no gender difference
  - Adult form has 3:2 male predominance
- Ethnicity
  - Distribution is worldwide

Presentation

- Usually presents in childhood but may present in infancy or early adulthood
  - Less likely to occur in adults
- Lesions limited to larynx in majority of cases
  - Extension through tracheobronchial tree into lung occurs in 5%
- Symptoms include hoarseness, inspiratory stridor, and rarely respiratory obstruction
- In children, tend to grow rapidly and recur repeatedly after surgery
  - Adult laryngeal papillomas are usually self-limiting
- Spontaneous regression may occur at puberty
- Rarely spread to lungs and give rise to infiltrating squamous cell carcinoma

Treatment

- Endoscopic surgical resections

Prognosis

- Clinical course is unpredictable, with periods of active disease and remissions
- Most common extralaryngeal spread is to oral cavity, followed by trachea and bronchi
- Extralaryngeal spread occurs in 30% of children and about 15% of adults
- Endobronchial and pulmonary dissemination occurs in 5% of patients
- Onset in neonatal period is associated with poor prognosis, with greater need for tracheotomy and likelihood of death
- No histological features correlate with prognosis
- Irradiation increases the risk of cancer development

Route of Infection

- HPV is transmitted to child from maternal genital infection during vaginal delivery
- Cesarian section does not completely prevent infection

MACROSCOPIC FEATURES

General Features

- Grape-like excrescences, typically involving larynx
- Exophytic, branching, pedunculated, or sessile masses

Key Facts

Terminology
- Multiple squamous papillomas, usually in larynx, occasionally extending into trachea and bronchi, caused by human papillomavirus (HPV) infection

Etiology/Pathogenesis
- Human papillomaviruses types 6 and 11 are associated with lesions

Clinical Issues
- Most common benign epithelial tumors of larynx
- Bimodal age distribution; 1st peak before 5 years (juvenile form), and 2nd peak at 20-40 years of age (adult form)
- In children, tend to grow rapidly and recur repeatedly after surgery
- Treatment: Endoscopic surgical resections
- Clinical course is unpredictable, with periods of active disease and remissions
- Onset in neonatal period is associated with poor prognosis, with a greater need for tracheotomy and likelihood of death
- No histological features correlate with prognosis

Macroscopic Features
- Generally small lesions, 1-5 mm

Microscopic Pathology
- Finger-like or frond-like projections of squamous mucosa containing thin fibrovascular cores
- Viral changes such as koilocytes and binucleation can be seen
- Dysplasia is rarely seen and should be reported

- Pink or red with finely lobulated surface

Sections to Be Submitted
- Multiple sections need to be taken when there is extralaryngeal spread, especially when lung is involved

Size
- Generally small lesions, 1-5 mm

Endoscopic Appearance
- Pedunculated tan-white polypoid excrescences in mucosa of airway, with variable compromise of its lumen
- Surfaces of lesions may be smooth or slightly verrucoid
- Lesions bleed with minor trauma

MICROSCOPIC PATHOLOGY

Histologic Features
- Finger-like or frond-like projections of squamous mucosa containing thin fibrovascular cores
- Basal cell hyperplasia is usually present, extending up to middle 1/3 of epithelium
- Maturation of squamous epithelium toward surface
- Viral changes (koilocytes, binucleation) can be seen in upper portion of epithelium
- Mitoses (usually in basal or parabasal cells) and dyskeratotic cells may be present
- Only minimal keratinization is present
- Dysplasia is rarely seen and should be reported

DIFFERENTIAL DIAGNOSIS

Verrucous Carcinoma
- Thicker squamous fronds with marked keratosis
- Invasion seen as blunt pushing edge

Papillary Squamous Cell Carcinoma
- Architecturally similar to papillomatosis but cytologically malignant

DIAGNOSTIC CHECKLIST

Clinically Relevant Pathologic Features
- Histologic features do not predict recurrence or malignant transformation
  - Smoking and irradiation are risk factors for malignant transformation
  - Repeated recurrences are thought to be due to virus reservoir in normal-appearing mucosa

Pathologic Interpretation Pearls
- Papillomas have very characteristic appearance, which tends to remain the same despite multiple recurrences
- DNA aneuploidy and Ki-67 proliferative index may predict disease recurrence and extension; however, these are not performed routinely

SELECTED REFERENCES

1. Lin HW et al: Malignant transformation of a highly aggressive human papillomavirus type 11-associated recurrent respiratory papillomatosis. Am J Otolaryngol. 31(4):291-6, 2010
2. Martins RH et al: Laryngeal papillomatosis: morphological study by light and electron microscopy of the HPV-6. Braz J Otorhinolaryngol. 74(4):539-43, 2008
3. Stephen JK et al: An epigenetically derived monoclonal origin for recurrent respiratory papillomatosis. Arch Otolaryngol Head Neck Surg. 133(7):684-92, 2007
4. Coope G et al: Juvenile laryngeal papillomatosis. Prim Care Respir J. 15(2):125-7, 2006
5. Manjarrez ME et al: Detection of human papillomavirus and relevant tumor suppressors and oncoproteins in laryngeal tumors. Clin Cancer Res. 12(23):6946-51, 2006

LARYNGOTRACHEAL PAPILLOMATOSIS

Microscopic Features

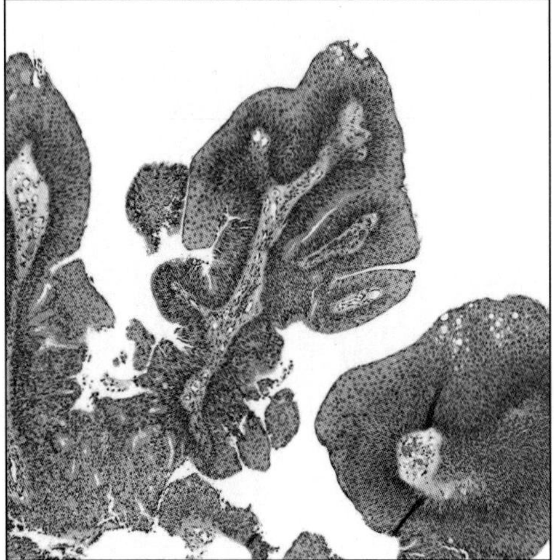
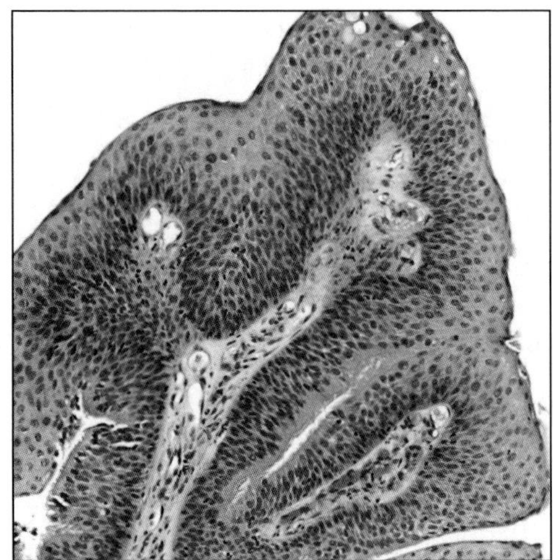

(Left) *Low-power view shows the characteristic papillary projections in this squamous papilloma removed from a 3 year old who had multiple such surgeries in the past 2 years. There are several papillary projections with branching cores covered by epithelium, which is fairly uniform in thickness. Note the tangential cut in the lower right corner. No submucosa is present.* ***(Right)*** *Intermediate-power photomicrograph shows maturing squamous epithelium covering the fibrovascular cores.*

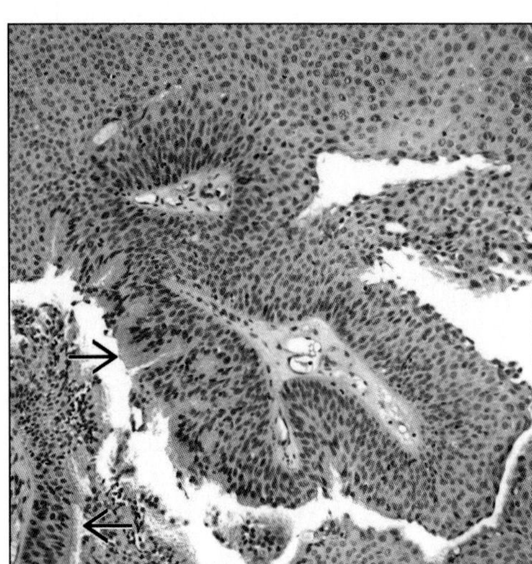
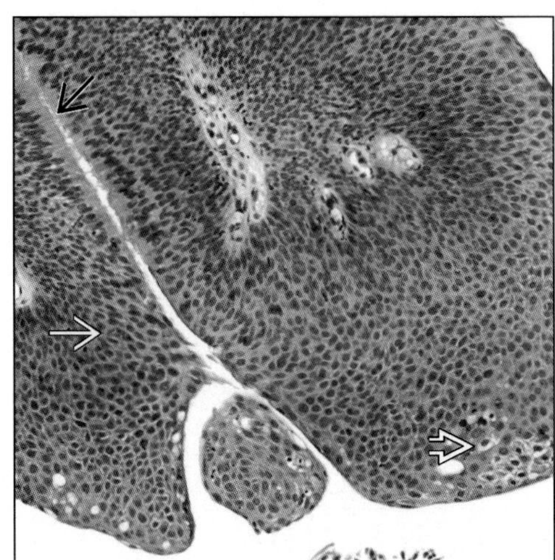

(Left) *Intermediate-power view shows the typical stratified squamous epithelium with surface maturation. Note the foci of residual respiratory-type epithelium.* ***(Right)*** *This photomicrograph highlights the transition between respiratory and squamous epithelium. There is some variation in nuclear size in the squamous epithelium with koilocytes near the surface. Note the delicate fibrovascular core containing capillaries and minimal chronic inflammation.*

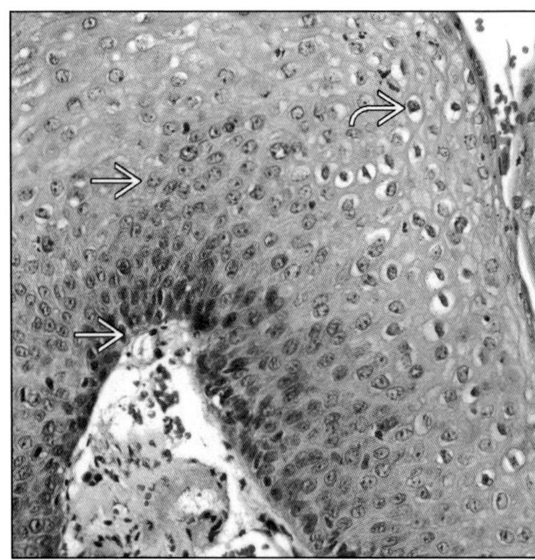
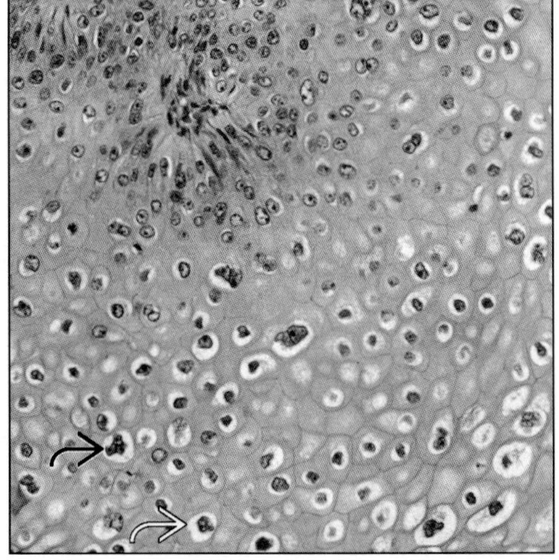

(Left) *High-power image shows thickened basal layers in the lower 1/3 of the squamous epithelium lining the papilloma. The upper layers show koilocytosis with occasional binucleated cells.* ***(Right)*** *High-power image shows an area of a papilloma with marked koilocytosis (irregular hyperchromatic nuclei and perinuclear halos) indicating human papilloma virus infection as the etiology of the lesion. Note the lack of inflammation and mitosis.*

Differential Diagnosis

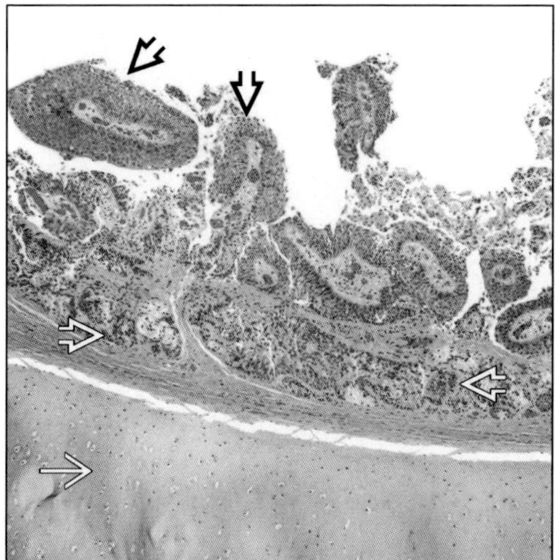

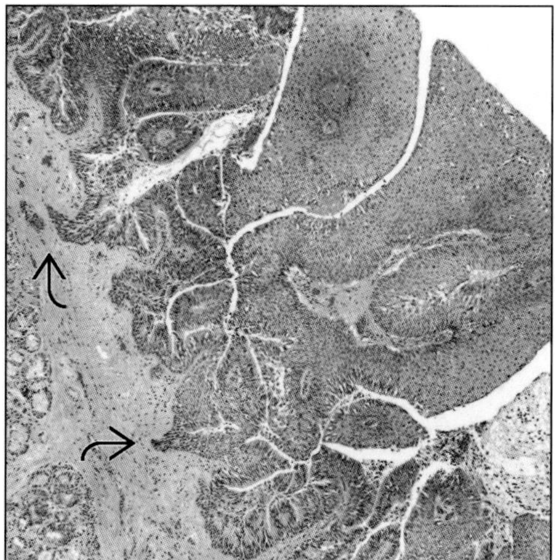

(Left) *This image is from a 12 year old with a long history of multiple laryngotracheal papillomas that were resected over the last 10 years. Section of the trachea shows multiple squamous papillomas ⇨, bronchial glands ➡, and cartilage ➡.* ***(Right)*** *Intermediate-power image shows thick dysplastic basal epithelium with areas suspicious for early invasive squamous cell carcinoma ↗. Bronchial glands are to the left in this field.*

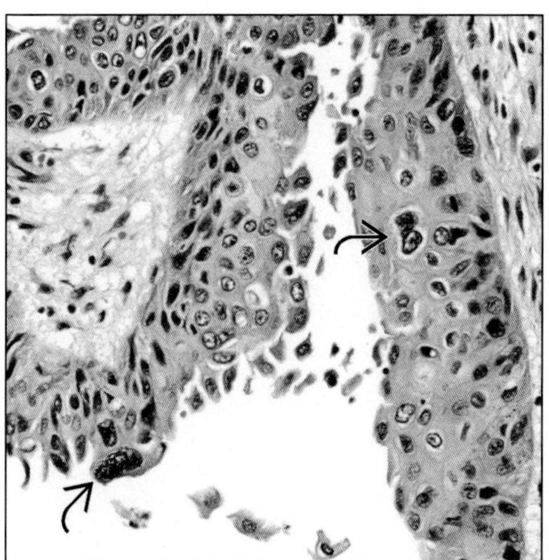

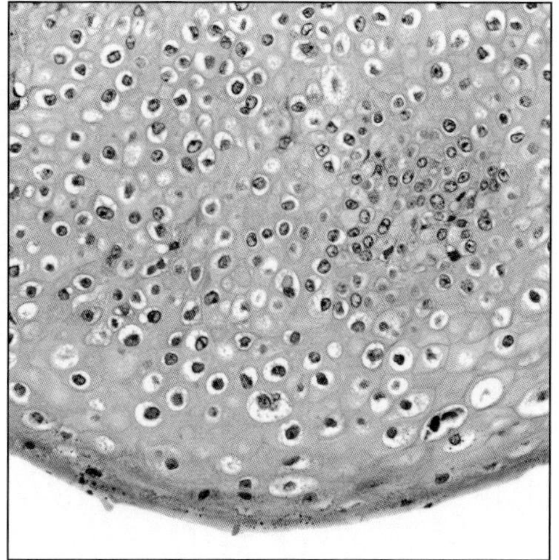

(Left) *High-power image shows markedly dysplastic squamous mucosa lining the papillomas in this area. Note full thickness dysplasia with enlarged, hyperchromatic, and irregular nuclei ↗.* ***(Right)*** *Intermediate-power image from the same patient shows prominent koilocytosis. Comparison of several areas from this lesion showed marked progression from benign to severe dysplasia/carcinoma in situ as seen on the left image, emphasizing the importance of adequate sampling of these lesions.*

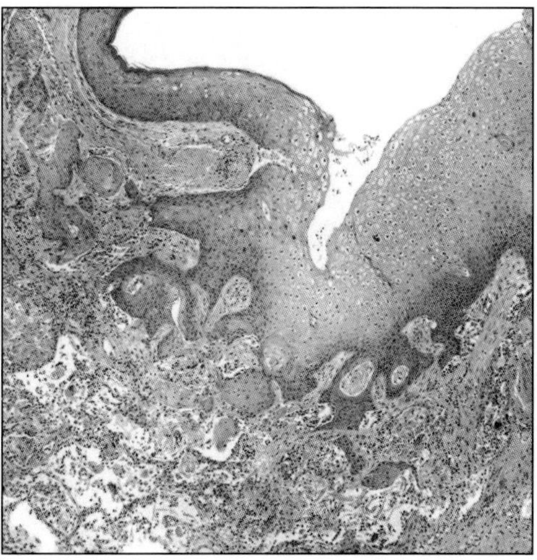

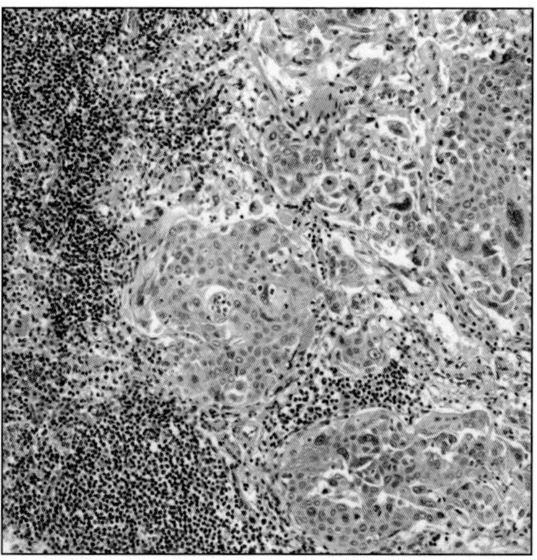

(Left) *This section of lung shows well-differentiated squamous cell carcinoma, which was found at autopsy. The image shows a cystic space formed by the carcinoma, which is invading into the underlying lung tissue.* ***(Right)*** *Intermediate-power image shows metastatic squamous cell carcinoma in a lymph node from a patient (at autopsy). The carcinoma, as seen here, is a rare complication of recurrent papillomatosis.*

Mediastinum

Neoplasm, Benign

Neoplasm, Malignant Primary

CYSTIC TERATOMA OF THE HEART

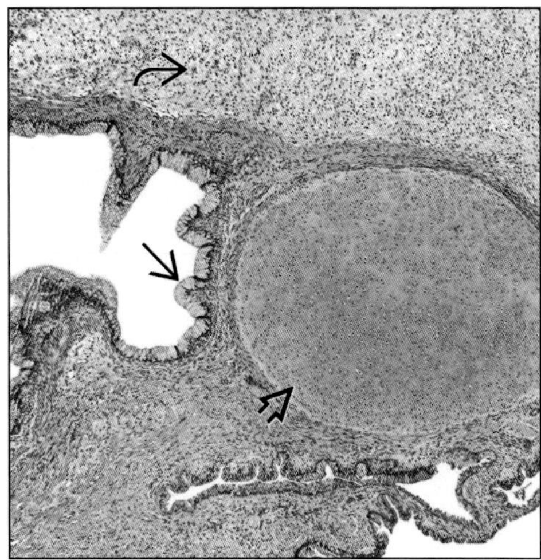

Low-power photomicrograph of a teratoma of the heart in a newborn shows cysts lined by epithelium ➔, a nodule of cartilage ➔, and neural tissue ➔. The patient had presented with a large tumor.

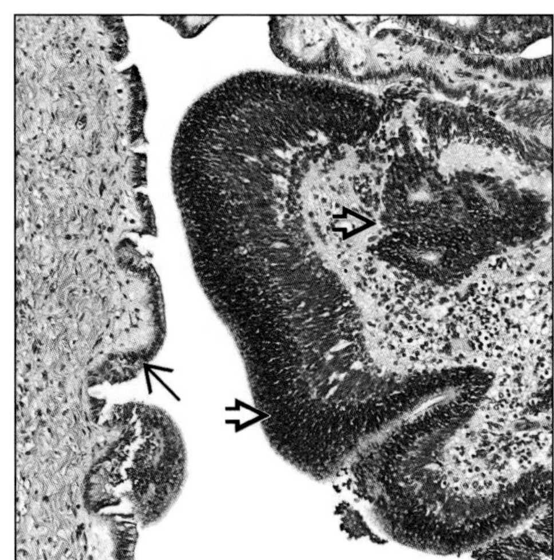

A cystic teratoma of the heart with mature epithelium ➔ and immature neural tissue ➔ is shown here at intermediate power.

TERMINOLOGY

Synonyms

- Immature teratoma, germ cell tumor

Definitions

- Tumor composed of all 3 germ cell layers: Ectoderm, mesoderm, and endoderm

CLINICAL ISSUES

Epidemiology

- Incidence
  - Rare cardiac and pericardial tumor
  - 2nd most common cardiac tumor in fetus and neonate, after rhabdomyoma

Site

- Much more common in pericardium; rarely intracardiac

Presentation

- Typically presents in newborn
- May be diagnosed in utero by ultrasound
- Symptoms are due to mass effect of tumor or fluid in pericardial space
- May be fetal hydrops or stillbirth
- Neonate presents with respiratory difficulty, cyanosis, &/or congestive heart failure
- If pericardial effusion is large, there may be cardiac tamponade

Treatment

- Surgical resection of tumor
- Intrapericardial tumors are resected easily
- Intracardiac teratomas are often unresectable

Prognosis

- Depends on size and resectability
- Recurrences have been reported
- Malignant transformation, although rare, caries a poor prognosis

IMAGE FINDINGS

Echocardiographic Findings

- Heterogeneous and encapsulated mass
- Tumors in pericardial cavity are commonly attached to pulmonary artery and aorta
- Intracardiac tumors arise from atrial or ventricular wall and protrude into cardiac chamber

MACROSCOPIC FEATURES

General Features

- Has both cystic and solid components, which appear multilobulated

Size

- Pericardial tumors may be as large as 15 cm
- Intracardiac tumors are usually 2-9 cm

Sections to Be Submitted

- 1-2 sections per cm of tumor to detect any malignant component
- Sample all grossly variable areas

MICROSCOPIC PATHOLOGY

Histologic Features

- Tumor is composed of multiple immature and mature tissue elements
  - Immature tissue elements are haphazardly arranged
    - Elements vary in proportions
- Immature neural tissue is often present
- Cystic spaces seen in tumor are often lined by epithelium, either respiratory type or squamous
- Choroidal tissue is commonly seen
- Other tissues may also be present, such as

Key Facts

Terminology

- Tumor composed of all 3 germ cell layers: Ectoderm, mesoderm, and endoderm

Clinical Issues

- 2nd most common cardiac tumor in fetus and neonate, after rhabdomyoma
- Location: Much more common in pericardium; rarely intracardiac
- Typically presents in newborn
- Symptoms are due to mass effect of tumor or fluid in pericardial space
- Treatment is surgical resection of tumor
- Prognosis depends on size and resectability

Microscopic Pathology

- Tumor is composed of immature mesenchyme, epithelium, and neural tissue, haphazardly arranged and in varying proportions

---

  - Neural tissue
  - Cartilage
  - Bone
  - Skeletal muscle
  - Adipose tissue
  - Pancreas
  - Thyroid
- Grading of teratoma, as described for tumors arising in ovary, is not applicable to pericardial/cardiac teratoma

Cytologic Features

- If cardiac tamponade is present due to pericardial effusion, it may be tapped and sent for cytological evaluation
- Pericardial fluid is serous and may contain mesothelial cells
- Would be highly unusual to aspirate tumor itself, since most cardiac tumors are resected if at all possible

DIFFERENTIAL DIAGNOSIS

Malignant Germ Cell Tumor

- Malignancy may occur in a teratoma
- Embryonal carcinoma and yolk sac tumors are most common
- Morphologic features of malignant germ cell tumors are the same regardless of where they occur in the body

DIAGNOSTIC CHECKLIST

Clinically Relevant Pathologic Features

- Immature cystic teratoma is considered a benign tumor
- Rarely, malignant germ cell component may be present

Pathologic Interpretation Pearls

- Frozen section diagnosis is possible on the rare occasion it is requested
- Immature neural tissue is commonly present; however, its amount is not graded

SELECTED REFERENCES

1. Fagiana AM et al: Management of a fetal intrapericardial teratoma: a case report and review of the literature. Congenit Heart Dis. 5(1):51-5, 2010
2. Avni FE et al: Tumours of the fetal body: a review. Pediatr Radiol. 39(11):1147-57, 2009
3. Isaacs H Jr: Fetal hydrops associated with tumors. Am J Perinatol. 25(1):43-68, 2008
4. Uzun O et al: Cardiac tumours in children. Orphanet J Rare Dis. 2:11, 2007
5. Singh J et al: Some more about intrapericardial teratomas in perinatal period. J Pediatr Surg. 41(4):877-8; author reply 878, 2006

IMAGE GALLERY

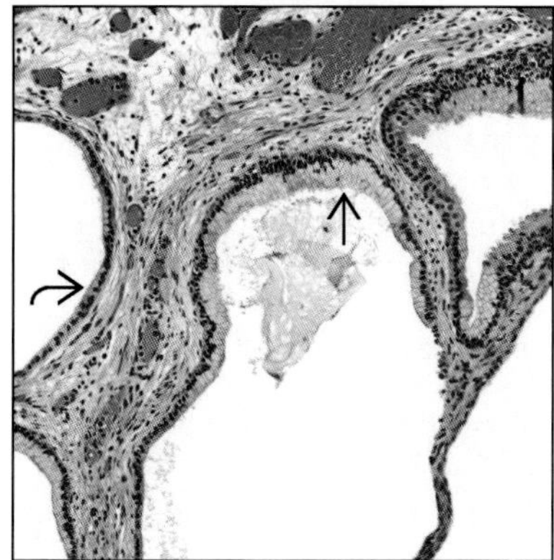

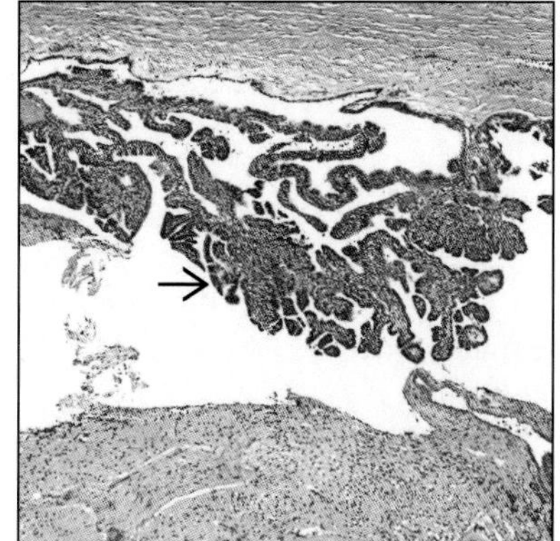

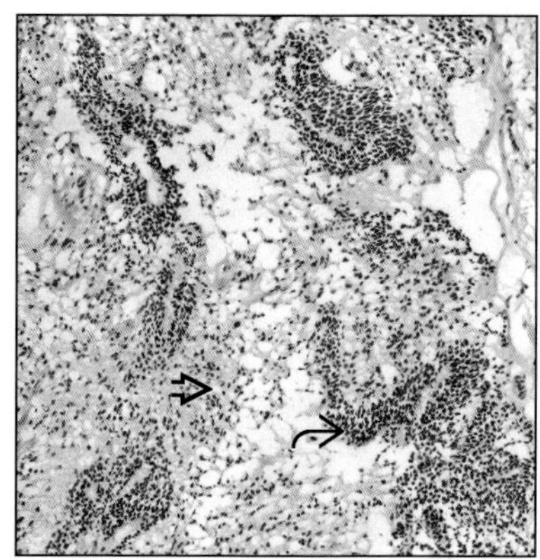

*(**Left**) Irregularly shaped cysts are lined by flat ⇨ to columnar ⇨ mucinous epithelium. (**Center**) Papillary fronds of choroidal tissue ⇨ fill a cystic space. Neural tissue is seen at the bottom of the field. (**Right**) Initial diagnosis in this case was made using a frozen section, illustrated here. Immature neural tissue ⇨ can be recognized easily within loose mesenchyme ⇨.*

THYMOMA

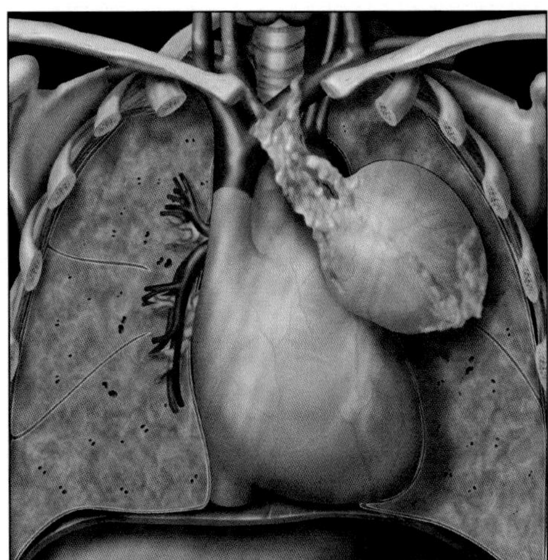

Schematic representation of the chest cavity shows a round to ovoid, well-circumscribed thymoma in the anterior mediastinal compartment on top of the pericardium and protruding onto the left hemithorax.

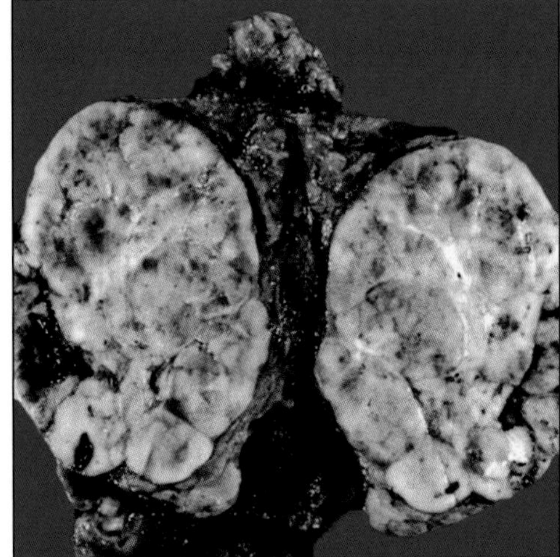

Gross appearance of bisected thymoma shows a well-circumscribed, fleshy, lobulated mass composed of tan-white, homogeneous, rubbery tissue with focal areas of congestion and hemorrhage.

TERMINOLOGY

Abbreviations

- Thymic epithelial neoplasm (TEM)

Synonyms

- Primary thymic epithelial neoplasm

Definitions

- Primary thymic epithelial neoplasm composed of thymic epithelial cells admixed in varying proportions with immature T-lymphocytes

ETIOLOGY/PATHOGENESIS

Pathogenesis

- Unknown
- Close association with myasthenia gravis and other autoimmune disorders

CLINICAL ISSUES

Presentation

- Chest pain
- Shortness of breath
- Paraneoplastic syndrome (myasthenia gravis, hypogammaglobulinemia, pure red cell aplasia, etc.)
- Superior vena cava syndrome
- Asymptomatic in up to 30% of cases
- Incidental finding on routine chest x-ray or during coronary artery bypass surgery

Natural History

- Majority of thymomas are very low-grade malignant neoplasms with generally indolent behavior
- Size and status of capsular integrity are 2 important determinant factors for prognosis
  - Invasive tumors are associated with more aggressive behavior
- Incompletely excised tumors have tendency to recur locally and spread along chest cavity
- Recurrences can take place many years after initial resection (i.e., > 10-15 years)
- Most common sites for metastases are lung, pleura, and thoracic lymph nodes
- Extrathoracic metastases are extremely rare (< 5% of cases)

Treatment

- Complete surgical excision for noninvasive tumors
- Radiation therapy for incompletely resected tumors
- Surgical excision + postoperative radiation therapy for invasive tumors
- Repeat surgical excision + radiation for recurrent tumors
- Combination chemotherapy for advanced stage and metastatic tumors
- Best chance for cure is complete surgical excision with negative margins

Prognosis

- Most important prognostic factor is clinical staging (Koga modified Masaoka scheme)
- Stage I and II: 80-90% survival at 15 years
- Stage III: 70% survival at 15 years
- Stage IV: 60% survival at 5 years
- Stages I and II include infiltration of capsule and minimal invasion of perithymic fat
  - Collectively regarded as "noninvasive" tumors; confined to anterior mediastinum
- Stage III and IV include infiltration of adjacent or neighboring structures, implants, and distant metastases
  - Collectively regarded as "invasive"

IMAGE FINDINGS

General Features

- Best diagnostic clue

THYMOMA

Key Facts

Clinical Issues

- Majority of thymomas are very low-grade malignant neoplasms with generally indolent behavior
- Status of capsular integrity is most important determinant factor for prognosis

Microscopic Pathology

- WHO classification system is based predominantly on cell type, cytologic atypia, and proportion of lymphocytes to epithelial cells: Thymoma type A, AB, B1, B2, B3, and thymic carcinoma
- 2 basic cell types are recognized: Spindle/oval and round/epithelioid cells
  - Type A thymoma: Composed of oval/spindle cells with scattered nuclear chromatin and inconspicuous or absent nucleoli without mitotic activity
  - Type AB thymoma: Composed of oval/spindle cells identical to those seen in type A but admixed with abundant small lymphocytes
  - Type B1 thymoma: Composed of round/epithelioid cells with single small eosinophilic nucleolus and abundant cytoplasm, admixed with numerous small T-lymphocytes
  - Type B2 thymoma: Composed of approximate equal admixture of round epithelial cells with small lymphocytes
  - Type B3 thymoma: Composed of sheets of large epithelioid cells admixed with scant lymphocytes
- Thymic carcinoma (type C thymoma): Characterized by overt cytologic features of malignancy and absence of organotypical thymic features; resembles carcinomas at other sites

  - Smooth or lobulated anterior mediastinal mass
- Location
  - Generally anterior mediastinum
  - May also occur in posterior mediastinum
  - May arise ectopically in pulmonary hilum, pleura, or head and neck
- Size
  - Usually between 4-15 cm

Radiographic Findings

- Round or oval anterior mediastinal mass
- Usually centered over heart; best seen on lateral view
- Linear and peripheral calcifications in capsule (10% of patients)

MR Findings

- T1WI: Isointense relative to muscle
- T2WI: Hyperintense, approaching signal of fat

CT Findings

- CECT best imaging tool for thymoma
- Oval or lobulated mass within anterior mediastinum
- Homogeneous enhancement is common in small tumors
- Heterogeneous enhancement more common in large tumors
- Thin and linear calcifications seen within capsule in 1/3 of patients
- Cystic changes and necrosis common in larger tumors
- Obliteration of mediastinal fat planes or mediastinal structures seen in invasive tumors

MACROSCOPIC FEATURES

General Features

- Generally well-circumscribed, encapsulated, solid tumor
- Homogeneous tan-white, rubbery tissue on cut surface
- Lobulated cut surface
- May be cystic and multilocular
- May contain calcifications in capsule or within tumor
- Rarely can be multifocal
- Can be ectopically located in posterior mediastinum, lung, neck, or pleura
- Can show areas of necrosis and hemorrhage
- Invasive tumors usually compromise adjacent structures, including large vessels, pericardium, pleura
- Distant metastases are rare

Sections to Be Submitted

- At least 1 section per cm of tumor greatest diameter
- Take additional sections if tumor shows variegated appearance
- Sample solid areas in cyst walls in multicystic tumors
- Always include sections of inked outer surface of specimen
- Coordination with surgeon should be sought to establish "true" margins to be sampled
- Any structures attached to specimen (i.e., pleura, lung, large vessels) should be inked and sampled separately as they represent "true" margins

MICROSCOPIC PATHOLOGY

Histologic Features

- Histologic classification is controversial
- Currently 2 systems are in use: Suster & Moran classification and WHO schema
- Suster & Moran classification: Based on degree of organotypical differentiation, divided into 3-tiered system
  - Well differentiated (thymoma)
  - Moderately differentiated (atypical thymoma)
  - Poorly differentiated (thymic carcinoma)
- WHO system is based primarily on cell type, cytologic atypia, and proportion of lymphocytes to epithelial cells
  - WHO type A: Composed of spindle cells without cytologic atypia
  - WHO type AB: Composed of spindle cells admixed with abundant lymphocytes
  - WHO type B1: Composed of round epithelioid cells admixed with abundant lymphocytes

THYMOMA

  - WHO type B2: Composed of round epithelioid cells admixed with equal amount of lymphocytes
  - WHO type B3: Composed predominantly of epithelial cells with cytologic atypia
- WHO classification has a series of other distinctive histologic types that do not fit into standard categories
  - "Metaplastic" thymoma
  - Multifocal thymoma
  - Microscopic thymoma
  - Micronodular thymoma
  - Anaplastic thymoma
- Older ("traditional") classification by Bernatz et al from Mayo Clinic is still used today by many; divides thymomas based on their cell composition
  - Lymphocyte-rich thymoma
  - Mixed lymphoepithelial thymoma
  - Epithelial-rich thymoma
  - Spindle cell thymoma

Cytologic Features

- 2 basic cell types are recognized
  - Oval/spindle cells (type A, AB)
  - Round/epithelioid cells (types B1-3)
- Type A thymoma is composed of oval or spindle cells with scattered nuclear chromatin and inconspicuous or absent nucleoli and no mitotic activity
  - Spindle cell thymoma usually contains few lymphocytes
  - Majority of spindle cell thymomas are low grade and encapsulated
  - Invasive or atypical spindle cell thymoma can follow aggressive behavior
  - Distant metastases and death can occur in some cases of spindle cell thymoma
- Type AB thymoma is composed of oval or spindle cells identical to those in type "A" but admixed with abundant small lymphocytes
  - Spindle cells do not display mitotic activity
  - Lymphocytes admixed with epithelial cells are of T-cell type
  - Tumors usually contain admixture of lymphocyte-rich with lymphocyte-poor areas
  - Tumors may be composed exclusively of lymphocyte-rich areas and be confused with B1 thymoma
- Type B1 thymoma is composed of round/epithelioid cells with single small eosinophilic nucleolus and abundant cytoplasm, admixed with numerous small T-lymphocytes
  - Small lymphocytes predominate and overshadow epithelial cells
  - Contains frequent perivascular spaces and areas of "medullary" differentiation
  - Equivalent to "lymphocyte-rich" or "lymphocyte-predominant" in traditional classification (Mayo Clinic)
- Type B2 thymoma is composed of approximately equal admixture of round epithelial cells with small lymphocytes
  - Epithelial cells may show mild degree of atypia and enlargement of nuclei
  - Admixtures with B1 areas may be seen in about 30% of cases
  - Equivalent to "mixed lymphoepithelial" thymoma of traditional classification (Mayo Clinic)
- Type B3 thymoma is composed of sheets of large epithelioid cells admixed with scant lymphocytes
  - Epithelial cells are characterized by nuclear enlargement with dense chromatin pattern and prominent nucleoli
  - Mitotic figures can be encountered in epithelial cells
  - Cell nuclei show tendency to adopt raisin-like configuration
  - Cytoplasm of tumor cells is usually abundant and eosinophilic with sharp cell borders
  - Tendency for epithelial cells to palisade around perivascular spaces
  - Tumor cells can also be oval or spindled with similar nuclear features
- Type A thymomas may exhibit unusual growth patterns
  - Hemangiopericytic growth pattern
  - Micronodular growth pattern with lymphoid B-cell hyperplasia
  - Biphasic pattern with pseudosarcomatous stroma ("metaplastic" thymoma)
  - Skin adnexal-like ("adenoid") growth pattern
  - Sclerosing growth pattern
  - Rosette-forming growth pattern
- Type B thymomas may exhibit unusual features
  - Extensive multilocular thymic cyst-like changes
  - Areas of infarction, hemorrhage, and necrosis
  - Massive infiltration by plasma cells in stroma
  - Clear cell changes
  - "Starry sky" appearance simulating lymphoma
- Type C thymoma (thymic carcinoma) is characterized by overt cytologic evidence of malignancy and absence of organotypical features of thymic differentiation
  - Diagnosis of exclusion
  - Requires demonstration of absence of tumor elsewhere clinically and radiographically

Lymphatic/Vascular Invasion

- Very rare; unknown significance but generally associated with worse prognosis

Margins

- Very difficult to determine without assistance of surgeon
- True resection margins need to be inked or tagged by surgeon before submitting to pathology
- Inked anterior surface does not represent "margin" unless it was invading at time of surgery
- True margins need to be inked for proper assessment

Lymph Nodes

- Thymoma rarely metastasizes to lymph nodes
- Majority of lymph node metastases in thymoma are to mediastinal nodes
- Other intrathoracic lymph nodes may also be involved more rarely by metastatic thymoma

DIFFERENTIAL DIAGNOSIS

Lymphoblastic Lymphoma

- Does not show scattered keratin-positive cells admixed with immature T-lymphocytes
- Shows rapid growth with sudden onset of symptoms
  - Thymoma is slow-growing tumor with slowly progressive symptoms
- Most common age for lymphoblastic lymphoma is childhood and adolescence
  - Most common age for thymoma is in middle-aged adults; rare in children and adolescents

Acquired Multilocular Thymic Cyst

- Multilocular cysts do not contain discrete areas attached to walls of cysts showing typical type B thymoma
  - Type A thymoma can undergo massive cystic changes, but cells lining the cysts are spindle cells
- Shows small cuboidal or squamous epithelial cells lining the cysts in continuity with dilated Hassall corpuscles
- Shows prominent lymphoid follicular hyperplasia and severe acute and chronic inflammation with cholesterol cleft granulomas

Hemangiopericytoma/Solitary Fibrous Tumor

- Spindle cells in solitary fibrous tumors are not keratin-positive but are are CD34, Bcl-2, and CD99 positive
- Show characteristic linear pattern of stromal collagenization resulting in deposition of rope-like collagen separating spindle cells
- Devoid of immature T cells
  - Spindle cell thymoma may contain variable number of immature T cells admixed with epithelial cells

Neuroendocrine Carcinomas

- Positive for neuroendocrine markers
  - Rosette-like structures in thymoma are positive for cytokeratin
- Thymic carcinoids usually show increased mitotic activity and tumor cell necrosis
- Tumor cells in carcinoids show characteristic stippled ("salt and pepper") chromatin pattern
- Other features of thymic carcinoids include nested growth pattern ("zellballen") and formation of trabeculae, ribbons, and festoons

DIAGNOSTIC CHECKLIST

Clinically Relevant Pathologic Features

- Encapsulation/circumscription
- Presence or absence of cytologic atypia in epithelial cells
- Size of tumor
- Clinical stage
- Presence or absence of myasthenia gravis

Pathologic Interpretation Pearls

- Great variation in histologic appearance due to tumor heterogeneity
- Identification of scattered keratin-positive neoplastic cells in lymphocyte-rich tumors
- Hemorrhage and necrosis may be seen in encapsulated, low-grade, well-differentiated tumors; not to be mistaken for ominous sign
- Capsular invasion is most significant prognostic factor
- Rarely, thymoma may be devoid of a capsule; should not be overinterpreted as invasion
- Types A, AB, B1, and B2 in WHO classification observe similar behavior; prognosis is determined by status of capsular integrity
- Type B3 thymoma in WHO classification has slightly more aggressive biologic behavior with frequent invasion at time of diagnosis and earlier recurrences

SELECTED REFERENCES

1. Casey EM et al: Clinical management of thymoma patients. Hematol Oncol Clin North Am. 22(3):457-73, 2008
2. Gupta R et al: Evidence-based pathology and the pathologic evaluation of thymomas: transcapsular invasion is not a significant prognostic feature. Arch Pathol Lab Med. 132(6):926-30, 2008
3. Marchevsky AM et al: Evidence-based pathology and the pathologic evaluation of thymomas: the World Health Organization classification can be simplified into only 3 categories other than thymic carcinoma. Cancer. 112(12):2780-8, 2008
4. Moran CA et al: The World Health Organization (WHO) histologic classification of thymomas: a reanalysis. Curr Treat Options Oncol. 9(4-6):288-99, 2008
5. Rossi G et al: Thymoma classification: does it matter? Histopathology. 53(4):483-4, 2008
6. Suster S et al: Histologic classification of thymoma: the World Health Organization and beyond. Hematol Oncol Clin North Am. 22(3):381-92, 2008
7. Verghese ET et al: Interobserver variation in the classification of thymic tumours--a multicentre study using the WHO classification system. Histopathology. 53(2):218-23, 2008
8. Wick MR: Prognostic factors for thymic epithelial neoplasms, with emphasis on tumor staging. Hematol Oncol Clin North Am. 22(3):527-42, 2008
9. Suster S et al: Thymoma classification: current status and future trends. Am J Clin Pathol. 125(4):542-54, 2006
10. Suster S: Diagnosis of thymoma. J Clin Pathol. 59(12):1238-44, 2006
11. Suster S et al: Problem areas and inconsistencies in the WHO classification of thymoma. Semin Diagn Pathol. 22(3):188-97, 2005
12. Travis WD et al. Pathology and genetics of tumors of the lung, pleura, thymus and heart. In World Health Organization Classification of Tumors. Lyon: IARC Press. 145-71, 2004
13. Marchevsky AM et al: Protocol for the examination of specimens from patients with thymic epithelial tumors located in any area of the mediastinum. Arch Pathol Lab Med. 127(10):1298-303, 2003
14. Rieker RJ et al: Histologic classification of thymic epithelial tumors: comparison of established classification schemes. Int J Cancer. 98(6):900-6, 2002
15. Moran CA et al: On the histologic heterogeneity of thymic epithelial neoplasms. Impact of sampling in subtyping and classification of thymomas. Am J Clin Pathol. 114(5):760-6, 2000

THYMOMA

Immunohistochemistry

Antibody	Reactivity	Staining Pattern	Comment
AE1/AE3	Positive	Cytoplasmic	Stains only neoplastic thymic epithelial cells
p63	Positive	Nuclear	Stains neoplastic thymic epithelial cells in all histologic types
CK19	Positive	Cytoplasmic	Stains neoplastic cells in all histologic types of thymoma
CD1a	Positive	Cytoplasmic	Stains immature T-lymphocytes
TdT	Positive	Nuclear	Stains immature T-lymphocytes
CD3	Positive	Cytoplasmic	Stains T-lymphocytes
CD99	Positive	Cytoplasmic	Stains immature T-lymphocytes
CD20	Positive	Cytoplasmic	May be positive in spindle cells in thymoma (WHO types A and AB) and also highlights small subpopulation of B-lymphocytes
Bcl-2	Positive	Cytoplasmic	May be positive in spindle cell thymoma (WHO types A and AB)
CD5	Negative	Cytoplasmic	Negative in epithelial cells of most thymomas, except WHO B3
CD117	Negative	Cytoplasmic	Negative in epithelial cells of most thymomas; stains germ cells and mast cells within tumor

Histologic Classification Systems for Thymoma

Suster & Moran Classification	WHO 2004 Schema
Well-differentiated thymic epithelial neoplasm (**thymoma**)	WHO type A (spindle cell)
	WHO type AB (spindle cell with abundant lymphocytes)
	WHO type B1 (lymphocyte-predominant)
	WHO type B2 (lymphoepithelial)
Moderately differentiated thymic epithelial neoplasm (**atypical thymoma**)	WHO type B3 (epithelial-rich)
Poorly differentiated thymic epithelial neoplasm (**thymic carcinoma**)	Thymic carcinoma

Classification of Thymoma According to Grades of Differentiation (Suster & Moran)

Diagnosis	Differentiation Grade	Features
Thymoma	Well-differentiated thymic neoplasm	Preservation of organotypical features of thymic differentiation; no cytologic evidence of atypia
Atypical thymoma	Moderately differentiated thymic neoplasm	Partial preservation of organotypical features of differentiation of the thymus; mild to moderate cytologic atypia
Thymic carcinoma	Poorly differentiated thymic neoplasm	Loss of organotypical features of differentiation of the thymus; overt cytologic evidence of malignancy

16. Suster S et al: Micronodular thymoma with lymphoid B-cell hyperplasia: clinicopathologic and immunohistochemical study of eighteen cases of a distinctive morphologic variant of thymic epithelial neoplasm. Am J Surg Pathol. 23(8):955-62, 1999
17. Suster S et al: Primary thymic epithelial neoplasms: spectrum of differentiation and histological features. Semin Diagn Pathol. 16(1):2-17, 1999
18. Suster S et al: Thymoma, atypical thymoma, and thymic carcinoma. A novel conceptual approach to the classification of thymic epithelial neoplasms. Am J Clin Pathol. 111(6):826-33, 1999
19. Suster S et al: Thymoma with pseudosarcomatous stroma: report of an unusual histologic variant of thymic epithelial neoplasm that may simulate carcinosarcoma. Am J Surg Pathol. 21(11):1316-23, 1997
20. Suster S et al: Primary thymic epithelial neoplasms showing combined features of thymoma and thymic carcinoma. A clinicopathologic study of 22 cases. Am J Surg Pathol. 20(12):1469-80, 1996
21. Suster S et al: Malignant thymic neoplasms that may mimic benign conditions. Semin Diagn Pathol. 12(1):98-104, 1995
22. Dawson A et al: Observer variation in the histopathological classification of thymoma: correlation with prognosis. J Clin Pathol. 47(6):519-23, 1994
23. Koga K et al: A review of 79 thymomas: modification of staging system and reappraisal of conventional division into invasive and non-invasive thymoma. Pathol Int. 44(5):359-67, 1994
24. Suster S et al: Cystic thymomas. A clinicopathologic study of ten cases. Cancer. 69(1):92-7, 1992
25. Suster S et al: Thymic carcinoma. A clinicopathologic study of 60 cases. Cancer. 67(4):1025-32, 1991
26. Wick MR: Assessing the prognosis of thymomas. Ann Thorac Surg. 50(4):521-2, 1990

Cell Types in Thymoma

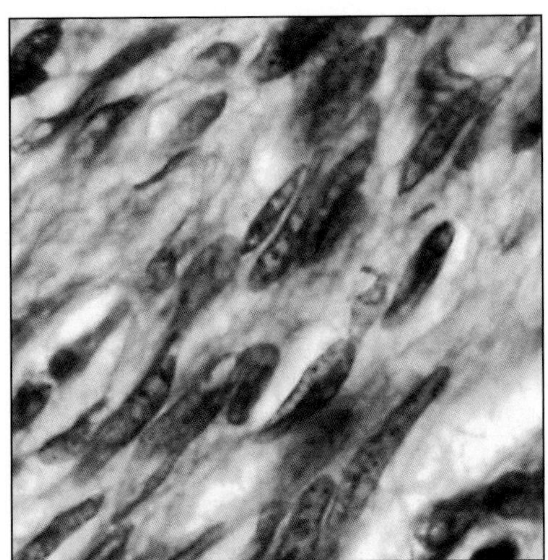

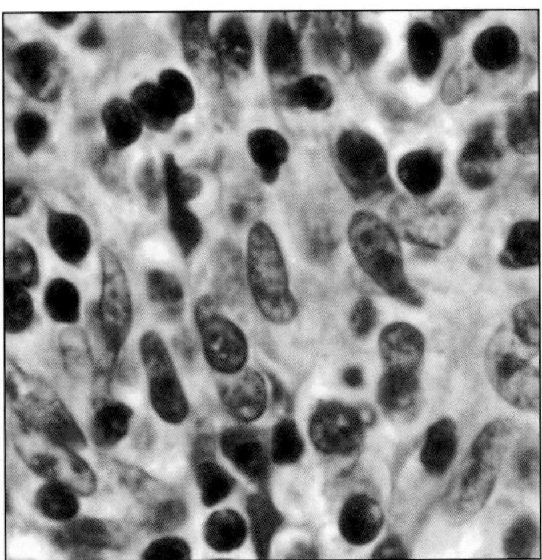

*(**Left**) Type A thymoma is composed of spindle cells with elongated nuclei showing dispersed chromatin pattern and absent or very inconspicuous nucleoli and an indistinct rim of lightly eosinophilic to amphophilic cytoplasm. (**Right**) Type AB thymoma is composed of a similar proliferation of spindle cells with elongated nuclei showing dispersed chromatin pattern. The cells are essentially identical to those seen in type A except they are surrounded by abundant lymphocytes.*

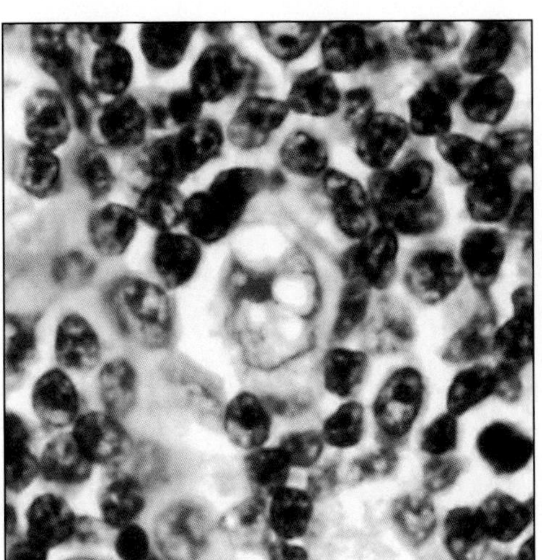

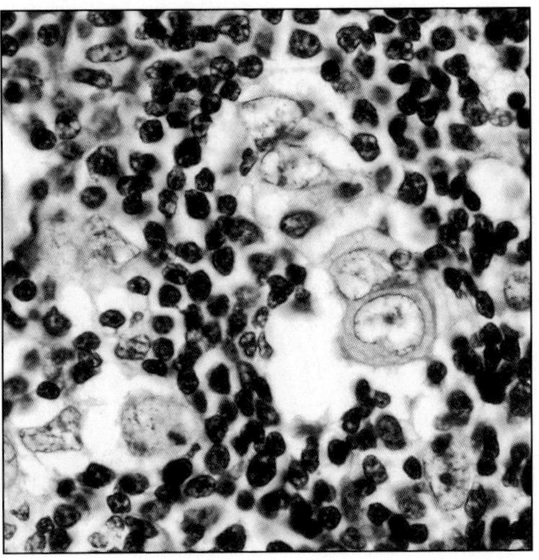

*(**Left**) Type B1 thymoma is composed of large round epithelioid cells with large vesicular nuclei that contain a single prominent eosinophilic nucleolus and are surrounded by an indistinct rim of amphophilic cytoplasm. (**Right**) Type B2 thymoma shows round epithelioid cells that may be slightly larger than those seen in B1 thymomas but essentially show similar nuclear features. Notice that there are more epithelial cells per lymphocyte than in type B1.*

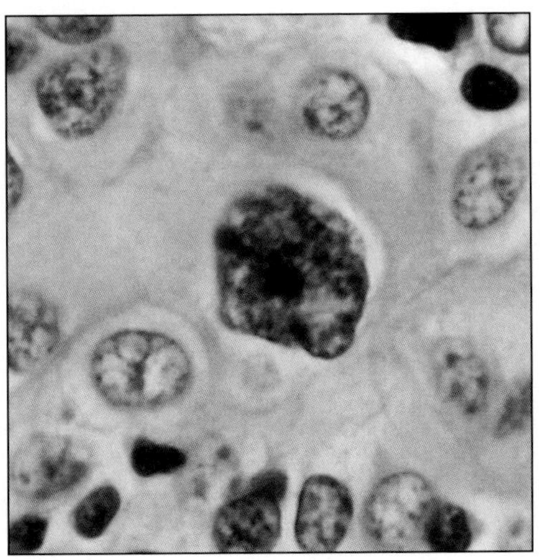

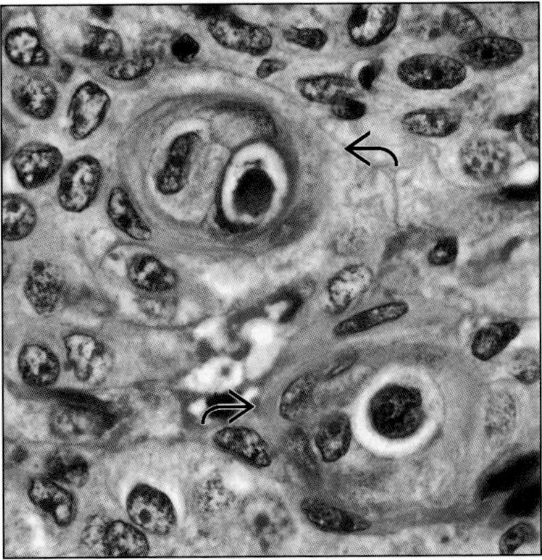

*(**Left**) Type B3 thymoma shows sheets of large epithelioid to polygonal cells with enlarged nuclei, marked increase in nuclear chromatin, prominent nucleoli, and abundant eosinophilic cytoplasm with sharp cell borders. (**Right**) Type B3 thymoma may show foci of abortive squamous differentiation, displaying large round to polygonal cells with large nuclei and prominent nucleoli. Notice the tight apposition and molding of the cells forming abortive squamous eddies ⮫.*

Spindle Cell Thymoma (WHO Type A)

(Left) *Spindle cell thymoma (WHO type A) shows fascicles of bland-appearing spindle cells admixed with a few scattered small lymphocytes.* ***(Right)*** *High-power view of a spindle cell thymoma (WHO type A) shows spindle cells with elongated nuclei that contain scattered chromatin and lack nucleoli. The cells are characterized by a scant rim of indistinct amphophilic cytoplasm. This spindle cell proliferation can closely resemble a spindle cell mesenchymal neoplasm.*

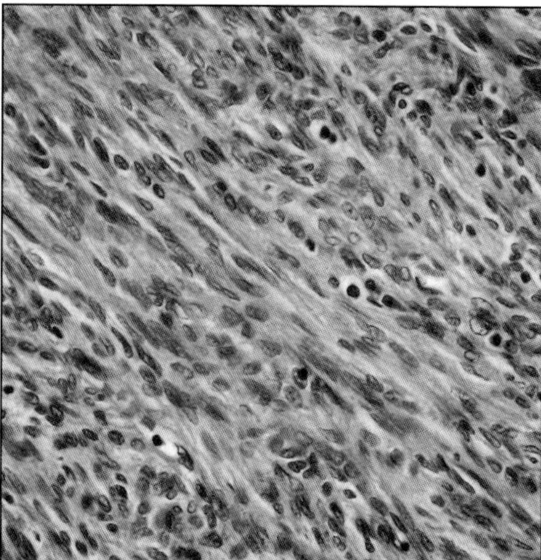

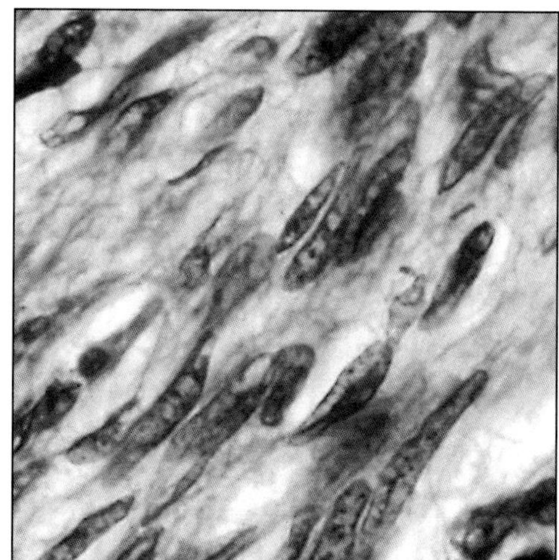

(Left) *A short storiform pattern is appreciated in this example of spindle cell thymoma (WHO type A). Notice the sprinkling of small lymphocytes in the background. This growth pattern can be confused with a fibrohistiocytic neoplasm or a solitary fibrous tumor of the mediastinum.* ***(Right)*** *Spindle cell thymoma (WHO type A) shows a striking microcystic pattern of growth with small, abortive, gland-like structures. The microcysts are primarily composed of dilated perivascular spaces.*

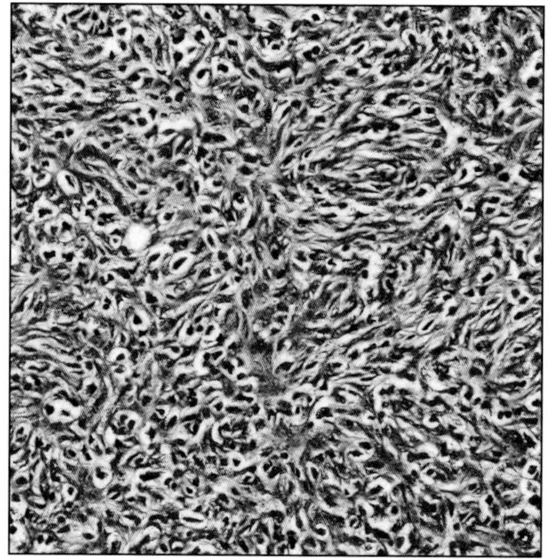

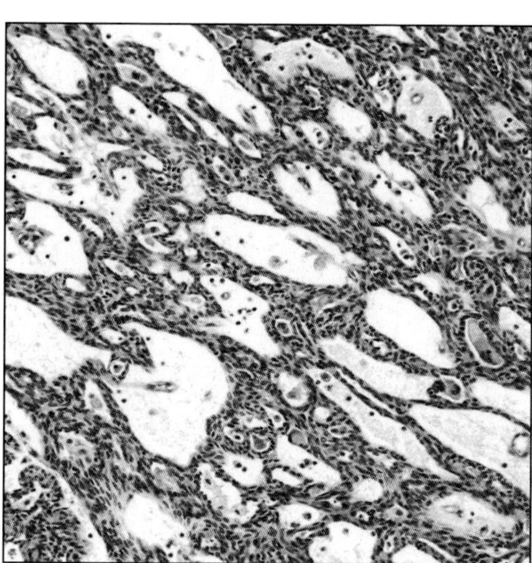

(Left) *Spindle cell thymoma (WHO type A) shows a macrocystic pattern of growth with large, irregular cystic spaces lined by the thymic epithelial cells. The macrocysts are caused by confluence and coalescence of smaller, dilated perivascular spaces.* ***(Right)*** *Spindle cell thymoma (WHO type A) shows capsular invasion by tumor ⇨. Notice the solid nodule traversing the fibrous capsule of the thymus that is still attached to the underlying main tumor mass by a short pedicle ➔.*

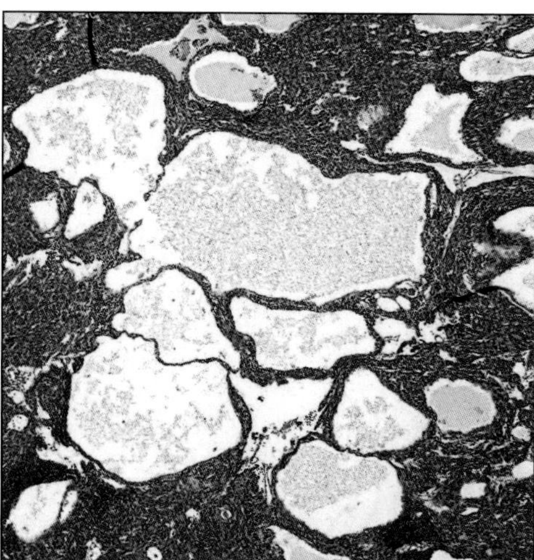

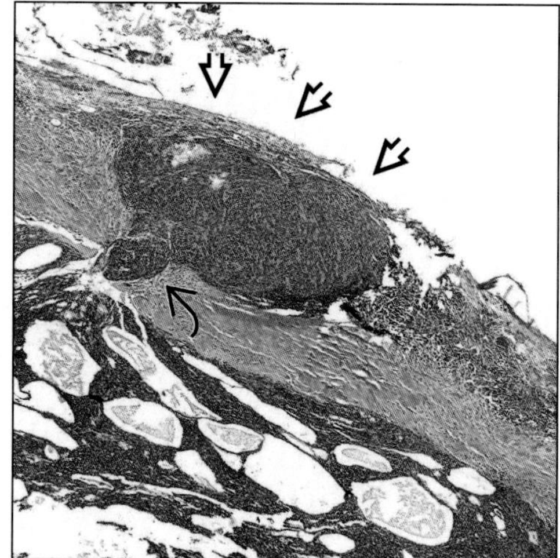

Unusual Variants of Spindle Cell Thymoma

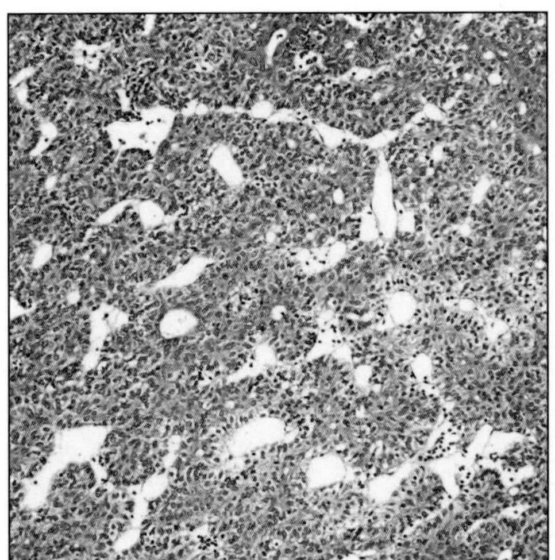

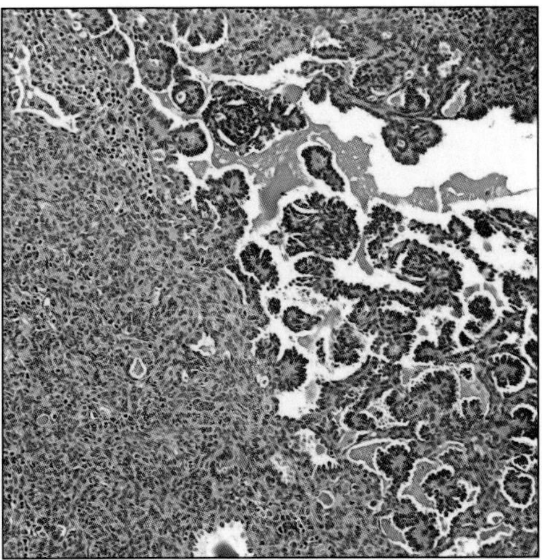

(Left) *Spindle cell thymoma (WHO type A) shows a striking hemangiopericytoma-like vascular pattern. Notice numerous small to medium-sized vascular spaces displaying open lumens and occasional branching of vessels.* ***(Right)*** *Spindle cell thymoma (WHO type A) shows prominent papillary structures (right half of field) that gradually merge with solid spindle cell component on the left side. These tumors can be confused with metastatic papillary carcinoma.*

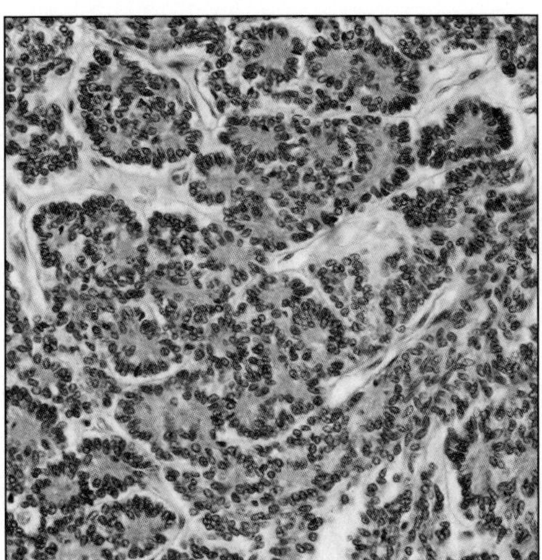

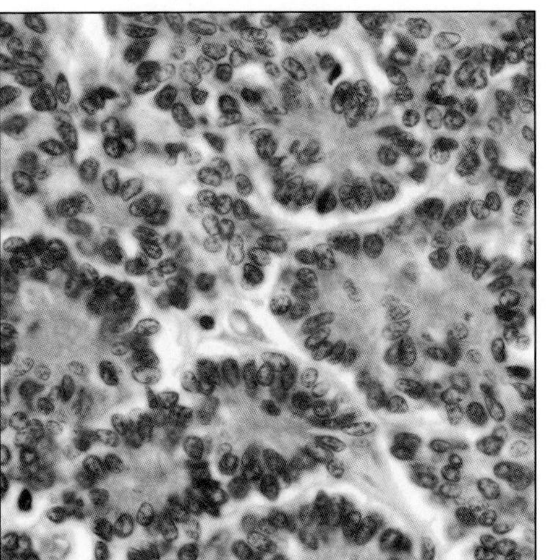

(Left) *Spindle cell thymoma (WHO type A) shows numerous small, rosette-like structures with striking palisading of nuclei in the periphery and central cores that contain amorphous material.* ***(Right)*** *High-power view of spindle cell thymoma with epithelial rosettes shows rosette-like structures displaying peripheral palisading of nuclei and central cores containing pink amorphous material. These tumors may be confused with primary or metastatic neuroendocrine neoplasms.*

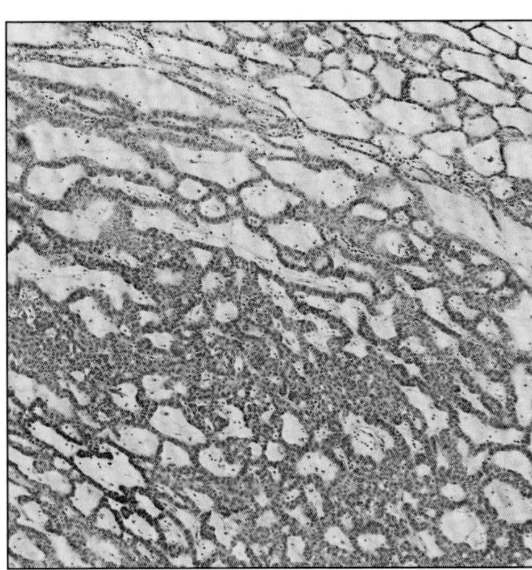

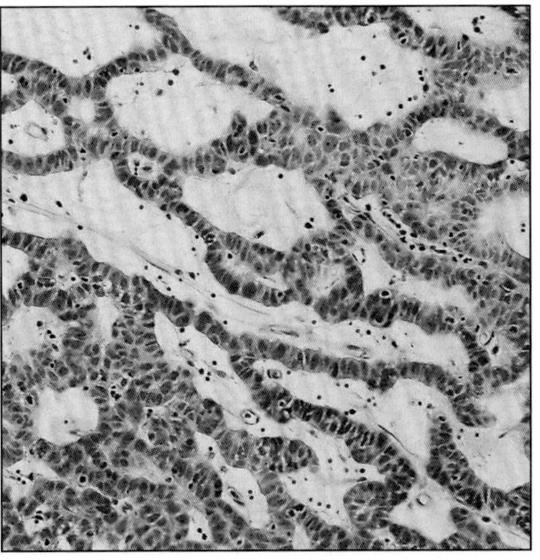

(Left) *Spindle cell thymoma (WHO type A) shows a delicate lace-like pattern composed of cords and rows of single cells adopting a net-like configuration reminiscent of a benign skin adnexal tumor.* ***(Right)*** *High-power view of spindle cell thymoma shows an adenoid, lace-like arrangement of tumor cells. The cells are oval to spindled and adopt a palisaded appearance. A few scattered small lymphocytes are also present. The image is reminiscent of a benign skin adnexal tumor.*

THYMOMA

Unusual Variants of Spindle Cell Thymoma

*(**Left**) Micronodular thymoma with lymphoid B-cell hyperplasia shows discrete, small nodules against a background of small lymphocytes in the stroma. (**Right**) High power of a micronodule in micronodular thymoma shows cells with oval nuclei surrounded by an indistinct rim of amphophilic cytoplasm. The cells surrounding the nodule are polyclonal B-lymphocytes. This image can be confused with a metastatic carcinoma to mediastinal lymph node.*

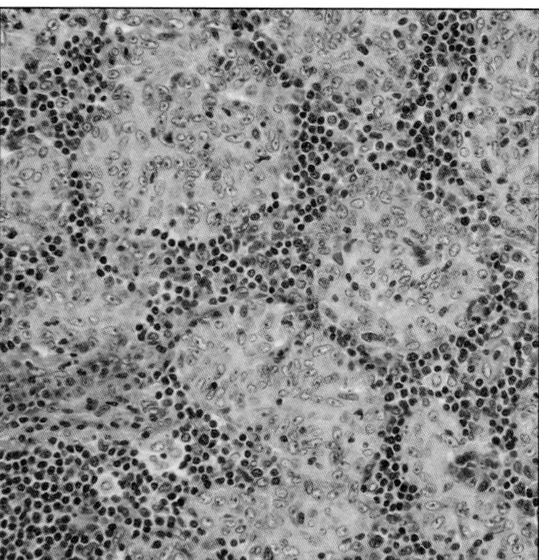

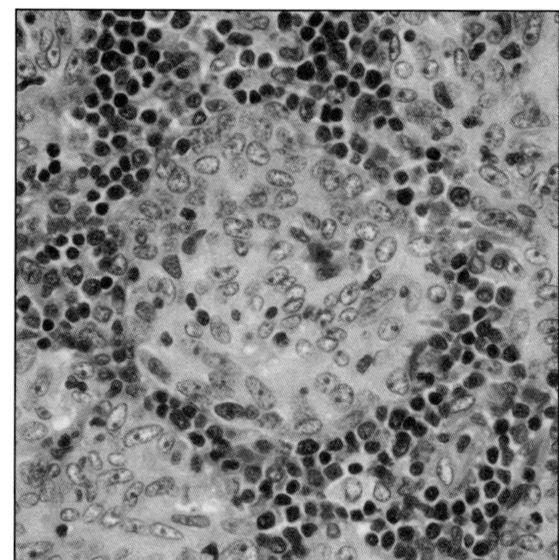

*(**Left**) Micronodular thymoma with lymphoid B-cell hyperplasia shows a hyperplastic lymphoid follicle with reactive germinal center ⮫. The solid nodule beneath is composed mainly of spindle to oval cells with scant cytoplasm. (**Right**) Spindle cell thymoma (WHO type A) shows massive dilatation of the perivascular spaces with abundant hyalinization and sclerosis. Notice fibroepitheliomatous appearance caused by strands of epithelial cells circumscribing hyalinized stroma.*

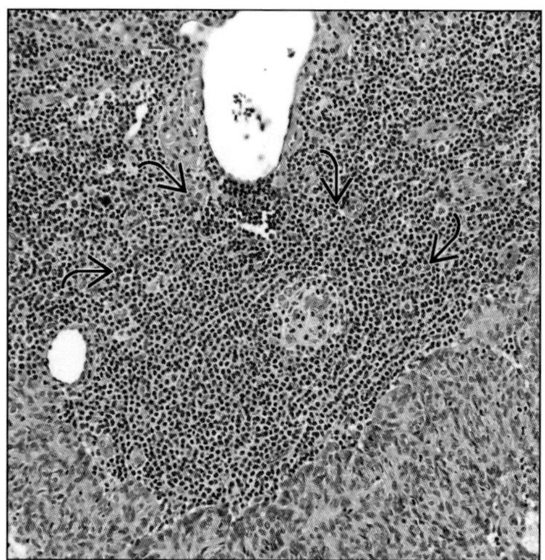

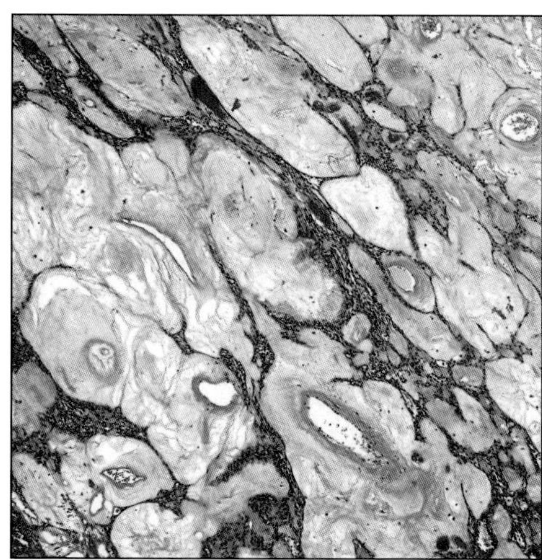

*(**Left**) Rhabdomyomatous variant of thymoma shows a biphasic appearance on scanning magnification. There are strands and cords of oval to spindle epithelial tumor cells circumscribing clusters of large eosinophilic cells. (**Right**) High power of rhabdomyomatous thymoma shows large "rhabdoid" cells in the center characterized by small oval nuclei surrounded by an ample rim of densely eosinophilic cytoplasm. These cells express desmin and correspond to "myoid" cells of the thymus.*

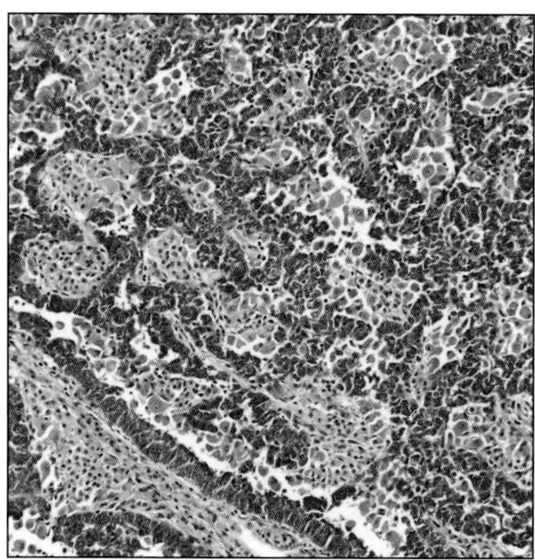

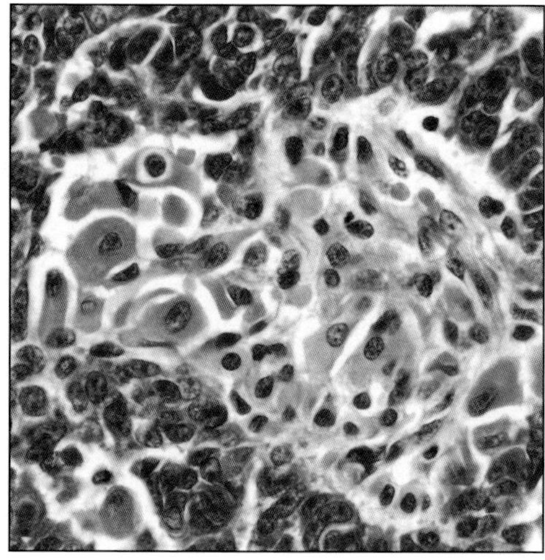

"Metaplastic" Thymoma with Pseudosarcomatous Stroma

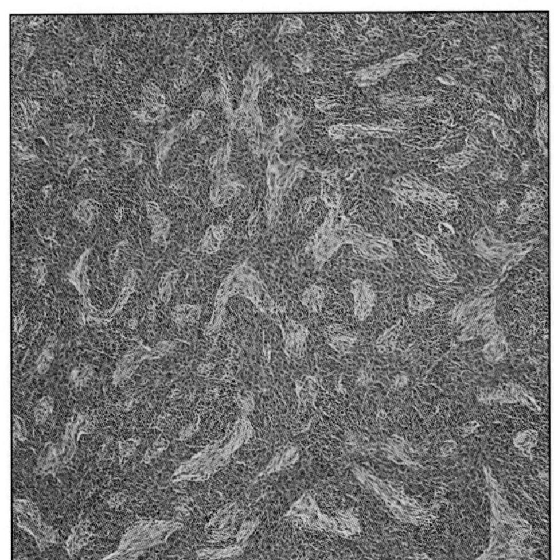

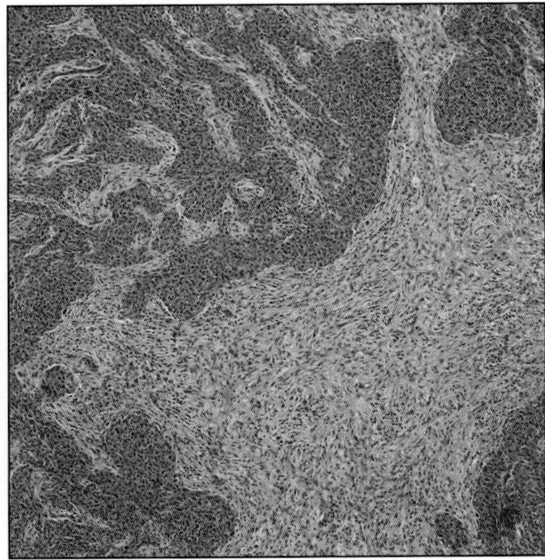

*(**Left**) Spindle cell thymoma with pseudosarcomatous stroma (so-called "metaplastic" thymoma) shows a sieve-like architecture with anastomosing cords and trabeculae of epithelial tumor cells circumscribing stromal areas containing a spindle cell population. (**Right**) Thymoma with pseudosarcomatous stroma shows a sharp demarcation between the epithelial component (periphery) and the spindle cell stromal component (center).*

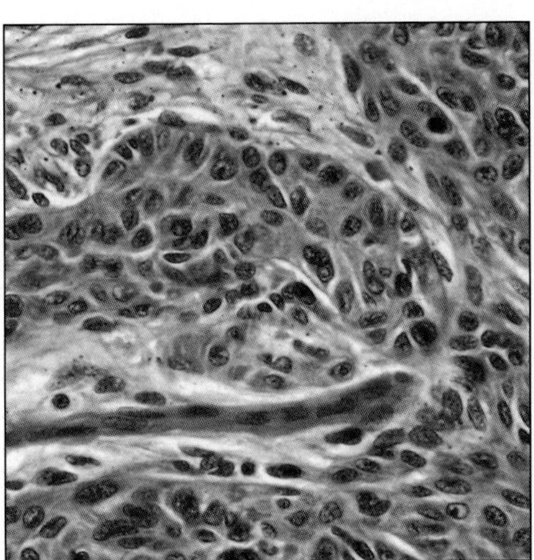

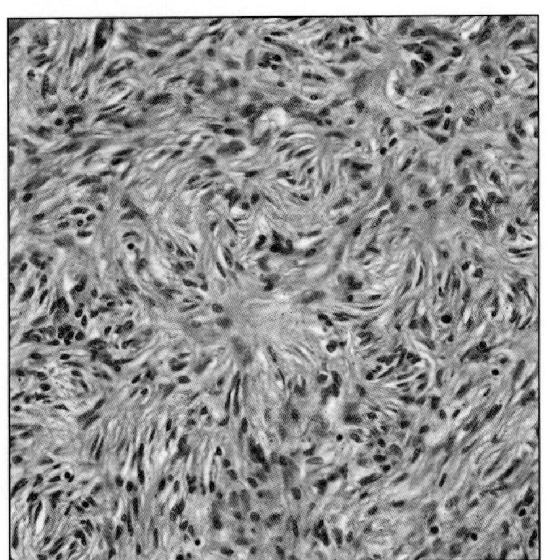

*(**Left**) High magnification of epithelial component is shown in thymoma with pseudosarcomatous stroma ("metaplastic" thymoma). Notice the large, oval to round nuclei with prominent nucleoli. (**Right**) High magnification of stromal component of spindle cell thymoma with pseudosarcomatous stroma shows a storiform pattern of growth. Notice the bland appearance of the spindle cells, the absence of nuclear pleomorphism and mitoses, and the lack of necrosis.*

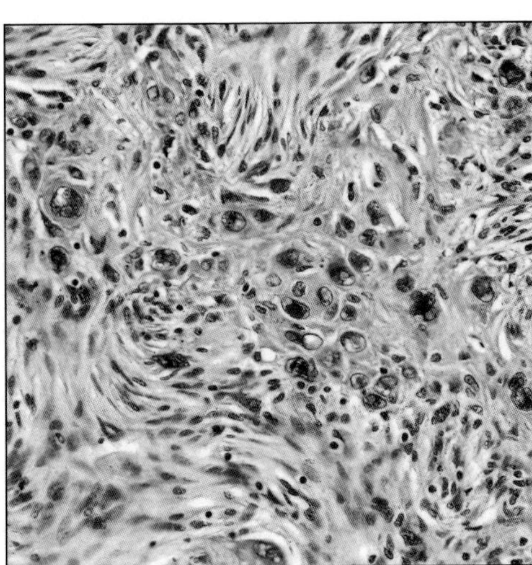

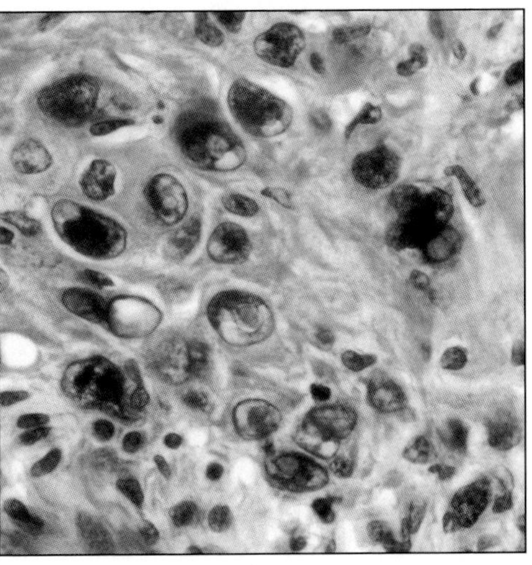

*(**Left**) Epithelial component in thymoma with pseudosarcomatous stroma ("metaplastic" thymoma) shows marked cytologic atypia in many of the tumor cells. Notice that the spindle cell stroma surrounding the tumor cell island lacks mitotic activity and nuclear pleomorphism. (**Right**) High magnification of atypical epithelial component in thymoma with pseudosarcomatous stroma ("metaplastic" thymoma) shows enlarged tumor cells with large nuclei and prominent nucleoli.*

Lymphocyte-Rich Spindle Cell Thymoma (WHO Type AB)

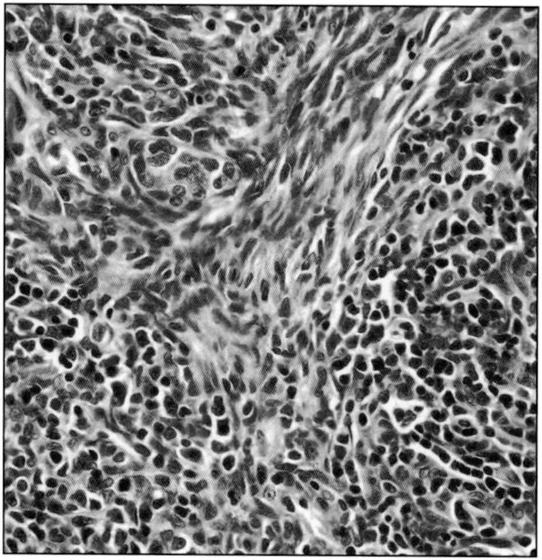

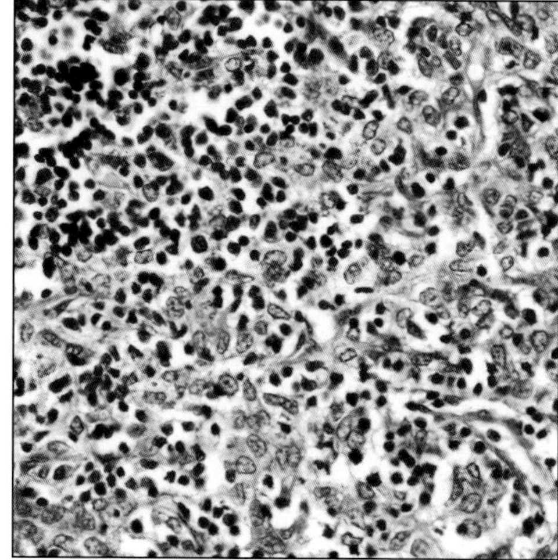

(Left) *Lymphocyte-rich spindle cell thymoma (WHO type AB) shows storiform fascicle of spindle cells (center) with few lymphocytes surrounded by areas that contain scattered spindle cells admixed with numerous lymphocytes.* ***(Right)*** *High power of lymphocyte-rich spindle cell thymoma (WHO type AB) shows scattered small spindle epithelial cells admixed with numerous scattered small lymphocytes. The small spindle cells show identical nuclear features to those in the fascicular areas.*

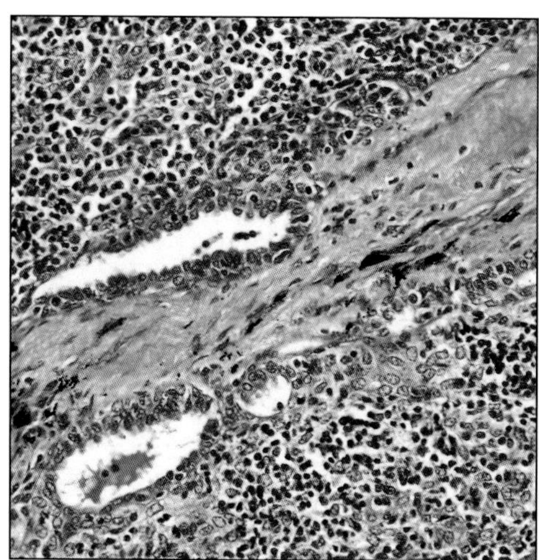

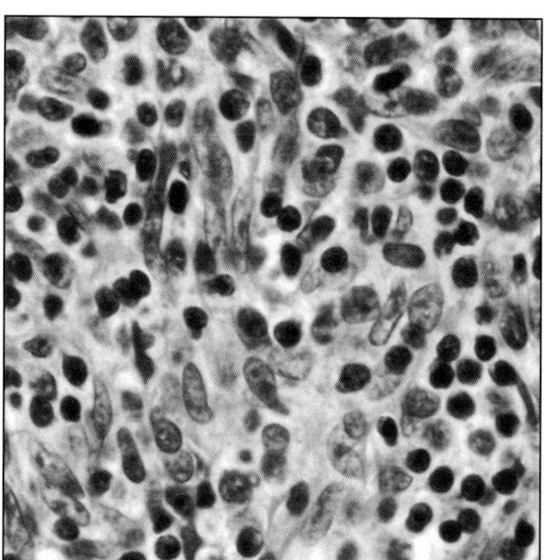

(Left) *Lymphocyte-rich spindle cell thymoma shows focal glandular structures admixed with the spindle cell population. Similar gland-like structures are commonly seen in conventional spindle cell thymoma and should not be mistaken for metastatic adenocarcinoma.* ***(Right)*** *High power of lymphocyte-rich spindle cell thymoma shows oval to spindle-shaped nuclei with dispersed chromatin and absent or inconspicuous nucleoli identical to those of conventional spindle cell thymoma.*

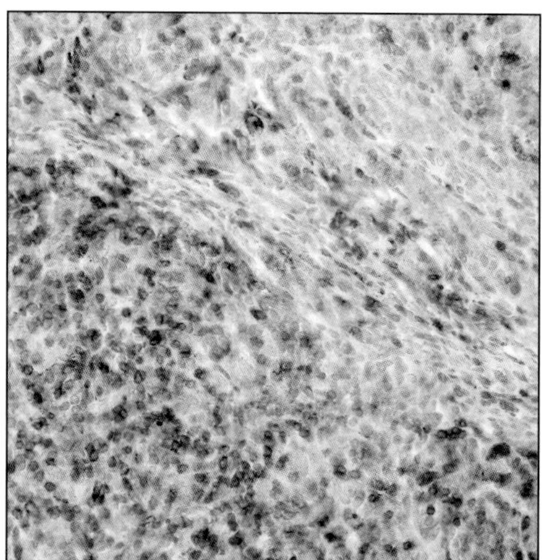

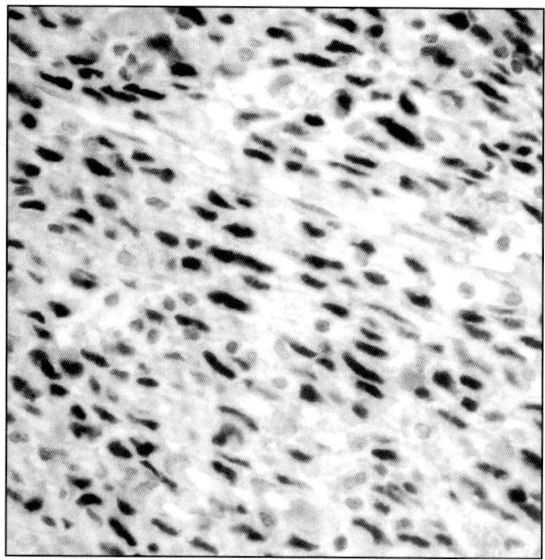

(Left) *Immunohistochemical staining of lymphocyte-rich spindle cell thymoma (WHO type AB) for the lymphoid marker CD1a highlights numerous immature T-lymphocytes admixed with the spindle cells.* ***(Right)*** *Immunohistochemical staining of lymphocyte-rich spindle cell thymoma (WHO type AB) with p63 antibody shows strong nuclear positivity in the spindle thymic epithelial cells. Notice that the stain highlights the elongated, oval to spindle shape of the nuclei in the tumor cells.*

Lymphocyte-Rich Thymoma (WHO Type B1)

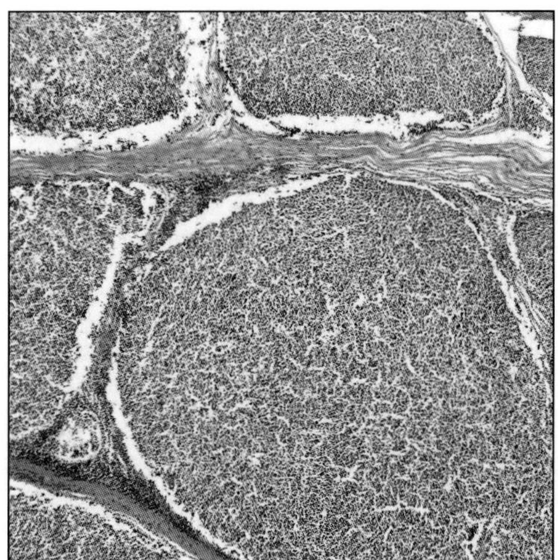

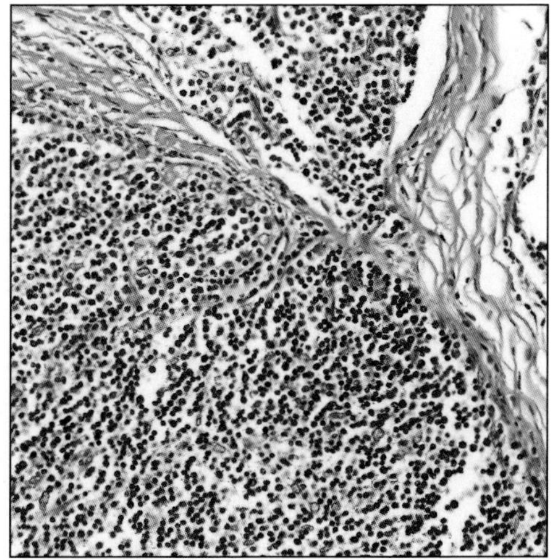

(Left) *Lymphocyte-rich thymoma (WHO type B1) shows round lobules of tumor tissue containing abundant lymphocytes. The lobules are circumscribed by broad bands of fibroconnective tissue.* ***(Right)*** *Higher magnification of round cellular lobule in lymphocyte-rich thymoma (WHO type B1) shows a predominantly lymphoid cell population. The lobules are separated by thin bands of fibrocollagenous tissue. These tumors can be easily mistaken for lymphocytic lymphomas.*

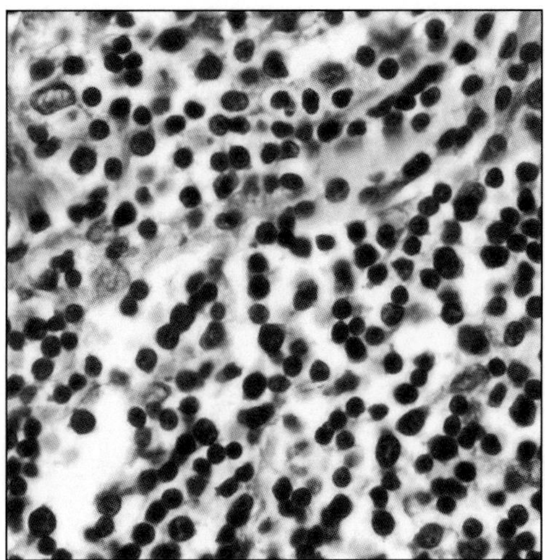

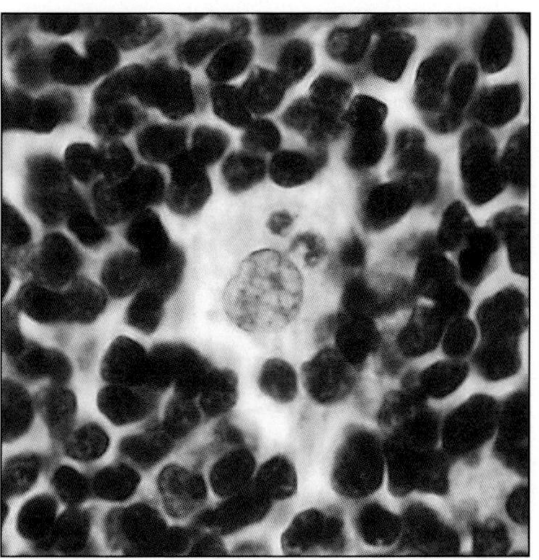

(Left) *High magnification of lymphocyte-rich thymoma (WHO type B1) shows a monotonous population of small lymphocytes with only rare scattered cells with larger nuclei and indistinct rim of cytoplasm.* ***(Right)*** *High magnification of lymphocyte-rich thymoma (WHO type B1) shows a large neoplastic epithelial cell in the center surrounded by a dense population of small lymphocytes.*

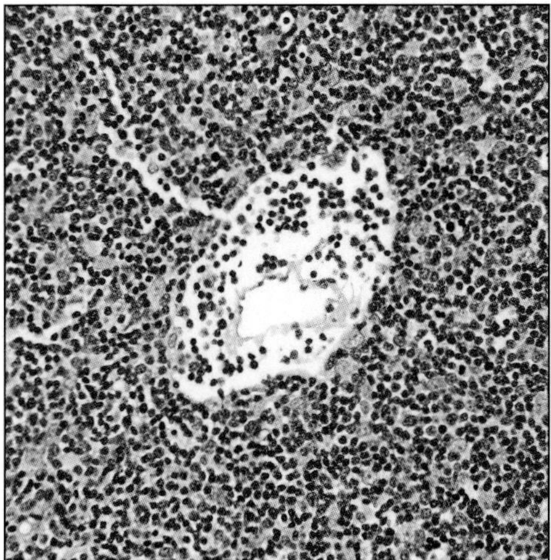

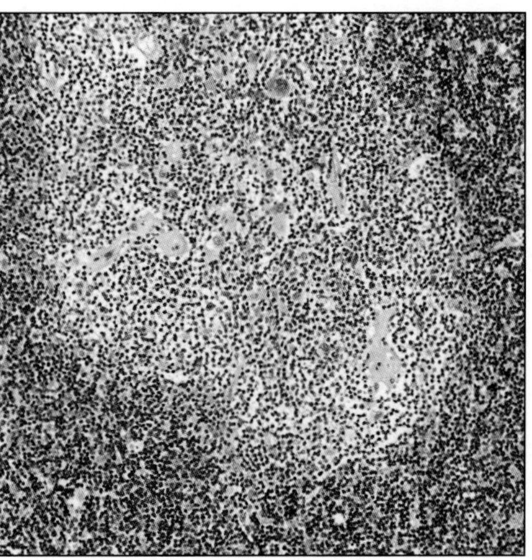

(Left) *Lymphocyte-rich thymoma (WHO type B1) shows a dilated perivascular space (center of the field) filled with scattered small lymphocytes. Notice the small vessel lumen "floating" inside the empty perivascular space.* ***(Right)*** *Lymphocyte-rich thymoma (WHO type B1) shows an area of "medullary" differentiation (center). This area is sparsely cellular and contains fewer lymphocytes than the surrounding parenchyma, as well as areas of hyalinization with abortive Hassall corpuscles.*

THYMOMA

Unusual Features in Lymphocyte-Rich Thymoma

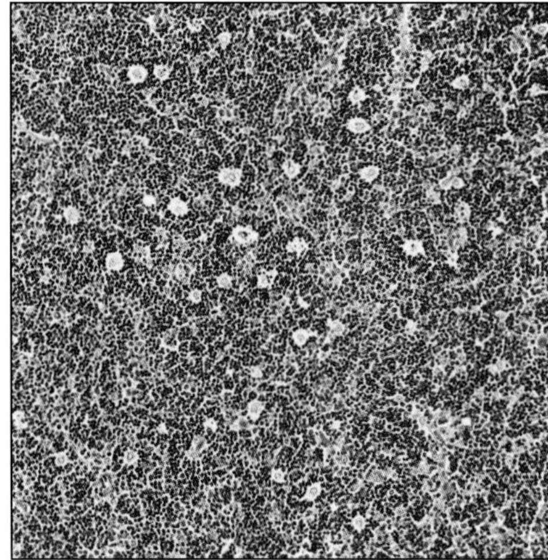

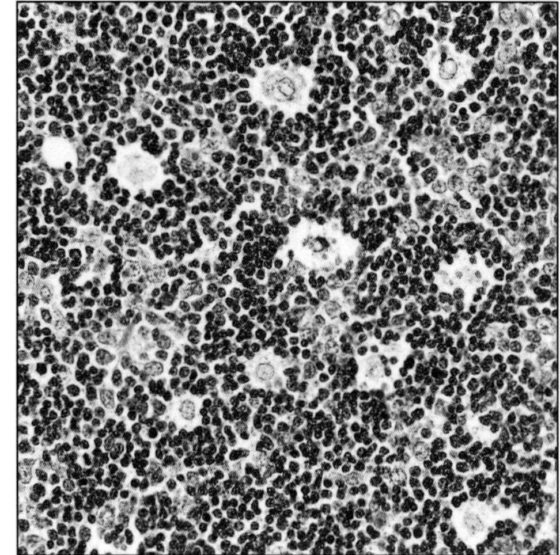

(Left) *Lymphocyte-rich thymoma (WHO type B1) shows prominent "starry sky" appearance. These tumors can be easily confused with lymphoblastic lymphoma, which are also often characterized by this histologic appearance.* ***(Right)*** *Lymphocyte-rich thymoma (WHO type B1) shows "starry sky" appearance represented by the large cells surrounded by clear spaces. The "starry sky" appearance is caused by an abundance of tingible-body macrophages.*

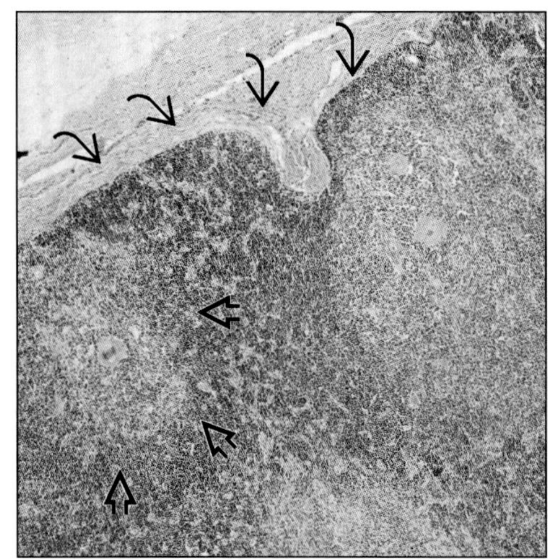

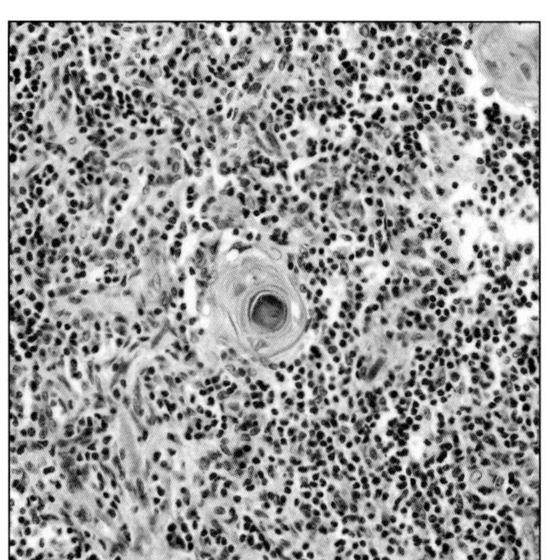

(Left) *Lymphocyte-rich thymoma (WHO type B1) shows well-developed and sharply defined areas that resemble the normal cortex → circumscribing lighter areas that resemble the thymic medulla ⇨. Tumors with these features were termed "organoid" and "predominantly cortical" thymoma in prior terminology.* ***(Right)*** *High-power view shows a Hassall corpuscle within an area of "medullary" differentiation in lymphocyte-rich thymoma (WHO type B1; "organoid" thymoma).*

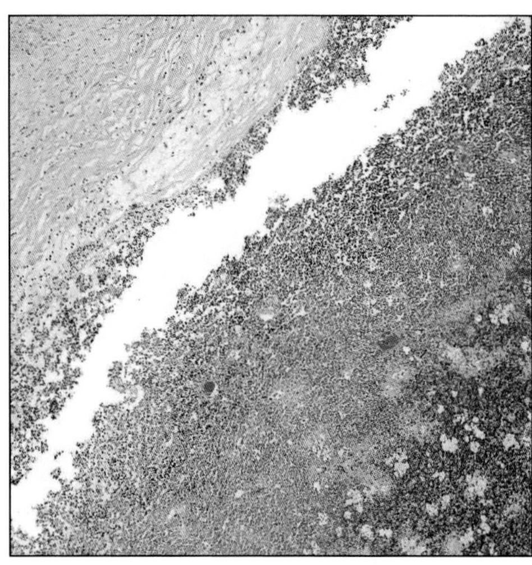

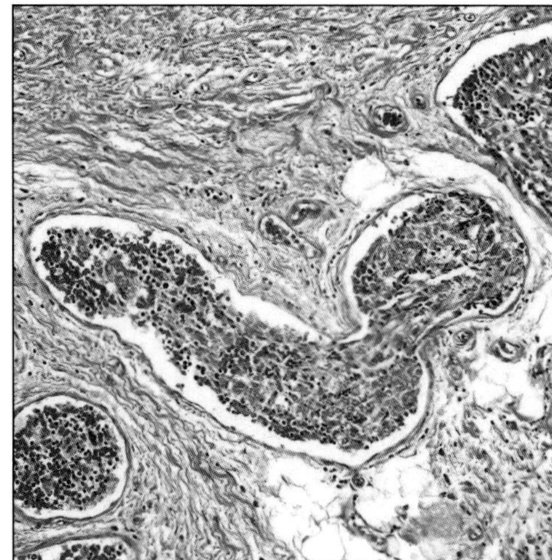

(Left) *Area of necrosis and infarction is seen in lymphocyte-rich (WHO type B1) thymoma. This is caused by vaso-occlusive phenomena in the vicinity of the infarcted areas of tumors with cystic changes. This should not be mistaken for a sign of malignancy or more aggressive behavior.* ***(Right)*** *Focus of vascular invasion in lymphocyte-rich thymoma (WHO type B2) is shown. The significance of this finding is unknown, but it is believed to be associated with more aggressive behavior.*

Lymphocyte-Rich Thymoma (WHO Type B2)

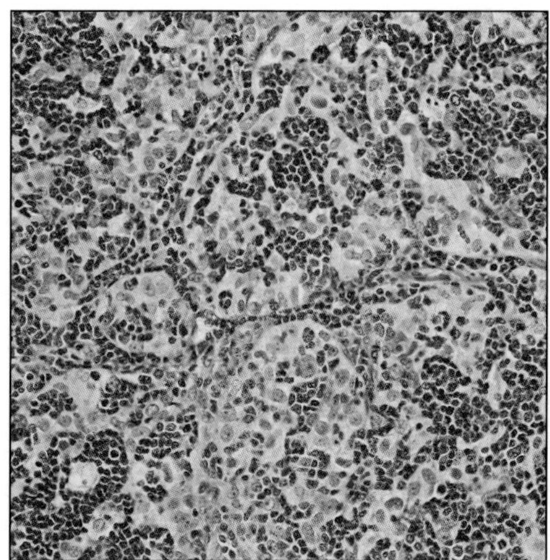

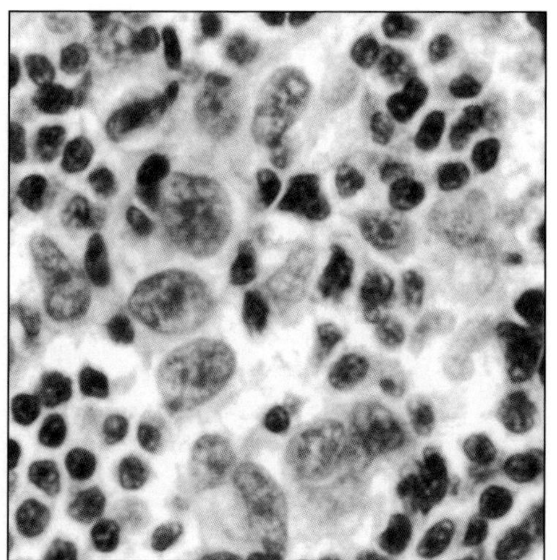

(Left) *Mixed lymphoepithelial (WHO type B2) thymoma shows approximately equal admixture of lymphocytes with neoplastic epithelial cells.* ***(Right)*** *Higher magnification of mixed lymphoepithelial thymoma (WHO type B2) shows abundant large, round to oval epithelial cells displaying vesicular nuclei with prominent eosinophilic nucleoli and an indistinct rim of amphophilic cytoplasm. Note the variation in size and shape of the epithelial cells.*

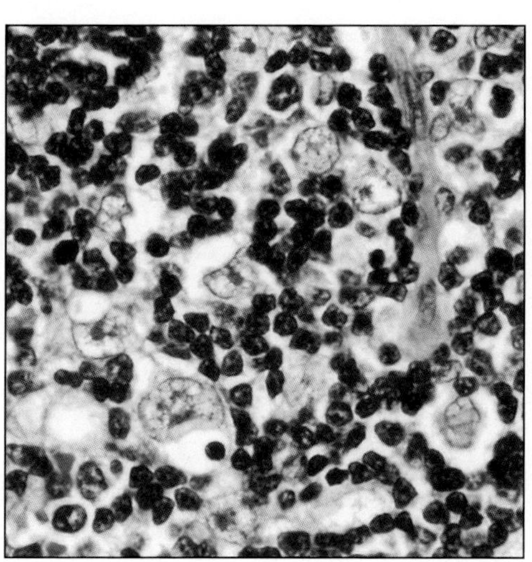

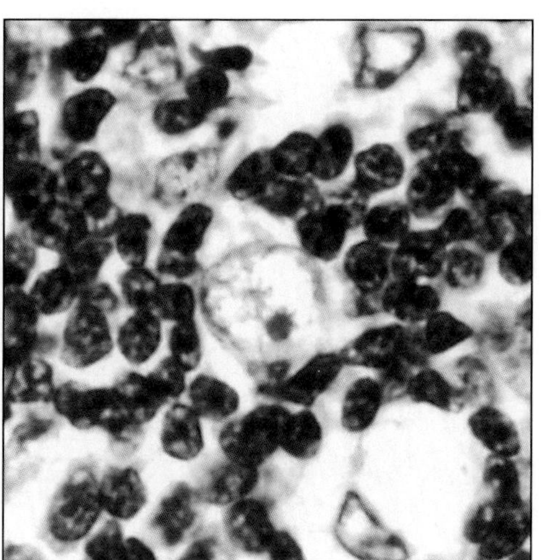

(Left) *Another example of mixed lymphoepithelial thymoma (WHO type B2) shows a large number of thymic epithelial cells admixed with small lymphocytes.* ***(Right)*** *High power of mixed lymphoepithelial thymoma (WHO type B2) shows a large epithelial cell in the center surrounded by small lymphocytes. The large cell in the center of the field shows a vesicular nucleus with prominent eosinophilic nucleolus.*

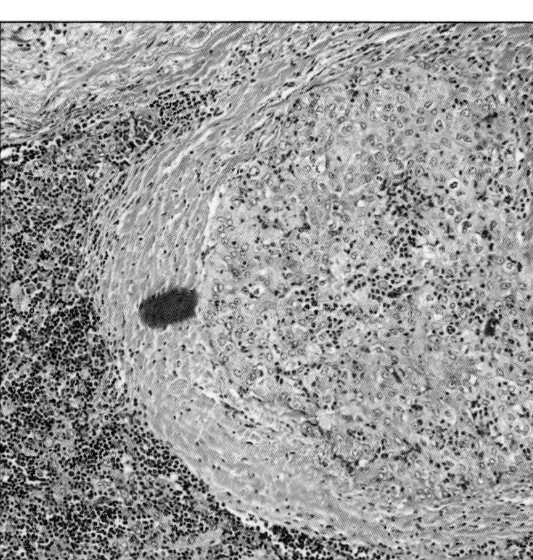

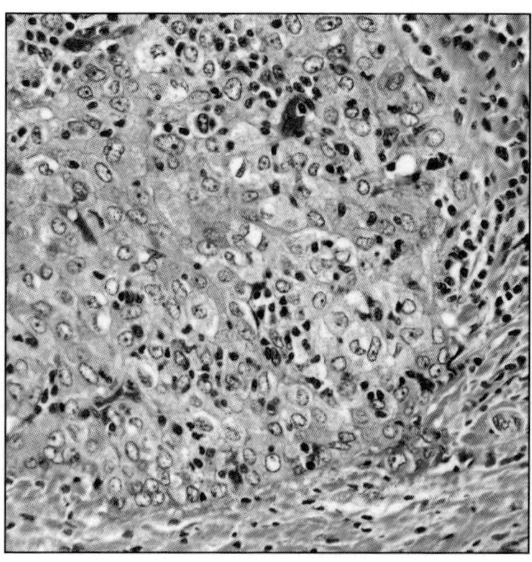

(Left) *Combinations of thymoma WHO type B2 and B3 are seen in approximately 30% of cases. The nodule on the right corresponds to a focus of atypical thymoma (WHO B3). The areas on the left show lymphoepithelial thymoma (WHO type B2) and contain a higher density of small lymphocytes.* ***(Right)*** *Higher magnification shows a nodule with atypical thymoma (WHO type B3) in a combined thymoma, type B2 + B3. Notice the large size of the epithelial cells.*

Immunohistochemical Features

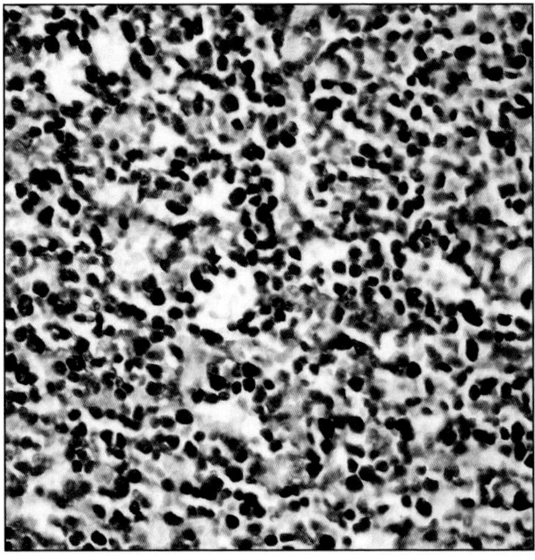

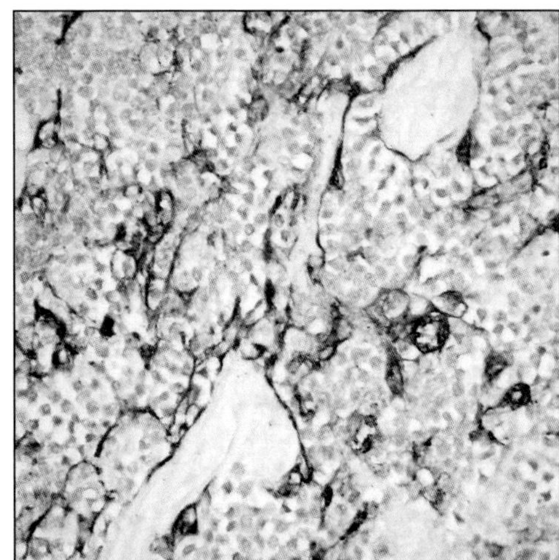

(Left) *Lymphocyte-rich thymoma with "starry sky" appearance simulating lymphoblastic lymphoma shows striking nuclear positivity in small lymphocytes for TdT and should not be confused with lymphoblastic lymphoma.* ***(Right)*** *Immunoperoxidase stain for cytokeratin AE1/AE3 in lymphocyte-rich thymoma simulating lymphoblastic lymphoma shows scattered isolated keratin-positive tumor cells. Identification of keratin-positive cell population is critical to make the correct diagnosis.*

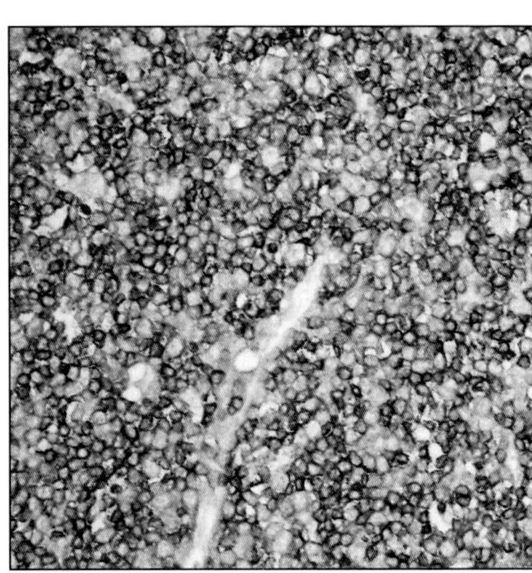

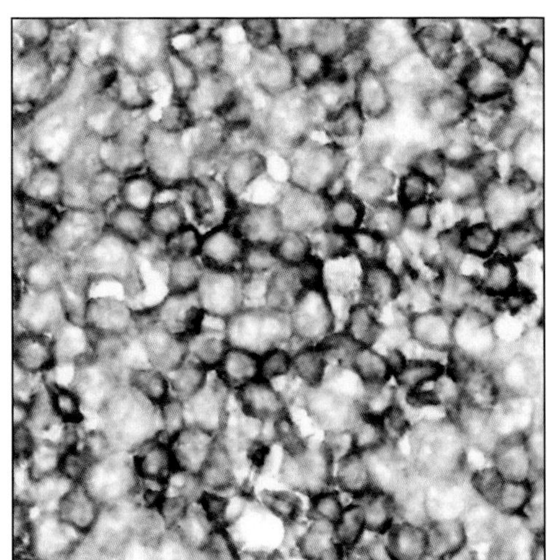

(Left) *Strong membrane positivity for CD3 is observed in this lymphocyte-rich thymoma (WHO type B1). A similar pattern of staining would also be expected for CD1a, a marker of immature T cells.* ***(Right)*** *Positive CD99 staining of the tumor cells is seen in this lymphocyte-rich thymoma (WHO type B1). CD99 is a marker of T-lymphoblasts and can be used in lieu of CD1a or TdT for the demonstration of immature T-lymphoblastic cells in lymphocyte-rich thymomas.*

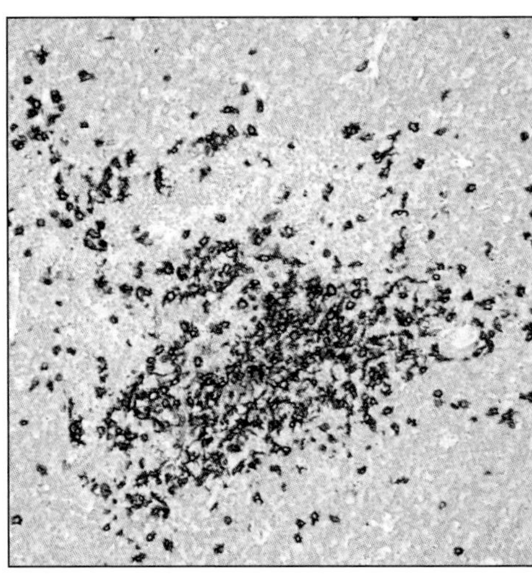

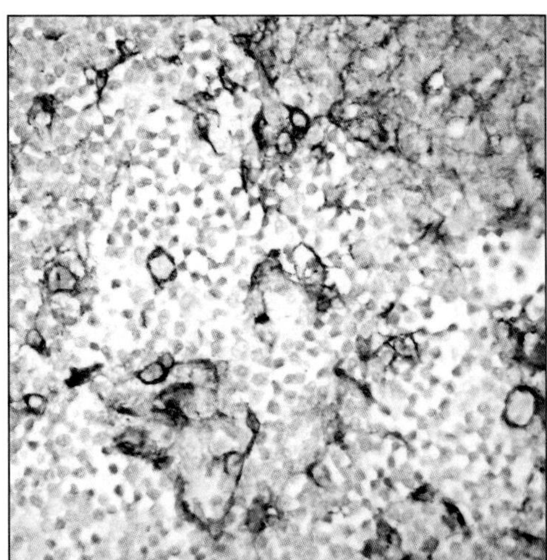

(Left) *This cluster of small lymphocytes is seen to stain with CD20, a B-cell marker. This represents residual islands of the native thymic B-cell lymphoid cell population that can give rise to MALT lymphomas in the thymus.* ***(Right)*** *Lymphocyte-rich thymoma (WHO type B1) shows a network of scattered keratin-positive thymic epithelial cells against a background of small lymphocytes. The scattered nature of the keratin-positive cells identifies them as the neoplastic epithelial component.*

Thymoma, Miscellaneous

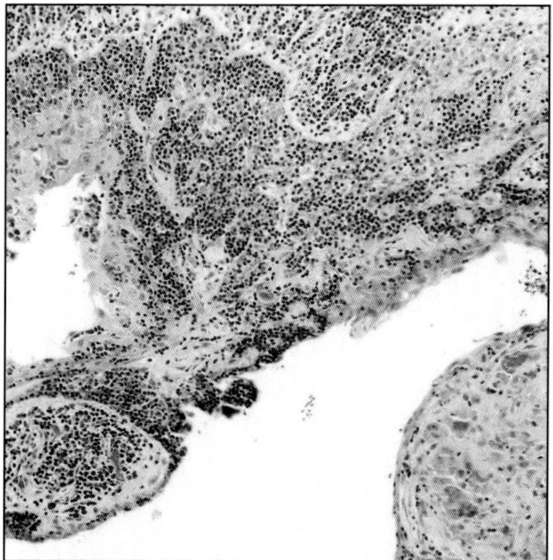

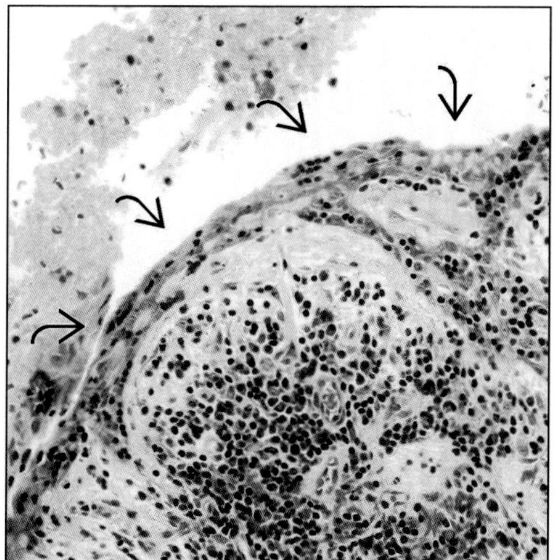

(Left) *Lymphocyte-rich (WHO type B1) thymoma shows secondary multilocular cystic changes in the surrounding, uninvolved, residual thymus. The epithelial lining of the cysts is in continuity with dilated Hassall corpuscles and devoid of cytologic atypia.* ***(Right)*** *High power in lymphocyte-rich thymoma shows secondary multilocular thymic cyst-like changes. Notice hemorrhage and inflammation in the wall of the cyst and the flattened squamous epithelial lining* ➚.

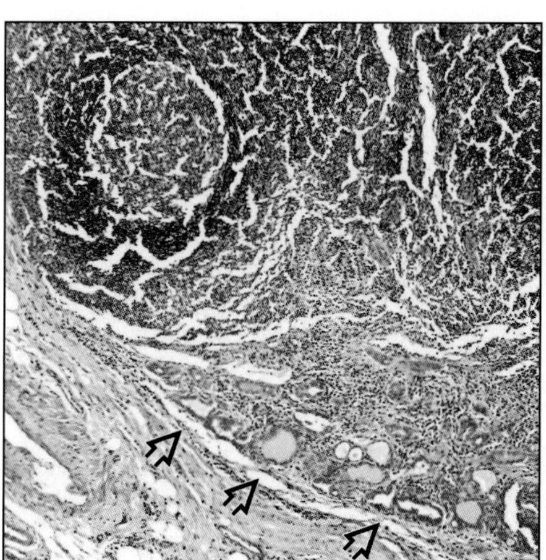

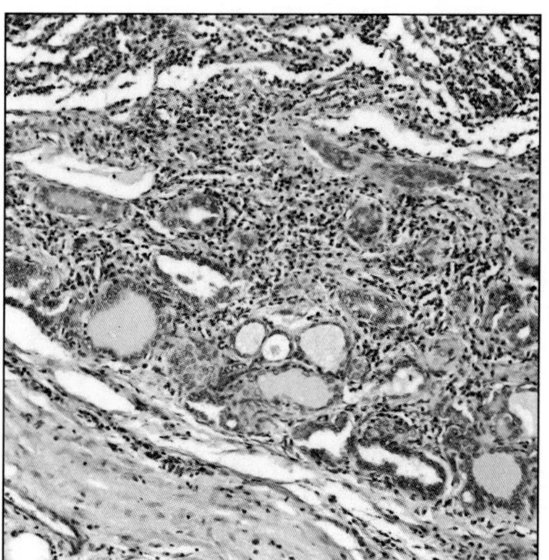

(Left) *Metastasis of spindle cell thymoma to a mediastinal lymph node is seen. Notice the gland-like structures* ➨ *in the lymph node sinus percolating into the node adjacent to a follicle with a germinal center.* ***(Right)*** *High-power view of lymph node metastasis from spindle cell thymoma (WHO type A) to mediastinal lymph node is shown. Notice solid nests of spindle cells admixed with cyst-like structures within lymph node sinus.*

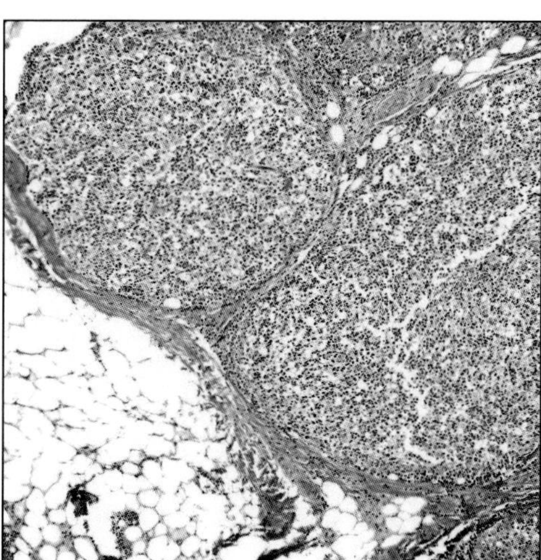

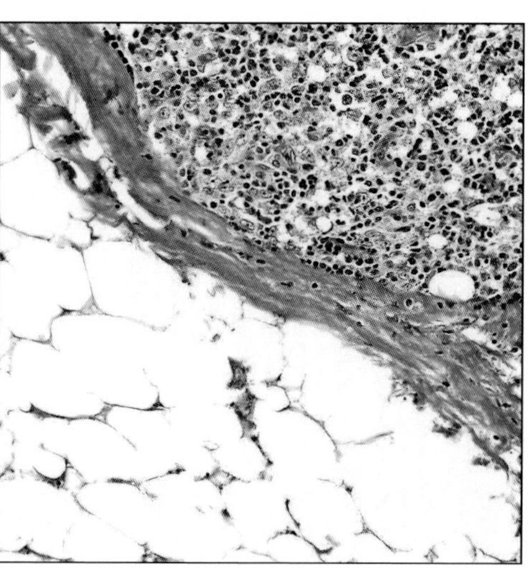

(Left) *Invasion of the capsule into mediastinal fat is noted in this example of mixed lymphoepithelial thymoma (WHO type B2). Notice preservation of the lobular architecture. This focus would be considered microinvasion (stage IIA) in the modified Masaoka staging (Koga et al). The tumor would be thus classified as "noninvasive" because it does not yet invade neighboring organs.* ***(Right)*** *High-power view shows microinvasive lymphoepithelial thymoma infiltrating perithymic fat.*

Cardiovascular

Neoplasm, Benign

RHABDOMYOMA

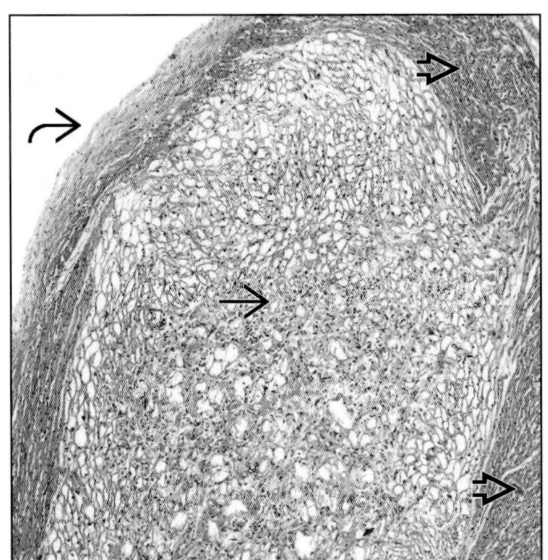

Cardiac hamartoma in a newborn shows the pale tumor ➔, which is located in the myocardium ⇨, causing a bulge into the cavity ↗. The tumor is well circumscribed but not encapsulated.

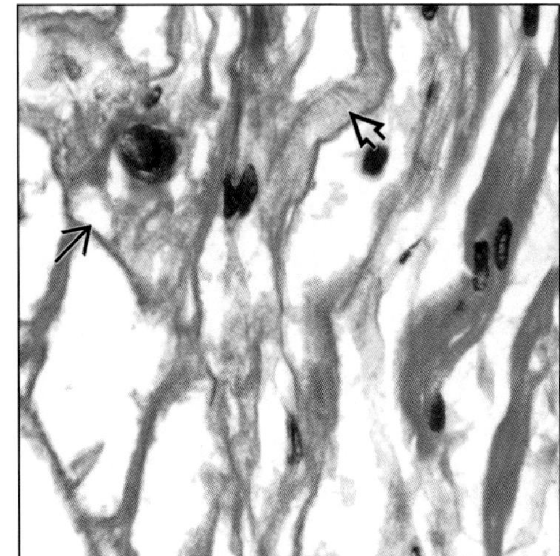

At high magnification, some tumor cells are vacuolated while others are eosinophilic with cross striations ⇨. Note the spider cell ➔ upper left, with central nucleus and cytoplasmic strands.

TERMINOLOGY

Definitions

- Congenital hamartoma of heart strongly associated with tuberous sclerosis

ETIOLOGY/PATHOGENESIS

Genetic Association

- 90% of cardiac rhabdomyomas are associated with tuberous sclerosis; the rest are sporadic or associated with congenital heart disease
- Tuberous sclerosis is autosomal dominant in 1/3 and sporadic in 2/3
- Causative mutation is in gene *TSC1/TSC2*

CLINICAL ISSUES

Presentation

- Occasionally diagnosed in utero when investigating fetal hydrops or cardiac arrhythmia
- After birth, symptoms (such as hypoxic spells and cardiac failure) are related to obstruction of blood flow
- Arrhythmias occur in about 1/3 of patients

Treatment

- Surgical resection is indicated only in those with significant symptoms

Prognosis

- Large size and hydrops are associated with poor neonatal outcome
- Majority regress spontaneously
- Overall prognosis is related to severity of tuberous sclerosis lesions

Incidence

- All cardiac tumors are rare, but rhabdomyoma is most common accounting for 60% of tumors in infants and children
- Incidence is 1 in 6,000 live births
- All cases present before age 25 years

IMAGE FINDINGS

Ultrasonographic Findings

- Solid hyperechoic masses in ventricular myocardium or ventricular septum; may protrude into and distort the chamber

MACROSCOPIC FEATURES

Gross Features

- Firm, white, well-circumscribed nodules, 1 mm to several centimeters in size
- Can be single or multiple
- In sporadic cases, tumors tend to be single and larger
- Occur most frequently in left ventricle or ventricular septum
- May occur in myocardium or may protrude into chamber

MICROSCOPIC PATHOLOGY

Histologic Features

- Tumor is composed of sheets of vacuolated cells that are rich in glycogen and are thus strongly PAS(+)
- Spider cells, although pathognomic, are few; these are large cells with central nuclei and radial extensions from nuclei to the periphery
- Tumor cells contain variable numbers of myofibrils; cross striations can be identified on high power
- There is no nuclear atypia, mitosis, or necrosis

RHABDOMYOMA

Key Facts

Etiology/Pathogenesis
- 90% of cardiac rhabdomyomas are associated with tuberous sclerosis

Clinical Issues
- Most common cardiac tumor; large size and hydrops associated with poor outcome; majority regress spontaneously

Macroscopic Features
- Firm, white, well-circumscribed nodules, 1 mm to several centimeters in size
- Most frequent in left ventricle/ventricular septum

Microscopic Pathology
- Tumor composed of large vacuolated cells; spider cells are pathognomic; tumor cells are positive for PAS and muscle markers such as actin, desmin, myoglobin

ANCILLARY TESTS

Histochemistry
- Periodic acid-Schiff
  - Reactivity: Positive
  - Staining pattern
    - Cytoplasmic

Immunohistochemistry
- Tumor cells are positive for muscle markers such as actin, desmin, myoglobin
- Spider cells are ubiquitin positive, a protein in the apoptosis pathway, which may explain spontaneous regression of cardiac rhabdomyomas

DIFFERENTIAL DIAGNOSIS

Histiocytoid Cardiomyopathy
- Tumor nodules are small
- Cells are large but do not form well-circumscribed tumors; cytoplasm is more granular and eosinophilic

Myxoma
- More common in adults; most on left side of interatrial septum
- Small stellate cells with abundant cytoplasm and indistinct borders, arranged singly, in cords, or in vasoformative ring structures within large amount of gelatinous stroma

Glycogen Storage Disease
- Can mimic vacuolated cells of rhabdomyoma
- Have abundant glycogen but do not form well-circumscribed nodules

DIAGNOSTIC CHECKLIST

Clinically Relevant Pathologic Features
- Mitotic rate
  - No mitosis or expression of proliferation markers such as Ki-67, which indicates that these are hamartomas

Pathologic Interpretation Pearls
- Spider cells
- Large cells with vacuolated cytoplasm

SELECTED REFERENCES

1. Jain D et al: Benign cardiac tumors and tumorlike conditions. Ann Diagn Pathol. 14(3):215-30, 2010
2. Isaacs H: Perinatal (fetal and neonatal) tuberous sclerosis: a review. Am J Perinatol. 26(10):755-60, 2009
3. Ramírez-Marrero MA et al: Early complete regression of multiple cardiac tumors suggestive of cardiac rhabdomyomas. Rev Esp Cardiol. 62(6):708-9, 2009
4. Dereddy NR et al: Resection of ventricular rhabdomyomas in infants presenting with cardiac failure. Cardiol Young. 18(6):635-7, 2008

IMAGE GALLERY

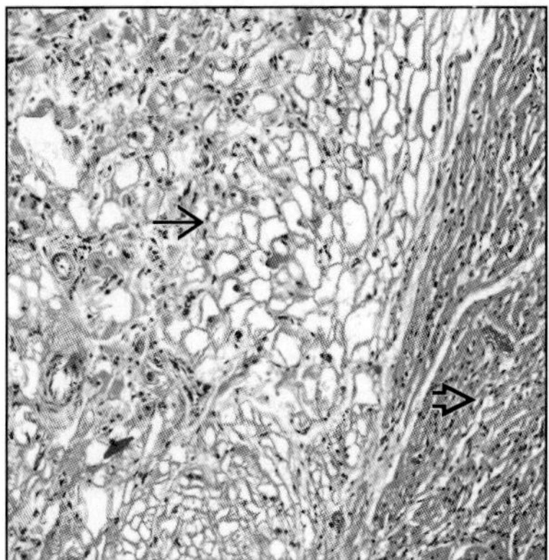
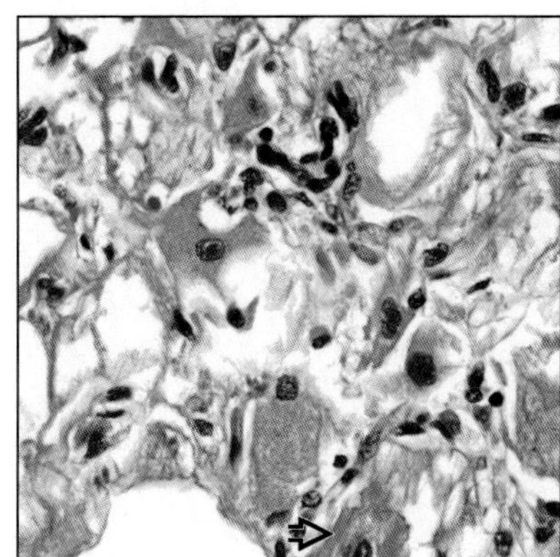
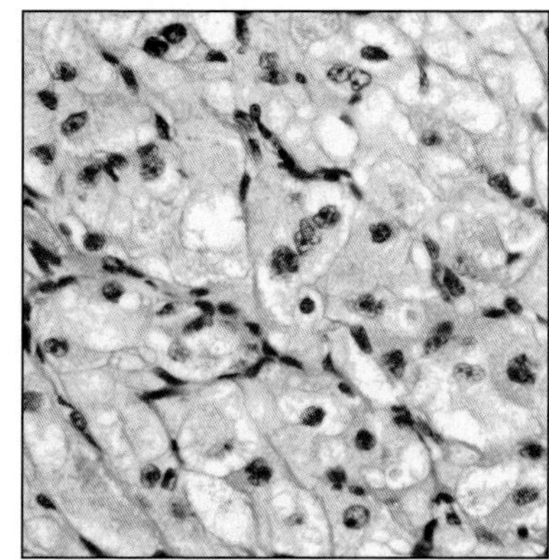

*(**Left**) H&E shows rhabdomyoma with vacuolated cells ⇒. Note the adjacent uninvolved myocardium ⇨ to the right. (**Center**) High-power view of cardiac rhabdomyoma shows a mixture of vacuolated and pink cells. Cross striations ⇨ can be identified in some of the cells. (**Right**) The main differential diagnostic consideration is histiocytoid cardiomyopathy, shown here at high power. The cells are more uniformly eosinophilic than those seen in cardiac rhabdomyoma.*

FIBROMA

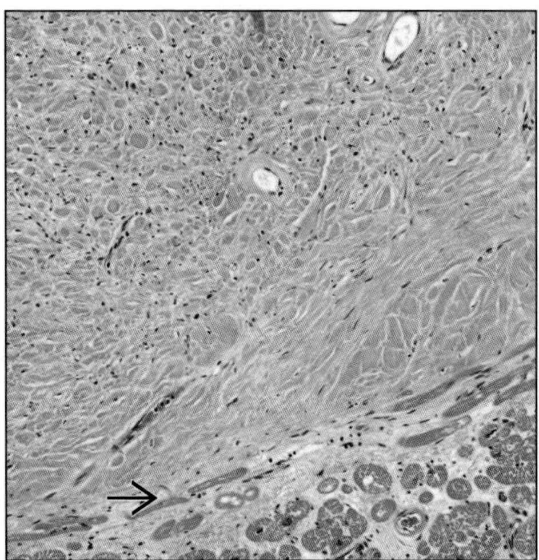
Low-power view of a cardiac fibroma shows a well-demarcated tumor compressing adjacent myocytes ➔. The tumor is relatively uniform and hypocellular. There is no hemorrhage or necrosis.

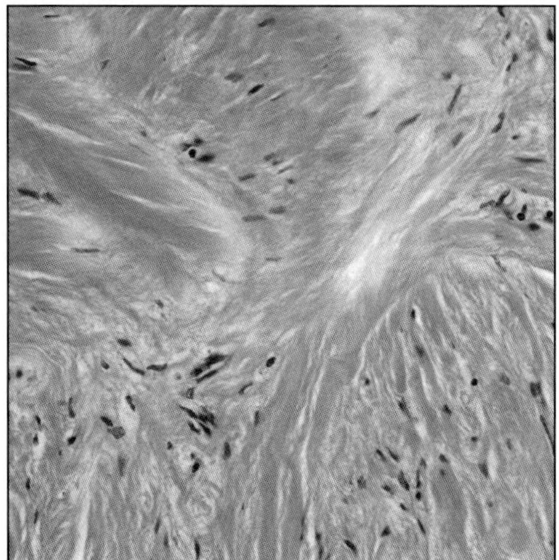
High-power view shows a bland hypocellular and hypovascular tumor composed of spindle cells and fibrous tissue, including collagen bundles. There is no dysplasia, mitosis, or necrosis.

TERMINOLOGY

Definitions

- Benign tumor of the heart composed of fibroblasts and collagen
- It is still controversial whether fibroma is a hamartoma or neoplasm

ETIOLOGY/PATHOGENESIS

Genetic Association

- About 4% of tumors are associated with basal cell nevus (Gorlin) syndrome
- *PTCH1* mutations are associated with Gorlin syndrome
- Loss of *PTCH1* loci found in a case of sporadic cardiac fibroma
- No β-catenin mutation identified

CLINICAL ISSUES

Presentation

- 2nd most common type of pediatric cardiac tumor after rhabdomyoma
- Usually detected in infancy or in utero
  - 1/3 are detected by 1 year of age
- May present with cardiomegaly, heart failure, ventricular arrhythmias, or sudden death
- 1/3 are asymptomatic; tumor is discovered incidentally on imaging

Treatment

- Definitive treatment is surgical excision
- Tumor can be shelled out, but this leaves behind small bits of tumor
  - May lead to recurrence, but many patients do well even with partial resection
- For very large tumors, heart transplantation may be needed

Prognosis

- Good outcome for most patients
- Cardiac fibromas do not regress

IMAGE FINDINGS

Echocardiography

- Usually large mass which is noncontractile, solid, and has heterogeneous echogenicity

MACROSCOPIC FEATURES

General Features

- Solitary mass located in interventricular septum or free wall of the ventricles
- Size ranges from 2-10 cm
- All are nonencapsulated, may be well circumscribed or infiltrative
- Cut surface is dense white; often central calcification due to poor vascularization of center of tumor
- No necrosis, hemorrhage or cysts
- Grossly resembles leiomyoma

MICROSCOPIC PATHOLOGY

Histologic Features

- Resembles fibromatosis histologically
- Composed of spindle cells
- More cellular in infants; adults have more collagen
- Elastic fibers are present in > 1/2 of the tumors
- Chronic inflammation may be present in tumor
- Elastic van Gieson is positive

FIBROMA

Key Facts

Terminology

- Benign tumor of the heart composed of fibroblasts and collagen

Clinical Issues

- 2nd most common type of pediatric cardiac tumor (after rhabdomyoma)
- Good outcome after surgical excision

Macroscopic Features

- Solitary mass, 2-10 cm, in interventricular septum or free wall of the ventricles
- Nonencapsulated, well circumscribed or infiltrative
- Cut surface is dense white; often central calcification

Microscopic Pathology

- Resembles fibromatosis, composed of bland spindle cells positive for SMA

ANCILLARY TESTS

Immunohistochemistry

- Muscle markers such as smooth muscle actin and desmin positive
- Vimentin is diffusely positive; myogenin negative

DIFFERENTIAL DIAGNOSIS

Inflammatory Myofibroblastic Pseudotumor

- Rare tumor composed of myofibroblastic cells and variable amount of mostly chronic inflammation consisting of plasma cells and lymphocytes

Organized Thrombus

- Mural mass with prominent hemosiderin
- No infiltration into cardiac muscle

Myxoma with Fibrosis

- More common in adults
- Mural lesion, not intramuscular
- Fibrous tissue, hemosiderin, some stellate cells

Fibrosarcoma

- Tumor occurring mostly in adults, but may occasionally affect children or adolescents; fibroma is mainly seen in newborns or neonates < 6 months old
- Prominent atypia, mitoses, and foci of necrosis

Rhabdomyoma

- Large vacuolated tumor cells, "spider cells"
  - Secondary to accumulation of glycogen

DIAGNOSTIC CHECKLIST

Clinically Relevant Pathologic Features

- Age distribution
  - Seen in newborns and young infants
- Gross appearance
  - Well circumscribed or infiltrative but amenable to resection
- Mitotic rate; no mitoses

Pathologic Interpretation Pearls

- Intramyocardial tumor mainly composed of mature fibrous tissue
- No pleomorphism, hemosiderin, necrosis or mitosis
- Inflammation not a significant component
- SMA(+), may be desmin(+) as well

SELECTED REFERENCES

1. Castillo JG et al: Characterization and management of cardiac tumors. Semin Cardiothorac Vasc Anesth. 14(1):6-20, 2010
2. Jain D et al: Benign cardiac tumors and tumorlike conditions. Ann Diagn Pathol. 14(3):215-30, 2010
3. Yinon Y et al: Fetal cardiac tumors: a single-center experience of 40 cases. Prenat Diagn. 30(10):941-9, 2010
4. Burke A et al: Pediatric heart tumors. Cardiovasc Pathol. 17(4):193-8, 2008
5. Rivera-Dávila AD et al: Primary cardiac and pericardial tumors. Bol Asoc Med P R. 100(4):48-54, 2008

IMAGE GALLERY

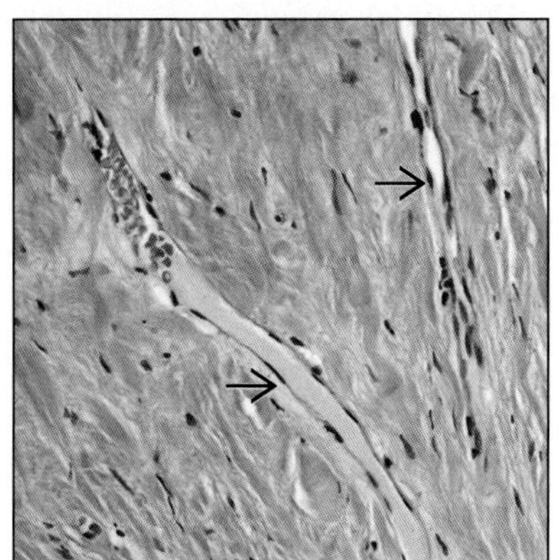

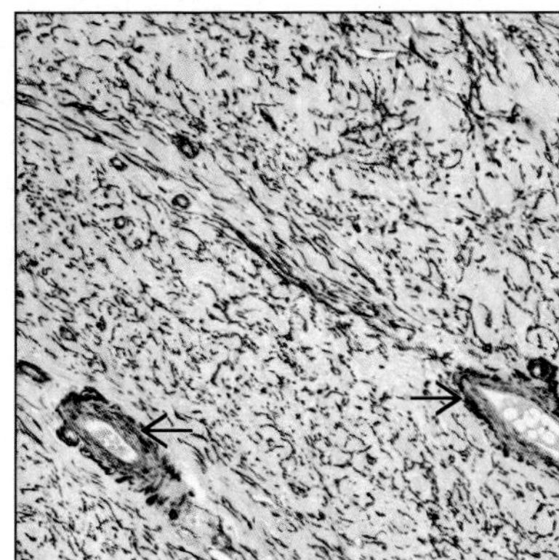

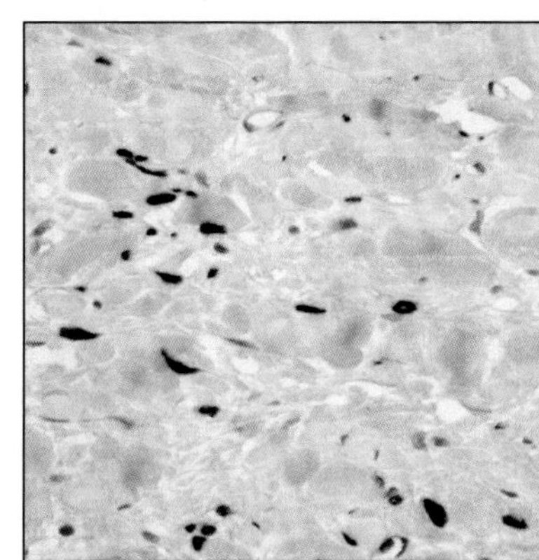

*(**Left**) Bland, uniform spindle cells are seen on this high-power image. There is abundant collagen and thin-walled blood vessels ⇒. Note the lack of mitosis, atypia, and entrapped myocytes. (**Center**) IHC stain for smooth muscle actin shows positive staining in lesional cells. Note the positive blood vessel walls ⇒, which serve as internal control. (**Right**) IHC stain for desmin shows focal nuclear positivity in lesional cells. Dense collagen fibers are negative.*

HISTIOCYTOID CARDIOMYOPATHY

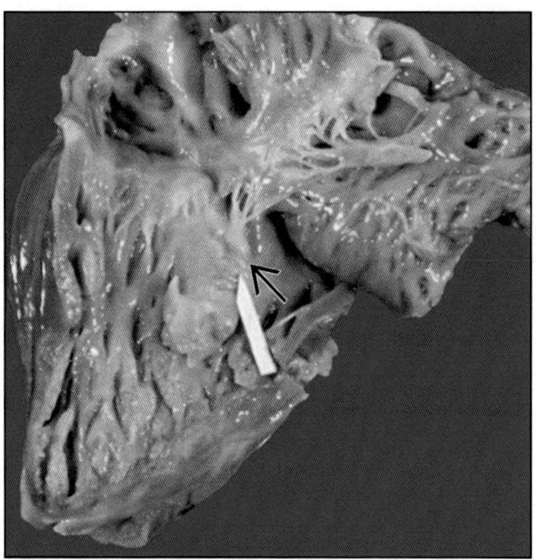

In this gross photograph of a heart, there are multiple subendocardial nodules present on the intraventricular septum ➔.

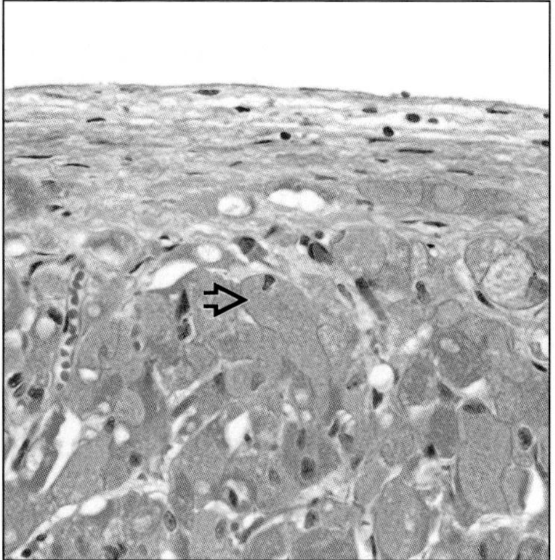

This subendocardial nodule is composed of large, polygonal, histiocytoid-like cells ➲.

TERMINOLOGY

Abbreviations

- Histiocytoid cardiomyopathy (HC)

Synonyms

- Arachnocytosis of myocardium
- Congenital cardiomyopathy
- Infantile cardiomyopathy
- Infantile cardiomyopathy with histiocytoid changes
- Infantile xanthomatous cardiomyopathy
- Foamy myocardial transformation
- Focal lipid cardiomyopathy
- Isolated cardiac lipidosis
- Myocardial or conduction system hamartoma

Definitions

- Rare distinctive arrhythmogenic disorder characterized morphologically by focal collections of altered histiocytoid myocytes
- Associated with hamartomatous/neoplastic lesion of Purkinje cells of cardiac conduction system

ETIOLOGY/PATHOGENESIS

Unproven Theories

- Viral infection
- Myocardial ischemia
- Toxic exposure
- Metabolic disorders
  - Glycogen storage disease
  - Cardiac lipidosis
- Mitochondrial disorder
  - Mitochondrial cytochrome *b* gene
  - MERRF mitochondrial DNA mutation
  - *Sox6* mutation
- X-linked chromosomal abnormality
  - Associated with microphthalmia linear skin defect

CLINICAL ISSUES

Epidemiology

- Age
  - Occurs predominantly in 1st 2 years of life
    - 20% diagnosed in 1st month
    - 60% diagnosed in 1st year
    - < 3% diagnosed after 2 years of life
    - No reported cases after 3 years of life
- Gender
  - Female preponderance of 3:1
- Ethnicity
  - Caucasian (80%)
  - African-American (15%)
  - Latin-American (3%)
  - Oriental (extremely rare)

Presentation

- Spectrum of uncontrolled/malignant arrhythmias
  - Paroxysmal atrial tachycardia
  - Atrial fibrillation
  - Ventricular fibrillation
  - Ventricular tachycardia
  - Premature atrial contractions
  - Premature ventricular contraction
  - Wolff-Parkinson-White syndrome
  - Right or left bundle branch block
- Flu-like symptoms
- Cardiomegaly
- Associated anomalies
  - Cardiac malformation (16%)
    - Ventricular and atrial septal defects
    - Hypoplastic left heart syndrome
    - Endocardial fibroelastosis
  - Extracardiac anomalies (17%)
    - Corneal opacities
    - Microcephaly
    - Cataract
    - Aphakia
    - Hydrocephalus

HISTIOCYTOID CARDIOMYOPATHY

Key Facts

Terminology

- Rare distinctive arrhythmogenic disorder associated with hamartomatous/neoplastic lesion of Purkinje cells of cardiac conduction system

Clinical Issues

- Spectrum of uncontrolled/malignant arrhythmias
- Occurs predominantly in 1st 2 years of life
- Female preponderance is 3:1
- Caucasian (80%)
- African-American (15%)

Macroscopic Features

- Cardiomegaly (95%)
- Subendocardial yellow-tan nodules/plaques
  - Single or multiple
  - Seen in both ventricles, septum, and on all 4 cardiac valves

Microscopic Pathology

- Multifocal, ill-defined islands of large polygonal cells
  - Superabundance of swollen mitochondria: Push diminished myofibrils to periphery of cell

Ancillary Tests

- 2 significantly downregulated sets of genes aligned sequentially along genome
- Strong decreases in IL-33 expression
  - Downregulation of *IL-33-IL1RL1/p38-MAPK/S100A8-S100A9* axis
  - Leads to reduced activation of NF-κB complex, negatively impacting the myocardium

- Agenesis of corpus callosum
- Cleft palate
- Laryngeal web
- Linear skin defect
- Renal cyst

  - Extracardiac histiocytoid cells in exocrine and endocrine glands (7%)
  - Combined cardiac and extracardiac anomalies (4%)
- ~ 20% present as sudden death

Treatment

- Options
  - Surgical intervention
  - Electrophysiological mapping
  - Ablation of arrhythmogenic foci
  - Cardiac transplant (extensive disease)

Prognosis

- Survival rate of approximately 80%
- Fatal if left untreated
- Has improved in last 2 decades

MACROSCOPIC FEATURES

General Features

- Cardiomegaly (95%)
- Subendocardial yellow-tan nodules/plaques
  - Single or multiple
  - Ranging in size from 1-15 mm
  - Mainly seen beneath the endocardium
    - Lesions follow distribution of bundle branches of conduction system
  - Also found in
    - Ventricles
    - Atria
    - Papillary muscles
    - Septum
    - On all 4 cardiac valves
  - Rarely seen in inner myocardium and subepicardial areas
- Lesions may be grossly inapparent as nodules
- Multiple cross sections of myocardium may show mottled appearance with irregular, ill-defined, yellowish-tan areas

MICROSCOPIC PATHOLOGY

Histologic Features

- Multifocal, ill-defined islands of large polygonal myocytes
  - Range in size from 20-40 μm
  - Granular eosinophilic foamy cytoplasm
  - Small round to oval-shaped nucleus
  - Occasional nucleoli
  - Cytoplasmic appearance due to extensive accumulation of mitochondria
    - Histiocytoid appearance
  - Distributed along bundle branches of the conduction system
- Sinoatrial and atrioventricular nodes are involved in majority of cases

Ultrastructural Features

- Poorly developed intercellular junctions
  - Scattered desmosomes
  - Intercalated discs
- Cytoplasm
  - Superabundance of swollen mitochondria
    - Push diminished myofibrils to periphery of cell
    - Disorganized cristae
    - Dense membrane bounded granules
  - Has lipid droplets of variable size
  - Has leptometric fibers

ANCILLARY TESTS

Molecular Genetics

- 2 significantly down-regulated sets of genes aligned sequentially along the genome
  - *S100A8*, *S100A9*, and *S100A12* at 1q21.3
  - *IL1RL1* (ST2), *IL18R1*, and *IL18RAP* at 2q12.1a
- Strong decreases in *IL-33* expression

HISTIOCYTOID CARDIOMYOPATHY

- Down regulation of *IL-33-IL1RL1/p38-MAPK/S100A8-S100A9* axis
  - Leads to reduced activation of NF-κB complex, negatively impacting myocardium

DIFFERENTIAL DIAGNOSIS

Sudden Infant Death Syndrome (SIDS)

- Diagnosis of exclusion

Mitochondrial Cardiomyopathy

- Shows no discrete nodules
- All myocytes are affected but to variable degree
- Mitochondria are significantly abnormal in shape
  - Enlarged
  - Vary in size
  - Increased number of cristae
    - Cross section shows arrangement in concentric circular fashion (like growth rings of a tree) surrounding occasional dense bodies

Rhabdomyoma

- Shows typical "spider cells"
- Not clinically associated with cardiac arrhythmias
  - Associated with tuberous sclerosis

SELECTED REFERENCES

1. Shehata B et al: Identification of candidate genes for histiocytoid cardiomyopathy (HC) using whole genome expression analysis: analyzing material from the HC registry. Pediatr Dev Pathol. Epub ahead of print, 2011
2. Jain D et al: Histiocytoid cardiomyopathy: does it exist in the fetal-age group? Cardiovasc Pathol. Epub ahead of print, 2010
3. Edston E et al: Histiocytoid cardiomyopathy and ventricular non-compaction in a case of sudden death in a female infant. Int J Legal Med. 123(1):47-53, 2009
4. Finsterer J et al: Is mitochondrial disease the common cause of histiocytoid cardiomyopathy and non-compaction? Int J Legal Med. 123(6):507-8, 2009
5. Gelberg HB: Purkinje fiber dysplasia (histiocytoid cardiomyopathy) with ventricular noncompaction in a savannah kitten. Vet Pathol. 46(4):693-7, 2009
6. Abramovitz M et al: Optimization of RNA extraction from FFPE tissues for expression profiling in the DASL assay. Biotechniques. 44(3):417-23, 2008
7. Burke A et al: Pediatric heart tumors. Cardiovasc Pathol. 17(4):193-8, 2008
8. Finsterer J: Histiocytoid cardiomyopathy: a mitochondrial disorder. Clin Cardiol. 31(5):225-7, 2008
9. Ghavami S et al: S100A8/A9 at low concentration promotes tumor cell growth via RAGE ligation and MAP kinase-dependent pathway. J Leukoc Biol. 83(6):1484-92, 2008
10. Aksglaede L et al: [Histiocytoid cardiomyopathy. A rare cause of ventricular tachycardia and sudden cardiac death in small children.] Ugeskr Laeger. 168(1):61-2, 2006
11. Gilbert-Barness E et al: Pathogenesis of cardiac conduction disorders in children genetic and histopathologic aspects. Am J Med Genet A. 140(19):1993-2006, 2006
12. Shehata BM et al: Benign tumours with myocyte differentiation. In Travis WD et al: World Health Organization Classification of Tumors: Pathology and Genetics; Tumours of the Lung, Pleura, Thymus and Heart. Lyon: IARC Press. 254-59, 2004
13. Vallance HD et al: A case of sporadic infantile histiocytoid cardiomyopathy caused by the A8344G (MERRF) mitochondrial DNA mutation. Pediatr Cardiol. 25(5):538-40, 2004
14. Shehata BM et al: Histiocytoid cardiomyopathy: three new cases and a review of the literature. Pediatr Dev Pathol. 1(1):56-69, 1998
15. Bird LM et al: Female infant with oncocytic cardiomyopathy and microphthalmia with linear skin defects (MLS): a clue to the pathogenesis of oncocytic cardiomyopathy? Am J Med Genet. 53(2):141-8, 1994
16. Gelb AB et al: Infantile histiocytoid cardiomyopathy--myocardial or conduction system hamartoma: what is the cell type involved? Hum Pathol. 24(11):1226-31, 1993
17. Kearney DL et al: Pathologic features of myocardial hamartomas causing childhood tachyarrhythmias. Circulation. 75(4):705-10, 1987

HISTIOCYTOID CARDIOMYOPATHY

Microscopic and Ultrastructural Features

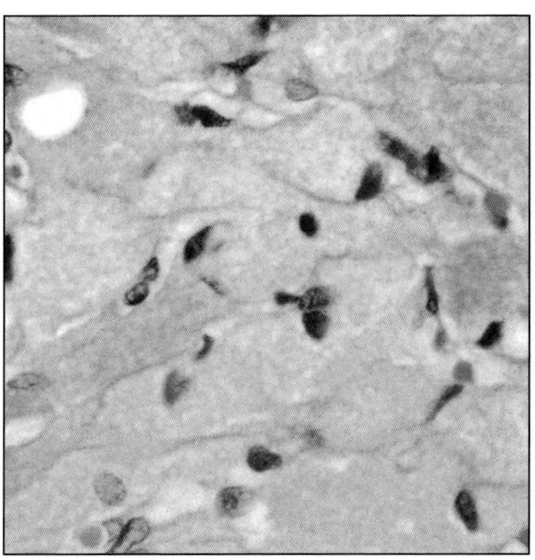

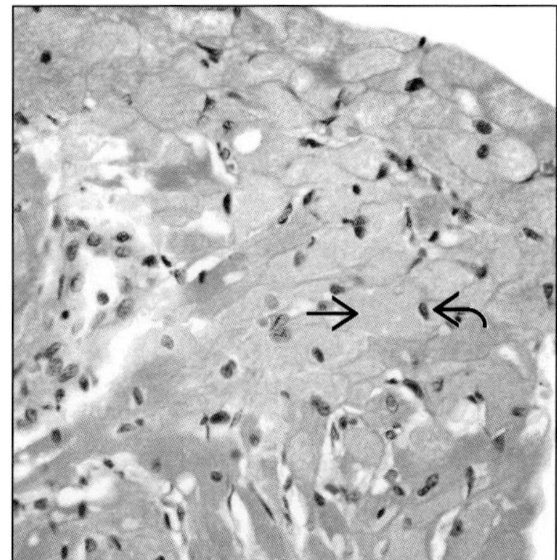

(Left) *Enlarged myocytes have a histiocytoid appearance due to their pale, foamy cytoplasm in this example of histiocytoid cardiomyopathy.* ***(Right)*** *Sheets of histiocytoid cardiomyopathy cells show abundant foamy cytoplasm →, small nuclei ↪, and occasional prominent nucleoli (not shown). The eosinophilic foamy cytoplasm is related to the abundant mitochondria.*

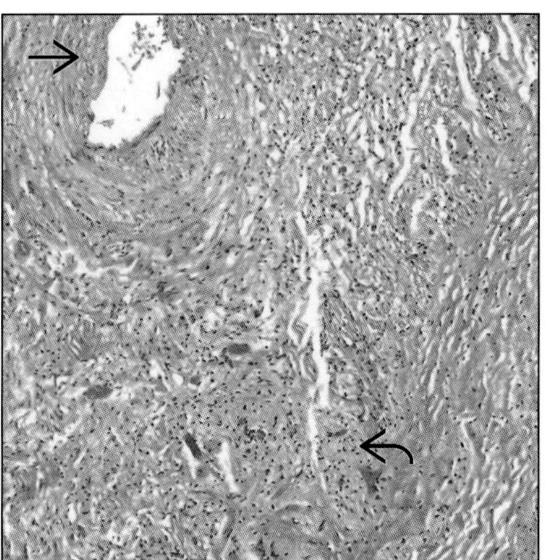

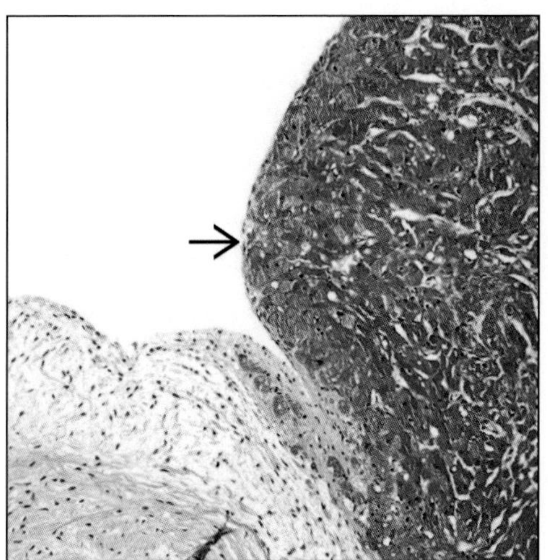

(Left) *This sinoatrial node is heavily infiltrated by histiocytoid cardiomyopathy cells ↪. Note the artery in the upper left corner →.* ***(Right)*** *A histiocytoid cardiomyopathy nodule → on the top of a cardiac valve is highlighted by this trichrome stain.*

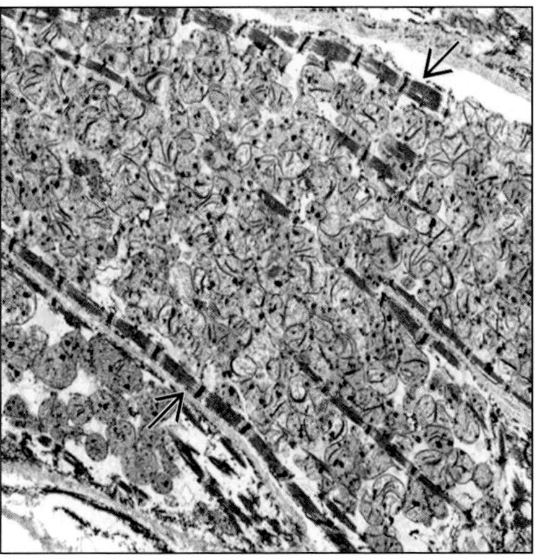

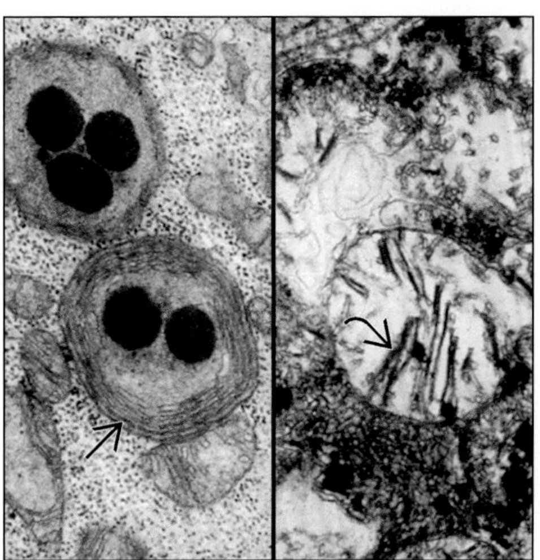

(Left) *Electron micrograph image shows abundant mitochondria pushing the myofibrils → to the periphery of the cells.* ***(Right)*** *Electron micrography image compares mitochondrial cardiomyopathy (left) containing cisterna arranged in concentric circles → around dense bodies to histiocytoid cardiomyopathy (right) containing swollen mitochondria with slightly disorganized cisterna ↪.*

Alimentary Canal

Neoplasm, Benign

Neoplasm, Malignant Primary

Protocol for the Examination of Specimens from Patients with Neuroendocrine Tumors of the Appendix

Protocol for the Examination of Specimens from Patients with Gastrointestinal Stromal Tumors

GINGIVAL GRANULAR CELL TUMOR OF THE NEWBORN

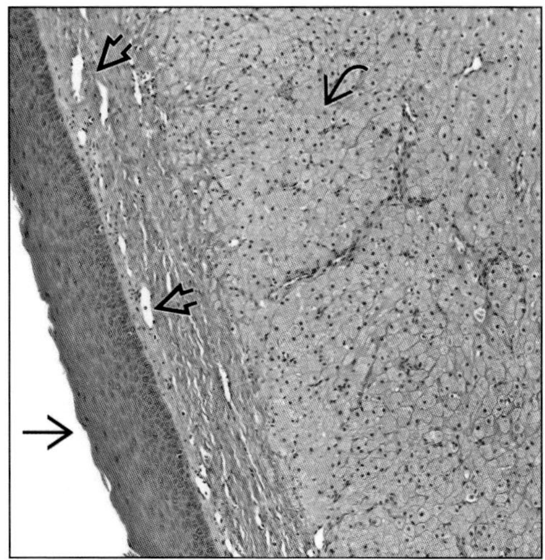

Hematoxylin & eosin shows a keratinized squamous epithelium ➔, numerous vascular channels within the collagenous connective tissue layer ➔, and the stroma with granular cells ➔.

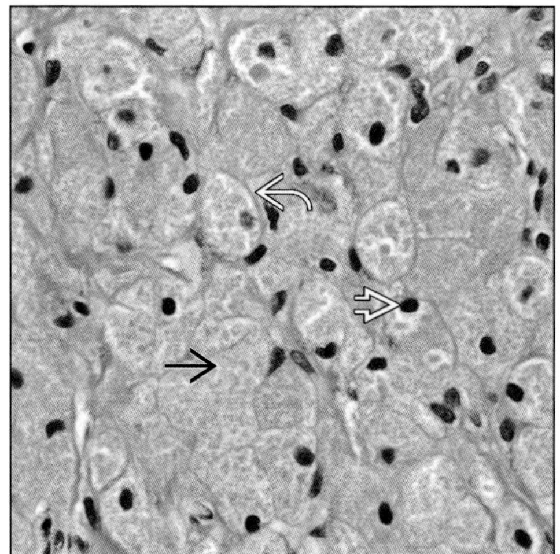

Hematoxylin & eosin shows granular cells with abundant eosinophilic granular cytoplasm ➔, distinct cell membranes ➔, and single, small, round, basophilic nuclei ➔.

TERMINOLOGY

Synonyms

- Congenital epulis, congenital granular cell myoblastoma, granular cell fibroblastoma, Neumann tumor

Definitions

- Rare benign mesenchymal tumor originating from oral cavity in newborns
- Thought to be different entity from other granular cell tumors

ETIOLOGY/PATHOGENESIS

Etiology

- Exact mechanism of pathogenesis is still not clear
- Maternal hormonal stimulus proposed
- Histogenesis is debated; proposed cells of origin include
  - Odontogenic epithelium
  - Undifferentiated mesenchymal cells
  - Fibroblasts
  - Pericytes
  - Smooth muscle cells
  - Histiocytes

CLINICAL ISSUES

Epidemiology

- Incidence
  - Rare pediatric tumor
  - Approximately 200 cases have been reported in literature
- Age
  - Congenital
- Gender
  - Female predominance (M:F = 1:8-10)

Site

- Most commonly arises from maxillary anterior alveolar ridge
- May occur along mandibular alveolar ridge (maxillary to mandibular ratio is 3:1)
- Uncommon tongue involvement

Presentation

- Round to ovoid, often pedunculated nodule, covered by smooth mucosal surface protruding from mouth
- Lesion can cause
  - Difficulty swallowing
    - In utero, may lead to polyhydramnios
  - Difficulty breathing
- Usually not associated with bone, dental abnormalities, or with other congenital malformations

Natural History

- No further growth after birth
- Small lesions may regress spontaneously

Treatment

- Surgical approaches
  - Complete local excision is indicated when lesion is obstructing feeding or respiration
  - Conservative surgical removal with CO_2 laser is alternative approach
- Conservative treatment is indicated for small, nonsymptomatic lesions

Prognosis

- Good prognosis
  - Absence of local recurrence even after incomplete excision

IMAGE FINDINGS

Ultrasonographic Findings

- Well-defined, round, hyperechoic mass protruding from anterior oral cavity

GINGIVAL GRANULAR CELL TUMOR OF THE NEWBORN

Key Facts

Terminology
- Rare benign mesenchymal tumor originating from oral cavity in newborns
- Congenital epulis, congenital granular cell myoblastoma, granular cell fibroblastoma, Neumann tumor
- Thought to be different entity from other granular cell tumors

Clinical Issues
- Female predominance (M:F = 1:8-10)
- Most commonly arises from maxillary anterior alveolar ridge
- No further growth after birth
- Small lesions may regress spontaneously
- Complete local excision > indicated when lesion is obstructing feeding or respiration
- Absence of local recurrence even after incomplete excision

Macroscopic Features
- Usually solitary, multiple in 5-16% of cases

Diagnostic Checklist
- Unlike granular cell tumor in adults, granular cell tumor of newborns shows
  - Lack of pseudoepitheliomatous hyperplasia of overlying squamous epithelium
  - Prominent vascular connective tissue
  - S100(-)
- Granular cells have abundant granular eosinophilic cytoplasm, arranged in islands, strands, or syncytial masses
- ± perivascular lymphocytic and histiocytic infiltrate

- Branching pattern of feeder vessels

MR Findings
- Not specific for diagnosis
- Helpful in determining characteristics and extent of tumor for preoperative planning
  - Ovoid-round, well-defined mass usually arising from maxillary or mandibular alveolar ridge
  - Isointense to muscle ± post-contrast enhancement on T1-weighted images
  - Inhomogeneous signal intensity with central isointensity & hypo-/hyperintense peripheral rim on T2 images

CT Findings
- Moderately enhancing tumor in paramedian to midline anterior oral cavity
- Lesion base has its base on maxillary or mandibular gum

MACROSCOPIC FEATURES

General Features
- Firm, protuberant, multilobulated, ± pedunculated, nonencapsulated, pink-tan mass
- Usually solitary; multiple in 5-16% of cases
- Cut surface tends to be tan-yellow, smooth, and glistening

Sections to Be Submitted
- 1-2 cassettes with full-thickness sections of lesion

Size
- Variable: A few mm to 9 cm

MICROSCOPIC PATHOLOGY

Histologic Features
- Nonencapsulated, well-circumscribed tumor
- Composed of homogeneous polygonal large cells
  - Abundant eosinophilic, granular cytoplasm
  - Distinct cell membranes
  - Arranged in strands, islands, or syncytial masses
  - Single, small, round, centrally/eccentrically located nuclei
- Peripheral collagenous connective tissue layer with numerous vascular channels
- Overlying keratinized squamous epithelium with no pseudoepitheliomatous hyperplasia
- ± perivascular collection of lymphocytes and histiocytes

DIFFERENTIAL DIAGNOSIS

Granular Cell Histiocytic Reactions
- Inflammatory cells other than perivascular lymphocytes and histiocytes

Oropharyngeal Teratoma (Epignathus)
- Well-differentiated cell lines derived from all 3 germ cell layers
- Elevated levels of AFP

Maxillary Melanotic Neuroectodermal Tumor of Infancy
- Biphasic pattern
  - Small, round, neuroblast-like cells
  - Epithelioid cells with eosinophilic cytoplasm containing variable amounts of melanin
- Epithelioid cells are HMB-45(+)

Congenital Fibrous Epulis
- Overlying layer of squamous epithelium ± irregular acanthosis and parakeratosis
- Mild subepithelial inflammatory infiltration with small blood vessels
- Irregular bundles of connective tissue
- Variable amount of spindle cells with oval-fusiform nuclei

Pyogenic Granuloma
- Proliferating endothelial cells separated by edematous stroma to include inflammatory cells

GINGIVAL GRANULAR CELL TUMOR OF THE NEWBORN

Immunohistochemistry

Antibody	Reactivity	Staining Pattern	Comment
Vimentin	Positive	Cytoplasmic	
NSE	Positive	Cytoplasmic	
CD68	Positive	Cell membrane & cytoplasm	
S100	Negative		Opposite staining pattern as other granular cell tumors
Desmin	Negative		
Laminin	Negative		
CK-PAN	Negative		
HLA-DR	Negative		
Myoglobin	Negative		
ER	Negative		
PR	Negative		

Dermoid Cyst

- Cyst lined by keratinized squamous epithelium with intraluminal keratin

DIAGNOSTIC CHECKLIST

Pathologic Interpretation Pearls

- Unlike granular cell tumor in adults, granular cell tumor of newborns shows
  - Prominent vascular connective tissue ± perivascular collection of lymphocytes and histiocytes
  - Lack of pseudoepitheliomatous hyperplasia of overlying squamous epithelium
  - S100(-)
- Granular cells have abundant granular eosinophilic cytoplasm, arranged in islands, strands, or syncytial masses

SELECTED REFERENCES

1. Kim YD et al: Congenital epulis: prenatal ultrasonographic and postnatal MR features with pathologic correlation. Oral Surg Oral Med Oral Pathol Oral Radiol Endod. 106(5):743-8, 2008
2. Kumar B et al: Neonatal oral tumors: congenital epulis and epignathus. J Pediatr Surg. 43(9):e9-11, 2008
3. Fister P et al: A newborn baby with a tumor protruding from the mouth. Diagnosis: congenital gingival granular cell tumor. Acta Dermatovenerol Alp Panonica Adriat. 16(3):128-30, 2007
4. Sakai VT et al: Complete spontaneous regression of congenital epulis in a baby by 8 months of age. Int J Paediatr Dent. 17(4):309-12, 2007
5. Tandon P et al: Congenital epulis of the newborn: a case report with review of literature. Indian J Pathol Microbiol. 50(3):593-4, 2007
6. Kanotra S et al: Congenital epulis. J Laryngol Otol. 120(2):148-50, 2006
7. Messina M et al: Prenatal diagnosis and multidisciplinary approach to the congenital gingival granular cell tumor. J Pediatr Surg. 41(10):E35-8, 2006
8. Olson JL et al: Congenital epulis. J Craniofac Surg. 16(1):161-4, 2005
9. Raissaki MT et al: Congenital granular cell tumor (epulis): postnatal imaging appearances. J Comput Assist Tomogr. 29(4):520-3, 2005
10. Song WS et al: A case report of congenital epulis in the fetus. J Oral Maxillofac Surg. 63(1):135-7, 2005
11. Bilen BT et al: Obstructive congenital gingival granular cell tumour. Int J Pediatr Otorhinolaryngol. 68(12):1567-71, 2004
12. Parmigiani S et al: A rare case of multiple congenital epulis. J Matern Fetal Neonatal Med. 16 Suppl 2:55-8, 2004
13. Shaw L et al: Congenital epulis: three-dimensional ultrasonographic findings and clinical implications. J Ultrasound Med. 23(8):1121-4, 2004
14. Roy S et al: Congenital epulis: prenatal imaging with MRI and ultrasound. Pediatr Radiol. 33(11):800-3, 2003
15. Uğraş S et al: Immunohistochemical study on histogenesis of congenital epulis and review of the literature. Pathol Int. 47(9):627-32, 1997
16. Shipp TD et al: The ultrasonographic appearance and outcome for fetuses with masses distorting the fetal face. J Ultrasound Med. 14(9):673-8, 1995
17. Takahashi H et al: Immunohistochemical study of congenital gingival granular cell tumor (congenital epulis). J Oral Pathol Med. 19(10):492-6, 1990
18. Tucker MC et al: Gingival granular cell tumors of the newborn. An ultrastructural and immunohistochemical study. Arch Pathol Lab Med. 114(8):895-8, 1990
19. Stewart CM et al: Oral granular cell tumors: a clinicopathologic and immunocytochemical study. Oral Surg Oral Med Oral Pathol. 65(4):427-35, 1988
20. Lack EE et al: Gingival granular cell tumor of the newborn (congenital "epulis"): ultrastructural observations relating to histogenesis. Hum Pathol. 13(7):686-9, 1982

Radiologic and Microscopic Features

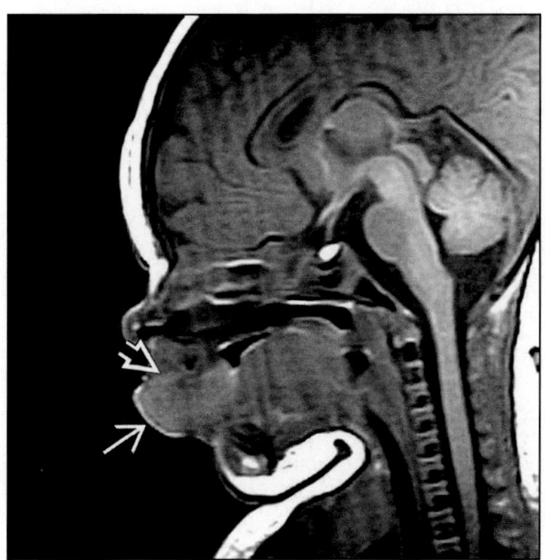

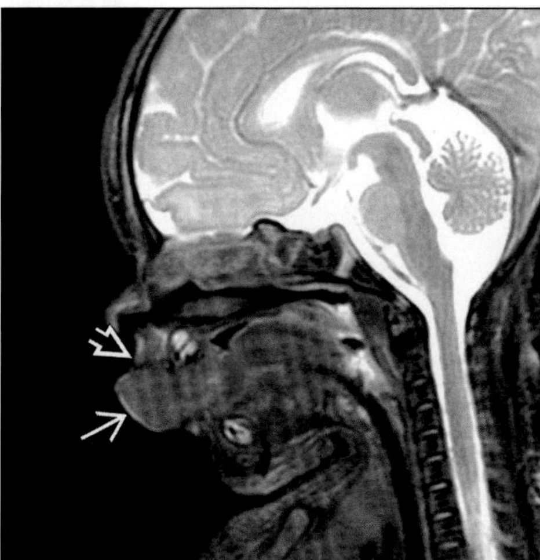

(Left) *Sagittal T1 nonenhanced MR shows an intermediate signal mass arising from the maxillary gum area. The granular cell tumor appears smooth, well-defined, and projects anteriorly away from the oral cavity airway.* ***(Right)*** *Sagittal T2 MR reveals a hypointense gingival granular cell tumor protruding from the maxillary gum.*

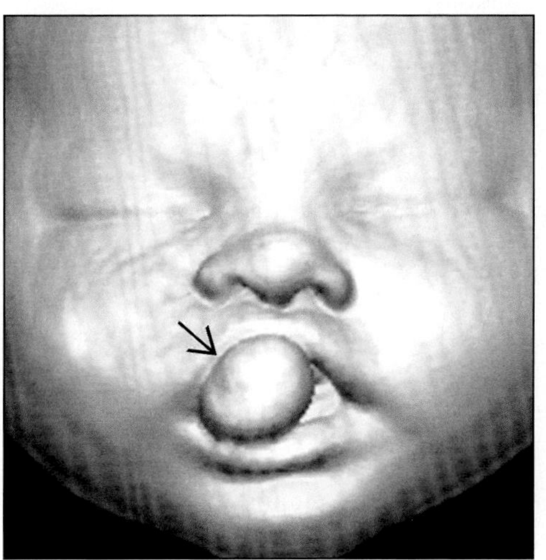

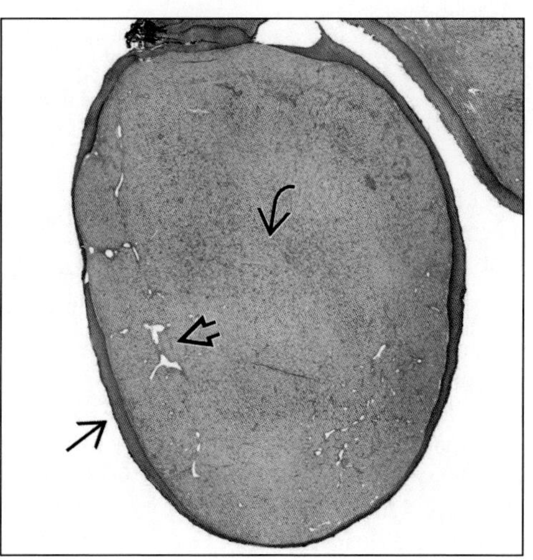

(Left) *3D surface-rendered CT shows a paramedian tumor projecting anteriorly from the maxillary gum area. Gingival granular cell tumor is a benign lesion occurring in female newborns (M:F = 1:8); maxillary gums (maxilla:mandible = 4:1).* ***(Right)*** *Hematoxylin & eosin shows at low magnification a nonencapsulated, well-circumscribed tumor composed of a keratinized squamous epithelium, vascular collagenous tissue layer, and homogeneous stroma.*

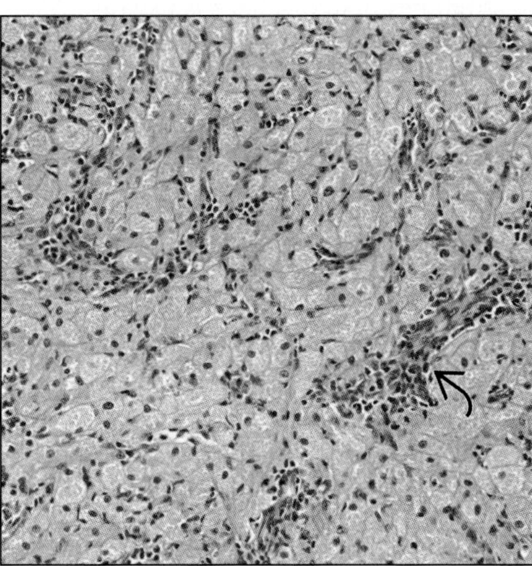

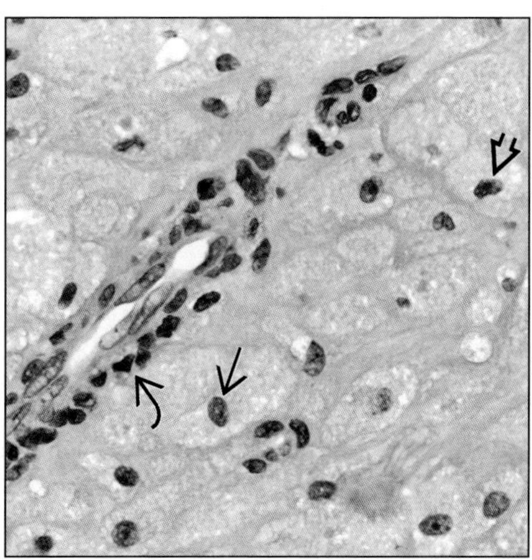

(Left) *Hematoxylin & eosin shows stroma with granular cells and perivascular collection of lymphocytes.* ***(Right)*** *Hematoxylin & eosin shows in a higher magnification a perivascular lymphocytic infiltrate and granular cells with centrally and eccentrically located nuclei.*

LYMPHATIC MALFORMATION

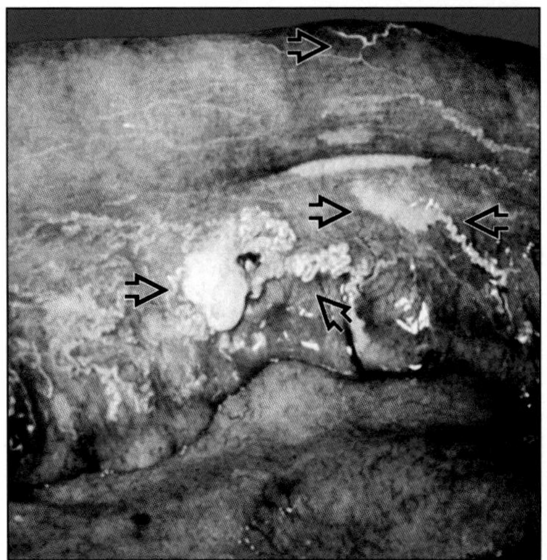

Gross photograph shows markedly dilated lymphatic channels ➪ on the serosa of the small intestine. (Courtesy J. Yardley, MD.)

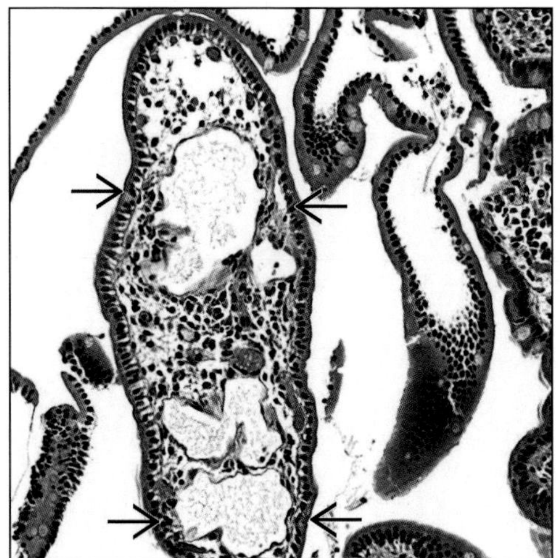

Hematoxylin & eosin shows the tip of an intestinal villus with dilated lacteals ➔ seen within the lamina propria in this case of intestinal lymphangiectasia.

TERMINOLOGY

Abbreviations

- Primary intestinal lymphangiectasia (PIL)

Synonyms

- Primary intestinal lymphangiectasia = Waldmann disease
- Generalized lymphangiomatosis = cystic angiomatosis

Definitions

- Lymphangioma: Benign neoplasm originating from focal proliferation of lymphatic channels
- Generalized lymphangiomatosis: Rare disorder characterized by diffuse proliferation of lymphatic vessels
- Primary intestinal lymphangiectasia: Dilated lacteals and lymphatic channels in small bowel leading to protein-losing enteropathy

ETIOLOGY/PATHOGENESIS

Etiology

- Lymphangioma
  - Maldevelopment of embryonic lymphangiogenesis is most acceptable etiology
  - Failure of communication between lymphatic and venous vessels > blind lymphatic vessels > dilatation > cystic tumor
  - Dysregulation of angiogenesis may contribute to lymphangioma growth and progression
- Primary intestinal lymphangiectasia
  - Unknown

Genetics

- *VEGFRC, VEGFR3, PROX1, FOXC2, SOX18* genes are involved in lymphagiogenesis
- Syndromes associated with primary intestinal lymphangiectasia
  - Yellow nail syndrome
  - Klippel-Trenaunay syndrome
  - Hennekan syndrome
  - Neurofibromatosis type 1
  - Turner syndrome
  - Noonan syndrome

CLINICAL ISSUES

Epidemiology

- Incidence
  - Lymphangiomas of alimentary canal are extremely rare
  - Primary intestinal lymphangiectasia is rare; exact incidence is unknown
- Age
  - Majority of intraabdominal lymphangiomas become symptomatic before 5 years of age
  - Generalized lymphangiomatosis occurs in 1st and 2nd decades of life
  - Primary intestinal lymphangiectasia is usually diagnosed in children before 3 years of age
- Gender
  - Intraabdominal lymphangiomas in pediatric patients have slight male predominance (~ 2:1 ratio)
  - Generalized lymphangiomatosis has no gender predilection

Site

- Intraabdominal lymphangiomas commonly occur in mesentery, omentum, retroperitoneum
  - Occasionally occur in visceral organs (esophagus, stomach, small and large bowels, pancreas, spleen, liver)
- Generalized lymphangiomatosis can affect any organ, except central nervous system
- Primary intestinal lymphangiectasia most commonly occurs in small intestine

Presentation

- Lymphangioma: Related to site and size of tumor

LYMPHATIC MALFORMATION

Key Facts

Terminology
- Lymphangioma is benign neoplasm that arises from focal proliferation of lymphatic channels
- Generalized lymphangiomatosis is rare disorder characterized by diffuse proliferation of lymphatic vessels
- Primary intestinal lymphangiectasia: Dilated lacteals and lymphatic channels in small bowel leading to protein-losing enteropathy

Etiology/Pathogenesis
- *VEGFRC*, *VEGFR3*, *PROX1*, *FOXC2*, *SOX18* genes are involved in lymphangiogenesis

Clinical Issues
- Primary intestinal lymphangiectasia most commonly occurs in small intestine

Microscopic Pathology
- Surgical resection margins are of great importance in lymphangioma
- Lymphangioma and PIL are microscopically identical
  - Variably sized, thin-walled spaces lined by flat endothelial cells within mucosa, submucosa, and serosa
  - Loose myxoid stroma surrounds lymphatic spaces
  - Lymphoid aggregates are often seen within wall of lymphatic spaces
  - PIL often contains foamy macrophages

Diagnostic Checklist
- Biopsy findings must be correlated with clinical history, as dilated lacteals are nonspecific

  - Incidental finding
  - Abdominal distension
  - Cystic mass on palpation
  - Bowel obstruction
  - Acute abdomen
- Generalized lymphangiomatosis: Depends on primarily affected site
  - Spleen: Splenomegaly, left upper quadrant pain
  - Lungs: Dyspnea, wheezing
  - Bones: Asymptomatic, local pain, pathologic fracture
- Primary intestinal lymphangiectasia
  - Pitting edema (peripheral, usually unilateral, moderate-severe)
  - Lymphedema
  - Serous effusion (pleural effusions, pericarditis, chylous ascites)
  - Malabsorption, protein-losing enteropathy
    - Hypoproteinemia: Hypoalbuminemia, hypogammaglobulinemia
    - Fat-soluble vitamin deficiencies
  - Lymphopenia
  - Hypocalcemia
  - Abdominal pain
  - Nausea, vomiting, diarrhea, steatorrhea
  - Inability to gain weight; weight loss
  - Growth retardation

Endoscopic Findings
- Lymphangioma
  - Smooth, submucosal polypoid lesion
- Primary intestinal lymphangiectasia
  - Dilatation of intestinal lacteals
  - White, edematous villi with overlying chylo-like substance
  - ± chylous distension of subserosal intestinal and mesenteric lymphatics
  - Focal lesions might not be identified; video capsule endoscopy may be indicated

Laboratory Tests
- Primary intestinal lymphangiectasia
  - Albumin and γ-globulin levels
  - Complete blood count
  - Fat-soluble vitamin levels
  - Calcium

Natural History
- Primary intestinal lymphangiectasia
  - Protein loss leads to hypoproteinemia and lymphopenia, which leads to infectious complications

Treatment
- Options, risks, complications
  - Lymphangioma
    - Complete surgical resection is treatment of choice
    - Laparoscopic approach is preferred
    - Laparotomy exposes patient to adhesions and associated complications
  - Generalized lymphangiomatosis
    - No specific treatment; usually palliative
  - Primary intestinal lymphangiectasia
    - High-protein, low-fat diet with medium-chain triglyceride supplementation
    - Use of octreotide may be of benefit
    - Surgery has been used in some cases, typically when more segmental
    - Steroids have been tried with inconsistent results
    - Albumin may be needed to treat hypoproteinemia

Prognosis
- Lymphangioma
  - High recurrence rate with incomplete resection
  - Potential for proliferative or locally infiltrating course
- Generalized lymphangiomatosis
  - Prognosis depends on extent of disease and involved organs
  - Usually poor
  - Death frequently occurs due to respiratory failure secondary to infection/chylous accumulation
- Primary intestinal lymphangiectasia
  - Chronic debilitating disease
  - Chronic lymphedema

LYMPHATIC MALFORMATION

IMAGE FINDINGS

Ultrasonographic Findings

- Lymphangioma
  - Unilocular/multilocular anechoic mass
- Primary intestinal lymphangiectasia
  - Thickening of intestinal wall
  - Distension of intestinal loops
  - Plical hypertrophy
  - Mesenteric edema

CT Findings

- Lymphangioma
  - Nonenhancing, extramucosal mass with homogeneous attenuation
  - Generalized lymphangiomatosis
    - Well-defined cystic lesions
    - Visceral and osseous lesions often show contrast enhancement on CT scan
- Primary intestinal lymphangiectasia
  - Diffuse, nodular small bowel edema and wall thickening
  - Small bowel distension
  - ± "halo" sign: Outer ring of high CT attenuation surrounding lower attenuation inner ring

MACROSCOPIC FEATURES

General Features

- Lymphangioma
  - Submucosal polypoid, generally solitary cystic lesion
- Primary intestinal lymphangiectasia
  - Yellow-white dilated lymphatic channels on intestinal serosa

MICROSCOPIC PATHOLOGY

Histologic Features

- Lymphangioma and PIL are microscopically similar
  - Variably sized, thin-walled spaces lined by flat endothelial cells within mucosa, submucosa, &/or serosa
    - Loose myxoid stroma surrounds lymphatic spaces
    - In lymphangioma, dilated lymphatics are often seen within mesentery
  - Lymphoid aggregates, smooth muscle, and scattered blood vessels are often seen within wall of lymphatic spaces
  - Edematous submucosa and villi may be present in PIL
  - Mild to moderate blunting of villi may be present in PIL
  - PIL often contains foamy macrophages
  - Diffuse dilation of lacteals within small bowel mucosa is typically seen in PIL
- Diffuse lymphangiomatosis
  - Identical to lymphangioma on biopsy

Margins

- Surgical resection margins are of great importance in lymphangioma

Predominant Pattern/Injury Type

- Cystic

Predominant Cell/Compartment Type

- Lymphatics

DIFFERENTIAL DIAGNOSIS

Secondary Lymphangiectasia

- May be due to constrictive pericarditis, local obstruction (tumor), radiation, or cardiac surgery
- Identical to PIL in biopsy, only distinguished by history

Hemangioma

- Numerous, dilated blood-filled spaces within mucosa and submucosa

Hemangiolymphangioma

- Composed of both lymphatics and blood vessels

Celiac Disease

- Blunt villi or intraepithelial lymphocytes missing from PIL
- Lymphatic dilatation is not present within mucosa and submucosa

Crohn Disease

- Will have inflammatory component missing from PIL
  - ± segmental ulceration
  - ± sarcoid-type granulomas

DIAGNOSTIC CHECKLIST

Pathologic Interpretation Pearls

- Biopsy findings must be correlated with clinical history, as dilated lacteals are nonspecific

SELECTED REFERENCES

1. Blei F: Congenital lymphatic malformations. Ann N Y Acad Sci. 1131:185-94, 2008
2. Vignes S et al: Primary intestinal lymphangiectasia (Waldmann's disease). Orphanet J Rare Dis. 3:5, 2008
3. Weeda VB et al: Mesenteric cystic lymphangioma: a congenital and an acquired anomaly? Two cases and a review of the literature. J Pediatr Surg. 43(6):1206-8, 2008
4. Al-Salem AH: Lymphangiomas in infancy and childhood. Saudi Med J. 25(4):466-9, 2004
5. Hebra A et al: Mesenteric, omental, and retroperitoneal cysts in children: a clinical study of 22 cases. South Med J. 86(2):173-6, 1993

LYMPHATIC MALFORMATION

Microscopic Features

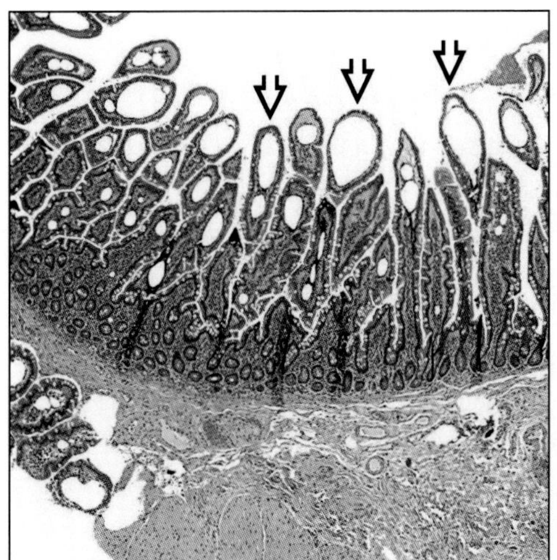

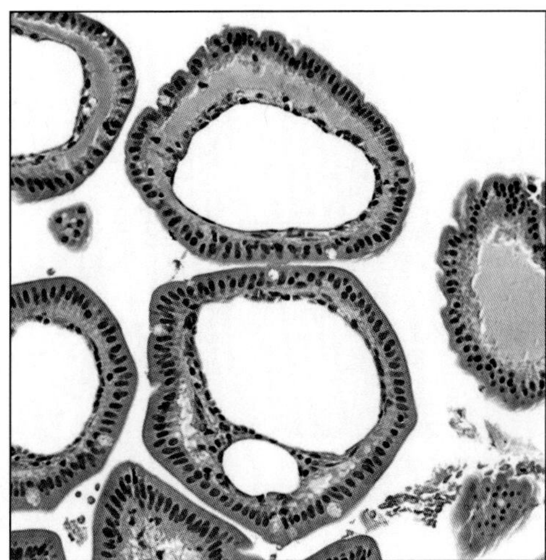

(Left) Hematoxylin & eosin shows a low-power view of the small bowel mucosa with diffuse dilation of lacteals. ***(Right)*** Hematoxylin & eosin shows a high-power view of dilated lacteals. Although not specific, this finding is typical of primary intestinal lymphangiectasia. Identical changes can also be seen in secondary lymphangiectasia.

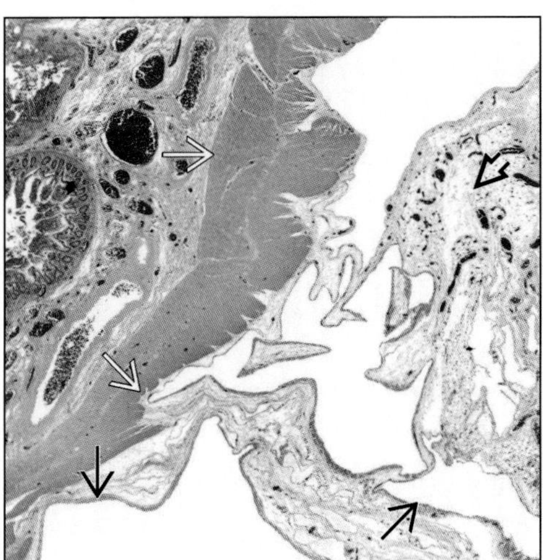

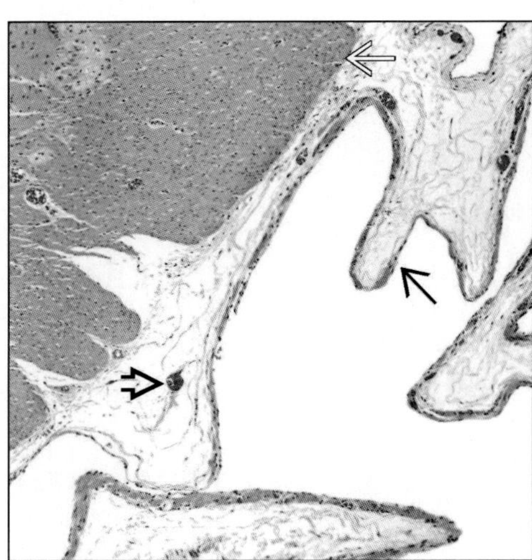

(Left) Low-power view shows a lymphangioma with irregularly dilated lymphatic spaces within the small bowel serosa, surrounded by loose myxoid stroma. The lymphatic spaces extend into the muscularis propria. ***(Right)*** High-power view shows dilated lymphatic spaces lined by a single layer of flattened endothelium within the serosa adjacent to the muscularis propria. The walls of the spaces are edematous and show scattered blood vessels.

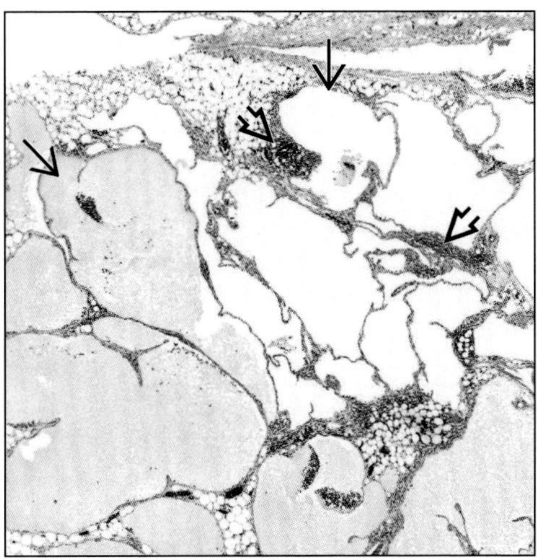

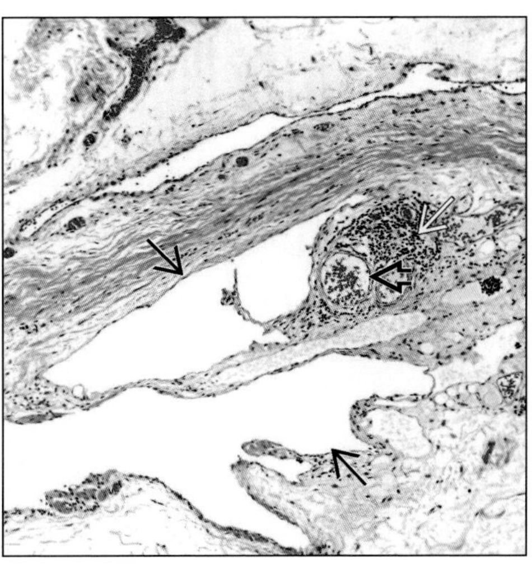

(Left) Low-power view shows a mesenteric lymphangioma with numerous variably sized, irregular lymphatic spaces filled with an amorphous faintly eosinophilic material. Lymphoid aggregates are seen focally in the walls of some of the spaces and in the intervening mesentery. ***(Right)*** Hematoxylin & eosin shows a high-power view of a mesenteric lymphangioma with lymphoid aggregates and blood vessels within the wall of dilated lymphatic spaces.

JUVENILE POLYPS

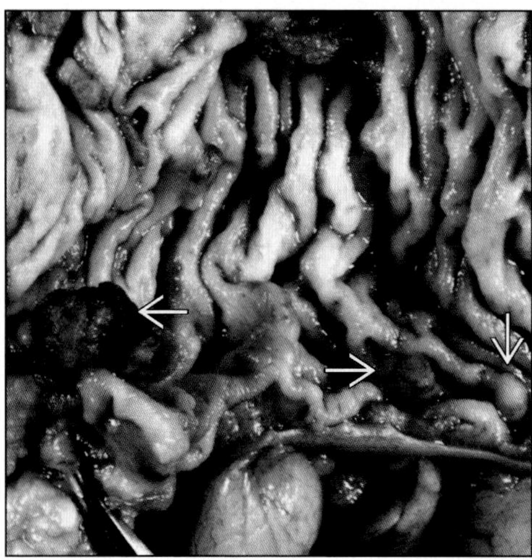

Gross photograph shows a colonic resection in a JPS patient. Several variably sized, spherical polyps ➡ can be seen on the mucosa.

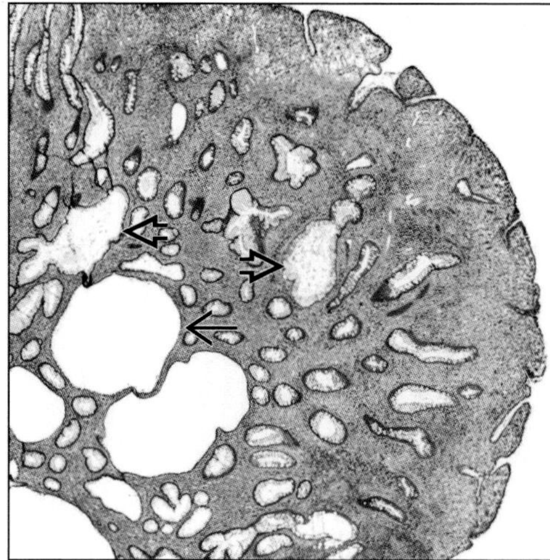

Hematoxylin & eosin shows a low-power view of a juvenile polyp. Note the spherical shape with cystically dilated crypts ⇨, some of which contain mucin ⇨.

TERMINOLOGY

Definitions

- Polypoid collection of gastrointestinal glands/crypts surrounded by prominent edematous &/or inflamed stroma
  - 1 type of hamartomatous polyp
- Juvenile polyposis syndrome (JPS)
  - ≥ 5 juvenile polyps in colon
  - Extracolonic juvenile polyps
  - Any hamartomatous polyp in patient with family history of JPS
  - Subtypes
    - Juvenile polyposis coli: Multiple polyps restricted to colon
    - Juvenile gastrointestinal polyposis: Multiple polyps from stomach to rectum
    - Familial juvenile polyposis of stomach: Restricted to stomach

ETIOLOGY/PATHOGENESIS

Genetics

- JPS is autosomal dominant
- ~ 50% of JPS families have mutations in 1 of 2 genes
  - *SMAD4* (a.k.a. *DPC4*)
  - *BMPR1A* (bone morphogenic protein receptor 1A)

CLINICAL ISSUES

Epidemiology

- Incidence
  - Most common polyp in children
  - Pediatric incidence of sporadic juvenile polyps ~ 1-2%
- Age
  - Peak incidence 2-4 years
  - Sporadic juvenile-type polyps can occur at any age
- Gender
  - M = F for isolated polyps
  - M > F for multiple polyps/JPS

Site

- Most occur in colon but may occur throughout GI tract

Presentation

- Hematochezia, melena
  - May occur in JPS but not usually with sporadic polyps

Endoscopic Findings

- JPS: Numerous polyps (up to hundreds)

Natural History

- Sporadic polyps
  - May occur at any age; clinically indolent
- JPS
  - Usually presents in 1st 2 decades of life
  - Increased risk of gastrointestinal cancer
    - Relative risk of colorectal carcinoma ~ 34

Treatment

- Surgical approaches
  - Resection may be performed for very heavy polyp burden &/or dysplasia/neoplasia in JPS
- Neoplasia screening
  - Endoscopy at least every 3 years for JPS patients
  - If only a few polyps are found, endoscopic removal is appropriate

MACROSCOPIC FEATURES

General Features

- Small, usually pedunculated polyps
  - Most ~ 1 cm in diameter; may be up to several cm
  - Pink, spherical, sometimes appear lobulated
    - Cystically dilated crypts/glands may be visible as gray patches

JUVENILE POLYPS

Key Facts

Terminology

- 1 type of hamartomatous polyp
- May be seen in juvenile polyposis syndrome (JPS)

Etiology/Pathogenesis

- JPS is autosomal dominant
  - Mutations in *SMAD4* or *BMPR1A* seen in ~ 50% of JPS families

Clinical Issues

- Most common polyp in children

Microscopic Pathology

- Surface erosion &/or ulcers common

Diagnostic Checklist

- Histologically identical polyps can be seen in other hamartomatous polyposis syndromes

MICROSCOPIC PATHOLOGY

Histologic Features

- Variably dilated, irregularly shaped crypts or glands
  - Lining epithelium is specific to site (i.e., gastric glands in stomach, crypts in colon)
  - May be markedly dilated and mucin-filled
  - Crypts in colonic polyps may appear serrated (reminiscent of hyperplastic polyp)
- Prominent stroma surrounds crypts/glands
  - Mixed inflammatory infiltrate (may be very prominent); lymphoid aggregates &/or follicles possible
  - Dilated superficial capillaries
  - Smooth muscle fibers sparse, if present at all
- Surface erosion &/or ulcers common
  - Superficial stroma may be replaced by granulation tissue when deeper ulcers present
- Gastric examples may be indistinguishable from more common gastric hyperplastic polyps
- Dysplasia (if present) similar to that seen in other settings
  - Nuclear hyperchromasia, crowding, stratification
  - Architectural abnormalities (crowding of crypts/ glands, cribriform architecture)
- "Ganglioneuromatous" neural proliferation may be seen in lamina propria &/or submucosa

DIAGNOSTIC CHECKLIST

Clinically Relevant Pathologic Features

- Gross appearance
  - Round (spherical), usually pedunculated polyp with cystic spaces

Pathologic Interpretation Pearls

- Histologically identical polyps can be seen in other hamartomatous polyposis syndromes
  - Cowden syndrome
  - Bannayan-Riley-Ruvalcaba syndrome
  - Cronkhite-Canada syndrome
    - Polyps are sessile in this setting
- Always search for epithelial dysplasia in juvenile polyps
  - Most common in large (> 1 cm) polyps
  - May occur as dysplastic focus in recognizable juvenile polyp or as "adenoma" without any residual juvenile features

SELECTED REFERENCES

1. Zbuk KM et al: Hamartomatous polyposis syndromes. Nat Clin Pract Gastroenterol Hepatol. 4(9):492-502, 2007
2. Lowichik A et al: Gastrointestinal polyposis in childhood: clinicopathologic and genetic features. Pediatr Dev Pathol. 6(5):371-91, 2003

IMAGE GALLERY

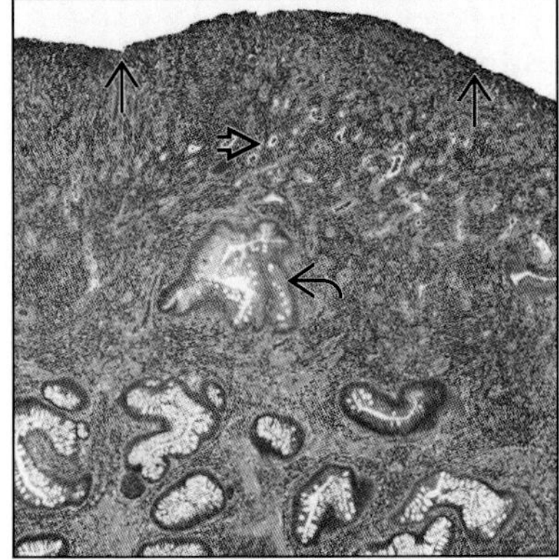
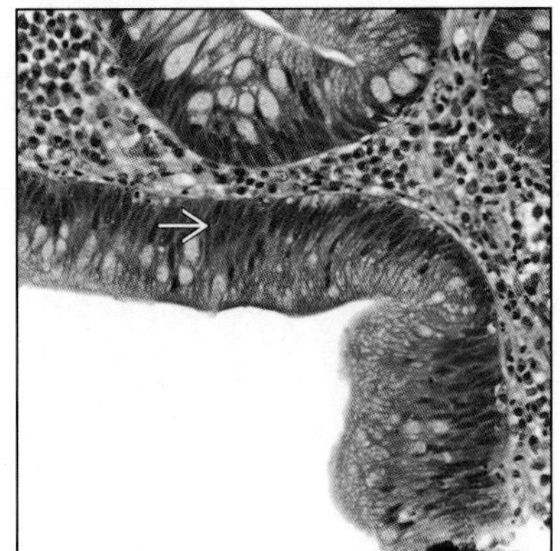
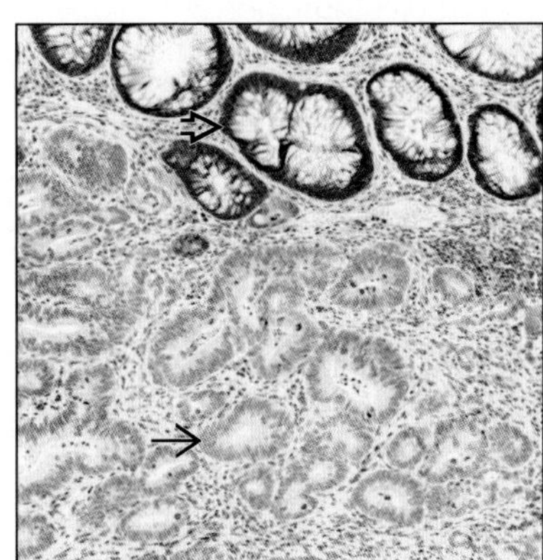

*(**Left**) Hematoxylin & eosin shows a juvenile polyp with surface erosion ⮕. The superficial lamina propria has been replaced by granulation tissue ⮕ and some of the irregular crypts appear serrated ⮕. (**Center**) Hematoxylin & eosin shows low-grade dysplasia in a juvenile polyp. Note the hyperchromatic, stratified nuclei ⮕. (**Right**) SMAD4 immunostain in a juvenile polyp shows loss of nuclear staining in the dysplastic component ⮕. The same polyp also harbored a focus of invasive adenocarcinoma. Nondysplastic epithelium ⮕ retains nuclear staining.*

FAMILIAL ADENOMATOUS POLYPOSIS

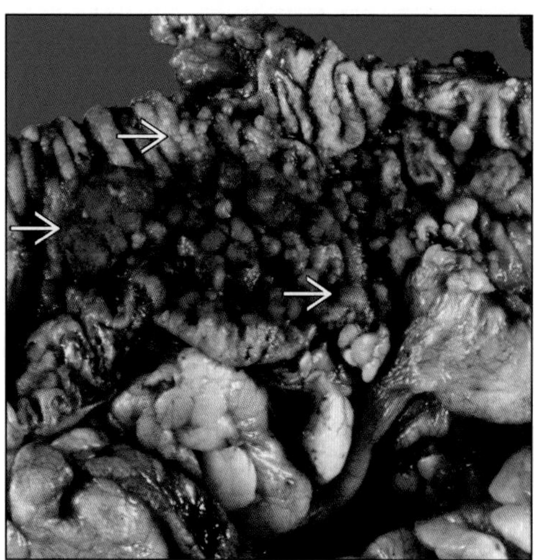

Gross photograph of a colectomy specimen from an FAP patient shows dozens of variably sized polyps ➔ carpeting the mucosa.

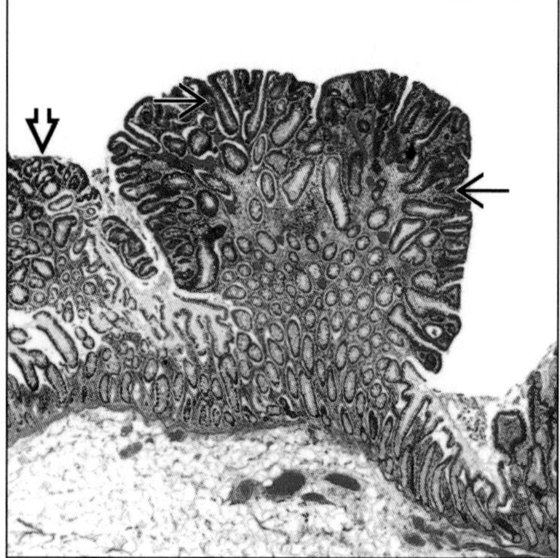

Hematoxylin & eosin shows a low-power view of an adenoma from a patient with FAP. Note the hyperchromasia and crowding of the superficial crypts ➔. A 2nd smaller adenoma ➔ is nearby.

TERMINOLOGY

Abbreviations

- Familial adenomatous polyposis (FAP)

Synonyms

- Familial polyposis coli
- Gardner syndrome (GS)
  - Variant of FAP with conspicuous extracolonic manifestations
    - Duodenal (especially periampullary) adenomas and gastric fundic gland polyps (± dysplasia)
    - Osteomas, desmoid fibromas, skin tumors, endocrine tumors, ocular and tooth abnormalities
- Turcot syndrome
  - Variant of FAP in which patients also have brain tumors (medulloblastomas)
  - May also refer to Lynch syndrome/hereditary nonpolyposis colon cancer patients with brain tumors (gliomas)

Definitions

- FAP: Autosomal dominant syndrome with > 100 colonic adenomas
- Attenuated FAP (AFAP): Hereditary cancer syndrome with < 100 colonic polyps
  - Most often < 30 adenomas that tend to be located in right colon

ETIOLOGY/PATHOGENESIS

Genetics

- Autosomal dominant and highly penetrant
  - Germline mutation in *APC* (adenomatous polyposis coli) gene (5q21-q22)
    - Tumor suppressor involved in *Wnt* signaling pathway (downregulates β-catenin)
    - Loss of tumor suppressor activity allows mutations in other key genetic loci (e.g., *TP53*, *RAS*)
    - Loss of 2nd (non-germline-mutated) allele → development of tumors ("2-hit hypothesis")
  - Specific mutations → specific FAP phenotypes
    - Variations in penetrance and mutation site → different manifestations (e.g., extraintestinal tumors in GS vs. FAP)
    - AFAP has *APC* mutations near proximal or distal ends of gene
- FAP phenotype may also arise from spontaneous, noninherited *APC* mutations (1/5 to 1/3 of cases)

CLINICAL ISSUES

Epidemiology

- Incidence
  - Approximately 0.005-0.015%
    - Most common genetic polyposis syndrome, but accounts for < 1% of all colon carcinomas
- Age
  - Wide range of age at presentation, from 2 months to > 70 years
    - Most present by age 20
    - AFAP rarely presents in children
  - Adenomas typically appear during 2nd decade of life
  - Mean age of adenocarcinoma development = 5th decade but may occur as early as 2nd decade
  - Extragastrointestinal manifestations may appear earlier than adenomas and be presenting feature
- Gender
  - M = F

Presentation

- Symptoms relatively rare
  - Rectal bleeding, intussusception possible (particularly with large polyps)
  - Electrolyte loss may occur when polyposis is very extensive

FAMILIAL ADENOMATOUS POLYPOSIS

Key Facts

Terminology
- FAP: Autosomal dominant, > 100 colonic adenomas
- AFAP: < 100 colonic polyps
- GS: FAP with prominent extraintestinal manifestations

Etiology/Pathogenesis
- Germline mutation in *APC* gene (5q21-q22)

Clinical Issues
- Adenomas typically appear during 2nd decade of life
- Lethal by 5th decade if untreated
- Skin, bone, and soft tissue tumors in GS often clinically obvious but may not be recognized as syndromic
- Early endoscopic screening must be offered to confirmed patients as well as affected first-degree relatives (mutation carriers) and family members with inconclusive genetic results

Macroscopic Features
- Polyps are sessile, usually < 1 cm

Microscopic Pathology
- Most are tubular adenomas; villous adenomas rare
- Early lesion: Single crypt ("unicryptal") adenoma

Diagnostic Checklist
- *APC* mutations seen in 60-90% of FAP patients
- Family members of newly diagnosed patient must also be genetically tested
- Patients with FAP phenotype but no *APC* mutation identified should be tested for *MYH* mutation

---

- Skin, bone, and soft tissue tumors in GS often clinically obvious but may not be recognized as syndromic
- Periampullary polyps can obstruct common bile duct → acute pancreatitis
- If/when carcinoma develops, symptoms typical of sporadic carcinoma (bleeding, pain, mass)

Endoscopic Findings
- Colon usually "carpeted" by > 100 (possibly thousands) of polyps on colonic mucosa
  - Usually sessile and < 1 cm but larger & pedunculated polyps possible
  - Polyp distribution: Left > right in full-blown FAP
    - AFAP may show left-sided sparing
- Fundic gland polyps in stomach

Natural History
- Colorectal cancer inevitable without colectomy (100% risk by age 60)
  - Risk ↑ with age and number of polyps
    - Few polyps progress to cancer, but large polyp burden leads to high risk

Treatment
- Surgical approaches
  - Affected individuals (with proven mutation and adenomas) → prophylactic colectomy by age 25
    - Total colectomy with ileal pouch-anal anastomosis (IPAA)
    - Subtotal colectomy with ileo-rectal anastomosis (less useful due to cancer risk in residual rectum)
    - Subsequent screening of residual rectum or ileal pouch still necessary
  - Extraintestinal tumors (e.g., desmoid fibromas) may also be surgically resected
- Drugs
  - COX-2 inhibitors may inhibit adenoma development in remainder of GI tract after prophylactic colectomy
    - Not 100% effective at cancer prevention and polyps reemerge after treatment cessation
- Endoscopic screening
  - Must begin by age 10 for confirmed patients as well as affected first-degree relatives (mutation carriers)
    - Family members with inconclusive genetic results should also be screened
  - Both upper and lower GI tract must be screened
  - Complete colonoscopy important (left colon may be spared in attenuated FAP)

Prognosis
- By early 3rd decade, cancer risk ~ 5%
- Lethal by 5th decade if untreated

MACROSCOPIC FEATURES

General Features
- Colonic manifestations
  - FAP: 100s to 1,000s of polyps carpet colonic mucosa
  - AFAP: < 100 polyps, right > left
- Extracolonic gastrointestinal manifestations
  - Gastric polyps (most commonly fundic gland polyps)
    - Occur earlier & are more likely to contain dysplasia in FAP patients than general population
    - Gastric cancer rare
  - Small intestinal adenomas
    - Most occur in periampullary region of duodenum
    - Occur later than colorectal adenomas in FAP patients, but earlier than in general population
    - May progress to carcinoma (common cause of death in patients after colectomy)
  - Biliary tract
    - Hepatoblastomas may occur in male infants
    - Biliary tree & gallbladder carcinomas possible
- Extragastrointestinal manifestations (part of GS when extensive)
  - Desmoid tumor ("Gardner fibroma")
    - Occur in up to 1/3 of FAP patients
    - Most common in retroperitoneum, mesentery, abdominal wall; may arise at sites of trauma or prior surgery

- Benign but locally aggressive; 2nd leading cause of death after colorectal carcinoma (intestinal/ureteral obstruction, etc.)
- Difficult to eradicate, requiring multiple surgeries

- Osteomas
  - Commonly affect skull (especially mandible & maxilla → facial deformity) and long bones
- Ocular abnormalities
  - Congenital hypertrophy of retinal pigment epithelium (CHRPE)
  - Pigmented lesions of retina; may be seen in infants → earliest finding specific for FAP
- Skin tumors
  - Epidermoid & sebaceous cysts on face, scalp, extremities
  - Neurofibromas, lipomas, leiomyomas, fibromas, pigmented lesions
- Tooth abnormalities
  - Missing teeth, supernumerary teeth, impactions, root abnormalities
- Endocrine tumors
  - Pancreatic endocrine neoplasms, pituitary tumors
  - Thyroid tumors (most commonly papillary); M:F = 1:17

- Diagnostic criteria for FAP (any of the following)
  - > 100 colorectal adenomas
    - < 100 adenomas (typically 1-50) in AFAP
  - Germline *APC* mutation
  - Family history of FAP with at least 1 of
    - Desmoid, osteoma, epidermoid cyst

Sections to Be Submitted

- For colectomies, adenomas should be extensively sampled and larger polyps explored for invasive carcinoma
  - Careful lymph node dissection necessary when invasive carcinoma found

MICROSCOPIC PATHOLOGY

Histologic Features

- Adenomas and carcinoma
  - Histologically identical to sporadic lesions, with crowded, hyperchromatic, and pseudostratified epithelial nuclei
  - Most colonic polyps are tubular adenomas; villous adenomas rare
  - Gastric fundic gland polyps may have dysplasia
- Early lesion: Single crypt ("unicryptal") adenoma
  - Expands to become oligocryptal and eventually becomes grossly/endoscopically visible polyp
- Fibromatosis/desmoid tumors
  - Elongated spindle cells separated by intervening collagen fibers
  - Immunohistochemically positive for β-catenin (nuclear staining)
- Other tumors
  - Histologically identical to sporadic counterparts (lipomas, leiomyomas, osteomas, etc.)

DIFFERENTIAL DIAGNOSIS

MYH-associated Polyposis

- Human MutY homologue gene (*MYH* or *MutYH*)
  - Base excision DNA repair gene located on chromosome 1p
  - Repairs oxidative damage to DNA → defects allow mutations in *APC* and *RAS*
- Similar phenotype to FAP
  - Increased risk of carcinoma (even when no colonic polyps present)
- Autosomal recessive inheritance (mutations in both alleles needed for polyposis phenotype)

Juvenile Polyposis Syndrome

- Autosomal dominant syndrome characterized by multiple (> 5) pedunculated hamartomatous polyps
  - Inflammatory stroma containing irregular, dilated crypts
  - Most juvenile polyps lack cytological dysplasia

Cronkhite-Canada Syndrome

- Nongenetic polyposis syndrome with controversial malignancy association
  - Polyps histologically identical to juvenile polyps, involving GI tract from stomach through colon

DIAGNOSTIC CHECKLIST

Clinically Relevant Pathologic Features

- *APC* mutations seen in 60-90% of FAP patients
  - Clinical diagnosis should be followed by sequencing of *APC* gene in search for mutation
- Family members of newly diagnosed patient must also be tested for the same mutation
  - If mutation absent and family member asymptomatic, no further screening (e.g., endoscopy) necessary
  - When family mutation is unknown, screening of family members necessary even with negative *APC* mutation analysis
- Patients with FAP phenotype but no *APC* mutation identified should be tested for *MYH* mutation

SELECTED REFERENCES

1. Alkhouri N et al: Familial adenomatous polyposis in children and adolescents. J Pediatr Gastroenterol Nutr. 51(6):727-32, 2010
2. Desai TK et al: Syndromic colon cancer: lynch syndrome and familial adenomatous polyposis. Gastroenterol Clin North Am. 37(1):47-72, vi, 2008
3. Groen EJ et al: Extra-intestinal manifestations of familial adenomatous polyposis. Ann Surg Oncol. 15(9):2439-50, 2008
4. Coffin CM et al: Gardner fibroma: a clinicopathologic and immunohistochemical analysis of 45 patients with 57 fibromas. Am J Surg Pathol. 31(3):410-6, 2007
5. Galiatsatos P et al: Familial adenomatous polyposis. Am J Gastroenterol. 101(2):385-98, 2006

Microscopic Features and Ancillary Techniques

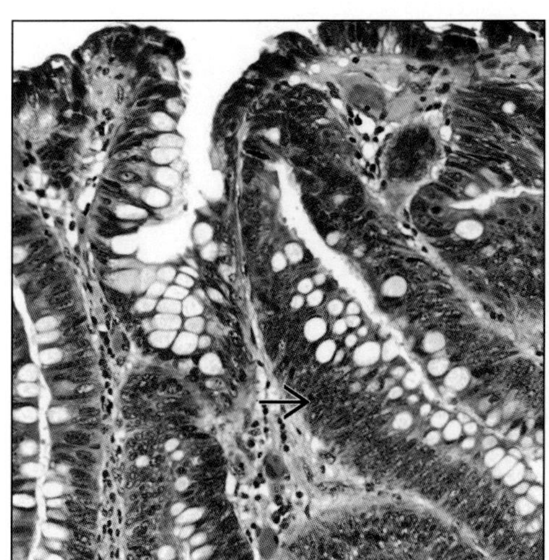

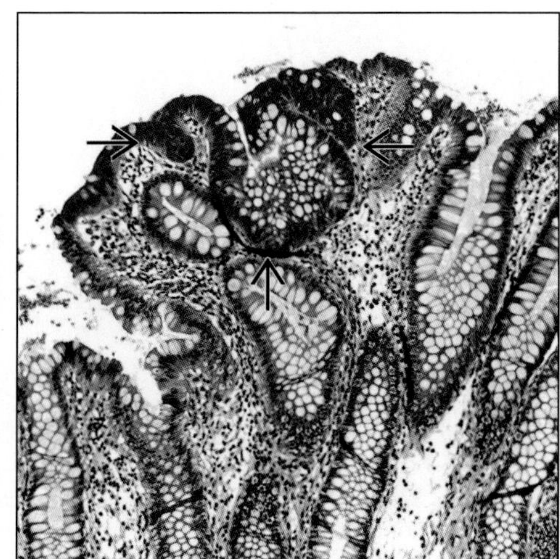

(Left) *Hematoxylin & eosin shows a high-power view of an adenoma from a patient with FAP. It is indistinguishable from a sporadic adenoma. Note elongated, hyperchromatic, and crowded nuclei → in the dysplastic epithelium.* ***(Right)*** *Hematoxylin & eosin shows an oligocryptal adenoma → from a patient with FAP. Such lesions are invisible on gross examination.*

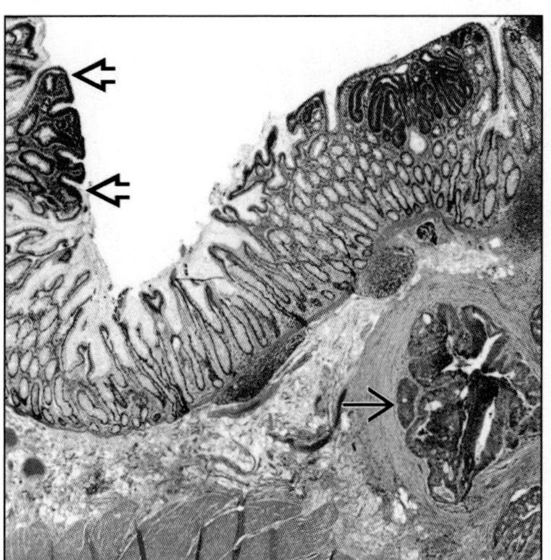

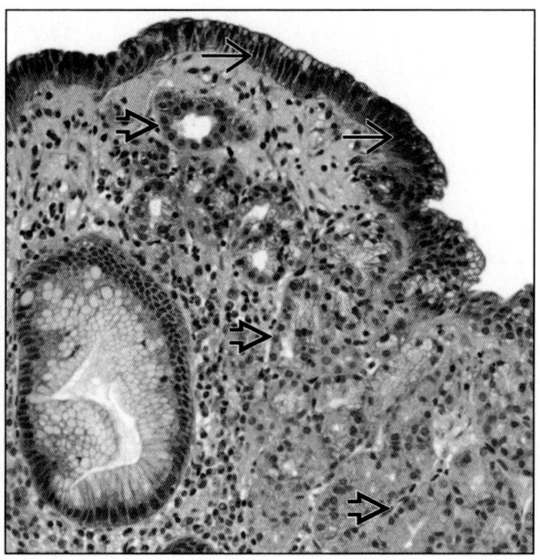

(Left) *Hematoxylin & eosin shows a low-power view of an invasive adenocarcinoma → arising in a patient with FAP. Note the presence of a tiny adenoma ⇨ in the adjacent mucosa.* ***(Right)*** *Hematoxylin & eosin shows a focus of epithelial dysplasia → in a gastric fundic gland polyp found in a patient with FAP. Note crowded oxyntic glands ⇨ immediately below the surface epithelium. Other areas of the polyp had cystically dilated oxyntic glands.*

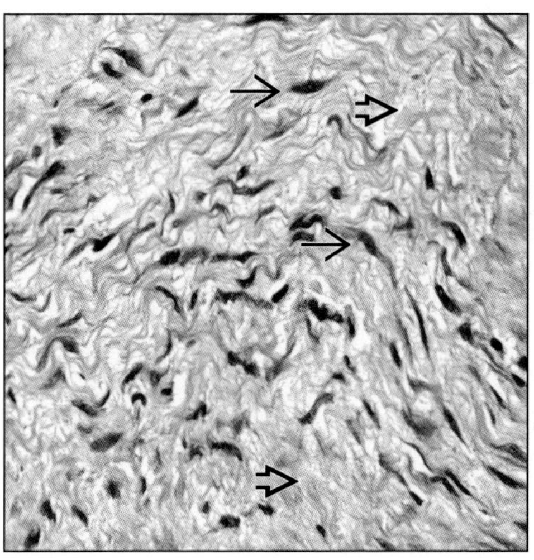

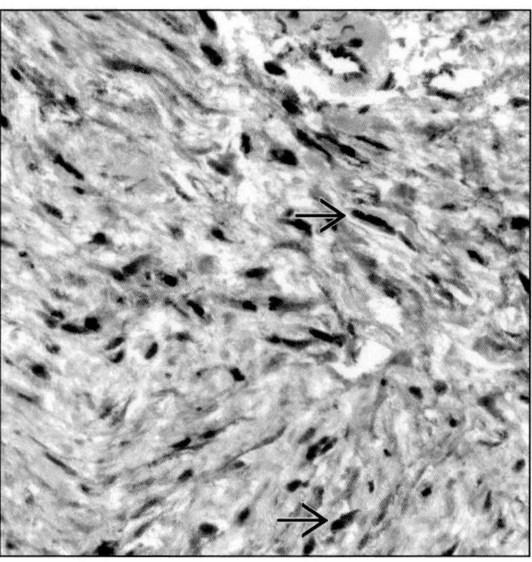

(Left) *This GS-related desmoid tumor has darkly staining, spindled fibroblast nuclei → with intervening collagen fibers ⇨ that surround and separate the nuclei. Most such tumors are unencapsulated.* ***(Right)*** *β-catenin immunohistochemical stain of a desmoid tumor shows nuclear staining → in at least a subset of cells.*

PEUTZ-JEGHERS POLYPS

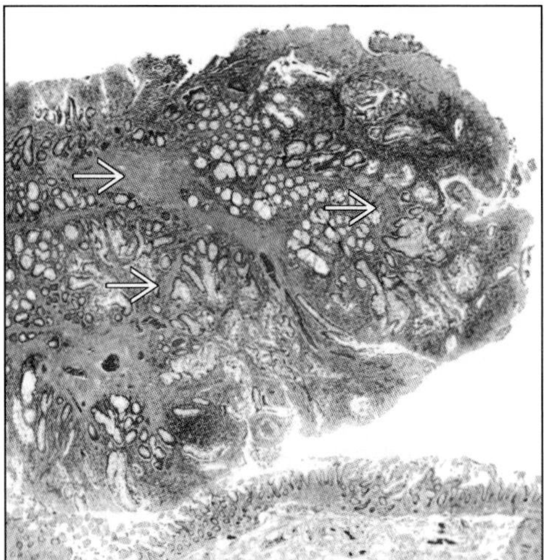

Low-power photomicrograph shows an ileal PJP. Note arborizing smooth muscle bundles ➔ that divide groups of crypts into a lobulated architecture.

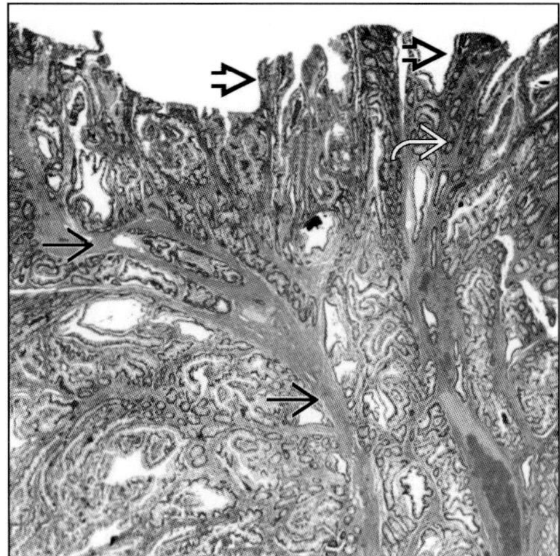

Medium-power photomicrograph of PJP shows well-organized smooth muscle ➔ and "papillary" or villiform surface ➔. Some of the muscle bundles ➔ reach the mucosal surface.

TERMINOLOGY

Abbreviations

- Peutz-Jeghers (PJ)
- Peutz-Jeghers polyp (PJP)

Definitions

- PJ syndrome
  - Characteristic hamartomatous polyps in gastrointestinal (GI) tract
  - Pigmented (melanotic) areas in perioral region (lips, buccal mucosa) and elsewhere
  - Increased risk of GI, breast, pancreas, and certain genital tract tumors
- PJP may also occur sporadically

ETIOLOGY/PATHOGENESIS

Genetics

- Autosomal dominant
- Up to 70% of PJ syndrome patients have germline mutations in *STK11*
  - Also known as *LKB1*
  - Chromosome 19p13.3
  - Involved in chromatin remodeling, cell cycle, Wnt signaling pathway
    - Mutations result in mTOR pathway abnormalities/dysregulation
- Truncating mutations result in most severe phenotype

CLINICAL ISSUES

Epidemiology

- Incidence
  - Estimated at 1/25,000 to 1/300,000
- Age
  - ~2/3 of patients diagnosed in 2nd-3rd decade
    - Diagnosis often delayed until 1st hamartomatous polyp identified
  - Most others present in 1st decade

Presentation

- Pigmented lesions
  - Oral/perioral most common
    - > 90% involve lips
    - Buccal mucosa involved in ~ 80%
  - Other sites
    - Skin around mouth and nose
    - Fingers
    - Soles of feet
    - Eyelids
  - Melanotic areas may not be visible in infancy and may fade with age
- Bleeding
  - Hematochezia with colonic polyps
  - Hematemesis with gastric and duodenal polyps
  - May result in anemia
- Abdominal pain
  - Large polyps (or clusters of polyps) can cause GI obstruction
  - Polyps may lead to intussusception
- Prolapse of rectal polyps
- Tumors
  - Colorectal carcinoma
  - Pancreatic carcinoma
  - Gastric and small intestinal carcinoma
  - Breast cancer
  - Genital tract tumors
    - Sex cord tumor with annular tubules (SCTAT) of ovary
    - Large cell calcifying Sertoli cell tumor of testis
    - Minimal deviation adenocarcinoma (adenoma malignum) of uterine cervix
- Other manifestations outside GI tract
  - Polyps in urinary bladder, renal pelvis, nasobronchial tree
  - Skeletal abnormalities (clubfoot, scoliosis)

PEUTZ-JEGHERS POLYPS

Key Facts

Terminology
- PJ syndrome characterized by GI polyps, pigmented mucocutaneous lesions, and increased risk of cancer
- PJP may also occur sporadically

Etiology/Pathogenesis
- Up to 70% of PJ syndrome patients have germline mutations in *STK11* on chromosome 19p13.3

Clinical Issues
- Pigmented lesions
- Abdominal pain, bleeding, intussusception, obstruction
- Markedly increased risk of cancer in PJ syndrome
  - Relative risk of all carcinomas ~ 15%
- Patients require close surveillance with polypectomy; resection for malignancy, obstruction

Macroscopic Features
- GI polyps may be solitary or multiple
- Polyps can occur in clusters but do not carpet mucosa

Microscopic Pathology
- Hamartomatous polyps with arborizing smooth muscle bundles and possible epithelial dysplasia
- Other distinctive tumors
  - SCTAT in ovary
  - Large cell calcifying Sertoli cell tumor or intratubular large cell hyalinizing Sertoli cell neoplasia in testis
  - Minimal deviation adenocarcinoma of uterine cervix

Treatment
- Surgical approaches
  - Resection for
    - Malignant tumors
    - PJP with epithelial dysplasia
    - Intussusception or obstruction
    - Intractable bleeding or prolapse of large polyps
- Endoscopic polypectomy
- Screening of first-degree relatives
  - Melanotic pigmented lesions
  - Precocious puberty (may indicate ovarian/testicular tumors)
  - Upper and lower endoscopic examination (including push enteroscopy) beginning at age 12
  - Pancreatic imaging (e.g., endoscopic ultrasound)
  - Mammograms beginning at age 18
  - Pelvic exam/Pap smear for cervical tumors
  - Serum CA-125 measurement beginning at age 25
- Genetic testing for asymptomatic first-degree relatives

Prognosis
- Markedly increased risk of cancer in PJ syndrome
  - Less risk than in patients with familial adenomatous polyposis
  - Relative risk of all carcinomas ~ 15%
  - Colon
    - Diagnosed at mean age of ~ 46%
    - 39% cumulative risk
  - Stomach
    - 29% cumulative risk
  - Small intestine
    - 13% cumulative risk
  - Pancreas
    - 36% cumulative risk
  - Breast
    - 54% absolute risk
  - Genital
    - 21% absolute risk for ovary, 10% for uterine cervix, 9% for testis
- Some evidence that even patients with sporadic PJP have elevated cancer risk

Diagnostic Criteria
- PJ syndrome may be diagnosed when
  - PJP number > 5
  - Any PJP are found in a patient with characteristic mucocutaneous pigmentation
  - Either PJP or mucocutaneous pigmentation is found in a patient with family history of PJ syndrome

MACROSCOPIC FEATURES

General Features
- GI polyps may be solitary or multiple
  - Polyps do not carpet mucosa as in familial adenomatous polyposis
  - Often occur in clusters
- Lobulated, cauliflower-like appearance

Size
- GI polyps variably sized
  - Small polyps usually sessile
  - Larger polyps typically pedunculated

Sites
- Polyps occur in jejunum > ileum > duodenum > colon > stomach (in order of decreasing frequency)

MICROSCOPIC PATHOLOGY

Histologic Features
- PJP
  - Hamartomatous polyp
    - Characterized by normal mucosal elements in disarray
    - Type of epithelium depends on site in GI tract
  - Arborizing smooth muscle bundles are key feature visible at low power
    - Separate crypts/glands into lobules surrounded by muscle
    - Small foci of displaced epithelial elements surrounded by smooth muscle fibers may mimic invasive adenocarcinoma

PEUTZ-JEGHERS POLYPS

- Best exemplified in small intestinal polyps; colonic and gastric may have less prominent muscle component
  - Surface erosion or ulcer common
  - Epithelial dysplasia may be present
    - Morphologically identical to sporadic adenomatous dysplasia
    - Elongated, crowded, hyperchromatic nuclei with increased mitotic activity
- Pigmented lesions
  - Epithelial/epidermal acanthosis
  - Prominent basal melanin
- SCTAT
  - Found in ~ 1/3 of PJ syndrome patients
    - Some observers think SCTAT occurs in essentially all female PJ syndrome patients
  - Often multiple, bilateral tumors
  - Tumors composed of characteristic tubules of cells with peripheral nuclei and central clear zone
  - Tubule lumens contain inspissated, eosinophilic hyaline material
- Sertoli cell tumors
  - Occur in young boys and may be bilateral
  - May produce estrogen
  - Large cell calcifying Sertoli cell tumor can be seen in PJ syndrome or in other conditions
    - Intratubular large cell hyalinizing Sertoli cell neoplasia seen primarily in setting of PJ syndrome
- Minimal deviation adenocarcinoma of uterine cervix
  - "Adenoma malignum"
  - Low-grade appearance, but highly aggressive behavior
  - Malignant glands infiltrate without stromal response
  - > 50% associated with *STK11* mutations

DIFFERENTIAL DIAGNOSIS

Juvenile Polyp

- Macroscopic appearance very similar
- Surface erosion very common
- Lacks arborizing smooth muscle
  - No lobular arrangement
  - Caveat: PJP from mucosal sites that tend to have less prominent muscle (e.g., colon) can strongly resemble juvenile polyps
- Cystically dilated crypts/glands characterize juvenile polyps
- Juvenile polyps have loose, edematous lamina propria with mixed inflammatory cell infiltrate
- Different genetic abnormalities in syndromic juvenile polyps (juvenile polyposis syndrome)
  - *SMAD4* and *BMPR1A* mutations characterize juvenile polyposis syndrome

Mucosal Prolapse Polyp

- Tend to occur in colon where fecal stream is solid (left colon, especially sigmoid and rectum)
- Smooth muscle component not as organized as in PJP
  - No characteristic arborization
  - Tiny slips of smooth muscle often "pinch" basal crypts, creating "pointed" appearance
- Large mucosal prolapse polyps in rectum can be confusing

DIAGNOSTIC CHECKLIST

Clinically Relevant Pathologic Features

- Age distribution
- Organ distribution
- Gross appearance

Pathologic Interpretation Pearls

- Arborizing smooth muscle bundles very characteristic of PJP
- Lobular arrangement of epithelial structures (crypts/glands) created by muscle bundles
- PJP may resemble juvenile or mucosal prolapse polyps
  - Disorganized muscle and muscle fibers surrounding individual crypts favor mucosal prolapse
  - Loose, edematous lamina propria with cystically dilated crypts/glands favors juvenile polyp
- PJP may or may not have epithelial dysplasia
- Do not mistake epithelial displacement for invasive adenocarcinoma
- Sporadic PJP somewhat controversial but may have same cancer risk as syndromic cases

SELECTED REFERENCES

1. Sekino Y et al: Solitary Peutz-Jeghers type hamartomatous polyps in the duodenum are not always associated with a low risk of cancer: two case reports. J Med Case Reports. 5(1):240, 2011
2. van Lier MG et al: High cancer risk and increased mortality in patients with Peutz-Jeghers syndrome. Gut. 60(2):141-7, 2011
3. Salloch H et al: Truncating mutations in Peutz-Jeghers syndrome are associated with more polyps, surgical interventions and cancers. Int J Colorectal Dis. 25(1):97-107, 2010
4. Burkart AL et al: Do sporadic Peutz-Jeghers polyps exist? Experience of a large teaching hospital. Am J Surg Pathol. 31(8):1209-14, 2007
5. de Leng WW et al: Nasal polyposis in Peutz-Jeghers syndrome: a distinct histopathological and molecular genetic entity. J Clin Pathol. 60(4):392-6, 2007
6. Mehenni H et al: Molecular and clinical characteristics in 46 families affected with Peutz-Jeghers syndrome. Dig Dis Sci. 52(8):1924-33, 2007
7. Hearle N et al: Frequency and spectrum of cancers in the Peutz-Jeghers syndrome. Clin Cancer Res. 12(10):3209-15, 2006
8. Amos CI et al: Genotype-phenotype correlations in Peutz-Jeghers syndrome. J Med Genet. 41(5):327-33, 2004
9. Entius MM et al: Molecular genetic alterations in hamartomatous polyps and carcinomas of patients with Peutz-Jeghers syndrome. J Clin Pathol. 54(2):126-31, 2001
10. Petersen VC et al: Misplacement of dysplastic epithelium in Peutz-Jeghers Polyps: the ultimate diagnostic pitfall? Am J Surg Pathol. 24(1):34-9, 2000
11. Wang ZJ et al: Allelic imbalance at the LKB1 (STK11) locus in tumours from patients with Peutz-Jeghers' syndrome provides evidence for a hamartoma-(adenoma)-carcinoma sequence. J Pathol. 188(1):9-13, 1999

Microscopic Features

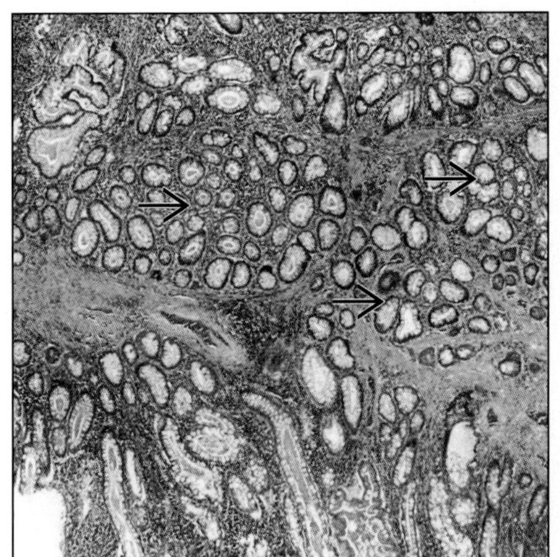

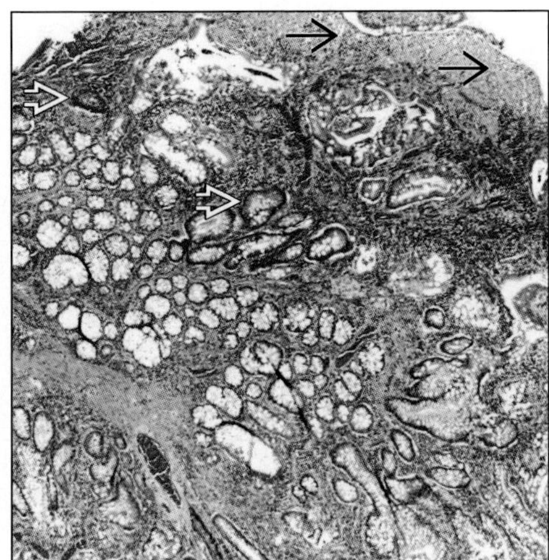

(Left) *Medium-power photomicrograph of a small intestinal PJP illustrates its hamartomatous nature, with normal mucosal elements in a disorganized arrangement. The clusters of crypts are separated into lobules → by the smooth muscle.* ***(Right)*** *This PJP has surface erosion →, a common finding that can induce reactive atypia of the adjacent epithelium ⇨.*

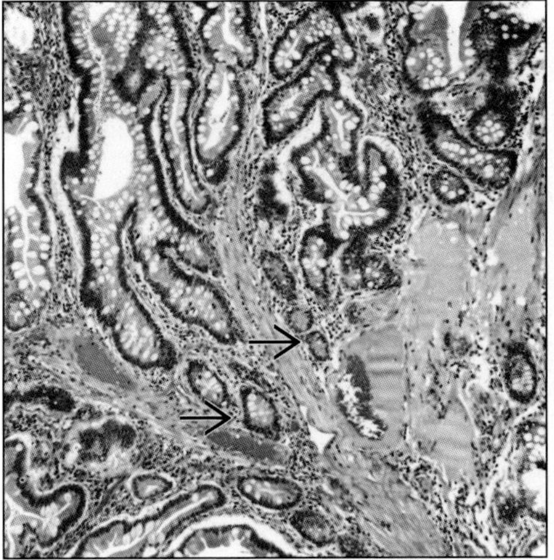

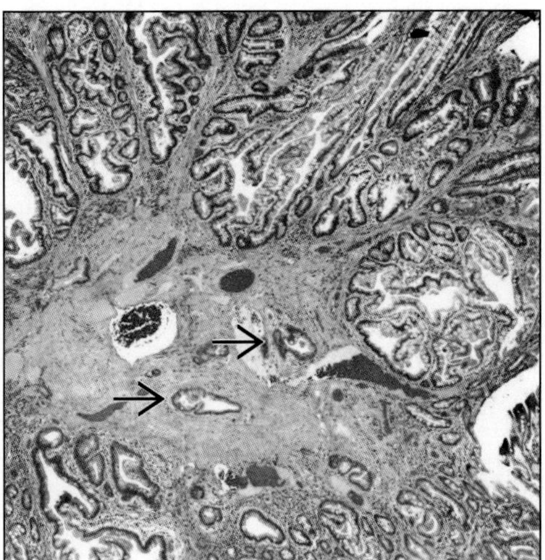

(Left) *High-power photomicrograph of a PJP shows the lack of smooth muscle fibers surrounding individual crypts →. Instead, the arborizing muscle bundles are relatively compact as they traverse the mucosa. More disorganized muscle fibers surrounding individual crypts would favor a mucosal prolapse polyp.* ***(Right)*** *This PJP contains "displaced" epithelium → in the muscle bundles, a finding that can mimic invasive adenocarcinoma.*

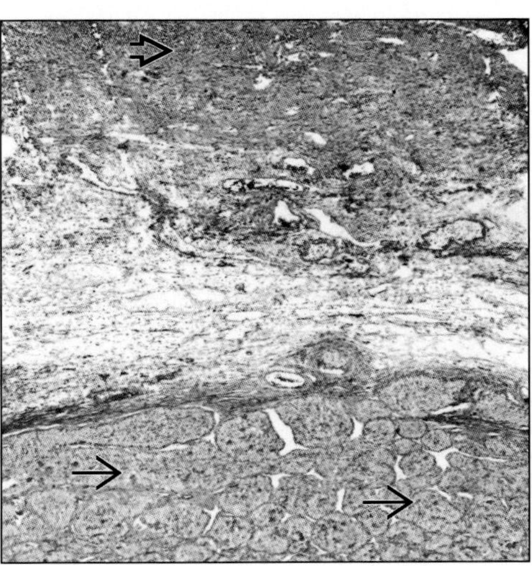

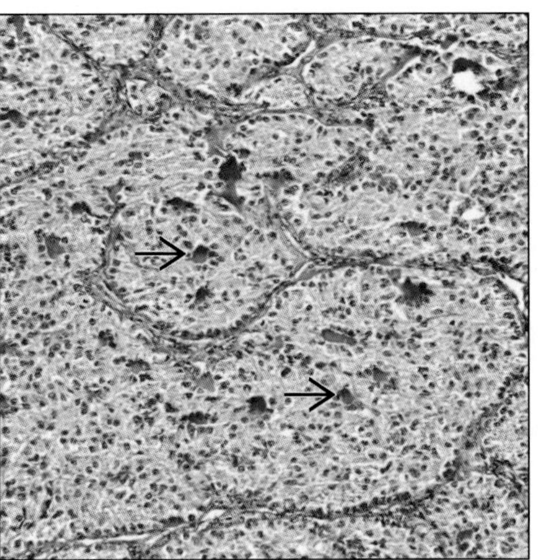

(Left) *This ovarian tumor is a sex cord tumor with annular tubules (SCTAT) → from a patient with PJ syndrome. Normal ovarian stroma ⇨ can be seen at the top of the photomicrograph.* ***(Right)*** *This high-power view of a SCTAT illustrates the circumscribed nests composed of cells with peripheral nuclei. The tumor cells form tubules → that are filled with eosinophilic hyaline material.*

INFLAMMATORY POLYPS

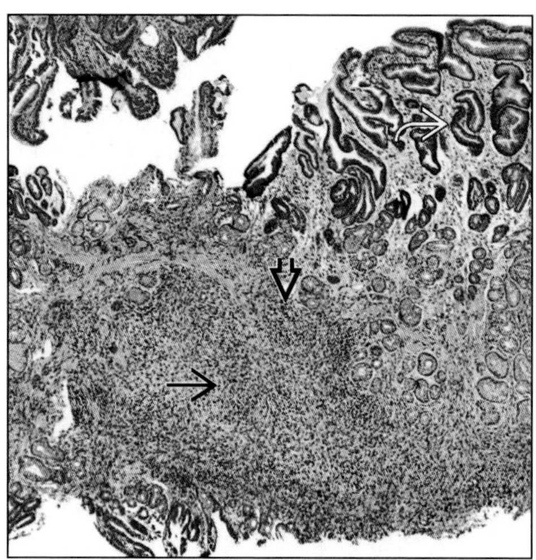

This gastric IFP is centered in the submucosa ➙. The muscularis mucosae ➯ is focally disrupted, and the overlying mucosa is reactive ➘. (Courtesy H. Appelman, MD.)

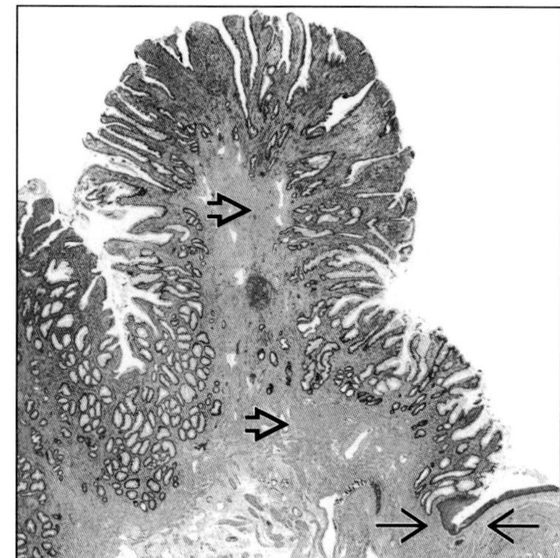

This large ICP is in close proximity to the anal transition zone ➙. Note abundant fibers of the muscularis mucosae ➯ that extend into the polyp. (Courtesy H. Appelman, MD.)

TERMINOLOGY

Abbreviations

- Inflammatory fibroid polyp (IFP)
- Inflammatory cloacogenic polyp (ICP)
- Cap polyp (CP)
- Inflammatory pseudopolyp (IPP)

Definitions

- IFP
  - Benign submucosal proliferation of vascular fibrous tissue with admixed inflammatory cells
  - Composed of bland spindle cells (lesional cells) in a loose, edematous stroma
- ICP
  - Intensely inflamed, polypoid, prolapsed mucosa with secondary reactive/regenerative epithelial changes
    - Benign, but may mimic malignancy or inflammatory bowel disease (IBD)
- CP
  - Characteristic benign inflammatory polyp with "cap" of necroinflammatory exudate
- IPP
  - Inflamed, regenerative mucosa protruding above surrounding mucosa &/or ulcer bed
    - Hence, "**pseudo**polyp"
    - Overlap with generic term "inflammatory polyp"

ETIOLOGY/PATHOGENESIS

IFP

- Platelet-derived growth factor receptor α (*PDGFRA*) gene mutations
  - Mutations in exon 18 → gastric IFP
  - Mutations in exon 12 → small intestinal IFP
- May have dendritic cell origin
- Some familial cases identified ("Devon polyposis")

ICP

- Mucosal prolapse
  - Often seen in setting of solitary rectal ulcer syndrome (SRUS)
    - Dysfunction of puborectalis muscle during defecation
    - Leads to straining at stool and prolapse of mucosa

CP

- Unknown etiology
  - Some may be related to mucosal prolapse
  - Many polyps (dozens) can occur throughout GI tract ("cap polyposis")
- Polyps with similar appearance may be found in other settings (in IBD, at anastomotic sites, etc.)

IPP

- Intense mucosal inflammation
  - Most commonly in setting of IBD
  - Other causes possible (ischemia, infection, etc.)

CLINICAL ISSUES

Epidemiology

- Incidence
  - IFP, ICP, and CP all relatively rare
  - IPP common in setting of IBD
- Age
  - All entities occur in wide age range, including pediatric patients

Site

- IFP: Most common in stomach (especially antrum)
  - Rare in small intestine and colon
- ICP: Distal-most rectum/anal transition zone
  - At or near dentate line
- CP: Most common in distal colon (sigmoid/rectum) but can occur throughout GI tract in cap polyposis
  - Also seen at anastomotic sites

INFLAMMATORY POLYPS

Key Facts

Terminology
- IFP: Submucosal proliferation of vascular fibrous tissue with inflammation
- ICP: Polypoid, prolapsed mucosa with reactive/ regenerative epithelial changes
- CP: Benign inflammatory polyp with necroinflammatory "cap"
- IPP: Inflamed, regenerative mucosa protruding above surrounding mucosa ± ulcer

Etiology/Pathogenesis
- IFP: *PDGFRA* gene mutations
- ICP and some CP: Mucosal prolapse
- IPP: Most common in setting of IBD

Clinical Issues
- IFP: Gastric outlet obstruction
- ICP: Rectal bleeding, pain, tenesmus
- CP: Diarrhea, mucoid stool, bleeding, tenesmus
- IPP: Usually not inherently symptomatic

Microscopic Pathology
- IFP: Collection of highly vascularized spindle cells with eosinophils and lymphoplasmacytic infiltrate
  - Blood vessels may have "onion-skin" appearance
  - CD34(+)
- ICP: Prominent smooth muscle bundles replace normal lamina propria elements
  - Reactive/regenerative epithelial changes common
- CP: Characteristic "cap" of fibroinflammatory exudate with underlying granulation tissue
- IPP: Regenerative mucosa with distorted crypts

- IPP: Colon most common, classically associated with IBD
  - Similar polyps can occur anywhere in GI tract with inflammation

Presentation
- IFP
  - Gastric outlet obstruction
  - Small intestinal examples may cause obstruction or intussusception
  - May be incidentally discovered (particularly rare colonic lesions)
  - Hemorrhage possible from overlying mucosal injury
- ICP
  - Rectal bleeding, pain, tenesmus
- CP/cap polyposis
  - Diarrhea, mucoid stool, bleeding, tenesmus
  - Some cases of cap polyposis accompanied by extensive protein loss & hypoproteinemia
- IPP
  - Usually not inherently symptomatic → symptoms from underlying condition (e.g., IBD)

Treatment
- Symptom dependent
  - All may be managed conservatively if asymptomatic or minimally symptomatic
  - Excision/resection for clinically problematic lesions
    - May be endoscopically removed or surgically resected

Prognosis
- All 4 entities benign with no risk of malignant transformation

MACROSCOPIC FEATURES

General Features
- IFP
  - Based in submucosa
    - May disrupt muscularis mucosae and extend into mucosa
    - Can impinge on underlying muscularis propria
  - Fairly well demarcated
  - Size: Usually < 5 cm (1-4 cm typical)
- ICP
  - Polypoid lesion at dentate line
    - Variably sized → "ICP" term usually reserved for larger examples
    - Small polyps with similar features usually diagnosed more descriptively (e.g., "polypoid prolapsed mucosa" or "prolapse-type changes")
  - May make a large mass, mimicking neoplasm
- CP
  - Sessile or low pedunculated
  - Size: ≤ 2 cm
- IPP
  - Sessile or pedunculated
  - Size: Rarely > 2 cm
  - Projects above surrounding ulcers

MICROSCOPIC PATHOLOGY

Histologic Features
- IFP
  - Collection of highly vascularized spindle cells with mixed inflammation
    - Stroma often edematous
    - Eosinophils very prominent, with accompanying lymphoplasmacytic population
    - Lymphoid aggregates occasionally present
    - Neutrophils not prominent
    - Larger blood vessels may have "onion-skin" appearance (best seen in gastric examples)
  - Well demarcated, but no capsule
  - Overlying mucosa often has intense reactive changes
    - Spindle cell proliferation may disrupt muscularis mucosae and encroach on overlying mucosa
  - CD34(+) on immunohistochemistry
- ICP
  - Prominent smooth muscle bundles replace normal lamina propria elements

INFLAMMATORY POLYPS

- Reflect etiology (mucosal prolapse)
- Surround and "pinch" basal crypts
- Can mimic an infiltrative process
  - Villiform surface
  - Reactive/regenerative epithelial changes common
    - May impart hyperplastic &/or adenomatous appearance to crypts
  - Crypts displaced into submucosa by prolapse → "colitis cystica profunda"
- CP
  - Characteristic "cap" of fibroinflammatory exudate with underlying granulation tissue
  - Regenerative, dilated, and tortuous crypts beneath cap
- IPP
  - Regenerative mucosa with distorted crypts
    - Intensely regenerative epithelium can be confused with dysplasia, particularly in setting of IBD
  - Often eroded or ulcerated surface
    - Small IPP may be entirely composed of granulation tissue ("granulation tissue polyp")
  - Crypts may resemble those of hyperplastic polyp and may have acute cryptitis

DIFFERENTIAL DIAGNOSIS

Hyperplastic Polyp

- Lacks muscular element of prolapse-related polyps (ICP, CP)
- May be inflamed, but usually not to extent seen in IPP or CP

Adenoma

- Contains bona fide epithelial dysplasia
- Prolapsed adenomas in distal rectum can be problematic
  - Features of both adenoma and ICP present

Polyposis Syndromes

- Extensive IPP in cases of colitis, as well as cap polyposis, can mimic cancer-associated polyposis syndromes
- Most polyposis syndromes have characteristic polyp appearance (e.g., Peutz-Jeghers syndrome) &/or adenomatous polyps (e.g., familial adenomatous polyposis)
- Background inflammatory disease (e.g., IBD) a helpful histological clue for extensive IPP
- Family history may be helpful

Gastrointestinal Stromal Tumor (GIST)

- Spindle cells in IFP can resemble GIST
- GIST usually centered in muscularis propria not submucosa
- GIST composed of more uniform spindle cell population without prominent inflammatory infiltrate
- Lesional cells in IFP negative for C-kit (CD117)
  - Mast cells in inflammatory infiltrate of IFP will be C-kit positive

Schwannoma

- Spindle cell tumor that can resemble IFP
- Like GIST, schwannoma usually centered in muscularis propria
- Typically surrounded by "cuff" of nodular lymphoid infiltrate
- S100 positive by immunohistochemistry

DIAGNOSTIC CHECKLIST

Pathologic Interpretation Pearls

- IFP
  - Prominent eosinophils and "onion skin" vessels are clues to diagnosis
- ICP
  - "Pointed" or "diamond-shaped" basal crypts reflect compression by smooth muscle bundles → mucosal prolapse
- CP
  - Fibrinopurulent "cap" over reactive crypts is key feature
- IPP
  - Intense regenerative epithelial changes must not be confused with dysplasia

SELECTED REFERENCES

1. Rittershaus AC et al: Benign gastrointestinal mesenchymal BUMPS: a brief review of some spindle cell polyps with published names. Arch Pathol Lab Med. 135(10):1311-9, 2011
2. Lasota J et al: Gain-of-function PDGFRA mutations, earlier reported in gastrointestinal stromal tumors, are common in small intestinal inflammatory fibroid polyps. A study of 60 cases. Mod Pathol. 22(8):1049-56, 2009
3. Rossi G et al: PDGFR expression in differential diagnosis between KIT-negative gastrointestinal stromal tumours and other primary soft-tissue tumours of the gastrointestinal tract. Histopathology. 46(5):522-31, 2005
4. Ng KH et al: Cap polyposis: further experience and review. Dis Colon Rectum. 47(7):1208-15, 2004
5. Ozolek JA et al: Inflammatory fibroid polyps of the gastrointestinal tract: clinical, pathologic, and molecular characteristics. Appl Immunohistochem Mol Morphol. 12(1):59-66, 2004
6. Pantanowitz L et al: Inflammatory fibroid polyps of the gastrointestinal tract: evidence for a dendritic cell origin. Am J Surg Pathol. 28(1):107-14, 2004
7. Rodríguez-Leal GA et al: Inflammatory cloacogenic polyp and solitary rectal ulcer syndrome resemble rectal adenocarcinoma. Am J Gastroenterol. 90(8):1362-3, 1995
8. Washington K et al: Inflammatory cloacogenic polyp in a child: part of the spectrum of solitary rectal ulcer syndrome. Pediatr Pathol. 13(4):409-14, 1993
9. Lobert PF et al: Inflammatory cloacogenic polyp. A unique inflammatory lesion of the anal transitional zone. Am J Surg Pathol. 5(8):761-6, 1981

Microscopic Features

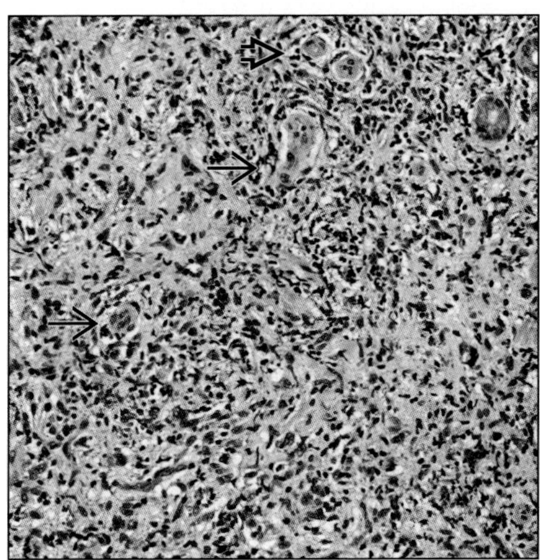

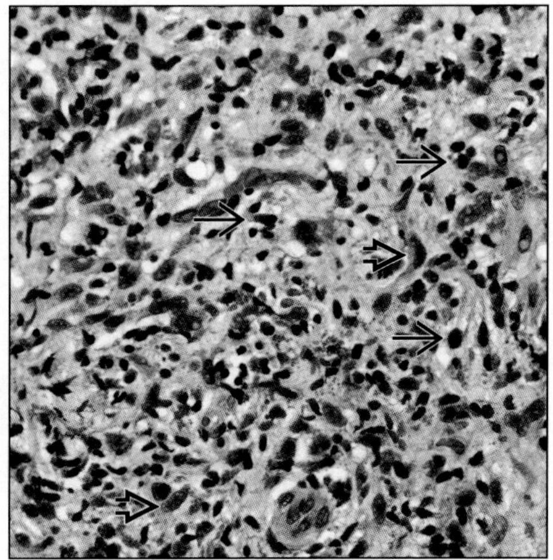

(Left) *This IFP has a prominent inflammatory infiltrate in an edematous background. Several blood vessels ➡ are visible, some with a subtle "onion skin" appearance ➡ imparted by surrounding spindle cells. (Courtesy H. Appelman, MD.)* ***(Right)*** *At high magnification, the prominent eosinophils ➡ in this IFP are easily visible, as are the lesional spindle cells ➡. (Courtesy H. Appelman, MD.)*

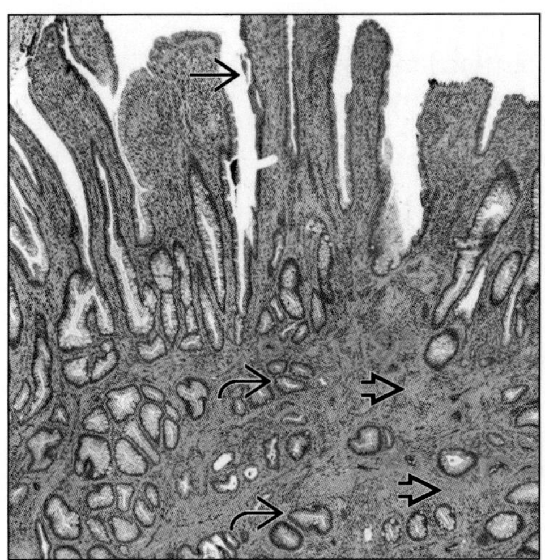

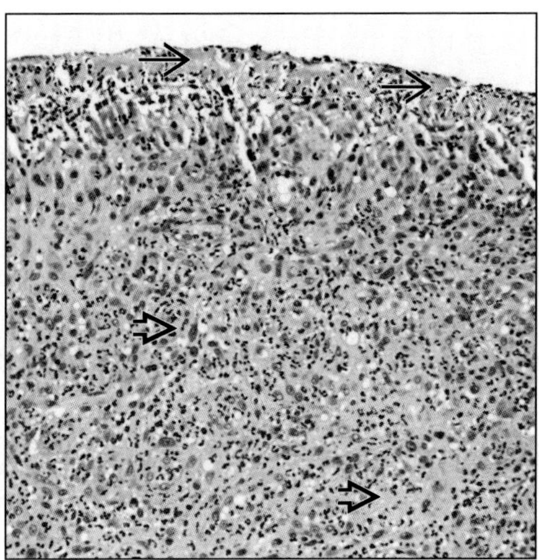

(Left) *This ICP has a villiform surface ➡, with smooth muscle around the basal crypts ➡, displacing normal lamina propria. Many of the crypts have the "pointed" or diamond-shaped ➡ appearance of mucosal prolapse. Care must be taken not to misinterpret this as infiltration of the muscle by a carcinoma. (Courtesy H. Appelman, MD.)* ***(Right)*** *The "cap" of a CP is composed of a fibrinopurulent surface exudate ➡ with underlying granulation tissue ➡. (Courtesy H. Appelman, MD.)*

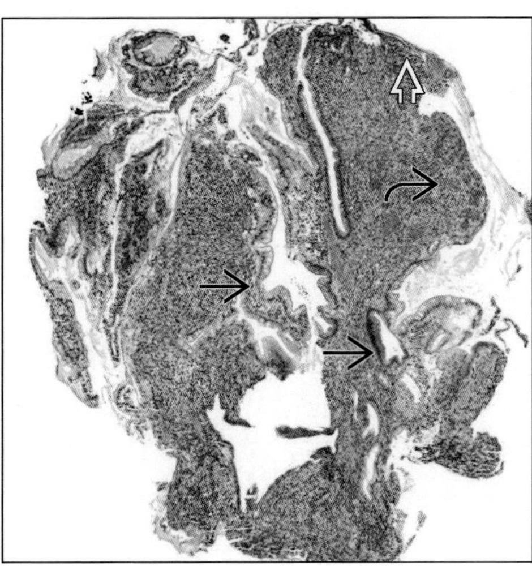

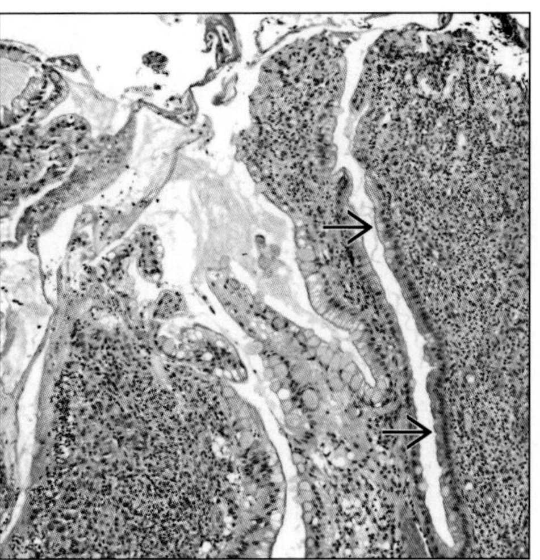

(Left) *This IPP from a patient with ulcerative colitis has distorted crypts ➡ and a surface erosion ➡. The lamina propria contains numerous inflammatory cells and has a granulation tissue-like appearance ➡. (Courtesy H. Appelman, MD.)* ***(Right)*** *At higher magnification, the regenerative epithelium ➡ of this IPP is visible. The nuclear hyperchromasia and mucin depletion can mimic dysplasia, particularly in the setting of inflammatory bowel disease. (Courtesy H. Appelman, MD.)*

CRONKITE-CANADA SYNDROME

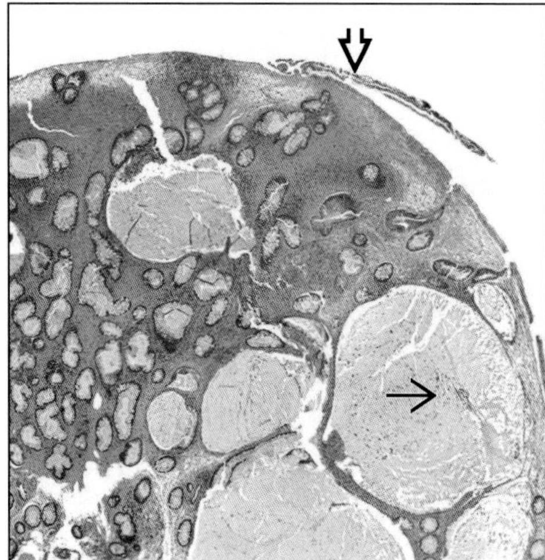

CCS polyp from the colon, with dilated crypts ➔ and eroded surface ⇨, is essentially identical to a juvenile-type polyp. (Courtesy B. McKenna, MD.)

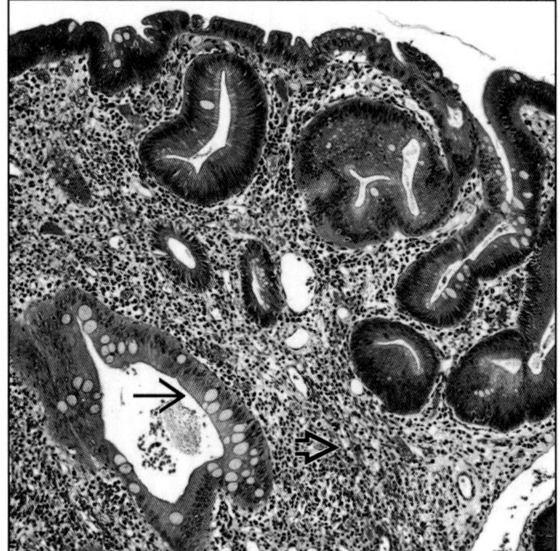

Higher power view shows a colonic CCS polyp. The epithelium lining the variably dilated crypts ➔ is recognizably intestinal. Note mixed lamina propria inflammation ⇨. (Courtesy B. McKenna, MD.)

TERMINOLOGY

Abbreviations

- Cronkhite-Canada syndrome (CCS)

Definitions

- Noninherited syndrome
  - Hamartomatous polyps throughout most of gastrointestinal tract
  - Often accompanied by protein-losing enteropathy
  - Extragastrointestinal (ectodermal) manifestations
- "Juvenile polyposis of infancy"
  - Syndrome with manifestations similar to CCS occurring in infants
  - Patients lack family history of polyposis (unlike conventional juvenile polyposis syndrome)

ETIOLOGY/PATHOGENESIS

Uncertain

- Possible environmental factor(s)
  - Japanese patients overrepresented; also occurs in Europe and United States
- Other potential etiological factors postulated

CLINICAL ISSUES

Epidemiology

- Incidence
  - Rare
    - Reported cases number in hundreds
- Age
  - Middle adulthood (5th-6th decade)

Presentation

- Diarrhea
  - May result in electrolyte abnormalities
- Weight loss
  - Malabsorption, protein-losing enteropathy possible
- Hematochezia
- Abdominal pain
  - Intestinal obstruction possible
- Ectodermal manifestations
  - Alopecia (scalp and body)
  - Hyperpigmentation
  - Onychodystrophy
  - Vitiligo

Endoscopic Findings

- Polyps occur throughout most of gastrointestinal tract
  - Esophagus spared

Treatment

- Supportive
  - Electrolyte replacement
  - Nutritional support
- Surgery
  - May be necessary in cases with intractable bleeding, obstruction, malignancy

Prognosis

- As many as 20% of patients reported to develop adenocarcinoma
  - Malignant potential controversial
    - Unclear whether dysplasia & neoplasia is connected to syndrome or coincidental
  - Carcinoma usually develops in colon; much less common in stomach
  - May arise in polypoid or nonpolypoid mucosa
- ~ 50% mortality
  - Typically from chronic wasting, anemia, bleeding, infection

MACROSCOPIC FEATURES

General Features

- Mucosa appears diffusely nodular with superimposed discrete polyps
  - Polyps may be sessile or pedunculated

Key Facts

Clinical Issues

- Rare, noninherited syndrome
- Usually presents in middle adulthood
- Hamartomatous polyps, protein-losing enteropathy and ectodermal manifestations
- As many as 20% of patients reported to develop adenocarcinoma
- ~ 50% mortality

Microscopic Pathology

- Intestinal CCS polyps essentially indistinguishable from juvenile polyps
- Mucosa between discrete polyps diffusely nodular, with similar histological features to those seen in polyps
- Gastric CCS polyps essentially identical to gastric hyperplastic polyps

  - Cystically dilated spaces may impart "mucinous" appearance to cut surfaces

MICROSCOPIC PATHOLOGY

Histologic Features

- Intestinal CCS polyps essentially indistinguishable from juvenile polyps
  - Dilated, irregularly shaped crypts or glands
  - Prominent inflammatory infiltrate in edematous lamina propria
- Mucosa between discrete polyps diffusely nodular, with similar histological features to those seen in polyps
- Gastric CCS polyps essentially identical to gastric hyperplastic polyps

DIFFERENTIAL DIAGNOSIS

Hyperplastic Polyps

- Sporadic hyperplastic polyps in colon may resemble CCS polyps
- No association with malabsorption or protein-losing enteropathy

Juvenile Polyposis

- Hereditary syndrome, usually presents early in life
  - Associated with *SMAD4* or *BMPR1A* mutations
- Polyps histologically similar to CCS
  - More commonly pedunculated
  - Intervening mucosa normal in juvenile polyposis
- No ectodermal manifestations

DIAGNOSTIC CHECKLIST

Clinically Relevant Pathologic Features

- Symptom complex
  - Hamartomatous polyps combined with extragastrointestinal manifestations
    - Malabsorption, protein-losing enteropathy
    - Ectodermal manifestations

Pathologic Interpretation Pearls

- Hamartomatous polyps involve stomach through colon, esophagus spared
- Essentially indistinguishable from mucosal polyps seen in juvenile polyposis
- Intervening mucosa between discrete polyps has similar histological features

SELECTED REFERENCES

1. Ward EM et al: Review article: the non-inherited gastrointestinal polyposis syndromes. Aliment Pharmacol Ther. 16(3):333-42, 2002
2. Burke AP et al: The pathology of Cronkhite-Canada polyps. A comparison to juvenile polyposis. Am J Surg Pathol. 13(11):940-6, 1989

IMAGE GALLERY

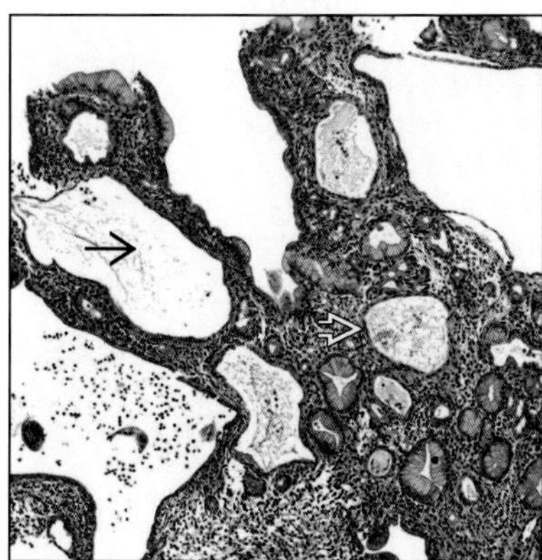

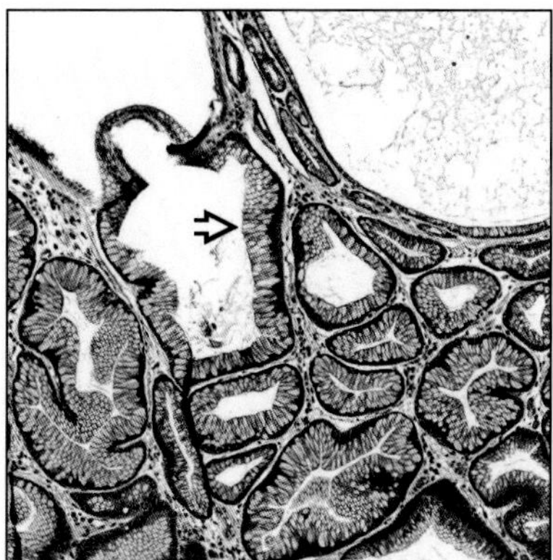

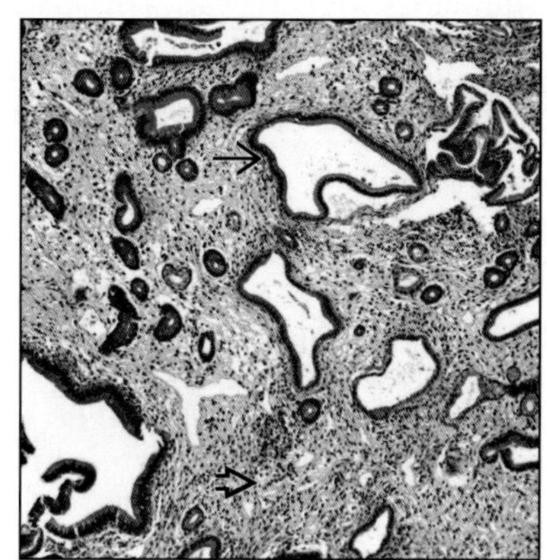

(Left) *This gastric CCS polyp has cystically dilated pits ⇒ and glands ➡ with inflamed and edematous lamina propria. (Courtesy H. Appelman, MD and J. Greenson, MD.)* ***(Center)*** *Closer view of gastric CCS polyp shows abundant foveolar-type mucin cells ➡, identical to those seen in gastric hyperplastic polyps. (Courtesy H. Appelman, MD and J. Greenson, MD.)* ***(Right)*** *A duodenal CCS polyp has characteristic edematous lamina propria ➡ with mixed inflammation, as well as cystically dilated crypts ⇒. (Courtesy H. Appelman, MD and J. Greenson, MD.)*

NEUROENDOCRINE TUMORS

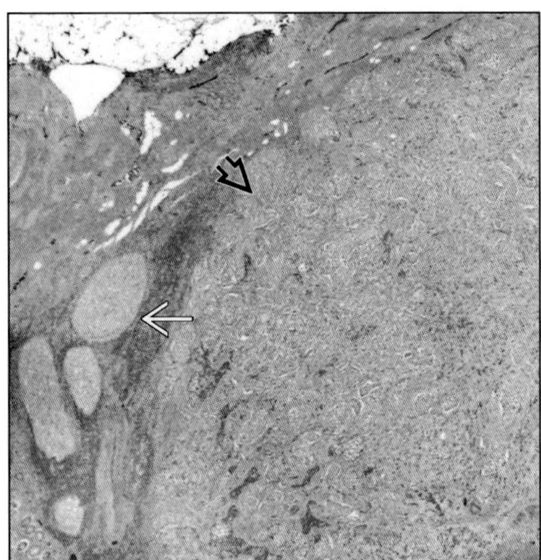

Appendiceal tip involved by a classic carcinoid tumor ➯ is seen. Note the difference in patterns presented by normal lymphoid follicles, commonly found in the tip of appendices ➡ and the carcinoid tumor.

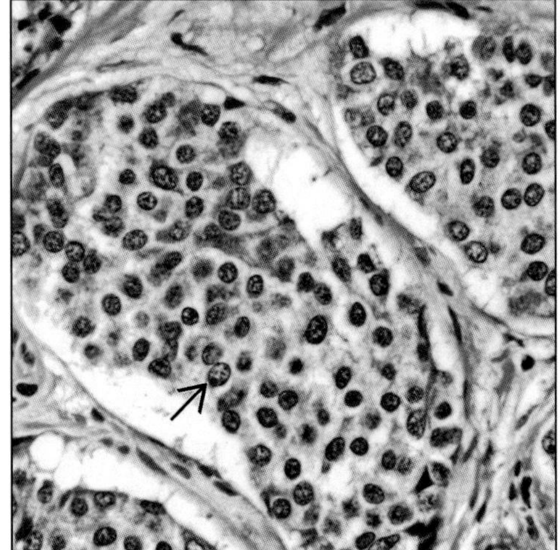

Carcinoid tumor composed of polygonal, uniform cells shows amphophilic cytoplasm and round nuclei with stippled ("salt and pepper") chromatin ➙. No mitotic figures are identified.

TERMINOLOGY

Abbreviations

- Neuroendocrine tumor (NET)

Synonyms

- Neuroendocrine neoplasm
- Endocrine neoplasm

Definitions

- Heterogeneous group of malignant neoplasms characterized by presence of epithelial and neuroendocrine differentiation with prognosis predicated on tumor type
- Well-differentiated neuroendocrine tumor
  - Carcinoid tumor (typical and atypical)
  - Neuroendocrine tumor (grades 1 and 2)
  - Neuroendocrine carcinoma (low and intermediate grades)
- Poorly differentiated neuroendocrine carcinoma
  - Small-cell carcinoma undifferentiated neuroendocrine carcinoma (SCUNC)
  - Large-cell neuroendocrine carcinoma
  - Neuroendocrine tumor (grade 3)
  - Neuroendocrine carcinoma (high grade)
- Terminology for NETs varies by anatomic site

ETIOLOGY/PATHOGENESIS

Etiology

- Most NETs in childhood are sporadic

Genetics

- May be familial and associated with
  - Multiple endocrine neoplasia type 1 (MEN1)
  - Neurofibromatosis type 1 (NF1)
  - von Hippel-Lindau syndrome (VHL)
  - Tuberous sclerosis syndrome

CLINICAL ISSUES

Epidemiology

- Incidence
  - Uncommon in pediatric population
- Age
  - Incidence increases with age
  - Usually occurs in older children and adolescents

Site

- NETs arising from the diffuse endocrine system can occur in any organ of the body
- In children and young adults, NET commonly arises in lung, breast, and appendix

Presentation

- Varies depending on location, size of tumor, and presence of metastases
- Most tumors are incidental findings
- Carcinoid syndrome
  - Symptoms include
    - Vasomotor flushing
    - Episodic hypotension
    - Diarrhea
  - Rarely occurs in children
  - Associated with involvement of liver by metastatic disease
- Paraneoplastic syndrome
  - Occasionally occurs with small cell carcinoma of lung and may include
    - Cushing syndrome, Lambert-Eaton syndrome, Schwartz-Bartter syndrome

Laboratory Tests

- Neurohormonal substances that may be measurable in serum or 24-hour urine include
  - 5-serotonin and metabolites
    - 5-hydroxytryptophan
    - 5-hydroxyindole acetate
  - Catecholamines, metanephrine, calcitonin

Key Facts

Terminology
- Heterogeneous group of malignant neoplasms characterized by presence of epithelial and neuroendocrine differentiation with prognosis predicated on tumor type

Etiology/Pathogenesis
- Most NETs in childhood are sporadic

Clinical Issues
- Uncommon in pediatric population
- Incidence increases with age
- Usually occurs in older children and adolescents
  - In children and young adults, NET commonly arises in lung, breast, and appendix
- Presentation varies depending on location, size of tumor, and presence of metastases
- Most NETs in childhood are low-grade neoplasms
- NETs may recur locally or metastasize
  - Overall, approximately 10-20% of NETs in children are metastatic at diagnosis
  - Metastatic disease often involves regional lymph nodes, liver, and bones

Diagnostic Checklist
- All NETs show stippled ("salt and pepper") chromatin
- Differentiation among types predicated on degree of nuclear pleomorphism, extent of mitotic activity, and presence of necrosis
- All NETs are submucosal tumors showing variety of growth patterns, including organoid, trabecular, ribbons, cribriform, or solid growth ± fibrovascular stroma

  - Gastrin, glucagon, insulin, ACTH, GHRH

Natural History
- Most NETs in childhood are low-grade neoplasms
- NETs may recur locally or metastasize
  - Overall, approximately 10-20% of NETs in children are metastatic at diagnosis
  - Metastatic disease often involves regional lymph nodes, liver, and bones

Treatment
- Surgical approaches
  - Depend on size and site of tumor
  - Complete surgical resection of tumor is treatment of choice and relates to outcome
  - Nodal sampling is performed for staging
- Adjuvant therapy
  - Adjunctive chemotherapy is used for metastatic disease

Prognosis
- Prognostic factors include size, depth of invasion, histology, and stage
- Carcinoid tumor
  - Indolent biology with excellent behavior generally cured following complete surgical resection
- Atypical carcinoid tumor
  - Prognosis is dependent on extent of disease at presentation
  - Often metastasizes
- Small cell undifferentiated neuroendocrine carcinoma (SCUNC)
  - Poor
  - Metastases are common

MACROSCOPIC FEATURES

General Features
- Carcinoid tumor
  - Submucosal nodular or polypoid mass
    - Tan-white appearance
    - Varying in size from a few mm up to 3 cm in diameter
  - Surface ulceration generally absent
- Atypical carcinoid
  - Submucosal nodular or polypoid mass
    - Tan-white appearance
    - Varying in size from a few mm up to 4 cm in diameter
  - Surface ulceration may be present
- SCUNC
  - Submucosal mass usually with surface ulceration

MICROSCOPIC PATHOLOGY

Histologic Features
- Carcinoid tumor
  - Submucosal tumor arranged in organoid, trabecular, ribbons, or solid growth pattern with fibrovascular stroma
  - Uniform cells with eosinophilic cytoplasm
    - Centrally located round nuclei
    - Low nuclear to cytoplasmic ratio
    - Stippled ("salt and pepper") nuclear chromatin pattern
  - Absence of pleomorphism, mitoses, necrosis
  - Glands &/or squamous differentiation can be seen
  - Surface ulceration uncommon
  - Vascular, lymphatic, and perineural invasion absent
- Atypical carcinoid
  - Submucosal tumor in organoid, trabecular, ribbons, cribriform, or solid growth pattern with prominent fibrovascular stroma
    - Infiltrative growth when present may include neurotropism and lymphovascular invasion
  - Hypercellular with mild to marked nuclear pleomorphism
    - Round to oval nuclei
    - Stippled ("salt and pepper") nuclear chromatin
    - Nuclei can be centrally or eccentrically (plasmacytoid) located
    - Nucleoli may be prominent

NEUROENDOCRINE TUMORS

Immunohistochemistry

Antibody	Reactivity	Staining Pattern	Comment
Synaptophysin	Positive	Cytoplasmic	Positive in nearly all cases
Chromogranin-A	Positive	Cytoplasmic	Positive in most cases
CD56	Positive	Cell membrane	Sensitive but not specific
CD57	Positive	Cell membrane	
NSE	Positive	Cytoplasmic	Sensitive but not specific
Calcitonin	Positive	Cytoplasmic	Atypical carcinoid (primary and metastatic) calcitonin immunoreactive in > 80%
AE1/AE3	Positive	Cytoplasmic	
CK8/18/CAM5.2	Positive	Cytoplasmic	

- Eosinophilic to clear to oncocytic cytoplasm
- Mitoses uncommon but can be seen, including atypical forms
- Necrosis may be focally identified
- Glands, squamous differentiation, and neural-type rosettes can be identified
- Surface ulceration may be prominent

- SCUNC
  - Submucosal tumor arranged in solid nests, sheets, or ribbons with absence of fibrovascular stromal component
  - Hypercellular with hyperchromatic, pleomorphic, oval to spindle-shaped nuclei
    - Increased nuclear to cytoplasmic ratio
    - Stippled ("salt and pepper") nuclear chromatin with absent to inconspicuous nucleoli
    - "Crush" artifact frequent
    - Nuclear molding identified
  - Nondescript cytoplasm and indistinct cell borders
  - Glands, squamous differentiation, and neural-type rosettes can be identified
  - Abundant mitoses, including atypical forms
  - Confluent foci of necrosis and individual cell necrosis common
  - Surface ulceration present
  - Neurotropism and lymphovascular invasion common

DIFFERENTIAL DIAGNOSIS

Thyroid Medullary Carcinoma

- Thyroid-based mass
- Overlapping light microscopic and immunohistochemical findings with atypical carcinoid
  - Serum calcitonin levels almost invariably elevated in thyroid medullary carcinoma and almost always within normal limits in atypical carcinoid

Malignant Melanoma

- Presence of S100 protein and melanocytic immunomarkers (HMB-45, melan-A, tyrosinase)
- Absent cytokeratin and neuroendocrine marker immunoreactivity

Malignant Lymphoma

- Presence of hematolymphoid immunomarkers
- Absent cytokeratin and neuroendocrine marker immunoreactivity

Gastrointestinal Adenocarcinoma

- Atypical cytology
- Chromogranin and synaptophysin negative

DIAGNOSTIC CHECKLIST

Pathologic Interpretation Pearls

- All NETs show stippled ("salt and pepper") chromatin
- Differentiation among types predicated on degree of nuclear pleomorphism, extent of mitotic activity, and presence of necrosis
- All NETs are submucosal tumors showing variety of growth patterns, including organoid, trabecular, ribbons, cribriform, or solid growth ± fibrovascular stroma

SELECTED REFERENCES

1. Sarvida ME et al: Neuroendocrine tumors in children and young adults: rare or not so rare. Endocrinol Metab Clin North Am. 40(1):65-80, vii, 2011
2. Klimstra DS et al: Pathology reporting of neuroendocrine tumors: application of the Delphic consensus process to the development of a minimum pathology data set. Am J Surg Pathol. 34(3):300-13, 2010
3. Vinik AI et al: Neuroendocrine tumors: a critical appraisal of management strategies. Pancreas. 39(6):801-18, 2010
4. Oberg K: Genetics and molecular pathology of neuroendocrine gastrointestinal and pancreatic tumors (gastroenteropancreatic neuroendocrine tumors). Curr Opin Endocrinol Diabetes Obes. 16(1):72-8, 2009
5. Gustafsson BI et al: Bronchopulmonary neuroendocrine tumors. Cancer. 113(1):5-21, 2008
6. Moraes TJ et al: Pediatric pulmonary carcinoid: a case report and review of the literature. Pediatr Pulmonol. 35(4):318-22, 2003
7. D'Aleo C et al: Carcinoid tumors of the appendix in children: two case reports and review of the literature. Pediatr Hematol Oncol. 18(5):347-51, 2001
8. Parham DM: Neuroectodermal and neuroendocrine tumors principally seen in children. Am J Clin Pathol. 115 Suppl:S113-28, 2001

Microscopic and Immunohistochemical Features

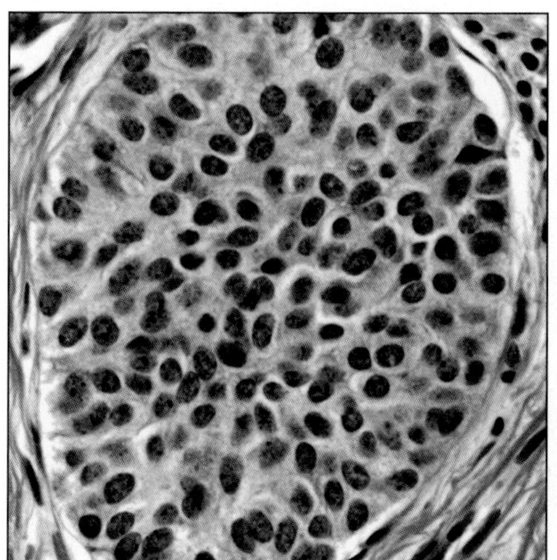

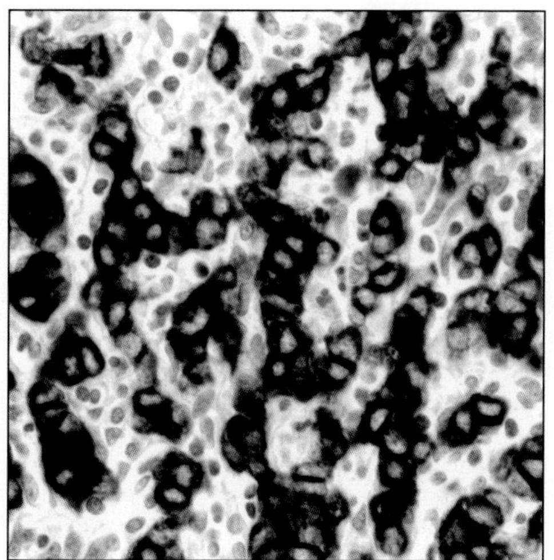

(Left) *At high magnification, cytomorphologic features of carcinoid include uniform round to oval nuclei with characteristic dispersed ("salt and pepper") nuclear chromatin and absence of nuclear pleomorphism, mitotic activity, and necrosis.* ***(Right)*** *Lesional cells are diffusely immunoreactive for cytokeratin (CAM5.2). The extent of cytokeratin reactivity varies from case to case and even within the same case, such that cytokeratin staining may be diffusely present or only focally seen.*

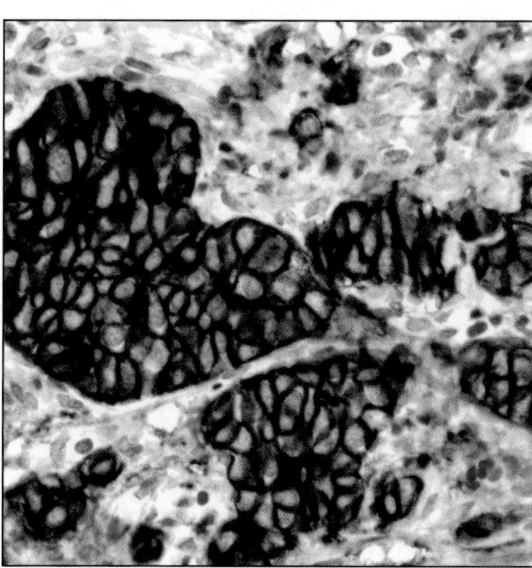

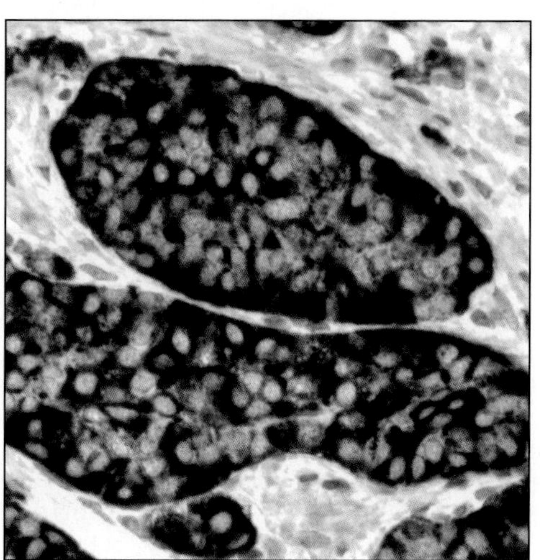

(Left) *In addition to epithelial markers, carcinoid tumors also include diffuse immunoreactivity for chromogranin.* ***(Right)*** *Lesional cells are diffusely immunoreactive for synaptophysin. Light microscopic features, including character of nuclear chromatin pattern, absence of significant pleomorphism, & mitotic activity, coupled with the presence of immunostaining for epithelial markers & neuroendocrine markers, points to a neuroendocrine-type neoplasm.*

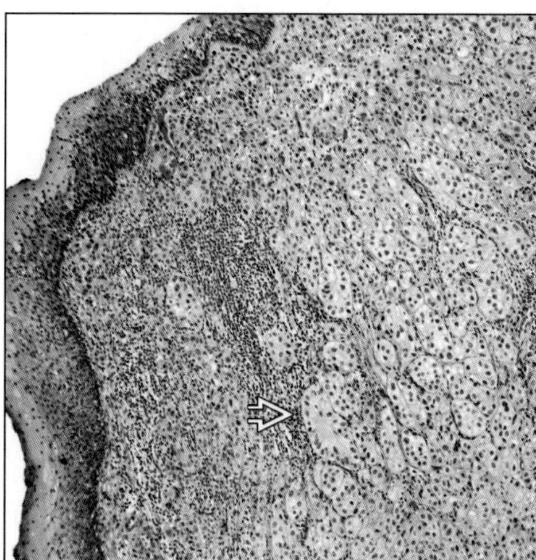

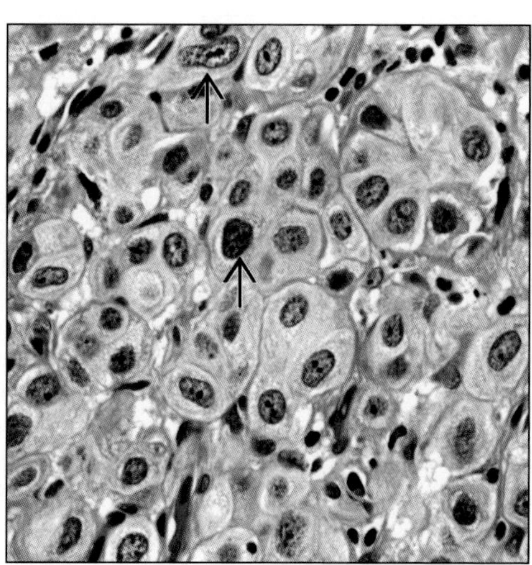

(Left) *Atypical carcinoid ⇨ appears as a submucosal cellular infiltrate with organoid growth and fibrovascular stroma.* ***(Right)*** *At high magnification, the cell nest pattern is present, composed of cells with round to oval nuclei, dispersed ("salt and pepper") nuclear chromatin, inconspicuous to small nucleoli, and eosinophilic cytoplasm. Variable but identifiable nuclear pleomorphism is present →, but there is an absence of mitotic figures and necrosis.*

GASTROINTESTINAL STROMAL TUMOR

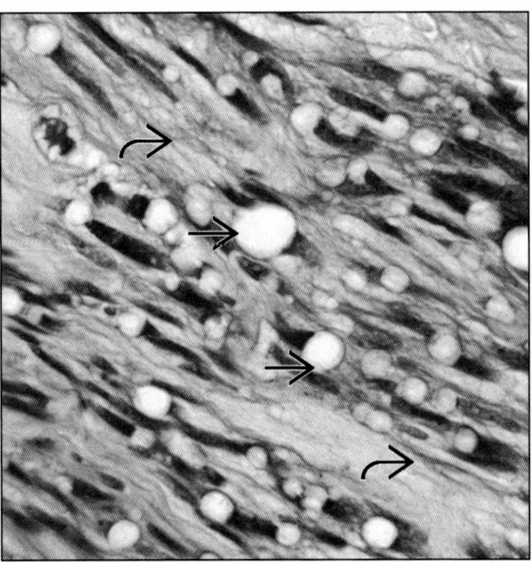

In addition to prominent paranuclear vacuoles ➔, note the brightly eosinophilic fibrillary cytoplasm ➔, both features reminiscent of smooth muscle differentiation.

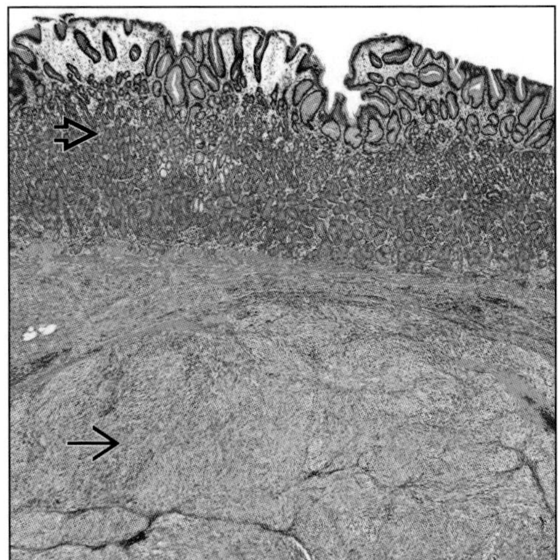

At low magnification, this gastric GIST ➔ involves the muscularis propria of the gastric body. The lesion is lobulated and well marginated. The gastric mucosa ➔ is not involved.

TERMINOLOGY

Abbreviations

- Gastrointestinal stromal tumor (GIST)

Synonyms

- Gastrointestinal smooth muscle tumors (used interchangeably in literature before year 2000)
- Gastrointestinal pacemaker cell tumor

Definitions

- Generally *KIT* or *PDGFRA* mutation: Driven mesenchymal tumors with CD117 and CD34 positivity
  - Wild type *KIT* (no mutation)
    - More common in pediatric population and those with neurofibromatosis type 1 (NF1)
  - Arise from interstitial cells of Cajal
    - Gastrointestinal pacemaker cells

ETIOLOGY/PATHOGENESIS

Molecular Genetics

- Constitutive activating *KIT* mutation
  - 80% of tumors
  - Activating mutations in exons 11, 9, 13, and 17
- *PDGFRA* activation mutations
  - 4-18% of tumors
  - *PDGFRA* gene is adjacent to *KIT* locus
  - Mutations in exons 18, 12, and 14
- Approximately 10% of GIST lack *KIT* or *PDGFRA* mutations

CLINICAL ISSUES

Epidemiology

- Incidence
  - About 4,500 new cases per year in USA
- Age
  - Commonly diagnosed between the ages 6-18 years
  - Cases associated with Carney triad or NF1
    - Seen in children > 10 years old
- Gender
  - No predilection in most series
  - Strong female predilection in Carney triad-associated cases
- Ethnicity
  - Overrepresentation of malignant examples reported in African-Americans

Site

- Stomach most common site in pediatric population
  - > 80% of cases
  - May be multifocal or solitary
  - All Carney triad-associated cases arise in stomach
- Primary extraintestinal (mesentery, omentum, retroperitoneum) is rare
  - Most lesions in mesentery are considered metastases/direct spread from GI tract
  - Lesions of omentum considered as contiguous with stomach

Presentation

- Gastrointestinal bleeding
  - Most common presentation
- GI obstruction
- Abdominal pain
- Incidental
  - During surgery, imaging studies, or endoscopy
- Small percentage of cases is associated with Carney triad or NF1
  - GIST associated with Carney triad
    - Tend to be epithelioid gastric GISTs
    - Lack *KIT* and *PDGFRA* mutations
    - Lack succinate dehydrogenase B expression (in contrast to most GISTs)
  - Carney triad consists of
    - GIST
    - Pulmonary chondroma

Key Facts

Terminology
- Generally *KIT* or *PDGFRA* mutation-driven mesenchymal tumor
- Wild type *KIT* (no mutation) more common in pediatric population
- Arise from intersitial cells of Cajal

Etiology/Pathogenesis
- Constitutive activating *KIT* mutation
- *PDGFRA* activation mutations

Clinical Issues
- Small percentage of cases associated with Carney triad or NF1
- Pediatric population has overall better prognosis
- Stomach is most common site in pediatric population
- May be multifocal or solitary
- Several guidelines exist used to determine risk of aggressive behavior

Microscopic Pathology
- Uniform spindle cells or epithelioid cells
- Fascicles, storiform or nested
- Nuclear pleomorphism is rare
- Eosinophilic cytoplasm
- Perinuclear vacuoles common

Ancillary Tests
- CD117 positive
  - Diffuse cytoplasmic or dot-like positivity
  - Can be negative in treated tumor
- CD34 positivity in 70%
- Vimentin positive

    - Extraadrenal paragangliomas
  - GIST associated with NF1
    - Interaction between *KIT* gene product and *NF1* gene product
    - Tumors have CD117 immunolabeling but no *KIT* gene mutations
    - Tumors often multiple
    - GISTs arise in small intestine

Treatment
- Surgical approaches
  - Complete resection, regardless of site
- Drugs
  - Imatinib mesylate (Gleevec): Inhibits tyrosine kinases (e.g., Kit)
  - Newer drugs
    - Used for acquired resistance to imatinib (attributed to secondary *KIT* or *PDGFRA* mutations) or initial lack of response
    - Sunitinib malate (SU11248): Used for patients with *KIT* exon 9 mutations, others
    - Additional drugs in development

Prognosis
- Determining risk of aggressive behavior
  - Several guidelines exist
  - Grouped by tumor size and mitotic count into
    - Benign
    - Uncertain malignant potential
    - High malignant potential
    - Other terminology includes low, intermediate, and high risk
- Patient age and tumor location
  - Pediatric population has overall better prognosis
    - Even if metastases are present

MACROSCOPIC FEATURES

General Features
- Usually well-marginated lesions with their epicenters in muscularis propria

MICROSCOPIC PATHOLOGY

Histologic Features
- Cellular spindle cell tumor
  - Fascicles, whorled or storiform
  - Monotonous nuclei
    - Nuclear pleomorphism is uncommon
  - Palisading
  - Perinuclear vacuoles
    - May indent nucleus
  - Eosinophilic cytoplasm
  - Some cases have multinucleated cells
- Epithelioid GIST
  - Sheets or nests of cells
  - Large, round, polygonal cells
  - Perinuclear vacuoles
  - Eosinophilic or clear cytoplasm
  - May have a chondromyxoid background
  - Carney triad cases typically epithelioid
- Reports of skeletal muscle differentiation in post-treatment lesions

Cytologic Features
- Uniform spindle cells on aspirates
- Performing immunolabeling on aspiration samples can be diagnostic

ANCILLARY TESTS

Immunohistochemistry
- CD117 positivity
  - Diffuse cytoplasmic positivity
  - May be dot-like or membranous
  - Can be negative in treated tumor
- CD34 positivity in 70%
- Vimentin positive
- Muscle cell markers are variably positive
- Data accumulating on PDGFRA antibodies
- Additional more specific markers
  - Protein kinase C theta (PKC-θ)
  - DOG1 (deleted on GIST 1)

Electron Microscopy

- Dense core neurosecretory granules on ultrastructure

DIFFERENTIAL DIAGNOSIS

Solitary Fibrous Tumor

- Vanishingly rare in GI tract
  - Classically encountered in pleura
- Spindle cell lesion, hemangiopericytoma-like vascular pattern
  - Uniform angulated cells in "patternless" pattern
  - Minimal inflammation
- CD34(+), Bcl-2(+), CD117(-)
- No *KIT* mutations
- Usually benign
  - Some malignant examples

Gastrointestinal Schwannoma

- Usually in muscularis propria of stomach
  - Spindle cells with focal palisading
  - May have infiltrative pattern
  - Minimal vascular changes
  - Negligible mitotic activity
- Prominent lymphoid cuff
- Intralesional lymphoplasmacytic inflammation
- S100(+), CD117(-)
- No *KIT* mutations
  - Differs from somatic soft tissue schwannoma by lacking *NF2* mutations
- Benign

Mesenteric Fibromatosis

- Epicenter in mesentery with extension into muscularis propria
- Infiltrative growth pattern
  - Poorly marginated
- Pale cells, abundant collagen, prominent small vessels
  - Mesenteric examples have ectatic thin-walled vessels
  - Mesenteric examples can have storiform pattern
  - Lesional cells have eosinophilic cytoplasm, delicate nuclear membranes, small uniform nucleoli
- Usually CD34(-), some cases have cytoplasmic CD117, nuclear β-catenin (GISTs lack nuclear β-catenin)
- β-catenin and *APC* gene mutations
- No *KIT* mutations
- Benign but prone to local recurrences

Melanoma

- Metastases tend to spread to small bowel
  - Can be detected in lacteals on mucosal biopsy specimens
  - Occasional anal and esophageal primaries
- Typically more pleomorphic than GIST
  - May be pigmented
  - Intranuclear cytoplasmic invaginations (pseudoinclusion)
- CD117 often positive, but also S100 protein, other melanocytic markers
  - Spindle cell melanomas often lack "specific" melanocytic immunohistochemical markers
- About 20% of mucosal melanomas have *KIT* mutations and respond to treatment
- Aggressive lesions

SELECTED REFERENCES

1. Benesch M et al: Gastrointestinal stromal tumours in children and young adults: a clinicopathologic series with long-term follow-up from the database of the Cooperative Weichteilsarkom Studiengruppe (CWS). Eur J Cancer. 47(11):1692-8, 2011
2. Verschuur A et al: [Gastrointestinal stromal tumours in pediatrics: a summary of the literature on this orphan disease.] Bull Cancer. 98(1):79-86, 2011
3. Benesch M et al: Gastrointestinal stromal tumors (GIST) in children and adolescents: A comprehensive review of the current literature. Pediatr Blood Cancer. 53(7):1171-9, 2009
4. Menon-Andersen D et al: Population pharmacokinetics of imatinib mesylate and its metabolite in children and young adults. Cancer Chemother Pharmacol. 63(2):229-38, 2009
5. Pappo AS et al: Pediatric gastrointestinal stromal tumors. Hematol Oncol Clin North Am. 23(1):15-34, vii, 2009
6. Antonescu CR: Targeted therapies in gastrointestinal stromal tumors. Semin Diagn Pathol. 25(4):295-303, 2008
7. Espinosa I et al: A novel monoclonal antibody against DOG1 is a sensitive and specific marker for gastrointestinal stromal tumors. Am J Surg Pathol. 32(2):210-8, 2008
8. Guler ML et al: Expression of melanoma antigens in epithelioid gastrointestinal stromal tumors: a potential diagnostic pitfall. Arch Pathol Lab Med. 132(8):1302-6, 2008
9. Lasota J et al: Clinical significance of oncogenic KIT and PDGFRA mutations in gastrointestinal stromal tumours. Histopathology. 53(3):245-66, 2008
10. Sauseng W et al: Clinical, radiological, and pathological findings in four children with gastrointestinal stromal tumors of the stomach. Pediatr Hematol Oncol. 24(3):209-19, 2007
11. Miettinen M et al: Gastrointestinal stromal tumors in patients with neurofibromatosis 1: a clinicopathologic and molecular genetic study of 45 cases. Am J Surg Pathol. 30(1):90-6, 2006
12. Miettinen M et al: Gastrointestinal stromal tumors: review on morphology, molecular pathology, prognosis, and differential diagnosis. Arch Pathol Lab Med. 130(10):1466-78, 2006
13. Miettinen M et al: Gastrointestinal stromal tumors of the stomach in children and young adults: a clinicopathologic, immunohistochemical, and molecular genetic study of 44 cases with long-term follow-up and review of the literature. Am J Surg Pathol. 29(10):1373-81, 2005
14. Fletcher CD et al: Diagnosis of gastrointestinal stromal tumors: A consensus approach. Hum Pathol. 33(5):459-65, 2002
15. Kindblom LG et al: Gastrointestinal pacemaker cell tumor (GIPACT): gastrointestinal stromal tumors show phenotypic characteristics of the interstitial cells of Cajal. Am J Pathol. 152(5):1259-69, 1998

Microscopic and Immunohistochemical Features

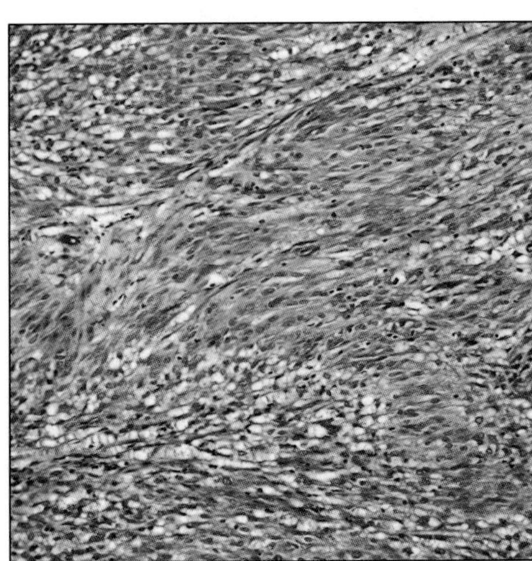

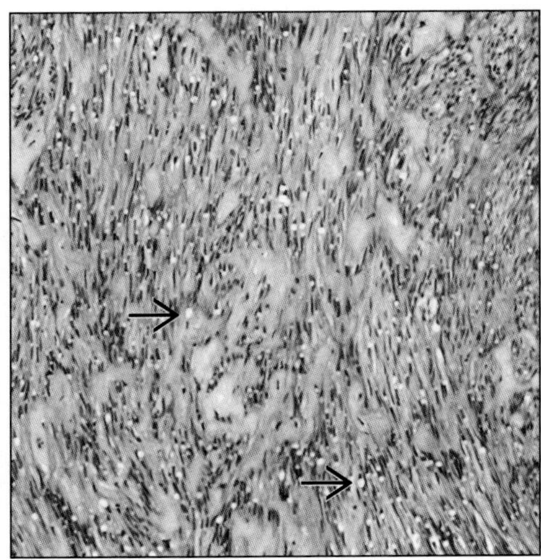

(Left) *This spindle cell gastric GIST has high cellularity and would be expected to have a high mitotic rate. Such appearances are often associated with an unfavorable outcome.* ***(Right)*** *In this image of a spindle cell gastric GIST, paranuclear vacuoles ➙, usually associated with benign behavior, are numerous.*

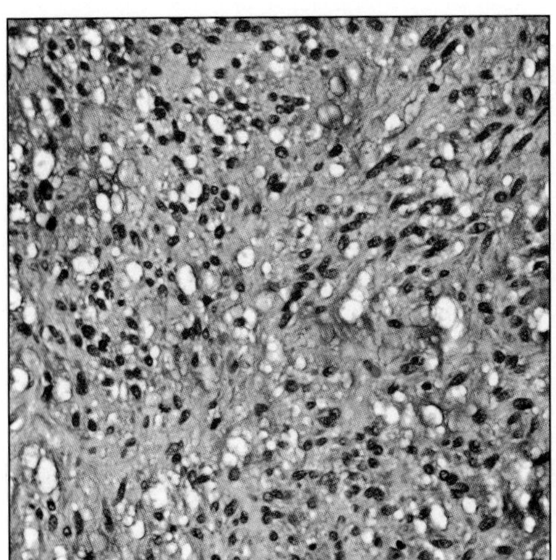

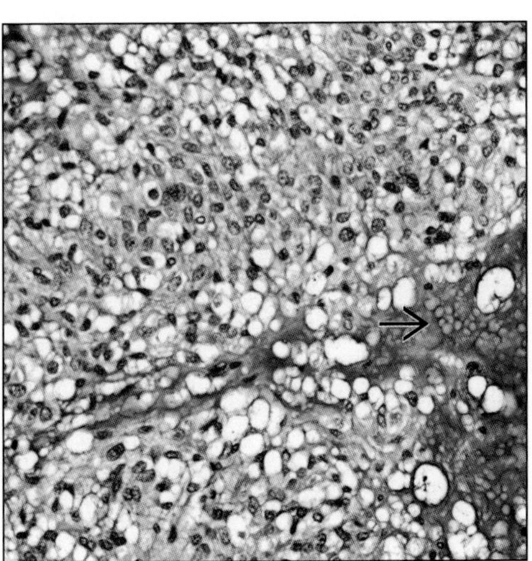

(Left) *This epithelioid gastric GIST tumor has uniform tumor cells with prominent vacuoles. The cellularity of this lesion is relatively low, such that there is minimal nuclear overlap. Patients whose tumors have such features typically have a favorable outcome.* ***(Right)*** *Note the cytologic features of this epithelioid gastric GIST. The nuclei are uniform without prominent nucleoli, and there is a chondromyxoid background ➙.*

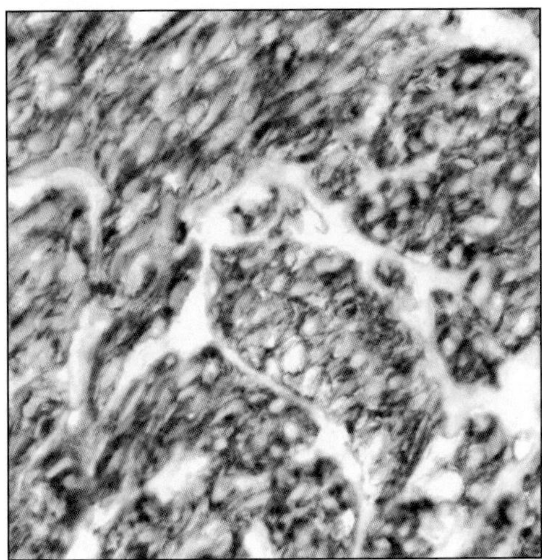

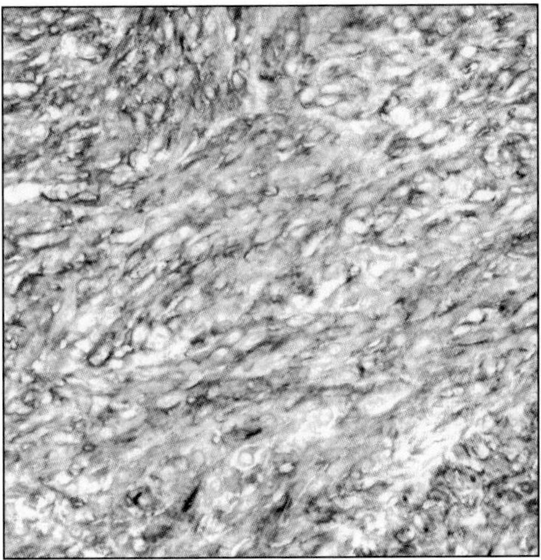

(Left) *CD117 shows membranous and cytoplasmic labeling in a gastric spindle cell GIST. CD117 is extremely useful in confirming an impression of GIST but is not specific for GIST; for example, melanomas commonly express CD117 in a membranous pattern.* ***(Right)*** *CD34 shows cytoplasmic labeling in a gastric spindle cell GIST. About 80% of gastric GISTs express CD34, more than those in the small bowel (about 60%).*

PROTOCOL FOR APPENDIX NET SPECIMENS

Appendix: Excision (Appendectomy) or Resection

Surgical Pathology Cancer Case Summary (Checklist)

Specimen (select all that apply)

___ Appendix
___ Cecum
___ Right colon
___ Terminal ileum
___ Other (specify): ___________________________
___ Not specified

Procedure

___ Appendectomy
*Length: _________ cm
* Appendectomy and right colectomy
*Length of appendix: _________ cm
*Length of colonic segment: ________ cm
___ Other (specify): ___________________________

Specimen Integrity

___ Intact
___ Fragmented
*Number of pieces in fragmented specimens: ___
___ Other (specify): ___________________________

****Specimen Size (if applicable)***

*Specify: _________ (length) x _________ cm

Tumor Site

___ Proximal half of appendix
___ Distal half of appendix
___ Diffusely involving appendix
___ Appendix, not otherwise specified
___ Unknown
___ Other (specify): ___________________________

Tumor Size

Greatest dimension: _________ cm
*Additional dimensions: _________ x _________ cm
___ Cannot be determined

Histologic Type

___ Carcinoid
___ Atypical carcinoid
___ Other (specify): ___________________________

****Alternate Histologic Classification***

*___ Well-differentiated endocrine tumor, benign behavior
*___ Well-differentiated endocrine tumor, uncertain behavior
*___ Well-differentiated endocrine carcinoma

****Histologic Grade*****

*___ Not applicable
*___ GX: Cannot be assessed
*___ G1: Low grade
*___ G2: Intermediate grade
*___ Other (specify): ___________________________

Mitotic Rate

Specify: ___/10 high-power fields (HPF)

PROTOCOL FOR APPENDIX NET SPECIMENS

___ Cannot be determined

Microscopic Tumor Extension

___ Cannot be assessed
___ No evidence of primary tumor
___ Tumor invades lamina propria
___ Tumor invades submucosa
___ Tumor invades muscularis propria
___ Tumor invades subserosal tissue without involvement of visceral peritoneum
___ Tumor extends into mesoappendix
___ Tumor penetrates serosa (visceral peritoneum)
___ Tumor directly invades adjacent structures (specify: ___________________)
___ Tumor penetrates to the surface of the visceral peritoneum (serosa) and directly invades adjacent structures (specify: ___________________)

Margins

Proximal margin

___ Cannot be assessed
___ Uninvolved by tumor
___ Involved by tumor

Distal margin (not applicable for appendectomy specimens)

___ Not applicable
___ Cannot be assessed
___ Uninvolved by tumor
___ Involved by tumor

Mesenteric (mesoappendiceal) margin

___ Cannot be assessed
___ Uninvolved by tumor
Distance of tumor from closest mesenteric margin: ________ mm or ________ cm
___ Involved by tumor

***Circumferential (radial) margin**

*___ Not applicable
*___ Cannot be assessed
*___ Uninvolved by tumor
*___ Involved by tumor (tumor present 0-1 mm from margin)

If all margins uninvolved by neuroendocrine tumor:
Distance of tumor from closest margin: ________ mm
Specify margin: ___________________

Lymph-Vascular Invasion

___ Not identified
___ Present
___ Indeterminate

*Perineural Invasion

*___ Not identified
*___ Present
*___ Indeterminate

Pathologic Staging (pTNM)

TNM descriptors (required only if applicable) (select all that apply)

___ m (multiple primary tumors)
___ r (recurrent)
___ y (post treatment)

Primary tumor (pT)

___ pTX: Primary tumor cannot be assessed
___ pT0: No evidence of primary tumor
___ pT1: Tumor ≤ 2 cm in greatest dimension
___ pT1a: Tumor ≤ 1 cm in greatest dimension

PROTOCOL FOR APPENDIX NET SPECIMENS

___ pT1b: Tumor > 1 cm but ≤ 2 cm

___ pT2: Tumor > 2 cm but ≤ 4 cm or with extension to the cecum

___ pT3: Tumor > 4 cm or with extension to the ileum

___ pT4: Tumor directly invades other adjacent organs or structures, e.g., abdominal wall and skeletal muscle

Regional lymph nodes

___ Cannot be assessed

___ pN0: No regional lymph node metastasis

___ pN1: Metastasis in regional lymph nodes

___ No nodes submitted or found

Number of lymph nodes examined

Specify: _________

___ Number cannot be determined (explain): ___________________________

Number of lymph nodes involved

Specify: _________

___ Number cannot be determined (explain): ___________________________

Distant metastasis

___ Not applicable

___ pM1: Distant metastasis

*Specify site(s), if known: ___________________________

*Ancillary Studies (select all that apply)

*___ Ki-67 index

*___ ≤ 2%

*___ > 2-20%

*___ > 20%

*___ Other (specify): ___________________________

*___ Not performed

*Additional Pathologic Findings (select all that apply)

*___ Tumor necrosis

*___ Acute appendicitis

*___ Other (specify): ___________________________

*Data elements with asterisks are not required. These elements may be clinically important but are not yet validated or regularly used in patient management. **For poorly differentiated neuroendocrine carcinomas, the College of American Pathologists (CAP) checklist for carcinoma of the appendix should be used. Adapted with permission from College of American Pathologists, "Protocol for the Examination of Specimens from Patients with Neuroendocrine Tumors (Carcinoid Tumors) of the Appendix." Web posting date February 2011, www.cap.org.

Gastrointestinal Stromal Tumor (GIST): Biopsy

Surgical Pathology Cancer Case Summary (Checklist)

Procedure

___ Core needle biopsy
___ Endoscopic biopsy
___ Other (specify): ____________________________
___ Not specified

****Specimen Size***

*Greatest dimension: _________ cm
*Additional dimensions: _________ x _________ cm
*___ Cannot be determined

Tumor Site

Specify: ____________________________
___ Not specified

****Tumor Size***

*Greatest dimension: _________ cm
*Additional dimensions: _________ x _________ cm
*___ Cannot be determined

GIST Subtype

___ Spindle cell
___ Epithelioid
___ Mixed
___ Other (specify): ____________________________

Mitotic Rate

Specify: _________ /50 high-power fields (HPF)

****Necrosis***

*___ Not identified
*___ Present
  *Extent: _________ %
*___ Cannot be determined

Histologic Grade

___ GX: Grade cannot be assessed
___ G1: Low grade; mitotic rate ≤ 5/50 HPF
___ G2: High grade; mitotic rate > 5/50 HPF

Risk Assessment

___ None
___ Very low risk
___ Low risk
___ Intermediate risk
___ High risk
___ Overtly metastatic
___ Cannot be determined

Distant Metastasis

___ Cannot be assessed
___ Distant metastasis
  Specify site(s), if known: ____________________________

Additional Pathologic Findings

Specify: ____________________________

Ancillary Studies (select all that apply)

Immunohistochemical studies

___ KIT (CD117)

___ Positive

___ Negative

___ Others (specify): ____________________

___ Not performed

Molecular genetic studies (e.g., KIT or PDGFRA mutational analysis)

___ Submitted for analysis; results pending

___ Performed, see separate report: ____________________

___ Performed

Specify method(s) and results: ____________________

___ Not performed

Pre-biopsy Treatment (select all that apply)

___ No therapy

___ Systemic therapy performed

Specify type: ____________________

___ Therapy performed, type not specified

___ Unknown

**Treatment Effect*

*Specify percentage of viable tumor: ________ %

**Data elements with asterisks are not required. These elements may be clinically important but are not yet validated or regularly used in patient management. Adapted with permission from College of American Pathologists, "Protocol for the Examination of Specimens from Patients with Gastrointestinal Stromal Tumor." Web posting date February 2011, www.cap.org.*

Gastrointestinal Stromal Tumor (GIST): Resection

Surgical Pathology Cancer Case Summary (Checklist)

Procedure

___ Excisional biopsy

___ Resection

Specify type (e.g., partial gastrectomy): ____________________

___ Metastasectomy

___ Other (specify): ____________________

___ Not specified

Tumor Site

Specify (if known): ____________________

___ Not specified

Tumor Size

Greatest dimension: ________ cm

*Additional dimensions: ________ x ________ cm

___ Cannot be determined

Tumor Focality

___ Unifocal

___ Multifocal

Specify number of tumors: ________

Specify size of tumors: ____________________

GIST Subtype

___ Spindle cell

___ Epithelioid

___ Mixed

___ Other (specify): ____________________

Mitotic Rate

Specify: ________ /50 HPF

**Necrosis*

*___ Not identified

*____ Present

*Extent: _________ %

*____ Cannot be determined

Histologic Grade

____ GX: Grade cannot be assessed

____ G1: Low grade; mitotic rate ≤ 5/50 HPF

____ G2: High grade; mitotic rate > 5/50 HPF

Risk Assessment

____ None

____ Very low risk

____ Intermediate risk

____ High risk

____ Overtly malignant/metastatic

____ Cannot be determined

Margins

____ Cannot be assessed

____ Negative for GIST

Distance of tumor from closest margin: _________ cm

____ Margin(s) positive for GIST

Specify margin(s): __________________________

Pathologic Staging (pTNM)

TNM descriptors (required only if applicable) (select all that apply)

____ m (multiple)

____ r (recurrent)

____ y (post treatment)

Primary tumor (pT)

____ pTX: Primary tumor cannot be assessed

____ pT0: No evidence for primary tumor

____ pT1: Tumor ≤ 2 cm

____ pT2: Tumor > 2 cm but ≤ 5 cm

____ pT3: Tumor > 5 cm but ≤ 10 cm

____ pT4: Tumor > 10 cm in greatest dimension

Regional lymph nodes (pN)

____ Not applicable

____ pM1: Distant metastasis

*Specify site(s) if known: __________________________

*Additional Pathologic Findings

*Specify: __________________________

Ancillary Studies (select all that apply)

Immunohistochemical studies

____ KIT (CD117)

____ Positive

____ Negative

____ Others (specify): __________________________

____ Not performed

Molecular genetic studies (e.g., KIT or PDGFRA mutational analysis)

____ Submitted for analysis; results pending

____ Performed, see separate report: __________________________

____ Performed

Specify method(s) and results: __________________________

____ Not performed

PROTOCOL FOR GASTROINTESTINAL STROMAL TUMORS

Pre-resection Treatment (select all that apply)

___ No therapy

___ Previous biopsy or surgery

Specify: ___________________________

___ Systemic therapy performed

Specify type: ___________________________

___ Therapy performed, type not specified

___ Unknown

****Treatment Effect***

*Specify percentage of viable tumor: ________ %

**Data elements with asterisks are not required. These elements may be clinically important but are not yet validated or regularly used in patient management. Adapted with permission from College of American Pathologists, "Protocol for the Examination of Specimens from Patients with Gastrointestinal Stromal Tumor." Web posting date February 2011, www.cap.org.*

Liver/Pancreas

Neoplasm, Benign

Neoplasm, Borderline

Neoplasm, Malignant Primary

Protocol for the Examination of Specimens from Patients with Carcinoma of the Exocrine Pancreas

Protocol for the Examination of Specimens from Patients with Hepatoblastoma

Protocol for the Examination of Specimens from Patients with Hepatocellular Carcinoma

CAVERNOUS HEMANGIOMA

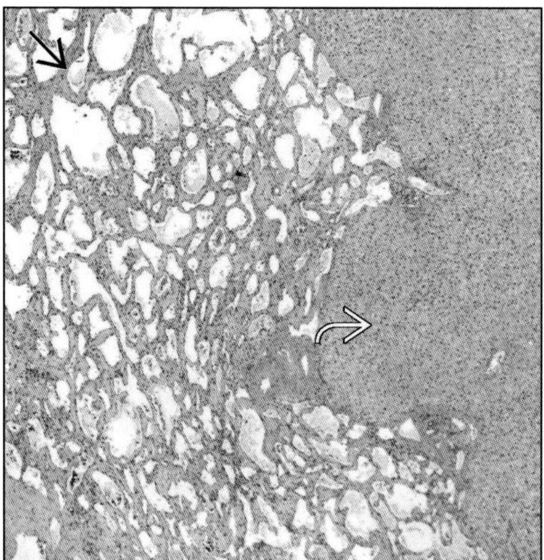

Hematoxylin & eosin shows an interface between normal liver parenchyma ➔ and cavernous hemangioma, a well-circumscribed lesion composed of variably sized vascular spaces ➔.

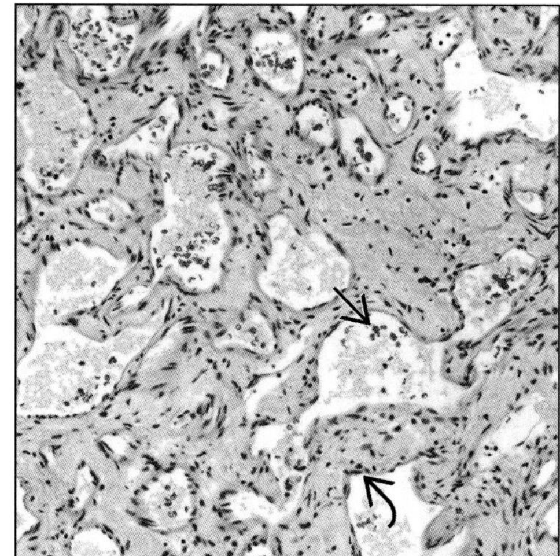

High-power view of a cavernous hemangioma demonstrates blood-filled spaces ➔ lined by single layers of flat endothelial cells resting in a fibromyxoid stroma ➔.

TERMINOLOGY

Abbreviations

- Cavernous hemangioma (CH)

Synonyms

- Cavernoma, sclerosing hemangioma

Definitions

- Benign vascular tumor

CLINICAL ISSUES

Epidemiology

- Incidence
  - Most common benign tumor of liver in 1st year of life
  - Rarely seen in children older than 3 years
- Gender
  - Female predominance (F:M = 5:1)

Site

- Most commonly seen in right lobe of liver

Presentation

- Incidental finding
- Abdominal distension
- Hepatomegaly
- Kasabach-Merritt syndrome
  - Consumptive coagulopathy
  - ± cutaneous hemangiomas

Laboratory Tests

- CBC
  - Anemia and thrombocytopenia in patients with Kasabach-Merritt syndrome

Natural History

- Grows rapidly in 1st year of life
- Becomes stable around age 1
- Recedes spontaneously with time
  - Variable time of involution
    - Approximately 75% of lesions tend to heal completely between 5-7 years of age

Treatment

- Conservative approach is treatment of choice in most cases
  - Steroids may be used to reduce immature hemangioma tissue
  - α-2a interferon has been demonstrated to be efficient in reducing large hemangiomas
  - α-2a interferon is considered treatment of choice for cases of Kasabach-Merritt syndrome
- Surgical intervention may be eventually needed
  - When conservative approach is incapable of controlling disease
  - In cases of cardiac failure secondary to arteriovenous shunt
  - In cases of uncertain diagnosis
  - Lobe resection is indicated in cases of focal tumor
  - Ligature of hepatic artery is indicated in cases of bipolar tumors

Prognosis

- Benign lesion with no potential for malignant transformation
- Larger lesions may lead to hemodynamic disorder
  - Death may occur due to high output cardiac failure secondary to arteriovenous shunting
- Increased morbidity and mortality in patients presenting with Kasabach-Merritt syndrome

IMAGE FINDINGS

General

- Tc-99m SPECT is most specific and sensitive method
  - Red cell accumulation on delayed images

Key Facts

Terminology
- Cavernous hemangioma (CH)

Clinical Issues
- Most common benign tumor of liver in 1st year of life
- Female predominance (F:M = 5:1)
- Most commonly seen in right lobe of liver
- Grows fast in 1st year of life
- Recedes spontaneously with time
- Conservative approach is treatment of choice in most cases
- Larger lesions may lead to hemodynamic disorder

Macroscopic Features
- Well-circumscribed, variably sized tumor

Microscopic Pathology
- Variably sized vascular spaces lined by single layer of bland-looking endothelial cells

Immunohistochemistry

Antibody	Reactivity	Staining Pattern	Comment
CD34	Positive	Cell membrane & cytoplasm	Highlights endothelial cells; rarely necessary for diagnosis of CH
CD31	Positive	Cell membrane	Highlights endothelial cells; rarely necessary for diagnosis of CH

MACROSCOPIC FEATURES

General Features
- Well-circumscribed, variably sized tumor
- Hemorrhagic areas ± central fibrosis
- Usually solitary
  - Occasionally seen as multiple lesions (diffuse hemangiomatosis)

MICROSCOPIC PATHOLOGY

Histologic Features
- Variably sized vascular spaces lined by a single layer of bland-looking endothelial cells
- Fibromyxoid stroma
  - ± extensive fibrosis (sclerosing hemangioma)
- Well demarcated from surrounding liver

DIFFERENTIAL DIAGNOSIS

Arteriovenous Malformation
- Direct communication between arteries and veins
  - No intervening capillary bed
- No angiogenesis is observed
- Unlike vascular malformation, hemangioma is composed of a proliferation of endothelial cells

Lymphangioma
- Composed of dilated lymphatic spaces

Peliosis Hepatis
- Dilated blood-filled spaces without endothelial lining

Infantile Hemangioendothelioma
- Bile ductules and hepatocytes are often seen within tumor

SELECTED REFERENCES

1. Isaacs H Jr: Fetal and neonatal hepatic tumors. J Pediatr Surg. 42(11):1797-803, 2007
2. Prokurat A et al: Hemangioma of the liver in children: proliferating vascular tumor or congenital vascular malformation? Med Pediatr Oncol. 39(5):524-9, 2002

IMAGE GALLERY

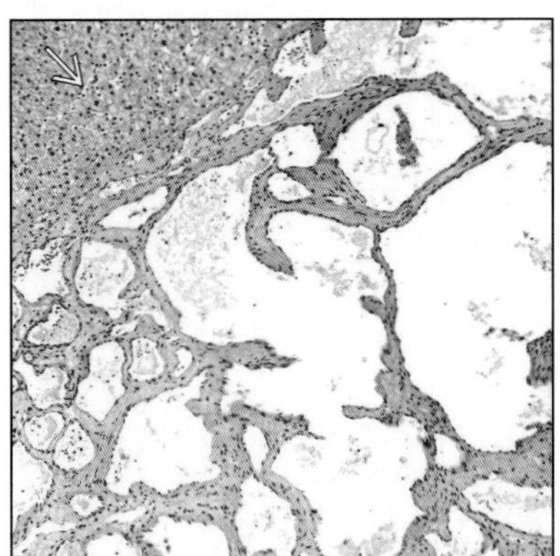

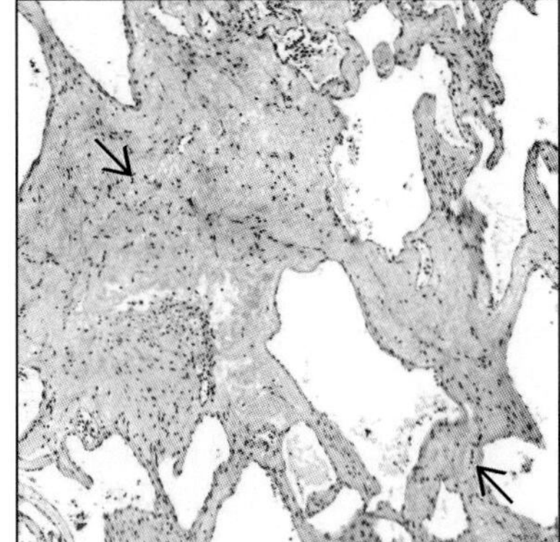

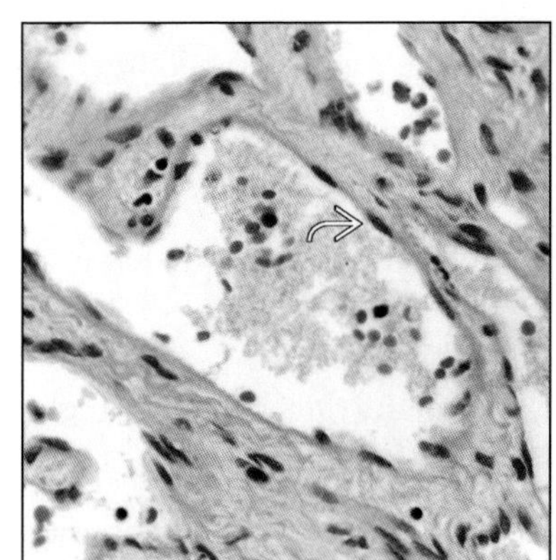

(Left) *Hematoxylin & eosin shows large vascular spaces surrounded by normal hepatic parenchyma ➡.* ***(Center)*** *Hematoxylin & eosin shows vascular spaces separated by fibrous-myxoid stroma ➡. The thickness of the stroma may vary even within the same lesion. Some cavernous hemangiomas (sclerosing hemangioma) may demonstrate extensively fibrotic stroma (not shown).* ***(Right)*** *High-power view demonstrates a single layer of flattened, bland-appearing endothelial cells ➡.*

MESENCHYMAL HAMARTOMA

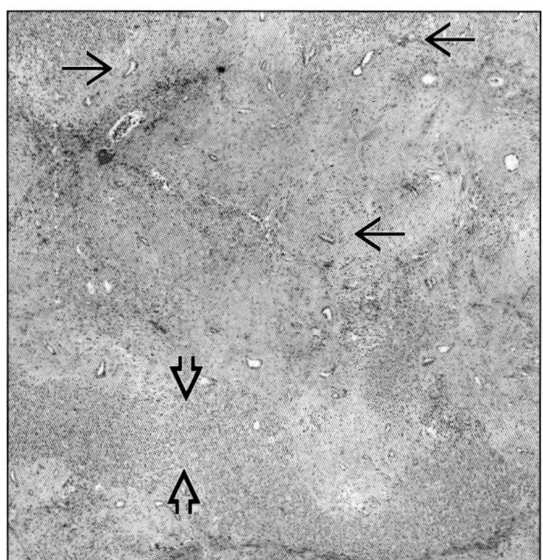

Hematoxylin & eosin shows a low-power view of nodular lesions composed of branching bile ducts immersed in myxomatous, loose connective tissue ⇒, separated by unremarkable hepatocytes ⇨.

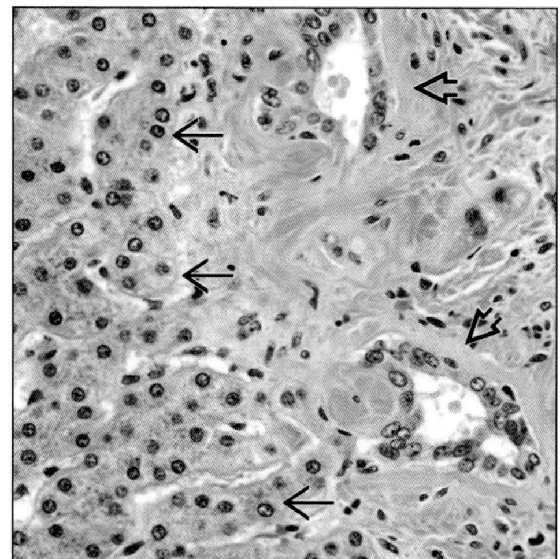

Hematoxylin & eosin shows a high-power view of irregularly shaped, branching bile ducts ⇨. Hamartomatous nodules are surrounded by normal-appearing hepatocytes ⇒.

TERMINOLOGY

Definitions

- Rare benign lesion of liver with predilection for infants

ETIOLOGY/PATHOGENESIS

Etiology

- Uncertain
- Regarded as congenital malformation of ductal plates
- Thought to arise from connective tissue of portal tracts
- Cysts may form from ischemic degeneration of tumor mesenchymal tissue

Genetics

- Recurrent translocations involving chromosome 19q
- Isolated cases associated with tuberous sclerosis

CLINICAL ISSUES

Epidemiology

- Incidence
  - 3rd most common liver tumor in infants/young children
- Age
  - Most commonly occurs in first 2 years of life
- Gender
  - Slight male predominance

Site

- Right lobe of liver is affected in most cases
- Majority of lesions are peripherally located

Presentation

- Asymptomatic (incidental finding)
- Abdominal distention
- Hepatomegaly
- Anorexia (due to tumor compression of stomach)
- Respiratory distress (mass effect)
- Obstructive jaundice (centrally located lesions)

Natural History

- Tumor enlargement thought to occur secondary to accumulation of fluid within cysts
- Potential for malignant transformation into embryonal sarcoma (rare)
- Spontaneous regression can occur

Treatment

- Options, risks, complications
  - Complete surgical excision is warranted
- Surgical approaches
  - Excision of tumor including additional rim of unremarkable hepatic parenchyma

Prognosis

- Lesion is cured by complete surgical excision
- Large, hypervascular lesions may rupture leading to fatal hemorrhage

IMAGE FINDINGS

Ultrasonographic Findings

- Solitary or multiple, well-defined, and variably sized anechoic cysts
- Intervening solid echogenic areas
- Calcifications are usually absent

MR Findings

- Multiseptated mass with fluid-filled cysts
- Cysts show high signal on T1- and low signal on T2-weighted sequences
- ± displacement of major intraabdominal vessels

CT Findings

- Well-circumscribed, partially cystic mass
- Heterogeneous appearance
- Calcifications are usually absent

Key Facts

Clinical Issues

- 3rd most common liver tumor in infants and young children
- Most commonly occurs in 1st 2 years of life
- Right lobe is affected in most cases
- Lesion is cured by complete surgical excision

Macroscopic Features

- Well-circumscribed/encapsulated solid-cystic mass
- Usually solitary and large

Microscopic Pathology

- Nodular pattern of growth
- Myxomatous, loose stroma
- Proliferation of irregular-shaped branching bile ducts separated by unremarkable hepatocytes
- Variable-sized cysts lined by low cuboidal epithelium
- ± extramedullary hematopoiesis

Diagnostic Checklist

- α-fetoprotein may be elevated

MACROSCOPIC FEATURES

General Features

- Well-circumscribed, encapsulated, partially cystic
- Usually solitary, large and tan colored

MICROSCOPIC PATHOLOGY

Histologic Features

- Nodular pattern of growth
- Myxomatous, loose stroma
- Proliferation of irregular-shaped branching bile ducts separated by unremarkable hepatocytes
- Variable-sized cysts lined by low cuboidal epithelium
- Low-power appearance may resemble fibroadenoma of breast
- ± extramedullary hematopoiesis
- Surrounding normal hepatic parenchyma

DIFFERENTIAL DIAGNOSIS

Hepatoblastoma

- Atypical hepatocytes and stroma

Infantile Hemangioendothelioma

- Nodular proliferation of irregular, interconnected vascular channels

Malignant Embryonal Sarcoma

- Atypical stroma and tumor cells; numerous mitotic figures
- Occurs in older children (~ 8 years old)

Parasitic Cysts

- Absent branching bile duct proliferation
- Parasite is usually identified within cyst

DIAGNOSTIC CHECKLIST

Pathologic Interpretation Pearls

- Nodular growth pattern
- Bland-looking, loose stroma usually shows concentric arrangement around bile ducts
- α-fetoprotein may be elevated

SELECTED REFERENCES

1. Rajaram V et al: DNA sequence of the translocation breakpoints in undifferentiated embryonal sarcoma arising in mesenchymal hamartoma of the liver harboring the t(11;19)(q11;q13.4) translocation. Genes Chromosomes Cancer. 46(5):508-13, 2007
2. Ye BB et al: Mesenchymal hamartoma of liver: magnetic resonance imaging and histopathologic correlation. World J Gastroenterol. 11(37):5807-10, 2005
3. Emre S et al: Liver tumors in children. Pediatr Transplant. 8(6):632-8, 2004
4. Yen JB et al: Hepatic mesenchymal hamartoma. J Paediatr Child Health. 39(8):632-4, 2003

IMAGE GALLERY

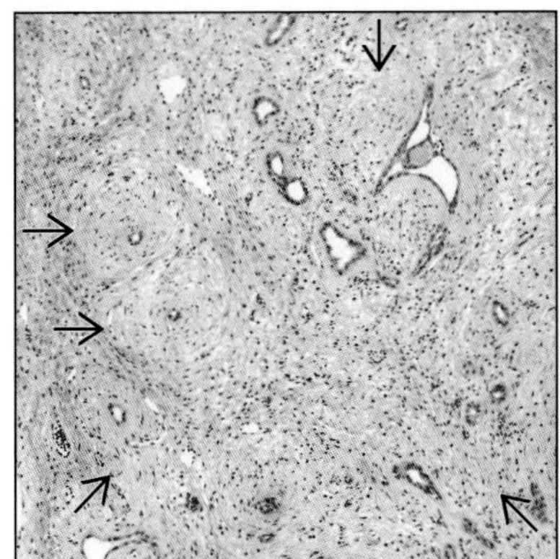

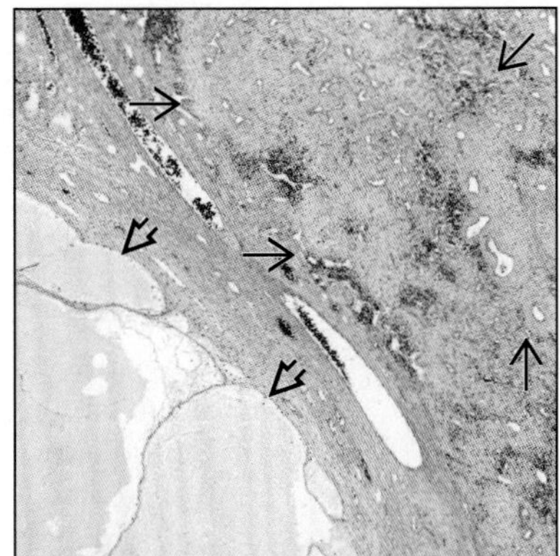

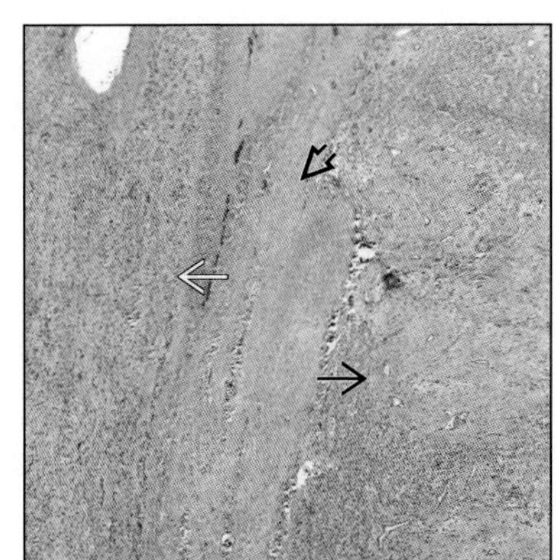

(Left) *Hematoxylin and eosin shows a low-power view of concentric arrangement of the stroma around bile ducts ⇒.* ***(Center)*** *Hematoxylin & eosin shows the interface between variably sized thin-walled cysts ⊳ and hamartomatous nodules ⇒ comprised of a proliferation of branching bile ducts and surrounding mesenchyma.* ***(Right)*** *Hematoxylin & eosin shows a well-circumscribed mesenchymal hamartoma ⇒ separated from normal hepatic parenchyma ➡ by a capsule ⊳.*

FOCAL NODULAR HYPERPLASIA

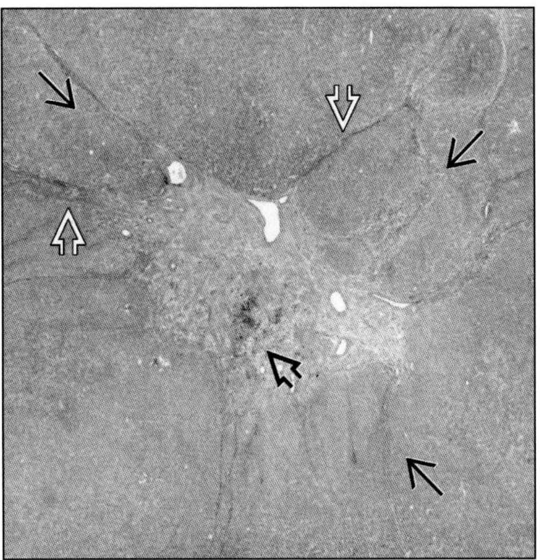

Hematoxylin & eosin shows a low-power view of incomplete hepatocyte nodules ⇨ separated by fibrous septae ➡ radiating from a central scar ⇨.

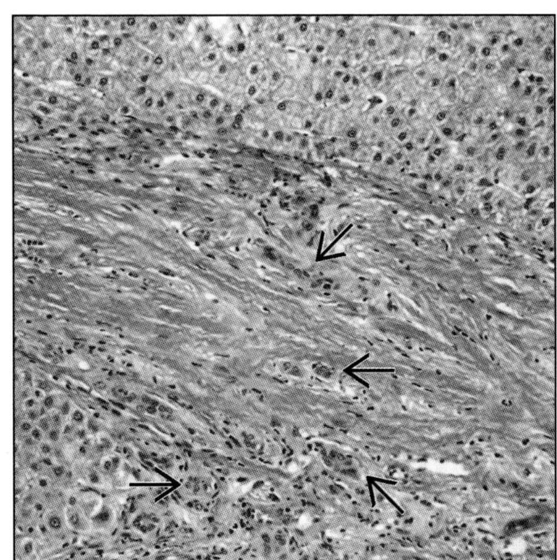

Hematoxylin & eosin shows a high-power view of bile ductular proliferation ⇨ within radiating collagenous septa.

TERMINOLOGY

Abbreviations

- Focal nodular hyperplasia (FNH)

Synonyms

- Hepatic pseudotumor
- Solitary hyperplastic nodule
- Benign hepatoma

ETIOLOGY/PATHOGENESIS

Etiology

- Uncertain
- Controversial monoclonal vs. polyclonal nature
- Regarded as hyperplastic response of hepatocytes to arterial malformation

CLINICAL ISSUES

Epidemiology

- Incidence
  - Rare in children
  - Isolated cases have been associated with glycogen storage disease type 1a
- Age
  - Variable, may range from 2-13 years
- Gender
  - No gender predominance

Presentation

- Asymptomatic; incidental finding
- Abdominal mass

Laboratory Tests

- Serum α-fetoprotein (AFP)
  - Levels usually within normal range

Natural History

- Asymptomatic lesions may remain stable
- ± spontaneous regression

Treatment

- Options
  - Should be assessed individually
  - Asymptomatic cases
    - Conservative approach: Follow-up with repeat ultrasound
  - Symptomatic/complicated cases
    - Surgical resection
    - ± liver transplantation

Prognosis

- Overall, good prognosis

MACROSCOPIC FEATURES

General Features

- Usually solitary and small (< 5 cm)
- Well-defined, tan-brown, nodular mass
- Central scar (characteristic but not always present)
- Normal liver parenchyma outlines lesion

MICROSCOPIC PATHOLOGY

Histologic Features

- Incomplete nodules of uniform hepatocytes separated by central radiating fibrous septa
  - Bile ductule proliferation within fibrous septa ± mixed acute and chronic inflammation
  - ± bile stasis, glycogen, and Mallory bodies within hepatocytes
  - Few/absent interlobular portal tracks
- Central scar is composed of dense collagen and thick-walled arteries

Key Facts

Terminology

- Benign epithelial tumor-like lesion composed of hepatocellular nodules outlined by central radiating fibrous septa

Clinical Issues

- Rare in children
- No gender predominance

Macroscopic Features

- Usually solitary and small nodular mass (< 5 cm)
- Normal liver parenchyma outlines lesion
- Central scar (characteristic but not specific and not always present)

Microscopic Pathology

- Bile ductule proliferation, mixed acute and chronic inflammation within fibrous septae
- Few/absent interlobular bile ducts and portal vein

DIFFERENTIAL DIAGNOSIS

Hepatocellular Adenoma

- Most commonly occurs in childbearing age women
- Associated with oral contraceptive therapy and sex hormone imbalances
- Lack bile ductular proliferation and portal tracts within adenoma
- Lack fibrous septae with thick-walled vessels

Mesenchymal Hamartoma

- (Partially) cystic mass
- Proliferation of irregular-shaped bile ducts haphazardly distributed in stroma, surrounded by normal liver parenchyma
- Lack fibrous septae

Regenerative Nodule

- Multiple hepatocellular nodules
- Distorted portal tracts within nodules
- Unremarkable fibrosis

Nodular Regenerative Hyperplasia

- Multiple nodules of hepatocytes diffusely spread throughout liver
- Rim of hepatocyte atrophy in edges of nodules
- Lack fibrous septae

Well-Differentiated Hepatocellular Carcinoma

- Thickened (> 3 hepatocytes thick) &/or irregular cell plates
- Pseudoglandular, acinar architecture
- Increased nuclear to cytoplasmic ratio

Fibrolamellar-Hepatocellular Carcinoma

- Comprised of large, neoplastic hepatocytes with prominent nucleoli
- Bile staining

SELECTED REFERENCES

1. Assy N et al: Characteristics of common solid liver lesions and recommendations for diagnostic workup. World J Gastroenterol. 15(26):3217-27, 2009
2. Sato Y et al: Hepatic stellate cells are activated around central scars of focal nodular hyperplasia of the liver--a potential mechanism of central scar formation. Hum Pathol. 40(2):181-8, 2009
3. Somech R et al: Focal nodular hyperplasia in children. J Pediatr Gastroenterol Nutr. 32(4):480-3, 2001

IMAGE GALLERY

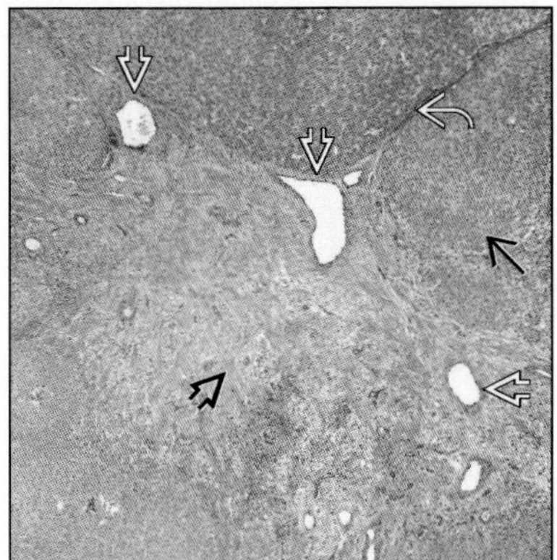

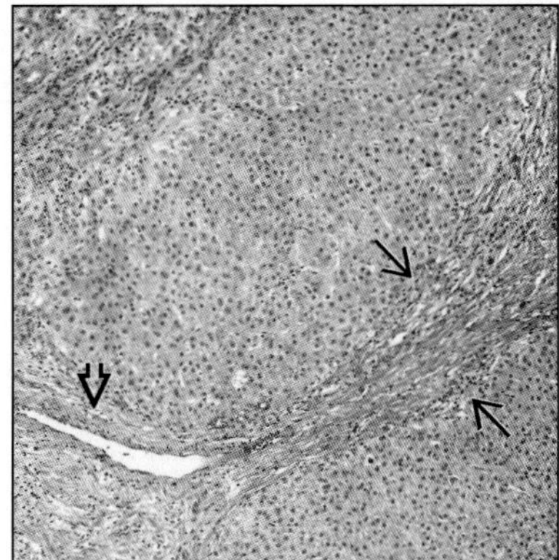

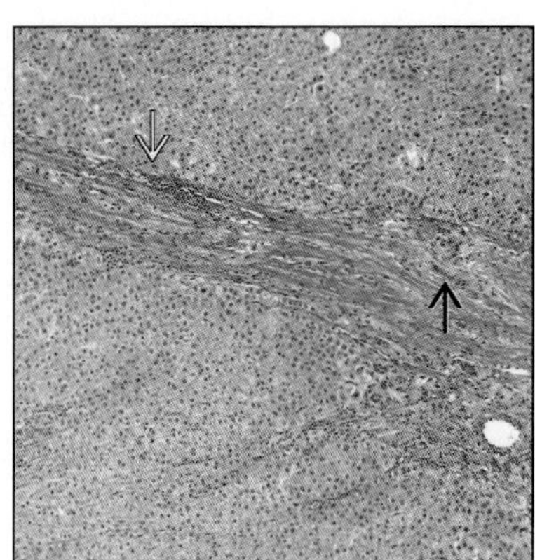

*(**Left**) Hematoxylin & eosin shows a central scar ⇨ composed of dense collagen and thick-walled vessels ➡ from which radiating septae ➡ delineate incomplete hepatocyte lobules →. (**Center**) Hematoxylin & eosin shows a thick-walled vessel ⇨ present at the periphery of the central scar and radiating septa with focal chronic inflammation →. (**Right**) Hematoxylin & eosin shows bile duct proliferation → and chronic inflammation ➡ within septa.*

NODULAR REGENERATIVE HYPERPLASIA

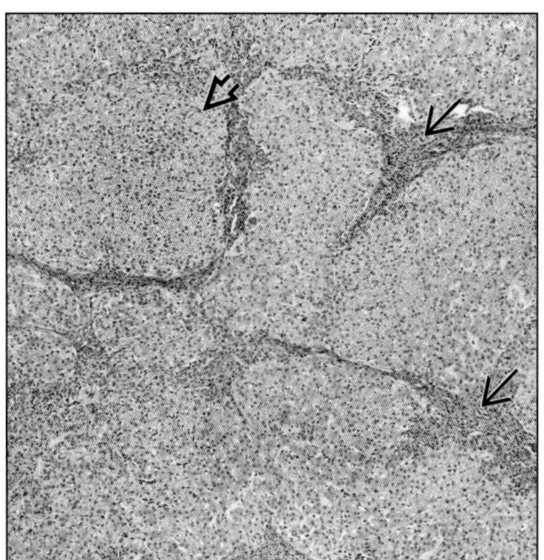

Hematoxylin & eosin shows liver parenchyma with multiple nodules composed of regenerating hepatocytes (pale areas) ⇨ separated by atrophic hepatic parenchyma with an eosinophilic appearance →.

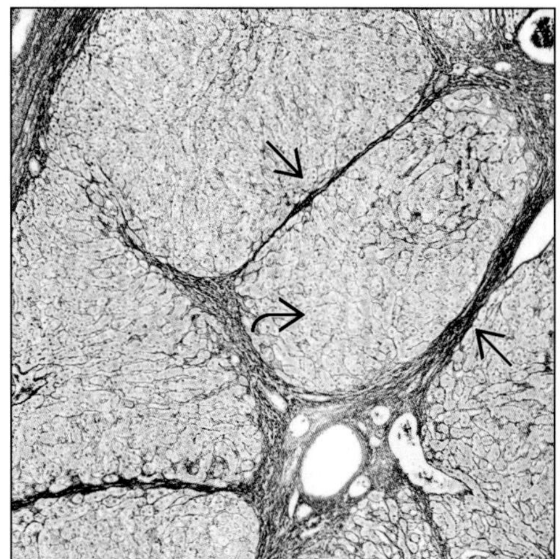

Reticulin stain outlines nodular parenchyma architecture → and highlights increased hepatocyte plate thickness in regenerative hepatocytes ↷.

TERMINOLOGY

Abbreviations

- Nodular regenerative hyperplasia (NRH)

Synonyms

- Nodular transformation
- Partial nodular transformation
- Noncirrhotic nodulation

Definitions

- Benign epithelial neoplasm composed of hyperplastic hepatocytes similar to surrounding liver parenchyma

ETIOLOGY/PATHOGENESIS

Environmental Exposure

- NRH has been associated with anticonvulsant, immunosuppressive, and chemotherapeutic drugs

Etiology

- Uncertain
- Regarded as a primary generalized proliferative disorder of the liver
- Vascular disorders leading to central hepatic ischemia and secondary proliferation of hepatocytes in the portal region have been hypothesized
- Associated with congenital malformations, hematologic abnormalities, neoplasms, metabolic and collagen diseases

CLINICAL ISSUES

Epidemiology

- Incidence
  - Rare in infants and children
- Age
  - Most commonly occurs in teenagers
  - May present between 5-20 years of age
  - Median age of reported pediatric cases: 8 years old
- Gender
  - No sex predilection

Presentation

- Incidental finding
- Hepatomegaly
- ± splenomegaly
- ± features of portal hypertension

Laboratory Tests

- Liver function tests are usually normal

Natural History

- No or low malignant potential

Treatment

- Options
  - Clinical follow-up is warranted to watch for potential future complications

Prognosis

- **Benign, irreversible condition**
- Potential complications related to portal hypertension

IMAGE FINDINGS

General Features

- Nodular appearance may resemble neoplasia
- Liver size may be normal, enlarged, or reduced

MACROSCOPIC FEATURES

General Features

- Multiple, variably sized, coalescent nodules

NODULAR REGENERATIVE HYPERPLASIA

Key Facts

Etiology/Pathogenesis
- Uncertain

Clinical Issues
- Rare in infants and children
- **Benign**

Microscopic Pathology
- Diffuse hepatocyte nodules
- **No remarkable fibrosis between nodules**

Ancillary Tests
- Reticulin highlights increased hepatocyte plate thickness in regenerative areas

Top Differential Diagnoses
- Focal nodular hyperplasia
- Hepatocellular carcinoma (fibrolamellar variant)
- Hepatocellular adenoma
- Cirrhosis
- Congenital hepatic fibrosis

MICROSCOPIC PATHOLOGY

Histologic Features
- Diffuse nodular appearance of hepatic parenchyma, more pronounced in portal areas
  - Nodules comprise hyperplastic regenerating hepatocytes
  - Increased hepatocyte plate thickness in regenerative areas
- **No fibrosis between nodules**
- Nodules are separated by atrophic hepatic parenchyma

ANCILLARY TESTS

Histochemistry
- Reticulin
  - Reactivity: Positive
  - Staining pattern
    - Outlines nodular architecture of parenchyma and highlights increased hepatocyte plate thickness in regenerative areas
- Masson trichrome stain
  - Unremarkable perinodular fibrous expansion

DIFFERENTIAL DIAGNOSIS

Focal Nodular Hyperplasia
- **Central scar**
- Incomplete nodules separated by radiating fibrous septa

Hepatocellular Carcinoma (Fibrolamellar Variant)
- Most commonly occurs in older children or in early adulthood
- Bile staining
- Composed of large, neoplastic hepatocytes with prominent nucleoli

Hepatocellular Adenoma
- Most commonly occurs in women of childbearing age
- Associated with oral contraceptive therapy and sex hormone imbalances

Cirrhosis
- Hepatic nodules separated by fibrous bands
- Bile duct proliferation
- Cholestasis

Congenital Hepatic Fibrosis
- Dense fibrous bands surrounding nodules composed of unremarkable hepatocytes
- Bile ductular proliferation

SELECTED REFERENCES

1. Moran CA et al: Nodular regenerative hyperplasia of the liver in children. Am J Surg Pathol. 15(5):449-54, 1991

IMAGE GALLERY

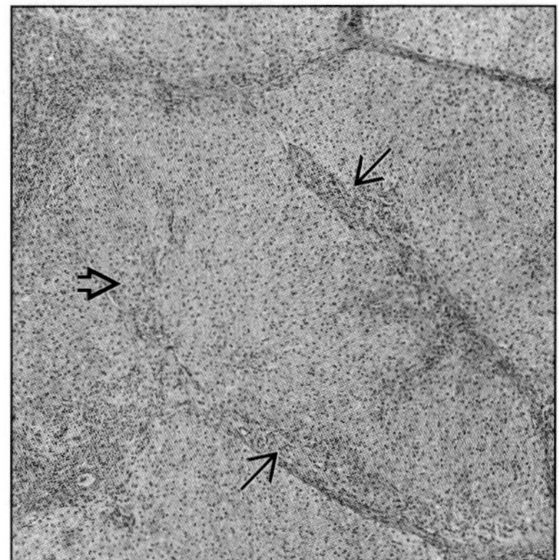

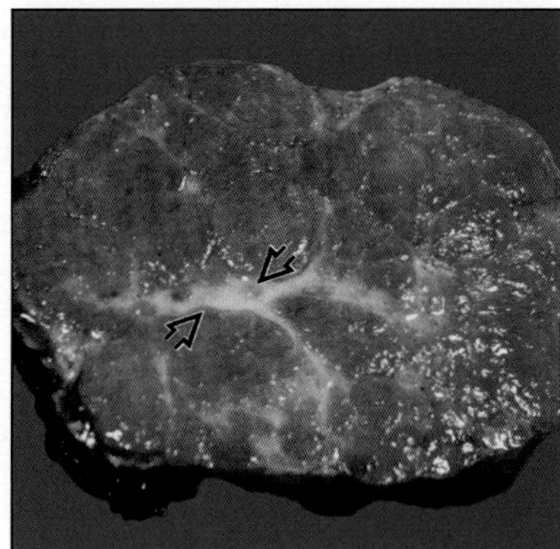

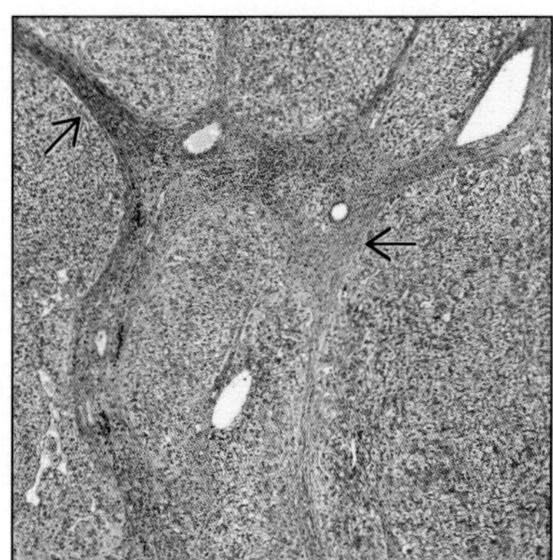

*(**Left**) NRH is composed of multiple nodules of regenerating hepatocytes with pale cytoplasm ⇨ surrounded by rims of atrophic hepatocytes →. Note the absence of perinodular fibrosis. (**Center**) Gross photograph of focal nodular hyperplasia (FNH) in a partial hepatectomy specimen is shown for comparison. A central scar ⇨, a common feature of FNH, is not seen in NRH. (**Right**) Masson trichrome in focal nodular hyperplasia highlights fibrous septae between hepatic nodules →. In contrast, NRH does not show intervening fibrosis.*

PANCREATOBLASTOMA

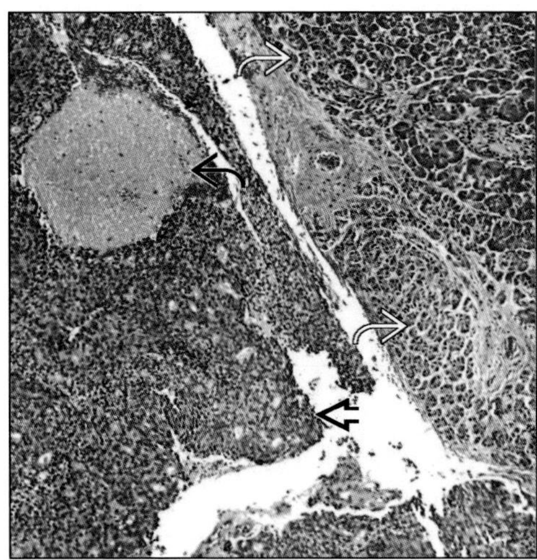

Pancreatoblastoma shows acinar arrangement ⊳ and focal necrosis ⊳. Compared to the adjacent normal pancreatic parenchyma ⊳, neoplastic cells have a primitive, basophilic appearance.

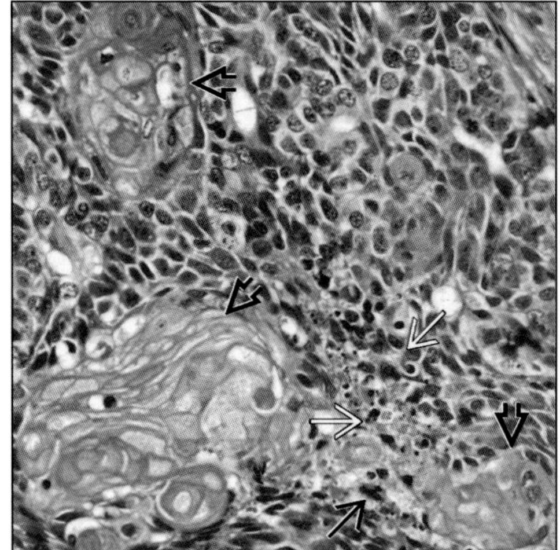

Hematoxylin & eosin shows a densely cellular, mitotically active ⊳ pancreatoblastoma exhibiting karyorrhexis, tumor cell necrosis ⊳, and characteristic squamous corpuscles ⊳.

TERMINOLOGY

Abbreviations

- Pancreatoblastoma (PB)

Synonyms

- Pancreaticoblastoma
- Infantile pancreatic carcinoma

ETIOLOGY/PATHOGENESIS

Developmental Anomaly

- Arises from pluripotent stem cells that recapitulate the embryogenesis of pancreas and sustain the ability to differentiate into all 3 pancreatic cell types

Genetics

- LOH of chromosome 11p15.5, often of maternal origin
- Mutations in β-catenin/*APC* pathway
- Abnormal *SMAD4/DPC4* gene, with loss of Dpc4 expression
- Isolated cases associated with Beckwith-Wiedemann syndrome and familial adenomatous polyposis of colon

CLINICAL ISSUES

Epidemiology

- Incidence
  - Rare pancreatic neoplasm of childhood
    - Comprises 0.5% of pancreatic nonendocrine tumors
- Age
  - Most commonly occurs in 1st decade of life
- Gender
  - Slight male predominance (M:F = 1.14:1)
- Ethnicity
  - More common in Asians than Caucasians

Presentation

- Upper abdominal mass, ± pain
- Diarrhea/vomiting
- Weight loss
- Jaundice

Laboratory Tests

- Serum α-fetoprotein (AFP)
  - Often elevated
    - Decreases following tumor resection

Treatment

- Surgical approaches
  - Complete surgical resection is first-line treatment for localized tumors
    - Preoperative chemotherapy may reduce tumor volume and allow surgical resection
- Adjuvant therapy
  - Chemo- and radiotherapy are indicated to treat locally unresectable tumor, metastatic disease, or local recurrences of PB

Prognosis

- Tend to be less aggressive in infants and children compared to adults
- Good prognosis in absence of metastasis
  - > 15% of patients present with metastatic disease at diagnosis
    - Liver is most common site of metastases
- Risk of local recurrence even after complete surgical resection

MACROSCOPIC FEATURES

General Features

- Well circumscribed, lobulated
- Usually encapsulated, large, and solitary
- Tan-gray, soft cut surface, separated by fibrous bands
- ± necrosis, hemorrhage, and calcification
- Most commonly occurs in pancreatic head

PANCREATOBLASTOMA

Key Facts

Terminology
- Pancreatoblastoma (PB)
- Malignant epithelial neoplasm with varied patterns, predominantly acinar, and characteristic squamoid corpuscles separated by fibrous stromal bands

Etiology/Pathogenesis
- Mutations in β-*catenin/APC* pathway
- Abnormal *SMAD4/DPC4* gene: Loss of Dpc4 expression

Clinical Issues
- Rare pancreatic neoplasm of childhood
- Most commonly occurs in 1st decade of life
- Slight male predominance (M:F = 1.14:1)
- Serum α-fetoprotein (AFP) elevated in majority of patients
- Complete surgical resection is first-line treatment for localized tumors
- Tend to be less aggressive in infants and children compared to adults
- Liver is most common site of metastases

Macroscopic Features
- Most common in pancreatic head
- Usually encapsulated, large, and solitary

Top Differential Diagnoses
- Acinar cell carcinoma
- Solid-pseudopapillary tumor
- Pancreatic endocrine neoplasms

Diagnostic Checklist
- Squamoid corpuscles
- Nuclear β-catenin positive

Immunohistochemistry

Antibody	Reactivity	Staining Pattern	Comment
α-fetoprotein	Positive	Cytoplasmic	Acinar component, if serum AFP is elevated
Chymotrypsin	Positive	Cytoplasmic	Acinar component ~ 100% of cases
Trypsin	Positive	Cytoplasmic	Acinar component ~ 100% of cases
Lipase	Positive	Cytoplasmic	Acinar component ~ 100% of cases
CK-PAN	Positive	Cytoplasmic	Acinar component
Chromogranin-A	Positive	Cytoplasmic	Endocrine component
Synaptophysin	Positive	Cytoplasmic	Endocrine component
β-catenin	Positive	Nuclear	Abnormal nuclear accumulation of β-catenin gene product when β-*catenin* gene is mutated
SMAD4	Negative		When *SMAD4* gene is mutated

MICROSCOPIC PATHOLOGY

Histologic Features
- Variably dense cellularity
- Nested, sheet-like, acinar, and solid growth patterns
  - Acinar, endocrine, ductal components
- Squamoid corpuscles or nests
- Intervening fibrous stroma between lobules
- Occasional heterologous components (e.g., cartilage, bone, and osteoid)

DIFFERENTIAL DIAGNOSIS

Acinar Cell Carcinoma
- Usually occurs in late adulthood
- Absence of squamoid corpuscles
- Acinar pattern without fibrous stromal bands
- Usually CEA and AFP negative

Solid-Pseudopapillary Tumor
- Usually occurs in childbearing-age females
- Absence of squamoid corpuscles
- Pseudopapillae
- Vimentin and CD10 positive
- Nuclear β-catenin positive in most cases
- CEA, lipase, CK7, and CK19 negative

Pancreatic Endocrine Neoplasms
- Absence of squamoid corpuscles
- Positive for specific pancreatic and gastroenteric hormones, e.g., gastrin, insulin, glucagon

DIAGNOSTIC CHECKLIST

Pathologic Interpretation Pearls
- Distinct acinar and squamoid cell differentiation
- Nuclear β-catenin positive

SELECTED REFERENCES

1. Gu WZ et al: Childhood pancreatoblastoma: clinical features and immunohistochemistry analysis. Cancer Lett. 264(1):119-26, 2008
2. Saif MW: Pancreatoblastoma. JOP. 8(1):55-63, 2007
3. Dhebri AR et al: Diagnosis, treatment and outcome of pancreatoblastoma. Pancreatology. 4(5):441-51; discussion 452-3, 2004
4. Défachelles AS et al: Pancreatoblastoma in childhood: clinical course and therapeutic management of seven patients. Med Pediatr Oncol. 37(1):47-52, 2001
5. Klimstra DS et al: Pancreatoblastoma. A clinicopathologic study and review of the literature. Am J Surg Pathol. 19(12):1371-89, 1995

Microscopic Features

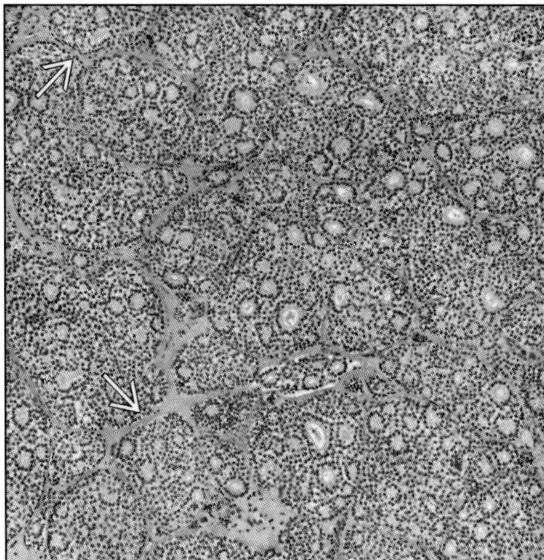

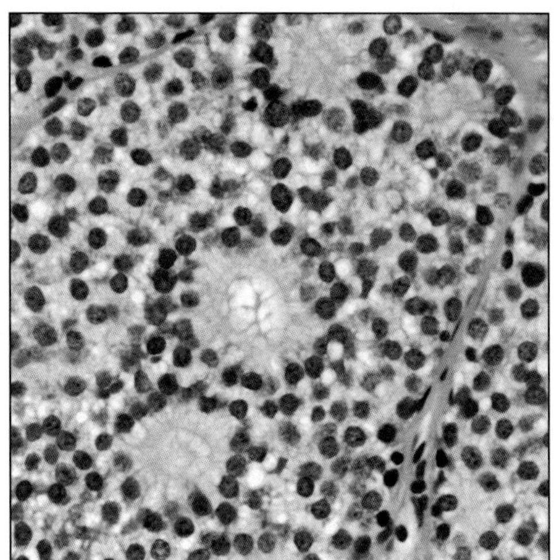

(Left) *Pancreatoblastoma with acinar differentiation and nested growth pattern separated by bands of fibrous tissue → is shown. Identical growth patterns can be present in acinar cell carcinomas and pancreatic endocrine neoplasms, but characteristic squamoid corpuscles are only seen in pancreatoblastoma.* ***(Right)*** *High-power view of acinar structures shows medium-sized, bland-appearing cells. Characteristics of neoplastic cells vary in different areas of pancreatoblastoma.*

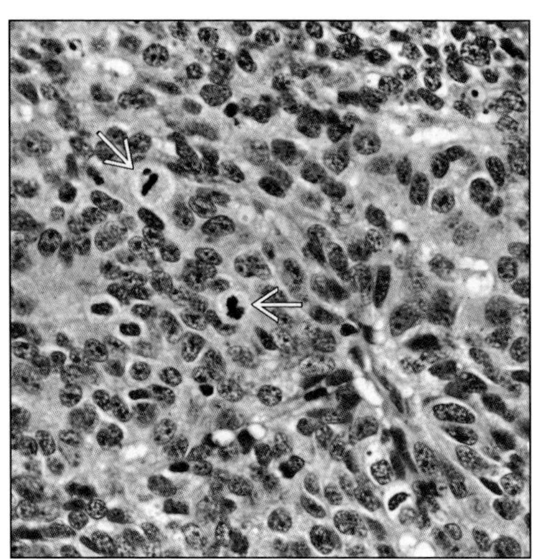

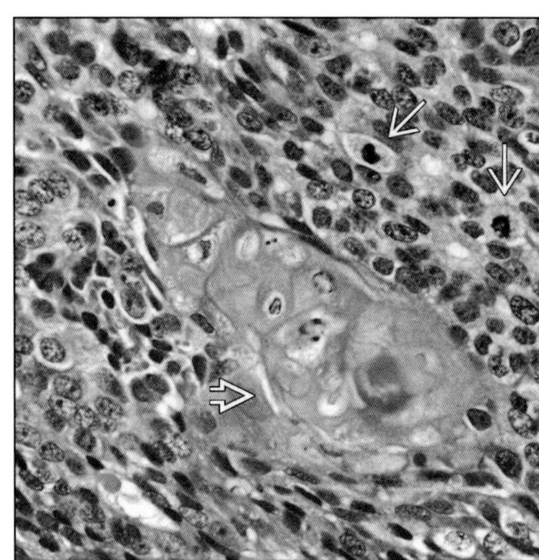

(Left) *In this example of a pancreatoblastoma, there are markedly enlarged, pleomorphic nuclei with clumped chromatin and prominent nucleoli. Numerous mitotic figures → are also noted. Despite dense cellularity, vague acinar structures are still apparent.* ***(Right)*** *High-power view shows a keratinized squamous corpuscle ⇨. The surrounding neoplasm is mitotically active →, high grade, and displays a vaguely acinar arrangement of neoplastic cells.*

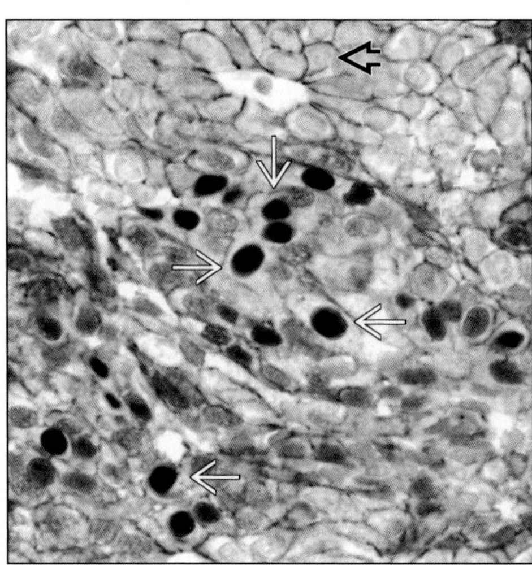

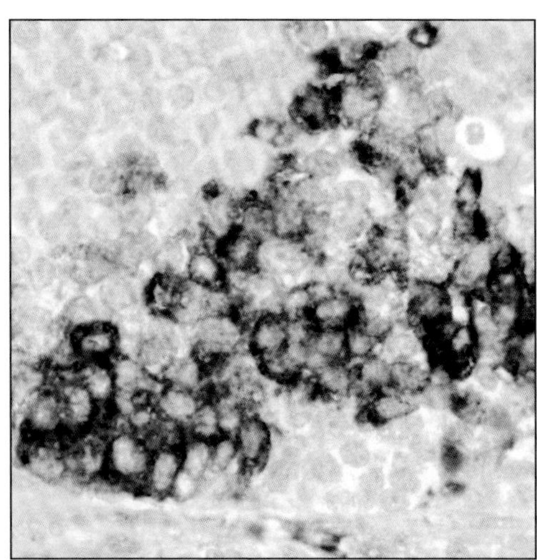

(Left) *Immunohistochemical staining for β-catenin in a pancreatoblastoma shows nuclear accumulation of β-catenin →. Some neoplastic cells show membranous β-catenin labeling but are negative for nuclear accumulation ⇨, likely reflecting a mosaic pattern of β-catenin gene mutation in this case.* ***(Right)*** *Immunohistochemical staining for AFP shows strong cytoplasmic positivity on neoplastic cells. AFP staining is most sensitive when serum AFP is elevated.*

Microscopic Features

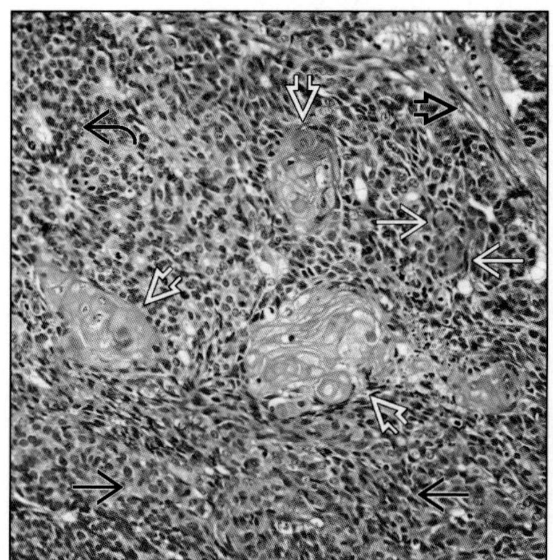

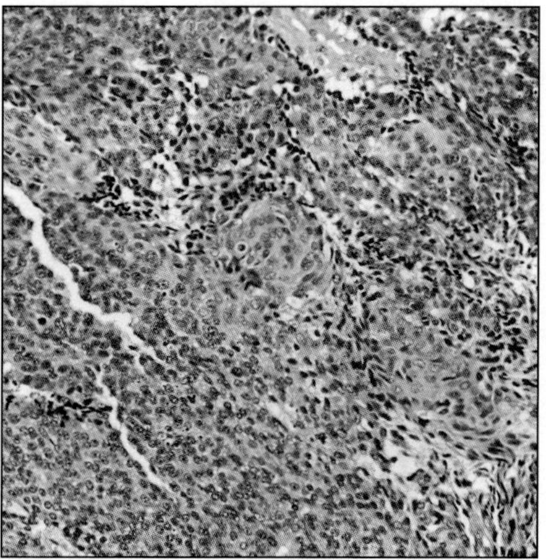

(Left) *H&E shows a hypercellular pancreatoblastoma, which exhibits sheet-like ⇒ and acinar ⇒ growth patterns. Keratinized squamoid corpuscles ⇒ are interspersed within the tumor. Focal dyskeratotic cells ⇒ are noted. Neoplastic cells are separated by fibrous bands ⇒.* ***(Right)*** *H&E shows a pancreatoblastoma with a predominantly sheet-like arrangement of neoplastic cells.*

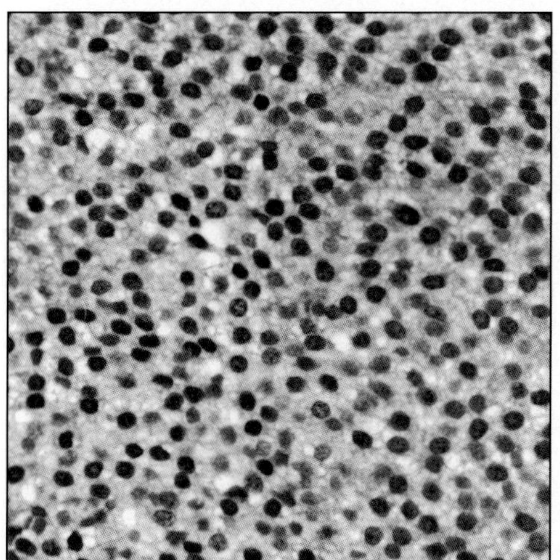

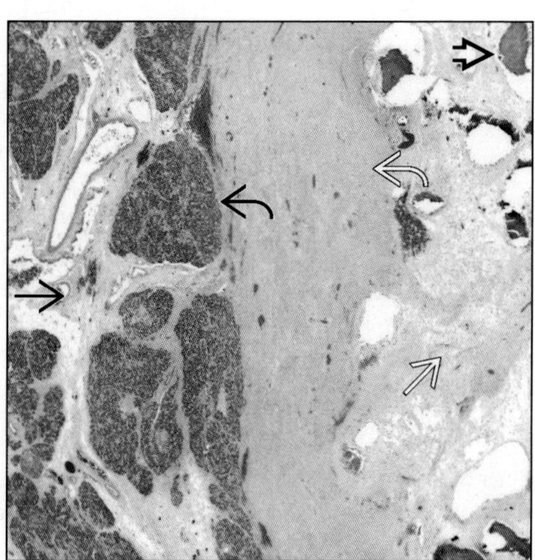

(Left) *H&E shows neoplastic cells with abundant amphophilic cytoplasm and ill-defined cell borders, arranged in a predominantly solid pattern. The nuclei are round to oval, with finely stippled chromatin and inconspicuous nucleoli.* ***(Right)*** *Pancreatoblastoma status post chemotherapy demonstrates changes consistent with treatment effect, including edema ⇒, fibrosis ⇒, and calcification ⇒. Adjacent nonneoplastic pancreatic parenchyma ⇒ shows interspersed fibrosis ⇒.*

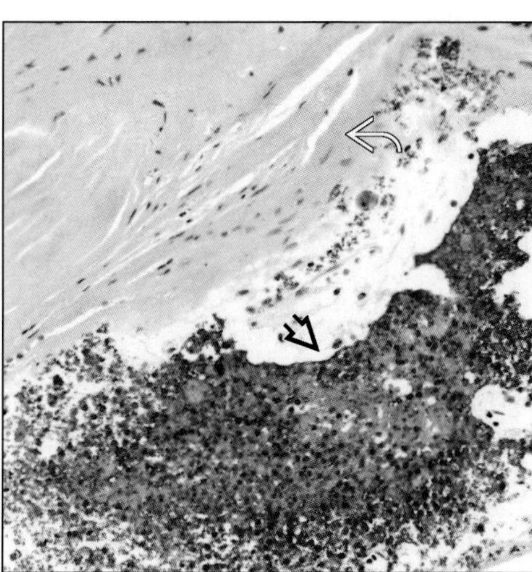

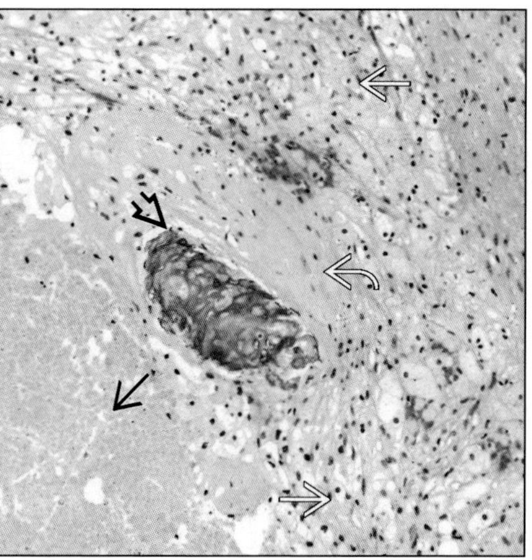

(Left) *H&E shows a pancreatoblastoma status post adjuvant chemotherapy. The residual tumor is composed of necrotic cellular debris arranged in a loosely cohesive, vaguely recognizable acinar pattern ⇒. Note the adjacent fibrotic reaction ⇒.* ***(Right)*** *H&E shows a residual keratinized squamoid corpuscle ⇒ following chemotherapeutic treatment. Note the adjacent edema ⇒, fibrosis ⇒, and focal area of necrosis ⇒.*

NESIDIOBLASTOSIS

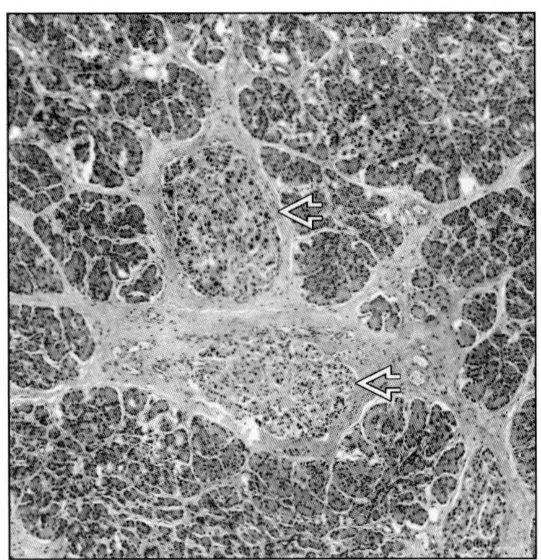

Low-power view of nesidioblastosis shows large, irregularly shaped islets ➡ within an otherwise unremarkable pancreatic parenchyma.

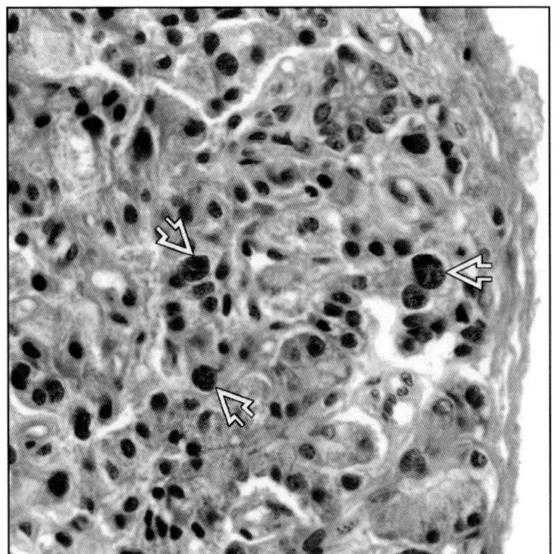

High-power view of nesidioblastosis shows large islet cells with enlarged hyperchromatic nuclei ➡.

TERMINOLOGY

Synonyms

- Islet cell dysmaturation syndrome (ICDS)

Definitions

- Proliferation of pancreatic islet cells (single or in clusters) associated with recurrent, persistent, and symptomatic hyperinsulinemic hypoglycemia
- **Nesidioblastosis may be focal or diffuse**

ETIOLOGY/PATHOGENESIS

Genetics

- Mutations in *ABCC8* (coding for SUR1) and *KCNJ11* (coding for *Kir6.2),* components of the β cell potassium channel
  - Focal nesidioblastosis is associated with paternally inherited *ABCC8* and with loss of heterozygosity (LOH) of chromosome 11p15
- Mutations in glucokinase, glutamate dehydrogenase, 3-hydroxyacyl-CoA dehydrogenase genes

CLINICAL ISSUES

Epidemiology

- Incidence
  - ~ 1 in 2,500 to 1 in 50,000 births/year
- Age
  - **Most commonly occurs in neonates and infants**
    - 1st year of life

Presentation

- Recurrent, persistent, and symptomatic hyperinsulinemic hypoglycemia
- Macrosomia, hepatomegaly, and plethora at birth

Laboratory Tests

- Hypoglycemia
- Elevated insulin levels in presence of hypoglycemia
  - Serum insulin levels may not be absolutely elevated
- Elevated plasma C-peptide
- Lack of urinary ketones on urinalysis

Treatment

- Therapy of choice depends on whether disease is focal or diffuse
- Conservative management
  - Frequent feeding
  - Intravenous glucose infusions
  - Administration of diazoxide, nifedipine, octreotide, glucagon, cortisone
- Surgical approaches
  - Partial, subtotal, or near total (95%) pancreatectomy
    - Indicated when conservative management fails to control hyperinsulinemia
    - Most effective in cases of unifocal nesidioblastosis
    - Extensive surgeries complicated by exocrine pancreatic insufficiency &/or glucose intolerance/ diabetes mellitus
- Preoperative localization of lesion(s) should be attempted
  - PET/CT; transhepatic catheterization of pancreatic veins; intraarterial calcium stimulation with pancreatic arteries hormone sampling can be used for this purpose

Prognosis

- Hypoglycemic episodes often do not improve with age
  - Clinical &/or surgical intervention is warranted
- Overall, multifocal and diffuse lesions tend to have worst response to treatment

MACROSCOPIC FEATURES

General Features

- Pancreas is usually unremarkable
- In focal nesidioblastosis, small uni-, bi-, or multifocal nodule(s) may be identified

NESIDIOBLASTOSIS

Key Facts

Clinical Issues

- Most commonly occurs in neonates and infants (1st year of life)
- Presents as recurrent and persistent hyperinsulinemic hypoglycemia
- Elevated insulin to glucose ratio
- Serum insulin levels may not be absolutely elevated

Diagnostic Checklist

- Immunohistochemistry and comparison to age-matched controls may be needed to diagnose discrete diffuse lesions
- Ample sampling on frozen section is recommended
  - Different pancreatic areas should be sampled and specimens compared

MICROSCOPIC PATHOLOGY

Histologic Features

- Hyperplasia and hypertrophy of pancreatic β cells
  - **Diffuse nesidioblastosis**
    - Enlargement and hyperchromasia of β cell nuclei distributed throughout the pancreas
    - Ductuloinsular complexes (association of pancreatic ductules with adjacent β cells)
    - Variably sized and shaped islets distributed throughout the acinar tissue
    - Immunohistochemistry and comparison to age-matched controls may be needed to diagnose discrete diffuse lesions
  - **Focal nesidioblastosis**
    - Abnormal islet aggregation
    - Focal or multifocal nodular lesions
    - Clusters of large β cells with enlarged hyperchromatic nuclei (a.k.a. focal adenomatosis or adenomatous hyperplasia)
    - β cell clusters are separated by acinar cells
    - Lesion contains other pancreatic endocrine cells (e.g., δ, α)
    - Ductuloinsular complexes are usually present

ANCILLARY TESTS

Frozen Sections

- Ample sampling is recommended
  - Different pancreatic areas should be sampled and specimens compared

Immunohistochemistry

- Hyperplastic β cells in nesidioblastosis show cytoplasmic immunopositivity for insulin
  - Insulin immunolabeling may be similar or slightly weaker within lesion than in adjacent pancreatic tissue

DIFFERENTIAL DIAGNOSIS

Insulinoma

- Composed only of β cells
- β cell clusters may extend into adjacent pancreatic parenchyma
- Trabecular, solid, or acinar growth pattern

SELECTED REFERENCES

1. Delonlay P et al: Neonatal hyperinsulinism: clinicopathologic correlation. Hum Pathol. 38(3):387-99, 2007
2. Goossens A et al: Diffuse and focal nesidioblastosis. A clinicopathological study of 24 patients with persistent neonatal hyperinsulinemic hypoglycemia. Am J Surg Pathol. 13(9):766-75, 1989

IMAGE GALLERY

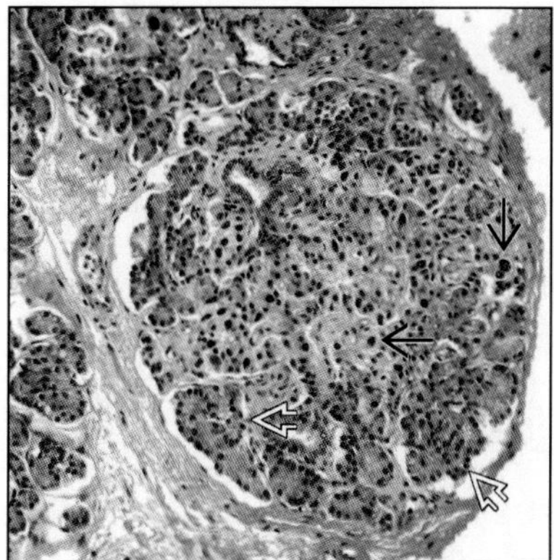

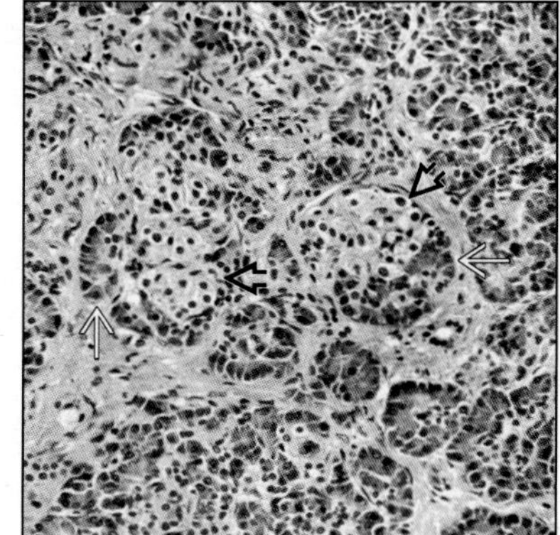

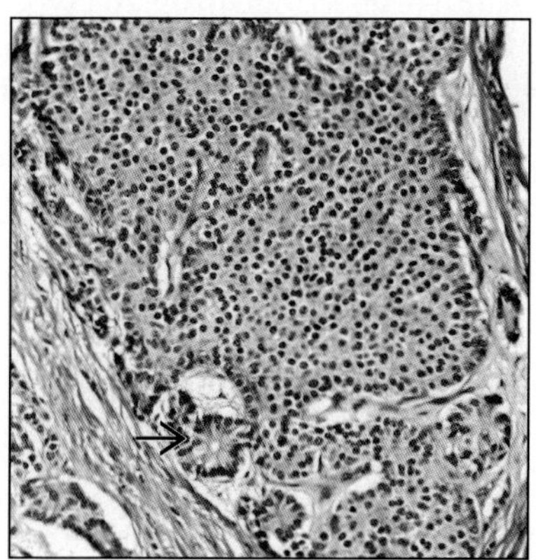

(Left) *Focal nesidioblastosis shows clusters of large β cells with enlarged hyperchromatic nuclei →. In this lesion, pancreatic acinar cells are interspersed with the β-cell clusters ➡. **(Center)** Nesidioblastosis showing clusters of hypertrophic β cells ⇨ admixed with rims of pancreatic acinar cells ➡. **(Right)** This insulinoma shows a solid and acinar → growth pattern. Note the monotonous nuclei.*

ISLET CELL ADENOMA

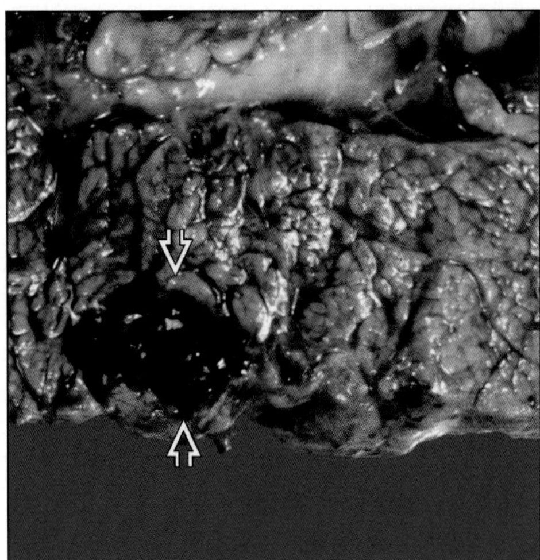

Gross photograph shows a well-circumscribed, dark red-brown insulinoma ➡ in the body of pancreas.

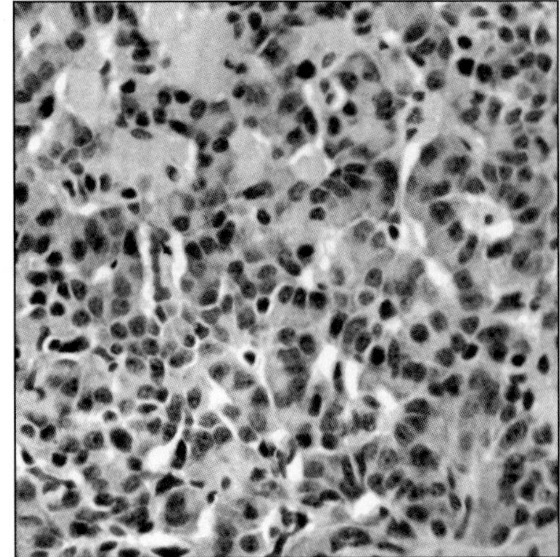

Hematoxylin & eosin shows a high-power view of an insulinoma with neoplastic cells with moderate amphophilic cytoplasm and bland nuclei arranged in a trabecular pattern.

TERMINOLOGY

Synonyms

- Pancreatic endocrine neoplasm (PEN)
- Well-differentiated endocrine carcinoma of pancreas
- APUDoma

Definitions

- Neoplasms of islet cells, which may be
  - **Functional** (hormonal hypersecretion leading to clinical syndromes)
    - Insulinoma (most common): β cell
    - Glucagonoma: α cell
    - Gastrinoma: G cell
    - Somatostatinoma: Δ cell
    - VIPoma
  - **Nonfunctional**

ETIOLOGY/PATHOGENESIS

Etiology

- Solitary tumors are usually sporadic
  - May be associated with chromosomal alterations
- Multiple tumors may be associated with
  - Multiple endocrine neoplasia type 1
  - von Hippel-Lindau syndrome
- Rare cases associated with tuberous sclerosis

CLINICAL ISSUES

Epidemiology

- Incidence
  - Uncommon in children
    - Insulinoma is most common functional PEN in children

Site

- May occur anywhere throughout pancreas
  - Functional tumors most common in head and tail
  - Nonfunctional tumors usually occur in tail
- Gastrinoma may occur in duodenum

Presentation

- **Insulinoma**
  - Hypoglycemia and associated symptoms
- **Glucagonoma**
  - Necrolytic migratory erythema, weight loss, stomatitis, diabetes
- **Gastrinoma**
  - Zollinger-Ellison syndrome (diarrhea, peptic ulcers)
- **Somatostatinoma**
  - Cholelithiasis, hypochlorhydria, diabetes
- **VIPoma**
  - Verner-Morrison syndrome (watery diarrhea, achlorhydria, hypokalemia)
- Nonfunctional tumors are usually incidentally found
  - Some may present with abdominal distension, pain, and nausea

Laboratory Tests

- Serum elevation of related functional hormones
- Chromogranin-A may be elevated

Treatment

- Surgical resection is treatment of choice for solitary tumors
- Associated clinical syndromes may require specific treatment

Prognosis

- Worse in large (> 2 cm), poorly differentiated, and mitotically active tumors
- Metastatic potential cannot be determined based only on microscopic features of tumors

MACROSCOPIC FEATURES

General Features

- Well-circumscribed, red-tan cut surface

ISLET CELL ADENOMA

Key Facts

Terminology
- Functional (hormonal hypersecretion leading to clinical syndromes)
- Nonfunctional

Clinical Issues
- Uncommon in children
- Insulinoma is most common functional PEN in children
- Serum elevation of related functional hormones

Microscopic Pathology
- Islet cells arranged in nests, trabeculae, or glands

Diagnostic Checklist
- Immunohistochemical stain may not correlate with serum hormone elevations
- Some tumors express more than 1 hormone
- Intensity and pattern on immunohistochemical stain may vary between tumors and within same tumor

Immunohistochemistry

Antibody	Reactivity	Staining Pattern	Comment
Synaptophysin	Positive	Cytoplasmic	Usually diffuse staining
Chromogranin-A	Positive	Cytoplasmic	Usually focal and inconsistent staining
CK8/18/CAM5.2	Positive	Cytoplasmic	
Insulin	Positive	Cytoplasmic	In insulinomas
Glucagon	Positive	Cytoplasmic	Usually inconsistent staining in glucagonomas
Gastrin	Positive	Cytoplasmic	In gastrinomas
VIP	Positive	Cytoplasmic	In VIPomas

- Variable size: Functional tumors are usually smaller than nonfunctional ones
- ± fibrosis or cystic changes

MICROSCOPIC PATHOLOGY

Histologic Features
- Islet cells arranged in nests, trabeculae, or glands
  - Abundant eosinophilic to amphophilic cytoplasm
  - Round to oval nuclei with coarse, stippled chromatin
  - Inconspicuous nucleoli
- Variable amount of hyalinized stroma and mitotic figures
- ± amyloid deposits (insulinoma)
- ± psammoma bodies (somatostatinoma)

DIFFERENTIAL DIAGNOSIS

Pancreatoblastoma
- Display squamoid corpuscles

Acinar Cell Carcinoma
- Acinar differentiation
- Chymotrypsin, trypsin, and lipase positive

SELECTED REFERENCES

1. Jaksic T et al: A 20-year review of pediatric pancreatic tumors. J Pediatr Surg. 27(10):1315-7, 1992
2. Grosfeld JL et al: Pancreatic tumors in childhood: analysis of 13 cases. J Pediatr Surg. 25(10):1057-62, 1990

IMAGE GALLERY

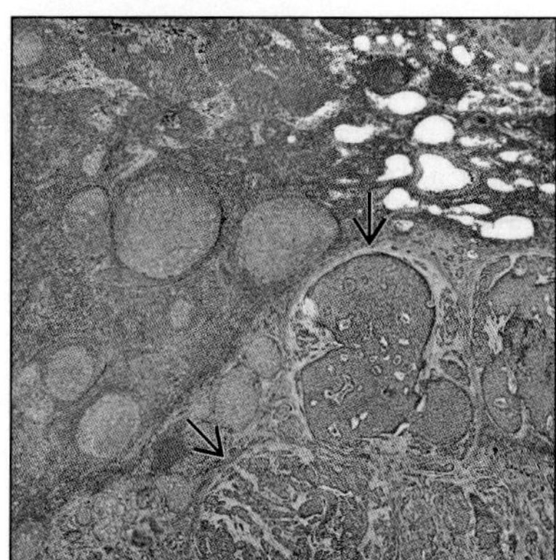

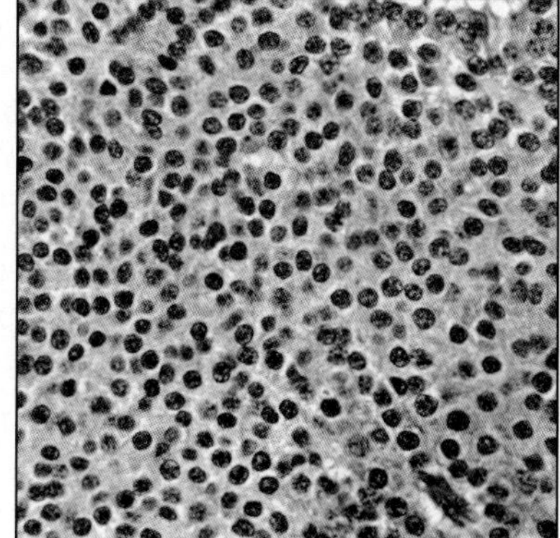

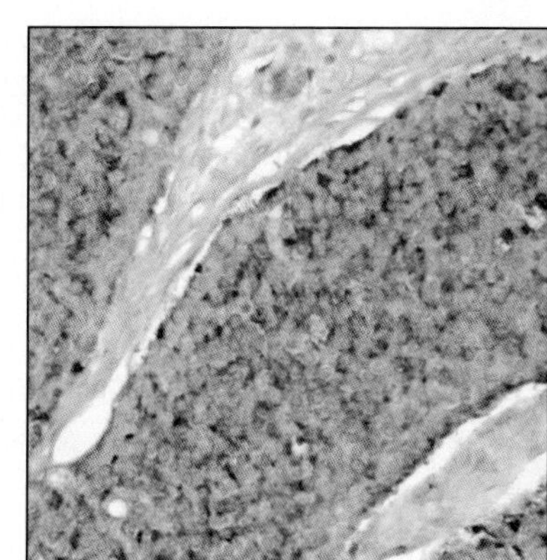

(Left) *Hematoxylin and eosin shows a low-power view of metastatic deposits of gastrinoma ⇒ within a lymph node. The nests of tumor cells are separated by hyalinized stroma.* ***(Center)*** *Hematoxylin & eosin shows a high-power view of a gastrinoma with eosinophilic cytoplasm and bland monomorphic nuclei with coarse, stippled ("salt and pepper") chromatin.* ***(Right)*** *Gastrin stained section of gastrinoma shows diffuse reactivity in a cytoplasmic distribution.*

HEPATOBLASTOMA

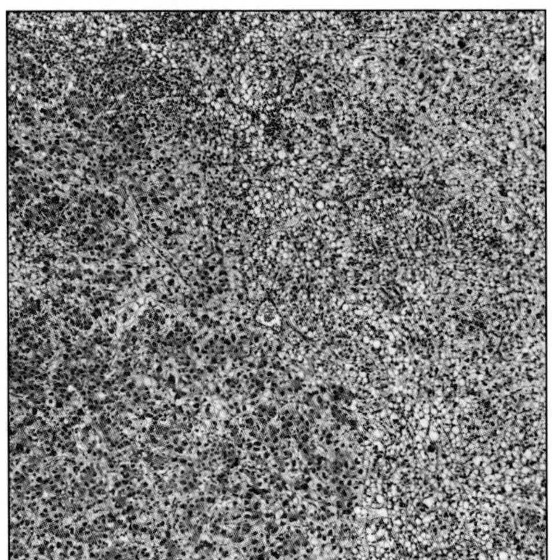

Hematoxylin & eosin shows a low-power view of a pure fetal hepatoblastoma with alternating light and dark areas.

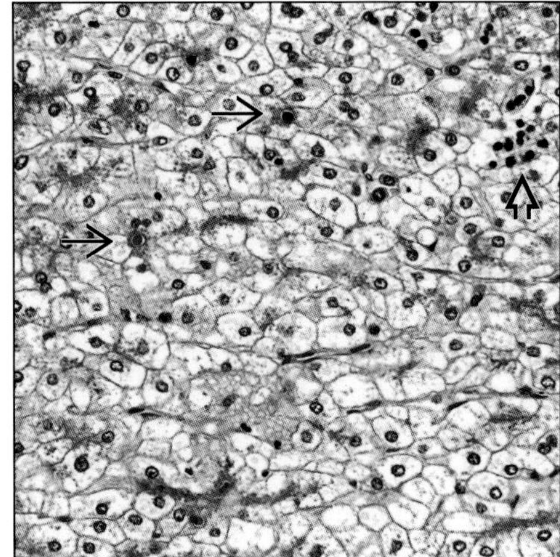

High-power view shows a pure fetal hepatoblastoma, recapitulating fetal hepatocytes. Note the cluster of extramedullary hematopoiesis ⇨ and cholestatic foci →.

TERMINOLOGY

Abbreviations

- Hepatoblastoma (HB)

Definitions

- Primary pediatric hepatic malignancy composed of cells that resemble developing fetal and embryonic liver

ETIOLOGY/PATHOGENESIS

Developmental Anomaly

- Arises from pluripotent stem cells that sustain ability of differentiating into both hepatocytes and biliary epithelial cells
- Association with several congenital malformations, metabolic, and pathophysiologic abnormalities
- Association with genetic syndromes, such as familial adenomatous polyposis (FAP) of the colon, Beckwith-Wiedemann syndrome, Li-Fraumeni syndrome, and trisomy 18
- Familial hepatoblastoma cases have been documented

Genetics

- β-catenin mutation-associated Wnt pathway activation in 70-90% of hepatoblastoma
- Inactivation of *APC* gene (5q21-q22) in 10% of sporadic hepatoblastomas
- Loss of heterozygosity on chromosomes 11p, 1q and 1p

Environmental Factors

- Low birth weight (< 1,000 g)

CLINICAL ISSUES

Epidemiology

- Age
  - Most common malignant liver neoplasm in children
    - 88% in children < 5 years and 3% > 15 years
- Gender
  - Male predominance (2:1)

Site

- Right lobe of liver (most common site)

Laboratory Tests

- Increased serum α-fetoprotein in 75-96% of patients
  - Useful marker of response to therapy and recurrence
  - Neonates < 6 months of age have normally elevated α-fetoprotein

Treatment

- Surgical approaches
  - Complete resection of tumor is first-line treatment
    - 1/3 to 1/2 have resectable disease at presentation
  - Orthotopic liver transplant (nonmetastatic unresectable neoplasm)
- Adjuvant therapy
  - Adjuvant and neoadjuvant combination chemotherapy converts > 50% of inoperable tumors to resectable tumors
    - HB is sensitive to cytostatic and cytotoxic drugs

Prognosis

- Resectability and tumor stage are most important prognostic factors in survival
- Pure fetal hepatoblastoma with low mitotic rate (≤ 2 mitosis/10 HPFs) = favorable prognosis
- Small undifferentiated cell pattern confers worse prognosis

MACROSCOPIC FEATURES

General Features

- Solitary or multifocal heterogeneous mass
- Appearance varies depending on predominant histologic pattern

HEPATOBLASTOMA

Key Facts

Terminology
- Primary hepatic malignancy with diverse patterns of differentiation, including epithelial, mesenchymal, and a varied combination of them

Clinical Issues
- Most common pediatric hepatic neoplasm in Western countries
- Commonly affects children younger than 5 years
- Right lobe of liver (most common site)
- Metastatic disease in approximately 20% of patients at diagnosis, majority to lungs
- Elevated serum AFP in most cases

Macroscopic Features
- Usually solitary
- Appearance varies depending on predominant histologic pattern

Microscopic Pathology
- **Epithelial subtype**
  - Fetal pattern
  - Embryonal pattern
  - Combined fetal and embryonal patterns
  - Macrotrabecular pattern
  - Small cell undifferentiated type
- **Mixed epithelial-mesenchymal type**

Diagnostic Checklist
- Pure fetal epithelial hepatoblastoma
  - Low power "dark and light appearance"
- Macrotrabecular hepatoblastoma
  - Broad trabeculae throughout tumor

  - Fetal pattern areas resemble normal liver
  - Embryonal and small cell patterns are fleshy to gelatinous, pale pink or gray-tan
  - Mesenchymal, osteoid-like areas are firm, fibrous, or calcified

Sections to Be Submitted
- At least 1 cassette/centimeter to ensure correct classification of histologic pattern

MICROSCOPIC PATHOLOGY

Histologic Features
- **Epithelial subtype**
  - Fetal pattern
    - Uniform hepatocytes arranged in trabeculae 2-3 cells thick
    - Alternating light and dark areas based on cytoplasmic content of glycogen
    - Extramedullary hematopoiesis
  - Embryonal pattern
    - Primitive cells arranged in sheets, nests, trabeculae, acinar configuration, or pseudorosettes
    - Increased mitotic activity
    - ± extramedullary hematopoiesis
  - Macrotrabecular pattern
    - Cells arranged in trabeculae > 10 cells thick throughout tumor
  - Small cell undifferentiated type (SCUD)
    - Dyscohesive, uniform, round cells arranged in sheets or showing diffuse growth
    - Scant basophilic cytoplasm, hyperchromatic nuclei, inconspicuous nucleoli
    - Increased mitotic activity
- **Mixed epithelial-mesenchymal subtype**
  - Variable combination of mesenchymal and epithelial components
  - Nonteratoid mesenchymal elements
    - Osteoid-like, myxoid, fibrous
  - Teratoid mesenchymal elements
    - Skeletal muscle, bone
    - Keratinized squamous epithelium
    - Neuroid-melanocytic
    - Intestinal epithelium

DIFFERENTIAL DIAGNOSIS

Hepatocellular Carcinoma (HCC)
- Should be differentiated from macrotrabecular hepatoblastoma
- HCC most commonly occur in older children (> 5 years)
- HCC lacks "light and dark appearance" and extramedullary hematopoiesis

Hepatic Adenoma
- Should be differentiated from epithelial subtype (fetal pattern)
- Hepatic adenoma most commonly occurs in childbearing-aged women
- Hepatic adenoma lacks "light and dark appearance"

Metastatic Hepatic Tumors
- Small blue cell tumors (e.g., neuroblastoma, neuroendocrine tumors, lymphoma) should be differentiated from SCUD and embryonal HB

Normal Liver Parenchyma
- Nuclear &/or cytoplasmic immunoreactivity for β-catenin in hepatoblastoma

SELECTED REFERENCES

1. Meyers RL et al: Predictive power of pretreatment prognostic factors in children with hepatoblastoma: a report from the Children's Oncology Group. Pediatr Blood Cancer. 53(6):1016-22, 2009
2. Finegold MJ et al: Protocol for the examination of specimens from pediatric patients with hepatoblastoma. Arch Pathol Lab Med. 131(4):520-9, 2007

HEPATOBLASTOMA

Microscopic Features

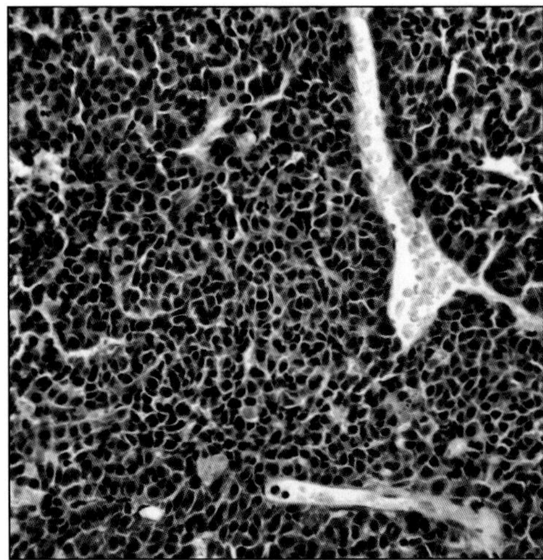

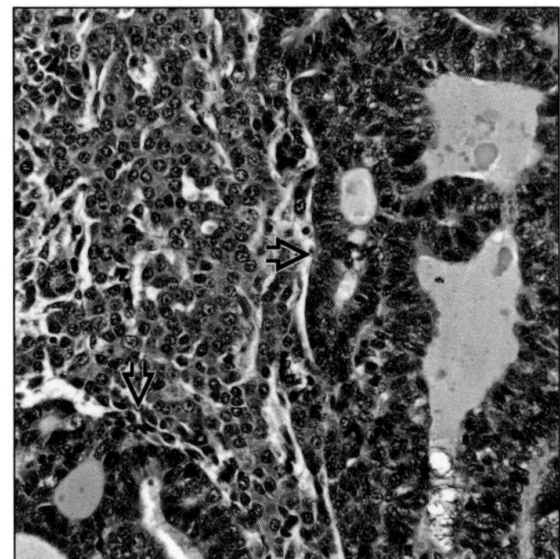

(Left) *H&E shows a hepatoblastoma composed of embryonal epithelial cells with scant basophilic cytoplasm, pleomorphic nuclei, and increased nuclear to cytoplasmic ratio growing in sheets and vague nested structures.* ***(Right)*** *Embryonal epithelial cells arranged in glandular structures ⊳ are illustrated in this example of a hepatoblastoma.*

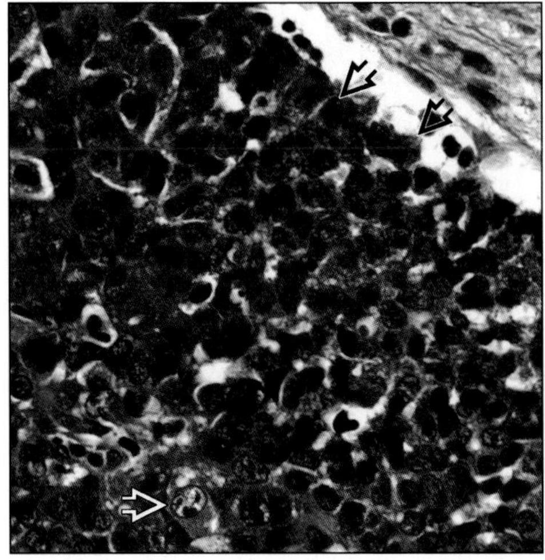

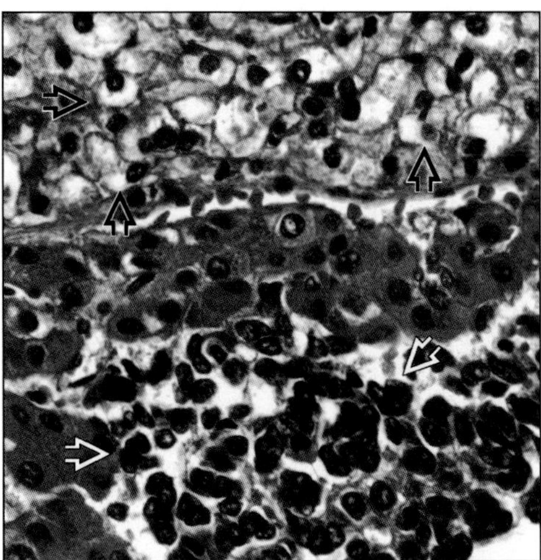

(Left) *Embryonal epithelial cells of this hepatoblastoma are seen ➡ merging into a focus of small undifferentiated cells ⊳, which have a "small round blue cell tumor" pattern. The presence of foci of small undifferentiated cells grants a poorer prognosis.* ***(Right)*** *Small undifferentiated and dyscohesive cells ➡ with scant cytoplasm are shown adjacent to more typical fetal epithelial cells with abundant clear cytoplasm ⊳ for comparison.*

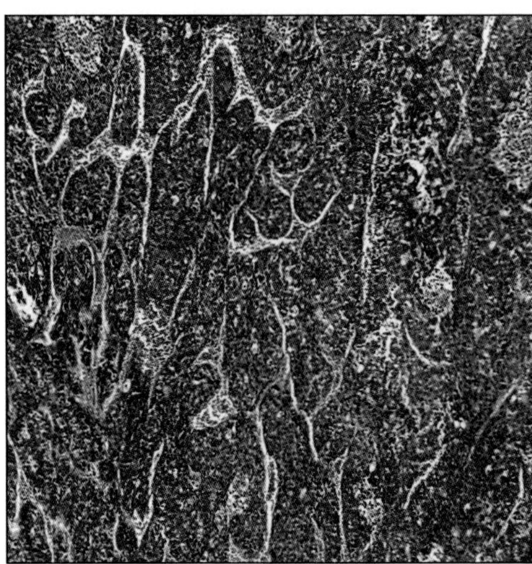

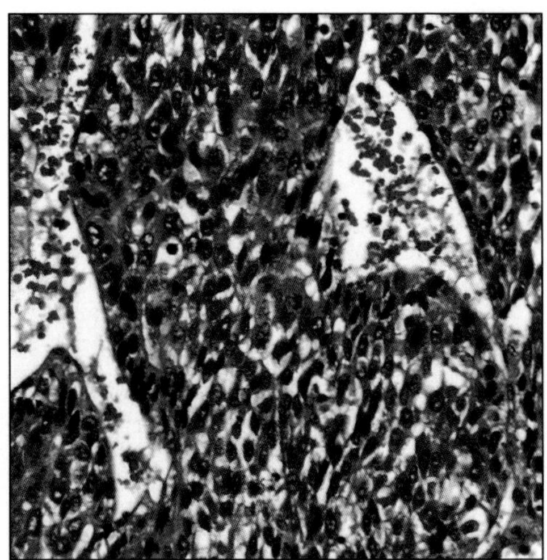

(Left) *Low-power view shows hepatoblastoma with a macrotrabecular pattern of growth. This hepatoblastoma subtype should be differentiated from hepatocellular carcinoma.* ***(Right)*** *High magnification shows a macrotrabecular growth pattern composed of embryonal epithelial cells. Cells arranged in > 10 cell-thick trabeculae may be either fetal epithelial or embryonal epithelial and can be seen throughout hepatoblastomas with macrotrabecular growth patterns.*

Microscopic and Gross Features

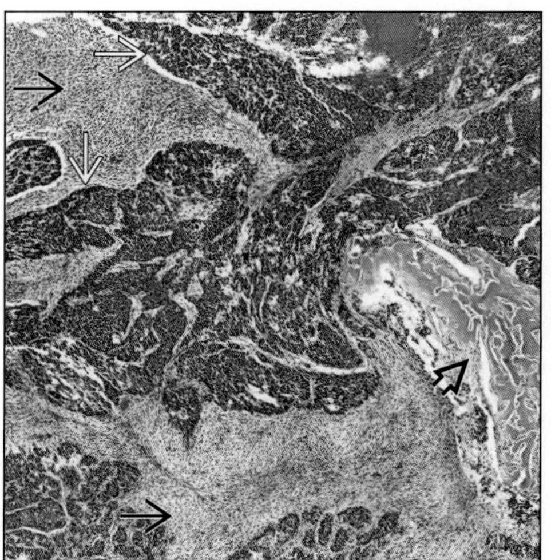

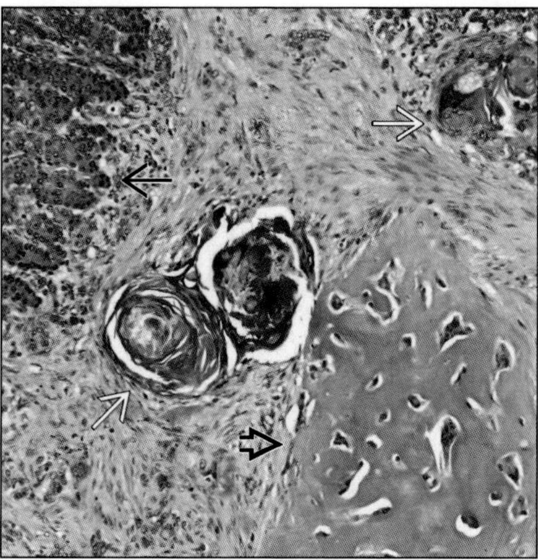

(Left) Low-power view of a mixed epithelial and mesenchymal hepatoblastoma shows an embryonal epithelial pattern ➔, spindled mesenchymal component ➔, and a focus of osteoid-like element ➔. **(Right)** Higher magnification of mixed epithelial and mesenchymal hepatoblastoma shows focal osteoid-like tissue ➔ within fibrous stroma. The neoplastic epithelial cells are arranged in cords ➔ and squamoid nests ➔.

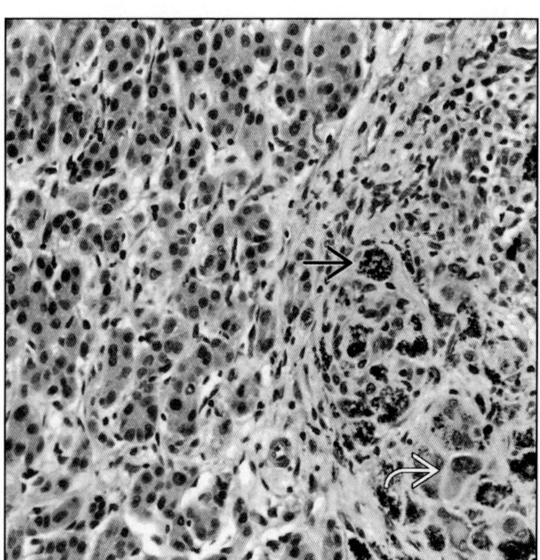

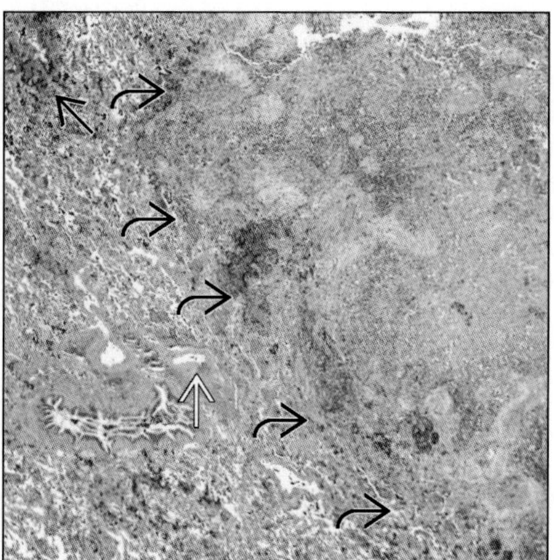

(Left) This mixed epithelial and mesenchymal hepatoblastoma with teratoid features has neoplastic epithelial cells adjacent to melanin pigment ➔ and ganglion-like cells ➔. Teratoid features have no prognostic significance. **(Right)** Metastatic hepatoblastoma to the lung is shown. Note the relatively well-circumscribed ➔, hemorrhagic ➔, perivascular ➔ proliferation of heterogeneous neoplastic cells within the lung parenchyma.

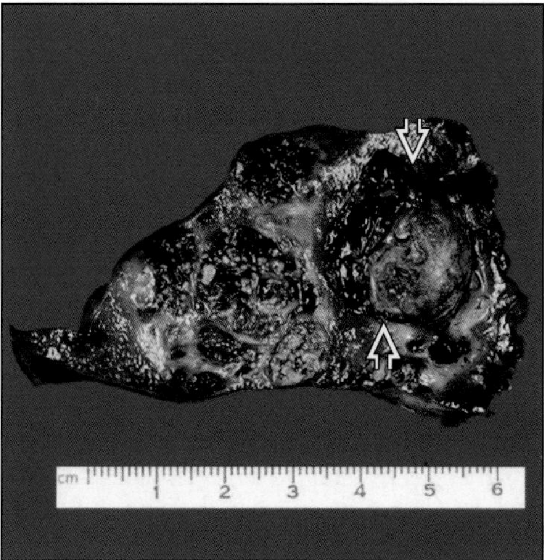

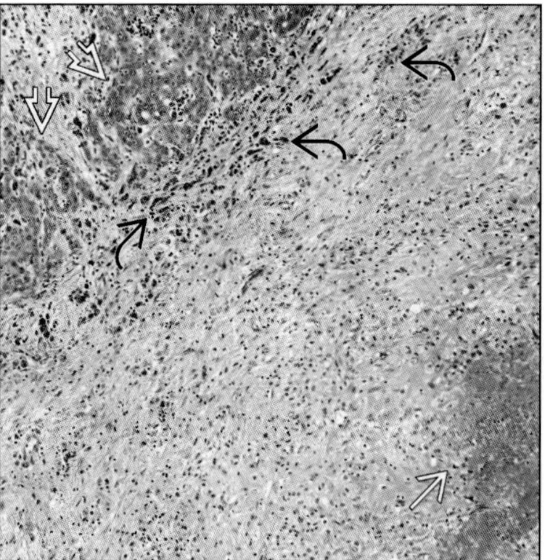

(Left) Gross photograph shows a mixed epithelial and mesenchymal hepatoblastoma ➔ treated with preoperative chemotherapy. **(Right)** This hepatoblastoma shows extensive treatment effect, including fibrosis, hemorrhage ➔, and necrosis ➔. Note the nodules of viable neoplastic embryonal epithelial cells in an acinar configuration ➔.

HEMANGIOENDOTHELIOMA

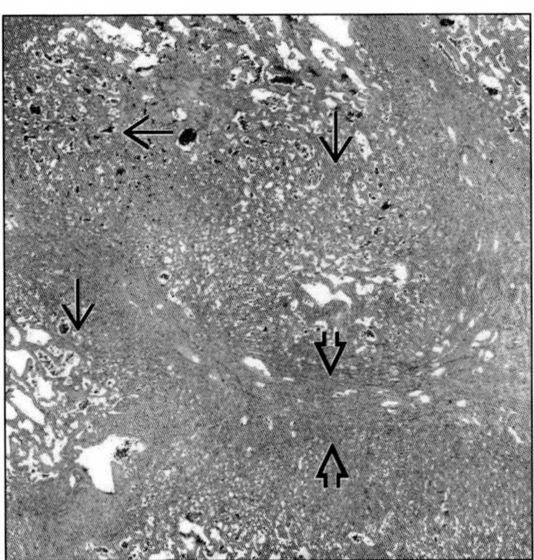

Hematoxylin & eosin shows a nodular proliferation of variably sized vascular spaces ➔ separated by collagenous stroma ➔.

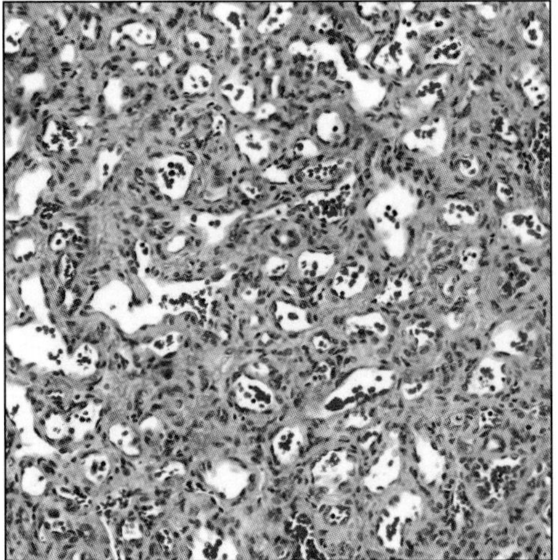

Hematoxylin & eosin shows small to medium, irregularly shaped vascular spaces lined by single layers of bland-looking endothelial cells. No mitotic figures are identified.

TERMINOLOGY

Synonyms

- Infantile hepatic hemangioendothelioma
- Type I hemangioendothelioma
  - Infantile hepatic hemangioma
- Type II hemangioendothelioma
  - Referred to by some authors as hepatic angiosarcoma (controversial nomenclature)

CLINICAL ISSUES

Epidemiology

- Incidence
  - Most common pediatric vascular neoplasm of liver
- Age
  - Most commonly occurs in infancy or early childhood
    - Majority diagnosed in 1st 6 months of life
- Gender
  - Female predominance (~ 2:1)
- Ethnicity
  - Most frequent in Caucasians

Presentation

- Asymptomatic abdominal mass
- Hepatomegaly
- Nausea/vomiting
- Failure to thrive
- Congestive heart failure
- Kasabach-Merritt syndrome
  - Consumptive coagulopathy
  - Associated with vascular neoplasms
- Hypothyroidism (catabolism of thyroid hormone by tumor)
- May be associated with Beckwith-Wiedemann syndrome, renal agenesis, and meningomyelocele

Natural History

- Type I hemangioendothelioma may regress spontaneously

Treatment

- Options
  - Corticosteroid therapy
  - Interferon-α
  - Complete surgical resection
  - Multiagent chemotherapy (not standardized)
  - Radiotherapy

Prognosis

- Overall good, especially for solitary, asymptomatic tumors, which respond to treatment
- Multifocal, large tumors may be associated with hepatic or cardiac failure
- Cellularity, cytologic atypia, and mitotic activity are related to aggressive behavior
  - Worst prognosis for type II hemangioendothelioma

MACROSCOPIC FEATURES

General Features

- Poorly circumscribed, cystic and solid lesion
- Usually multifocal
- Alternating fibrotic and hemorrhagic foci

MICROSCOPIC PATHOLOGY

Histologic Features

- Nodular proliferation of irregular, interconnected vascular channels
- 2 histological subtypes, which often overlap
- Type I
  - Irregularly dilated vascular spaces lined by single layers of bland-looking endothelial cells
    - Rare mitotic activity
  - Collagenous stroma separates vascular spaces

HEMANGIOENDOTHELIOMA

Key Facts

Terminology

- Infantile hepatic hemangioendothelioma

Clinical Issues

- Most common pediatric vascular neoplasm of liver
- Majority diagnosed in 1st 6 months of life
- Female predominance (~ 2:1 ratio)
- Type I hemangioendothelioma may regress spontaneously
- Multifocal, large tumors may be associated with hepatic or cardiac failure

Diagnostic Checklist

- **Type I hemangioendothelioma**
  - Bland-looking endothelial cell lining
- **Type II hemangioendothelioma**
  - Large, pleomorphic endothelial cells, usually with atypical nuclei
  - Benign in nature; may behave aggressively

Immunohistochemistry

Antibody	Reactivity	Staining Pattern	Comment
CD31	Positive	Cell membrane	Endothelial cells
CD34	Positive	Cell membrane	Endothelial cells
FVIIIRAg	Positive	Cytoplasmic	Endothelial cells

  - Bile ductules and hepatocytes are often seen within tumor (especially near its periphery)
  - ± extramedullary hematopoiesis
  - ± thrombosis, necrosis, hemorrhage, calcification, fibrosis
- Type II
  - Vascular spaces lined by hypercellular, pleomorphic, large endothelial cells with hyperchromatic, atypical nuclei
    - Irregular intraluminal branching and budding
    - Variable mitotic activity
  - Lack bile ductules within tumor

DIFFERENTIAL DIAGNOSIS

Hepatic Angiosarcoma

- Rare in infancy and early childhood
- Slit-like vascular spaces lined by atypical, spindle-shaped endothelial cells outlining broad hepatic cords
- Frequent mitotic activity
- Usually FVIIIRAg negative

Cavernous Hemangioma

- All age groups
- Large vascular spaces lined by flat, bland-appearing endothelial cells outlining hypocellular fibrous septae
- Septae projection within vascular spaces

SELECTED REFERENCES

1. North PE et al: Vascular tumors of infancy and childhood: beyond capillary hemangioma. Cardiovasc Pathol. 15(6):303-17, 2006
2. Emre S et al: Liver tumors in children. Pediatr Transplant. 8(6):632-8, 2004
3. Maksimak M et al: Hemangioendothelioma of the hepatobiliary system: the classic and the unusual. J Pediatr Gastroenterol Nutr. 10(1):131-7, 1990
4. Noronha R et al: Hepatic angiosarcoma in childhood. A case report and review of the literature. Am J Surg Pathol. 8(11):863-71, 1984

IMAGE GALLERY

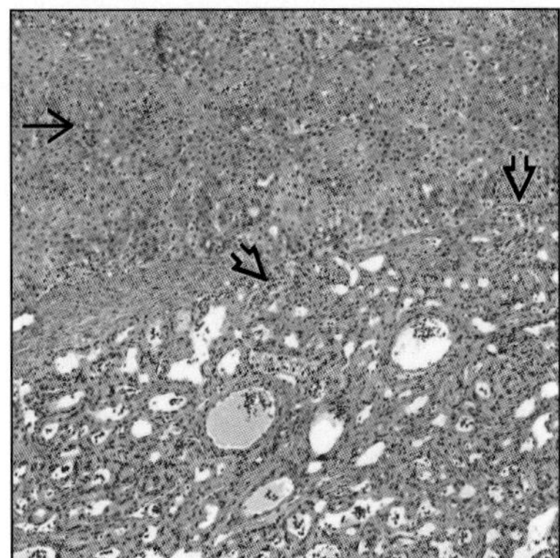

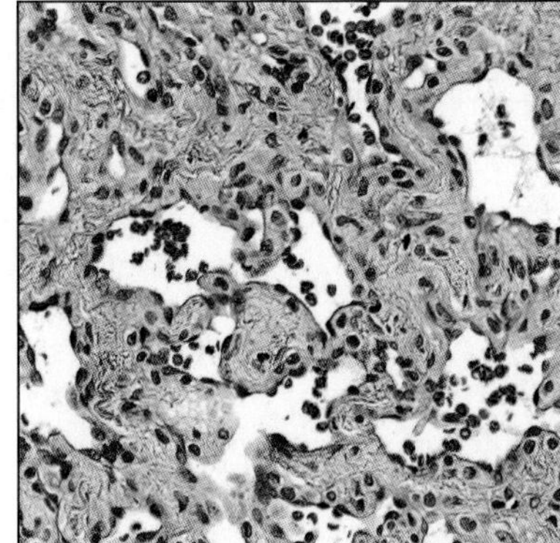

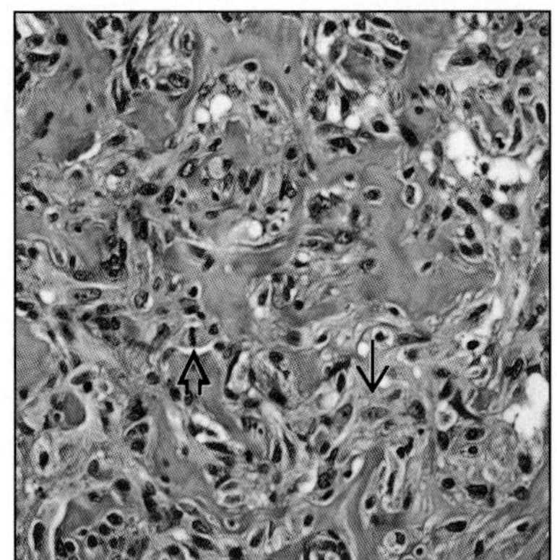

(Left) *Hematoxylin & eosin shows bile ducts ⊳ and hepatocytes → in the periphery of a hemangioendothelioma.* ***(Center)*** *Hematoxylin & eosin shows a high-power view of a hemangioendothelioma with vascular spaces lined by bland endothelial cells. The bland endothelial appearance and rare mitotic activity differentiate this lesion from angiosarcoma.* ***(Right)*** *Hematoxylin & eosin shows an angiosarcoma with atypical → and mitotically active endothelial cells ⊳. (Courtesy C. Sjostrom, MD.)*

HEPATOCELLULAR CARCINOMA

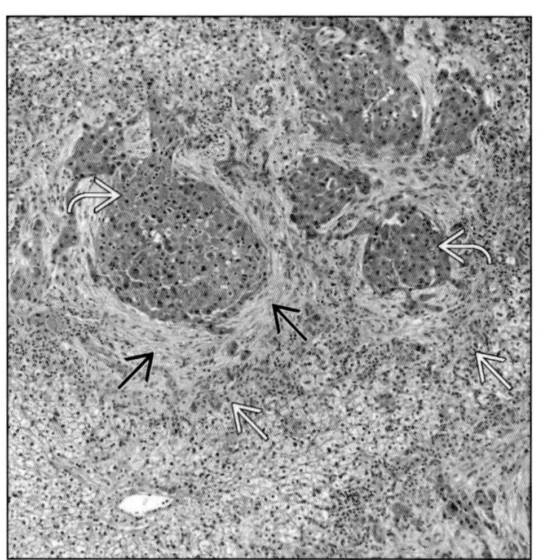

Fibrolamellar hepatocellular carcinoma composed of nests of large, eosinophilic hepatocytes ➡ is separated by loose collagenous bands ➡ and intervening small bile duct proliferation ➡.

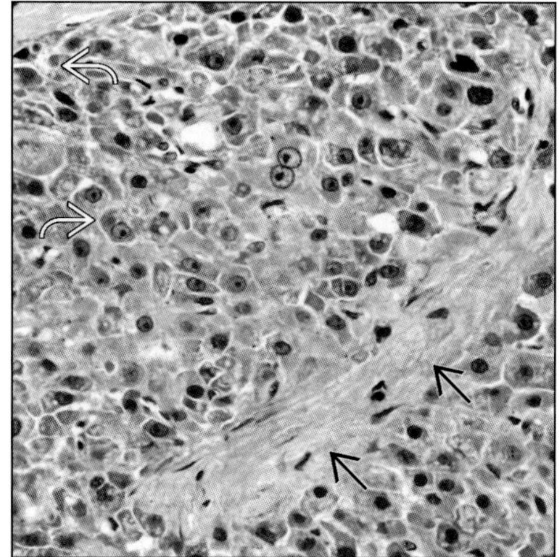

Hematoxylin & eosin shows neoplastic hepatocytes of a FL-HCC exhibiting large vesicular nuclei. Tumor cells are intersected by hyaline collagenous bands ➡. Intracytoplasmic bile is noted ➡.

TERMINOLOGY

Definitions

- Conventional hepatocellular carcinoma (HCC)
  - Rare entity in pediatrics
- Fibrolamellar hepatocellular carcinoma (FL-HCC)
  - Distinct subtype of HCC
    - Different clinical and histologic features from conventional HCC

ETIOLOGY/PATHOGENESIS

Infectious Agents

- Hepatitis B virus induces malignant transformation of hepatocytes

Genetics

- Disease association to HCC
  - **Type 1 tyrosinemia**
    - Accumulation of succynilacetone (carcinogenic potential)
  - **Glycogen storage disease types 1A and 3**
    - Development of hepatic adenoma (precursor lesion to HCC)
  - **α-1-antitrypsin deficiency**
    - Accumulation of mutant protein in endoplasmic reticulum
    - Development of hepatic adenoma (precursor lesion to HCC)
  - **Hereditary hemochromatosis**
    - Biliary atresia
    - Cirrhosis (precursor lesion to HCC)

FL-HCC

- Absence of risk factors associated with HCC
- Majority arise in noncirrhotic liver

CLINICAL ISSUES

Epidemiology

- Incidence
  - HCC
    - Rare malignancy in children
    - Higher incidence in Asia and Africa (hepatitis B)
  - FL-HCC
    - Uncommon hepatic neoplasia
    - Represents < 3% of HCC
    - More common in West than in Asia and Africa
- Age
  - HCC usually affects individuals > 35 years
  - FL-HCC mostly occurs between 5-35 years old

Presentation

- Abdominal pain
- Hepatomegaly
- Weakness
- Weight loss

Laboratory Tests

- Serum α-fetoprotein (AFP)
  - Elevated in HCC
  - Normal in FL-HCC

Treatment

- Surgical approaches
  - Complete resection of tumor is first line of treatment
    - Often impossible in HCC due to advanced stage of disease at diagnosis
  - Liver transplantation may be attempted for nonmetastatic, unresectable tumors
- Adjuvant therapy
  - HCC is relatively chemoresistant

Prognosis

- HCC

HEPATOCELLULAR CARCINOMA

Key Facts

Terminology
- Conventional hepatocellular carcinoma (HCC)
- Fibrolamellar hepatocellular carcinoma (FL-HCC)
  - Distinct subtype of HCC
  - Different clinical and histologic features from conventional HCC

Etiology/Pathogenesis
- FL-HCC
  - Not related to the same risk factors associated to HCC
  - Majority of FL-HCC arise in noncirrhotic liver

Clinical Issues
- HCC
  - Rare in children
  - Resectability is most important prognostic feature, regardless of histologic subtype
  - Relatively chemoresistant
- FL-HCC
  - Most commonly occurs between 5-35 years old
  - Does not have more favorable prognosis than other HCC histologic variants in children

Macroscopic Features
- HCC is usually multiple and may involve hepatic lobes bilaterally
- **FL-HCC is usually solitary and large with central scar**

Immunohistochemistry

Antibody	Reactivity	Staining Pattern	Comment
Hep-Par1	Positive	Cytoplasmic	Stains ~ 90% of HCC; also stains benign hepatocytes
CEA-P	Positive		Canalicular staining pattern; may be absent in poorly differentiated tumors
CD10	Positive		Canalicular staining pattern
Glypican-3	Positive	Cell membrane	~ 70-80% of cases; assists in differential diagnosis of HCC vs. benign hepatocellular neoplasms

  - Resectability of tumor is most important prognostic feature, regardless of histologic subtype
  - Multifocal tumors bear high risk of local relapse even if completely resected
- FL-HCC
  - Unlike in adults, FL-HCC does not have more favorable prognosis than HCC in children

MACROSCOPIC FEATURES

General Features
- HCC
  - Usually multiple ± bilateral lobe involvement
- FL-HCC
  - Usually solitary with central scar

MICROSCOPIC PATHOLOGY

Histologic Features
- HCC
  - Varied growth patterns (trabecular, acinar, solid)
  - Large polygonal cells
    - Granular eosinophilic cytoplasm
    - Increased nuclear to cytoplasmic ratio
  - ± multinucleated tumor giant cells
  - Intracytoplasmic/intraluminal bile
  - Graded as well, moderately, or poorly differentiated
  - Cytologic variants include pleomorphic, clear cell, and sarcomatoid (spindle cell)
- FL-HCC
  - Large hepatocytes arranged in nests, sheets, or trabeculae separated by hypocellular hyaline collagenous bands
    - Oncocytic cytoplasm
    - Large nuclei with prominent nucleoli
    - ± cytoplasmic hyaline inclusions or cytoplasmic pale inclusions
  - **Noncirrhotic hepatic background**

DIFFERENTIAL DIAGNOSIS

Hepatoblastoma
- Most cases occur in children younger than 3 years
- Neoplastic hepatocytes recapitulate developing fetal liver

Hepatocellular Adenoma
- Most commonly occur in females of childbearing age
- Bland-looking hepatocytes arranged in 1-2 cell-thick plates
- Glypican-3 (GPC3) negative

Metastatic Hepatic Tumors
- e.g., adenocarcinoma, neuroendocrine tumors
- Lack bile production
- Hep-Par1 negative

SELECTED REFERENCES

1. Blum HE et al: Hepatocellular carcinoma: an update. Arch Iran Med. 10(3):361-71, 2007

HEPATOCELLULAR CARCINOMA

Microscopic Features

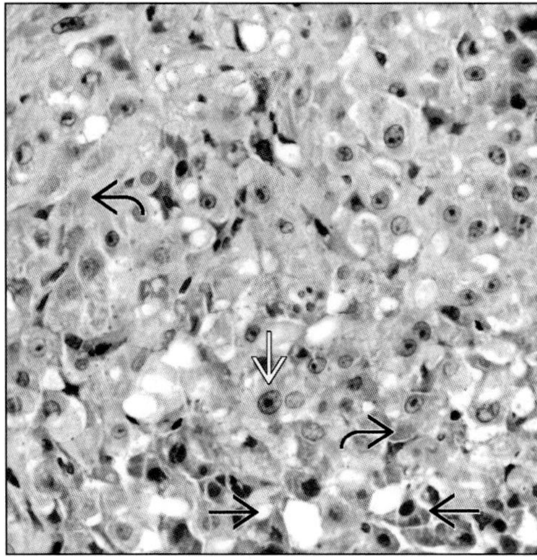

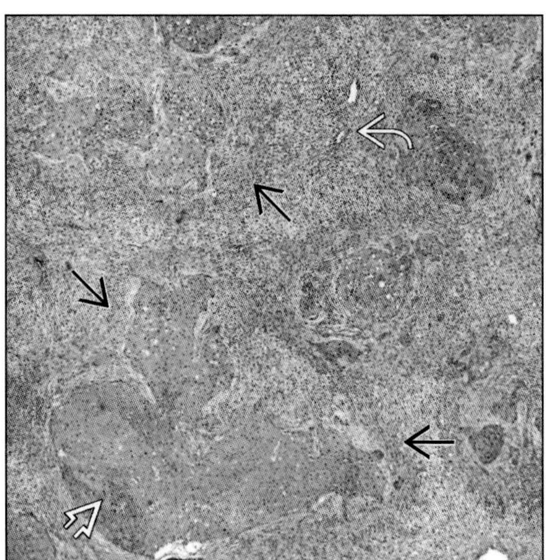

(Left) *FL-HCC composed of polygonal hepatocytes with granular eosinophilic cytoplasm shows scattered hyaline globules ▷. Neoplastic cells exhibit large, slightly pleomorphic nuclei with prominent nucleoli ➡. The tumor has solid and acinar growth patterns ➔. No mitotic figures are identified.* ***(Right)*** *Low-power view shows a FL-HCC composed of nests of neoplastic hepatocytes ➡, rimmed by proliferating bile ductules ➔ and intervening islands of normal hepatocytes ▷.*

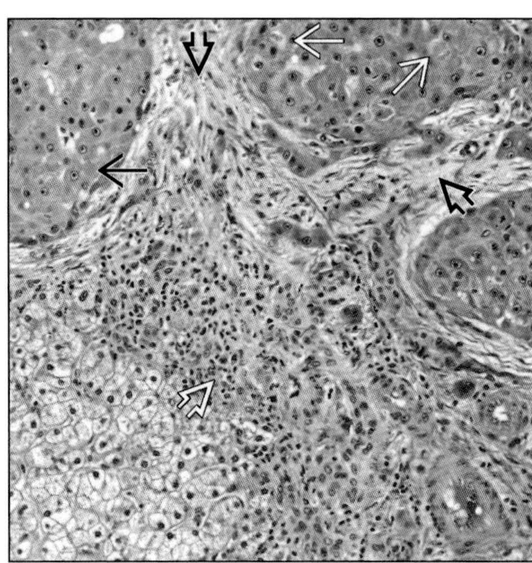

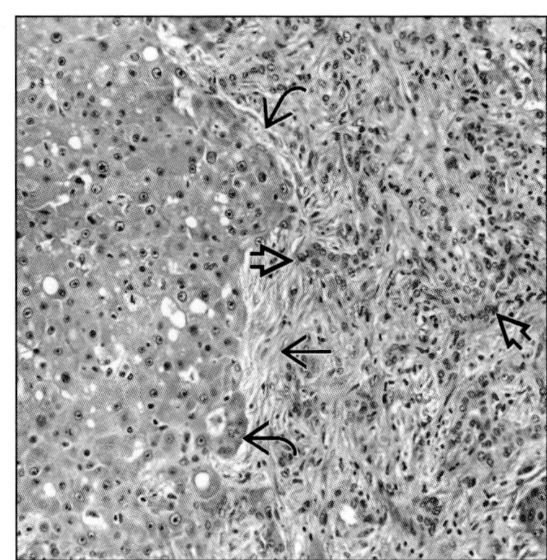

(Left) *FL-HCC shows nests of oncocytic hepatocytes arranged in solid and acinar patterns. Intracanalicular bile ➡ and intracytoplasmic eosinophilic globules ➔ are focally present. This subtype of HCC has abundant lamellar hyaline collagenous bands ➩ interspersed with tumor cells. Note bile duct proliferation ➡.* ***(Right)*** *FL-HCC arranged in solid and vaguely acinar patterns ▷ is seen. Neoplastic cells are surrounded by proliferating bile ducts ➩ and lamellar fibrous bands ➔.*

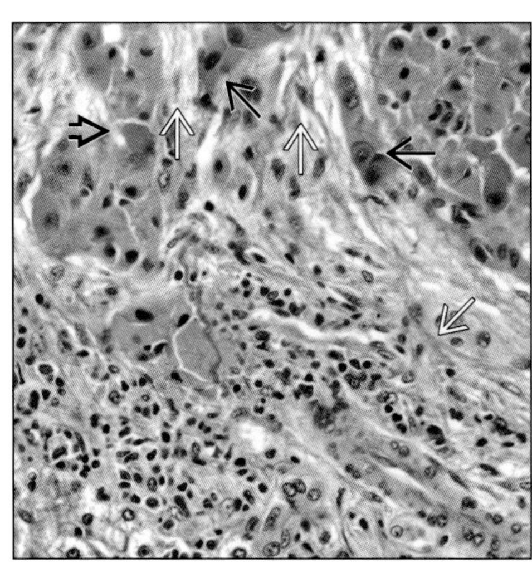

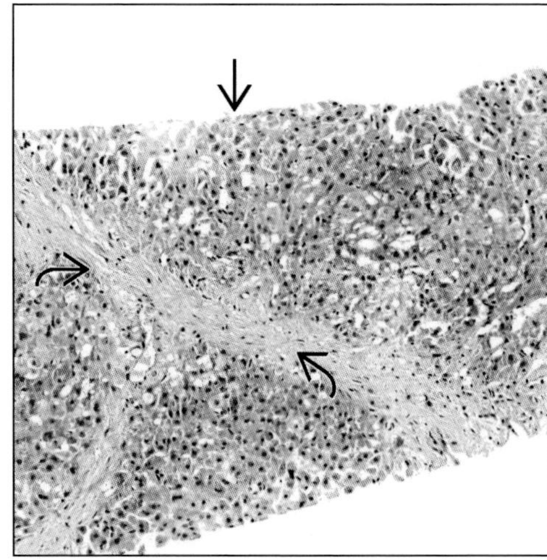

(Left) *Hematoxylin & eosin shows high-power view of a FL-HCC with an intracytoplasmic eosinophilic hyaline globule ➩. These globules are frequently positive for PAS and are PAS-diastase resistant. Lamellar hyalinized fibrous bands ➡ separate neoplastic cells ➔.* ***(Right)*** *Hematoxylin & eosin shows low-power view of a liver core biopsy from a FL-HCC, demonstrating compact nests of neoplastic hepatocytes ➔ intersected by thick, hypocellular fibrous collagenous bands ▷.*

Microscopic Features and Ancillary Techniques

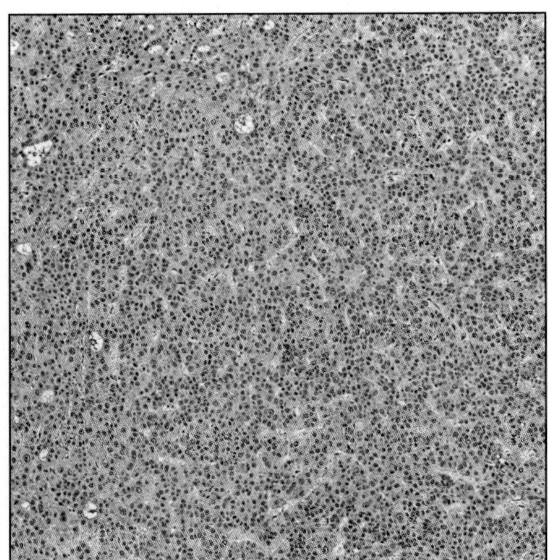

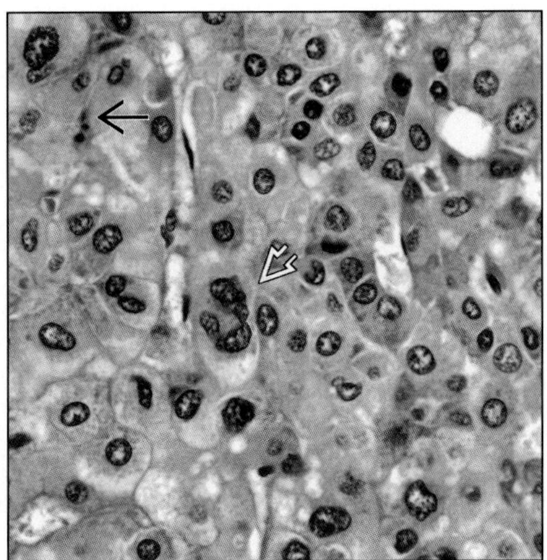

(Left) *Hematoxylin & eosin shows a low-power view of a conventional HCC exhibiting trabecular growth pattern.* ***(Right)*** *Hematoxylin & eosin shows high-power view of a moderately differentiated HCC composed of large, polygonal neoplastic cells with granular eosinophilic cytoplasm and large pleomorphic nuclei featuring coarse, clumped chromatin. A multinucleated tumor giant cell is evident in the center of the field ➡. Characteristic intracanalicular bile is focally present ➔.*

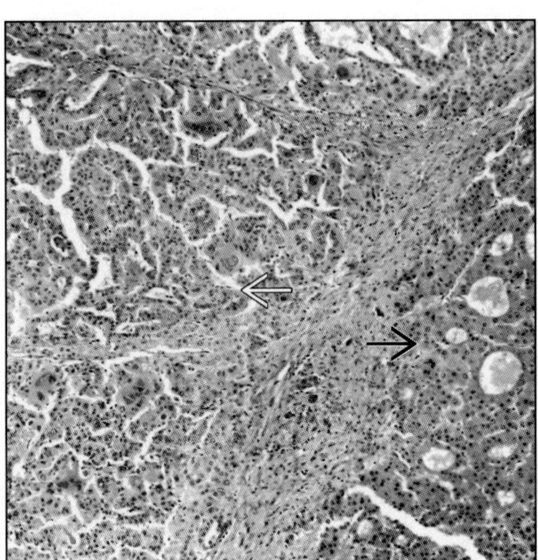

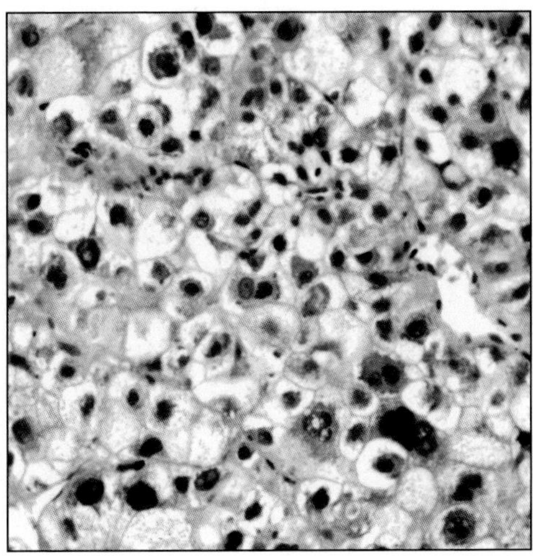

(Left) *Hematoxylin & eosin shows low-power view of a moderately differentiated HCC exhibiting both trabecular ➡ and acinar architecture ➔ in the same tumor.* ***(Right)*** *Hematoxylin & eosin shows a clear cell variant of HCC composed of large polygonal cells with prominent clear cytoplasm, which arises from artifactual loss of cytoplasmic glycogen or fat during sample processing. This variant should be differentiated from metastatic adenocarcinomas exhibiting clear cytoplasm.*

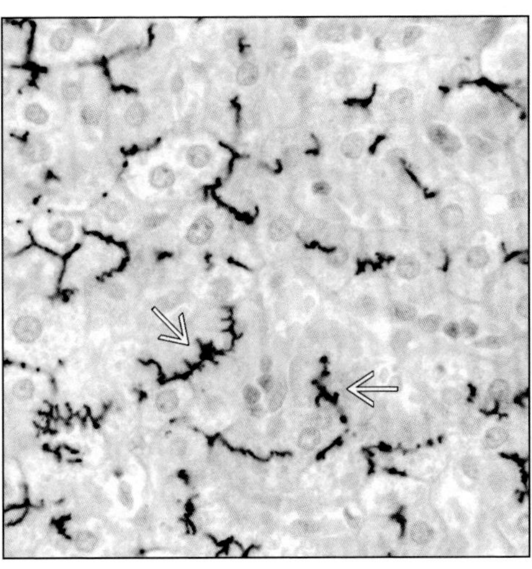

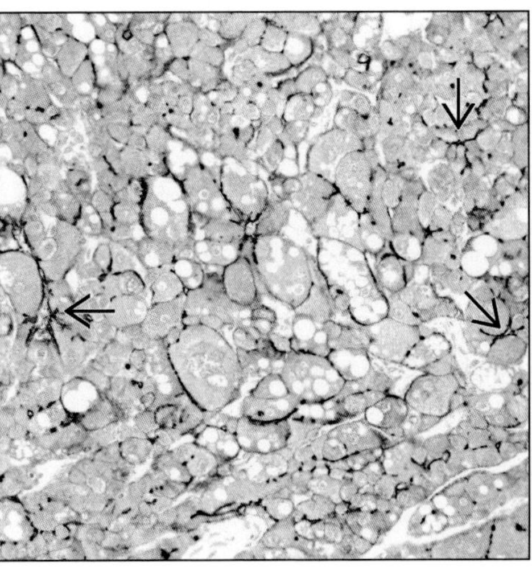

(Left) *Immunohistochemical staining for monoclonal CD10 in a conventional HCC shows a characteristic canalicular staining pattern ➡. Both neoplastic and nonneoplastic hepatocytes may exhibit this staining pattern, which is not observed in metastatic carcinomas or cholangiocarcinomas.* ***(Right)*** *IHC stain for polyclonal CEA in a HCC shows canalicular staining pattern ➔, which may be absent in poorly differentiated tumors.*

PROTOCOL FOR EXOCRINE PANCREAS TUMOR SPECIMENS

Pancreas (Exocrine): Resection

Surgical Pathology Cancer Case Summary (Checklist)

Specimen (select all that apply)

___ Head of pancreas
___ Body of pancreas
___ Tail of pancreas
___ Duodenum
___ Stomach
___ Common bile duct
___ Gallbladder
___ Spleen
___ Adjacent large vessels
  ___ Portal vein
  ___ Superior mesenteric vein
  ___ Other large vessel (specify): ___________________________
___ Other (specify): ___________________________
___ Not specified
___ Cannot be determined

Procedure

___ Pancreaticoduodenectomy (Whipple resection), partial pancreatectomy
___ Pancreatoduodenectomy (Whipple resection), total pancreatectomy
___ Partial pancreatectomy, pancreatic body
___ Partial pancreatectomy, pancreatic tail
___ Other (specify): ___________________________
___ Not specified

Tumor Site (select all that apply)

___ Pancreatic head
___ Uncinate process
___ Pancreatic body
___ Other (specify): ___________________________
___ Not specified

Tumor Size

Greatest dimension: _________ cm
*Additional dimensions: _________ x _________ cm
___ Cannot be determined

Histologic Type (select all that apply)

___ Ductal adenocarcinoma
___ Mucinous noncystic carcinoma
___ Signet ring cell carcinoma
___ Adenosquamous carcinoma
___ Undifferentiated (anaplastic) carcinoma
___ Undifferentiated carcinoma with osteoclast-like giant cells
___ Mixed ductal-endocrine carcinoma
___ Serous cystadenocarcinoma
  ___ Noninvasive
  ___ Invasive
___ Intraductal papillary-mucinous carcinoma
  ___ Noninvasive
  ___ Invasive
___ Acinar cell carcinoma
___ Acinar cell cystadenocarcinoma
___ Mixed acinar-endocrine carcinoma

___ Other (specify): ___________________________

Histologic Grade (ductal carcinoma only)

___ Not applicable
___ GX: Cannot be assessed
___ G1: Well differentiated
___ G2: Moderately differentiated
___ G3: Poorly differentiated
___ G4: Undifferentiated
___ Other (specify): ___________________________

Microscopic Tumor Extension (select all that apply)

___ Cannot be assessed
___ No evidence of primary tumor
___ Carcinoma in situ
___ Tumor is confined to pancreas
___ Tumor invades ampulla of Vater or sphincter of Oddi
___ Tumor invades duodenal wall
___ Tumor invades peripancreatic soft tissues
　　*___ Tumor invades retroperitoneal soft tissue
　　*___ Tumor invades mesenteric adipose tissue
　　*___ Tumor invades mesocolon
　　*___ Tumor invades other peripancreatic soft tissue (specify): ___________________________
　　___ Tumor invades extrapancreatic common bile duct
___ Tumor invades other adjacent organs or structures (specify): ___________________________

Margins (select all that apply)

___ Cannot be assessed
___ Margins uninvolved by invasive carcinoma
　　Distance of invasive carcinoma from closest margin: _________ mm
　　*Specify margin (if possible): ___________________________
___ Margins uninvolved by carcinoma in situ
___ Margin(s) involved by carcinoma in situ
　　___ Carcinoma in situ present at common bile duct margin
　　___ Carcinoma in situ present at pancreatic parenchymal margin
___ Margin(s) involved by invasive carcinoma
　　___ Uncinate process (retroperitoneal) margin (nonperitonealized surface of uncinate process)
　　___ Distal pancreatic margin
　　___ Common bile duct margin
　　___ Proximal pancreatic margin
　　___ Other (specify): ___________________________
*___ Invasive carcinoma involves posterior retroperitoneal surface of pancreas

Treatment Effect (applicable to carcinomas treated with neoadjuvant therapy) (select all that apply)

___ No prior treatment
___ Present
　　*___ No residual tumor (complete response, grade 0)
　　*___ Marked response (grade 1, minimal residual cancer)
　　*___ Moderate response (grade 2)
___ No definite response identified (grade 3, poor or no response)
___ Not known

Lymph-Vascular Invasion

___ Not identified
___ Present
___ Indeterminate

PROTOCOL FOR EXOCRINE PANCREAS TUMOR SPECIMENS

Pathologic Staging (pTNM)

TNM descriptors (required only if applicable) (select all that apply)

___ m (multiple primary tumors)

___ r (recurrent)

___ y (post treatment)

Primary tumor (pT)

___ pTX: Cannot be assessed

___ pT0: No evidence of primary tumor

___ pTis: Carcinoma in situ

___ pT1: Tumor limited to pancreas, ≤ 2 cm in greatest dimension

___ pT2: Tumor limited to pancreas, > 2 cm in greatest dimension

___ pT3: Tumor extends beyond pancreas but without involvement of celiac axis or superior mesenteric artery

___ pT4: Tumor involves celiac axis or superior mesenteric artery

Regional lymph nodes (pN)

___ pNX: Cannot be assessed

___ pN0: No regional lymph node metastasis

___ pN1: Regional lymph node metastasis

___ No nodes submitted or found

Number of lymph nodes examined

Specify: _________

___ Number cannot be determined (explain): __________________________

Number of lymph nodes involved

Specify: _________

___ Number cannot be determined (explain): __________________________

Distant metastasis (pM)

___ Not applicable

___ pM1: Distant metastasis

*Specify site(s), if known: __________________________

**Additional Pathologic Findings (select all that apply)*

*___ None identified

*___ Pancreatic intraepithelial neoplasia (highest grade: PanIN _________)

*___ Chronic pancreatitis

*___ Acute pancreatitis

*___ Other (specify): __________________________

**Ancillary Studies*

*Specify: __________________________

**Clinical History (select all that apply)*

*___ Neoadjuvant therapy

*___ Familial pancreatitis

*___ Familial pancreatic cancer syndrome

*___ Other (specify): __________________________

*___ Not specified

**Data elements with asterisks are not required. These elements may be clinically important but are not yet validated or regularly used in patient management. Adapted with permission from College of American Pathologists, "Protocol for the Examination of Specimens from Patients with Carcinoma of the Exocrine Pancreas." Web posting date February 2011, www.cap.org. Protocol applies to all epithelial tumors of the exocrine pancreas. Endocrine tumors and tumors of the ampulla of Vater are not included.*

Stage Groupings

Stage	Tumor	Node	Metastasis
0	Tis	N0	M0
IA	T1	N0	M0
IB	T2	N0	M0
IIA	T3	N0	M0
IIB	T1	N1	M0
	T2	N1	M0
	T3	N1	M0
III	T4	Any N	M0
IV	Any T	Any N	M1

Adapted from 7th edition AJCC Staging Forms.

PROTOCOL FOR HEPATOBLASTOMA SPECIMENS

Hepatoblastoma (Pediatric Liver)

Resection

Procedure

___ Right lobectomy
___ Extended right lobectomy
___ Medial segmentectomy
___ Left lateral segmentectomy
___ Total left lobectomy
___ Explanted liver
___ Other (specify): ___________________________
___ Not specified

Tumor Site

___ Right lobe
___ Left lobe
___ Right and left lobes
___ Other (specify): ___________________________
___ Not specified

Tumor Size (specify for each nodule)

Greatest dimension: _________ cm
*Additional dimensions: _________ x _________ cm
___ Cannot be assessed

****Tumor Focality (within liver)***

*___Unifocal
*___Multifocal
*___Indeterminate
*___Cannot be assessed

Histologic Type

___ Hepatoblastoma, epithelial type, fetal pattern (mitotically inactive)
___ Hepatoblastoma, epithelial type, fetal pattern (mitotically active)
___ Hepatoblastoma, epithelial type, fetal and embryonal pattern
___ Hepatoblastoma, epithelial type, macrotrabecular pattern
___ Hepatoblastoma, epithelial type, small cell undifferentiated pattern
*Percentage of tumor with this histologic feature: _________
___ Hepatoblastoma, mixed epithelial and mesenchymal type without teratoid features
___ Hepatoblastoma, mixed epithelial and mesenchymal type with teratoid features
___ Hepatoblastoma, rhabdoid type
___ Hepatoblastoma, other (specify): ___________________________
___ Other (specify): ___________________________

Histologic Grade

___ Favorable (purely epithelial, fetal subtype, mitotically inactive with $\leq$ 2 mitoses in 10 40x objective fields; stage 1)
___ Less favorable (all subtypes other than those designated "favorable" or "unfavorable")
___ Unfavorable (small cell undifferentiated or rhabdoid as predominant or sole histopathologic subtype; any stage)

Margins (select all that apply)

Macroscopic extent of tumor at operation
___Tumor extends into adjacent organ(s)
___Tumor extends into adjacent soft tissue
___ Diaphragm
___ Abdominal wall
___ Other (specify): ___________________________
___ Intraoperative tumor spill

Resection margin

___ Cannot be assessed
___ Uninvolved by invasive tumor
Distance of invasive tumor from closest margin: ________ mm OR ________ cm
Specify margin(s): ___________________________
___ Involved by invasive tumor
Specify margin(s): ___________________________

Capsular surface
___ Cannot be assessed
___ Uninvolved by invasive tumor
Distance of invasive tumor from closest surface: ________ mm OR ________ cm
Specify margin: ___________________________
___ Involved by invasive tumor

*Lymph-Vascular Invasion (select all that apply)

*___ Not identified
*___ Portal vein invasion present
*___ Hepatic vein invasion present
*___ Present within tumor nodules
*___ Present in vessels of parenchyma outside of tumor nodules
*___ Indeterminate

Lymph Nodes

___ Cannot be assessed
___ Regional lymph node metastasis not identified
___ Regional lymph node metastasis present
Specify location, if known: ___________________________
Specify: Number of lymph nodes examined: ________
Number of lymph nodes involved by tumor: ________

Distant Metastases

___ Not applicable
___ Distant metastasis present (includes metastasis to lymph nodes in the following locations: Inferior phrenic, distal to hilum, hepatoduodenal ligament, or caval region)
*Specify site(s), if known: ___________________________

Staging (Children's Oncology Group) (select all that apply)

___ Stage I
Complete resection, margins grossly and microscopically negative for tumor
___ Stage II
Microscopic residual tumor present
___ Microscopic residual tumor present at hepatic resection margin
___ Microscopic residual tumor present at extrahepatic resection margin
___ Intraoperative tumor spill
___ Stage III
Gross residual tumor present
___ Macroscopic tumor visible at resection margin(s)
___ Lymph node metastasis present
___ Stage IV
Metastatic disease present
___ Primary tumor completely resected
___ Primary tumor not completely resected

*Additional Pathologic Findings (select all that apply)

*___ None identified
*___ Cirrhosis/fibrosis
*___ Iron overload
*___ Hepatitis (specify type): ___________________________
*___ Other (specify): ___________________________

Other (specify): ____________________

**Data elements with asterisks are not required. These elements may be clinically important but they are not yet validated or regularly used in patient management. Adapted with permission from College of American Pathologists, "Protocol for the Examination of Specimens from Patients with Hepatoblastoma." Web posting date October 2009, www.cap.org.*

Hepatocellular Carcinoma: Hepatic Resection

Surgical Pathology Cancer Case Summary (Checklist)

Specimen (select all that apply)

___ Liver

___ Gallbladder

___ Other (specify): ___________________________

___ Not specified

Procedure (select all that apply)

___ Wedge resection

___ Partial hepatectomy

  *___ Major hepatectomy (≥ 3 segments)

  *___ Minor hepatectomy (< 3 segments)

___ Other (specify): ___________________________

___ Not specified

Tumor Size

Greatest dimension: _________ cm

*Additional dimensions: _________ x _________ cm

___ Cannot be determined

Tumor Focality

___ Solitary (specify location): ___________________________

___ Multiple (specify location): ___________________________

Histologic Type

___ Hepatocellular carcinoma

___ Fibrolamellar hepatocellular carcinoma

___ Undifferentiated carcinoma

___ Other (specify): ___________________________

___ Carcinoma, type cannot be determined

Histologic Grade

___ Not applicable

___ GX: Cannot be assessed

___ GI: Well differentiated

___ GII: Moderately differentiated

___ GIII: Poorly differentiated

___ GIV: Undifferentiated/anaplastic

___ Other (specify): ___________________________

Tumor Extension (select all that apply)

___ Tumor confined to liver

___ Tumor involves a major branch of portal vein

___ Tumor involves 1 or more hepatic vein(s)

___ Tumor involves visceral peritoneum

___ Tumor directly invades gallbladder

___ Tumor directly invades other adjacent organs (specify): ___________________________

Margins (select all that apply)

Parenchymal margin

___ Cannot be assessed

___ Uninvolved by invasive carcinoma

  Distance of invasive carcinoma from closest margin: _________ mm

  Specify margin: ___________________________

___ Involved by invasive carcinoma

Other margin

Specify margin: ___________________________

PROTOCOL FOR HEPATOCELLULAR CARCINOMA SPECIMENS

____ Cannot be assessed
____ Uninvolved by invasive carcinoma
____ Involved by invasive carcinoma

Lymph-Vascular Invasion

Macroscopic venous (large vessel) invasion (V)
____ Not identified
____ Present
____ Indeterminate

Microscopic (small vessel) invasion (L)
____ Not identified
____ Present
____ Indeterminate

**Perineural Invasion*

*____ Not identified
*____ Present
*____ Indeterminate

Pathologic Staging (pTNM)

TNM descriptors (required only if applicable) (select all that apply)
____ m (multiple primary tumors)
____ r (recurrent)
____ y (post treatment)

Primary tumor (pT)
____ pTX: Cannot be assessed
____ pT0: No evidence of primary tumor
____ pT1: Solitary tumor without vascular invasion
____ pT2: Solitary tumor with vascular invasion or multiple tumors, none > 5 cm
____ pT3a: Multiple tumors > 5 cm
____ pT3b: Single tumor or multiple tumors of any size involving a major branch of portal vein or hepatic veins
____ pT4: Tumor(s) with direct invasion of adjacent organs other than gallbladder or with perforation of visceral peritoneum

Regional lymph nodes (pN)
____ pNX: Cannot be assessed
____ pN0: No regional lymph node metastasis
____ pN1: Regional lymph node metastasis
____ No nodes submitted or found

Number of lymph nodes examined
Specify: ________
____ Number cannot be determined (explain): ________________________

Number of lymph nodes involved
Specify: ________
____ Number cannot be determined (explain): ________________________

Distant metastasis (pM)
____ Not applicable
____ pM1: Distant metastasis
*Specify site(s), if known: ________________________

**Additional Pathologic Findings (select all that apply)*

*Fibrosis score
*____ Cirrhosis/severe fibrosis (Ishak score 5-6) (F1)
*____ None to moderate fibrosis (Ishak score 0-4) (F2)
*____ Hepatocellular dysplasia
*____ Low-grade dysplastic nodule
*____ High-grade dysplastic nodule
*____ Steatosis
*____ Iron overload

*____ Chronic hepatitis (specify etiology): __________________________

*____ Other (specify): __________________________

*____ None identified

*Ancillary Studies

*Specify: __________________________

*Clinical History (select all that apply)

*____ Cirrhosis

*____ Hepatitis C infection

*____ Hepatitis B infection

*____ Alcoholic liver disease

*____ Obesity

*____ Hereditary hemochromatosis

*____ Other (specify): __________________________

*____ Not known

**Data elements with asterisks are not required. These elements may be clinically important but are not yet validated or regularly used in patient management. Adapted with permission from College of American Pathologists, "Protocol for the Examination of Specimens from Patients with Hepatocellular Carcinoma." Web posting date February 2011, www.cap.org.*

Stage Groupings

Stage	Tumor	Node	Metastasis
I	T1	N0	M0
II	T2	N0	M0
IIIA	T3a	N0	M0
IIIB	T3b	N0	M0
IIIC	T4	N0	M0
IVA	Any T	N1	M0
IVB	Any T	Any N	M1

Adapted from 7th edition AJCC Staging Forms.

Genitourinary

Neoplasm, Benign

Neoplasm, Malignant Primary

Protocol for the Examination of Specimens from Patients with Wilms Tumors

Protocol for the Examination of Specimens from Patients with Malignant Germ Cell and Sex Cord-Stromal Tumors of the Testis

Protocol for the Examination of Specimens from Patients with Carcinoma of the Ovary

MESOBLASTIC NEPHROMA

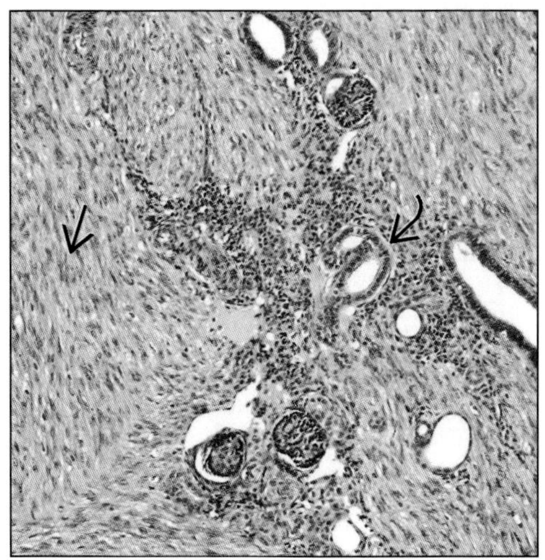

Low-power view shows bland uniform spindle cells ⇒ (characteristic of classic type of CMN) infiltrating and entrapping renal structures ⇒.

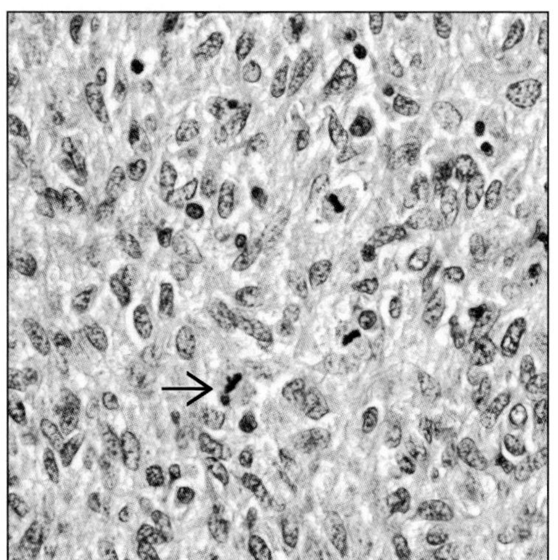

High-power view shows plump spindle cells with atypia and a high mitotic rate ⇒, characteristic of cellular variant of CMN.

TERMINOLOGY

Abbreviations

- Congenital mesoblastic nephroma (CMN)

Definitions

- Spindle cell neoplasm of kidney, composed of myofibroblasts
- Subtypes/variants: Classic, cellular, and mixed

ETIOLOGY/PATHOGENESIS

Genetics

- Classic variant has no consistent genetic abnormality and may represent infantile fibromatosis of kidney
- Cellular variant has t(12;15)(p13;q25) chromosomal translocation resulting in *ETV6-NTRK3* gene fusion
  - Same translocation as seen in infantile fibrosarcoma
- No gene fusion demonstrated in mixed pattern
- Occasional association of CMN with Beckwith-Wiedemann syndrome

CLINICAL ISSUES

Presentation

- Most common renal tumor of infancy
  - Presents as abdominal mass; may be associated with polyhydramnios, premature delivery, and nonimmune hydrops
  - Hypertension (due to renin production by entrapped renal elements) may be present

Treatment

- Surgical approaches
  - Complete nephrectomy is necessary due to infiltrative nature of classic variant

Prognosis

- Majority cured with surgery and have excellent outcome
  - Recurrences and metastases occur in ~ 5-10% of patients, risk factors for which are incomplete excision, cellular histology, stage III or higher, and involvement of intrarenal or sinus vessels

MACROSCOPIC FEATURES

General Features

- Solitary, unilateral, characteristically whorled or trabeculated; gray-white to yellow with rather indistinct tumor-kidney interface and softly bulging cut surface
- Cysts, hemorrhage, and necrosis common and have no prognostic significance
- Tumor tends to arise centrally within kidney and extensively involves renal sinus

Sections to Be Submitted

- Tumor-kidney interface, medial extent of tumor
- 1 section per cm of maximum tumor dimension is recommended

MICROSCOPIC PATHOLOGY

Histologic Features

- Classic variant (24% of cases): Intersecting bundles of spindle cells with minimal atypia and infrequent mitoses
  - Tumor infiltrates extensively into adjacent renal parenchyma
    - Thus, wide margins are necessary
  - Dysplastic trapped tubules and islands of cartilage are often seen
- Cellular variant (66% of cases): Pushing border, dense cells, mitoses, and "sarcomatous" appearance

MESOBLASTIC NEPHROMA

Key Facts

Terminology
- Congenital mesoblastic nephroma (CMN)
- Spindle cell neoplasm of kidney, composed of myofibroblasts
- Subtypes/variants: Classic, cellular, and mixed

Etiology/Pathogenesis
- Cellular variant has t(12;15)(p13;q25) chromosomal translocation resulting in *ETV6-NTRK3* gene fusion
  - Same translocation as seen in infantile fibrosarcoma
- Occasional association of CMN with Beckwith-Wiedemann syndrome

Clinical Issues
- Most common renal tumor of infancy
- Majority cured with surgery and have excellent outcome
- Increased risk of local recurrence with incomplete excision

Microscopic Pathology
- Classic variant (24% of cases): Intersecting bundles of spindle cells with minimal atypia and infrequent mitoses
- Cellular variant (66% of cases): Pushing border, dense cells, mitoses, and "sarcomatous" appearance

Top Differential Diagnoses
- Clear cell sarcoma of kidney
- Wilms tumor
- Metanephric fibroma
- Rhabdoid tumor of kidney

- Mixed (10-20% of cases): Both histologic patterns seen in different areas

Predominant Pattern/Injury Type
- Infiltrative
  - Nonencapsulated tumor composed of spindle cells

Predominant Cell/Compartment Type
- Myofibroblast

DIFFERENTIAL DIAGNOSIS

Metanephric Fibroma
- Metanephric fibroma has tubules with surrounding loose mesenchyme as integral part of tumor
  - Classic CMN entraps renal tubules

Clear Cell Sarcoma of Kidney (CCSK)
- Cellular variant of CMN lacks "chicken-wire" vascular pattern of CCSK
- CMN is positive for desmin &/or actin-sm and vimentin; CCSK is positive for vimentin only
- Presence of renal dysplasia (e.g., cartilage) diagnostic for CMN
- Presence of variant patterns of CCSK (e.g., myxoid, sclerosing, epithelioid, palisading)
- > 1 year old and presence of metastases (other than lung) support CCSK

Wilms Tumor
- Very rare in infants, especially those under 6 months of age
- Blastema-predominant WT has very high mitotic rate, with numerous apoptotic cells
- Compressed pseudocapsule in contrast to extensively infiltrating CMN

Rhabdoid Tumor of Kidney
- Occasionally CMN can have unusually prominent nuclei, in which case immunohistochemical stain for INI1 (BAF47), positive nuclear staining in CMN, and absent staining in rhabdoid tumor are diagnostic

DIAGNOSTIC CHECKLIST

Clinically Relevant Pathologic Features
- Invasive pattern and subtype

Pathologic Interpretation Pearls
- Vast majority of patients < 1 year old, at which age other pediatric renal tumors are less common
- Cellular variant has sarcomatous appearance but complete resection is often curative
- Surgical margins need to be evaluated carefully, especially medial (renal hilar) margin

SELECTED REFERENCES

1. Bandyopadhyay R et al: Unusual morphology in mesoblastic nephroma. Pediatr Surg Int. 25(1):109-12, 2009
2. Gupta R et al: Cellular mesoblastic nephroma in an infant: report of the cytologic diagnosis of a rare paediatric renal tumor. Diagn Cytopathol. 37(5):377-80, 2009
3. Sebire NJ et al: Paediatric renal tumours: recent developments, new entities and pathological features. Histopathology. 54(5):516-28, 2009
4. Barroca H: Fine needle biopsy and genetics, two allied weapons in the diagnosis, prognosis, and target therapeutics of solid pediatric tumors. Diagn Cytopathol. 36(9):678-84, 2008
5. van den Heuvel-Eibrink MM et al: Characteristics and survival of 750 children diagnosed with a renal tumor in the first seven months of life: a collaborative study by the SIOP/GPOH/SFOP, NWTSG, and UKCCSG Wilms tumor study groups. Pediatr Blood Cancer. 50(6):1130-4, 2008
6. Ahmed HU et al: Part I: Primary malignant non-Wilms' renal tumours in children. Lancet Oncol. 8(8):730-7, 2007
7. Huang CC et al: Classification of malignant pediatric renal tumors by gene expression. Pediatr Blood Cancer. 46(7):728-38, 2006
8. Bisceglia M et al: Congenital mesoblastic nephroma: report of a Case with review of the most significant literature. Pathol Res Pract. 196(3):199-204, 2000
9. Schild RL et al: Diagnosis of a fetal mesoblastic nephroma by 3D-ultrasound. Ultrasound Obstet Gynecol. 15(6):533-6, 2000

MESOBLASTIC NEPHROMA

Gross and Microscopic Features

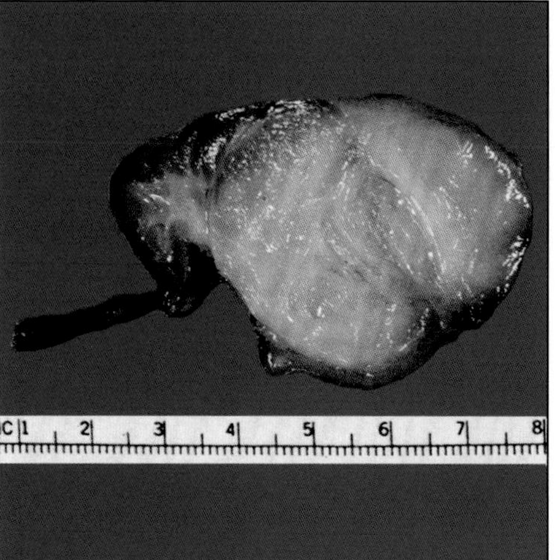

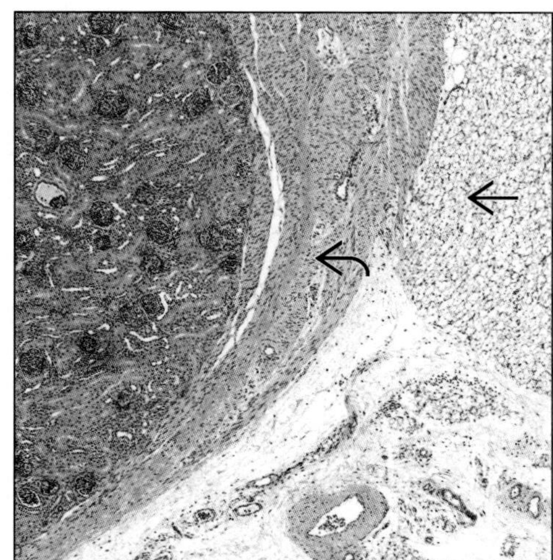

(Left) *Gross photograph shows a nephrectomy specimen from a 7 week old. The cut surface shows a white-tan infiltrating tumor (classic variant of CMN) with residual renal parenchyma seen on the left.* ***(Right)*** *This low-power magnification shows a classic variant of congenital mesoblastic nephroma infiltrating fat → and growing over the capsule ↪.*

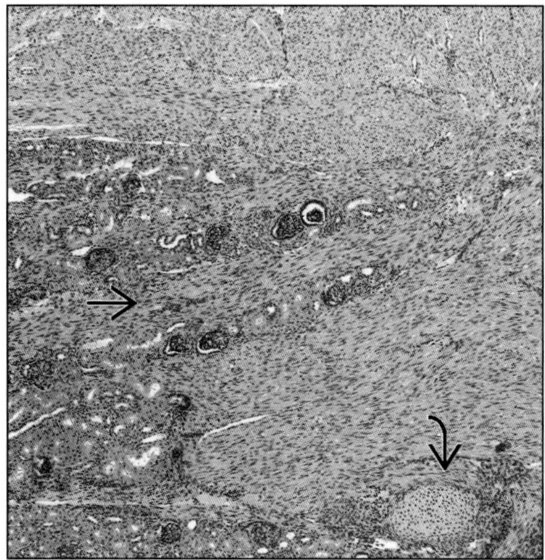

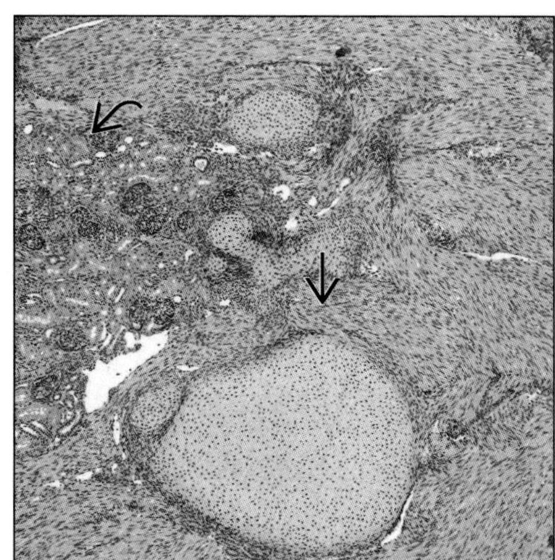

(Left) *Low-power view shows classic variant of CMN infiltrating into adjacent renal parenchyma, forming finger-like projections →. Metaplastic cartilage ↪ is present on the lower right.* ***(Right)*** *Islands of metaplastic cartilage → are present in this classic variant of congenital mesoblastic nephroma. Adjacent immature renal parenchyma ↪ is seen on the left.*

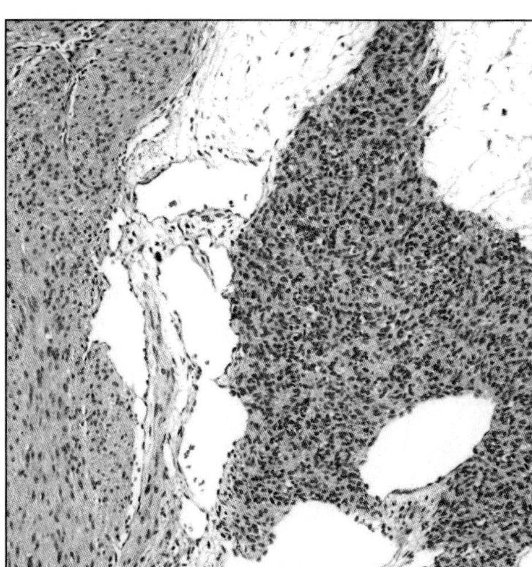

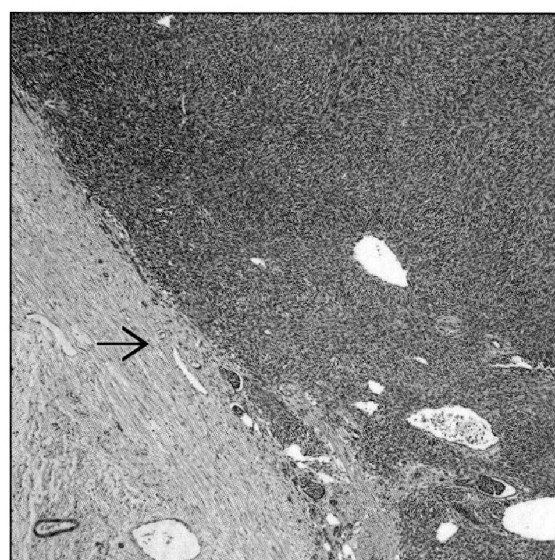

(Left) *Mixed classic (left) and cellular (right) congenital mesoblastic patterns are seen on this intermediate-power view.* ***(Right)*** *This low-power view of a cellular variant of congenital mesoblastic nephroma shows the pushing edge of the tumor → in contrast with the infiltrating edge of a classic variant.*

Differential Diagnosis

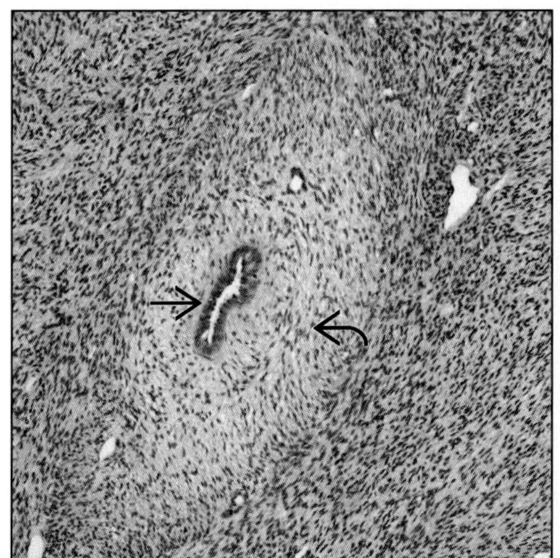

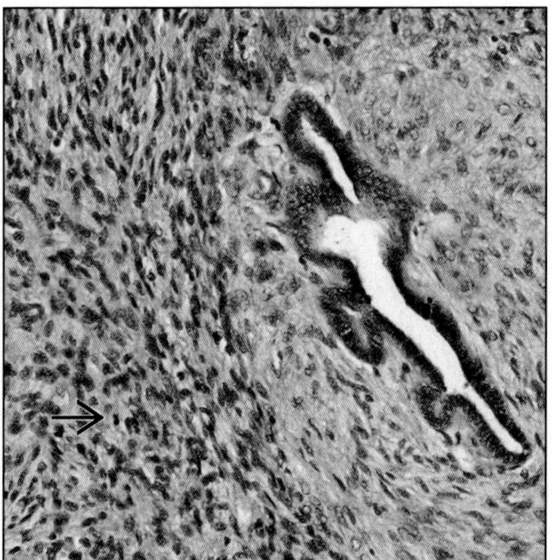

(Left) *This photomicrograph of metanephric fibroma shows a cellular spindle cell tumor with a tubule ➔ surrounded by loose mesenchyme ↩.* ***(Right)*** *At high power, mitotic figure ➔ can be seen in the cellular spindle cell component in this case of metanephric adenoma.*

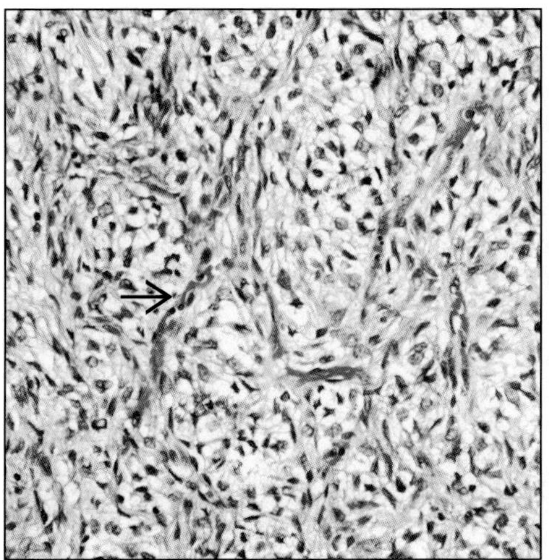

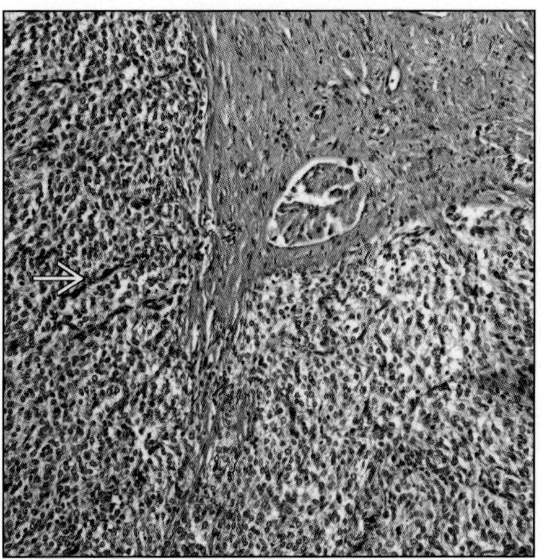

(Left) *This photomicrograph shows the classic pale cells separated by a fine network of capillaries ➔ in a case of clear cell sarcoma of the kidney.* ***(Right)*** *This example of a clear cell sarcoma is a tumor lacks the typical clear cell appearance but still shows the classic vascular pattern ➔.*

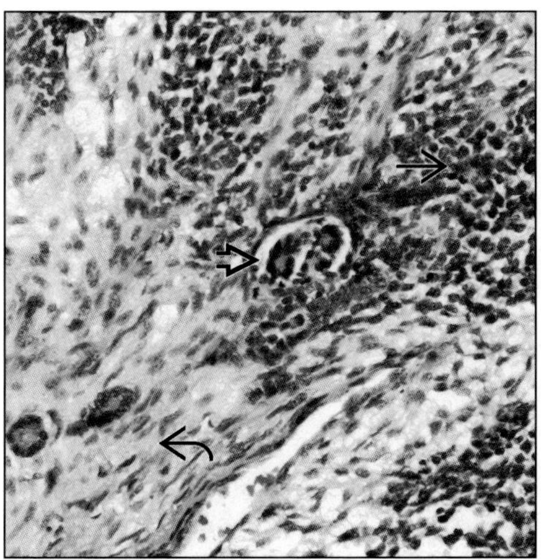

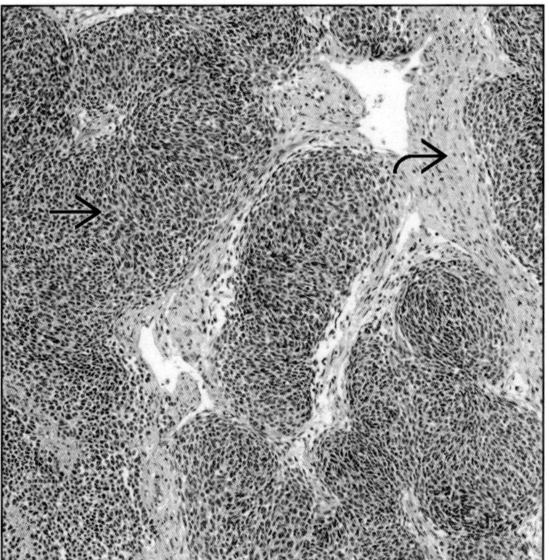

(Left) *This Wilms tumor shows the classic triphasic pattern with blastema ➔, epithelial components ⇨, and stroma ↩.* ***(Right)*** *This is a blastema-predominant ➔ Wilms tumor with a minor component of stroma ↪, forming darker and lighter areas in contrast to the uniform appearance seen in congenital mesoblastic nephroma.*

NEPHROGENIC REST AND NEPHROBLASTOMATOSIS

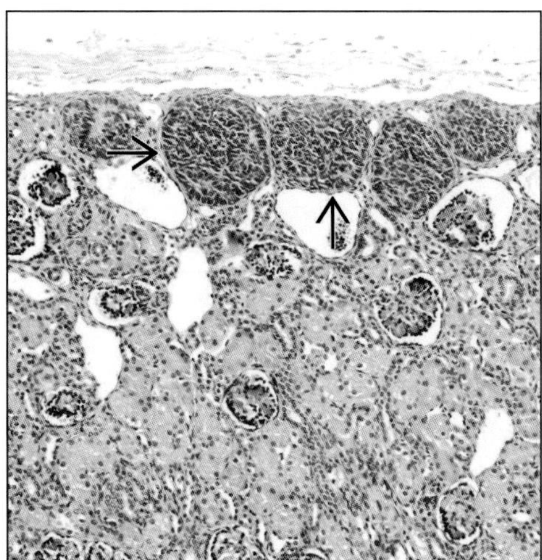

Intermediate-power view of an uninvolved kidney from a 3 year old with Wilms tumor shows several perilobar rests in a row under the capsule ➡, which are unencapsulated and noninfiltrative.

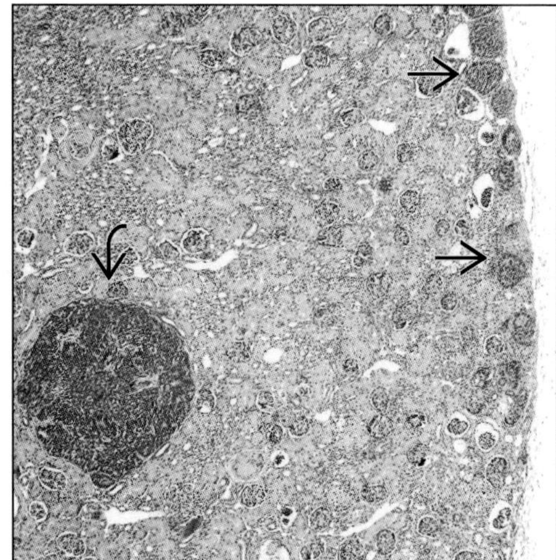

Low-power view shows perilobar nephrogenic rests in the subcapsular area ➡ and a focus of intralobar rest in the deep cortex ➡. The foci are expansile (hyperplastic rests).

TERMINOLOGY

Abbreviations

- Intralobar nephrogenic rest (ILNR)
- Perilobar nephrogenic rest (PLNR)

Definitions

- Abnormally persistent foci of embryonal cells in kidney with the potential to develop into Wilms tumor (WT)
- When multifocal or diffuse, term nephroblastomatosis is used

ETIOLOGY/PATHOGENESIS

Developmental Anomaly

- ILNR and PLNR have different genetic defects
- Perilobar rests occur in hemihypertrophy, Beckwith-Wiedemann syndrome, some sporadic tumors, and occasionally with cystic renal dysplasia and rarely with congenital mesoblastic nephroma
- Intralobar rests are seen with WAGR (Wilms tumor, aniridia, genitourinary malformation, mental retardation) and Denys-Drash syndromes
- Both subtypes thought to be precursor lesion of Wilms tumor

CLINICAL ISSUES

Presentation

- Abnormal imaging finding or, more often, found in kidneys resected for Wilms tumor

Natural History

- Rests may be dormant, sclerosing, or hyperplastic
- Majority regress over time and become fibrotic
- Some give rise to Wilms tumor
- Massive nephroblastomatosis may also regress over time
- When found in nephrectomy done for Wilms tumor, indicates increased risk of Wilms tumor developing in contralateral kidney; close follow-up with radiologic imaging of remaining kidney is needed

Treatment

- Drugs
  - Massive bilateral nephroblastomatosis may require chemotherapy
  - Nephrogenic rests require no treatment

Prognosis

- Massive nephroblastomatosis responds well to chemotherapy

MACROSCOPIC FEATURES

General Features

- Nephroblastomatosis gives rise to reniform enlargement of kidney(s) appearing as pale, markedly thickened cortex on cut surface
- Perilobar nephrogenic rests appear as small (generally < 1 cm), round to oval, pale areas in subcapsular region
- Intralobar nephrogenic rests appear as pale, ill-defined areas in deeper cortex

MICROSCOPIC PATHOLOGY

Histologic Features

- Perilobar rests are unencapsulated but well defined and round to oval in shape
- Ill-defined intralobar rests intermingle with renal parenchyma
- Consist of variable amounts of blastemic, epithelial, and stromal components which, on high power, may be indistinguishable from Wilms tumor
- Hyperplastic rests have frequent mitoses and apoptotic cells, but no frank necrosis or anaplasia

Key Facts

Terminology

- Intralobar nephrogenic rest (ILNR) and perilobar nephrogenic rest (PLNR)
- Abnormally persistent foci of embryonal cells in kidney with potential to develop into Wilms tumor (WT); when multifocal or diffuse, term nephroblastomatosis is used

Clinical Issues

- Rests may be dormant, sclerosing, or hyperplastic
- Some give rise to Wilms tumor

Microscopic Pathology

- Consist of variable amounts of blastemic, epithelial, and stromal components which, on high power, may be indistinguishable from Wilms tumor

Top Differential Diagnoses

- Wilms tumor

Predominant Cell/Compartment Type

- Renal cortex, perilobar or intralobar

DIFFERENTIAL DIAGNOSIS

Wilms Tumor

- Larger (usually 5 cm or more) and often has compressed connective tissue forming pseudocapsule as well as areas of necrosis &/or hemorrhage
- Invasion into veins, renal capsule, or hilar fat supports diagnosis of Wilms tumor

DIAGNOSTIC CHECKLIST

Pathologic Interpretation Pearls

- Triphasic composition is similar to Wilms tumor
- Most nephrogenic rests are small, unencapsulated lesions

SELECTED REFERENCES

1. Vicens J et al: Diffuse hyperplastic perilobar nephroblastomatosis. Pediatr Dev Pathol. 12(3):237-8, 2009
2. Witt O et al: 13-cis retinoic acid treatment of a patient with chemotherapy refractory nephroblastomatosis. J Pediatr Hematol Oncol. 31(4):296-9, 2009
3. Alessandri JL et al: Perlman syndrome: report, prenatal findings and review. Am J Med Genet A. 146A(19):2532-7, 2008
4. Fukuzawa R et al: Wilms tumour histology is determined by distinct types of precursor lesions and not epigenetic changes. J Pathol. 215(4):377-87, 2008
5. Owens CM et al: Bilateral disease and new trends in Wilms tumour. Pediatr Radiol. 38(1):30-9, 2008
6. Vuononvirta R et al: Perilobar nephrogenic rests are nonobligate molecular genetic precursor lesions of insulin-like growth factor-II-associated Wilms tumors. Clin Cancer Res. 14(23):7635-44, 2008
7. Wagner N et al: A novel Wilms' tumor 1 gene mutation in a child with severe renal dysfunction and persistent renal blastema. Pediatr Nephrol. 23(9):1445-53, 2008
8. Fukuzawa R et al: Molecular pathology and epidemiology of nephrogenic rests and Wilms tumors. J Pediatr Hematol Oncol. 29(9):589-94, 2007
9. Perlman EJ et al: Hyperplastic perilobar nephroblastomatosis: long-term survival of 52 patients. Pediatr Blood Cancer. 46(2):203-21, 2006
10. Perlman EJ: Pediatric renal tumors: practical updates for the pathologist. Pediatr Dev Pathol. 8(3):320-38, 2005
11. Cozzi F et al: Conservative management of hyperplastic and multicentric nephroblastomatosis. J Urol. 172(3):1066-9; discussion 1069-70, 2004
12. Hennigar RA et al: Clinicopathologic features of nephrogenic rests and nephroblastomatosis. Adv Anat Pathol. 8(5):276-89, 2001

IMAGE GALLERY

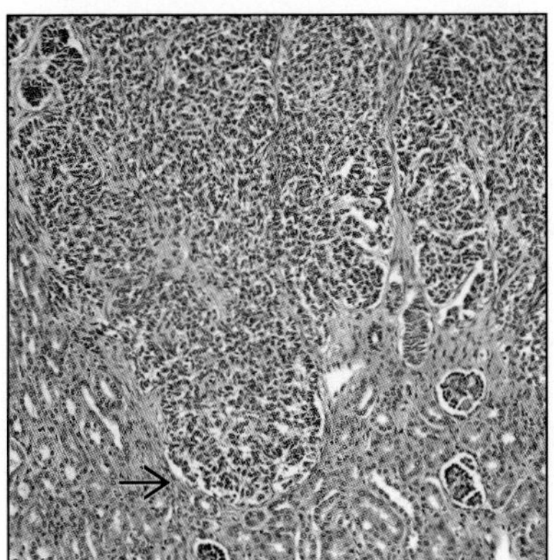

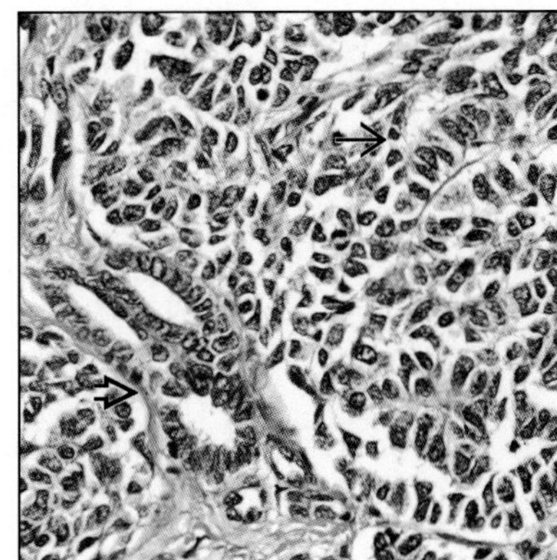

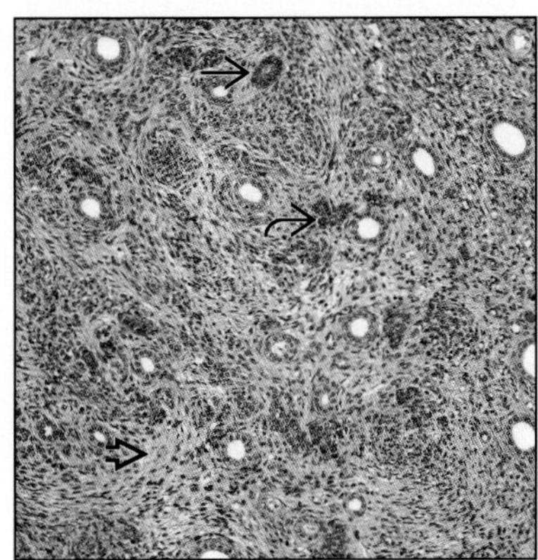

(Left) *Low power from a 1 year old with bilateral enlargement of kidneys shows massive nephroblastomatosis with an infiltrative border ⇒. Note absence of pseudocapsule.* ***(Center)*** *High power of hyperplastic nephrogenic rest shows blastema ⇒ and epithelial components ⇒, which are indistinguishable from Wilms tumor at this power.* ***(Right)*** *Intermediate power shows intralobar rest composed of blastema ⇒, epithelium ⇒, and stroma ⇒, intermingled with renal tissue.*

RHABDOID TUMOR

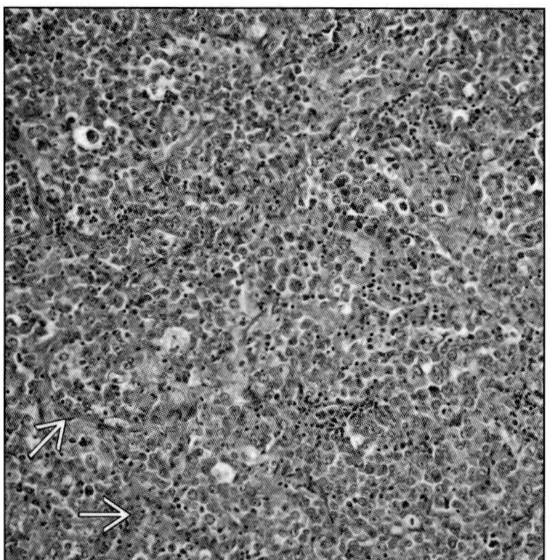

Sheets of loosely cohesive tumor cells with large nuclei and abundant eosinophilic cytoplasm are shown. A delicate network of fibrovascular septae ➡ can also be appreciated.

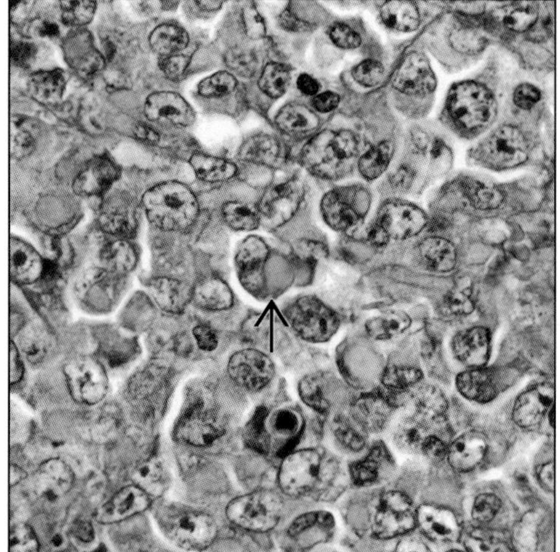

High-power view highlights mononuclear tumor cells with pleomorphic nuclei, conspicuous nucleoli, and intracytoplasmic eosinophilic hyaline inclusions ➡.

TERMINOLOGY

Synonyms

- Malignant rhabdoid tumor
- Rhabdomyosarcomatoid neoplasm
- Rhabdomyosarcomatous Wilms tumor
  - Originally thought to represent a variant of Wilms tumor

Definitions

- Highly malignant pediatric tumor of unknown origin with extremely poor prognosis
- Represents approximately 2% of pediatric renal neoplasms
- Similar tumor described in brain (atypical teratoid/rhabdoid tumor)

CLINICAL ISSUES

Epidemiology

- Age
  - 0-9 years (mean: 16.8 months)
  - > 90% diagnosed by 3 years of age
- Gender
  - M > F (1.5:1)

Site

- Kidney
  - Tumor originally described in kidney
  - Later recognized in extrarenal locations
    - Central nervous system (atypical teratoid/rhabdoid tumor)
    - Soft tissue

Presentation

- Abdominal fullness
- Large bulky abdominal mass
- Hypercalcemia
  - Tumor production of parathyroid hormone-related protein or prostaglandin E2
  - Corrects with removal of tumor
  - No prognostic significance
- Fever
- Hematuria
- High tumor stage at presentation
  - Up to 75% present with stage III, IV, or V disease
- Association with early brain metastases and primary intracranial masses
  - Medulloblastoma
  - Primitive neuroectodermal tumor
  - Cerebellar and brainstem astrocytomas
  - Ependymoma
- Frequent metastases to lung, abdomen, liver, brain, and bone

Treatment

- Surgical approaches
  - Nephrectomy
- Radiation
  - To tumor bed
- Multi-agent chemotherapy
  - Often have poor response
- Combination of surgery, multi-agent chemotherapy, and radiotherapy coupled with autologous stem cell transplantation appears promising

Prognosis

- Extremely poor prognosis with aggressive behavior
  - Mortality rate > 80%
- 24% 5-year survival rate
  - Increasing survival with increasing age at diagnosis
- Predictors of poor prognosis include
  - Younger age at diagnosis
  - Higher tumor stage
  - Presence of CNS lesions

IMAGE FINDINGS

General Features

- Large intrarenal mass involving renal hilum

RHABDOID TUMOR

Key Facts

Terminology

- Highly malignant pediatric tumor of unknown origin with extremely poor prognosis

Clinical Issues

- > 90% diagnosed by 3 years of age
- High tumor stage at presentation
- Many present with concurrent CNS neoplasm

Macroscopic Features

- Well circumscribed and unencapsulated
- Foci of hemorrhage and necrosis

Microscopic Pathology

- Sheets of monotonous, loosely cohesive large ovoid to polygonal cells
- Tumor cells exhibit rhabdoid features
  - Intracytoplasmic inclusions

Ancillary Tests

- SNF5 (INI1/BAF47) negative immunostaining considered specific
  - Reliable surrogate marker of *SNF5/INI1* gene deletion or inactivating mutations

Top Differential Diagnoses

- Epithelioid sarcomas
  - Typically arises in distal extremities of adults
  - Frequent *SNF5/INI1* gene inactivation results in loss of SNF5 nuclear immunostaining
- Wilms tumor (nephroblastoma) with rhabdoid features
  - Most common malignant renal neoplasm of children
  - Positive SNF5 nuclear immunostaining

- Rhabdoid tumor is often indistinguishable from Wilms tumor
  - May see subcapsular fluid collection, which is unusual in Wilms tumor
- Invasion of renal vein and inferior vena cava may be seen

Ultrasonographic Findings

- Large lobulated mass
- Heterogeneous echogenicity

MR Findings

- Large centrally located lobulated tumor
- Areas of hemorrhage and necrosis surround tumor lobules

CT Findings

- Large heterogeneous mass that replaces or involves kidney

MACROSCOPIC FEATURES

General Features

- Well-circumscribed and unencapsulated
- Soft, pale, gray-tan bulging cut surface
- Foci of hemorrhage and necrosis
- Involves renal medulla
- Frequently involves renal vein

Size

- 3-17 cm in diameter (mean: 9.6 cm)
- May replace entire kidney

MICROSCOPIC PATHOLOGY

Microscopic Features

- Sheets of monotonous loosely cohesive large, ovoid to polygonal cells
  - High nuclear grade
    - Moderate nuclear pleomorphism
    - Vesicular chromatin
    - Prominent central eosinophilic nucleoli
- Tumor cells exhibit rhabdoid features
  - Abundant eosinophilic cytoplasm
  - Intracytoplasmic inclusions
    - Tangled intermediate filaments
- Frequent mitotic figures
- Infiltrative and diffuse pattern of growth
  - Often replaces entire kidney
  - Alveolar, trabecular, and dyscohesive patterns may also be seen

Histologic Variants

- 1 to multiple variants may be present with classical pattern
- Most comprise only a minority of overall tumor
- Variant patterns include
  - Sclerosing (most common)
  - Epithelioid
  - Spindled
  - Lymphomatoid
  - Vascular
  - Pseudopapillary
  - Cystic

ANCILLARY TESTS

Immunohistochemistry

- SNF5 (INI1/BAF47) negativity considered to be specific among malignant rhabdoid tumors
  - Reliable surrogate marker of *SNF5/INI1* gene deletions or inactivating mutations
  - Not considered to be 100% specific
    - Reports of *SNF5/INI1* gene alterations with loss of SNF5 immunostaining in epithelioid sarcomas and undifferentiated sarcomas with more favorable prognosis
- No evidence of myoblastic differentiation
- Positive for EMA, cytokeratin, α-1-antichymotrypsin, and vimentin

Cytogenetics

- Abnormalities of chromosome 22
  - Monosomy 22

RHABDOID TUMOR

Immunohistochemistry

Antibody	Reactivity	Staining Pattern	Comment
CK8/18/CAM5.2	Positive	Cytoplasmic	
AE1/AE3	Positive	Cytoplasmic	
EMA	Positive	Cell membrane & cytoplasm	
Vimentin	Positive	Cytoplasmic	
SNF5	Negative		a.k.a. INI1 and BAF47
Myogenin	Negative		

- 22q deletions
- *SNF5/INI1* gene deletions and mutations (22q11.2)
- Germline mutations described

Molecular Genetics

- Characterized by *SNF5/INI1* gene mutations
  - Tumor suppressor gene
  - Member of the chromatin remodeling SWI/SNF multiprotein complex
  - Results in loss of SNF5 nuclear immunostaining

DIFFERENTIAL DIAGNOSIS

Epithelioid Sarcomas

- Typically arises in distal extremities of adults
- Rarely occurs in patients under 10 years
- Less aggressive behavior
- May also occur in proximal extremities and trunk
- Painless, slow-growing nodule
- Usually located in dermis or subcutis
- Large cell "proximal type" variant may have rhabdoid features
- Frequent *SNF5/INI1* gene inactivation results in loss of SNF5 nuclear immunostaining
  - Frequency still significantly lower than that observed in rhabdoid tumor
- EMA, cytokeratin, vimentin, CD34 (50%), and β-catenin immunopositivity
  - CD34 and β-catenin immunostaining not observed in rhabdoid tumor

Renal Cell Carcinoma with Rhabdoid Differentiation

- Rarely observed in children
- More frequently observed in older populations
- Positive SNF5 nuclear immunostaining

Wilms Tumor (Nephroblastoma) with Rhabdoid Features

- Most common malignant renal neoplasm of children
- Characteristically triphasic
- Hypercalcemia, hematuria, and fever less frequent clinical features
  - Positive SNF5 nuclear immunostaining

Rhabdomyosarcoma

- Reactivity for muscle specific markers
- Positive SNF5 nuclear immunostaining

Mesoblastic Nephroma with Focal Rhabdoid Features

- Tumor cells negative for epithelial markers
- Positive SNF5 nuclear immunostaining
- May also present with hypercalcemia
- Chromosomal abnormalities frequently present

Clear Cell Sarcoma

- Distinguish from sclerosing pattern
- Tumor cells negative for epithelial markers
- Positive SNF5 nuclear immunostaining

Desmoplastic Small Round Cell Tumor

- Desmin positive (90%)
- NSE positive (80%)
- Positive SNF5 nuclear immunostaining

DIAGNOSTIC CHECKLIST

Pathologic Interpretation Pearls

- Diagnosis of extrarenal tumors and tumors with variant histology can be difficult
  - Combination of aggressive behavior, poor response to intensive chemotherapy, and lack of INI1 staining favor diagnosis of rhabdoid tumor

SELECTED REFERENCES

1. Kohashi K et al: Infrequent SMARCB1/INI1 gene alteration in epithelioid sarcoma: a useful tool in distinguishing epithelioid sarcoma from malignant rhabdoid tumor. Hum Pathol. 40(3):349-55, 2009
2. Kreiger PA et al: Loss of INI1 expression defines a unique subset of pediatric undifferentiated soft tissue sarcomas. Mod Pathol. 22(1):142-50, 2009
3. Wu X et al: Rhabdoid tumour: a malignancy of early childhood with variable primary site, histology and clinical behaviour. Pathology. 40(7):664-70, 2008
4. Amar AM et al: Clinical presentation of rhabdoid tumors of the kidney. J Pediatr Hematol Oncol. 23(2):105-8, 2001
5. Vujanić GM et al: Rhabdoid tumour of the kidney: a clinicopathological study of 22 patients from the International Society of Paediatric Oncology (SIOP) nephroblastoma file. Histopathology. 28(4):333-40, 1996
6. Weeks DA et al: Rhabdoid tumor of kidney. A report of 111 cases from the National Wilms' Tumor Study Pathology Center. Am J Surg Pathol. 13(6):439-58, 1989

Radiologic and Microscopic Features

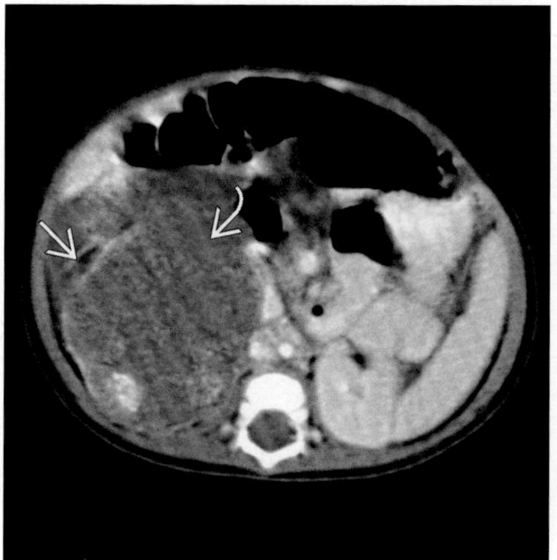

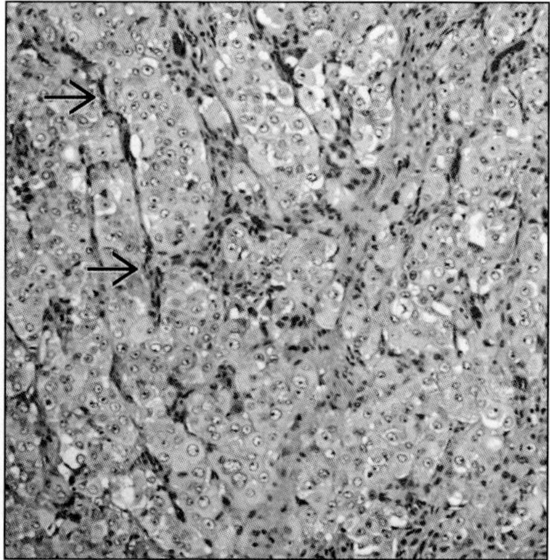

(Left) *Axial contrast-enhanced CT shows a large heterogeneous mass ➔ replacing the right kidney with areas of subcapsular fluid ➔ that help distinguish rhabdoid tumor from Wilms tumor. No brain tumors were found in this patient.* ***(Right)*** *Hematoxylin & eosin shows tumor cells with large pleomorphic nuclei, conspicuous nucleoli, and abundant pale eosinophilic cytoplasm arranged in a trabecular pattern of growth. A delicate fibrovascular stroma separates the tumor trabeculae ➔.*

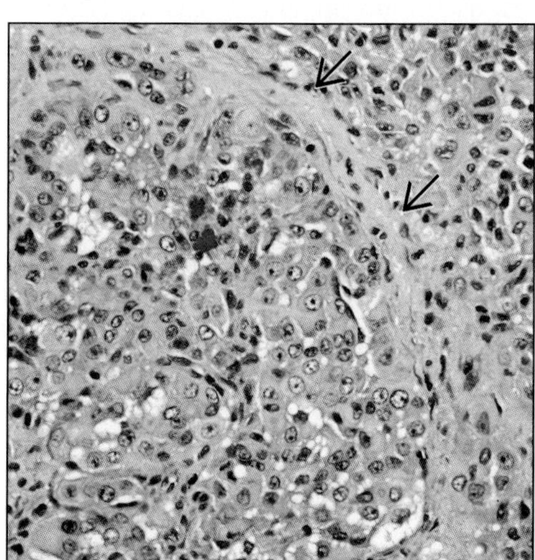

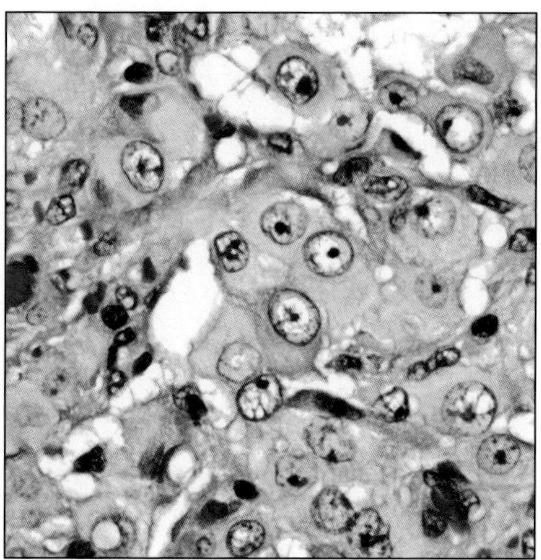

(Left) *Hematoxylin & eosin stained section shows loosely cohesive tumor cells set amongst a fibrovascular stroma ➔.* ***(Right)*** *High-power view shows mononuclear tumor cells with large nuclei, conspicuous nucleoli, and vesicular chromatin. The nucleus is eccentrically placed due to the abundant amount of pale eosinophilic cytoplasm imparting a rhabdoid appearance to the tumor cells.*

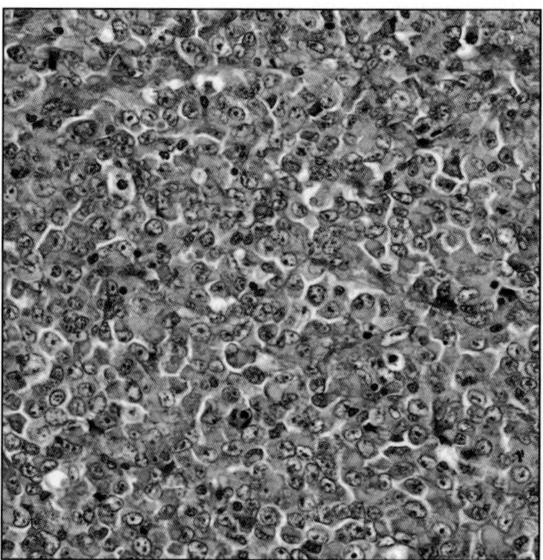

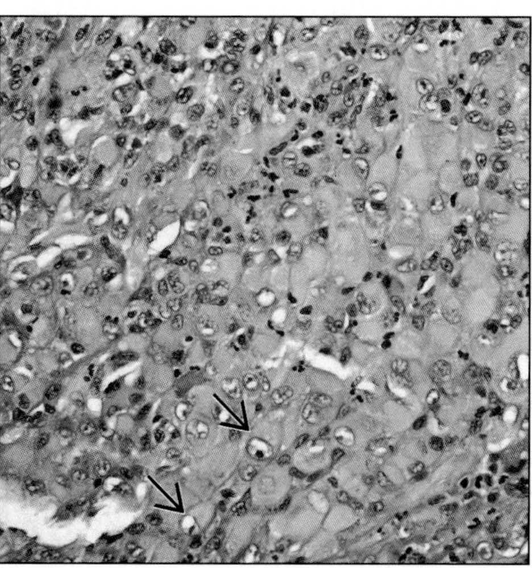

(Left) *Medium-power view shows sheets of loosely cohesive tumor cells with eccentrically placed nuclei and abundant eosinophilic cytoplasm.* ***(Right)*** *Epithelioid sarcoma with rhabdoid features is shown for reference. Note the large epithelioid cells ➔ with abundant eosinophilic cytoplasm and eccentrically placed nuclei reminiscent of rhabdoid cells.*

CLEAR CELL SARCOMA

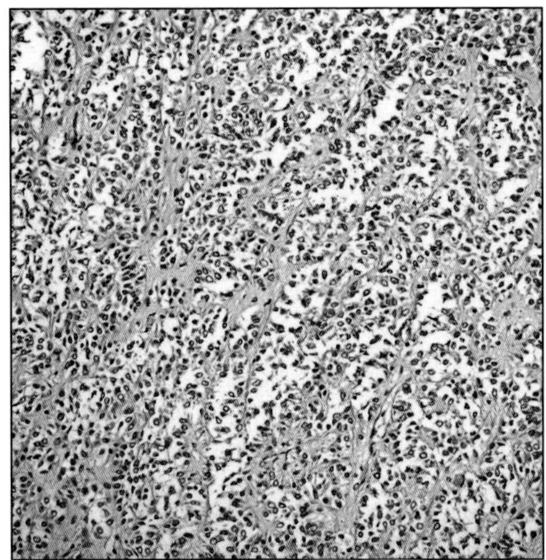

Classic pattern of CCSK shows the loosely spaced and often dyscohesive cells attached to the delicate fibrovascular septae.

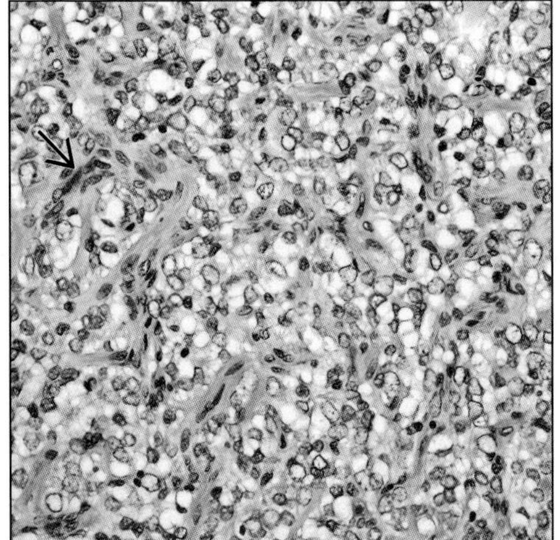

Classic pattern of CCSK at high power shows tumor cells with clear to vesicular nuclei and pale to clear cytoplasm with indistinct cell borders separated by delicate fibrovascular septae ➔.

TERMINOLOGY

Abbreviations

- Clear cell sarcoma of kidney (CCSK)

Synonyms

- Bone-metastasizing renal tumor

Definitions

- Uncommon malignant renal neoplasm of childhood with poor prognosis
- Formerly regarded as morphologic variant of Wilms tumor

CLINICAL ISSUES

Epidemiology

- Incidence
  - ~ 20 new cases/year in USA
  - Comprise ~ 4% of childhood renal tumors
- Age
  - 2 months to 14 years
    - Mean age of 3 years
    - Highest incidence in years 2 and 3
    - Congenital cases reported
- Gender
  - Male predominance (M:F = 2:1)

Presentation

- Large unicentric renal mass
- Lymph node metastases common at presentation (29%)
- Hematuria
- Hypertension

Treatment

- Surgical approaches
  - Unilateral nephrectomy
- Adjuvant therapy
  - Doxorubicin, dactinomycin, and vincristine (4th National Wilms Tumor Study regimen)
  - Treatment with doxorubicin shown to improve outcome
- Radiation
  - Tumor bed radiation therapy

Prognosis

- Aggressive clinical course
- Frequent metastases
  - Ipsilateral renal hilar lymph nodes most common site at presentation
  - Bone, lung, and abdomen/retroperitoneum most common sites of recurrence
- Independent prognostic factors
  - Treatment with doxorubicin
    - Improves outcome
  - Revised stage 1 (5th National Wilms Tumor Study criteria)
    - 98% overall survival rate
  - Patient age
    - Improved outcome in patients ages 2-4 years
  - Presence of tumor necrosis
    - Adverse factor for survival
    - Only histological variable

IMAGE FINDINGS

General Features

- Radiologic features are common to all malignant renal neoplasms

MACROSCOPIC FEATURES

General Features

- Large, unicentric renal mass
- Well circumscribed
- Most commonly located in renal medulla
- Tan-gray mucoid cut surface

CLEAR CELL SARCOMA

Key Facts

Terminology

- Uncommon malignant renal neoplasm of childhood with poor prognosis

Clinical Issues

- Comprise ~ 4% of childhood renal tumors
- Frequent metastases
  - Lymph node metastases common at presentation (29%)
  - Bone, lung, and abdomen/retroperitoneum most common sites of recurrence
- Aggressive clinical course
- Independent prognostic factors
  - Treatment with doxorubicin
  - Revised stage 1 (NWTS 5 criteria)
  - Patient age
  - Presence of tumor necrosis

Microscopic Pathology

- Classic pattern
  - Nests and cords of cells separated by arborizing fibrovascular septa
- Variant patterns frequently observed

Ancillary Tests

- Tumor cells immunoreactive for vimentin only

Top Differential Diagnoses

- Wilms tumor (blastemal predominant)
  - WT1(+)
- Peripheral neuroectodermal tumor
  - CD99(+)
  - Characteristic cytogenetics t(11;22)
- Congenital mesoblastic nephroma
  - Characteristic cytogenetics, t(12;15)

- Frequent foci of cystic change, hemorrhage, and necrosis
- Rare extension into renal vein

Size

- Mean diameter of 11.3 cm (range: 2.3-24 cm)

MICROSCOPIC PATHOLOGY

Microscopic Features

- Classic pattern
  - Nests and cords of cells separated by arborizing fibrovascular septa
  - Septae may be thin and delicate or cellular
  - Nests/cords contain plump-ovoid cells with indistinct cell borders
  - Round nuclei with fine chromatin without prominent nucleoli
  - Necrosis
    - Independent factor for adverse prognosis
  - Entrapped renal tubules along periphery
- Variant patterns (listed in order of observed frequency)
  - Myxoid
  - Sclerosing
  - Cellular
  - Epithelioid trabecular
  - Palisading (Verocay-body)
  - Spindled
  - Storiform
  - Anaplastic
    - Defined by nuclear hyperchromasia, nuclear gigantism, and atypical mitoses
- Histologic variants do not affect prognosis

ANCILLARY TESTS

Immunohistochemistry

- Tumor cells immunoreactive for vimentin only
- CD34 and FVIIIRAg highlight thin septal capillaries
- p53 immunostaining in anaplastic cases
- Low Ki-67 staining indices (mean of 21%)

DIFFERENTIAL DIAGNOSIS

Wilms Tumor (Blastemal Predominant)

- Rarely metastasizes to bones
- Overlapping nuclei with coarse chromatin and molding
- Focal tubule formation
- WT1(+)
- Focal cytokeratin positivity
- Patchy vimentin reactivity

Peripheral Neuroectodermal Tumor

- CD99(+)
- Focal cytokeratin positivity
- Characteristic cytogenetics t(11;22)

Congenital Mesoblastic Nephroma

- May resemble spindle cell variant of CCSK
- Vimentin and actin immunoreactive
- Occasional desmin immunoreactivity
- Characteristic cytogenetics, t(12;15)

SELECTED REFERENCES

1. Argani P et al: Clear cell sarcoma of the kidney: a review of 351 cases from the National Wilms Tumor Study Group Pathology Center. Am J Surg Pathol. 24(1):4-18, 2000
2. Amin MB et al: Clear cell sarcoma of kidney in an adolescent and in young adults: a report of four cases with ultrastructural, immunohistochemical, and DNA flow cytometric analysis. Am J Surg Pathol. 23(12):1455-63, 1999
3. Parikh SH et al: Clear cell sarcoma of the kidney: an unusual presentation and review of the literature. J Pediatr Hematol Oncol. 20(2):165-8, 1998
4. Looi LM et al: An immunohistochemical study comparing clear cell sarcoma of the kidney and Wilms' tumor. Pathology. 25(2):106-9, 1993

CLEAR CELL SARCOMA

Microscopic Features

(Left) Nests of tumor cells with clear to amphophilic cytoplasm are separated by delicate fibrovascular septae in this classic pattern of clear cell sarcoma of the kidney. (Right) Spindle cell pattern of CCSK is shown. A purely spindle cell clear cell sarcoma of the kidney raises the differential of a variety of sarcomas, such as congenital mesoblastic nephroma. Immunoreactivity for vimentin only will help distinguish a CCSK from a congenital mesoblastic nephroma.

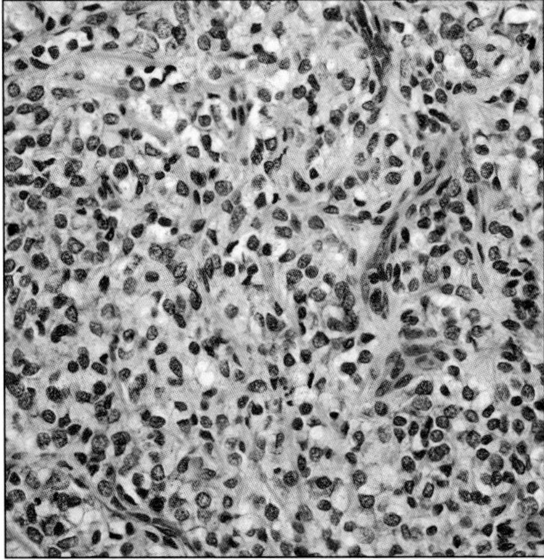

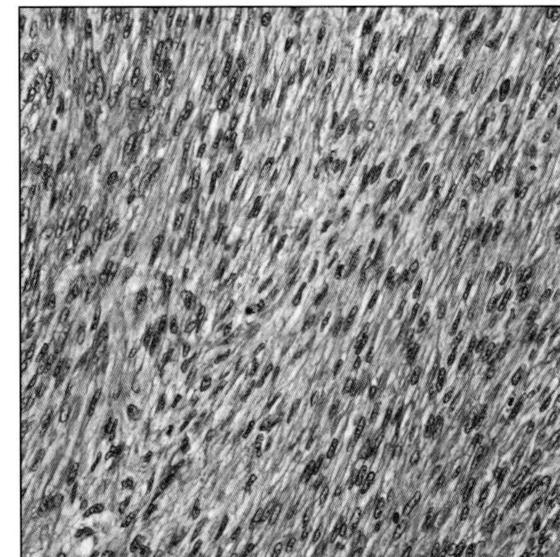

(Left) Medium-power view of a clear cell sarcoma of the kidney demonstrates areas of spindle cell to storiform pattern of growth. Typically, with adequate sampling, areas of more classic patterns of growth can be found. (Right) Palisading pattern of clear cell sarcoma of the kidney is shown and can very closely resemble the pattern of growth observed in a schwannoma. Negative S100 immunoreactivity and extensive sampling for more classic areas will help rule out this possibility.

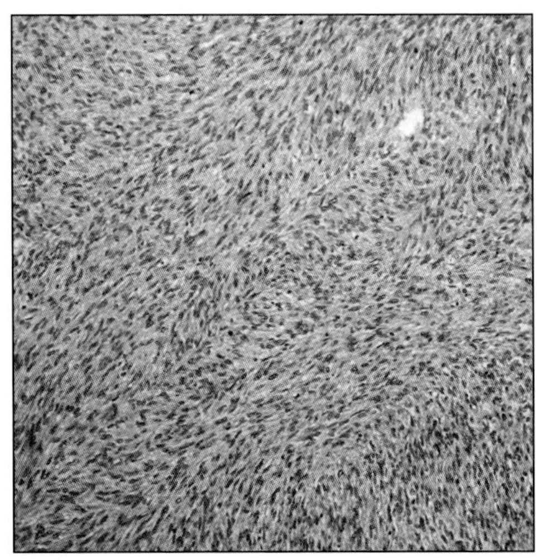

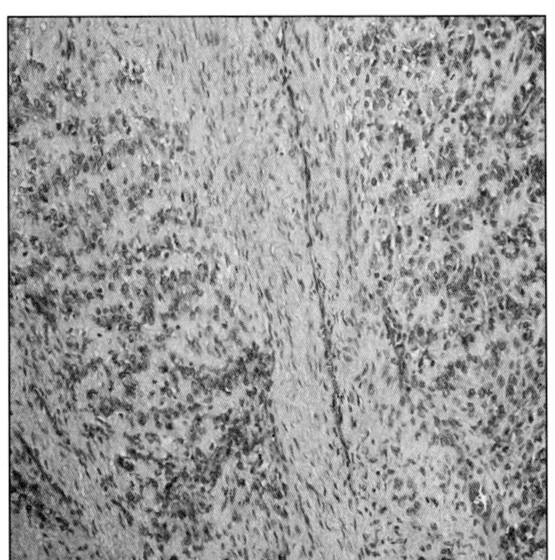

(Left) Medium-power view of a clear cell sarcoma of the kidney shows areas of hyaline sclerosis ⮫ with entrapped tubules → and spindle cell patterns of growth ⇨. (Right) High-power view of a clear cell sarcoma of the kidney demonstrates a focus of hyaline sclerosis. This pattern can be prominent, and it may require broad sampling to identify areas of more classic patterns.

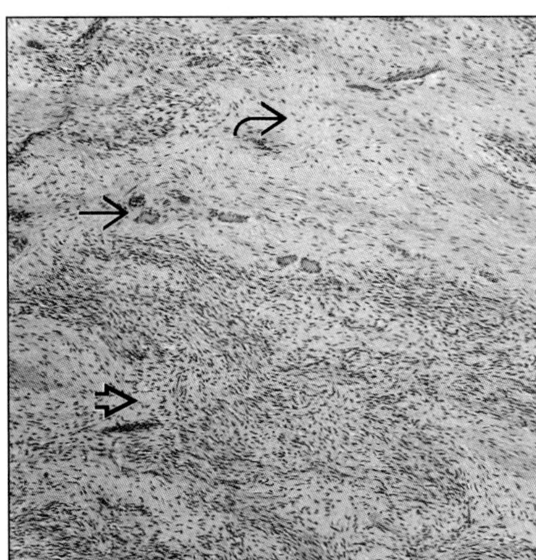

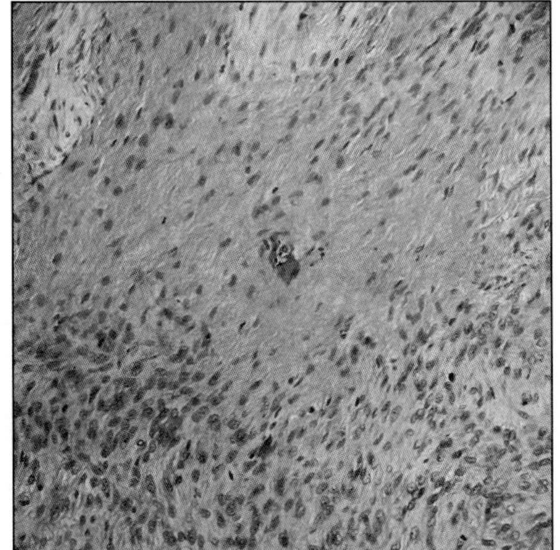

Microscopic Features

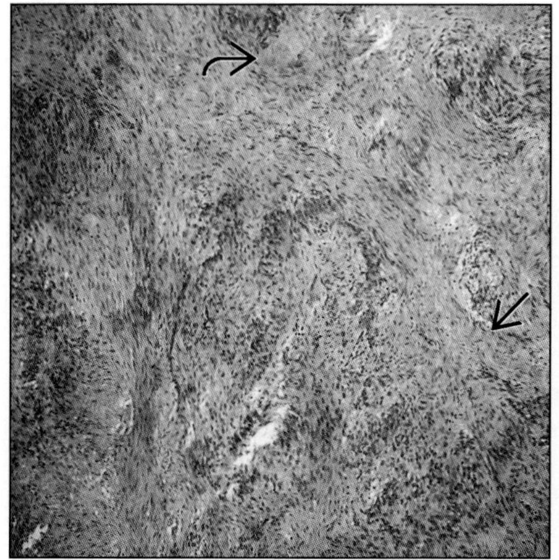

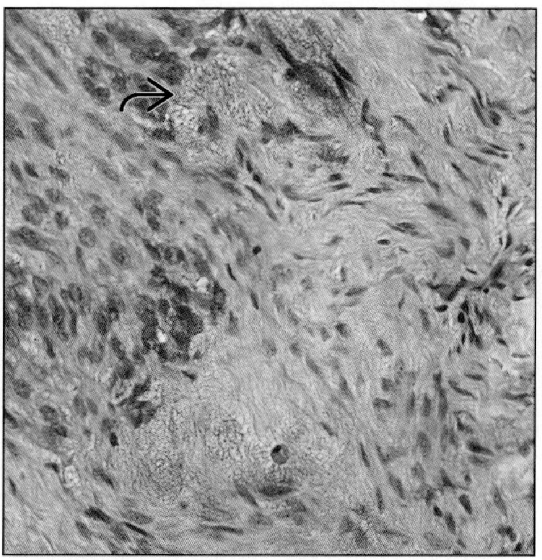

(Left) *Medium-power view of this clear cell sarcoma of the kidney shows numerous foci of myxoid material* ⤻ *interspersed by hyalinized and thickened septae* →. ***(Right)*** *Pools of myxoid material* ⤻ *are seen in this clear cell sarcoma of the kidney at high power. Nests of round to spindle-shaped tumor cells are also present.*

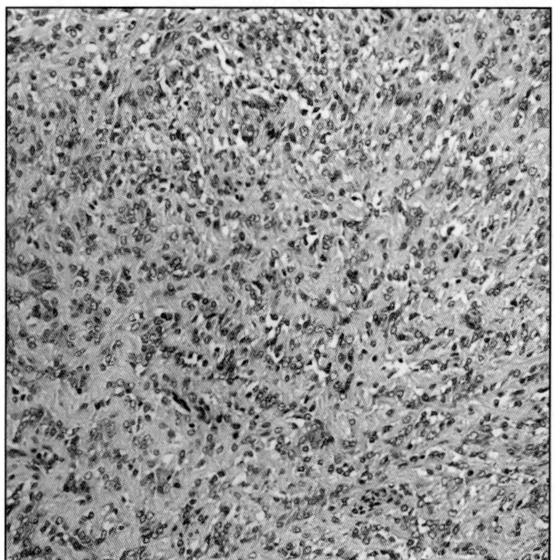

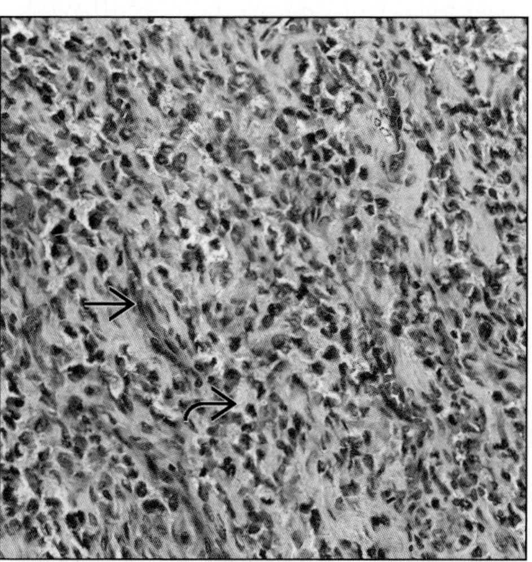

(Left) *A trabecular pattern of growth is seen in this CCSK from medium power. This pattern, when prominent, may resemble a carcinoma.* ***(Right)*** *Scattered, dyscohesive tumor cells are shown in this CCSK. Many of the tumor cells show prominent eosinophilic cytoplasm reminiscent of a rhabdoid tumor of the kidney. The characteristic small pools of mucin* ⤻, *thin fibrovascular septae* →, *lack of high-grade nuclei, and lack of conspicuous nucleoli will help distinguish this tumor as a CCSK.*

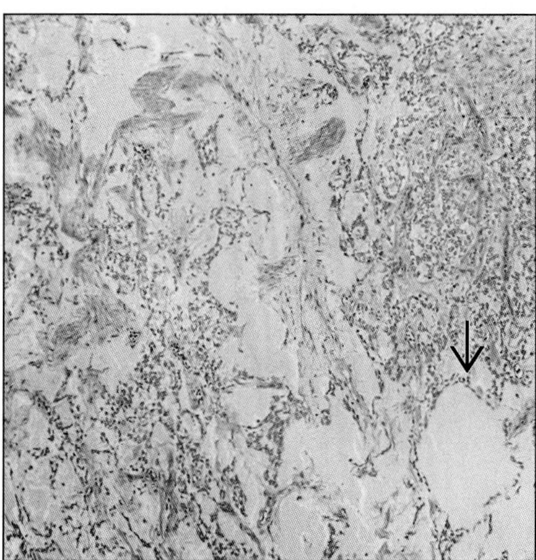

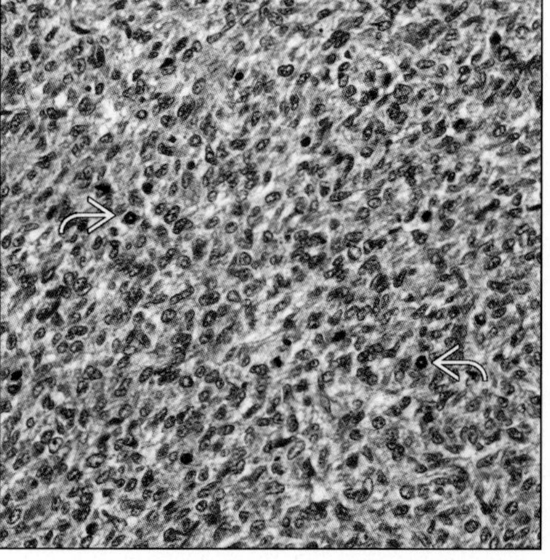

(Left) *Medium-power view shows a CCSK with numerous prominent cysts* → *containing pools of amorphous-myxoid material. Other areas (not shown) showed well-formed cysts amongst a more classic pattern of growth.* ***(Right)*** *Medium-power view of a CCSK shows the increased cellularity, nuclear hyperchromasia, mild-moderate pleomorphism, and numerous atypical mitotic figures* ➡ *that are consistent with the anaplastic pattern of growth.*

WILMS TUMOR

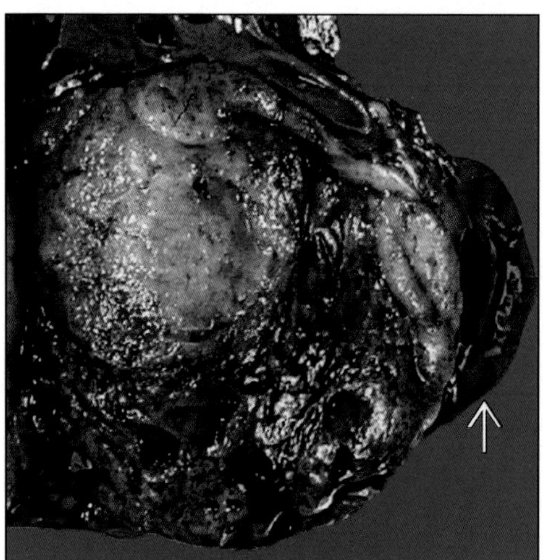

Gross appearance of a Wilms tumor shows a well-circumscribed, soft, tan mass, with areas of hemorrhage bulging from the native renal parenchyma ➡. Examination of the renal sinus is important.

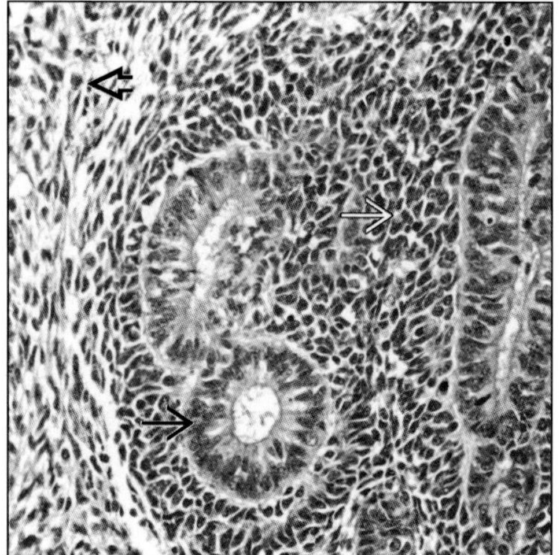

Typical triphasic morphology of Wilms tumor is shown. Note the blastemal ➡, epithelial ➡, and stromal ➡ components.

TERMINOLOGY

Abbreviations

- Wilms tumor (WT)

Synonyms

- Nephroblastoma

Definitions

- Malignant embryonal neoplasm derived from nephrogenic blastema cells, typically showing multiphasic patterns of differentiation

ETIOLOGY/PATHOGENESIS

Developmental Anomaly

- Approximately 10% are associated with syndromic conditions, including
  - WAGR syndrome (**W**ilms tumor, **a**niridia, **g**enitourinary malformations, mental **r**etardation)
  - Denys-Drash syndrome (Wilms tumor, mesangial sclerosis, pseudohermaphroditism)
  - Beckwith-Wiedemann syndrome (Wilms tumor, hemihypertrophy, macroglossia, omphalocele, visceromegaly)
  - Familial nephroblastoma
  - Others
    - Trisomy 18, Perlman syndrome, Bloom syndrome, Fraser syndrome, Klippel-Trenaunay syndrome

WT1 Gene Deletions or Point Mutations

- *WT1* gene is localized to chromosome 11p13
- *WT1* gene alterations are consistently present in WAGR and Denys-Drash syndromes
- Among sporadic nephroblastomas, deletions in focus are present in 1/3 and mutations in 10% of cases only
  - *WT1*-mutant tumors also show β-catenin (*CTNNB1*) mutations, activating Wnt signaling pathway
- Tumors with *WT1* mutations usually have stromal-prominent histology and presence of rhabdomyogenesis
  - Often associated with intralobar nephrogenic rests (ILNR)
- Such tumors common in both East Asians and whites

WT2 Gene Alterations

- 11p15 is location for putative *WT2* gene
- 11p15 alterations are common in Beckwith-Wiedemann syndrome
  - Insulin growth factor 2 (*IGF2*) gene and closely related H19 locus located within *WT2* region
  - Normally, only paternal allele-specific *IGF2* expressed (imprinting), because of differential methylation status of *H19* in paternal and maternal alleles
- Loss of imprinting (LOI) of *IGF2* and hypermethylation of *H19*-related genes identified in 33-50% of Wilms tumors
- Tumors with LOI are usually stroma poor
  - Often associated with perilobar nephrogenic rests (PLNR)
- Such tumors are rare in East Asians

Tumor-Specific Loss of Heterozygosity (LOH) for Chromosomes 1p and 16q

- Present in a proportion of Wilms tumors with favorable histology
  - Indicator of significantly increased risk of aggressive behavior
    - Current COG treatment protocols recommend more aggressive treatment for favorable histology Wilms tumors with LOH

CLINICAL ISSUES

Epidemiology

- Incidence

WILMS TUMOR

Key Facts

Etiology/Pathogenesis

- Approximately 10% are associated with syndromic conditions

Clinical Issues

- Peak incidence: 2-4 years; 98% of cases in children < 10 years of age
- Account for > 80% of renal tumors in children
- Overall survival currently > 90%
- Most significant unfavorable factors include high stage at presentation and diffuse anaplasia (unfavorable histology)
- 4% of WT are bilateral
- Identification of nephrogenic rests in resected kidney indicates greater probability of bilateral WT

Macroscopic Features

- Cut surface often shows soft consistency and is uniformly pale gray, tan, or pink and can resemble brain tissue

Microscopic Pathology

- Triphasic pattern consisting of undifferentiated blastema and epithelial and stromal components
- Features of anaplasia include markedly increased (3x) tumor cell nuclei with hyperchromasia and multipolar mitotic figures
- Only diffuse anaplasia is clinically/therapeutically important; therefore, differentiation from focal anaplasia is essential
- Anaplasia correlates with resistance to chemotherapy and with *P53* mutations in tumor

  - 1/8,000 children
    - Accounts for > 80% of renal tumors in children
- Age
  - Peak incidence: 2-4 years
    - 98% of cases in children < 10 years of age
    - Rare in infants < 6 months of age
    - Very uncommon in adults

Presentation

- Abdominal mass is most common presentation
  - Often detected by parents while bathing or clothing child
- Pain, hematuria, hypertension, acute abdominal crisis are other common presentations
- 4% of WTs are bilateral
  - Children with bilateral tumors typically present a year earlier than children with unilateral tumors

Treatment

- In general, Children's Oncology Group (COG) advocates primary resection
  - Further therapy is determined by stage and presence of anaplasia or "unfavorable histology"
  - Post-nephrectomy, stage I, and favorable histology stage II tumors given vincristine and dactinomycin (18 weeks)
  - Stage II tumors with LOH and stage III tumors given vincristine, dactinomycin, and doxorubicin (triple therapy) (24 weeks)
    - Stage III patients receive radiotherapy in addition to chemotherapy
    - Stage III tumors demonstrating LOH receive standard triple therapy regimen plus cyclophosphamide and etoposide
  - Stage IV tumors given triple therapy (24 weeks) together with abdominal radiotherapy for local residual disease &/or whole-lung radiotherapy if lung metastases visualized on chest radiography
  - Patients with stage II-IV Wilms with diffuse anaplasia treated more aggressively
    - Cyclophosphamide/carboplatin/etoposide and vincristine/doxorubicin/cyclophosphamide (30 weeks) plus radiation therapy
    - Stage I tumors with diffuse anaplasia treated like nonanaplastic tumors
  - Adjuvant chemotherapy now avoided for young patients (< 2 years) with small (< 550 g nephrectomy weight) stage I favorable histology Wilms tumor
    - Pathologic evaluation of lymph nodes an essential requirement for this approach
- Société Internationale d'Oncologie Pédiatrique (SIOP) advocates preoperative therapy followed by surgical resection; further therapy determined by response to prior therapy
  - Before resection, patients without metastasis receive vincristine and dactinomycin (4 weeks); those with metastases receive vincristine, dactinomycin, and doxorubicin (6 weeks)
  - Additional therapy given is based on residual tumor in nephrectomy specimen
    - Stage I residual disease: Additional vincristine and dactinomycin (4 weeks)
    - Stage II and III residual tumors: Adjuvant vincristine, dactinomycin, and doxorubicin (27 weeks)
    - Stage II with lymph node metastasis and all stage III patients: Additional radiotherapy
    - Children with stage IV Wilms tumor initially started on 3-drug regimen; those with incomplete remission switched to ifosfamide, carboplatin, etoposide, and doxorubicin

Prognosis

- In spite of differences in management, survivals are similar with both the COG and SIOP protocols
- Overall survival currently > 90%
- Most significant unfavorable factors include high stage at presentation and diffuse anaplasia (unfavorable histology)
- Majority of pre-therapy Wilms tumors with blastemal predominance are very sensitive to therapy

- Blastemal-type post-therapy tumors are considered resistant to chemotherapy and treated as anaplastic tumors in SIOP protocols
- Nephrogenic rests
  - Foci of persistent nephrogenic cells that resemble developing kidney
  - Perilobar nephrogenic rests are located at periphery of renal lobule
    - Tend to be multiple with well-defined borders and blastema predominant
    - Can be seen in disease-free kidneys
  - Intralobar nephrogenic rests are located within renal lobule
    - Usually single and stroma predominant
    - Typically seen only in kidneys with WT
  - Nephrogenic rests are seen in 41% of unilateral WT and 95% of bilateral WT
  - Identification of nephrogenic rests in resected kidney indicates greater probability of bilateral WT

MACROSCOPIC FEATURES

General Features

- Most tumors are unicentric
  - 7% are multicentric, and 5% are bilateral
- Usually sharply demarcated from surrounding renal parenchyma
  - Tumors are surrounded by compressed renal and perirenal tissue creating a pseudocapsule
- Cut surface often shows soft consistency, can resemble brain tissue, and is uniformly pale gray, tan, or pink
- Tumors with prominent stromal component are firm with a whorled cut surface
- Foci of hemorrhage and necrosis and cystic change are common

Specimen Handling and Sections to be Submitted

- All pediatric renal tumor specimens must be weighed
  - Weight determines decisions about therapy in some cases, e.g., no chemotherapy in younger patients with stage I tumor and total kidney weight < 550 g
- Before opening specimen, perihilar and perirenal lymph nodes should be identified and sampled
  - Lack of pathologic evaluation of lymph nodes excludes some (otherwise qualifying) patients from "no chemotherapy required" approach
- Areas with suspected ruptures should be inked in colors different from color choice for true margin
- Specimen should be fixed overnight, after taking sample for tumor banking and other special studies
- Sampling from renal sinus and margins of resection are essential for adequate staging
- Most sections taken from tumor must include tumor-renal parenchyma interface to evaluate tumor borders
- Documenting exact site from which each block is obtained is necessary
  - Often critical for evaluating focal vs. diffuse anaplasia and for addressing staging issues in some cases

MICROSCOPIC PATHOLOGY

Histologic Features

- Most characteristic: Triphasic pattern consisting of undifferentiated blastema and epithelial and stromal components
  - Many tumors have only biphasic or monophasic features
- Most components in Wilms tumor correspond to structures at various stages of nephrogenesis
- **Blastemal cells**: Small, closely packed, mitotically active cells with scant cytoplasm, overlapping nuclei, evenly distributed coarse chromatin, and usually small nucleoli
  - Can resemble other "small round blue cell tumors" of childhood
  - Blastema can be arranged in serpentine, nodular, or diffuse pattern
  - Tumors with diffuse blastemal pattern often have infiltrative margins, unlike most other types of Wilms tumor
- **Epithelial components**: Ranging from primitive rosette-like tubules to well-formed maturing and mature tubules; ill-formed glomerular structures and variable papillary architecture
  - Tubules are lined by primitive columnar or cuboidal cells with elongated nuclei
  - Mucinous, squamous, neural, or endocrine differentiation may occasionally be present
- **Stromal component**: Loose myxoid and fibroblastic spindled cells are commonly seen
  - WT stroma can differentiate along the line of almost any soft tissue type
  - Occasionally, fat, cartilage, bone, ganglion cells, or neuroglia are also seen
  - Rarely, differentiation toward soft tissue types is mature and diffuse
    - Tumors with combinations of stromal and epithelial differentiation have been termed "teratoid WT"
- **Anaplasia**: WTs are categorized into "favorable" and "unfavorable" histology based on absence or presence of anaplasia
  - Large hyperchromatic nuclei that are at least 3x larger than blastemal nuclei
    - Enlarged nuclei in skeletal muscle fibers found in stroma are not evidence of anaplasia
  - Large hyperdiploid mitotic figures
    - Do not confuse anaplasia with normal-sized mitotic figures that appear multipolar due to artifact
  - Approximately 5-6% of WTs show anaplasia
    - Anaplasia is rare in infants younger than 1 year of age
    - Unfavorable histology is seen in 13% of tumors from children older than 5 years
  - Anaplasia correlates with resistance to chemotherapy and with *P53* mutations in tumor
  - Only diffuse anaplasia clinically/therapeutically important; therefore, differentiation from focal anaplasia essential

- Extensive sampling is important: 1 section per cm of tumor or 1 section per 20 g of tumor
  - Anaplasia is considered focal when present only
    - In single/multiple sharply localized regions
    - Within primary intrarenal tumor, surrounded by nonanaplastic tumor
    - With no severe nuclear unrest (pleomorphism and hyperchromasia) in rest of tumor
    - And not present in intravascular tumor

Lymphatic/Vascular Invasion

- Invasion of renal sinus veins or lymphatics considered stage II in both COG and SIOP staging systems
  - Intrarenal vascular invasion does not upstage tumor

ANCILLARY TESTS

Immunohistochemistry

- Immunoreactive for WT1 protein
  - Immunoreactivity usually limited to blastemal and epithelial elements; stroma negative
  - Blastemal cells may label for desmin but not other muscle markers like actin, myogenin, MYOD1
  - Vimentin and cytokeratin negative or focally positive in blastema: Cytokeratin usually positive in epithelial components
    - CK7 may also be positive in more differentiated epithelial cells
  - pax-2 usually positive

DIFFERENTIAL DIAGNOSIS

Other Small Blue Cell Tumors

- Differentiation from blastemal Wilms tumor
  - Presence of nuclear molding, early tubular differentiation with organized nuclear alignment around early lumina is typical of blastema
    - Presence of true tubular lumina always favors Wilms tumor
  - Immunostains may be required in small biopsies to exclude other possibilities, including neuroblastoma, rhabdomyosarcoma, and PNET

Immature Teratoma

- Differentiation from Wilms tumor with extensive heterologous differentiation (so-called teratoid Wilms)
  - Teratoma shows organized (organ-like) differentiation (e.g., ciliated epithelium with smooth muscle and cartilage)
  - Wilms tumor is characterized by random juxtaposition of different tissue types
  - Presence of nephrogenic blastema with true tubules and other nephrogenic patterns supports diagnosis of Wilms tumor

Metanephric Adenoma

- Differentiation from epithelial-predominant Wilms tumor
  - Uniform, nonoverlapping nuclei with delicate chromatin and inconspicuous nucleoli and lack of mitotic figures in metanephric adenoma
  - Immunostain for WT1 may be negative or weak and focally positive in metanephric adenoma vs. usually strong and diffuse in Wilms tumor
  - CD57 is positive

Papillary Renal Cell Carcinoma (Type 1, Solid Glomeruloid Variant)

- Differentiation from epithelial-predominant Wilms tumor with papillary areas
  - Papillary RCC often with foamy macrophages
  - Glomeruloid tufts in tumor occasionally with higher grade cytology, including more prominent nucleoli, compared to cells forming tubules
  - AMACR and CK7 diffuse and strongly positive and WT1 usually negative in papillary RCC
    - In Wilms tumor, AMACR negative, CK7 usually negative or focally positive, and WT1 diffuse and strong positive

DIAGNOSTIC CHECKLIST

Clinically Relevant Pathologic Features

- Gross appearance
  - Most Wilms tumors, other than those with diffuse blastemal pattern, are well circumscribed
    - Differentiates them radiologically and grossly from more aggressive pediatric tumors like rhabdoid tumor of kidney, as well as most mesoblastic nephromas

Pathologic Interpretation Pearls

- Reporting of presence or absence of anaplasia is an essential component of surgical pathology report on Wilms tumor
  - Diffuse anaplasia, when present, is usually apparent in most tumor sections
  - Anaplasia at any margin or in extrarenal sites is considered diffuse anaplasia
  - Anaplasia present in random biopsy (although rarely performed) is considered diffuse anaplasia
- Identification of nephrogenic rests in resected kidney indicates a greater probability of bilateral WT

SELECTED REFERENCES

1. Vujanić GM et al: The pathology of Wilms' tumour (nephroblastoma): the International Society of Paediatric Oncology approach. J Clin Pathol. 63(2):102-9, 2010
2. Davidoff AM: Wilms' tumor. Curr Opin Pediatr. 21(3):357-64, 2009
3. Huang CC et al: Predicting relapse in favorable histology Wilms tumor using gene expression analysis: a report from the Renal Tumor Committee of the Children's Oncology Group. Clin Cancer Res. 15(5):1770-8, 2009
4. Cerrato F et al: Different mechanisms cause imprinting defects at the IGF2/H19 locus in Beckwith-Wiedemann syndrome and Wilms' tumour. Hum Mol Genet. 17(10):1427-35, 2008
5. Sonn G et al: Management of Wilms tumor: current standard of care. Nat Clin Pract Urol. 5(10):551-60, 2008
6. Dome JS et al: Treatment of anaplastic histology Wilms' tumor: results from the fifth National Wilms' Tumor Study. J Clin Oncol. 24(15):2352-8, 2006

WILMS TUMOR

Staging of Pediatric Renal Tumors (Children's Oncology Group)

Stage	Main Pathologic Feature	Details of Pathologic Findings
I	Tumor limited to kidney and completely resected	Renal capsule intact
		No invasion of lymphatics or veins of renal sinus
		No prior biopsy
		No metastases
		Margins negative
II	Tumor extends beyond kidney but completely resected	Tumor penetrates renal capsule
		Tumor invades lymphatics or veins in renal sinus
		Tumor invades renal vein, but vein margin negative
		No metastases
		Margins negative
III	Residual tumor or nonhematogenous metastases confined to abdomen	Involves abdominal lymph nodes
		Peritoneal contamination or implants
		Tumor spillage of any degree occurring before or during surgery
		Gross residual tumor in abdomen
		Biopsy of tumor (including fine needle aspiration)
		Resection margin involved by tumor
IV	Hematogenous metastases or spread beyond abdomen	
V	Bilateral renal tumors	Tumor on each side to be staged separately and reported as substage on that side (e.g., stage V; substage III [right], substage I [left])

Revised SIOP Working Classification of Nephroblastoma after Neo-Adjuvant Therapy

Stage	Risk Level	Residual Tumor Type
I	Low-risk tumors	Cystic, partially differentiated nephroblastoma
		Completely necrotic nephroblastoma
II	Intermediate-risk tumors	Nephroblastoma, epithelial type, stromal type, mixed type, or regressive type
		Nephroblastoma, focal anaplasia
III	High-risk tumors	Nephroblastoma, blastemal type
		Nephroblastoma, diffuse anaplasia

7. Grundy PE et al: Loss of heterozygosity for chromosomes 1p and 16q is an adverse prognostic factor in favorable-histology Wilms tumor: a report from the National Wilms Tumor Study Group. J Clin Oncol. 23(29):7312-21, 2005
8. Fukuzawa R et al: Epigenetic differences between Wilms' tumours in white and east-Asian children. Lancet. 363(9407):446-51, 2004
9. Vujanić GM et al: Revised International Society of Paediatric Oncology (SIOP) working classification of renal tumors of childhood. Med Pediatr Oncol. 38(2):79-82, 2002
10. Green DM et al: Treatment with nephrectomy only for small, stage I/favorable histology Wilms' tumor: a report from the National Wilms' Tumor Study Group. J Clin Oncol. 19(17):3719-24, 2001
11. Beckwith JB: National Wilms Tumor Study: an update for pathologists. Pediatr Dev Pathol. 1(1):79-84, 1998
12. Beckwith JB: Nephrogenic rests and the pathogenesis of Wilms tumor: developmental and clinical considerations. Am J Med Genet. 79(4):268-73, 1998
13. Faria P et al: Focal versus diffuse anaplasia in Wilms tumor--new definitions with prognostic significance: a report from the National Wilms Tumor Study Group. Am J Surg Pathol. 20(8):909-20, 1996
14. Green DM et al: Treatment outcomes in patients less than 2 years of age with small, stage I, favorable-histology Wilms' tumors: a report from the National Wilms' Tumor Study. J Clin Oncol. 11(1):91-5, 1993
15. Breslow N et al: Prognostic factors in nonmetastatic, favorable histology Wilms' tumor. Results of the Third National Wilms' Tumor Study. Cancer. 68(11):2345-53, 1991
16. Beckwith JB et al: Histopathology and prognosis of Wilms tumors: results from the First National Wilms' Tumor Study. Cancer. 41(5):1937-48, 1978

Radiologic and Gross Features

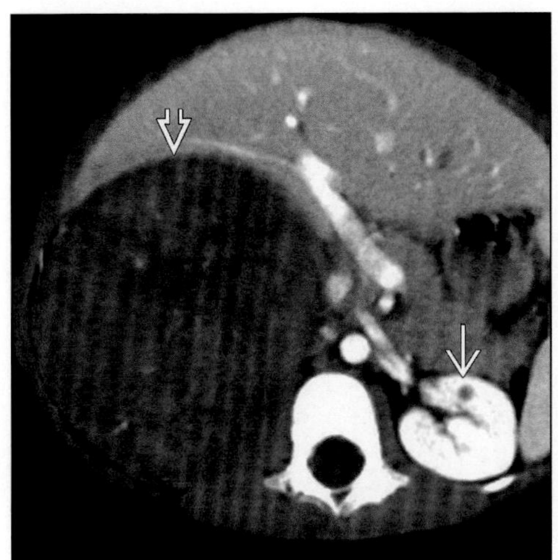

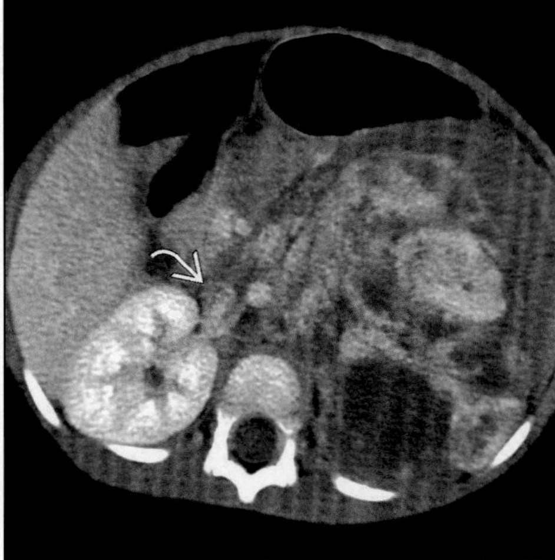

(Left) *Axial CECT shows a large, poorly enhancing Wilms tumor in the right flank ➡ and a small low-density area in the contralateral kidney ➡, which was a synchronous Wilms tumor.* ***(Right)*** *Axial CECT shows inferior extension of the tumor, displacement of the aorta and mesenteric vessels, and an additional low-density thrombus in the vena cava ➡.*

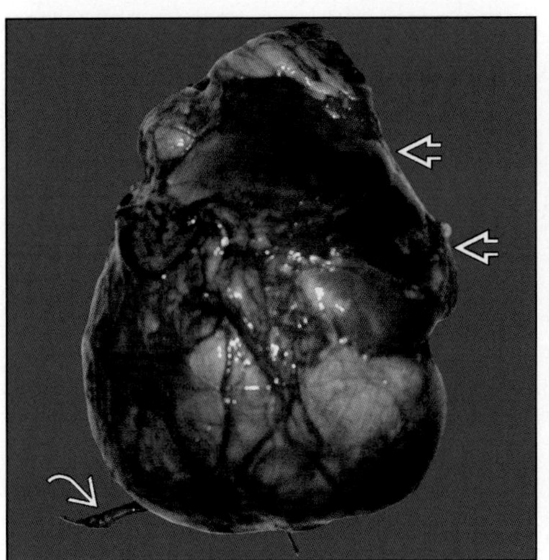

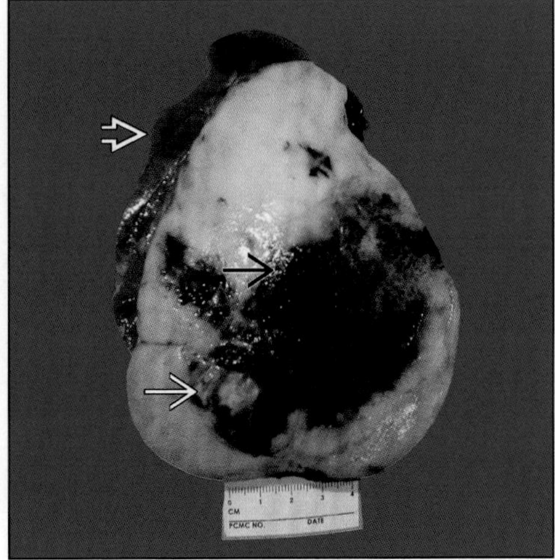

(Left) *Total nephrectomy specimen shows an area of relatively intact residual kidney ➡ and ureter ➡. Wilms tumors often weigh more than 500 grams. (Courtesy L. Erickson, PA.)* ***(Right)*** *Wilms tumor shows areas of hemorrhage ➡ and necrosis ➡. The tan-pink tumor can resemble cerebral cortex in consistency. Note the uninvolved portion of the kidney ➡. (Courtesy L. Erickson, PA.)*

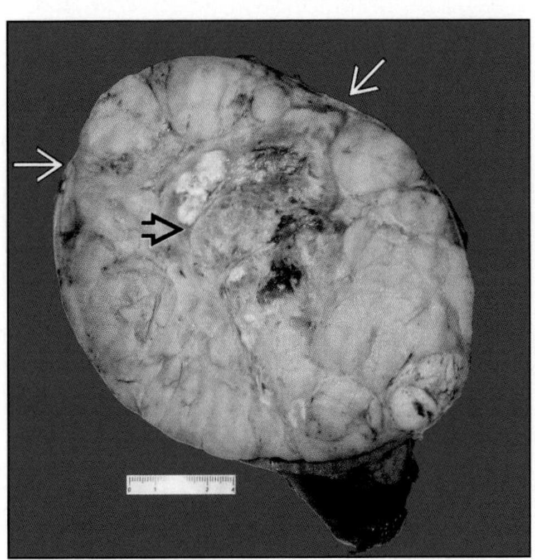

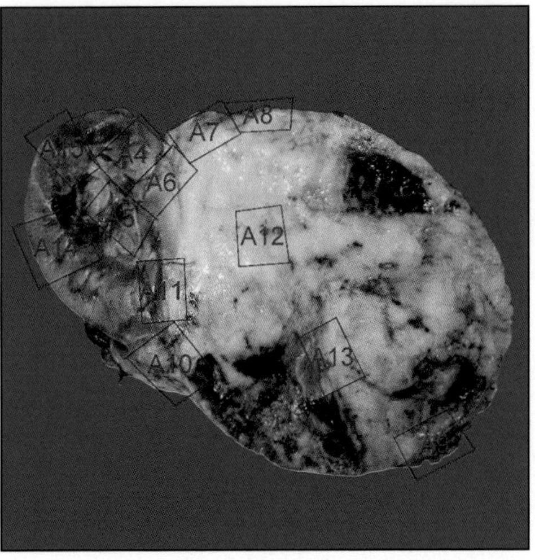

(Left) *Section shows Wilms tumor post formalin fixation. This tumor has an inflammatory pseudocapsule ➡ and areas of hemorrhage and necrosis ➡. (Courtesy L. Erickson, PA.)* ***(Right)*** *Wilms tumor shows an example of section mapping. It is important to sample normal kidney in order to document nephrogenic rests. Areas of suspected rupture should also be examined histologically, for example section A9. (Courtesy L. Erickson, PA.)*

WILMS TUMOR

Microscopic Features

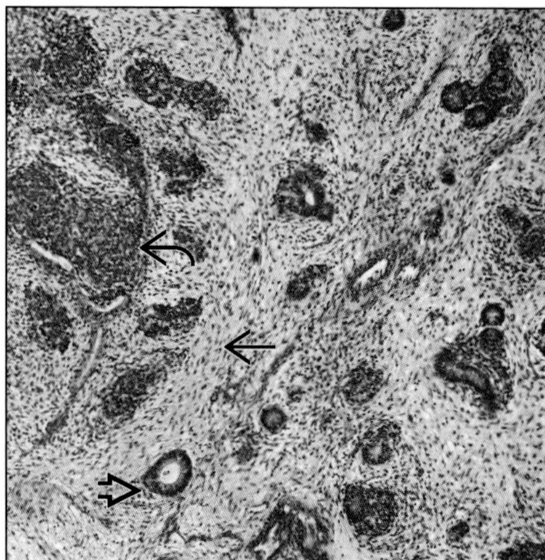

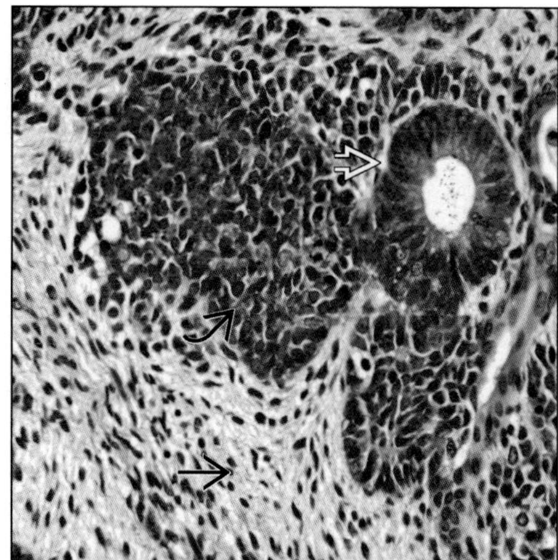

*(Left) This H&E section shows a Wilms tumor with triphasic histology. Note the epithelial ⇨, blastemal ↗, and stromal components →. **(Right)** High-power view shows a Wilms tumor with triphasic histology, including the epithelial ⇨, blastemal ↗, and stromal components →. Be aware that biphasic and monophasic tumors also occur. All 3 components need not be present to make a diagnosis of Wilms tumor.*

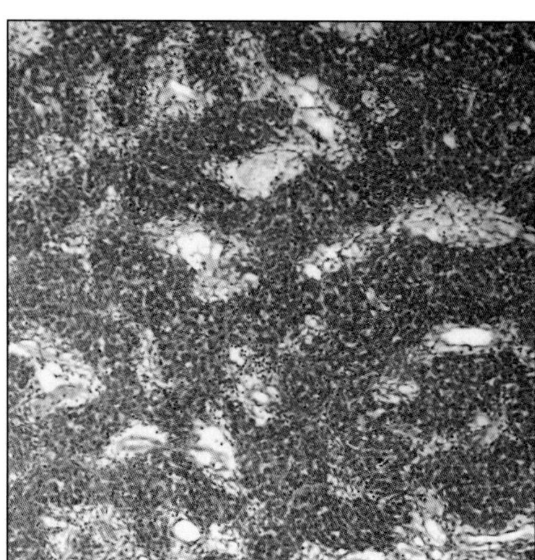

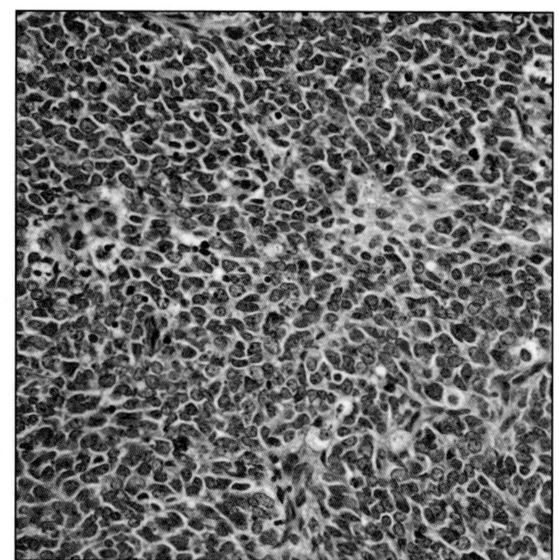

*(Left) Blastema-predominant Wilms tumor is shown. Blastema can be arranged in a diffuse, nodular, or serpentine pattern. **(Right)** Blastema consists of small, closely packed, mitotically active cells with scant cytoplasm, overlapping nuclei, evenly distributed coarse chromatin, and usually small nucleoli.*

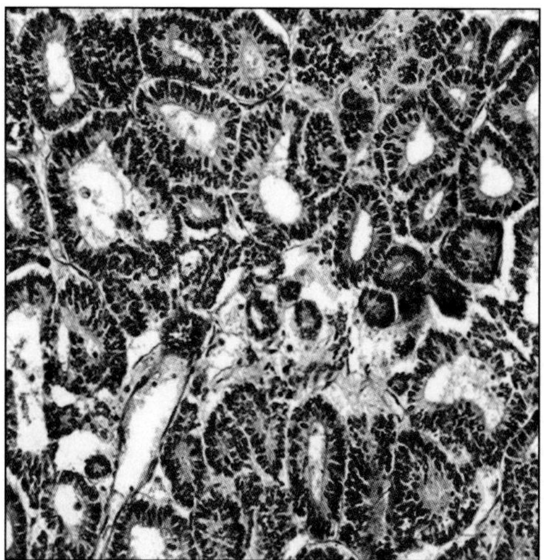

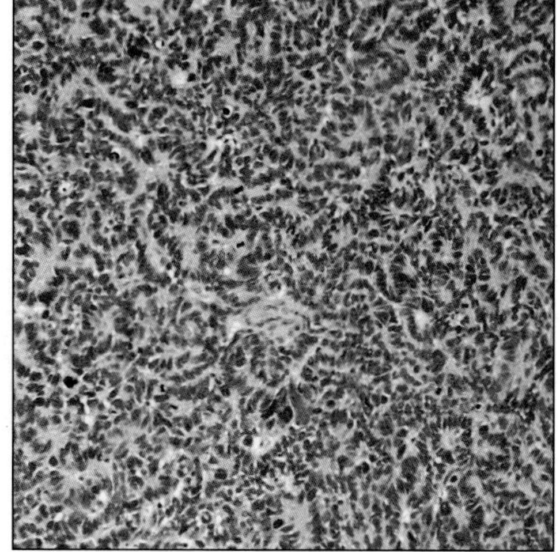

*(Left) Epithelial areas in Wilms tumors most often show tubular differentiation of variable degrees, ranging from poorly developed tubular structures embedded in blastema to tubules showing well-formed lumina, usually lined by primitive and mitotically active cells. **(Right)** In this epithelial-predominant Wilms tumor, the nuclei of the epithelial component consist of tubular structures with primitive columnar to cuboidal cells. The nuclei may show molding and are typically elongated.*

Microscopic Features

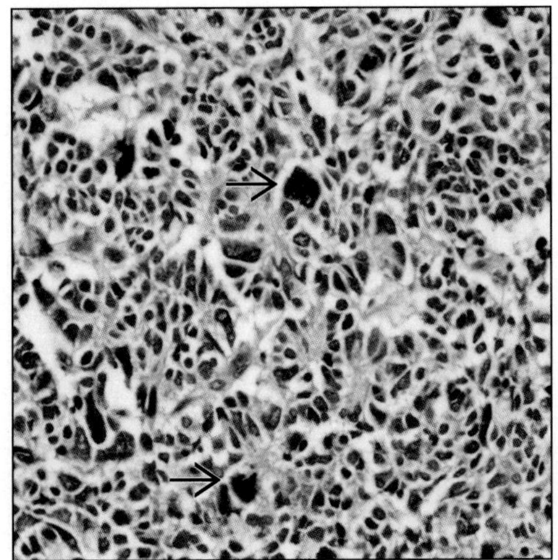

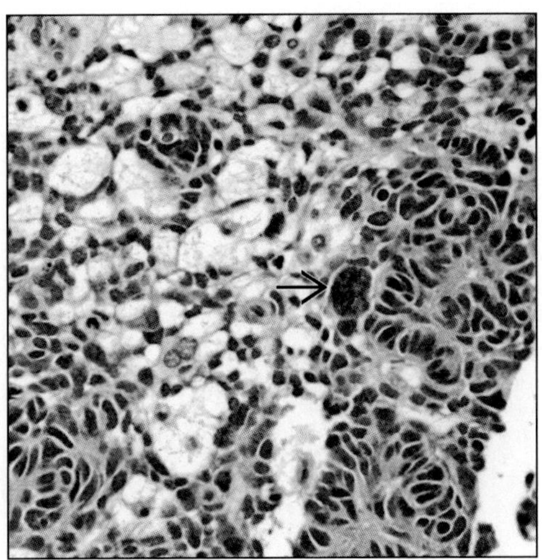

(Left) *Wilms tumors are classified as having favorable or unfavorable histology based on the absence or presence of anaplasia. Anaplasia is defined as the presence of large hyperchromatic nuclei ⇒ and multipolar mitotic figures.* ***(Right)*** *This Wilms tumor shows unfavorable histology. Note the enlarged nucleus ⇒, which is also hyperchromatic. Enlarged nuclei that are not hyperchromatic should not be considered evidence of anaplasia.*

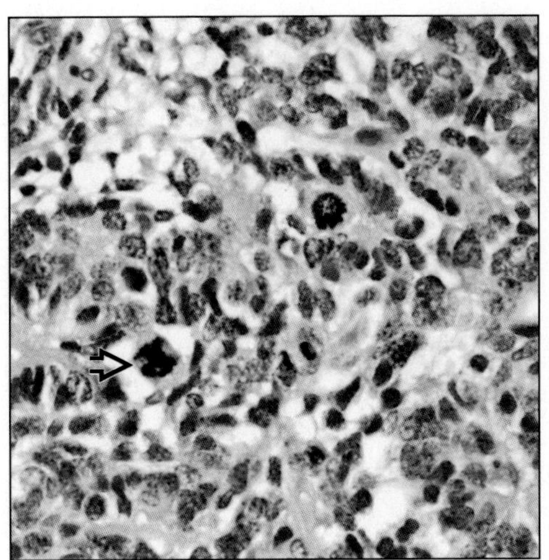

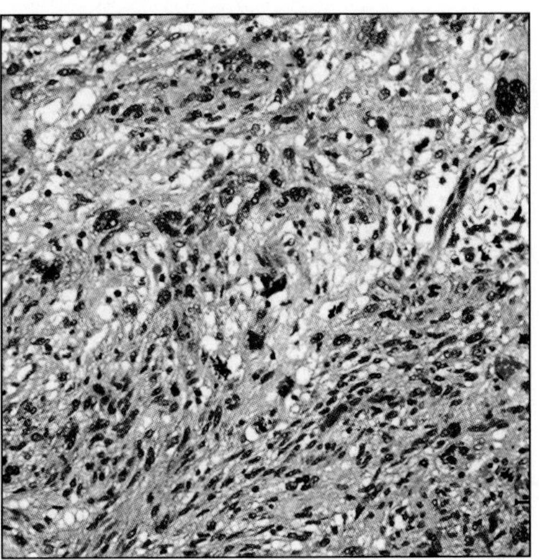

(Left) *This Wilms tumor shows unfavorable histology. Note the large multipolar mitotic figure ⇨. Mitotic figures that are not enlarged should not be considered evidence of anaplasia.* ***(Right)*** *Anaplasia may be present in any or all of the 3 components of Wilms tumor. This image shows anaplastic features in the mesenchymal element of a tumor. Focal vs. diffuse anaplasia essentially does not convey the relative amount but the distribution and location of anaplasia.*

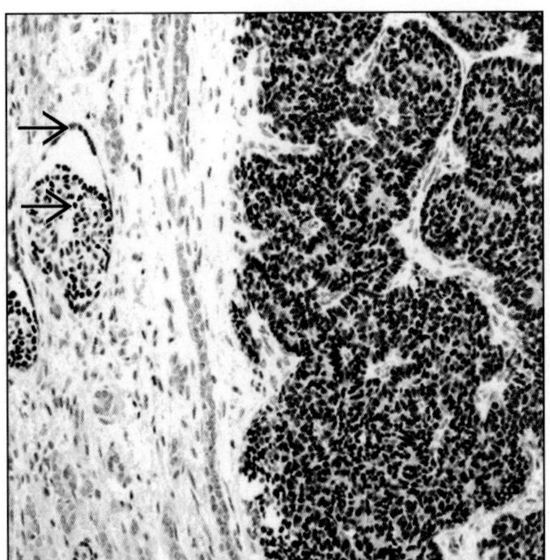

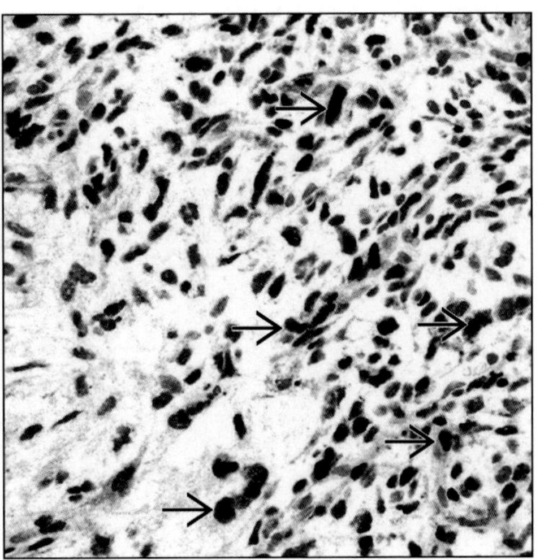

(Left) *WT1 staining usually shows diffuse nuclear positivity in the blastemal and epithelial areas of the tumor, with the stroma being negative. Note the positive reaction in the glomerular mesangium and Bowman capsule lining ⇒ that acts as an internal control for WT1.* ***(Right)*** *Most anaplastic tumors show P53 gene mutations, corresponding to immunohistochemical overexpression ⇒ in the majority of cases. P53 mutations have been associated with resistance to chemotherapy.*

WILMS TUMOR

Microscopic Features

(Left) Post-therapy tumors often show large areas with foamy ⇨ or hemosiderin-laden macrophages. Rare differentiated tubules may be present in such areas, and these are regarded as regressive changes ➡. *(Right)* Post-therapy WT shows histiocytic response ⇨, few "cell rests" →, and residual blastemal elements ➡. SIOP requires determination of the proportion of blastemal elements in the viable areas for risk stratification and further therapy.

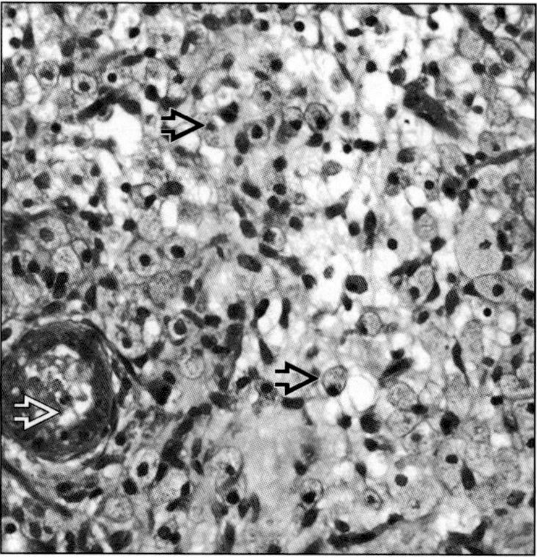

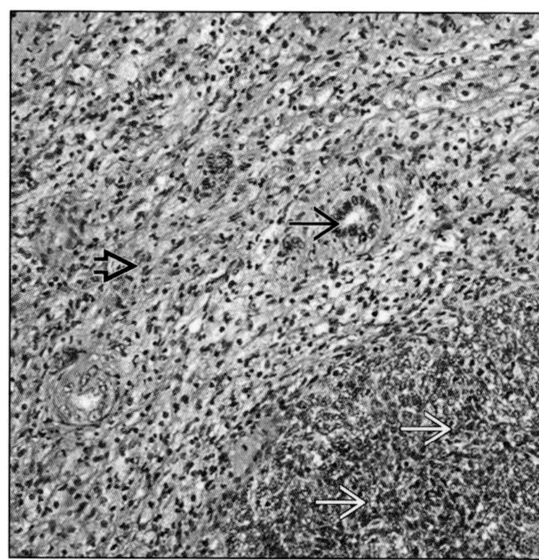

(Left) A majority of post-therapy WTs show extensive fibrosis. Relatively mature-appearing tubules in such a background are regarded as epithelial rests ⇨ and not considered in the classification of post-therapy tumors. *(Right)* While squamous differentiation may be seen in pre-treatment cases, this is a more common feature in post-chemotherapy residual tumors ⇨.

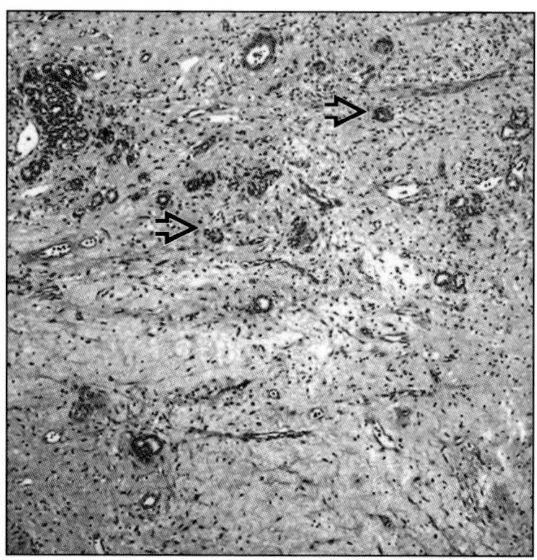

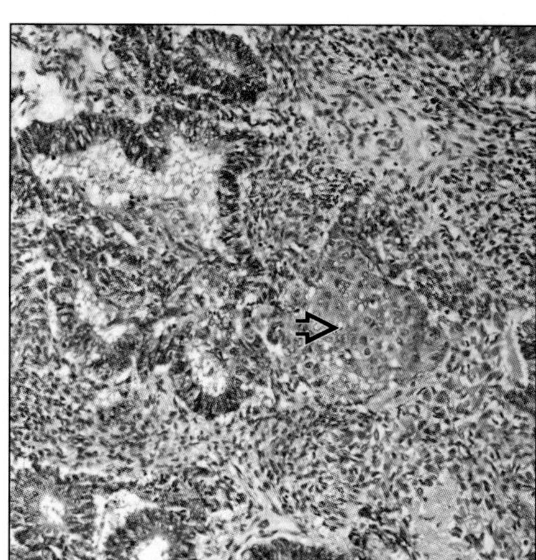

(Left) Commonly, the stromal component consists of loose myxoid ⇨ and fibroblastic spindle cells; however, WT stroma can differentiate along many types of soft tissue. Smooth muscle, skeletal muscle →, fat, cartilage, bone, and neural components may be identified. *(Right)* The stroma of this Wilms tumor contains skeletal muscle differentiation →. Enlarged nuclei in skeletal muscle fibers are not evidence of anaplasia.

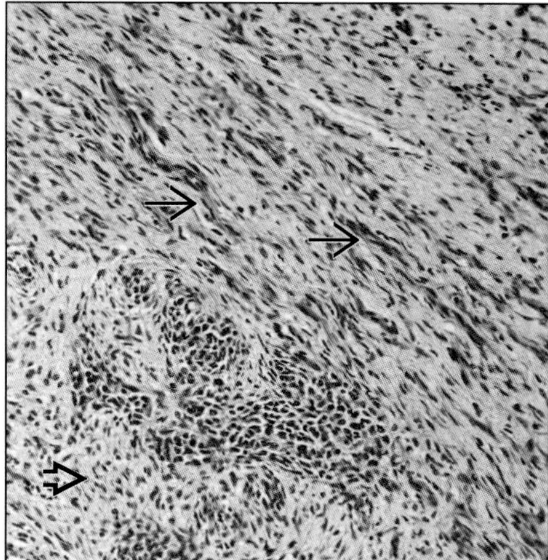

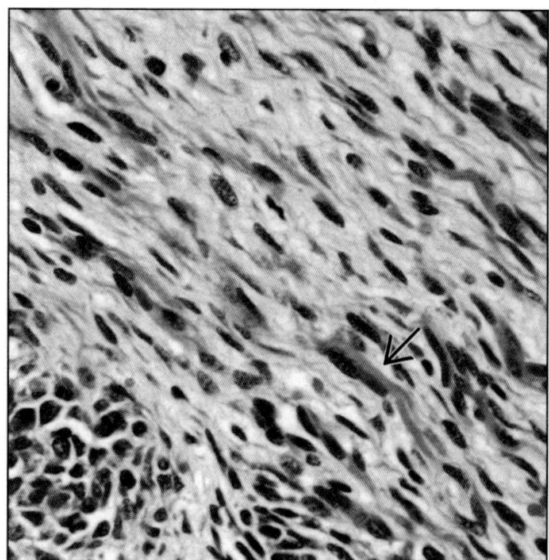

Microscopic Features

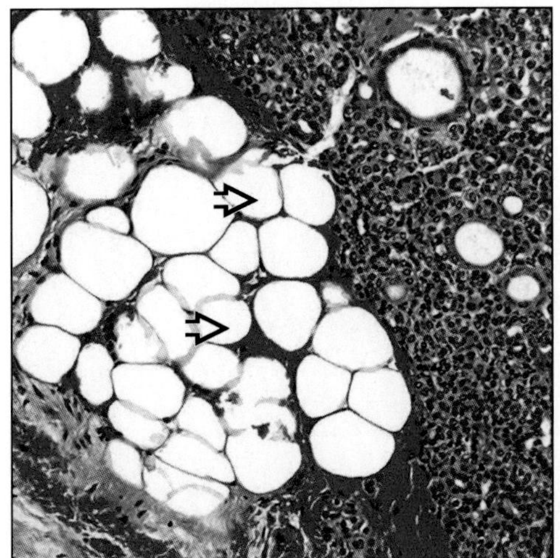

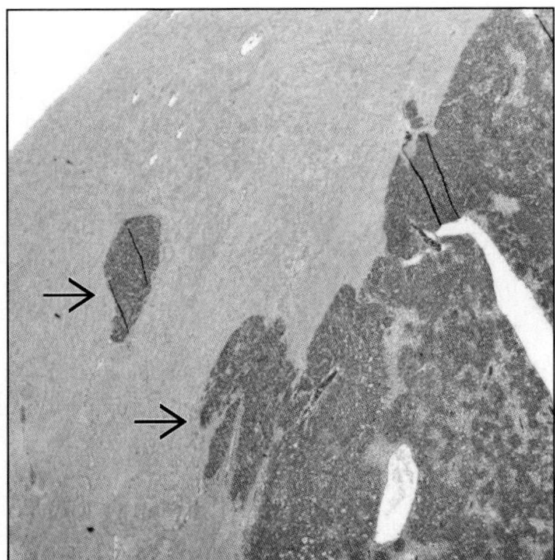

(Left) *Undifferentiated, myxoid, fibroblastic, myofibroblastic, adipocytic ⇨, smooth muscle, cartilage, bone, and neuroglial type cells are the other stromal components that may be present in WT.* ***(Right)*** *This H&E section shows penetration of the pseudocapsule →. Although this tumor extends locally outside of the kidney, it is still considered to be a stage II tumor, as it was completely resected.*

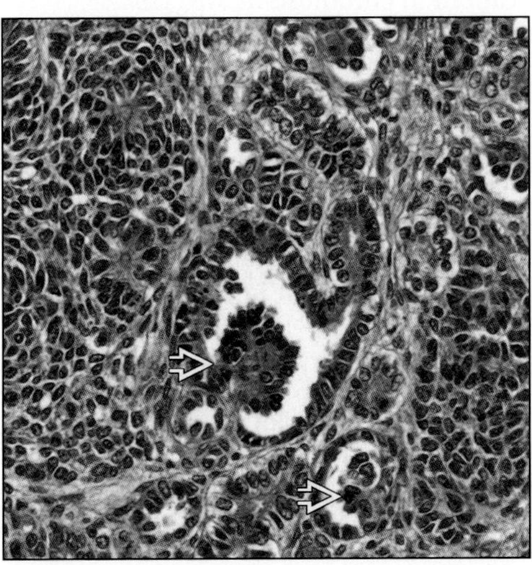

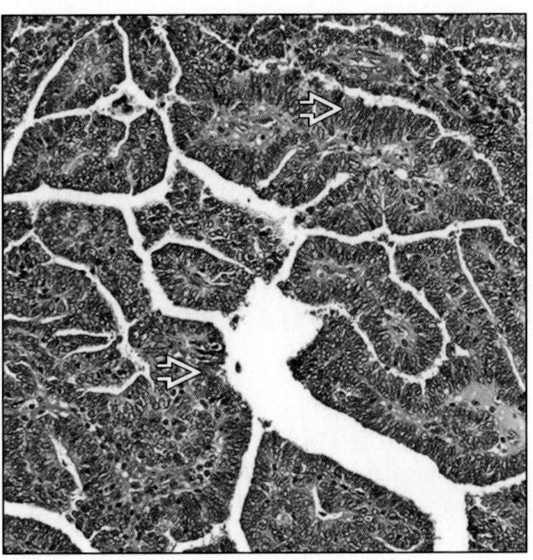

(Left) *Glomerular differentiation in Wilms tumor may range from primitive or attempted glomerular formations ➡ to almost mature glomeruli closely resembling those of normal kidneys.* ***(Right)*** *Papillary formations are also common in epithelial areas. Very often, the lining cells appear primitive ➡, but differentiation to more mature cells may also be seen, particularly in patients who have received prior chemotherapy.*

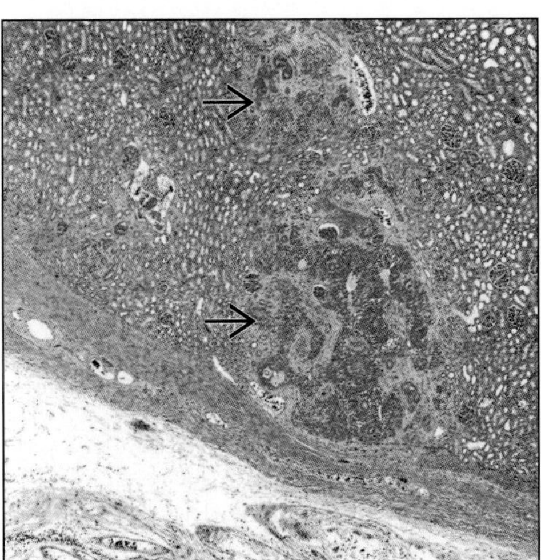

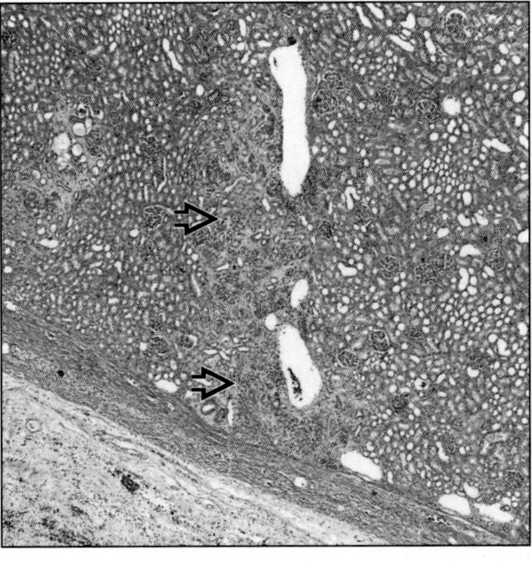

(Left) *Nephrogenic rests → are foci of cells that resemble the developing kidney. They may be perilobar or intralobar in location.* ***(Right)*** *The examination of uninvolved kidney for the presence of nephrogenic rests ⇨ is important. The presence of nephrogenic rests indicates a greater possibility of bilateral WT.*

MITF/TFE FAMILY TRANSLOCATION-ASSOCIATED CARCINOMA

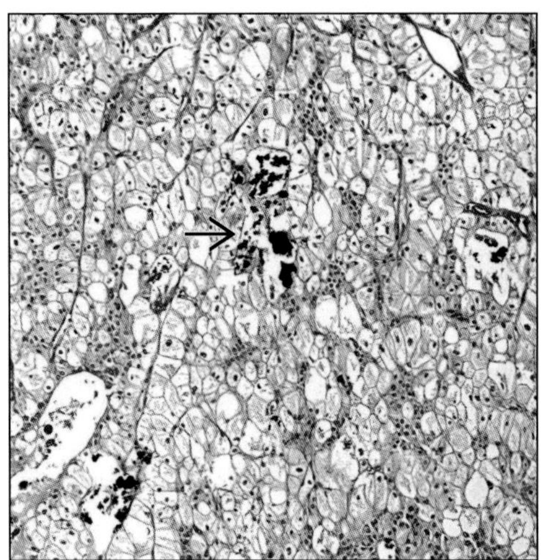

Photomicrograph of a TFE3 renal carcinoma shows nests of clear cells separated by delicate vasculature. Voluminous cytoplasm and psammomatous calcifications ➡ are quite typical.

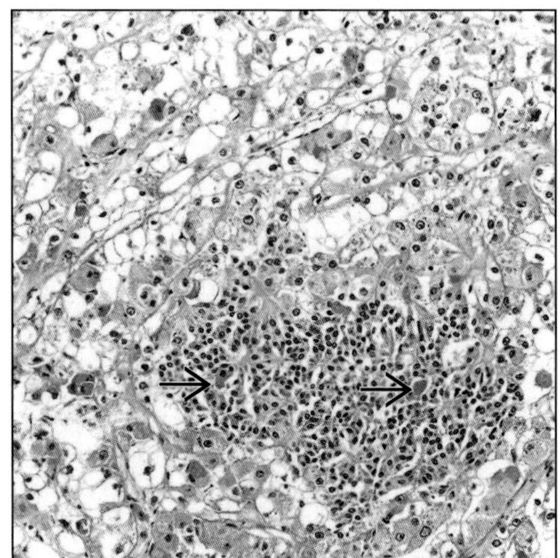

Typical microscopic features of TFEB renal carcinoma include sheets of cells separated by vascular septations and 2 cell types with the smaller cells surrounding hyaline material ➡.

TERMINOLOGY

Abbreviations

- Microphthalmia-associated transcription factor (*MiTF*), transcription factor binding to IGHM enhancer 3 (*TFE3*), transcription factor EB (*TFEB*) translocation-associated carcinoma

Synonyms

- Translocation-associated carcinoma, Xp11.2 and t(6;11) renal carcinomas, *TFE3* (Xp11.2) and *TFEB* [t(6;11)] carcinomas

Definitions

- Renal carcinomas characterized and defined by translocations involving MiTF/TFE family genes (*TFE3* or *TFEB*), and fusions to different genes at a number of different chromosomal locations, including
  - 17q25 (*ASPL*), 1q21 (*PRCC*), 1p34 (*PSF*), Xq12 (*nonO*), 17q23 (*CLTC*), 17q25 (*RCC17*), 3q23 (unknown), 11q12 (*alpha*)

ETIOLOGY/PATHOGENESIS

Molecular Abnormalities

- *TFE3*, *TFEB*, *TFEC*, and *MiTF* are members of MiTF-TFE family of basic helix-loop-helix zipper (bHLH-Zip) factors that bind DNA as homo- and heterodimers
- Members of this family believed to be involved in developmental and cellular processes in various cell types
  - *MiTF* in maturation of melanocytes of neural crest origin, retinal pigment epithelium, and bone marrow-derived mast cells and osteoclasts
  - *TFEB* in placental vascularization
  - *TFE3* in transforming growth factor β (TGF-b)-activated signal transduction and B-cell activation, as well as cooperation with *MiTF* and *TFEC* in osteoclast development
- *TFE3* gene localized to chromosome Xp11.2
- Reported chromosomal translocations and corresponding gene fusion identified in *TFE3* carcinomas
  - Alveolar soft part sarcoma chromosome region, candidate 1 gene *(ASPSCR1* or *ASPL)-TFE3*; t(X;17)(p11.2;q25)
    - *ASPL* (a.k.a. *ASPSCR1* or *PRCC2*) is novel gene of unknown function
    - Translocation similar to that in alveolar soft part sarcoma (ASPS)
    - However, translocation balanced in *TFE3* renal carcinoma, unlike the unbalanced translocation (loss of some genetic material) in ASPS
  - Papillary renal cell carcinoma (translocation-associated) gene *(PRCC)-TFE3*; t(X;1)(p11.2;q21)
    - *PRCC* is novel gene encoding major subunit of clathrin, a multimeric cytoplasmic organelle protein
  - PTB-associated splicing factor gene *(PSF)-TFE3*; t(X;1)(p11.2;p34)
  - *nonO-TFE3*; inv(X)(p11;q12)
    - *PSF* and *nonO* are splicing factor genes
  - Clathrin heavy chain 1 gene *(CLTC)-TFE3*; t(X;17)(p11.2;q23)
    - *CLTC* encodes a major subunit of clathrin
  - *RCC17-TFE3*; t(X;17)(p11.2;q25.3)
  - Unknown gene-*TFE3*; t(X;3)(p11;q23)
  - Different *TFE3* gene fusions consistently lead to overexpression of fusion protein relative to native *TFE3*, such that protein becomes detectable by immunohistochemical assay
- *TFEB* gene localized to chromosome 6p21
  - *TFEB* gene fused to *alpha* gene, an intron-less gene of unknown function on chromosome 11q12
    - Translocation fuses *alpha* gene with 1st intron of *TFEB* transcription factor gene
  - *Alpha-TFEB* fusion gene results in dysregulated expression of normal full-length TFEB protein detectable by immunohistochemistry

MITF/TFE FAMILY TRANSLOCATION-ASSOCIATED CARCINOMA

Key Facts

Terminology

- Renal carcinomas characterized and defined by translocations involving *MiTF/TFE* family genes (*TFE3* or *TFEB*) and with fusions to different, mostly well-characterized genes at a number of different chromosomal locations, including
  - 17q25 (*ASPL*), 1q21 (*PRCC*), 1p34 (*PSF*), Xq12 (*nonO*), 17q23 (*CLTC*), 17q25 (*RCC17*), 3q23 (unknown), 11q12 (*alpha*)

Clinical Issues

- Uncommon, but constitute a large proportion of renal cell carcinomas in pediatric age groups
- *TFE3* renal carcinomas among children, particularly *ASPL-TFE3* carcinomas, usually present at advanced stage
- Clinical course more aggressive in adults, with multiple reported deaths due to disease

Microscopic Pathology

- Carcinoma with high nuclear grade, prominent papillary &/or solid alveolar growth patterns, and composed of clear cells is most distinctive histopathologic appearance in Xp11 tumors
  - However, presence of cells with granular eosinophilic cytoplasm is not uncommon

Ancillary Tests

- These carcinomas are negative or only focally positive for epithelial markers and vimentin
- TFE3 and TFEB are highly sensitive and specific immunohistochemical markers for *TFE3* and *TFEB* renal carcinomas

Post-Chemotherapy

- Approximately 10-15% of cases in children with prior exposure to chemotherapy
  - Exposure usually during 1st and 2nd decades of life for other childhood malignancies or SLE
  - Interval between chemotherapy and development of renal carcinoma ranges between 2-13 years
  - Exact mechanism for post-chemotherapy development of these tumors not known
  - Possible contributing factor
    - Relatively increased proliferation in growing pediatric kidney rendering it more sensitive to mutagenic effects of chemotherapeutic agents

CLINICAL ISSUES

Epidemiology

- Incidence
  - Renal cell carcinomas account for < 5% of pediatric renal neoplasms
    - Although uncommon, translocation-associated renal carcinomas constitute large proportion of renal cell carcinomas in pediatric age group
  - Few cases described in adults with the oldest being in a 78-year-old man
    - However, in a large recent consecutive series from Japan, comprised 1.6% of all RCCs in adults and 15% of RCCs in patients < 45 years of age
    - Because of marked differences in number of RCCs in adults and children, absolute total number of cases in adults likely greater than in children
- Gender
  - As more cases are being reported, there seems to be no definite sex bias

Presentation

- Pediatric and young adult patients are usually symptomatic at presentation, and only a few cases are incidentally discovered
- Most common symptom is hematuria, followed by abdominal mass, abdominal pain, and weight loss
- Rare atypical presentations in adults include heavily calcified renal mass, outflow obstruction with consequent pyelonephritis, misdiagnosis as renal cyst or nephrolithiasis

Treatment

- Optimal treatment approach remains to be determined
- Reported cases have been managed similarly to conventional renal cell carcinoma

Prognosis

- *TFE3* renal carcinomas among children, particularly *ASPL-TFE3* carcinomas, usually present at advanced stage
  - In spite of high stage at presentation, including lymph node metastasis, based on relatively short follow-up, clinical behavior usually not aggressive
- Among the relatively small number of reported cases in adults, clinical course more aggressive, with multiple reported deaths due to disease
- Sites of metastasis include lymph nodes, lung, liver, spine, and adrenal gland
- All reported cases of *TFEB* renal carcinoma have been organ-confined tumors, and none has recurred or metastasized
  - However, clinical follow-up information limited

MACROSCOPIC FEATURES

General Features

- Mostly well circumscribed but nonencapsulated
  - Some tumors with irregular infiltrative outlines, with perirenal and renal sinus extensions
  - Rarely, pseudocapsule is present, and it may show calcifications
- Cut surface tan-yellow, often showing hemorrhage and necrosis; similar to clear cell renal cell carcinoma

Size

- 2.7-21 cm, reported mean: 6.8 cm

MICROSCOPIC PATHOLOGY

Histologic Features

- While morphologic features often correlate with translocation type, significant morphologic overlap between different translocation groups
- Carcinoma with high nuclear grade, prominent papillary &/or solid alveolar growth patterns, and composed of clear cells is most distinctive histopathologic appearance in Xp11 tumors
- However, presence of cells with granular eosinophilic cytoplasm is not uncommon
- Histology of Xp11 translocation carcinomas with specific chromosomal translocations often have characteristic features
  - *ASPL-TFE3* carcinoma usually shows
    - Cells with voluminous, clear to eosinophilic cytoplasm; discrete cell borders, vesicular nuclear chromatin, and prominent nucleoli
    - Tumor cells often are dyscohesive, which leads to alveolar and pseudopapillary architecture
    - True papillary formations are also not uncommon and rarely may be predominant architectural pattern
    - Psammoma bodies are almost universal and sometimes extensive; usually form upon characteristic hyaline nodules
  - *PRCC-TFE3* carcinoma typically shows
    - Less abundant cytoplasm
    - Few psammoma bodies and hyaline nodules
    - More nested and compact architecture
    - Some nests with central lumina forming acinar pattern
    - Papillary architecture is common; present either merging with or sharply defined from the acinar areas
    - Usually, but not always, lower nuclear grade than *ASPL-TFE3* tumors
- Unusual histologic features
  - Biphasic population of larger clear cells and smaller cells clustered around nodular hyaline material similar to t(6;11) translocation renal cell carcinoma
  - Pleomorphic giant cells
  - Focal "hobnailed" pattern
  - Fascicles of neoplastic spindle cells
- Morphologic features of other Xp11 translocation carcinomas (*PSF-TFE3, nonO-TFE3, CLTC-TFE3*) not well defined because of few reported cases
- Alpha-*TFEB* carcinomas with t(6;11)(p21;q12) usually with
  - Nests, sheets, and tubules of cells separated by thin vascular septae
  - Papillary architecture is uncommon but may be focally to extensively present in some tumors
  - Most tumor cells with abundant clear cytoplasm, well-defined cell borders, and round nuclei
    - Nuclei usually uniform but often with prominent nucleoli
  - Some tumors with variable proportion of granular eosinophilic cytoplasm
  - Usually minor subpopulation of smaller cells with high nuclear to cytoplasmic ratio and dense nuclear chromatin
    - Typically clustered around nodules of hyaline basement membrane material
    - Hyaline material may not be present in some of the smaller cell areas or may be entirely absent
  - Similar, biphasic morphology may rarely also be seen in Xp11 (*TFE3*) carcinomas

Predominant Pattern/Injury Type

- Neoplastic

Predominant Cell/Compartment Type

- Epithelial

ANCILLARY TESTS

Immunohistochemistry

- Unlike common RCCs, these carcinomas are negative or only focally positive for cytokeratins and epithelial membrane antigen (EMA/MUC1)
- Vimentin is usually negative but may be weakly and focally positive
- CD10, RCC antigen, AMACR, and E-cadherin are usually positive in *TFE3* carcinomas
- CD10 and RCC antigen are usually absent or only focally positive in *TFEB* tumors
- *TFE3* is highly sensitive and specific marker for Xp11 translocation-associated carcinomas
  - Diffuse nuclear labeling reported to have sensitivity of 97.5% and specificity of 99.6%
  - ASPS also shows diffuse and strong nuclear reactivity
  - Very rare cases of adrenal cortical carcinoma reported to be positive
  - Other renal cell tumors and large number of nonrenal tumors tested have been negative
- *TFEB* is highly sensitive and specific marker for 6;11 translocation-associated carcinomas
  - Lymphocytes sometimes may show weak nuclear reactivity
- Melanocytic markers Melan-A(MART-1) and HMB-45 frequently positive in *TFEB* carcinoma
- Melan-A(MART-1) and HMB-45 rarely expressed in *TFE3* tumors, particularly those with *PSF-TFE3* and *CLTC-TFE3* fusions

Electron Microscopy

- *TFE3* renal carcinomas
  - Evidence of epithelial differentiation present varying from cell junctions, well-formed glandular lumens containing microvilli, and basement membranes
  - Intracytoplasmic fat and glycogen are present, similar to conventional renal cell carcinoma
  - In *PRCC-TFE3* carcinoma, intracisternal microtubules similar to those in melanoma are sometimes present
  - In *ASPL-TFE3* carcinoma, abundant electron-dense granules similar in size and shape to those seen in alveolar soft part sarcoma are present

        - Rare instance of well-formed rhomboid crystals characteristic of alveolar soft part sarcoma reported
- *TFEB* renal carcinomas
    - Polygonal cells rich in mitochondria, with scattered membrane-bound granules and varying amount of glycogen
    - Occasional cell junctions; true desmosomes not prominent
    - Distinctive extracellular pools of duplicated basement membrane material surrounded by smaller tumor cells
        - Multilamellar appearance of basement membrane material at higher magnification

DIFFERENTIAL DIAGNOSIS

Clear Cell Renal Cell Carcinoma

- High-grade clear cell carcinoma with large solid alveoli vs. *ASPL-TFE3* carcinoma
    - Transition to more typical lower grade, smaller acinar growth pattern is often present
    - Cells with voluminous cytoplasm are uncommon
    - Psammomatous calcifications are rarely, if ever, seen
    - Immunostains for PAN-CK(AE1/AE3), CAM5.2, and EMA/MUC1 are positive, and AMACR and TFE3 are negative
- Clear cell carcinoma vs. *TFEB* renal carcinoma
    - Clear cell carcinoma lacks biphasic pattern of large epithelioid cells and clusters of smaller cells
    - Immunostains for PAN-CK(AE1/AE3), CAM5.2, EMA/MUC1, CD10, and vimentin are usually diffusely positive
    - TFEB is negative

Papillary Renal Cell Carcinoma

- Foamy macrophages are frequent in papillary cores
- PAN-CK(AE1/AE3), CAM5.2, CK7, and AMACR are positive
- TFE3 and TFEB are negative

Clear Cell-Papillary Renal Cell Carcinoma

- Nuclei are low grade and arranged in linear pattern away from basement membrane
- Tumors are often cystic
- On immunostaining, these are CK7, CA9, and HMCK(34βE12) positive
- AMACR and CD10 mostly negative

DIAGNOSTIC CHECKLIST

Pathologic Interpretation Pearls

- Renal tumors with clear cell cytology with voluminous cytoplasm should always raise differential diagnostic consideration of translocation-associated carcinoma
    - Possibility is particularly high in younger patients
    - Level of suspicion should be higher in cases
        - Not showing areas typical of lower grade clear cell renal cell carcinoma morphology
        - Showing any papillary architecture
    - Immunohistochemical staining for epithelial markers (cytokeratins and EMA/MUC1) in such cases must be performed
        - Negative or only focal positivity of these stains further strengthens possibility of translocation-associated carcinoma
- Tumors resembling high-grade clear cell renal cell carcinoma, but showing prominent psammomatous calcifications, also require exclusion of translocation-associated renal carcinoma
    - Psammomatous calcifications, particularly when numerous, very unusual finding in clear cell renal cell carcinoma

SELECTED REFERENCES

1. Komai Y et al: Adult Xp11 translocation renal cell carcinoma diagnosed by cytogenetics and immunohistochemistry. Clin Cancer Res. 15(4):1170-6, 2009
2. Camparo P et al: Renal translocation carcinomas: clinicopathologic, immunohistochemical, and gene expression profiling analysis of 31 cases with a review of the literature. Am J Surg Pathol. 32(5):656-70, 2008
3. Geller JI et al: Translocation renal cell carcinoma: lack of negative impact due to lymph node spread. Cancer. 112(7):1607-16, 2008
4. Argani P et al: Xp11 translocation renal cell carcinoma in adults: expanded clinical, pathologic, and genetic spectrum. Am J Surg Pathol. 31(8):1149-60, 2007
5. Argani P et al: Translocation carcinomas of the kidney after chemotherapy in childhood. J Clin Oncol. 24(10):1529-34, 2006
6. Argani P et al: Renal carcinomas with the t(6;11)(p21;q12): clinicopathologic features and demonstration of the specific alpha-TFEB gene fusion by immunohistochemistry, RT-PCR, and DNA PCR. Am J Surg Pathol. 29(2):230-40, 2005
7. Argani P et al: Primary renal neoplasms with the ASPL-TFE3 gene fusion of alveolar soft part sarcoma: a distinctive tumor entity previously included among renal cell carcinomas of children and adolescents. Am J Pathol. 159(1):179-92, 2001
8. Weterman MJ et al: Nuclear localization and transactivating capacities of the papillary renal cell carcinoma-associated TFE3 and PRCC (fusion) proteins. Oncogene. 19(1):69-74, 2000
9. Sidhar SK et al: The t(X;1)(p11.2;q21.2) translocation in papillary renal cell carcinoma fuses a novel gene PRCC to the TFE3 transcription factor gene. Hum Mol Genet. 5(9):1333-8, 1996
10. Suijkerbuijk RF et al: Identification of a yeast artificial chromosome that spans the human papillary renal cell carcinoma-associated t(X;1) breakpoint in Xp11.2. Cancer Genet Cytogenet. 71(2):164-9, 1993
11. Tomlinson GE et al: Cytogenetics of a renal cell carcinoma in a 17-month-old child. Evidence for Xp11.2 as a recurring breakpoint. Cancer Genet Cytogenet. 57(1):11-7, 1991
12. de Jong B et al: Cytogenetics of a renal adenocarcinoma in a 2-year-old child. Cancer Genet Cytogenet. 21(2):165-9, 1986

Gross and Microscopic Features

*(**Left**) Typical gross appearance of a TFE3 renal carcinoma shows a well-circumscribed tumor with tan-yellow cut surface. Many tumors, however, show invasion into perinephric fat ⊳. (**Right**) Well-circumscribed TFE3 renal carcinoma is shown. Most MiTF renal carcinomas are well circumscribed, without a distinct tumor capsule. However, satellite nodules into the surrounding parenchyma are quite common. Some TFE3 carcinomas show a pseudocapsule ⊳, often with calcifications.*

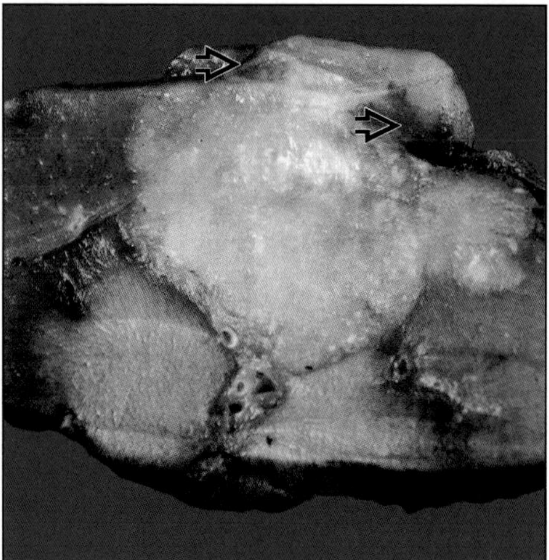

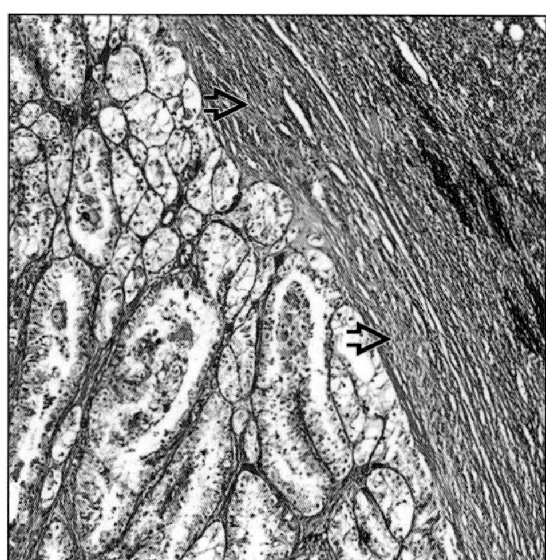

*(**Left**) Hematoxylin & eosin stain shows characteristic light microscopic features of a TFE3 renal carcinoma. The presence of numerous psammomatous calcifications → in a tumor resembling high-grade clear cell RCC should always be investigated for a TFE carcinoma. (**Right**) Solid alveolar architectural pattern in a TFE3 carcinoma, as seen here, is quite common, and the thin branching septations may raise the possibility of a high-grade clear cell renal cell carcinoma.*

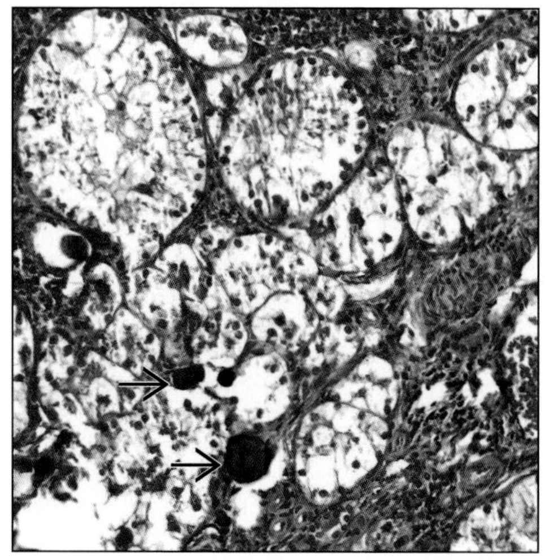

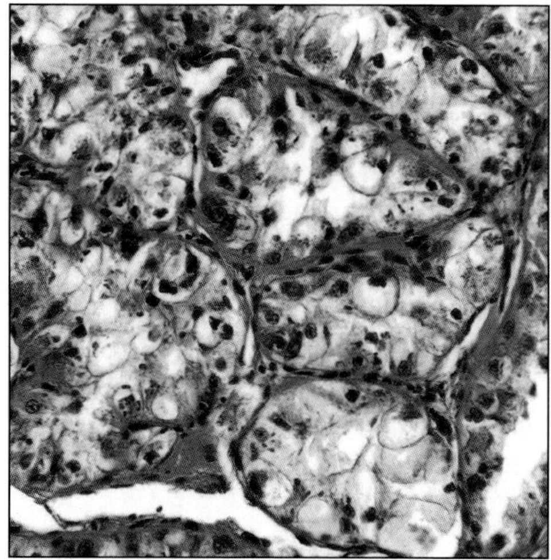

*(**Left**) Papillary architecture in TFE3 renal carcinoma is quite common. Clear cell cytology with papillary architecture →, psammomatous calcifications ↗, and cells with voluminous cytoplasm ⊳ strongly point toward the diagnosis of a TFE3 carcinoma, rather than a clear cell RCC. (**Right**) A high-magnification view of TFE3 carcinoma with papillary architecture shows voluminous clear cytoplasm and high-grade nuclei. Intracytoplasmic hyaline globules → are also occasionally seen.*

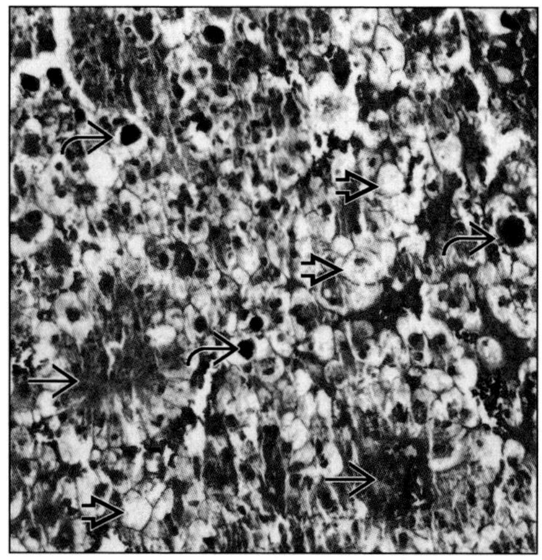

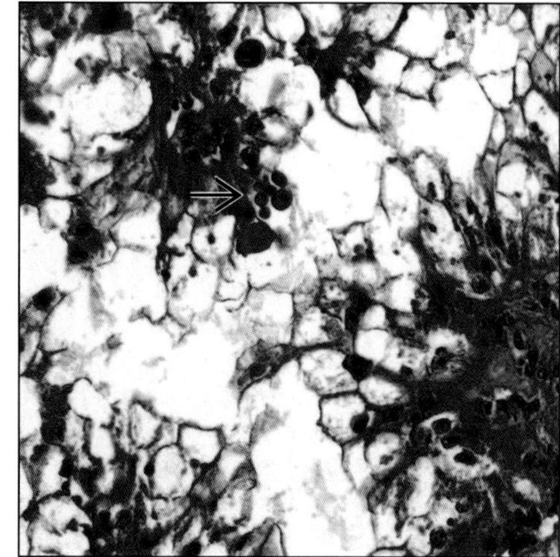

Microscopic Features and Ancillary Techniques

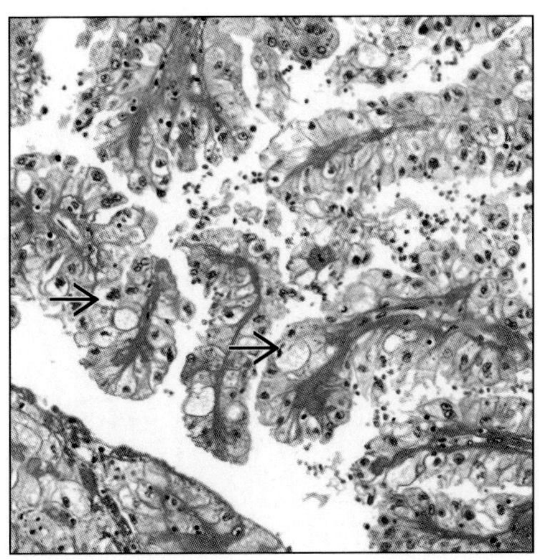

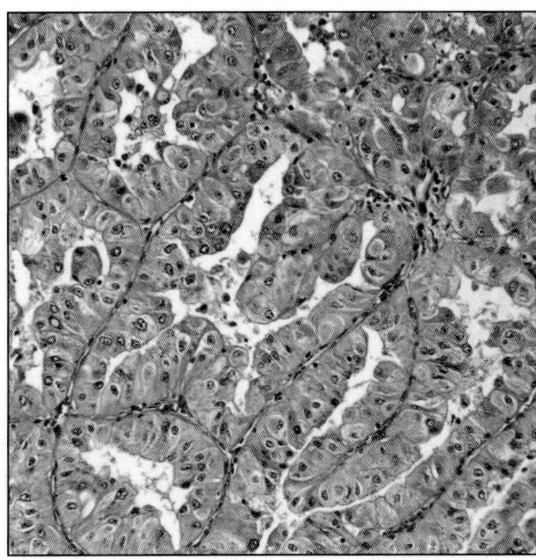

(Left) *Most TFE3 tumors may show pseudopapillary architecture with dyscohesive solid acini, but true papillary architecture is not uncommon. The voluminous cytoplasm in some of the cells ➔ is a prominent pointer toward translocation-associated carcinoma.* ***(Right)*** *While clear cell cytology is common in TFE3 carcinomas, some tumors may show prominent to predominant, and, rarely, almost exclusive cytoplasmic eosinophilia.*

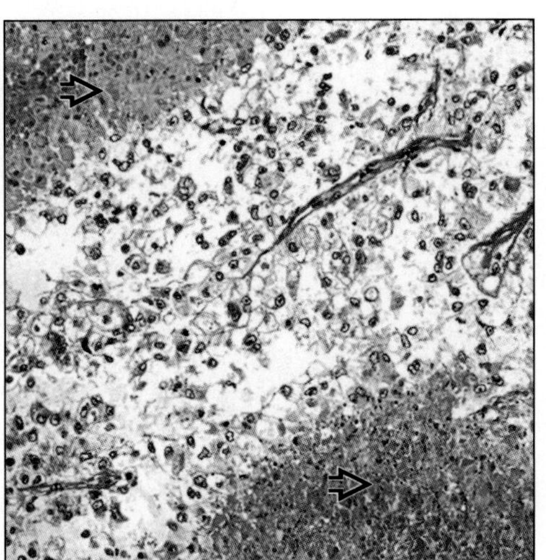

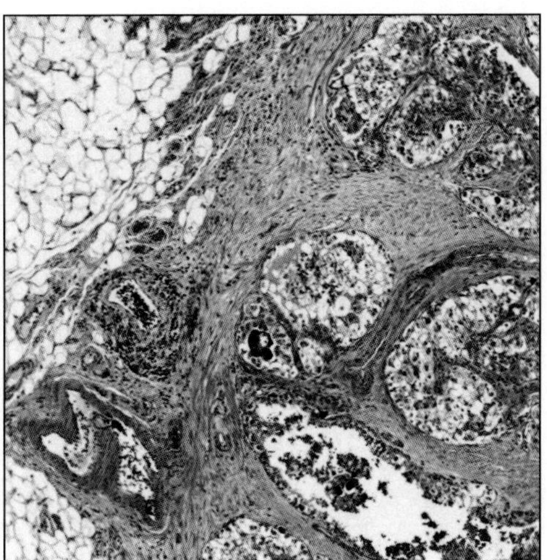

(Left) *Coagulative tumor necrosis ⇨ and hemorrhage are commonly observed in TFE renal carcinoma. These findings are often noted even in gross specimens. This photomicrograph is a reflection of such commonly observed gross findings.* ***(Right)*** *This photomicrograph shows perinephric fat invasion in a TFE3 carcinoma. TFE3 renal carcinomas often present at high tumor stage. However, compared to the adults, high stage does not necessarily predict aggressive outcome in children.*

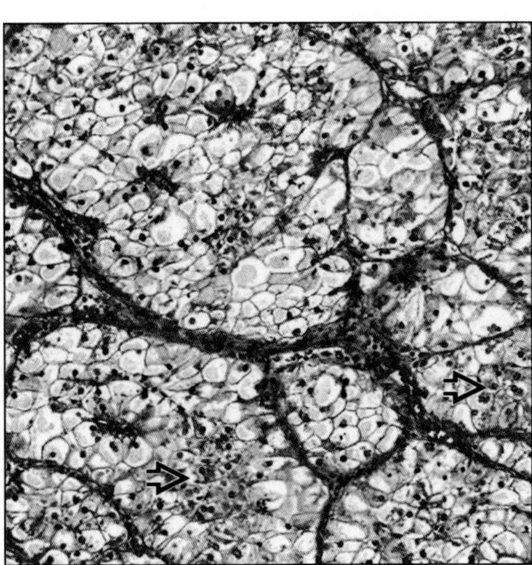

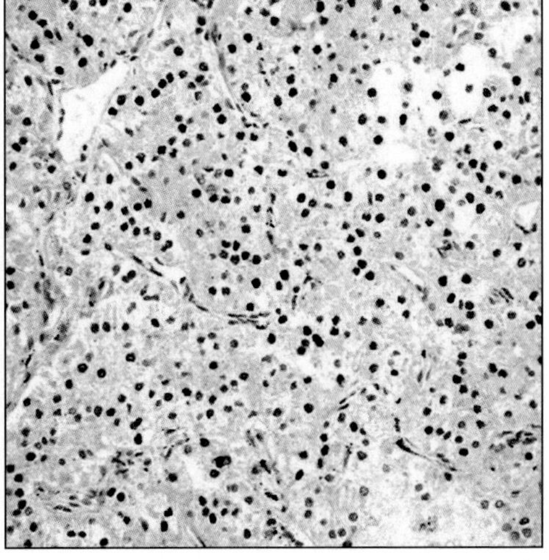

(Left) *Solid alveolar growth pattern is not uncommon in TFE3 renal carcinoma. The solid alveoli may show central cell dyscohesion ⇨ and morphologically mimic alveolar soft part sarcoma. Such a growth pattern is commonly associated with ASPL-TFE3 gene fusion.* ***(Right)*** *This image depicts TFE3 immunohistochemical staining in a ASPL-TFE3 carcinoma. Diffuse and strong nuclear positivity for TFE3 is characteristic of all types of Xp11 renal carcinomas, irrespective of the fusion gene partner.*

Microscopic Features and Ancillary Techniques

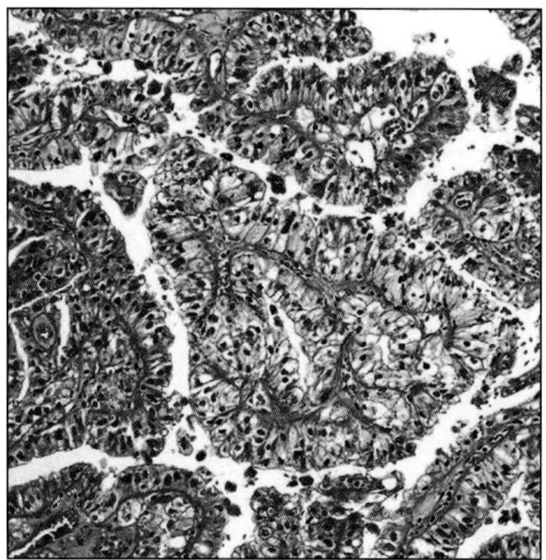

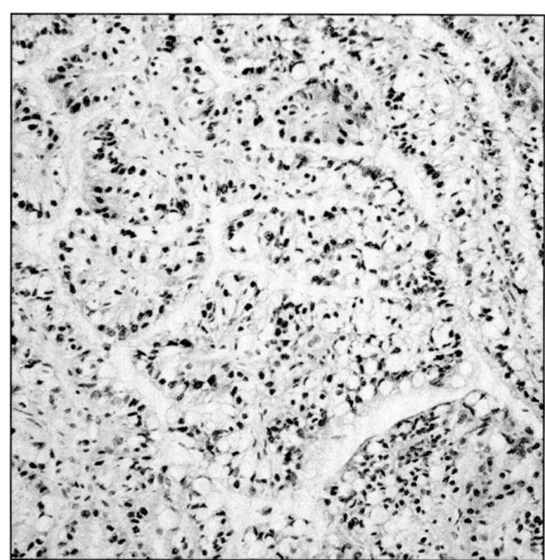

(Left) *This TFE3 renal carcinoma depicts prominent papillary architecture. Papillary architecture with prominent clear cell and high-grade cytology should always raise the differential diagnostic possibility of a translocation-associated renal carcinoma.* ***(Right)*** *TFE3 immunoreactivity is seen in a TFE3 renal carcinoma with prominent papillary architecture. Diffuse TFE3 positivity is highly specific and sensitive for TFE3 carcinoma; it correlates very well with Xp11.2 (TFE3 gene) translocation.*

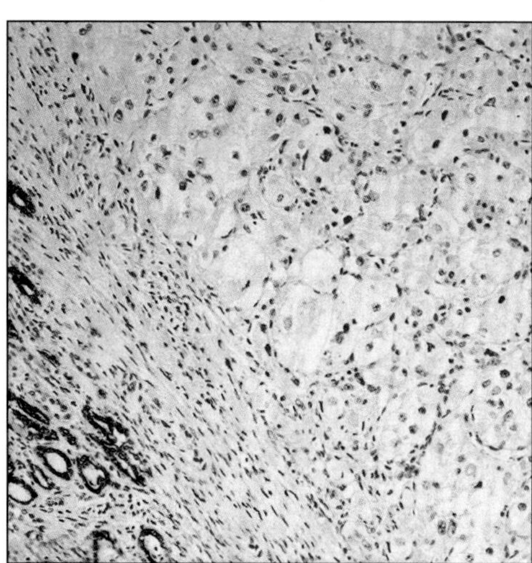

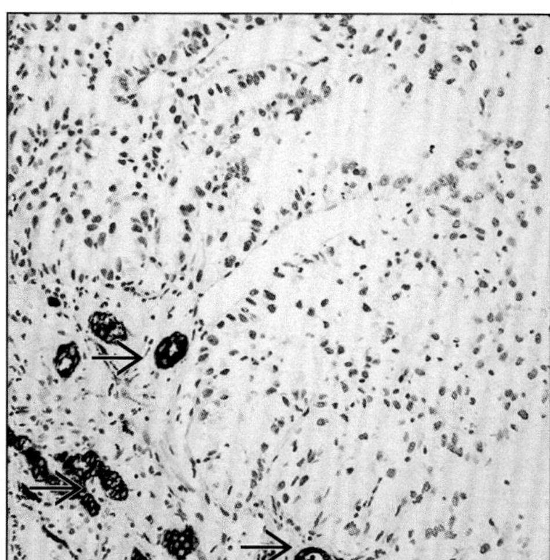

(Left) *Immunostaining for PAN-CK(AE1/AE3) in TFE3 carcinoma is usually negative.* ***(Right)*** *Unlike other renal tumors, translocation-associated renal carcinomas are negative or only focally and weakly positive for cytokeratins and EMA/MUC1. Tumors with clear cells, voluminous cytoplasm, with or without papillary architecture, and lacking staining for epithelial markers strongly point toward TFE3 renal carcinoma. Note the positive internal control* ➔.

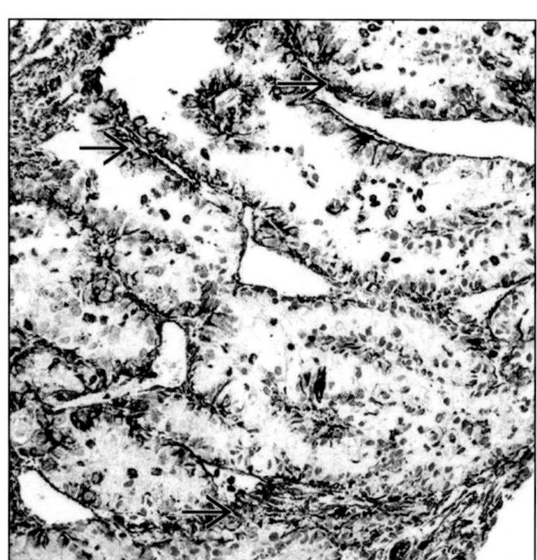

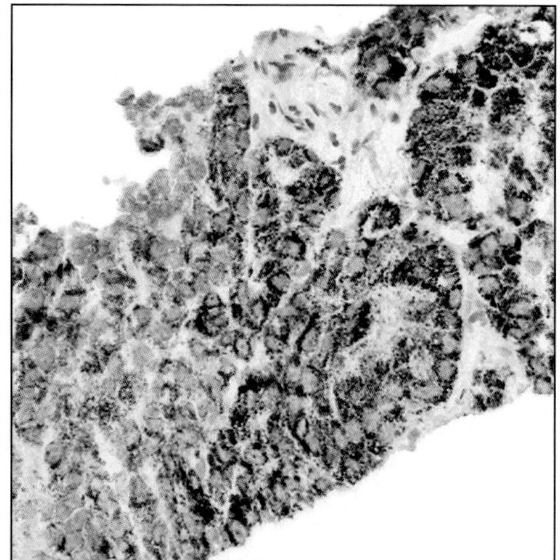

(Left) *Vimentin immunostain shows rare tumor cells positive in a TFE3 renal carcinoma. Note the diffuse and strong positivity in the fibrovascular septa* ➔. *Diffuse and strong positivity for vimentin is rare in MiTF/TFE family translocation-associated carcinomas.* ***(Right)*** *AMACR usually shows diffuse positivity in translocation-associated carcinomas. Negativity for CK7 and diffuse positivity for AMACR can help in differentiating these tumors from both the clear cell and papillary RCC.*

Microscopic Features and Ancillary Techniques

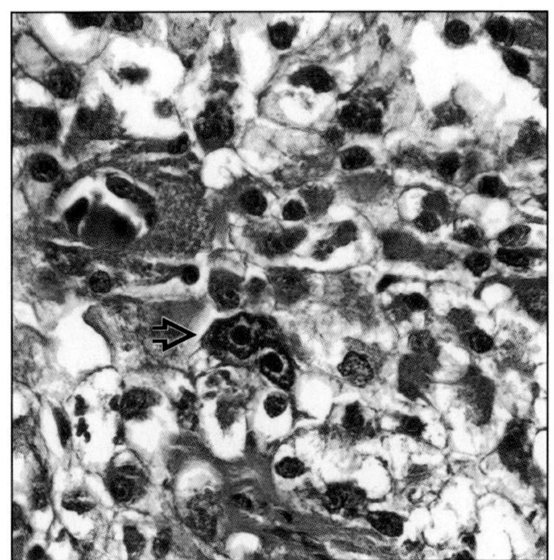

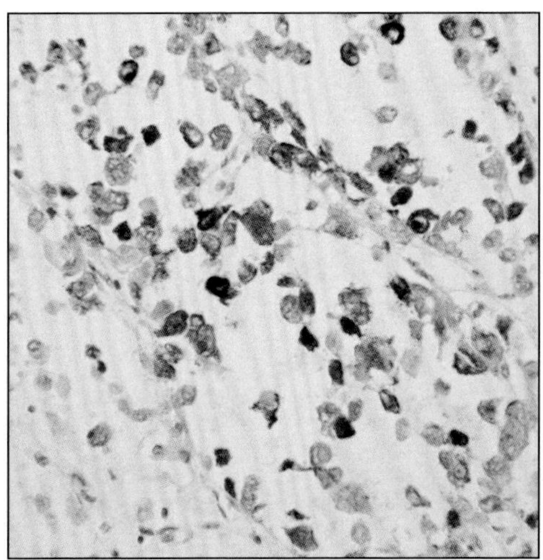

(Left) *Some translocation-associated renal carcinomas, particularly those in adults, may occasionally show marked focal cytologic atypia ⊡ and presence of pleomorphic giant cells.* ***(Right)*** *While melanocytic markers HMB-45 and Melan-A(MART-1) are frequently positive in TFEB renal carcinomas, rare cases of TFE3 tumors may also show focal positivity, particularly those with PSF-TFE3 and CLTC-TFE3 fusions. This image depicts HMB-45 positivity in a TFE3 renal carcinoma.*

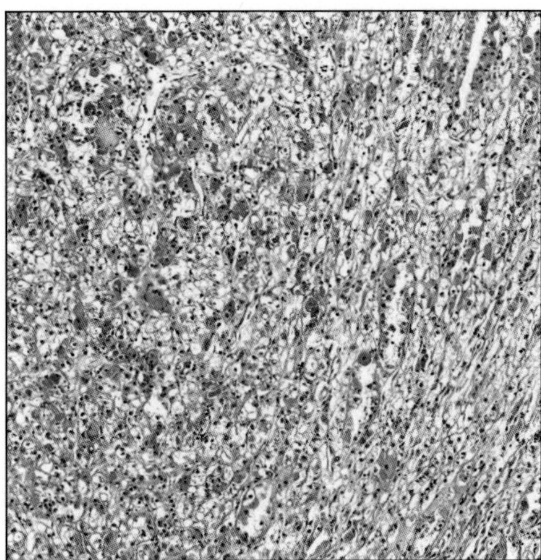

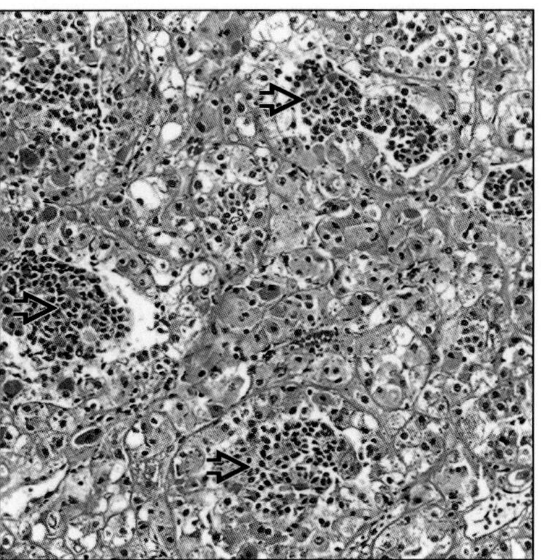

(Left) *A low-magnification view of a TFEB [t(6;11)] renal carcinoma shows nests, sheets, and tubules of cells, predominantly with clear cytoplasm, separated by thin vascular septae.* ***(Right)*** *However, the most characteristic feature of TFEB renal carcinoma is a biphasic morphology. Dispersed among the larger cells are clusters and islands of smaller cells ⊡ with high nuclear to cytoplasmic ratio and somewhat denser-appearing nuclear chromatin.*

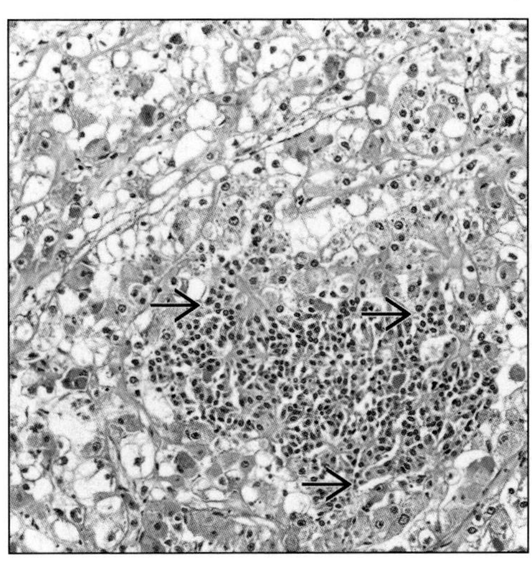

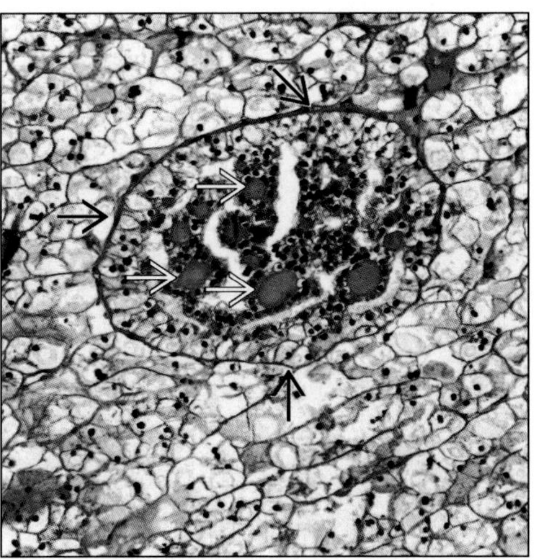

(Left) *The collections of smaller cell population in TFEB tumors may show irregular outlines ⊡ but may be sharply delimited in some instances.* ***(Right)*** *This smaller cell population in a TFEB renal carcinoma is present within the confines of a tubular structure ⊡ lined by larger epithelioid cells similar to the rest of the tumor. The smaller cells are arranged around small nodules of hyaline material ⊡ that is ultrastructurally shown to be basement membrane material.*

MITF/TFE FAMILY TRANSLOCATION-ASSOCIATED CARCINOMA

Microscopic Features and Ancillary Techniques

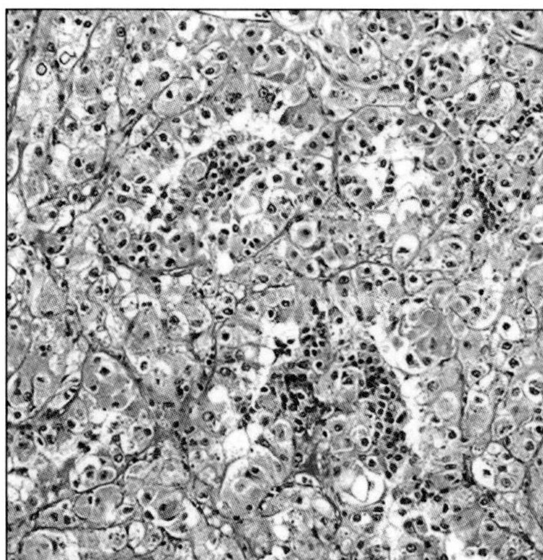

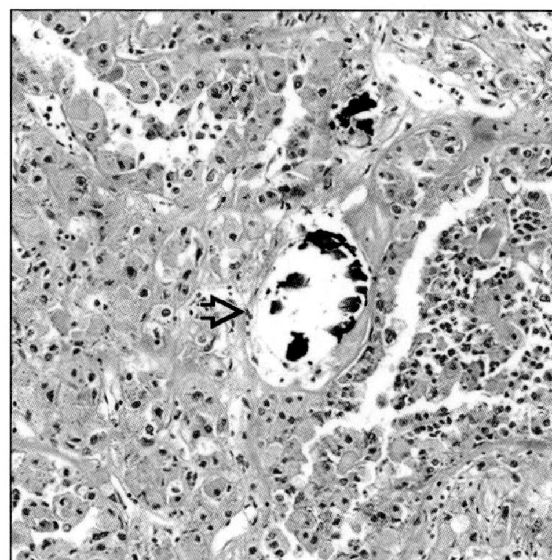

(Left) *While the nodules of basement membrane material within the smaller cell clusters are typically abundant in a given tumor, in some cases such hyaline nodules may be quite rare and difficult to find.* ***(Right)*** *Focal calcification is seen in a t(6;11) renal carcinoma ⮚. Compared to the TFE3 tumors, psammomatous calcifications in TFEB carcinomas are quite rare and may be completely absent.*

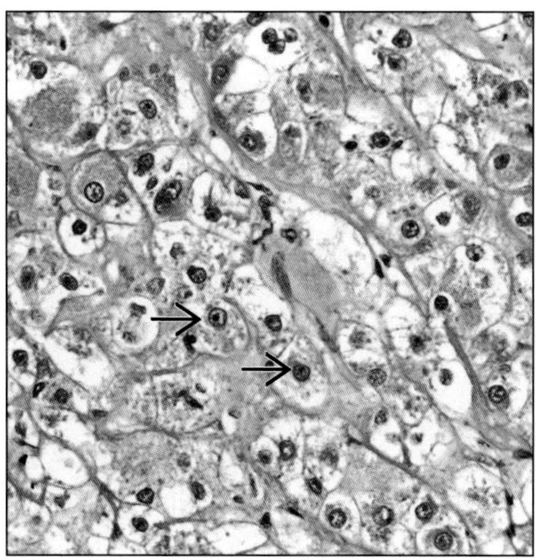

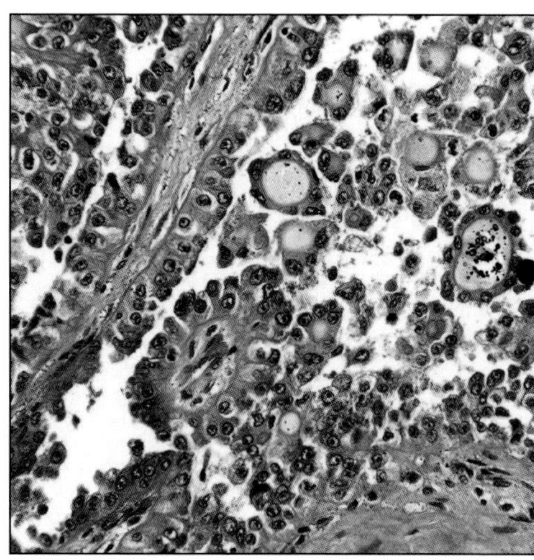

(Left) *While most tumors show an admixture of cells with clear and eosinophilic cytoplasm, some TFEB tumors are predominantly or almost exclusively composed of cells with eosinophilic cytoplasm. Most tumors do not show significant nuclear pleomorphism, but the presence of prominent nucleoli → is not uncommon.* ***(Right)*** *Focal papillations are seen in many of the TFEB renal carcinomas, but prominent papillary architecture may be observed in some cases.*

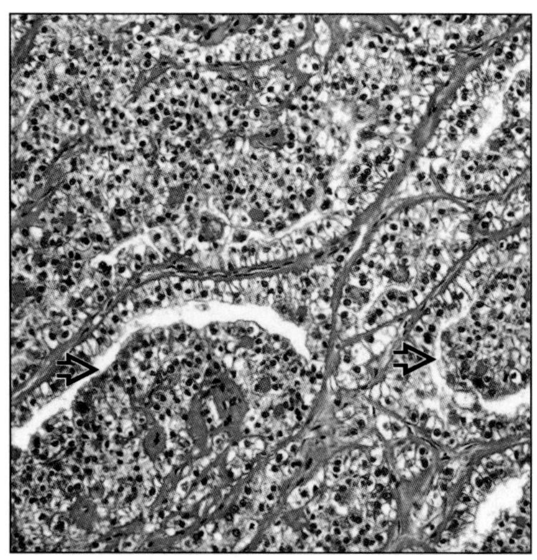

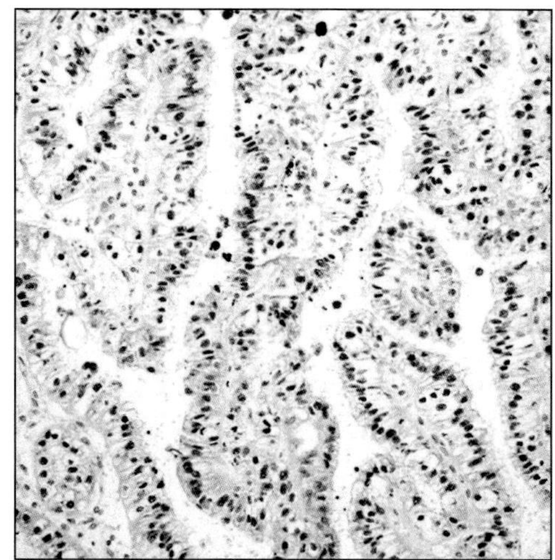

(Left) *This TFEB renal carcinoma has focal papillations ⮚ in a background with a predominantly nested growth pattern.* ***(Right)*** *TFEB immunostaining shows diffuse nuclear positivity in a TFEB renal carcinoma. As with TFE3 immunostain in Xp11.2 carcinomas, TFEB immunostain is highly specific for t(6;11) tumors. Both these antibodies show no cross-reactivity with each other. TFEB immunostain may also show focal nuclear staining in some lymphocytes.*

Microscopic Features and Ancillary Techniques

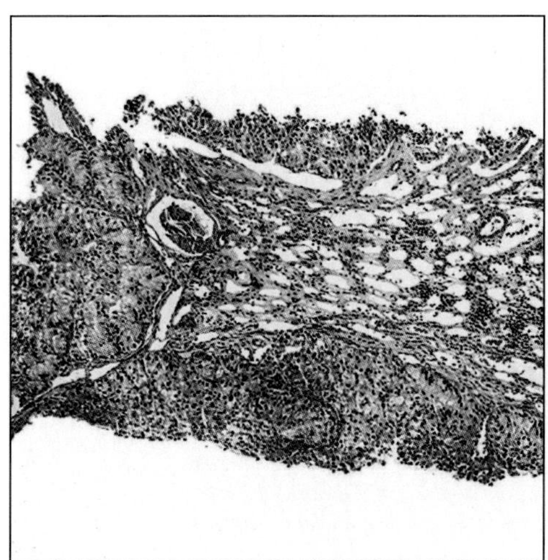

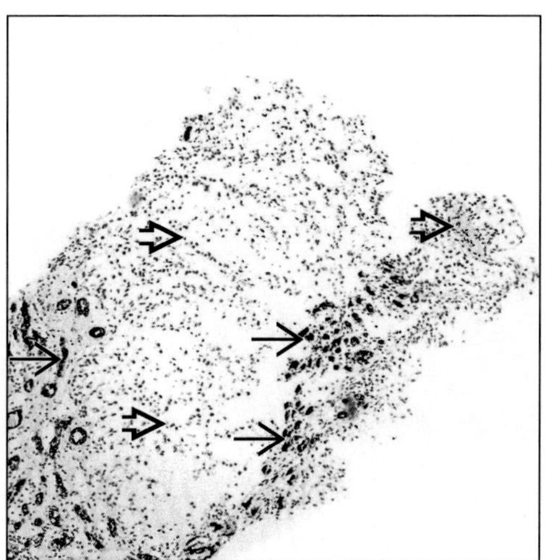

(Left) *Solid nests, variable papillary architecture, clear cell cytology, and voluminous cytoplasm in a renal tumor should alert one to the possibility of a translocation-associated carcinoma. Attention to these findings may lead to accurate diagnosis even on needle biopsies of the kidney.* ***(Right)*** *The suspicion of TFE carcinoma is further strengthened by the absence of immunoreactivity ⇨ for epithelial markers (PAN-CK[AE1/AE3] in this instance), with appropriate internal control →.*

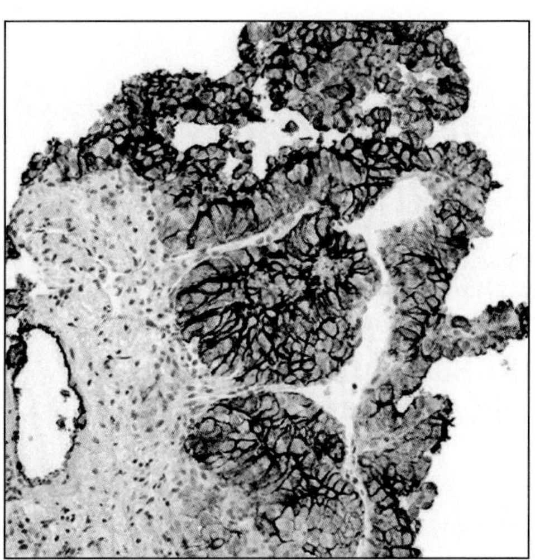

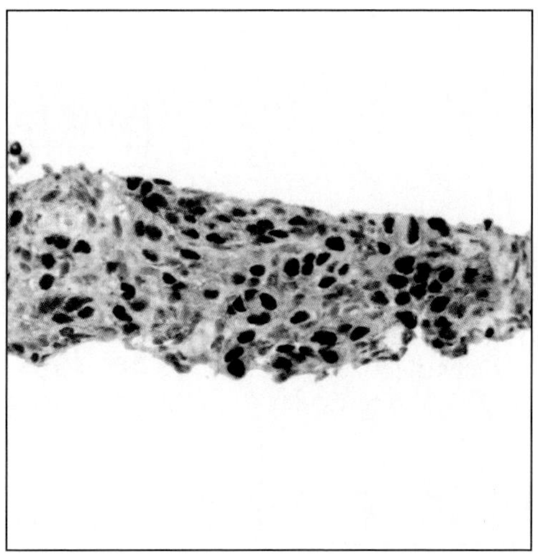

(Left) *CD10 usually shows diffuse positivity in TFE3 renal carcinomas. However, the staining is usually weak and more focal in TFEB tumors.* ***(Right)*** *TFE3 immunoreactivity is observed in a needle core biopsy of a renal mass in a 35-year-old man. Although the lack of staining for cytokeratins (including CK7) and diffuse positivity for AMACR and CD10 increase the morphologic suspicion of a TFE carcinoma, only diffuse nuclear reactivity with the TFE antibodies will confirm the diagnosis.*

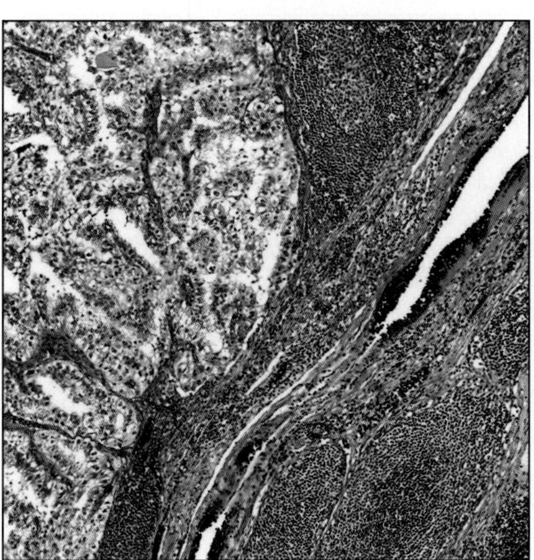

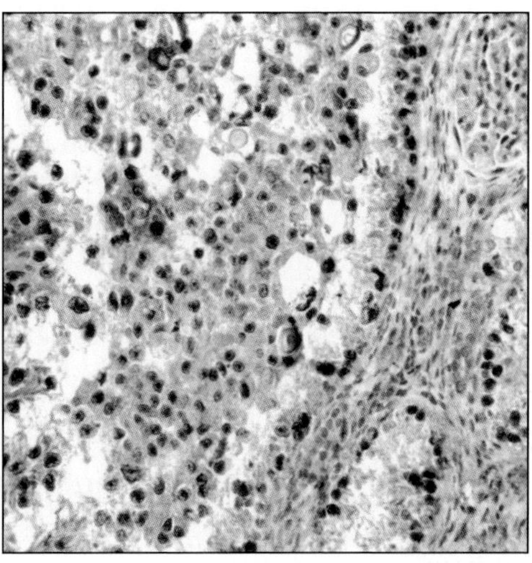

(Left) *This image shows a TFE3 renal carcinoma metastatic to a lymph node. Metastatic sites include lymph nodes, lung, liver, spine, and adrenal gland. Lymph node metastases are quite common, both in children and adults. Children with lymph node metastases, however, maintain a favorable prognosis (at least in the short term), whereas the same does not hold true in adults with metastases.* ***(Right)*** *Diffuse nuclear immunoreactivity for TFE3 in a metastatic lymph node mass confirms the diagnosis.*

DYSGERMINOMA

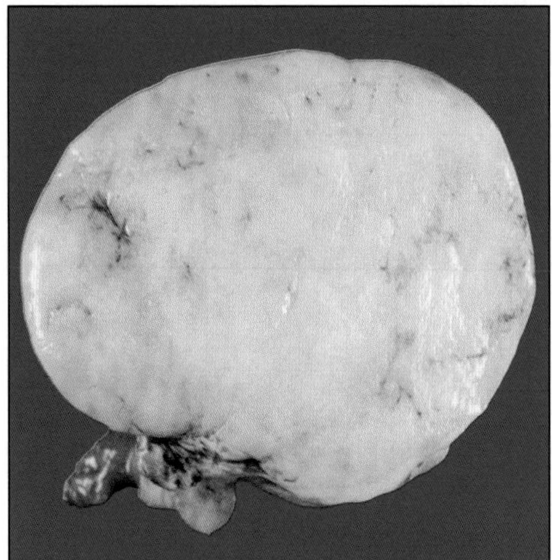

Gross photograph of dysgerminoma demonstrates the solid, tan cut surface. Cystic degeneration, hemorrhage, or necrosis may be present.

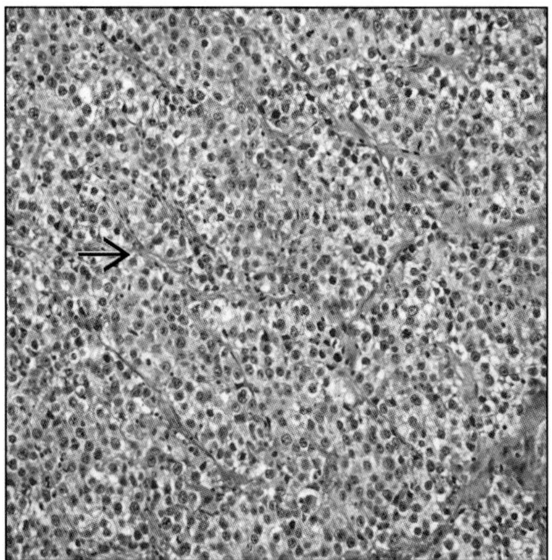

Hematoxylin & eosin demonstrates sheets of cells separated by thin fibrous septae ⇒. Tumor cells are of uniform size and have clear to finely granular cytoplasm.

TERMINOLOGY

Synonyms

- Ovarian seminoma

Definitions

- Ovarian germ cell tumor

ETIOLOGY/PATHOGENESIS

Developmental Anomaly

- 5% arise in abnormal gonads, such as gonadal dysgenesis, gonadoblastoma (50%), and testicular feminization syndrome

CLINICAL ISSUES

Epidemiology

- Incidence
    - 6% of childhood ovarian neoplasms
    - Most present in adolescence and early adult life

Site

- Right (50%), left (33-35%), bilateral (10-17%)

Presentation

- Abdominal pain &/or enlargement
- Can be found incidentally (pregnancy)
- Can present with elevated serum human chorionic gonadotropin
- Rarely associated with hypercalcemia

Natural History

- Local spread or metastasis (via lymphatics)
- May rupture when large

Treatment

- Chemotherapy with surgical removal

Prognosis

- Survival rate is 95%

MACROSCOPIC FEATURES

General Features

- Round, oval, or lobulated gray-white solid tumor with smooth fibrous capsule
- Lobulated gray-tan cut surface
- Areas of hemorrhage or necrosis may be seen

Sections to Be Submitted

- Extensive sampling recommended, especially of less typical areas (i.e., cystic areas, if present)

Size

- Up to 50 cm (5 kg tumor reported)

MICROSCOPIC PATHOLOGY

Histologic Features

- Nests and sheets of uniform large round cells (15-25 μm) with abundant, clear to finely granular cytoplasm, prominent nucleoli, and well-defined cell borders
    - Some variation in cell size is usually seen
    - Detectable mitotic activity
- Prominent fibrous septae with lymphocytic infiltrate
    - Granulomatous reaction can be seen
- Multinucleated syncytiotrophoblasts may be present
- Tubular or cord-like pattern may be seen
- Hyalinization may be very prominent
- Focal necrosis, hyaline change in vessels, germinal centers, or granulomatous foci may be present

Predominant Pattern/Injury Type

- Solid
- Sheets

DYSGERMINOMA

Key Facts

Terminology
- Ovarian germ cell tumor

Etiology/Pathogenesis
- 5% arise in abnormal gonads, such as gonadal dysgenesis, gonadoblastoma (50%), and testicular feminization syndrome

Clinical Issues
- Most present in adolescence and early adult life

Macroscopic Features
- Round, oval, or lobulated gray-white solid tumor with smooth fibrous capsule

Microscopic Pathology
- Nests and sheets of uniform large round cells (15-25 μm), with abundant, clear to finely granular cytoplasm, prominent nucleoli, and well-defined cell borders
- Prominent fibrous septae with lymphocytic infiltrate

Immunohistochemistry

Antibody	Reactivity	Staining Pattern	Comment
PLAP	Positive	Cell membrane	
CD117	Positive	Cytoplasmic	
HCG	Positive	Cytoplasmic	Only in syncytiotrophoblastic cells
EMA	Negative	Not applicable	

Predominant Cell/Compartment Type
- Germ, seminomatous

ANCILLARY TESTS

Histochemistry
- Periodic acid Schiff with diastase digestion
  - Reactivity: Negative
- Periodic acid-Schiff
  - Positive, cytoplasmic staining pattern

DIFFERENTIAL DIAGNOSIS

Clear Cell Carcinoma
- Absent prominent lymphocytic infiltrate
- Epithelial tumor shows strong positivity for cytokeratins

Embryonal Carcinoma
- Prominent clefts, alveoli, cell-lined spaces, and larger cells with marked pleomorphism
- Irregular nuclei with more than 1 prominent nucleolus
- CD30(+)

Malignant Lymphoma
- More pronounced nuclear pleomorphism
- Leukocyte common antigen positive and PLAP(-)

SELECTED REFERENCES

1. Roth LM et al: Recent advances in the pathology and classification of ovarian germ cell tumors. Int J Gynecol Pathol. 25(4):305-20, 2006
2. Baker PM et al: Immunohistochemistry as a tool in the differential diagnosis of ovarian tumors: an update. Int J Gynecol Pathol. 24(1):39-55, 2005
3. McCluggage WG: Ovarian neoplasms composed of small round cells: a review. Adv Anat Pathol. 11(6):288-96, 2004
4. Schwartz PE: Surgery of germ cell tumours of the ovary. Forum (Genova). 10(4):355-65, 2000
5. Matias-Guiu X et al: Clear cell tumors of the female genital tract. Semin Diagn Pathol. 14(4):233-9, 1997

IMAGE GALLERY

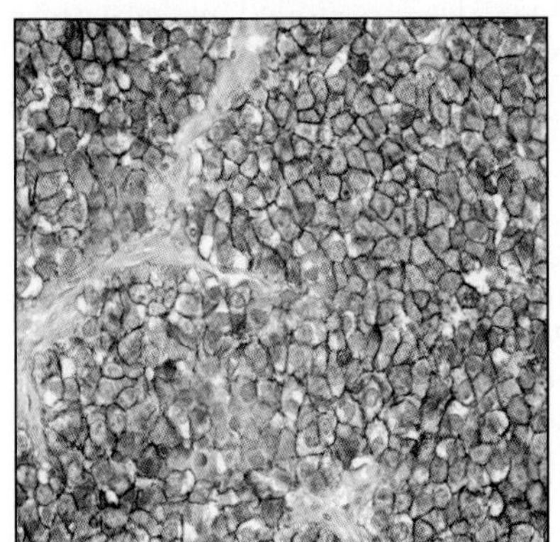

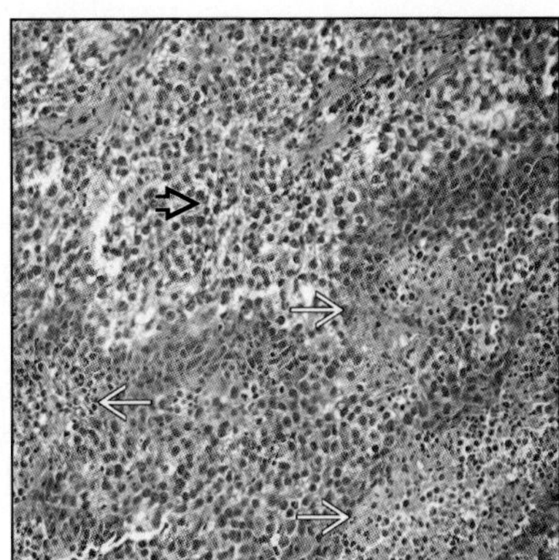

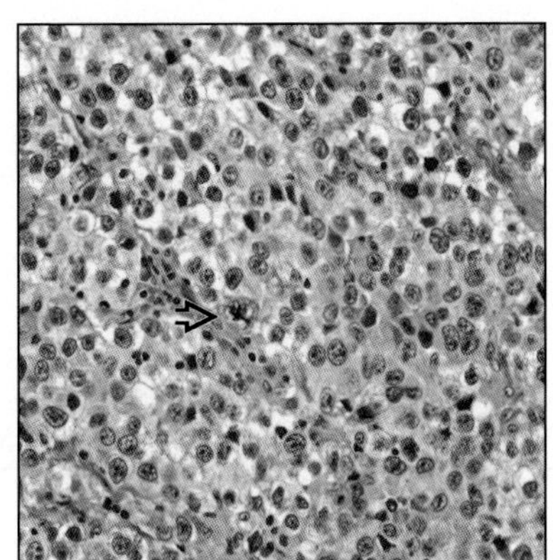

(Left) CD117 demonstrates uniform membranous staining of lesional cells. *(Center)* Hematoxylin & eosin shows sheets of tumor cells with areas of necrosis ➡ within a viable tumor ⇨. The presence of necrosis does not have an adverse prognosis as in other neoplastic entities. *(Right)* Hematoxylin & eosin of dysgerminoma show cells with central nuclei and 1 or few prominent nucleoli. Mitoses may be numerous, including atypical forms ⇨.

YOLK SAC TUMOR

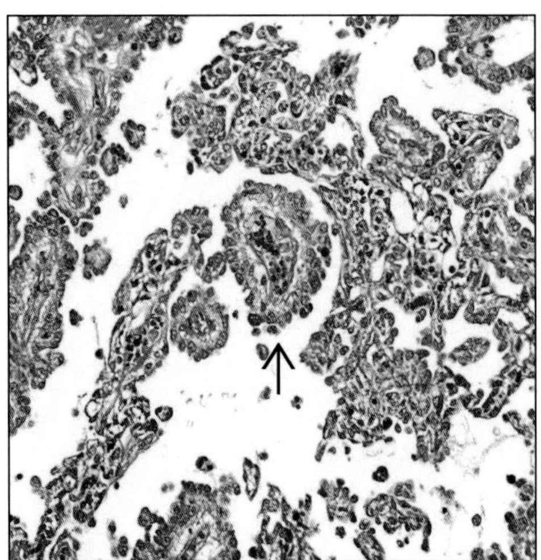

Schiller-Duval body ⇒ is present. This structure is a capillary lined by a layer of cells. It is considered diagnostic but not a requirement for diagnosis of yolk sac tumor.

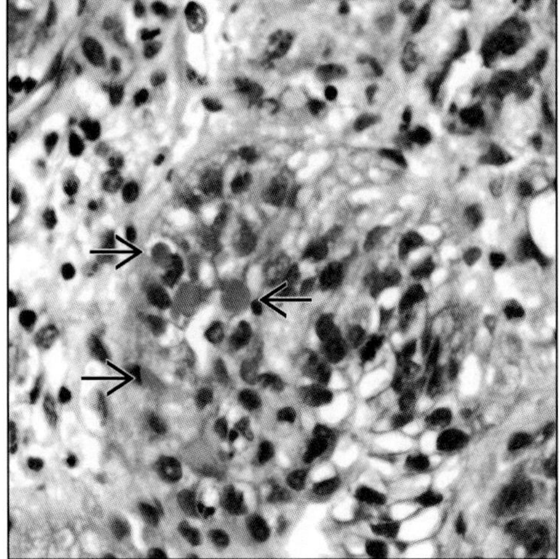

Prominent hyaline globules ⇒ are present inside and outside of cells. These globules are periodic acid-Schiff(+), diastase resistant.

TERMINOLOGY

Abbreviations

- Yolk sac tumor (YST)

Synonyms

- Endodermal sinus tumor

Definitions

- Germ cell neoplasm

CLINICAL ISSUES

Epidemiology

- Incidence
  - 2nd most common germ cell tumor after dysgerminoma
- Age
  - Median age of presentation: 18 years

Presentation

- Abdominal mass
  - Almost always unilateral
  - Rupture or torsion occurs in about 10% of patients
- Elevated serum α-fetoprotein, usually > 1,000 ng/mL
- Presents either as pure form or as component of mixed malignant germ cell tumor

Treatment

- Combination of salpingo-oophorectomy and adjuvant combination chemotherapy

Prognosis

- Complete cure for all stages in > 80% of patients

IMAGE FINDINGS

General Features

- Size
  - Usually > 10 cm (size variation: 3-30 cm)

MACROSCOPIC FEATURES

General Features

- Encapsulated, firm, smooth or lobulated, gray-yellow, solid and cystic with necrosis and hemorrhage

MICROSCOPIC PATHOLOGY

Histologic Features

- Wide range of histologic patterns; 1 or 2 may predominate in same tumor
- Micro and macrocystic
  - Small and large cystic spaces forming honeycomb pattern, lined by flat, pleomorphic cells with hyperchromatic nuclei with brisk mitotic activity
- Solid
  - Sheets of small polygonal cells with clear cytoplasm and large vesicular/pyknotic nuclei with prominent nucleoli
- Alveolar-glandular
  - Alveolar spaces lined by 1 or more layers of cuboidal or columnar cells with large nuclei, cellular aggregates, or myxomatous stroma in background
- Polyvesicular vitelline
  - Variably sized vesicles surrounded by dense stroma and lined by columnar or cuboidal cells and partly by flat cells
- Hepatoid
  - Solid sheets or cords of polygonal cells with abundant eosinophilic and granular cytoplasm resembling hepatocytes (not a predominant pattern)
- Glandular or primitive endodermal
  - Primitive endodermal cells forming glands or sheets within connective tissue
  - Degree of differentiation varies from primitive to well differentiated, may resemble mature enteric epithelium
- Papillary

YOLK SAC TUMOR

Key Facts

Terminology
- Endodermal sinus tumor
- Germ cell neoplasm

Clinical Issues
- Elevated serum α-fetoprotein, usually > 1,000 ng/mL
- 2nd most common germ cell tumor after dysgerminoma
- Presents either as pure form or as component of mixed malignant germ cell tumor

Macroscopic Features
- Encapsulated, firm, smooth or lobulated, gray-yellow, solid and cystic with necrosis and hemorrhage

Microscopic Pathology
- Most tumors exhibit reticular architecture reflecting extraembryonic differentiation
- Composed of irregular spaces lined by epithelial cells with glycogen-rich cytoplasm and large hyperchromatic nuclei with prominent nucleoli; mitoses are numerous
- Perivascular formations known as Schiller-Duval bodies
  - Capillaries lined by cuboidal to columnar cells with surrounding capsular space lined by single layer of flat cells; considered diagnostic but not required for diagnosis
- Presence of brightly eosinophilic intra- and extracellular hyaline granules

Immunohistochemistry

Antibody	Reactivity	Staining Pattern	Comment
α-fetoprotein	Positive	Cytoplasmic	
CK-PAN	Positive	Cytoplasmic	
α-1-antitrypsin	Positive	Cytoplasmic	
CEA-P	Positive	Cytoplasmic	In areas of enteric differentiation
EMA	Negative		

  - Papillary structures composed of connective tissue cores lined by pleomorphic cells; connective tissue may be hyalinized

Predominant Pattern/Injury Type
- Reticular
  - Irregular spaces lined by epithelial cells with glycogen-rich cytoplasm & large hyperchromatic nuclei with prominent nucleoli; mitoses are numerous

Predominant Cell/Compartment Type
- Schiller-Duval bodies: Capillaries lined by cuboidal to columnar cells with surrounding capsular space lined by single layer of flat cells
- Presence of brightly eosinophilic intra- and extracellular hyaline granules

ANCILLARY TESTS

Histochemistry
- PAS-diastase
  - Reactivity: Positive
  - Diastase resistant
  - Staining pattern: In eosinophilic granules

DIFFERENTIAL DIAGNOSIS

Clear Cell Carcinoma
- More common in older age group, lack of honeycomb and microcystic pattern, tubular spaces are lined by hobnail cells; solid areas are composed of large cells with clear cytoplasm and small nuclei

Embryonal Carcinoma
- Lack of specific patterns seen in yolk sac tumor; tumor cells are larger with more abundant cytoplasm and pleomorphic nuclei with prominent nucleoli

Dysgerminoma
- Cells with clear to lightly eosinophilic cytoplasm and round large nuclei, tumor cells are negative for α-fetoprotein and keratin

Endometrioid Carcinoma
- Yolk sac tumor may resemble secretory type endometrial glands

SELECTED REFERENCES

1. Dällenbach P et al: Yolk sac tumours of the ovary: an update. Eur J Surg Oncol. 32(10):1063-75, 2006
2. McCluggage WG et al: Immunohistochemistry as a diagnostic aid in the evaluation of ovarian tumors. Semin Diagn Pathol. 22(1):3-32, 2005
3. Ulbright TM: Germ cell tumors of the gonads: a selective review emphasizing problems in differential diagnosis, newly appreciated, and controversial issues. Mod Pathol. 18 Suppl 2:S61-79, 2005
4. Kawai M et al: Alpha-fetoprotein in malignant germ cell tumors of the ovary. Gynecol Oncol. 39(2):160-6, 1990

YOLK SAC TUMOR

Gross and Microscopic Features

(Left) Gross photograph shows oval tumor, tan to gray, with solid and cystic areas and visible foci of hemorrhage. The external surface of these tumors is usually smooth. Microcystic appearance is seen when polyvesicular vitelline component is present. ***(Right)*** *Low power of yolk sac tumor shows endodermal sinus pattern ⇒ and focal myxomatous pattern ⇗.*

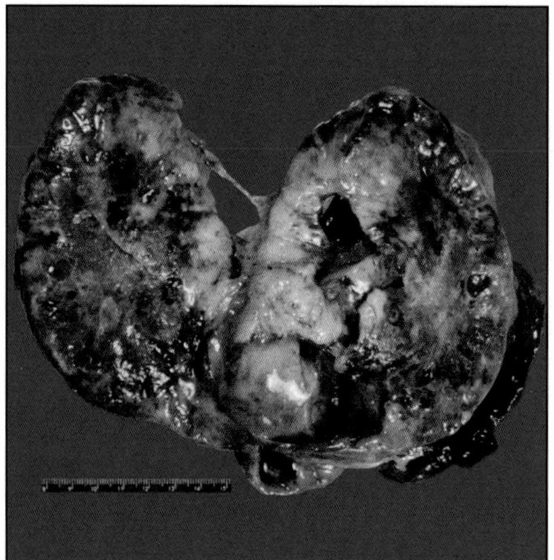

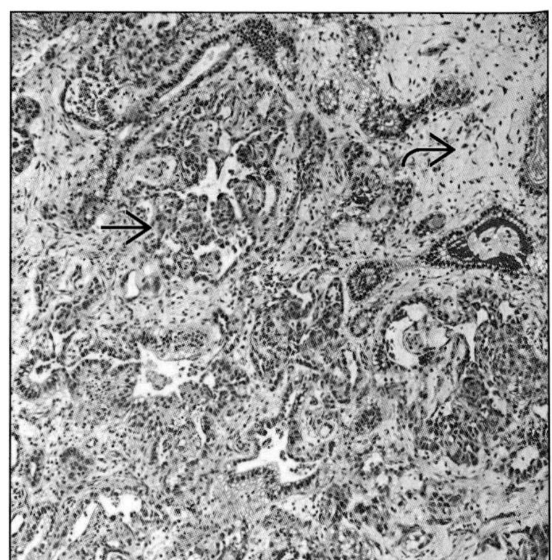

(Left) High magnification of yolk sac tumor demonstrates prominent papillary architecture and hyalinized cores ⇒. Lining cells can exhibit a significant cellular and nuclear pleomorphism and mitotic activity. The hyalinization may be variable and not as prominent as in this image. This papillary pattern may be the predominant pattern within the tumor. ***(Right)*** *Yolk sac tumor shows microcystic pattern with some variation of size.*

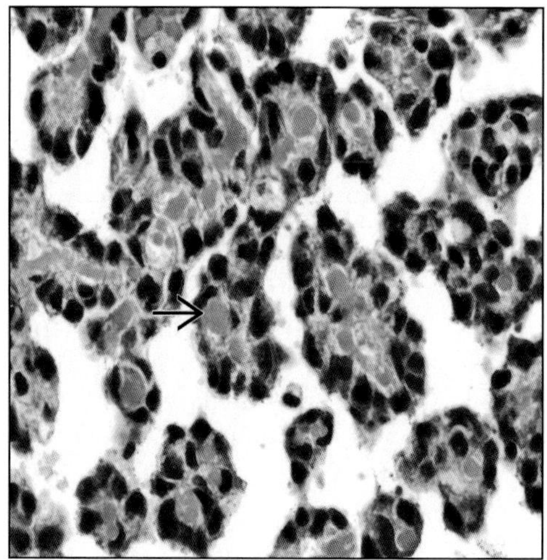

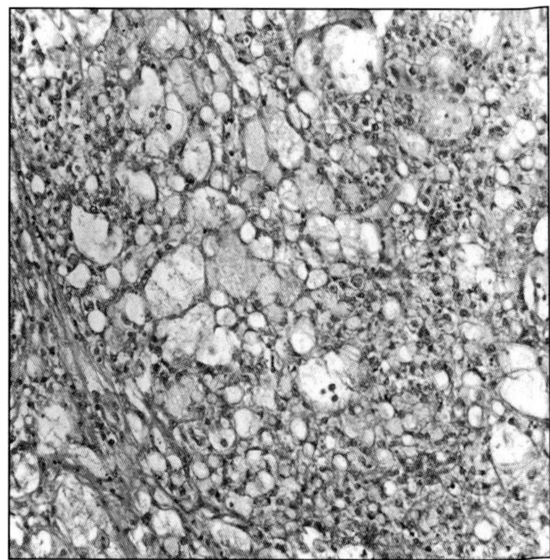

(Left) Low-power view shows polyvesicular vitelline pattern with numerous spaces lined by a single layer of cuboidal cells ⇒ and surrounded by cellular stroma. The lining cells may show luminal vacuolation. There is a variation between the cyst size and shape. There are instances when the entire tumor shows this pattern and is thus designated as polyvesicular vitelline tumor. ***(Right)*** *Yolk sac tumors are diffusely immunoreactive for α-fetoprotein. This image demonstrates strong cytoplasmic positivity of most tumor cells.*

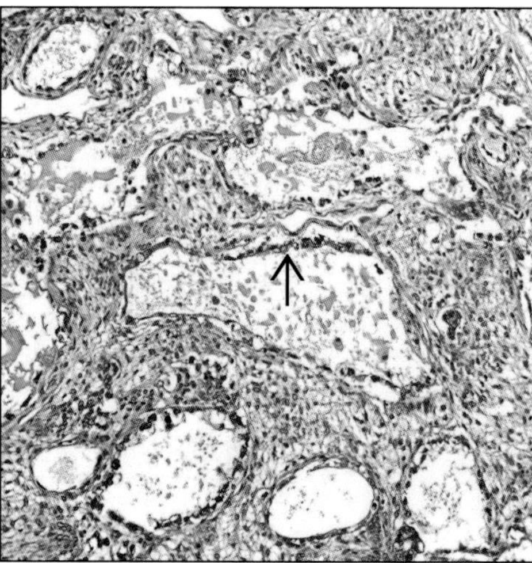

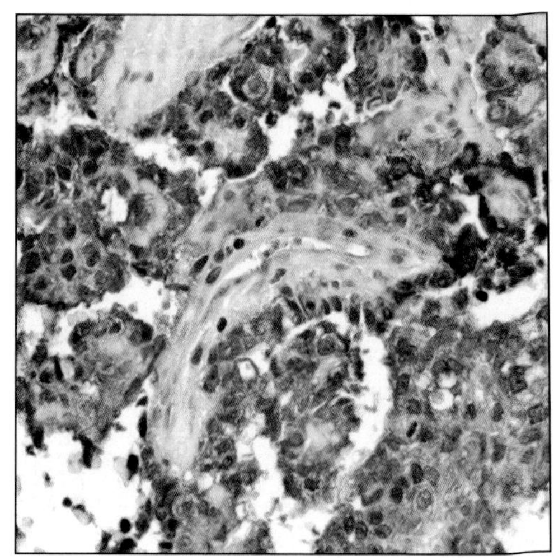

Microscopic Features

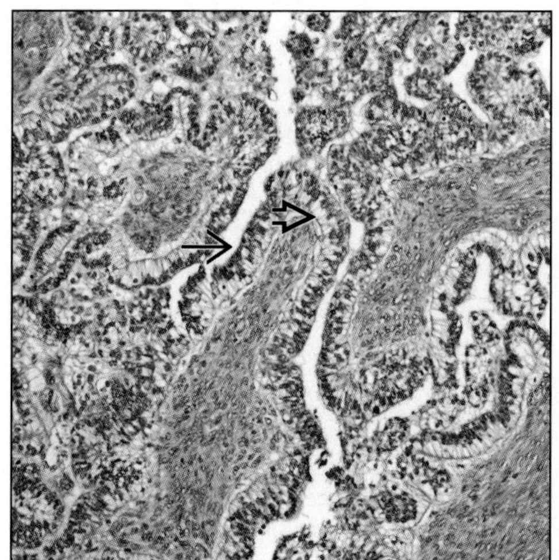

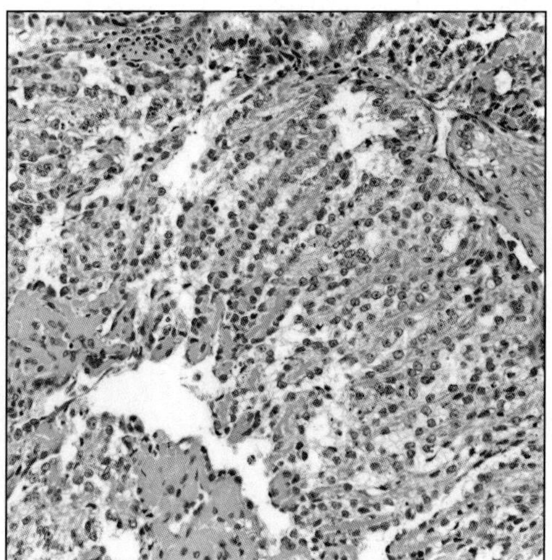

(Left) *Low power shows yolk sac tumor with prominent endometrioid-like glandular pattern. Glands are lined by tall columnar cells ⇒ with subnuclear vacuoles ⇨. Endometrioid adenocarcinoma is one of the differential diagnoses. Presence of other yolk sac components aids in establishing the right diagnosis.* ***(Right)*** *Low-power magnification of prominent papillary-type yolk sac tumor demonstrates numerous papillae with hyaline cores.*

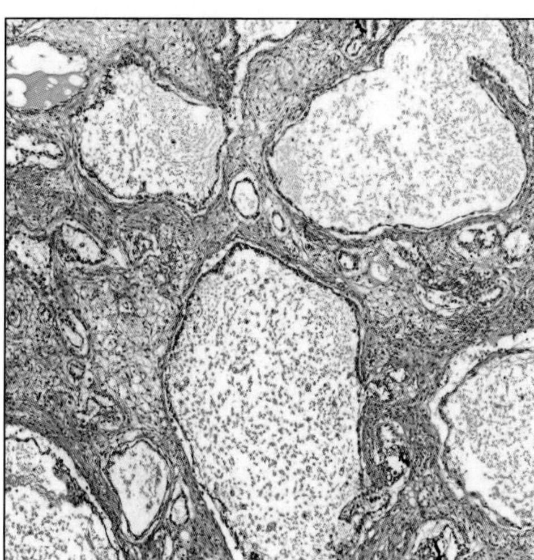

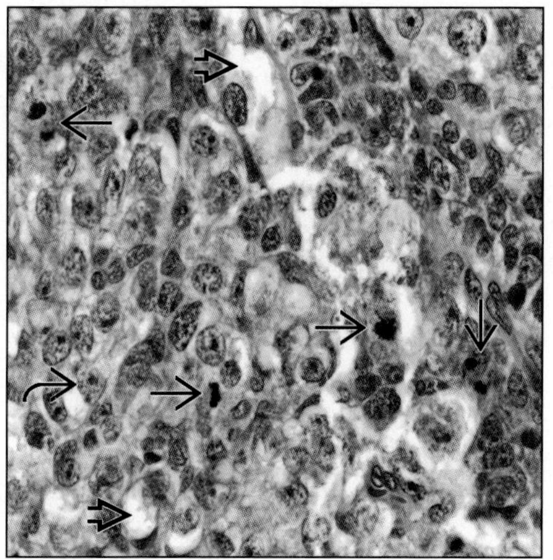

(Left) *Yolk sac tumor with numerous cystic spaces represents the polyvesicular vitelline variant. This image demonstrates dramatic variability of the cyst size. When these cysts are large enough, they can be appreciated grossly.* ***(Right)*** *High-power magnification shows yolk sac tumor with numerous mitoses ⇒. Some of the cells demonstrate clear (glycogen-rich) cytoplasm ⇨. Also of note are hyperchromatic nuclei with prominent nucleoli ⇗.*

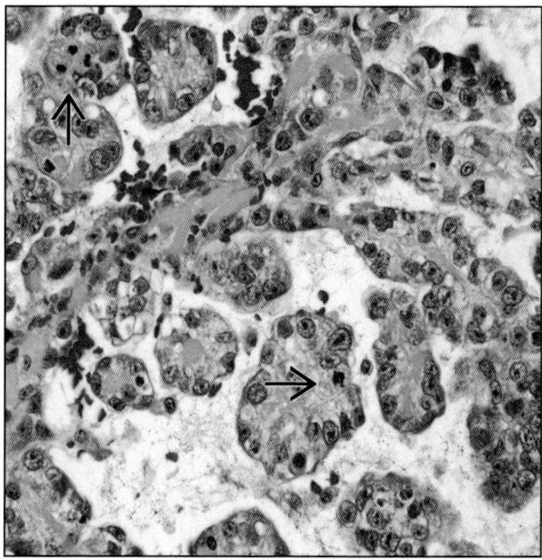

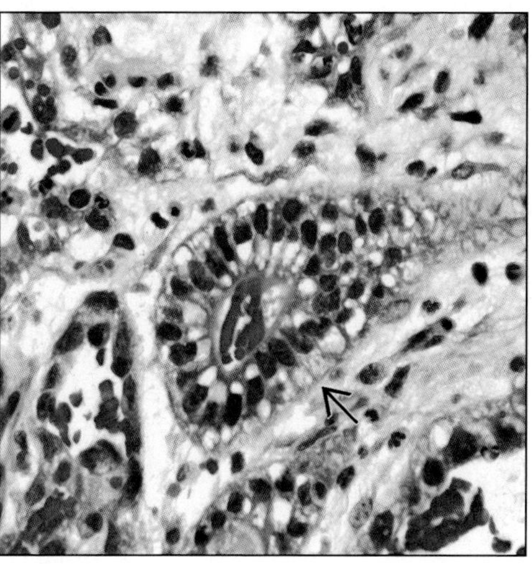

(Left) *Papillae in this image show variably hyalinized cores. Lining cells are highly atypical, with prominent nucleoli and mitoses ⇒.* ***(Right)*** *High-power magnification shows Schiller-Duval body ⇒ in the myxoid background. Cells lining the capillary reveal prominent subnuclear vacuoles.*

TERATOMAS

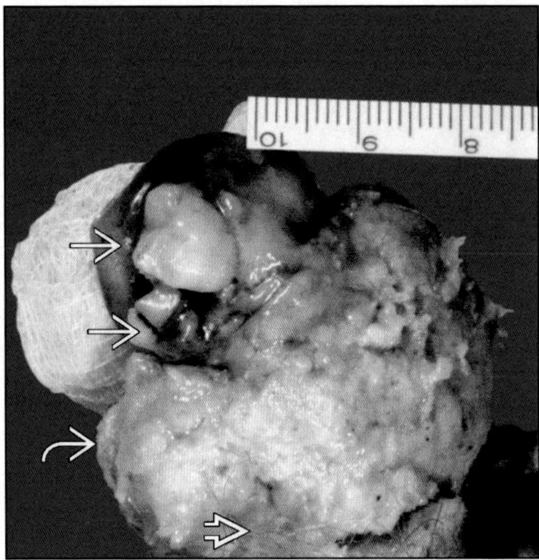

The inner lining of mature cystic teratoma is seeded with teeth ➡. The rest of the cyst lining is covered by grumous sebaceous material ➡ intermixed with occasional hair ➡.

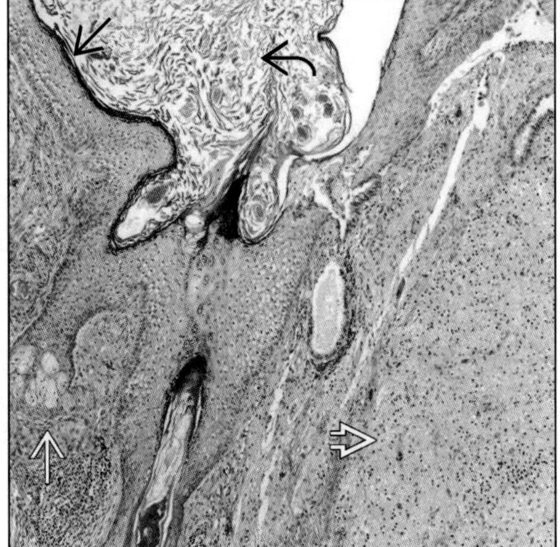

This image shows a mature teratoma. Note the mature squamous epithelium ➡ with prominent acellular keratotic debris ➡. Underneath the epithelium are a sebaceous unit ➡ and mature neural tissue ➡.

TERMINOLOGY

Synonyms

- Mature cystic teratoma
- Dermoid cyst

Definitions

- Germ cell neoplasm consisting of 2 or 3 embryonic layers (ectoderm, mesoderm, endoderm) in any combination
- Presence of any immature tissue is diagnostic of immature teratoma

CLINICAL ISSUES

Epidemiology

- Incidence
  - Mature teratomas
    - 2/3 of all ovarian tumors in patients under 15 years of age
  - Immature teratomas
    - 2-3% of ovarian teratomas
    - Occur predominantly in children
    - Frequent component of malignant germ cell tumor
    - Contralateral dermoid cyst or another benign tumor in 10% of cases
  - Struma ovarii
    - Most common in 5th decade
    - Rarely seen in pediatric population

Site

- Unilateral
- Bilateral in 15% of cases
- Contralateral to malignant germ cell tumor in 5-10% of cases

Presentation

- Abdominal mass
- Abdominal pain
  - Asymptomatic in 25%
- Torsion or rupture may occur, leading to hemoperitoneum and acute abdomen

Laboratory Tests

- Low-level elevation of α-fetoprotein (AFP)
  - Rarely exceeds 1,000 ng/mL
  - Higher levels suggestive of yolk sac tumor
- Other tumor markers that may be elevated
  - Human chorionic gonadotropin
  - Neuron-specific enolase
  - Carcinoembryonic antigen
  - Thyroid hormones (struma ovarii)

Treatment

- Surgical approaches
  - Ovarian cystectomy

Prognosis

- Mature teratomas
  - Benign tumors
  - Malignant transformation in 1-2% of cases
    - Most in postmenopausal women
- Immature teratomas
  - Benign behavior in pediatric population
  - Surgery is curative with immature teratoma of any grade
  - Presence of yolk sac tumor component is only valid predictor of recurrence

IMAGE FINDINGS

Radiographic Findings

- Mature cystic teratomas
  - Central areas of low density surrounded by ring of increased capsular density
- Calcified tissues including bone and teeth may help render radiographic diagnosis

TERATOMAS

Key Facts

Clinical Issues
- Immature teratomas
  - Benign behavior in pediatric population
- Abdominal pain
- Asymptomatic in 25%

Macroscopic Features
- Mature teratomas
  - Almost always cystic
  - Cysts filled with sebaceous material and hair
  - Teeth are seen in about 1/3 of cases
  - Rokitansky protuberance (solid nodule, composed of fat with teeth or bone, usually protrudes into lumen)
- Immature teratomas
  - Usually large (18 cm)
  - Encapsulated, predominantly solid
  - Solid areas: Soft, fleshy, gray to pink, frequently with areas of hemorrhage and necrosis

Microscopic Pathology
- Mature teratomas
  - Ectodermal elements: Epidermis, pilosebaceous structures, teeth, sweat glands, neural tissue
- Immature teratomas
  - Mixture of mature and immature elements
- Endodermal elements: Thyroid tissue, respiratory and gastrointestinal structures
- Mesodermal elements: Adipose tissue, smooth muscle, bone, and cartilage

Diagnostic Checklist
- Important to exclude presence of yolk sac tumor or dysgerminoma

MACROSCOPIC FEATURES

General Features
- **Mature teratomas**
  - Almost always cystic
  - Cysts filled with sebaceous material and hair
  - Cyst contents liquid at body temperature, solid at room temperature
  - Teeth are seen in about 1/3 of cases
  - Solid nodule (Rokitansky protuberance)
    - Composed of fat with teeth or bone
    - Protrudes into lumen
  - Mature tissues may be seen
    - Brain, bone, cartilage, fat, mucinous cysts, and thyroid
  - Partially developed organs rarely identified
  - Can be solid
- **Immature teratomas**
  - Usually large (18 cm)
  - Encapsulated
  - Predominantly solid
  - Solid areas
    - Soft and fleshy
    - Gray to pink
    - Frequent areas of hemorrhage and necrosis
  - Mature teratoma cysts found in 26% of cases
    - Cysts with mucinous/serous/bloody fluid
    - Hair may be present

Sections to Be Submitted
- Solid areas

Size
- 0.5-40 cm (average: 15 cm)

MICROSCOPIC PATHOLOGY

Mature Teratoma
- Ectodermal elements
  - Epidermis and sweat glands
  - Pilosebaceous structures
  - Neural tissue
  - Teeth
- May see other ectodermal derivatives
  - Cerebrum
  - Cerebellum
  - Choroid plexus
  - Retina
- Endodermal elements
  - Respiratory and gastrointestinal structures
  - Thyroid tissue
- Mesodermal elements
  - Smooth and striated muscle
  - Adipose tissue
  - Bone and cartilage
- Rarely identified tissues
  - Adrenal, pituitary, pancreatic, renal, thymic, mammary, and prostatic tissue
- Mitotic figures can be identified in fetal tissues
  - Fetal cartilage and cerebellar tissue showing increased density and mitotic activity can be present; not diagnostic of immature teratoma
- Benign tumors may develop
  - Carcinoid, struma, adrenal adenoma, prolactinoma, glomus tumor, sebaceous adenoma, and nevus

Immature Teratoma
- Mixture of mature and immature elements
- Immature elements can consist of
  - Neuroepithelial rosettes and tubules
  - Mitotically active glia
  - Areas that resemble neuroblastoma or glioblastoma
- Islands of immature cartilage, bone, skeletal muscle, and glandular structures
- Endodermal elements, including hepatic tissue and intestinal-type epithelium, may give rise to yolk sac tumor
- Mature tissue identical to those of mature teratoma
- Grading based on amount of immature neural tissue
  - Grade 1 tumors
    - < 1 low-power field in any 1 slide
  - Grade 2 tumors
    - 2-3 low-power fields in any 1 slide

TERATOMAS

Immunohistochemistry			
Antibody	**Reactivity**	**Staining Pattern**	**Comment**
GFAP	Positive	Cytoplasmic	Neuroectodermal tissue
NSE	Positive	Cytoplasmic	Neuroectodermal tissue
S100P	Positive	Cytoplasmic	Neuroectodermal tissue
Synaptophysin	Positive	Cytoplasmic	Neuroectodermal tissue
NGFR	Positive	Cytoplasmic	Neuroectodermal tissue
α-fetoprotein	Positive	Cytoplasmic	Intestinal-type glands and hepatic tissue
TTF-1	Positive	Cytoplasmic	Struma ovarii

- Grade 3 tumors
  - 4 or more low-power fields in any 1 slide
- Implants or metastases
  - Mostly immature
  - Can consist of mature glial tissue

Struma Ovarii

- Thyroid tissue is predominant or sole component
- Normal thyroid tissue that resembles thyroid follicular adenoma
- May be associated with
  - Dermoid cyst, carcinoid tumor, Brenner tumor, or mucinous tumor

DIFFERENTIAL DIAGNOSIS

Yolk Sac Tumor with Glandular and Hepatoid Differentiation

- Glandular pattern shows nests of primitive endodermal glands surrounded by connective tissue
  - Differentiation varies from primitive to well differentiated
- Hepatoid pattern is composed of cells resembling hepatocytes
  - More primitive appearance may resemble immature teratoma
- Generous sampling will yield other yolk sac patterns
- Elevated serum AFP is seen in yolk sac tumors with normal to slightly elevated levels in teratomas

Primitive Neuroectodermal Tumor (PNET)

- Lack of other teratomatous elements
- Neuroectodermal tumors are positive for GFAP and CD99
- Molecular studies for *EWS/FLI-1* transcript due to t(11;22) (q24;q12) characterize PNET

Malignant Mesodermal Mixed Tumor

- Typically in older women
- Composed of sarcomatous and carcinomatous elements
  - Carcinoma is adenocarcinoma, squamous cell carcinoma, or adenosquamous carcinoma
  - Sarcomatous elements include leiomyosarcoma, chondrosarcoma, rhabdomyosarcoma, fibrosarcoma, and undifferentiated sarcomatous tissue
- Neuroectodermal elements are rare

Well-Differentiated Endometrioid Carcinoma

- Extensive squamous differentiation in carcinoma can be seen
- Malignant glandular component is present when sampled well
- Carcinomas usually present in older women

DIAGNOSTIC CHECKLIST

Pathologic Interpretation Pearls

- Exclude presence of yolk sac tumor or dysgerminoma
- When hepatic or intestinal-type tissue present in immature teratomas, search for yolk sac tumor component

SELECTED REFERENCES

1. Marina NM et al: Complete surgical excision is effective treatment for children with immature teratomas with or without malignant elements: A Pediatric Oncology Group/ Children's Cancer Group Intergroup Study. J Clin Oncol. 17(7):2137-43, 1999
2. Heifetz SA et al: Immature teratomas in children: pathologic considerations: a report from the combined Pediatric Oncology Group/Children's Cancer Group. Am J Surg Pathol. 22(9):1115-24, 1998
3. Bonazzi C et al: Pure ovarian immature teratoma, a unique and curable disease: 10 years' experience of 32 prospectively treated patients. Obstet Gynecol. 84(4):598-604, 1994
4. Comerci JT Jr et al: Mature cystic teratoma: a clinicopathologic evaluation of 517 cases and review of the literature. Obstet Gynecol. 84(1):22-8, 1994
5. O'Connor DM et al: The influence of grade on the outcome of stage I ovarian immature (malignant) teratomas and the reproducibility of grading. Int J Gynecol Pathol. 13(4):283-9, 1994
6. Kleinman GM et al: Primary neuroectodermal tumors of the ovary. A report of 25 cases. Am J Surg Pathol. 17(8):764-78, 1993
7. Masih K et al: Gonadal teratomas: a study of 206 cases. Indian J Pathol Microbiol. 36(4):495-8, 1993
8. Steeper TA et al: Solid ovarian teratomas: an immunocytochemical study of thirteen cases with clinicopathologic correlation. Pathol Annu. 19 Pt 1:81-92, 1984

Microscopic Features

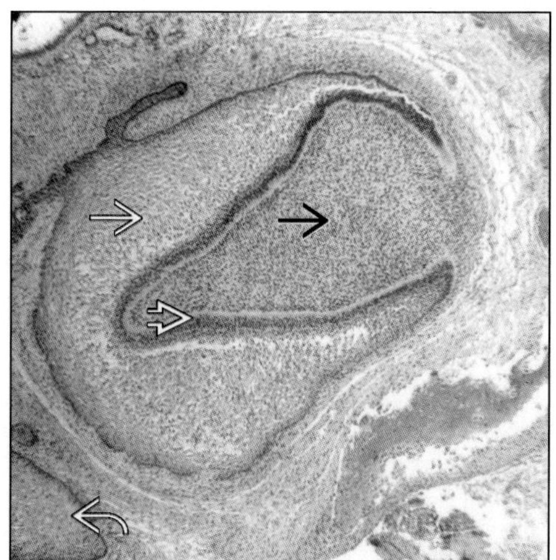

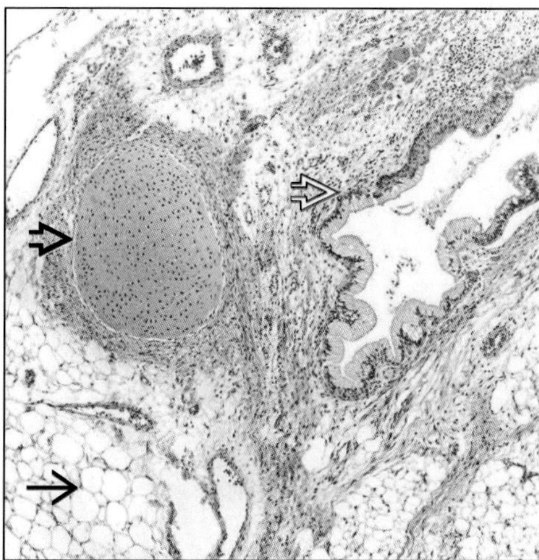

(Left) *Low-power view shows a mature teratoma with a cross section of tooth. Dental papilla → and enamel organ are easily recognized →. The enamel organ contains layers of ameloblasts and odontoblast that form a prominent line →. Left lower corner of this image shows squamous epithelial lining →.* ***(Right)*** *Low power of mature teratoma demonstrates mature, easily recognized tissues including cartilage →, adipose →, and glandular →.*

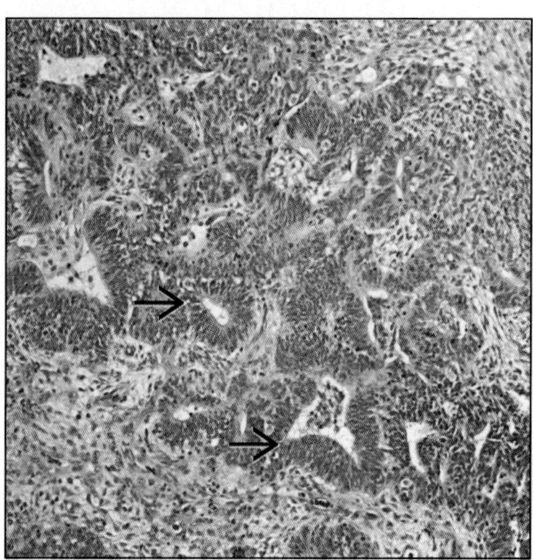

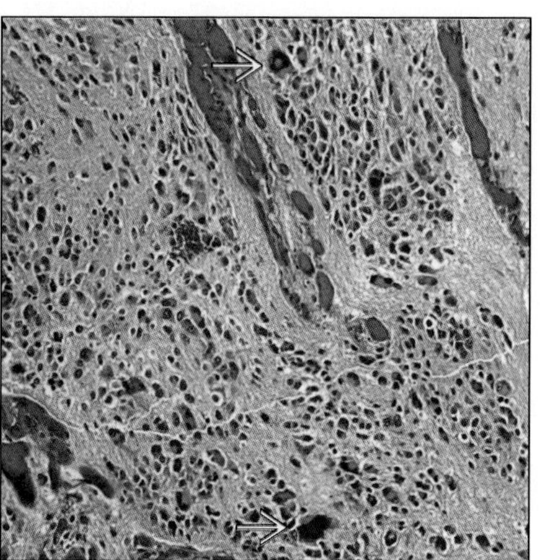

(Left) *Low-power image demonstrates immature teratoma with prominent immature neuroectodermal elements. These elements are comprised of neuroepithelial tubules → with haphazard distribution. On occasions these tubules might resemble rosettes seen in primitive neurectodermal tumors.* ***(Right)*** *This image also demonstrates immature teratoma composed of neural tissue. In this case, however, the immature neural elements consist of sheets of large and atypical cells →.*

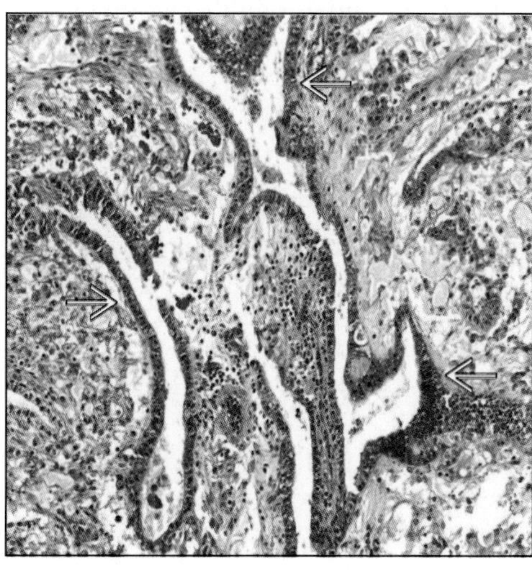

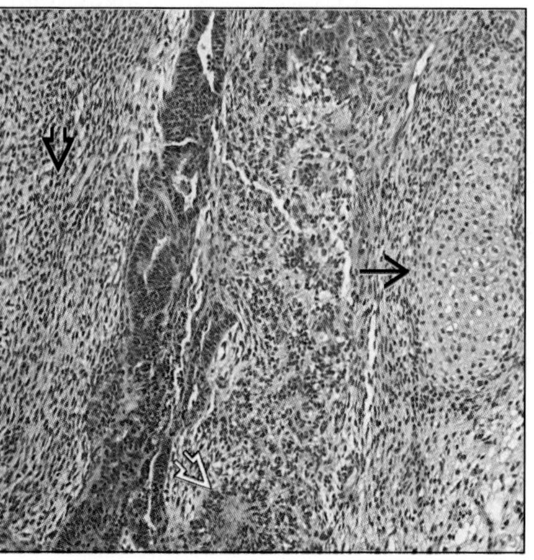

(Left) *Section of immature teratoma demonstrates prominent glandular proliferation →. The immature glandular component, combined with loose and lacy stroma, resembles yolk sac tumor. Yolk sac tumor may arise in immature teratoma, therefore it is important to exclude its presence by careful sampling.* ***(Right)*** *Low-power view of immature teratoma shows several immature components: Cartilage →, mesenchyme →, and neuroepithelial rosettes →.*

JUVENILE GRANULOSA CELL TUMOR

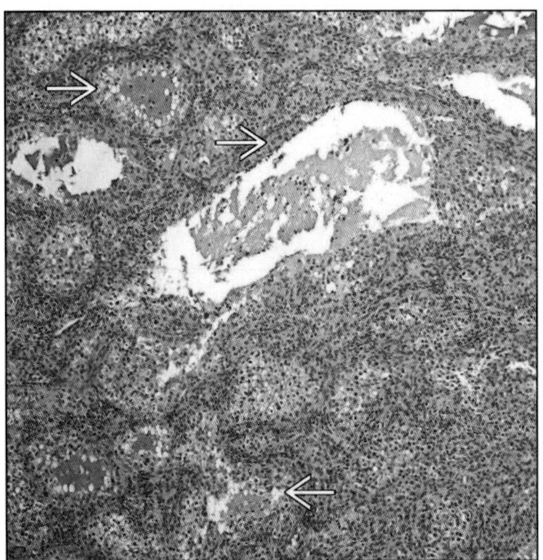

Low magnification of juvenile granulosa cell tumor demonstrates multiple follicles of different size and shape, filled with basophilic material ➡.

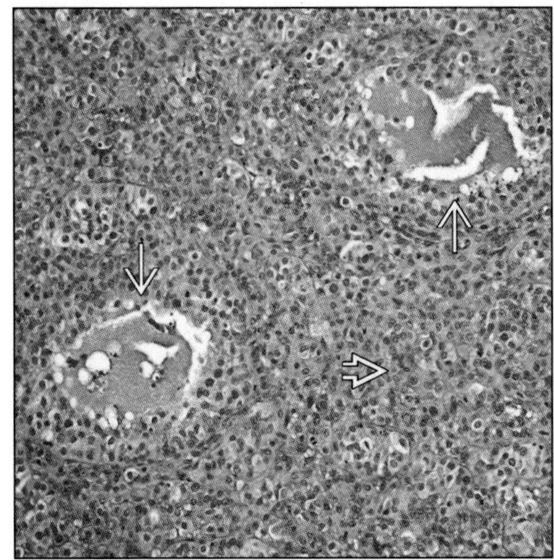

This juvenile granulosa cell tumor exhibits both cellular areas ➡ and follicles ➡.

TERMINOLOGY

Abbreviations

- Juvenile granulosa cell tumor (JGCT)

CLINICAL ISSUES

Epidemiology

- Incidence
  - 50% are prepubertal

Presentation

- Approximately 80% present with sexual precocity
- Abdominal pain
- Associated with Ollier disease (enchondromatosis) and Maffucci syndrome (enchondromatosis and hemangiomatosis)
- Unilateral; rarely bilateral (2% of cases)
- Spread beyond ovaries is unusual

Treatment

- Surgical approaches
  - Salpingo-oophorectomy

Prognosis

- Good prognosis with low recurrence rate

MACROSCOPIC FEATURES

General Features

- Solid and cystic neoplasm (can present as uniformly cystic or solid)
  - Average size: 12 cm
  - Solid component may be yellow, tan, or gray
  - Areas of necrosis and hemorrhage may be present

MICROSCOPIC PATHOLOGY

Histologic Features

- Minimal to marked nuclear atypia
- Variable mitotic rate (5.5-7/10 HPF)

Predominant Pattern/Injury Type

- Cellular neoplasm with follicle formation
  - Follicles of variable size and shape
  - Lumens contain eosinophilic or basophilic secretions
  - Lining cells vary in thickness

Predominant Cell/Compartment Type

- Granulosa cells
  - Round with hyperchromatic nuclei and abundant eosinophilic cytoplasm
  - Lack of nuclear grooves in most cases, unlike adult granulosa cell tumor
- Theca cells
  - Usually luteinized with lipid-staining cytoplasm
  - More spindled than granulosa cells

ANCILLARY TESTS

Cytogenetics

- Trisomy 12
  - Demonstrated by FISH
  - Detected in the majority of cases
  - Considered to be a nonrandom abnormality

DIFFERENTIAL DIAGNOSIS

Anaplastic Juvenile Granulosa Cell Tumor

- Striking nuclear atypia with orderly architecture
- Areas resembling undifferentiated carcinoma

Adult Granulosa Cell Tumor (AGCT)

- Regular follicles

JUVENILE GRANULOSA CELL TUMOR

Key Facts

Etiology/Pathogenesis
- Trisomy 12 demonstrated by FISH

Clinical Issues
- Approximately 80% present with sexual precocity
- Associated with Ollier disease (enchondromatosis) and Maffucci syndrome (enchondromatosis and hemangiomatosis)

Macroscopic Features
- Solid and cystic neoplasm (can present as uniformly cystic or solid)

Microscopic Pathology
- Follicles of variable size and shape
- Granulosa cells are round with hyperchromatic nuclei and abundant eosinophilic cytoplasm
- Lack of nuclear grooves in most cases, unlike in adult granulosa cell tumor

Immunohistochemistry

Antibody	Reactivity	Staining Pattern
Inhibin	Positive	Cytoplasmic
CD99	Positive	Cell membrane
Calretinin	Positive	Cytoplasmic

- Call-Exner bodies
- Nuclear grooves and lack of luteinization

Yolk Sac Tumor
- Poly-vesicular variant of yolk sac tumor may resemble JGCT
- α-fetoprotein is negative in JGCT

Thecoma
- Rarely seen before age 30
- Lacks follicles as seen in JGCT
- Reticulin stain helpful in highlighting granulosa cells of JGCT

Clear Cell Carcinoma
- Older age group
- Lack of inhibin

Small Cell Carcinoma
- Neoplastic cells with scant cytoplasm
- Hypercalcemia
- Negative calretinin and inhibin, positive cytokeratin

SELECTED REFERENCES

1. Kaur H et al: Juvenile granulosa cell tumor of the ovary presenting with pleural effusion and ascites. Int J Clin Oncol. 14(1):78-81, 2009
2. Leyva-Carmona M et al: Ovarian juvenile granulosa cell tumors in infants. J Pediatr Hematol Oncol. 31(4):304-6, 2009
3. Dudani R et al: Juvenile granulosa cell tumor of testis: case report and review of literature. Am J Perinatol. 25(4):229-31, 2008
4. Deavers MT et al: Ovarian sex cord-stromal tumors: an immunohistochemical study including a comparison of calretinin and inhibin. Mod Pathol. 16(6):584-90, 2003
5. Gell JS et al: Juvenile granulosa cell tumor in a 13-year-old girl with enchondromatosis (Ollier's disease): a case report. J Pediatr Adolesc Gynecol. 11(3):147-50, 1998
6. Bouffet E et al: Juvenile granulosa cell tumor of the ovary in infants: a clinicopathologic study of three cases and review of the literature. J Pediatr Surg. 32(5):762-5, 1997
7. Schofield DE et al: Trisomy 12 in pediatric granulosa-stromal cell tumors. Demonstration by a modified method of fluorescence in situ hybridization on paraffin-embedded material. Am J Pathol. 141(6):1265-9, 1992
8. Scully RE: Juvenile granulosa cell tumor. Pediatr Pathol. 8(4):423-7, 1988

IMAGE GALLERY

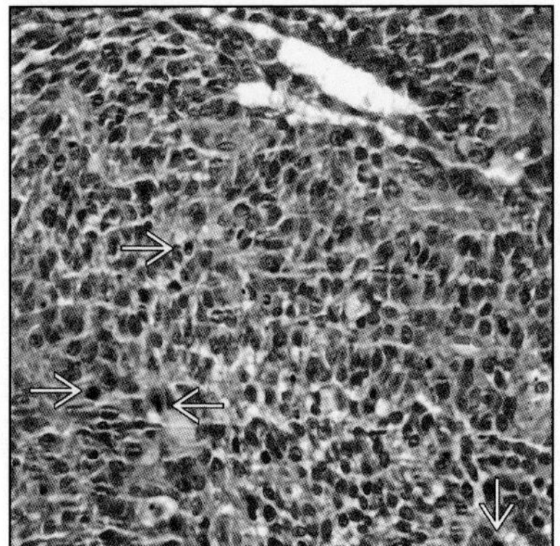

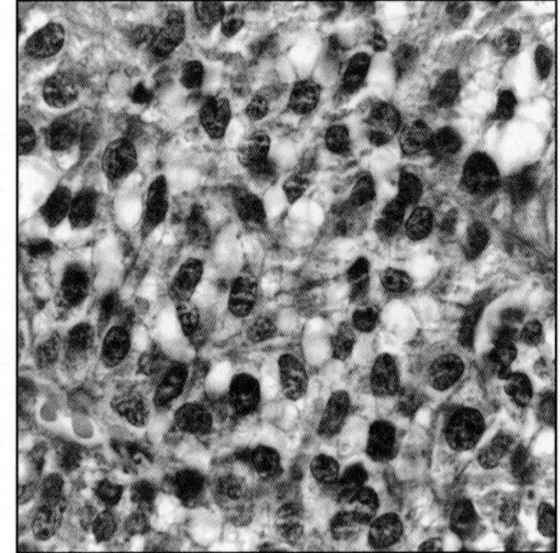

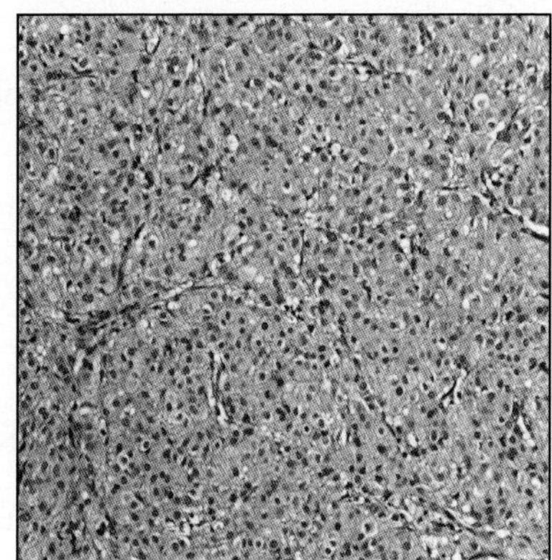

(Left) *High power of juvenile granulosa cell tumor highlights cellular areas with frequent mitotic figures* ➡. *(Center)* *High magnification of juvenile granulosa cell tumor shows round cells with abundant cytoplasm and lack of nuclear grooves.* *(Right)* *This image of juvenile granulosa cell tumor shows only solid area that is composed of luteinized cells with abundant cytoplasm.*

THECOMA-FIBROMA

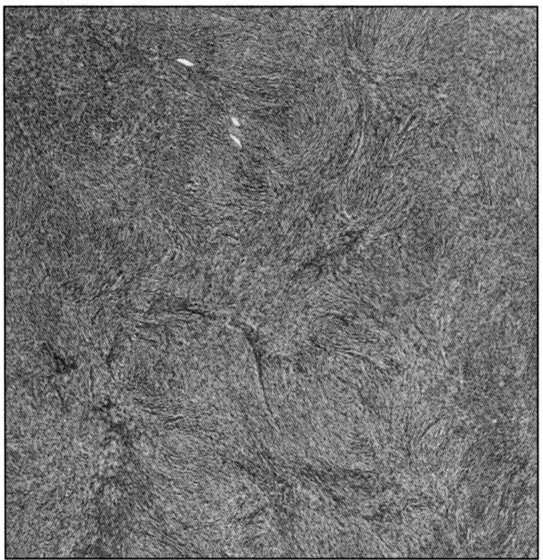

Hematoxylin & eosin of fibroma shows a fascicular arrangement of spindle cells with minimal amount of cytoplasm.

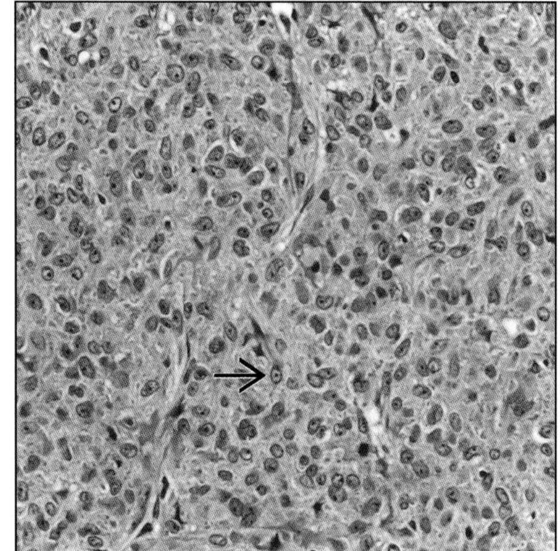

Hematoxylin & eosin of thecoma cells that have a moderate amount of amphophilic cytoplasm illustrates nuclei that have open chromatin and small nucleoli ⇒. There is no atypia or mitotic activity.

TERMINOLOGY

Definitions

- Sex cord-stromal tumors

CLINICAL ISSUES

Epidemiology

- Age
  - Most frequent in middle-aged women
  - Rare in pediatric population

Site

- Can be bilateral (approximately 8% of fibromas, 3% of thecomas)

Presentation

- Fibroma
  - Rarely as Meig syndrome: Ascites and pleural effusion
  - Rarely associated with nevoid basal cell carcinoma syndrome (NBCCS) a.k.a. Gorlin syndrome
- Thecoma
  - Hormone secreting with estrogenic and androgenic changes

Treatment

- Surgical excision is appropriate treatment

Prognosis

- Both are benign with excellent prognosis

MACROSCOPIC FEATURES

Fibroma

- ≤ 6 cm in size; solid, firm, well circumscribed, white to yellow cut surface
- Areas of edema, cyst formation, and rarely necrosis and hemorrhage may be present
- Focal calcifications might occur (more common in NBCCS)

Thecoma

- 5-10 cm in size; solid with yellow cut surface; occasionally white
- Cystic change, hemorrhage, necrosis, and focal calcification can be present

MICROSCOPIC PATHOLOGY

Histologic Features

- Fibromas and thecomas have overlapping features
  - Tumors that contain features of both entities should be classified as fibro-thecomas

Fibroma

- Spindle cell proliferation in fascicular and storiform pattern
- Spindle cells might be separated by hyalinized collagen
- Intercellular edema may be seen
- Spindle cells might contain small amount of lipid
- Mitoses are rare; < 3/10 HPF
  - When > 4 mitoses/10 HPF, it is considered mitotically active cellular fibroma

Thecoma

- Sheets of round to spindle cells with moderate to large amount of pale, sometimes vacuolated cytoplasm (cytoplasm is lipid-rich)
- Fibroblasts producing collagen are interspersed throughout
- Nuclei lack atypia or mitoses
  - Mild nuclear atypia with bizarre nuclei might be rarely seen
  - Severe atypia, high mitotic activity, and malignant behavior should point to different tumor classification
- Hyalinized and calcified areas may be present

THECOMA-FIBROMA

Key Facts

Clinical Issues
- Rare in pediatric population
- Both fibroma and thecoma are benign with excellent prognosis

Microscopic Pathology
- Fibromas and thecomas have overlapping features
- Tumors that contain features of both entities should be classified as fibro-thecomas
- Fibroma
  - Spindle cell proliferation in fascicular and storiform pattern
  - Mitoses are rare; < 3/10 HPF
- Thecoma
  - Sheets of round to spindle cells with moderate to large amount of pale sometimes vacuolated cytoplasm (cytoplasm is lipid-rich)
  - Nuclei lack atypia or mitoses

Immunohistochemistry

Antibody	Reactivity	Staining Pattern	Comment
Inhibin	Positive	Cytoplasmic	Both fibroma and thecoma
Calretinin	Positive	Cytoplasmic	Both fibroma and thecoma
CK-PAN	Negative		
EMA	Negative		

DIFFERENTIAL DIAGNOSIS

Fibroma
- Massive edema and stromal hyperplasia
  - Bilateral, entrapped follicles are present; minimal collagen formation
- Fibrosarcoma
  - Moderate to severe nuclear atypia with increased mitotic rate of > 4/10 HPF
- Sclerosing stromal tumor
  - Cellular areas are surrounded by edematous stroma
  - 2 types of cells are present: Spindle cells and round to oval lutein cells

Thecoma
- Steroid cell tumor
  - Minimal spindle cell component and large polygonal cells with abundant eosinophilic cytoplasm
- Stromal hyperthecosis
  - Almost always bilateral
  - Background of normal stromal cells with nests of lutein cells
- Luteinized granulosa cell tumor
  - Characteristic nuclear features and presence of nonluteinized areas should aid in separating this tumor from thecoma

SELECTED REFERENCES

1. Chechia A et al: Incidence, clinical analysis, and management of ovarian fibromas and fibrothecomas. Am J Obstet Gynecol. 199(5):473, 2008
2. Nocito AL et al: Ovarian thecoma: clinicopathological analysis of 50 cases. Ann Diagn Pathol. 12(1):12-6, 2008
3. Irving JA et al: Cellular fibromas of the ovary: a study of 75 cases including 40 mitotically active tumors emphasizing their distinction from fibrosarcoma. Am J Surg Pathol. 30(8):929-38, 2006
4. Dal Cin P et al: Fibrosarcoma versus cellular fibroma of the ovary. Am J Surg Pathol. 22(4):508-10, 1998

IMAGE GALLERY

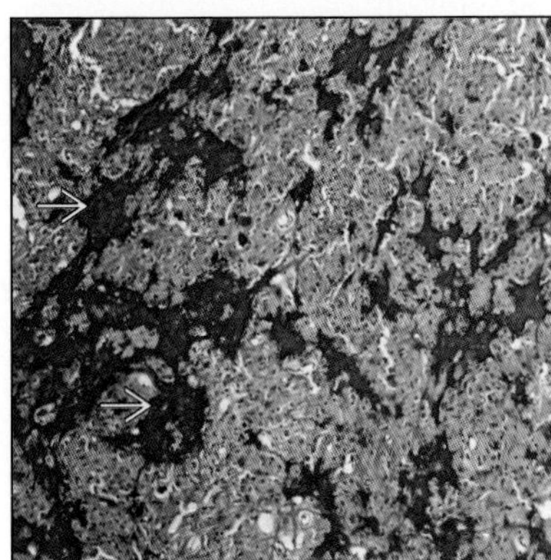

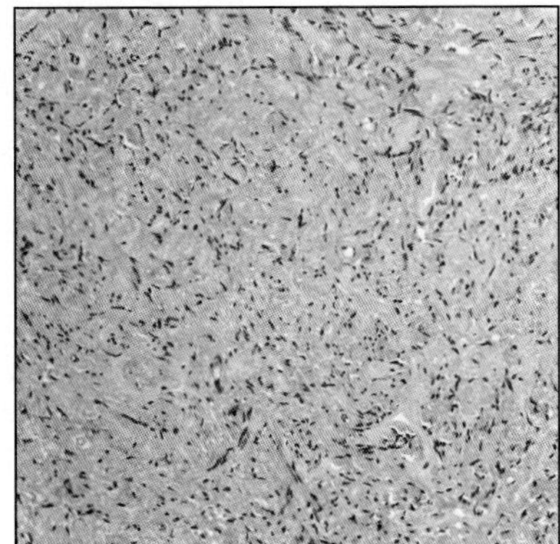

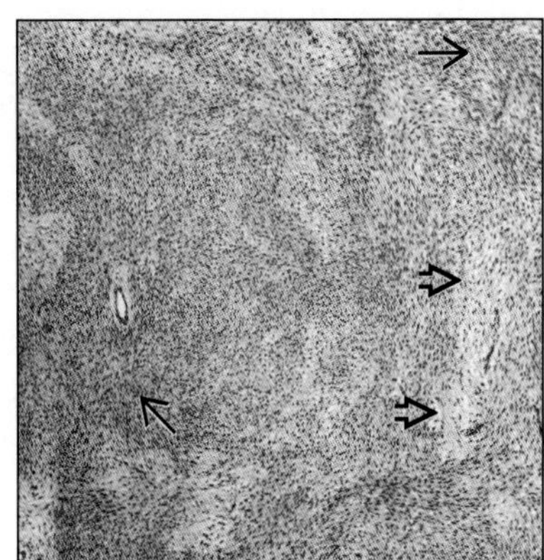

(Left) *Hematoxylin & eosin shows thecoma with prominent areas of calcifications ➡.* ***(Center)*** *Hematoxylin & eosin of fibroma shows a lesion with scant cellularity and a prominent hyalinization.* ***(Right)*** *Hematoxylin & eosin of fibroma shows cellular areas ➡ among edematous and less cellular stroma ➡. Massive edema is a differential diagnosis for fibroma. In massive edema there is a preservation of follicles and other normal ovarian structures, whereas in fibromas they are displaced.*

SERTOLI-LEYDIG CELL TUMORS

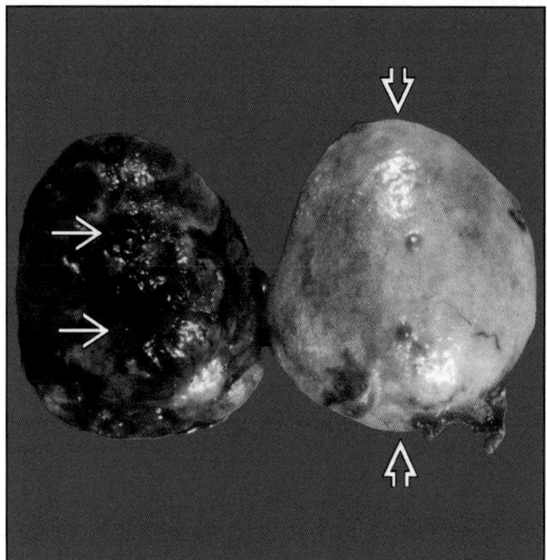

Gross photograph of SLCT shows outer surface ➡ and cut surface ➡ that is solid, slightly lobulated, pale yellow, and with focal areas of hemorrhage.

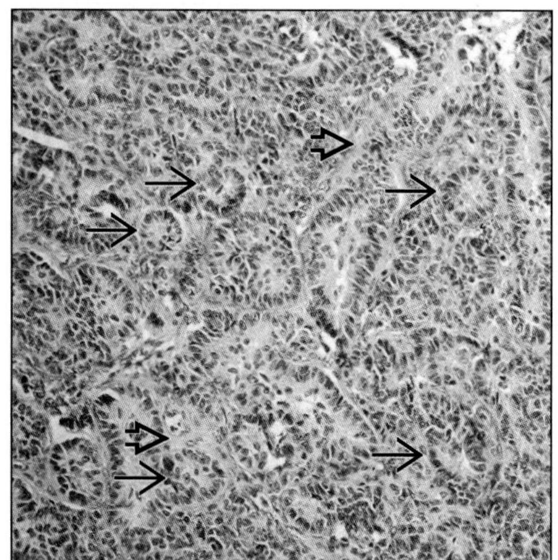

Image of well-differentiated SLCT demonstrates numerous tubules of Sertoli cells →. There is a minimal amount of intervening stroma between the tubules ⇨.

TERMINOLOGY

Abbreviations

- Sertoli-Leydig cell tumor (SLCT)

Definitions

- Sex cord-stromal/steroid cell tumor that can present in patients with androgen insensitivity syndrome

CLINICAL ISSUES

Epidemiology

- Incidence
  - < 0.5% of all ovarian tumors
- Age
  - 75% occur in women younger than 30 years (mean age: 25 years)
  - Retiform types tend to occur at mean age of 15 years

Presentation

- Abdominal pain
- Virilization in about 1/2 of cases
- Elevated α-fetoprotein can be seen

Treatment

- Surgical resection
- Chemotherapy is used when tumors present at advanced stage

Prognosis

- Most are benign (when stage I)
  - Stage II tumors have poor prognosis
- If they recur, it is within 1st 2 years
- Malignant tumors spread within abdomen and without distant metastases

MACROSCOPIC FEATURES

General Features

- Solid, lobulated, pale yellow cut surface
- May have cystic component, especially when heterologous elements are present
- Poorly differentiated tumors may have necrosis and hemorrhage

Size

- Mean size: 13 cm

MICROSCOPIC PATHOLOGY

Histologic Features

- Well differentiated (10% of tumors)
  - Hollow or solid tubules (oval or round) of cuboidal to columnar Sertoli cells
    - Lumens usually do not contain any secretions
    - Sertoli cell nuclei are round with minimal amount of cytoplasm, without nucleoli, atypia, or mitotic figures
  - Intervening stroma contains nests of Leydig cells
    - Leydig cells contain abundant amount of eosinophilic cytoplasm
    - Reinke crystals can be seen in about 20% of cases
- Intermediate differentiation tumors (45-50% of tumors)
  - Tubules, nests, or sheets of immature (dark cells with small, round, oval, or angular nuclei) Sertoli cells
    - Mitotic figures are present
  - Leydig cells are seen among Sertoli cells and stroma
- Poorly differentiated (sarcomatoid) (10% of tumors)
  - Spindled cells that may resemble fibrosarcoma
    - Numerous mitotic figures are present (> 10/10 HPF)
  - Nests of Leydig cells can be seen
- Retiform (15% of tumors)

SERTOLI-LEYDIG CELL TUMORS

Key Facts

Terminology
- Sex cord-stromal and steroid cell tumor

Etiology/Pathogenesis
- Can present in patients with androgen insensitivity syndrome

Clinical Issues
- < 0.5% of all ovarian tumors
- Most are benign (when stage I)

Macroscopic Features
- Solid, lobulated, yellowish cut surface
- Mean size is ~ 13 cm
- May have cystic component, especially when heterologous elements are present

Microscopic Pathology
- Well differentiated (10%)
- Tubules of cuboidal to columnar cells (Sertoli cells)
- Tubules are mostly hollow, oval, or round; may be dilated
- Sertoli cell nuclei are round, without nucleoli, atypia, or mitotic activity
- Nests of Leydig cells in intervening stroma
- Leydig cells contain abundant amount of eosinophilic cytoplasm (Reinke crystals can be seen in about 20% of cases)
- Intermediate differentiation tumors (45-50%)
- Poorly differentiated (sarcomatoid) (10%)
    - Spindled cells that may resemble fibrosarcoma
- Retiform (15%)
- With heterologous elements (20%)

    - Tubular structures that resemble rete of ovary or testis
    - Tubules contain papillary or polypoid structures
        - Some tubules are small and round with prominent hyalinized cores
        - Some tubules may be extensively branched and mimic atypical proliferative serous tumors
- SLCT with heterologous elements (20% of tumors)
    - Heterologous elements include
        - Mucinous glands: Lined by well-differentiated mucinous epithelium that can be benign, borderline, or of low-grade malignancy
        - Fetal cartilage, embryonal rhabdomyosarcoma

Immunohistochemistry
- Positive for inhibin, calretinin, low-molecular weight cytokeratins, progesterone, and androgen receptors

Genetics
- SLCTs lack *SRY* gene

DIFFERENTIAL DIAGNOSIS

Endometrioid Carcinoma
- Positive for EMA/MUC1 and CK7 and negative for inhibin and calretinin
- Contain glands that are larger than Sertoli tubules and often have mucin secretions

Adult Granulosa Cell Tumor
- SLCTs lack Call-Exner bodies and nuclear grooves
- Granulosa cell tumors have micro- or macrofollicular pattern

Krukenberg Tumor
- Tubules of Krukenberg tumor show more atypia and signet ring cells that are mucicarmine positive
- Cells lining the tubules of Krukenberg tumor exhibit atypia and pleomorphism to much greater extent than SLCTs

Carcinoid Tumor
- Stroma of carcinoid tumors is less cellular and more fibromatous than in SLCTs
- Carcinoid tumors show immunoreactivity for chromogranin and synaptophysin

Ependymoma
- Has pseudorosettes and stains positive for glial fibrillary acidic protein

Teratoma
- Presence of mucinous heterologous elements might be confused with teratoma, but adequate sampling should aid in arriving to correct diagnosis
- Teratomas lack Sertoli and Leydig cells and usually have prominent ectodermal component

DIAGNOSTIC CHECKLIST

Clinically Relevant Pathologic Features
- Retiform subtypes are associated with more likelihood of malignant behavior

SELECTED REFERENCES

1. Talerman A et al: Sertoli-Leydig cell tumor of the ovary. Int J Gynecol Pathol. 4(2):171-2, 1985
2. Young RH et al: Ovarian Sertoli cell tumors: a report of 10 cases. Int J Gynecol Pathol. 2(4):349-63, 1984
3. Zaloudek C et al: Sertoli-Leydig tumors of the ovary. A clinicopathologic study of 64 intermediate and poorly differentiated neoplasms. Am J Surg Pathol. 8(6):405-18, 1984
4. Roth LM et al: Sertoli-Leydig cell tumors: a clinicopathologic study of 34 cases. Cancer. 48(1):187-97, 1981
5. Tavassoli FA et al: Sertoli tumors of the ovary. A clinicopathologic study of 28 cases with ultrastructural observations. Cancer. 46(10):2281-97, 1980

SERTOLI-LEYDIG CELL TUMORS

Microscopic Features

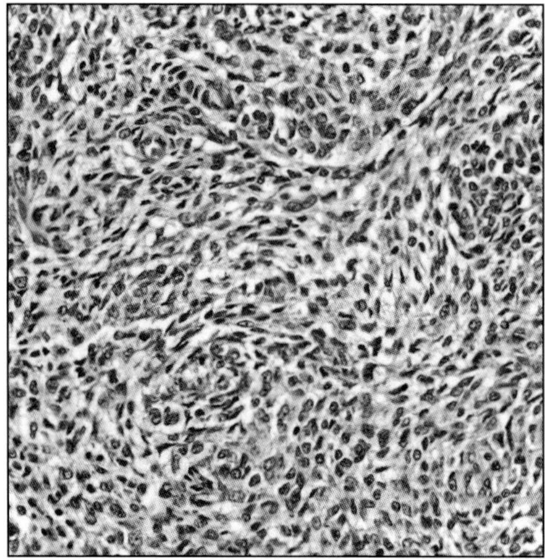

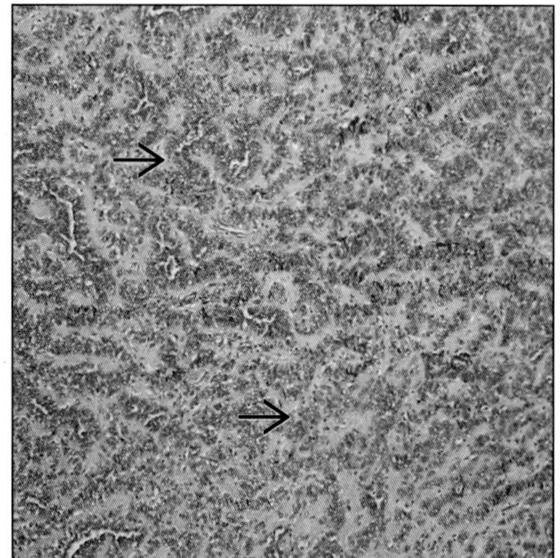

(Left) *This high-power image demonstrates poorly differentiated SLCT. This pattern of fascicular spindle cells might mimic undifferentiated tumors or sarcomas, and therefore it is important to sample the tumor well to find more differentiated areas. Cells show nuclear atypia and there is increased mitotic activity.* ***(Right)*** *Thin cords ⇒ are a prominent feature in this intermediate SLCT. Cords are composed of Sertoli cells and are highlighted by intervening hyalinized stroma.*

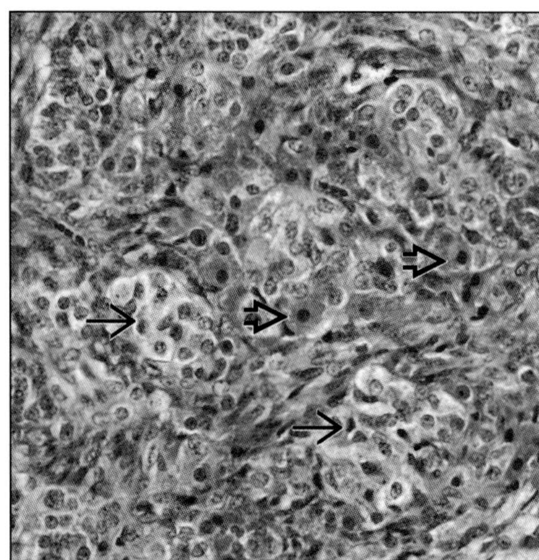

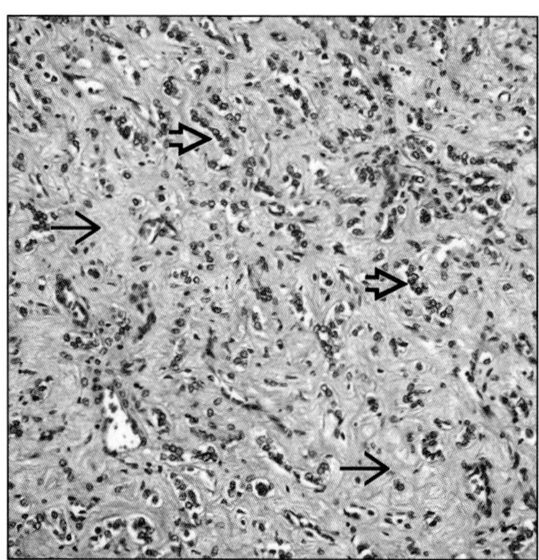

(Left) *High-power photograph shows intermediate SLCT with nests of Sertoli cells ⇒ and intervening Leydig cells ⇨. Leydig cells in comparison to Sertoli cells have abundant eosinophilic cytoplasm and centrally placed nuclei. Crystals of Reinke may be identified in some of the Leydig cells.* ***(Right)*** *This low power image of SLCT demonstrates prominent hyalinized stroma ⇒ and thin cords of Sertoli cells ⇨.*

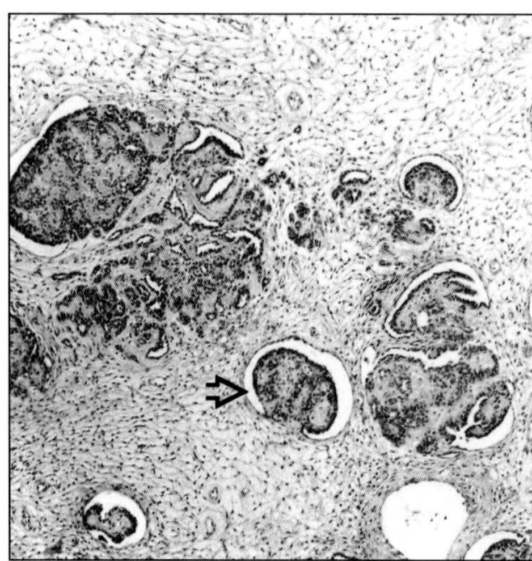

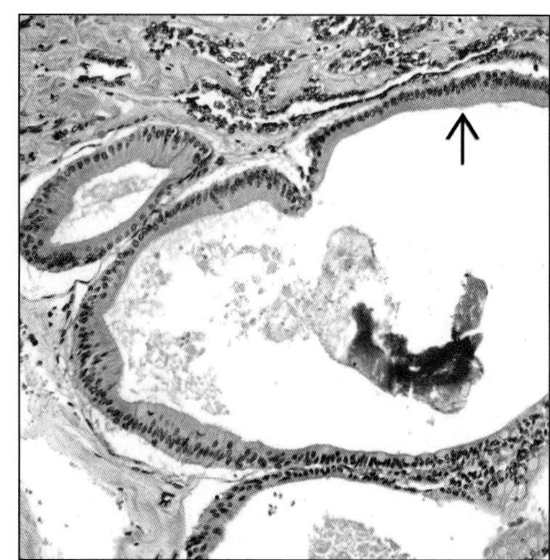

(Left) *This retiform SLCT has distinct papillary structures ⇨ embedded in dense fibrous stoma. These tumors tend to present earlier than other variants of SLCTs and might be mimickers of other ovarian neoplasms including serous borderline tumors and yolk sac tumors.* ***(Right)*** *This SLCT shows prominent heterologous elements composed of cysts lined by a single layer of mucinous epithelium ⇒. The cyst lining can be of well-differentiated gastric or intestinal type.*

Microscopic Features

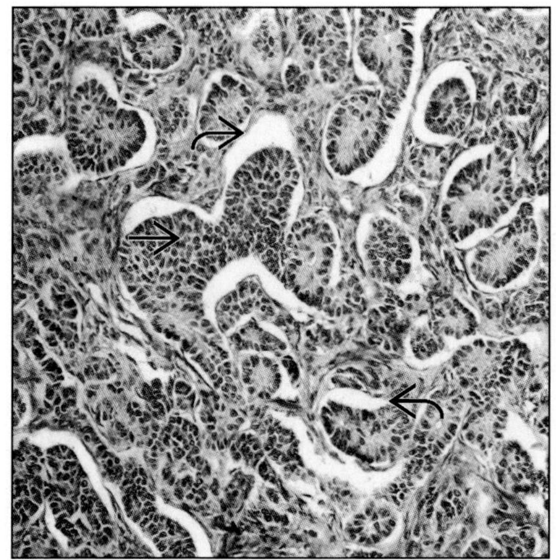

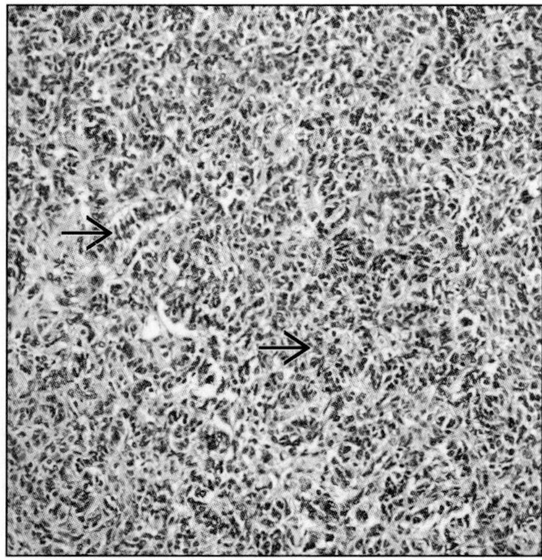

(Left) *Hematoxylin & eosin of retiform SLCT shows numerous cords → embedded within dense fibrous stroma. There is also prominent clefting ↪. Stroma may vary from paucicellular and hyalinized to densely cellular and immature. Cords are composed of epithelial cells with varying degree of stratification and nuclear atypia.* ***(Right)*** *This image of SLCT of intermediate differentiation shows minimal intervening stroma and suggestion of cords → of Sertoli cells.*

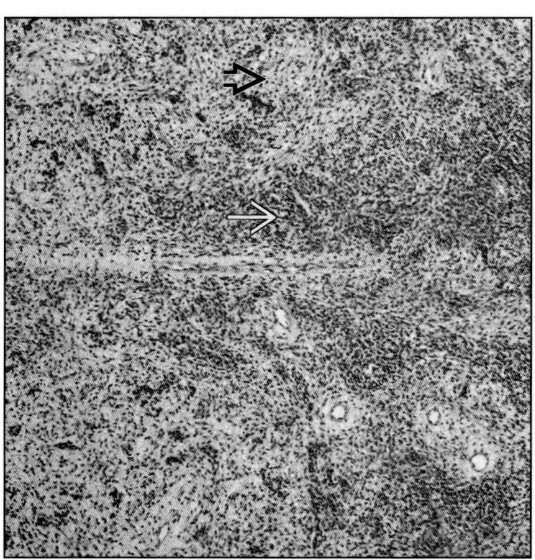

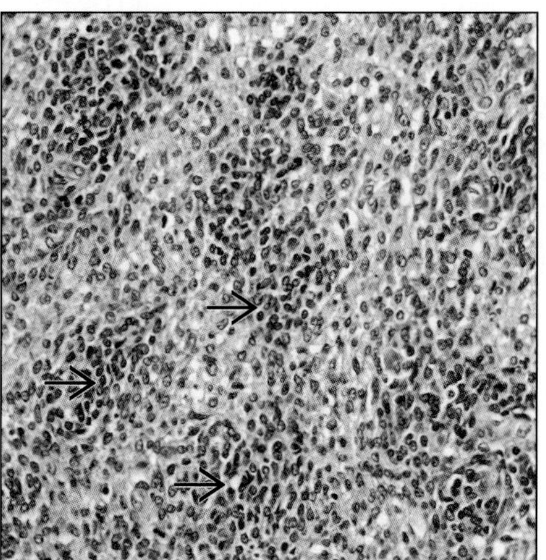

(Left) *Low magnification of SLCT demonstrates 2 distinct areas. Cellular ➡ and edematous (less cellular) ⇨ areas can be appreciated. This appearance might mimic other sex cord-stromal tumors, in particular fibrothecoma.* ***(Right)*** *High magnification provides a closer look at contrasting areas of different cellularity. Cellular nests → are intersected by less cellular stromal cells. In contrast to fibrothecomas, cells are round and show more significant atypia.*

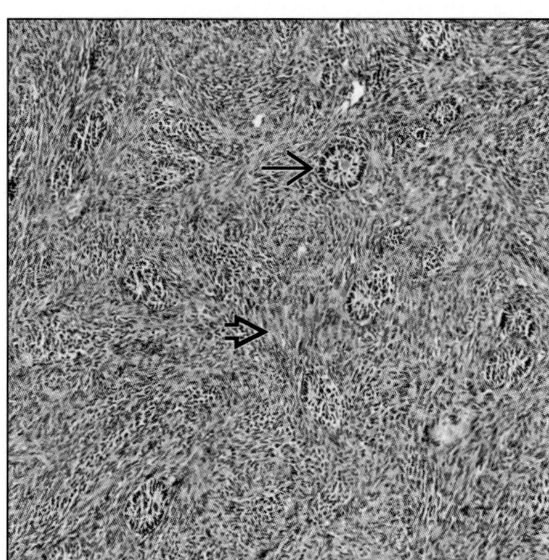

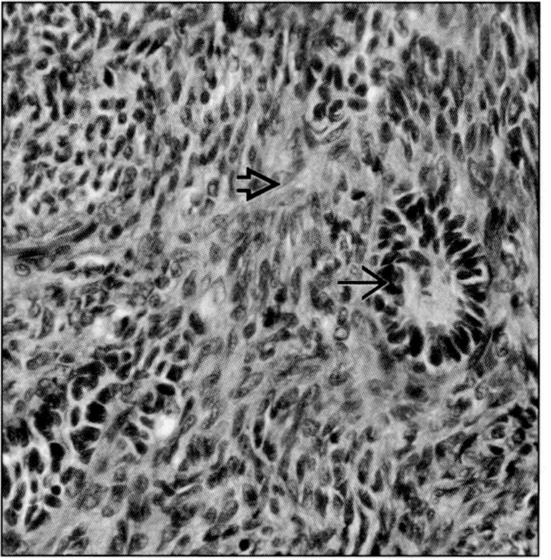

(Left) *Low-power view of intermediate to poorly differentiated SLCT demonstrates predominantly spindled stromal proliferation ⇨ with occasional tubules →. This appearance may be mimicked by some metastatic carcinomas with tubular gland pattern. Immunohistochemical stains and clinical history are helpful in this differential.* ***(Right)*** *This is a high magnification of moderately to poorly differentiated SLCT with tubules → and dense spindled stroma ⇨.*

BOTRYOID RHABDOMYOSARCOMA

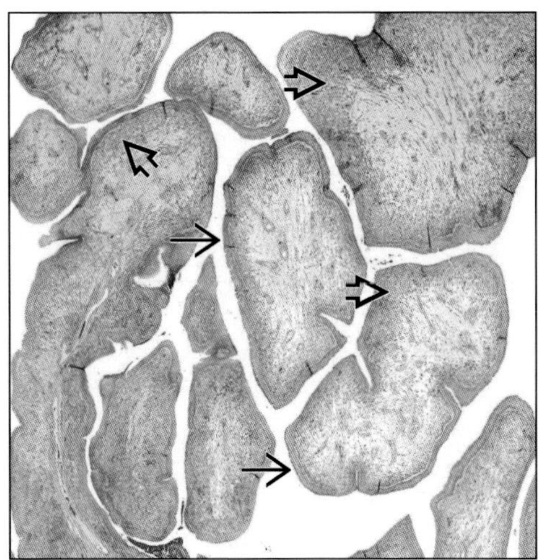

Low-power view demonstrates papillary configuration. Papillae are lined by epithelium ➔ and the cambium layer is seen as a darker layer underneath ➲.

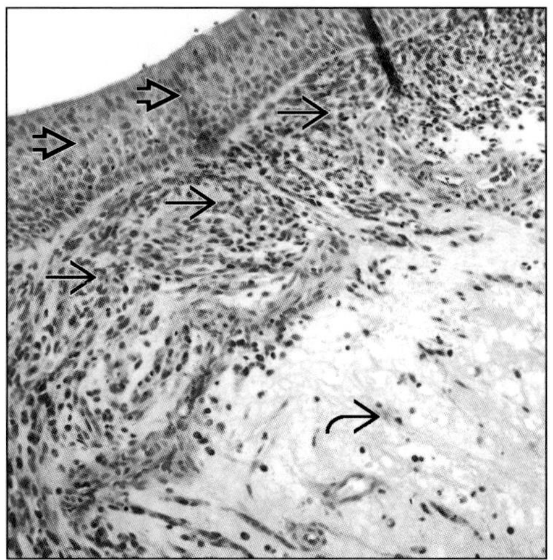

High magnification highlights the cambium layer ➔ that lies underneath the epithelial lining ➲ and above the edematous and less cellular zone ↗.

TERMINOLOGY

Synonyms

- Embryonal rhabdomyosarcoma
  - Subtype of embryonal rhabdomyosarcoma
- Sarcoma botryoides

CLINICAL ISSUES

Epidemiology

- Incidence
  - Most common vaginal cancer in infants and young children
- Age
  - 90% occur in females < 5 years of age
    - Mean age at diagnosis: 2 years
  - Can be seen in young adults

Site

- Vagina
  - Anterior wall
- Other sites
  - Cervix
  - Bladder

Presentation

- Vaginal mass
  - Appear as papillae, small nodules; pedunculated or sessile soft, polypoid masses
- May protrude through vaginal introitus
- Vaginal bleeding

Natural History

- Invasion of local structures
- Regional lymph node metastases
- Distant metastases

Treatment

- Combination of surgery, chemotherapy, and radiation

Prognosis

- Excellent
- Cure rates between 90-95%

MACROSCOPIC FEATURES

General Features

- Soft, tan or gray
- Nodular
- Grape-like mass

MICROSCOPIC PATHOLOGY

Histologic Features

- Cambium layer
  - Densely cellular zone beneath epithelium
  - Composed of small primitive cells, rhabdomyoblasts
    - Variable appearance from round to polyhedral with scant to more abundant eosinophilic cytoplasm
    - Strap cells with cross striations can be interspersed among more primitive cells
    - Frequent mitoses are present
- Less cellular edematous zone adjacent to cambium layer
- Hyaline cartilage may be seen

DIFFERENTIAL DIAGNOSIS

Fibroepithelial Polyp (Mesodermal Stromal Polyp)

- Mean age at diagnosis: 40 years (range from newborn to 77 years)
- Size varies from 0.5-4 cm
- Contains edematous fibrovascular stroma covered by stratified squamous epithelium
  - Stroma contains variable fibroblasts

BOTRYOID RHABDOMYOSARCOMA

Key Facts

Clinical Issues
- Most common vaginal cancer in infants and young children
- About 90% occur in females < 5 years of age (can be seen in young adults)
- Vagina (along anterior wall)
- Vaginal mass that can protrude through vaginal introitus
- Cure rates between 90-95%

Macroscopic Features
- Soft, tan or gray, nodular, grape-like mass

Microscopic Pathology
- Cambium layer is densely cellular zone beneath epithelium
- Rhabdomyoblasts vary in appearance from round to polyhedral with scant to more abundant eosinophilic cytoplasm

Immunohistochemistry

Antibody	Reactivity	Staining Pattern	Comment
Desmin	Positive	Cytoplasmic	Rhabdomyoblasts
MYOD1	Positive	Nuclear	Rhabdomyoblasts; may not be present in all tumors
Myogenin	Positive	Nuclear	Rhabdomyoblasts; may not be present in all tumors
Myoglobin	Positive	Cytoplasmic	Rhabdomyoblasts

- 1/2 of these polyps contain large cytologically atypical stromal cells with hyperchromatic, pleomorphic nuclei, abundant cytoplasm, and tapered cytoplasmic processes
- Mitoses are variable but mostly low
- Lacks cambium layer
- Lacks invasion of overlying squamous epithelium
- Absence of skeletal muscle differentiation

Rhabdomyoma
- Rare benign tumor
- More common in women of reproductive age
  - Average age at diagnosis: About 45 years
- Presents as solitary, polypoid to nodular mass
- Size varies from 1-11 cm in diameter
- Composed of benign-appearing fetal or adult-type skeletal muscle cells
  - Cells are spindle to oval with abundant granular eosinophilic cytoplasm
- Surrounding fibrous stroma is variable in quantity
- Lacks cambium layer

Müllerian Papilloma
- Complex papillary projections
- Lined by flat cuboidal epithelium
- Cores of loose fibrovascular tissue
- Cytologic atypia and mitoses are absent

SELECTED REFERENCES

1. Riedlinger WF et al: Myogenic markers in the evaluation of embryonal botryoid rhabdomyosarcoma of the female genital tract. Pediatr Dev Pathol. 8(4):427-34, 2005
2. Qualman SJ et al: Intergroup Rhabdomyosarcoma Study: update for pathologists. Pediatr Dev Pathol. 1(6):550-61, 1998
3. Hays DM et al: Sarcomas of the vagina and uterus: the Intergroup Rhabdomyosarcoma Study. J Pediatr Surg. 20(6):718-24, 1985
4. Hays DM et al: Rhabdomyosarcoma of the female urogenital tract. J Pediatr Surg. 16(6):828-34, 1981

IMAGE GALLERY

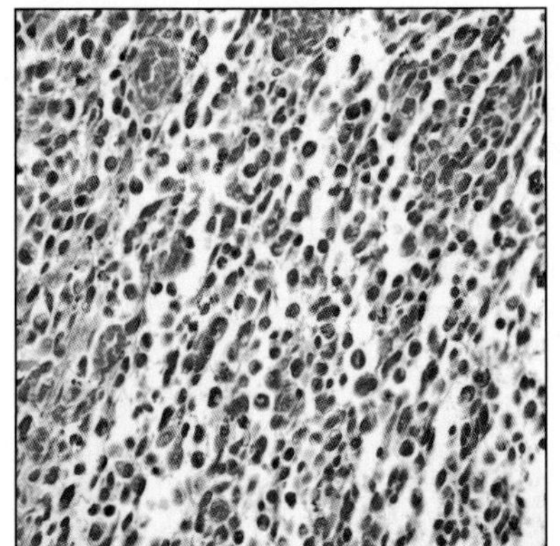

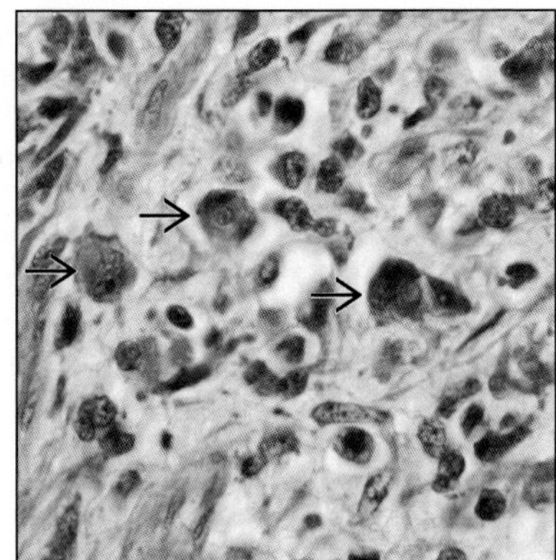

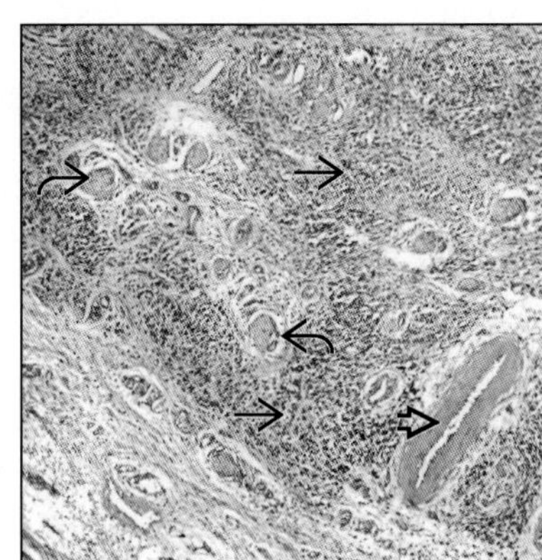

(Left) *Cambium cell layer is composed of sheets of small, round cells with minimal amount of cytoplasm.* ***(Center)*** *High-power magnification shows rhabdomyoblasts ➡ with eosinophilic cytoplasm. Rhabdomyoblasts vary in morphology from round to strap-shaped and contain eosinophilic cytoplasm with cross striations, which might not be seen in some cases.* ***(Right)*** *Small primitive cells ➡ infiltrate tissue around vessel ⇨ and nerves ↗.*

GONADOBLASTOMA

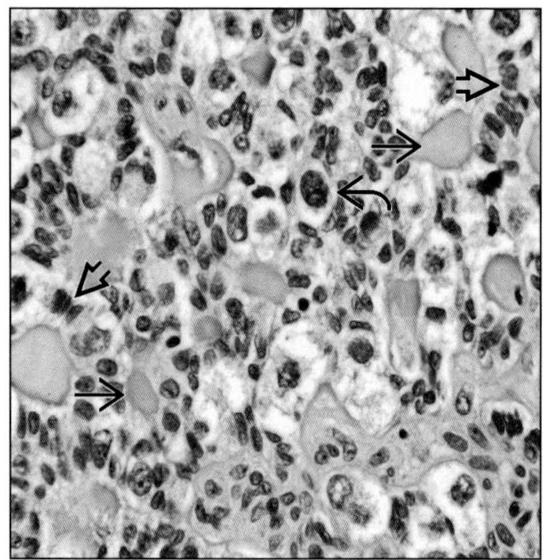

High-power view of cellular nest shows prominent hyaline globules ➔ surrounded by primitive Sertoli and granulosa cells ➔. Germ cells can be recognized by their large, round, centrally placed nuclei ➔.

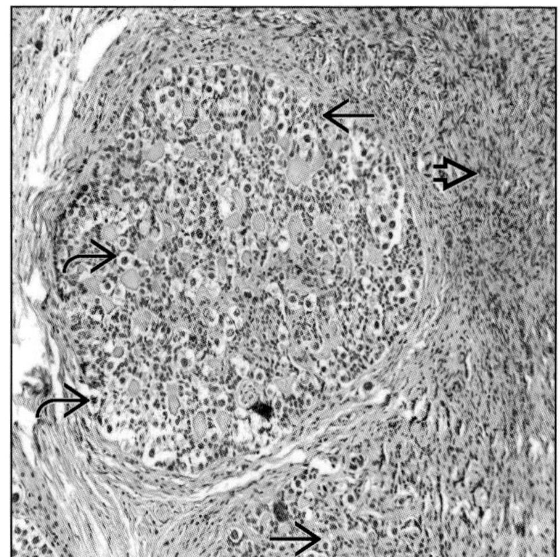

Low-power view of gonadoblastoma shows cellular nests ➔ embedded in dense fibrous stroma ➔. Different cell components are recognized; especially large germ cells with clear cytoplasm ➔.

TERMINOLOGY

Definitions

- Mixed germ cell tumor composed of germ cells and sex cord-stromal derivatives

ETIOLOGY/PATHOGENESIS

Developmental Anomaly

- Associated with pure or mixed gonadal dysgenesis or in male pseudohermaphrodites
  - Most occur in genetic males who are phenotypically female
    - Underlying abnormality may be 46XY pure gonadal dysgenesis or mixed gonadal dysgenesis associated with 45X or 46XY karyotype
- *GBY* region of Y chromosome has been implicated

CLINICAL ISSUES

Epidemiology

- Incidence
  - Very rare tumor
- Age
  - Occurs before the age of 20 years

Presentation

- Primary amenorrhea
- Developmental abnormalities of genitalia
- Association with virilization or estrogen secretion
- Discovered as gonadal tumor

Prognosis

- Pure gonadoblastomas are benign
- Considered in situ malignant germ cell tumor due to frequently encountered malignancy in germ cell component

MACROSCOPIC FEATURES

General Features

- Solid
- Soft to firm
- Gray or yellow to brown
- Smooth lobulated surface
- Calcifications (50% of cases)

Size

- Usually < 8 cm
- 25% of tumors are microscopic

MICROSCOPIC PATHOLOGY

Histologic Features

- Nests of variable size and shape embedded in dense fibrous stroma
  - Nests are comprised of
    - Large, round germ cells with vesicular nuclei, prominent nucleoli, and abundant cytoplasm
    - Germ cells are similar in morphology and immunohistochemical profile to dysgerminoma cells
    - Exhibit increased mitotic activity
    - Immature Sertoli and granulosa cells are arranged around pink hyaline bodies, around germ cells, or rim periphery of cellular nest
    - In surrounding fibrous stroma, Leydig or lutein cells can be identified in about 2/3 of cases
  - Calcifications vary from focal to extensive
    - Present in about 80% of cases
  - Stroma surrounding nests varies in cellularity from scant to cellular
- 1/2 of cases are overgrown by mixed germ cell tumor component
  - Component of dysgerminoma is seen in 80% of cases

GONADOBLASTOMA

Key Facts

Terminology

- Mixed germ cell tumor composed of germ cells and sex cord-stromal derivatives

Etiology/Pathogenesis

- Associated with pure or mixed gonadal dysgenesis or in male pseudohermaphrodites

Clinical Issues

- Very rare tumor
- Due to high incidence of malignant component, it is considered an in situ malignant germ cell tumor

Microscopic Pathology

- Nests of variable size and shape embedded in dense fibrous stroma
- Calcifications vary from focal to extensive (present in about 80% of cases)

Immunohistochemistry

Antibody	Reactivity	Staining Pattern	Comment
Inhibin	Positive	Cytoplasmic	Positive in Sertoli, granulosa, Leydig or lutein cells
CD117	Positive	Cytoplasmic	Positive in germ cells
OCT4	Positive	Nuclear	Positive in germ cells

  - Involvement is variable, from small foci to extensive overgrowth
- Other tumor components include
  - Yolk sac
  - Embryonal carcinoma
  - Choriocarcinoma
  - Immature teratoma

DIFFERENTIAL DIAGNOSIS

Pure Dysgerminoma

- Lacks distinct nested germ cell arrangement
- Lacks Sertoli and granulosa cell components

Sex Cord Tumor with Annular Tubules

- Lacks germ cell component

Mixed Germ Cell-Sex Cord-Stromal Tumor

- Occurs in normal gonads
- Germ cells and sex cord derivatives are admixed with each other forming 3 different histologic patterns
  - Cords or trabeculae surrounded by connective tissue
  - Tubular structures lacking lumen surrounded by connective tissue
  - Germ cell aggregates surrounded by sex cord elements
- Has less uniform appearance
- No nest-like pattern
- Absence of calcifications or hyalinization

SELECTED REFERENCES

1. Salo P et al: Molecular mapping of the putative gonadoblastoma locus on the Y chromosome. Genes Chromosomes Cancer. 14(3):210-4, 1995
2. Troche V et al: Neoplasia arising in dysgenetic gonads. Obstet Gynecol Surv. 41(2):74-9, 1986
3. Khalid BA et al: Dysgerminoma--gonadoblastoma and familial 46XY pure gonadal dysgenesis: case report and review of the genetics and pathophysiology of gonadal dysgenesis and H-Y antigen. Aust N Z J Obstet Gynaecol. 22(3):175-9, 1982
4. Talerman A: The pathology of gonadal neoplasms composed of germ cells and sex cord stroma derivatives. Pathol Res Pract. 170(1-3):24-38, 1980
5. Scully RE: Gonadoblastoma. A review of 74 cases. Cancer. 25(6):1340-56, 1970

IMAGE GALLERY

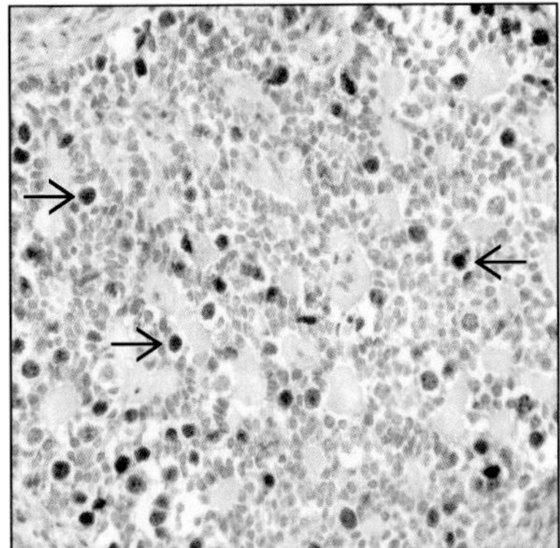

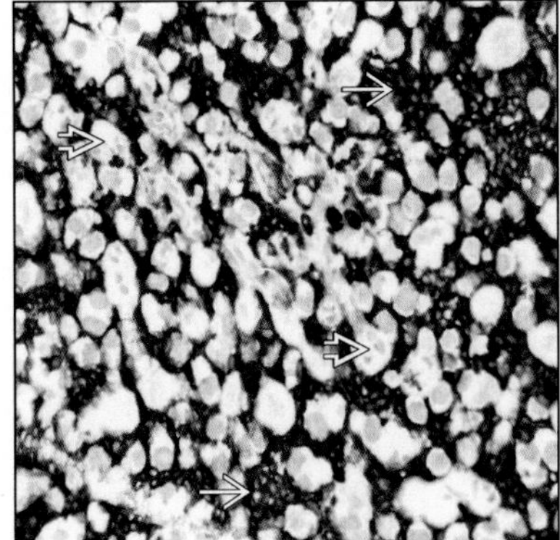

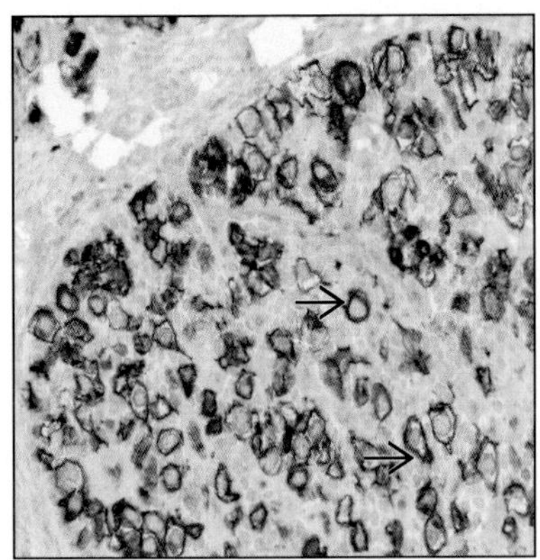

(Left) *POU5F1 highlights germ cells scattered throughout the cellular nest ⇨. In about 1/2 of cases, gonadoblastoma is overgrown by dysgerminoma, in which case immunohistochemical stain POU5F1 would show sheets of positive germ cells with no other intervening component.* ***(Center)*** *Inhibin stain shows positive immunoreactivity of Sertoli and granulosa cells ➡. Nonreactive spaces are germ cells ⇨.* ***(Right)*** *CD117 demonstrates strong cytoplasmic staining of germ cells ⇨.*

PROTOCOL FOR WILMS TUMOR SPECIMENS

Wilms Tumor

Kidney: Resection for Pediatric Renal Tumor

Procedure

___ Partial nephrectomy
___ Radical nephrectomy
___ Bilateral partial nephrectomies
___ Other (specify): ____________________________
___ Not specified

Specimen Size

Kidney dimensions: _________ x _________ x _________ cm
Weight: _________ g

Specimen Laterality

___ Right
___ Left
___ Not specified

****Tumor Site(s) (select all that apply)***

*___ Upper pole
*___ Middle
*___ Lower pole
*___ Other (specify): ____________________________
*___ Not specified

Tumor Size

Greatest dimension: _________ cm
*Additional dimensions: _________ x _________ cm
___ Cannot be determined
For specimens with multiple tumors, specify greatest dimension of each additional tumor:
Greatest dimension tumor #2: _________ cm
Greatest dimension tumor #3: _________ cm
Other (specify): ____________________________

Tumor Focality

___ Unifocal
___ Multifocal
Number of tumors in specimen (specify): _________
___ Indeterminate
___ Cannot be assessed

Macroscopic Extent of Tumor

Gerota fascia
___ Gerota fascia intact
___ Gerota fascia disrupted
___ Indeterminate
___ Cannot be assessed

Renal sinus (select all that apply)
___ Renal sinus involvement by tumor not identified
___ Tumor minimally extends into renal sinus soft tissue
___ Tumor extensively involves renal sinus soft tissue
___ Tumor involves lymph-vascular spaces in renal sinus

Renal vein
___ Renal vein invasion present
___ Renal vein invasion not identified
___ Indeterminate
___ Cannot be assessed

Adjacent organ involvement (select all that apply)
- ___ Tumor extension into adjacent organ present (specify organ: ___________________________)
- ___ Tumor extension into adjacent organ not identified
- ___ Indeterminate
- ___ Cannot be assessed

Histologic Type (select all that apply)

___ Wilms tumor, favorable histology
___ Wilms tumor, focal anaplasia
___ Wilms tumor, diffuse anaplasia
___ Congenital mesoblastic nephroma, classical
___ Congenital mesoblastic nephroma, cellular
___ Congenital mesoblastic nephroma, mixed
___ Clear cell sarcoma
___ Rhabdoid tumor
___ Other (specify): ___________________________
___ Malignant neoplasm, type indeterminate

**Nephrogenic Rests (select all that apply)*

*___ Nephrogenic rests not identified
*___ Nephrogenic rests present
- *___ Nephrogenic rests, intralobar
- *___ Nephrogenic rests, perilobar
  - *___ Diffuse, hyperplastic
  - *___ Multifocal
  - *___ Focal
- *___ Nephrogenic rests, unclassified

*___ Cannot be assessed

Margins (select all that apply)

___ Cannot be assessed
___ Margin involvement by tumor not identified
- Distance of tumor from closest margin: _________ mm OR _________ cm
- Specify margin: ___________________________

___ Margin(s) involved by tumor
- ___ Gerota fascia
- ___ Renal vein
- ___ Inferior vena cava
- ___ Ureter
- ___ Other (specify): ___________________________

Lymph Nodes

___ Regional lymph node metastasis not identified
___ Regional lymph node metastasis present (specify site [if known]: ___________________________)
___ No nodes submitted or found

Number of lymph nodes examined
- Specify: _________
- ___ Number cannot be determined (explain): ___________________________

Number of lymph nodes involved
- Specify: _________
- ___ Number cannot be determined (explain): ___________________________

Distant Metastasis†

___ Not applicable
___ Distant metastasis present
- *Specify site(s) if known: ___________________________

PROTOCOL FOR WILMS TUMOR SPECIMENS

Children's Oncology Group Staging System for Pediatric Renal Tumors Other Than Renal Cell Carcinoma (select all that apply under appropriate stage)

____ Stage I: Tumor limited to kidney and completely resected

- ____ Penetration of renal capsule by tumor not identified
- ____ Tumor involvement of extrarenal or renal sinus lymph-vascular spaces not identified
- ____ Tumor metastasis to lymph nodes not identified

____ Stage II: Tumor extends beyond kidney but completely resected

- ____ Tumor extends beyond renal capsule but with negative resection margin
- ____ Tumor involvement of extrarenal or renal sinus lymph-vascular spaces present
- ____ Tumor involves renal vein but has not been transected and is not attached to vein wall at resection margin
- ____ Tumor extensively involves renal sinus soft tissue

____ Stage III: Residual tumor

- ____ Tumor present at margin(s) of resection
- ____ Tumor capsular rupture identified
- ____ Tumor spill before or during surgery identified
- ____ Piecemeal excision of tumor (removal of tumor in > 1 piece)
- ____ Metastatic tumor in regional lymph nodes identified
- ____ History of renal tumor biopsy before definitive surgery

____ Stage IV: Metastatic disease

- ____ Hematogenous metastases or lymph node metastases outside abdominopelvic region (beyond renal drainage system, e.g., lung, liver)

____ Stage V

- ____ Bilateral renal involvement at diagnosis (each side should also be staged separately, according to above criteria, as I to IV)
  Specify (both): Right kidney stage: _________ Left kidney stage: _________

***Additional Pathologic Findings**

*Specify: ____________________________

**Data elements with asterisks are not required. These elements may be clinically important but are not yet validated or regularly used in patient management. Protocol applies to all renal tumors of childhood except renal cell carcinoma. Use adult kidney protocol for renal cell carcinoma. Note: For bilateral tumors, complete a separate checklist for each kidney. Adapted with permission from College of American Pathologists, "Protocol for the Examination of Specimens from Pediatric Patients with Wilms Tumors." Web posting date February 2011, www.cap.org.*
†Note: Distant metastasis category includes both hematogenous metastasis or lymph node metastasis outside the abdomen-pelvic region (beyond the renal drainage system).

PROTOCOL FOR MALIGNANT GCT AND SEX CORD-STROMAL TUMOR SPECIMENS

Testis

Radical Orchiectomy

Serum Tumor Markers (select all that apply)

*___ Unknown
*___ Serum marker studies within normal limits
*___ Alpha-fetoprotein (AFP) evaluation
*___ Beta-subunit of human chorionic gonadotropin (b-hCG) elevation
*___ Lactate dehydrogenase (LDH) elevation

Specimen Laterality

___ Right
___ Left
___ Both
___ Not specified

Tumor Focality

___ Unifocal
___ Multifocal

Tumor Size

Greatest dimension of main tumor mass: _________ cm
*Additional dimensions: _________ x _________ cm
Greatest dimensions of additional tumor nodules: _________ cm, _________ cm, etc.
___ Cannot be determined

Macroscopic Extent of Tumor

___ Confined to testis
___ Invades hilar soft tissues
___ Invades tunica vaginalis (perforates mesothelium)
___ Invades epididymis
___ Invades spermatic cord
___ Other (specify): ___________________________

Histologic Type (select all that apply)

___ Intratubular germ cell neoplasia, unclassified only
___ Seminoma, classic type
___ Seminoma with associated scar
___ Seminoma with syncytiotrophoblastic cells
___ Mixed germ cell tumor
(Specify components and approximate percentages): ___________________________
___ Embryonal carcinoma
___ Yolk sac tumor
___ Choriocarcinoma, biphasic
___ Choriocarcinoma, monophasic
___ Placental site trophoblastic tumor
___ Teratoma
___ Teratoma with secondary somatic-type malignant component
(Specify type): ___________________________
___ Monodermal teratoma, carcinoid
___ Monodermal teratoma, primitive neuroectodermal tumor
___ Monodermal teratoma, other (specify): ___________________________
___ Spermatocytic seminoma
___ Spermatocytic seminoma with a sarcomatous component
___ Mixed germ cell-sex cord-stromal tumor, gonadoblastoma
___ Mixed germ cell-sex-cord stromal tumor, others
(Specify): ___________________________
___ Testicular scar

PROTOCOL FOR MALIGNANT GCT AND SEX CORD-STROMAL TUMOR SPECIMENS

____ Scar only
____ Scar with intratubular germ cell neoplasia
____ Sex cord-stromal tumor
____ Leydig cell tumor
____ Sertoli cell tumor
____ Classic
____ Sclerosing
____ Large cell calcifying
____ Granulosa cell tumor
____ Adult type
____ Juvenile type
____ Mixed, with components
(Specify components and approximate percentages): ____________________________
____ Unclassified
____ Malignant neoplasm, type cannot be determined
____ Other (specify): ____________________________

Margins

Spermatic cord margin
____ Cannot be assessed
____ Uninvolved by tumor
____ Involved by tumor

Other margin(s)
____ Cannot be assessed
____ Uninvolved by tumor (specify): ____________________________
____ Involved by tumor (specify): ____________________________
____ Not applicable

Microscopic Tumor Extension (select all that apply)

*____ Rete testis
*____ Epididymis
*____ Hilar fat
____ Spermatic cord
____ Tunica vaginalis (perforates mesothelium)
____ Scrotal wall
____ None of the above

Lymph-Vascular Invasion

____ Absent
____ Present
____ Indeterminate

Pathologic Staging (pTNM)

TNM descriptors (required only if applicable) (select all that apply)
____ m (multiple)
____ r (recurrent)
____ y (post-treatment)

Primary tumor (pT)
____ pTX: Cannot be assessed
____ pT0: No evidence of primary tumor
____ pTis: Intratubular germ cell neoplasia (carcinoma in situ)
____ pT1: Tumor limited to testis and epididymis without vascular/lymphatic invasion
Tumor may invade tunica albuginea but not tunica vaginalis
____ pT2: Tumor limited to testis and epididymis with vascular/lymphatic invasion
Or tumor extending through tunica albuginea with involvement of tunica vaginalis
____ pT3: Tumor invades spermatic cord ± vascular/lymphatic invasion
____ pT4: Tumor invades scrotum ± vascular/lymphatic invasion

Regional lymph nodes (pN)

___ pNX: Cannot be assessed

___ pN0: No regional lymph node metastasis

___ pN1: Metastasis with a lymph node mass ≤ 2 cm in greatest dimension

Or ≤ 5 positive nodes, none > 2 cm in greatest dimension

___ pN2: Metastasis with a lymph node mass > 2 cm but ≤ 5 cm in greatest dimension

Or > 5 nodes positive, none > 5 cm

Or evidence of extranodal extension of tumor

___ pN3: Metastasis with a lymph node mass > 5 cm in greatest dimension

___ No nodes submitted or found

Number of lymph nodes examined

Specify: ________

___ Number cannot be determined (explain): __________________________

Number of lymph nodes involved

Specify: _________

___ Number cannot be determined (explain): ___________________________

Distant metastasis (pM)

___ Not applicable

___ pM1: Distant metastasis present

___ pM1a: Nonregional nodal or pulmonary metastasis

___ pM1b: Distant metastasis other than to nonregional lymph nodes and lung

*Specify site(s) if known: ___________________________

*Serum Tumor Markers (S)

*___ SX: Serum marker studies not available or performed

*___ S0: Serum marker study levels within normal limits

*___ S1: LDH < 1.5 x N† **and** hCG < 5,000 mIU/mL **and** AFP < 1,000 ng/mL

*___ S2: LDH 1.5-10 x N **or** hCG 5,000-50,000 mIU/mL **or** AFP 1,000-10,000 ng/mL

*___ S3: LDH > 10 x N **or** > hCG 50,000 **or** AFP > 10,000 ng/mL

*Additional Pathologic Findings (select all that apply)

*___ None identified

*___ Intratubular germ cell neoplasia

*___ Hemosiderin-laden macrophages

*___ Atrophy

*___ Other (specify): ___________________________

**Data elements with asterisks are not required. These elements may be clinically important but are not yet validated or regularly used in patient management. Adapted with permission from College of American Pathologists, "Protocol for the Examination of Specimens from Patients with Malignant Germ Cell and Sex Cord-Stromal Tumors of the Testis." Web posting date February 2011, www.cap.org. †N indicates the upper limit of normal for the LDH assay.*

PROTOCOL FOR OVARIAN CARCINOMA SPECIMENS

Ovary

Oophorectomy, Salpingo-Oophorectomy, Subtotal Oophorectomy or Removal of Tumor in Fragments, Hysterectomy with Salpingo-Oophorectomy

Specimen (select all that apply)

___ Right ovary
___ Left ovary
___ Right fallopian tube
___ Left fallopian tube
___ Uterus
___ Cervix
___ Omentum
___ Peritoneum
___ Other (specify): ____________________________
___ Not specified
___ Cannot be determined

Procedure (select all that apply)

___ Right oophorectomy
___ Left oophorectomy
___ Right salpingo-oophorectomy
___ Left salpingo-oophorectomy
___ Bilateral salpingo-oophorectomy
___ Subtotal right oophorectomy
___ Subtotal left oophorectomy
___ Supracervical hysterectomy
___ Hysterectomy
___ Omentectomy
___ Peritoneal biopsies
___ Other (specify): ____________________________
___ Not specified

Lymph Node Sampling

___ Performed
___ Not performed
___ Not known

Specimen Integrity

Right ovary

___ Not applicable
___ Capsule intact
___ Capsule ruptured
___ Fragmented
___ Other (specify): ____________________________

Left ovary

___ Not applicable
___ Capsule intact
___ Capsule ruptured
___ Fragmented
___ Other (specify): ____________________________

Primary Tumor Site (select all that apply)

___ Right ovary
___ Left ovary
___ Bilateral ovarian involvement
___ Not specified

Ovarian Surface Involvement

___ Present
___ Absent
___ Uncertain/cannot be determined

Tumor Size

Right ovary (if applicable)
Greatest dimension: _________ cm
*Additional dimensions: _________ x _________ cm
___ Cannot be determined

Histologic Type (select all that apply)

___ Serous, borderline tumor
___ Serous, carcinoma
___ Mucinous, borderline tumor, intestinal type
___ Mucinous, borderline tumor, endocervical type (seromucinous type)
___ Mucinous carcinoma
___ Endometrioid borderline tumor
___ Endometrioid carcinoma
___ Clear cell borderline tumor
___ Clear cell carcinoma
___ Transitional cell borderline tumor
___ Transitional cell carcinoma
___ Brenner tumor, malignant type
___ Squamous cell carcinoma
___ Mixed epithelial borderline tumor
Specify types and percentages: ___________________________
___ Mixed epithelial carcinoma
Specify types and percentages: ___________________________
___ Undifferentiated carcinoma
___ Carcinosarcoma (malignant Müllerian mixed tumor)
___ Granulosa cell tumor
___ Other sex cord-stromal tumor (specify type): ___________________________
___ Malignant germ cell tumor
Specify types and percentages: ___________________________
___ Other(s) (specify): ___________________________

Histologic Grade

World Health Organization (WHO) grading system
(Applies to all carcinomas, including serous carcinomas)
___ GX: Cannot be assessed
___ G1: Well differentiated
___ G2: Moderately differentiated
___ G3: Poorly differentiated
___ G4: Undifferentiated
2-tier grading system
(May be applied to serous carcinomas and immature teratomas only)
___ Low grade
___ High grade
___ Other (specify): ___________________________
___ Not applicable

Implants (only applies to advanced stage serous/seromucinous borderline tumors) (select all that apply)

___ Not applicable/not sampled
Noninvasive implant(s)
___ Not present
___ Present (specify sites): ___________________________

*Type of noninvasive implant(s)
*___ Epithelial
*___ Desmoplastic

Invasive implant(s)
___ Not present
___ Present (specify sites): ___________________________

Extent of Involvement of Other Tissues/Organs (select all that apply)

___ Right ovary
___ Involved
___ Not involved
___ Not applicable

___ Left ovary
___ Involved
___ Not involved
___ Not applicable

___ Right fallopian tube
___ Involved
___ Not involved
___ Not applicable

___ Left fallopian tube
___ Involved
___ Not involved
___ Not applicable

___ Omentum
___ Involved
___ Not involved
___ Not applicable

___ Uterus
___ Involved (specify location: ___________________________)
___ Not involved
___ Not applicable

___ Peritoneum
___ Involved
___ Not involved
___ Not applicable

___ Other organs/tissues (specify): ___________________________

**Treatment Effect (applicable to carcinomas treated with neoadjuvant therapy)*

*___ No definite or minimal response identified (poor or no response)
*___ Marked response (minimal residual cancer)

**Lymph-Vascular Invasion*

*___ Not identified
*___ Present
*___ Indeterminate

Pathologic Staging (pTNM) [FIGO])

TNM descriptors (required only if applicable) (select all that apply)
___ m (multiple primary tumors)
___ r (recurrent)
___ y (post-treatment)

Primary tumor (pT)
___ pTX [--]: Cannot be assessed
___ pT0 [--]: No evidence of primary tumor
___ pT1 [I]: Tumor limited to ovaries (1 or both)
___ pT1a [IA]: Tumor limited to 1 ovary; capsule intact, no tumor on ovarian surface

No malignant cells in ascites or peritoneal washings#

___ pT1b [IB]: Tumor limited to both ovaries; capsule intact, no tumor on ovarian surface

No malignant cells in ascites or peritoneal washings

___ pT2 [II]: Tumor involves 1 or both ovaries with pelvic extension &/or implants

___ pT2a [IIA]: Extension &/or implants on uterus &/or tube(s)

No malignant cells in ascites or peritoneal washings

___ pT2b [IIB]: Extension to other pelvic tissues

No malignant cells in ascites or peritoneal washings

___ pT2c [IIC]: Pelvic extension &/or implants (T2a or T2b/IIa or IIb)

With malignant cells in ascites or peritoneal washings

___ pT3 &/or N1 [III]: Tumor involves one or both ovaries with confirmed peritoneal metastasis outside pelvis

Including liver capsule metastasis &/or regional lymph node metastasis [N1]

___ pT3a [IIIA]: Microscopic peritoneal metastasis beyond pelvis (no macroscopic tumor)

___ pT3b [IIIB]: Macroscopic peritoneal metastasis beyond pelvis

≤ 2 cm in greatest dimension

___ pT3c &/or N1 [IIIC]: Peritoneal metastasis beyond pelvis

> 2 cm in greatest dimension &/or regional lymph node metastasis

Regional lymph nodes (pN)

___ pNX: Cannot be assessed

___ pN0: No regional lymph node metastasis

___ pN1 [IIIC]: Regional lymph node metastasis

___ No nodes submitted or found

Number of lymph nodes examined

Specify: ________

___ Number cannot be determined (explain): ________________________

Number of lymph nodes involved

Specify: ________

___ Number cannot be determined (explain): ________________________

Distant metastasis (pM)

___ Not applicable

___ pM1 [IV]: Distant metastases (excludes peritoneal metastasis)†

*Specify site(s), if known: ________________________

*Additional Pathologic Findings (select all that apply)

*___ None identified

*___ Endometriosis

*___ Ovarian

*___ Extraovarian

*___ Endosalpingiosis

*___ Other(s)

*Specify site(s) and type(s): ________________________

*Ancillary Studies

*Specify: ________________________

*Clinical History (select all that apply)

*___ *BRCA1/2* family history

*___ Hereditary breast/ovarian cancer

*___ Other (specify): ________________________

**Data elements with asterisks are not required. These elements may be clinically important but are not yet validated or regularly used in patient management. #Nonmalignant ascites is not classified. The presence of ascites does not affect staging unless malignant cells are present. †Note: If pleural effusion is present, there must be a positive cytology for a stage IV designation. Parenchymal liver metastasis is classified as stage IV disease, whereas liver capsule metastasis is classified as stage III disease. Adapted with permission from College of American Pathologists, "Protocol for the Examination of Specimens from Patients with Carcinoma of the Ovary." Web posting date: February 2011, www.cap.org.*

Hematopoietic

Neoplasm, Borderline

Neoplasm, Malignant Primary

Protocol for the Examination of Specimens from Patients with Hematopoietic Neoplasms Involving Bone Marrow

Protocol for the Examination of Specimens from Patients with Hodgkin Lymphoma

Protocol for the Examination of Specimens from Patients with Non-Hodgkin Lymphoma

HEMOPHAGOCYTIC SYNDROME

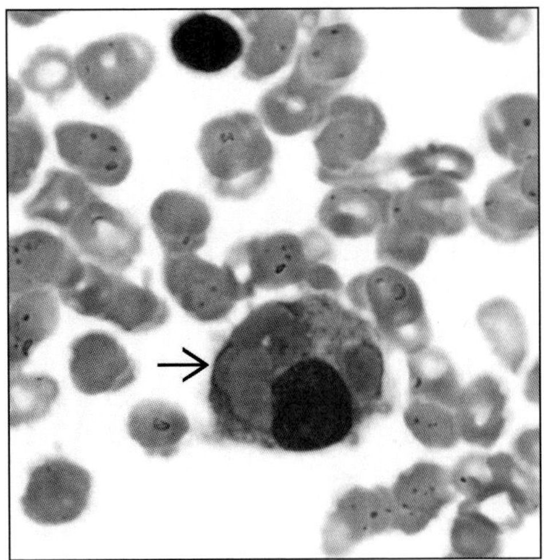

Bone marrow aspirate smear shows a histiocyte that has engulfed multiple erythrocytes ⇒. Although not seen in this example, a clear halo often surrounds the engulfed erythrocyte, platelet, or leukocyte.

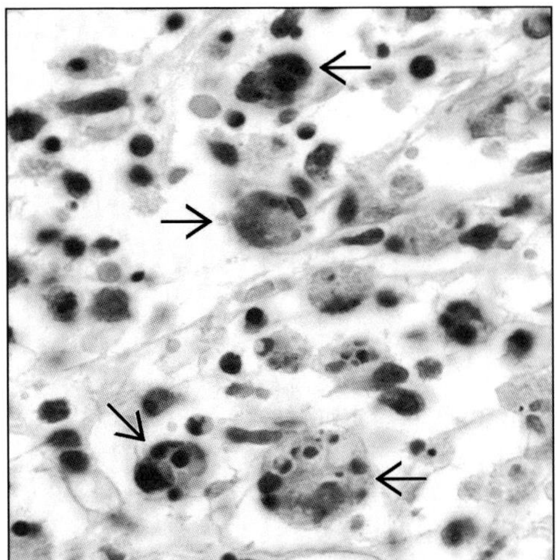

Histiocytes ⇒, as depicted here, can also be seen engulfing platelets, leukocytes, and erythrocytes.

TERMINOLOGY

Abbreviations

- Hemophagocytic syndrome (HS)

Synonyms

- Hemophagocytic lymphohistiocytosis (HLH)

Definitions

- Severe life-threatening hyperinflammatory condition with characteristic signs, symptoms, and laboratory findings
- Highly fatal disease of children

ETIOLOGY/PATHOGENESIS

Primary (Genetic) HLH

- **Familial HLH**
  - Autosomal recessive or X-linked inheritance
  - Multiple gene mutations described
  - Perforin (*PRF1*) gene mutations
    - Cytotoxic granule protein
    - Involved in introduction of cytotoxic effector molecules into cytoplasm of target cells
    - Accounts for 20-40% of familial HLH
    - Most often present in early childhood
  - *UNC13D/MUNC13-4* gene mutations
    - Mutations disrupt normal release of granules from cytotoxic T cells
    - Accounts for 17-30% of familial HLH
  - *STX11* gene mutations
    - Rare
    - Described only in patients of Turkish origin
- **Immune deficiency-associated HLH**
  - Chediak-Higashi syndrome
    - Characterized by albinism, coagulopathy, neurological symptoms, and pyogenic infections
    - Abnormally large granules in histiocytes, NK-cells, and cytotoxic lymphocytes
    - *CHS1/LYST* gene mutation
    - Impaired vesicle transport
    - Impaired NK- and T-cell cytotoxicity
    - 85% enter accelerated phase, indistinguishable from HLH patients
  - Griscelli syndrome
    - Rare autosomal recessive disorder
    - Characterized by albinism and neurological defects
    - *RAB27A* and *MYO5A* gene mutations
    - *RAB27A* gene mutations only associated with HLH
    - Severely impaired cytotoxic activity
    - Impaired vesicle docking
  - X-linked lymphoproliferative syndrome
    - Syndrome associated with development of lymphoma, hypogammaglobulinemia, and HLH
    - *SH2D1A* gene mutations
    - Impaired signal transduction and lymphocyte activation
    - Increased chance of developing HLH following viral infections
  - Wiskott-Aldrich syndrome
    - X-linked recessive disorder
    - Characterized by eczema, thrombocytopenia, and recurrent infections
    - *WASP* gene mutations
    - Mutations disrupt development of functional secretory synapses and cell trafficking
    - Impaired NK-cell cytotoxicity
  - Other immunodeficiencies associated with HLH
    - Severe combined immunodeficiency
    - Omenn syndrome
    - DiGeorge syndrome
- Distinguishing primary HLH from acquired HLH is often impossible

Acquired HLH

- Often associated with infections
  - Viral infections

HEMOPHAGOCYTIC SYNDROME

Key Facts

Terminology
- Severe life-threatening hyperinflammatory condition with characteristic signs, symptoms, and laboratory findings

Etiology/Pathogenesis
- **Familial HLH**
  - Autosomal recessive or X-linked inheritance
  - Multiple gene mutations described
- **Immune deficiency-associated HLH**
  - Chediak-Higashi syndrome
  - Griscelli syndrome
  - X-linked lymphoproliferative syndrome
  - Wiskott-Aldrich syndrome
- **Acquired HLH**
  - Often associated with infections
  - May occur with certain malignancies
  - May occur in association with autoimmune diseases

Clinical Issues
- 0.12 in 100,000 children per year (familial form)
- Cardinal symptoms
  - Prolonged, high-grade fever
  - Splenomegaly
  - Hepatosplenomegaly
  - Cytopenias
- ~ 5% 1-year overall survival rate without treatment
- Familial HLH, invariably fatal without treatment

Microscopic Pathology
- Hemophagocytosis
- Phagocytosis of red blood cells, white blood cells, and platelets

---

    - Most often of herpes group (EBV, CMV, HHV-6, HHV-8, VZV, and HSV)
    - HIV, parvovirus, adenovirus, hepatitis virus
  - Bacterial, spirochetal, and fungal-associated infections
  - Leishmaniasis
  - Genetic forms of HLH may also be triggered by infections
- May occur with certain malignancies
  - Cutaneous lymphomas
  - Anaplastic large cell lymphoma
  - EBV-positive lymphoproliferative disorder of childhood
  - EBV genome often detected in T-/NK-cell lymphoma-associated cases
- May occur in association with autoimmune diseases
  - Systemic juvenile idiopathic arthritis
    - Estimated to occur in 7% of patients
  - Adult onset Still disease
  - Lupus erythematosus
  - **Macrophage activation syndrome**
    - Considered a special form of HLH
    - Occurs in children and adults with autoimmune diseases
    - Less severe cytopenias
    - More pronounced coagulopathy
    - Severe cardiac impairment
    - Defective NK-cell function
    - Triggered by viruses and drugs
- Rare reports of HLH associated with sickle cell disease

Pathophysiology
- Defective cytotoxic T-cell and NK-cell activity
  - Impaired elimination of cellular targets
  - Impaired downregulation of immune response
- Defective apoptotic activity
- Excessive activation of lymphocytes and macrophages
- Sustained immune activation
  - Persistently high cytokine levels responsible for clinical picture of HLH
- Profound cytokine activation results in organ dysfunction

CLINICAL ISSUES

Epidemiology
- Incidence
  - 0.12 in 100,000 children per year (familial form)
- Age
  - Acquired HLH
    - Occurs in all age groups
  - Familial HLH
    - Children (70-80% < 1 year of age)

Presentation
- Cardinal symptoms
  - Prolonged, high-grade fever
  - Splenomegaly
  - Hepatosplenomegaly
  - Cytopenias
  - Often occur in setting of acute infection
- Less common symptoms
  - Lymphadenopathy
  - Rash
  - Jaundice
  - Neurologic signs and symptoms
    - Seizures, cranial nerve palsies
  - Pulmonary effusions
- Anorexia
- Failure to thrive
- **Characteristic laboratory values**
  - Hypertriglyceridemia
  - Elevated LDH
  - Hyperferritinemia
  - Elevated transaminases
  - Hyperbilirubinemia
  - Hypofibrinogenemia
  - Increased soluble CD25 (IL-2 receptor)
    - Valuable marker of disease
    - Marker of increased T-lymphocyte activation
  - Decreased to absent natural killer-cell activity
    - Correlates with known genetic defects associated with HLH
  - Cytopenias affecting at least 2 cell lineages

- Elevated prothrombin time and partial thromboplastin time and thrombin time

Laboratory Tests

- Complete blood count
- Liver enzymes
- Bilirubin
- Lipid profile
- Ferritin
- Coagulation profile
- Fibrinogen
- Bone marrow study
- Lumbar puncture
- Infectious work-up

Natural History

- Uncontrolled hyperinflammation leads to sustained neutropenia and death

Treatment

- Drugs
  - Corticosteroids
    - Dexamethasone (preferred in pediatric protocols)
    - High-dose prednisolone (genetic HLH and pediatric MAS)
  - Cyclosporin A
  - Immunoglobulins
    - Mainly used in adults
  - Etoposide
  - Liposomal amphotericin B
    - Leishmania-associated HLH
- Stem cell transplantation
  - Only curative method in genetic HLH
- Combination therapies
  - Dexamethasone, cyclosporin A, and etoposide
  - Corticosteroids with immunoglobulins
    - Adults with less severe disease
  - Corticosteroids ± cyclosporin A
    - Autoimmune disease-associated HLH
- HLH-94 protocol
  - Dexamethasone, cyclosporin A, VP-16, and intrathecal methotrexate combined with stem cell transplantation
  - 3-year overall survival rate of 50-70%
- HLH-2004 protocol
  - Aggressive treatment with dexamethasone, etoposide, cyclosporin A, intrathecal methotrexate
  - Stem cell transplant in children with familial disease or disease that is persistent, reactivated or unresponsive to therapy
- Emerging therapies
  - Anti-cytokine medications
    - Anti-TNF-α, anti-INF-γ, anti-IL-6, anti-IL-18
    - Still under study
  - Should not replace established protocols

Prognosis

- ~ 5% 1-year overall survival rate without treatment
- Familial HLH, invariably fatal without treatment

MICROSCOPIC PATHOLOGY

Microscopic Features

- Hemophagocytosis
  - Phagocytosis of red blood cells, white blood cells, and platelets
  - May be observed in
    - Spleen, lymph nodes, CSF, and liver
  - Most commonly observed in the bone marrow
- Bone marrow examination
  - Normal trilineage maturation
  - Normo to hypercellularity
  - Hemophagocytosis
    - Not required for diagnosis
    - May be absent initially

DIFFERENTIAL DIAGNOSIS

Infection in Immunocompetent Patient

- Signs and symptoms generally not as pronounced as in HLH
- Typically lack organomegaly and cytopenias
- Lack many of biochemical parameters associated with HLH

Acute Leukemia

- Similar initial clinical symptoms
- Rule out with peripheral blood and bone marrow evaluation

Langerhans Cell Histiocytosis

- Hepatosplenomegaly, fever, and cytopenias may be present
- Typically show bone lesions
- Characteristic rash
- Distinct histological picture
  - CD1a(+) Langerhans cells
  - Inflammatory infiltrate (eosinophils, neutrophils, and lymphocytes)
  - Phagocytic histiocytes

Metabolic Disease

- May show organomegaly, liver dysfunction, and high triglycerides
- Lack cytopenias and prolonged fever

DIAGNOSTIC CHECKLIST

Pathologic Interpretation Pearls

- Consider HLH when patient presents with
  - Prolonged fever unresponsive to antibiotics
  - Hepatosplenomegaly
  - Cytopenias

SELECTED REFERENCES

1. Arceci RJ: When T cells and macrophages do not talk: the hemophagocytic syndromes. Curr Opin Hematol. 15(4):359-67, 2008

HEMOPHAGOCYTIC SYNDROME

Diagnostic Criteria for HLH

Diagnosis is Established by Fulfilling 1 or 2 of the Following Criteria

Molecular Diagnosis Known to Cause HLH

OR

Signs and Symptoms (5 out of the following criteria)

- (a) Fever
- (b) Splenomegaly
- (c) No evidence of malignancy
- (d) Cytopenias (≥ 2 hematopoietic cell lineages on CBC)
  - (i) Hemoglobin < 90 g/L (< 10 g/L in infants < 4 weeks of age)
  - (ii) Platelets < 100 x 10^9/L
  - (iii) Neutrophils < 1.0 x 10^9/L
- (e) Hypertriglyceridemia &/or hypofibrinogenemia
  - (i) Fasting triglycerides at least 3.0 mmol/L (≥ 265 mg/dL)
- (f) Hemophagocytosis in bone marrow or spleen or lymph nodes
- (g) Low or absent NK-cell activity
- (h) Ferritin at least 500 μg/L
- (i) Soluble CD25 at least 2,400 U/mL

Adapted from the Treatment Protocol of the 2nd International HLH study, 2004.

HLH Classification and Disease Associations

Primary and Acquired HLH

Primary (Genetic) HLH

- Familial HLH
- Immune deficiency-associated HLH
  - (a) Chediak-Higashi syndrome
  - (b) Griscelli syndrome
  - (c) X-linked lymphoproliferative syndrome
  - (d) Wiskott-Aldrich syndrome
  - (e) Less common causes
    - (i) SCID
    - (ii) Omenn syndrome
    - (iii) DiGeorge syndrome

Acquired HLH

- Infections
  - (a) Viral (herpes viruses), bacterial, and fungal
- Malignancies
  - (a) Cutaneous lymphoma
  - (b) Anaplastic large cell lymphoma
  - (c) EBV(+) lymphoproliferative disorder of childhood
- Autoimmune diseases

2. Bryceson YT et al: Defective cytotoxic lymphocyte degranulation in syntaxin-11 deficient familial hemophagocytic lymphohistiocytosis 4 (FHL4) patients. Blood. 110(6):1906-15, 2007
3. Henter JI et al: HLH-2004: Diagnostic and therapeutic guidelines for hemophagocytic lymphohistiocytosis. Pediatr Blood Cancer. 48(2):124-31, 2007
4. Janka GE: Familial and acquired hemophagocytic lymphohistiocytosis. Eur J Pediatr. 166(2):95-109, 2007
5. Janka GE: Hemophagocytic syndromes. Blood Rev. 21(5):245-53, 2007
6. Filipovich AH: Hemophagocytic lymphohistiocytosis and related disorders. Curr Opin Allergy Clin Immunol. 6(6):410-5, 2006
7. Henter JI: Biology and treatment of familial hemophagocytic lymphohistiocytosis: importance of perforin in lymphocyte-mediated cytotoxicity and triggering of apoptosis. Med Pediatr Oncol. 38(5):305-9, 2002
8. Fadeel B et al: Familial hemophagocytic lymphohistiocytosis: too little cell death can seriously damage your health. Leuk Lymphoma. 42(1-2):13-20, 2001

HEMOPHAGOCYTIC SYNDROME

Microscopic Features

*(**Left**) Bone marrow core biopsy from low power highlights florid HLH. There appear to be numerous multinucleated cells ➡ that upon closer inspection represent florid hemophagocytosis. (**Right**) Bone marrow aspirate smear seen under oil immersion demonstrates hemophagocytosis. Note the histiocyte that has engulfed several erythrocytes ➡ and multiple platelets ➡.*

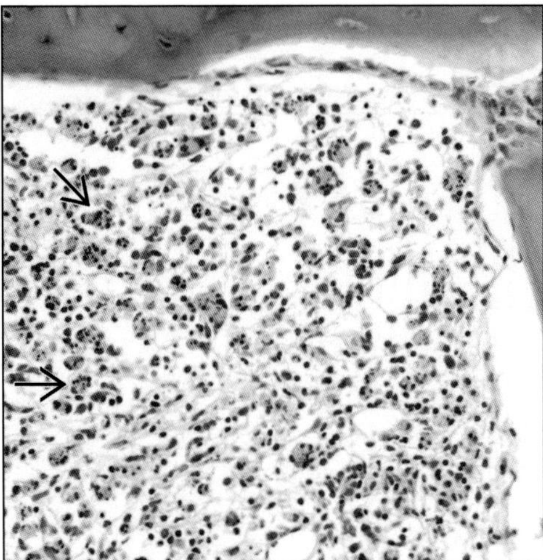

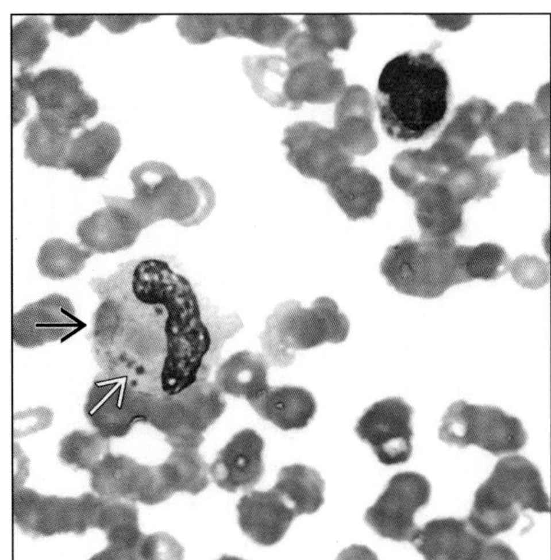

*(**Left**) A bone marrow aspirate shows a histiocyte engulfing both platelets ➡ and erythrocytes ➡. The clear halos ➡ surrounding the engulfed cells are often seen and are an indication of true hemophagocytosis, which can often be confused with a cell simply overlapping the histiocyte. (**Right**) A histiocyte is seen engulfing an erythrocyte ➡ along with fungal organisms ➡ in this case of disseminated histoplasmosis secondary to chronic steroid treatment for sarcoidosis.*

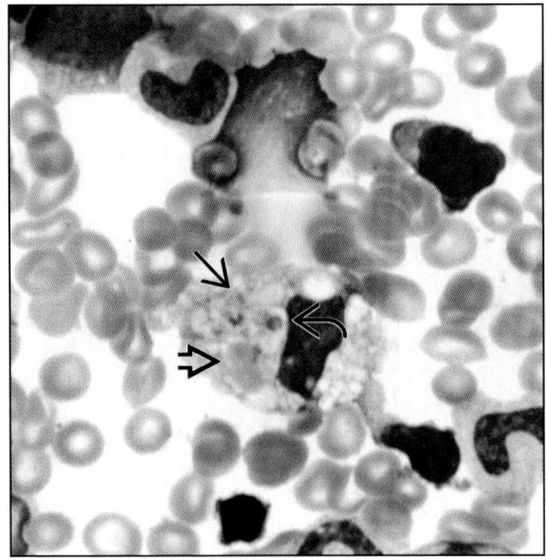

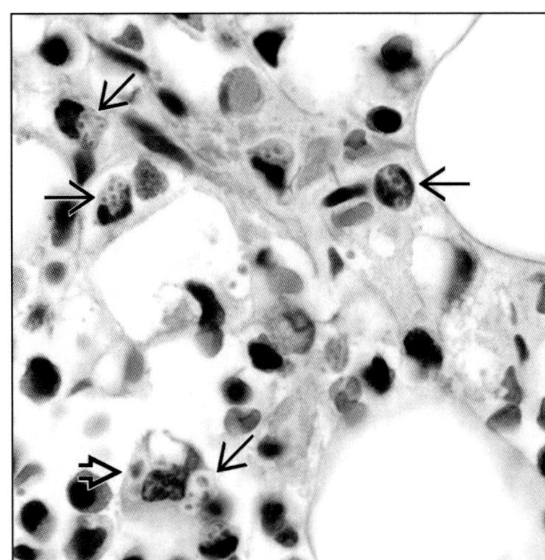

*(**Left**) A histiocyte is shown engulfing a nucleated red blood cell ➡ along with fungal organisms ➡ in this case of disseminated histoplasmosis with associated HLH. At first glance the organisms may be confused with platelets. (**Right**) Prominent HLH was observed in the bone marrow of this patient with ALK(+) anaplastic large cell lymphoma. Numerous histiocytes were seen engulfing platelets, leukocytes, and red blood cells ➡.*

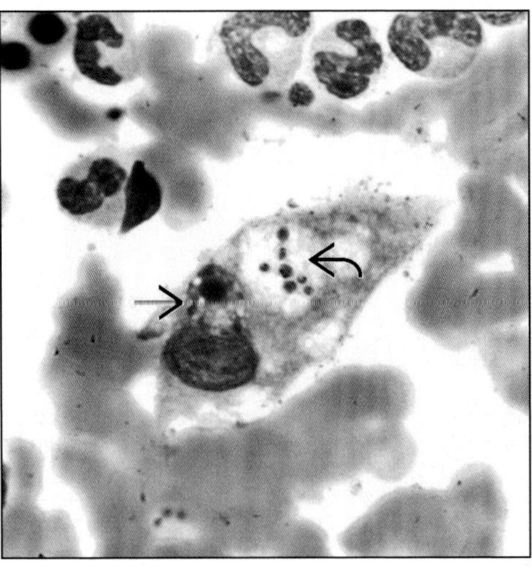

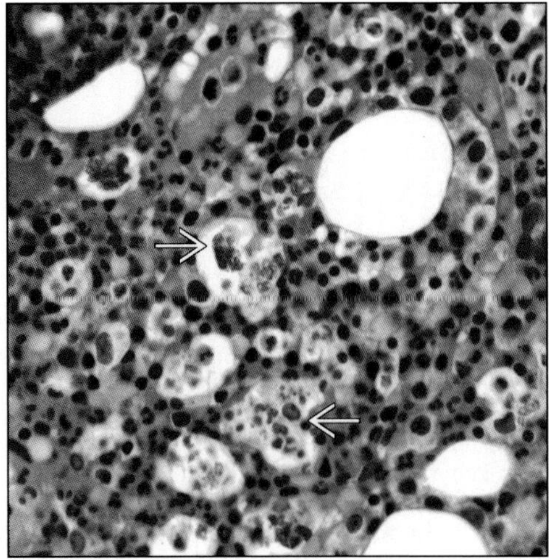

Microscopic Features

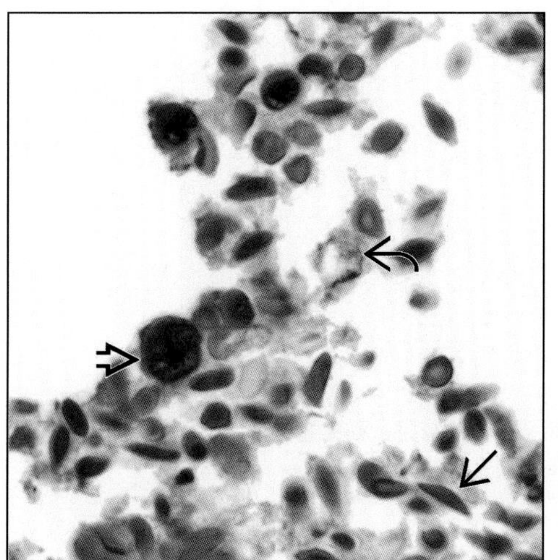

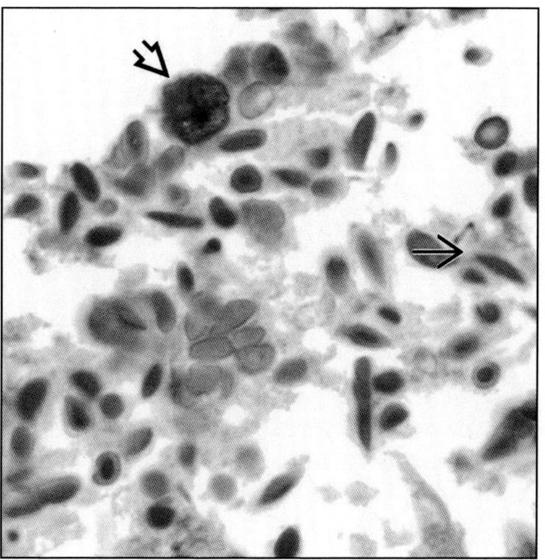

(Left) *Hemophagocytosis is shown in a patient with sickle cell disease. Note the scattered sickle cells →, hemophagocytosis →, and hemosiderin pigment →.* ***(Right)*** *Bone marrow aspirate smear is seen under oil immersion in a patient with sickle cell disease. Sickle cells are easily identified →. In addition, multiple histiocytes are seen engulfing the abnormal erythrocytes →.*

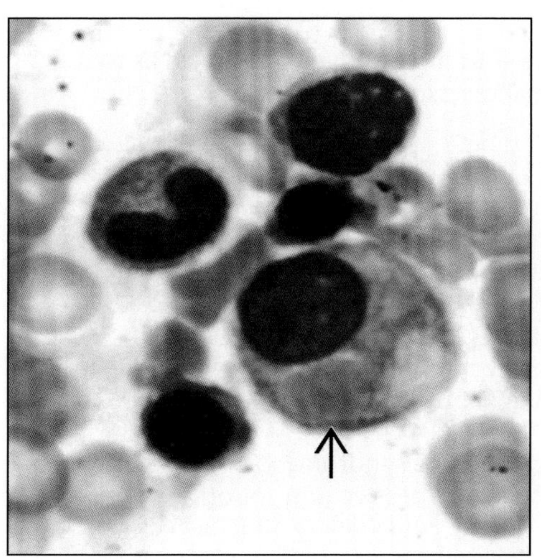

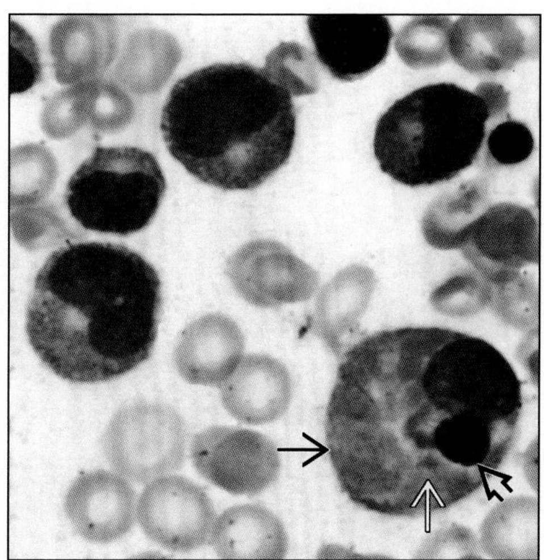

(Left) *This bone marrow aspirate smear was taken from a pediatric patient with a highly aggressive and fatal NK-cell lymphoma. The hemophagocytosis →, as depicted here, was a very striking feature in this case.* ***(Right)*** *In this bone marrow aspirate smear taken from a pediatric patient with a highly aggressive and fatal NK-cell lymphoma, the histiocyte has engulfed multiple red blood cells →, a lymphocyte →, and a small platelet →.*

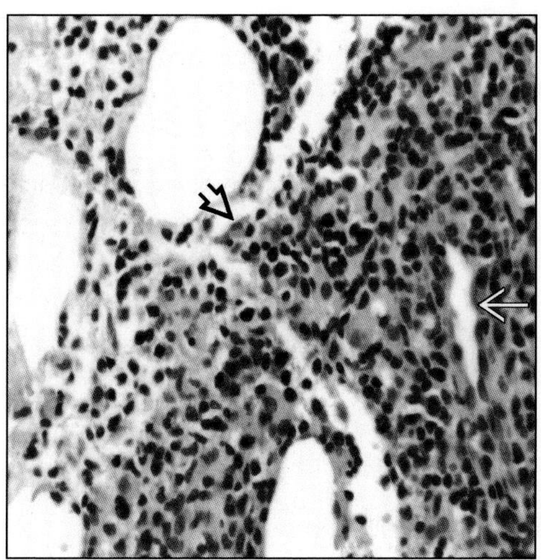

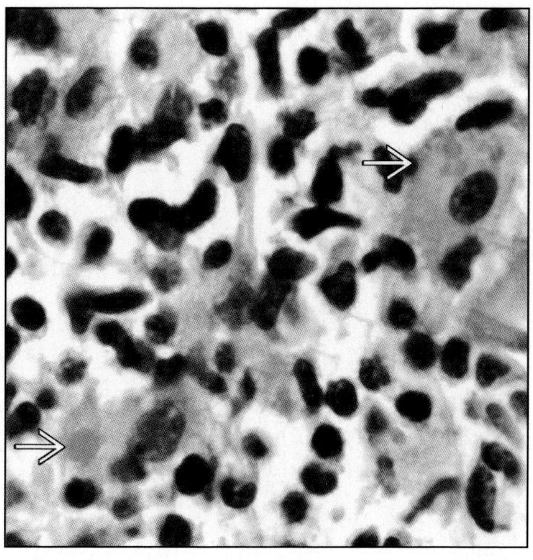

(Left) *H&E stained section of a skin punch biopsy from a pediatric patient with an aggressive & fatal NK-cell lymphoma shows malignant NK cells surrounding a vascular structure →. Focal hemophagocytosis → was present in all examined skin biopsies, a liver biopsy, and throughout the bone marrow.* ***(Right)*** *High-power view of malignancy-associated hemophagocytosis → is seen in a skin punch biopsy of a pediatric patient with NK-cell lymphoma.*

OVERVIEW OF LYMPHOPROLIFERATIVE DISORDERS ASSOCIATED WITH PID

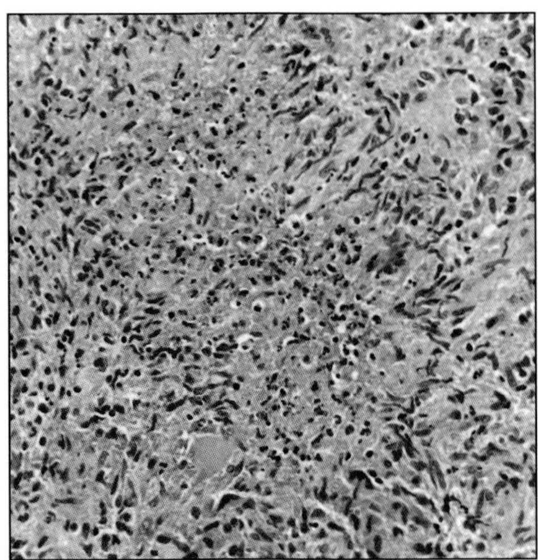

Chronic granulomatous inflammation involving lymph node in a patient with common variable immunodeficiency (CVID) is shown.

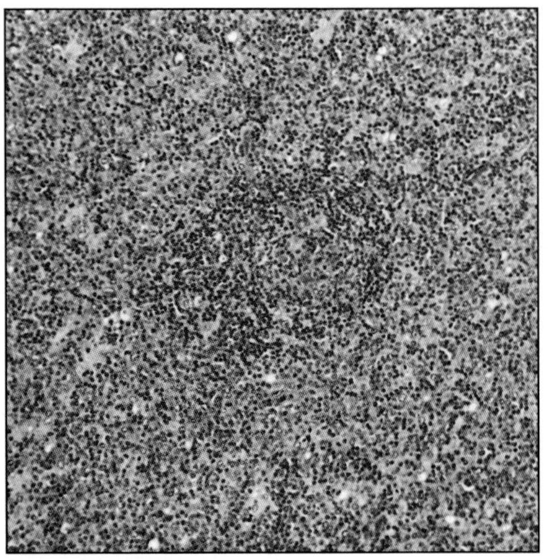

H&E shows B-cell lymphoma with polymorphous features in a patient with ataxia-telangiectasia (AT).

TERMINOLOGY

Definitions

- Lymphomas and lymphoma-like lesions arising in clinical setting of primary immunodeficiency
  - Primary immunodeficiency disorders are heterogeneous group of genetic diseases that result in immunocompromised state

Abbreviations

- Primary immunodeficiency disorders (PID)

Synonyms

- Primary immune disorders
- Congenital immunodeficiency diseases (disorders)

EPIDEMIOLOGY

Incidence

- Variable incidence of clinically evident PID in USA
  - Cumulative incidence: 1 in 10,000
  - Incidence likely higher but some diseases are not evident clinically
- Lymphoproliferative disorders (LPDs) associated with PID
  - LPDs are most common neoplasms in patients with PID
    - Up to 75% of all neoplasms in a given PID
  - Risk of developing LPD varies by type of PID, ranging 0.7-15% (accurate estimation is difficult due to low incidence)

Age Range

- PIDs are more common in pediatric age group
  - Exception: Common variable immunodeficiency disease (CVID) occurs in adults
- Median age of LPD onset: 7.1 years (per Immunodeficiency Cancer Registry)
  - Recent increase in LPDs at older ages due to better survival of PID patients

Gender

- More common in males; true for X-linked as well as for autosomal recessive disorders

ETIOLOGY/PATHOGENESIS

Etiology

- Gene mutations account for many PIDs
  - X-linked hyper-IgM syndrome (XHIGM): *CD40* or CD40 ligand (*CD40LG*)
  - Autoimmune lymphoproliferative syndrome (ALPS): *FAS* or FAS ligand (*FASLG*)
  - Ataxia-telangiectasia (AT): *ATM*
  - Nijmegen breakage syndrome (NBS): *NBS1* (nibrin)
- Complex abnormalities account for other PIDs
  - Wiskott-Aldrich syndrome exhibits defective function of T cells, B cells, neutrophils, and macrophages

Pathogenesis

- Basis for increased risk of hematologic neoplasms is poorly understood, likely multifactorial
  - Epstein-Barr virus infection drives subset of LPDs in PID settings
  - Defective DNA mismatch repair involved in AT and NBS
  - Possible underlying immune defect against cancer cells

CLINICAL IMPLICATIONS

Clinical Presentation

- Patients with PID often present with recurrent infection
  - Fever, fatigue, infectious-mononucleosis-like syndrome

- Lymphadenopathy &/or hepatosplenomegaly occur in ALPS and X-linked lymphoproliferative syndrome (XLP)
  - In XLP, fulminant infectious mononucleosis (FIM) can occur, which is marked by fever, rash, generalized lymphadenopathy, and hepatomegaly

Site

- LPDs in PID often present in extranodal sites

Treatment

- Reduced risk of LPD after allogeneic stem cell transplant in PIDs
- Limited data due to rarity of PIDs and lack of randomized trials
- Recommendation is to treat with histologic subtype-specific protocol
- Possible role for immunoregulatory therapy (e.g., interferon-α 2b)

Prognosis

- Related to both underlying PID and type of LPD
  - Most LPDs in PID patients are clinically aggressive
  - Self limited, ALPS; clinically indolent, common variable immunodeficiency (CVID)
- Newer antimicrobial therapies that allow more aggressive treatments have improved prognosis
- Fatal hemophagocytic syndrome can occur in EBV-driven infectious mononucleosis
  - Occurs in XLP and severe combined immunodeficiency (SCID)

MICROSCOPIC FINDINGS

Nonneoplastic Lesions in Lymph Nodes

- Spectrum of morphologic abnormalities
- Subtle alterations may require immunophenotyping
- Common findings
  - Lymphoid depletion
  - Atrophic follicles with progressive depletion of germinal centers
  - Depletion of small lymphocytes in paracortical region with increase in histiocytes and plasma cells
  - Similar findings observed in spleen and tonsils at autopsy
- Secondary changes
  - Chronic granulomatous inflammation secondary to infections
  - Florid reactive hyperplasia
  - Atypical hyperplasia
- Fatal infectious mononucleosis (FIM) resulting from EBV infection (XLP, SCID)
  - Extreme atypical hyperplasia
  - Polymorphous lymphoid cells with plasmacytoid and immunoblastic differentiation
  - Systemic uncontrolled proliferation of abnormal B cells
  - Frequent hemophagocytic syndrome, most readily identified on bone marrow aspirates
- Waxing and waning lymphoproliferations (CVID)
  - Variable morphology showing follicular hyperplasia and paracortical expansion with many EBV(+) cells
  - Characteristic nodular lymphoid hyperplasia in gastrointestinal tract
- Autoimmune lymphoproliferative syndrome
  - Expansion of CD4(-), CD8(-) T cells (so-called double negative cells)
  - Increased CD5(+) polyclonal B cells
  - Prominent follicular hyperplasia
- X-linked hyper-IgM syndrome
  - Extensive accumulation of IgM-producing plasma cells in extranodal sites without malignant transformation
  - Peripheral blood B-cells express only IgM and IgD

Precursor Lesions

- Broad morphologic spectrum
- Increasingly dominant clonal population, from polyclonal, to oligoclonal, to monoclonal
- Monoclonal expansions may or may not progress to major persistent lesions

Neoplastic Lesions

- Increased risk of developing leukemias, lymphomas, and nonhematopoietic tumors (lymphoma > leukemia)
- In general, morphology and immunophenotype similar to lymphomas in immunocompetent hosts
- Polymorphous cytologic features commonly seen
- Non-Hodgkin lymphoma (NHL)
  - Overall, B-cell more common than T-cell lymphomas
    - Exception: In ataxia-telangiectasia, T-cell lymphoma/leukemia is common
  - Diffuse large B-cell lymphoma (DLBCL) is most common NHL in PID patients
    - Immunophenotype similar to DLBCLs in immunocompetent patients
    - If EBV(+): Focal expression or absence of CD20 and CD79a; aberrant CD30(+)
  - Many cases are polymorphous with plasmacytoid differentiation
  - Frequently EBV(+)
  - Burkitt lymphoma is more common in XLP than in other PIDs
- Hodgkin lymphoma (HL)
  - 2nd most common LPD per Immunodeficiency Cancer Registry
    - ~ 10% of all lymphomas in PID patients
  - Classical HL most common in PID patients
    - Lymphocyte depleted and mixed cellularity types more common due to feeble immune response
    - HRS cells: CD15(+/-), CD30(+), pax-5(+, dim), CD45/LCA(-)
  - NLPHL relatively uncommon except in patients with ALPS

CLASSIFICATION

Immunodeficiencies

- Combined T- and B-cell immunodeficiencies
  - Severe combined immunodeficiency (SCID)
  - X-linked hyper-IgM syndrome
- Predominantly antibody deficiencies

OVERVIEW OF LYMPHOPROLIFERATIVE DISORDERS ASSOCIATED WITH PID

- Common variable immunodeficiency (CVID)
- Other well-defined immunodeficiency syndromes
  - Ataxia-telangiectasia (AT)
  - Nijmegen breakage syndrome (NBS)
  - Wiskott-Aldrich syndrome (WAS)
- Diseases of immune dysregulation
  - Autoimmune lymphoproliferative syndrome (ALPS)
  - X-linked lymphoproliferative disorder (XLP)
- Congenital defects of phagocyte number, function, or both
- Defects in innate immunity
- Autoinflammatory disorders
- Complement deficiencies

DIAGNOSTIC TESTS

Laboratory Tests to Diagnose PID

- Multiple tests may be required to establish diagnosis of PID; however, testing for LPD in PID is same as in immunocompetent hosts
- Complete blood count
- Immunophenotyping of T and B cells
- Serum protein electrophoresis and immunofixation
- Measurement of serum levels of vitamins, cytokines, ligands, and immunoglobulins
- In vitro functional assays
- Testing for autoantibodies
- Molecular genetic testing for gene mutations

Molecular Genetic Testing to Diagnose LPD

- Antigen receptor gene rearrangement
  - Gene clonality useful for establishing diagnosis of LPD; may not predict clinical behavior
    - Polyclonal LPD can be fatal, such as in fatal infectious mononucleosis; monoclonal LPD can be indolent
  - Monoclonal immunoglobulin heavy and light chain gene rearrangements present in overt B-cell lymphomas, limited information on T-cell clonality
- EBV DNA
  - EBV infection common in many LPDs in PID
  - Demonstration of EBV possible at molecular level using specific probes
  - EBV terminal repeat analysis may be helpful in establishing monoclonality
- Oncogenes
  - Defects related to primary immune defect: *FAS* mutation in ALPS, mutations in gene encoding *SAP/SLAM* in XLP
  - Defects occurring during course of LPDs: Inversions &/or translocations of T-cell receptor (*TCR*) genes in AT
- Chromosomal translocations
  - Limited information available
  - AT: In normal state, ~ 10% of lymphocytes have aberrations corresponding to *TCR* genes and *TCL-1*

DIFFERENTIAL DIAGNOSIS FOR NONNEOPLASTIC LESIONS

Neoplastic Hematologic Lesions in PID

- Critical to determine whether LPD is benign or malignant since benign lesions can histologically mimic lymphoma
- Immunophenotyping and molecular studies are useful for this purpose

Benign Lymphoid Tissue in Neonates

- Morphologic spectrum in normal newborns may be difficult to distinguish from PID-related changes
- Lymph nodes at birth are primarily composed of small primary B-follicles in cortex and poorly developed paracortex

Lymphoid Depletion in Longstanding Infections

- Lymphoid depletion in non-PID babies with longstanding infections can be difficult to distinguish from lymphoid depletion in PID

Angioimmunoblastic T-cell Lymphoma

- Overlapping features: Lymphoid depletion, paracortical expansion, polymorphous cell population
- Distinguishing features: AITL occurs mainly in elderly, T cells in PID do not express CD10, Bcl-6, or CXCL13

Castleman Disease, Hyaline Vascular Type

- Overlapping features: Atrophic follicles with lymphocyte depletion and hypervascularity
- Distinguishing features: Clinical history; lymph nodes are not enlarged in PID and lack features such as twinning and "onion skin" appearance

DIFFERENTIAL DIAGNOSIS FOR NEOPLASTIC LESIONS

PID-associated LPDs

- In general, LPDs in PID are histologically and immunophenotypically indistinguishable from lesions arising in immunocompetent hosts
- Differential diagnosis is same as for lesions in immunocompetent hosts
- Clinical history is critical for establishing PID setting

DIAGNOSTIC CHECKLIST

Clinically Relevant Pathologic Features

- Presentation of LPD usually early in life
- Propensity to involve extranodal sites; high frequency of EBV infection
- Broad morphologic and biologic spectrum of lymphoproliferations
- Knowledge of preexisting PID is critical

OVERVIEW OF LYMPHOPROLIFERATIVE DISORDERS ASSOCIATED WITH PID

Epidemiology and Clinical Features of PID

Category	Disease	Inheritance	Population	Frequency (%)	Clinical Features
T- and B-cell immunodeficiencies	SCID	AR, X	1 in 100,000 live births	1-5	Severe recurrent infections
	XHIGM	X	1 in 20,000,000 live male births	1-2	Pancytopenia, hepatobiliary tract disease, *Pneumocystis jiroveci* infections, diarrhea
Antibody deficiencies	CVID	AD, S	1 in 10-50,000 live births	21-31	Variable phenotype, recurrent bacterial infections
	IgA deficiency	AD, S	1 in 700 individuals of European origin	> 50 (most common)	Prone to bacterial infections
Immune dysregulation	XLP	X	400 documented cases	< 1	EBV infections trigger clinical and immunologic abnormalities
	ALPS	AD, AR	Unknown	< 1	Present in infancy with autoimmune cytopenias, autoimmune diseases
Other syndromes	WAS	X	1 in 250,000 live male births	1-3	Thrombocytopenia with small platelets, eczema
	AT	AR	1 in 40-100,000 live births	2-8	Cerebellar degeneration with progressive ataxia, oculocutaneous telangiectasia
	NBS	AR	1 in 100,000 live births	1-2	Microcephaly, café au lait spots, hypersensitivity to ionizing radiation

SCID = severe combined immunodeficiency; XHIGM = X-linked hyper-IgM syndrome; CVID = common variable immunodeficiency; XLP = X-linked lymphoproliferative syndrome; ALPS = autoimmune lymphoproliferative syndrome; WAS = Wiskott-Aldrich syndrome; AT = ataxia-telangiectasia; NBS = Nijmegen breakage syndrome; AD = autosomal dominant; AR = autosomal recessive; X = X-linked; S = sporadic.

Malignancies in PID*

Category	Disease	Malignancy Rate (%)	Median Age (Years)	Gender (M to F)	Hematologic	Nonhematologic
T- and B-cell immunodeficiencies	SCID	1.5	1.6	3.3 to 1	EBV-associated, FIM, NHL, HL, leukemias	Renal and pulmonary leiomyomata
	XHIGM	7.8	7.2		EBV-associated (DLBCL, HL), LGL leukemia	NA
Antibody deficiencies	CVID	2.5 (onset < 16 years), 8.5 (onset > 16 years)	23	1.3 to 1	NHL (50%); EBV-associated (DLBCL, HL), SLL, MALT lymphoma, LPL, PTCL (2-7%)	Epithelial tumors (39%; stomach, breast, bladder, cervix, vulva)
	IgA deficiency	Rare	NA	NA	HL, leukemia or lymphoma (25%)	NA
Immune dysregulation	XLP	30	NA	NA	EBV associated (FIM, DLBCL, Burkitt), aplastic anemia	NA
	ALPS	10-20	< 1	NA	Increased risk of NHL (50x) and HL (10x); NLPHL, classical HL, DLBCL, Burkitt, PTCL (3-10%)	NA
Other syndromes	WAS	13	6.2	M only	EBV associated (DLBCL, HL)	Cerebellar astrocytoma, Kaposi sarcoma, muscle tumors
	AT	33	8.5	1.7 to 1	Nonleukemic clonal T-cell proliferations, DLBCL, Burkitt, T-PLL (young adults), T-ALL/LBL (age: 1-5 years), HL (10-30%)	Epithelial tumors
	NBS	Rare	NA	NA	DLBCL, PTCL, T-ALL/LBL, HL (28-36%)	Brain tumors

**Data based on Immunodeficiency Cancer Registry; FIM = fatal infectious mononucleosis; NHL = non-Hodgkin lymphoma; HL = Hodgkin lymphoma; NA = information not available; LGL = large granular lymphocyte; SLL = small lymphocytic lymphoma; MALT = mucosa-associated lymphoid tissue; LPL = lymphoplasmacytic lymphoma; PTCL = peripheral T-cell lymphoma; NLPHL = nodular lymphocyte predominant HL; ALL/LBL = acute lymphoblastic leukemia/lymphoblastic lymphoma.*

OVERVIEW OF LYMPHOPROLIFERATIVE DISORDERS ASSOCIATED WITH PID

Microscopic and Immunohistochemical Features

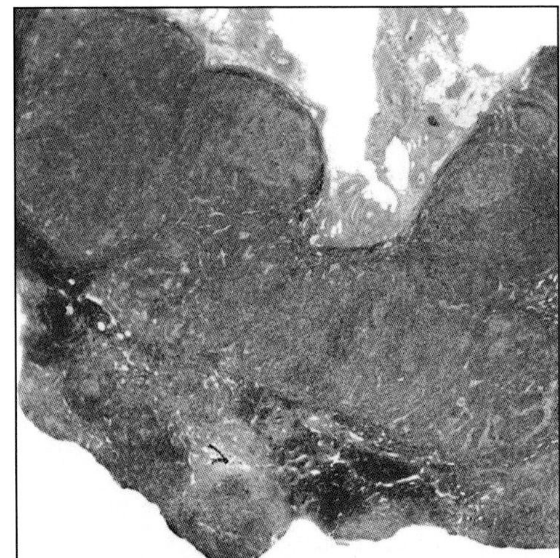

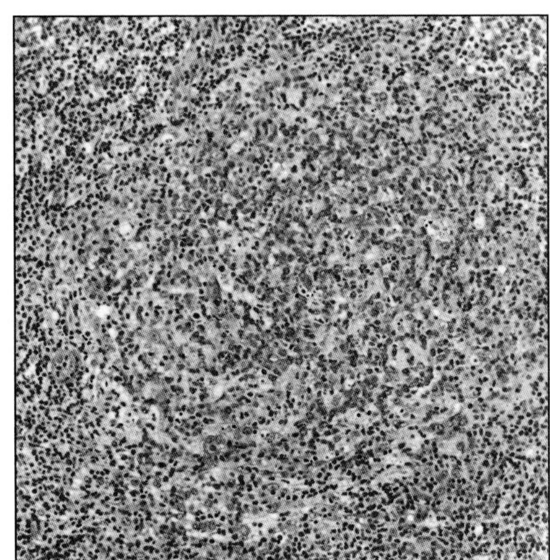

(Left) *Lymph node biopsy specimen shows atypical paracortical hyperplasia in a CVID patient. The overall nodal architecture is distorted but not effaced. The paracortical regions are expanded, vascular proliferation is present, and sinuses are patent.* ***(Right)*** *Lymph node shows atypical paracortical hyperplasia in a CVID patient. Higher magnification of paracortical region shows a heterogeneous cell population. There was no evidence of T- or B-cell clonality by PCR analysis.*

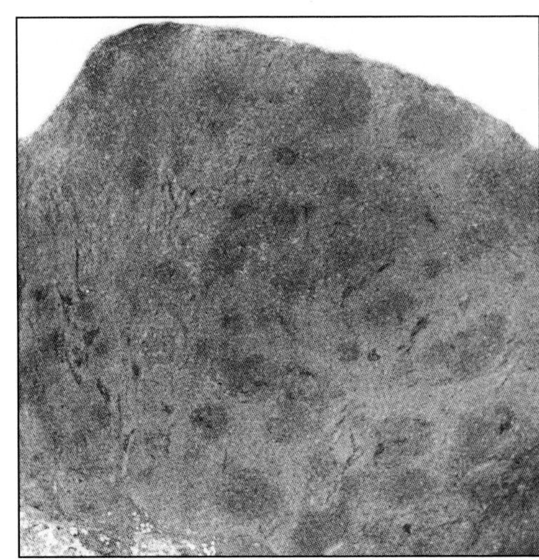

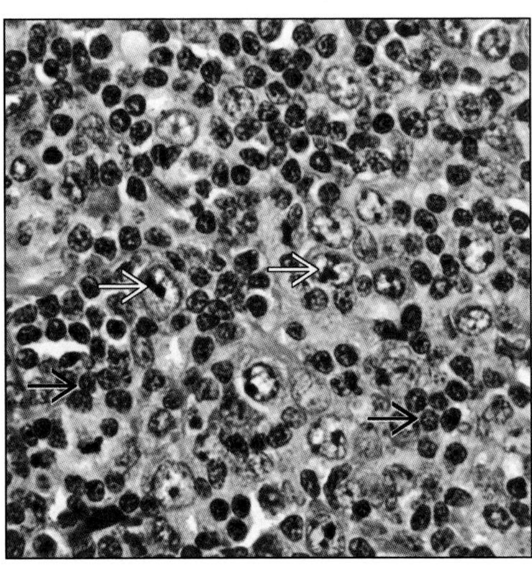

(Left) *Lymph node involved by polymorphous B-cell lymphoproliferative disorder (LPD) in a patient with AT is shown. Note the effacement of the interfollicular region. Monoclonal immunoglobulin heavy chain gene rearrangement was detected by PCR.* ***(Right)*** *H&E shows lymph node involved by polymorphous B-cell LPD in an AT patient. The interfollicular region shows a polymorphic lymphoid infiltrate of predominantly medium-sized lymphocytes ⇨ admixed with large transformed cells ➡.*

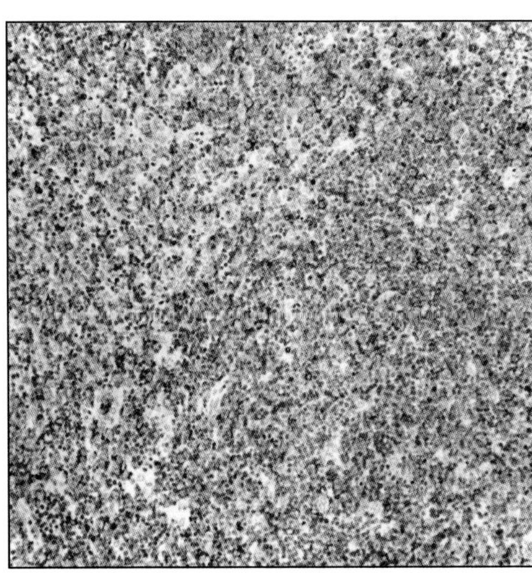

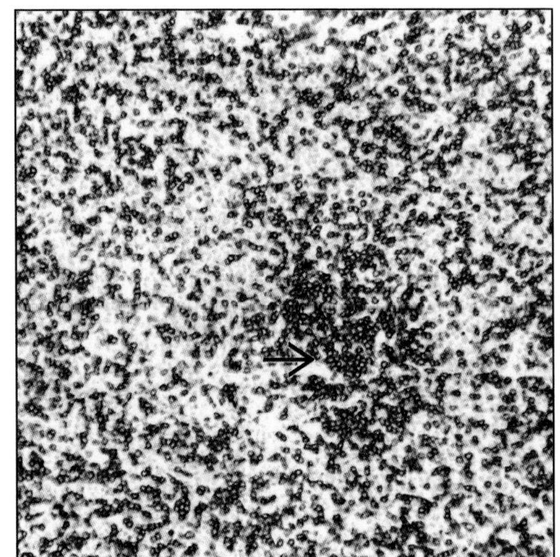

(Left) *Lymph node involved by polymorphous B-cell LPD in an AT patient is shown. Most lymphocytes are CD20(+) and show primarily interfollicular staining pattern. By flow cytometry, B cells were CD19(+), CD20(+), and dim monotypic immunoglobulin kappa(+).* ***(Right)*** *Lymph node involved by polymorphous B-cell LPD in an AT patient is shown. The atypical cells are CD3(-). There is a marked increase of CD3(+) T-lymphocytes in a dystrophic follicle ⇨.*

Microscopic and Immunohistochemical Features

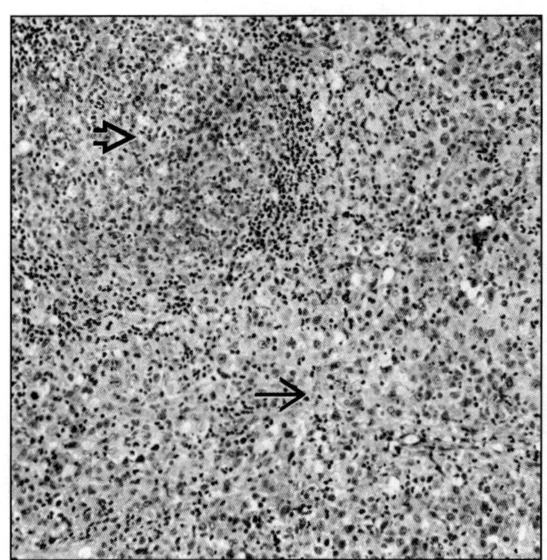

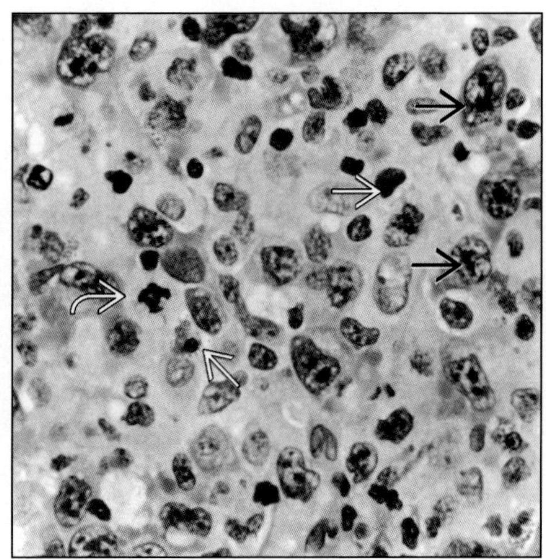

(Left) *Lymph node involved by diffuse large B-cell lymphoma (DLBCL) with an interfollicular pattern ➔ is shown in a patient with Wiskott-Aldrich syndrome (WAS). A reactive follicle is also present ➔.* ***(Right)*** *H&E shows lymph node involved by DLBCL in a WAS patient. The neoplastic cells ➔ are predominantly intermediate to large sized with irregular nuclear contours, prominent nucleoli, and abundant cytoplasm. There are scattered interspersed eosinophils ➔, and a mitotic figure ➔ is present.*

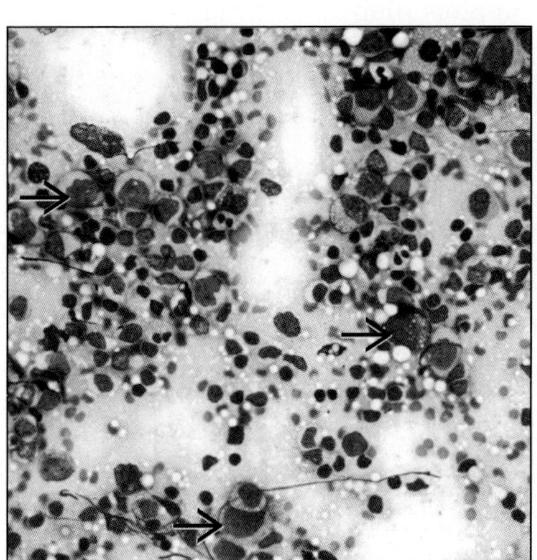

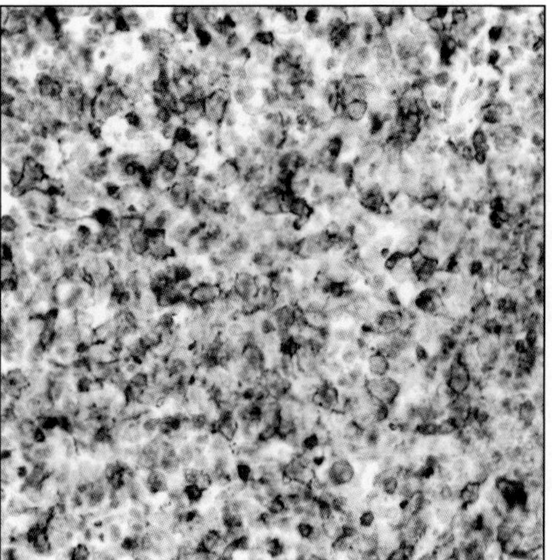

(Left) *Touch imprint of lymph node involved by DLBCL in a WAS patient is shown. Note the many large cells ➔. A mixed inflammatory cell infiltrate is also present in the background.* ***(Right)*** *Lymph node involved by DLBCL in a WAS patient is shown. Anti-CD20 antibody highlights large atypical B cells. Flow cytometric immunophenotyping showed that the B cells were CD19(+), CD20(+), and monotypic immunoglobulin κ light chain(+).*

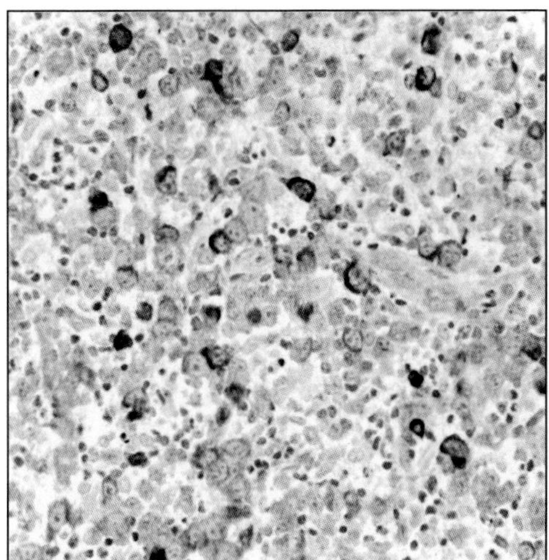

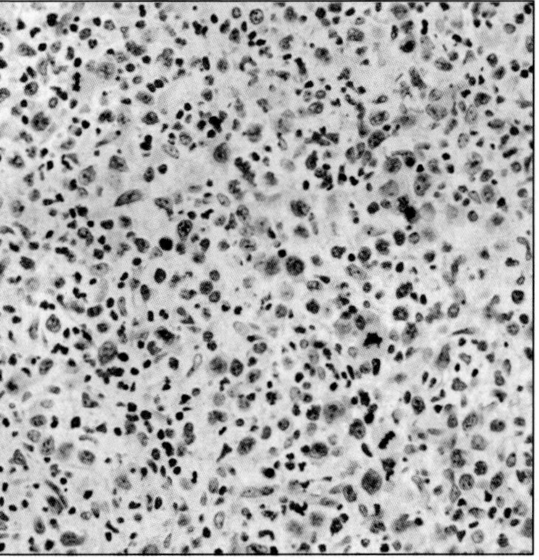

(Left) *Lymph node involved by DLBCL in a WAS patient is shown. The large neoplastic cells are immunoglobulin κ light chain(+), shown by immunohistochemistry.* ***(Right)*** *Lymph node involved by DLBCL in a WAS patient is shown. The large neoplastic cells are immunoglobulin λ light chain(-) by immunohistochemistry.*

AUTOIMMUNE LYMPHOPROLIFERATIVE SYNDROME

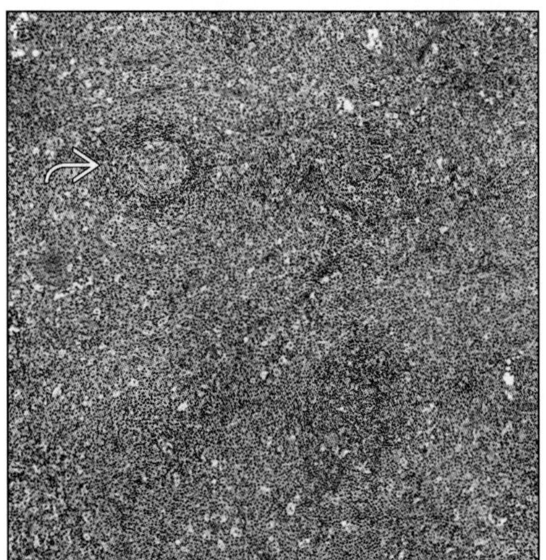

The paracortex of the lymph node in this case of autoimmune lymphoproliferative syndrome (ALPS) is markedly expanded. Small lymphoid follicles are also present ➡.

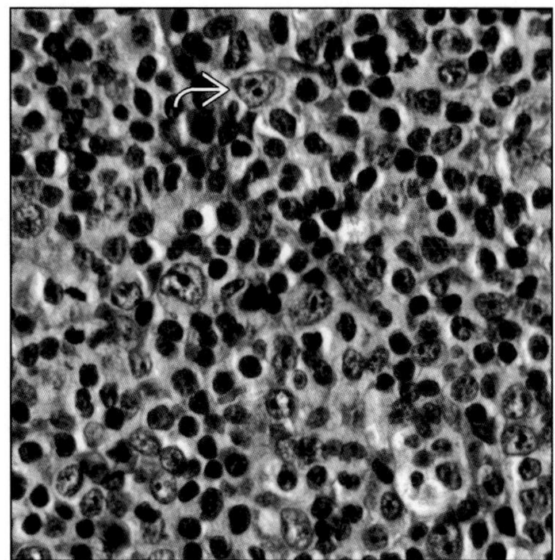

ALPS involving a lymph node shows the paracortex populated by small lymphocytes and many large immunoblasts with prominent nucleoli ➡.

TERMINOLOGY

Abbreviations

- Autoimmune lymphoproliferative syndrome (ALPS)

Definitions

- Disease of disrupted lymphocyte homeostasis as result of defective Fas-mediated apoptosis

ETIOLOGY/PATHOGENESIS

Genetic Mutations in FAS Pathway

- FAS pathway mutations cause ALPS
- *FAS* mutations are usually heterozygous
- Multiple types have been described
- **Type I**: Accounts for approximately 65% of all ALPS cases
  - 3 type I subtypes
    - Ia: Germline mutations in *FAS* (*TNFRSF6, CD95, APO1*) gene
    - Ib: Germline mutations in FAS ligand (*FASLG*) gene
    - Is: Somatic mutations in *FAS* gene
- **Type II**: Germline mutations in gene encoding caspase 10
- **Type III**: No identifiable genetic mutations in FAS pathway
  - Accounts for approximately 20-30% of all ALPS cases
- **Type IV**: Very rare
  - Gain-of-function mutation in *NRAS*
  - Patients have ALPS phenotype but normal Fas-mediated apoptosis
- ALPS is multistep process requiring more than a single genetic hit for clinical expression
- In most cases, mutations are inherited in autosomal dominant fashion
  - Therefore, penetrance is 100% at cellular level
  - Penetrance for clinical phenotype of ALPS is variable
    - Significant proportion of family members can have mutation without phenotype of ALPS
    - Additional factors must contribute to expression of disease

CASPASE 8 Mutations

- Once considered part of ALPS
- Present with lymphadenopathy and defective Fas-mediated apoptosis
- Profound apoptotic defects in B, T, and NK cells
- Patients often have mucocutaneous herpes virus infections
- Therefore, *CASP8* mutations are now considered to represent a distinct disease

CLINICAL ISSUES

Presentation

- Chronic nonmalignant lymphoproliferation, often appearing in 1st year of life
  - Chronic &/or recurrent lymphadenopathy in ~ 80% of patients
  - Splenomegaly ± hypersplenism in ~ 85% of patients
  - Hepatomegaly in ~ 45% of patients
  - Lymphocytic interstitial pneumonia
- Autoimmune diseases in ~ 70% of patients
  - Cytopenias are most frequent
    - Autoimmune hemolytic anemia
    - Immune thrombocytopenia
    - Autoimmune neutropenia
    - > 1 lineage is often affected
  - Evans syndrome
    - Originally described in 1951
    - Autoimmune destruction of erythrocytes and platelets
    - Subset of these patients has ALPS
  - Other less common autoimmune phenomena in ALPS include
    - Skin rash: Often of urticarial nature

AUTOIMMUNE LYMPHOPROLIFERATIVE SYNDROME

Key Facts

Etiology/Pathogenesis

- Disease of disrupted lymphocyte homeostasis as result of defective Fas-mediated apoptosis
- Many mutations have been identified in ALPS
- Type I: Accounts for approximately 65% of all ALPS cases; 3 subtypes
  - Ia: Germline mutations in *FAS* gene
  - Ib: Germline mutations in *FASLG* gene
  - Is: Somatic mutations in *FAS* gene
- Type II: Germline mutations in gene encoding caspase 10
- Type III: Accounts for approximately 20-30% of all ALPS cases
  - No identifiable genetic mutations in *FAS* pathway
- Type IV: Very rare; gain-of-function mutation in *NRAS*

Clinical Issues

- Chronic nonmalignant lymphoproliferation
  - Lymph nodes, spleen, liver
- Autoimmune disease
- Increased risk for lymphoma

Microscopic Pathology

- Marked paracortical expansion with increased DNT cells

Ancillary Tests

- Flow cytometry
  - Increased DNT cells: TCR-α/β(+), CD3(+), CD4(-), CD8(-)
- Apoptosis assay: Defective FAS-induced apoptosis in ALPS types Ia and Ib

    - Autoimmune hepatitis
    - Autoimmune glomerulonephritis
    - Autoimmune thyroiditis
    - Uveitis and Guillain-Barré syndrome
    - Vasculitis and panniculitis
    - Autoimmune colitis
    - Autoimmune cerebellar syndrome
    - Patients followed into adulthood have increased risk of pulmonary fibrosis
- ALPS patients have increased risk of malignancies of various types
  - Increased risk of Hodgkin lymphoma and non-Hodgkin lymphoma
    - 51x increased risk of Hodgkin lymphoma
    - 14x increased risk of non-Hodgkin lymphoma
    - Usually not related to Epstein-Barr virus infection
  - Increased risk of carcinomas
    - Thyroid, breast, liver, tongue, skin
  - Increased risk of leukemias
  - Some ALPS patients present with multiple neoplasms (thyroid/breast adenomas, gliomas)
- Presentation related to type of genetic mutation
  - Homozygous or compound heterozygous *FAS* mutations lead to
    - Severe lymphoproliferation before, at, or shortly after birth
    - Patients typically succumb to lymphoproliferation &/or autoimmunity at early age
  - Mutations in any domain of Fas lead to same clinical phenotype of ALPS
    - Lymphoma is most often associated with mutations affecting intracellular domains of Fas

Laboratory Tests

- Peripheral blood lymphocytosis
- Serum
  - Elevated concentrations of IgG, IgA, and IgE; normal or decreased concentration of IgM
  - Increased levels of interleukin (IL)-10
  - Increased levels of vitamin B12
- Autoimmune antibodies
  - Autoantibodies to red cells, platelets, and neutrophils are often found
  - Anti-smooth muscle and anti-phospholipid antibodies can be positive
  - Anti-nuclear antibodies and rheumatoid factor can be positive
- Flow cytometric immunophenotyping of peripheral blood shows increased double negative T cells
  - Double negative T cells (DNT) = TCR-α/β(+), CD3(+), CD4(-), CD8(-)
    - Normal range: DNT cells have been expressed as percentage of total lymphocytes; total T cells and TCR-α/β(+) T cells in various studies
    - Normal range may differ according to patient age and flow cytometry gating strategy
    - DNT cells are increased if > 1% of total T cells (peripheral blood)
    - Markedly increased (3-60%) DNTs in peripheral blood is very specific for ALPS
    - Present in all subtypes of ALPS
    - Found in peripheral blood, lymph nodes, spleen, and other tissues
    - Role of DNT cells in ALPS, and whether these cells are pathogenic or merely a marker of disease, remains to be determined
  - Other flow cytometry findings
    - Increased TCR-γ/δ(+) DNT cells
    - Increased CD8(+), CD57(+) T cells
    - Increased CD5(+) B cells
    - Increased HLA-DR(+) T cells
    - Decreased CD27(+) B cells
    - Decreased CD4(+), CD25(+) regulatory T cells
  - DNT can be increased in other autoimmune diseases
    - Usually low-level increase of DNT in these diseases
    - Systemic lupus erythematosus
    - Immune thrombocytopenic purpura
  - *FAS* mutations in 100% of DNT population in somatic ALPS patients suggest that these cells contribute to disease pathogenesis
- In vitro Fas-mediated apoptosis assays are helpful for diagnosis of ALPS

AUTOIMMUNE LYMPHOPROLIFERATIVE SYNDROME

- Isolate peripheral blood mononuclear cells from ALPS patient
- Activate T cells with mitogen and expand with IL-2 in culture for 28 days
- Expose T cells to anti-Fas IgM antibody
  - Normal T cells: Rapid cell death and apoptosis
  - ALPS T cells: No or impaired cell death
- Type of ALPS mutation yields different results for in vitro Fas-mediated apoptosis
  - Type I: Often exhibit defective FAS-induced apoptosis
  - Types II and III: No defective FAS-induced apoptosis
- Molecular genetic assays
  - *FAS*
    - *FAS* germline mutations identified throughout entire coding region and exons/introns of *FAS*
    - Sequencing of entire coding region and intron/exon boundaries of *FAS* gene detects ~ 90% of mutations
    - *FAS* somatic mutation detection often performed on sorted DNT cells
  - *FASLG*
    - Sequence analysis of entire coding region of *FASLG* gene is available clinically
  - *CASP10*
    - Sequence analysis of entire coding region of *CASP10* gene is available clinically

Natural History

- Nonmalignant lymphoproliferative manifestations in ALPS often regress or improve over time
- Autoimmunity shows no permanent remission with advancing age
- Risk for development of lymphoma appears to be lifelong

Treatment

- Some patients with ALPS require no treatment
- Hemolytic anemia and thrombocytopenia
  - Prednisone
  - Immunosuppressant
    - Mycophenolate mofetil (CellCept)
    - Sirolimus (rapamycin)
  - Only a few patients respond to intravenous immunoglobulin
  - Rituximab: Anti-CD20 monoclonal chimeric antibody
    - Percentage of ALPS patients are predisposed to develop common variable immunodeficiency disease (CVID) upon rituximab treatment
    - Reserved for patients who fail all other therapies
  - Splenectomy to control autoimmune cytopenias is discouraged
    - ALPS patients have increased risk of developing postsplenectomy sepsis despite vaccination and antibiotic prophylaxis
    - No long-term effect to control cytopenia(s)
- Bone marrow (hematopoietic stem cell) transplantation carries risks
  - Reduced-intensity transplant can reduce transplant-associated risks

Prognosis

- Refer to natural history

Recently Proposed Diagnostic Criteria for ALPS

- Major
  - Chronic nonmalignant lymphoproliferation
    - > 6 months
    - Splenomegaly &/or lymphadenopathy of at least 2 nodal groups
  - Marked elevation of peripheral blood DNTs of at least 5%
  - Defective in vitro Fas-mediated apoptosis
  - Identifiable genetic mutation, germline or somatic
    - *FAS, FASL, CASP10, NRAS*
- Minor
  - Autoimmune cytopenias
    - Thrombocytopenia, neutropenia, &/or hemolytic anemia
    - Proven to be immune-mediated by autoantibody detection or response to immunosuppressive agent
  - Moderate elevation in DNTs
  - Elevated serum IgG
  - Elevated serum IL-10
  - Elevated serum vitamin B12
  - Elevated plasma Fas ligand level
- Diagnosis established if
  - 3 major criteria present or
  - 2 major + 2 minor criteria present

IMAGE FINDINGS

Radiographic Findings

- Imaging studies detect lymphadenopathy or hepatosplenomegaly
- Lymphoproliferations in ALPS are FDG PET avid
- Cannot distinguish benign from malignant; therefore, biopsy needed

MICROSCOPIC PATHOLOGY

Lymph Nodes

- Marked expansion of paracortical (T-cell) zones
  - Lymphocytes show various stages of immunoblastic transformation
    - Small, intermediate, and large lymphocytes; often with clear cytoplasm
    - Increased immunoblasts
    - Mitotic figures increased
  - Small plasma cells without atypia are common
  - Eosinophils or neutrophils are typically absent
  - Reduced or absent tingible body macrophages
  - Some cases may show prominent postcapillary venules
- Germinal centers show spectrum of reactive changes ranging from
  - Florid follicular hyperplasia
    - Tingible body macrophages can be prominent
  - Progressive transformation of germinal centers (PTGC)

- Atrophic follicles with regressive changes (Castleman-like)
- Changes resembling Rosai-Dorfman disease can occur

Spleen

- Expanded white pulp
  - Reactive follicular hyperplasia
  - Reactive marginal zone hyperplasia
- Expanded red pulp
  - Increased DNT cells
  - Immunoblasts
  - Polytypic plasma cells

Bone Marrow

- ± interstitial lymphoid aggregates
  - Large lymphoid cells

Liver

- Portal tract triaditis
- DNT cells can be increased

ANCILLARY TESTS

Immunohistochemistry

- Lymph node or other tissue site
  - Increased DNT cells
    - TCR-α/β(+), CD3(+), CD4(-), CD8(-)
    - CD45RO(-), CD45RA(+), CD25(-)
  - Large subset of T cells are CD57(+), TIA(+), and perforin (+)
  - Small subset of T cells are CD4(+)
  - Small subset of T cells are CD8(+)
  - CD16(-), CD56(-) assessed in frozen tissue
- Follicles express polytypic Ig light chains
  - B-cell antigens (+), Bcl-6(+), Bcl-2(-)
- Plasma cells express polytypic Ig light chains
- Tests for Epstein-Barr virus (EBV) are usually negative
  - EBV-LMP1(-)
  - EBER(-) by in situ hybridization

Flow Cytometry

- Can be performed on cell suspension of lymph node or other tissue site
  - Increased DNT cells

Molecular Genetics

- No evidence of monoclonal *TCR* gene rearrangements
- No evidence of monoclonal *Ig* gene rearrangements
- No distinctive chromosomal translocations
- *FAS* gene mutations

DIFFERENTIAL DIAGNOSIS

Common Variable Immunodeficiency Disease (CVID)

- Specific genetic mutations are unknown, but CVID is likely to be heterogeneous
- Cases with low/absent B cells and low serum concentrations of immunoglobulin (Ig) are usually not confused with ALPS
  - ALPS patients often have normal or increased number of B cells
- Cases with presence of B cells can cause difficulty in differential diagnosis
  - Lymph node
    - Reactive follicular hyperplasia
    - Paracortical expansion without increased DNT cells
    - Often many EBV(+) cells in paracortical areas
    - Frequently associated with granulomatous inflammation of infectious causes
    - Some cases can show atypical lymphoid hyperplasia with markedly expanded B- and T-cell populations
  - Gastrointestinal tract
    - Nodular lymphoid hyperplasia, some with monoclonal Ig rearrangement
  - Nodular lymphoid hyperplasia and granulomas can be seen in many organs
    - Lung, spleen, skin, liver, bone marrow, endocrine organs, brain, etc.

X-linked Lymphoproliferative Syndrome (XLP)

- Mutations in *SH2D1A* gene
- Patients do not manifest significant immune defects until exposure to EBV
- 75% of patients develop fulminant infectious mononucleosis
  - Lymph node shows changes of fulminant infectious mononucleosis
    - Increased immunoblasts and plasma cells
    - Significant necrosis
  - Often associated with hemophagocytic lymphohistiocytosis
  - Most patients succumb to hepatic necrosis &/or bone marrow failure
  - Survivors are at risk for subsequent hypogammaglobulinemia, lymphoma, hemophagocytic syndrome, and aplastic anemia
- Laboratory findings
  - Serologic tests for EBV IgM antibodies (+)
  - Quantitative EBV-specific polymerase chain reaction (+)

Wiskott-Aldrich Syndrome (WAS)

- X-linked; *WASP* mutations
  - WASP is key regulator of signaling and cytoskeletal reorganization in hematopoietic cells
- Clinical presentation
  - Thrombocytopenia
  - Immunodeficiency, eczema
  - Autoimmune manifestations
    - Autoimmune hemolytic anemia, cutaneous vasculitis, arthritis, and nephropathy
  - High susceptibility to developing tumors
- Histologic features of lymph node
  - In early phase of disease, often shows follicular hyperplasia
  - Later stage of disease often shows progressive depletion of germinal centers
  - Paracortical lymphocyte depletion with the following
    - Increased immunoblasts (transformed cells)

- Increased eosinophils and atypical plasma cells
- Extramedullary hematopoiesis

Evans Syndrome

- Originally described as patient with 2 autoimmune cytopenias
  - Platelets and erythrocytes
- Now clear that some patients with this syndrome have ALPS
- All patients with Evans syndrome should be tested for defects in Fas-mediated apoptosis

Autoimmune Diseases

- Low-level increases in DNTs in blood occur in autoimmune diseases
  - Can lead to misdiagnosis as ALPS
- Full autoimmune work-up will show evidence that suggests specific autoimmune disease
- No defects in Fas-mediated apoptosis

Peripheral T-cell Lymphoma (PTCL)

- In most cases, lymph node is completely replaced by PTCL
- Neoplastic cells in PTCL are often associated with eosinophils
- Immunophenotype: PTCL cells are commonly CD4(+), CD8(-) or CD4(-), CD8(+)
- EBV(+) in some types of PTCL
- Monoclonal *TCR* gene rearrangements

DIAGNOSTIC CHECKLIST

Clinically Relevant Pathologic Features

- Lymphadenopathy and hepatosplenomegaly
- Autoimmune diseases
  - Cytopenias are most common
  - Various organs can be involved
- Defective apoptosis leading to expansion of antigen-specific lymphocyte populations
  - Defects are related to gene mutations (mainly of FAS pathway)
- Most mutations are congenital, with germline mutations in *FAS*, *FASL*, and *CASP10*
  - Somatic mutations of *FAS* also occur
  - In some patients, known mutations have not been found

Pathologic Interpretation Pearls

- Lymph nodes show marked paracortical expansion
  - Lymphocytes show various stages of immunoblastic transformation
    - Mitotic figures can be numerous
  - Varying degrees of follicular hyperplasia or regressive changes
  - Immunophenotyping shows increased DNT cells in paracortex
  - Changes resembling Rosai-Dorfman disease can occur
  - Increased risk of Hodgkin and non-Hodgkin lymphoma
- Immunophenotyping of peripheral blood is helpful
  - Increased DNT cells (> 1%)
    - DNT cells = TCR-α/β(+), CD3(+), CD4(-), CD8(-), CD45RA(+); CD45RO(-)
  - Increased TCR-γ/δ(+) DNT cells
  - Increased CD8(+) and CD57(+) T cells
  - Increased CD5(+) B cells and HLA-DR(+) T cells
  - Decreased CD27(+) B cells
  - Decreased CD4(+), CD25(+) regulatory T cells

SELECTED REFERENCES

1. Dowdell KC et al: Somatic FAS mutations are common in patients with genetically undefined autoimmune lymphoproliferative syndrome. Blood. 115(25):5164-9, 2010
2. Seif AE et al: Identifying autoimmune lymphoproliferative syndrome in children with Evans syndrome: a multi-institutional study. Blood. 115(11):2142-5, 2010
3. Teachey DT et al: Advances in the management and understanding of autoimmune lymphoproliferative syndrome (ALPS). Br J Haematol. 148(2):205-16, 2010
4. Bosticardo M et al: Recent advances in understanding the pathophysiology of Wiskott-Aldrich syndrome. Blood. 113(25):6288-95, 2009
5. Bristeau-Leprince A et al: Human TCR alpha/beta+ CD4-CD8- double-negative T cells in patients with autoimmune lymphoproliferative syndrome express restricted Vbeta TCR diversity and are clonally related to CD8+ T cells. J Immunol. 181(1):440-8, 2008
6. Seif A et al: Testing patients with Evans syndrome for the autoimmune lymphoproliferative syndrome (ALPS): results of a large multi-institutional clinical trial (ASPHO supplement). Pediatric Blood & Cancer. 50: S22-S23, 2008
7. Maric I et al: Histologic features of sinus histiocytosis with massive lymphadenopathy in patients with autoimmune lymphoproliferative syndrome. Am J Surg Pathol. 29(7):903-11, 2005
8. Straus SE et al: The development of lymphomas in families with autoimmune lymphoproliferative syndrome with germline Fas mutations and defective lymphocyte apoptosis. Blood. 98(1):194-200, 2001
9. Jackson CE et al: Autoimmune lymphoproliferative syndrome with defective Fas: genotype influences penetrance. Am J Hum Genet. 64(4):1002-14, 1999
10. Jackson CE et al: Autoimmune lymphoproliferative syndrome, a disorder of apoptosis. Curr Opin Pediatr. 11(6):521-7, 1999
11. Lim MS et al: Pathological findings in human autoimmune lymphoproliferative syndrome. Am J Pathol. 153(5):1541-50, 1998
12. Elenitoba-Johnson KS et al: Lymphoproliferative disorders associated with congenital immunodeficiencies. Semin Diagn Pathol. 14(1):35-47, 1997
13. Sander CA et al: Lymphoproliferative lesions in patients with common variable immunodeficiency syndrome. Am J Surg Pathol. 16(12):1170-82, 1992
14. Snover DC et al: Wiskott-Aldrich syndrome: histopathologic findings in the lymph nodes and spleens of 15 patients. Hum Pathol. 12(9):821-31, 1981

Microscopic Features

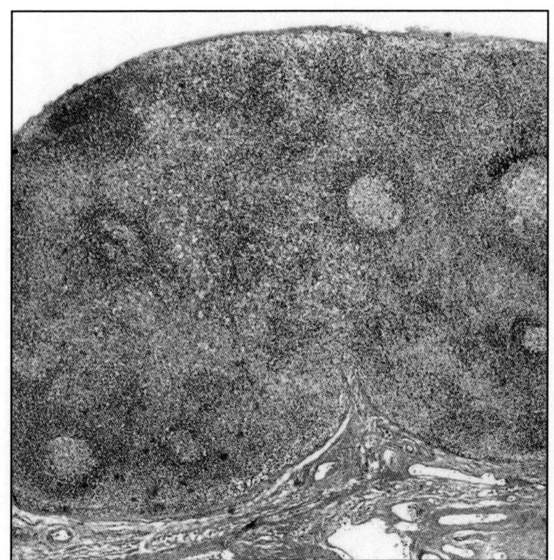

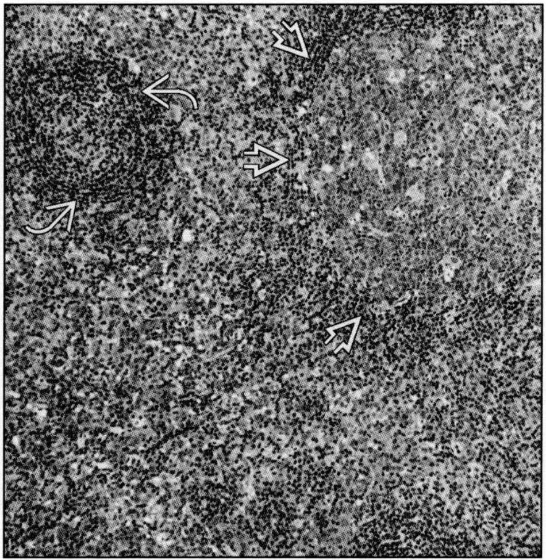

(Left) *This lymph node involved by ALPS is relatively small, and the overall architecture is maintained. The paracortical regions are expanded, and follicular hyperplasia is also present.* ***(Right)*** *This image shows a hyperplastic follicle and an adjacent small follicle with regressive changes in a lymph node involved by ALPS. The follicles in ALPS lymph nodes often exhibit a spectrum of changes, ranging from hyperplastic to regressive (Castleman-like).*

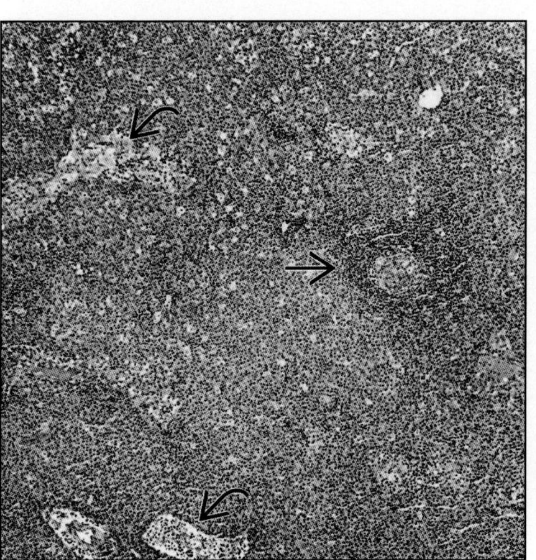

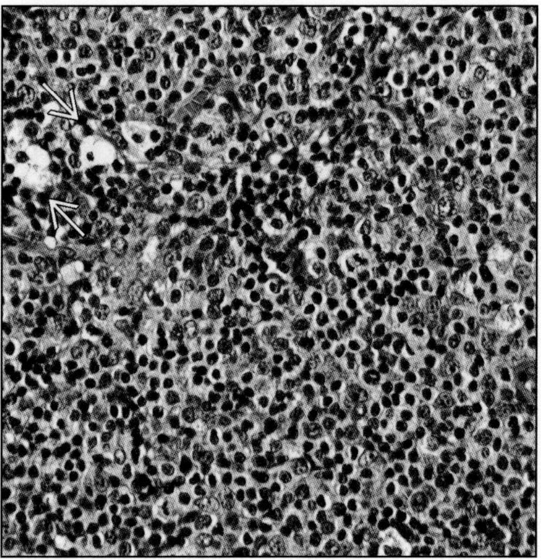

(Left) *In this case of ALPS with lymph node involvement, there is marked hyperplasia and expansion in the paracortex. Lymph node sinuses are patent, and a small but hyperplastic follicle is also shown.* ***(Right)*** *The lymphocytes in the paracortex often show reduced apoptosis manifested histologically by the presence of rare tingible body macrophages.*

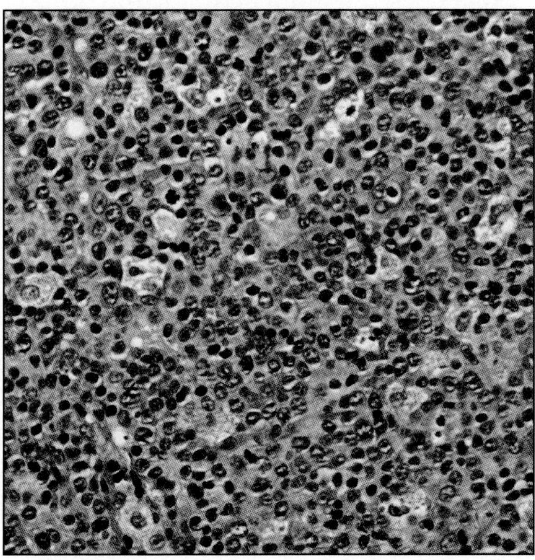

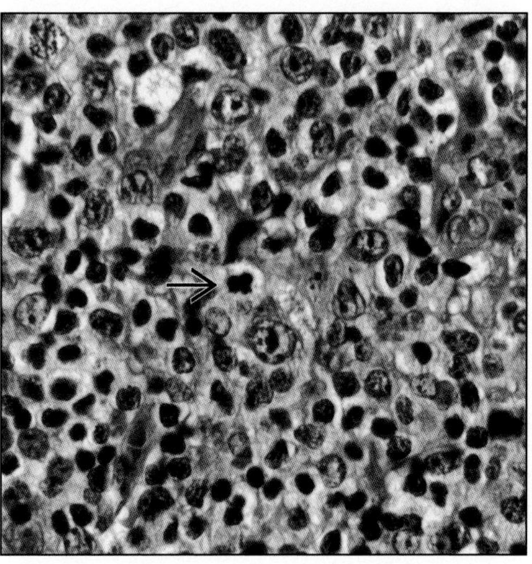

(Left) *High-power magnification of a reactive germinal center in a non-ALPS case shows normal apoptosis, including many tingible body macrophages.* ***(Right)*** *High-magnification view shows immunoblasts and mitotic figures in the paracortex. Mitotic figures can be conspicuous in ALPS, and a high proliferation rate shown by Ki-67 immunostaining also can be high (not shown).*

Microscopic Features

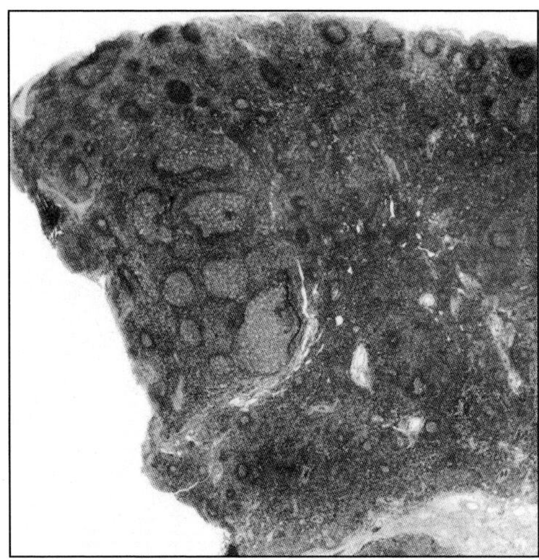

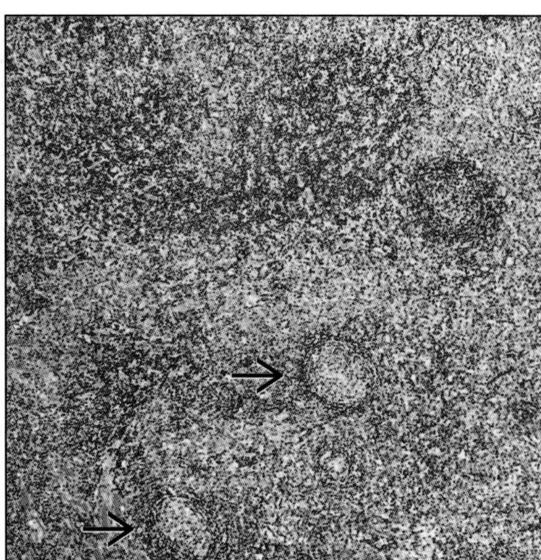

(Left) *The overall architecture of the lymph node in this case of ALPS is preserved. At this low-power magnification, marked follicular hyperplasia is easily appreciated. Paracortical hyperplasia is also present but is better seen at higher power magnification.* ***(Right)*** *This image shows paracortical expansion and small reactive follicles ⇒ in a lymph node involved by ALPS.*

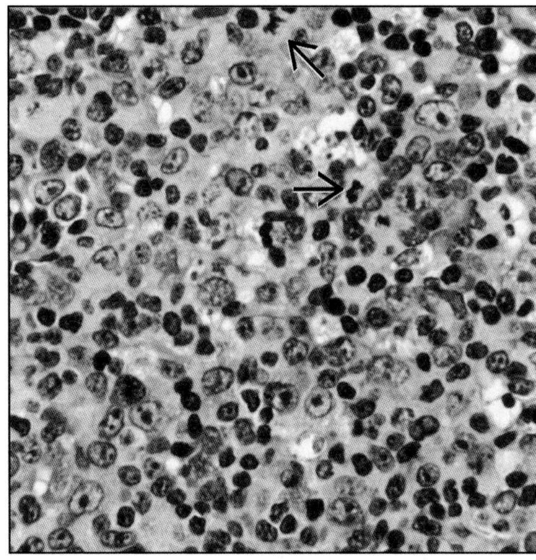

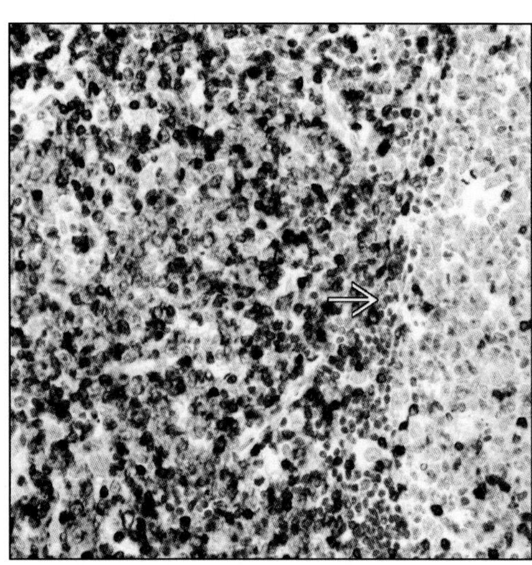

(Left) *This high magnification of the paracortical region of a lymph node in an ALPS case shows a mixture of cell types, including small lymphocytes, histiocytes, and immunoblasts with prominent nucleoli. Mitotic figures are present ⇒.* ***(Right)*** *Most T cells in the paracortical region of ALPS cases are CD3(+) and negative for CD4 and CD8 (not shown). A CD3(-) reactive follicle ➡ is also present.*

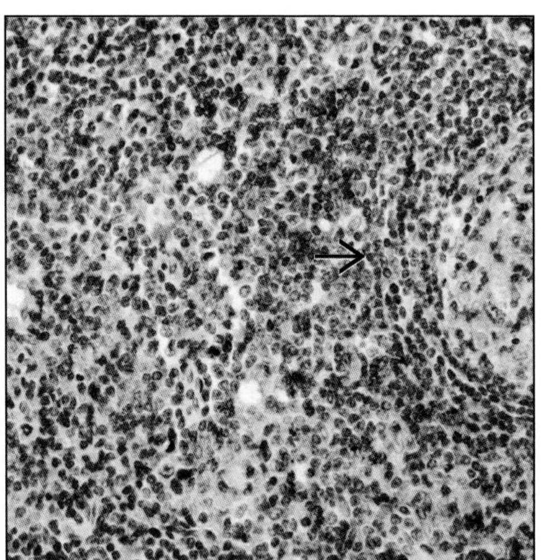

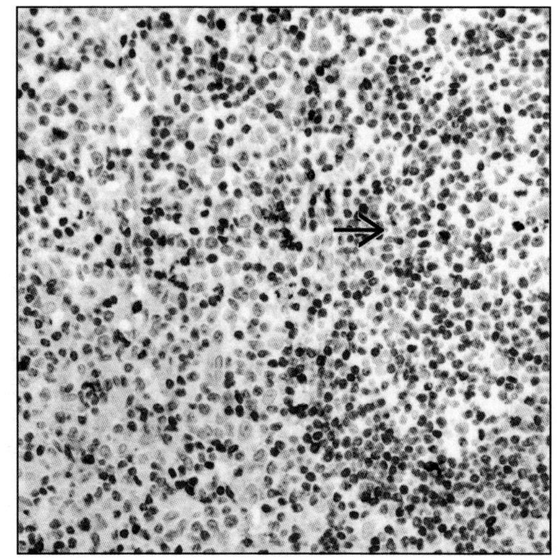

(Left) *Some T cells and histiocytes in the paracortex of this lymph node involved by ALPS are dimly CD4(+), but most of the T cells are CD4(-). A reactive follicle ⇒ is also present.* ***(Right)*** *Most T cells in the paracortical region of lymph nodes involved by ALPS are also CD8(-). A reactive follicle ⇒ is present.*

Microscopic Features

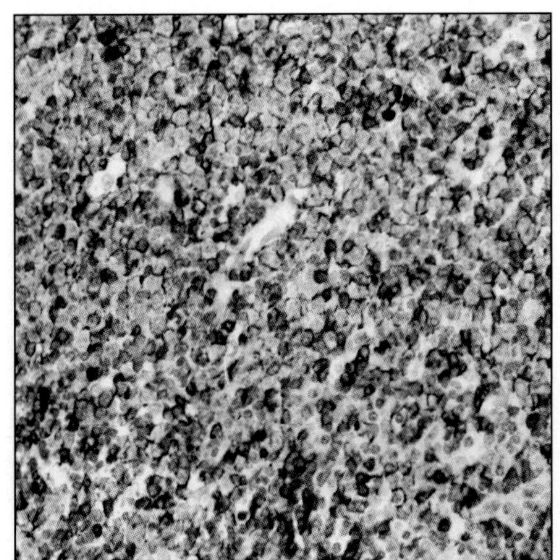

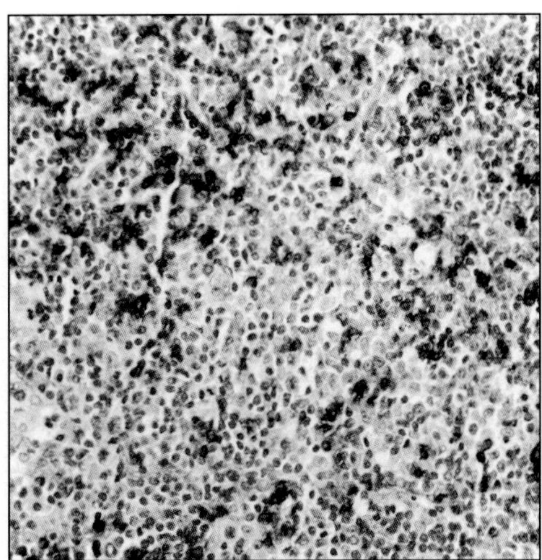

(Left) *Most T cells in the paracortical region of this lymph node are CD45RA(+). Increased T cells that are CD45RA(+) and CD45RO(-) are typically present in lymph nodes of ALPS patients.* ***(Right)*** *Most T cells in the paracortical region of this lymph node involved by ALPS are CD45RO(-).*

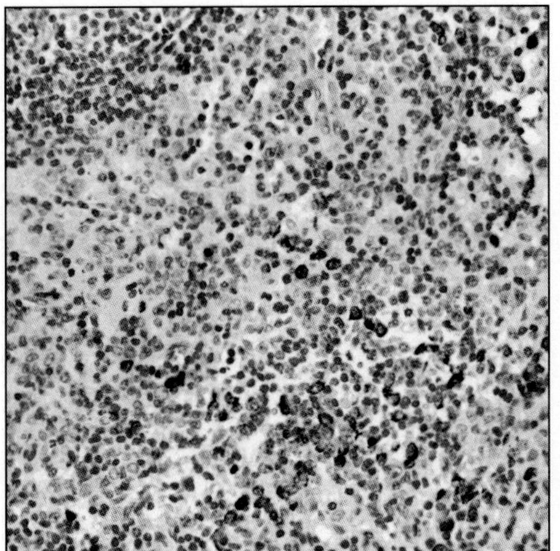

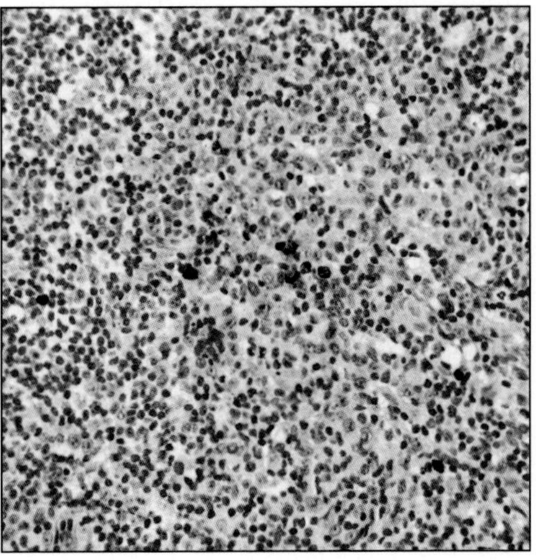

(Left) *Small plasma cells without atypia are commonly present in the paracortical region of ALPS lymph nodes and express polytypic immunoglobulin light chains. Kappa immunohistochemical stain is shown here.* ***(Right)*** *Small plasma cells without atypia are commonly present in the paracortical region of ALPS lymph nodes and express polytypic immunoglobulin light chains. Lambda immunohistochemical stain is shown here.*

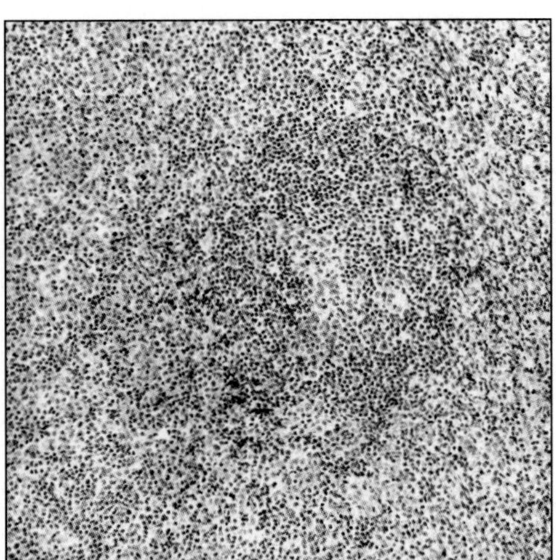

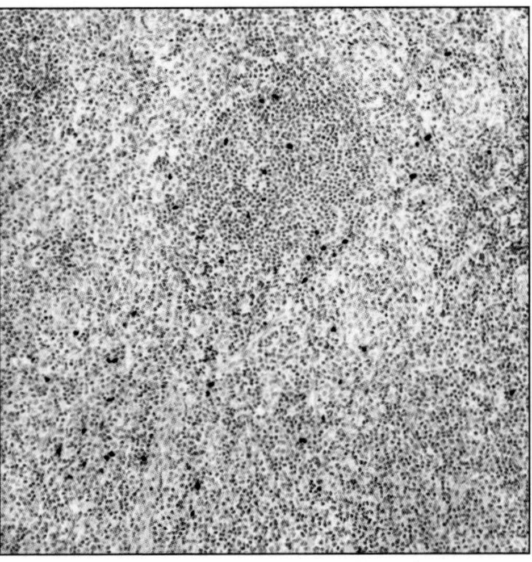

(Left) *In situ hybridization is usually negative for Epstein-Barr virus encoded RNA (EBER) in ALPS lymph nodes, as shown in this image.* ***(Right)*** *Scattered TdT(+) lymphoid cells can be present in the paracortical regions of ALPS lymph nodes, especially in patients of a very young age.*

AUTOIMMUNE LYMPHOPROLIFERATIVE SYNDROME

Microscopic Features

(Left) In some cases of ALPS, such as the one shown here, the paracortical areas are markedly expanded and confluent, demonstrating a diffuse proliferation pattern. These cases can raise the differential diagnosis with peripheral T-cell lymphoma. **(Right)** Increased postcapillary high endothelial venues are often observed in the paracortical regions of lymph nodes from patients with ALPS.

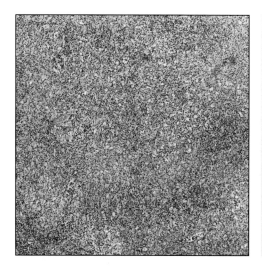

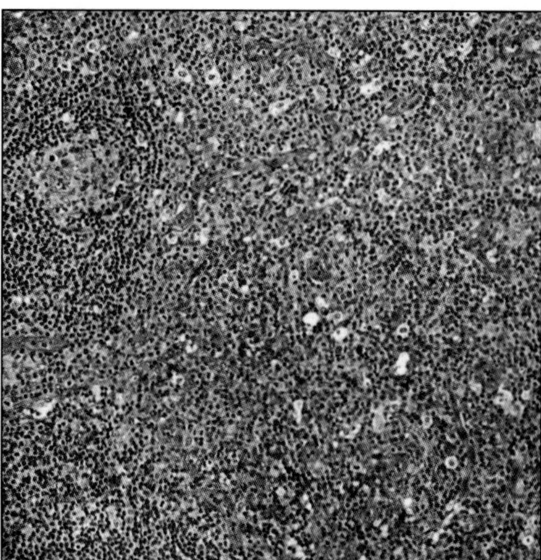

(Left) CD3 highlights many T cells in the expanded paracortex in this ALPS lymph node. In this field, the T cells surround a regressed follicle ➔. **(Right)** CD20 highlights small follicles, with most of the B cells being confined to the follicles in ALPS lymph nodes.

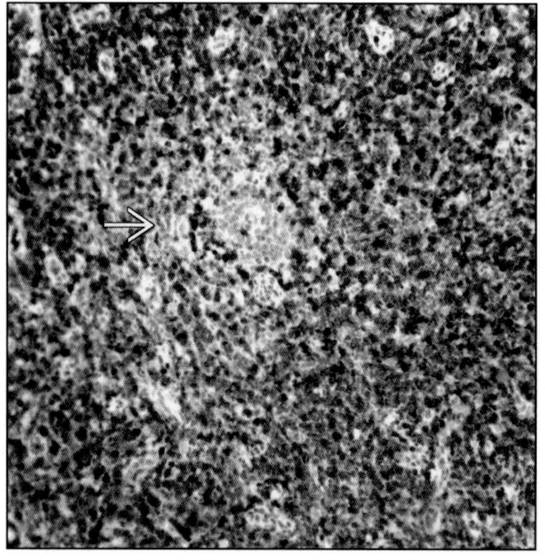

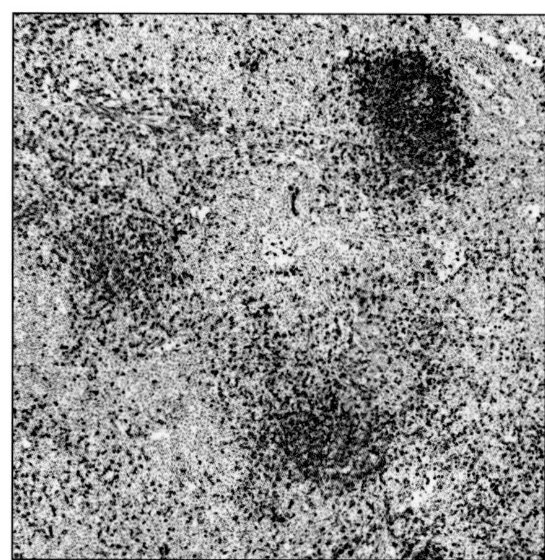

(Left) CD4 highlights scattered T cells and some histiocytes in this ALPS lymph node. Most of the T cells are CD4(-) and CD8(-) (not shown). **(Right)** CD8 highlights very few T cells in this ALPS lymph node. Most of the T cells are CD8(-) and CD4(-) (not shown).

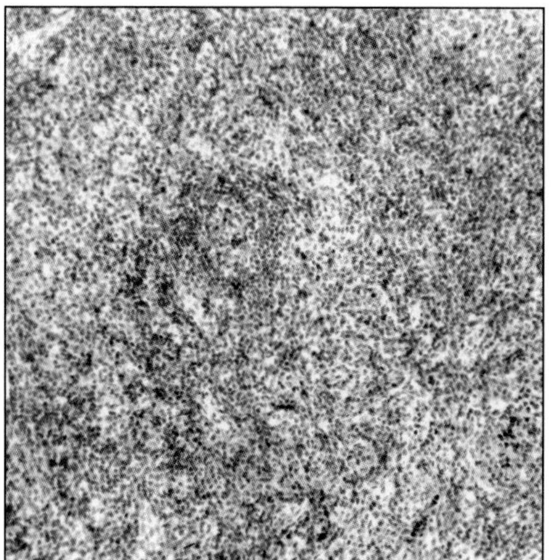

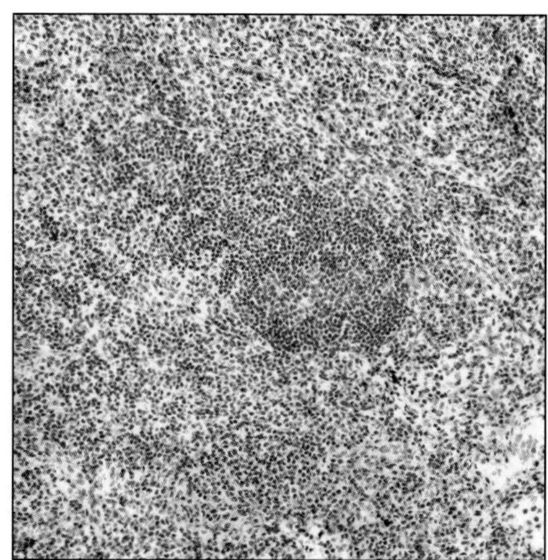

Flow Cytometric Immunophenotyping

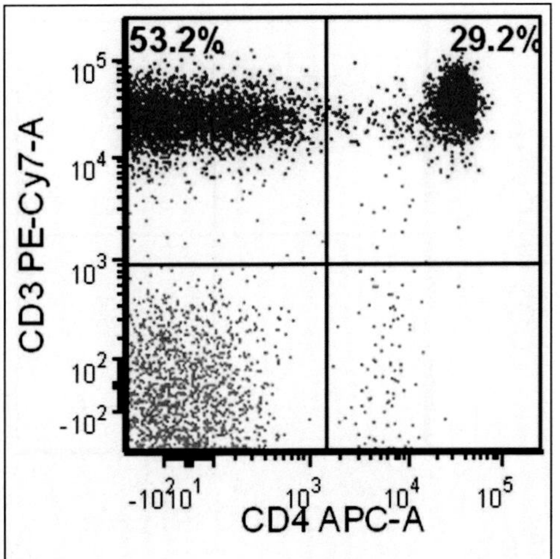

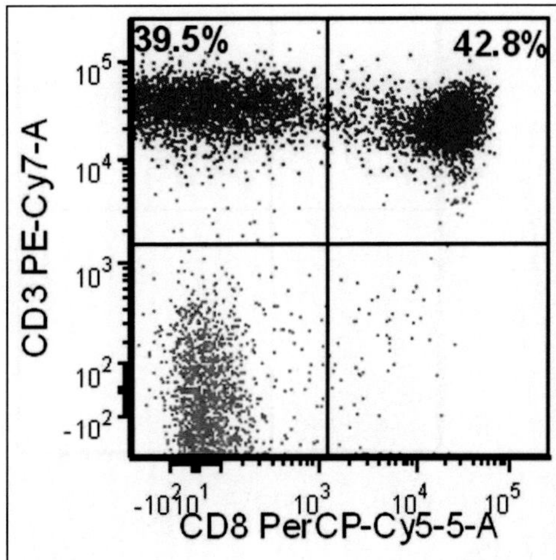

(Left) *Flow cytometry analysis of peripheral blood (PB) in an ALPS patient shows 29.2% CD4(+) T cells.* ***(Right)*** *Flow cytometry analysis of PB in an ALPS patient shows 42.8% CD8(+) T cells. These percentages of CD4(+) and CD8(+) cells do not add up to 100%, indicative of the presence of double-negative T cells.*

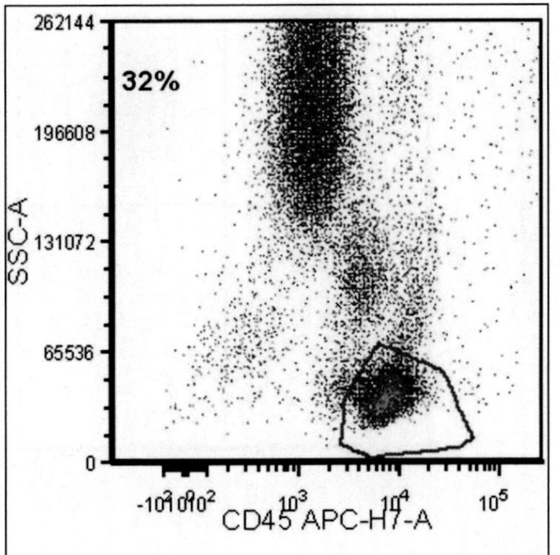

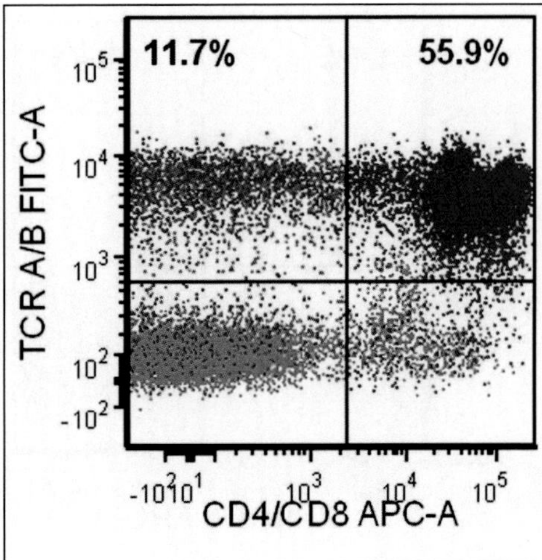

(Left) *Flow cytometric immunophenotyping panels designed for regular blood testing are often gated on total lymphocytes, based on side scatter/CD45. This approach is not optimal for analysis in patients with ALPS.* ***(Right)*** *In this case of ALPS, the gating is based on the lymphocyte gate, and DNT cells represent 11.7% of total lymphocytes. DNT cells are TCR-α/β(+), CD4(-), CD8(-). CD4 & CD8 antibodies are labeled with the same fluorochrome to detect CD4(-), CD8(-) cells.*

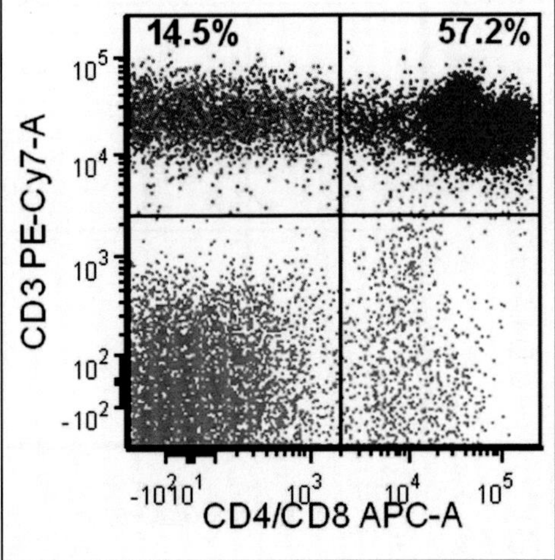

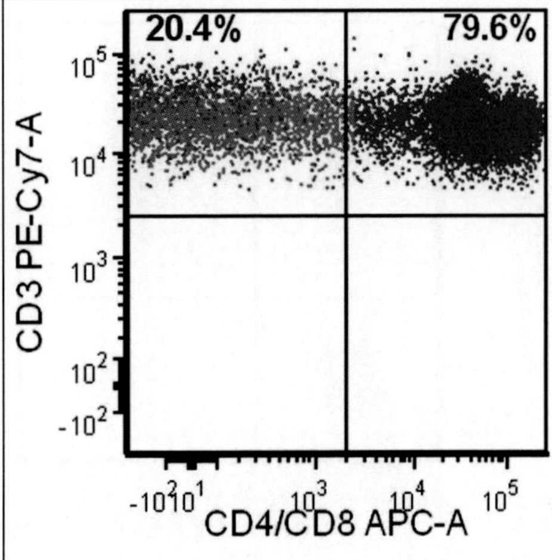

(Left) *Flow cytometry analysis of PB in an ALPS patient shows gating based on lymphocyte gate. DNT cells are CD3(+), TCR-α/β(+), CD4(-), and CD8(-) (in fuchsia color). Note that not all the CD3(+), CD4(-), CD8(-) cells are TCR-α/β(+) DNT; some are γ/δ(+) DNT cells.* ***(Right)*** *CD3(+) T cells are gated in this analysis of PB in an ALPS patient. The percentage of cells that are CD3(+), CD4(-), CD8(-) is different from that obtained by gating on total lymphocytes (20.4% vs. 14.5%).*

Flow Cytometric Immunophenotyping

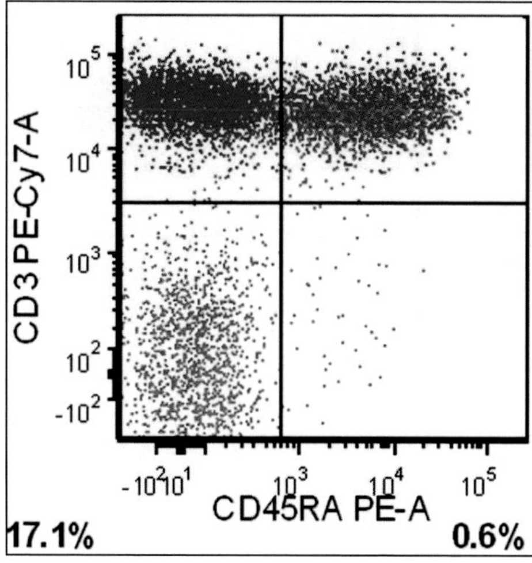

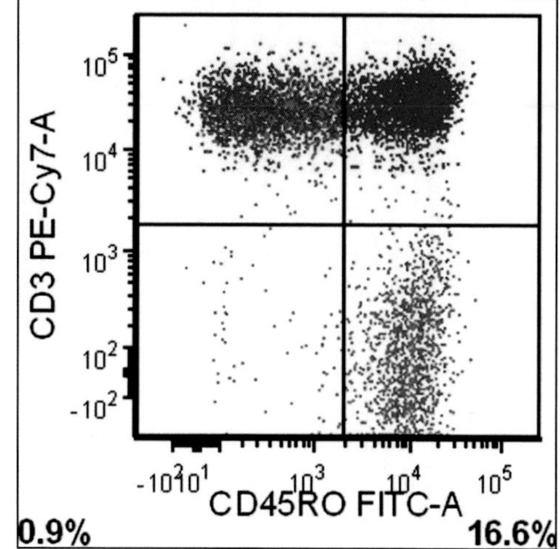

(Left) *Peripheral blood of ALPS patient shows that double-negative T (DNT) cells (highlighted in fuchsia color) are CD45RA(+).* ***(Right)*** *Peripheral blood of ALPS patient shows that the DNT cells (highlighted in fuchsia color) are CD45RO(-).*

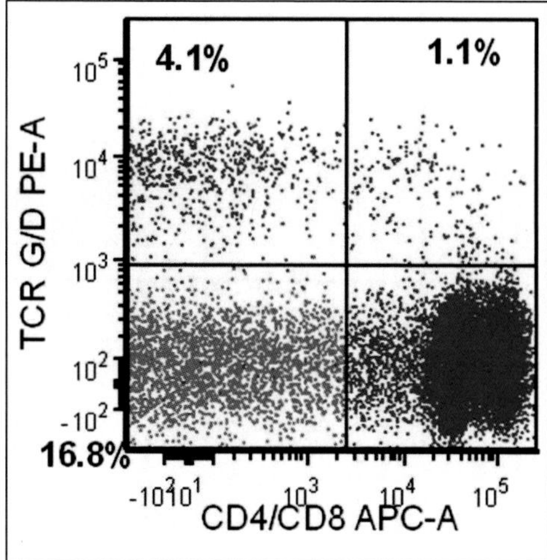

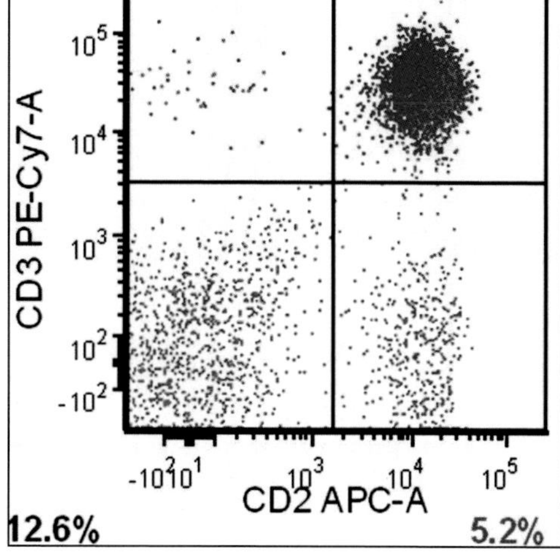

(Left) *Peripheral blood of ALPS patient shows TCR-γ/δ(+), CD4(-), CD8(-) T cells. A component of CD3(+), CD4(-), CD8(-) cells are also increased in ALPS (4.1% of total T cells in this case).* ***(Right)*** *Peripheral blood of ALPS patient shows DNT cells with normal expression of CD2 and CD5 (not shown).*

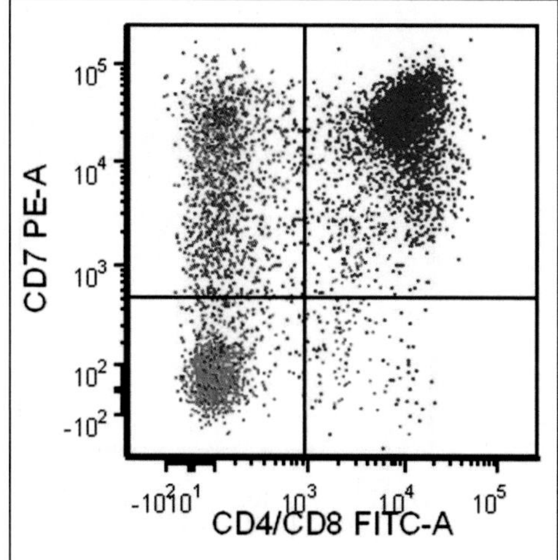

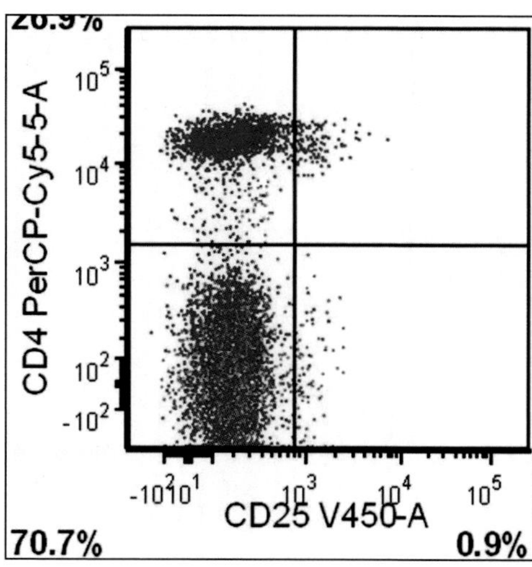

(Left) *Peripheral blood of ALPS patient shows DNT cells that are heterogeneous with decreased expression of CD7. CD7 expression on T cells also can be downregulated in inflammatory conditions.* ***(Right)*** *Peripheral blood of ALPS patient shows very few CD4(+), CD25(+) regulatory T cells. DNT cells are typically CD25(-), another feature of ALPS.*

Flow Cytometric Immunophenotyping

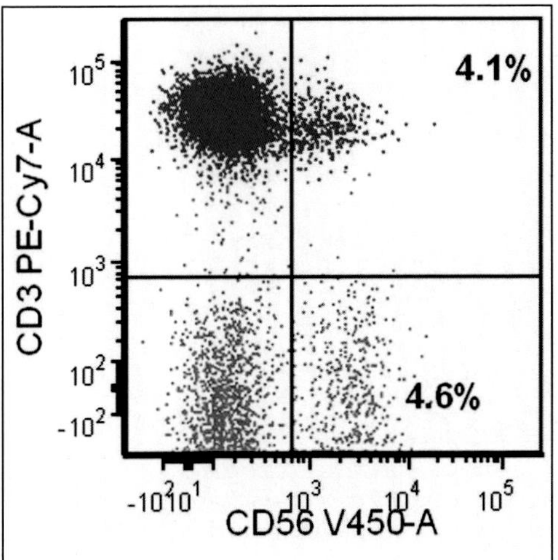

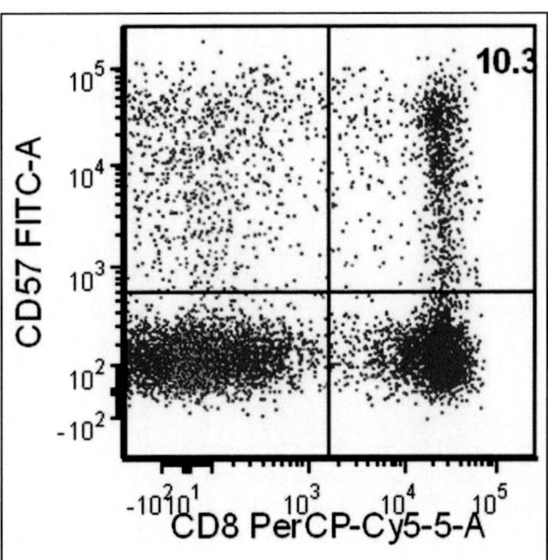

(Left) *Peripheral blood of ALPS patient shows a normal number of NK cells that are CD3(-) and CD56(+). NK cells in ALPS patients are often normal in number (4.6% of total lymphocytes in this case).* ***(Right)*** *Peripheral blood of ALPS patient shows large granular lymphocytes that are CD3(+), CD8(+), and CD57(+). Large granular lymphocytes are often increased in ALPS (10.3% of T cells in this case).*

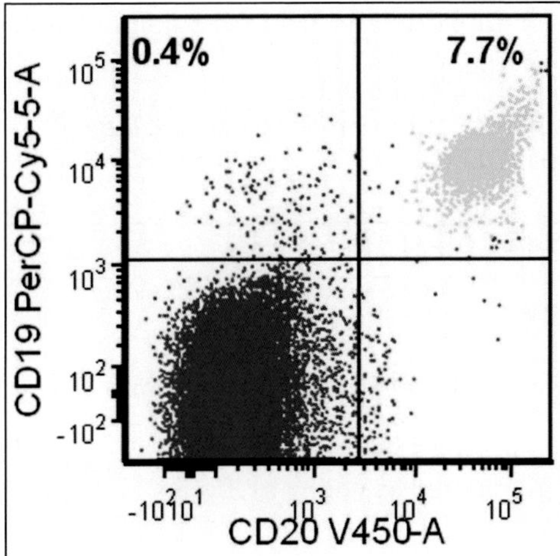

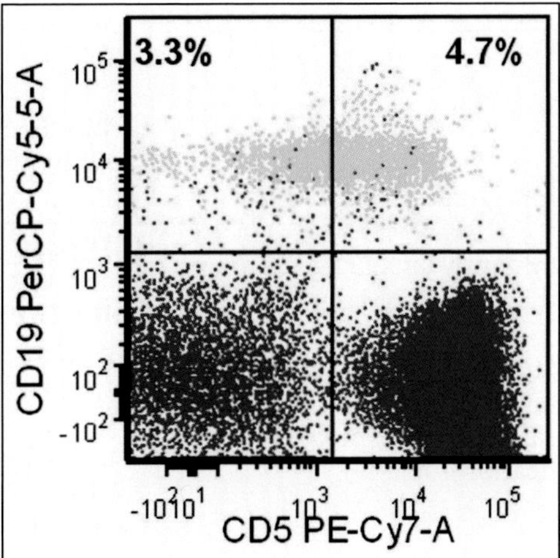

(Left) *Flow cytometry analysis of peripheral blood in an ALPS patient who had a normal to increased absolute number of B cells is shown. This differs from common variable immunodeficiency patients who have reduced B cells.* ***(Right)*** *Flow cytometry analysis of peripheral blood in an ALPS patient shows an increased number of CD5(+) B cells. CD5(+) B cells are often increased in ALPS patients. In this case, CD5(+) B cells represented > 50% of total B cells.*

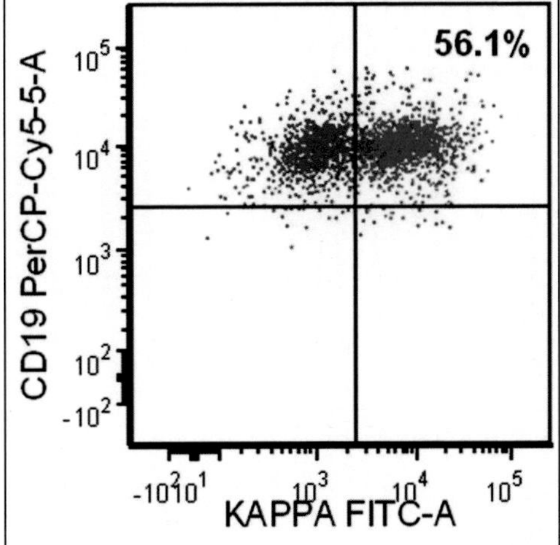

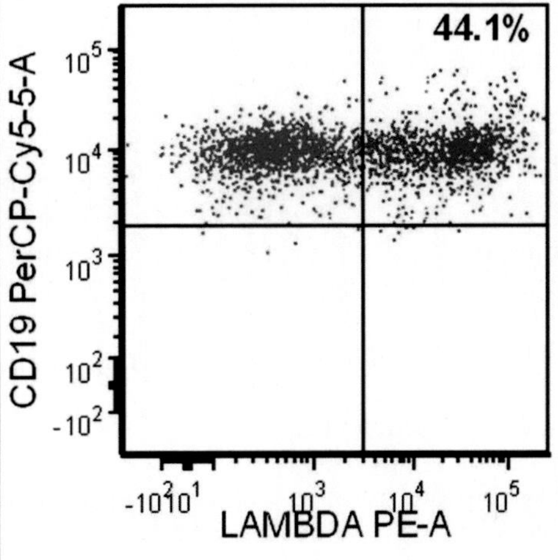

(Left) *Peripheral blood of an ALPS patient shows that the B cells are polytypic as assessed by kappa and lambda light chain expression. Kappa B cells are highlighted in red and lambda are highlighted in blue.* ***(Right)*** *Peripheral blood of an ALPS patient shows that the B cells are polytypic as assessed by kappa and lambda light chain expression. Kappa B cells are highlighted in red while lambda B cells are highlighted in blue.*

PEDIATRIC FOLLICULAR LYMPHOMA

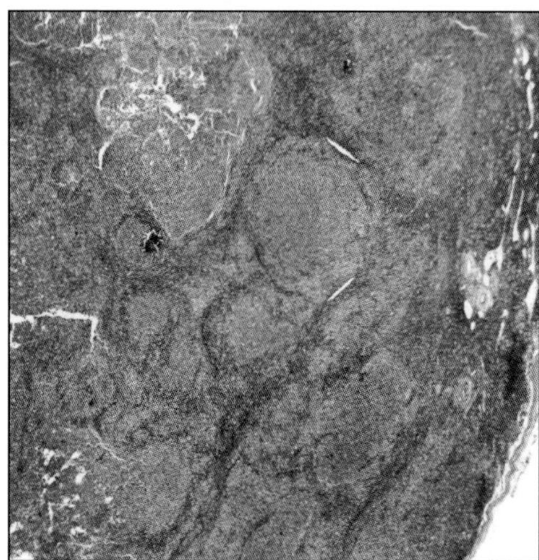

H&E stained section of a lymph node from an adolescent male involved by follicular lymphoma shows compact neoplastic follicles that lack polarization and tingible body macrophages.

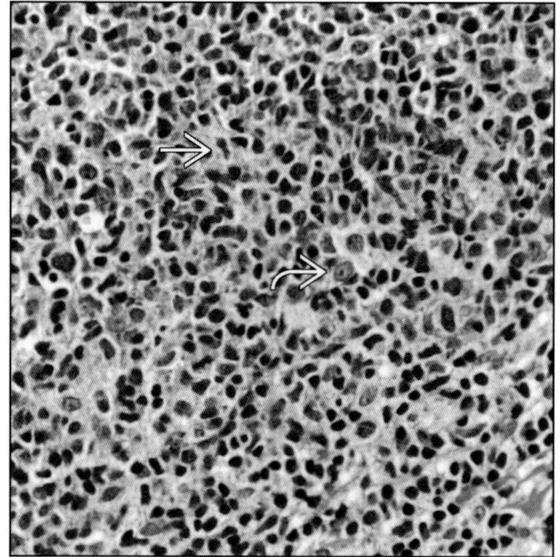

A neoplastic follicle is shown in this case of pediatric follicular lymphoma. Note a mixture of neoplastic large centroblasts ➔ and smaller centrocytes ➔ that often display twisted nuclei.

TERMINOLOGY

Abbreviations

- Pediatric follicular lymphoma (pFL)

Synonyms

- Follicular center cell lymphoma, grades 1-3 (REAL classification)
- Follicular lymphoma, predominantly small cleaved cell, mixed small cleaved and large cell, or large cell (Working Formulation)
- Centroblastic/centrocytic lymphoma (Kiel classification)
- Nodular lymphoma, poorly differentiated, mixed, or histiocytic (Rappaport classification)

Definitions

- Variant of FL that shares many similar features but shows some unique clinical, cytogenetic, molecular, and immunophenotypic characteristics
- Mature B-cell neoplasm composed of germinal (follicle) center lymphocytes (centrocytes and centroblasts) in variable mixture

ETIOLOGY/PATHOGENESIS

Pathogenesis

- Less well understood than in adults
- Bcl-2 overexpression as result of t(14;18)(q32;q21)/*IgH-BCL2* gene rearrangement
  - Smaller proportion have *BCL2* translocations (more often in older children)
    - Bcl-2 inhibits programmed cell death, giving Bcl-2(+) lymphoma cells a survival advantage
  - Most pFLs are negative for Bcl-2 protein
    - Associated with lower stage disease and older age
- *BCL6* gene rearrangements thought to play a role
- Mutations or deletions of the *P53* tumor suppressor gene have been implicated in the progression of adult FL
  - Their role in pFL is still unclear
- Pathogenesis may be more similar to diffuse large B-cell lymphoma (DLBCL)

CLINICAL ISSUES

Epidemiology

- Incidence
  - < 3% of childhood non-Hodgkin lymphomas
- Age
  - Median age range: 7.5-11.7 years
  - Can occur in children as young as 3 years
- Gender
  - Male:female ratio of 4:1

Site

- Commonly involve lymph nodes of head and neck, tonsils, and Waldeyer ring
- Extranodal occurrence at a variety of sites
  - Gastrointestinal tract
  - Parotid gland
  - Kidney
  - Epididymis
  - Skin
  - Testis
    - Propensity for testicular involvement reported
- More commonly localized

Presentation

- Typically present with early-stage disease
  - Localized lymphadenopathy

Treatment

- Adjuvant therapy
  - Combination chemotherapy
    - Rituximab plus CHOP (cyclophosphamide, doxorubicin, vincristine, and prednisone)

PEDIATRIC FOLLICULAR LYMPHOMA

Key Facts

Terminology
- Variant of FL that shares many similar features but shows some unique clinical, cytogenetic, and immunophenotypic characteristics

Clinical Issues
- < 3% of childhood non-Hodgkin lymphomas
- Median age range: 7.5-11.7 years
- Male:female ratio = 4:1
- Commonly involve lymph nodes of the head and neck, tonsils, and Waldeyer ring
- Propensity for testicular involvement reported
- Typically present with early-stage disease

Microscopic Pathology
- Pediatric FL should fulfill histologic criteria of adult FL

Ancillary Tests
- Positive for B-cell markers: CD19(+), CD20(+), CD79a(+), pax-5(+)
- Low propensity for Bcl-2 expression in pFLs
- Low frequency of t(14;18)(q32;q21) in pFLs
- Flow cytometry helpful in demonstrating clonality
- Southern blot and PCR may also be helpful in establishing clonality

Top Differential Diagnoses
- Follicular hyperplasia
- Pediatric marginal zone lymphoma
- Diffuse large B-cell lymphoma
- Lymphoblastic lymphoma
- Burkitt lymphoma
- Chronic orchitis

  - Surgical excision alone in localized disease has been advocated

Prognosis
- Considered curable in most cases

MACROSCOPIC FEATURES

General Features
- Enlarged lymph node or lymphoid tissue with nodular appearance

MICROSCOPIC PATHOLOGY

Histologic Features
- Pediatric FL should fulfill histologic criteria of FL
  - Strict criteria required to distinguish from the much more common benign follicular hyperplasia
- Neoplastic follicles are composed of centrocytes and centroblasts
  - Variable cytologic predominance according to grade of tumor
    - Low grade (grades 1 and 2)
    - Grade 1: 0-5 centroblasts per high-power field on average
    - Grade 2: 6-15 centroblasts per high-power field on average
    - Grade 3: > 15 centroblasts or immunoblasts per high-power field on average; 3A: Centrocytes present; 3B: Follicles composed entirely of large blastic cells
    - Some high-grade cases have sparse centrocytes
  - ~ 75% of pFL are grades 2 or 3
- Key findings include
  - Total or extensive replacement of nodal architecture
  - Usually shows large expansile follicular growth pattern
  - Crowding of nodules with little interposed lymphoid tissue
  - Even distribution of nodules throughout node or lesion
  - Uniformity in size and shape of nodules
  - Neoplastic follicles lack polarization
  - Neoplastic follicles lack tingible body macrophages
  - Paucity of reactive lymphoid cells in interfollicular areas (plasma cells and immunoblasts)
    - Immunostains may be helpful to highlight
  - Cytologically atypical cells in the interfollicular regions similar to those in follicles
  - Monomorphous appearance of cytologically atypical cells in neoplastic follicles
  - Neoplastic follicles may coexist with reactive follicles in same lymph node
- May progress from follicular to diffuse architectural growth pattern
- Bone marrow biopsy specimen may show paratrabecular aggregates
  - Other patterns may be present, but rare without paratrabecular pattern

ANCILLARY TESTS

Immunohistochemistry
- Positive for B-cell markers: CD19(+), CD20(+), CD79a(+), pax-5(+)
- Low propensity for Bcl-2 expression in pFLs
  - ~ 30% express Bcl-2 protein
  - Most FL of the testis are Bcl-2(-)
- CD10(+) and Bcl-6(+) in most cases
- Follicular dendritic meshworks usually present
  - CD21(+), CD23(+), CD35(+), &/or CNA.42(+)
- T-cell antigens(-), cyclin-D1(-), TdT(-)
- Variable proliferation rate as determined with Ki-67
  - Low-grade FL usually has low proliferation rate (< 20%)
  - Distribution of ki-67 positive cells is more uniform
- Role of p53 expression in pFL remains unclear

Flow Cytometry
- Monotypic surface immunoglobulin(+)
- Heavy chains: IgM(+) or IgG(+), and IgD(-)
  - IgD(+) in rim of occasional residual mantle zone lymphocytes

PEDIATRIC FOLLICULAR LYMPHOMA

- CD19(+), CD20(+), CD22(+), and CD79a(+)
- Usually CD10(+)
  - Occasional downregulation of CD10 in peripheral blood and bone marrow
- T-cell antigens (-)
- TdT(-)

Cytogenetics

- Low frequency of t(14;18)(q32;q21) in pFLs
  - Unclear role for testing for this translocation
- Other rare cytogenetic abnormalities include i(17q) and *BCL6* rearrangement

Molecular Genetics

- Determination of *IgH* gene rearrangements by southern blot and PCR may be helpful in establishing clonality
  - Most breakpoints in *BCL2* on chromosome 18 occur on MBR (major breakpoint region)
  - PCR assays can sensitively detect most of these breakpoints
  - FISH assays, unlike PCR, can assess all breakpoints but are less sensitive
  - Other minor breakpoints: Mcr (minor cluster region), icr (intermediate cluster region), etc.
- Important to remember that
  - PCR can detect *BCL2-IgH* fusion sequences in people without evidence of FL
    - Frequency of (+) result correlates with increasing age
    - Finding suggests that other molecular mechanisms are required for lymphomagenesis

DIFFERENTIAL DIAGNOSIS

Follicular Hyperplasia (FH)

- Predominantly cortical distribution of follicles
- Reactive follicles are variable in size and shape
- Expansion of the interfollicular areas (interfollicular hyperplasia) often accompanies FH
- Immunophenotype and molecular studies show polytypic B cells
- Ki-67 positive cells may show polarization with sharp demarcation along edge of follicle
- Staining for Bcl-2 may not be helpful as most pFLs are Bcl-2 negative

Pediatric Marginal Zone Lymphoma

- Similar clinical and morphologic features
- Immunophenotypic studies are often useful in this differential diagnosis
- Neoplastic B cells are CD5(-) and CD10(-)
- Follicular dendritic cell markers can be used to highlight follicle colonization

Diffuse Large B-cell Lymphoma (DLBCL)

- Diffuse arrangement of large cells with variable composition
  - Centroblastic, immunoblastic, pleomorphic, lymphocyte/histiocyte-rich
- B-cell lineage: CD19(+), CD20(+), CD5(-), CD10(+/-), Bcl-6(+/-)
- DLBCL more common in children than FL

Lymphoblastic Lymphoma

- Distinguish FL of testis from secondary lymphoblastic lymphoma
  - Most testicular lymphomas in children are secondary to Burkitt lymphoma or lymphoblastic lymphoma
- Immunophenotype
  - Immature B- or T-cell immunophenotype
    - TdT(+)

Burkitt Lymphoma

- Distinguish FL of the testis from secondary Burkitt lymphoma
  - Most testicular lymphomas in children are secondary to Burkitt lymphoma or lymphoblastic lymphoma
- Mature B-cell immunophenotype with very high proliferation index
  - CD10(+), CD19(+), CD20(+), Bcl-6(+), Bcl-2(-), sIg(+), Ki-67(+) in > 95%
  - Often show starry sky pattern
- Neoplastic cells show diffuse pattern of growth with little to no pleomorphism

Chronic Orchitis

- Distinguish from FL of testis
- Histologic features may resemble classic FL
- May require demonstration of clonality by flow cytometry or molecular methods

SELECTED REFERENCES

1. Kumar R et al: Rituximab in combination with multiagent chemotherapy for pediatric follicular lymphoma. Pediatr Blood Cancer. 57(2):317-20, 2011
2. Setty BA et al: Rare pediatric non-hodgkin lymphoma. Curr Hematol Malig Rep. 5(3):163-8, 2010
3. Agrawal R et al: Pediatric follicular lymphoma: a rare clinicopathologic entity. Arch Pathol Lab Med. 133(1):142-6, 2009
4. Jaglowski SM et al: Lymphoma in adolescents and young adults. Semin Oncol. 36(5):381-418, 2009
5. Bacon CM et al: Primary follicular lymphoma of the testis and epididymis in adults. Am J Surg Pathol. 31(7):1050-8, 2007
6. Heller KN et al: Primary follicular lymphoma of the testis: excellent outcome following surgical resection without adjuvant chemotherapy. J Pediatr Hematol Oncol. 26(2):104-7, 2004
7. Lu D et al: Primary follicular large cell lymphoma of the testis in a child. Arch Pathol Lab Med. 125(4):551-4, 2001
8. Swerdlow SH: Small B-cell lymphomas of the lymph nodes and spleen: practical insights to diagnosis and pathogenesis. Mod Pathol. 12(2):125-40, 1999

Microscopic Features and Differential Diagnosis

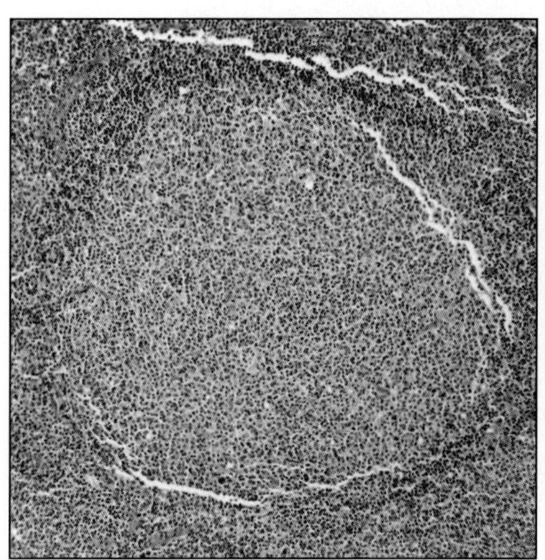

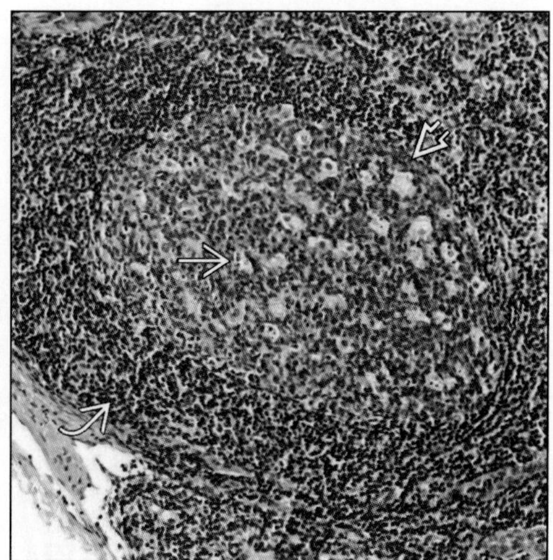

(Left) *A large neoplastic follicle is shown in this case of pediatric FL. Histologic features should resemble FL of adults; neoplastic follicles of similar size and shape that lack polarization, distinct mantle zones, and often lack tingible body macrophages as highlighted here.* ***(Right)*** *A benign reactive secondary follicle is shown for comparison. Note the prominent and polarized mantle zone ➢ and germinal center ➢ with abundant tingible body macrophages ➢.*

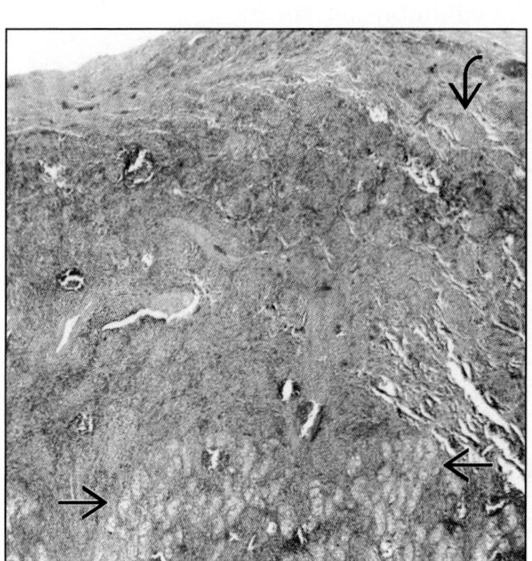

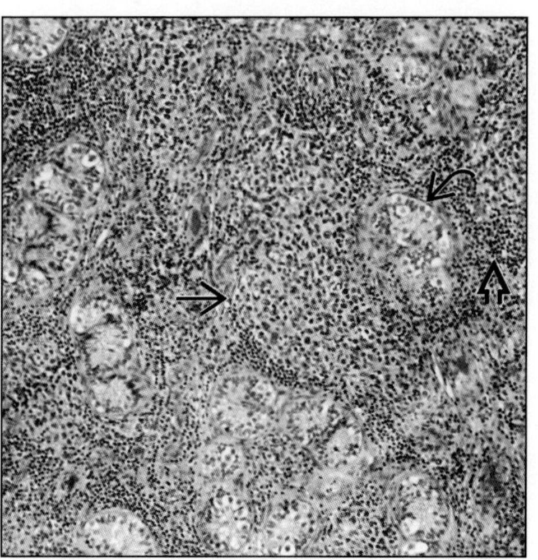

(Left) *Follicular lymphoma of the testis in an adolescent male is shown. Neoplastic nodules ➢ are seen extending from the capsule down into the testicular parenchyma with some residual seminiferous tubules present ➢.* ***(Right)*** *Neoplastic nodules ➢ are seen infiltrating throughout the testis in this case of FL, disrupting and distorting the usual testicular architecture. Small mature T-cells ➢ are also intermixed amongst the seminiferous tubules ➢ and neoplastic nodules.*

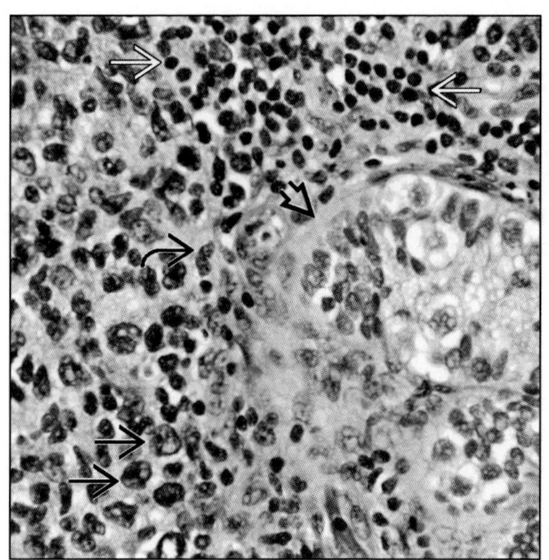

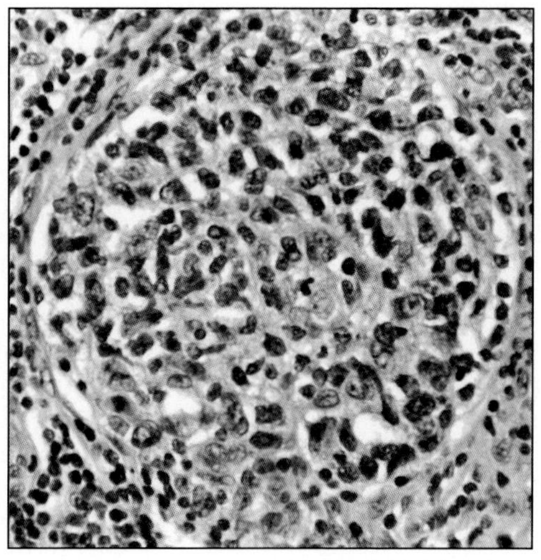

(Left) *High-power view of FL of the testis shows the neoplastic cells, which include large centroblasts ➢ and smaller centrocytes ➢ adjacent to a seminiferous tubule ➢. Small round nonneoplastic T cells (CD3 stain not shown) are also present in the background ➢.* ***(Right)*** *A neoplastic nodule is shown in this pediatric case of FL of the testis. Bcl-2 immunostaining was negative (not shown). FISH for the t(14;18) was also negative; however, clonality was demonstrated by PCR.*

DIFFUSE LARGE B-CELL LYMPHOMA

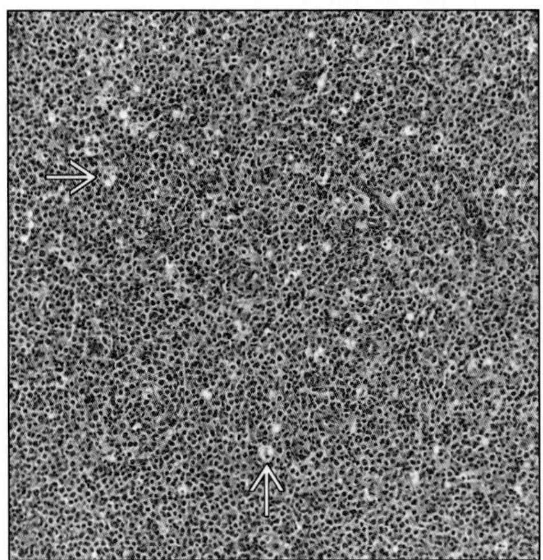

Sheets of large B cells with some tingible body macrophages ➡ are shown in this DLBCL. This starry sky appearance also seen in BL is not specific and only reflects a high degree of proliferation.

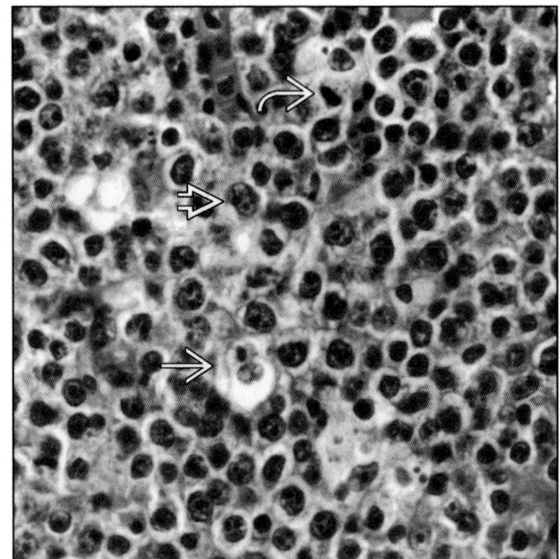

DLBCL with a high proliferation index is evidenced by scattered tingible body macrophages ➡ and mitotic figures ➡. Note the large nuclei and single to multiple nucleoli ➡ of the large cells.

TERMINOLOGY

Abbreviations

- Diffuse large B-cell lymphoma (DLBCL)

Definitions

- Diffuse proliferation of large neoplastic B cells
  - Large cell defined as at least the size of a tissue histiocyte or 2x the size of a normal lymphocyte
  - Variety of morphologic variants
    - Centroblastic
    - Immunoblastic
    - Anaplastic
  - All morphologic variants have similar aggressive behavior
  - Molecular subgroups
    - Germinal center B-cell-like (GCB)
    - Activated B-cell-like (ABC)
    - Distinction of molecular subgroups not currently required
  - Immunophenotypic subgroups
    - CD5(+) DLBCL
    - GCB
    - Non-GCB
    - Distinction of immunophenotypic subgroups not currently required
  - Important diagnostic subtype in pediatric population
    - T-cell/histiocyte-rich large B-cell lymphoma (THRLBCL)

ETIOLOGY/PATHOGENESIS

Infectious Agents

- Not thought to play a significant role
- Commonly EBV(-)

Immunodeficiency/Immunosuppression

- Inherited immune deficiency is significant risk factor
- DLBCL is most common subtype of immunodeficiency-associated lymphomas

Dysregulated Cell Proliferation

- Frequently show higher expression rates of *c-M*yc
- More frequent translocations involving *c-Myc*; t(8;14)
- Translocation t(14;18)(q32;q21) and *BCL6* abnormalities are very rare in pediatric DLBCLs

CLINICAL ISSUES

Epidemiology

- Incidence
  - Children and young adults can be affected
    - Account for 10-20% of pediatric non-Hodgkin lymphomas
  - Predominantly disease of older adults
- Age
  - Rarely diagnosed in children < 4 years of age
- Gender
  - Male:female ratio of 2:1

Presentation

- Enlarging mass in nodal or extranodal sites
  - Nodal disease is more common
  - Localized disease is more common
- Lower frequency of bone marrow and central nervous system involvement
- Frequent B symptoms (fever, night sweats, or weight loss)

Treatment

- Multiagent chemotherapy
  - Short, dose-intense courses
- Treatment strategies similar to those of Burkitt lymphoma
- Role of monoclonal antibodies (i.e., rituximab) as a part of therapy have yet to be determined

DIFFUSE LARGE B-CELL LYMPHOMA

Key Facts

Terminology
- Diffuse proliferation of large neoplastic B cells
- Variety of morphologic variants: Centroblastic, immunoblastic, and anaplastic
- All morphologic variants have similar aggressive behavior

Clinical Issues
- Account for 10-20% of pediatric non-Hodgkin lymphomas
- Rarely diagnosed in children < 4 years
- Enlarging mass in nodal or extranodal sites
  - Nodal and localized disease are more common
- Treatment strategies and outcomes similar to those of Burkitt lymphoma

Microscopic Pathology
- Irrespective of location, DLBCL diffusely replaces normal architecture
- TCHRLBCL shows individually scattered cells in background of T cells and histiocytes

Top Differential Diagnoses
- Burkitt lymphoma (BL)
- Anaplastic large cell lymphoma (ALCL)
- Primary mediastinal (thymic) large B-cell lymphoma
- Follicular lymphoma
- B-lymphoblastic lymphoma
- Nodular lymphocyte predominant Hodgkin lymphoma (NLPHL)
- Small round blue cell tumors of childhood

Prognosis
- High response and cure rates (> 90%)
- Outcome similar to patients with Burkitt lymphoma

MACROSCOPIC FEATURES

General Features
- Enlarged lymph node with fleshy, tan cut surface

MICROSCOPIC PATHOLOGY

Histologic Features
- **Diffuse large B-cell lymphoma**
  - Irrespective of location, DLBCL diffusely replaces normal architecture
  - Centroblastic morphologic variant
    - Most common in pediatric DLBCL
    - Medium to large-sized lymphoid cells
    - Oval to round nuclei with vesicular chromatin and 2-4 nuclear membrane-bound nucleoli
    - Variable amounts of amphophilic to basophilic cytoplasm
  - Immunoblastic morphologic variant
    - Medium to large-sized lymphoid cells
    - Oval to round nuclei with a single centrally located nucleolus
    - Variable amounts of basophilic cytoplasm
    - Plasmablastic features (eccentrically located nucleus) can be seen
  - Anaplastic morphologic variant
    - Extremely rare
    - Large to very large cells
    - Bizarre pleomorphic nuclei
    - May resemble Hodgkin &/or Reed-Sternberg cells and cells of anaplastic large cell lymphoma
- **T-cell/histiocyte-rich large B-cell lymphoma**
  - Diffuse to nodular growth pattern with effacement of lymph node architecture
  - Individually scattered neoplastic large B cells
    - Do not form aggregates or sheets
    - Tumor cells vary in size, commonly resemble centroblasts and may resemble cells associated with Hodgkin lymphoma
  - Neoplastic B cells are in a background of nonneoplastic small T cells
  - Scattered bland, nonepithelioid histiocytes
  - Histologic progression to DLBCL can be seen

ANCILLARY TESTS

Immunohistochemistry
- Pan-B-cell antigens (+)
  - CD19, CD20, CD22, CD79a
- CD10 and Bcl-6 are frequently positive (GCB immunophenotype)
- FOXP1(+/-), Bcl-2(+/-)
- CD30(-/+), usually weak and partial
- Proliferation fraction (MIB-1/Ki-67) is usually high
- Use of immunohistochemical panels to predict outcome has no demonstrated value in pediatric DLBCL
- GCB immunophenotype accounts for most pediatric DLBCL
  - CD10(+) &/or Bcl-6(+) without IRF-4/MUM1
- Algorithms proposed to identify GCB and non-GBC types
  - Hans et al
  - Choi et al
- Neoplastic B cells of THRLBCL lack CD15, CD30, and CD138
  - May express Bcl-2 and EMA

DIFFERENTIAL DIAGNOSIS

Burkitt Lymphoma (BL)
- Distinguishing atypical BL from DLBCL can be difficult
- Most common DLBCL immunophenotype is identical to that of BL; CD10(+), Bcl-6(+), Bcl-2(-)
- Starry sky pattern and higher proliferation index in BL
- Extranodal involvement more common in BL

DIFFUSE LARGE B-CELL LYMPHOMA

- FISH analysis for t(8;14) or alternative *MYC* translocations

Anaplastic Large Cell Lymphoma (ALCL)

- Effacement of lymph node architecture with intrasinusoidal involvement common
- Tumor cells are of cytotoxic T-cell origin
- Expresses T-cell antigens (CD3[-] in some cases), CD30, and ALK

Primary Mediastinal (Thymic) Large B-cell Lymphoma

- Young females
- Anterosuperior mediastinal mass
- Locally aggressive with local compressive effects
- Large cells with pale cytoplasm (often is retraction artifact) and sclerosis (compartmentalization)
- Thymic components, such as Hassall corpuscles, may be identified
- Positive for pan-B-cell markers
- CD30 often (+) but usually weak &/or focal (~ 75%)
- CD23 (70%), Bcl-6, and MUM1 (most cases)
- From practical point of view, difficult to diagnose by histologic findings alone
  - Clinical correlation is essential for diagnosis

Follicular Lymphoma

- Rare in children
- Usually presents as high-grade (3a or 3b) in children
- Follicular growth pattern, presence of centrocytes and follicular dendritic cells will help distinguish from DLBCL

B-lymphoblastic Lymphoma

- Precursor B phenotype; TdT(+)
- Lymph node involvement by lymphoblastic lymphoma is more commonly of precursor T-cell origin

Nodular Lymphocyte Predominant Hodgkin Lymphoma (NLPHL)

- Distinguishing TCHRLBCL from NLPHL can be difficult
- Immunophenotype of tumor cells in NLPHL is similar; CD20(+), CD79a(+), Bcl-6(+)
- Nodular growth pattern in NLPHL
  - Large spherical meshworks of CD21(+) follicular dendritic cells
  - Filled with small B cells
  - Numerous CD4, CD57 and PD-1(+) T cells are also present

Small Round Blue Cell Tumors of Childhood

- Overlapping morphologic features
- Clinical correlation and use of an appropriate IHC panel will assist in diagnosis (e.g., CD20, CD45, TdT, desmin, myogenin, synaptophysin, chromogranin, keratin, CD99, FLI-1)

Plasmablastic Lymphoma

- Large neoplastic cells, most of which resemble immunoblasts or plasmablasts
- Plasma cell-associated markers expressed (CD138, CD38, Vs38c, and EMA)
- CD56 frequently positive
  - CD56 expression is rare in DLBCL
- Almost always negative for CD20 and pax-5
- CD45 (LCA) weak or negative
- Some cases positive for some T-cell markers, including CD4 and CD7
- EBV frequently positive (~ 75%)
- Commonly associated with immunodeficiency

B-cell Lymphoma, Unclassifiable, with Features Between DLBCL and BL

- Features of high-grade lymphoma
  - High proliferation rate
  - Apoptosis/necrosis
  - "Starry sky" pattern
- Shows either an immunophenotype typical of BL with atypical morphology or typical BL morphology with atypical immunophenotype
- Subset of cases have translocations involving *MYC*, *BCL2*, &/or *BCL6* (double- and triple-hit lymphomas)

Undifferentiated Carcinoma

- Cohesive tumor cells
  - May be best appreciated on FNA smear preparations
- Distinguish with appropriate IHC panel

SELECTED REFERENCES

1. Meyer PN et al: Immunohistochemical methods for predicting cell of origin and survival in patients with diffuse large B-cell lymphoma treated with rituximab. J Clin Oncol. 29(2):200-7, 2011
2. Choi WW et al: A new immunostain algorithm classifies diffuse large B-cell lymphoma into molecular subtypes with high accuracy. Clin Cancer Res. 15(17):5494-502, 2009
3. Hochberg J et al: Adolescent non-Hodgkin lymphoma and Hodgkin lymphoma: state of the science. Br J Haematol. 144(1):24-40, 2009
4. Reiter A et al: Recent advances in the understanding and management of diffuse large B-cell lymphoma in children. Br J Haematol. 142(3):329-47, 2008
5. Camara DA et al: Immunoblastic morphology in diffuse large B-cell lymphoma is associated with a nongerminal center immunophenotypic profile. Leuk Lymphoma. 48(5):892-6, 2007
6. Hans CP et al: Confirmation of the molecular classification of diffuse large B-cell lymphoma by immunohistochemistry using a tissue microarray. Blood. 103(1):275-82, 2004
7. Lim MS et al: T-cell/histiocyte-rich large B-cell lymphoma: a heterogeneous entity with derivation from germinal center B cells. Am J Surg Pathol. 26(11):1458-66, 2002
8. Lazzarino M et al: Primary mediastinal B-cell lymphoma with sclerosis: an aggressive tumor with distinctive clinical and pathologic features. J Clin Oncol. 11(12):2306-13, 1993

Microscopic Features

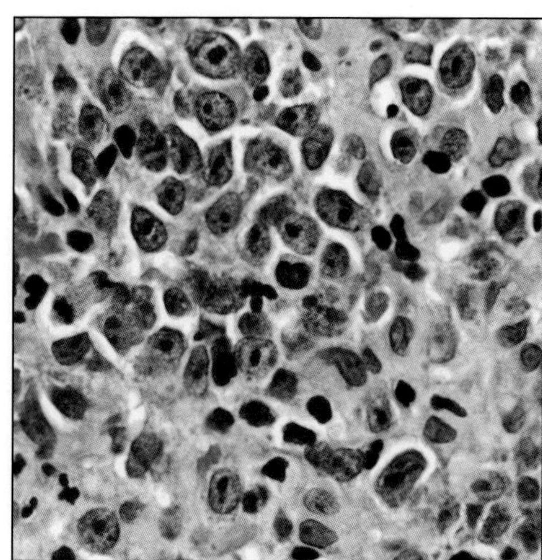

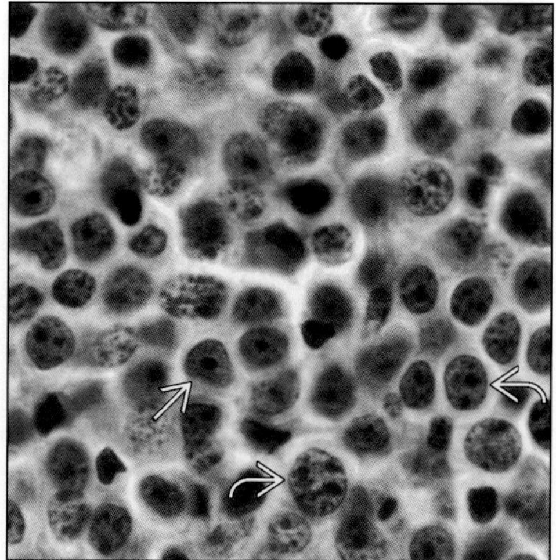

(Left) *Immunoblastic variant of DLBCL is composed of monotonous large cells with central nucleoli & a plasmacytoid appearance. (Courtesy F. Vega, MD, PhD.)* ***(Right)*** *Centroblastic variant of DLBCL shows a mixture of both centroblasts ➢ & immunoblasts →. Centroblasts are characterized by multiple nuclear membrane-bound nucleoli. This variant is the most common among pediatric DLBCLs, though morphologic subtyping is not currently required for treatment.*

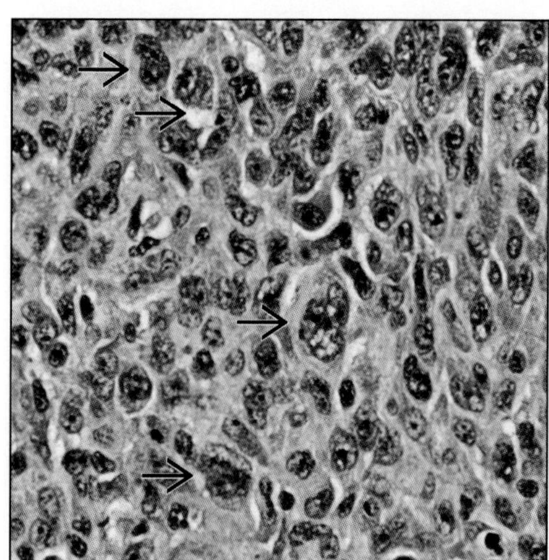

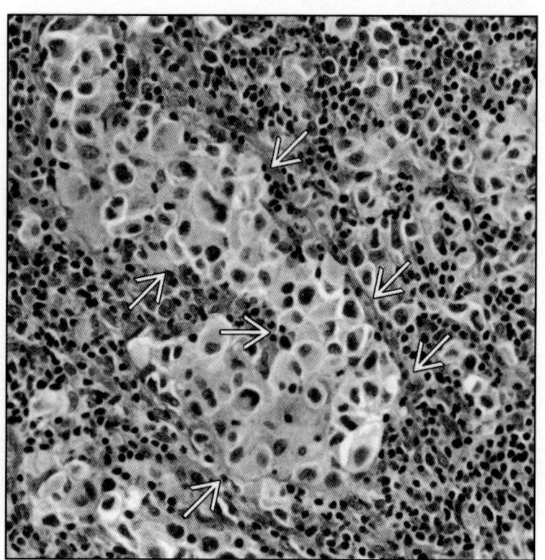

(Left) *The anaplastic variant of DLBCL is characterized by pleomorphic neoplastic cells, mostly large with irregular nuclei, vesicular chromatin, and distinct nucleoli →. This neoplasm was positive for CD20 and CD30. (Courtesy F. Vega, MD, PhD.)* ***(Right)*** *Note the presence of large tumor cells within the sinuses → in this case of DLBCL, anaplastic variant. The neoplasm was positive for CD20, CD30, and CD45 (LCA) and was negative for CD3 and CD15. (Courtesy F. Vega, MD, PhD.)*

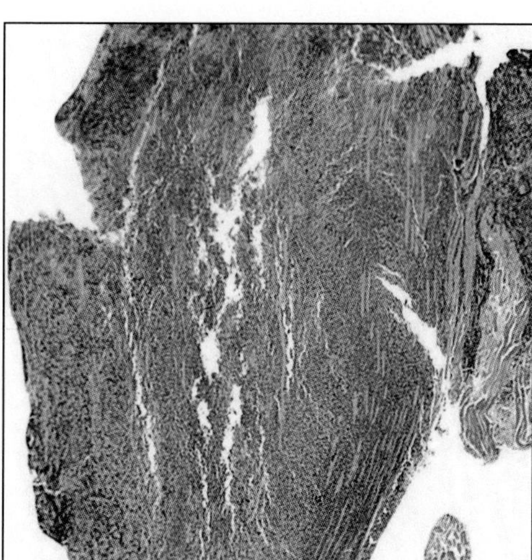

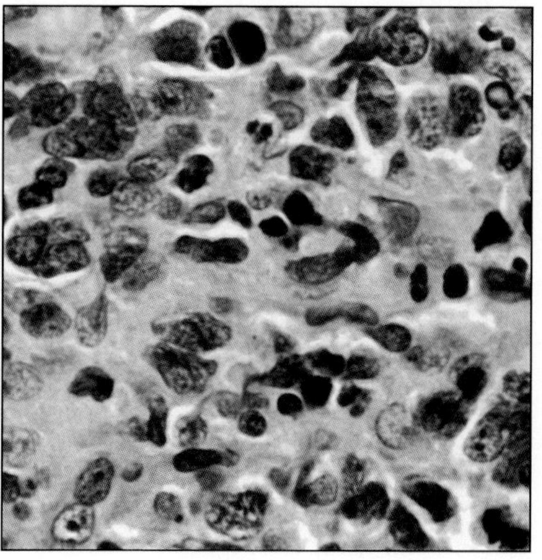

(Left) *A pterygoid mass in a 14-year-old female shows sheets of mononuclear cells infiltrating skeletal muscle. The differential includes many of the small round blue cell tumors.* ***(Right)*** *A pterygoid mass in a young female shows sheets of atypical large cells that stained positive for CD10, CD20, CD79a, and Bcl-6 with a proliferation index of 80-90%. Though the immunophenotype suggests BL, the proliferation index and morphology are most consistent with a DLBCL, anaplastic variant.*

DIFFUSE LARGE B-CELL LYMPHOMA

Microscopic Features and Ancillary Techniques

(Left) An enlarged right cervical lymph node in a 14-year-old male shows complete effacement of the lymph node by numerous small lymphocytes and histiocytes with occasional large atypical cells ➔ that expressed CD20, Bcl-6, pax-5, OCT2, and BOB1 without expression of CD15 and CD30 consistent with TCHRLBCL. ***(Right)*** *Scattered large CD20(+) B cells are shown in this case of TCHRLBCL from an enlarged right cervical lymph node in a 14-year-old male.*

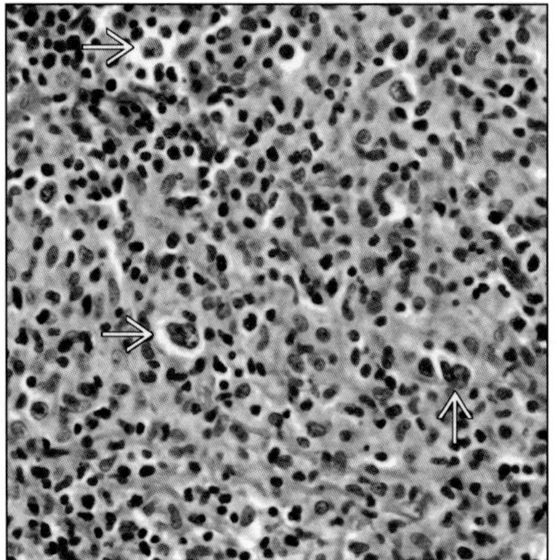

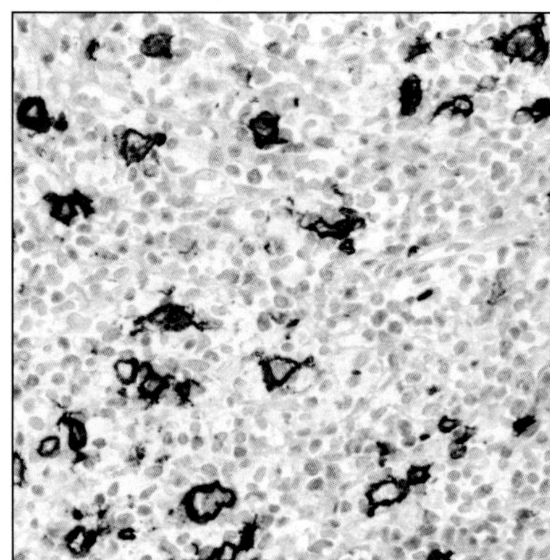

(Left) The large cells in this case of TCHRLBCL show positive nuclear staining for pax-5. The cells also stained positive for CD20, Bcl-6, OCT2, and BOB1. ***(Right)*** *The differential of TCHRLBCL includes NLPHL. Staining for PD-1 (shown here) can help in this differential. In TCHRLBCL PD-1 is negative in the expanded neoplastic areas. Some positive-staining cells may be present, but are typically associated with residual follicles as shown in this example ➔.*

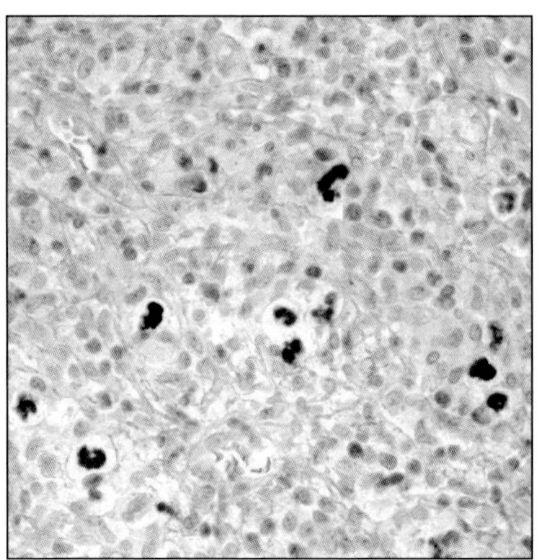

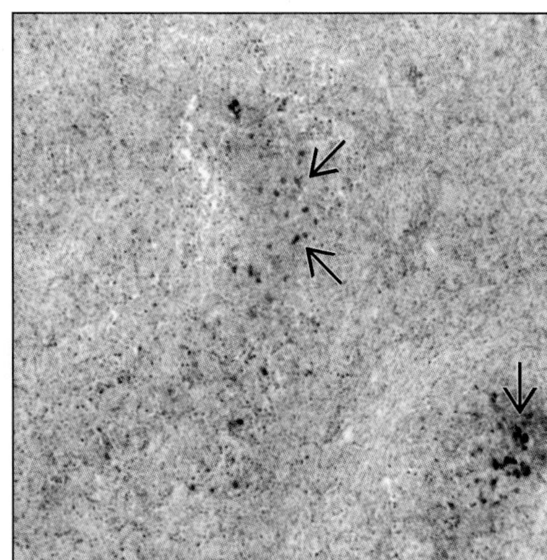

(Left) CD45 highlights sheets of large cells in this DLBCL that also stained positive for CD20 and Bcl-6. ***(Right)*** *Ki-67 (MIB-1) is an important stain to perform in the workup of DLBCL. Evaluation of the proliferation index will help in the differential diagnosis (e.g., atypical BL vs. DLBCL) and though commonly used to help predict prognosis in adults, it may not be as helpful in this regard in pediatric DLBCLs.*

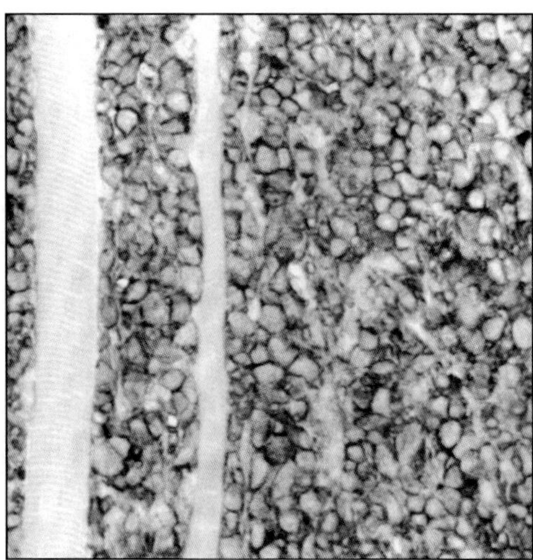

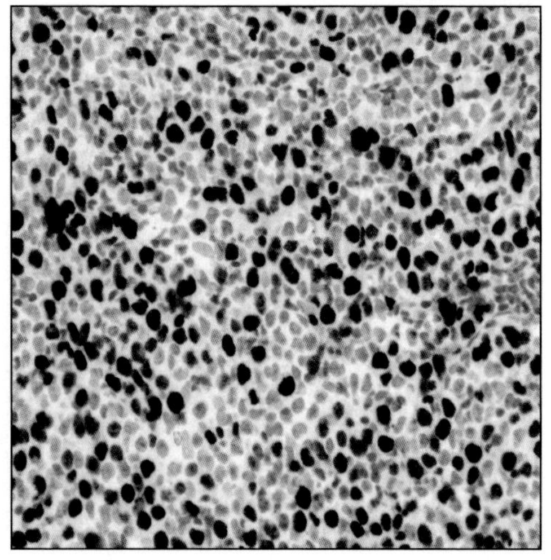

Differential Diagnosis

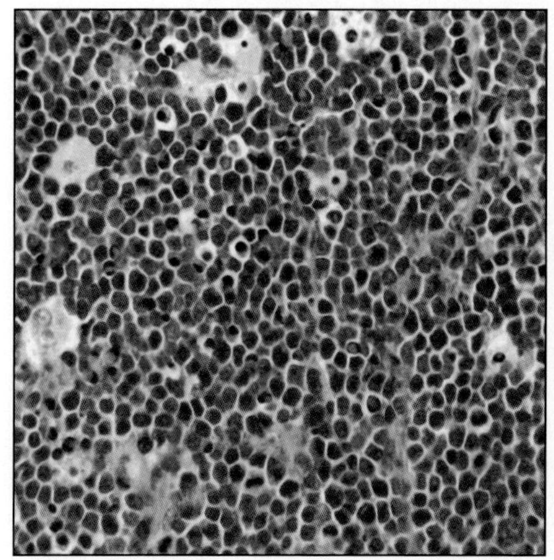

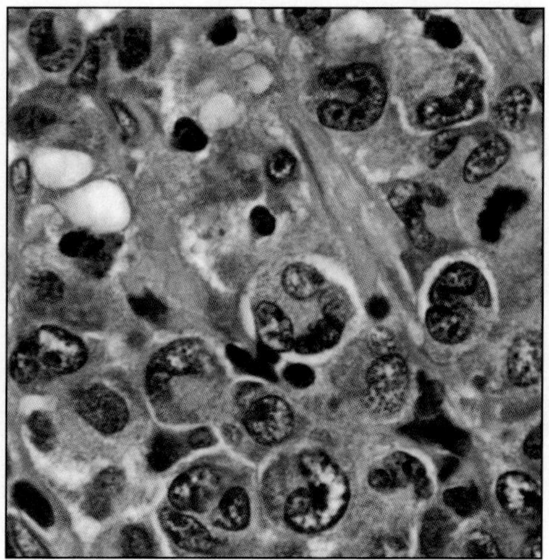

(Left) *An example of BL with sheets of intermediate-sized blue cells and scattered tingible body macrophages is shown for comparison. Note the more compact arrangement, less conspicuous nucleoli, dispersed chromatin, and lack of abundant cytoplasm that are more characteristic of BL.* ***(Right)*** *An example of ALCL that shows the typical "hallmark cells" is shown for comparison. An IHC panel that includes pan-T-cell markers, CD30, and ALK1 will help make the diagnosis.*

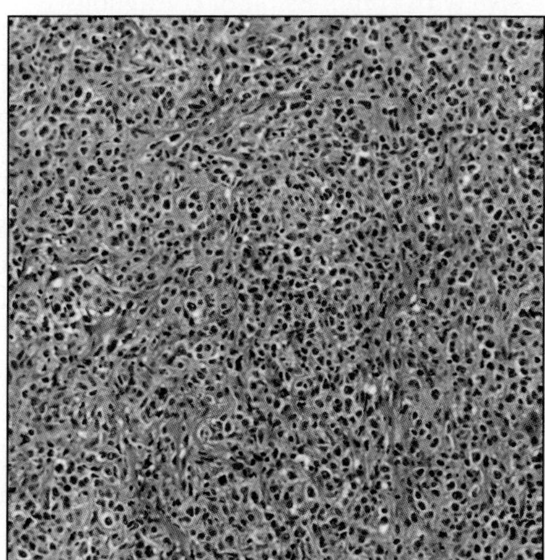

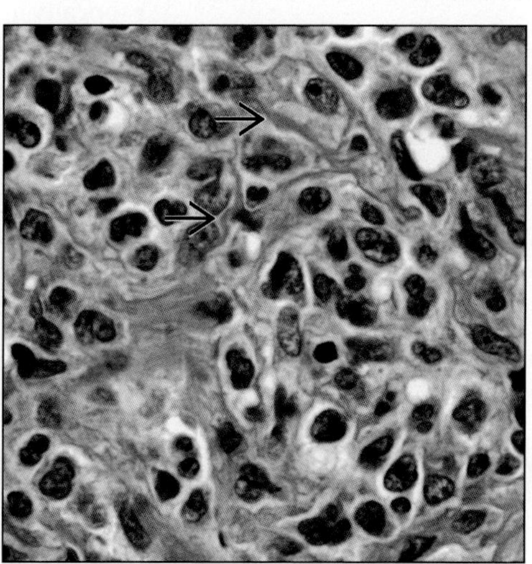

(Left) *The differential of DLBCL arising in the mediastinum often includes PMLBCL as shown here. Clinical correlation in conjunction with morphology and an IHC panel that includes CD30 will help with this differential.* ***(Right)*** *A high-power view of PMLBCL is shown for comparison. Note the fine sclerotic bands* ➔ *that compartmentalize the large B cells, which have pleomorphic nuclei, vesicular chromatin, conspicuous nucleoli, and retracted cytoplasm.*

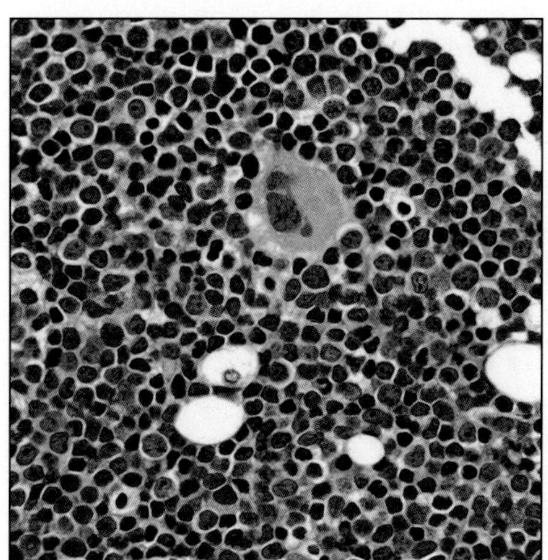

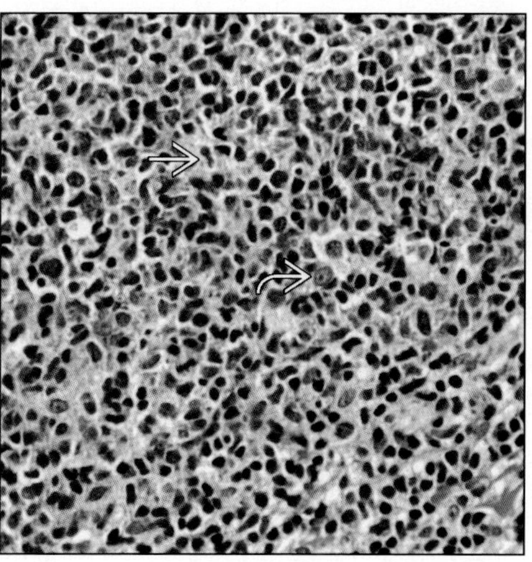

(Left) *B-LBL more commonly shows intermediate-sized cells with fine chromatin and inconspicuous nucleoli as shown here in a bone marrow core biopsy. An IHC panel including both pan-B-cell markers and TdT will help make the correct diagnosis.* ***(Right)*** *A neoplastic follicle in this case of pediatric FL is shown for comparison. Note the mixture of neoplastic large centroblasts* ➔ *and smaller twisted centrocytes* ➔ *that are characteristic of this diagnosis.*

PRIMARY MEDIASTINAL (THYMIC) LARGE B-CELL LYMPHOMA

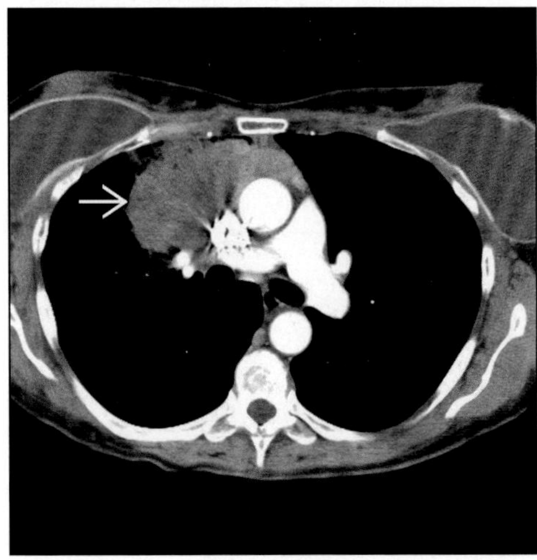

CT scan of a young woman who presented with a large anterior mediastinal mass ➡ shows an example of primary mediastinal large B-cell lymphoma (PMLBCL).

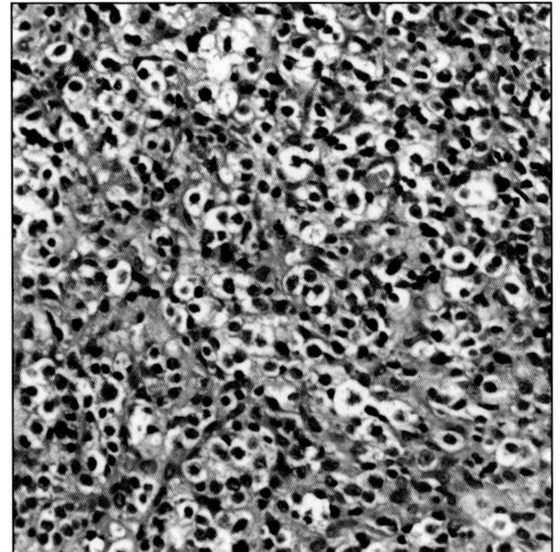

PMLBCL is composed of large cells with pale cytoplasm (retraction artifact) and fine sclerosis compartmentalizing the tumor cells. The neoplastic cells were CD20(+) (not shown).

TERMINOLOGY

Abbreviations

- Primary mediastinal (thymic) large B-cell lymphoma (PMLBCL)

Synonyms

- Mediastinal large B-cell lymphoma
- Thymic large B-cell lymphoma

Definitions

- Diffuse large B-cell lymphoma (DLBCL) arising in mediastinum of putative thymic B-cell origin

ETIOLOGY/PATHOGENESIS

Cell of Origin

- Thymic B cell is presumed

CLINICAL ISSUES

Epidemiology

- Incidence
  - 2% of all non-Hodgkin lymphomas
- Age
  - Most frequent from 20-35 years
- Gender
  - M:F ratio = 1:2

Presentation

- Enlarging mass in anterior-superior mediastinum
- Often manifests as bulky disease defined as > 10 cm in diameter
  - ~ 75% of patients
- B symptoms in 20-30%
- PMLBCL patients have distinctive serum chemistry profile
  - Low serum β2 microglobulin and high lactate dehydrogenase (LDH) levels
- Locally aggressive with compression of contiguous organs
  - Superior vena cava syndrome occurs in up to 30% of patients
- Frequent infiltration of local structures and organs
  - Lung parenchyma, chest wall, pleura, and pericardium
- Extrathoracic disease at diagnosis is rare
- Bone marrow infiltration at presentation is also rare
- Extrathoracic sites are often involved at relapse
  - Central nervous system, liver, adrenals, ovaries, and kidneys

Treatment

- Drugs
  - Systemic chemotherapy is required; many regimens can be used
    - R-CHOP, rituximab, cyclophosphamide, hydroxydaunorubicin (doxorubicin), Oncovin (vincristine), prednisone
    - MACOPB, methotrexate, leucovorin, doxorubicin, cyclophosphamide, vincristine, prednisone, bleomycin
    - DA-EPOCH+R, etoposide, prednisone, vincristine, cyclophosphamide, doxorubicin plus rituximab
    - HyperCVAD-R, high-dose cyclophosphamide, vincristine, doxorubicin, cytarabine, methotrexate, rituximab
  - If risk factors are present, central nervous system prophylaxis is recommended
    - High-dose methotrexate therapy
- Radiation
  - Involved field therapy can be used for patients with bulky disease

Prognosis

- 60-70% chance of cure with appropriate therapy
  - Outcome similar to that of patients with nodal DLBCL

Key Facts

Terminology
- Diffuse large B-cell lymphoma (DLBCL) arising in mediastinum of putative thymic B-cell origin

Clinical Issues
- Most frequent from 20-35 years
- M:F ratio = 1:2
- Enlarging mass in anterior-superior mediastinum
- Frequent infiltration of mediastinal structures and organs
- Prognosis is similar to patients with other types of DLBCL
  - 60-70% chance of cure with appropriate therapy

Microscopic Pathology
- Diffuse to vaguely nodular growth pattern usually associated with variable degrees of sclerosis
- Interstitial sclerosis with compartmentalization of tumor cells
- Hodgkin-like or Reed-Sternberg-like cells can be present

Ancillary Tests
- CD20(+), CD45/LCA(+), IRF-4/MUM1(+/-)
- CD30(+) ~ 75%, usually weak &/or focal
- CD10(-), CD15(-), cyclin-E(-)
- Monoclonal *Ig* gene rearrangements

Top Differential Diagnoses
- Nodular sclerosis Hodgkin lymphoma
- B-cell lymphoma, unclassifiable, with features intermediate between DLBCL and CHL
- Diffuse large B-cell lymphoma
- T-lymphoblastic leukemia/lymphoma

- Recurrences are almost always seen in 1st 2 years of follow-up

IMAGE FINDINGS

Radiographic Findings
- Large mass in anterior-superior mediastinum
- Often FDG PET scan positive

MACROSCOPIC FEATURES

General Features
- Unusual for mass to be resected based on size and location
- In resection specimens, residual thymus gland may be identified
- Currently, diagnosis is often established by needle biopsy

MICROSCOPIC PATHOLOGY

Histologic Features
- Diffuse to vaguely nodular growth pattern usually associated with variable degrees of sclerosis
- Interstitial sclerosis surrounds and compartmentalizes small groups of tumor cells
- Broad collagenous bands divide tumor into large nodules
- Intermediate to large lymphoid cells
  - Pale cytoplasm, often result of retraction artifact
  - HRS-like cells can be present
- Reactive infiltrate of small T lymphocytes and histiocytes
  - ± plasma cells and eosinophils
- Thymic components, such as Hassall corpuscles, may be identified
  - If present, supports thymic involvement and diagnosis of PMLBCL

Cytologic Features
- Large lymphoma cells are present in fine needle aspiration smears
  - Not readily distinguishable from other types of large B-cell lymphoma
  - Extensive sclerosis can reduce yield of neoplastic cells aspirated

ANCILLARY TESTS

Immunohistochemistry
- Positive for common pan-B-cell markers
  - CD19, CD20, CD22, CD79a
- Positive for B-cell transcription factors
  - BOB1, OCT2, PU.1, pax-5
- CD45/LCA(+), p63(+) in ~ 95%
- CD30(+/-) in ~ 75% of cases
  - Expression is usually weak &/or focal
- IRF-4/MUM1(+) in ~ 75%
- CD23(+/-), MAL(+/-)
- Bcl-2(+/-), Bcl-6(+/-); staining intensity can be variable
- CD10(-), CD15(-)
- T-cell antigens(-)
- EBV-LMP is usually negative
- Cyclin-D1(-), cyclin-E(-)

Flow Cytometry
- B-cell immunophenotype
- Discordance in B-cell receptor expression is common in PMLBCL
  - Surface Ig(-) and CD79a(+)
- Variable loss of HLA class I and II (HLA-DR) molecules

Cytogenetics
- Comparative genomic hybridization
  - Common regions of gain
    - Gains in 9p24 ~ 75% and 2p15 ~ 50%
    - Gains in chromosome X and in 12q31
    - *JAK2* at 9p24 is not mutated
  - Common regions of loss
    - 1p, 3p, 13q, 15q, and 17p

PRIMARY MEDIASTINAL (THYMIC) LARGE B-CELL LYMPHOMA

- Well-characterized chromosomal translocations are rare/absent in PMLBCL
  - *CCND1*, *BCL2*, *BCL6*, and *MYC*

In Situ Hybridization

- EBER(-)

Molecular Genetics

- Monoclonal *Ig* gene rearrangements
- No monoclonal T-cell receptor gene rearrangements
- High frequency of *BCL6* gene mutations
- *SOCS1* mutations in subset of cases
- High levels of expression of
  - IL-13 receptor
  - JAK2 and STAT1

Gene Expression Profiling

- Studies have shown overlap in gene expression profile between PMLBCL and classical Hodgkin lymphoma
  - Signature is distinct from nodal DLBCLs
    - Either germinal center B-cell or activated B-cell types

Activation of NF-κB

- Nuclear location of c-REL
- Cytoplasmic expression of TRAF1
- Combination of nuclear c-REL with expression of TRAF1 is highly specific for PMLBCL

DIFFERENTIAL DIAGNOSIS

Nodular Sclerosis (NS) Classical Hodgkin Lymphoma (CHL)

- Usually young patients
- Slight female predominance
- Mediastinal involvement in ~ 80%
- Histologic features
  - Nodular growth pattern with fibrosis
    - Dense collagenous bands surround nodules
    - Collagenous bands are polarizable
  - Variable numbers of large Hodgkin/lacunar and Reed-Sternberg (HRS) cells
  - Many inflammatory cells present
    - Eosinophils, neutrophils, plasma cells
- Many histologic variants of nodular sclerosis CHL have been described
  - Based on number of neoplastic cells, extent and nature of fibrosis, and inflammatory background
  - Syncytial variant is most relevant
    - Sheets of large HRS cells can mimic DLBCL
    - Often large areas of necrosis
    - Immunophenotype typical of CHL
- Immunophenotype of CHL
  - CD30(+), CD15(+/-)
  - pax-5(+) with characteristic weaker (dim) expression than reactive B cells
  - CD20(-/+), CD79a(-/+)
    - Weakly &/or variably positive in 20% of cases
  - Other B-cell transcription factors absent or dimly expressed
  - CD45/LCA(-), EMA usually negative
  - Small subset (~ 5%) of CHL can express T-cell antigens
- Molecular genetic features
  - Monoclonal *IgH* gene rearrangements (+)
    - Best detected by single cell PCR analysis
    - Can be positive by standard PCR methods in cases with many HRS cells
  - No evidence of monoclonal *TCR* gene rearrangements

B-cell Lymphoma with Features Intermediate Between DLBCL and CHL

- Lymphoma with clinical, morphologic, &/or immunophenotypic features between DLBCL and CHL
- Usually young patients
- Male predominance
- Mediastinum is most commonly involved
  - Supraclavicular lymph nodes can be involved
- Histologic features
  - Areas of confluent sheets of pleomorphic large tumor cells resembling DLBCL
  - Other areas can show scattered large cells resembling HRS cells in CHL
- Mixed immunophenotype
  - Expression of common markers of CHL
    - CD30(+) all cases &/or CD15(+/-)
    - pax-5(+) and IRF-4/MUM1(+)
  - Expression of markers usually absent in CHL
    - CD45/LCA(+), CD20(+) uniform and strong, and C79a(+)
    - OCT2(+), BOB1(+)
  - Cells with this "mixed immunophenotype" constitute predominant neoplastic cell population
- Molecular genetic features
  - Most cases have monoclonal *IgH* gene rearrangements
  - Few cases reported have *BCL6* rearrangements

Diffuse Large B-cell Lymphoma

- Older adults, but also occurs in children and young adults
- Histologic features
  - Diffuse growth pattern
  - Large neoplastic cells (centroblasts &/or immunoblasts)
  - Large anaplastic cells can be present; known as anaplastic variant
    - These neoplasms may have intrasinusoidal growth pattern
    - CD30(+/-)
  - Large pleomorphic cells with features of HRS-like cells can be present
  - Sclerosis is frequent in extranodal sites
- Immunophenotype
  - CD19(+), CD20(+), CD22(+), CD79a(+)
  - pax-5(+), OCT2(+), BOB1(+)
  - CD10(+) and Bcl-6(+) in variable proportion of cases
  - CD30(-/+); if positive, often weak and focal except anaplastic variant
  - CD45/LCA(+), CD15(-)
  - Monotypic Ig(+)

        - Cytoplasmic, in cases with plasmacytoid differentiation
        - Surface; best shown by flow cytometry
- Molecular genetic features
    - Monoclonal *IgH* gene rearrangements positive
    - t(14;18)(q32;q21)/*IgH-BCL2*(+) in ~ 20-30%
    - t(3;14)(q27;q32) or other partners with *BCL6* in ~ 20-30%
    - *MYC* translocations or gene rearrangements in ~ 10-15%
- Gene expression profiling has shown 2 subsets
    - Germinal center B cell
    - Activated B cell
        - This subset has poorer prognosis

T-lymphoblastic Leukemia/Lymphoma

- Adolescents and young adults
- Male predominance
- High leukocyte count and bone marrow involvement common
- Large mediastinal mass in ~ 75% of patients
- Histologic features
    - Diffuse pattern
        - "Starry sky" appearance is present in 10-20% of cases
    - Small to medium-sized lymphoblasts with fine ("dusty") nuclear chromatin
    - High mitotic activity
    - Sclerosis can be present, compartmentalizing lymphoma cells in groups
        - This feature can mimic PMLBCL
- Immunophenotype
    - Immature T-cell lineage
        - TdT(+) in almost all cases
        - Variable expression of CD1a, CD2, CD3, CD4, CD5, CD7, and CD8
        - CD34(+/-), CD99(-/+)
- Molecular genetics
    - Monoclonal T-cell receptor gene rearrangements
    - Monoclonal *IgH* gene rearrangements also common
        - Known as "lineage infidelity"

DIAGNOSTIC CHECKLIST

Clinically Relevant Pathologic Features

- Age: 20-35 years
- Gender: Female predominance
- Localization: Anterior mediastinum
- No systemic lymphadenopathy at presentation

Pathologic Interpretation Pearls

- Morphology: Sclerosis
- Immunophenotype characteristic
    - CD45/LCA(+), CD20(+)
    - CD30(+) variable and weak
    - IRF-4/MUM1(+/-), Bcl-2(+/-), Bcl-6(+/-)
    - EBV(-), CD10(-), T-cell markers(-)

Problems with Current Definition of PMLBCL

- Criteria for diagnosis are in large part clinical in patients with DLBCL
    - Location of disease
    - Age and sex of patient
- Cases of nodal DLBCL can involve mediastinal lymph nodes
    - In small biopsy specimens, PMLBCL and nodal DLBCL can be indistinguishable
- In effect, this makes the category of PMLBCL somewhat impure
    - ~ 25% of all cases classified as PMLBCL may instead be nodal DLBCL
- Immunophenotypic or molecular makers that specifically recognize PMLBCL and can be assessed routinely in clinical laboratories are needed

SELECTED REFERENCES

1. Hoeller S et al: BOB.1, CD79a and cyclin E are the most appropriate markers to discriminate classical Hodgkin's lymphoma from primary mediastinal large B-cell lymphoma. Histopathology. 56(2):217-28, 2010
2. Pervez S et al: Mediastinal lymphomas: primary mediastinal (thymic) large B-cell lymphoma versus classical Hodgkin lymphoma, histopathologic dilemma solved? Pathol Res Pract. 206(6):365-7, 2010
3. Salama ME et al: The value of CD23 expression as an additional marker in distinguishing mediastinal (thymic) large B-cell lymphoma from Hodgkin lymphoma. Int J Surg Pathol. 18(2):121-8, 2010
4. Faris JE et al: Primary mediastinal large B-cell lymphoma. Clin Adv Hematol Oncol. 7(2):125-33, 2009
5. Mottok A et al: Inactivating SOCS1 mutations are caused by aberrant somatic hypermutation and restricted to a subset of B-cell lymphoma entities. Blood. 114(20):4503-6, 2009
6. Zinzani PL et al: Rituximab combined with MACOP-B or VACOP-B and radiation therapy in primary mediastinal large B-cell lymphoma: a retrospective study. Clin Lymphoma Myeloma. 9(5):381-5, 2009
7. Rodríguez J et al: Primary mediastinal B-cell lymphoma: treatment and therapeutic targets. Leuk Lymphoma. 49(6):1050-61, 2008
8. Rodig SJ et al: Expression of TRAF1 and nuclear c-Rel distinguishes primary mediastinal large cell lymphoma from other types of diffuse large B-cell lymphoma. Am J Surg Pathol. 31(1):106-12, 2007
9. Weniger MA et al: Gains of REL in primary mediastinal B-cell lymphoma coincide with nuclear accumulation of REL protein. Genes Chromosomes Cancer. 46(4):406-15, 2007
10. Calaminici M et al: CD23 expression in mediastinal large B-cell lymphomas. Histopathology. 45(6):619-24, 2004
11. Pileri SA et al: Primary mediastinal B-cell lymphoma: high frequency of BCL-6 mutations and consistent expression of the transcription factors OCT-2, BOB.1, and PU.1 in the absence of immunoglobulins. Am J Pathol. 162(1):243-53, 2003
12. Lamarre L et al: Primary large cell lymphoma of the mediastinum. A histologic and immunophenotypic study of 29 cases. Am J Surg Pathol. 13(9):730-9, 1989

PRIMARY MEDIASTINAL (THYMIC) LARGE B-CELL LYMPHOMA

Radiologic and Microscopic Features

*(**Left**) Chest radiograph shows a large mediastinal mass in this case of primary mediastinal large B-cell lymphoma. (**Right**) Residual thymic tissue ➚ can be associated with PMLBCL ➙ in excisional biopsy specimens. The identification of thymic tissue is helpful as it supports PMLBCL and is evidence against systemic nodal diffuse large B-cell lymphoma at this site.*

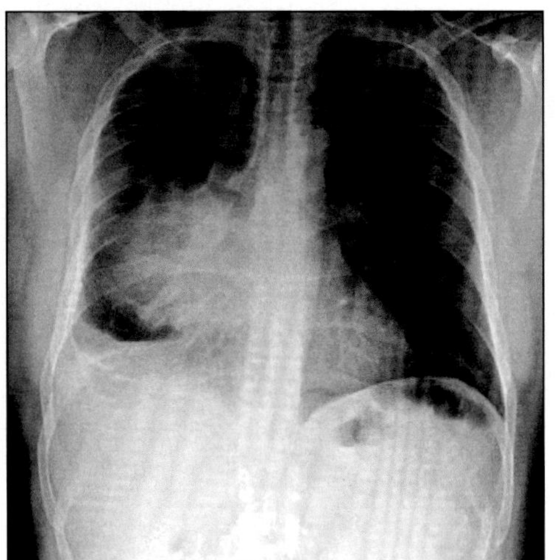

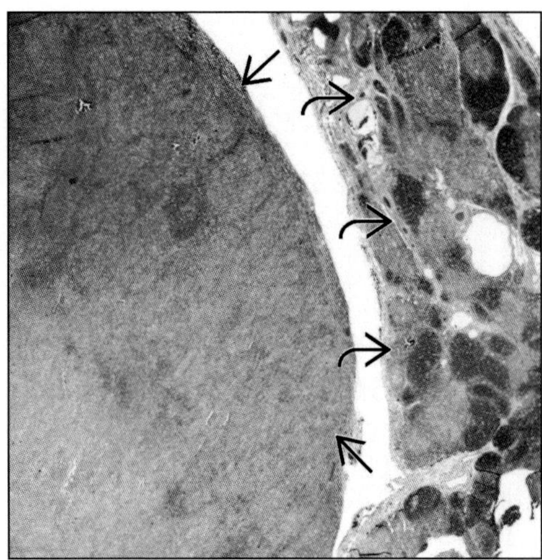

*(**Left**) Primary mediastinal large B-cell lymphoma is shown. The neoplasm has a nodular pattern with nodules partially surrounded by fibrosis ➙. The neoplastic cells were CD20(+), focally CD30(+), CD3(-), and CD10(-) (not shown). (**Right**) Primary mediastinal large B-cell lymphoma is shown. This case is composed of a relatively homogeneous population of medium-sized tumor cells with scattered large and pleomorphic tumor cells ➙.*

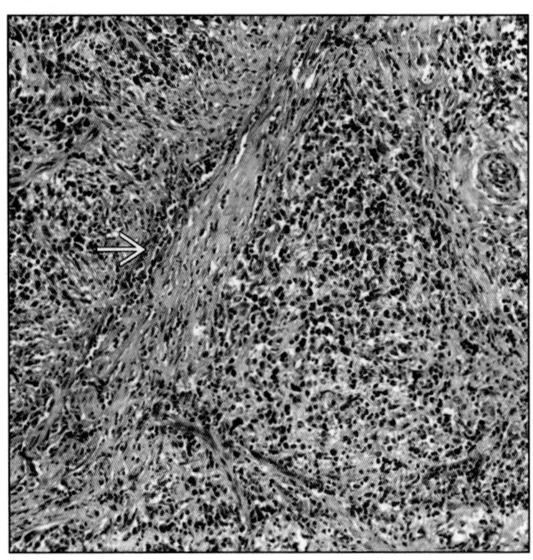

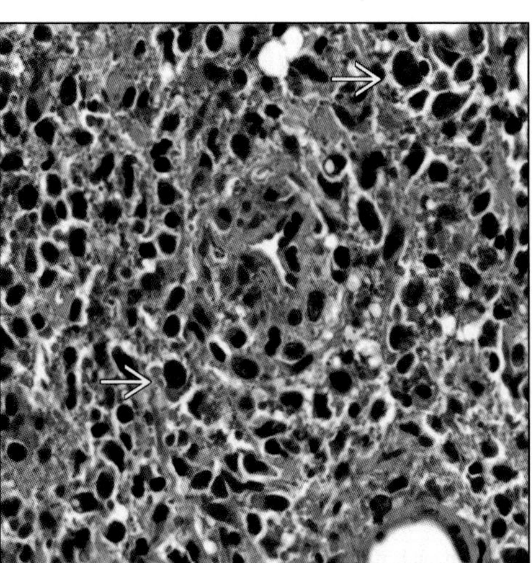

*(**Left**) Scattered large neoplastic cells are present in a background of small lymphocytes resembling T-cell/histiocyte-rich large B-cell lymphoma. In other areas, sheets of large tumor cells were present (not shown). (**Right**) This case of PMLBCL is composed of medium-sized tumor cells with angulated nuclei and scattered large pleomorphic tumor cells ➙ in a background of interstitial fibrosis.*

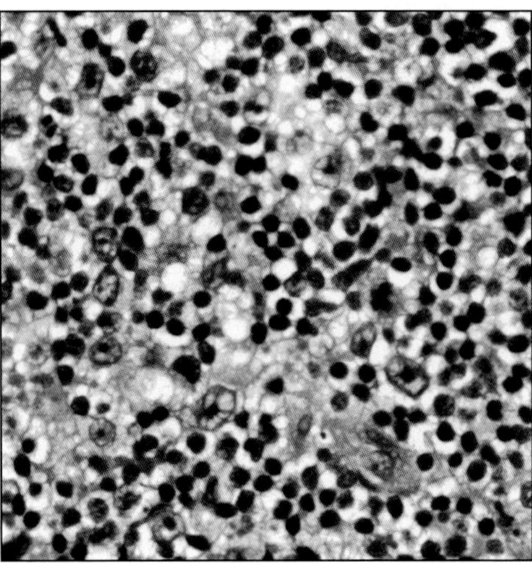

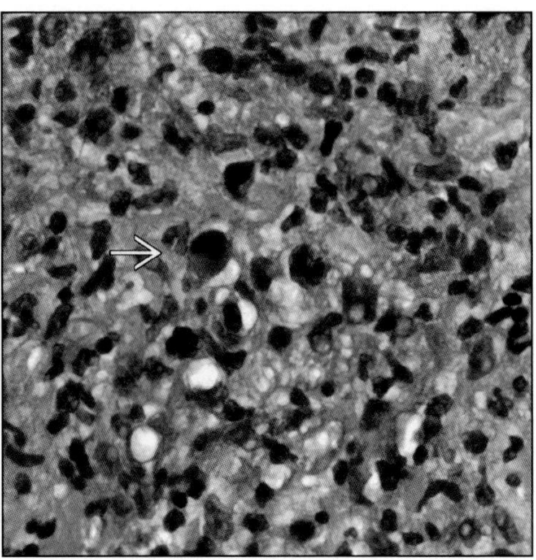

Microscopic Features

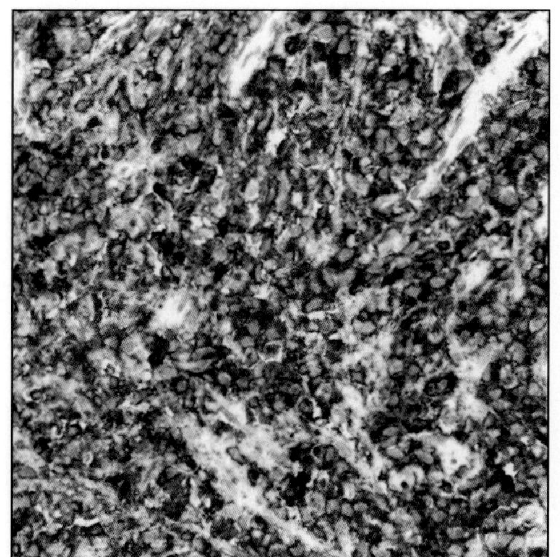

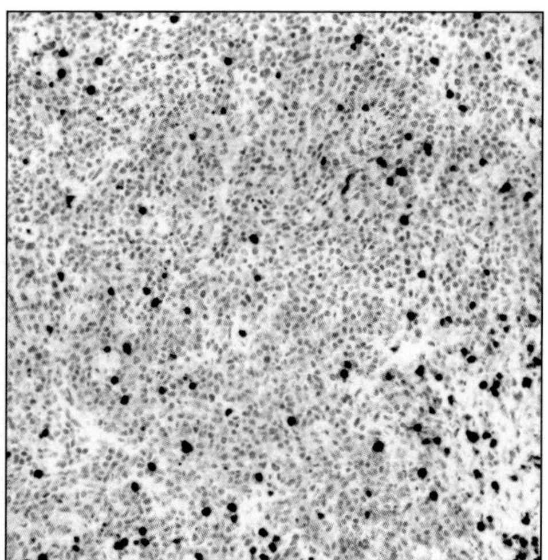

(Left) *The tumor cells are strongly and uniformly positive for CD20 as well as other B-cell markers (not shown).* ***(Right)*** *The tumor cells are usually negative for T-cell markers, including CD3. PMLBCL are also usually negative for CD10, CD15, and EBER (not shown).*

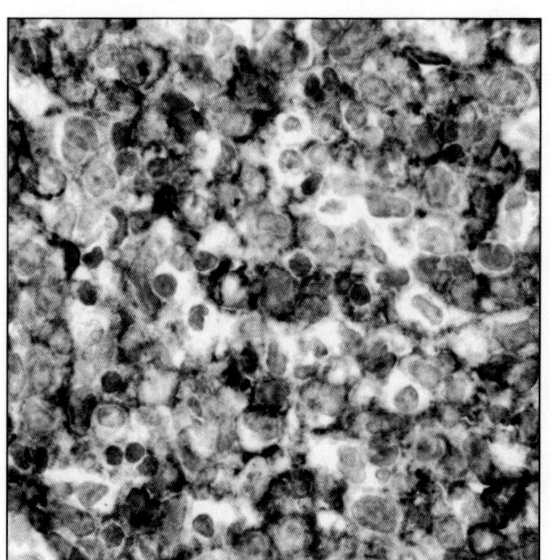

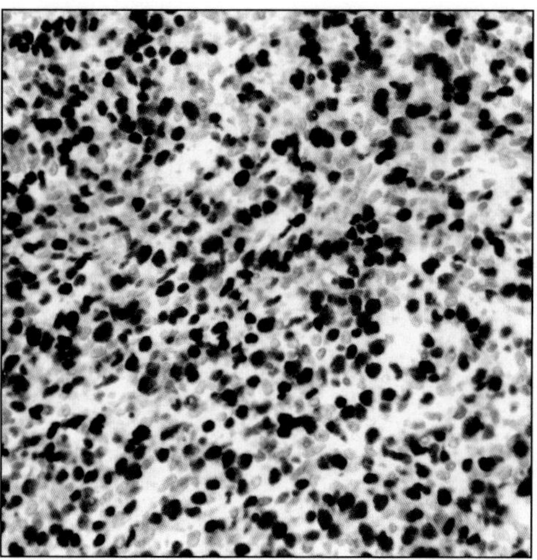

(Left) *The tumor cells in this case are strongly but focally positive for CD30. The quality of this positivity is different from that found in classical Hodgkin lymphoma (bright and homogeneous).* ***(Right)*** *The tumor cells in this case are brightly and uniformly IRF-4/MUM1(+). This antigen is expressed in most cases (~ 75%) of PMLBCL.*

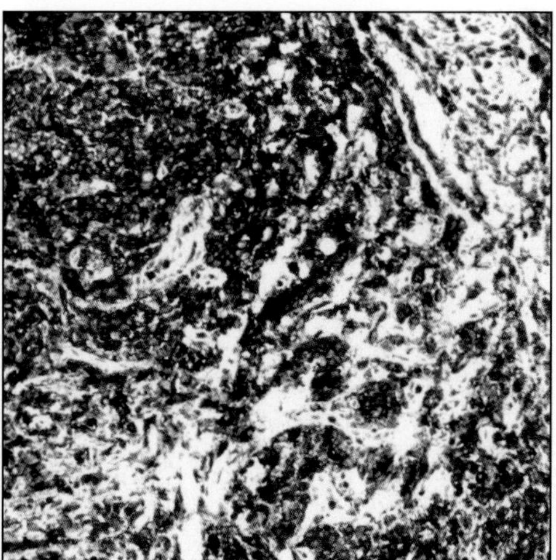

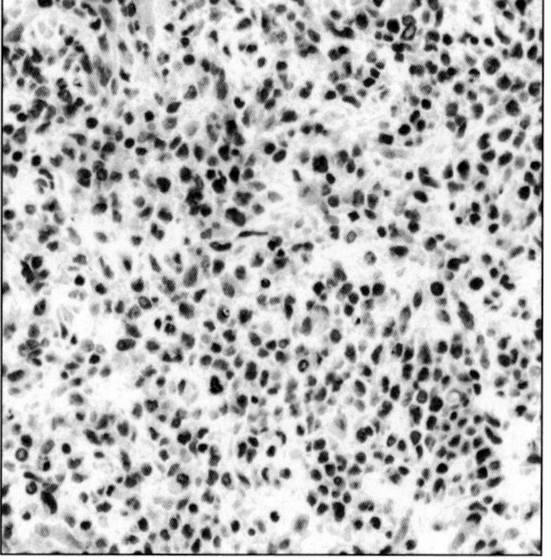

(Left) *The tumor cells are strongly CD45/LCA positive in this case.* ***(Right)*** *The tumor cells are negative for TdT. TdT is positive in lymphoblastic lymphomas/leukemias of B- and T-cell lineages. T-cell lymphoblastic lymphoma/leukemia typically occurs as a mediastinal mass, often with superior vena cava obstruction in adolescents and young adult men.*

PRIMARY MEDIASTINAL (THYMIC) LARGE B-CELL LYMPHOMA

Microscopic Features

(Left) Needle biopsy specimen shows 2 cores of tissue. Needle biopsy, often performed with fine needle aspiration and flow cytometry immunophenotyping, is a very common method for establishing the diagnosis of PMLBCL. **(Right)** This field shows abundant thin strands of sclerosis ⇨ that partially surround and compartmentalize the neoplastic cells.

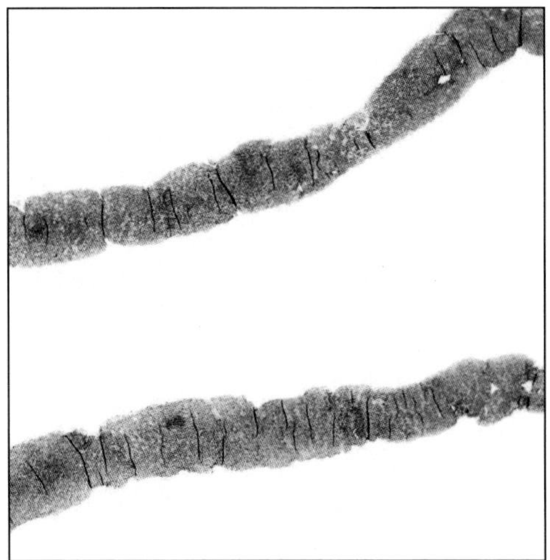

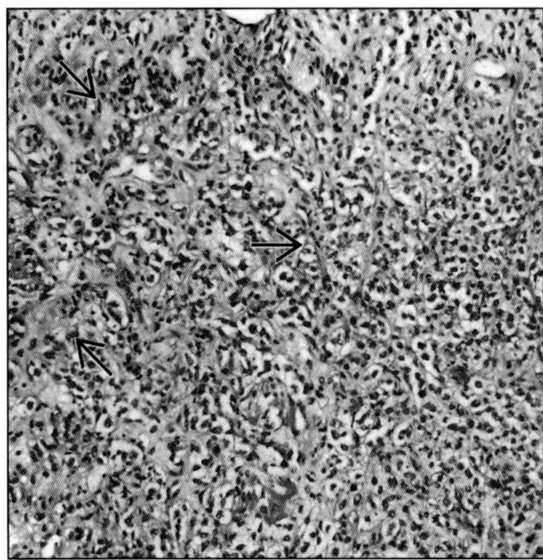

(Left) In this field, the neoplastic cells are large and exhibit artifactual retraction of the cytoplasm, imparting a clear appearance. A thin band of sclerosis ➡ is also present in this field. **(Right)** The neoplastic cells are brightly CD20(+). CD20 expression in classical Hodgkin lymphoma is usually dim and variable, unlike the pattern shown here.

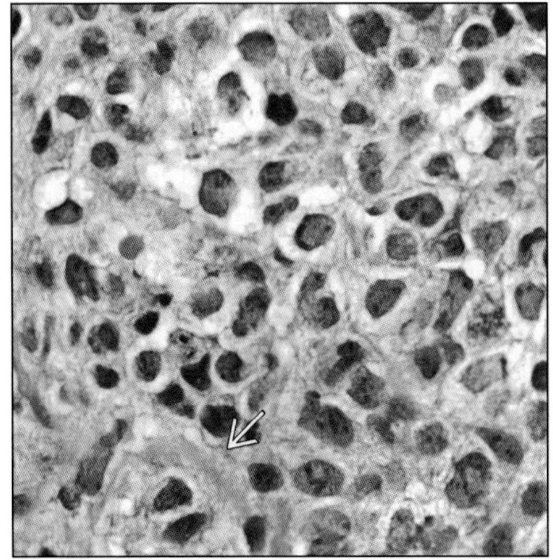

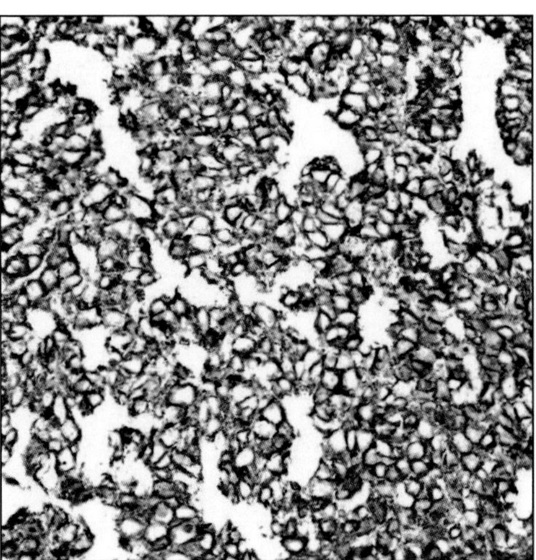

(Left) The neoplastic cells are dimly CD30(+). This pattern of CD30 expression is common in PMLBCL and not seen in most cases of classical Hodgkin lymphoma. **(Right)** The neoplastic cells are CD3(-). Small reactive T cells are CD3(+) and serve as an internal control for this immunostain.

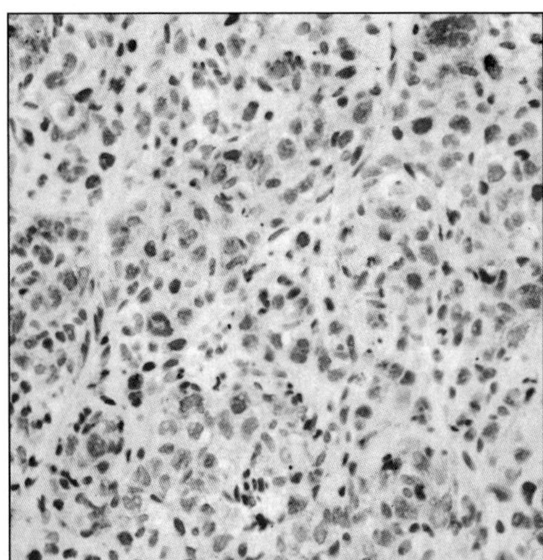

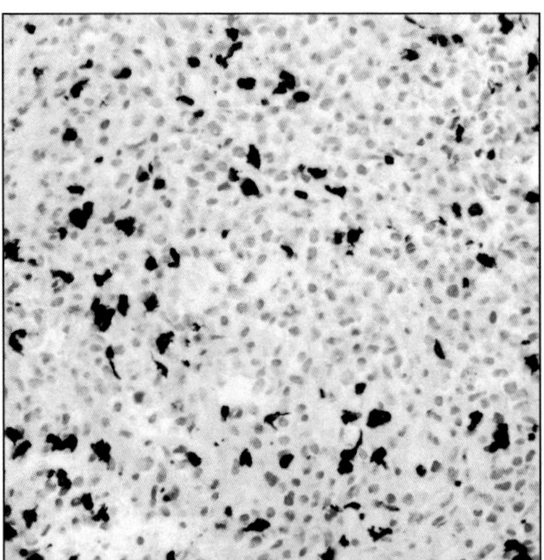

Differential Diagnosis

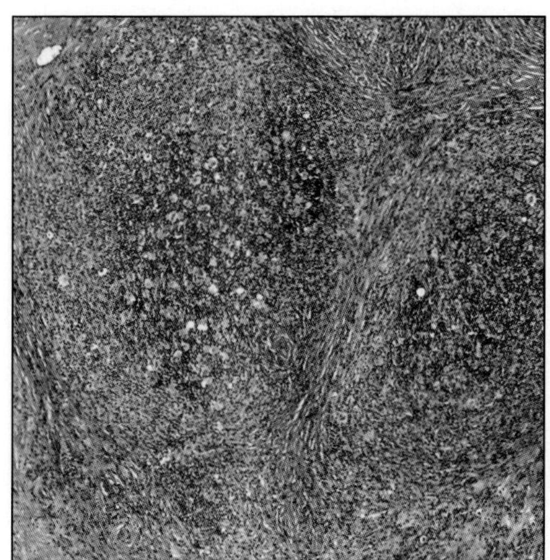

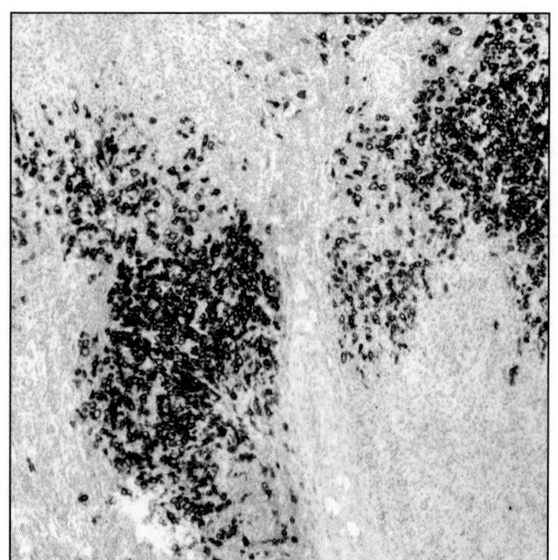

(Left) *This is a case of nodular sclerosis Hodgkin lymphoma (NSHL). The neoplasm is nodular with nodules surrounded by collagen bands.* ***(Right)*** *Inside the nodules of NSHL, the large tumor cells are uniformly and strongly CD30(+) (shown). The neoplastic cells were also pax-5(+) and CD15(+), and were CD20(-) and CD45/LCA(-) (not shown). This immunophenotype supports the diagnosis of NSHL.*

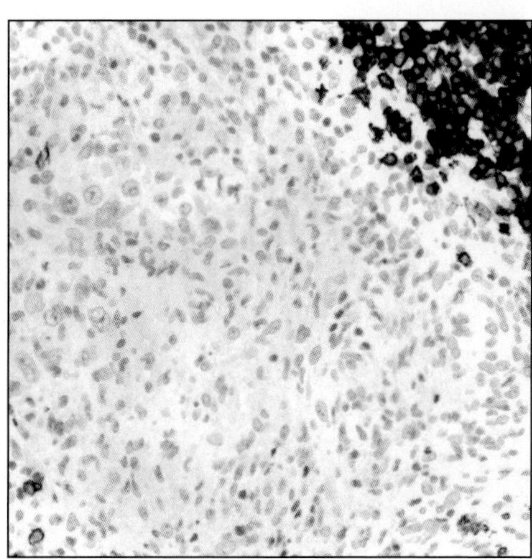

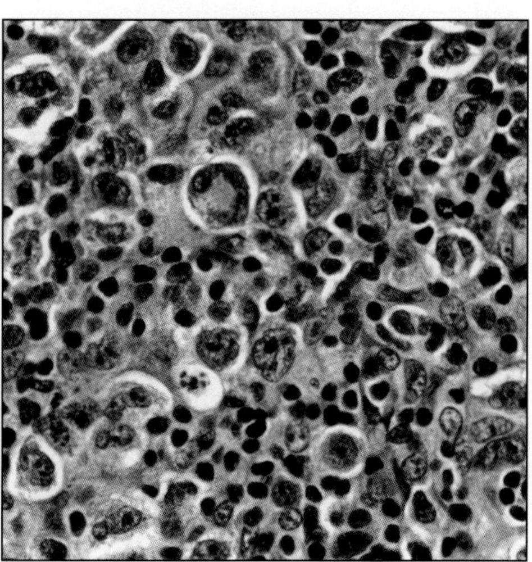

(Left) *In classical Hodgkin lymphoma, tumor cells are characteristically negative for CD45/LCA. Note presence of reactive lymphoid cells (right upper corner) that are CD45/LCA(+).* ***(Right)*** *This case of syncytial variant NSHL shows sheets of large neoplastic cells with few eosinophils in the background. Note presence of many large pleomorphic tumor cells. Tumor cells were CD30(+), CD15(+), pax-5(+) and EBER(+), and CD3(-), CD20(-), and CD45/LCA(-) (not shown).*

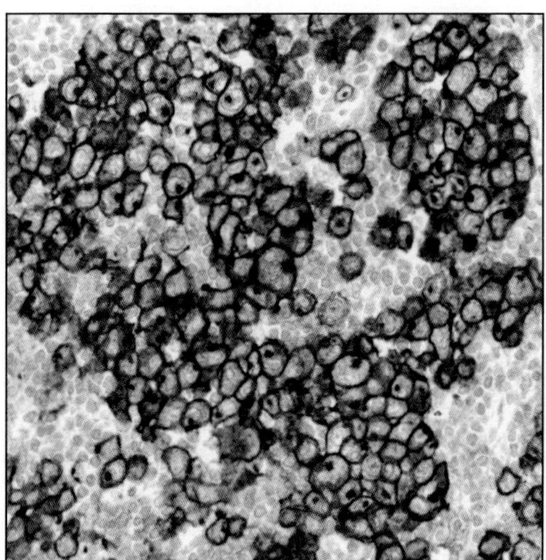

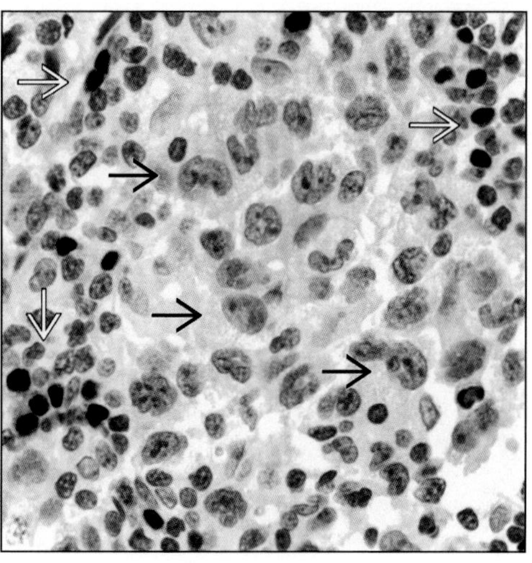

(Left) *Syncytial variant of NSHL shows sheets of large neoplastic cells strongly and uniformly CD30(+).* ***(Right)*** *In classical Hodgkin lymphoma, the tumor cells are characteristically weakly positive for pax-5 ⇒. Note the presence of reactive small B cells strongly pax-5(+) ➡.*

PRIMARY MEDIASTINAL (THYMIC) LARGE B-CELL LYMPHOMA

Differential Diagnosis

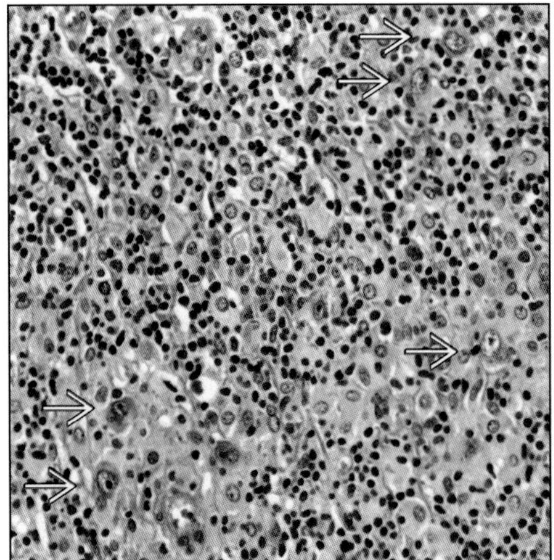

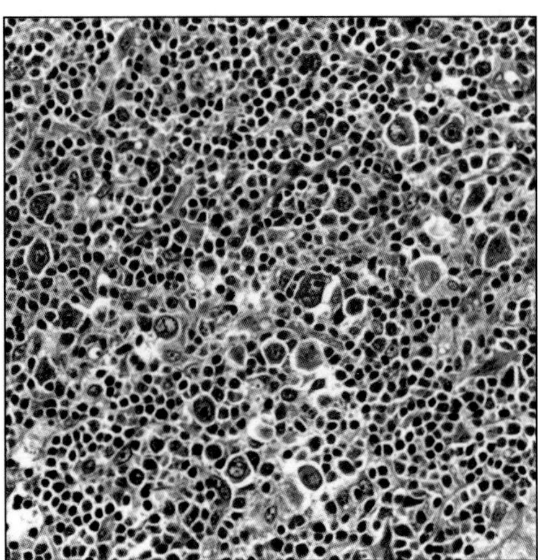

(Left) *A case of B-cell lymphoma, unclassifiable, with features intermediate between diffuse large B-cell lymphoma and classical Hodgkin lymphoma (DLBCL/CHL) is characterized by scattered large tumor cells with large eosinophilic nucleoli ➡ in a background of numerous small lymphocytes.* ***(Right)*** *This case of DLBCL/CHL shows areas of scattered large neoplastic cells in a background of small lymphocytes resembling CHL. In other areas, there are sheets of large tumor cells resembling DLBCL.*

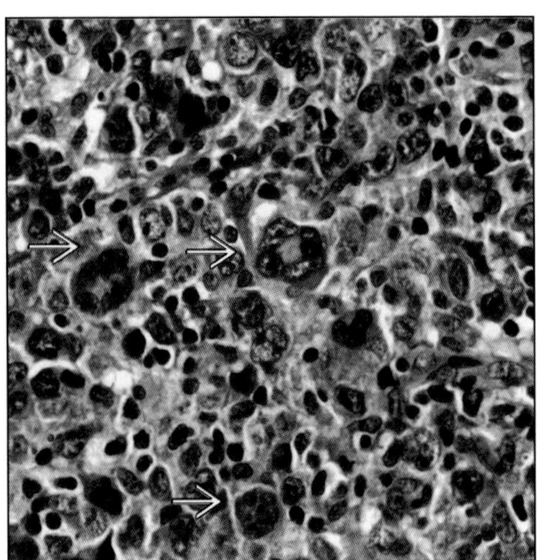

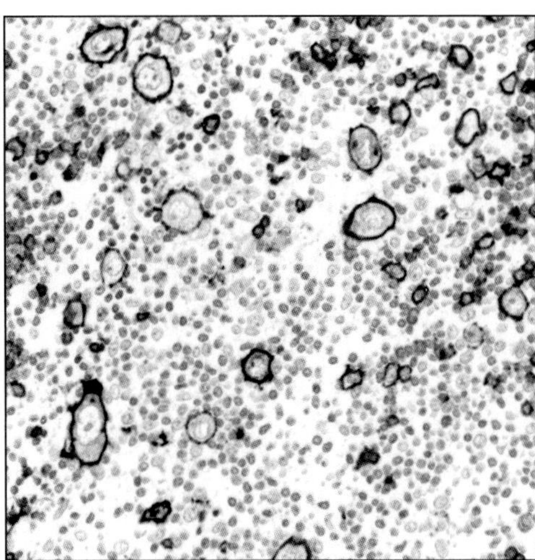

(Left) *This case of DLBCL/CHL is composed of large and very pleomorphic tumor cells, some of which are multinucleated ➡.* ***(Right)*** *The tumor cells in this case of DLBCL/CHL are brightly CD20(+). Although CD20 may be weakly and focally positive in a subset of CHL, strong and uniform expression is unusual. This case also has diffuse areas of tumor cells resembling DLBCL.*

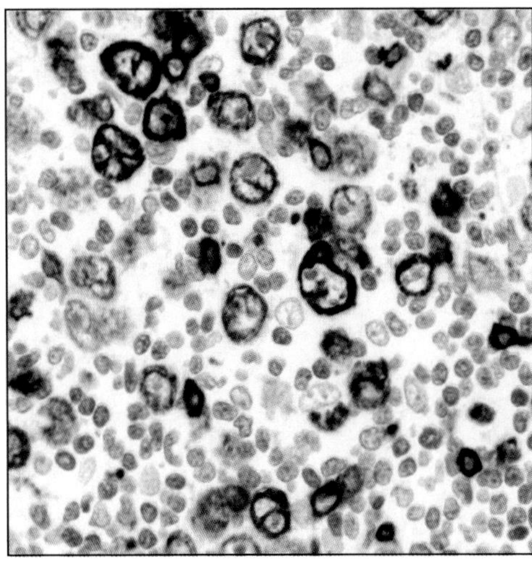

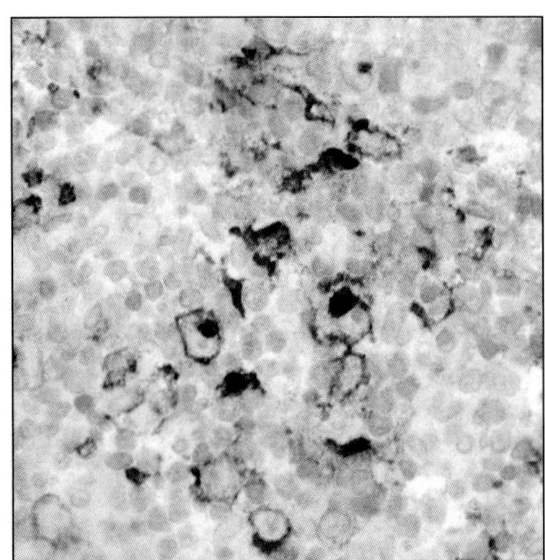

(Left) *In this case of DLBCL/CHL, the tumor cells are brightly CD79a(+). CD79a is uncommonly expressed in CHL. This case also has diffuse areas resembling DLBCL.* ***(Right)*** *DLBCL/CHL shows focal positivity for CD30. Note that the tumor cells show variable degrees of CD30 expression, and the variable size of the neoplastic cells is also highlighted by CD30. CHL is usually characterized by a strong and uniform positivity for CD30. The tumor cells are also usually large in size.*

Differential Diagnosis

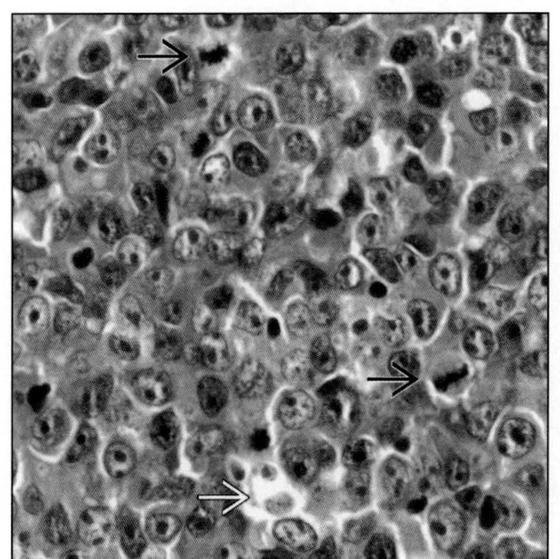

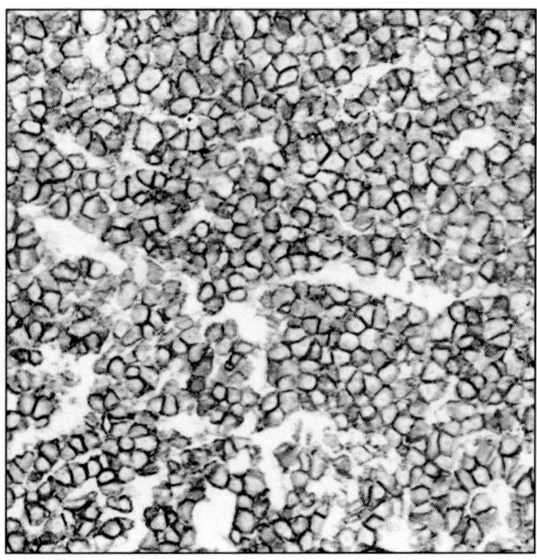

(Left) *Diffuse large B-cell lymphoma (DLBCL), immunoblastic variant, shows large immunoblasts compared with the size of histiocyte nuclei ➡. Immunoblasts have a single, central, prominent nucleolus. Note the presence of several mitoses ➡.* ***(Right)*** *In this case of DLBCL, immunoblastic variant, the neoplastic cells are strongly CD20(+).*

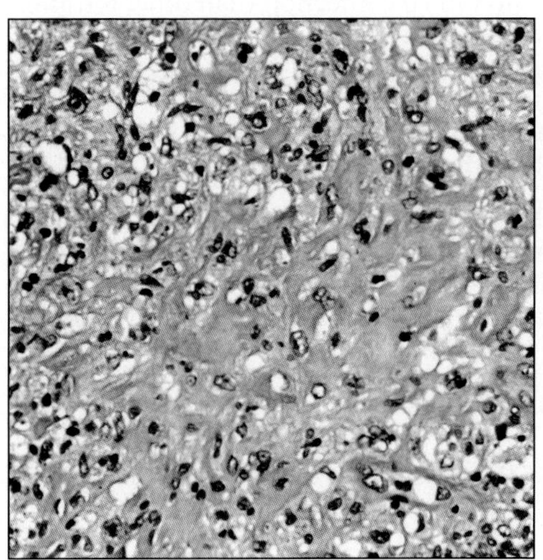

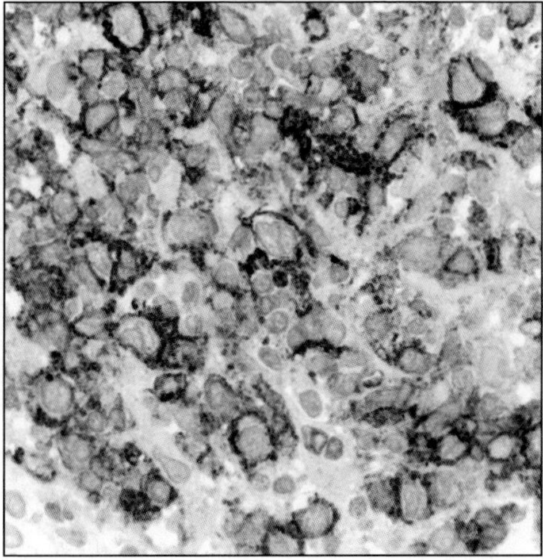

(Left) *DLBCL, centroblastic variant, associated with marked sclerosis is shown. The centroblasts are large with vesicular nuclear chromatin and cleaved nuclei. Sclerosis is frequently seen in cases of DLBCL involving extranodal sites.* ***(Right)*** *Nodal DLBCL, centroblastic variant, shows large tumor cells that are CD10(+). PMLBCL is characteristically negative for CD10.*

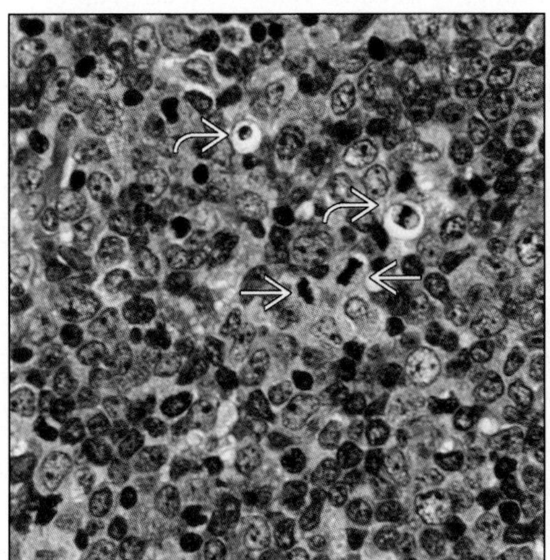

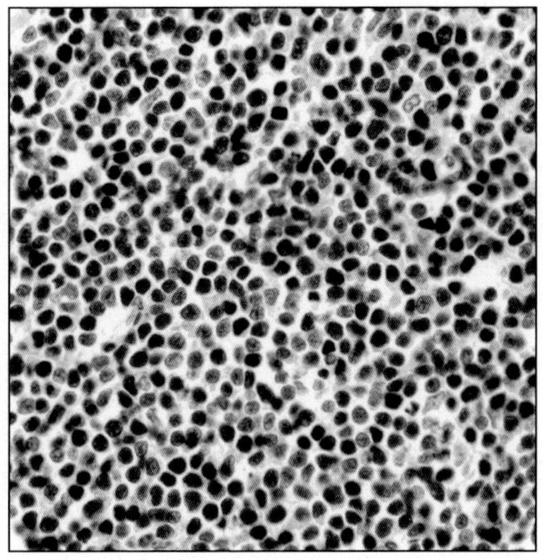

(Left) *T-lymphoblastic leukemia/lymphoma is composed of lymphoblasts with irregular nuclear contours, fine chromatin (blastic appearance), small nucleoli, and a high mitotic rate. Note presence of several mitoses ➡ and apoptotic bodies ➡.* ***(Right)*** *TdT shows T-lymphoblastic leukemia/lymphoma. The lymphoblasts are usually TdT(+). Tumor cells also express T-cell antigens, such as CD1a, CD2, CD3, CD4, CD5, CD7, and CD8 in accord with their stage of differentiation.*

BURKITT LYMPHOMA

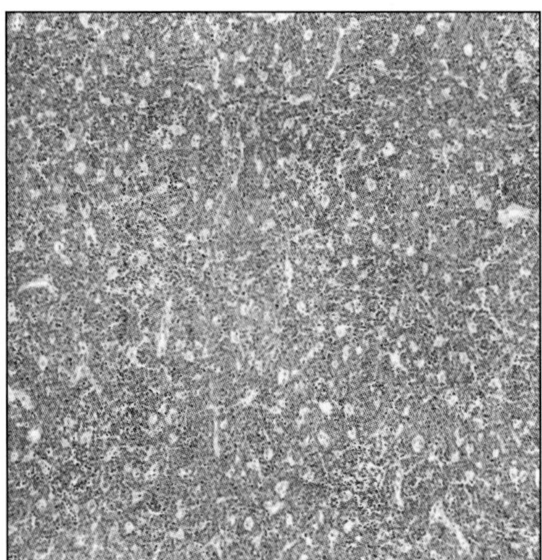

The characteristic diffuse pattern of growth with a "starry sky" pattern is shown. The "starry sky" pattern is indicative of a high proliferation index and is not specific for Burkitt lymphoma.

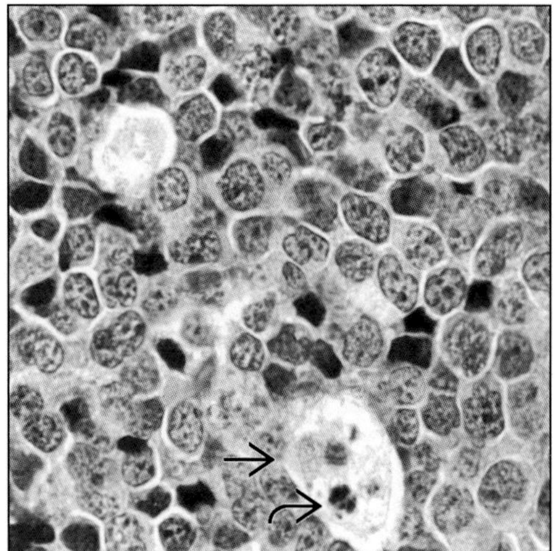

High-power view highlights a macrophage ➡ engulfing an apoptotic cell ↪. The scattered pale-appearing macrophages are what impart the "starry sky" pattern seen on low-power views.

TERMINOLOGY

Abbreviations

- Burkitt lymphoma (BL)

Definitions

- Aggressive B-cell non-Hodgkin lymphoma with extremely high proliferation index and characteristic translocation involving chromosome 8q24 (*MYC*)
- 3 clinical variants are recognized
  - Endemic BL
  - Sporadic BL
  - Immunodeficiency-associated BL

ETIOLOGY/PATHOGENESIS

Infectious Agents

- **Endemic BL**
  - EBV present in nearly all cases (98%)
    - Increased viral loads and early infection are known risk factors for tumor development
  - Strong epidemiological link with holoendemic *Plasmodium falciparum* malaria and EBV infection
    - Thought to be polymicrobial disease associated with interaction of 2 pathogens (*P. falciparum* and EBV)
    - Thought to be related to an exhausted EBV-specific T-cell response, reactivation of latently infected memory B cells, &/or chronic B-cell activation/stimulation
    - Arboviruses and plant tumor promoters (*Euphorbia tirucalli*) are other possible cofactors
- **Sporadic BL**
  - EBV present in subset of cases (20-30%)
  - Low socioeconomic status and early EBV infection associated with higher incidence of EBV positive sporadic BL
- **Immunodeficiency-associated BL**
  - EBV present in subset of cases (30-40%)
  - More common in HIV infection than other forms of immunosuppression
    - Can occur with high CD4 T-cell counts in HIV infection
  - May be related to polyclonal B-cell activation seen in both HIV infection and malaria

Cytogenetics

- Chromosomal translocations involving *MYC* (8q24) are key in all types of BL
- Provides dramatic growth advantage to affected cell

CLINICAL ISSUES

Epidemiology

- Incidence
  - **Endemic BL**
    - 4-10 cases/100,000 children
    - M > F (2:1)
    - Occurs primarily in equatorial Africa and Papua, New Guinea
    - Most common malignant neoplasm in children under 15 years
  - **Sporadic BL**
    - 0.3 cases/100,000
    - M > F (3:1)
    - Occurs in industrialized nations
    - More common in Caucasians than Asian or African-Americans (10:1)
    - Represents 40% of all childhood lymphomas
  - **Immunodeficiency-associated BL**
    - Incidence is low
    - Overall incidence of lymphoma in HIV(+) patients is decreasing in era of highly active antiretroviral therapy

Site

- **General**
  - Extranodal sites (most often involved)
  - Lymph node presentation more common in adults

BURKITT LYMPHOMA

Key Facts

Terminology
- Aggressive B-cell non-Hodgkin lymphoma with extremely high proliferation index and characteristic translocation involving chromosome 8q24 (*c-Myc*)
- 3 clinical variants (endemic BL, sporadic BL, immunodeficiency-associated BL)

Clinical Issues
- Often present with bulky disease/high tumor burden
- Leukemic presentation is rare

Microscopic Pathology
- Diffuse proliferation of medium-sized blastic tumor cells
- Proliferation index of nearly 100%
- "Starry sky" pattern

Ancillary Tests
- Immunophenotype
  - C10(+), CD19(+), CD20(+), Bcl-6(+), Ki-67(+ > 95%); TdT(-), Bcl-2(-)
- Recommended IHC panel
  - CD10, CD20, Bcl-6, Bcl-2, Ki-67
- MYC translocation partners include 14q32, 2p11, and 22q11

Top Differential Diagnoses
- Diffuse large B-cell lymphoma
- B- or T-lymphoblastic leukemia/lymphoma
- B-cell lymphoma, unclassifiable, with features intermediate between DLBCL and BL
- Small round blue cell tumors
- Myeloid sarcoma

  - Waldeyer ring and mediastinum (rare)
- **Endemic BL**
  - Jaw and other facial bones (50-60%)
  - Breast and abdomen
  - Bone marrow in < 10%
  - Typically lack leukemic presentation
- **Sporadic BL**
  - Abdominal mass (most common)
    - Ileocecal region
  - Ovaries, kidneys, breasts
  - Jaw tumors (rare)
- **Immunodeficiency-associated BL**
  - Nodal and bone marrow involvement are frequent

Presentation
- Often present with bulky disease/high tumor burden
  - Advanced stage III/IV
- Symptoms often present for only a few weeks
- Leukemic presentation is rare
  - Burkitt leukemia variant (acute lymphocytic leukemia; L3, FAB classification)
  - Present with peripheral blood and bone marrow involvement

Laboratory Tests
- Lactate dehydrogenase (LDH)
  - Stage and serum LDH levels correlate with tumor burden
  - LDH < 400 U/L correlates with stage I or II disease
  - LDH > 400 U/L correlates with advanced stage III or IV disease

Treatment
- Cyclical intensive chemotherapy and aggressive intrathecal prophylaxis
  - May experience tumor lysis syndrome
- Addition of rituximab may be beneficial
- Cure rates of up to 90% in low-stage disease and 60-80% in advanced disease
- Relapse typically occurs 1 year from diagnosis

Prognosis
- Endemic and sporadic BL
  - Highly aggressive
  - Curable
  - Better prognosis for children than adults

MACROSCOPIC FEATURES

General Features
- Tan-yellow cut surface
- ± hemorrhage and necrosis

MICROSCOPIC PATHOLOGY

Microscopic Features
- Microscopic features of clinical variants are identical
- Diffuse proliferation of medium-sized blastic tumor cells
  - Squared-off borders with retracted cytoplasm (fixation artifact)
  - Round nuclei with finely clumped and dispersed chromatin
  - Multiple paracentric nucleoli
  - Deeply basophilic cytoplasm ± vacuoles
- Numerous mitotic figures
  - Proliferation index of nearly 100%
- "Starry sky" pattern
  - Imparted by numerous benign macrophages
  - Related to high proliferation index/high cell turnover
  - Florid granulomatous pattern may be present
- BL with plasmacytoid differentiation
  - Eccentric basophilic cytoplasm
  - Single central nucleolus
  - Occasionally observed in children
  - More common in immunodeficiency states
- Atypical BL
  - More pleomorphic nuclei
  - More prominent nucleoli
  - Share a similar gene expression profile to classic BL
  - Distinguish from diffuse large B-cell lymphoma (DLBCL) and B-cell lymphoma, unclassifiable with features intermediate between DLBCL and BL

BURKITT LYMPHOMA

ANCILLARY TESTS

Cytogenetics

- *MYC* translocations at band 8q24
  - Partners include
    - *IgH* (14q32) in 80%
    - κ light chain (2p11) in 15%
    - λ light chain (22q11) in 5%
    - Non-Ig partners are rare
  - Not specific for BL
- 10% of cases may lack demonstrable *MYC* translocation by FISH
  - Translocation often shown by other techniques
  - If negative, other characteristics must be present to make diagnosis
- Other genetic and epigenetic alterations involve
  - *BAX*, p16, p53, p73, p130/Rb2, and *BCL6*
  - Additional (complex) cytogenetics more common in adults
    - Distinguish from DLBCL and B-cell lymphoma, unclassifiable with features intermediate between DLBCL and BL
  - Additional abnormalities correlate with poorer prognosis

In Situ Hybridization

- Epstein-Barr virus encoded RNA (EBER)
  - Convenient method for detecting EBV in BL
  - EBNA1 antigen is also expressed (type I latency pattern)

Gene Expression Profiling

- Gene expression signature unique to BL and distinct from DLBCL in most cases

Immunophenotype

- Express
  - Moderate to strong levels of IgM and surface light chains
  - B-cell associated antigens (CD19, CD20, CD22, CD79a)
  - CD10, CD38, CD43, CD45, Bcl-6
    - Germinal center B-cell phenotype (CD10[+], Bcl-6[+], MUM1[-])
  - Ki-67/MIB-1 (95% or higher positivity)
- Do not express
  - Bcl-2 (rarely show weak staining)
    - More often seen in adults
    - If present, must show other characteristic features of BL (morphology and *Ig/MYC* translocation) and lack *BCL2* or *BCL6* translocations to be classified as BL
  - TdT
  - MUM1/IRF-4 (positive in a subset)
- **Recommended IHC panel**
  - CD10, CD20, Bcl-6, Bcl-2, Ki-67

DIFFERENTIAL DIAGNOSIS

Diffuse Large B-cell Lymphoma

- Proliferation of large neoplastic cells with pleomorphic nuclei and vesicular chromatin
- Lacks "starry sky" pattern
- Proliferation (Ki-67) rate < 90%
- Differentiating from atypical BL can be difficult

B- or T-lymphoblastic Leukemia/Lymphoma (LBL)

- T-LBL often involves lymph nodes and mediastinum
- B-LBL in children typically present as an acute leukemia
- Blastic chromatin with inconspicuous nucleoli
- TdT(+)

B-cell Lymphoma, Unclassifiable, with Features Intermediate Between DLBCL and BL

- More commonly show complex cytogenetics
- May have non-*Ig* gene as translocation partner with *MYC*
- Immunophenotype or morphology that would be considered atypical for BL
- More commonly encountered in adults
- Diagnosis should not be made
  - In cases of morphologically typical DLBCL with *MYC* rearrangement
  - In otherwise typical BL in which *MYC* rearrangement cannot be demonstrated

Small Round Blue Cell Tumors

- Ewing sarcoma/peripheral neuroectodermal tumors
  - Lack B-cell antigens and express CD99 and keratin in a subset
- Neuroblastomas
  - Lack diffuse "starry sky" pattern of growth
  - Lack B-cell antigens and express NSE, S100
- Rhabdomyosarcomas
  - Lack diffuse "starry sky" pattern of growth
  - Express muscle-associated markers

Myeloid Sarcoma

- More immature chromatin
- Expresses myeloid-associated antigens
- Subset may express CD19 and pax-5

MALPRACTICE CONSIDERATIONS

Diagnostic Accuracy

- Essential to prevent under- or overtreatment
- More aggressive treatment needed for BL
- Adult patients with BL may not be cured with traditional DLBCL therapy (R-CHOP)
- Adults with BL benefit from more aggressive therapy
- Distinguishing BL from DLBCL is often more difficult in older patients

STAGING

Clinical Staging System for Childhood Non-Hodgkin Lymphoma (Murphy et al)

- Stage I
  - Single tumor or single anatomic area excluding mediastinum and abdomen

BURKITT LYMPHOMA

Immunohistochemistry

Antibody	Reactivity	Staining Pattern	Comment
CD10	Positive	Cell membrane	
CD19	Positive	Cell membrane	
CD20	Positive	Cell membrane	
CD22	Positive	Cell membrane	
CD79-α	Positive	Cell membrane	
Bcl-6	Positive	Nuclear	
Ki-67	Positive	Nuclear	Positive in ≥ 95% of cells
Bcl-2	Negative		
TdT	Negative		
CD44	Negative		
CD138	Negative		
IRF-4	Negative		May be positive in as many as 25%
EBV-LMP	Negative		In situ hybridization studies for EBER are recommended, as BL does not express LMP1 or EBNA2

Differential Diagnosis of Burkitt Lymphoma

Diagnosis	Histology	IHC	Molecular	Clinical
Burkitt lymphoma	Diffuse pattern of growth with "starry sky" pattern	Expresses pan B-cell markers, CD10(+), Bcl-6(+), Ki-67 > 95%, and Bcl-2(-)	*MYC* rearrangements t(8;14), t(2;8), or t(8;22); tend to have few genetic alterations in addition to MYC (simple karyotype)	Propensity for specific locations (ileocecal regions or jaw)
B-cell lymphoma, unclassifiable, with features intermediate between DLBCL and Burkitt lymphoma	Overlapping features; typically either show histologic features of BL with atypical immunophenotype or show immunophenotype of BL with atypical histology	Expresses pan B-cell markers, CD10(+), Bcl-6(+), Bcl-2(+/-), and Ki-67 < 95%	*Ig* and non-*Ig MYC* rearrangements; *MYC* and *BCL2* rearrangements (consider double hit lymphoma); complex karyotypes common	Often presents with widespread extranodal disease
Diffuse large B-cell lymphoma	Large neoplastic B-cells with pleomorphic nuclei and vesicular chromatin	Expresses pan B-cell markers, CD10(+/-), Bcl-6(+/-), Bcl-2(+/-), and Ki-67 < 90%	*MYC* rearrangement (-/+), *BCL6* rearrangement (+/-), &/or *BCL2* rearrangement (+/-)	Presents with nodal and extranodal disease
B-lymphoblastic leukemia/lymphoma	Immature chromatin with inconspicuous nucleoli and scant cytoplasm	TdT(+) with B-cell markers	Lack *MYC* rearrangements	Often present as an acute leukemia

- Stage II
  - Single extranodal tumor with regional lymph node involvement
  - ≥ 2 nodal areas on same side of diaphragm
  - 2 single tumors ± regional lymph node involvement on same side of diaphragm
  - Primary gastrointestinal tract tumor, usually in ileocecal area, ± involvement of associated mesenteric lymph nodes only, grossly completely resected
- Stage III
  - 2 single tumors or ≥ 2 nodal areas on opposite sides of diaphragm
  - All primary intrathoracic tumors (mediastinal, pleural, thymic)
  - All extensive intraabdominal disease, unresectable
  - All paraspinal or epidural tumors, regardless of other tumor sites
- Stage IV
  - Any of the above with initial central nervous system or bone marrow involvement

SELECTED REFERENCES

1. Jaglowski SM et al: Lymphoma in adolescents and young adults. Semin Oncol. 36(5):381-418, 2009
2. Kenkre VP et al: Burkitt lymphoma/leukemia: improving prognosis. Clin Lymphoma Myeloma. 9 Suppl 3:S231-8, 2009
3. Rowe M et al: Burkitt's lymphoma: the Rosetta Stone deciphering Epstein-Barr virus biology. Semin Cancer Biol. 19(6):377-88, 2009
4. Ferry JA: Burkitt's lymphoma: clinicopathologic features and differential diagnosis. Oncologist. 11(4):375-83, 2006
5. Murphy SB et al: Non-Hodgkin's lymphomas of childhood: an analysis of the histology, staging, and response to treatment of 338 cases at a single institution. J Clin Oncol. 7(2):186-93, 1989

BURKITT LYMPHOMA

Microscopic Features

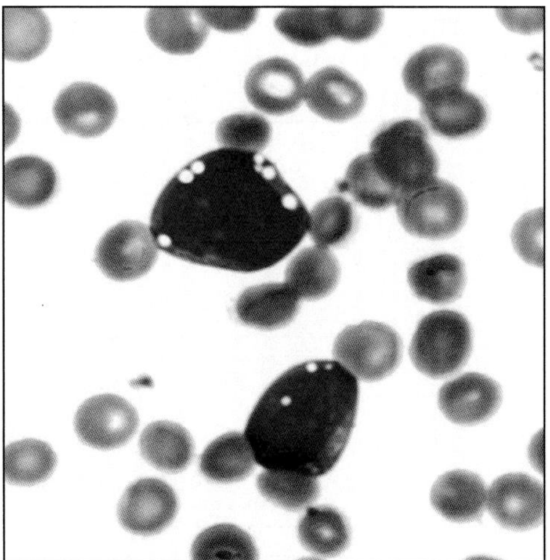

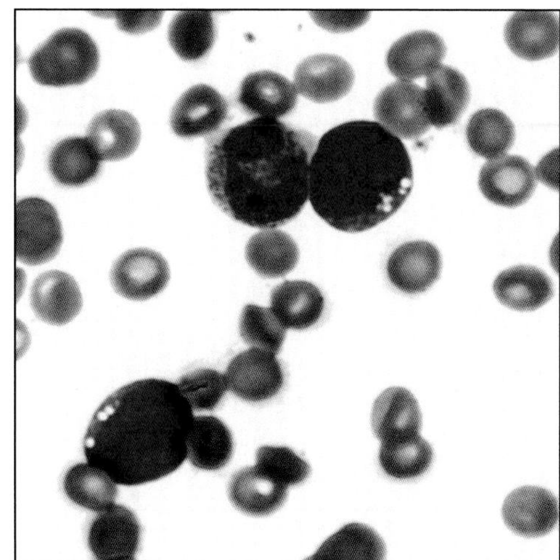

(Left) *Leukemic presentation of Burkitt lymphoma, although rare, can be seen. Burkitt lymphoma cells often show cytoplasmic vacuoles, which can be helpful in differentiating them from B- and T-lymphoblastic leukemias.* ***(Right)*** *The circulating Burkitt lymphoma cells are intermediate in size and typically larger than mature B cells. Note the dispersed chromatin with variably conspicuous nucleoli and cytoplasmic vacuoles.*

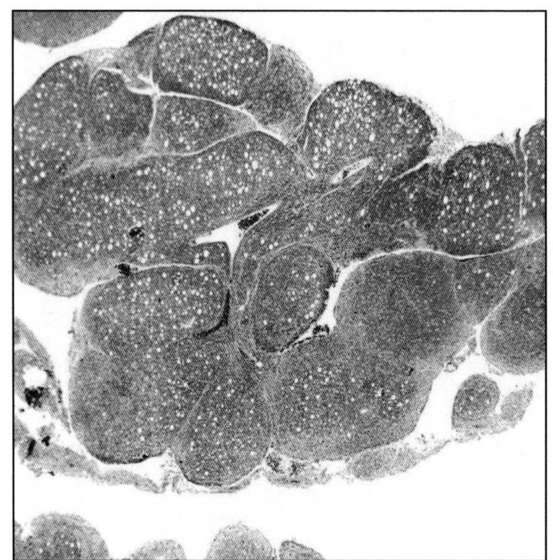

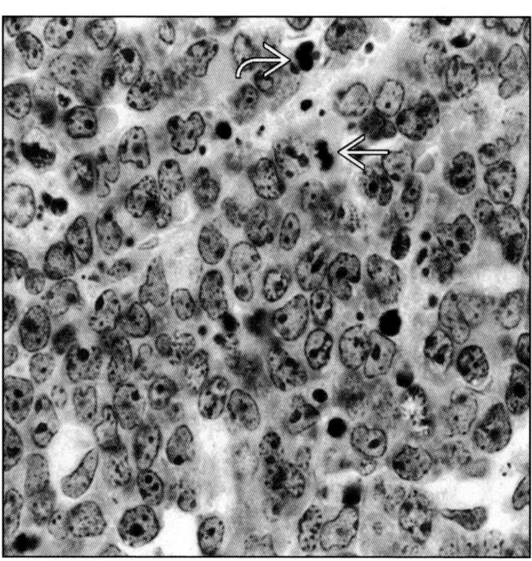

(Left) *Low-power view shows sporadic BL that has completely replaced the mesenteric adipose tissue. The "starry sky" pattern, although visible, was related to residual adipocytes.* ***(Right)*** *Atypical BL with pleomorphic nuclei and more prominent nucleoli is shown. Although the differential would include diffuse large B-cell lymphoma, the immunophenotype, extremely high proliferation index, and cytogenetic features were typical of BL. Note the apoptotic debris ➦ and mitotic figure ➔.*

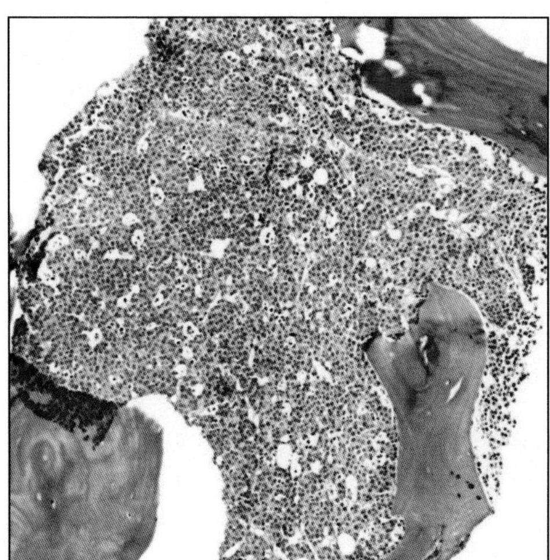

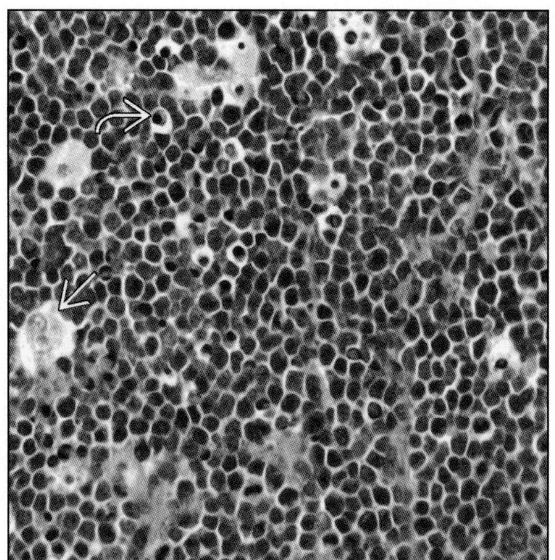

(Left) *Burkitt lymphoma shows complete replacement of the bone marrow. Note the diffuse pattern of growth with a vaguely "starry sky" pattern.* ***(Right)*** *Medium-power view of BL highlights the intermediate size of the cells with slight retraction of the cytoplasm, which imparts a squared-off appearance to the cells. Note the scattered macrophages ➔ and apoptotic cells ➦ that are indicative of high proliferative activity.*

Ancillary Tests and Differential Diagnosis

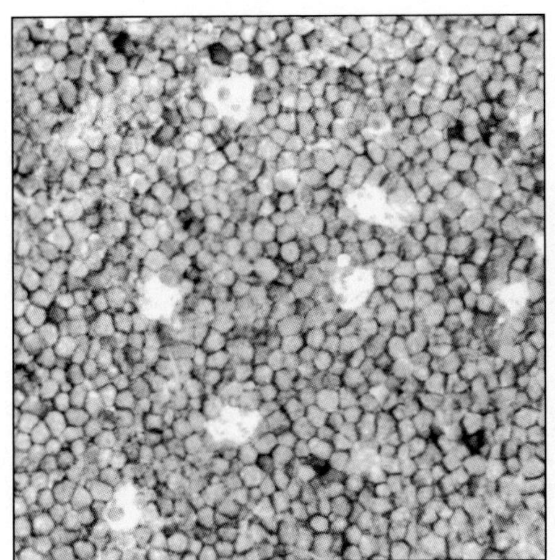

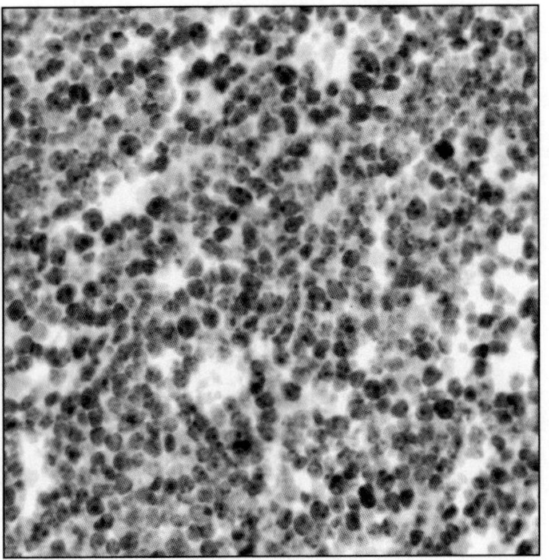

(Left) *Uniform expression of CD20 is shown in this classic example of Burkitt lymphoma.* ***(Right)*** *Ki-67 immunostaining of this classic example of BL shows an extremely high proliferation index with nearly 100% of the neoplastic cells showing positive nuclear reactivity.*

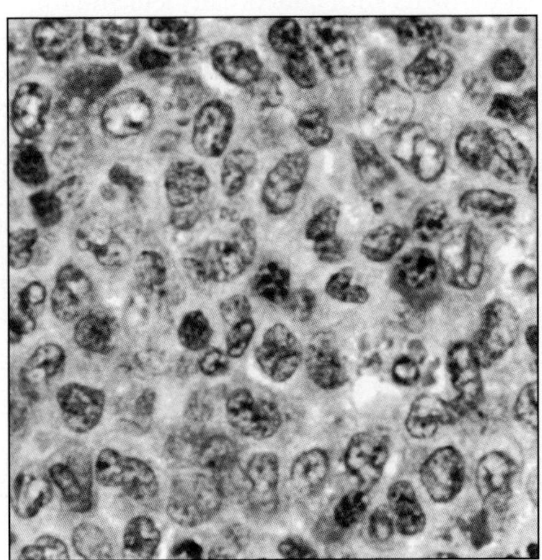

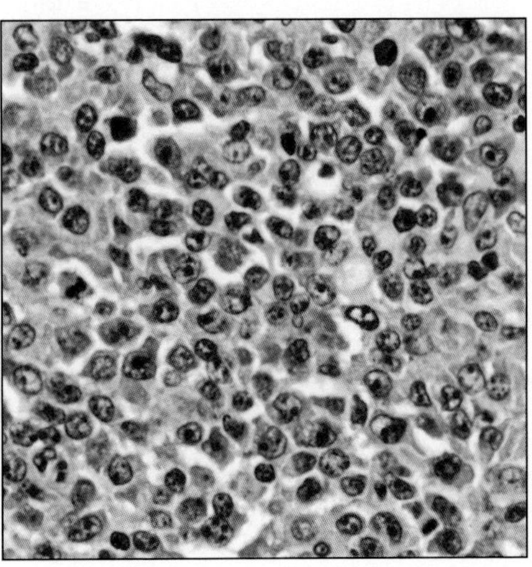

(Left) *High-power view of a myeloid sarcoma is shown. Note the larger, more pleomorphic nuclei with monocytoid features and inconspicuous nucleoli.* ***(Right)*** *An example of diffuse large B-cell lymphoma (DLBCL) is shown. Note the more pleomorphic nuclei, more prominent nucleoli, vesicular chromatin, and variable amounts of amphophilic cytoplasm that are more typical of DLBCL than of Burkitt lymphoma.*

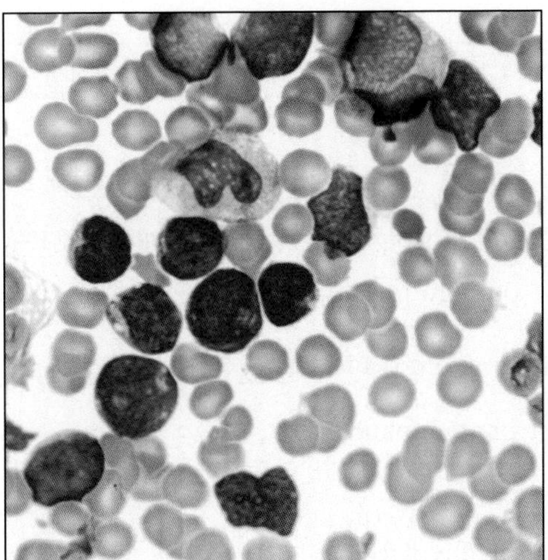

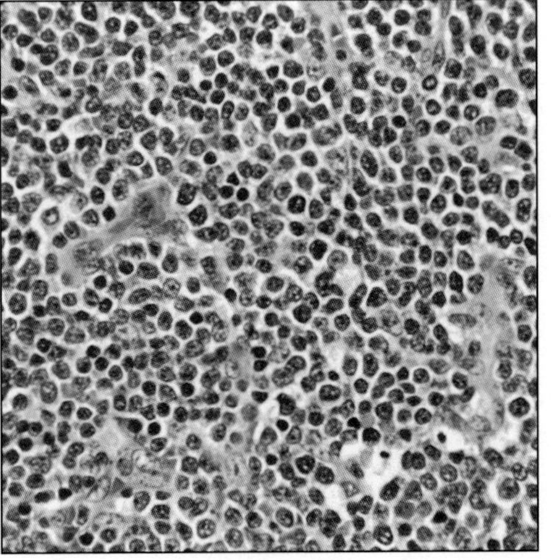

(Left) *T-lymphoblastic leukemia (T-LBL) is shown. Although there can be overlapping features between the leukemic presentations of BL and T-LBL, the lack of cytoplasmic vacuoles, deeply basophilic cytoplasm, and more variable-sized and shaped nuclei are more typical of T-LBL.* ***(Right)*** *T-lymphoblastic lymphoma is shown. Although a diffuse proliferation of tumor cells with a "starry sky" pattern can be seen, the diagnosis can easily be made with immunostains.*

B-LYMPHOBLASTIC LEUKEMIA/LYMPHOMA

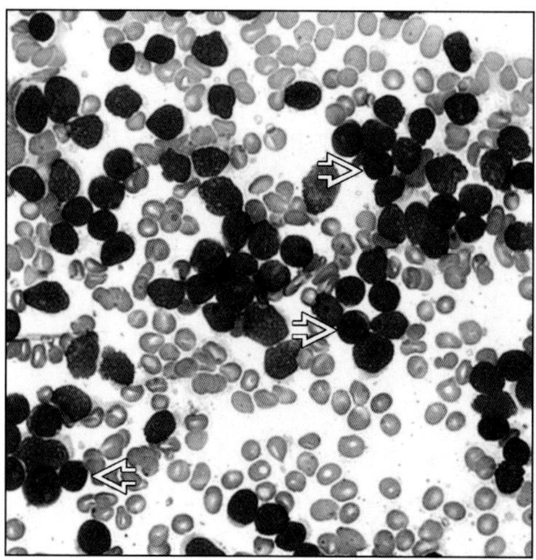
Typical small uniform lymphoblasts (L1 blasts) are seen in this bone marrow smear from a 3-year-old boy with a new diagnosis of B-LL. Rare mature lymphocytes ➡ are seen among lymphoblasts.

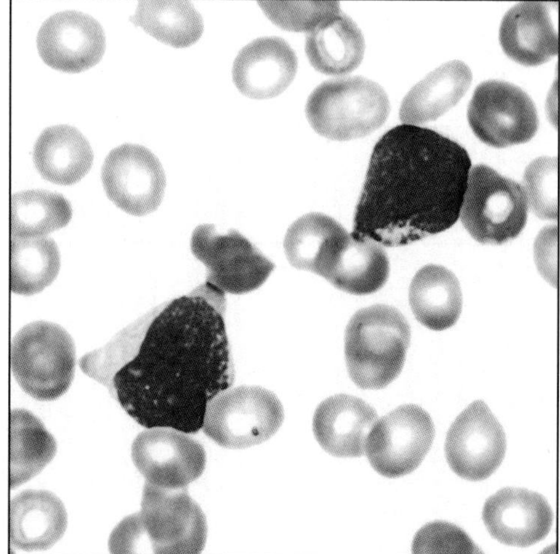
Peripheral blood smear from a 12-year-old girl with B-LL reveals large blasts (L2 blasts) with coarse cytoplasmic azurophilic granules, which may be seen in acute lymphoblastic leukemia (ALL) with t(9;22).

TERMINOLOGY

Abbreviations

- B-lymphoblastic leukemia/lymphoma (B-LL)

Synonyms

- B-cell acute lymphoblastic leukemia/lymphoma (B-ALL/B-LBL)

Definitions

- B-LL is neoplasm of precursors (lymphoblasts) committed to B-cell lineage
- When blood and bone marrow are extensively involved, "acute lymphoblastic leukemia" (B-LL) is appropriate term
- When disease is confined to mass with absent or minimal blood and marrow involvement, term "lymphoblastic lymphoma" (B-LBL) is used
- If patient presents with mass lesion, blood, and marrow involvement, ≥ 25% blasts in marrow defines leukemia (B-LL)
- Blasts express immature markers: CD34 and TdT

ETIOLOGY/PATHOGENESIS

Etiology

- B-LL arises in either hematopoietic stem cell or B-cell progenitor

Pathogenesis

- Genetic factors
  - Genetic abnormalities can result in constitutively activated oncogenes, activated kinase activity, or altered transcriptional regulation
  - Many ALLs are thought to be congenital
  - Genetic alterations in preleukemic cells in utero are proposed as initiating events
    - Presence of *TV6-RUNX6* (a.k.a. *TEL-AML1*) gene fusion or hyperdiploidy in neonatal blood spots on Guthrie cards
    - Monozygotic twins with concordant leukemia share same genetic abnormalities
  - 2nd hit may be required for developing overt leukemia
    - Most cases of ALL with *TV6-RUNX1* fusion have deletion of nonarranged *TV6* allele; latter is subclonal and probably occurs postnatally
    - Leukemia can develop many years after identification of *TV6-RUNX1* fusion
  - Increased incidence in patients with inherited genetic disorders
    - Down syndrome
    - Neurofibromatosis type 1 (NF1)
    - Bloom syndrome
    - Ataxia telangiectasia
- Environmental factors linked to increased incidence
  - Exposure to intrauterine ionizing radiation
  - Exposure to ionizing radiation
  - Exposure to pesticides
  - Post-chemotherapy

CLINICAL ISSUES

Epidemiology

- Incidence
  - B-LL is most common childhood neoplasm
  - Incidence is estimated at 1-4.75/100,000 persons per year
  - 80-85% of ALL is of B-cell origin
- Age
  - 75% of cases present before age 6
- Gender
  - Slight male predominance

Site

- Bone marrow is primary site
- Blood is typically involved
- CNS, lymph nodes, liver, spleen, and testis are often involved

B-LYMPHOBLASTIC LEUKEMIA/LYMPHOMA

Key Facts

Terminology

- B-LL is neoplasm of precursors (lymphoblasts) committed to B-cell lineage

Etiology/Pathogenesis

- B-LL arises in either hematopoietic stem cell or B-cell progenitor
- Many ALLs are thought to be congenital
- Cytogenetic abnormalities can result in constitutively activated oncogenes, activated kinase activity, or altered transcriptional regulation
- Increased risk in patients exposed to ionizing radiation, pesticides, &/or chemotherapy

Clinical Issues

- B-LL is most common childhood neoplasm
- 80-85% of ALL cases are of B-cell origin
- 75% of cases occur before age 6
- Most present with constitutional symptoms
- Bone pain, arthralgias, or CNS symptoms common
- 20% patients may have "preleukemic" state with cytopenia 2-9 months before overt leukemia
- Intensive chemotherapy protocols are mainstay treatment
- Intrathecal prophylactic therapy routinely done to prevent CNS relapse
- Patients with "very high risk" may benefit from allogeneic SCT
- Excellent prognosis; complete remission rate over 95% in children and 60-85% in adults
- Complex prognostic systems including clinical, biologic, cytogenetic findings, and response to therapy

- Skin, soft tissue, bone, and lymph nodes are primary sites of involvement in B-LBL

Presentation

- Constitutional symptoms
  - Fever
  - Night sweats
  - Weight loss
- Symptoms related to anemia, thrombocytopenia, or neutropenia
  - Fatigue
  - Bleeding tendency
  - Neutropenic fever
- Signs and symptoms related to leukemic infiltrate
  - Bone pain
  - Arthralgias
  - CNS symptoms
  - Frequent hepatosplenomegaly
  - Lymphadenopathy may be present

Laboratory Tests

- CBC findings
  - Variable white blood cell (WBC) count
    - 50% of patients have WBC < 10 x 10^9/L (low)
    - 30% of patients have WBC between 10-50 x 10^9/L
    - 20% of patients have WBC > 50 x 10^9/L
  - Anemia & thrombocytopenia almost always present
  - 20% of patients may have "preleukemic" state with cytopenia 2-9 months before overt leukemia
  - Rarely patients present with asymptomatic eosinophilia

Treatment

- Intensive chemotherapy protocols are mainstay treatment
  - Patients are stratified as standard risk or high risk based on clinical, biologic prognostic factors, and cytogenetic findings
  - Patients are further stratified at end of induction based on response to therapy and minimal residual disease (MRD) assessment
- Intrathecal prophylactic therapy ± cranial radiation routinely done to prevent CNS relapse
- Stem cell/bone marrow transplantation
  - Autologous stem cell transplant (SCT) not effective
  - Patients with the following "very high risk" findings may benefit from allogeneic SCT
    - Failure to achieve complete remission after 5 weeks of therapy
    - t(9;22) or t(4;11) positive
    - WBC count > 100 x 10^9/L
- Supportive therapy for cytopenia(s)
- Personalized therapy is improving with advances in cytogenetic, molecular, pharmacogenomics studies

Prognosis

- Overall prognosis
  - Excellent; complete remission rate over 95% in children and 60-85% in adults
  - Cure rate is ~ 80% in children and < 50% in adults
  - Infants with *MLL* gene rearrangement generally have poor prognosis
  - Adolescents and young adults have better outcome treated with pediatric protocols than with adult protocols
  - CNS and testis are sanctuary for leukemic cells and are common relapse sites
- Clinical and biologic prognostic factors
  - Favorable factors
    - Age 1-10 years
    - Female
    - WBC < 50 x 10^9/L
    - Common type of ALL by immunophenotype
    - No CNS disease
  - Unfavorable factors
    - < 1 or > 10 years
    - Male
    - WBC > 50 x 10^9/L
    - Lack of CD10 expression by immunophenotyping
    - Presence of CNS disease
- Cytogenetic abnormalities as prognostic predicators
  - Favorable
    - Hyperdiploidy (> 50 chromosomes, especially with trisomy 4, 10, 17)
    - t(12;21) or *TV6-RUNX6* fusion

- Unfavorable
  - Hypodiploidy (< 45 chromosomes)
  - t(9;22) or *BCR-ABL1* fusion
  - *MLL* rearrangement; t(4;11) or *MLL-AF4* fusion
  - Intrachromosomal *RUNX1* amplification
  - Complex abnormalities
- Intermediate
  - t(5;14) or *IL3-IGH* fusion
  - T(1;19) or *TCF3-PBX1*(a.k.a. *E2A-PBX1*) fusion
  - Normal karyotype
  - Any other abnormalities not in favorable or unfavorable findings

- Response to therapy as prognostic predicator
  - Favorable
    - No morphologically detectable blasts at day 7 or 14 marrow
    - Morphologic remission at end of induction
    - Good peripheral blood response to week of systemic steroid prior to multiagent chemotherapy
  - Unfavorable
    - Morphologically detectable blasts at day 7 or 14 marrow
    - Requirement for 2 or more cycles of induction chemotherapy to achieve complete morphologic remission
    - Poor peripheral blood response to week of systemic steroid therapy
- MRD assessment
  - Low risk for relapse
    - Low MRD (< 10^{-3}) at day 8 or 15
    - Low MRD (< 10^{-3}) at end of induction
  - High risk for relapse
    - High MRD (> 10^{-3}) at day 8 or 15
    - High MRD (> 10^{-3}) at end of induction
- Gene expression analysis
  - Defines distinctive ALL subsets
  - Helps to separate patients who may be resistant to certain chemotherapy agents
  - Helps to predict early response and MRD
- Pharmacogenomics
  - Can predict how rapidly & effectively individual patients metabolize certain chemotherapeutic agents

MICROSCOPIC PATHOLOGY

Histologic Features

- Blood
  - Blasts are usually present in peripheral blood
  - Blasts vary in size from small to large
  - L1 blasts: Small blasts with scant cytoplasm, condensed chromatin, and indistinctive nucleoli
  - L2 blasts: Large blasts with moderate cytoplasm, dispersed chromatin, and variable nucleoli
  - May have coarse azurophilic cytoplasmic granules
- Bone marrow
  - Hypercellular marrow, usually extensively replaced by lymphoblasts
  - Blasts are fairly uniform in bone marrow
  - Core biopsy shows extensive replacement by lymphoblasts
  - Core biopsy may show "starry sky" pattern due to high proliferation/cell turnover
  - Patchy or diffuse preserved hematopoietic cells
  - Rarely marrow necrosis; ALL is most common neoplasm to present as diffuse necrosis in BM

ANCILLARY TESTS

Immunohistochemistry

- Often used when flow cytometric analysis is not available
  - CD34, TdT to confirm immaturity of blasts
  - CD19, CD79a, and CD20 to identify B-cell lineage

Flow Cytometry

- Degree of differentiation determines immunophenotype of blasts
  - Earliest stage blasts (early precursor B-LL) express CD19, cytoplasmic CD79a, cytoplasmic CD22, and TdT; such ALLs occur in infancy
  - Intermediate stage blasts (common B-LL) express CD10, CD19, surface CD79a, surface CD22, and TdT
  - Most mature stage blasts (pre-B-LL) express cytoplasmic μ chains (c-μ), CD34 often negative
- CD34 and CD20 expression variable
- CD45 can be negative but is typically weak
- Approximately 20-30% of cases also express myeloid-associated antigen markers CD15, CD13, and CD33
- CD13 expression is often seen in B-LL with t(12;21)
- CD13 & CD33 expression often seen in B-LL with t(9;22)
- Switch in immunophenotype during therapy is very common, usually gain or loss of myeloid markers

Cytogenetics

- Abnormalities in majority of B-LL/B-LBL cases
- Recurrent genetic abnormalities as defined by the World Health Organization include
  - t(12;21)(p13;q22) *TV6-RUNX1* (a.k.a. *TV6-RUNX1*); most common fusion in pediatric ALL
  - t(1;19)(q23;p13.3) *TCF3-PBX1 (E2A-PBX1)*
  - t(9;22)(q34;q11.2) *BCR-ABL1*
  - t(v;11q23) *MLL* rearranged; especially ALL in neonates/infants
  - t(5;14)(q31;q32) *IL3-IgH*, associated with eosinophilia
  - Hyperdiploidy (> 50 chromosomes)
  - Hypodiploidy (< 46 chromosomes)

PCR

- Almost all cases have clonal rearrangement of *IGH* gene
- Majority of cases also have clonal rearrangement of T-cell receptor (*TCR*) gene

DIFFERENTIAL DIAGNOSIS

Hematogones

- Can be numerous in children, especially during recovery after BM insults
- Immunophenotype
  - Demonstrates gradual gain of CD20 expression

Genetic Subtypes of B-lymphoblastic Leukemia

Aberration	Frequency	Prognosis	Unique Findings
t(12;21)(p13;q22); *ETV6-RUNX1*	25% in children; rare in adults	Very favorable with high cure rate; relapse usually occurs later than for other types of ALL	Common in children, not seen in infants, rare in adults; cryptic translocation; FISH or molecular test required for detection; translocation arises in utero, leukemia may develop years later; typically CD20(-); frequently expresses myeloid-associated antigen CD13
Hyperdiploidy (> 50 but < 66 chromosomes)	25% in children; rare in adults	Favorable, particularly good with trisomy 4, 10, and 17	Common in children, not seen in infants, rare in adults; CD45 often negative
t(9;22)(q34;q11.2); *BCR-ABL1*	2-4% in children; 25% in adults	Worst prognosis among patients with ALL	More common in adult ALL cases; rarely associated with T-ALL phenotype; frequent expression of myeloid-associated antigens CD13 and CD33; CD25 is highly associated with t(9;22) B-LL; may see coarse azurophilic cytoplasmic granules
t(v;11q23); *MLL* rearranged	Most common in infants < 1 year of age	Poor prognosis, particularly poor in infants < 6 months of age	Less common in older children, increased incidence with age into adulthood; may occur in utero; typically presents with very high WBC count; high frequency of CNS involvement at diagnosis; often CD10(-) and CD15(+); *MLL* gene has many fusion partners with *AF4* on chromosome 4q21 in majority of cases; *ENL* gene on chromosome 19p13 and *AF9* on chromosome 9p22 are common in remaining cases
Hypodiploidy (< 46 chromosomes)	5%; seen in both children and adults	Poor prognosis, particularly with less than 44 chromosomes	No unique morphologic, immunophenotypic, or cytochemical features
t(1;19)(q23;p13.3); *TCF3-PBX1*	6%; less common in adults	Intermediate with intensive therapy	Often has pre-B cell phenotype (CD19[+], CD10[+], cytoplasmic μ chain [cμ] [+]; absent or subset CD34 expression)
t(5;14)(q31;q32); *IL3-IGH*	Rare; < 1% of cases; seen in both children and adults	Not different from other ALL	Typically associated with increased circulating nonneoplastic eosinophils; clinical presentation, cytomorphology, immunophenotype, and prognosis are similar to other ALL; patient may present with asymptomatic eosinophilia

- Gradual loss of CD10, TdT, and CD34
- Lack of aberrant antigen expression

Burkitt Lymphoma (BL)

- BL is mature, high-grade B-cell lymphoma
- Lymphoma cells are large with unique punctate cytoplasmic vacuoles
- BL expresses surface immunoglobulin and lacks immature markers CD34 or TdT

Other Leukemias

- Immunophenotyping is helpful to distinguish B-LL from other leukemias

Small Round Blue Cell Tumors of Childhood

- Consider desmoplastic small round cell tumor, rhabdomyosarcoma, medulloblastoma, neuroblastoma, and Ewing sarcoma/primitive neuroectodermal tumor among others
- Distinguish from B-LBL with appropriate immunohistochemical panel &/or flow cytometry study

SELECTED REFERENCES

1. Faderl S et al: Adult acute lymphoblastic leukemia: concepts and strategies. Cancer. 116(5):1165-76, 2010
2. Pieters R et al: Biology and treatment of acute lymphoblastic leukemia. Hematol Oncol Clin North Am. 24(1):1-18, 2010
3. Reichard K: Precursor B- and T-cell acute lymphoblastic leukemia/lymphoma (aka lymphoblastic leukemia/ lymphoma). In Foucar K et al: Bone Marrow Pathology. Chicago: ASCP Press. 590-615, 2010
4. Vrooman LM et al: Childhood acute lymphoblastic leukemia: update on prognostic factors. Curr Opin Pediatr. 21(1):1-8, 2009
5. Attarbaschi A et al: Minimal residual disease values discriminate between low and high relapse risk in children with B-cell precursor acute lymphoblastic leukemia and an intrachromosomal amplification of chromosome 21: the Austrian and German acute lymphoblastic leukemia Berlin-Frankfurt-Munster (ALL-BFM) trials. J Clin Oncol. 26(18):3046-50, 2008
6. Borowitz MJ et al: B lymphoblastic leukemia/lymphoma with recurrent genetic abnormalities. In Swerdlow SH et al: WHO Classification of Tumours of Haematopoietic and Lymphoid Tissues. Lyon: IARC Press. 171-175, 2008
7. Borowitz MJ et al: B lymphoblastic leukemia/lymphoma, not otherwise specified. In Swerdlow SH et al: WHO Classification of Tumours of Haematopoietic and Lymphoid Tissues. Lyon: IARC Press. 168-170, 2008
8. Flotho C et al: A set of genes that regulate cell proliferation predicts treatment outcome in childhood acute lymphoblastic leukemia. Blood. 110(4):1271-7, 2007
9. Zhou J et al: Quantitative analysis of minimal residual disease predicts relapse in children with B-lineage acute lymphoblastic leukemia in DFCI ALL Consortium Protocol 95-01. Blood. 110(5):1607-11, 2007
10. Greaves M: Infection, immune responses and the aetiology of childhood leukaemia. Nat Rev Cancer. 6(3):193-203, 2006
11. Greaves MF et al: Origins of chromosome translocations in childhood leukaemia. Nat Rev Cancer. 3(9):639-49, 2003
12. Yeoh EJ et al: Classification, subtype discovery, and prediction of outcome in pediatric acute lymphoblastic leukemia by gene expression profiling. Cancer Cell. 1(2):133-43, 2002
13. Gaynon PS et al: Early response to therapy and outcome in childhood acute lymphoblastic leukemia: a review. Cancer. 80(9):1717-26, 1997
14. Smith M et al: Uniform approach to risk classification and treatment assignment for children with acute lymphoblastic leukemia. J Clin Oncol. 14(1):18-24, 1996

Variant Microscopic Features and Differential Diagnosis

*(**Left**) L2 lymphoblasts are present in a lymphoblastic leukemia patient. The large size of the blasts mimics acute myeloid leukemic cells. Immunophenotyping was required to establish the diagnosis. (**Right**) Bone marrow aspirate smear from a patient with B-LL and t(9;22) reveals blasts with scant to moderate cytoplasm and cytoplasmic blebbing, mimicking megakaryoblasts. Immunophenotyping reveals lymphoblasts with CD13 and CD33 coexpression, often seen in B-LL with t(9;22).*

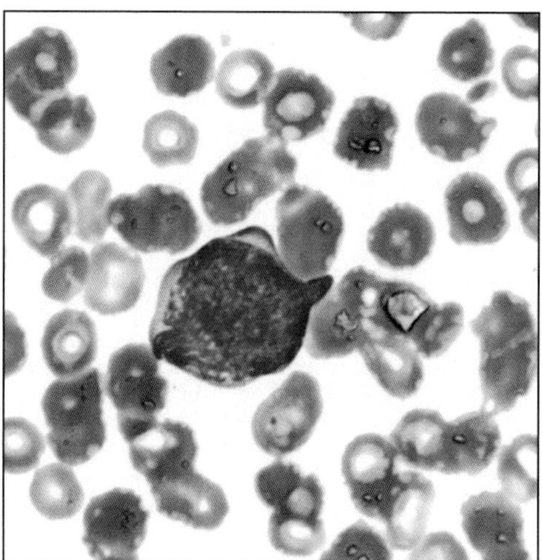

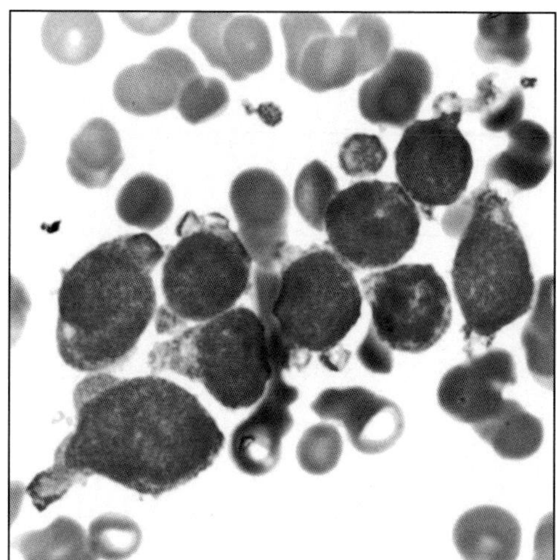

*(**Left**) Bone marrow aspirate smear from a 12-year-old girl with B-LL and t(9;22) is shown. The blasts depicted here demonstrate coarse cytoplasmic azurophilic granules, which may be seen in B-LL with t(9;22). (**Right**) Bone marrow clot section illustrates typical histologic features of ALL. The densely packed leukemic cells completely effaced marrow. Lymphoblasts have scant cytoplasm, round to slightly folded nuclei, finely dispersed chromatin, and small to prominent nucleoli.*

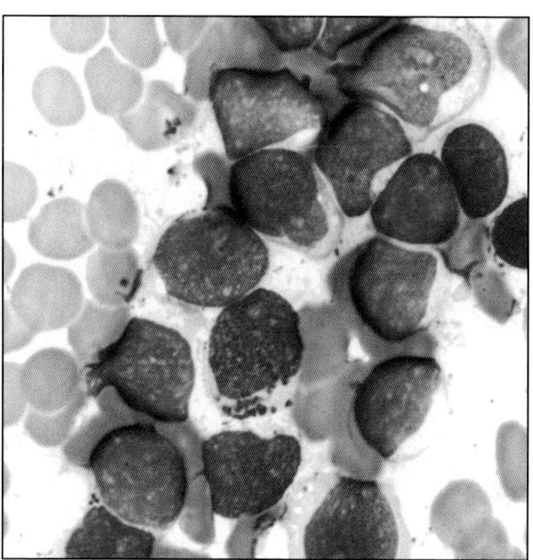

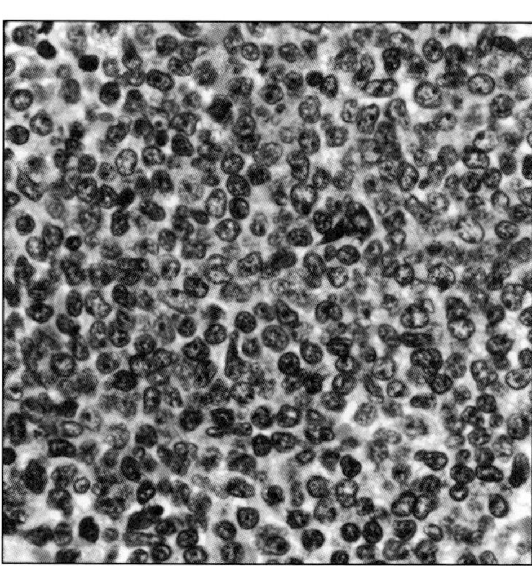

*(**Left**) Touch preparation of lymph node from a patient with newly diagnosed Burkitt lymphoma shows the characteristic uniform, medium-sized cells with slightly coarse chromatin, deep blue cytoplasm, and punctate cytoplasmic vacuoles. (**Right**) Tissue section of a lymph node of Burkitt lymphoma reveals uniform lymphoma cells with rigid cell borders, scattered mitosis, and a high fraction of apoptosis. Benign macrophages with ingested apoptotic tumor cells create a "starry sky" pattern.*

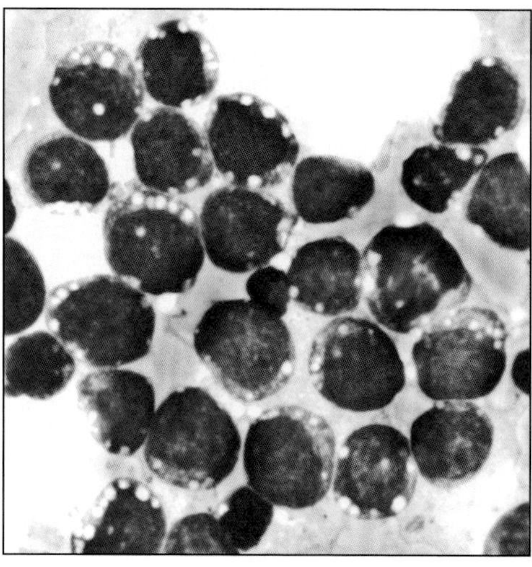

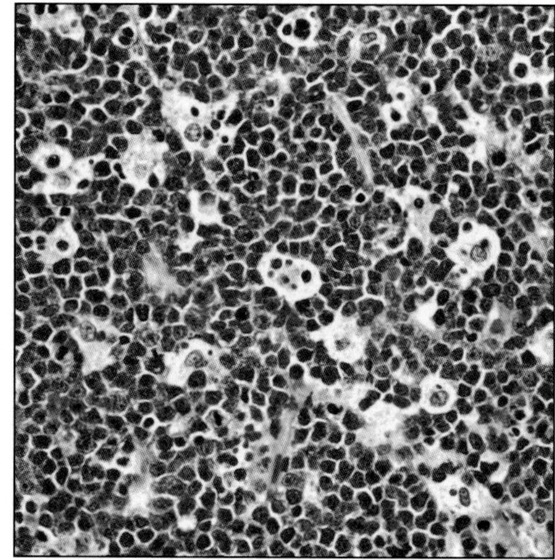

Variant Microscopic Features and Prognostic Tests

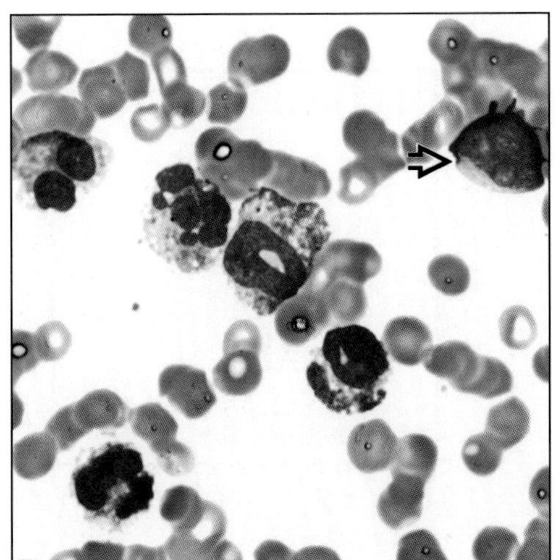

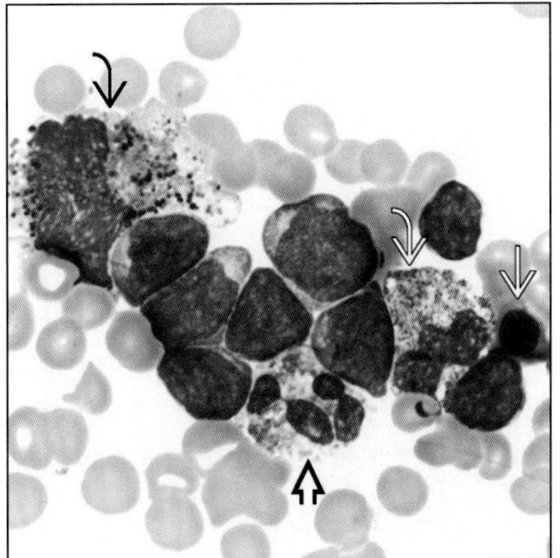

*(**Left**) A lymphoblast ➲ is accompanied by marked eosinophilia in the peripheral blood from a patient with B-lymphoblastic leukemia (B-LL). Eosinophilia is the characteristic feature in ALL with t(5;14), which was identified by routine karyotyping. (**Right**) Bone marrow aspirate shows a cluster of blasts surrounded by a mature eosinophil ➲, an eosinophil precursor with basophilic granules ➲, a segmented neutrophil ➲, and an erythroid precursor ➔.*

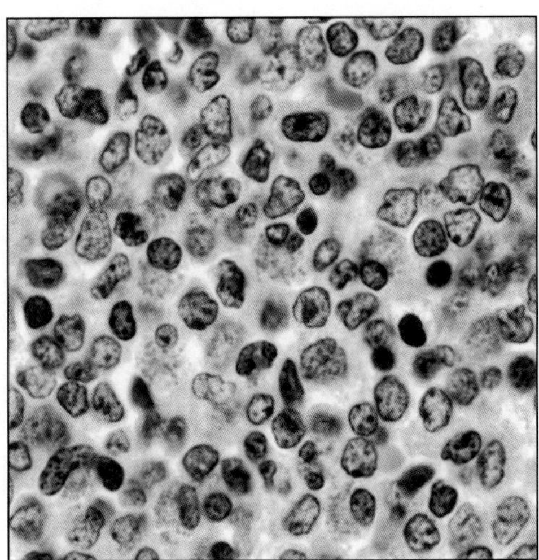

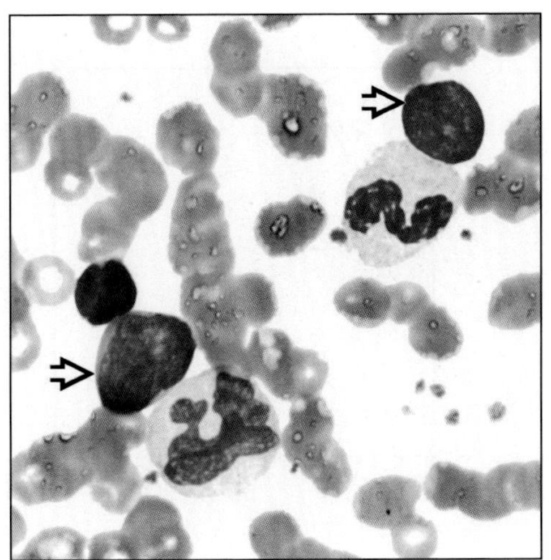

*(**Left**) Bone marrow clot section reveals extensive effacement of marrow by lymphoblasts. Numerous eosinophils and eosinophilic precursors are also seen. (**Right**) 2 lymphoblasts ➲ are accompanied by a segmented neutrophil, a mature lymphocyte, a monocyte, and multiple platelets. "Preclinical" B-LL was suspected by radiographic study in this 7-year-old boy. Complete blood count revealed numerous blasts without cytopenias.*

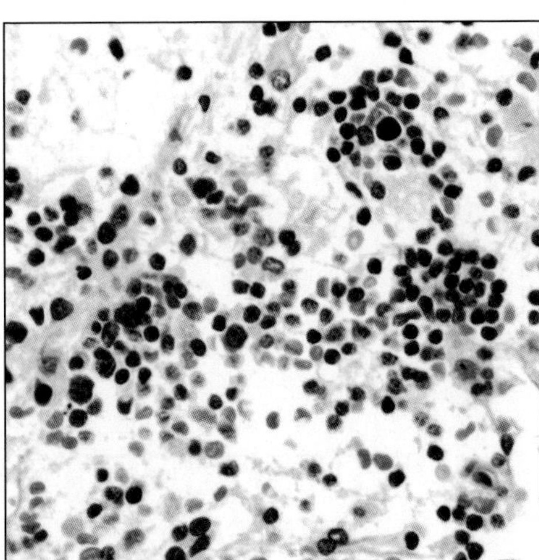

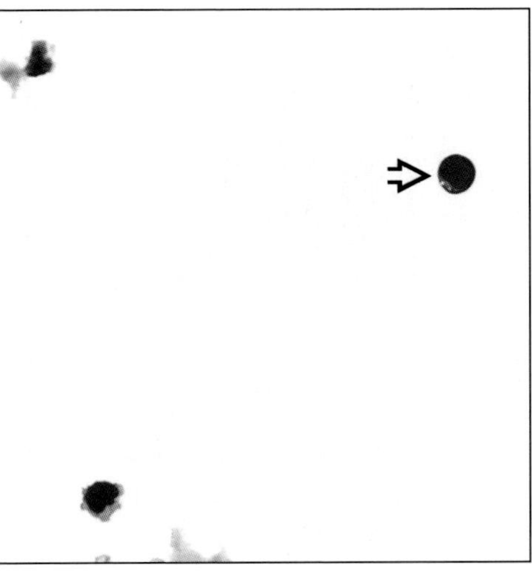

*(**Left**) Day 15 marrow is routinely biopsied as part of the protocols in ALL patients for prognosis. Focal residual disease is identified in addition to rare megakaryocytes and extensive post-chemotherapy marrow damage. The presence of significant residual disease is associated with adverse outcome. (**Right**) Cerebrospinal fluid (CSF) is routinely obtained before intrathecal therapy in ALL patients. The presence of blasts ➲ in CSF is associated with an adverse outcome.*

Ancillary Techniques and Differential Diagnosis

*(**Left**) The prototypical immunophenotype of B lymphoblasts include positive CD19, CD10, HLA-DR, and terminal deoxynucleotidyl transferase (TdT), and variable CD34, CD20, and weak CD45. The blasts ⇨ depicted here express both CD19 and CD10. (**Right**) CD45 is typically weak in B-LL ⇨. CD45 can be negative in a subset of cases. A small population of mature lymphocytes with bright CD45 is present ➚.*

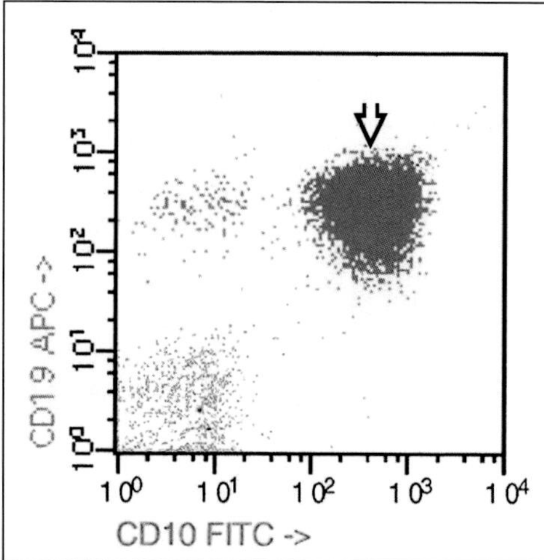

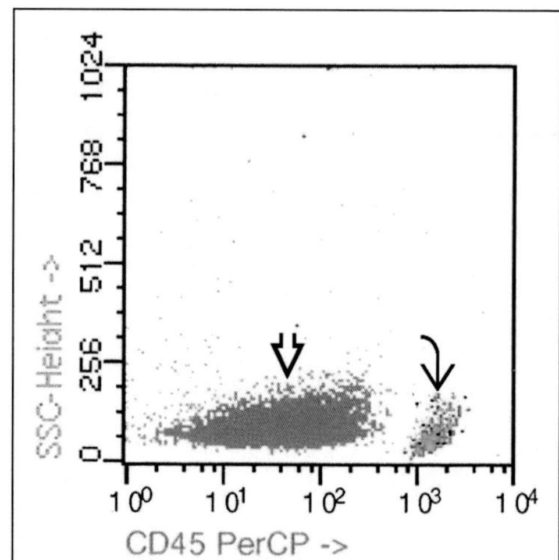

*(**Left**) Lymphoblasts express variable CD34. The lymphoblasts depicted here are positive for CD34 and negative for T-cell marker CD2 ⇨. A small population of CD2(+) T cells is seen here ➚. (**Right**) Lymphoblasts are typically positive for cytoplasmic CD79-a and TdT, as depicted here ⇨. TdT is a nuclear enzyme that can be assessed by flow cytometry after membranes are permeated.*

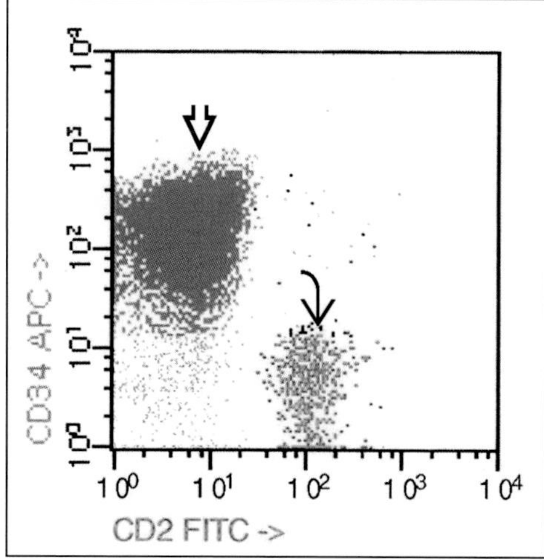

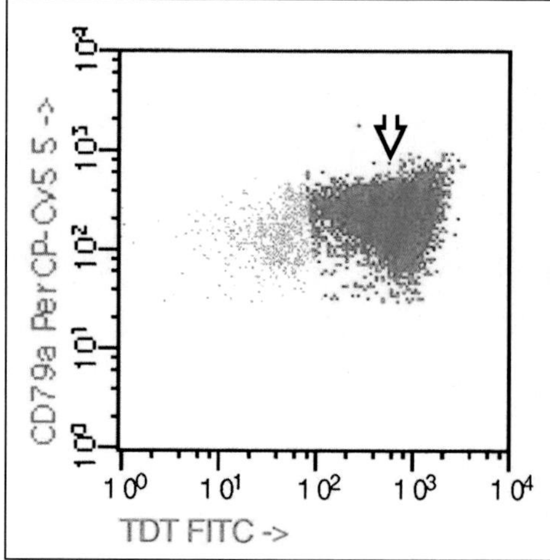

*(**Left**) HLA-DR is typically positive in B lymphoblastic leukemia (B-LL). The lymphoblasts depicted here are positive for HLA-DR and negative for T-cell marker CD7 ⇨. A small population of CD7(+) T cells is also seen ➚. (**Right**) The most helpful finding in differentiating hematogones from B-LL is the spectrum of expression from negative to positive for CD20, as shown here ➚. It is indicative of continuous maturation. Leukemic lymphoblasts typically form a tight cluster.*

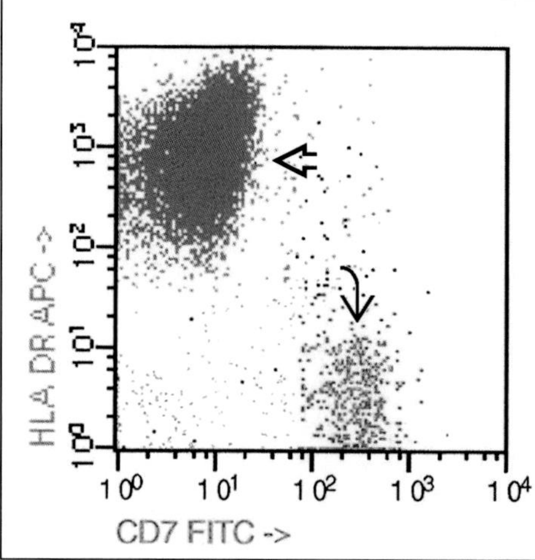

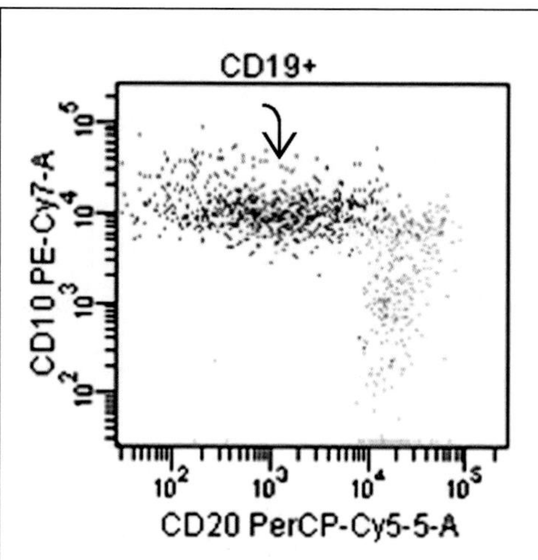

Ancillary Techniques

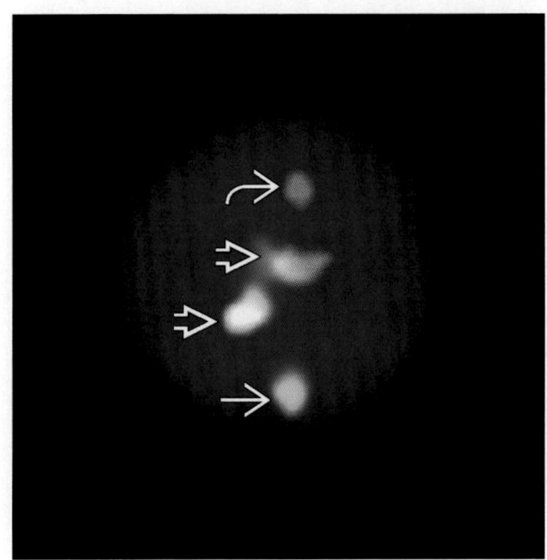

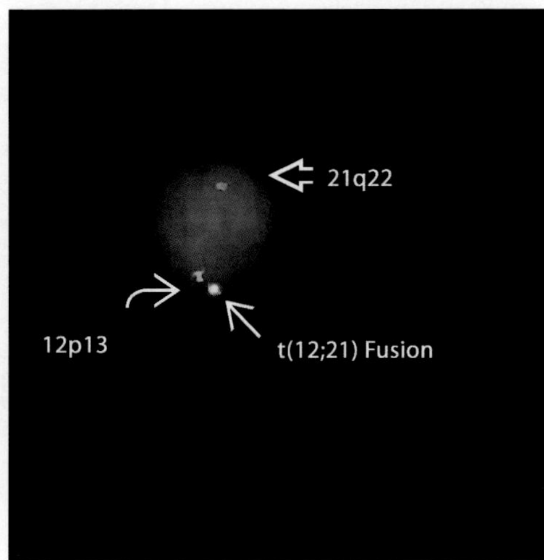

(Left) *Dual-color, dual-fusion fluorescence in situ hybridization (FISH) on interphase lymphoblastic nucleus demonstrates 2 copies of t(9;22) or BCR/ABL1 fusion. A normal copy of chromosome 9 and 22 is seen. t(9;22) is associated with adverse prognosis.* ***(Right)*** *Dual-color, dual-fusion FISH probes demonstrate the presence of t(12;21) TV6-RUNX1 fusion, a normal copy of 12p13/TV6 and 21q22/RUNX1 gene. One fusion signal is considered an atypical*

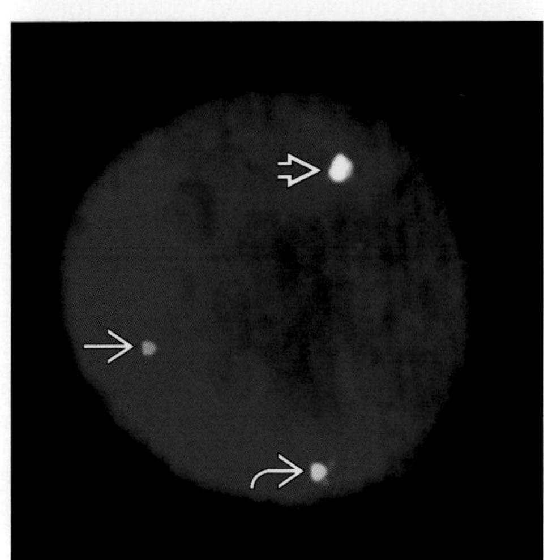

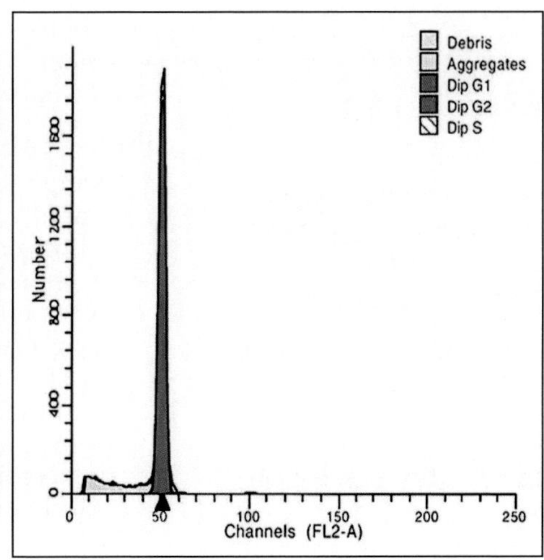

(Left) *Break-apart probe for MLL gene is located on chromosome 11q23. The normal MLL copy has fused red and green signals. The rearranged MLL gene is broken into 1 red and 1 green with unknown partner gene.* ***(Right)*** *DNA content is measured by flow cytometric analysis. A single peak with diploid DNA content from a normal control is depicted in this histogram.*

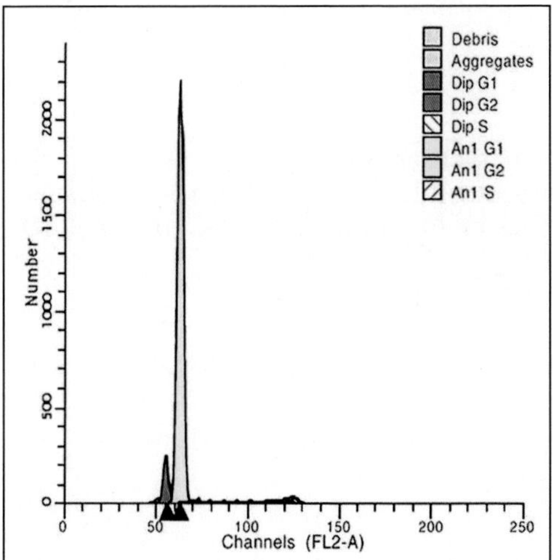

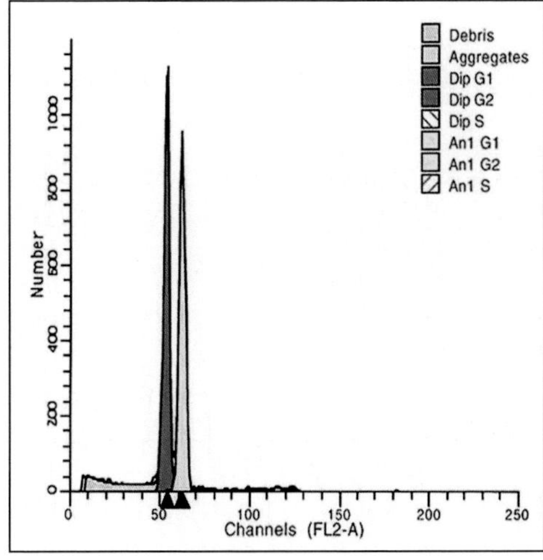

(Left) *In this patient sample, abnormal DNA content is shown as the prominent yellow peak. It represents aneuploid DNA content. A small red peak is also seen, representing residual normal hematopoietic cells with diploid DNA content.* ***(Right)*** *DNA index of 1.16 (i.e., hyperdiploidy) is calculated as the normal (red):patient (yellow) DNA content ratio in a mixed study. Conventional karyotyping is used to determine which chromosomes are duplicated.*

T-LYMPHOBLASTIC LEUKEMIA/LYMPHOMA

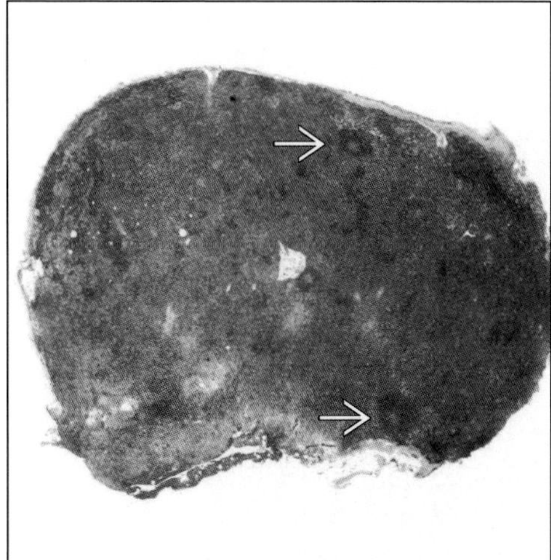

H&E shows lymph node with subtotal replacement by T-lymphoblastic lymphoma/leukemia. A few preserved lymphoid follicles ➔ can be seen.

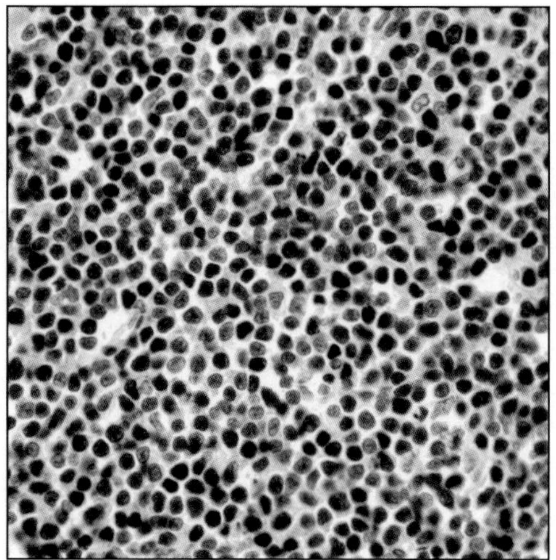

T-lymphoblastic lymphoma/leukemia involving lymph node is shown. TdT is strongly positive in the nuclei of the neoplastic cells.

TERMINOLOGY

Abbreviations

- T-lymphoblastic leukemia/lymphoma (T-LBL)

Synonyms

- Precursor T-cell lymphoblastic lymphoma/leukemia
- T-cell lymphoblastic lymphoma/acute lymphoblastic leukemia

Definitions

- Neoplasm of lymphoblasts committed to T-cell lineage
- Distinction between lymphoma and leukemia is arbitrary; by convention
- T-lymphoblastic lymphoma
    - Presentation with involvement of thymus, lymph nodes, &/or extranodal sites
    - No or minimal involvement of peripheral blood (PB) or bone marrow (BM)
- T-lymphoblastic leukemia (T-ALL)
    - Presentation with involvement of PB and BM

ETIOLOGY/PATHOGENESIS

Genetic

- Recurrent genetic aberrations that block precursor T-cell differentiation and survival
    - T-LBL is genetically heterogeneous disease
    - Number of translocations, deletions, and gene mutations have been shown
- Possible in utero origin in subset of cases

CLINICAL ISSUES

Epidemiology

- Incidence
    - 85-90% of lymphoblastic tumors presenting as lymphoma are of T-cell lineage
- Age
    - Median: 17 years for adolescents and 25 years for adults
- Gender
    - Sex ratio: 70% male, 30% female

Presentation

- T-lymphoblastic lymphoma
    - Rapidly growing anterior mediastinal mass (~ 75% of patients)
        - ± pleural effusions
        - Superior vena cava syndrome can occur
    - Lymphadenopathy is typically supradiaphragmatic (~ 50% of patients)
    - Extranodal presentation (~ 35% of patients)
        - Frequent sites: Skin, tonsils, liver, spleen, central nervous system, and testes
    - Most patients present with stage III or IV disease (~ 75% of patients)
- T-ALL
    - High leukocyte count
    - Lymphadenopathy and hepatosplenomegaly are common

Treatment

- Drugs
    - Aggressive chemotherapy
        - Cyclophosphamide, vincristine, doxorubicin, and dexamethasone/methotrexate/ara-C (hyperCVAD regimen)
        - High rates of complete response
- Radiation
    - Mediastinal radiation for bulky disease

Prognosis

- 5-year disease-free survival
    - Children: 65-75%
    - Adults: 40-60%

Key Facts

Terminology
- T-LBL is neoplasm of lymphoblasts committed to T-cell lineage
- Distinction between lymphoma and leukemia is arbitrary; by convention
  - T-lymphoblastic lymphoma: Presentation with disease in thymus, lymph nodes, &/or extranodal sites
  - T-lymphoblastic leukemia: Presentation with involvement of PB and BM

Clinical Issues
- Median age: 17 years for adolescents and 25 years for adults
- Sex ratio: 70% male, 30% female
- Stage III or IV disease (~ 75% of patients)
- Rapidly growing anterior mediastinal mass (~ 75% of patients)
- Lymphadenopathy is typically supradiaphragmatic

Microscopic Pathology
- Diffuse pattern of infiltration
  - "Starry sky" pattern in 10-20% of cases
- Small to medium-sized lymphoblasts with fine nuclear chromatin
- Lymphoblasts can infiltrate extranodal tissues in single-file pattern

Ancillary Tests
- Immunophenotype
  - T-cell antigens (+), TdT(+)
  - CD1a(+), CD10(+) in pre-T and cortical T stages
- Monoclonal *TCR* gene rearrangements

IMAGE FINDINGS

Radiographic Findings
- Anterior mediastinal mass can be shown by various modalities
- FDG-avid PET scan

MICROSCOPIC PATHOLOGY

Histologic Features
- Lymph node
  - Diffuse pattern of involvement
  - Complete or subtotal replacement of architecture
  - In cases with subtotal effacement
    - Preferential involvement of paracortical regions
    - Preserved lymphoid follicles
  - Tumor cells can infiltrate capsule and pericapsular tissue in single-file arrangement
  - "Starry sky" pattern in 10-20% of cases
  - Fibrous bands through tumor can impart nodular appearance
- Bone marrow
  - By convention
    - Lymphoma with < 25% of bone marrow involved
    - T-ALL: Extensive bone marrow disease
- Extranodal sites
  - Tumor cells often infiltrate fibrous tissue in single-file pattern

Cytologic Features
- In PB and BM aspirate smears
  - L1 blasts: Small with high nuclear to cytoplasm ratio and visible but not prominent nucleoli
  - L2 blasts: Intermediate size with prominent nucleoli and more abundant cytoplasm
  - Lymphoblasts usually are devoid of cytoplasmic granules
- In histologic sections of lymph nodes or extranodal sites
  - Lymphoblasts are small to medium-sized with scant cytoplasm
  - High mitotic activity
  - Convoluted or round nuclear contours
  - Immature (blastic) nuclear chromatin
    - "Dusty" or "salt and pepper" chromatin
    - Usually indistinct nucleoli
    - In small subset of cases, nucleoli are distinct and visible (so-called L2 variant)
- Rare cases of T-LBL are associated with eosinophilia
  - Either in PB and BM or intermixed with lymphoma cells in tissues

Predominant Cell/Compartment Type
- Hematopoietic, lymphoid

ANCILLARY TESTS

Immunohistochemistry
- T-cell antigens (+)
  - Cytoplasmic expression precedes surface expression
    - Cytoplasmic and surface antigen expression can be detected by immunohistochemistry
    - Routine flow cytometry detects surface antigen expression
    - Therefore, potential for discordance
- TdT(+), CD1a(+), CD10(+) in pre-T and cortical T stages
- CD34(+/-), CD99(+/-), CD117/C-Kit(-/+)
- CD45/LCA(+) at later stage of differentiation, TAL-1(+, ~ 50%)
- Ig(-), CD19(-), CD20(-), CD22(-)
  - CD79a(+/-)
- Proliferation rate usually high but variable
  - Ki-67 ~ 50-90%

Immunofluorescence
- TdT(+) in nuclear pattern in most cases
- This method can be used to assess T- and B-cell antigens
  - In large part, immunofluorescence has been replaced by flow cytometry

T-LYMPHOBLASTIC LEUKEMIA/LYMPHOMA

Flow Cytometry

- T-cell antigens are expressed in sequence as precursor T cells mature
  - T-LBL and T-ALL arise from precursor cell "frozen" in differentiation
  - T-ALL cases are more immature than T-LBL cases
- Pro-T (T-I)
  - CD7(+), cytoplasmic (c) CD3(+), CD34(+/-), CD2(-), CD5(-), CD4(-)/CD8(-), CD1a(-), surface(s) CD3(-)
- Pre-T (T-II)
  - TdT(+), CD7(+), cCD3(+), CD34(+/-), CD2(+), CD5(+), CD4(+/-)/CD8(+/-), CD1a(-), sCD3(-)
- Cortical T (T-III)
  - TdT(+), CD7(+), cCD3(+), CD2(+), CD5(+), CD4(+)/CD8(+), CD1a(+), sCD3(-), CD34(-)
- Mature T (T-IV)
  - CD7(+), cCD3(+), CD2(+), CD5(+), CD4(+) or CD8(+), CD1a(-), sCD3(+), CD34(-)
- Small subset of LBL may be of natural killer cell lineage
  - CD16(+), CD56(+), CD57(+), or CD94a(+)
  - CD2(+/-), CD7(+/-), CD3(-), CD5(-)
- TdT(+) in nuclear pattern in most cases
  - Cell permeabilization is required to assess by flow cytometry
- CD13(-/+) or CD33(-/+) in 20-30% of cases

Cytogenetics

- Normal karyotype in 30-40% of cases
- Common abnormalities at chromosome loci 14q11.2, 7q35, and 7p14-15
  - Location of T-cell receptors α and δ, β, and γ, respectively
  - Translocations juxtapose proto-oncogene with *TCR* resulting in overexpression
  - 1p32 *TAL1*
    - < 1% in infants, 7% in children, 12% in adults
    - t(1;14)(p32;q11)
  - 10q24 *HOX11*
    - 7% in children, 30% in adults
    - t(10;14)(q24;q11)
    - Early cortical stage; CD4(+)/CD8(+)
    - Better prognosis than other T-LBL types
  - 5q35 *HOX11L2*
    - 20% in children, 10-15% in adults
    - Pro-T stage
  - 9q34.3 *NOTCH1*
    - Translocations involving *NOTCH1* are rare: t(7;9)(q34;q34.3)
    - t(7;9)(q34;q34.3) results in truncated and active form of gene
- Other translocations
  - *NUP214/ABL1*
    - 8% adults
    - Both are on 9q34
    - Amplification with formation of episomal elements
  - 19p13 *LYL1*
    - 1.5% children, 2.5% adults
  - *MLL/ENL*/t(11;19)(q23;p13.3)
    - 0.3% children, 0.5% adults
  - Other *ABL1* translocations
    - *ETV6/ABL1*/t(9;12)(q34;p13)
    - *EML1/ABL1*/t(9;14)(q34;q32)
    - In vitro inhibition by ABL1 kinase inhibitors
    - *BCR/ABL1*/t(9;22)(q34;q11.2) rare in T-LBL
- Deletion of chromosome 9p
  - Deleted in 70% of T-LBL
  - Corresponds to loss of tumor suppressor gene *CDKN2A* (inhibitor of CDK4)
  - Leads to loss of G1 control of cell cycle

Molecular Genetics

- Gene rearrangements
  - Monoclonal T-cell receptor (*TCR*) gene rearrangements in almost all cases
    - Rearrangement of *TCR*δ occurs 1st
    - Followed by rearrangements of *TCR* γ, β, and α
  - Monoclonal *IgH* gene rearrangements in 20% of cases
- 1p32 *TAL1*
  - Interstitial deletions of *TAL1* locus are more common than t(1;14)(p32;q11)
- *NOTCH1* mutations are common
  - 58% of T-LBL carry mutation
    - Heterodimerization domain (HD): 27%
    - PEST domain: 15%
    - HD and PEST domains: 16%
  - *NOTCH1* activation signal can be abrogated by inhibition of γ-secretase
  - Protein regulates T-cell development
  - *PTEN* mutated in γ-secretase-resistant T-LBL

Gene Expression Profiling

- Studies have shown that T-LBL can be subdivided into multiple molecular signatures
  - These signatures correspond to cytogenetic subgroups
  - Signatures are also present in cases with normal cytogenetics

T-LBL with Eosinophilia

- Associated with abnormalities of *FGFR1*
- Most common: *ZNF198-FGFR1*/t(8;13)(p11;q12)
- Patients present with
  - Peripheral blood eosinophilia
  - Bone marrow myeloid hyperplasia with eosinophilia
  - ± morphologic evidence of dysplasia
- T-LBL (and rarely B-lymphoblastic leukemia/lymphoma [B-LBL]) is common in patients with *ZNF198-FGFR1*
- Patients subsequently develop myeloid malignancy
  - Acute myeloid leukemia most common
  - Myelodysplastic syndromes or myeloproliferative neoplasms also reported

DIFFERENTIAL DIAGNOSIS

B-lymphoblastic Leukemia/Lymphoma

- Most (~ 90%) cases present as B-lymphoblastic leukemia
  - ~ 10% of B-lymphoblastic tumors present as lymphoma
- Morphologically identical to T-LBL

- Convoluted or round nuclear contours
- Immature (blastic) chromatin
- Numerous mitotic figures

- Immunophenotype needed to distinguish B- from T-LBL
  - Pan-B-cell antigens (+) in B-LBL
    - CD19(+), CD20(+/-), CD22(+/-), pax-5(+)
  - ~ 10% of T-LBL are CD79a(+)
    - Potential pitfall when using limited panel
  - TdT(+), CD10(+/-): Similar to T-LBL
- Cytogenetics and molecular genetics
  - *BCR-ABL1*/t(9;22)(q34;q11.2) in approximately 30% of B-LBL cases
    - Mostly in adults
  - Monoclonal *IgH* gene rearrangements

Burkitt Lymphoma

- 3 types: Endemic (African), sporadic, and immunodeficiency-related
- Usually arises in extranodal sites
- Sporadic type occurs in Western nations
  - Ileocecal region of gastrointestinal tract very common
  - Mediastinum is rarely involved
- Morphologic features differ from T-LBL
  - Prominent "starry sky" pattern in virtually all cases
  - Monotonous, medium-sized cells with 2-5 distinct nucleoli
  - Very high mitotic and apoptotic rates
  - In smears: Moderate to abundant, deeply basophilic cytoplasm with many vacuoles
- Immunophenotype
  - Surface IgM(+), CD10(+), CD19(+)
  - CD20(+), CD22(+), CD79a(+)
  - Ki-67 > 99%, Bcl-6(+)
  - T-cell antigens(-), TdT(-), Bcl-2(-)
- Cytogenetics and molecular genetics
  - Translocations involving *MYC*
    - *MYC-IgH*/t(8;14)(q24;q32)
    - *Ig κ-MYC*/t(2;8)(p11;q24)
    - *MYC-Ig λ*/t(8;22)(q24;q11)
  - Monoclonal *IgH* gene rearrangements

Thymoma

- Presents as mediastinal mass as does T-LBL
- Lymphocyte-rich variants of thymoma are particularly troublesome
  - Many small thymic lymphocytes with immature cytologic features
  - Thymic lymphocytes are immature T cells similar to T-LBL
- Features helpful in differential diagnosis
  - Mitotic activity in thymoma is low to moderate and not high as in T-LBL
  - Thymic epithelial cells can be appreciated in lymphocyte-rich thymoma
    - Scattered intermediate to large cells with thin nuclear membranes
- Immunophenotype
  - Keratin (+) "interlocking" pattern of thymic epithelial cells in thymoma
- Molecular genetics
  - No evidence of monoclonal *TCR* gene rearrangements

Myeloid Sarcoma

- Tumor mass of myeloid blasts at extramedullary site
- Adults: Median age = 6th decade
- Can occur as
  - 1st manifestation or relapse of acute myeloid leukemia
  - Blastic transformation of myelodysplastic syndromes (MDS), myeloproliferative neoplasms (MPN), or MDS/MPN
- Mediastinum is unusual site for myeloid sarcoma
- Immunophenotype
  - CD33(+), CD68(+), CD117(+)
  - MPO(+), lysozyme (+)
  - CD3(-), CD5(-)
- Cytogenetics and molecular genetics
  - ± acute myeloid leukemia-type chromosomal changes (e.g., monosomy 7, trisomy 8, etc.)
  - Acute myeloid leukemia-type translocations can be present in myeloid sarcoma
  - No evidence of monoclonal *TCR* gene rearrangements

Blastoid Variant of Mantle Cell Lymphoma

- Tumor cells can appear lymphoblastoid with immature chromatin and high mitotic rate
- Immunophenotype
  - Surface Ig(+), CD19(+), CD20(+)
  - Cyclin-D1(+), CD5(+)
  - CD10(-), TdT(-)
- Cytogenetics and molecular genetics
  - *CCND1/IgH*/t(11;14)(q13;q32)
  - Monoclonal *IgH* gene rearrangements
  - No evidence of monoclonal *TCR* gene rearrangements

Ewing Sarcoma/Peripheral Neuroectodermal Tumor (ES/PNET)

- ES/PNET does not present as anterior superior mediastinal mass
- LBL can present as 1 or more lytic bone lesions and be misinterpreted as ES/PNET
  - More common for B-LBL than for T-LBL
- Immunophenotype
  - CD99(+) in common with T-LBL
  - ES/PNET does not express T-cell or B-cell antigens
- t(11;22)(q24;q12), t(21;22)(q22;q12), t(1;16)(q11;q11)
- Cytogenetics and molecular genetics
  - *EWS/FLI1*/t(11;22)(q24;q12) and other abnormalities involving *EWS* gene
  - No evidence of monoclonal *TCR* gene rearrangements

Small (Oat) Cell Carcinoma

- Primary lung neoplasm, but metastases can cause prominent mediastinal lymphadenopathy
- Patient population: Adults with history of smoking
- Small cell carcinoma is composed of cohesive tumor cells larger than lymphoblasts
- Immunophenotype
  - Keratin (+), chromogranin (+/-), synaptophysin (+/-)

  - CD3(-), CD5(-), TdT(-)

Merkel Cell Carcinoma

- Patient population: Elderly patients who present with skin lesions
- Does not present as mediastinal mass
- Merkel cell carcinoma is composed of cohesive tumor cells larger than lymphoblasts
- Immunophenotype
  - Keratin (+), cytokeratin 20 (+, often perinuclear)
  - T-cell antigens (-), TdT(-)

Rhabdomyosarcoma

- Alveolar rhabdomyosarcoma is type most likely to be confused with T-LBL
- Can present initially as extensive BM disease mimicking T-ALL
- Immunophenotype
  - Muscle markers (+)
  - T-cell antigens (-), TdT(-)
- Cytogenetics and molecular genetics
  - *PAX3-FOXO1*/t(2;13)(q35;q14) or *PAX7-FOXO1*/t(1;13)(p36;q14)
  - *PAX3-NCOA1*/t(2;2)(p23;q35) and *PAX3-NCOA2*/t(2;8)(q35;q13)

Acute Undifferentiated Leukemia (AUL)

- Can morphologically mimic T-ALL
- Unlike T-ALL, AUL does not express lineage-specific antigens
- Immunophenotyping of AUL must be comprehensive to exclude other entities

Mixed Phenotype Acute Leukemia (MPAL)

- Diagnostic criteria for MPAL are strict
- Criteria include
  - Bilineage: 2 distinct blast populations, 1 of which would meet criteria for AML even if < 20% **or**
  - Biphenotypic: Single blast population that meets criteria for T-/B-ALL and also expresses myeloid/monocytic markers
  - MPAL with t(9;22)(q34;q11.2); *BCR-ABL1*
  - MPAL with t(v;11q23), *MLL* rearranged
  - MPAL, B/myeloid or T/myeloid, not otherwise specified

Dermatofibrosarcoma Protuberans (DFSP)

- Does not present as anterior mediastinal mass
- Very rarely spreads to lymph nodes or BM
- Involves dermis of skin
- Most patients with DFSP are adults 20-50 years of age
- DFSP in dermis infiltrates in single file similar to T-LBL
- Immunophenotype
  - DFSP and T-LBL can be CD34(+)
  - DFSP is TdT(-), T-cell antigens (-)
- Cytogenetics and molecular genetics
  - *COL1A1-PDGFRβ*/t(17;22)(q22;q13) in ~ 90% of cases

DIAGNOSTIC CHECKLIST

Clinically Relevant Pathologic Features

- T-LBL is disease that primarily affects adolescents and young adults
- Male predominance
- Presenting symptoms and signs related to
  - Anterior mediastinal mass
  - Supradiaphragmatic lymphadenopathy
  - BM and PB involvement

Pathologic Interpretation Pearls

- Important morphologic features of T-LBL
  - Preferential involvement of paracortical regions of lymph node
  - Small to medium-sized cells with immature (blastic) nuclear chromatin
  - Single-file pattern of infiltration in extranodal tissues
  - High mitotic activity
- Important immunophenotypic features
  - TdT(+), T-cell antigens (+)
  - CD1a(+/-), CD10(+/-), CD34(+/-)
  - Immunophenotype corresponds to precursor T cell "frozen" in differentiation

SELECTED REFERENCES

1. Burkhardt B: Paediatric lymphoblastic T-cell leukaemia and lymphoma: one or two diseases? Br J Haematol. 149(5):653-68, 2010
2. Fortune A et al: T-lymphoblastic leukemia/lymphoma: a single center retrospective study of outcome. Leuk Lymphoma. 51(6):1035-9, 2010
3. Jackson CC et al: 8p11 myeloproliferative syndrome: a review. Hum Pathol. 41(4):461-76, 2010
4. Pieters R et al: Biology and treatment of acute lymphoblastic leukemia. Hematol Oncol Clin North Am. 24(1):1-18, 2010
5. Marks DI et al: T-cell acute lymphoblastic leukemia in adults: clinical features, immunophenotype, cytogenetics, and outcome from the large randomized prospective trial (UKALL XII/ECOG 2993). Blood. 114(25):5136-45, 2009
6. Teitell MA et al: Molecular genetics of acute lymphoblastic leukemia. Annu Rev Pathol. 4:175-98, 2009
7. Han X et al: Precursor T-cell acute lymphoblastic leukemia/lymphoblastic lymphoma and acute biphenotypic leukemias. Am J Clin Pathol. 127(4):528-44, 2007
8. Armstrong SA et al: Molecular genetics of acute lymphoblastic leukemia. J Clin Oncol. 23(26):6306-15, 2005
9. Weng AP et al: Activating mutations of NOTCH1 in human T cell acute lymphoblastic leukemia. Science. 306(5694):269-71, 2004
10. Dabaja BS et al: The role of local radiation therapy for mediastinal disease in adults with T-cell lymphoblastic lymphoma. Cancer. 94(10):2738-44, 2002
11. Nathwani BN et al: Lymphoblastic lymphoma: a clinicopathologic study of 95 patients. Cancer. 48(11):2347-57, 1981

Microscopic Features

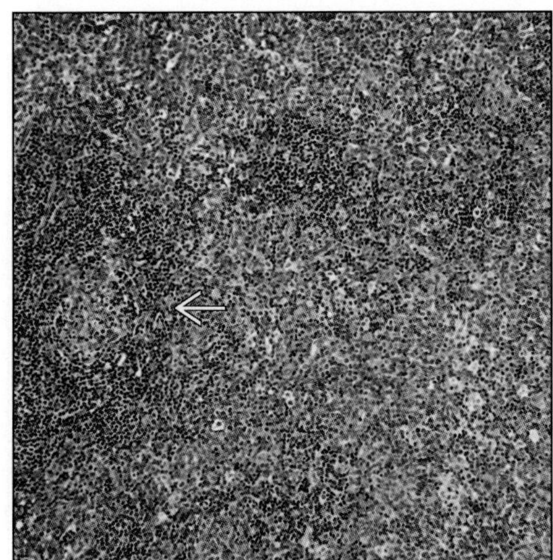

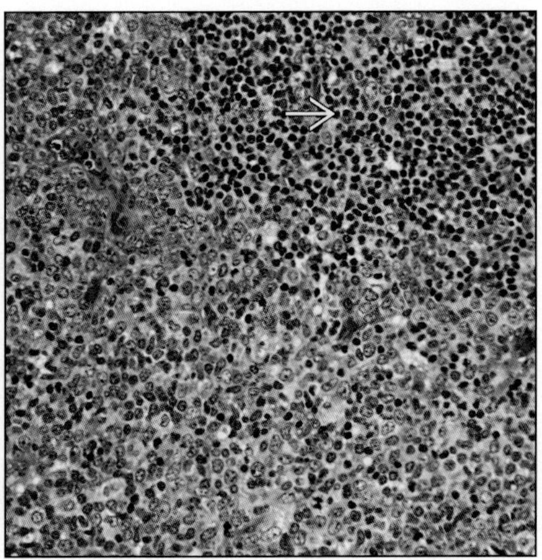

(Left) *Hematoxylin & eosin shows lymphoblasts subtotally replacing lymph node in this case of T-lymphoblastic lymphoma/leukemia. Note the residual follicle present along the left edge of the field* ➡*.* ***(Right)*** *A case of T-lymphoblastic lymphoma/leukemia with subtotal replacement of a lymph node is shown. The neoplastic lymphoblasts are larger than normal lymphocytes and have fine chromatin and scant cytoplasm. Note residual small lymphocytes at upper right* ➡*.*

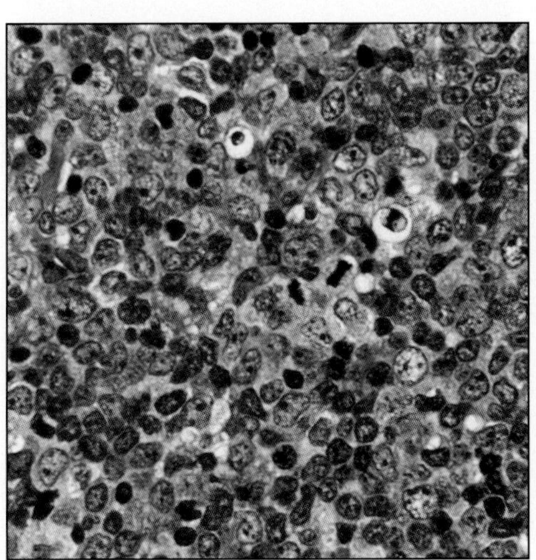

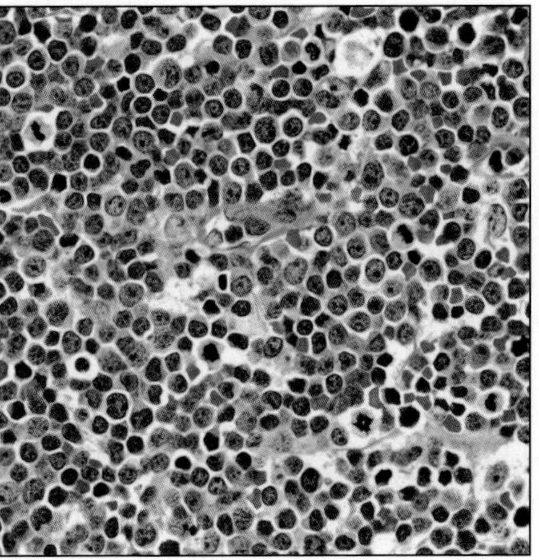

(Left) *T-lymphoblastic lymphoma/leukemia involving lymph node is shown. The neoplastic lymphoblasts have fine (immature) chromatin, small nucleoli, and a high mitotic rate.* ***(Right)*** *T-lymphoblastic lymphoma/leukemia involving lymph node is shown. The lymphoblasts are medium-sized with irregular nuclei, fine chromatin, inconspicuous nucleoli, and a high mitotic rate.*

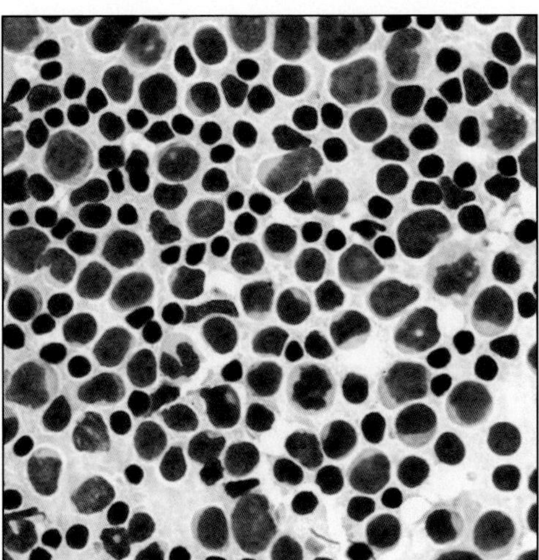

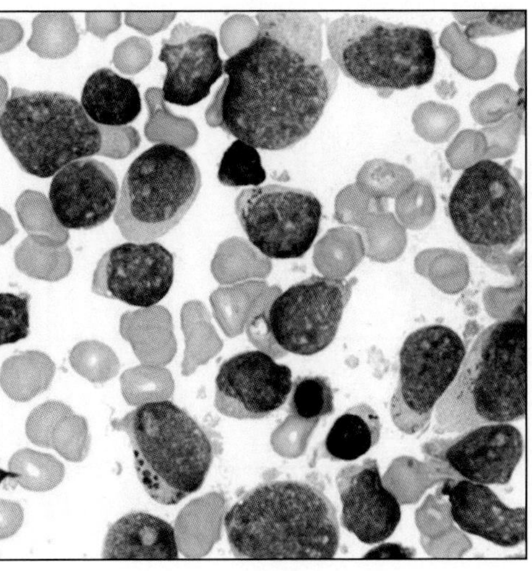

(Left) *T-lymphoblastic lymphoma/leukemia involving lymph node is shown. Touch imprint shows small to medium-sized lymphoblasts with fine chromatin and indistinct nucleoli. Mature small lymphocytes are also present in the background.* ***(Right)*** *Wright-Giemsa stain of bone marrow aspirate smear shows lymphoblasts with high nuclear to cytoplasmic ratio, fine chromatin, small nucleoli, and basophilic cytoplasm. Note that some blasts have cytoplasmic azurophilic granules.*

Diagrammatic and Flow Cytometry Features

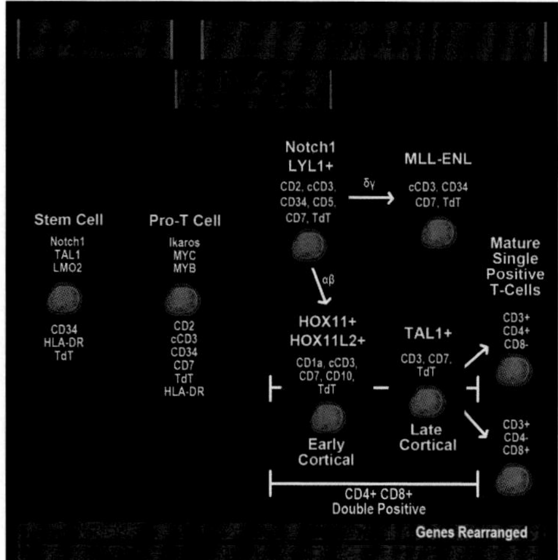

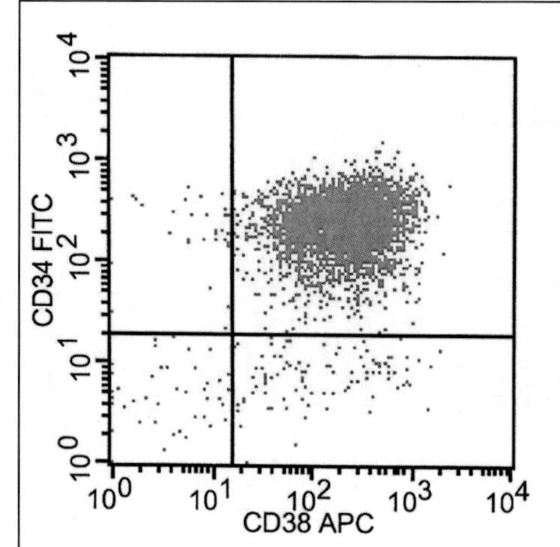

(Left) *Schematic shows the sequential stages of precursor T-cell differentiation. The immunophenotype of T-lymphoblastic lymphoma/leukemia (T-LBL) corresponds to a "frozen" stage of precursor T-cell differentiation.* ***(Right)*** *Flow immunophenotypic studies show that T-LBL blasts express CD34 and CD38.*

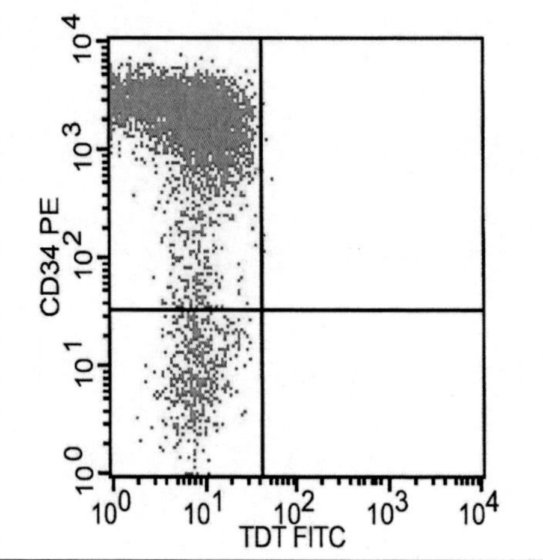

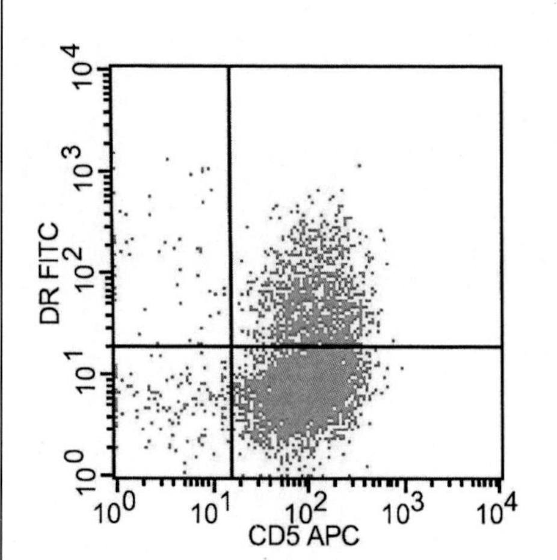

(Left) *Flow immunophenotypic studies show that T-LBL blasts are negative for TdT and positive for CD34.* ***(Right)*** *Flow immunophenotypic studies show that T-LBL blasts express CD5 and partial HLA-DR.*

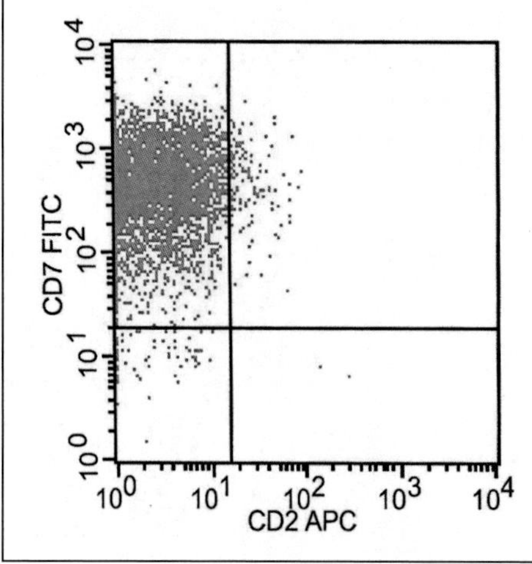

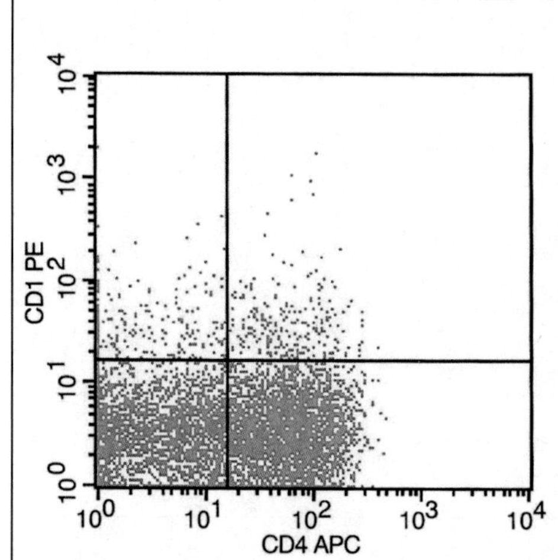

(Left) *Flow immunophenotypic studies show that T-LBL blasts express CD7 and are negative for CD2.* ***(Right)*** *Flow immunophenotypic studies show that this hypodiploid T-LBL with rearrangement involving 17p/TP53 expresses CD4 and partially expresses CD1.*

Immunohistochemistry and Differential Diagnosis

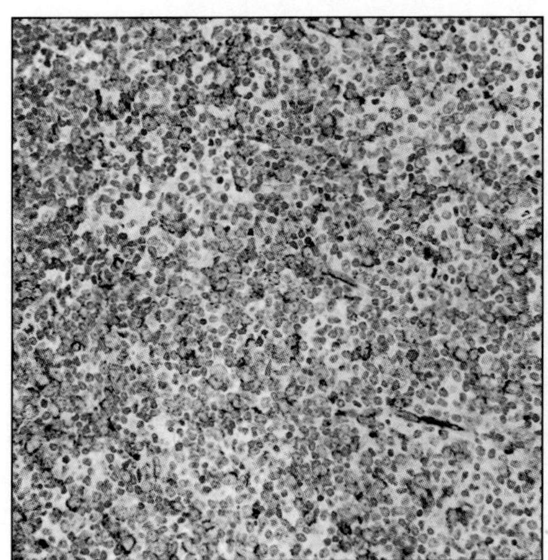

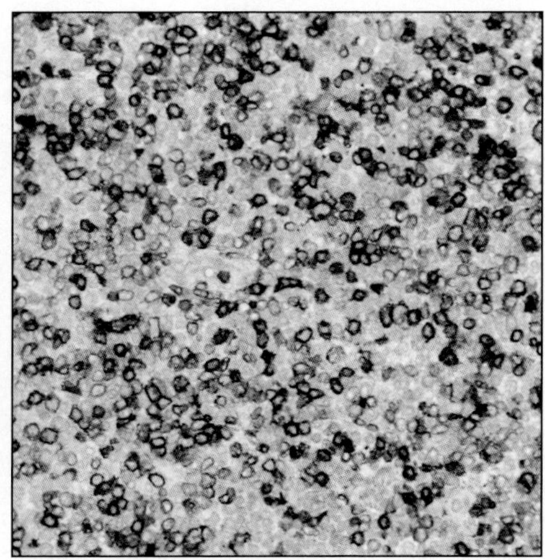

(Left) *A case of T-lymphoblastic lymphoma/leukemia involving lymph node is shown. CD34 is expressed by a subset of lymphoblasts in this case.* ***(Right)*** *A case of T-lymphoblastic lymphoma/leukemia involving a lymph node is shown. CD3 is positive with variable intensity in many lymphoblasts in this case.*

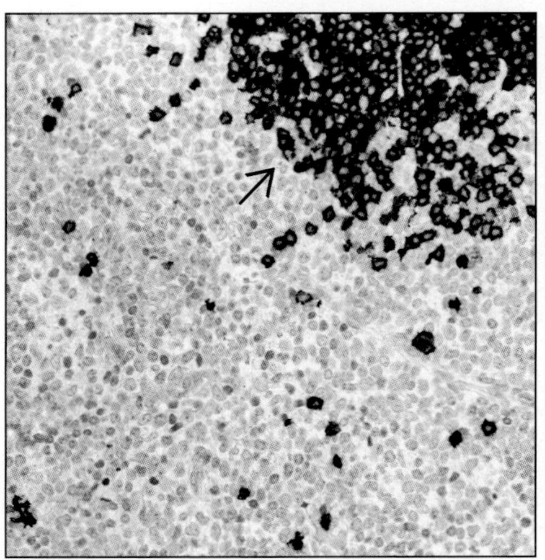

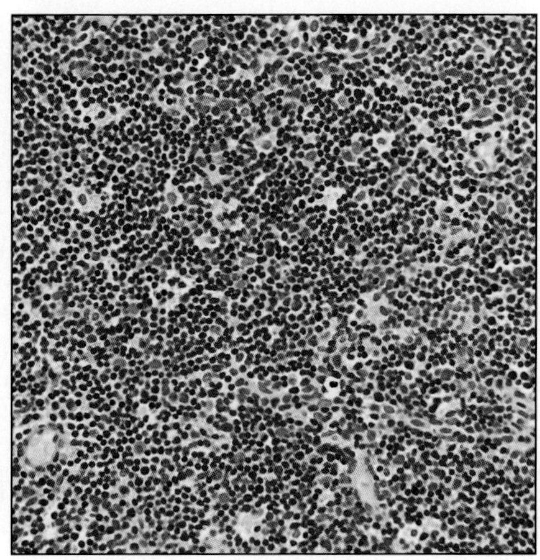

(Left) *CD20 stain is negative in the lymphoblasts in this case of T-lymphoblastic lymphoma/leukemia that involves a lymph node. A residual follicle is CD20(+) ⇒.* ***(Right)*** *This case of thymoma is composed of a high content of small lymphocytes and relatively few thymic epithelial cells that are difficult to appreciate in this field. Note the absence of mitotic figures in this neoplasm.*

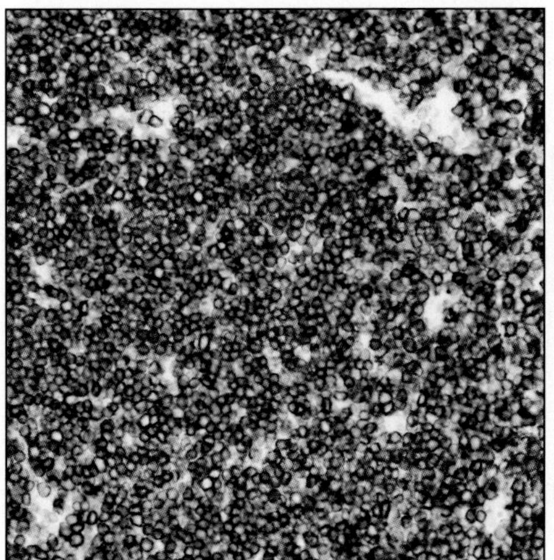

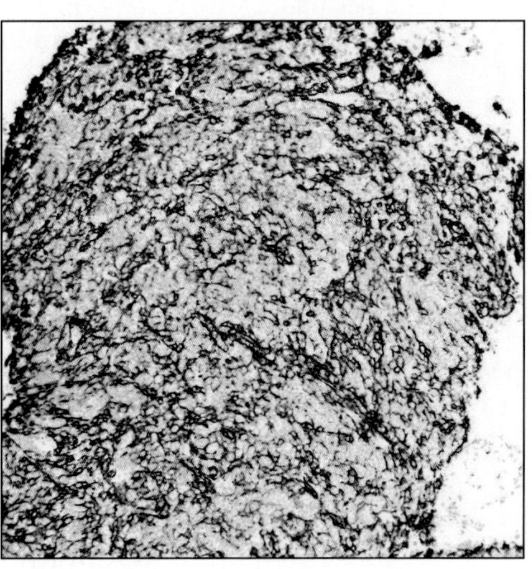

(Left) *CD3 immunostaining is strongly positive, highlighting the high content of the small T lymphocytes in this case of thymoma.* ***(Right)*** *A keratin immunohistochemical stain shows an interlocking pattern of positive-staining epithelial cells in this case of lymphocyte-predominant thymoma.*

ANAPLASTIC LARGE CELL LYMPHOMA, ALK+

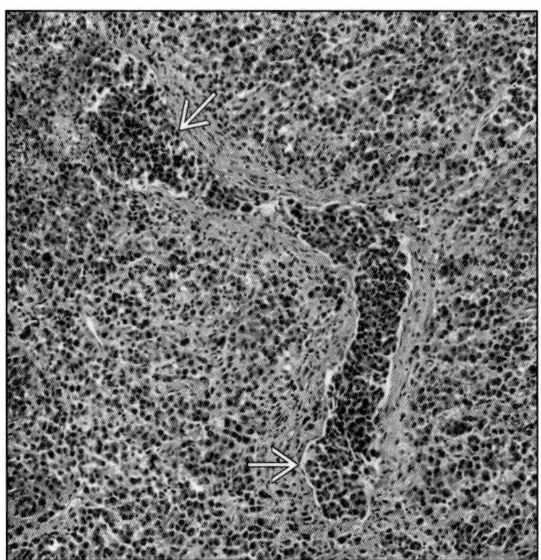

The characteristic sinusoidal pattern of growth ➡ is shown in this case of ALK(+) ALCL.

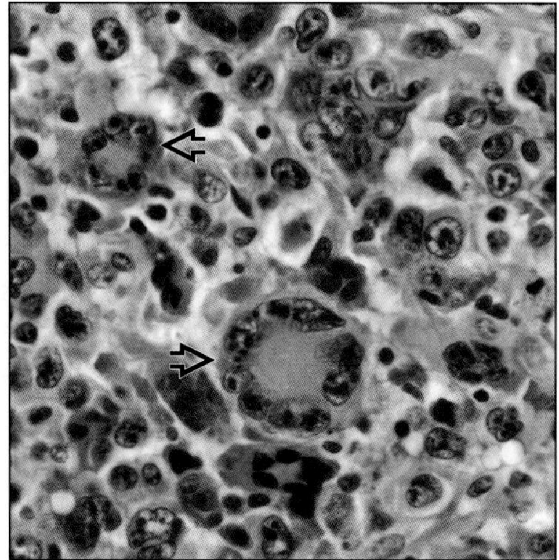

Several "wreath cells" ⇨ along with numerous neoplastic mononuclear cells are shown in this ALK(+) ALCL.

TERMINOLOGY

Abbreviations

- Anaplastic large cell lymphoma (ALCL)

Synonyms

- Ki-1 lymphoma

Definitions

- CD30(+) lymphoma of T- or null cell lineage with distinct histologic features and chromosomal translocation commonly involving *ALK* on chromosome 2p23 and *NPM* on chromosome 5q35

ETIOLOGY/PATHOGENESIS

Chromosomal Rearrangements

- Lead to enhanced ALK activity
- Partner genes promote dimerization of ALK molecules
- Allow ALK kinase to phosphorylate and become constitutively activated
- Activate downstream pathways
- Leads to oncogenic progression

CLINICAL ISSUES

Epidemiology

- Incidence
  - 20-30% of all non-Hodgkin lymphomas in pediatric population
    - 80-90% of all cases are ALK(+) ALCL
  - 2% of adult non-Hodgkin lymphomas in United States
- Age
  - Male predominance

Site

- Most common sites
  - Skin
  - Bone
  - Soft tissue
  - Lung
  - Liver

Presentation

- B-symptoms
  - Fever
  - Weight loss
  - Night sweats
- Most patients present with advanced stage III/IV disease
- Extranodal involvement common (60%)
- Bone marrow involvement (5-30%)
- Central nervous system (rare)

Treatment

- Intensive chemotherapy
  - CHOP (cyclophosphamide, hydroxydaunorubicin [doxorubicin], oncovin [vincristine] and prednisone) (first-line approach)
- Radiation therapy
  - Can be used as important complement to CHOP therapy
- ALK targeted therapy
  - Crizotinib
    - Currently undergoing clinical trials

Prognosis

- 5-year survival = 90%
  - Good complete response rates and overall survival compared with other types of T-cell lymphoma
  - ALK(+) ALCL have significantly higher 5-year survival rate as compared with ALK(-) ALCL

MACROSCOPIC FEATURES

General Features

- Enlarged lymph nodes
- Homogeneous tan-white cut surface

ANAPLASTIC LARGE CELL LYMPHOMA, ALK+

Key Facts

Terminology
- CD30(+) lymphoma of T- or null cell lineage with distinct histologic features and chromosomal abnormalities involving 2p23 and ALK

Clinical Issues
- 20-30% of all non-Hodgkin lymphomas in pediatric population
  - 80-90% of all cases are ALK(+) ALCL
- Most patients present with advanced stage III/IV disease
- Extranodal involvement common (60%)

Microscopic Pathology
- Common histologic variant (80%)
  - Large anaplastic cells that invade lymph node sinuses and exhibit cohesive appearance
- Histologic variants of ALCL
  - Lymphohistiocytic (5-10%)
  - Small cell (5-10%)
  - Sarcomatoid (1%)

Ancillary Tests
- Characterized by chromosomal translocations involving *ALK* gene at 2p23
- ALK fusion proteins described in other neoplasms

Top Differential Diagnoses
- ALK(-) ALCL
- Classical Hodgkin lymphoma (cHL)
- Diffuse large B-cell lymphoma (DLBCL)
- Cutaneous CD30(+) lymphoproliferative disorders

- ± necrosis

MICROSCOPIC PATHOLOGY

Histologic Features
- Common/classical variant
  - 80% of all cases
  - Large anaplastic cells that invade lymph node sinuses and exhibit a cohesive appearance
  - May mimic metastatic involvement of lymph node by solid tumor
  - Erythrophagocytosis can be seen in some cases
  - Mitotic figures and apoptotic cells are usually numerous
  - "Starry sky" pattern can be seen
  - Areas of necrosis
- Neoplastic cells: Large, irregular, and bizarre
  - Often with polylobated nuclei
- Cytological spectrum of neoplastic cells from small to large
  - Cell size variability helpful in distinguishing ALCL from classical Hodgkin lymphoma
- "Hallmark" cells characteristic
  - Large cells with eccentric horseshoe- or kidney-shaped nuclei
  - Prominent paranuclear eosinophilic Golgi region
  - Abundant cytoplasm that may be clear, basophilic, or eosinophilic
  - Nuclei commonly contain 1 or more prominent nucleoli
- Other characteristic cells
  - Doughnut cells
  - Wreath cells
  - Reed–Sternberg-like cells
- Histologic variants of ALCL
  - Common/classical (80%)
  - Lymphohistiocytic (5-10%)
  - Small cell (5-10%)
  - Other rare variants (~ 1%)
    - Sarcomatoid
    - Eosinophil and neutrophil-rich
    - Giant cell-rich
    - Signet ring cell
- Variants stand alone or may be associated with common variant
- Cases may resemble small round blue cell tumors
  - Distinguish by immunohistochemical staining patterns (CD30[+], ALK[+])

Cytologic Features
- Fine needle aspirate smears
  - Dyscohesive neoplastic cells
  - Mitotic figures are usually easily identified
  - Morphologic variants of ALK(+) ALCL may be difficult to recognize in cytology smears

Predominant Pattern/Injury Type
- Diffuse
  - May show focal, partial, or complete involvement of lymph node

ANCILLARY TESTS

Immunohistochemistry
- Strongly and uniformly positive for CD30 and ALK
- Can be of T- or null cell lineage
  - In cases of T-cell lineage, aberrant T-cell immunophenotype is common
    - Most tumors do not express CD3, CD5, or T-cell receptors (suggests defective T-cell signaling)
    - CD4(+) more often than CD8(+)
  - Both T- and null-cell ALK(+) ALCL usually carry monoclonal rearrangements of the T-cell receptor genes
- Commonly express cytotoxic proteins such as TIA-1, granzyme B, and perforin
- Clusterin, epithelial membrane antigen EMA (a.k.a. MUC1), Mcl-1, FLI-1, and MYC are commonly expressed
- CD99 expression has been reported
- CD45 can be absent
  - Combination of EMA(+) and CD45(-) can lead to misdiagnosis of carcinoma

- Almost all cases are negative for keratin
- Ki-67 proliferation index (PI)
  - PI is routinely very high: > 75% in common variant, but lower in lymphohistiocytic and small cell variants
- Bcl-2(-)
- Type of ALK staining correlates with type of underlying genetic abnormality
  - Cytoplasmic and nuclear: t(2;5)
  - Cytoplasmic, not coarsely granular: Variant translocations
    - Except t(2;X) and t(2;17)
  - Cytoplasmic, coarsely granular: t(2;17)
  - Membranous: t(2;X)

Cytogenetics

- Characterized by chromosomal translocations involving *ALK* gene at 2p23
- Methods used for demonstrating *ALK* abnormalities
  - Conventional cytogenetics
  - Fluorescence in situ hybridization (FISH)
  - Reverse-transcriptase (RT) PCR
    - Most only detect t(2;5) or a few of variant translocations
  - Long-range PCR
  - Immunohistochemistry
  - ALK immunostaining or FISH is recommended for initial diagnosis
- Chromosomal translocations
  - 75-80% of cases t(2;5)(p23;q35)
    - t(2;5) juxtaposes nucleophosmin (*NPM*) gene at 5q35 with *ALK* gene at 2p23
    - t(2;5) drives expression of novel fusion protein NPM-ALK
  - Variant chromosomal abnormalities (25% of cases)
    - *ALK* gene rearranged with other genes
    - Tropomyosin 3 (*TPM3*), t(1;2)(p25;p23)
    - TRK-fused gene (*TFG*), t(2;3)(p23;q21)
    - *ATIC*, inv(2)(p23;q35)
    - Moesin (*MSN*), t(2;X)(p23; q11-12)
    - Clathrin heavy chain (*CLTCL*), t(2;17)(p23;q23)
    - Tropomyosin 4 (*TPM4*), t(2;19)(p23;q13.1)
    - *ALO17*, t(2;17)(p23;q25)
    - *MYH9*, t(2;22)(p23;q11.2)
  - Additional translocations involving ALK will be recognized in future
- ALK fusion proteins also described in
  - Inflammatory myofibroblastic tumors
  - Non-small cell lung cancer (11%)
  - Breast cancer (2.4%)
  - Colorectal cancer (2.4%)
  - Diffuse large B-cell lymphomas (subset)
  - Squamous cell carcinoma of esophagus

Electron Microscopy

- Innumerable filopodia on surface of neoplastic cells
- Abundant cytoplasm contains many free ribosomes and moderate numbers of mitochondria
- Type 2 neurosecretory granules (150-750 nm in size) can be seen in cytoplasm or clustered in Golgi region

DIFFERENTIAL DIAGNOSIS

ALK(-) ALCL

- Considered provisional entity in current 2008 World Health Organization (WHO) lymphoma classification system
- Lymphoma morphologically within spectrum of ALK(+) ALCL
  - Strong, uniform expression of CD30
  - Lack ALK protein expression
- ALK(+) and ALK(-) tumors have distinctive gene expression signatures and genomic imbalances
- Worse prognosis than ALK(+) ALCL
- More common in adults with no age preference
- Immunophenotypically ALK(-) ALCL shares many features with ALK(+) ALCL
  - Commonalities
    - CD30(+) (strongly and uniformly positive)
    - Aberrant T-cell immunophenotype
    - Expression of cytotoxic molecules (50%)
    - Clusterin positive
  - Differences
    - ALK(-)
    - Bcl-2(+) in many cases
    - EBV(+) (subset of cases)

Classical Hodgkin Lymphoma (cHL)

- Immunophenotype very helpful to confirm diagnosis of cHL
- Tumor cells in HL positive for
  - CD15
  - CD30
  - Pax-5/BSAP (nuclear and characteristically weak)
  - CD20 or CD79a in 20% of cases; variable
- Negative for
  - EMA
  - CD45 (LCA)
  - ALK
  - TIA-1 and other cytotoxic proteins
- In contrast, ALK(+) ALCL tumor cells are ALK(+) and pax-5/BSAP(-)

Diffuse Large B-cell Lymphoma (DLBCL)

- Some DLBCL positive for CD30
  - However, in those cases tumor cells are
    - Pax-5/BSAP(+)
    - ALK(-)
- Rare DLBCL expresses ALK and carries either t(2;5) or t(2;17)
  - Plasmablastic morphology
  - Positive for
    - CD138
    - CD4
    - IgA
    - ALK
  - Usually negative for
    - B-cell markers
    - CD30
    - T-cell markers

Immunohistochemistry

Antibody	Reactivity	Staining Pattern	Comment
ALK1	Positive	Nuclear & cytoplasmic	75% of t(2;5); tumors with variant 2p23 abnormalities have cytoplasmic or membranous pattern
CD2	Positive	Cell membrane	
CD4	Positive	Cell membrane	CD4(+) more common than CD8(+)
CD30	Positive	Cell membrane & cytoplasm	Strongly and uniformly positive
CD45	Positive	Cell membrane	Positive in 50% of cases
EMA/MUC1	Positive	Cell membrane	
Clusterin	Positive	Golgi zone	Positive in 80-90% of cases
TIA	Positive	Cytoplasmic	Granzyme B and perforin are also usually positive
CD3	Negative	Cell membrane & cytoplasm	CD3 and CD5 are usually negative
CD5	Negative	Cell membrane	CD3 and CD5 are usually negative
Bcl-2	Negative	Cytoplasmic	Often positive in ALK(-) ALCL

Cutaneous CD30(+) Lymphoproliferative Disorders

- Spectrum of neoplasms
  - Lymphomatoid papulosis (LyP)
  - Primary cutaneous ALCL
  - Secondary systemic ALCL involving skin
  - Primary or secondary cHL involving skin
  - CD30(+) large B-cell lymphoma
- Diagnosis depends on correlation of clinical and histologic findings
- LyP: Grouped or disseminated papules that regress spontaneously after a few weeks
  - 3 histologic subtypes (A, B, and C) represent spectrum with overlapping features
- Primary cutaneous ALCL usually presents as solitary nodule that rapidly grows and often ulcerates
  - Cutaneous ALCL usually positive for
    - CD30
    - T-cell markers (CD2, CD3, CD4) with variable loss of CD5 and CD7
    - Cytotoxic molecules (TIA-1, granzyme B, perforin)
  - Immunophenotypic differences between primary cutaneous ALCL and systemic ALCL
    - EMA usually negative in cutaneous ALCL
    - Expression of ALK extremely rare (or absent) in cutaneous ALCL
  - Reliable pathologic criteria not currently available to distinguish cutaneous ALCL from systemic ALK(-) ALCL
  - No criteria to predict which cases of cutaneous ALCL likely to disseminate to other sites

Others Tumors Expressing ALK Protein

- Expression of either ALK or ALK fusion proteins documented in several primary solid cancers
  - Inflammatory myofibroblastic tumors
  - Non-small cell lung cancer (11%)
  - Breast cancers (2.4%)
  - Colorectal cancers (2.4%)
  - Subset of DLBCL
  - Squamous cell carcinoma of esophagus
  - Neuroblastoma
  - Glioblastoma
  - Alveolar subtype of rhabdomyosarcoma

SELECTED REFERENCES

1. Das P et al: Anaplastic large cell lymphoma: a critical evaluation of cytomorphological features in seven cases. Cytopathology. 21(4):251-8, 2010
2. Gustafson S et al: Anaplastic large cell lymphoma: another entity in the differential diagnosis of small round blue cell tumors. Ann Diagn Pathol. 13(6):413-27, 2009
3. Lin E et al: Exon array profiling detects EML4-ALK fusion in breast, colorectal, and non-small cell lung cancers. Mol Cancer Res. 7(9):1466-76, 2009
4. Hirsch B et al: CD30-induced signaling is absent in Hodgkin's cells but present in anaplastic large cell lymphoma cells. Am J Pathol. 172(2):510-20, 2008
5. Savage KJ et al: ALK- anaplastic large-cell lymphoma is clinically and immunophenotypically different from both ALK+ ALCL and peripheral T-cell lymphoma, not otherwise specified: report from the International Peripheral T-Cell Lymphoma Project. Blood. 111(12):5496-504, 2008
6. Amin HM et al: Pathobiology of ALK+ anaplastic large-cell lymphoma. Blood. 110(7):2259-67, 2007
7. Medeiros LJ et al: Anaplastic large cell lymphoma. Am J Clin Pathol. 127(5):707-22, 2007
8. Gascoyne RD et al: ALK-positive diffuse large B-cell lymphoma is associated with Clathrin-ALK rearrangements: report of 6 cases. Blood. 102(7):2568-73, 2003
9. Falini B: Anaplastic large cell lymphoma: pathological, molecular and clinical features. Br J Haematol. 114(4):741-60, 2001
10. Rassidakis GZ et al: Differential expression of BCL-2 family proteins in ALK-positive and ALK-negative anaplastic large cell lymphoma of T/null-cell lineage. Am J Pathol. 159(2):527-35, 2001
11. Stein H et al: CD30(+) anaplastic large cell lymphoma: a review of its histopathologic, genetic, and clinical features. Blood. 96(12):3681-95, 2000
12. Falini B et al: ALK+ lymphoma: clinico-pathological findings and outcome. Blood. 93(8):2697-706, 1999
13. Falini B et al: Lymphomas expressing ALK fusion protein(s) other than NPM-ALK. Blood. 94(10):3509-15, 1999
14. Falini B et al: ALK expression defines a distinct group of T/null lymphomas ("ALK lymphomas") with a wide morphological spectrum. Am J Pathol. 153(3):875-86, 1998
15. Stein H et al: The expression of the Hodgkin's disease associated antigen Ki-1 in reactive and neoplastic lymphoid tissue: evidence that Reed-Sternberg cells and histiocytic malignancies are derived from activated lymphoid cells. Blood. 66(4):848-58, 1985

ANAPLASTIC LARGE CELL LYMPHOMA, ALK+

Microscopic Features

*(**Left**) High-power image shows the large and pleomorphic cells of ALCL. Hallmark cells ➔ are usually present. Note the kidney-shaped nuclei and eosinophilic Golgi region ➔. (**Right**) Low-power view shows the lymphohistiocytic variant of ALK(+) ALCL. Numerous pale-appearing histiocytes and clusters of small lymphocytes ➔ are noted. (Courtesy F. Vega, MD, PhD.)*

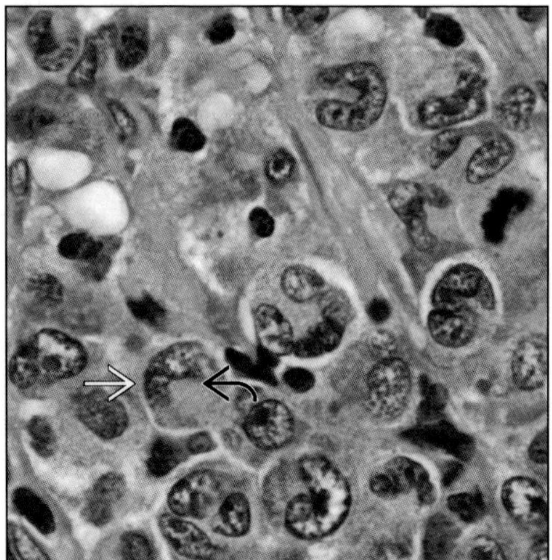

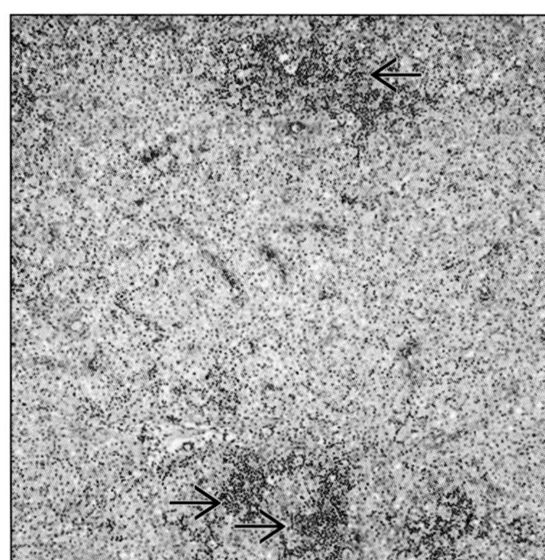

*(**Left**) The lymphohistiocytic variant of ALK(+) ALCL is associated with numerous reactive lymphocytes and histiocytes with relatively few large pleomorphic neoplastic cells. CD30 or ALK immunostain help in recognizing this variant. (**Right**) The small cell variant of ALK(+) ALCL is characterized by numerous small neoplastic cells. Large neoplastic cells ➔, although infrequent, are also seen. CD30 or ALK immunostain help in recognizing this variant. (Courtesy F. Vega, MD, PhD.)*

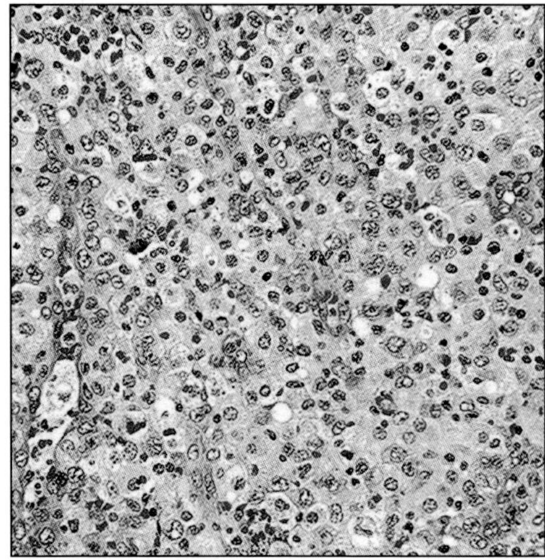

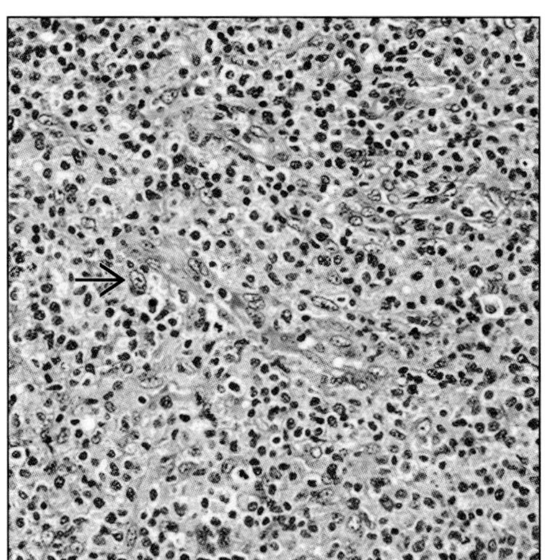

*(**Left**) In the monomorphic variant of ALK(+) ALCL, the neoplastic cells are intermediate to large and have a monomorphic appearance. CD30 or ALK immunostain help in recognizing this variant. (**Right**) Hematoxylin & eosin shows an ALK(+) ALCL, sarcomatoid variant. This variant is characterized by the presence of a subset of tumor cells with a spindle morphology. (Courtesy F. Vega, MD, PhD.)*

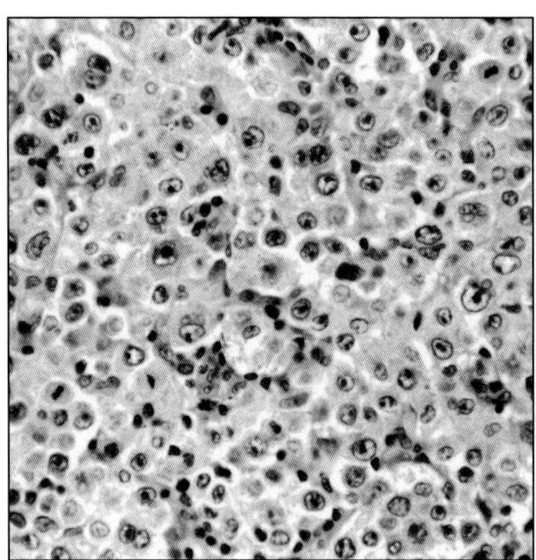

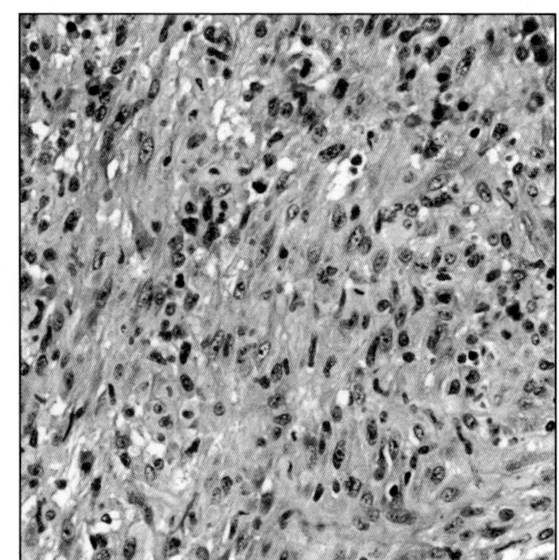

Ancillary Techniques

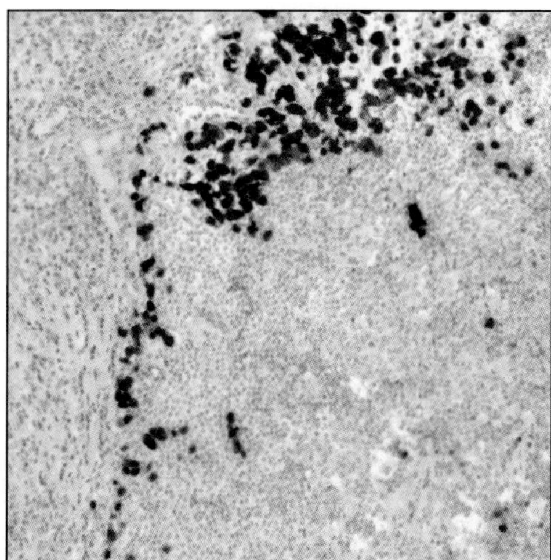

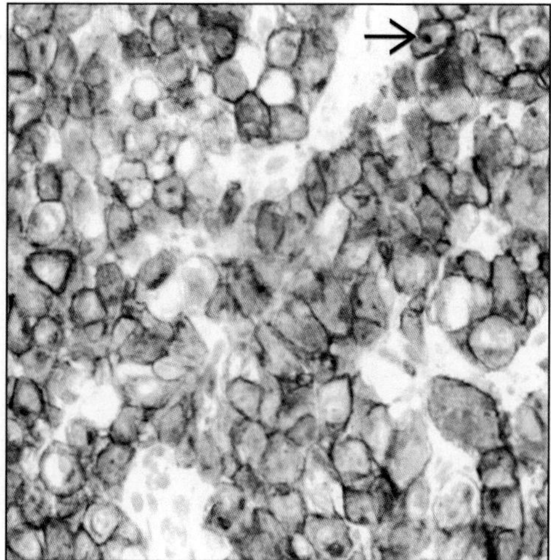

(Left) *ALK immunostain highlights a prominent sinusoidal growth of the tumor cells in ALK(+) ALCL. This pattern is particularly seen in lymph nodes not involved extensively. (Courtesy F. Vega, MD, PhD.)* ***(Right)*** *CD30 is strongly expressed by the neoplastic cells in ALK(+) and ALK(-) ALCL tumors. Note the characteristic membranous and paranuclear (Golgi) pattern ➔.*

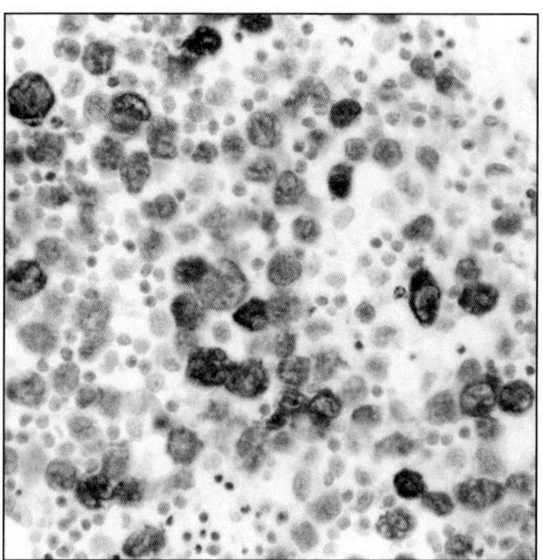

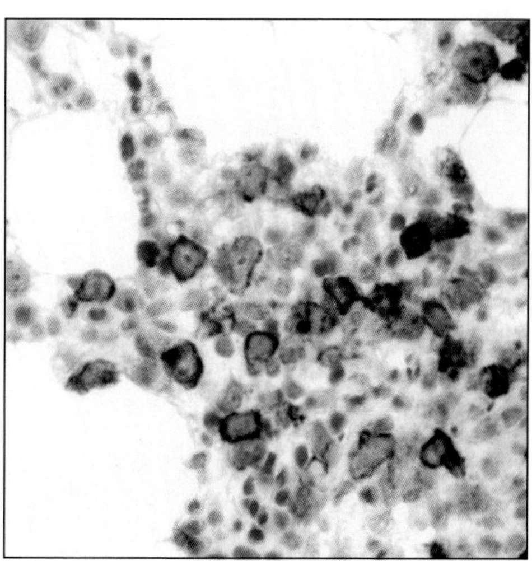

(Left) *In this case of ALK(+) ALCL, ALK immunostaining shows a cytoplasmic and weakly nuclear pattern indicating the presence of the t(2;5) (NPM-ALK).* ***(Right)*** *CD30 may help to identify ALCL in bone marrow. In some cases, few tumor cells are highlighted using immunostains. (Courtesy F. Vega, MD, PhD.)*

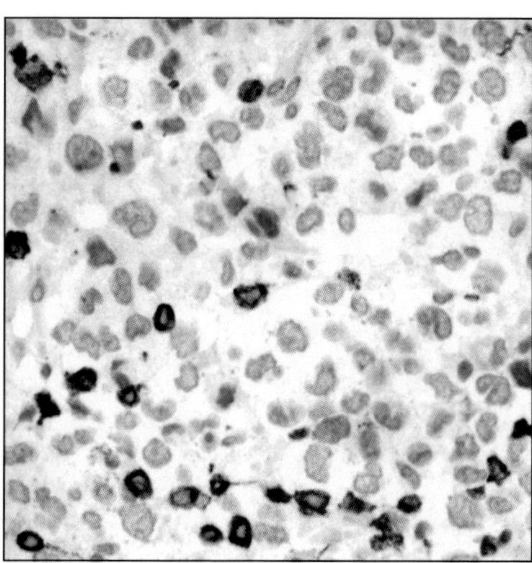

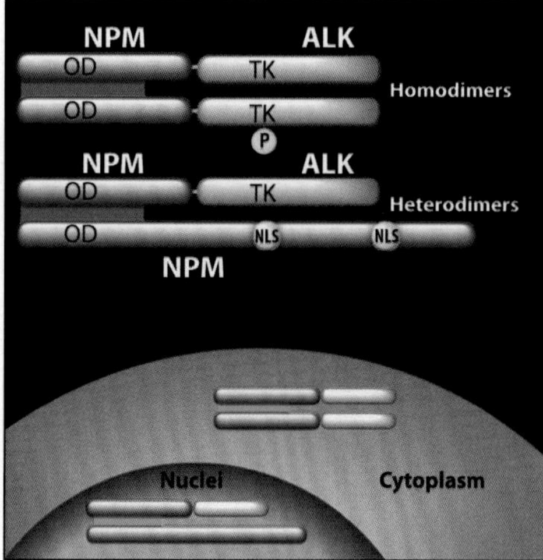

(Left) *Frequently, the tumor cells in ALK(+) and ALK(-) ALCL are CD3(-).* ***(Right)*** *NPM-ALK encodes a fusion protein that contains the tyrosine kinase (TK) domain of ALK. The oligomerization domain (OD) of NPM allows the formation of homodimers between NPM-ALK proteins and heterodimers NPM-ALK with wild type (WT) NPM. WT NPM has nuclear localization signals (NLS) that drive the heterodimers into the nucleus. Thus, in the presence of t(2;5), ALK immunostain is cytoplasmic and nuclear.*

Differential Diagnosis and Morphologic Variants

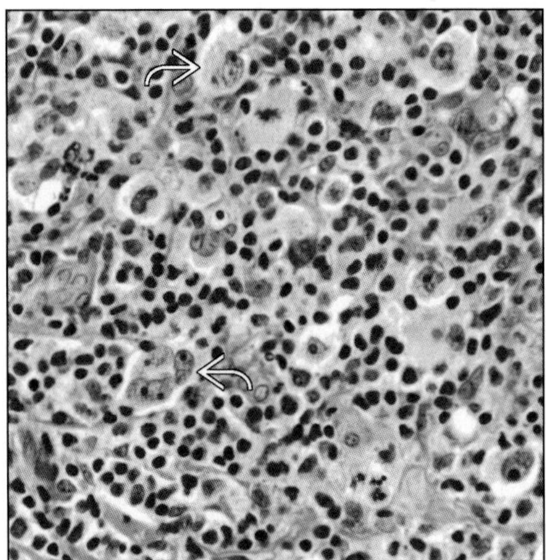

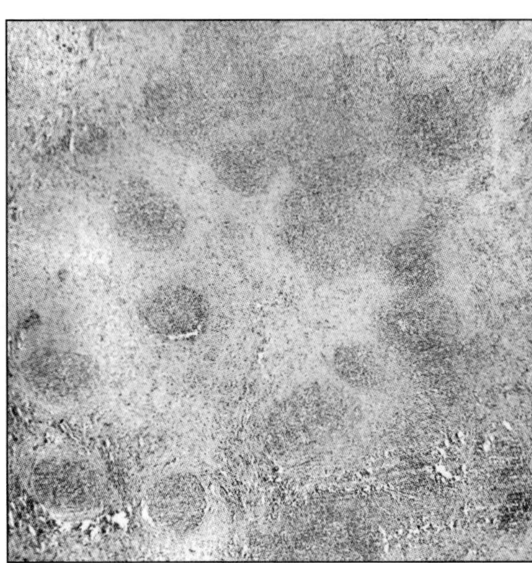

(Left) *This case of classical Hodgkin lymphoma shows numerous Hodgkin lymphoma cells with anaplastic features* ➦ *that closely resemble the hallmark cells of ALCL. Immunohistochemical stains and the background milieu help make the correct diagnosis.* ***(Right)*** *This case of ALK(+) ALCL shows a strong resemblance to classical Hodgkin lymphoma, nodular sclerosis type. Immunostains are helpful in distinguishing these cases from one another. (Courtesy C. Kjeldsberg, MD.)*

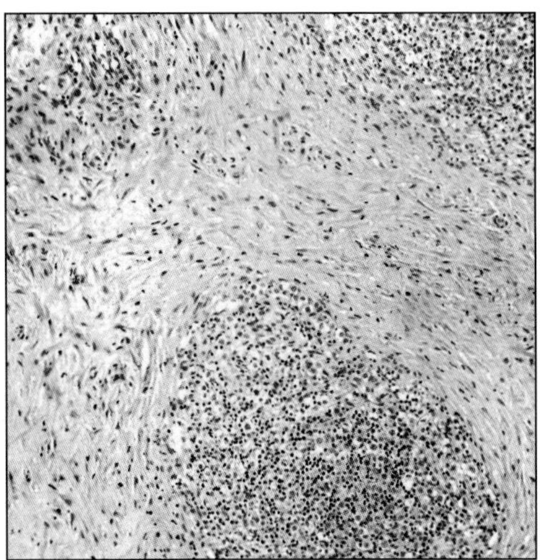

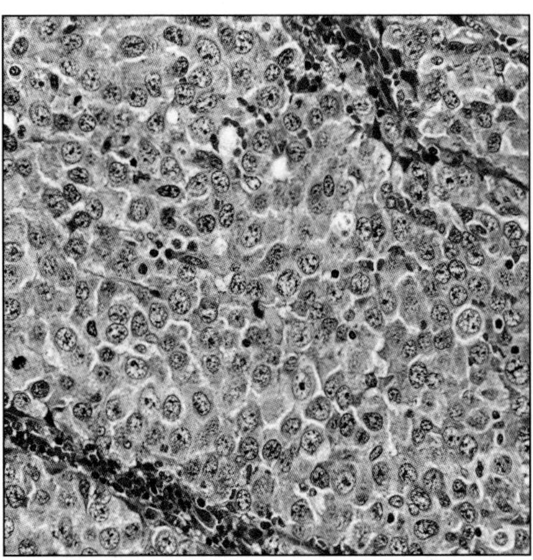

(Left) *Medium-power view shows a case of ALK(+) ALCL that closely resembles nodular sclerosis Hodgkin lymphoma. (Courtesy C. Kjeldsberg, MD.)* ***(Right)*** *The tumor cells in this case of DLBCL with t(2;17) have plasmablastic morphology and were positive for ALK (cytoplasmic, coarsely granular), CD79a (focally), and negative for CD30 and CD3. (Courtesy F. Vega, MD, PhD.)*

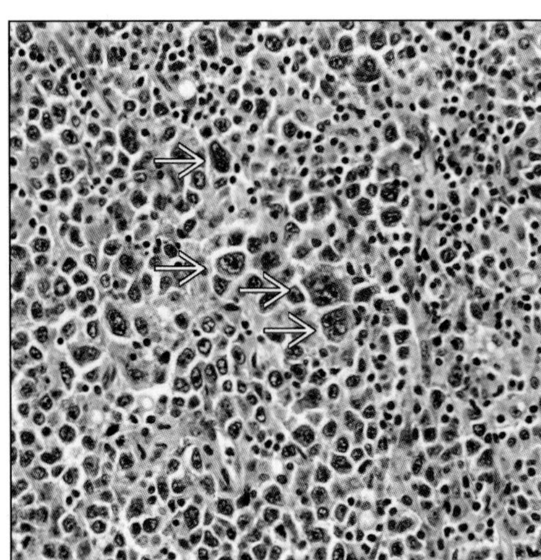

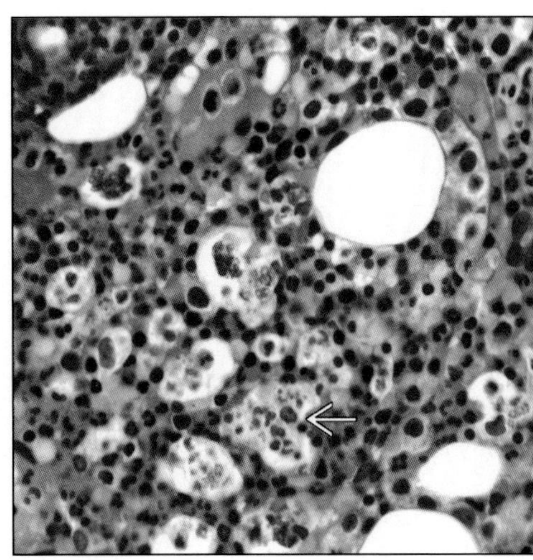

(Left) *In this case of DLBCL, the tumor cells have anaplastic morphology* ➔ *and were strongly and uniformly positive for CD30 and negative for CD20. pax-5/BSAP immunostain confirmed the diagnosis of DLBCL.* ***(Right)*** *Hemophagocytosis can be seen in patients with hematopoietic malignancies such as ALCL as illustrated in this case of ALK(+) ALCL with prominent hemophagocytosis* ➔ *in the bone marrow.*

Differential Diagnosis and Ancillary Studies

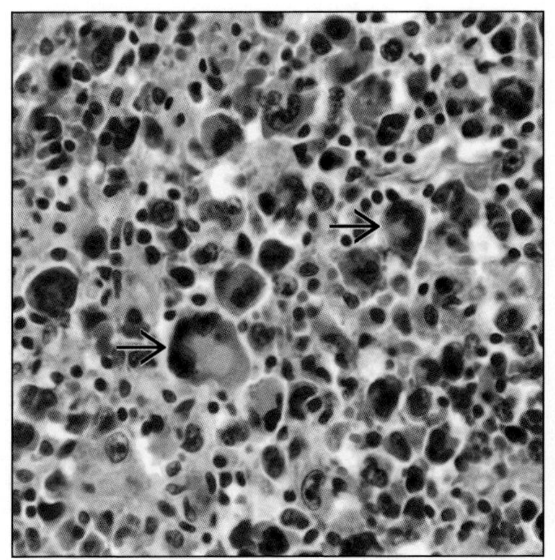

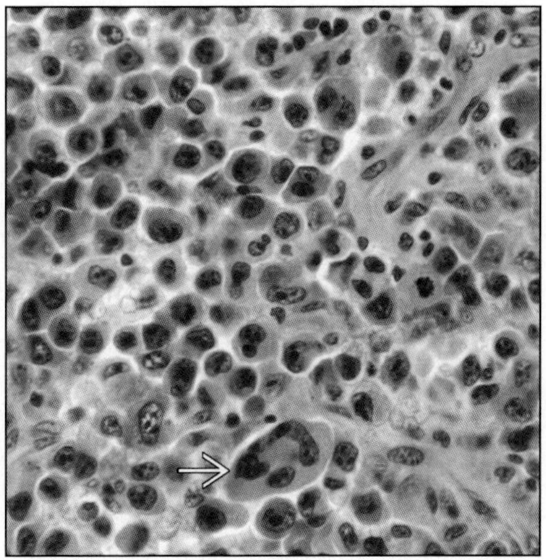

(Left) *This case of ALK(-) ALCL is morphologically indistinguishable from ALK(+) ALCL. Note the presence of hallmark cells ➔. The tumor cells were positive for CD30 and CD3 and negative for ALK.* ***(Right)*** *This case of ALK(-) ALCL is morphologically indistinguishable from ALK(+) ALCL. Note the presence of mononuclear cells and a wreath cell ➔, the latter of which tends to be more frequently observed in ALK(-) ALCL cases.*

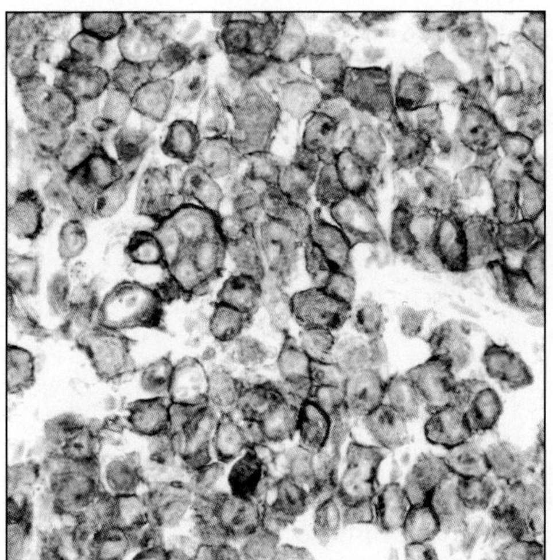

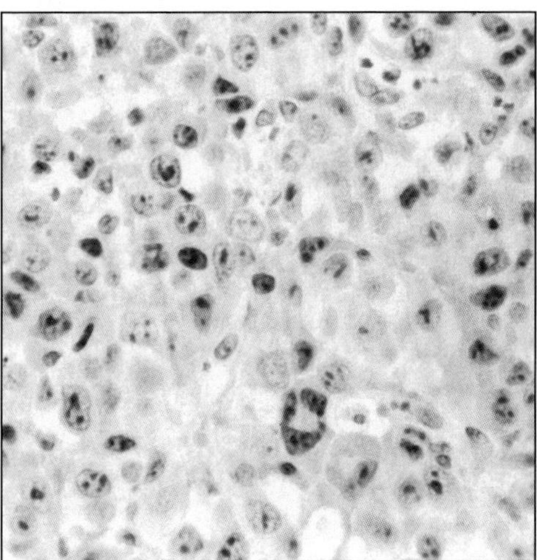

(Left) *Strong and uniform expression of CD30 was present in this case of ALK(-) ALCL.* ***(Right)*** *Complete absence of ALK protein expression is observed in this case of ALK(-) ALCL.*

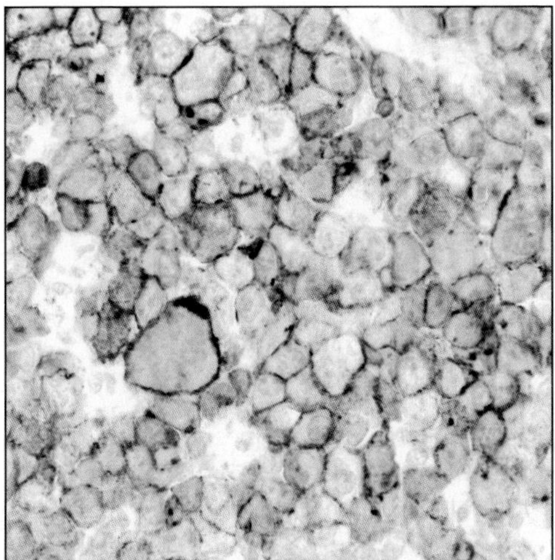

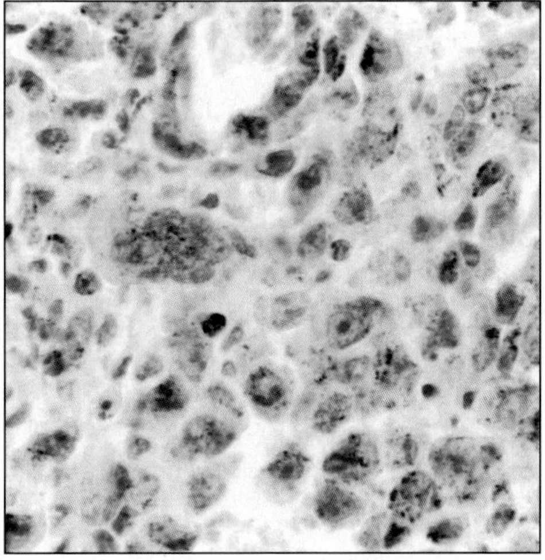

(Left) *CD2 is often expressed in both ALK(-) and ALK(+) cases of ALCL. Most tumors do not express CD3 or CD5.* ***(Right)*** *Cytotoxic proteins such as TIA-1(shown), granzyme B, and perforin are indicative of T-cell lineage and are expressed in both ALK(-) and ALK(+) ALCL cases. The staining pattern is coarsely granular and cytoplasmic. These stains can be helpful when many of the T-cell antigens are deleted.*

ACUTE MYELOID LEUKEMIA

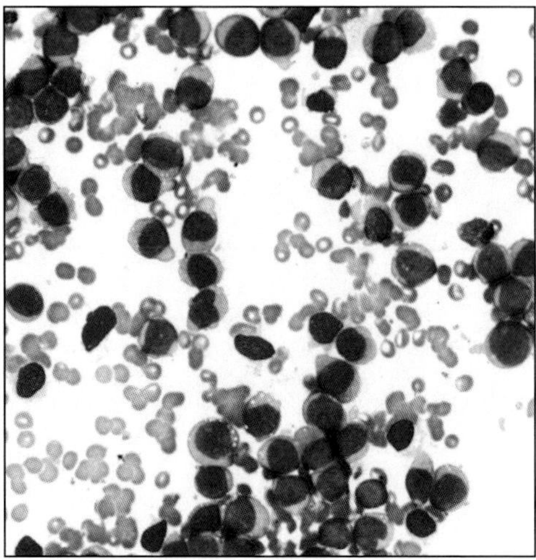

This case of acute monoblastic leukemia has effaced the entire bone marrow, typical of the behavior of AML in general. Clinical symptoms reflect this bone marrow failure. (Courtesy K. Reichard, MD.)

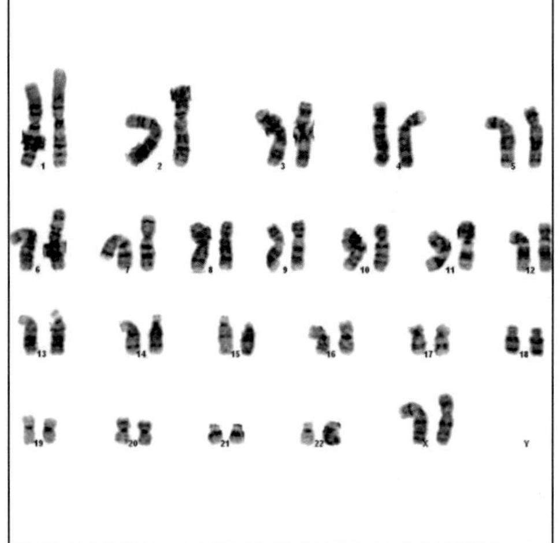

Karyotyping is required in the work-up of AML. As shown, a normal karyotype is seen in ~ 40-50% of all de novo cases of AML. Molecular studies may be pursued subsequently. (Courtesy K. Reichard, MD.)

TERMINOLOGY

Abbreviations

- Acute myeloid leukemia (AML)

Synonyms

- Acute myelogenous leukemia

Definitions

- Clonal hematopoietic neoplasm
- Blasts/blast equivalents comprise ≥ 20% of nucleated peripheral blood (PB) &/or bone marrow (BM) cells
  - Exceptions
    - AML with recurring genetic abnormality [t(15;17), t(8;21), inv(16)/t(16;16)]
    - Acute erythroid leukemia

Classification

- World Health Organization 2008 publication

EPIDEMIOLOGY

Age Range

- All ages affected; median age is 63 years
- Overall, proportion of acute leukemias that are AML increases with age
  - ~ 80% of adult acute leukemias are myeloid
- Some disease types are more prevalent in older adults
  - AML with myelodysplasia-related changes
- Some disease types are more prevalent in younger age groups
  - AML with recurring genetic abnormality [t(15;17), t(8;21), inv(16)/t(16;16), t(9;11)]
  - AML with t(1;22) occurs in infants and children < 3 years of age

Incidence

- 6,500 children and adolescents develop leukemia each year in the United States
  - AML comprises approximately 15-20% of all childhood leukemias
- 5-7 cases of AML/1,000,000 population/year

Natural History

- Clinically aggressive disease

ETIOLOGY/PATHOGENESIS

Constitutional Disorders

- Down syndrome
  - 10-20x increased risk for AML
  - > 500x increased risk for acute megakaryoblastic leukemia
- Fanconi anemia
  - Increased risk for developing AML
- Other inherited genetic disorders also predispose to development of AML
  - Klinefelter syndrome, Li-Fraumeni syndrome, severe congenital neutropenia (Kostmann syndrome), Shwachman-Diamond syndrome
  - Diamond-Blackfan syndrome, neurofibromatosis type 1, Noonan syndrome, dyskeratosis congenita, familial platelet disorders
  - Congenital amegakaryocytic thrombocytopenia, ataxia-telangiectasia, and Bloom syndrome

Acquired Disorders

- Aplastic anemia, myelodysplastic syndrome, amegakaryocytic thrombocytopenia, paroxysmal nocturnal hemoglobinuria

Environmental Exposure

- Radiation and chemotherapy
- Petroleum products, organic solvents (benzene), herbicides, and pesticides (organophosphates)

Underlying Hematopoietic Neoplasm

- Variable risk of progression to AML

- Myelodysplasia (MDS), myeloproliferative neoplasms (MPNs), MDS/MPN disorders

Pathogenesis of Leukemogenesis

- Accumulation of multiple genetic hits
- Class I and class II mutations
  - Class I: Pro-proliferative signal
    - e.g., *FLT3, JAK2, KIT*
  - Class II: Impairment of cellular maturation
    - e.g., *PML-RARA, CEBPA, RUNX1-RUNX1T1*

CLINICAL IMPLICATIONS

Clinical Presentation

- Symptoms related to bone marrow failure
  - Fatigue (anemia)
  - Bleeding (thrombocytopenia)
  - Infection (neutropenia)
- Extramedullary involvement
  - Skin lesions, gingival hyperplasia, myeloid sarcomas
- Abnormal CBC

Prognosis

- Overall 5-year survival has increased over past 2 decades to 60-65%
- Morphologic marrow response at different time points is important predictor of outcome
- Cytogenetics
  - Cytogenetic analysis considered one of the most important prognostic determinants in pediatric AML
    - 20% of children with AML do not have identifiable karyotypic alterations
  - Poor prognosis
    - AML with -5/del(5q), -7/del(7q) or complex karyotype (≥ 3 chromosome abnormalities)
    - AML with t(6;9)(p23;q34)
    - Additional chromosome aberrations acquired during disease course
- Molecular factors with poor prognosis
  - FMS-related tyrosine kinase 3-internal tandem duplication (*FLT3*-ITD) mutations
    - Only with normal karyotype (NK)-AML
    - More significant with high *FLT3*-ITD allelic ratios (> 0.4)
    - 20-25% of cases
    - Less common in younger patients
    - Point mutation in kinase domain of *FLT3* does not seem to have major influence on outcome
  - *KIT* mutations
    - When associated with core binding factor leukemias [t(8;21) and inv16/t(16;16)]
    - Significance is controversial in pediatric AML
  - Mixed lineage leukemia gene-partial tandem duplications (*MLL*-PTD)
  - Increased expression of *BAALC* with normal karyotype
  - 11q23 rearrangements
    - Most common in pediatric patients < 3 years of age
    - Detected in 50% of infants < 12 months
    - Incidence decreases in older children
  - *IDH1* and *IDH2* mutations
    - ~ 12% of NK-AML
    - Data in terms of significance are conflicting
- Molecular factors with improved prognosis
  - Nucleophosmin (*NPM1*) mutations
    - Favorable prognosis only with NK-AML and when *FLT3(-)*
    - 20-30% of all cases
    - Less common in childhood AML (8%)
    - Cytoplasmic expression of NPM1 is a surrogate marker for *NPM1* mutations
  - CCAAT/enhancer binding protein α (*CEBPA*) mutations
    - Provisional category of the 2008 WHO classification scheme
    - Comprises 17% of NK-AML
    - Favorable prognosis only with NK-AML
    - Test in *FLT3*(-), *NPM1*(-), NK-AML
  - Wilms tumor 1 (*WT1*) gene polymorphism (rs16754)
    - Significance of *WT1* mutations is controversial in pediatric age groups
- Additional factors associated with unfavorable prognosis
  - High white blood cell count
  - No response or no early response to induction therapy
  - Age > 10 years
    - Older children more likely to have unfavorable cytogenetics and FAB type M0, M1, M2, and M3
    - Children < 10 years more likely to have favorable cytogenetics and FAB types M4, M5, and M7
  - Non-Caucasian ethnicity
  - Obesity
  - Prior chemotherapy &/or radiation
  - Underlying hematopoietic neoplasm, e.g., MDS
  - Elevated LDH
  - Performance status
  - Minimal residual disease (MRD)
    - MRD positive at end of 1st induction (significantly worse prognosis)
    - 4.8x more likely to relapse and 3.1x more likely to die

Treatment

- Most protocols stratify therapy based upon cytogenetic, molecular, and response-based factors
  - Favorable-risk groups receive no transplant in 1st remission
  - Intermediate-risk groups use matched, related donor transplants if available
  - High-risk groups often use transplants from related or unrelated donors
- Acute promyelocytic leukemia and Down syndrome-associated leukemia in children < 4 years have completely separate care regimens and research protocols

MACROSCOPIC FINDINGS

General Features

- Myeloid sarcomas

ACUTE MYELOID LEUKEMIA

- Soft, fleshy, white-yellow, variable foci of necrosis

Specimen Handling

- Required elements in work-up of AML
  - PB &/or BM microscopic examination
  - Complete blood count
  - Flow cytometry
  - Cytogenetics
  - Sample for DNA/RNA extraction
  - Complete and accurate clinical history
    - Prior therapy
    - Prior hematologic neoplasm
- Additional elements to be considered on case-by-case basis
  - Cytochemistry
  - FISH
    - When karyotyping is inadequate
    - For cytogenetically cryptic abnormalities [e.g., inv(16)/t(16;16) and variant 11q23/*MLL* translocations]
  - Molecular genetics
    - Normal karyotype: *FLT3*, *CEBPA*, *NPM1* (others to be determined by institution)
    - Abnormal karyotype: Varies by institution, new discoveries, protocol requirement, etc.

MICROSCOPIC FINDINGS

Blasts and Blast Equivalents: General Features

- Meticulous attention must be paid to recognizing and counting blasts
- Which cells count as blasts/blast equivalents, and what are their cytologic features?
  - Myeloblasts
    - Cytoplasmic azurophilic granules, Auer rods
  - Monoblasts
    - Cytoplasmic, very fine, azurophilic granules; abundant blue-gray cytoplasm
  - Megakaryoblasts
    - May see cytoplasmic blebbing/shedding, but not specific
  - Promonocytes
    - Gray-blue cytoplasm, fine chromatin, variably conspicuous nucleoli, delicate nuclear grooves/ folds
  - Promyelocytes in acute promyelocytic leukemia (APL)
    - Single or bilobed nuclei, hypo- or hypergranular cytoplasm; may see cytoplasm packed with Auer rods
  - Erythroblasts are only enumerated when considering acute erythroid leukemia
    - Deeply basophilic cytoplasm, circumferential cytoplasmic vacuolization
- Enumeration of blast percent
  - In PB
    - % of circulating white blood cells
  - In uncomplicated BM
    - % of all nucleated cells excluding histiocytes, megakaryocytes, mast cells
  - In BM complicated by a 2nd hematologic neoplasm
    - % of all nucleated cells excluding coexisting tumor cells (e.g., plasma cells in myeloma, lymphoid cells in CLL)

Peripheral Blood

- Abnormal CBC
- Cytopenias
  - Anemia
  - Thrombocytopenia
  - Neutropenia
- Circulating blasts/blast equivalents
- Assess erythrocytes for evidence of disseminated intravascular coagulation

Bone Marrow Aspirate

- Requirements
  - Well stained
  - Adequate specimen
    - Cellular
    - Representative
    - Not hemodilute
    - If fibrotic or dry tap, assess touch preparation
- Enumerate blasts
- Assess for dysplasia in all lineages
  - Diagnostic criteria for AML with myelodysplasia-related changes
- Assess for increased/abnormal-appearing mast cells
  - Mastocytosis may be concurrent

Bone Marrow Core Biopsy

- Requirements
  - Similar to aspirate
  - Thin section
- Identify blasts
  - Utilize IHC if needed
  - Caveats
    - Not all blasts are CD34(+), particularly APL, megakaryocytic, monocytic, and erythroid blasts
    - IHC not as sensitive as flow cytometry
- Assess megakaryocytic dysplasia
- Evaluate for associated concurrent neoplasm
  - Mastocytosis
  - Other

Specialized Testing

- Cytochemical stains
  - Myeloperoxidase (MPO)
    - If positive, confirms myeloid lineage
    - If negative, does not exclude myeloid lineage
    - ~ 5% of acute monoblastic leukemias may show scattered MPO(+) granules
  - Nonspecific esterase (NSE)
    - If positive, confirms monocytic lineage
    - If negative, does not exclude monocytic lineage
- Flow cytometry
  - Should be performed in all new cases of AML
  - Establishes lineage
  - Establishes phenotype "fingerprint" for future monitoring
  - Blast markers
    - CD34: Not all blasts are CD34(+)
    - CD117: Also stains pronormoblasts, mast cells
    - TdT: Stains a subset of AMLs

- Myeloid markers
  - MPO, CD10, CD11b, CD13, CD33, CD117
- Monocytic markers
  - CD11c, CD14, CD36/CD64 coexpression, CD163, CD4 (weak), CD33 (bright)
- Megakaryocytic markers
  - CD31, CD41, CD42b, CD61
- Erythroid markers
  - Glycophorin A, hemoglobin A, CD71 (not specific)

- Immunohistochemistry
  - Useful if flow cytometry inadequate or not performed
  - Useful for enumerating blasts when aspirate is inadequate
  - In general, fewer antibodies are available compared with flow cytometry
    - Some are unique to IHC, however
    - CD68: Myeloid and monocytic
    - Lysozyme: Monocytic
    - CD31: Megakaryocytic lineage
- Cytogenetics
  - Should be performed in all new cases of AML
  - Submit in sodium heparin anticoagulant
  - Diagnostic (e.g., AML with recurring genetic abnormality)
  - Prognostic: Favorable, intermediate, and unfavorable risk groups
- FISH
  - Perform as needed depending on morphologic suspicion and cytogenetic findings
- Molecular genetics
  - Perform as per institution, protocol requirements, anticipated minimal residual disease testing
  - In general, NK-AMLs should be evaluated for *FLT3*, *CEBPA*, and *NPM1* mutations
  - Additional molecular mutations may be identified and require testing
  - EDTA anticoagulant is preferred for PCR-based assays (heparin is known inhibitor of PCR)
- Minimal residual disease testing
  - Methods include DNA- and RNA-based PCR assays and flow cytometry

REPORTING CRITERIA

Minimum Requirements

- Use WHO 2008 classification as possible
- Utilize synoptic reporting as possible
- Report results of ancillary studies
- Issue an integrated report to incorporate all diagnostic and prognostic data

Communication of Results

- New diagnosis, unsuspected relapse, suspected APL, associated disseminated intravascular coagulation
- Prompt, verbal notification of clinician(s)

DIFFERENTIAL DIAGNOSIS

Acute Lymphoblastic Leukemia

- Blasts are typically more round
- Immunophenotype will reveal B- or T-lineage markers

Leukemoid Reaction with Left Shift

- Blast population should not exceed 20%
- Will show a spectrum of maturational stages with toxic changes in mature forms
- Lack phenotypic aberrancies and cytogenetic abnormalities

Variant/Atypical Lymphocytosis

- Variant lymphocytes may resemble myeloid blasts
- Typically lack smooth dispersed blast chromatin
- Chromatin is more often "ropy" and heterogeneous
- Nucleoli may be present but usually do not appear large and "punched out"
- Immunophenotyping will reveal lymphoid lineage
- Characteristic in patients with EBV infectious mononucleosis (IM)
- Clinical history and viral serologies will also be helpful

Granulocyte Colony-Stimulating Factor (G-CSF)

- Blast count may exceed 20% in hypocellular specimen
- Transient phenomenon, nonclonal, no Auer rods

Blast Phase of Preexisting Myeloid Neoplasm

- Clinical history required

DIAGNOSTIC CHALLENGES

Use of G-CSF as a Component of AML Chemotherapy

- Determination of residual disease blast count difficult

Low Blast Count AML (< 20%)

- Diagnosis established by detecting recurring genetic abnormality: [t(15;17), t(16;16)/inv16, t(8;21)]

Hypocellular AML

- Document ≥ 20% blasts by IHC

Marked Increase in Erythroid Precursors

- High-grade MDS vs. erythroleukemia
  - Erythroleukemia tends to be composed mainly of erythroblasts
  - MDS often shows admixture of all stages of erythroid differentiation
- Exclude nonneoplastic disorders
  - Nutritional deficiency (vitamin B12, folate, copper)
  - Erythropoietin therapy

Fibrosis

- Often inaspirable
- Accurate blast count may require IHC: CD34, CD117
- Exclude transformation of prior hematologic malignancy

ACUTE MYELOID LEUKEMIA

AML Classification

Broad AML Category	Specific Subtypes
AML with recurring genetic abnormality	AML with t(8;21)(q22;q22); *RUNX1-RUNX1T1*
	AML with inv(16)(p13.1q11.2) or t(16;16)(p13.1;q11.2); *CBFB-MYH11*
	Acute promyelocytic leukemia with t(15;17)(q22;q21); *PML-RARA*
	AML with t(9;11)(p22;q23); *MLLT3-MLL*
	AML with t(6;9)(p23;q34); *DEK-NUP214*
	AML with inv(3)(q21q26) or t(3;3)(q21;q26); *RPN1-EVI1*
	AML with t(1;22)(p13;q13); *RBM15-MKL1*
	Provisional entity: AML with *NPM1* mutation
	Provisional entity: AML with *CEBPA* mutation
AML with myelodysplasia-related changes	
Therapy-related myeloid neoplasms	
AML, not otherwise specified	AML with minimal differentiation
	AML without maturation
	AML with maturation
	Acute myelomonocytic leukemia
	Acute monoblastic and monocytic leukemia
	Acute erythroid leukemia
	Acute megakaryoblastic leukemia
	Acute panmyelosis with myelofibrosis

Adapted from WHO 2008 classification.

AML Genetic Risk Classification

Risk Group	Cytogenetic Findings
Favorable	t(15;17)
	t(8;21)
	inv(16)/t(16;16)
	t(1;22)
Intermediate	t(9;11)
	Normal karyotype
	All cases not otherwise categorized as favorable or unfavorable
Unfavorable	Abn 3q excluding t(3;5)
	inv(3)/t(3;3)
	t(6;9)
	add(5q), del(5q) -5
	-7, add(7q)/del(7q)
	t(6;11)
	t(10;11)
	t(11q23) excluding 9;11 and 11;19
	t(9;22)
	-17/abn(17p)
	Complex (≥ 3) abnormalities

Chronic Myelomonocytic Leukemia vs. Acute Myelomonocytic Leukemia

- Requires good cytologic preparation and stain
- BM often shows higher proportion of immature cells than blood

SELECTED REFERENCES

1. Betz BL et al: Acute myeloid leukemia diagnosis in the 21st century. Arch Pathol Lab Med. 134(10):1427-33, 2010
2. Radhi M et al: Prognostic factors in pediatric acute myeloid leukemia. Curr Hematol Malig Rep. 5(4):200-6, 2010
3. Manola KN: Cytogenetics of pediatric acute myeloid leukemia. Eur J Haematol. 83(5):391-405, 2009

Microscopic Features

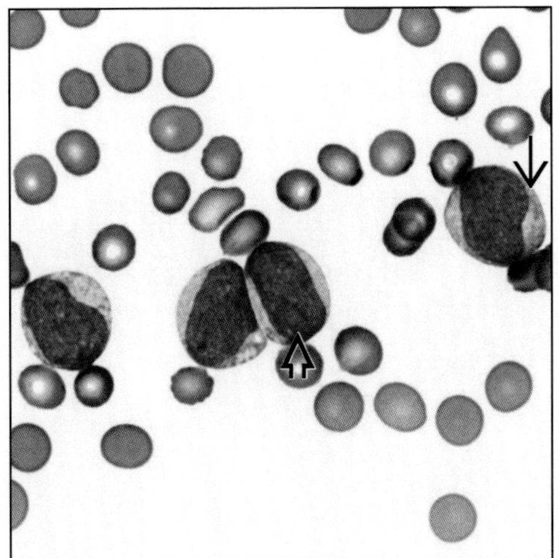

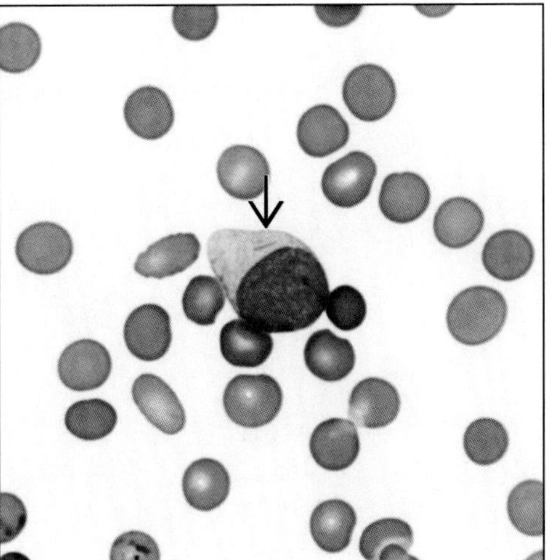

(Left) *This peripheral blood (PB) smear shows 4 myeloid blasts from a patient with newly diagnosed AML. The blasts illustrate typical myeloid morphology: Large size, prominent nucleoli* ⇨*, and moderate, lightly basophilic cytoplasm with a variable number of azurophilic granules* →*.* ***(Right)*** *Auer rods are a hallmark feature of a myeloid neoplasm* →*. They are said to represent a compact linear aggregation of MPO granules. Further investigation is required for final classification.*

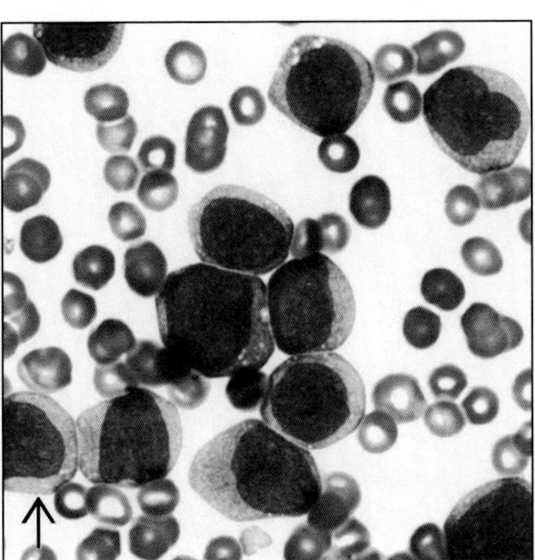

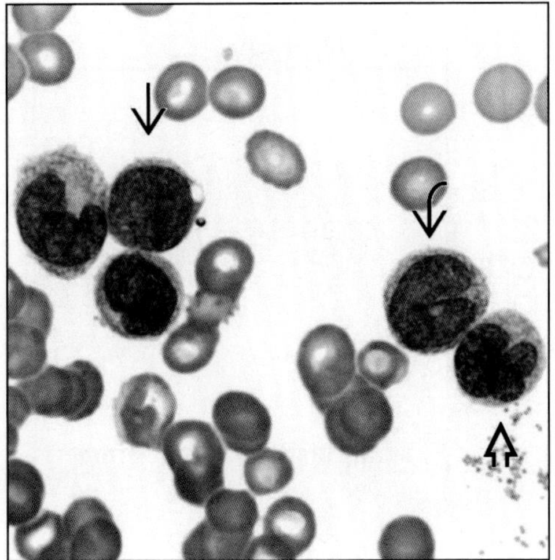

(Left) *This PB smear displays the typical cytology of monoblasts: Large with round nuclei, variably prominent nucleoli, and abundant cytoplasm, which may contain fine azurophilic granules* →*.* ***(Right)*** *This BM aspirate shows a spectrum of monocytic differentiation. Admixed is a blast* →*, abnormal monocytes* ⇨*, and a promonocyte* ↪*. Promonocytes show more dispersed chromatin, less nuclear convolution, delicate nuclear grooves, and variable nucleoli, and count as blast equivalents.*

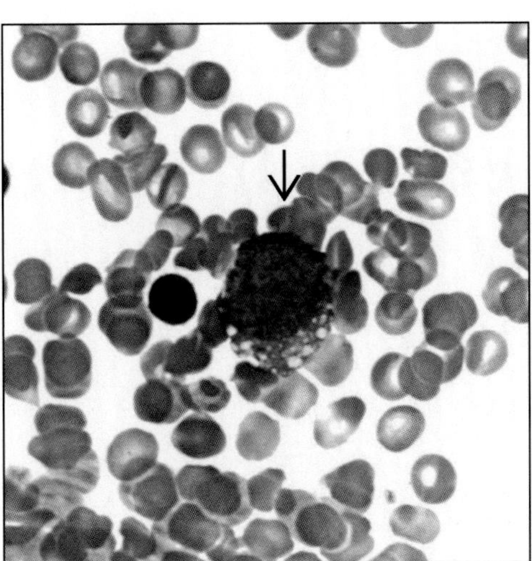

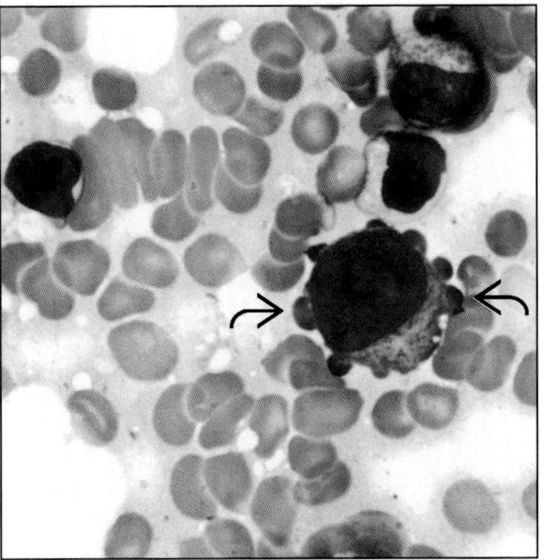

(Left) *This photomicrograph shows the typical features of a neoplastic erythroblast* →*. Erythroblasts are counted only as blasts when considering acute erythroid leukemia.* ***(Right)*** *Wright-stained bone marrow touch preparation from a young adult with a de novo acute megakaryocytic leukemia demonstrates a megakaryoblast with prominent cytoplasmic blebs* ↪*. (Courtesy M. Vasef, MD.)*

Ancillary Techniques

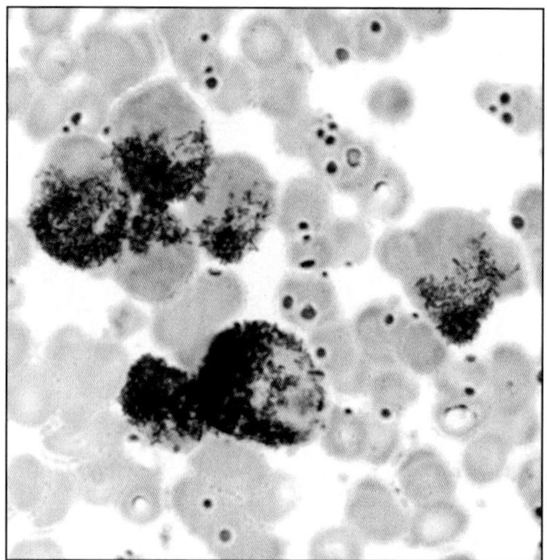

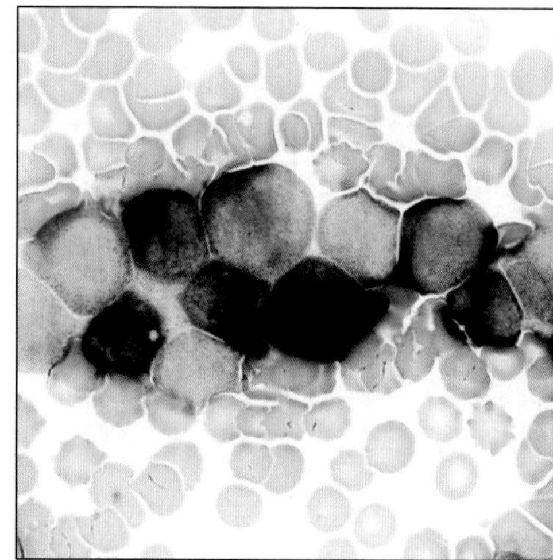

(Left) *This myeloperoxidase stain reveals marked and dense cytoplasmic granulation in blast-like cells confirming a diagnosis of acute promyelocytic leukemia (APL). In the cytologic hypogranular variant of APL, one may be surprised by the dense MPO positivity.* ***(Right)*** *This nonspecific esterase stain (brown) highlights the monoblasts in a case of acute monoblastic leukemia. Any degree of positivity is sufficient for monocytic differentiation. (Courtesy K. Reichard, MD.)*

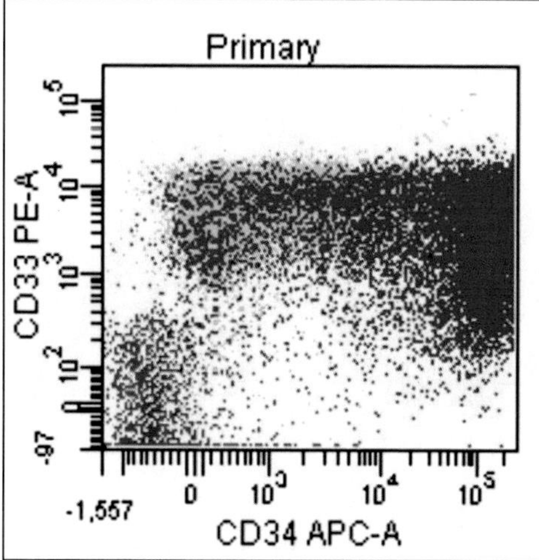

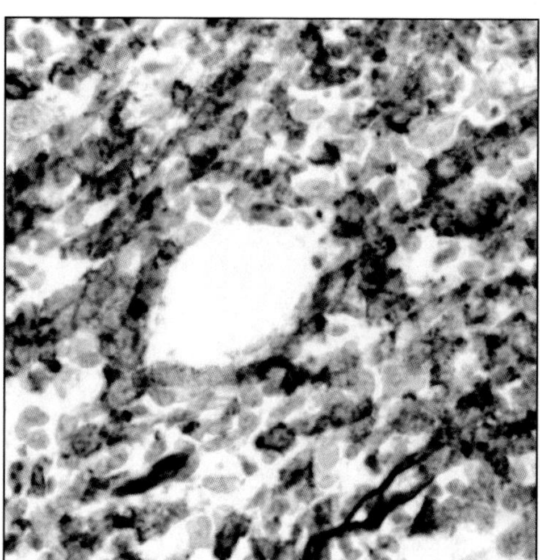

(Left) *Flow cytometry, a crucial component of the AML work-up, assigns lineage as well as establishes an antigen phenotype, which can be followed for residual disease testing. Neoplastic blasts (red) in this case are myeloid (CD33[+]) and confirmed blasts (CD34[+]).* ***(Right)*** *On occasion, flow cytometry is not available. IHC stains can verify an acute leukemia using lineage-specific and blast markers. CD34 reveals > 20% blasts in this acute leukemia. (Courtesy K. Reichard, MD.)*

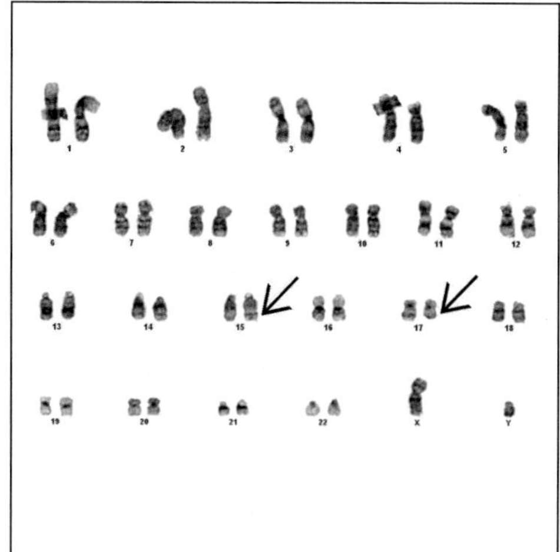

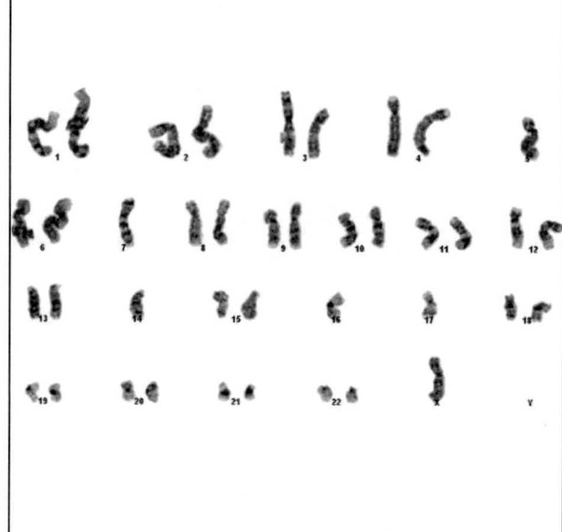

(Left) *Conventional cytogenetics is a necessary component of the AML work-up. Recurring genetic translocations with prognostic significance may be identified. This karyogram shows the t(15;17) ⇒ associated with acute promyelocytic leukemia.* ***(Right)*** *This karyogram indicates an abnormal highly complex karyotype in a case of de novo AML. A complex karyotype is variably defined (usually ≥ 3 abnormalities) and is associated with an unfavorable genetic risk. (Courtesy K. Reichard, MD.)*

Biopsy Features of AML

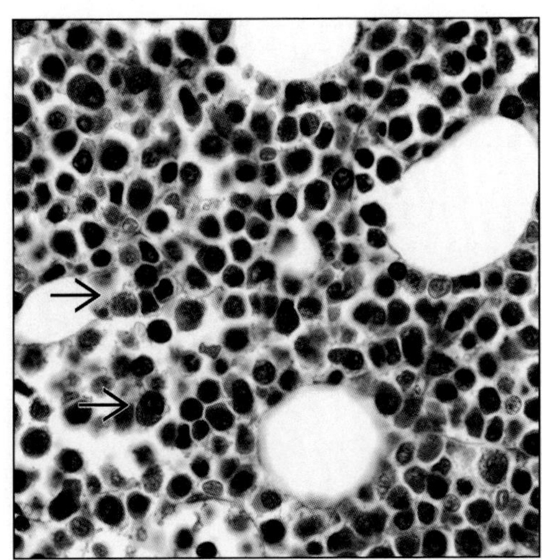

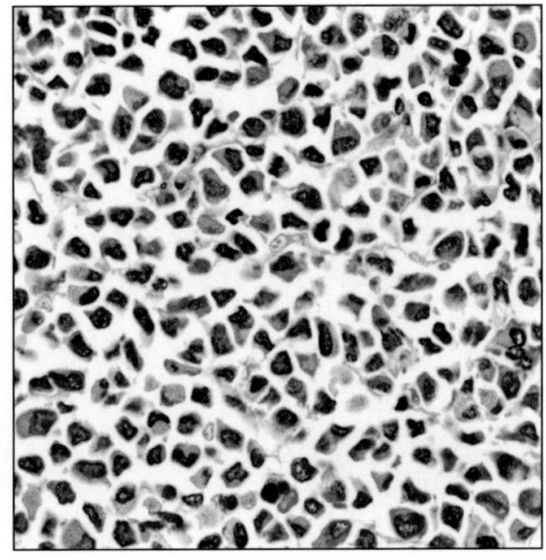

(Left) *This BM core biopsy illustrates the typical bone marrow-effacing findings in a case of acute myeloid leukemia. Sheets of large cells with blast-like chromatin are present. In addition, note the numerous admixed eosinophilic myelocytes ⇒.* ***(Right)*** *This BM core biopsy illustrates the features of APL, including abundant pink and heavily granulated cytoplasm. Although considered a low-blast count AML, APL typically presents with complete BM effacement, as in this case.*

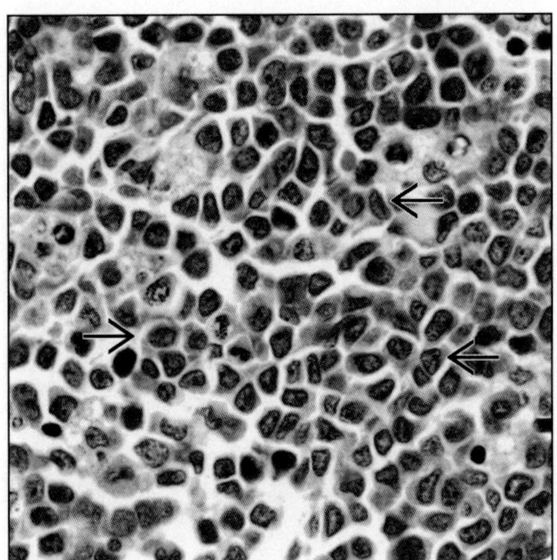

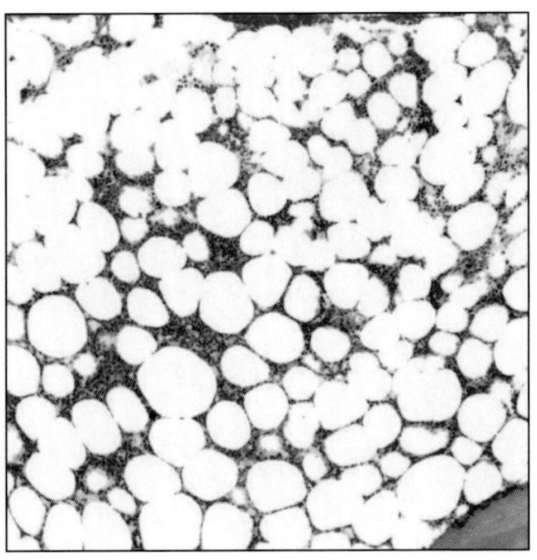

(Left) *This BM core shows the classic features of acute monoblastic leukemia. The cells are large with moderate cytoplasm and characteristic nuclear grooves ⇒.* ***(Right)*** *This is a tricky BM core biopsy due to the marked hypocellularity. Flow cytometry was suboptimal, but with IHC stains, it was revealed that all of these mononuclear cells are CD34(+) blasts. Hypocellular AML can be missed if not included on the differential diagnosis list. (Courtesy K. Reichard, MD.)*

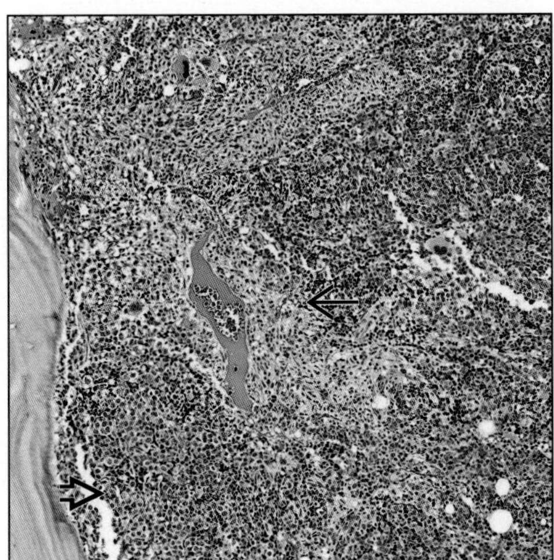

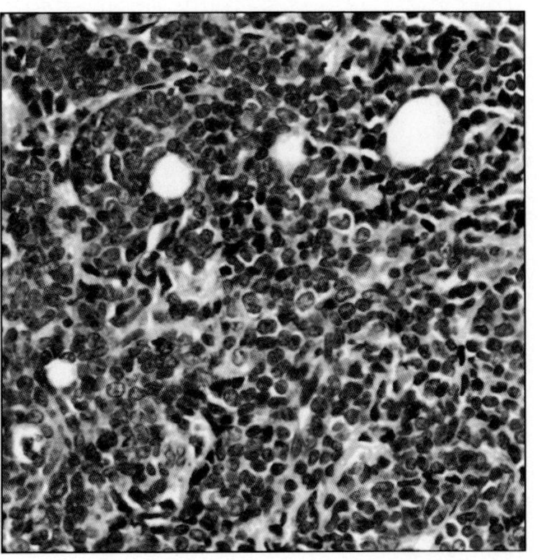

(Left) *AML may coexist with a concurrent hematologic neoplasm as in this case of AML and systemic mastocytosis. The neoplastic mast cells form compact aggregates ⇒ while the sheets of neoplastic myeloid blasts occupy the interstitial space ⇒.* ***(Right)*** *AML may have an initial presentation in an extramedullary location. In this example, a myeloid sarcoma was diagnosed after a breast mass biopsy for suspected carcinoma. At the time of presentation, the BM was < 10% involved.*

Microscopic Features and Flow Cytometry

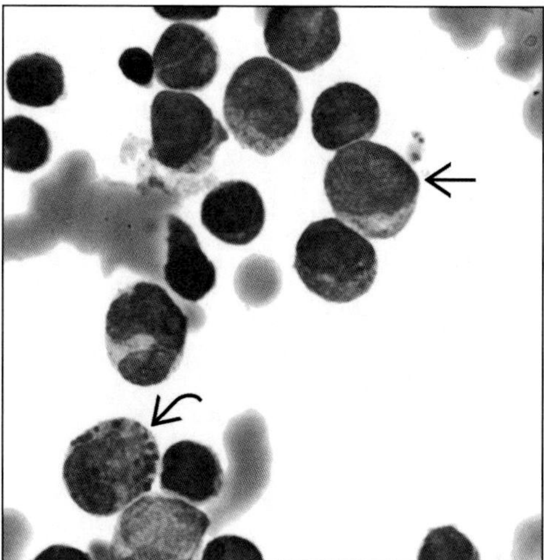

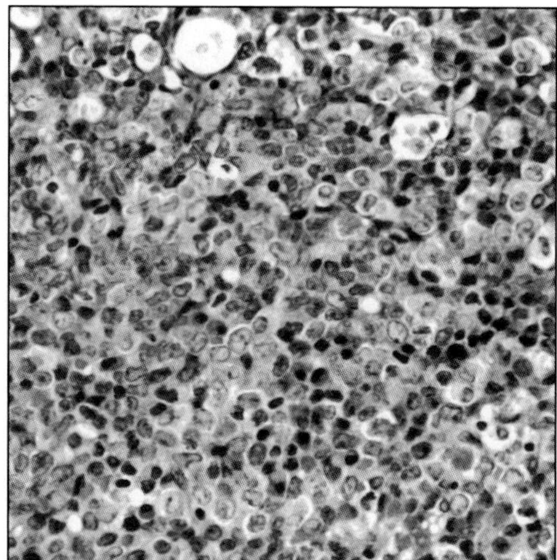

(Left) Most cases of AML with inversion 16 fit the morphologic criteria for acute myelomonocytic leukemia (FAB-M4): ≥ 20% myeloid blasts ⇒ and ≥ 20% monocytes. This subtype is also characterized by abnormal eosinophils that contain a combination of small eosinophilic granules and large basophilic granules ⇒. *(Right)* The core biopsy in this example of AML with inversion 16 shows sheets of blasts and increased eosinophils.

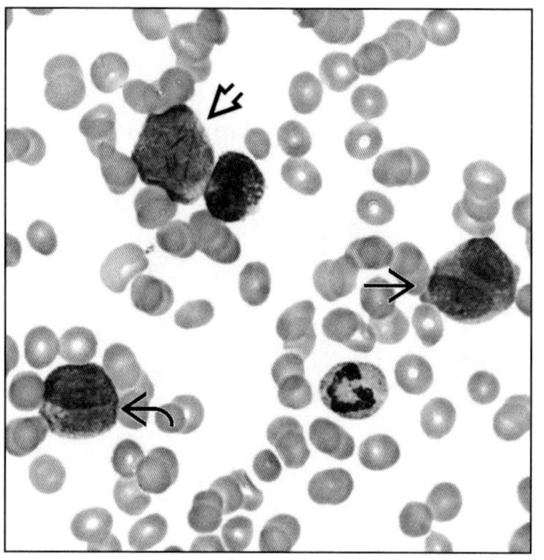

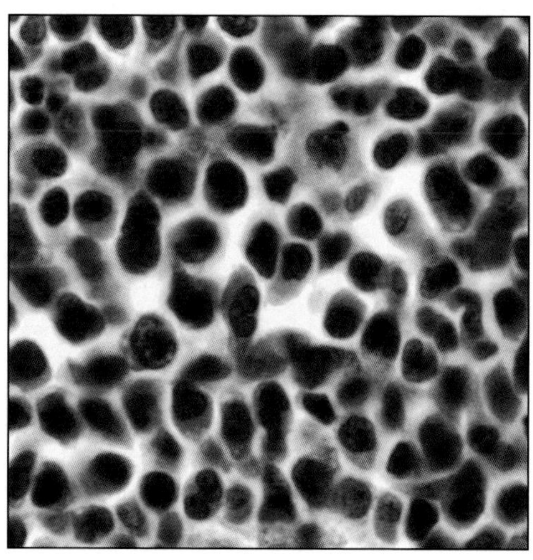

(Left) PB shows atypical promyelocytes (blast equivalents) in a case of APL that show folded/bilobed nuclei ⇒, prominent cytoplasmic granularity ⇒, and numerous Auer rods in some of the cells ⇒. *(Right)* Rare example of a myeloid sarcoma in a young patient with APL who had achieved morphologic and molecular remission. Examination of PB and BM showed no morphologic or molecular evidence of recurrent disease. This diagnosis was confirmed by IHC stains and FISH for t(15;17).

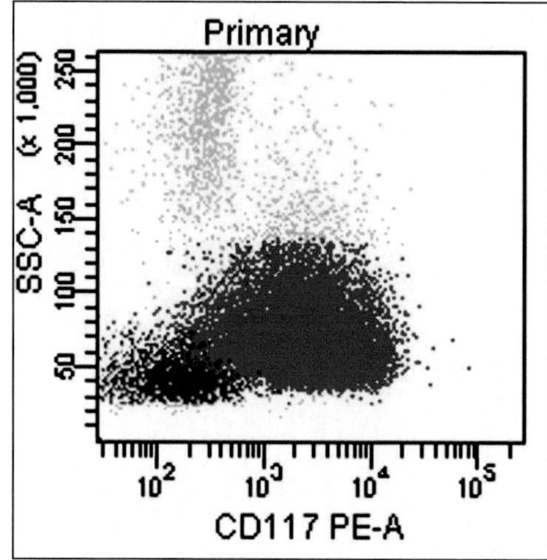

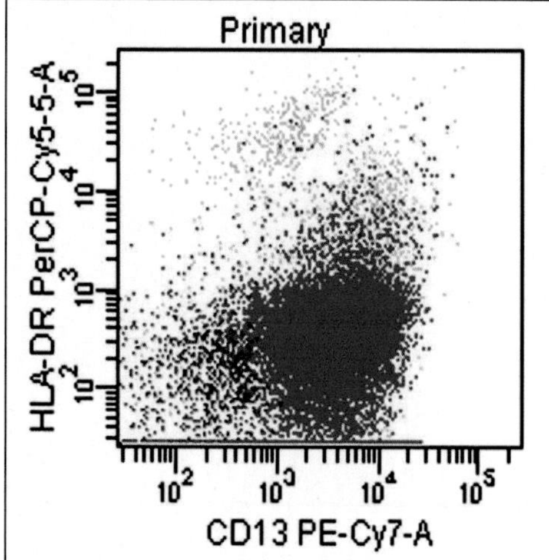

(Left) Flow cytometric analysis on a bone marrow specimen from a suspected case of acute promyelocytic leukemia demonstrates strong expression of CD117 (red population). This population was CD34 dim to negative. (Courtesy M. Vasef, MD.) *(Right)* Blasts/abnormal promyelocytes were CD13 positive (horizontal axis) and HLA-DR negative (vertical axis) in this case of APL. (Courtesy M. Vasef, MD.)

Differential Diagnosis

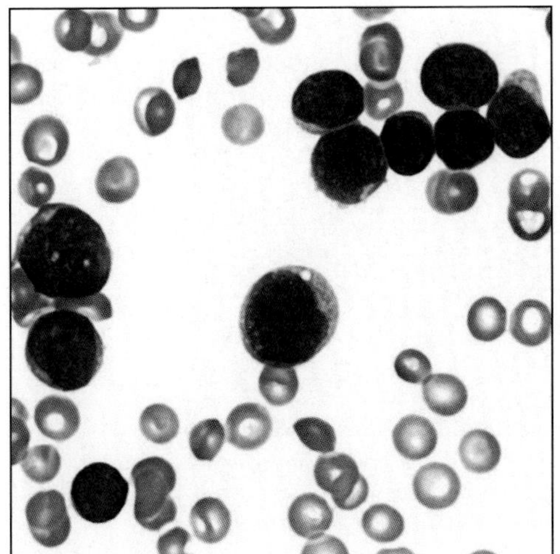

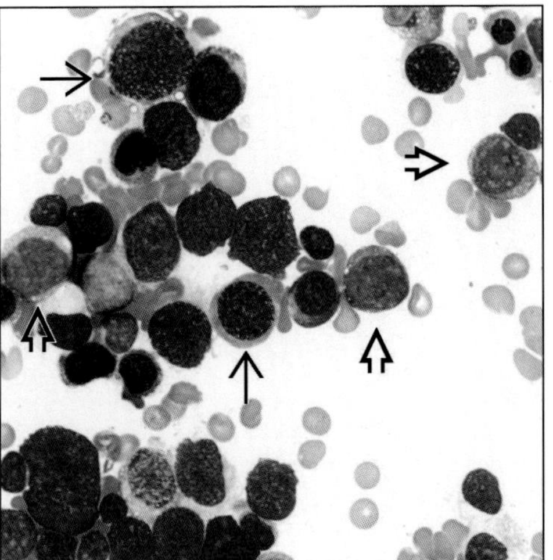

(Left) *Acute lymphoblastic leukemia is a differential diagnostic consideration for AML, particularly AML, NOS subtypes M0 and M1. Blasts tend to be smaller overall with scant agranular cytoplasm and inconspicuous nucleoli.* ***(Right)*** *This bone marrow aspirate smear shows a tricky case of markedly increased erythroid precursors* → *admixed with increased myeloid-appearing blasts* ⇨*. Such cases raise the possibility of acute erythroid leukemia.*

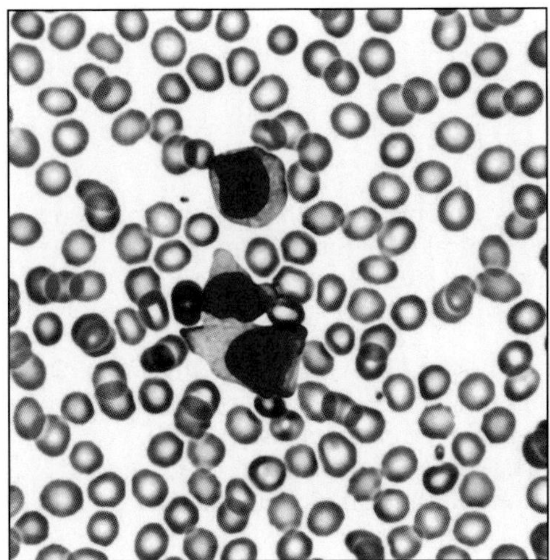

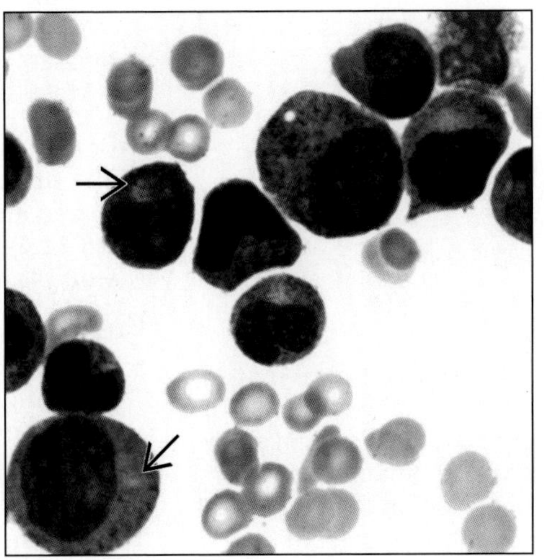

(Left) *Downey type II cells are intermediate-sized lymphocytes with mature smudged chromatin, inconspicuous nucleoli, and gray-blue cytoplasm that demonstrates peripheral basophilia. Cells are characteristic in patients with EBV IM. (Courtesy C. Wilson, MD, PhD.)* ***(Right)*** *BM aspirate smear shows left-shifted granulopoiesis in an adult on G-CSF. Note prominent paranuclear hof* →*, a common finding in nonneoplastic neutrophil regeneration. (Courtesy K. Foucar, MD.)*

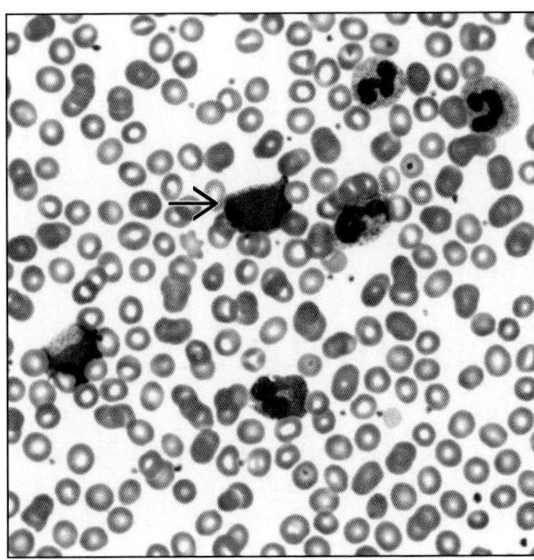

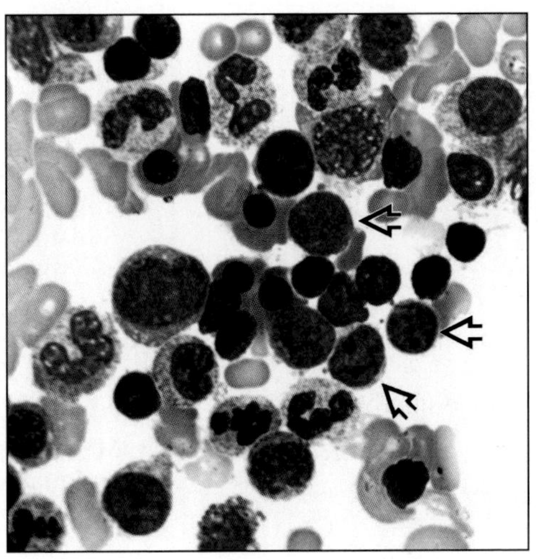

(Left) *Blood smear from a patient receiving recombinant G-CSF shows toxic changes and left shift to blasts* →*. Note that mature neutrophils predominate after early recovery occurs. (Courtesy K. Foucar, MD.)* ***(Right)*** *Bone marrow aspirate smear from a 3-year-old girl on G-CSF shows abundant maturing neutrophil lineage cells. Note numerous hematogones* ⇨ *(normal lymphoid cells), which are more numerous in specimens from young children. (Courtesy K. Foucar, MD.)*

MYELOID SARCOMA

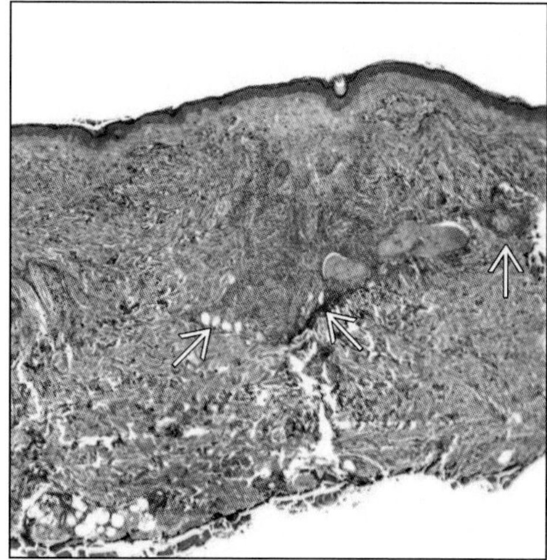

Section of skin at low power shows a patchy dense infiltrate ➡ of leukemic blasts in a patient with AML that showed monocytic differentiation.

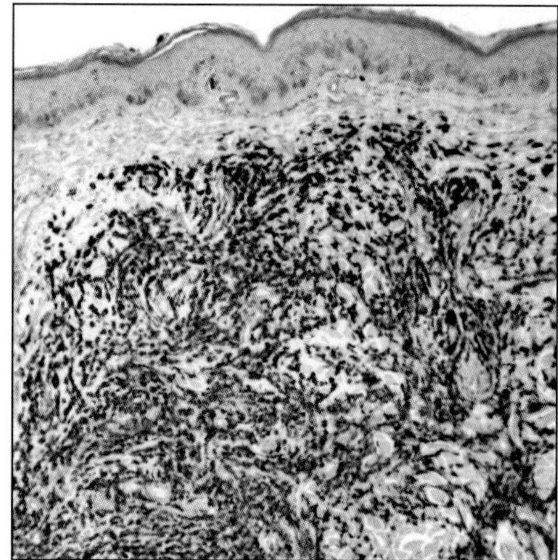

IHC staining by lysozyme in this section of skin highlights numerous leukemic blasts in this patient with previously diagnosed and treated AML. The findings are consistent with recurrent AML.

TERMINOLOGY

Abbreviations

- Myeloid sarcoma (MS)

Synonyms

- Extramedullary acute myeloid leukemia
- Extramedullary myeloid tumor
- Granulocytic sarcoma
- Chloroma

Definitions

- Rare manifestation of 1 or more myeloid tumor masses in extramedullary sites
- Myeloid blast infiltrates of any body site in a leukemic patient are not classified as myeloid sarcoma unless tumor masses show effaced tissue architecture
- MS is equivalent to a diagnosis of acute myeloid leukemia (AML)

ETIOLOGY/PATHOGENESIS

Developmental Anomaly

- Patients with certain inherited diseases have increased risk of developing AML/MS
  - Fanconi anemia, Down syndrome, Klinefelter syndrome, ataxia-telangiectasia, neurofibromatosis

Environmental Exposure

- Ionizing radiation
- Chemotherapy with cytotoxic agents and topoisomerase II inhibitors
- Chemicals (e.g., benzene, pesticides, herbicides)
- Cigarette smoking

CLINICAL ISSUES

Epidemiology

- Age
  - Wide age range (1 month to 89 years)
  - Median age: 56 years
- Gender
  - M:F = 1.2:1

Site

- Any site may be involved
- Most commonly involve skin (28-43%), lymph nodes (16-22%), and central nervous system (3-9%)
- Multiple anatomical sites (< 10% of cases)

Presentation

- May present de novo (27%) or concurrently with or following diagnosis of
  - AML, myeloproliferative neoplasm (MPN), or myelodysplastic syndrome (MDS)
- May be initial manifestation of AML relapse

Treatment

- High-dose anti-AML therapies as front-line approach
- Allogeneic or autologous bone marrow transplantation
  - High probability of long-term survival

Prognosis

- Autologous or allogeneic stem cell transplantation improves chances of prolonged survival and cure
- Prognosis does not appear to be affected by
  - Age, sex, anatomic site, presentation, clinical history (AML, MPN, MDS), histotype, phenotype, or cytogenetic findings

MACROSCOPIC FEATURES

Gross Pathology

- MS with granulocytic differentiation historically designated as chloroma (green coloration)
  - Result of verdoperoxide
  - Fades upon exposure to air within 2-3 hours

MYELOID SARCOMA

Key Facts

Clinical Issues
- Any site may be involved
- Most commonly involves skin (28-43%), lymph nodes (16-22%), and central nervous system (3-9%)

Microscopic Pathology
- Partial or complete effacement of tissue architecture by myeloid blasts that may or may not show features of maturation/differentiation
- Promyelocytic, myelomonocytic, or pure monoblastic differentiation can be seen

Ancillary Tests
- Immunohistochemistry is important for lineage determination and differential diagnosis
  - More commonly expresses CD33, CD34, CD43, CD68 (KP1), CD68 (PG-M1), CD99, CD117, lysozyme, and MPO
- Cytochemical stains performed on touch imprints may assist in lineage determination
  - Granulocytic lineage: Myeloperoxidase (+), chloracetate esterase (+)
  - Monocytic lineage: Nonspecific esterase (+)

Top Differential Diagnoses
- Aggressive lymphomas
- Blastic plasmacytoid dendritic cell neoplasm
- Histiocytic sarcoma
- Extramedullary hematopoiesis
- Small round cell tumors

MICROSCOPIC PATHOLOGY

Cytologic Features
- Touch imprints are very helpful
- Wright-Giemsa stain allows assessment of morphology
- Cytochemical stains (NSE, myeloperoxidase [MPO]) may be performed on unstained air-dried imprints

Microscopic Features
- Partial or complete effacement of tissue architecture by myeloid blasts that may or may not show features of maturation/differentiation
- Myeloid blasts
  - Medium to large-sized pleomorphic cells
    - Irregular nuclear contours
    - Thin nuclear membranes
    - Fine dispersed chromatin
    - Small nucleoli
    - Variable amounts of eosinophilic cytoplasm
- Promyelocytic, myelomonocytic, or pure monoblastic differentiation can be seen
  - Reniform nuclei suggest monocytic differentiation
- MS composed of predominantly megakaryoblasts or erythroblasts are rare
  - Often a manifestation of MS arising out of MPN
- Background of trilineage hematopoiesis or erythroid precursors or megakaryoblasts is rare
  - Typically seen in conjunction or in transformation from MPN

ANCILLARY TESTS

Immunohistochemistry
- Important for lineage determination and differential diagnosis
- More commonly expresses CD33, CD34, CD43, CD68 (KP1), CD68 (PG-M1), CD99, CD117, lysozyme, and MPO
- May also express CD4, CD30, CD56, terminal deoxynucleotidyl transferase (TdT), and glycophorin A
- Recommended panel may include
  - CD33, CD34, CD43, lysozyme, MPO, CD68, CD117, CD3, and CD20
  - Will successfully identify the vast majority of MS

Flow Cytometry
- Expresses a variety of myeloid-associated antigens
  - Granulocytic differentiation: CD11b(+), CD13(+), CD33(+), CD117(+), and MPO(+)
  - Monocytic differentiation: CD11c(+), CD14(+), bright CD33(+), bright CD64(+), and CD163(+)

Cytogenetics
- Conventional cytogenetics may be performed on fresh tissue
  - Evaluate for clonal evolution at relapse
  - Recurrent cytogenetic abnormalities may be detected
- Complex karyotype is associated with a worse prognosis
- A variety of chromosomal abnormalities have been identified
  - *MLL* rearrangements
  - *RUNX1-RUNX1T1*, t(8;21)(q22;q22)
    - Seen most commonly in childhood &/or in orbital lesions
    - Less frequent in adult series
  - Others include monosomy 7, trisomy 8, inv(16), trisomy 4, monosomy 16, del(16q), del(5q), del(20q), and trisomy 11

In Situ Hybridization
- Fluorescence in situ hybridization (FISH) may be performed on fresh or paraffin-embedded tissue
- Aberrations detected in about 55% of cases
- Recurrent chromosomal translocations more common in de novo cases
  - *RUNX1-RUNX1T1*, t(8;21)(q22;q22)
  - *PML-RARα*, t(15;17)(q22;q12)
  - *CBFβ-MYH11*, inv(16)/t(16;16)(p13.1q22)

Molecular Genetics
- RT-PCR can be used to identify some recurrent genetic abnormalities

  - *CBFβ-MYH11, PML-RARα, RUNX1-RUNX1T1*
- *JAK2* mutations can be identified in cases that arise from a MPN
- *BCR-ABL1* can be identified in cases that arise from chronic myelogenous leukemia (CML)
- *RAS* mutations can be identified in cases arising from chronic myelomonocytic leukemia (CMML)
- *FLT3, NPM1,* and *CEBPA* mutations may also be present

Cytochemistry

- Cytochemical stains performed on touch imprints may assist in lineage determination
  - Granulocytic lineage: Myeloperoxidase (+), chloracetate esterase (+)
  - Monocytic lineage: Nonspecific esterase (+)

DIFFERENTIAL DIAGNOSIS

Aggressive Lymphomas

- Lymphoblastic lymphoma
  - Immunophenotype by flow cytometry or immunohistochemistry will show B- or T-cell lineage
- Burkitt lymphoma
  - B-cell immunophenotype (CD10[+], CD20[+], CD79a[+], Bcl-6[+], sIg[+], Bcl-2[-])
  - High proliferation index (near 100%)
  - Characteristic translocation involving *MYC* with *IgH, kappa,* or *lambda*
- Diffuse large B-cell lymphoma (DLBCL)
  - Mature B-cell immunophenotype
  - Chromatin pattern typically more vesicular and mature
- Anaplastic large cell lymphoma (ALCL)
  - Prominent sinusoidal pattern
  - Distinct immunophenotype (T-cell antigens, CD30[+], ALK[+])
  - *ALK* gene translocations in ALK(+) ALCL

Blastic Plasmacytoid Dendritic Cell Neoplasm

- Usually presents with solitary or multiple skin lesions ± cytopenias
- 10-20% associated with or develop into AML
- Morphologically similar to MS
- Tumor cells do not react with MPO
- Expresses CD4, CD43, CD45RA, CD56, and plasmacytoid dendritic cell antigens (CD123, CD303, TCL1)
  - CD68(+) in 50% of cases
  - CD7 and CD33 expression is relatively common
  - Lysozyme and MPO negative

Histiocytic Sarcoma

- Substantial overlap between monocytic and histiocytic sarcoma
- Composed of mature tissue histiocytes by morphology and IHC
- No evidence of blood or bone marrow involvement in histiocytic sarcoma

Extramedullary Hematopoiesis

- Common in spleen, liver, and lymph nodes
- Shows trilineage hematopoiesis with maturation
- Not mass forming

Small Round Cell Tumors

- Rhabdomyosarcoma (RMS)
  - Distinguish with immunophenotypic markers (e.g., desmin, myogenin, MYOD1)
  - Cytogenetic abnormalities present in a subset of alveolar RMS
- Ewing/primitive neuroectodermal tumor
  - Distinguish with immunophenotypic markers (e.g., CD99, FLI1)
  - Characteristic translocation in 90-95% of cases; t(11;22)(q24;q12)
  - Other rare tumor-defining translocations detected by break-apart FISH probes for the *EWS* locus
- Desmoplastic small round cell tumor
  - Primitive small round blue cells embedded in abundant desmoplastic stroma
  - Distinguish with immunophenotypic markers (e.g., desmin, EMA, WT1)
- Medulloblastoma
  - Distinguish with immunophenotypic markers (e.g., synaptophysin, neurofilament, NSE)

DIAGNOSTIC CHECKLIST

Pathologic Interpretation Pearls

- Key findings that raise suspicion for MS include
  - Medium to large-sized blastic cells with folded nuclei, intracytoplasmic granules, and high mitotic rate
  - Green color of gross specimen

SELECTED REFERENCES

1. Campidelli C et al: Myeloid sarcoma: extramedullary manifestation of myeloid disorders. Am J Clin Pathol. 132(3):426-37, 2009
2. Alexiev BA et al: Myeloid sarcomas: a histologic, immunohistochemical, and cytogenetic study. Diagn Pathol. 2:42, 2007
3. Pileri SA et al: Myeloid sarcoma: clinico-pathologic, phenotypic and cytogenetic analysis of 92 adult patients. Leukemia. 21(2):340-50, 2007
4. Reinhardt D et al: Isolated myelosarcoma in children--update and review. Leuk Lymphoma. 43(3):565-74, 2002
5. Chang CC et al: Immunophenotypic profile of myeloid cells in granulocytic sarcoma by immunohistochemistry. Correlation with blast differentiation in bone marrow. Am J Clin Pathol. 114(5):807-11, 2000

Microscopic Features and Ancillary Techniques

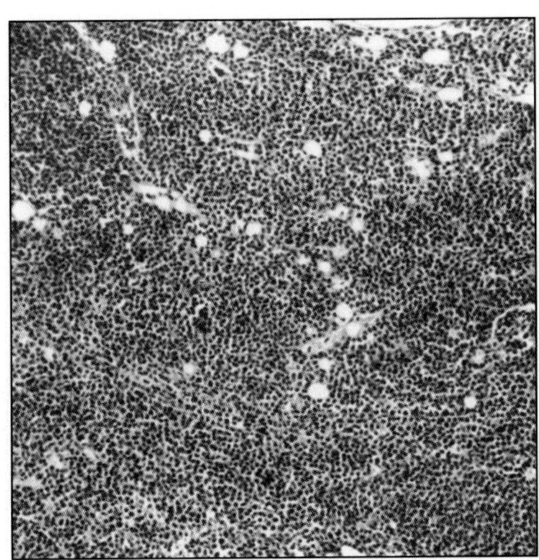

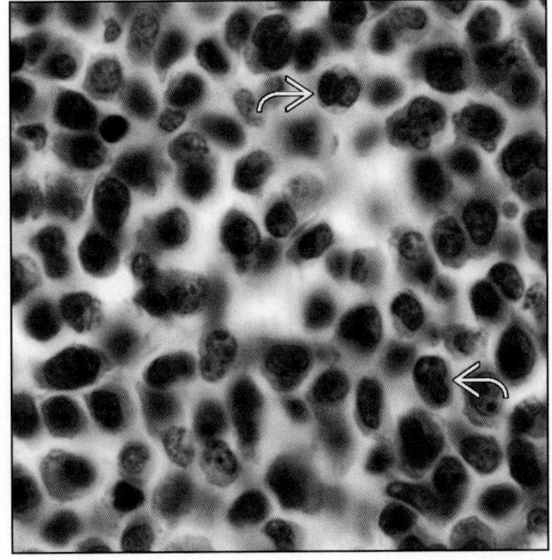

(Left) *Section from a bone lesion in a patient with APL previously in remission shows sheets of blasts (promyelocytes). Examination of PB and BM showed no morphologic or molecular evidence for APL.* ***(Right)*** *High-power view of MS in a patient with APL highlights the typical morphologic features: Folded/bilobed nuclei ➢ and abundant cytoplasm with granules. Diagnosis of this rare case was confirmed by FISH for t(15;17). PB and BM showed no evidence for APL.*

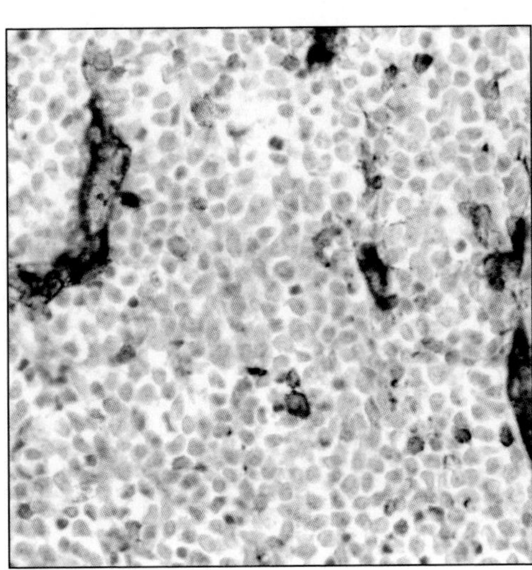

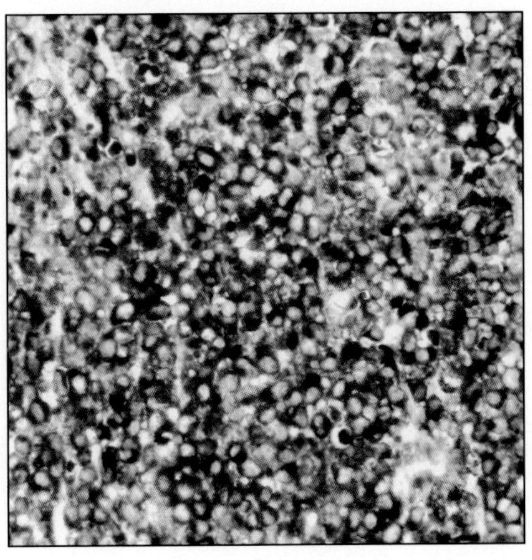

(Left) *IHC for CD34 shows negative staining in this MS with promyelocytic differentiation. It is important to note that CD34 cannot be used to rule out a diagnosis of MS as some blasts do not express CD34.* ***(Right)*** *IHC for myeloperoxidase shows strong reactivity in this MS taken from a bone lesion in a patient with APL in previous remission. Evaluation by FISH (not shown) for t(15;17) confirmed the diagnosis. Evaluation of PB and BM showed no evidence of disease.*

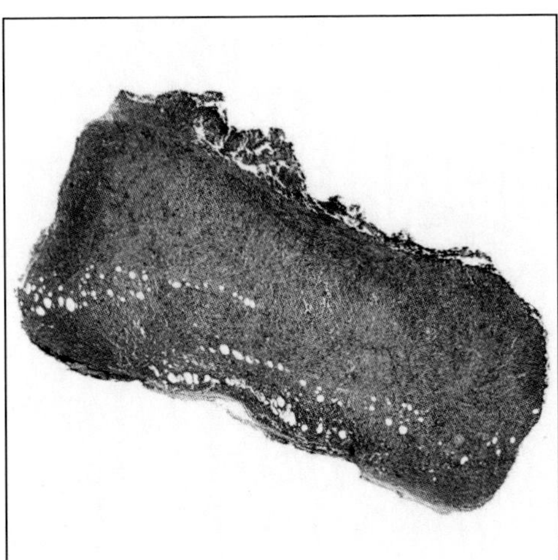

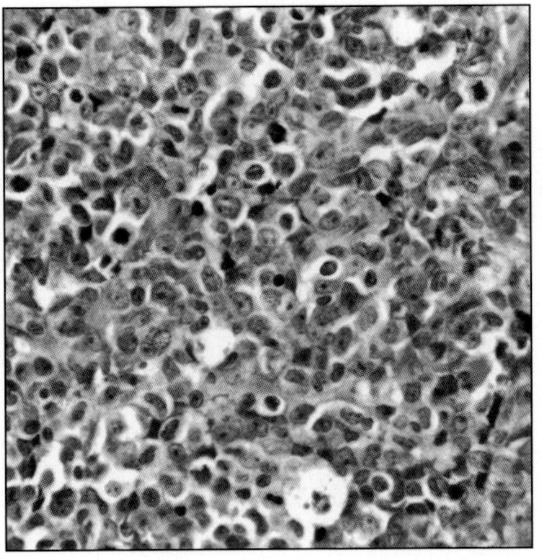

(Left) *Biopsy of a subcutaneous mass shows sheets of large cells, morphologically suspicious for blasts. Work-up with a panel of IHC stains will help confirm the diagnosis of MS and exclude other possible tumors.* ***(Right)*** *High-power view of a subcutaneous mass shows sheets of large cells with dispersed chromatin and conspicuous nucleoli. IHC stains (not shown) confirmed a diagnosis of MS. A subsequent BM evaluation showed increased myeloid blasts consistent with AML.*

MYELOID SARCOMA

Microscopic Features and Ancillary Techniques

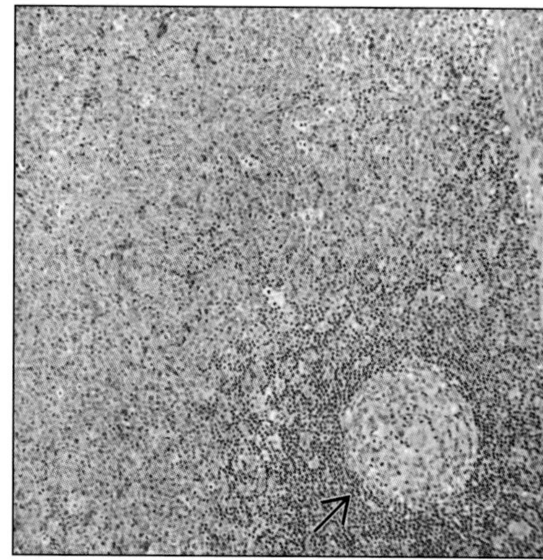

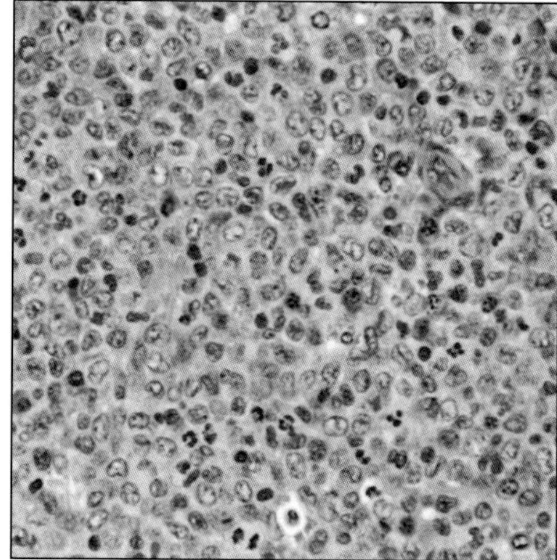

(Left) *Myeloid sarcoma may also present in lymph nodes, which raises the differential diagnosis of DLBCL and metastases. This lymph node shows sheets of large, pale-appearing cells that have effaced much of the lymph node architecture. A residual follicle* ➞ *is also noted.* ***(Right)*** *High-power view of MS involving a lymph node shows the typical large cells with pleomorphic nuclei and variably conspicuous nucleoli. IHC stains are key in confirming the diagnosis.*

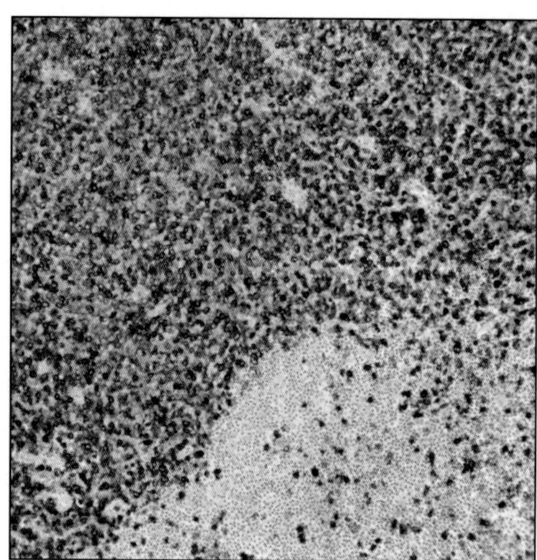

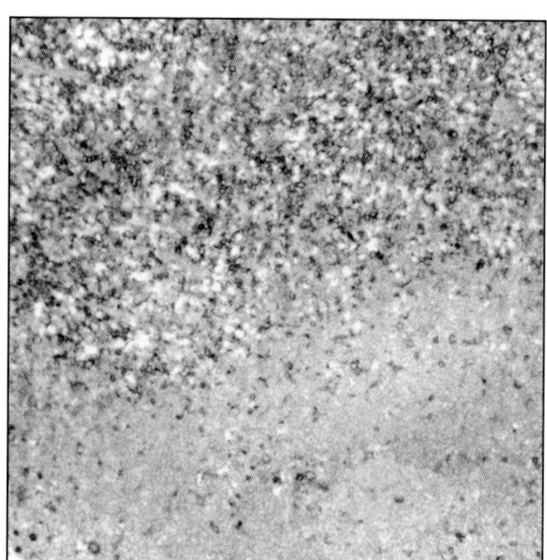

(Left) *IHC for lysozyme highlights sheets of leukemic blasts in this MS involving a lymph node. The pale, negative staining area represents a residual follicle.* ***(Right)*** *IHC for CD33 highlights the sheets of leukemic blasts in this MS involving a lymph node. The pale, negative staining area represents a residual follicle.*

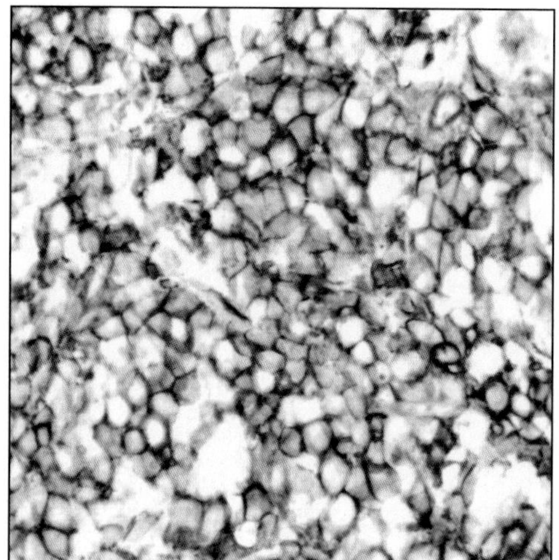

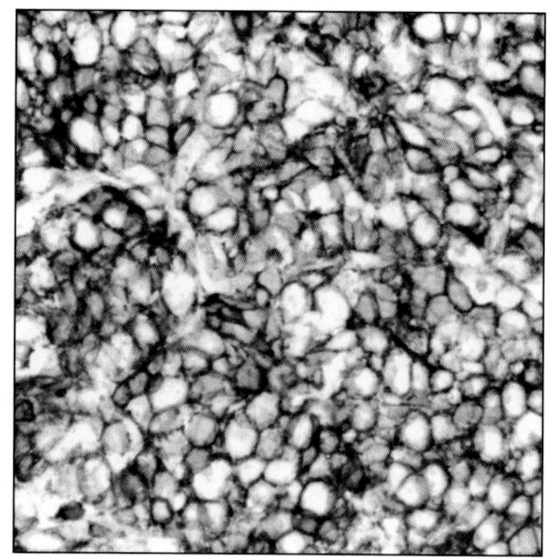

(Left) *IHC for CD34 can be helpful in making the diagnosis of MS; however, it is important to remember that not all blasts express CD34, and therefore a negative stain cannot exclude the diagnosis.* ***(Right)*** *CD43 is another commonly used stain in the work-up of MS and is considered along with lysozyme one of the most sensitive markers for this diagnosis. However, CD43 is not entirely specific.*

Differential Diagnosis

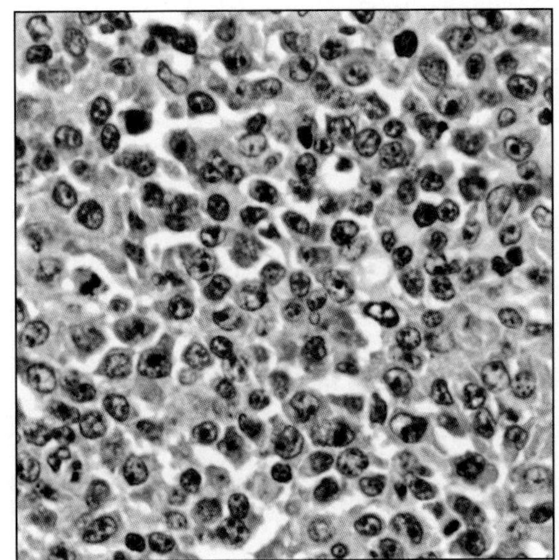

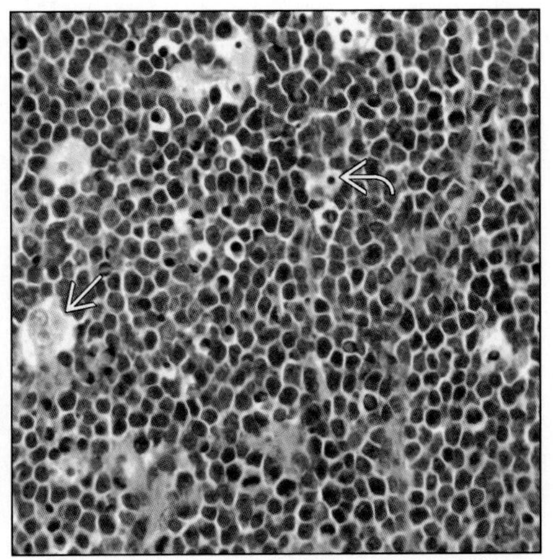

(Left) *An example of DLBCL is shown for comparison. Note the pleomorphic nuclei, prominent nucleoli, vesicular chromatin, and variable amounts of amphophilic cytoplasm. IHC stains are key to making the distinction from MS.* ***(Right)*** *An example of Burkitt lymphoma with typical morphologic features is shown for comparison. Note the intermediate size of the cells with little nuclear pleomorphism, slight retraction of the cytoplasm, and scattered macrophages ➡ and apoptotic cells ↷.*

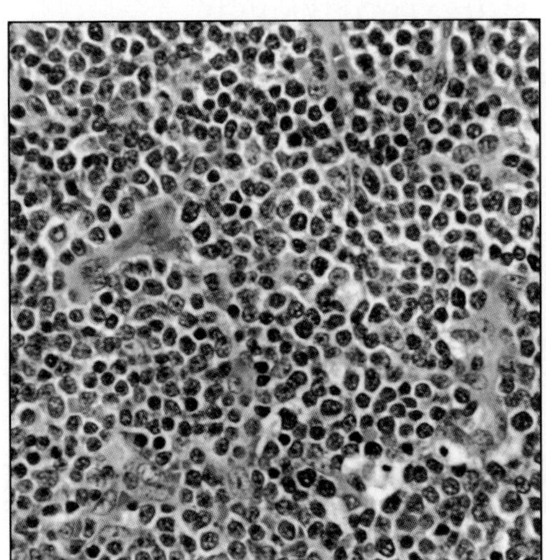

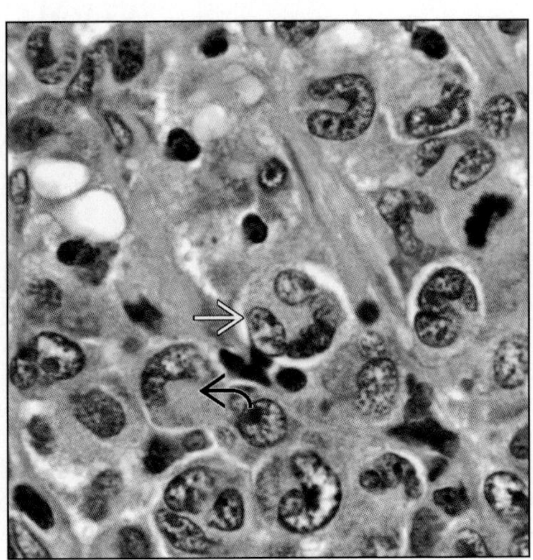

(Left) *T-lymphoblastic lymphoma is shown for comparison. The leukemic cells typically show less nuclear pleomorphism than myeloid blasts. The diagnosis can easily be made with a panel of immunostains &/or flow cytometry immunophenotyping.* ***(Right)*** *ALCL is another diagnostic consideration when sheets of large pleomorphic cells are present. Hallmark cells ➡ are usually present in ALCL. Note the kidney-shaped nuclei and eosinophilic Golgi region ↷.*

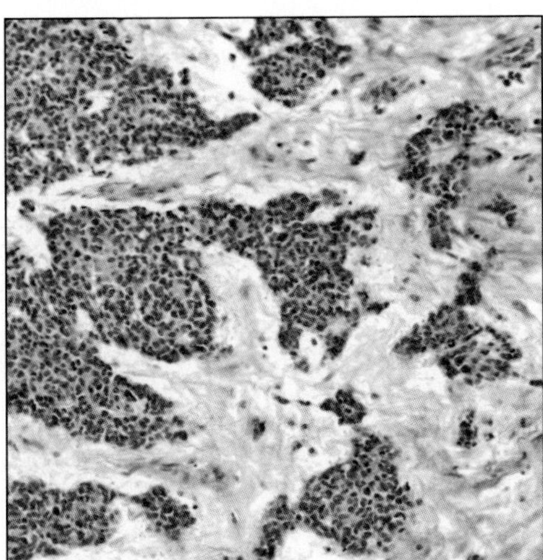

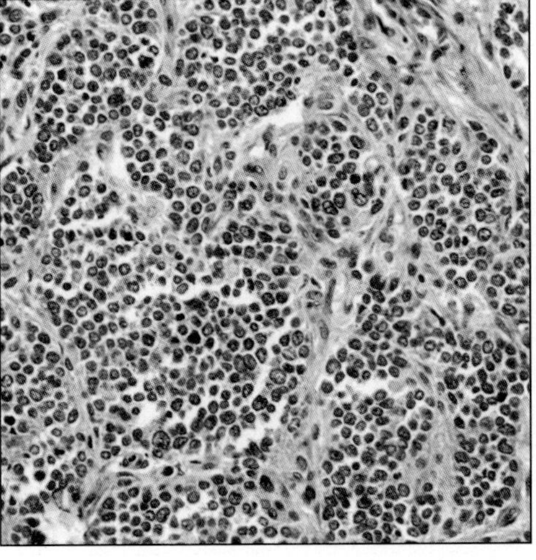

(Left) *An example of desmoplastic small round cell tumor demonstrates sharply demarcated nests of various size and shape surrounded by a desmoplastic stroma. IHC for desmin and WT1 will help confirm this diagnosis.* ***(Right)*** *This example of alveolar rhabdomyosarcoma (ARMS) shows nests of large cells separated by fibrovascular septa. Distinction of MS from the solid variant of ARMS can be challenging. IHC for desmin, myogenin, and MYOD1 will help confirm this diagnosis.*

MYELOID PROLIFERATIONS RELATED TO DOWN SYNDROME

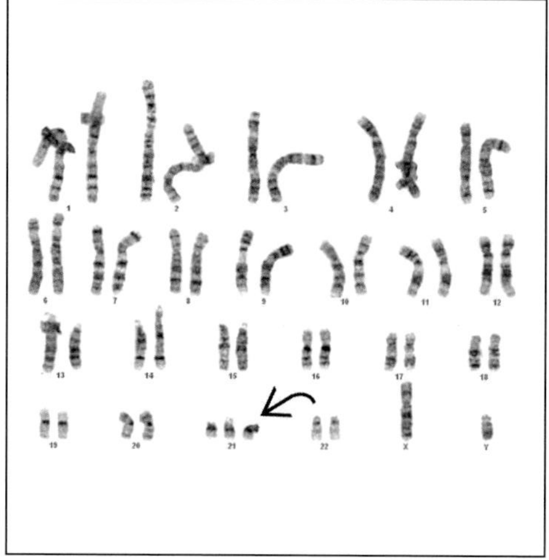

Myeloid proliferations in young children with constitutional trisomy 21 ⮫ have distinct clinical and biologic behavior. *GATA1* mutations are predictably present in this setting.

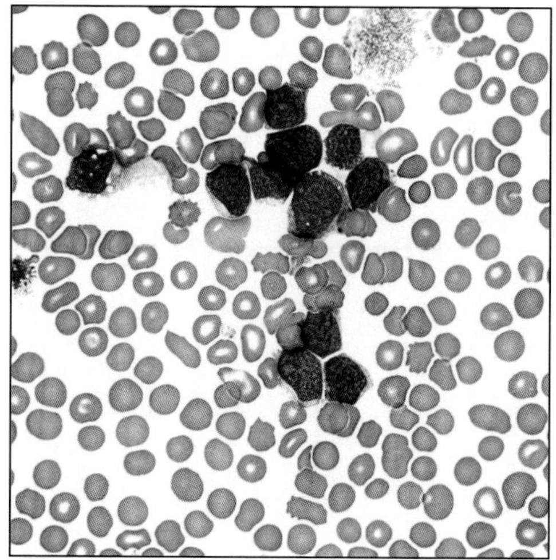

Circulating blasts are present in the peripheral blood of this 4-week-old male with Down syndrome, consistent with transient abnormal myelopoiesis. As expected, this state spontaneously resolved.

TERMINOLOGY

Definitions

- Down syndrome
  - Constitutional trisomy 21
  - Characterized by a number of congenital and developmental abnormalities, including (in neonate)
    - Hypotonia
    - Slanted palpebral fissures
    - Epicanthal folds
    - Single transverse palmar crease
    - Frequent cardiac anomalies
  - Rare individuals may be mosaics for trisomy 21
    - In these patients, subset of cells carry normal chromosome complement
    - Phenotypic effects may be mild, depending on prominence of trisomic cells
    - Very rarely, phenotypically normal mosaic individuals can be affected by myeloid proliferations
- Myeloid proliferations related to Down syndrome (MPRDS)
  - Major category of myeloid neoplasia in 2008 WHO classification
  - Includes 2 distinct entities
  - Transient abnormal myelopoiesis (TAM)
    - Unusual myeloid proliferation resembling acute myeloid leukemia (AML)
    - Resolves spontaneously
  - Myeloid leukemia associated with Down syndrome (MLADS)
    - In patients with Down syndrome, there is no prognostic or therapeutic distinction between states resembling myelodysplastic syndrome (MDS) and AML
    - Thus, MLADS incorporates both of these disease states without regard to blast percentage

ETIOLOGY/PATHOGENESIS

Normal Function of GATA1

- *GATA1* is located at Xp11.23
- Encodes transcription factor that binds to specific DNA sequences
  - Term *GATA1* derives from protein's recognition of sequences that contain the motif G-A-T-A
- Binding of GATA1 protein modulates transcription of associated genes
- Regulation by GATA1 is important in normal erythropoiesis and megakaryopoiesis
- *GATA1* encompasses 6 exons
  - Use of translation start site in exon 2 results in production of full-length GATA1 protein
    - This form of the protein predominates in normal cell

Role of GATA1 Mutation in MPRDS

- Acquired *GATA1* mutations are present in TAM and MLADS
  - Conversely, *GATA1* mutations are not observed in myeloid neoplasia outside clinical setting of Down syndrome
- These *GATA1* mutations result in decreased production of normal full-length GATA1 protein
  - Premature arrest of translation
  - Protein synthesis can instead proceed from alternative start site (methionine at position 83)
    - However, use of this alternative exon 3 start site leads to abbreviated ("short form") GATA1 protein
    - This form lacks amino terminal portion of protein essential for transcriptional activation of some genes
- Association between trisomy 21 and acquired *GATA1* mutations remains unexplained

MYELOID PROLIFERATIONS RELATED TO DOWN SYNDROME

Key Facts

Terminology

- Myeloid proliferations related to Down syndrome (MPRDS) encompasses transient abnormal myelopoiesis (TAM) and myeloid leukemia associated with Down syndrome (MLADS)
- TAM
  - Unusual myeloid proliferation resembling acute myeloid leukemia (AML)
  - Resolves spontaneously
- MLADS
  - Includes both early myelodysplastic syndrome (MDS)-like phase and subsequent frank leukemic state

Etiology/Pathogenesis

- Acquired *GATA1* mutations are present in TAM and MLADS

Clinical Issues

- 20-30% of patients who develop TAM later develop MLADS
- MLADS is associated with chemosensitivity and good prognosis

Top Differential Diagnoses

- "Conventional" AML in setting of Down syndrome
  - Patients with Down syndrome may also develop "conventional" AML
  - Usually older than age 5 at diagnosis
  - *GATA1* mutations are absent
- Reactive leukocytosis due to neonatal infection
- AML with t(1;22)(p13;q13)

Etiologic Relationship between TAM and MLADS

- Some studies have detected differences in gene expression profiles between TAM and MLADS blasts
- Blasts in MLADS often show clonal cytogenetic abnormalities in addition to constitutional trisomy 21
  - Trisomy 8 is commonly identified
  - In contrast, these additional clonal abnormalities are not characteristic of TAM

CLINICAL ISSUES

Epidemiology

- Incidence
  - Down syndrome affects approximately 1 in 800 newborns
  - TAM develops in at least 10% of newborns with Down syndrome
    - True incidence may be higher, since routine CBCs may not be performed in all cases
  - MLADS develops in 1-2% of patients with Down syndrome
    - Usually occurs by age 4 or 5
  - 20-30% of patients who develop TAM later develop MLADS

Presentation

- TAM
  - Acute blastemia
  - Hepatosplenomegaly
  - Average age at diagnosis is 3-7 days
    - Only exceptional cases present after 2 months of age
  - TAM has also been documented during fetal development
    - Can cause hydrops fetalis
- MLADS
  - May initially manifest as months-long state with many features similar to refractory cytopenia of childhood

Laboratory Tests

- Conventional cytogenetics
  - Confirms constitutional trisomy 21
- Flow cytometry
  - Similar findings in TAM and MLADS
  - Blasts express CD13, CD33, CD7, CD117, CD36, CD42, and CD61
    - Blasts in TAM are more likely to also express CD34, CD56, and CD41 than are blasts in MLADS
- Molecular analysis
  - Indicated to detect *GATA1* mutation if diagnosis as TAM or MLADS is not certain &/or to determine eligibility for treatment protocol

Prognosis

- TAM
  - Minority of patients die during TAM episode
    - Hepatic fibrosis significantly contributes to this mortality
  - If patients survive acute period of TAM, spontaneous remission is expected
    - However, 20-30% of these patients will later develop MLADS
    - Remaining patients experience durable remission
- MLADS
  - Good prognosis in young Down syndrome patients with *GATA1* mutations
    - Specific treatment protocols are indicated for this population

MICROSCOPIC PATHOLOGY

Morphologic Features of Blasts in TAM and MLADS

- Usually megakaryoblasts
  - Basophilic cytoplasm
  - Scant basophilic (MPO negative) granules
  - Cytoplasmic blebbing

Other Features of TAM

- Peripheral blood

MYELOID PROLIFERATIONS RELATED TO DOWN SYNDROME

Transient Abnormal Myelopoiesis vs. Myeloid Leukemia Associated with Down Syndrome

	Transient Abnormal Myelopoiesis (TAM)	Myeloid Leukemia Associated with Down Syndrome (MLADS)
Age at diagnosis	Neonates	Within 1st 4-5 years of life
Clinical behavior	Spontaneous remission within 3 months	Relatively good prognosis
Blast population	Virtually indistinguishable from MLADS	Usually megakaryoblastic
Cytogenetic findings	Constitutional trisomy 21	Trisomy 21, frequently with additional acquired clonal abnormalities
Molecular findings	*GATA1* mutation	*GATA1* mutation
Dysplasia	Present	Present

- Thrombocytopenia
- Generally impressive leukocytosis, though some cases have normal white blood cell count
- Blastemia

- Bone marrow
  - Erythroid and megakaryocytic dysplasia

Other Features of MLADS

- Peripheral blood
  - Pronounced dysplasia and macrocytosis are present in early stage of disease, even in absence of blasts
- Bone marrow
  - Trilineage dysplasia

DIFFERENTIAL DIAGNOSIS

"Conventional" AML in Setting of Down Syndrome

- Patients with Down syndrome may also develop "conventional" AML
  - Usually older than age 5 at diagnosis
  - *GATA1* mutations are absent

Acute Lymphoblastic Leukemia (ALL) in Setting of Down Syndrome

- Patients with Down syndrome also have greatly increased risk of developing ALL
- Routine immunophenotyping permits distinction between ALL and MPRDS

Reactive Leukocytosis Due to Neonatal Infection

- Acute blastemia of TAM is generally in excess of left shift associated with infection or inflammation, though overlap may occur
  - In uncertain cases, documentation of megakaryoblastic immunophenotype &/or *GATA1* mutation support a diagnosis of TAM
  - Clinical features of infection typically present

AML with t(1;22)(p13;q13)

- Megakaryoblastic leukemia that presents in infants and young children
  - These features overlap significantly with TAM and MLADS
- Though TAM and MLADS are restricted to children with Down syndrome, in rare cases (especially involving trisomy 21 mosaicism), diagnosis of Down syndrome will not yet be established when myeloid proliferation is recognized
  - Thus, conventional cytogenetic analysis, which will detect both trisomy 21 and t(1;22), is essential

GATA1-related X-linked Cytopenia

- Familial disorder characterized by inherited *GATA1* mutations and cytopenias of variable lineage
- Completely unrelated in all respects to Down syndrome and MPRDS
  - Thus, *GATA1*-related X-linked cytopenia only enters differential diagnosis if *GATA1* analysis is considered in isolation from clinical findings
  - However, Inherited *GATA1* mutations are most often missense mutations and therefore distinct from those seen in MPRDS

DIAGNOSTIC CHECKLIST

Pathologic Interpretation Pearls

- Bone marrow biopsy is generally not necessary in a case of uncomplicated TAM
  - All ancillary studies can be performed on peripheral blood blasts
  - In TAM, blast percentage is often lower in bone marrow than in peripheral blood
- Ongoing studies may further define role of molecular monitoring and treatment in TAM
  - Ideally, it would be possible to prospectively identify subset of TAM patients at risk for later MLADS

SELECTED REFERENCES

1. Kanezaki R et al: Down syndrome and GATA1 mutations in transient abnormal myeloproliferative disorder: mutation classes correlate with progression to myeloid leukemia. Blood. 116(22):4631-8, 2010
2. Roy A et al: Acute megakaryoblastic leukaemia (AMKL) and transient myeloproliferative disorder (TMD) in Down syndrome: a multi-step model of myeloid leukaemogenesis. Br J Haematol. 147(1):3-12, 2009

Microscopic Features

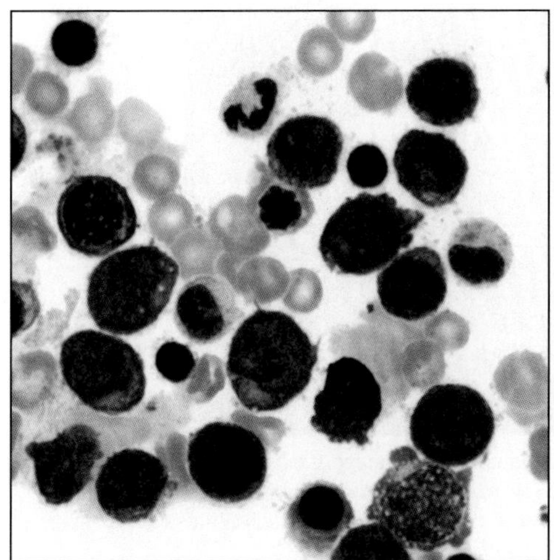

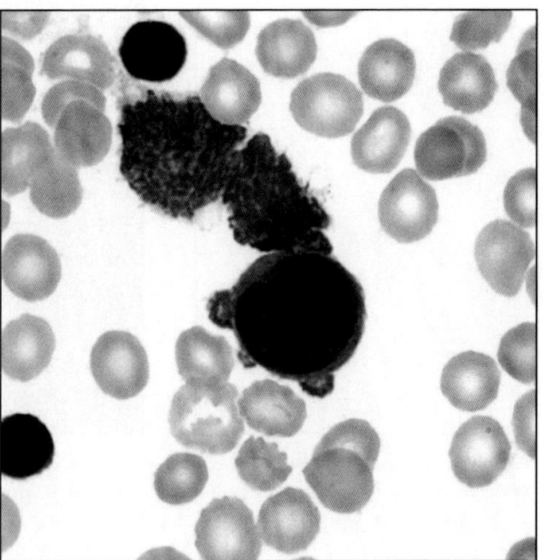

(Left) *Bone marrow aspirate smear from a 1-year-old male with Down syndrome and a prior history of resolved transient abnormal myelopoiesis with GATA1 mutation shows numerous megakaryoblasts, consistent with myeloid leukemia associated with Down syndrome.* ***(Right)*** *A megakaryoblast from a patient with myeloid leukemia associated with Down syndrome shows characteristic cytologic features, including basophilic cytoplasm and peripheral cytoplasmic "blebbing."*

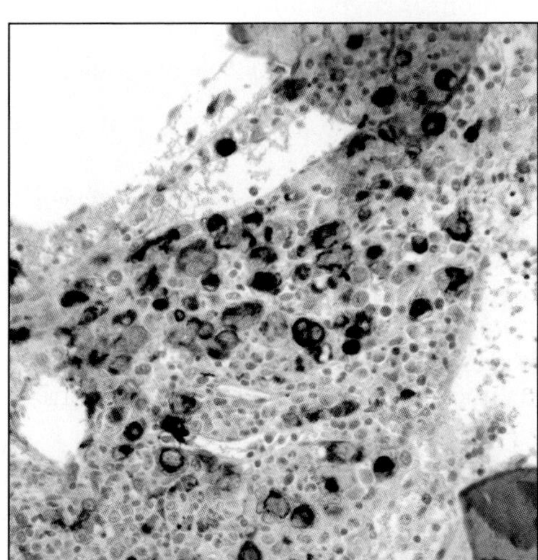

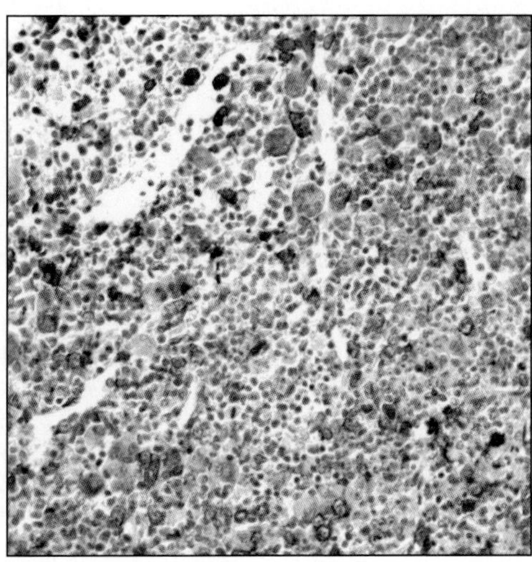

(Left) *CD31 highlights atypical megakaryocytes admixed with megakaryoblasts in a 20-month-old child with myeloid leukemia associated with Down syndrome. The child had a history of resolved transient myeloproliferative disorder.* ***(Right)*** *CD117 stains increased blasts in a case of myeloid leukemia associated with Down syndrome. This marker is very useful for tissue sections in this setting, as blasts in about 1/2 of such cases will be CD34 negative.*

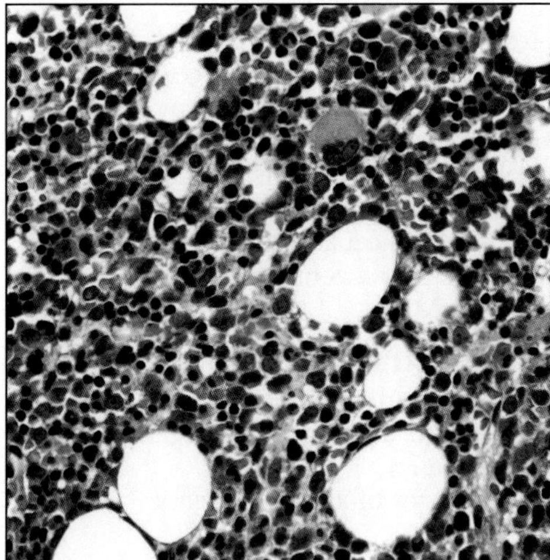

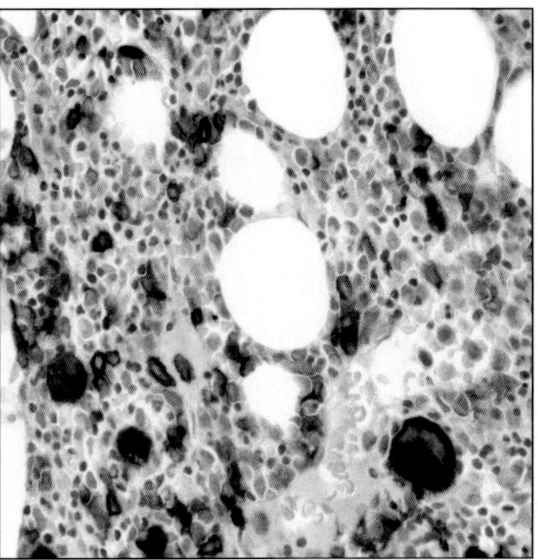

(Left) *Bone marrow core biopsy shows a blastic infiltrate with atypical megakaryocytes in a case of myeloid leukemia associated with Down syndrome. The karyotype showed multiple abnormalities in addition to the constitutional trisomy 21, including acquired trisomies of chromosomes 8, 14, and 19.* ***(Right)*** *CD42b stains atypical megakaryocytes and numerous megakaryoblasts in this patient with myeloid leukemia associated with Down syndrome. These patients have a relatively good prognosis.*

JUVENILE MYELOMONOCYTIC LEUKEMIA

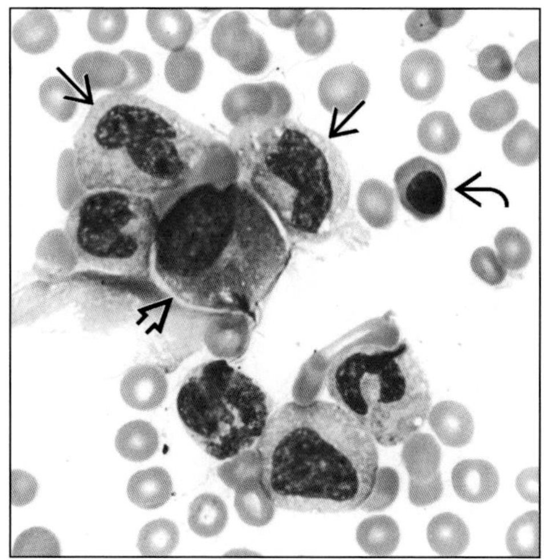

Peripheral blood from a patient with JMML shows some of the characteristic features of which include an absolute monocytosis ➡, left-shifted granulocytes ➡, and nucleated red blood cells ➡.

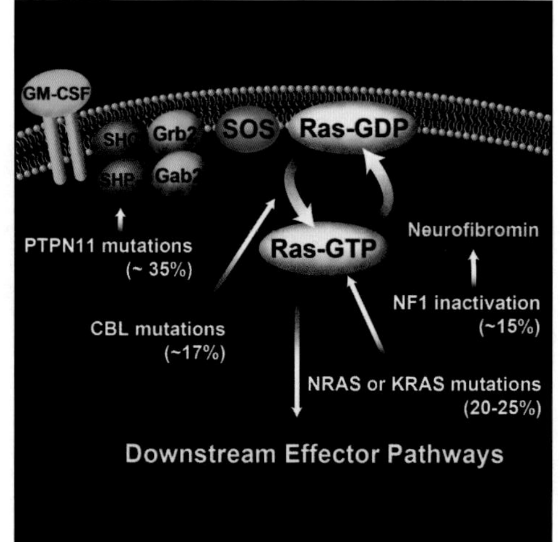

Illustration depicts the common mutations observed in sporadic cases of JMML along with their respective frequencies. All mutations result in the deregulation of the RAS/MAPK signaling pathway.

TERMINOLOGY

Abbreviations

- Juvenile myelomonocytic leukemia (JMML)

Synonyms

- Juvenile chronic myelomonocytic leukemia

Definitions

- Clonal hematopoietic disorder of childhood characterized by proliferation of predominantly granulocytic and monocytic lineages
  - Blasts plus promonocytes < 20% of cells in peripheral blood and bone marrow
  - Frequent erythroid and megakaryocytic abnormalities
  - Lacks *BCR-ABL1* or Ph chromosome
  - Characteristic mutations involving genes of RAS/MAPK pathway

ETIOLOGY/PATHOGENESIS

Molecular Background

- At least in part due to aberrant signal transduction resulting from mutations in components of RAS/MAPK signaling pathway
  - Proto-oncogenes including *PTPN11* and *RAS* (*NRAS* and *KRAS2*)
  - Tumor suppressor genes including *NF1* and *CBL*

De Novo, Nonsyndromic (Sporadic) Cases

- Somatic mutations in the following genes
  - *PTPN11* (35% of sporadic cases)
    - Encodes non-receptor tyrosine phosphatase protein SHP-2
    - Gain of function mutation results in activation of guanine nucleotide exchange factors (GNEFs) required for conversion of inactive GDP-RAS to active GTP-RAS
    - Results in continuous activation of RAS
    - Set of mutations is largely different compared to Noonan syndrome-associated JMML
  - *RAS* genes (*NRAS* and *KRAS2*) (20-25% of sporadic cases)
    - Role in transduction of extracellular signals to nucleus
    - Regulate cellular processes by switching between active GTP-RAS and inactive GDP-RAS forms
    - Amount of GTP-RAS is regulated by GNEFs and GTPase activating proteins (GAPs)
    - Active GTP-RAS activates RAF kinase, resulting in downstream proliferative effect
    - Activating point mutations are found in codons 12, 13, and 61 of *NRAS* and *KRAS*
  - *NF1* (15% of sporadic cases)
    - Encodes neurofibromin protein (GTPase activating protein for RAS)
    - Enhances hydrolysis of active GTP-RAS to inactive GDP-RAS
    - Mutations lead to increased GTP-RAS
  - *CBL* (17% of sporadic cases)
    - Encodes for E3 ubiquitin ligase
    - Marks activated receptor and non-receptor tyrosine kinases and other proteins for degradation
    - Mutations result in continuous activation of RAS
- All above mutations are largely mutually exclusive, suggesting that pathological activation of RAS-dependent pathways play a central role in the pathophysiology of JMML

Germline Predisposition Syndromes

- **Neurofibromatosis type 1 (NF1)** (10% of all cases)
  - Autosomal dominant or spontaneous (germline mutation in *NF1* gene)
  - 2nd event required for bi-allelic *NF1* gene inactivation
  - Clinical presentation
    - 6 or more "café au lait" macules

JUVENILE MYELOMONOCYTIC LEUKEMIA

Key Facts

Terminology
- Clonal hematopoietic disorder of childhood characterized by proliferation of predominantly granulocytic and monocytic lineages

Etiology/Pathogenesis
- Aberrant signal transduction resulting from mutations of components of RAS/MAPK signaling pathway (*PTPN11*, *RAS*, *NF1*, and *CBL* genes)

Clinical Issues
- Constitutional symptoms or evidence of infection
- Marked hepatosplenomegaly
- Lymphadenopathy

Top Differential Diagnoses
- Viral infections
- Acute myeloid leukemia (AML)
- Chronic myelogenous leukemia (CML)

Diagnostic Checklist
- Mandatory diagnostic criteria
  - Peripheral blood monocytosis > 1 x 10^9/L
  - Blasts (including promonocytes) < 20% of leukocytes in PB and BM
  - No Ph chromosome or *BCR-ABL1* fusion gene
- Additional criteria (≥ 2 required)
  - Hemoglobin F increased for age
  - Immature granulocytes in peripheral blood
  - WBC count > 10 x 10^9/L
  - In vitro GM-CSF hypersensitivity in myeloid progenitors
  - Clonal cytogenetic abnormality (i.e., monosomy 7)

    - 2 or more neurofibromas or 1 plexiform neurofibroma
    - Lisch nodules, axillary or inguinal freckling, &/or optic gliomas
- **Noonan syndrome**
  - Autosomal dominant or spontaneous (germline mutation in *PTPN11* gene in 50% of Noonan syndrome cases)
    - Hypothesis exists that mutations of *PTPN11* gene in Noonan syndrome have "weaker" transforming ability and therefore can be tolerated as germline events
  - JMML in the above setting behaves differently compared to sporadic cases
    - Occurs at very young age (infancy)
    - Tends to regress spontaneously
  - Clinical presentation
    - Facial dysmorphism, short stature, webbed neck, cardiac anomalies and varying levels of impaired cognition

CLINICAL ISSUES

Epidemiology
- Incidence
  - 1.3 cases/million children 0-14 years of age/year
    - < 2-3% of all leukemias in children
    - 20-30% of all cases of myelodysplastic and myeloproliferative disease in patients < 14 years of age
- Age
  - 1 month to adolescence
    - 75% in children < 3 years of age
- Gender
  - M:F = 2:1

Site
- Peripheral blood and bone marrow (always)
- Liver and spleen (virtually always)
- Lymph nodes, skin, and respiratory tract (common)
- Any tissue may be infiltrated

Presentation
- Constitutional symptoms or evidence of infection (most cases)
- Marked hepatosplenomegaly (95%)
- Lymphadenopathy (50%)
- Signs of bleeding (frequent)
- Skin rash (25%)
- Enlarged tonsils

Laboratory Tests
- Complete blood count (CBC)
  - Monocytosis > 1 x 10^9/L
  - Leukocytosis with left shift
  - Anemia and thrombocytopenia
- Markedly increased synthesis of hemoglobin F (50%)
- Polyclonal hypergammaglobulinemia
- Autoantibodies
- In vitro marked hypersensitivity of myeloid progenitor cells to GM-CSF

Treatment
- Hematopoietic stem cell transplant (HSCT)
  - Therapy-related mortality (15%)
  - Relapse is major cause of treatment failure (35%)
  - Graft vs. leukemia effect plays important role
- Splenectomy and high-dose chemotherapy are not recommended prior to patient receiving conditioning for HSCT unless clinically indicated for symptomatic relief
- Future targeted therapies are being investigated

Prognosis
- Cure rates of ~ 50% with HSCT
- Rapidly fatal if left untreated
  - 1-year median survival time without HSCT
  - Death from organ failure due to leukemic infiltration
- Rarely transforms into acute leukemia
- Most cases of Noonan syndrome-associated JMML presenting in neonatal period spontaneously resolve over 1st year of life

JUVENILE MYELOMONOCYTIC LEUKEMIA

- Well-established prognostic factors associated with short survival
  - Low platelet count (< 33 x 10^9/L)
  - Age > 2 years at diagnosis
  - High hemoglobin F at diagnosis
- Recently proposed prognostic factors
  - Lack of prognostic significance of specific genetic mutations (*PTPN11*, *RAS*, *NF1*, and *CBL*)
  - Microarray gene expression profiling studies (using DC model) identified 2 subclasses of patients (AML-like and non-AML-like) with significantly different clinical outcomes (10-year probability of survival: 7% vs. 74% respectively)
    - Gene expression-based classification seems to outperform all known clinical parameters in terms of prognostic relevance
  - Hypermethylation of *BMP4*, *CALCA*, *CDKN2B*, and *RARB* genes are associated with poor prognosis

MICROSCOPIC PATHOLOGY

Microscopic Features

- Peripheral blood (PB)
  - Absolute monocytosis (always)
  - Leukocytosis
    - Median WBC count 25-30 x 10^9/L
    - Mainly neutrophils, some promyelocytes and myelocytes
    - Blasts (including promyelocytes) usually < 5%, always < 20%
    - Eosinophilia and basophilia in minority of cases
    - Dysplasia minimal
  - Anemia
    - Nucleated red blood cells are common
    - Normocytic (most common)
    - Macrocytic (cases with monosomy 7)
    - Microcytic (cases with iron deficiency or acquired thalassemia phenotype)
  - Thrombocytopenia (common)
- Bone marrow aspirate and biopsy (BM)
  - Findings by themselves not diagnostic
  - Hypercellular BM with granulocytic proliferation
    - Erythroid precursors predominate in some cases
  - Monocytes less impressive than in PB (usually 5-10% of BM cells)
  - Blasts (including promyelocytes) < 20% of BM cells
    - Auer rods never present
  - Dysplasia minimal
    - Dysgranulopoiesis, including pseudo Pelger-Huet neutrophils or hypergranularity may be present
    - Erythroid precursors may be enlarged
  - Megakaryocytes often reduced in number
  - Reticulin fibrosis in some cases
- Other organs
  - Skin with leukemic infiltrate of myelomonocytic cells in superficial and deep dermis (common)
  - Lung with leukemic infiltrate in alveolar septa and alveoli
  - Spleen with leukemic infiltrate in red pulp, with predilection for trabecular and central arteries
  - Liver with leukemic infiltrate in sinusoids and portal tracts

Diagnostic Criteria

- WHO 2008 criteria
  - Peripheral blood monocytosis > 1 x 10^9/L
  - Blasts (including promonocytes) < 20% of leukocytes in PB and of nucleated BM cells
  - No Ph chromosome or *BCR-ABL1* fusion gene
  - Plus 2 or more of the following
    - Hemoglobin F increased for age
    - Immature granulocytes in PB
    - WBC count > 10 x 10^9/L
    - Clonal cytogenetic abnormality (i.e., monosomy 7)
    - In vitro GM-CSF hypersensitivity in myeloid cells
- More recent criteria incorporate somatic mutations (*PTPN11*, *RAS*, *NF1*, or *CBL*) and clinical diagnosis of NF1

ANCILLARY TESTS

Cytogenetics

- Normal karyotype (65%), monosomy 7 (25%), other abnormalities (10%)

Molecular Genetics

- Firm molecular diagnosis of JMML possible in 85-90%
- Molecular testing for specific mutations (*PTPN11*, *RAS*, *NF1*, or *CBL*)

DIFFERENTIAL DIAGNOSIS

Infectious Diseases

- Chronic viral infections (i.e., EBV, CMV, HHV6, and parvovirus) can cause sustained monocytosis and be associated with splenomegaly
  - Molecular studies, in vitro cultures and serologic tests may be helpful

Acute Myeloid Leukemia (AML)

- Distinguish from acute monocytic leukemia and acute myelomonocytic leukemia
- Blasts > 20% in PB or BM
- Presence of Auer rods excludes JMML and favors AML

Chronic Myelogenous Leukemia (CML)

- Presence of *BCR-ABL1* or Ph chromosome
- Peripheral basophilia invariably present
- Leukocytosis with fraction of monocytes usually < 3%

SELECTED REFERENCES

1. de Vries AC et al: Molecular basis of juvenile myelomonocytic leukemia. Haematologica. 95(2):179-82, 2010
2. Loh ML: Childhood myelodysplastic syndrome: focus on the approach to diagnosis and treatment of juvenile myelomonocytic leukemia. Hematology Am Soc Hematol Educ Program. 2010:357-62, 2010

Microscopic Features and Differential Diagnosis

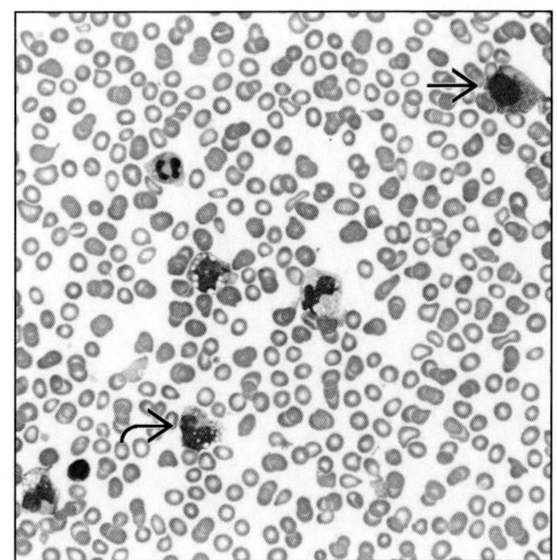

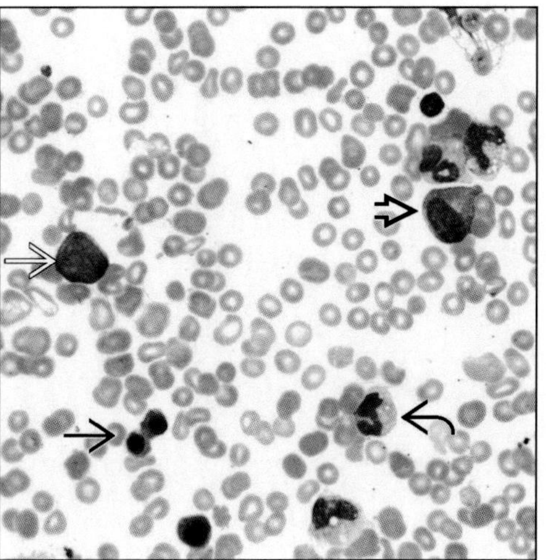

(Left) *Peripheral blood from medium power shows increased numbers of mature monocytes ⇨. Note the myelocyte → indicative of a left shift.* ***(Right)*** *High-power view of the peripheral blood from a patient with JMML shows many of the characteristic findings: Increased monocytes ⇨, left-shifted granulocytes ⇨, and occasional nucleated red blood cells →. A rare blast ➡ was also noted on the smear. Blasts and blast equivalents (promonocytes) are < 20% in PB and BM.*

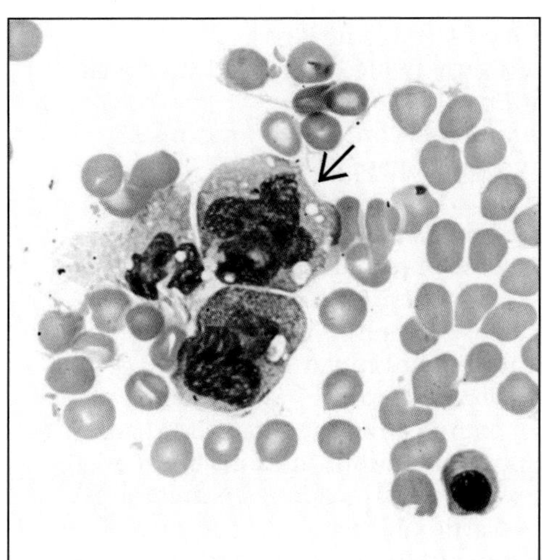

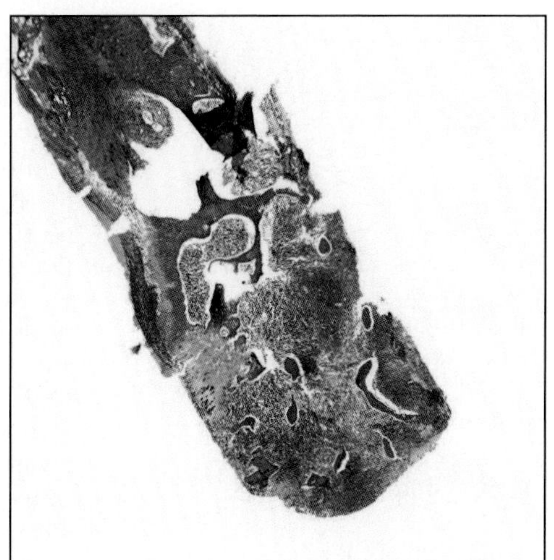

(Left) *Peripheral blood from a patient with JMML highlights an atypical-appearing monocyte →. Although dysplasia is often minimal in the PB and BM, some evidence of nuclear atypia and immaturity can be seen in the monocytes along with hypogranular and bilobed neutrophils.* ***(Right)*** *The core biopsy from a patient with JMML shows marrow hypercellularity, which included granulocytic and erythroid expansions. Monocytes also appeared increased but did not predominate.*

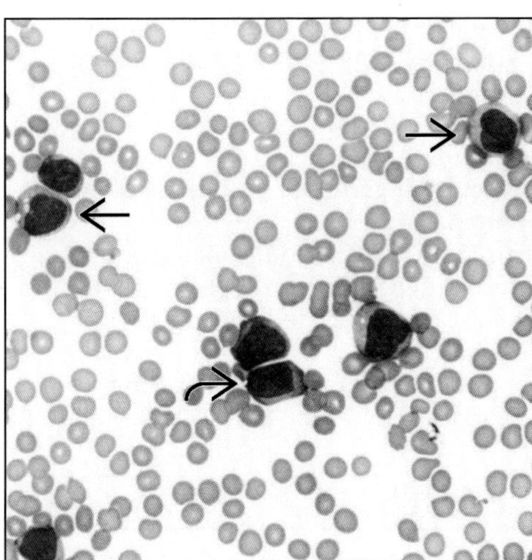

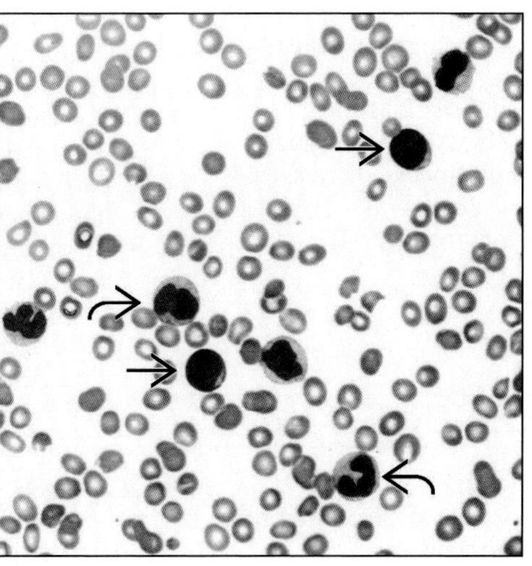

(Left) *Peripheral blood from a patient with acute monocytic leukemia (AML M5b) is shown for comparison. Note the predominance of monoblasts ⇨ and promonocytes →, which easily exceeded 20%.* ***(Right)*** *PB from a patient with acute myelomonocytic leukemia (AML M4) shows the presence of myeloid blasts →, which exceeded 20%, and a distinct population of mature monocytes ⇨. The presence of Auer rods (not shown) in blasts excludes JMML and favors AML.*

MASTOCYTOSIS

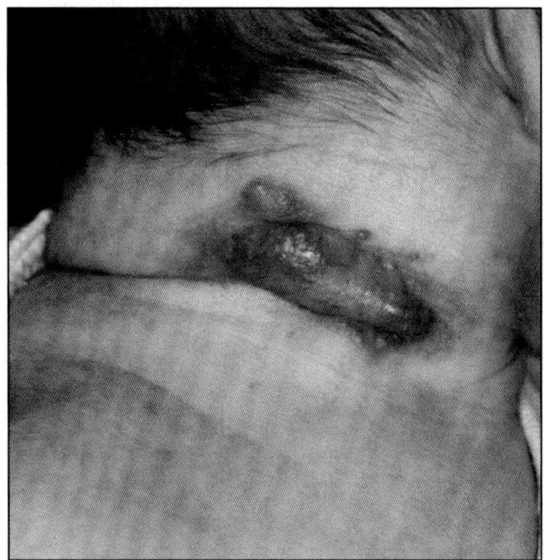

This newborn infant is seen with a mastocytoma of the skin that was present at birth on the right neck. Mastocytomas of the skin occur almost exclusively in infants. (Courtesy S. Vanderhooft, MD.)

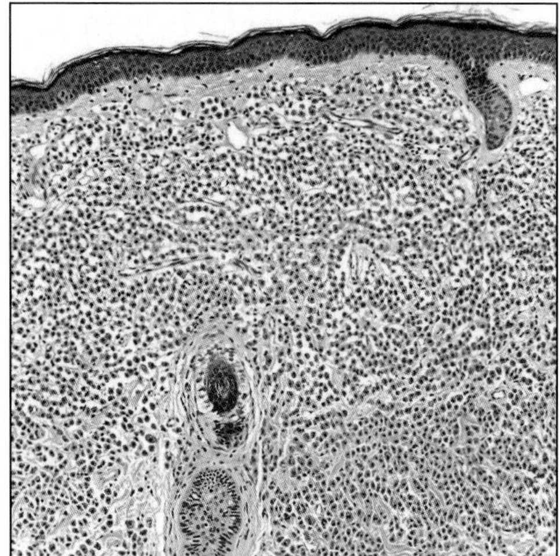

Mastocytoma of the skin in an infant shows a dense infiltrate of mast cells with epidermal sparring that at high power showed round nuclei with abundant eosinophilic cytoplasm.

TERMINOLOGY

Abbreviations

- Cutaneous mastocytosis (CM)
- Systemic mastocytosis (SM)

Synonyms

- Mast cell disease

Definitions

- Heterogeneous group of clonal, neoplastic mast cell proliferations that accumulate in 1 or more organ systems
- Subtypes based mainly on distribution of disease and clinical manifestations
  - **Cutaneous mastocytosis**: Mast cell infiltrates confined to skin
    - Urticaria pigmentosa (UP)/maculopapular cutaneous mastocytosis (MPCM)
    - Diffuse cutaneous mastocytosis
    - Mastocytoma of skin
  - **Systemic mastocytosis**: Involvement of at least 1 extracutaneous organ ± skin lesions
    - Indolent systemic mastocytosis (ISM)
    - Systemic mastocytosis with associated clonal hematological nonmast cell lineage disease (SM-AHNMD)
    - Aggressive systemic mastocytosis (ASM)
    - Mast cell leukemia (MCL)
    - Mast cell sarcoma (MCS)
    - Extracutaneous mastocytoma

ETIOLOGY/PATHOGENESIS

Molecular Background

- Frequently associated with somatic activating point mutations within *c-KIT* proto-oncogene
  - Encodes tyrosine kinase receptor for stem cell factor (SCF)
  - Various mutations result in ligand-independent activation of c-KIT tyrosine kinase
    - Constitutively activated c-KIT leads to clonal proliferation of mast cells
  - Most common mutation: *D816V* in exon 17 encoding tyrosine kinase domain
    - Identified in ≥ 95% of adults with SM when sensitive methods are used
    - Present in 35% of pediatric CM cases
    - Provides relative resistance to prototypical tyrosine kinase inhibitor imatinib
  - Other activating point mutations: *D816Y*, *D816H*, *D816F*, and *D816I* in exon 17 (rarely seen)
    - Frequency significantly higher in CM than in SM
  - Activating point mutations in exons 8, 9, and 11 (mutually exclusive with codon *816* mutations)
    - 44% of pediatric CM cases
- Pediatric CM historically regarded as reactive condition with transient dysregulation of local growth factors
  - Increasing evidence supports neoplastic nature associated with activating *c-KIT* mutations (as in adults)
    - Despite high rate of spontaneous regression (mechanism unknown)
- Rare familial cases with germline mutations of c-*KIT* have been reported
- In patients with SM-AHNMD, additional genetic defects are detected depending on type of AHNMD
- About 30% of SM cases associated with *TET2* mutations
  - *TET2* acts as putative tumor suppressor gene
  - 50% of those cases also carry *c-KIT* D816V mutation

CLINICAL ISSUES

Epidemiology

- Incidence
  - Very rare

MASTOCYTOSIS

Key Facts

Terminology

- Heterogeneous group of clonal, neoplastic proliferations of mast cells that accumulate in 1 or more organ systems
  - Cutaneous mastocytosis: Mast cell infiltrates confined to skin
  - Systemic mastocytosis: Involvement of at least 1 extracutaneous organ ± skin lesions

Etiology/Pathogenesis

- Frequently associated with somatic activating point mutations within *c-KIT* proto-oncogene
- About 30% of SM cases associated with *TET2* mutations

Clinical Issues

- 2/3 of cases occur in children (1st 2 years of life)
- Prognosis depends on disease category
  - Pediatric onset CM has favorable outcome
- Approximately 80% of patients with mastocytosis have evidence of skin involvement

Top Differential Diagnoses

- Reactive mast cell hyperplasia
- Congenital bullous diseases
- Cutaneous lymphoma
- Myelomastocytic leukemia
- Myeloid and lymphoid neoplasms with eosinophilia
- Child abuse

    - Lack of exact numbers with regard to frequency
    - Calculated incidence of 5-10 new cases per 1,000,000 population per year in various studies
  - CM
    - UP: Most common CM variant
    - Mastocytoma of skin (10-15% of pediatric CM cases)
    - Diffuse CM (rare)
  - SM
    - ISM: Most common SM variant (46% of SM cases)
    - SM-AHNMD (40% of SM cases)
    - ASM (12% of SM cases)
    - MCL, MCS, and extracutaneous mastocytoma are extremely rare
- Age
  - Occurs at any age
    - 2/3 occur in children in 1st 2 years of life
  - CM most common in children, less frequent in adults
    - 50% of affected children develop typical skin lesions before 6 months of age
    - May present at birth
  - SM generally diagnosed after 2nd decade of life, rare in pediatric population
- Gender
  - Slight male predominance in CM
  - M:F = 1:1-3 in SM

Site

- Approximately 80% of patients with mastocytosis have evidence of skin involvement
- CM: Mast cell infiltrates confined to skin
- SM: Involvement of at least 1 extracutaneous organ ± skin lesions
  - Bone marrow (BM) almost always involved
  - Skin lesions occur in ≥ 50% of cases, more often in those with indolent disease
  - Spleen, lymph nodes, liver, and gastrointestinal tract mucosa
  - Rarely peripheral blood (PB) shows leukemia
  - Any tissue may be affected

Presentation

- **CM**
  - Includes 3 distinct clinico-histopathological entities
  - Characterized by 2 main groups of symptoms
  - Skin lesions due to mast cell infiltrate and release of mediators (flushing, blistering, pruritus)
    - Lesions can urticate when stroked ("Darier" sign) in 1/2 of cases
  - Systemic symptoms due to release of mast cell mediators (histamine most significant)
    - Headache
    - GI manifestations including acid reflux disease, peptic ulcer disease, and diarrhea
    - Respiratory symptoms including shortness of breath and asthma exacerbations
    - Cardiovascular symptoms including tachycardia, hypotension, syncope, or, even rarely, shock
- **UP/MPCM**
  - Widespread distribution of tan macules and occasionally nodules or plaques
    - In children, lesions tend to be larger and papular
  - Most lesions show intraepidermal accumulation of melanin pigment
  - Sparing of palms, soles, face, and scalp
  - In children, typically involving head and lateral face
  - Number of lesions varies but does not predict presence of systemic disease
  - Rare special forms
    - Plaque form: Nonpigmented, plaque-forming lesions in young children
    - Nodular form: Brown nodules
    - Telangiectasia macularis eruptiva perstans (TMEP): Brown macules and erythema with telangiectasias on trunk and extremities
    - Blistering variant ("bullous mastocytosis"): Exaggeration of urticaria due to chymase cleaving dermal-epidermal junction (DEJ)
- **Diffuse CM**
  - Diffusely thickened skin with "orange peel" appearance and yellow-red discoloration
  - No discernible individual lesions

MASTOCYTOSIS

- In more severe variant, blistering may precede mast cell infiltration
    - Differential diagnosis with congenital bullous diseases
- More likely associated with severe systemic symptoms (higher concentrations of mast cells)
    - GI manifestations (including severe diarrhea), hypotension, or even shock

- **Mastocytoma of skin**
  - Single indurated red-brown macule, papule, plaque, or tumor measuring up to 4 cm in diameter
    - Multiple mastocytomas in different locations have been reported
  - Almost exclusively in infants
  - Slight predilection for trunk but also occurs on extremities, head, and neck
- **Systemic mastocytosis**
  - Includes 6 distinct clinico-histopathological entities
  - Symptoms grouped into few categories
  - Constitutional symptoms
    - Fatigue, weight loss, fever, diaphoresis
  - Skin manifestations
    - Pruritus, urticaria, dermographism
  - Mediator-related systemic events (due to release of histamine, eicosanoids, proteases, and heparin)
    - Same as CM systemic symptoms
  - Musculoskeletal complaints
    - Bone pain, osteopenia/osteoporosis, fractures, arthralgias, myalgias
  - Symptoms related to organ impairment due to mast cell infiltrates (absent in indolent but present in aggressive variants)
    - Splenomegaly (often minimal)
    - Lymphadenopathy and hepatomegaly (less frequent)
  - Hematological abnormalities
    - Anemia, leukocytosis, eosinophilia (frequent), neutropenia, and thrombocytopenia
    - BM failure only in aggressive or leukemic variants
    - Significant numbers of circulating mast cells are suggestive of MCL
    - 30-40% of SM has associated clonal hematological nonmast cell lineage disease (AHNMD) diagnosed before, simultaneously, or after SM diagnosis
    - Any defined myeloid or lymphoid malignancy possible, myeloid predominate (CMML most common)
- Differences in clinical presentation of different variants of SM will not be discussed as they are all rare in pediatric population

Laboratory Tests

- Serum total tryptase
  - Persistently elevated (> 20 ng/mL suggestive of SM, used as minor criterion for diagnosis)
    - Criterion not valid in SM-AHNMD
  - Normal to slightly elevated in patients with CM
    - Usually reserved for adult work-up of CM
- Histamine
  - May be very elevated in diffuse CM but are rarely part of routine work-up for CM

Treatment

- CM
  - Alleviate symptoms with antihistamines and topical steroids
  - Prevent episodes by avoiding mast cell degranulators
    - Physical stimuli (temperature changes, rubbing/friction, intense physical exertion)
    - Foods (spicy foods, citrus fruits, cheese, alcohol)
    - Medications (antibiotics, aspirin, lidocaine, etc.)
  - Educate and reassure families
- SM
  - Currently no cure
  - PKC412 tyrosine kinase inhibitor may be effective in treating SM with mutated *c-KIT*
- ASM, MCL, and MCS
  - Candidates for cytoreductive therapies

Prognosis

- Depends on disease category
- Pediatric onset CM has favorable outcome
  - Majority of cases have improvement of symptoms over time
    - Complete regression by adolescence in > 50%
    - Very low likelihood of progressive disease
  - Transformation to SM rare but more likely in diffuse CM than UP
- In adults, cutaneous lesions generally do not regress and are often associated with SM (usually ISM)
- SM
  - ISM usually normal life expectancy
  - Aggressive variants may survive only a few months
  - SM-AHNMD depends on associated hematological disorder
  - Predictors of worse prognosis for SM
    - Late onset of symptoms, absence of CM, thrombocytopenia, elevated LDH, anemia, BM hypercellularity, abnormal myeloid maturation patterns, PB smear abnormalities, elevated alkaline phosphatase, and hepatosplenomegaly
    - Percentage and morphology of mast cells in BM smears is independent predictor of survival

MICROSCOPIC PATHOLOGY

Microscopic Features

- Normal mast cells in tissue sections (H&E)
  - Loosely scattered
  - Round to oval nuclei with clumped chromatin and inconspicuous nucleoli
  - Low nuclear to cytoplasmic ratio with numerous cytoplasmic granules
- Normal mast cells on smear preparations (Romanowsky stains)
  - Medium-sized round to oval cells with round to oval nuclei and plentiful cytoplasm, containing densely packed metachromatic granules
    - Basophils: Smaller cells with segmented nuclei and larger and fewer granules
- Neoplastic mast cells
  - Cytology varies but abnormal features are almost always detected including spindling and hypogranularity

- More pronounced in high-grade lesions with occurrence of metachromatic blast cells being usual feature of mast cell leukemia
- Frequent bi- or multilobated nuclei ("promastocytes") usually indicate aggressive mast cell proliferation
- Mitotic figures in mast cells do occur but are infrequent even in aggressive or leukemic variants
  - Pattern of infiltrate may vary depending on tissue
  - Multifocal compact or diffuse compact mast cell infiltrates
    - Highly compatible with diagnosis
    - Additional immunohistochemical and molecular studies are still recommended
  - Diffuse interstitial infiltration pattern
    - Loosely scattered mast cells in absence of compact aggregates
    - Also observed in reactive mast cell hyperplasia and myelomastocytic leukemia
    - Additional immunohistochemical and molecular studies are necessary to establish diagnosis
- CM
  - **UP**
    - Aggregates of round to spindle-shaped mast cells in papillary and reticular dermis
    - Often in perivascular and periadnexal location
    - Mast cells are fewer in adults than in children
  - **Diffuse CM**
    - Band-like infiltrate of mast cells in papillary and upper reticular dermis
  - **Mastocytoma of skin**
    - Dense sheets of mature-appearing highly metachromatic mast cells in papillary and reticular dermis
    - May extend into subcutaneous tissues
    - Abundant cytoplasm
    - No cytologic atypia (distinguishes it from extremely rare mast cell sarcoma of skin)
    - Highest concentration of mast cells compared with other types of CM
- **SM: Bone marrow** (4 types of infiltrates)
  - **Multifocal**, sharply demarcated compact infiltrates of mast cells
    - Paratrabecular, perivascular, &/or parafollicular in location
    - "Mixed infiltrates" composed of mast cells, intermingled with lymphocytes, eosinophils, histiocytes, and fibroblasts
  - **Monomorphic** infiltrate with spindle-shaped mast cells that abut or stream along bony trabeculae
    - Significant reticulin fibrosis and thickening of adjacent bone are frequent
  - **Diffuse** replacement of BM by compact mast cell infiltrates
    - Usually mixture of spindle-shaped and round mast cells
    - Resembles sheets of fibroblasts
  - **Compact** infiltrates composed exclusively of round hypergranular mast cells (rare)
    - Tryptase positive round cell infiltration of BM (TROCI-BM)
  - Careful examination of BM not involved by mastocytosis is crucial
    - Unremarkable: ISM with skin and BM involvement or isolated BM mastocytosis
    - Extremely hypercellular due to proliferation of cells of nonmast cell lineages (reactive or coexisting hematopoietic neoplasm)
  - Reactive, nonclonal mast cell hyperplasia may accompany variety of hematological disorders (lymphoplasmacytic lymphoma and hairy cell leukemia)
- **SM: Lymph node**
  - Focal or diffuse infiltrates, often paracortical
  - Total effacement of lymph node architecture is rare
  - Hyperplasia of germinal centers, angioneogenesis, tissue eosinophilia, plasmacytosis, and reticulin/ collagen fibrosis may be present
- **SM: Spleen**
  - Red &/or white pulp may be involved
  - Eosinophilia and fibrosis are frequent
- **SM: Liver**
  - Small granulomatoid foci of mast cells within periportal tracts and loosely scattered mast cells within sinusoids
  - Widening and fibrosis of periportal areas
- **SM: Gastrointestinal (GI) tract mucosa**
  - Involvement frequently suspected clinically
  - Various patterns may be seen

Diagnostic Criteria

- CM
  - Skin lesions show typical clinical features of UP/ MPCM, diffuse cutaneous mastocytosis, or solitary mastocytoma
  - Mast cells in multifocal or diffuse pattern
  - Lack features/criteria of SM
- SM
  - Major criterion and 1 minor criterion or at least 3 minor criteria are present

ANCILLARY TESTS

Immunohistochemistry

- Normal mast cells express CD9, CD33, CD45, CD68, and CD117
  - Lack several myelomonocytic antigens including CD14, CD15, and CD16
  - Lack most T- and B-cell-related antigens
  - Tryptase expressed in virtually all mast cells irrespective of stage of maturation or neoplastic state
  - Chymase expressed in subpopulation of mast cells
    - Highly specific but less sensitive for atypical and immature mast cells than CD117
- Neoplastic mast cells have similar antigen profile to normal mast cells
  - In contrast, coexpress CD2 &/or CD25
    - Distinguish from CD2(+) T cells
    - CD25 expression may be inconsistent or even undetectable in well-differentiated SM or subgroup of MCL

MASTOCYTOSIS

Diagnostic Criteria for Systemic Mastocytosis*

Major Criterion**	Minor Criteria**
Multifocal, compact, dense mast cell infiltrates (≥ 15 mast cells in aggregates) in bone marrow or tissue sections	1) > 25% of mast cells show atypical, spindled, or immature morphologies in smears or tissue sections
	2) *D816V KIT* mutation present
	3) Mast cells show aberrant expression of CD2 &/or CD25
	4) Total serum tryptase level > 20 ng/mL***

*Adapted from WHO 2008 classification. **Diagnosis of SM made when major and 1 minor criterion or ≥ 3 minor criteria are present. ***Parameter not valid If AHNMD is present.*

Classification of Mastocytosis*

Categories	Comments
Cutaneous mastocytosis	Lacks features/criteria of SM
Systemic mastocytosis	Major and 1 minor or ≥ 3 minor criteria are present
Mast cell leukemia	≥ 20% mast cells in bone marrow; usually ≥ 10% mast cells in peripheral blood
Mast cell sarcoma	High-grade cytology; unifocal lesion; destructive; no evidence for SM
Extracutaneous mastocytoma	Low-grade cytology; unifocal lesion; nondestructive; no evidence for SM
Indolent systemic mastocytosis	Low mast cell burden; skin lesions typical
Aggressive systemic mastocytosis	≥ 1 of the following: Bone marrow dysfunction, hepatomegaly with liver function impairment, ascites, portal hypertension, skeletal involvement, splenomegaly, malabsorption, and weight loss
Systemic mastocytosis with associated clonal hematological nonmast cell lineage disease	Meets SM criteria and meets WHO criteria for clonal hematopoietic non-mast cell lineage disorder (i.e., MDS, MPN, AML, lymphoma)

Based on 2008 WHO classification scheme

DIFFERENTIAL DIAGNOSIS

Reactive Mast Cell Hyperplasia
- Lacks compact mast cell infiltrates, no atypical cytology, and no aberrant antigen expression
- May be seen in BM following toxic or inflammatory exposures

Congenital Bullous Diseases
- Blistering variants of UP and diffuse CM can clinically resemble bullous diseases
- No significant mast cell infiltrate on skin biopsy

Cutaneous Lymphoma
- Mast cells only mildly increased if any
- Evaluate with appropriate IHC panel

Myelomastocytic Leukemia
- Advanced myeloid neoplasm with elevated numbers of immature atypical mast cells
- Criteria for SM not met

Myeloid and Lymphoid Neoplasms with Eosinophilia
- Exclude *FIP1L1-PDGFRA* rearrangement in cases with PB and BM eosinophilia
- Serum tryptase and BM mast cells may be increased but typically less than SM
- Mast cells do not form large compact aggregates as in SM

Child Abuse
- CM can clinically resemble multiple bruises

SELECTED REFERENCES

1. Bodemer C et al: Pediatric mastocytosis is a clonal disease associated with D816V and other activating c-KIT mutations. J Invest Dermatol. 130(3):804-15, 2010
2. Klco JM et al: Molecular pathology of myeloproliferative neoplasms. Am J Clin Pathol. 133(4):602-15, 2010
3. Parker RI: Pediatric mast cell disease: what's the big (hematologic) deal? Pediatr Blood Cancer. 53(4):527-8, 2009
4. Uzzaman A et al: Pediatric-onset mastocytosis: a long term clinical follow-up and correlation with bone marrow histopathology. Pediatr Blood Cancer. 53(4):629-34, 2009
5. Briley LD et al: Cutaneous mastocytosis: a review focusing on the pediatric population. Clin Pediatr (Phila). 47(8):757-61, 2008
6. Metcalfe DD: Mast cells and mastocytosis. Blood. 112(4):946-56, 2008

Clinical and Microscopic Features

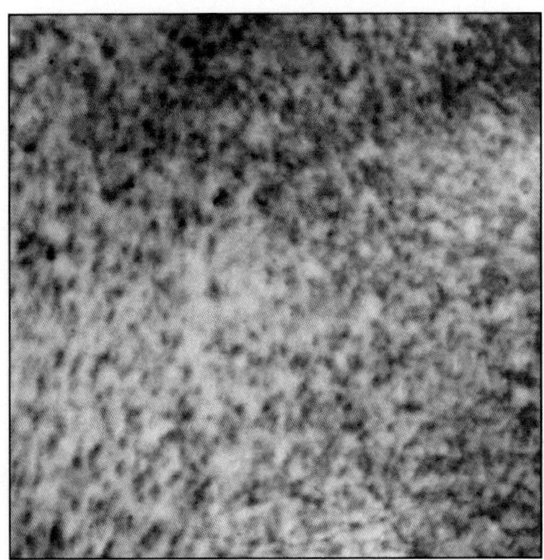

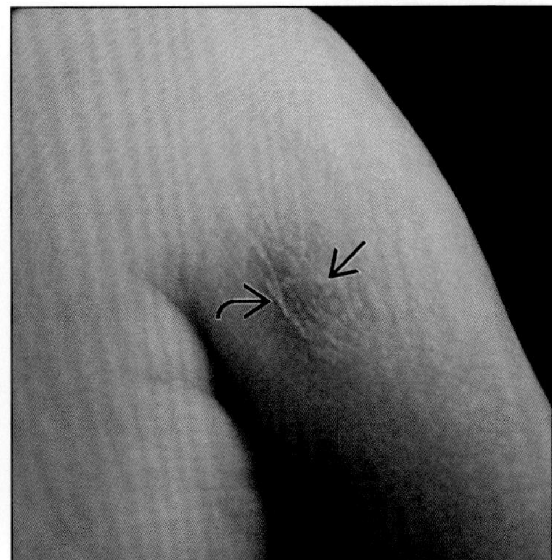

(Left) *Clinical image of maculopapular cutaneous mastocytosis is shown. Note the macular and maculopapular brown skin lesions. The pigmentation is usually caused by an intraepidermal accumulation of melanin. (Courtesy C. Bueso-Ramos, MD, PhD.)* ***(Right)*** *Brownish-red plaque ⇨ on the thumb of a 5-year-old boy shows a positive Darier sign where a linear wheal ⮫ has formed at the site of a scratch by the back end of a cotton swab. (Courtesy J. Hall, MD.)*

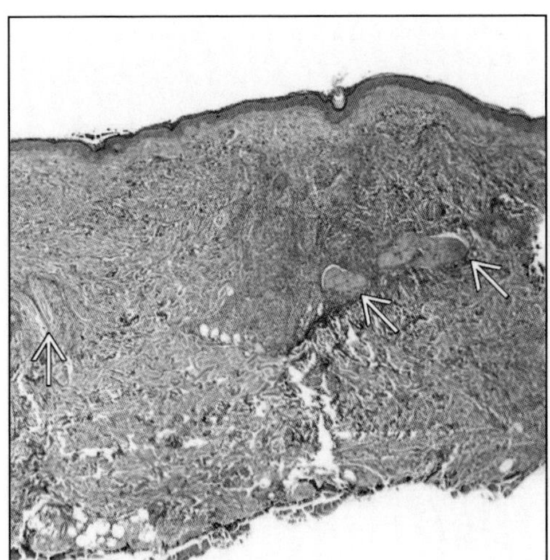

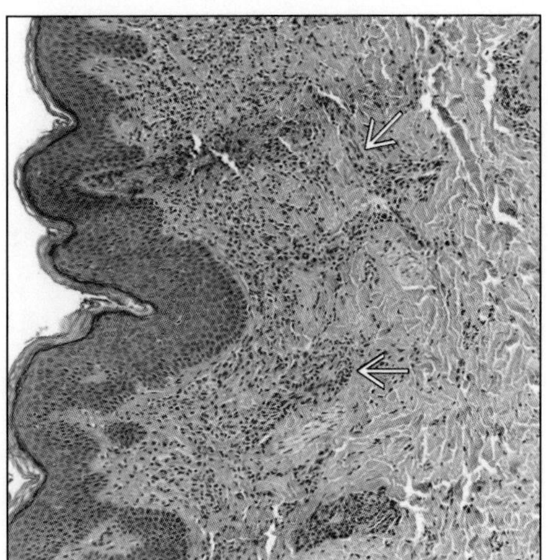

(Left) *Cutaneous mastocytosis is shown from low power to highlight the patchy mast cell infiltrates within the dermis. Some of the infiltrates are seen surrounding several adnexal structures ➡.* ***(Right)*** *Cutaneous mastocytosis is shown at medium power to highlight the dermal mast cell infiltrate ➡. The mast cells demonstrate variable cytologic features with some showing spindled nuclei and other areas showing more round nuclei. All contain abundant eosinophilic cytoplasm.*

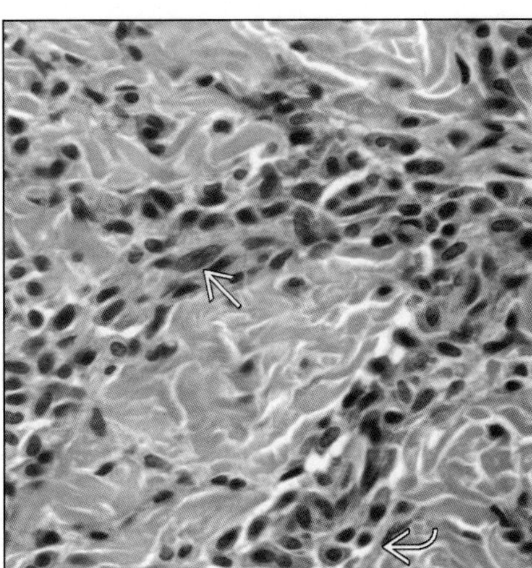

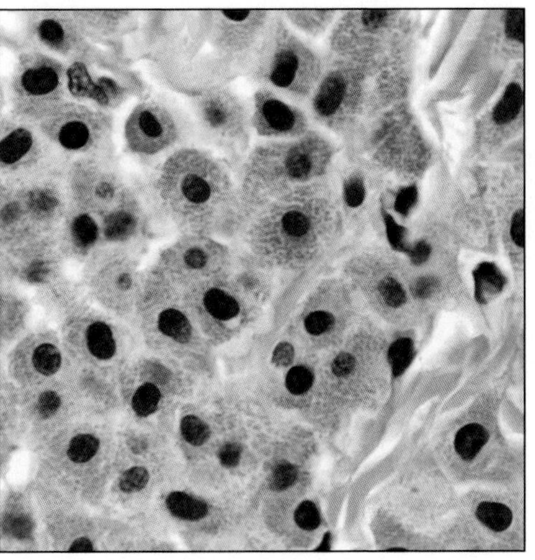

(Left) *Cutaneous mastocytosis with a variably dense dermal mast cell infiltrate is shown. This infiltrate in an adult should prompt staging to exclude systemic mastocytosis. Note the variable cytologic features, which include both spindled ➡ and round nuclei ⮫.* ***(Right)*** *High-power view of mastocytoma of the skin highlights the cytologic features, which in mastocytoma tend to be more commonly with round nuclei with abundant eosinophilic granular cytoplasm.*

MASTOCYTOSIS

Microscopic Features and Ancillary Techniques

*(**Left**) A bone marrow aspirate in a patient with SM shows scattered mast cells ⇒. Mast cells were readily identified away from the spicules whereas in many patients with a clinical suspicion of SM, careful inspection of the spicules for mast cells is required. (**Right**) A core biopsy from a patient with SM shows a cohesive aggregate of atypical mast cells ⇒. This finding meets both major (> 15 mast cells in aggregate) and minor (> 25% are of spindle-shaped) criteria for SM.*

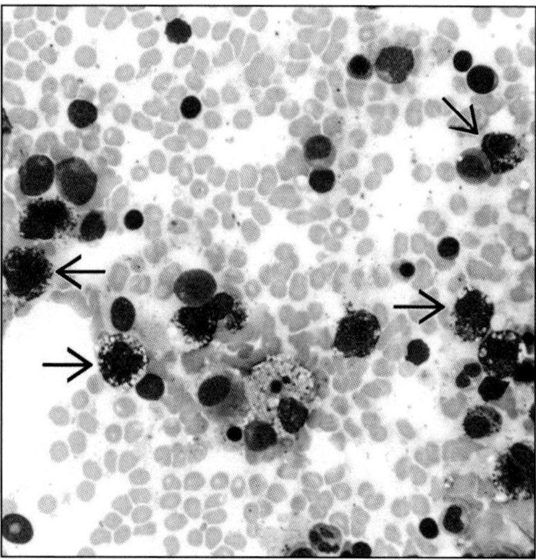

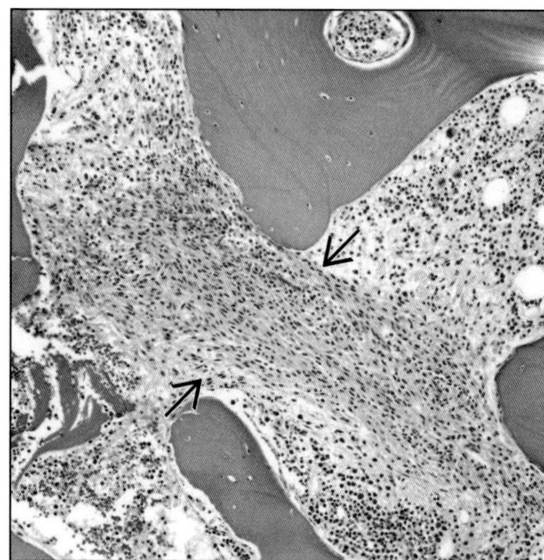

*(**Left**) Atypical mast cells forming a cohesive aggregate in a bone marrow core biopsy are shown at high power. Note the spindle-shaped nuclei ⇗ and the prominent cell borders ⇒ that are typical of mast cell infiltrates. (**Right**) Mast cell tryptase shows positive cytoplasmic reactivity in the mast cells that are seen forming an atypical cohesive aggregate in this core biopsy specimen. The findings are consistent with a diagnosis of SM.*

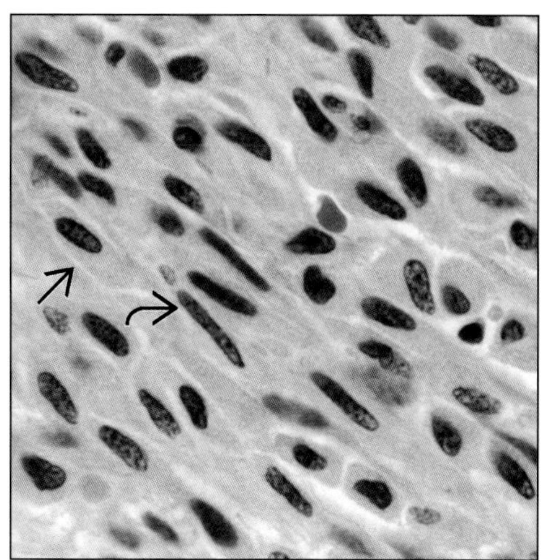

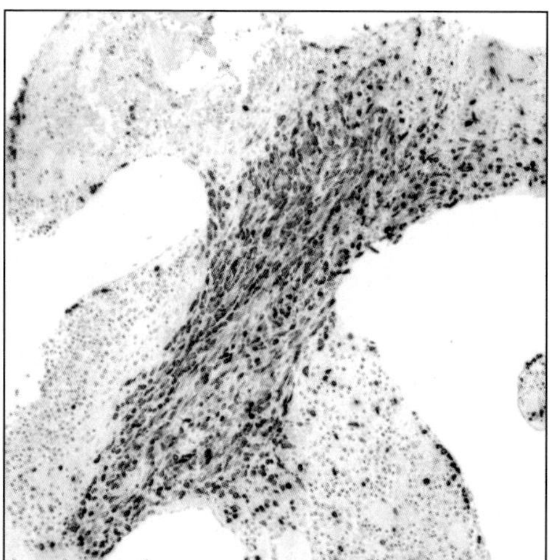

*(**Left**) Extracutaneous mastocytoma involving soft tissue of the shoulder is shown. Immunohistochemistry for CD2 highlights the mast cells. CD2 expression by mast cells is aberrant and supports mast cell neoplasia. (Courtesy C. Bueso-Ramos, MD, PhD.) (**Right**) IHC for CD25 shows a compact cluster of mast cells in this bone marrow biopsy specimen. Reactivity of mast cells with CD25 fulfills a minor diagnostic criterion for the diagnosis of SM. (Courtesy C. Bueso-Ramos, MD, PhD.)*

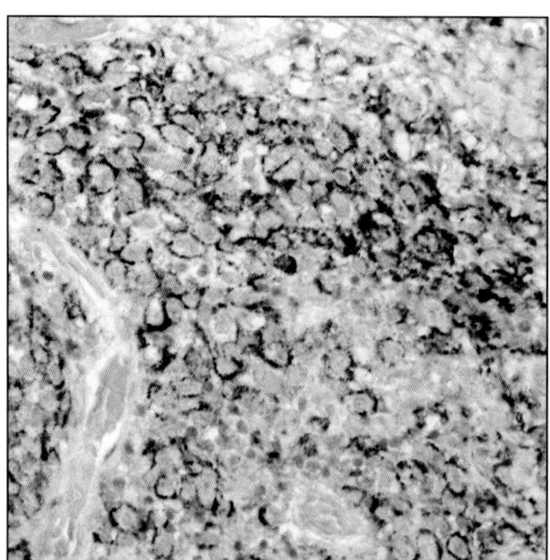

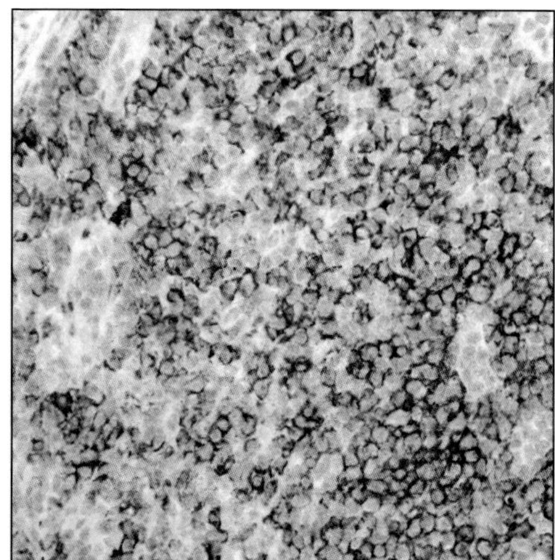

Microscopic Features and Differential Diagnosis

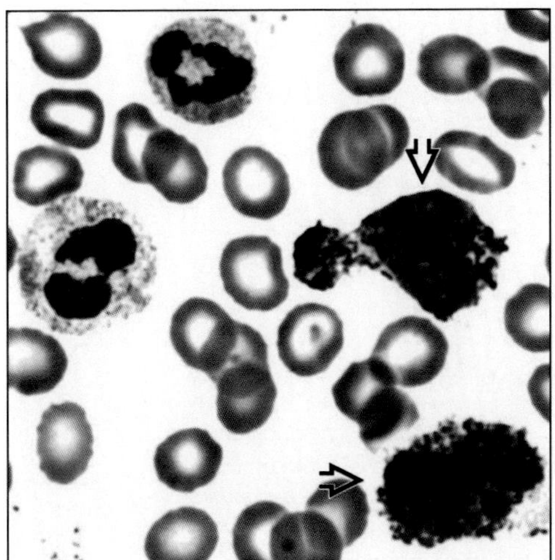

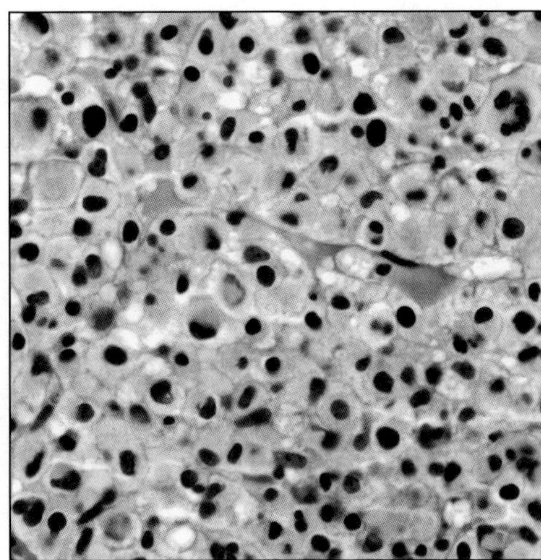

(Left) *2 circulating, well-granulated mast cells ➪ are seen in this PB smear from a patient with MCL. "Leukemic" MCL typically shows > 10% circulating mast cells. (Courtesy K. Reichard, MD.)* ***(Right)*** *Mast cell leukemia (MCL) is an aggressive form of mastocytosis and often a differential diagnostic consideration. In contrast to SM, the mast cells are more often round than spindled and account for ≥ 20% of BM aspirate nucleated cells. (Courtesy K. Reichard, MD.)*

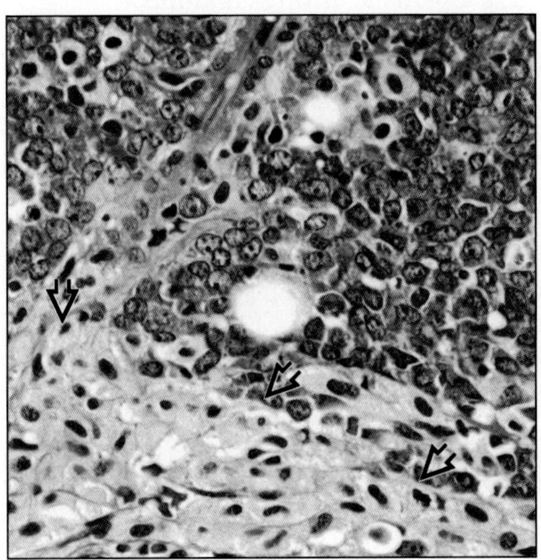

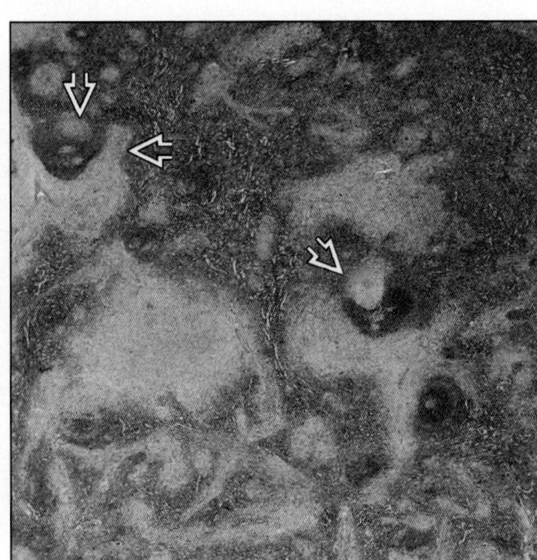

(Left) *The bone marrow shows a mast cell cluster ➪ adjacent to acute myeloid leukemia (AML) with t(8;21)(q22;q22) consistent with AHNMD. (Courtesy K. Reichard, MD.)* ***(Right)*** *Spleen in a patient with systemic mastocytosis (SM) is shown. Note perifollicular pale mast cell aggregates ➪. Characteristically patchy fibrosis is associated with, and can obscure, mast cells. (Courtesy C. Bueso-Ramos, MD, PhD.)*

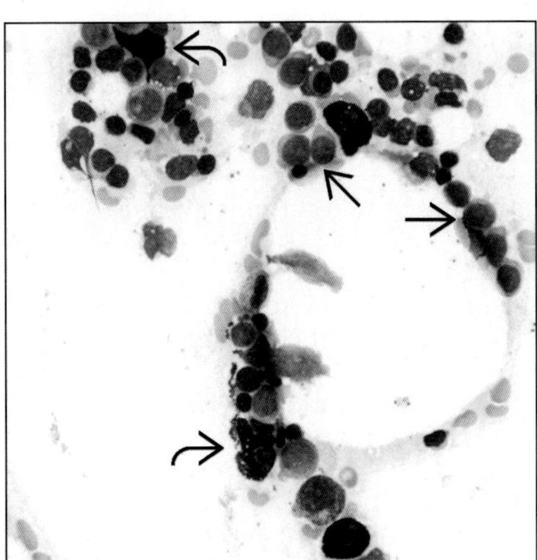

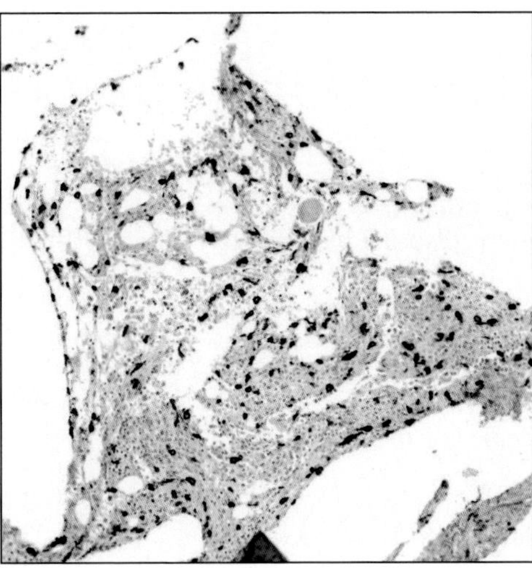

(Left) *Myelomastocytic leukemia is an exceedingly rare diagnosis. Myeloid blasts →, which typically predominate, are a key component of the diagnosis along with neoplastic mast cells ↷. (Courtesy K. Reichard, MD.)* ***(Right)*** *Mast cells are highlighted by CD117. Mast cell hyperplasia may occur after potent myeloablative chemotherapy or other massive toxic insult. In contrast to SM, mast cells do not form compact aggregates. (Courtesy K. Reichard, MD.)*

CHILDHOOD MYELODYSPLASTIC SYNDROME

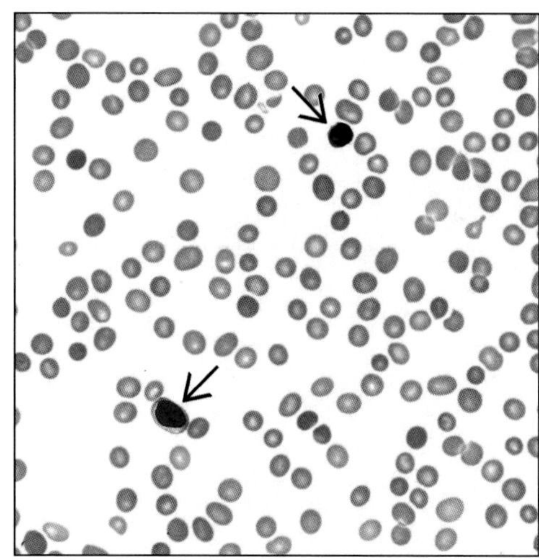

The peripheral blood smear from this 8-year-old boy with RCC shows significant pancytopenia with red cell anisocytosis and macrocytosis, predominantly lymphocytes ⇒ and no circulating blasts.

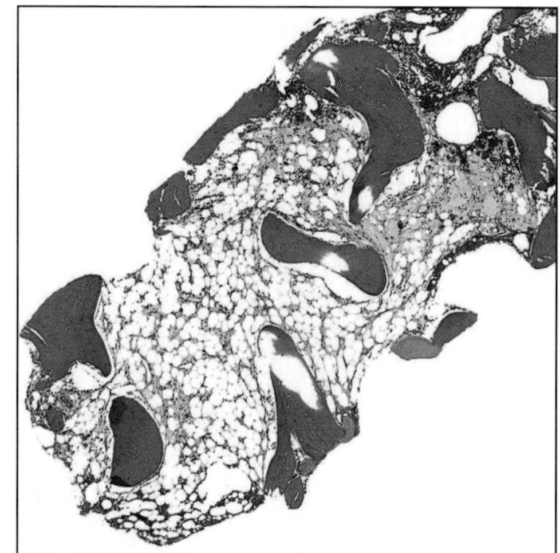

Trephine biopsy sections are markedly hypocellular (~ 5% cellularity) and show severe trilineage hypoplasia. Differentiating RCC from aplastic anemia in this type of case is difficult.

TERMINOLOGY

Abbreviations

- Myelodysplastic syndrome (MDS)

Synonyms

- Preleukemia

Definitions

- Myelodysplastic syndromes are a heterogeneous group of molecularly distinct entities that have
  - Peripheral blood with unexplained and persistent cytopenia(s)
    - < 20% blasts
    - < 1.0 X 10^9/L monocytes
  - Variable degrees of ineffective hematopoiesis
    - Simultaneous proliferation and apoptosis of hematopoietic cells
    - < 20% blasts in the marrow
  - Dysplasia in 1 or more myeloid lineages
    - Neutrophilic myeloid
    - Erythroid
    - Megakaryocytic
  - Increased risk for development of acute myeloid leukemia (AML)
- Childhood MDS is rare
  - Incidence is < 0.01/1000,000 individuals per year
  - Often associated with a genetic disorder or previous therapy
- Childhood MDS per 2008 WHO Classification of Tumors of Hematopoietic and Lymphoid Tissue
  - Includes primary (de novo) MDS only: Excludes secondary MDS
    - Congenital or acquired bone marrow failure disorders
    - Therapy-related MDS
    - Myeloid leukemia associated with Down syndrome
  - Refractory anemia of childhood (RCC): Provisional entity in WHO classification
    - Persistent cytopenia(s) during childhood
    - < 2% blasts in peripheral blood
    - < 5% blasts in bone marrow
    - Includes refractory cytopenia with unilineage dysplasia (RCUD)
    - Includes refractory cytopenia with multilineage dysplasia (RCMD)
    - Includes majority of cases of myelodysplastic syndrome, unclassifiable (MDS-U)
    - Reclassify into other MDS category if increased blasts develop
  - Classify similar to adult-type MDS **if** criteria for RCC are not fulfilled
    - Refractory anemia with excess blasts (RAEB)
    - Refractory anemia with ring sideroblasts (RARS): Exceedingly rare in children
    - MDS associated with isolated del (5q): Exceedingly rare in children
    - RCUD, RCMD, MDS-U should be classified as RCC

ETIOLOGY/PATHOGENESIS

Histogenesis

- Probably originates from primitive hematopoietic stem cell
  - Initiating mutation or transforming event is unknown
- Putative pathogenic mechanisms
  - Abnormal stem cell gives rise to clonal myelopoiesis
    - Influenced by haploinsufficiency and epigenetic changes
  - Ineffective hematopoiesis and apoptosis
    - Clonal myelopoiesis causes abnormal stromal response with altered immune and cytokine responses
    - Cytokines and immune system (particularly cytotoxic T cells) suppress proliferation and support apoptosis

CHILDHOOD MYELODYSPLASTIC SYNDROME

Key Facts

Terminology

- RCC: Provisional entity in 2008 WHO Classification
  - Persistent cytopenia(s) during childhood
  - < 2% blasts in peripheral blood
  - < 5% blasts in bone marrow
- Reclassify RCC into RAEB or AML if increased blasts develop
- MDS category similar to adults **if** criteria for RCC not fulfilled

Clinical Issues

- Childhood MDS
  - < 5% of hematopoietic neoplasms (< 14 years old)
  - RCC is most common subtype
- Prognosis
  - Monosomy 7 or complex karyotype has highest risk for disease progression
  - Trisomy 8 or normal karyotype may have long, stable course

Microscopic Pathology

- Minimal diagnostic criteria required
  - Dysplastic changes in 2 lineages (erythroid, granulocytic, megakaryocytic) or ≥ 10% dysplasia in single lineage
- 75% of RCC are hypocellular

Diagnostic Checklist

- Hypocellular MDS
  - Distinction from aplastic anemia or congenital bone marrow failure syndromes may be difficult
  - Finding of monosomy 7 is diagnostic of MDS
  - CD34 immunohistochemistry helps to identify blasts and subtype MDS

- Clonal evolution develops with additional mutations
  - Loss of tumor suppressor genes
  - Chromosome deletions
  - Inactivation by hypermethylation

CLINICAL ISSUES

Epidemiology

- Incidence
  - Childhood MDS
    - < 5% of hematopoietic neoplasms in children < 14 years old
  - RCC
    - 50% of childhood MDS
    - Most common subtype of MDS in children
    - More likely to have refractory neutropenia or refractory thrombocytopenia than refractory anemia
  - Refractory anemia with excess blasts (RAEB)
    - Children who have RCC and develop increased blasts should be reclassified into this category
- Age
  - All age groups of infants and children
- Gender
  - Boys and girls affected equally

Presentation

- Childhood MDS
  - Initial presentation of cytopenia(s)
    - Neutropenia &/or thrombocytopenia is most common
    - Subset with concurrent anemia
    - Isolated refractory anemia is uncommon
  - Most common symptoms include
    - Malaise
    - Bleeding
    - Fever
    - Infection
  - Lymphadenopathy without hepatosplenomegaly
    - If concurrent infection
  - No clinical signs or symptoms at presentation
    - ~ 20% of cases of RCC
  - Possible congenital abnormalities of different organ systems
    - Need to exclude congenital hematologic disorder

Laboratory Tests

- Complete blood count and peripheral blood smear review
- Bone marrow evaluation
- Cultures and serologies for infections
- Cytogenetic analysis
- Flow cytometric analysis or immunohistochemical evaluation
- Molecular and specialized tests to exclude underlying congenital syndromes
  - Chromosome breakage study
  - Telomere length or telomerase activity
  - Gene mutations

Treatment

- Careful observation until disease progression in absence of
  - Severe cytopenia(s)
  - Infections
  - Transfusion requirement
- Immunosuppressive therapy
  - For some cases of early bone marrow failure
  - Possibly more effective if small paroxysmal nocturnal hemoglobinuria (PNH) clone present
- Hematopoietic stem cell transplantation
  - Only curative therapy
    - RAEB
    - Indicated early for cases of RCC with monosomy 7 or complex karyotypes
    - Other abnormal karyotypes if suitable donor

Prognosis

- International Prognostic Scoring System (IPSS) for adults is of limited value in children
- RCC
  - Unknown if number of lineages involved is prognostically significant
  - Monosomy 7

CHILDHOOD MYELODYSPLASTIC SYNDROME

        - Highest risk for progression
        - Presence helps confirm diagnosis
    - Trisomy 8 or normal karyotype
        - May have long stable course
- RAEB
    - Distinction between RAEB-1 and RAEB-2 is of unclear clinical significance in children
    - May have slowly progressive disease
    - Complex karyotype
        - Highest risk for progression
- Advanced MDS
    - > 80% 5-year survival after allogeneic stem cell transplantation

MICROSCOPIC PATHOLOGY

Peripheral Blood

- Blast percentage
    - Based on 200-cell leukocyte differential count
        - < 2% in RCC
        - 2-19% in RAEB
- Anemia
    - 50% of RCC have hemoglobin level < 10 gm/dL
        - Most commonly macrocytic
        - Anisopoikilocytosis
        - Dimorphic red cell population
        - Circulating nucleated red blood cells
        - Coarse basophilic stippling
- Neutropenia
    - ≥ 10% neutrophils with dysplasia
        - Abnormal distribution and quality of cytoplasmic granules
        - Cytoplasmic hypogranulation
        - Pseudo Pelger-Huët nuclear anomaly, pelgeroid
        - Giant bands, neutrophil hypersegmentation
        - Presence of dysplasia helps to distinguish from aplastic anemia
    - 25% of RCC have markedly decreased number
        - May have insufficient neutrophils to evaluate for dysplasia
        - Evaluation of buffy coat specimen helps for identification of dysplastic neutrophils
- Thrombocytopenia
    - 75% of RCC
    - Occasional large and giant platelets
    - Agranular platelets

Bone Marrow

- Blast percentage in aspirate or touch preparations
    - Based on visual inspection and not flow cytometric analysis
    - Perform 500-cell leukocyte differential count
        - < 5% in RCC
        - 5-19% in RAEB
- Minimal diagnostic criteria required for RCC
    - Dysplastic changes in 2 lineages (erythroid, granulocytic, megakaryocytic) or
    - ≥ 10% dysplasia in single lineage
- RCC
    - 75% of cases are hypocellular (often 5-10% of normal age cellularity)
        - Left shifted erythropoiesis in patchy distribution
        - Usually a few clusters of ≥ 20 erythroid precursors
        - Increased proerythroblasts
        - Erythroid precursors have increased number of mitoses
        - Left shifted and markedly decreased granulopoiesis
        - Megakaryocytes are usually very low in number or absent
        - Identification of micromegakaryocytes helps in diagnosis
        - Lymphocytes may be increased
    - Normocellular or hypercellular
        - Often left shifted erythroid hyperplasia
        - Mild to moderately decreased granulopoiesis
        - Decreased, adequate, or increased megakaryocytes
- RAEB
    - Increased blasts or Auer rods
        - Includes all types of blasts or equivalents: Myeloblasts, monoblasts, promonocytes, megakaryoblasts
    - Often multilineage dysplasia
    - Myeloid series dysplasia
        - Abnormal localization of immature precursors (ALIP) in biopsies
        - Nuclear hyposegmentation
        - Pseudo Pelger-Huët nuclear anomaly
        - Abnormal distribution and quality of cytoplasmic granules
        - Left shift
    - Erythroid series dysplasia
        - Megaloblastic changes
        - Nuclear budding and bridging
        - Asynchronous nuclear to cytoplasmic maturation
        - Multinucleation, cloverleaf nuclei
        - Karyorrhexis, atypical mitoses
        - Vacuolated erythroblasts
    - Megakaryocytic series dysplasia
        - Atypical small or large monolobated megakaryocytes
        - Abnormal nuclear lobation
        - Multiple nuclei
        - Nucleoli
- Ring sideroblasts are extremely rare

ANCILLARY TESTS

Immunohistochemistry

- Perform on bone marrow core biopsy (or clot) sections
- CD34 for blasts; CD117 if blasts are CD34 negative
    - Quantify blasts; evaluate for aggregation or clustering
    - MDS subtype may be difficult to ascertain in hypocellular bone marrow
        - CD34 stain is important to evaluate for subtle blast population
- Myeloperoxidase or CD33
    - Quantify myeloid lineage
    - Evaluate for ALIP
- Hemoglobin A, glycophorin, or CD71
    - Quantify erythroid lineage
    - Evaluate for disruption of normal erythroid colony formation

- CD61 or CD41
  - Quantify megakaryocytes
  - Megakaryocytes are often decreased and difficult to visualize in hypocellular bone marrows
    - Helpful in detecting dysplastic megakaryocytes
    - Identification of micromegakaryocytes aids in confirming diagnosis of MDS, especially RCC

Flow Cytometry

- Evaluate for increased CD34 or CD117 positive blasts
- Myeloblasts with abnormal features
  - Coexpression of CD7, CD56, CD10, CD11b, or CD15
  - Absence of CD33, CD13 or HLA-DR
  - Abnormal intensity of antigen expression
    - For example, increased CD117 or CD13 on CD34(+) blast population
  - Absence of hematogone population
- Possible discordance with bone marrow blast percentages
  - Hemodilution (especially for fibrotic marrow)
  - Lysis of red blood cells, including some precursors
- Evaluate for aberrant lineage maturation patterns or antigen expression
  - Requires at least a 4-color analysis
  - Aberrant maturation patterns are often associated with morphologic findings
  - Findings suggestive of MDS
    - ≥ 3 aberrant features in erythroid, neutrophilic myeloid, or monocytic populations
    - Abnormally low side scatter by granulocytes due to cytoplasmic hypogranularity
    - Gain of abnormal antigens, i.e., abnormal CD56, CD19, CD7, CD5 on myeloid or monocytic cells
  - Reevaluate case over several months if highly suggestive for MDS by flow cytometric analysis and other findings are inconclusive

Cytogenetics

- Bone marrow conventional cytogenetic analysis
  - Requires adequate bone marrow aspirate specimen
    - May need to disaggregate trephine biopsy if fibrotic or packed marrow
    - Essential during initial evaluation to establish baseline karyotype
  - Identification of MDS associated abnormality
    - Helps to establish diagnosis
    - May not help to differentiate hypocellular MDS from aplastic anemia unless monosomy 7
    - Monosomy 7 is diagnostic of MDS
    - Provides prognostic information
  - Karyotypic abnormalities are detected in at least 50% of cases
    - Monosomy 7 and deletion 7q are the most frequent (40% of cases)
    - Trisomy 8 common
    - Monosomy 5 and del(5q) are uncommon
    - Most cases of RCC have a normal karyotype
  - Excludes low blast count acute myeloid leukemia
  - Trisomy 21 evaluation to exclude Down syndrome
    - MDS in Down syndrome is not included in childhood MDS category
- Fluorescence in situ hybridization (FISH)
  - Perform if insufficient conventional cytogenetic study (i.e., <20 metaphases)
  - Useful for hypocellular specimens
    - Can perform on bone marrow touch preparations, aspirate smears, or remaining cytogenetic cell pellet

DIFFERENTIAL DIAGNOSIS

Myeloid Leukemia Associated with Down Syndrome

- Encompasses both acute myeloid leukemia and MDS
  - Accounted for 20-25% of childhood MDS in previous classifications
- Preleukemic phase
  - Morphologic features similar to RCC
    - Dysplastic changes may be more pronounced than typical for RCC

Acquired Aplastic Anemia

- Megaloblastic or dysplastic features not typical at presentation
- Bone marrow is hypocellular with increased adipocytes
  - Lacks erythroid islands
    - Possible single small focus with < 10 cells showing maturation
    - Increased erythroblasts
  - Absent or markedly decreased granulocytic myelopoiesis
    - No significant dysplasia
    - Few small foci or scattered cells show maturation
  - Absent or markedly decreased megakaryocytes
    - No significant dysplasia or "micromegakaryocytes"
  - Small lymphoid aggregates or increased dispersed lymphocytes common
    - Associated mast cells
- May have morphologic features similar to RCC after immunosuppressive therapy
- Subset of aplastic anemia patients demonstrate clonal cytogenetic abnormalities
- Subset of patients progress to MDS

Inherited Bone Marrow Failure Disorders

- Fanconi anemia, dyskeratosis congenita, Shwachman-Diamond syndrome, amegakaryocytic thrombocytopenia, pancytopenia with radioulnar synostosis
- Features overlap morphologically with RCC
  - Need to exclude congenital syndrome
    - Clinical history and findings
    - Appropriate laboratory and molecular testing (i.e., chromosomal breakage studies, telomere length, telomerase activity)
- May progress to "secondary" MDS

Acquired Bone Marrow Failure Disorders

- Paroxysmal nocturnal hemoglobinuria (PNH)
  - Flow cytometric analysis for PNH clones is diagnostic
    - Small PNH clones may be seen in aplastic anemia and low-grade MDS with ultrasensitive testing

- Some studies suggest better response to immunosuppressive therapy if small PNH clones present
- Aplastic anemia during hematologic recovery

Low Blast Count Acute Myeloid Leukemia (AML)

- Cytogenetic, FISH, or molecular identification of 1 of the following recurrent genetic abnormalities is required
  - AML with inv(16)(p13.1q22), t(16;16)(p13.1q22); *CBFB-MYH11*
  - Acute promyelocytic leukemia with t(15;17)(q22;q12); *PML-RARA*
  - AML with t(8;21)(q22;q22); *RUNX1-RUNX1T1*
- Diagnostic of AML irrespective of blast percentage
- Auer rods in blasts more commonly seen in AML than in MDS

Reactive Disorders with Cytologic Dysplasia

- Nutritional deficiencies
  - Vitamin B12 or folate deficiency
  - Copper deficiency
- Medication or toxin effect
- Autoimmune disorders
  - Systemic lupus erythematosus
  - Autoimmune lymphoproliferative disorders
- Rheumatic diseases
- Metabolic disorders
  - Mevalonate kinase deficiency
- Infections
  - Particularly viruses
    - HIV, CMV
    - Hepatitis viruses
    - Parvovirus B19
    - 20% blast threshold for diagnosis of AML may not be applicable to children
- Ring sideroblasts are rare in childhood MDS
  - Consider a mitochondrial disorder or disorder of heme synthesis

Pathologic Interpretation Pearls

- Assessment for neutrophil and megakaryocytic dysplasia is essential
- Diagnosis of RCC may be made if dysplasia is not identified in ≥ 10% of cells in a single lineage
  - Lesser degree of dysplasia in at least 2 lineages will qualify for diagnosis
    - Erythroid, neutrophilic myeloid &/or megakaryocytic
    - Follow closely with repeat bone marrow evaluations before definitive diagnosis is rendered if normal karyotype
    - Provide data to refute other differential diagnostic considerations
- Bone marrow touch preparations are particularly helpful in RCC
  - Many cases have hypocellular bone marrows
    - Aspirate material is often insufficient for adequate morphologic &/or conventional cytogenetic evaluation
  - FISH studies can be performed to evaluate for MDS-related cytogenetic abnormalities
- "Secondary" MDS is much more common than de novo MDS in childhood
  - Most often therapy related
  - Secondary to congenital syndromes (including Down syndrome) or
  - Acquired bone marrow failure disorder
- Hematogones are often decreased in low-grade MDS

DIAGNOSTIC CHECKLIST

Clinically Relevant Pathologic Features

- Bone marrow specimens in RCC are often hypocellular
  - Distinction from aplastic anemia or congenital bone marrow failure syndromes may be difficult
    - Finding of monosomy 7 is diagnostic of MDS
    - Clinical correlation is essential
    - Specialized testing to exclude a congenital syndrome is warranted
    - Aplastic anemia and congenital bone marrow failure syndromes may progress to "secondary" MDS
  - Bone marrow evaluation
    - Immunohistochemical stains (CD34, CD117) are useful for blast identification and MDS classification
    - Step sections of the trephine biopsy help to identify micromegakaryocytes
    - Immunohistochemical stains for megakaryocytes aid in detecting dysplastic megakaryocytes
- Children with MDS may have slowly progressive disease
  - RAEB or AML with MDS changes and 20-29% blasts
    - May behave more like MDS than AML

SELECTED REFERENCES

1. Göhring G et al: Complex karyotype newly defined: the strongest prognostic factor in advanced childhood myelodysplastic syndrome. Blood. 116(19):3766-9, 2010
2. Shimamura A et al: Pathophysiology and management of inherited bone marrow failure syndromes. Blood Rev. 24(3):101-22, 2010
3. Yin CC et al: Recent advances in the diagnosis and classification of myeloid neoplasms--comments on the 2008 WHO classification. Int J Lab Hematol. 32(5):461-76, 2010
4. Hebeda KM et al: Changed concepts and definitions of myeloproliferative neoplasms (MPN), myelodysplastic syndromes (MDS) and myelodysplastic/myeloproliferative neoplasms (MDS/MPN) in the updated 2008 WHO classification. J Hematop. 2(4):205-10, 2009
5. Veltroni M et al: Advanced pediatric myelodysplastic syndromes: can immunophenotypic characterization of blast cells be a diagnostic and prognostic tool? Pediatr Blood Cancer. 52(3):357-63, 2009
6. Germing U et al: Epidemiology, classification and prognosis of adults and children with myelodysplastic syndromes. Ann Hematol. 87(9):691-9, 2008
7. Niemeyer CM et al: Myelodysplastic syndrome in children and adolescents. Semin Hematol. 45(1):60-70, 2008
8. Aktas D et al: Myelodysplastic syndrome associated with monosomy 7 in childhood: a retrospective study. Cancer Genet Cytogenet. 171(1):72-5, 2006

RCC and RAEB

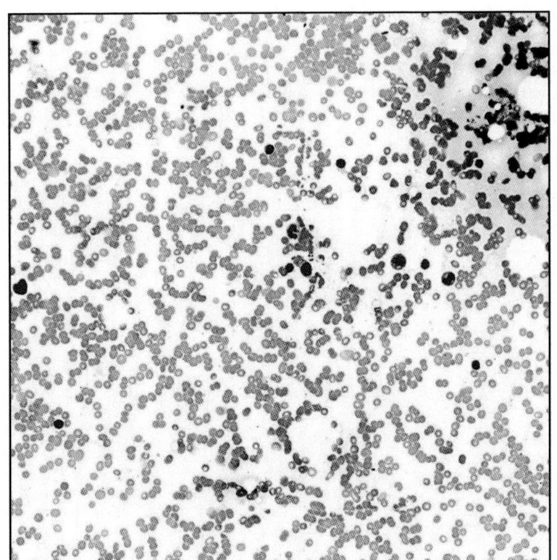

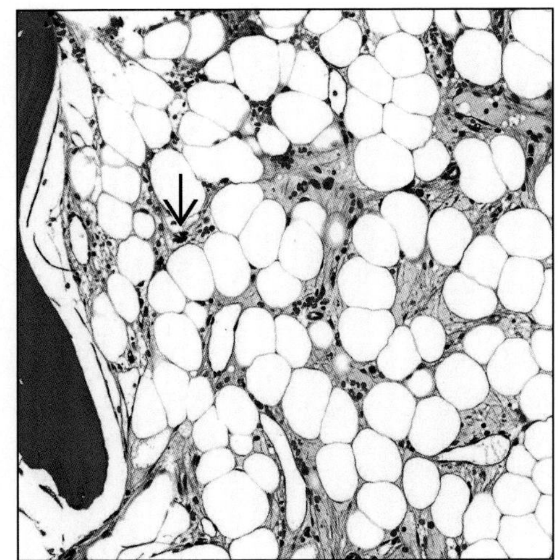

(Left) *Bone marrow aspirate smears from an 8-year-old boy have minimal hematopoietic cells for evaluation. Touch preparations are similar, while FISH analysis on the touch preparations identified monosomy 7 in 14% of cells.* ***(Right)*** *A higher power view of a core biopsy confirms markedly hypocellular bone marrow (~ 5% cellularity). No clusters of blasts are identified. Megakaryocytes are decreased but the identification of micromegakaryocytes ⮕ supports a diagnosis of MDS.*

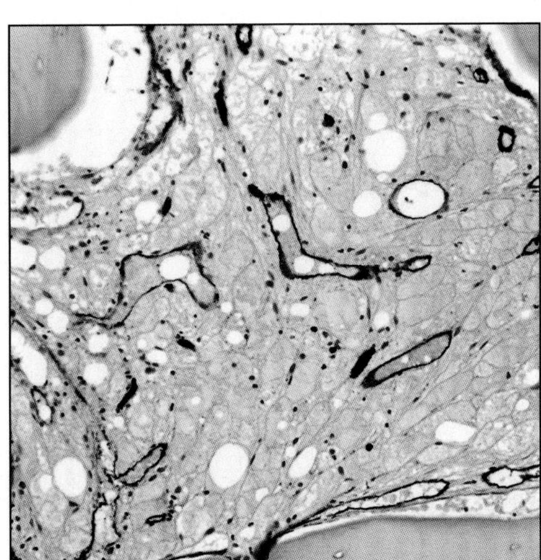

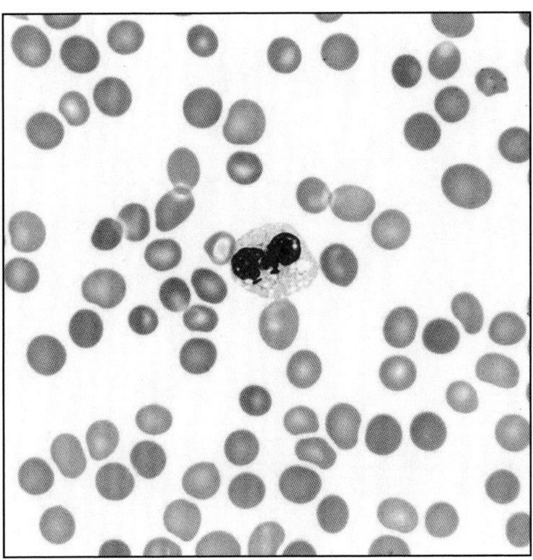

(Left) *A CD34 IHC stain highlights the vasculature and confirms the absence of a significant CD34(+) blast population. Stains for megakaryocytes are also useful to identify micromegakaryocytes.* ***(Right)*** *Repeat peripheral blood evaluation at 2 months in a suspected case of RCC continues to be pancytopenic but now shows circulating neutrophils with dysplastic features. The neutrophil shown here has cytoplasmic hypogranulation and a pseudo-Pelger-Huët-type nuclear anomaly.*

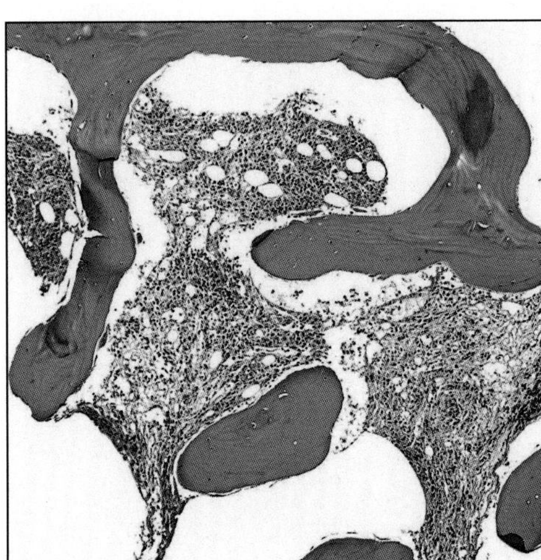

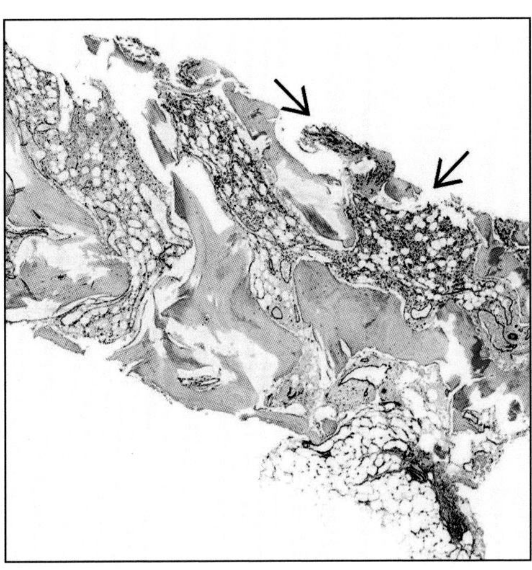

(Left) *The repeat trephine biopsy sections are variably cellular (10-70%) and have a M:E ratio of 1:1. Myelopoiesis and erythropoiesis are left shifted. Megakaryocytes are decreased.* ***(Right)*** *An immunohistochemical stain for CD34 highlights an increase in CD34(+) blasts. The blasts are present in greater numbers in the more cellular areas ⮕ with rare small aggregates of 3-5 blasts seen. The blasts comprised ~ 8% of the overall cellularity.*

CHILDHOOD MYELODYSPLASTIC SYNDROME

Childhood MDS and AML Transformation

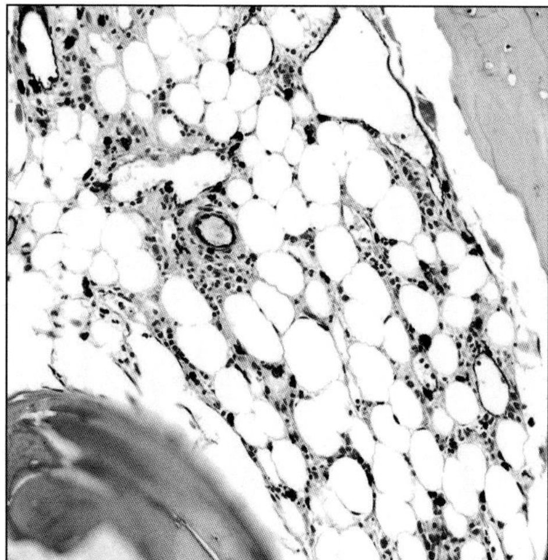

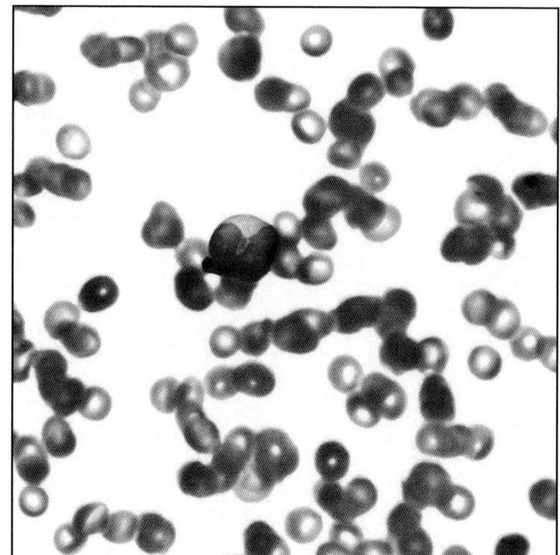

(Left) *The less cellular areas showed a slight increase in CD34(+) blasts. Monosomy 7 was identified in ~ 26% of cells by FISH analysis on touch preparations. This case is now classified as RAEB-1 instead of RCC, given the 8% blasts.* ***(Right)*** *A repeat peripheral blood smear performed at 2 months in a patient with RAEB-1 (8% CD34[+] blasts in marrow) now shows 2% circulating blasts with persistent macrocytic anemia and marked thrombocytopenia.*

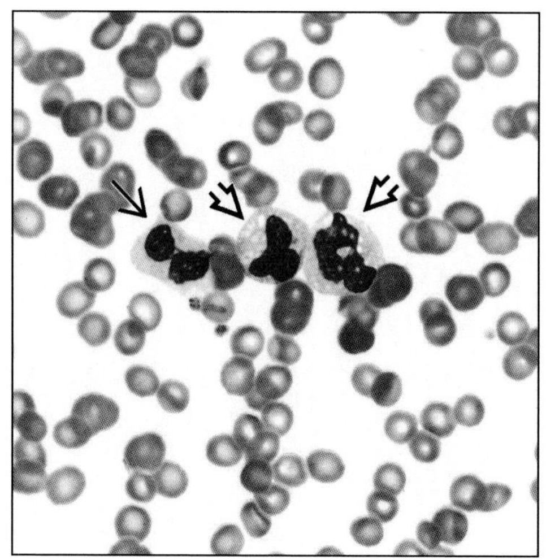

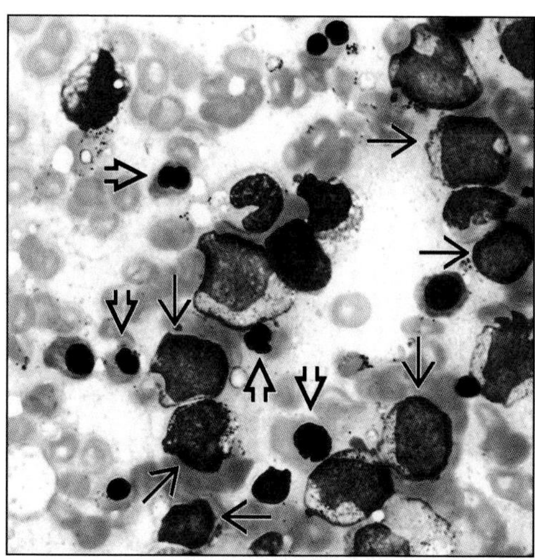

(Left) *In addition to circulating blasts, WBC count is normal and includes a greater number of neutrophils. The neutrophils are dysplastic and have cytoplasmic hypogranulation with pseudo Pelger-Huët nuclei ⇒ or abnormal nuclear segmentation ⇨.* ***(Right)*** *Aspirate smears are cellular with sufficient blasts ⇒ (~ 25%) diagnostic of transformation to acute myeloid leukemia. Background dyserythropoiesis ⇨ and decreased myeloid maturation is evident.*

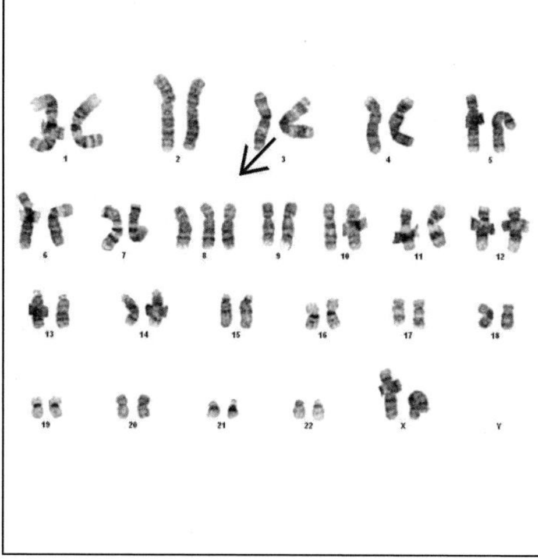

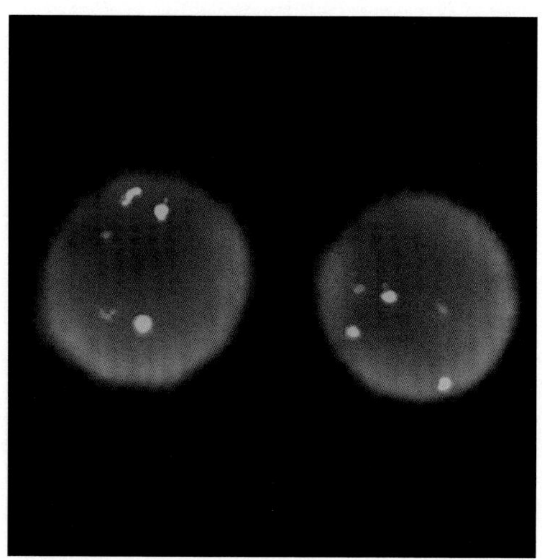

(Left) *Conventional cytogenetic study from a 4-year-old girl with relatively stable cytopenias shows an extra chromosome 8 ⇒ in 17 or 20 metaphases. Trisomy 8 is a recurrent abnormality in MDS and is associated with a long stable course similar to the identification of a normal karyotype.* ***(Right)*** *FISH analysis on an aspirate smear shows trisomy 8 with the 3 copies of chromosome 8 (CEP8 signals) shown in green. The 2 red signals represent normal 20q12 chromosomal regions.*

Bone Marrow Findings in Myelodysplasia

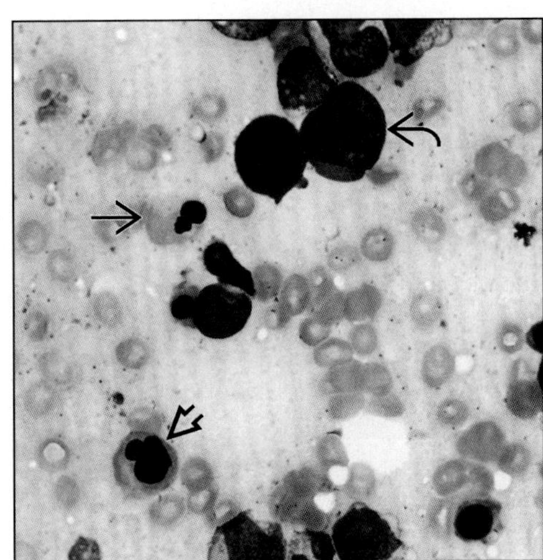

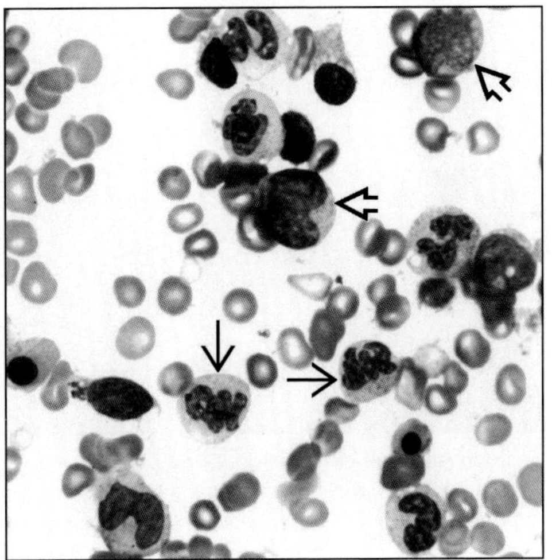

(Left) *This bone marrow aspirate has ≥ 10% dysplastic erythroid precursors, as manifested by nuclear budding ➡, hyperlobation ➡, and megaloblastic changes ➡. A left shift in erythroid maturation is common in childhood MDS.* ***(Right)*** *Dysgranulopoiesis in ≥ 10% of the myeloid lineage is the predominant finding in this MDS patient. Dysplastic features include irregular and abnormal nuclear segmentation ➡ and cytoplasmic hypogranulation ➡.*

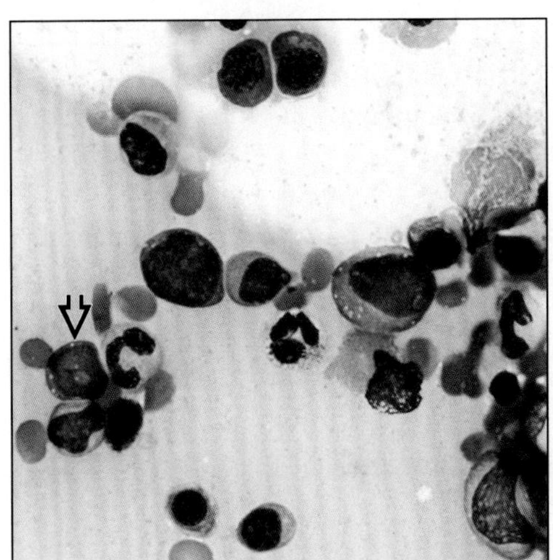

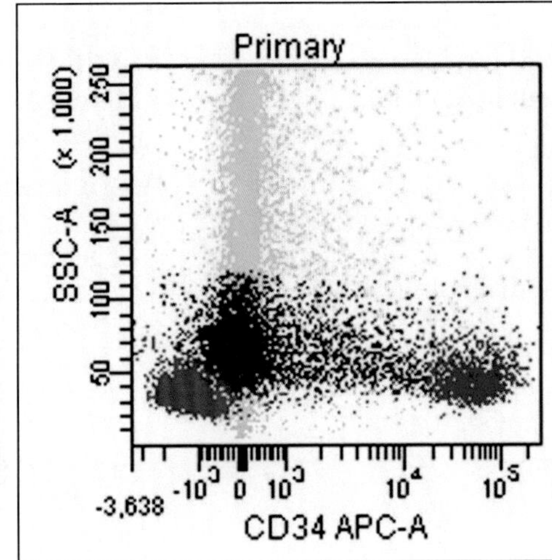

(Left) *Blasts in MDS may be small ➡ and are particularly difficult to identify in suboptimally prepared smears. Some cases of refractory anemia with excess blasts may not have prominent dysplastic features.* ***(Right)*** *An abnormally bright CD34(+) blast population (red) was detected by flow cytometric (FCM) analysis. Blast percentages should be based on visual inspection of the bone marrow rather than FCM analysis because of hemodilution and erythroid cell lysis of FCM specimens.*

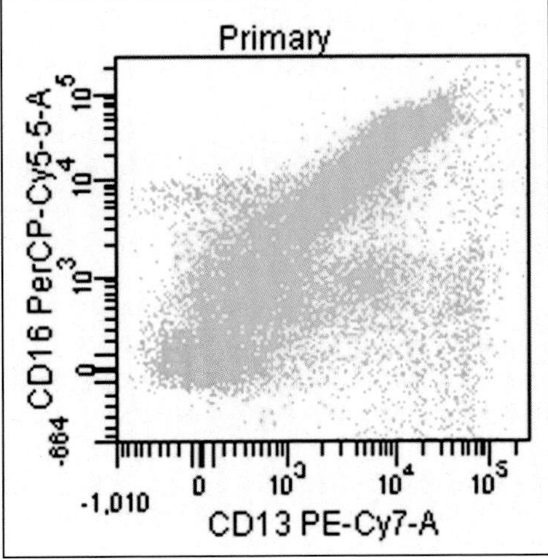

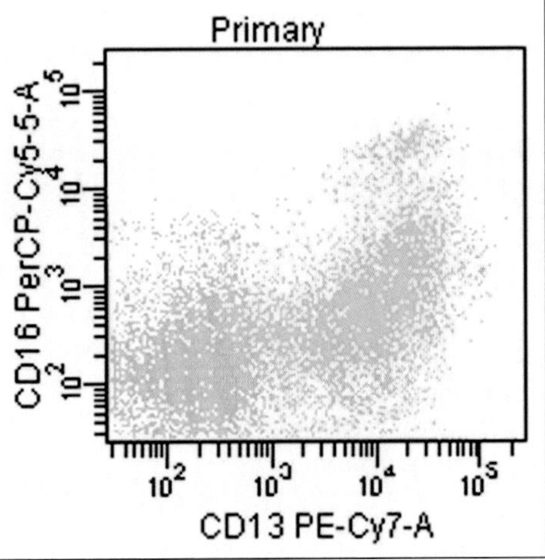

(Left) *Myeloid cells in MDS have abnormal maturation patterns that may be assessed by FCM. This histogram shows the CD13 vs. CD16 expression pattern of bone marrow granulocytes (yellow) in normal individuals. This pattern is sometimes referred to as a "Nike sign."* ***(Right)*** *The most common myeloid maturation abnormality found in MDS (after hypogranulation-altering side scatter characteristics) is decreased CD16 expression. Decreased CD11b is also frequently seen.*

NODULAR LYMPHOCYTE PREDOMINANT HODGKIN LYMPHOMA

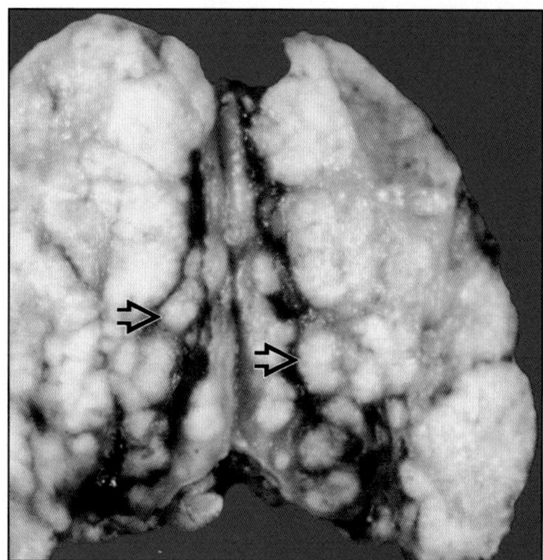

Nodular lymphocyte predominant Hodgkin lymphoma (NLPHL) in a lymph node shows multiple nodules of variable size ⇨ throughout the lymph node parenchyma.

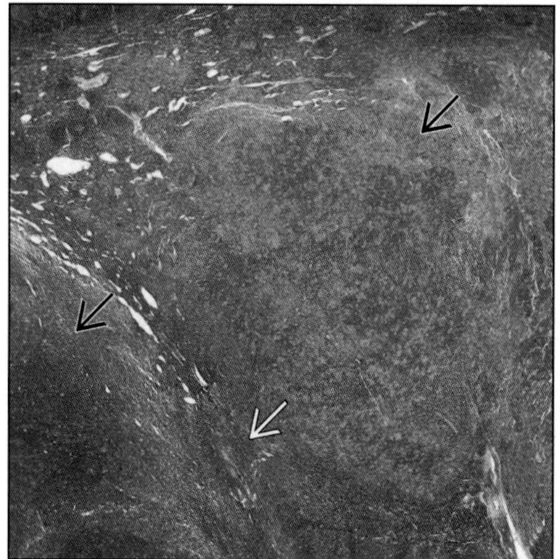

NLPHL involving lymph node is shown. The nodal architecture is effaced by multiple expansile nodules ⇨ with compressed interfollicular zones ➡. The nodules have a "moth-eaten" appearance.

TERMINOLOGY

Abbreviations

- Nodular lymphocyte predominant Hodgkin lymphoma (NLPHL)

Synonyms

- Nodular lymphocyte predominant Hodgkin disease (REAL, 1994)
- Lymphocytic-predominant Hodgkin disease (Rye, 1966)
- Lymphocytic &/or histiocytic predominance Hodgkin disease (Lukes and Butler, 1966)
- Paragranuloma (Jackson and Parker, 1944)

Definitions

- Nodular proliferation of scattered large neoplastic B cells associated with numerous inflammatory cells
  - Neoplastic cells are designated as lymphocyte-predominant (LP) cells
    - a.k.a. "popcorn" cells because of their hyperlobated nuclei with vesicular chromatin
    - Formerly called L&H (lymphocytic &/or histiocytic) cells
  - Neoplastic cells are usually confined within follicular dendritic cell meshworks
  - Background infiltrate of nonneoplastic small lymphocytes and histiocytes
    - Inflammatory cells greatly outnumber neoplastic LP cells
- Diffuse form of NLPHL
  - Term derived from Lukes and Butler classification, but its existence has been challenged
  - Most cases in this category have been reclassified as
    - T-cell/histiocyte-rich large B-cell lymphoma (THRLBCL)
    - NLPHL with diffuse THRLBCL-like areas
    - Classical Hodgkin lymphoma (CHL)
  - Rare cases of diffuse NLPHL probably exist, i.e., "moth-eaten" B-cell-rich pattern of NLPHL

ETIOLOGY/PATHOGENESIS

Postulated Normal Counterpart

- Germinal center B lymphocyte at centroblast stage of differentiation

Associated Lesions

- NLPHL is associated with progressive transformation of germinal centers (PTGC)
  - PTGC and NLPHL can involve same lymph node biopsy specimen
  - In past, PTGC often identified in staging laparotomy specimens of NLPHL patients
  - However, prospective studies of patients with PTGC show no increased risk of NLPHL

CLINICAL ISSUES

Epidemiology

- Incidence
  - 5-6% of all Hodgkin lymphomas
- Age
  - Median: 35 years
  - All age groups are affected
- Gender
  - Male to female ratio > 2:1

Site

- Lymph nodes
- Most commonly affected groups include cervical, axillary, or inguinal lymph nodes
  - Paraaortic and iliac lymph nodes less often involved
- Liver &/or spleen involved in ~ 10% of cases
- Mediastinum involved in ~ 7%
- Bone marrow rarely involved (~ 2%)
  - Bone marrow involvement is usually evidence of transformation to large B-cell lymphoma

Presentation

- Peripheral lymphadenopathy

NODULAR LYMPHOCYTE PREDOMINANT HODGKIN LYMPHOMA

Key Facts

Clinical Issues

- Peak incidence in 4th decade; affects all age groups
- Patients often present with stage I or II nodal disease
- Cervical, axillary, or inguinal lymph nodes
- Slow progression and frequent relapses
- Excellent prognosis
- ~ 3-5% of patients develop large B-cell lymphoma

Microscopic Pathology

- Nodular or nodular and diffuse patterns
- LP cells scattered in background of small lymphocytes and histiocytes
  - LP cells have vesicular chromatin, inconspicuous nucleolus, and thin nuclear membrane
- Mixture of different cell types gives "moth-eaten" pattern on low-power view
- No necrosis or thick fibrous bands
- Uninvolved lymph node shows reactive follicular hyperplasia &/or PTGC

Ancillary Tests

- Immunophenotype of LP cells
  - CD20(+), CD22(+), CD45/LCA(+), CD79a(+)
  - Bcl-6(+), pax-5(+), OCT2(+), BOB1(+)
  - CD15(-), CD30(-), EBV(-), Bcl-2(-)
- Single-cell PCR
  - LP cells carry monoclonal *IgH* gene rearrangements

Top Differential Diagnoses

- Lymphocyte-rich classical Hodgkin lymphoma
- T-cell/histiocyte-rich large B-cell lymphoma
- Progressive transformation of germinal centers
- Follicular lymphoma
- Nodular sclerosis Hodgkin lymphoma

  - Stage I or II in ~ 80% of patients
- B symptoms are uncommon (~ 10%)

Laboratory Tests

- Normal complete blood count; no leukemic phase
- Serum lactate dehydrogenase (LDH) or β-2-microglobulin levels rarely elevated

Natural History

- NLPHL is clinically indolent disease with frequent relapses
- Relapse-free survival curves show "staircase"
  - No plateau suggestive of cure
  - Early and late (> 10 years) relapses occur
  - Risk of relapse is independent of stage of disease or therapy
  - Relapse can be localized or generalized (~ 20%) disease
- ~ 3-5% of NLPHL transform to large B-cell lymphoma (LBCL)
  - Large B-cell lymphoma typically follows NLPHL but can coexist with or precede NLPHL
    - Subset of transformed cases resembles diffuse large B-cell lymphoma (DLBCL)
    - Clinically indolent when compared with de novo diffuse large B-cell lymphoma
  - 2nd subset resembles THRLBCL
- ~ 15% of patients die of disease with prolonged follow-up
  - Deaths related to therapy-refractory disease or 2nd malignancies
  - 2nd malignancies represent ~ 4% of all deaths
    - Acute leukemia (2%), non-Hodgkin lymphoma (1%), solid organ tumors (1%)

Treatment

- Options, risks, complications
  - "Watch and wait" has been advocated for pediatric patients with localized disease
- Drugs
  - Combination chemotherapy employed most often
  - Recommended regime: Doxorubicin, bleomycin, vinblastine, dacarbazine (ABVD)
  - Rituximab (anti-CD20) monoclonal antibody is often used
    - As part of ABVD regimen, upfront (R-ABVD)
    - At time of refractory disease
- Radiation
  - Localized disease may be treated with involved field radiation alone
    - This option is avoided in pediatric and adolescent patients to avoid injuring growth plates of bones

Prognosis

- Good prognosis with > 80% 10-year survival
  - Better survival for patients with low- vs. high-stage disease
  - Patients with NLPHL have better survival than patients with classical Hodgkin lymphoma
- Transformation to diffuse large B-cell lymphoma or THRLBCL is often associated with poorer prognosis
  - Bone marrow involvement is associated with aggressive clinical behavior
  - Prognosis may not be impacted if large B-cell lymphoma is localized and treated appropriately

IMAGE FINDINGS

Radiographic Findings

- Peripheral lymphadenopathy
- NLPHL lesions are not FDG PET avid

MICROSCOPIC PATHOLOGY

Histologic Features

- Complete or partial effacement of lymph node architecture
  - Nodular or nodular and diffuse patterns
  - Expansile nodules composed mostly of small lymphocytes and fewer histiocytes
    - Reactive lymphoid follicles usually absent within nodules
    - Absent or rare centrocytes or centroblasts within nodules

- Nodules larger than normal lymphoid follicles
- LP cells are large and scattered amongst abundant small lymphocytes and histiocytes
  - Represent ~ 1% of all cells
  - LP cells have variety of appearances
    - Multilobated "popcorn" cells with vesicular chromatin and multiple small nucleoli
    - Multinucleated or mummified cells
    - LP cells also can be round without multilobation
- Various architectural patterns have been described
  - Classical nodular pattern is most common
  - Serpiginous nodular pattern
    - Confluent irregular nodules
  - Nodular with extranodular LP cells
    - Pattern more commonly seen in patients with recurrence
  - Nodular pattern with T-cell-rich background
  - THRLBCL-like
    - Always associated with at least 1 typical nodule of NLPHL
    - Diffuse areas indistinguishable from primary THRLBCL
    - Most background lymphocytes are T cells and histiocytes
    - Absence of underlying follicular dendritic cell meshworks
    - Associated with B symptoms and higher clinical stage
  - Diffuse, B cell-rich with "moth-eaten" appearance
    - Uncommon pattern (< 5% of cases)
    - Most background lymphocytes are B cells
    - Underlying follicular dendritic cell meshworks positive
- Histiocytes may be epithelioid &/or form small granulomas
- Features common in classical Hodgkin lymphoma are usually absent in NLPHL
  - Eosinophils, neutrophils, and plasma cells are unusual
  - Classical Hodgkin and Reed-Sternberg (HRS) cells are absent or rare
  - Necrosis is rare; no fibrous bands around nodules
- Residual/uninvolved lymph node in biopsy specimens of NLPHL
  - Reactive follicular hyperplasia is usually present
  - PTGC commonly present
- Recurrent/relapsed NLPHL
  - Depletion of small lymphocytes with increased histiocytes
  - Fibrosis in up to 40% of cases with recurrence
  - Diffuse areas present; often increased in size

Cytologic Features

- Diagnosis of NLPHL difficult to establish in fine needle aspirate specimens
  - Nodular architecture difficult to appreciate in smears
  - Small lymphocytes, histiocytes, and large LP cells present
  - No granulocytes or plasma cells

Transformation of NLPHL to Large Cell Lymphoma

- Large cell lymphoma may coexist with or follow NLPHL
  - Large cells may form sheets, as in de novo diffuse large B-cell lymphoma, or be scattered, as in THRLBCL
- No consensus on pathologic criteria to distinguish between
  - NLPHL with diffuse THRLBCL-like areas vs. transformation to THRLBCL
- Transformation of NLPHL to THRLBCL can be diagnosed when
  - Diffuse areas of THRLBCL are identified, and
  - Patients have high-stage disease, including bone marrow involvement, &/or other clinical evidence of transformation, such as
    - High serum lactate dehydrogenase or β-2-microglobulin levels
    - Lytic bone lesions
  - Bone marrow involvement in patients with NLPHL is usually evidence of transformation
  - Extensive liver involvement is usually associated with transformation
- Transformation of NLPHL to diffuse large B-cell lymphoma
  - Sheets of large neoplastic cells outside nodules of NLPHL

ANCILLARY TESTS

Immunohistochemistry

- LP cells
  - CD20(+), CD22(+), CD79a(+), CD75(+)
  - pax-5(+), OCT2(+), BOB1(+), PU.1(+)
  - CD40(+), CD80(+), CD86(+)
  - Bcl-6(+), AID(+), SWAP-70(+)
  - CD45/LCA(+), Ki-67 (proliferation) high
  - EMA and MUM1(+) in ~ 50% of cases
  - IgD(+) in ~ 25% of cases
    - IgD correlates with younger patient age
  - Pan-T-cell antigens(-), Bcl-2(-)
  - CD15(-) and CD30(-)
    - CD30(+) LP cells reported in ~ 10% of NLPHL cases
    - CD30(+) reactive immunoblasts are common in NLPHL
    - CD15(+) LP cells very rare; often at time of relapse
  - Epstein-Barr virus (EBV)-LMP1(-)
    - Rare (< 1%) cases of NLPHL with EBV(+) LP cells reported in developed countries
- Background inflammatory infiltrate
  - Small lymphocytes are mixture of B and T cells
  - B cells
    - CD19(+), CD20(+), CD22(+), pax-5(+)
    - IgM(+), IgD(+)
    - CD10(-), Bcl-6(-)
  - T cells
    - CD2(+), CD3(+), CD5(+), CD7(+)
    - Form "rosettes" around LP cells

- Minor population of CD3(+) cells is of follicular T-helper cell lineage
  - CD3(+), CD4(+), CD57(+)
  - CD10(+), Bcl-6(+) < PD-1(+)
  - Form "rosettes" around LP cells in ~ 50% of cases
- Follicular dendritic cell meshworks are present in nodular areas
  - CD21(+), CD23(+), &/or CD35(+)
- Histiocytes
  - CD68(+)
- Recurrent/relapsed NLPHL
  - Depletion of background small B cells
  - Decreased or absent follicular dendritic cells
  - Increased numbers of background T cells and histiocytes
  - LP cells may express CD30 or rarely CD15

Flow Cytometry

- Polytypic B cells
- Mature T cells
  - CD4(+), CD8(+) T cells in ~ 50% of cases
- Large neoplastic cells are lost or overlooked in routine flow cytometric analysis

Cytogenetics

- Usually complex structural karyotypic aberrations
- Chromosome 3q27 (*BCL6* locus) involved in up to 60% of cases

In Situ Hybridization

- EBER(-) in LP cells
  - < 1% of NLPHL cases are EBER(+) in Western countries
  - EBV may be more common in LP cells of NLPHL in developing countries

PCR

- Monoclonal *IgH* or light chain gene rearrangements when using single-cell PCR analysis
- Rearrangements often not detectable using standard PCR or Southern blot methods and whole biopsy specimens

Array CGH

- 30-60% of cases may show gains or losses of chromosomes
  - Gains: Chromosomes 1, 2q, 3, 4q, 5q, 6, 8q, 11q, 12q, and X
  - Loss: Chromosome 17

Molecular Genetics

- Frequent somatic mutations of *IgH* variable region
  - Evidence of ongoing mutations
- *BCL6* gene rearrangements in ~ 50% of cases
  - *IgH* is most common partner
  - Other partners: Chromosome loci 2q23; 5q31, 6q22, 9q22, and 17p21

DIFFERENTIAL DIAGNOSIS

Lymphocyte-rich Classical Hodgkin Lymphoma, Nodular Variant

- Form of classical Hodgkin lymphoma with prominent nodular pattern that can closely mimic NLPHL
- Nodules composed of prominent mantle zones with atrophic or absent germinal centers
- HRS cells in mantle zones of enlarged lymphoid follicles
- Immunophenotype
  - HRS cells are CD15(+), CD30(+), EBV-LMP1(+/-), CD45/LCA(-)

T-cell/Histiocyte-rich Large B-cell (THRLBCL) Lymphoma

- Affects elderly patients; rare in children and adolescents
- B symptoms, high stage, and elevated serum LDH levels
- Usually not associated with reactive follicular hyperplasia or PTGC
- Diffuse growth pattern
- Large neoplastic cells represent < 10% of all cells in specimen

Nodular Sclerosis Hodgkin Lymphoma

- Uncommonly, cases of NLPHL are associated with fibrosis
  - Inguinal region is common site of fibrosis
  - Fibrosis is more often present at time of relapse
- Fibrosis in NLPHL is not birefringent/polarizable
  - Fibrous bands surrounding nodules are not present
- Immunophenotype
  - HRS cells are CD15(+), CD30(+), EBV-LMP1(+/-), CD45/LCA(-)

Follicular Lymphoma

- Usually stage IV disease on presentation
- Neoplastic follicles typically smaller than those seen in NLPHL
  - Neoplastic follicles commonly found in perinodal soft tissue
- Abundant neoplastic small and large centrocytes and large centroblasts
- Immunophenotype
  - CD10(+), Bcl-6(+), Bcl-2(+)
  - Flow cytometry immunophenotype shows monotypic B lymphocytes, CD10(+)

Progressive Transformation of Germinal Centers

- Rare patients can present with florid syndrome with generalized lymphadenopathy
- Lymph node architecture is preserved
- Markedly enlarged lymphoid follicles (often 3-4x larger than typical reactive follicle)
- Lymphoid follicles extensively colonized by mantle zone lymphocytes
  - Can infiltrate and obliterate germinal centers
- Enlarged follicles with underlying follicular dendritic cell meshwork

NODULAR LYMPHOCYTE PREDOMINANT HODGKIN LYMPHOMA

Immunohistochemistry

Antibody	Reactivity	Staining Pattern	Comment
CD45	Positive	Cell membrane	Almost always positive
Pan-B-cell Marker			
CD20	Positive	Cell membrane	Almost always positive
Transcription Factors			
pax-5	Positive	Nuclear	Stronger than reactivity in HRS cells of CHL
OCT2	Positive	Nuclear	Stronger than reactivity in HRS cells of CHL
BOB1	Positive	Nuclear	Stronger than reactivity in HRS cells of CHL
CHL Markers			
CD30	Negative	Nuclear & cytoplasmic	May rarely be positive; reactive immunoblasts are positive in interfollicular areas
CD15	Negative	Cytoplasmic	May rarely be positive in subset of cases
Germinal Center B-cell-associated Antigen			
Bcl-6	Positive	Nuclear	
Other Useful Markers			
EMA	Positive	Cell membrane	Positive in 50% of cases
EBER	Negative	Nuclear	Usually negative but may be positive in patients from underdeveloped countries
EBV-LMP	Negative	Cytoplasmic	Usually negative but may be positive in patients from underdeveloped countries

- LP cells are absent
- CD4(+), CD8(+) T cells are increased (similar to NLPHL)

Reactive Lymphoid Hyperplasia

- Lymph node architecture is preserved
- Well-defined germinal centers with polarization and distinct mantle zones
- Small and large centrocytes and centroblasts without atypia
- Tingible body macrophages usually abundant and prominent

DIAGNOSTIC CHECKLIST

Clinically Relevant Pathologic Features

- Clinically indolent disease that responds to therapy but frequently relapses
- Survival curves show early and late relapses without plateau
  - Suggests that no patients with NLPHL are "cured"

Pathologic Interpretation Pearls

- Expansile nodules with LP cells in small lymphocytic background
  - Pattern can be purely nodular or nodular and diffuse
  - Nodules are larger than lymphoid follicles of reactive conditions or follicular lymphoma
    - Most cells within nodules are reactive T and B cells
    - Histiocytes and follicular dendritic cell meshworks in nodules
    - LP cells represent < 1% of cells within nodules
- LP cells are B cells with germinal center-like immunophenotype

SELECTED REFERENCES

1. Biasoli I et al: Nodular, lymphocyte-predominant Hodgkin lymphoma: a long-term study and analysis of transformation to diffuse large B-cell lymphoma in a cohort of 164 patients from the Adult Lymphoma Study Group. Cancer. 116(3):631-9, 2010
2. Churchill HR et al: Programmed death 1 expression in variant immunoarchitectural patterns of nodular lymphocyte predominant Hodgkin lymphoma: comparison with CD57 and lymphomas in the differential diagnosis. Hum Pathol. 41(12):1726-34, 2010
3. Lee AI et al: Nodular lymphocyte predominant Hodgkin lymphoma. Oncologist. 14(7):739-51, 2009
4. Mourad WA et al: Morphologic, immunphenotypic and clinical discriminators between T-cell/histiocyte-rich large B-cell lymphoma and lymphocyte-predominant Hodgkin lymphoma. Hematol Oncol Stem Cell Ther. 1(1):22-7, 2008
5. Yang DT et al: Nodular lymphocyte predominant Hodgkin lymphoma at atypical locations may be associated with increased numbers of large cells and a diffuse histologic component. Am J Hematol. 83(3):218-21, 2008
6. Stamatoullas A et al: Conventional cytogenetics of nodular lymphocyte-predominant Hodgkin's lymphoma. Leukemia. 21(9):2064-7, 2007
7. Khoury JD et al: Bone marrow involvement in patients with nodular lymphocyte predominant Hodgkin lymphoma. Am J Surg Pathol. 28(4):489-95, 2004
8. Boudová L et al: Nodular lymphocyte-predominant Hodgkin lymphoma with nodules resembling T-cell/histiocyte-rich B-cell lymphoma: differential diagnosis between nodular lymphocyte-predominant Hodgkin lymphoma and T-cell/histiocyte-rich B-cell lymphoma. Blood. 102(10):3753-8, 2003

Microscopic Features

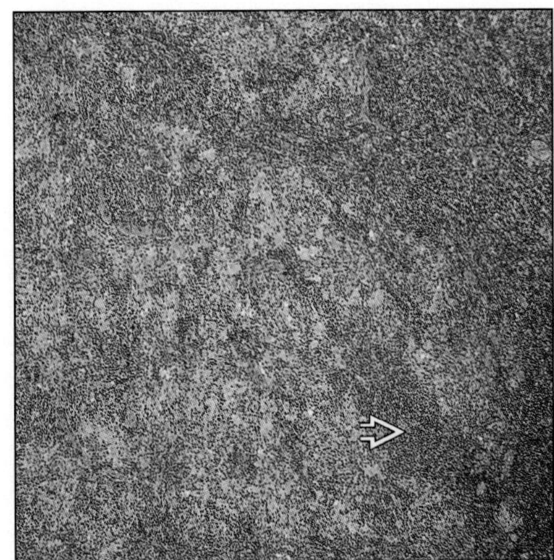

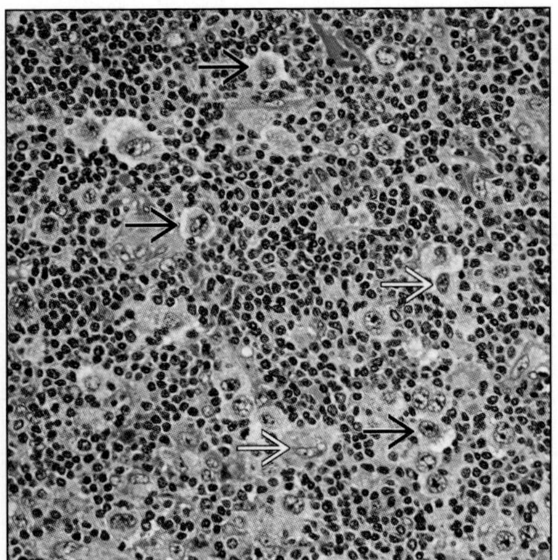

(Left) *Nodular lymphocyte predominant Hodgkin lymphoma (NLPHL) shows a large nodule with a "moth-eaten" pattern at low power due to the presence of larger cells in a background of small lymphocytes ➡.* ***(Right)*** *NLPHL involving lymph node is shown. At high power, the large neoplastic lymphocyte predominant (LP) cells ➡ are scattered among numerous small lymphocytes and a few histiocytes ➡.*

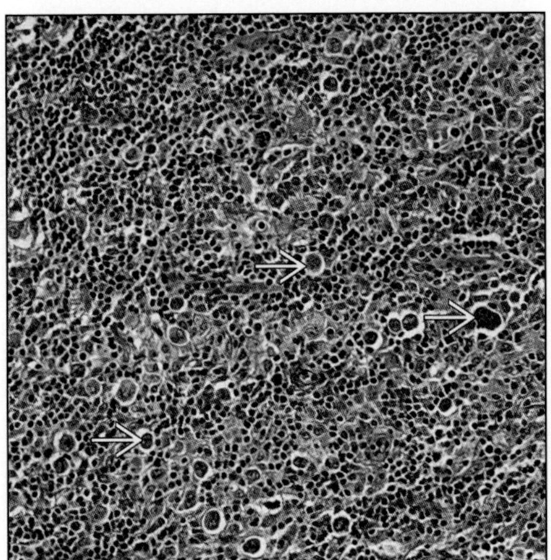

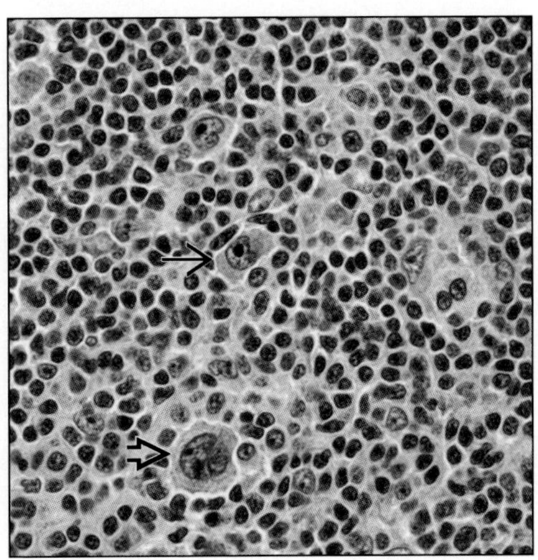

(Left) *Nodular lymphocyte predominant Hodgkin lymphoma (NLPHL) is shown. The cytology of the LP cells spans a spectrum. Some are mummified or have irregular nuclear contours, as in this case ➡.* ***(Right)*** *NLPHL involving lymph node shows various morphologic appearances of LP cells, including "popcorn" cells ➡ and one with a prominent nucleolus ➡, similar to the HRS cells of classical Hodgkin lymphoma.*

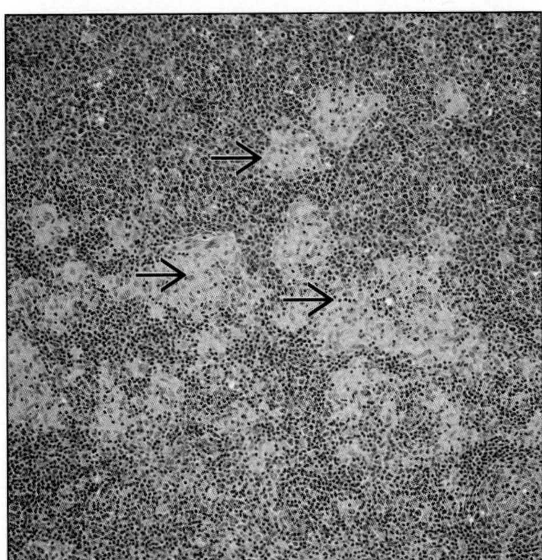

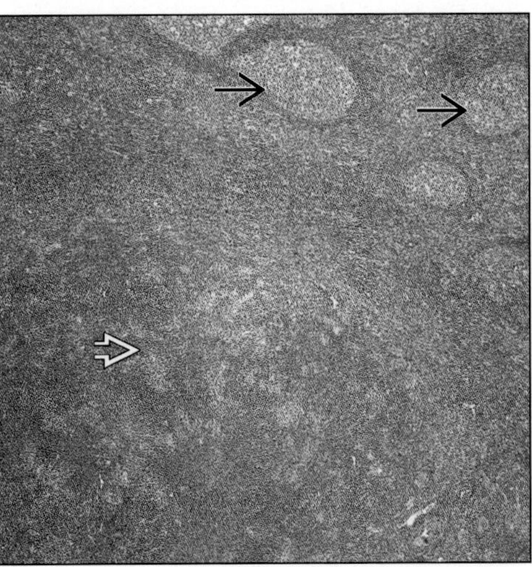

(Left) *Nodular lymphocyte predominant Hodgkin lymphoma shows small clusters of histiocytes forming noncaseating granulomata ➡.* ***(Right)*** *Hyperplastic lymphoid follicles ➡ as well as an expansile lymphoid follicle showing progressive transformation of germinal centers (PTGC) ➡ may be identified at the periphery of NLPHL. No atypical or LP cells were found in the follicle with PTGC.*

NODULAR LYMPHOCYTE PREDOMINANT HODGKIN LYMPHOMA

Immunohistochemical Features

*(**Left**) Nodular lymphocyte predominant Hodgkin lymphoma (NLPHL) shows large LP cells ⇨ as well as many of the small background lymphocytes as CD20(+). The small background lymphocytes are predominantly B cells in NLPHL. (**Right**) NLPHL involving lymph node is shown. The LP cells are strongly positive for pax-5 ⇨. In contrast, the HRS cells of classical Hodgkin lymphoma are dimly pax-5(+). Note also that LP cells can be multilobated.*

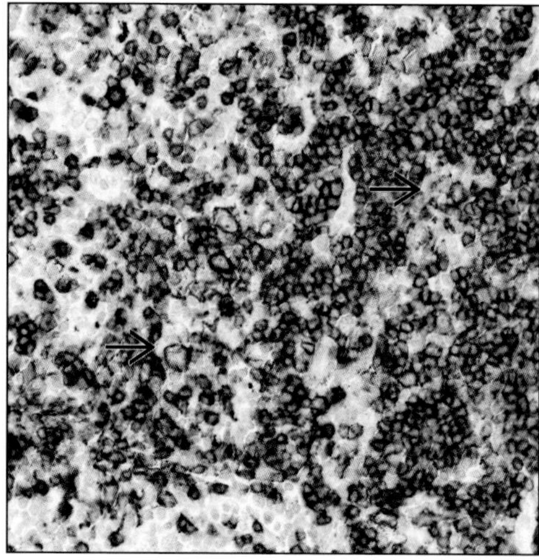

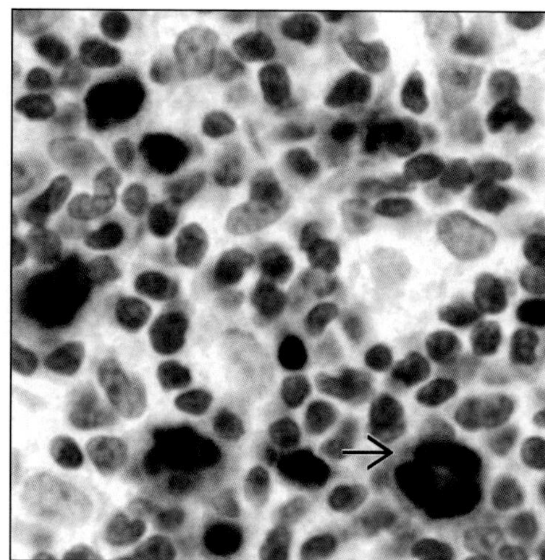

*(**Left**) Nodular lymphocyte predominant Hodgkin lymphoma (NLPHL) at low power shows that the neoplastic nodules ⇨ contain scattered small CD3(+) T cells ⇨. Most cells in the infiltrate are negative ⇨, suggesting that they are B lymphocytes. (**Right**) NLPHL involving lymph node shows small CD3(+) cells surrounding some LP cells, forming so-called rosettes ⇨.*

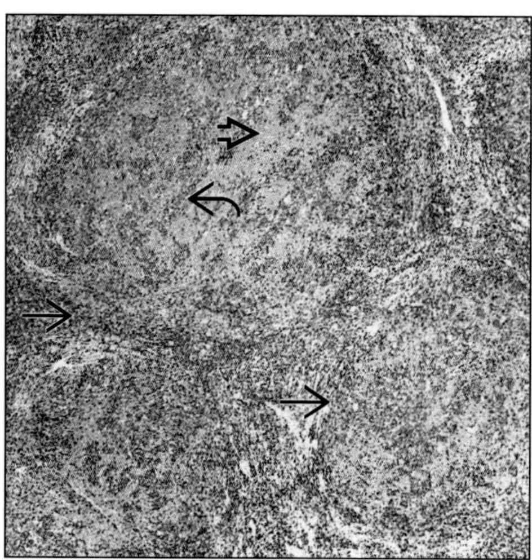

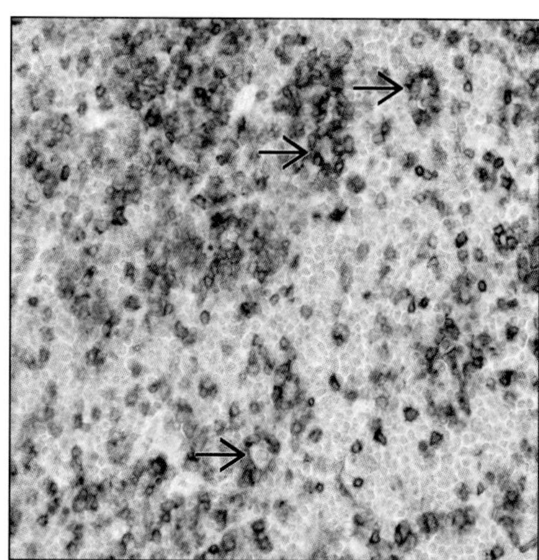

*(**Left**) Nodular lymphocyte predominant Hodgkin lymphoma (NLPHL) shows small CD57(+) T cells ⇨ surrounding 1 LP cell ⇨, forming a "rosette." CD3 is more sensitive than CD57 in identifying rosettes in NLPHL. (**Right**) NLPHL involving lymph node shows LP cells of NLPHL negative for CD30 ⇨. Interfollicular immunoblasts of intermediate size ⇨ are commonly CD30(+) in NLPHL and in reactive follicular hyperplasia.*

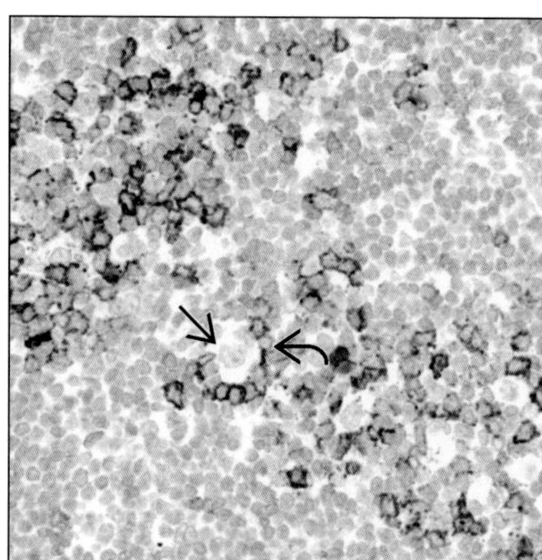

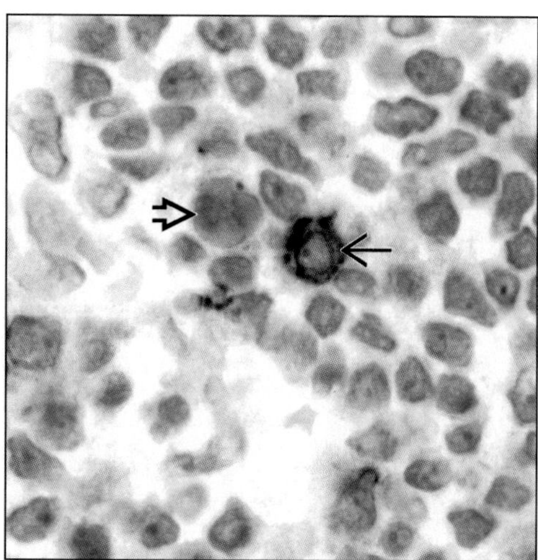

Immunohistochemical and Microscopic Features

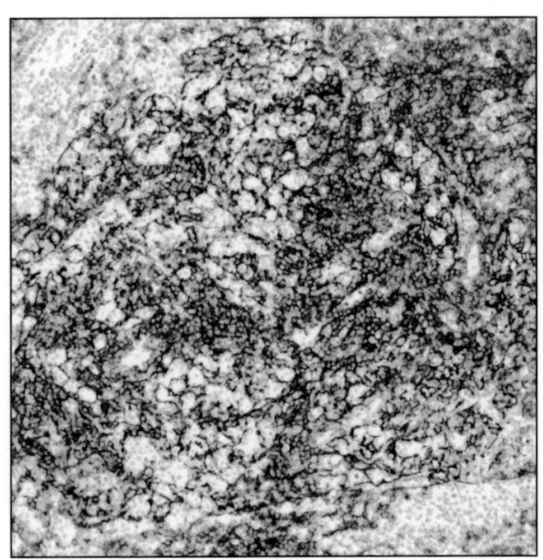

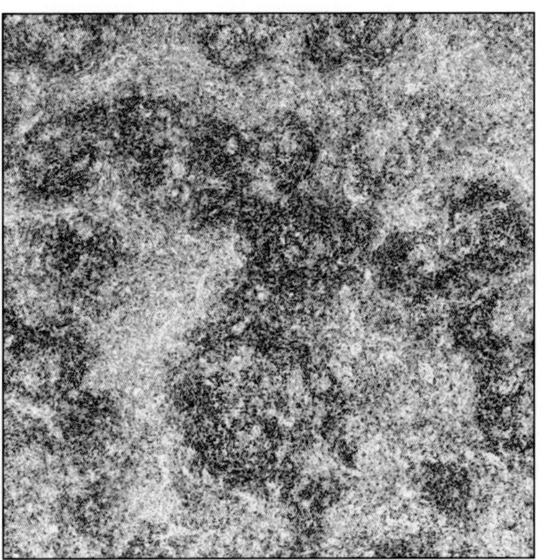

(Left) *Nodular lymphocyte predominant Hodgkin lymphoma (NLPHL) shows a classical nodular pattern. CD21 highlights a follicular dendritic cell meshwork underlying an enlarged nodule. This is the most common pattern identified in NLPHL.* ***(Right)*** *NLPHL, nodular serpiginous pattern, involving lymph node shows Pax-5 highlighting confluent nodules of B-lymphocytes, which convey a "serpiginous" pattern.*

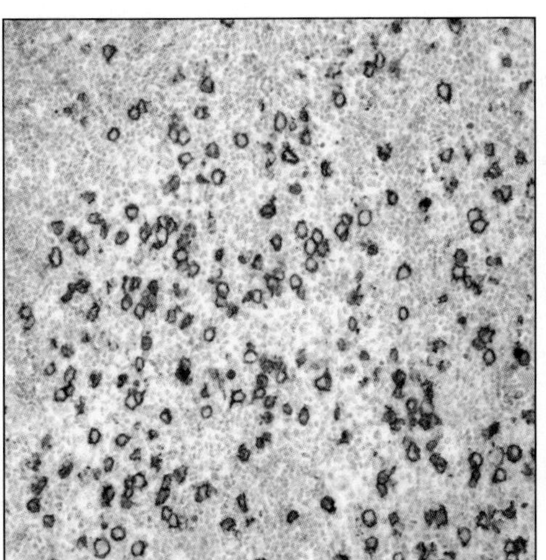

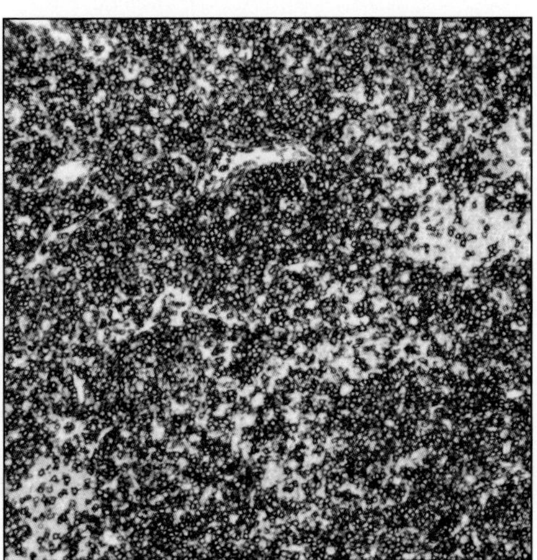

(Left) *Nodular lymphocyte predominant Hodgkin lymphoma (NLPHL), nodular T-cell-rich pattern is shown. CD20 immunohistochemistry highlights lymphocyte predominant (LP) cells in a nodule of NLPHL. The majority of small lymphocytes in the background are CD20(-).* ***(Right)*** *NLPHL, T-cell-rich pattern, involving lymph node shows CD3 immunohistochemistry highlighting numerous positive cells. This pattern is uncommon.*

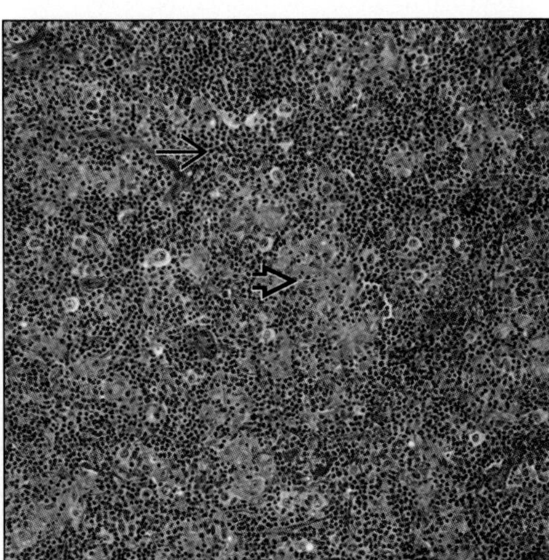

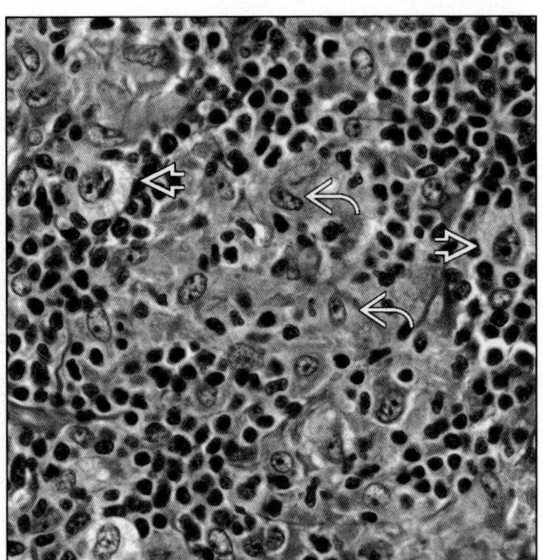

(Left) *Nodular lymphocyte predominant Hodgkin lymphoma (NLPHL), histiocyte-rich pattern is shown. Many cells in the background are histiocytes ⇨, which are admixed with small lymphocytes →.* ***(Right)*** *NLPHL, histiocyte-rich pattern, involving lymph node shows histiocytes ➡ that may form loose clusters. Only rare (~ 1%) LP cells ➡ are present.*

Transformation of NLPHL

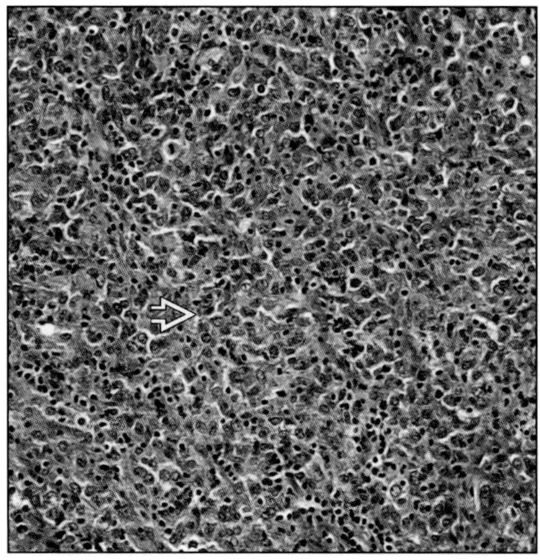

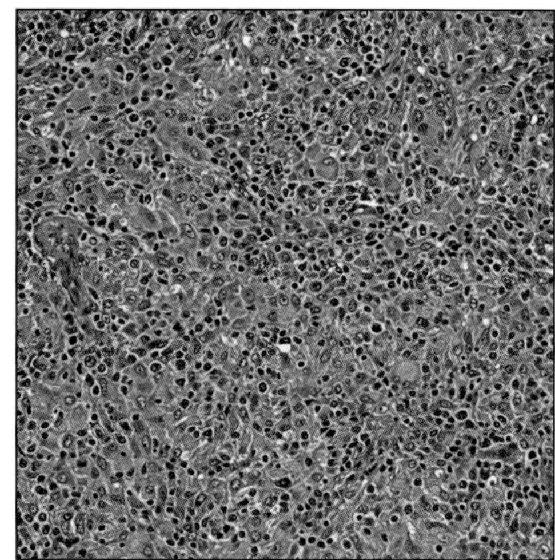

(Left) *Diffuse large B-cell lymphoma (DLBCL) arising from NLPHL shows the presence of sheets of large cells ⇨, which are diagnostic of transformation. NLPHL was identified in other parts of the lymph node.* ***(Right)*** *T-cell/ histiocyte-rich large B-cell lymphoma (THRLBCL) arising from NLPHL is shown. This pattern occurred after relapses of NLPHL and multiple chemotherapies. Compared with typical cases of NLPHL, histiocytes are more abundant, and lymphocytes are less abundant in THRLBCL.*

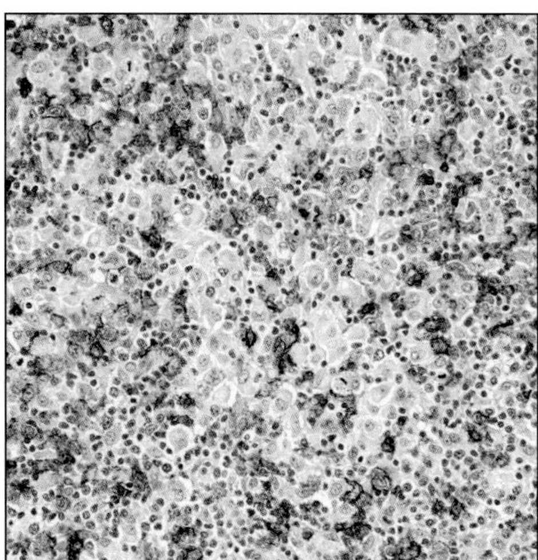

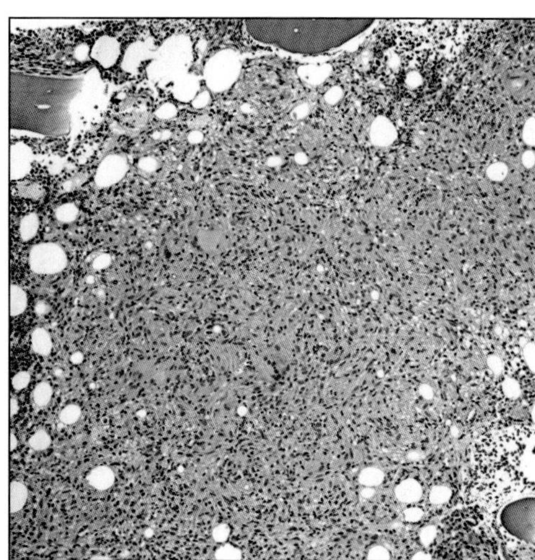

(Left) *T-cell/histiocyte-rich large B-cell lymphoma (THRLBCL) arising from transformation of NLPHL shows CD20 highlighting the neoplastic large cells and rare small reactive B-lymphocytes. Note that the B cells are markedly depleted in comparison with typical NLPHL.* ***(Right)*** *T-cell/histiocyte-rich large B-cell lymphoma (THRLBCL) arising from NLPHL shows bone marrow involvement by THRLBCL in a patient with NLPHL, indicating transformation of NLPHL.*

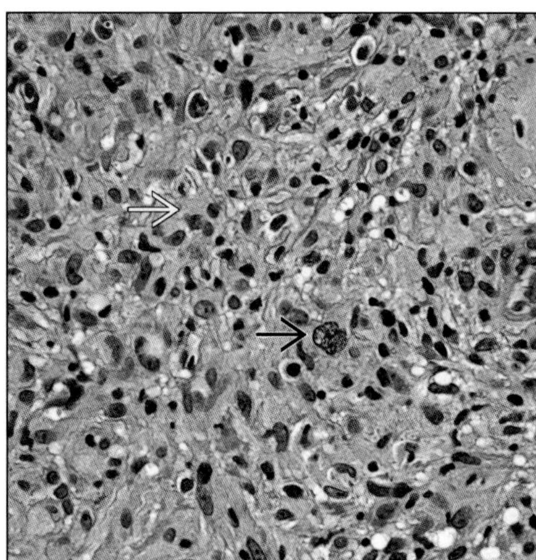

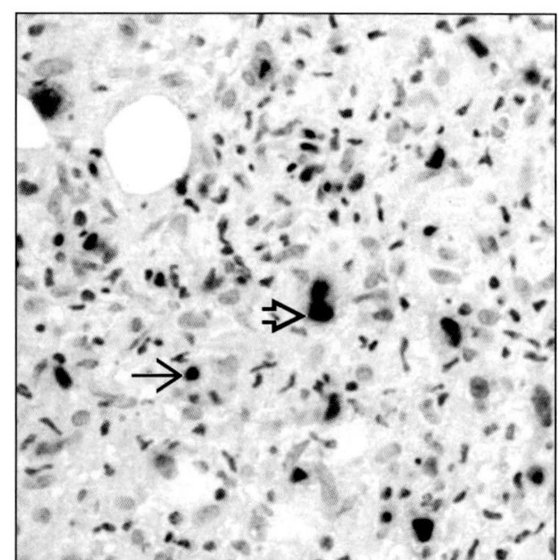

(Left) *T-cell/histiocyte-rich large B-cell lymphoma (THRLBCL) in bone marrow is shown. Bone marrow involvement by THRLBCL in a patient with NLPHL elsewhere indicates transformation of NLPHL. A large neoplastic cell → is surrounded by numerous histiocytes ⇨.* ***(Right)*** *T-cell/ histiocyte-rich large B-cell lymphoma (THRLBCL) in bone marrow shows a large neoplastic cell ⇨ as well as scattered small B cells → as Pax-5(+).*

Differential Diagnosis

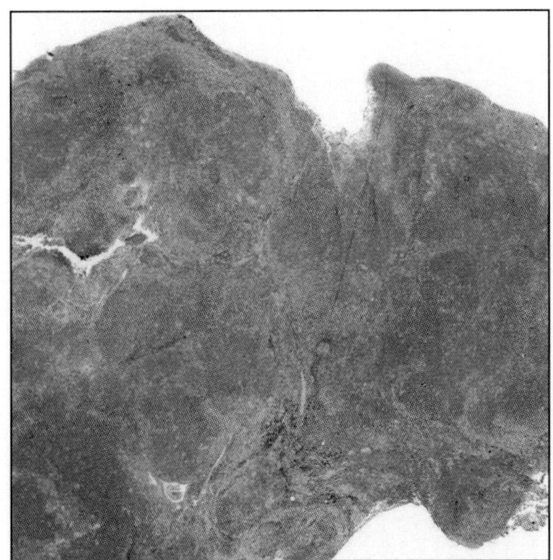

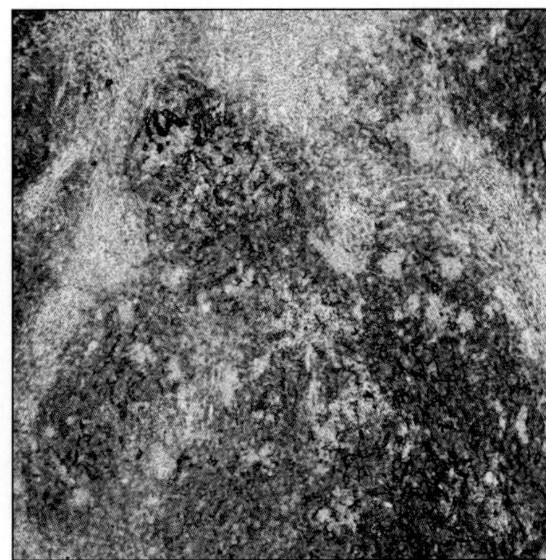

(Left) *Lymph node involved by lymphocyte-rich classical Hodgkin lymphoma (LRCHL), nodular variant shows a neoplasm resembling nodular lymphocyte predominant Hodgkin lymphoma (NLPHL) at low magnification. However, a "moth-eaten" pattern is not seen in this lymph node.* ***(Right)*** *LRCHL involving lymph node shows CD21 immunohistochemistry highlighting an expanded follicular dendritic cell meshwork.*

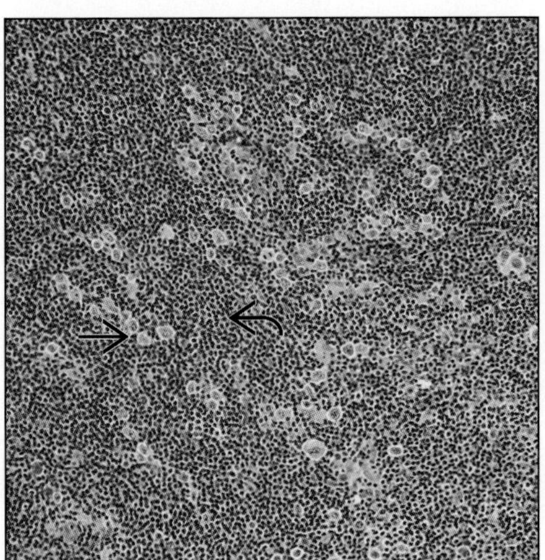

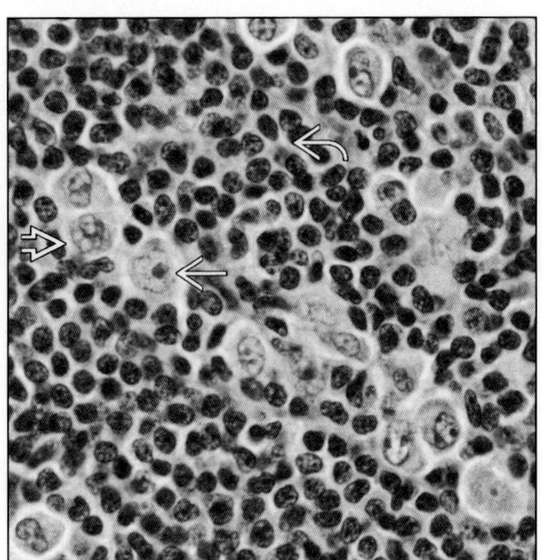

(Left) *Lymphocyte-rich classical Hodgkin lymphoma (LRCHL) shows Hodgkin and Reed-Sternberg (HRS) cells ⇒ scattered among numerous small reactive lymphocytes ⇒. Rare histiocytes are also noted.* ***(Right)*** *LRCHL involving lymph node is shown. HRS cells include cells with large multilobated vesicular nuclei ⇒ and large cells with prominent nucleoli ⇒. The background is composed predominantly of small lymphocytes ⇒.*

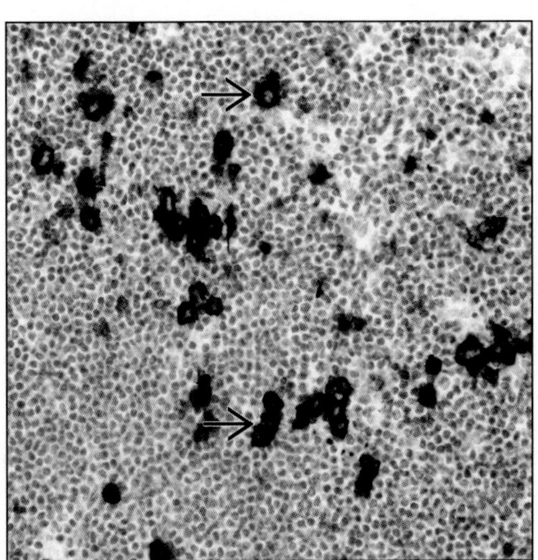

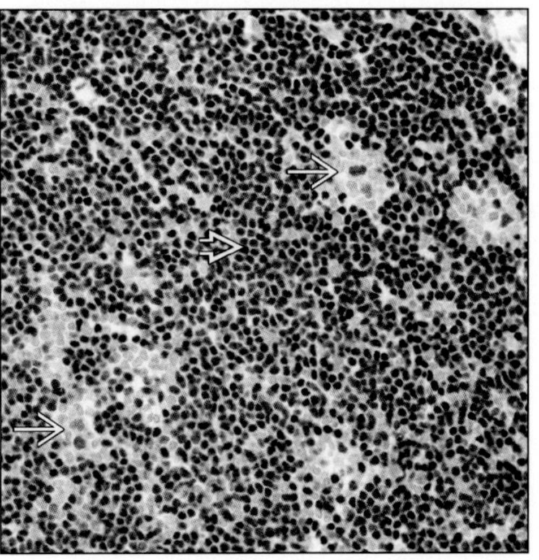

(Left) *Lymphocyte-rich classical Hodgkin lymphoma (LRCHL) is shown. The neoplastic cells are strongly CD30(+) ⇒, as any usual Hodgkin and Reed-Sternberg cell of classical Hodgkin lymphoma.* ***(Right)*** *LRCHL involving lymph node shows Pax-5 highlighting numerous small reactive B-lymphocytes, strongly positive ⇒ in the background, corresponding mainly to mantle zone lymphocytes. The neoplastic HRS cells ⇒ are weakly positive.*

NODULAR LYMPHOCYTE PREDOMINANT HODGKIN LYMPHOMA

Differential Diagnosis

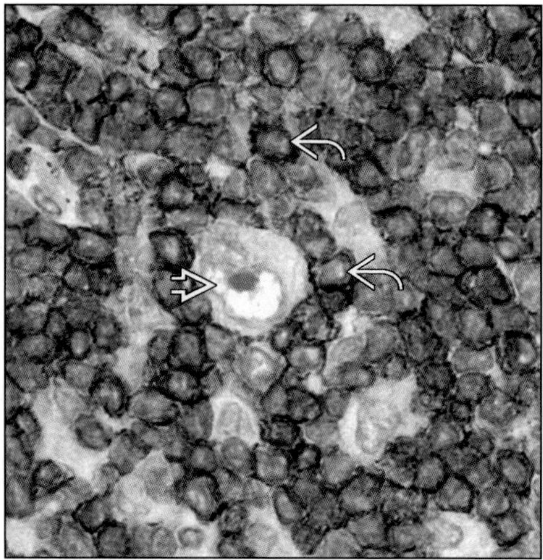

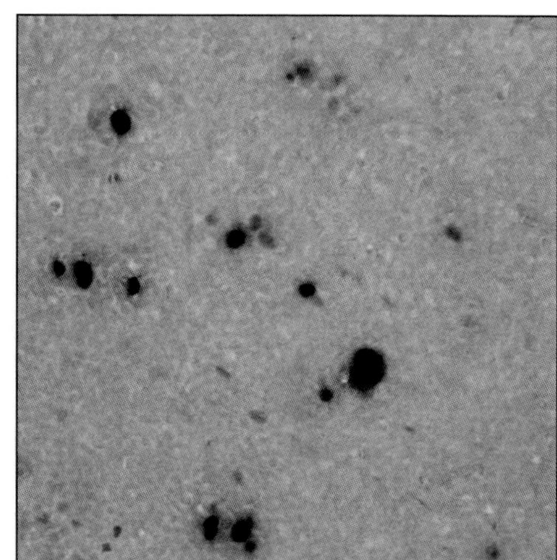

(Left) Lymphocyte-rich classical Hodgkin lymphoma (LRCHL) is shown. A Reed-Sternberg cell ➡ is CD45(-) whereas the surrounding small lymphocytes ➡ are CD45/LCA(+). CD45 is almost always negative in classical Hodgkin lymphoma. **(Right)** LRCHL involving lymph node is shown. In situ hybridization for EBV encoded RNA (EBER) highlights HRS cells. Approximately 20-40% of cases of LRCHL are EBV(+).

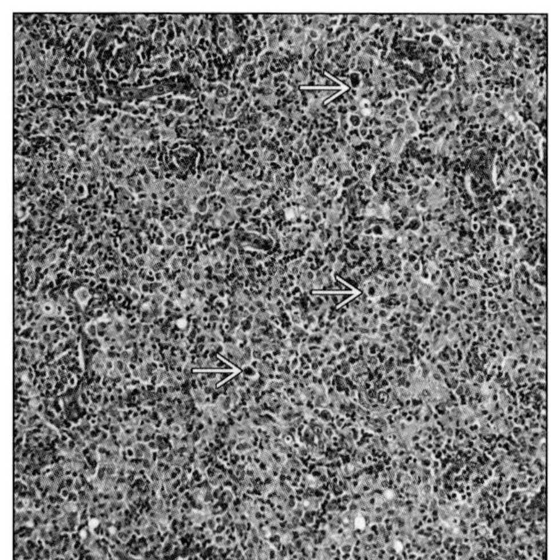

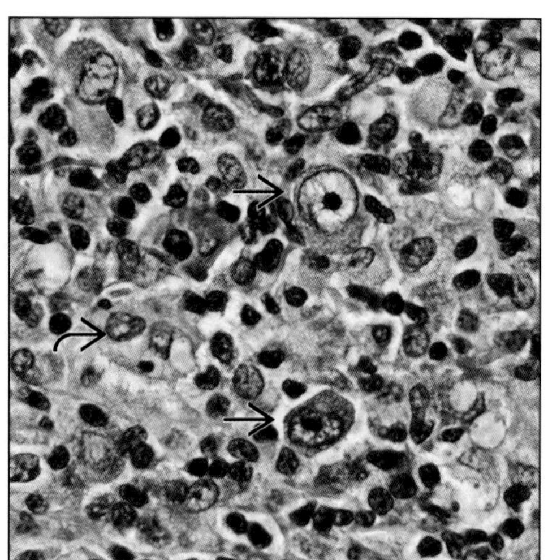

(Left) T-cell/histiocyte-rich large B-cell lymphoma (THRLBCL), involving lymph node shows diffuse infiltrate with large neoplastic cells ➡ scattered in a background of abundant small lymphocytes and histiocytes. **(Right)** THRLBCL involving lymph node shows neoplastic cells that are large with prominent nucleoli ➡ and may mimic HRS cells. Note numerous histiocytes ➡ in the background.

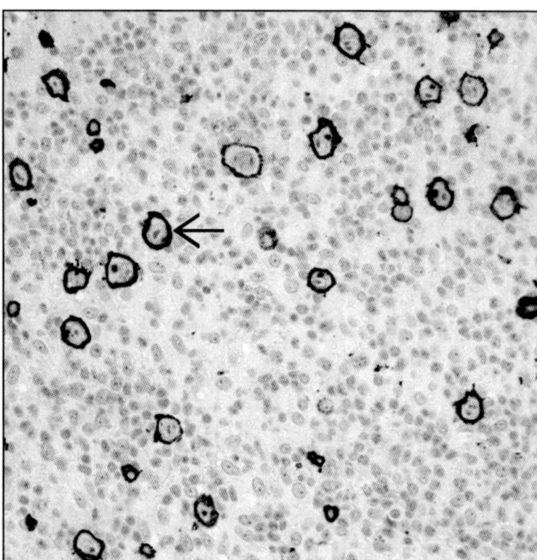

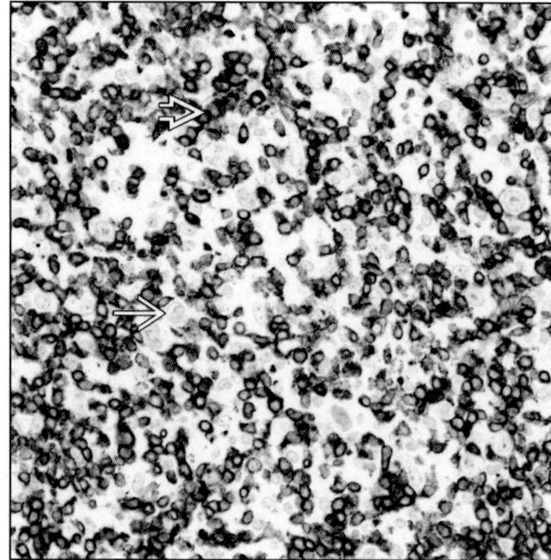

(Left) T-cell/histiocyte-rich large B-cell lymphoma (THRLBCL) shows large cells that are CD20(+) ➡. The majority of cells in the background are CD20(-) and probably correspond to T cells or histiocytes. **(Right)** THRLBCL involving lymph node shows a background composed of abundant T cells ➡ highlighted with CD3 that almost obscure scattered large neoplastic cells ➡.

Differential Diagnosis

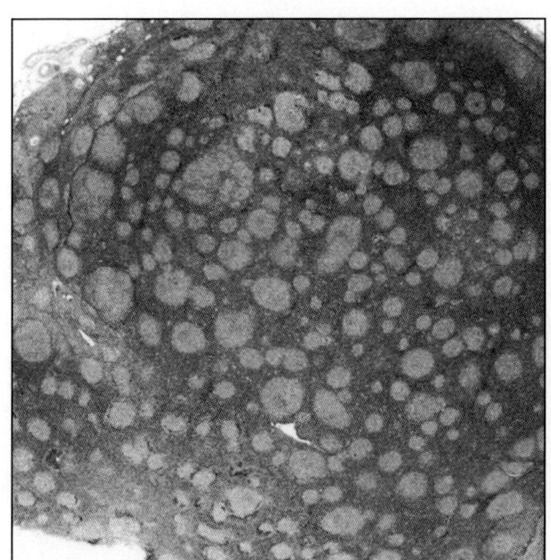

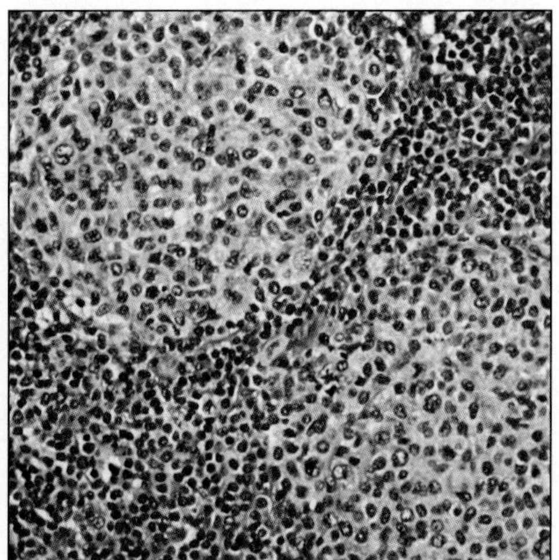

*(**Left**) Follicular lymphoma involving lymph node is shown. Unlike the nodules of NLPHL, the nodules of follicular lymphoma are smaller, more sharply delineated, and often lack mantle zones. (**Right**) Follicular lymphoma involving lymph node shows 2 neoplastic follicles composed of centrocytes with fewer centroblasts. No lymphocyte predominant (LP) cells are identified in follicular lymphoma.*

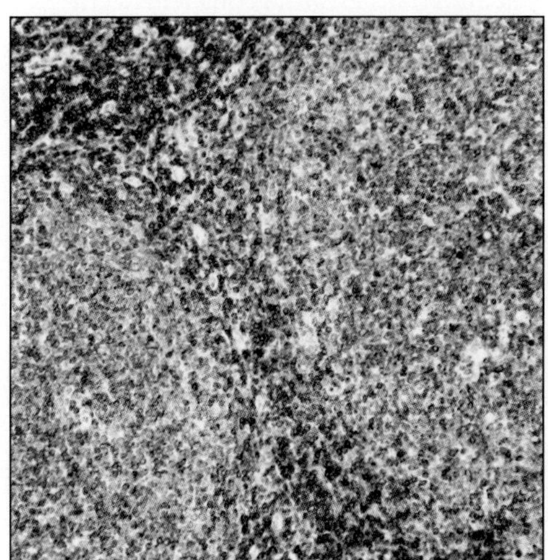

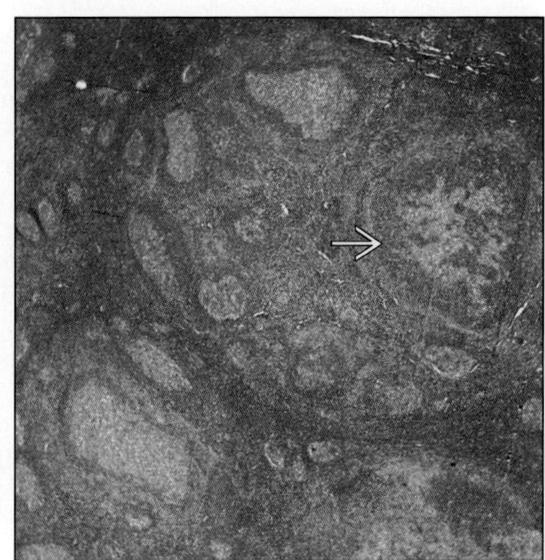

*(**Left**) Follicular lymphoma involving lymph node shows 2 Bcl-2(+) neoplastic follicles. (**Right**) Progressive transformation of germinal centers involving lymph node is shown. The follicles are large and irregular with prominent germinal centers. Mantle zone lymphocytes infiltrate into germinal centers, imparting an irregular outline to the germinal centers at low-power magnification ➔.*

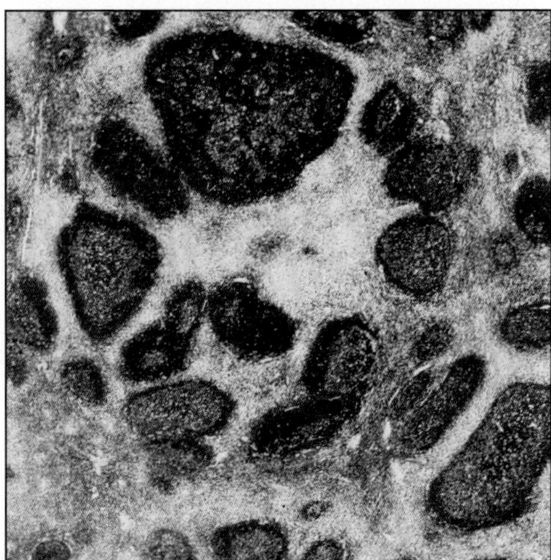

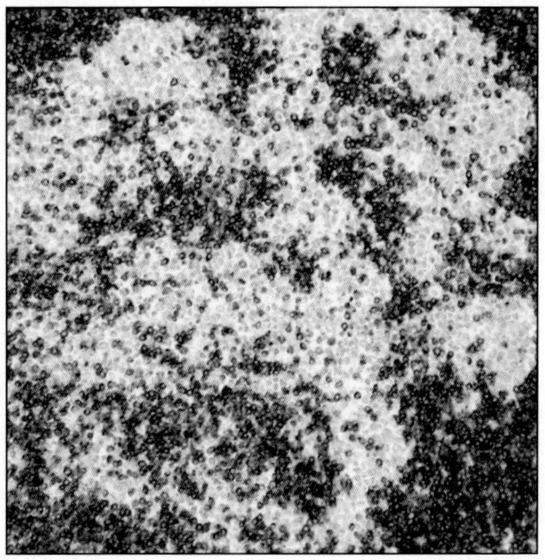

*(**Left**) Progressive transformation of germinal centers involving lymph node is shown. The follicles are composed of many CD20(+) B cells. The immunostain also highlights the variable, large size of transformed follicles. (**Right**) Progressive transformation of germinal centers involving lymph node shows reactive germinal center B cells in the transformed follicle that are Bcl-2(-), whereas mantle zone B and T cells are Bcl-2(+).*

CLASSICAL HODGKIN LYMPHOMA

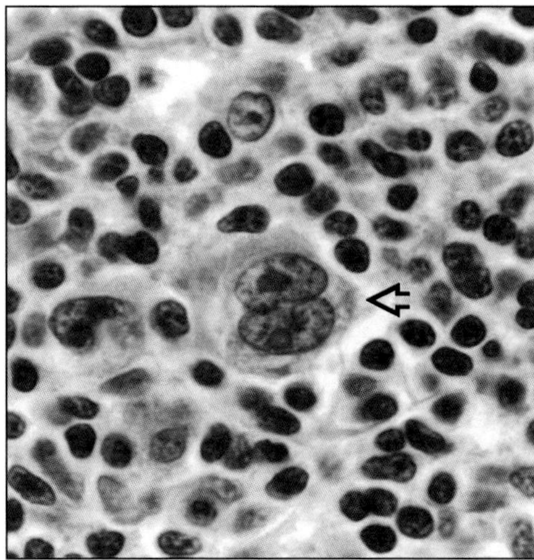

Characteristic Hodgkin Reed-Sternberg cell ⮞ shows large "mirror image" nuclei with thick nuclear membranes, vesicular chromatin, and prominent eosinophilic nucleoli.

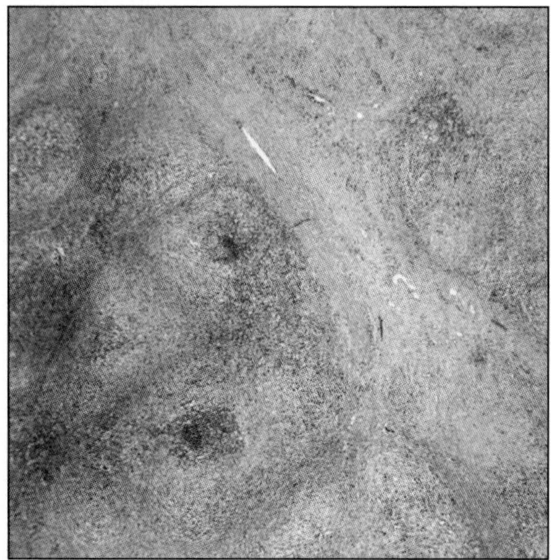

Characteristic low-power appearance of a lymph node involved by NS-CHL shows intersecting broad fibrous bands separating the cellular component into distinct and variably sized nodules.

TERMINOLOGY

Abbreviations

- Classical Hodgkin lymphoma (CHL)

Synonyms

- Hodgkin disease

Definitions

- Lymphoma of the young and old characterized by heterogeneous mixture of nonneoplastic inflammatory and accessory cells with minor component of large mononuclear and multinucleated tumor cells
  - Divided into 4 categories
    - Nodular sclerosis CHL (NS-CHL)
    - Mixed cellularity CHL (MC-CHL)
    - Lymphocyte-rich CHL (LR-CHL)
    - Lymphocyte-depleted CHL (LD-CHL)

ETIOLOGY/PATHOGENESIS

Infectious Agents

- EBV postulated to play role; however
  - Present in only a portion of cases
  - EBV(+) Hodgkin Reed-Sternberg (HRS) cells found in 40-50% of cases by in situ hybridization with EBV-encoded RNA (EBER)
  - Prevalence of EBV highest in MC-CHL, in higher clinical stages, and older patients
  - EBV positivity is seen in nearly 100% of HIV-infected patients
  - EBV positivity more common in tropical regions
  - History of infectious mononucleosis (IM) may predispose to Hodgkin lymphoma (HL)
- HIV infection and immunosuppression
  - Loss of immune surveillance

Germinal Center B-cell Origin

- Neoplastic cells
  - Have likely acquired disadvantageous *IgVH* gene mutations but did not undergo apoptosis
  - Have also acquired deregulated signaling pathways and transcription factors
    - NF-KB, Jak-Stat, PAX5, PIK3-Akt, Erk, AP1, Notch1, and receptor tyrosine kinases
  - Express a variety of tumor necrosis factor (TNF) receptor family members
    - TNF-α, lymphotoxin-α, CD30 ligand, CD40 ligand, RANK ligand
  - Express a variety of Th1 and Th2-related cytokines
    - Interleukin (IL)-2, IL-4, IL-5, IL-6, IL-9, IL-10, IL-12, IL-13, and interferon-γ
    - Unbalanced production of Th2 cytokines (i.e., IL-6, IL-10, IL-13)
  - Other expressed cytokines include
    - TARC, MDC, eotaxin, IL-3, IL-7, IL-8, inducible protein-1, GM-CSF, TGF-β
- Milieu of cytokines and receptors attract nonneoplastic inflammatory cells
  - Creates microenvironment that supports survival and proliferation of HRS cells

CLINICAL ISSUES

Epidemiology

- Incidence
  - 1 of the most frequent lymphomas in the Western world
  - Incidence: About 3-5 cases per 100,000 people per year
  - Account for 30% of all lymphomas
  - CHL accounts for 95% of all Hodgkin lymphomas (HL)
  - Incidence higher in patients with history of IM
- Age
  - Bimodal age curve
    - 1st peak at 15-35 years
    - 2nd peak at > 54 years

CLASSICAL HODGKIN LYMPHOMA

Key Facts

Terminology

- Lymphoma of the young and old characterized by heterogeneous mixture of nonneoplastic inflammatory and accessory cells with minor component of large mononuclear and multinucleated tumor cells

Clinical Issues

- Accounts for 95% of all Hodgkin lymphomas (HL)
- Cure rates of > 90% with modern treatment protocols

Microscopic Pathology

- Variable numbers of neoplastic and nonneoplastic inflammatory cells
- Hodgkin Reed-Sternberg cells (HRS cells)
  - Large pleomorphic nuclei with thick nuclear membranes that may appear as "mirror images" or may be multiple and interconnected
- HRS-cell variants
  - Lacunar cell, Hodgkin cell, mummified cell, anaplastic cell

Top Differential Diagnoses

- Nodular lymphocyte predominant Hodgkin lymphoma
- Infectious mononucleosis
- Large B-cell lymphomas
- Peripheral T-cell lymphoma
- Anaplastic large cell lymphoma
- Metastasis

- Gender
  - Male predominance in all types except NS-CHL

Site

- **General**
  - Cervical and supraclavicular lymph nodes (75% of cases)
  - Mediastinal, axillary, and paraaortic lymph nodes (frequent)
  - Mesenteric and epitrochlear lymph nodes (rare)
  - Splenic involvement (uncommon)
  - Bone marrow (~ 5%)
    - Indicates vascular invasion (stage IV disease)
- **NS-CHL** (~ 70% of cases)
  - Mediastinum &/or cervical lymph nodes (60-80%)
  - Splenic &/or lung (8-10%)
  - Bone marrow involvement (3%)
  - Liver (2%)
- **MC-CHL** (20-25% of cases)
  - Peripheral lymph nodes (frequent)
  - Spleen (30%)
  - Bone marrow (10%)
  - Liver (3%)
  - Mediastinum (uncommon)
- **LR-CHL** (5% of cases)
  - Peripheral lymph nodes (frequent)
  - Mediastinum (uncommon)
  - Typically lack bulky disease
- **LD-CHL** (< 1% of cases)
  - Retroperitoneal lymph nodes
  - Abdominal organs
  - Bone marrow

Presentation

- Peripheral lymphadenopathy
- Mediastinal mass
- B symptoms (fevers, night sweats, weight loss, pruritus, anorexia, fatigue, generalized weakness)
  - Reported in up to 40% of patients

Treatment

- Drugs
  - Multi-agent chemotherapy
- Radiation
  - Involved field radiotherapy
- Therapy for recurrent disease
  - High-dose chemotherapy and autologous stem cell transplant

Prognosis

- Overall, good prognosis
- Cure rates of > 90% with modern treatment protocols
- Histologic subtype less important as a predictive factor with current therapies
- Elevated serum levels of IL-6 and IL-10 associated with poor prognosis

MACROSCOPIC FEATURES

General Features

- Enlarged lymph node or mass with tan cut surface
- Whitish areas of fibrosis with vague nodularity typical of NS-CHL

MICROSCOPIC PATHOLOGY

Microscopic Features

- **General features**
  - Heterogeneous cell populations
    - Variable numbers of neoplastic and nonneoplastic inflammatory cells
  - Nonneoplastic cells
    - Represent an immune-mediated cellular reaction to neoplastic cells (cytokine driven)
    - Composition varies relative to histologic subtype
    - Admixture of lymphocytes (predominantly CD4[+] T cells), eosinophils, immunoblasts, plasma cells, neutrophils, histiocytes, and fibroblasts
  - Hodgkin Reed-Sternberg cells
    - Large pleomorphic nuclei with thick nuclear membranes that may appear as "mirror images" or may be multiple and interconnected

CLASSICAL HODGKIN LYMPHOMA

        - Each nucleus contains a single and prominent eosinophilic nucleolus
        - Eosinophilic or amphophilic cytoplasm
        - Often comprise no more than 1-3% of tumor volume
        - Pathognomic feature of HL
    - HRS cell variants
        - Lacunar cell: Retracted cytoplasmic membrane (artifact of formalin fixation)
        - Hodgkin cell: Single large round vesicular nucleus with single large eosinophilic nucleolus (considered a mononuclear HRS cell)
        - Mummified cell: Degenerated or apoptotic neoplastic cell
        - Anaplastic cell: Large and highly pleomorphic nuclei with coarse chromatin and prominent nucleoli
- **NS-CHL**
    - Distinct nodular growth pattern
        - Nodules surrounded by broad, interconnecting bands of fibrocollagenous tissue
    - Variable numbers of HRS cells, Hodgkin cells, and lacunar cells
    - Variable numbers of lymphocytes, eosinophils, and other nonneoplastic inflammatory cells
    - Cellular phase of NS-CHL
        - Abundance of lacunar cells with sparse bands of collagen
        - Lacunar cells congregate in center
        - ± necrosis
    - Fibrotic phase of NS-CHL
        - Extensive sclerosis with scant cellularity
    - Syncytial variant of NS-CHL
        - Formation of prominent aggregates/sheets of HRS cells &/or lacunar cells
        - Extreme form of cellular phase
        - Occurs in < 5% of cases
        - Exclude metastatic carcinoma and melanoma
- **MC-CHL**
    - Complete or near complete involvement of lymph nodes
    - Diffuse to vaguely nodular pattern of growth
        - Nodules are not surrounded by fibrous bands
    - Prominent mixed cellular infiltrate
        - Lymphocytes, plasma cells, eosinophils, histocytes, occasional neutrophils
        - Frequent HRS cells and Hodgkin cells
- **LR-CHL**
    - Nodular to diffuse pattern of growth
        - Nodules typically represent expanded mantle zone B cells
        - Small and regressed germinal centers may be seen in nodules
        - Nodules (follicular dendritic meshwork) may be highlighted by CD21
        - May resemble nodular lymphocyte predominant HL (NLPHL)
        - Lacks the lymphocytic and histiocytic "popcorn" cells of NLPHL
        - Intact germinal centers are infrequent in NLPHL
    - Predominance of lymphocytes
    - Few HRS and Hodgkin cells
    - Few to absent eosinophils and neutrophils
    - B symptoms are less frequent
- **LD-CHL**
    - Relative predominance of HRS cells in relation to background lymphocytes
    - Includes diffuse fibrosis and reticular subtypes
    - Most aggressive form of CHL
    - **Diffuse fibrosis subtype**
        - Poorly cellular and structureless lymph node
        - Replaced by fibrous tissue, scattered HRS cells, and residual lymphocytes
    - **Reticular subtype**
        - Hypercellular
        - Numerous large pleomorphic neoplastic cells (HRS cells or variants)
        - Distinguish from large cell lymphoma, histiocytic sarcoma, and anaplastic carcinoma

ANCILLARY TESTS

Immunohistochemistry

- Recommended panel
    - CD3, CD15, CD20, CD30, CD45
        - Distinguish CD15(+) granulocytes from CD15(+) HRS cells
        - Distinguish CD30(+) immunoblasts and histiocytes from CD30(+) mononuclear Hodgkin cells
        - CD3 is often difficult to evaluate and may require several adjacent HRS cells for accurate interpretation
    - If necessary pax-5, OCT2, and BOB1 may be performed

DIFFERENTIAL DIAGNOSIS

Nodular Lymphocyte Predominant Hodgkin Lymphoma (NLPHL)

- Distinguish from LR-CHL
- Background lymphocytes are mixture of B and T cells
- Intact germinal centers are infrequent in NLPHL
    - Progressive transformation of germinal center may be present
- Immunophenotype of neoplastic lymphocyte predominant (LP) cells
    - Positive: CD20, CD22, CD45, CD79a, Pax-5, OCT2, BOB1
    - Negative: CD15, CD30, EBV-LMP1
- Features common to CHL are usually absent
    - Eosinophils, neutrophils, and plasma cells are unusual
    - HRS cells are rare
    - Necrosis is rare; no fibrosis surrounding nodules

Infectious Mononucleosis

- Lymph node architecture more likely to be preserved
- Numerous immunoblasts with abundant apoptosis and tingible body macrophages
    - Immunoblasts may resemble HRS cells but will be immunophenotypically distinct
- Atypical/variant lymphocytes in peripheral blood

CLASSICAL HODGKIN LYMPHOMA

Immunohistochemistry

Antibody	Reactivity	Staining Pattern	Comment
CD15	Positive	Cell membrane	Golgi (paranuclear) staining is often observed; if negative, overnight staining may be required; not specific and is seen in granulocytes and a subset of peripheral T-cell lymphomas and rare B-cell lymphomas; expressed in 75-85% of cases
CD30	Positive	Cell membrane	Golgi staining is often observed; variable weak to strong staining is characteristic; not specific; expressed in ALCL (more often strong and uniform); PMLBCL, and in some carcinomas
pax-5	Positive	Nuclear	Staining is typically weaker than in neighboring B cells
IRF-4	Positive		
CD20	Negative		Positive in up to 40%; staining is often variable and patchy when present
CD45	Negative		Can be detected in about 7% of CHL
CD79-α	Negative		
EMA	Negative		Negative in > 90%
OCT2	Negative		Positive in < 10%
BOB1	Negative		Coexpressed with OCT2 in rare cases

- Serologic tests positive for EBV infection

Large B-cell Lymphomas

- Neoplastic cells may resemble Hodgkin cells but typically lack large eosinophilic nucleolus and thick nuclear membranes
- **Primary mediastinal (thymic) large B-cell lymphoma (PMLBCL)**
  - May be difficult to distinguish from NS-CHL of the mediastinum
  - Express B-cell antigens (CD19, CD20, CD22, CD79-a)
  - CD30 is expressed in > 80%
  - CD15 is rarely present
  - Lack surface Ig
- **T-cell/histiocyte-rich large B-cell lymphoma (THRLBCL)**
  - May also be difficult to distinguish from CHL
  - Express pan B-cell antigens and Bcl-6
  - CD30(+/-), EMA(+/-), CD15(-)
- Consider B-cell lymphoma, unclassifiable with features intermediate between diffuse large B-cell lymphoma and CHL (gray zone lymphoma)
  - Sparse inflammatory infiltrate
  - Neoplastic cells typically express
    - CD15, CD20 (uniform and strong), CD30, CD45, CD79-a, Bcl-6 (variable), pax-5, OCT2, and BOB1

Peripheral T-cell Lymphoma

- Many of the morphologic features can overlap
- Immunophenotyping of neoplastic cells is essential (T-cell panel)
  - Look for modulated T-cell antigen expression patterns
- Peripheral T-cell lymphomas can express both CD15 and CD30

Anaplastic Large Cell Lymphoma (ALCL)

- Distinguish from CHL with anaplastic cells
- CD30 expression is strong and uniform
- CD15 expression is rare
- Exclude with ALK, cytotoxic T-cell markers (granzyme B, perforin, TIA), CD45, EMA, and a thorough T-cell panel (CD2, CD3, CD4, CD5, CD7, CD8)
  - Interpret CD3 with caution (negative in > 75% of cases)
- Cytogenetic studies, if necessary, show t(2;5)(p23;q35)
  - 20-25% of ALK(+) ALCL lack t(2:5)(p23;q35)
- Most have clonally rearranged T-cell receptor genes

Metastasis

- Anaplastic carcinoma, embryonal carcinoma, melanoma, seminoma, and nasopharyngeal carcinoma may resemble syncytial variant of NS-CHL
- Exclude with thorough immunohistochemical panel as indicated

SELECTED REFERENCES

1. Aldinucci D et al: The classical Hodgkin's lymphoma microenvironment and its role in promoting tumour growth and immune escape. J Pathol. 221(3):248-63, 2010
2. Cader FZ et al: The contribution of the Epstein-Barr virus to the pathogenesis of childhood lymphomas. Cancer Treat Rev. 36(4):348-53, 2010
3. Carbone A et al: HIV-associated Hodgkin lymphoma. Curr Opin HIV AIDS. 4(1):3-10, 2009
4. Mani H et al: Hodgkin lymphoma: an update on its biology with new insights into classification. Clin Lymphoma Myeloma. 9(3):206-16, 2009
5. Skinnider BF et al: The role of cytokines in classical Hodgkin lymphoma. Blood. 99(12):4283-97, 2002
6. Marafioti T et al: Hodgkin and reed-sternberg cells represent an expansion of a single clone originating from a germinal center B-cell with functional immunoglobulin gene rearrangements but defective immunoglobulin transcription. Blood. 95(4):1443-50, 2000
7. Küppers R: Identifying the precursors of Hodgkin and Reed-Sternberg cells in Hodgkin's disease: role of the germinal center in B-cell lymphomagenesis. J Acquir Immune Defic Syndr. 21 Suppl 1:S74-9, 1999
8. Rüdiger T et al: Workshop report on Hodgkin's disease and related diseases ('grey zone' lymphoma). Ann Oncol. 9 Suppl 5:S31-8, 1998

Gross and Microscopic Features

*(**Left**) Gross photo shows a lymph node partially effaced by NS-CHL. Note the multiple tan-white nodules ➔ surrounded by thick fibrous bands ➔. (Courtesy C. Yin, MD, PhD.) (**Right**) FNA taken from an enlarged cervical lymph node shows a predominance of small lymphocytes and occasional HRS cells ➔. Note the large nuclei, prominent nucleoli, and abundant cytoplasm. The background cellular milieu of small lymphocytes and eosinophils (if present) can be very helpful.*

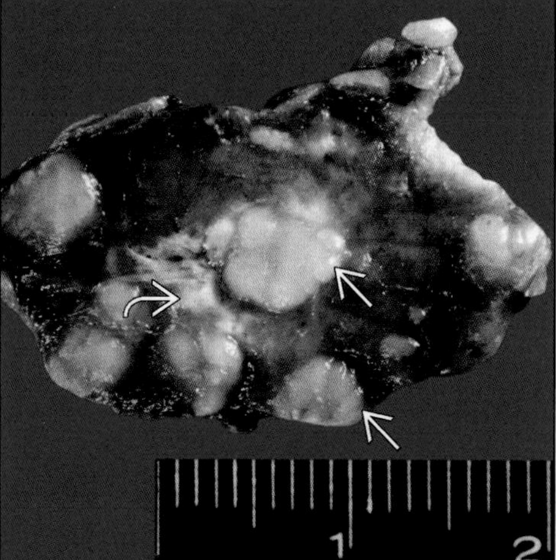

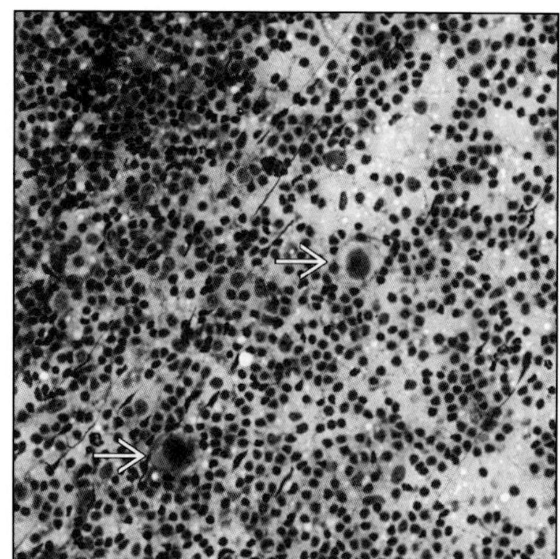

*(**Left**) High-power view of an FNA taken from an enlarged cervical lymph node shows a predominance of small lymphocytes and a characteristic HRS cell. (**Right**) High-power view shows 2 adjacent lacunar cells. The retracted cytoplasm, an artifact of formalin fixation, creates a clear area surrounding the nuclei.*

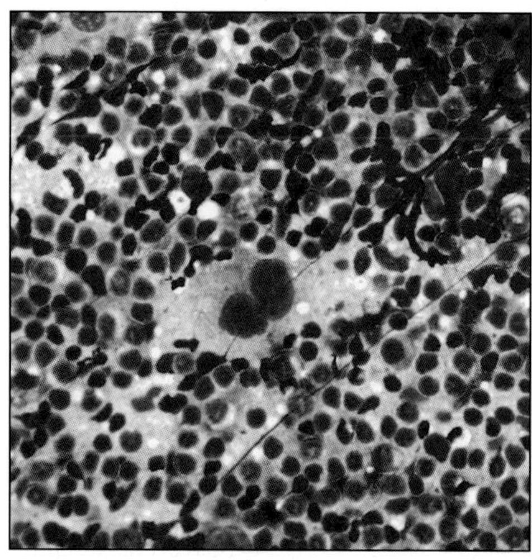

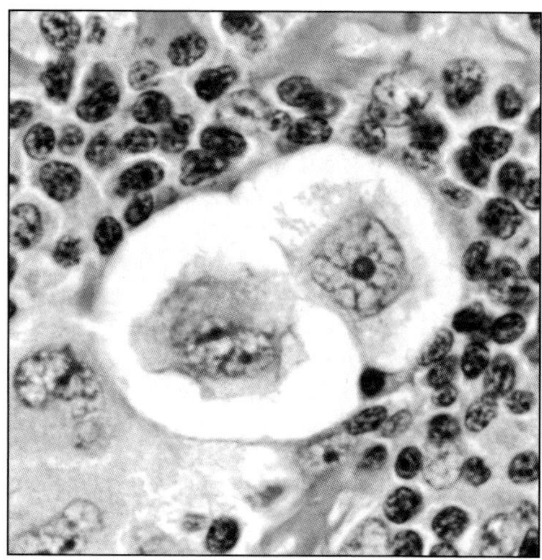

*(**Left**) An anaplastic variant HL cell is shown. The pattern of growth, cellular milieu, and tumor immunophenotype are helpful in making the distinction between CHL and ALCL. (**Right**) Syncytial variant of CHL shows large aggregates of mono- and multinucleate HL cells. Note the scattered eosinophils ➔. The background cellular milieu and immunophenotypic characteristics of the tumor cells are key in distinguishing this from other mimics such as diffuse large B-cell lymphoma and ALCL.*

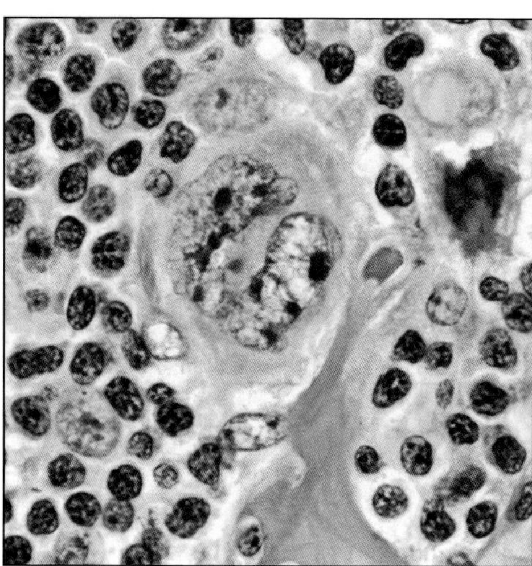

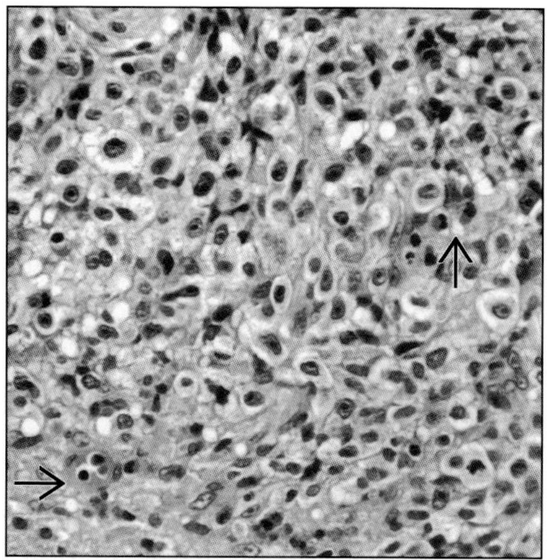

Microscopic Features

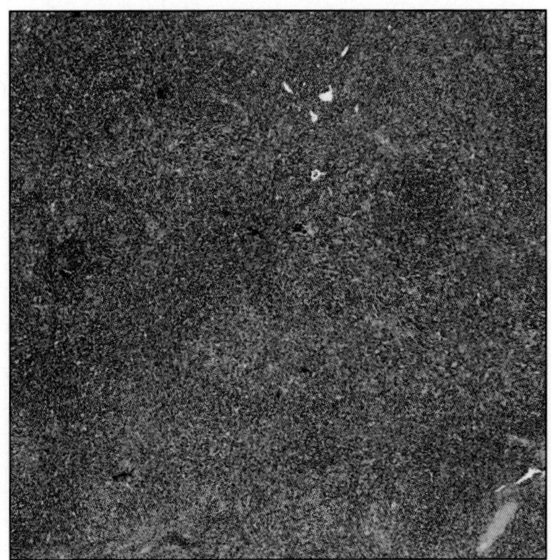

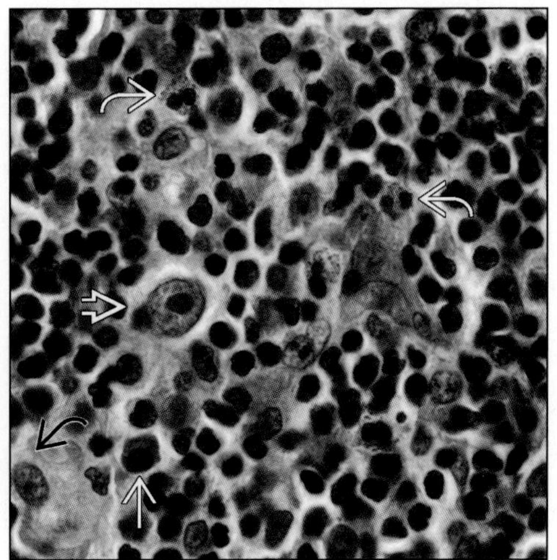

(Left) *Low-power view of MC-HL shows a diffuse to vaguely nodular pattern of growth without fibrosis.* ***(Right)*** *High-power view of MC-HL shows a cellular milieu very similar to that of NS-HL without the broad bands of fibrosis. Note the predominance of small lymphocytes with scattered eosinophils, an occasional plasma cell, and histiocyte. A distinct mononuclear HL cell with thick nuclear membranes and a single large nucleolus is also present.*

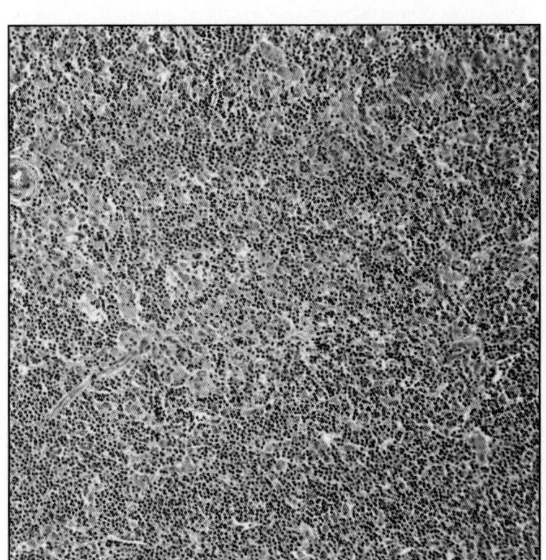

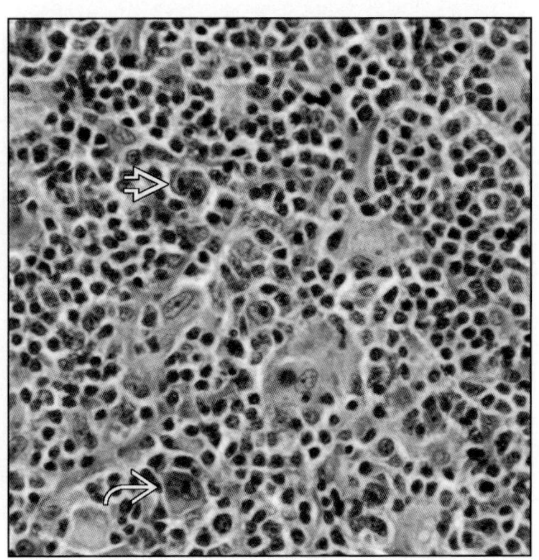

(Left) *Low-power view of LR-HL shows a lymph node completely effaced by a diffuse population of small lymphocytes.* ***(Right)*** *High-power view of LR-HL shows a predominance of small lymphocytes with occasional HRS and Hodgkin cells. Note the lack of eosinophils in the background cellular milieu.*

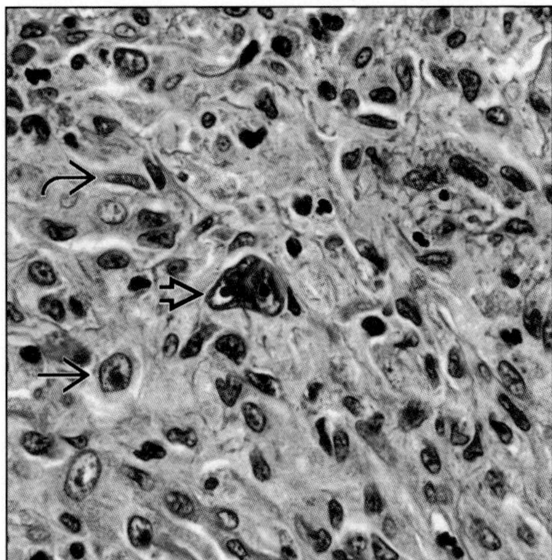

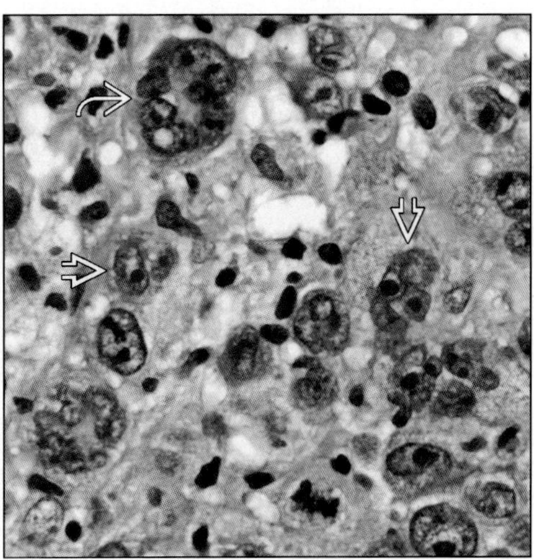

(Left) *LD-CHL involving a lymph node shows a HRS cell and Hodgkin cell admixed with fibroblasts imparting a spindle cell appearance, raising the differential diagnosis with sarcoma. (Courtesy C. Yin, MD, PhD.)* ***(Right)*** *LD-CHL, reticular variant, involves a lymph node. Many HRS cells, some with anaplastic features, are seen admixed with inflammatory cells and few lymphocytes. (Courtesy C. Yin, MD, PhD.)*

Microscopic Features and Ancillary Techniques

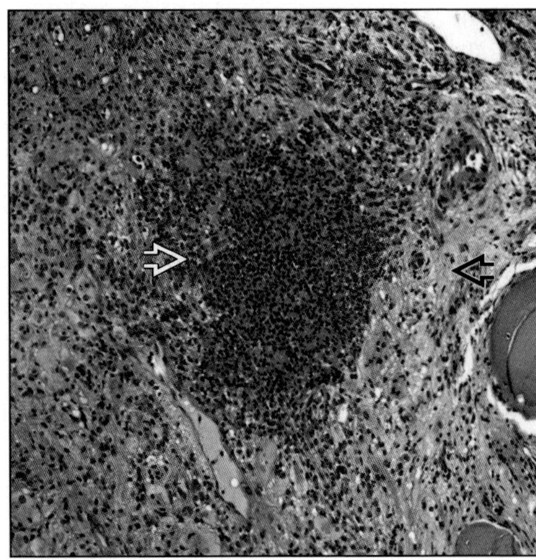

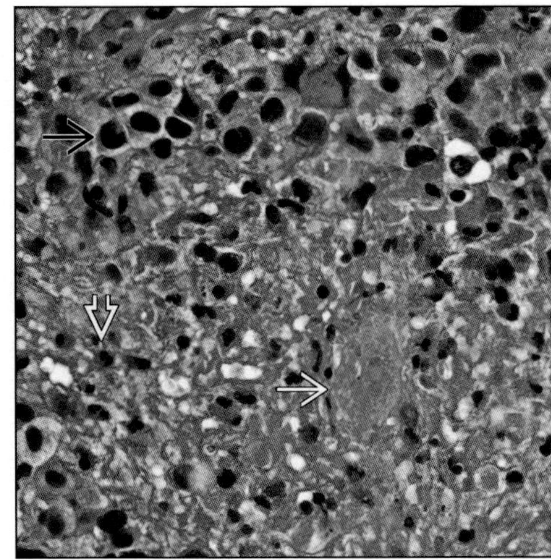

(Left) *NS-CHL involves the bone marrow. Histologic section shows effacement of bone marrow architecture due to stromal fibrosis ⇨ and an eosinophilic abscess ➡. (Courtesy C. Yin, MD, PhD.)* ***(Right)*** *Histologic section of NS-CHL involving the bone marrow shows HRS cells →. However, these cells can be scant or deceptively small. Marked eosinophilia ➡ and focal necrosis ➡ are also noted. (Courtesy C. Yin, MD, PhD.)*

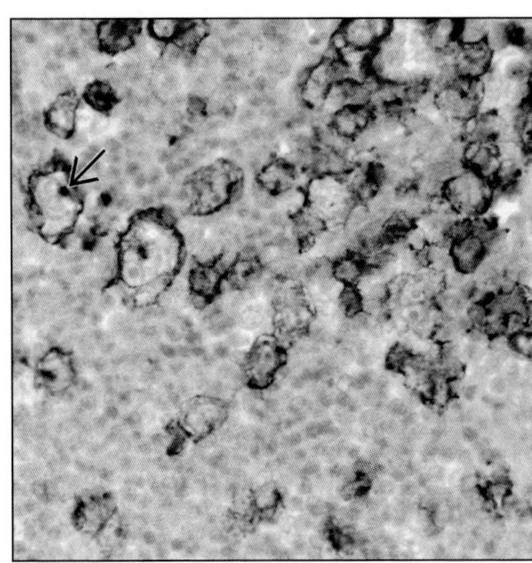

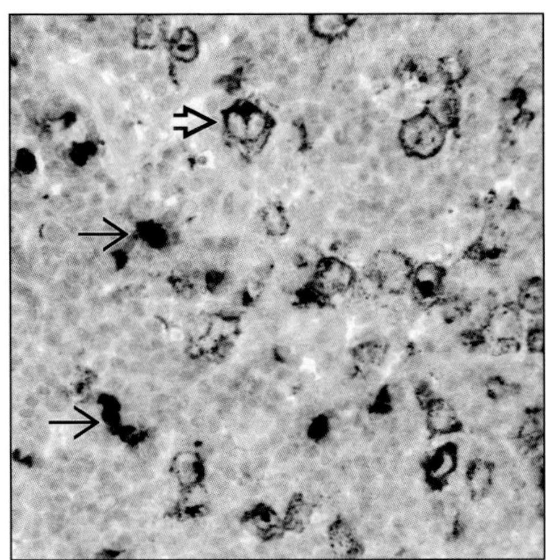

(Left) *CD30 immunostain performed on a lymph node involved by CHL shows the variable weak to strong membrane and Golgi reactivity → of the HRS cells. This pattern of reactivity can be helpful in making the distinction from the CD30(+) cells of ALCL, which typically show uniform strong reactivity.* ***(Right)*** *CD15 immunostain highlights both the HRS ⇨ and neighboring granulocytes →. Evaluation of CD15 can often be difficult due to the abundance of eosinophils in some cases.*

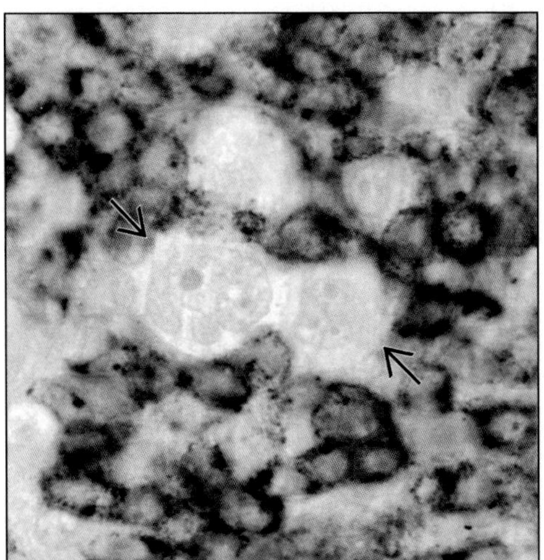

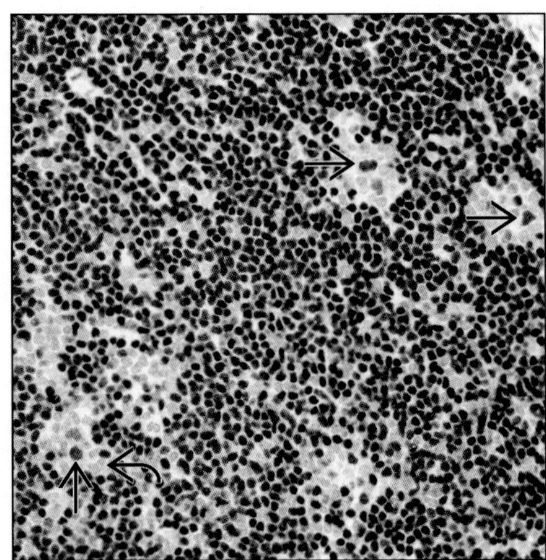

(Left) *Evaluation of CD3 reactivity in CHL often requires finding 2 adjacent HRS cells → to definitively exclude CD3 reactivity, which can be difficult given the numerous surrounding T cells.* ***(Right)*** *LR-CHL, nodular variant, involving a lymph node shows numerous small lymphocytes in the background that are pax-5(+) B cells. Scattered HRS → cells are more dimly pax-5(+) and are surrounded by rosettes of T cells that are negative for this immunostain ↩. (Courtesy S. Wang, MD.)*

Differential Diagnosis

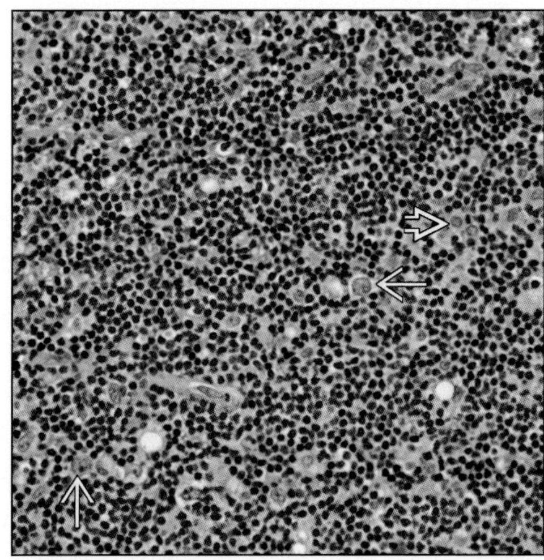

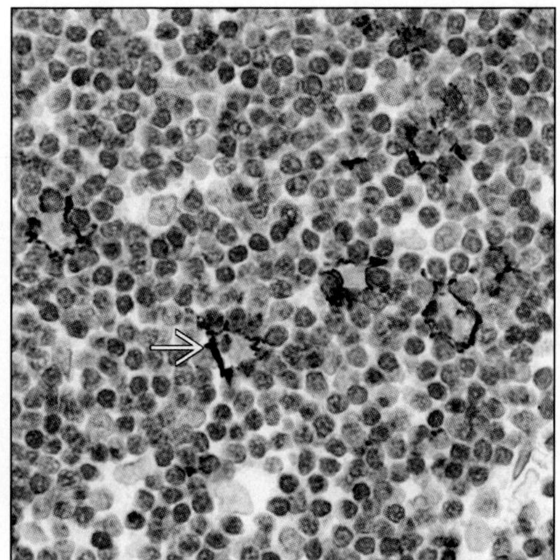

*(**Left**) Characteristic appearance of THRLBCL shows numerous small lymphocytes with occasional histiocytes ⇨ and large tumor cells ➡. Immunostains and the morphologic appearance of the tumor cells are helpful in making the distinction. (**Right**) IHC for CD20 performed in this lymph node involved by TCHRLBCL highlights the large neoplastic cells ➡ that strongly express CD20. Most of the small lymphocytes in the background represent reactive small T cells.*

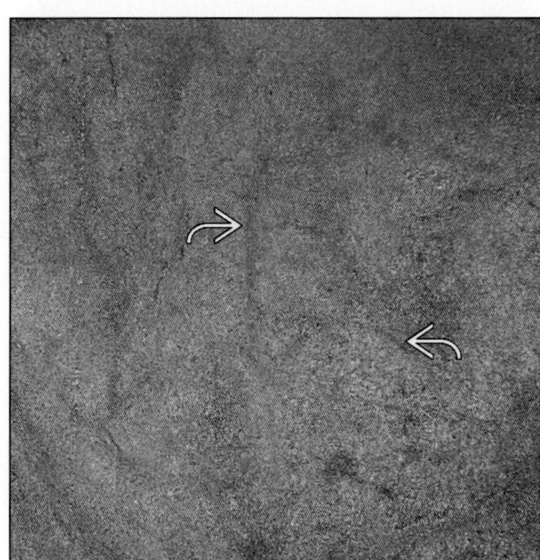

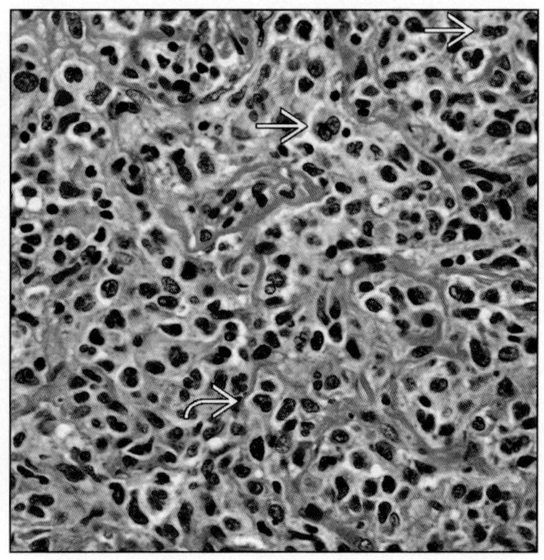

*(**Left**) PMLBCL shows thin bands of fibrosis ↪ imparting a vaguely nodular appearance in contrast to the broad bands of fibrosis seen in NS-CHL. (**Right**) PMLBCL shows thin delicate bands of fibrosis ↪ surrounding individual and small clusters of tumor cells. Occasional multilobated nuclei ➡ with distinct nucleoli are also present but lack the characteristic large eosinophilic nucleoli and immunoprofile of RS and Hodgkin cells.*

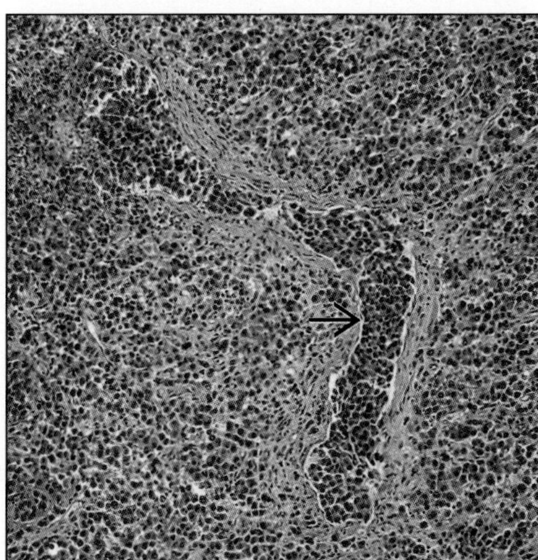

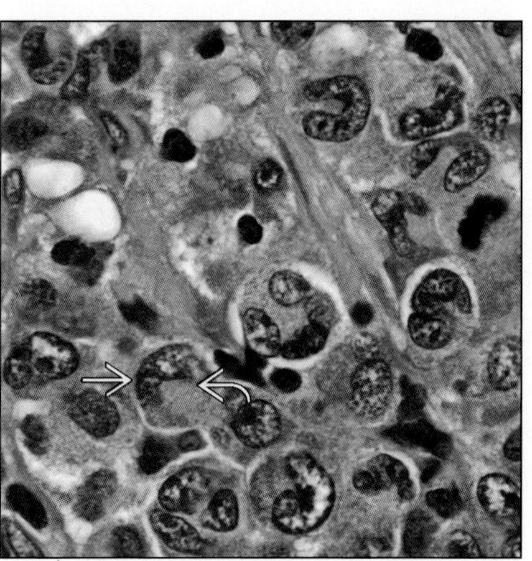

*(**Left**) The characteristic pattern of sinusoidal involvement → is shown in this case of ALK(+) ALCL. (**Right**) High-power image shows the large pleomorphic cells of ALCL. Hallmark cells ➡ are usually present. Note the kidney-shaped nuclei and eosinophilic Golgi region ↪. The diffuse and sinusoidal pattern of growth, along with the immunophenotype, will be helpful in making the distinction from CHL with a syncytial pattern of growth &/or anaplastic HL cells.*

PROTOCOL FOR BONE MARROW SPECIMENS

Bone Marrow: Aspiration, Core (Trephine) Biopsy

Surgical Pathology Cancer Case Summary (Checklist)

Specimen (select all that apply)

___ Peripheral blood smear
___ Bone marrow aspiration
___ Bone marrow aspirate clot (cell block)
___ Bone marrow core (trephine) biopsy
___ Bone marrow core touch preparation (imprint)
___ Other (specify): ___________________________
___ Not specified

Procedure (select all that apply)

___ Aspiration
___ Biopsy
___ Other (specify): ___________________________
___ Not specified

Aspiration Site (if performed) (select all that apply)

___ Right posterior iliac crest
___ Left posterior iliac crest
___ Sternum
___ Other (specify): ___________________________
___ Not specified

Biopsy Site (if performed) (select all that apply)

___ Right posterior iliac crest
___ Left posterior iliac crest
___ Other (specify): ___________________________
___ Not specified

Histologic Type

Note: The following is a partial list of the 2008 World Health Organization (WHO) classification and includes those neoplasms seen in bone marrow specimens

___ Histologic type cannot be assessed

Myeloproliferative neoplasms

___ Chronic myelogenous leukemia, *BCR-ABL1* positive
___ Chronic neutrophilia leukemia
___ Polycythemia vera
___ Primary myelofibrosis
___ Essential thrombocythemia
___ Chronic eosinophilic leukemia, not otherwise specified (NOS)
___ Mastocytosis (specify type): ___________________________
___ Myeloproliferative neoplasm, unclassifiable

Myeloid and lymphoid neoplasms with eosinophilia and abnormalities of PDGFRA, PDGFRB, and FGGR1

___ Myeloid or lymphoid neoplasm with *PDGFRA* rearrangement
___ Myeloid or lymphoid neoplasm with *FGFR1* abnormalities

Myelodysplastic/myeloproliferative neoplasms

___ Chronic myelomonocytic leukemia
___ Atypical chronic myeloid leukemia *BCR-ABL1* negative
___ Juvenile myelomonocytic leukemia
___ Myelodysplastic/myeloproliferative neoplasm, unclassifiable
___ Refractory anemia with ring sideroblasts associated with marked thrombocytosis†

Myelodysplastic syndromes

___ Refractory anemia
___ Refractory neutropenia
___ Refractory thrombocytopenia

____ Refractory anemia with ring sideroblasts
____ Refractory cytopenia with multilineage dysplasia
____ Refractory anemia with excessive blasts
____ Myelodysplastic syndrome associated with isolated del(5q)
____ Myelodysplastic syndrome, unclassifiable
____ Refractory cytopenia of childhood

Acute myeloid leukemia (AML) with recurrent genetic abnormalities

____ AML with t(8;21)(q22;22); *RUNX1-RUNX1T1*
____ AML with inv(16)(p13.1q22) or t(16;16)(p13.1;q22); *CBFB-MYH11*
____ Acute promyelocytic leukemia with t(15;17)(q22;q12); *PML-RARA*
____ AML with t(9;11)(p22;q23); *MLLT3-MLL*
____ AML with t(6;9)(p23;q34); *DEK-NUP214*
____ AML with inv(3)(q21q26.2) or t(3;3)(q21;q26.2); *RPN1-EVI1*
____ AML (megakaryoblastic) with t(1;22)(p13;q13); *RBM15-MKL1*
____ AML with mutated *NPM1*†
____ AML with mutated *CEBPA*†

Acute myeloid leukemia with myelodysplasia-related changes (select all that apply)

____ Multilineage dysplasia
____ Prior myelodysplastic syndrome
____ Myelodysplasia-related cytogenetic abnormalities

Therapy-related myeloid neoplasms

____ Therapy-related AML
____ Therapy-related myelodysplastic syndrome
____ Therapy-related myelodysplastic/myeloproliferative neoplasm

Acute myeloid leukemia, NOS

____ AML with minimal differentiation
____ AML without maturation
____ AML with maturation
____ Acute myelomonocytic leukemia
____ Acute monoblastic/monocytic leukemia
____ Acute erythroid leukemia
____ Acute megakaryocytic leukemia
____ Acute basophilic leukemia
____ Acute panmyelosis with myelofibrosis
____ AML, NOS#

Myeloid proliferations related to Down syndrome

____ Transient abnormal myelopoiesis
____ Myeloid leukemia associated with Down syndrome

Acute leukemias of ambiguous lineage

____ Acute undifferentiated leukemia
____ Mixed phenotype acute leukemia with t(9;22)(q34;q11.2); *BCR-ABL1*
____ Mixed phenotype acute leukemia with t(v;11q23); *MLL* rearranged
____ Mixed phenotype acute leukemia, B/myeloid, NOS
____ Mixed phenotype acute leukemia, T/myeloid, NOS
____ Mixed phenotype acute leukemia, NOS, rare types (specify type): ____________________________
____ Natural killer (NK) cell lymphoblastic leukemia/lymphoma†

Other myeloid leukemias

____ Blastic plasmacytoid dendritic cell neoplasm

Precursor lymphoid neoplasms

____ B lymphoblastic leukemia/lymphoma, NOS#
____ B lymphoblastic leukemia/lymphoma with t(9;22) (q34;q11.2); *BCR-ABL1*
____ B lymphoblastic leukemia/lymphoma with t(v;11q23); *MLL* rearranged
____ B lymphoblastic leukemia/lymphoma with t(12;21)(p13;q22); *TEL-AML1 (ETV6-RUNX1)*
____ B lymphoblastic leukemia/lymphoma with hyperdiploidy

PROTOCOL FOR BONE MARROW SPECIMENS

____ B lymphoblastic leukemia/lymphoma with hypodiploidy (hypodiploid ALL)
____ B lymphoblastic leukemia/lymphoma with t(5;14)(q31;q32); *IL3-IGH*
____ B lymphoblastic leukemia/lymphoma with t(1;19)(q23;p13.3); *E2A-PBX1 (TCF3-PBX1)*
____ T lymphoblastic leukemia/lymphoma

Mature B-cell neoplasms

____ Chronic lymphocytic leukemia/small lymphocytic lymphoma
____ B-cell prolymphocytic leukemia
____ Splenic B-cell marginal zone lymphoma
____ Hairy cell leukemia
____ Splenic B-cell lymphoma/leukemia, unclassifiable†
____ Splenic diffuse red pulp small B-cell lymphoma†
____ Hairy cell leukemia-variant†
____ Lymphoplasmacytic lymphoma
____ Plasma cell myeloma
____ Extranodal marginal zone lymphoma of mucosa-associated lymphoid tissue (MALT lymphoma)
____ Follicular lymphoma
____ Mantle cell lymphoma
____ Diffuse large B-cell lymphoma (DLBCL), NOS
____ T-cell/histiocyte-rich large B-cell lymphoma
____ Primary cutaneous DLBCL, leg type
____ Epstein-Barr virus (EBV)-positive DLBCL of the elderly†
____ DLBCL associated with chronic inflammation
____ Lymphomatoid granulomatosis
____ Anaplastic lymphoma kinase (ALK)-positive large B-cell lymphoma
____ Plasmablastic lymphoma
____ Large B-cell lymphoma arising in HHV8-associated multicentric Castleman disease
____ Burkitt lymphoma
____ B-cell lymphoma, unclassifiable, with features intermediate between diffuse large B-cell lymphoma and Burkitt lymphoma
____ B-cell lymphoma, unclassifiable, with features intermediate between diffuse large B-cell lymphoma and classical Hodgkin lymphoma
____ B-cell lymphoma, NOS
____ Other (specify): ____________________________

Mature T- and NK-cell neoplasms

____ T-cell lymphoma, subtype cannot be determined (not a category within the WHO classification)
____ T-cell prolymphocytic leukemia
____ T-cell large granular lymphocytic leukemia
____ Chronic lymphoproliferative disorder of NK cells†
____ Aggressive NK-cell leukemia
____ Adult T-cell leukemia/lymphoma
____ Extranodal NK/T-cell lymphoma, nasal type
____ Enteropathy-associated T-cell lymphoma
____ Hepatosplenic T-cell lymphoma
____ Mycosis fungoides
____ Peripheral T-cell lymphoma, NOS
____ Angioimmunoblastic T-cell lymphoma
____ Anaplastic large cell lymphoma, ALK(+)
____ Anaplastic large cell lymphoma, ALK(-)†

Hodgkin lymphoma

____ Nodular lymphocyte predominant Hodgkin lymphoma
____ Classical Hodgkin lymphoma

Histiocytic and dendritic cell neoplasms

____ Histiocytic sarcoma
____ Langerhans cell histiocytosis
____ Langerhans cell sarcoma
____ Interdigitating dendritic cell sarcoma

____ Follicular dendritic cell sarcoma
____ Disseminated juvenile xanthogranuloma
____ Histiocytic neoplasm, NOS

Post-transplant lymphoproliferative disorders (PTLD)##

Early lesions:
____ Plasmacytic hyperplasia
____ Infectious mononucleosis-like PTLD
____ Polymorphic PTLD
____ Monomorphic PTLD (B- and T/NK-cell types)
Specify subtype: ____________________
____ Classical Hodgkin lymphoma-type PTLD###
____ Other (specify): ____________________

*Additional Pathologic Findings

*Specify: ____________________

*Cytochemical/Special Stains

*____ Performed
*Specify stains and results: ____________________
*____ Not performed

Immunophenotyping (Flow Cytometry &/or Immunohistochemistry)

____ Performed, see separate report: ____________________
____ Performed
Specify method(s) and results: ____________________
____ Not performed

Cytogenetic Studies

____ Performed, see separate report: ____________________
____ Performed
Specify method(s) and results: ____________________
____ Not performed

*Fluorescence In Situ Hybridization

*____ Performed, see separate report: ____________________
*____ Performed
Specify method(s) and results: ____________________
*____ Not performed

*Molecular Genetic Studies

*____ Performed, see separate report: ____________________
*____ Performed
Specify method(s) and results: ____________________
*____ Not performed

*†These histologic types denote provisional entities in the 2008 WHO classification. #An initial diagnosis of "AML, NOS" or "B-lymphoblastic leukemia/lymphoma, NOS" may need to be given before the cytogenetic results are available or for cases that do not meet criteria for other leukemia subtypes. ##These disorders are listed for completeness, but not all of them represent frank lymphomas. ###Classical Hodgkin lymphoma type PTLD can be reported using either this protocol or the separate College of American Pathologists protocol for Hodgkin lymphoma. *Data elements with asterisks are not required. These elements may be clinically important but are not yet validated or regularly used in patient management. Adapted with permission from College of American Pathologists, "Protocol for the Examination of Specimens from Patients with Hematopoietic Neoplasms Involving the Bone Marrow." Web posting date February 2011, www.cap.org.*

PROTOCOL FOR HODGKIN LYMPHOMA SPECIMENS

Hodgkin Lymphoma: Biopsy, Resection

Surgical Pathology Cancer Case Summary (Checklist)

Specimen (select all that apply)

___ Lymph node(s)
___ Other (specify): ___
___ Not specified

Procedure

___ Biopsy
___ Resection
___ Other (specify): ___
___ Not specified

Tumor Site (select all that apply)

___ Lymph node(s), site not specified
___ Lymph node(s)
Specify site(s): ___
___ Other tissue(s) or organ(s) (specify): ___
___ Not specified

Histologic Type (based on 2008 WHO classification)

___ Nodular lymphocyte predominant Hodgkin lymphoma
___ Classical Hodgkin lymphoma
___ Classical Hodgkin lymphoma, histologic subtype cannot be determined
___ Nodular sclerosis classical Hodgkin lymphoma
___ Mixed cellularity classical Hodgkin lymphoma
___ Lymphocyte-rich classical Hodgkin lymphoma
___ Lymphocyte-depleted classical Hodgkin lymphoma
___ Hodgkin lymphoma, histologic subtype cannot be determined

****Pathologic Extent of Tumor (select all that apply)***

*___ Involvement of a single lymph node region
*Specify sites: ___
*___ Involvement of ≥ 2 lymph node regions on same side of diaphragm
*Specify sites: ___
*___ Involvement of lymph node regions on both sides of diaphragm
*Specify sites: ___
*___ Spleen involvement
*___ Liver involvement
*___ Bone marrow involvement
*___ Other site involvement
*Specify site(s): ___

****Additional Pathologic Findings***

*Specify: ___

Immunophenotyping (Immunohistochemistry)

___ Performed, see separate report: ___
___ Performed
Specify method(s) and results: ___
___ Not performed

****Clinical Prognostic Factors and Indices (select all that apply)***

*___ International Prognostic Score (IPS) (specify): ___
*___ B symptoms present
*___ Other (specify): ___

**Data elements with asterisks are not required. These elements may be clinically important but are not yet validated or regularly used in patient management. Adapted with permission from College of American Pathologists, "Protocol for the Examination of Specimens from Patients with Hodgkin Lymphoma." Web posting date October 2009, www.cap.org.*

Non-Hodgkin Lymphoma/Lymphoid Neoplasms: Biopsy, Resection

Surgical Pathology Cancer Case Summary (Checklist)

Specimen (select all that apply)

___ Lymph node(s)
___ Other (specify): ______________________
___ Not specified

Procedure

___ Biopsy
___ Resection
___ Other (specify): ______________________
___ Not specified

Tumor Site (select all that apply)

___ Lymph node(s), site not specified
___ Lymph node(s)
  Specify site(s): ______________________
___ Other tissue(s) or organ(s): ______________________
___ Not specified

Histologic Type

___ Histologic type cannot be assessed

Precursor lymphoid neoplasms

___ B-lymphoblastic leukemia/lymphoma, not otherwise specified (NOS)#
___ B-lymphoblastic leukemia/lymphoma with t(9;22)(q34;q11.2); *BCR-ABL1*
___ B-lymphoblastic leukemia/lymphoma with t(v;11q23); *MLL* rearranged
___ B-lymphoblastic leukemia/lymphoma with t(12;21)(p13;q22); *TEL-AML1* (*ETV6-RUNX1*)
___ B-lymphoblastic leukemia/lymphoma with hyperdiploidy
___ B-lymphoblastic leukemia/lymphoma with hypodiploidy (hypodiploid acute lymphoblastic leukemia/lymphoma [ALL])
___ B-lymphoblastic leukemia/lymphoma with t(5;14)(q31;q32); *IL3-IGH*
___ B-lymphoblastic leukemia/lymphoma with t(1;19)(q23;p13.3); *E2A-PBX1* (*TCF3-PBX1*)
___ T-lymphoblastic leukemia/lymphoma

Mature B-cell neoplasms

___ B-cell lymphoma, subtype cannot be determined (Note: Not a category within the WHO classification)
___ Chronic lymphocytic leukemia/small lymphocytic lymphoma
___ B-cell prolymphocytic leukemia
___ Splenic B-cell marginal zone lymphoma
___ Hairy cell leukemia
___ Splenic B-cell lymphoma/leukemia, unclassifiable†
___ Splenic diffuse red pulp small B-cell lymphoma†
___ Hairy cell leukemia-variant†
___ Lymphoplasmacytic lymphoma
___ Gamma heavy chain disease
___ Mu heavy chain disease
___ Alpha heavy chain disease
___ Plasma cell myeloma
___ Solitary plasmacytoma of bone
___ Extraosseous plasmacytoma
___ Extranodal marginal zone lymphoma of mucosa-associated lymphoid tissue (MALT lymphoma)
___ Nodal marginal zone lymphoma
___ Pediatric nodal marginal zone lymphoma†
___ Follicular lymphoma
___ Pediatric follicular lymphoma†
___ Primary intestinal follicular lymphoma†
___ Primary cutaneous follicle center lymphoma

PROTOCOL FOR NON-HODGKIN LYMPHOMA SPECIMENS

___ Mantle cell lymphoma
___ Diffuse large B-cell lymphoma (DLBCL), NOS
___ T-cell/histiocyte-rich large B-cell lymphoma
___ Primary DLBCL of central nervous system (CNS)
___ Primary cutaneous DLBCL, leg type
___ Epstein-Barr virus (EBV) positive DLBCL of the elderly†
___ DLBCL associated with chronic inflammation
___ Lymphomatoid granulomatosis
___ Primary mediastinal (thymic) large B-cell lymphoma
___ Intravascular large B-cell lymphoma
___ Anaplastic lymphoma kinase (ALK) positive large B-cell lymphoma
___ Plasmablastic lymphoma
___ Large B-cell lymphoma arising in HHV8-associated multicentric Castleman disease
___ Primary effusion lymphoma
___ Burkitt lymphoma
___ B-cell lymphoma, unclassifiable, with features intermediate between diffuse large B-cell lymphoma and Burkitt lymphoma
___ Other (specify): ______________________

Mature T- and NK-cell neoplasms

___ T-cell lymphoma, subtype cannot be determined (Note: Not a category within the WHO classification)
___ T-cell prolymphocytic leukemia
___ T-cell large granular lymphocytic leukemia
___ Chronic lymphoproliferative disorder of NK cells†
___ Aggressive NK-cell leukemia
___ Systemic EBV(+) T-cell lymphoproliferative disease of childhood
___ Hydroa vacciniforme-like lymphoma
___ Adult T-cell leukemia/lymphoma
___ Extranodal NK/T-cell lymphoma, nasal type
___ Enteropathy-associated T-cell lymphoma
___ Hepatosplenic T-cell lymphoma
___ Subcutaneous panniculitis-like T-cell lymphoma
___ Primary cutaneous anaplastic large cell lymphoma
___ Lymphomatoid papulosis
___ Primary cutaneous gamma-delta T-cell lymphoma
___ Primary cutaneous CD8(+) aggressive epidermotropic cytotoxic T-cell lymphoma†
___ Peripheral T-cell lymphoma, NOS
___ Angioimmunoblastic T-cell lymphoma
___ Anaplastic large cell lymphoma, ALK(+)
___ Anaplastic large cell lymphoma, ALK(-)†
___ Other (specify): ______________________

Histiocytic and dendritic cell neoplasms

___ Histiocytic sarcoma
___ Langerhans cell histiocytosis
___ Langerhans cell sarcoma
___ Interdigitating dendritic cell sarcoma
___ Fibroblastic reticular cell tumor†
___ Indeterminate dendritic cell tumor†
___ Disseminated juvenile xanthogranuloma

Post-transplant lymphoproliferative disorders (PTLD)##

Early lesions

___ Plasmacytic hyperplasia
___ Infectious mononucleosis-like PTLD
___ Polymorphic PTLD
___ Monomorphic PTLD (B- and T/NK cell types)
Specify subtype: ______________________

___ Classical Hodgkin lymphoma type PTLD###

*Pathologic Extent of Tumor (select all that apply)

*___ Involvement of a single lymph node region

*Specify site: ___________________________

*___ Involvement of ≥ 2 lymph node regions on same side of diaphragm

*Specify sites: ___________________________

*___ Spleen involvement

*___ Liver involvement

*___ Bone marrow involvement

*___ Other site involvement

*Specify site(s): ___________________________

*Additional Pathologic Findings

*Specify: ___________________________

Immunophenotyping (Flow Cytometry &/or Immunohistochemistry)

___ Performed, see separate report: ___________________________

___ Performed

*Specify method(s) and results: ___________________________

*___ Not performed

*Cytogenetic Studies

___ Performed, see separate report: ___________________________

___ Performed

*Specify method(s) and results: ___________________________

*___ Not performed

*Molecular Genetic Studies

___ Performed, see separate report: ___________________________

___ Performed

*Specify method(s) and results: ___________________________

*___ Not performed

*Clinical Prognostic Factors and Indices (select all that apply)

*___ International Prognostic Index (IPI) (specify): __________

*___ Follicular Lymphoma International Prognostic Index (FLIPI) (specify): __________

*___ B symptoms present

*___ Other (specify): ___________________________

*Data elements with asterisks are not required. These elements may be clinically important but are not yet validated or regularly used in patient management. †Denotes provisional entities in the 2008 WHO classification. #An initial diagnosis of "B lymphoblastic leukemia/lymphoma, NOS" may need to be given before the cytogenetic results are available. ##These disorders are listed for completeness, but not all of them represent frank lymphomas. ###Classical Hodgkin lymphoma type PTLD can be reported using either this protocol or the separate College of American Pathologists protocol for Hodgkin lymphoma. Adapted with permission from College of American Pathologists, "Protocol for the Examination of Specimens from Patients with Non-Hodgkin Lymphoma/Lymphoid Neoplasms." Web posting date June 2010, www.cap.org.

Reference

Antibody Index

Molecular Factors Index

ANTIBODY INDEX

Antibodies Discussed

Antibody Name/ Symbol	Antibody Description	Clones/Alternative Names	Chapters
α-1-antichymotrypsin	alpha 1 antichromotrypsin		Calcifying Fibrous Tumor
α-1-antitrypsin	alpha 1 antitrypsin	A1AT	Yolk Sac Tumor
α-fetoprotein	alpha 1 fetoprotein	AFP, Z5A06, Clone C3	Ependymoblastoma; Focal Nodular Hyperplasia; Hepatoblastoma; Hepatocellular Carcinoma; Juvenile Granulosa Cell Tumor; Mesenchymal Hamartoma; Pancreatoblastoma; Sertoli-Leydig Cell Tumors; Teratomas; Yolk Sac Tumor
β-2-microglobulin		B2-microglob	Nodular Lymphocyte Predominant Hodgkin Lymphoma
β-catenin	beta catenin; involved in regulation of cell adhesion and in signal transduction through Wnt pathway	B-catenin, CLONE 14, E-5, RB-9035Po, 17C2, 5H10	Adrenal Cortical Adenoma; Adrenal Cortical Carcinoma; Calcifying Fibrous Tumor; Craniopharyngioma; Desmoid Fibromatosis; Familial Adenomatous Polyposis; Fibroma; Fibromatosis Colli; Gardner Fibroma; Gastrointestinal Stromal Tumor; Hepatoblastoma; Infantile Fibrosarcoma; Infantile/ Juvenile Hyaline Fibromatosis; Inflammatory Myofibroblastic Tumor; Medulloblastoma; Myofibroma and Myofibromatosis; Nodular Fasciitis; Pancreatoblastoma; Papillary Thyroid Carcinoma; Pilomatricoma; Rhabdoid Tumor; Synovial Sarcoma; Wilms Tumor
β-catenin-nuclear	beta catenin nuclear		Desmoid Fibromatosis; Familial Adenomatous Polyposis; Gardner Fibroma; Hemangiopericytoma
β-tubulin	beta tubulin	B-tubulin, TUJ1	Pineal Parenchymal Tumors; Subependymal Giant Cell Tumor
κ light chain	kappa light chain	KAPPA	Autoimmune Lymphoproliferative Syndrome; Overview of Lymphoproliferative Disorders Associated with Primary Immune Deficiency
λ light chain	lambda light chain	LAMBDA	Autoimmune Lymphoproliferative Syndrome; Overview of Lymphoproliferative Disorders Associated with Primary Immune Deficiency
ACTH	adrenocorticotropic hormone		Adrenal Cortical Adenoma
Actin-HHF-35	actin, muscle (HHF35)	MSA, HHF-35	Hemangiopericytoma; Infantile Fibrosarcoma; Kaposiform Hemangioendothelioma; Mucoepidermoid Carcinoma; Myofibroma and Myofibromatosis; Rhabdomyosarcoma
Actin-sm	actin, smooth muscle	SMA, ASM-1, CGA7, 1A4, HUC1-1	Atypical Teratoid/Rhabdoid Tumor; Fibroma; Fibrous Umbilical Polyp; Gastrointestinal Stromal Tumor; Glomus Tumor; Hemangioma of Infancy; Hemangiopericytoma; Inclusion Body Fibromatosis; Infantile Fibromatosis; Infantile Fibrosarcoma; Inflammatory Myofibroblastic Tumor; Mesoblastic Nephroma; Myofibroma and Myofibromatosis; Neurothekeoma; Nodular Fasciitis; Pleomorphic Adenoma; Sialoblastoma
AE1/AE3	mixture of 2 anticytokeratin clones that detect a variety of both high-and low-molecular weight cytokeratins		Adamantinoma; Adrenal Cortical Carcinoma; Chordoma; Desmoplastic Small Round Cell Tumor; Glomus Tumor; Infantile Fibrosarcoma; Medulloblastoma; Melanotic Neuroectodermal Tumor of Infancy; MiTF/TFE Family Translocation-associated Carcinoma; Neuroendocrine Tumors; Papillary Thyroid Carcinoma; Pleuropulmonary Blastoma; Rhabdoid Tumor; Secretory Carcinoma; Thymoma

ANTIBODY INDEX

AFP	Alpha 1 fetoprotein	α-fetoprotein, Z5A06, Clone C3	Gingival Granular Cell Tumor of the Newborn; Hepatoblastoma; Pancreatoblastoma; Pineal Parenchymal Tumors; Teratomas
ALK	anaplastic lymphoma kinase 1	ALK1, 5A4, ALKC	Anaplastic Large Cell Lymphoma, ALK +; Calcifying Fibrous Tumor; Diffuse Large B-Cell Lymphoma; Inflammatory Myofibroblastic Tumor; Omental Mesenteric Hamartoma
ALK1	anaplastic lymphoma kinase 1	5A4, ALKC	Anaplastic Large Cell Lymphoma, ALK +; Calcifying Fibrous Tumor; Diffuse Large B-Cell Lymphoma; Inflammatory Myofibroblastic Tumor; Neuroblastoma and Ganglioneuroblastoma
AMACR	alpha-methylacyl-CoA racemase (AMACR)	13H4, P504S	MiTF/TFE Family Translocation-associated Carcinoma; Wilms Tumor
Androgen receptor	androgen receptor	AR441, F39.4.1, AR-N20, ANDROGEN RE	Gynecomastia Trichoepithelioma
APC	adenomatous polyposis coliprotein		Desmoid Fibromatosis; Familial Adenomatous Polyposis; Gardner Fibroma
Aromatase	key enzyme in the byosynthesis of estrogen		Gynecomastia
Basic fibroblast growth factor		FGF2, BFGF, BASIC FGF	Intravascular Papillary Endothelial Hyperplasia
Bcl-2	B-cell lymphoma 2; suppresses apoptosis in a variety of cell systems	ONCL2, BCL2/100/D5, 124, 124.3	Anaplastic Large Cell Lymphoma, ALK+; Burkitt Lymphoma; Diffuse Large B-Cell Lymphoma; Fibrous Histiocytoma; Hemangiopericytoma; Nodular Lymphocyte Predominant Hodgkin Lymphoma; Pediatric Follicular Lymphoma; Synovial Sarcoma; Thymoma; Trichoepithelioma
Bcl-6	B-cell CLL/lymphoma 6	LN22, GI191E/A8, N-3, PG-B6P, P1F6, 3FR-1	Burkitt Lymphoma; Classical Hodgkin Lymphoma; Diffuse Large B-Cell Lymphoma; Nodular Lymphocyte Predominant Hodgkin Lymphoma; Pediatric Follicular Lymphoma
BER-EP4	epithelial cell adhesion molecule	AUA1, VU-1D9, EPCAM, C10, HEA125	Trichoepithelioma
BOB1	B-cell OCT-binding protein 1	SC955, BOB.1	Classical Hodgkin Lymphoma; Diffuse Large B-Cell Lymphoma; Nodular Lymphocyte Predominant Hodgkin; Lymphoma; Primary Mediastinal (Thymic) Large B-cell Lymphoma
C-Kit	C-kit; tyrosine-protein kinase activity	CD117, C-19 (C-KIT), 104D2, 2E4, CKIT, A4502, H300, CMA-767	Desmoid Fibromatosis; Inflammatory Polyps; Mastocytosis
CA9	carbonic anhydrase IX	CAIX, ab1508, M75, NB100-417	MiTF/TFE Family Translocation-associated Carcinoma
Calcitonin	polypeptide hormone produced by parafollicular cells (C cells) of the thyroid	CALBINDIN28	Follicular Adenoma; Medullary Thyroid Carcinoma; Neuroendocrine Tumors; Papillary Thyroid Carcinoma
Caldesmon	actin interacting and calmodulin binding protein found in smooth muscle and other cell types		Myofibroma and Myofibromatosis
Calponin	thin filament-associated protein that is implicated in regulation and modulation of smooth muscle contraction	N3, 26A11, CALP, CNN1, SMCC, Sm Calp	Chondromyxoid Fibroma; Hemangiopericytoma; Inclusion Body Fibromatosis; Myofibroma and Myofibromatosis; Pleomorphic Adenoma
Calretinin	29 kDa calcium binding protein that is expressed in central and peripheral nervous system and in many normal and pathological tissues	DAK-CALRET, 5A5, CAL 3F5, DC8, AB149	Adrenal Cortical Carcinoma; Juvenile Granulosa Cell Tumor; Sertoli-Leydig Cell Tumors; Synovial Sarcoma; Thecoma-Fibroma
CAM5.2	cytokeratin 8/18 (CAM5.2)	5D3, Zym5.2, 5D3, CAM 5.2, KER 10.11, NCL-5D3	Choroid Plexus Tumors
Carcinoembryogenic antigen		CEA-M, mCEA, CEA-B18, CEA-D14, CEAGOLD 1, T84.6, CEA-GOLD 2, CEA 11, CEA-GOLD 3, CEA 27, CEAGOLD 4, CEA 41, CEA-GOLD 5, T84.1, CEA-M, A5B7, CEJ065, IL-7, T84.66, TF3H8-1, 0062, D14, alpha-7, PARLAM 1, ZC23, CEM010, A115, COL-1, AF4, 12.140.10, 11-7, M773, CEA-M431_31, CEJO65	Medullary Thyroid Carcinoma; Syringoma; Teratomas

ANTIBODY INDEX

CD1a	T-cell surface glycoprotein	JPM30, CD1A, O10, NA1/34	Chondroblastoma; Juvenile Xanthogranuloma; Langerhans Cell Histiocytosis; Thymoma
CD2	T-cell surface antigen, LFA2	271, MT910, AB75, LFA-2	Anaplastic Large Cell Lymphoma, ALK +; Autoimmune Lymphoproliferative Syndrome; B Lymphoblastic Leukemia/ Lymphoma; Mastocytosis; Primary Mediastinal (Thymic) Large B-Cell Lymphoma
CD3	T-cell receptor	F7238, A0452, CD3-P, CD3-M, SP7, PS1	Anaplastic Large Cell Lymphoma, ALK +; Autoimmune Lymphoproliferative Syndrome; Classical Hodgkin Lymphoma; Desmoplastic Small Round Cell Tumor; Diffuse Large B-Cell Lymphoma; Nodular Lymphocyte Predominant Hodgkin Lymphoma; Overview of Lymphoproliferative Disorders Associated with Primary Immune Deficiency; Primary Mediastinal (Thymic) Large B-Cell Lymphoma; T Lymphoblastic Leukemia/ Lymphoma; Thymoma
CD4	T-cell surface glycoprotein, L3T4	IF6, 1290, 4B12, 1F6, CD04	Acute Myeloid Leukemia; Anaplastic Large Cell Lymphoma, ALK+; Autoimmune Lymphoproliferative Syndrome; Burkitt Lymphoma; Classical Hodgkin Lymphoma; Diffuse Large B-Cell Lymphoma; Myeloid Sarcoma; T Lymphoblastic Leukemia/Lymphoma
CD5	T-cell surface glycoprotein Leu1, T1	NCL-CD5, 4C7, 54/B4, 54/F6	Anaplastic Large Cell Lymphoma, ALK +; Autoimmune Lymphoproliferative Syndrome; Childhood Myelodysplastic Syndrome; T Lymphoblastic Leukemia/ Lymphoma; Thymoma
CD7	T-cell antigen precursor Leu 9	272, CD7-272	Anaplastic Large Cell Lymphoma, ALK +; Autoimmune Lymphoproliferative Syndrome; B Lymphoblastic Leukemia/ Lymphoma; Diffuse Large B-Cell Lymphoma; Myeloid Sarcoma; T Lymphoblastic Leukemia/Lymphoma
CD8	T-cell coreceptor antigen, Leu 2, T-cytotoxic cells	M7103, C8/144, C8/144B	Autoimmune Lymphoproliferative Syndrome; Primary Mediastinal (Thymic) Large B-Cell Lymphoma
CD9	motility-related protein-1 (MRP-1)	72F16, BA-2	Mastocytosis
CD10	neutral endopeptidase	NCL-270, CALLA, neprilysin, neutral endopeptidase, NEP	B Lymphoblastic Leukemia/Lymphoma; Burkitt Lymphoma; Diffuse Large B-Cell Lymphoma; Hepatocellular Carcinoma; MiTF/TFE Family Translocation-associated Carcinoma; Pancreatoblastoma; Pediatric Follicular Lymphoma; Pleomorphic Adenoma; Primary Mediastinal (Thymic) Large B-Cell Lymphoma
CD13	plays role in growth of DC/macrophage progenitors and precursors		Acute Myeloid Leukemia; B Lymphoblastic Leukemia/Lymphoma; Childhood Myelodysplastic Syndrome
CD14	coreceptor for lipopolysaccharide binding protein	FMC32	Mastocytosis
CD15	reacts with Reed-Sternberg cells of Hodgkin disease and with granulocytes	VIM-2,3C4, LEU-M1, TU9, VIM-D5, MY1, CBD1, MMA, 3CD1, C3D1, Lewis x, SSEA-1	Anaplastic Large Cell Lymphoma, ALK+; Childhood Myelodysplastic Syndrome; Classical Hodgkin Lymphoma; Diffuse Large B-Cell Lymphoma; Inflammatory Myofibroblastic Tumor; Nodular Lymphocyte Predominant Hodgkin Lymphoma
CD16	Fc receptor of IgG		Childhood Myelodysplastic Syndrome; Mastocytosis
CD19	B-cell antigen		B Lymphoblastic Leukemia/Lymphoma; Burkitt Lymphoma
CD20	tumor necrosis factor SF8	BER-H2, KI-1, TNFRSF8	Anaplastic Large Cell Lymphoma, ALK +; Autoimmune Lymphoproliferative Syndrome; B Lymphoblastic Leukemia/ Lymphoma; Burkitt Lymphoma; Classical Hodgkin Lymphoma; Diffuse Large B-Cell Lymphoma; Myeloid Sarcoma;

			Nodular Lymphocyte Predominant Hodgkin Lymphoma; Overview of Lymphoproliferative Disorders Associated with Primary Immune Deficiency Pediatric Follicular Lymphoma; Primary Mediastinal (Thymic) Large B-Cell Lymphoma; T Lymphoblastic Leukemia/ Lymphoma; Thymoma
CD21	CR2, complement component receptor 2, Epstein-Barr virus receptor	IF8	Classical Hodgkin Lymphoma; Nodular Lymphocyte Predominant Hodgkin Lymphoma
CD22	B-cell receptor	FPC1, LEU 14	B Lymphoblastic Leukemia/Lymphoma; Burkitt Lymphoma; Classical Hodgkin Lymphoma; Diffuse Large B-Cell Lymphoma; Primary Mediastinal (Thymic) Large B-Cell Lymphoma
CD23	Fc ϵ RII, low-affinity IgE receptor, IGEBF	1B12, MHM6BU38	Primary Mediastinal (Thymic) Large B-Cell Lymphoma; Diffuse Large B-Cell Lymphoma
CD25	If-2 receptor alpha	2A3, 4C9	B Lymphoblastic Leukemia/Lymphoma; Hemophagocytic Syndrome; Mastocytosis
CD30	tumor necrosis factor SF8	BER-H2, KI-1, TNFRSF8	Anaplastic Large Cell Lymphoma, ALK +; Classical Hodgkin Lymphoma; Diffuse Large B-Cell Lymphoma; Inflammatory Myofibroblastic Tumor; Langerhans Cell Histiocytosis; Nodular Lymphocyte Predominant Hodgkin Lymphoma; Primary Mediastinal (Thymic) Large B-Cell Lymphoma
CD31	platelet endothelial cell adhesion molecule	JC/70, JC/70A, PECAM-1	Cavernous Hemangioma; Glomus Tumor; Hemangioendothelioma; Hemangioma of Infancy; Kaposiform Hemangioendothelioma; Malignant Peripheral Nerve Sheath Tumor; Myeloid Proliferations Related to Down Syndrome; Pseudoangiomatous Stromal Hyperplasia; Spindle Cell Hemangioma; Tufted Angioma
CD33	SIGLEC lectin 3	PWS44	Acute Myeloid Leukemia; B Lymphoblastic Leukemia/Lymphoma; Childhood Myelodysplastic Syndrome; Myeloid Sarcoma
CD34	hematopoietic progenitor cell antigen	MY10, IOM34, QBEND10, 8G12, 1309, HPCA-1, NU-4A1, TUK4, clone 581, BI-3c5	Acute Myeloid Leukemia; B Lymphoblastic Leukemia/Lymphoma; Calcifying Fibrous Tumor; Cavernous Hemangioma; Childhood Myelodysplastic Syndrome; Clear Cell Sarcoma; Desmoid Fibromatosis; Fibrous Umbilical Polyp; Gardner Fibroma; Gastrointestinal Stromal Tumor; Giant Cell Fibroblastoma/ Dermatofibrosarcoma Protuberans; Hemangioendothelioma; Hemangioma of Infancy; Hemangiopericytoma; Kaposiform Hemangioendothelioma; Malignant Melanoma; Myeloid Proliferations Related to Down Syndrome; Myeloid Sarcoma; Myofibroma and Myofibromatosis; Neurofibroma; Proliferative Fasciitis/Myositis; Pseudoangiomatous Stromal Hyperplasia; Rhabdoid Tumor; Synovial Sarcoma; T Lymphoblastic Leukemia/Lymphoma; Trichoepithelioma; Tufted Angioma
CD38	acute lymphoblastic T-cell antigen	SPC32, VS38, T10	Diffuse Large B-Cell Lymphoma
CD42b	platelet surface membrane glycoprotein that functions as a receptor for von Willebrand factor (VWF)	glycoprotein Ib, GP lb	Acute Myeloid Leukemia; Myeloid Proliferations Related to Down Syndrome
CD43	major sialoglycoprotein on surface of human T lymphocytes, monocytes, granulocytes, and some B lymphocytes	LEU-22, DF-T1, L60, MT1, sialophorin, leukosialin, SPN	Burkitt Lymphoma; Myeloid Sarcoma
CD44	CD 44 (cell adhesion receptor for hyaluronic acid HCAM)	HCAM, CD44H, B-F24, A3D8, 2C5, CD44S, F10-44.2, 156-3C11, DF1485, BBA10, VFF-14, CD44V10, CD44V3, 3G5, CD44V3-10-P, CD44V3-10, 3D2, CD44V4_5, CD44V5,	Burkitt Lymphoma

ANTIBODY INDEX

		VFF-8, VFF-7, 2F10, VFF-18, CD44V6, CD44V7, VFF-9, CD44V7_8, VFF-17	
CD45	leukocyte common antigen	LCA, PD7/26, 1.22/4.14, T29/33, RP2/18, PD7, 2D1, 2B11+PD7/26	Anaplastic Large Cell Lymphoma, ALK+; B Lymphoblastic Leukemia/Lymphoma; Classical Hodgkin Lymphoma; Desmoplastic Small Round Cell Tumor; Diffuse Large B-Cell Lymphoma; Ewing Sarcoma; Nodular Lymphocyte Predominant Hodgkin Lymphoma; Primary Mediastinal (Thymic) Large B-Cell Lymphoma; Retinoblastoma
CD45RA	isoform of CD45 expressed by naive T cells	4KB5, MT2, CD45RA, MB1	Autoimmune Lymphoproliferative Syndrome
CD45RO	isoform of CD45 located on memory T cells	ICH1-L, low molecular weight isoform LCA	Autoimmune Lymphoproliferative Syndrome
CD56	NCAM (neutral cellular adhesion molecule)	MAB735, ERIC-1, 25-KD11, 123C3, 24-MB2, BC56C04, 1B6, 14-MAB735, NCC-LU-243, MOC-1, NCAM	Diffuse Large B-Cell Lymphoma; Neuroblastoma and Ganglioneuroblastoma; Neuroendocrine Tumors; Synovial Sarcoma
CD57	β-1,3-glucuronyltransferase 1 (glucuronosyltransferase P)	LEU-7, NK1, HNK-1, TB01, B3GAT1	Diffuse Large B-Cell Lymphoma; Melanotic Neuroectodermal Tumor of Infancy; Neuroendocrine Tumors; Neurothekeoma; Nodular Lymphocyte Predominant Hodgkin Lymphoma; Wilms Tumor
CD61	cluster of differentiation found on thrombocytes corresponding to glycoprotein IIb/IIIa	Integrin, beta 3 (platelet glycoprotein IIIa), ITGB3, GP3A, GPIIIa, Y2/5, HPA	Acute Myeloid Leukemia; Childhood Myelodysplastic Syndrome; Myeloid Proliferations Related to Down Syndrome
CD63	tetraspan intracellular granule protein	NKI/C3, basophil activation test in allergy	Giant Cell Fibroblastoma/ Dermatofibrosarcoma Protuberans; Neurothekeoma
CD68	cytoplasmic granule protein of monocytes, macrophages	PG-M1, KP-1	Fibrous Histiocytoma; Gingival Granular Cell Tumor of the Newborn; Juvenile Myelomonocytic Leukemia; Juvenile Xanthogranuloma; Myeloid Sarcoma; Proliferative Fasciitis/Myositis
CD71	protein required for iron delivery from transferrin to cells	transferrin receptor protein 1 (TfR1)	Acute Myeloid Leukemia; Childhood Myelodysplastic Syndrome
CD79-a	immunoglobulin-associated alpha, MB1	MB-1, 11D10, 11E3, CD79A, HM47/A9, HM57, JCB117, CD79a, CD79-a	Anaplastic Large Cell Lymphoma, ALK +; Diffuse Large B-Cell Lymphoma; Primary Mediastinal (Thymic) Large B-Cell Lymphoma
CD79-α	immunoglobulin-associated alpha, MB1	MB-1, 11D10, 11E3, CD79A, HM47/ A9, HM57, JCB117, CD79a, CD79-α	Burkitt Lymphoma; Classical Hodgkin Lymphoma; Ewing Sarcoma; Primary Mediastinal (Thymic) Large B-Cell Lymphoma
CD95	fatty acid synthase; plays a role in regulating apoptosis	FAS, APO-1, CD95, UB2, B-10, FAS	Autoimmune Lymphoproliferative Syndrome
CD99	cell surface glycoprotein for migration, T cell adhesion, MIC2	CD99-MEMB, MIC2, 12E7, HBA71, O13, P30/32MIC2, M3601	Anaplastic Large Cell Lymphoma, ALK +; Burkitt Lymphoma; Desmoplastic Small Round Cell Tumor; Ewing Sarcoma; Inclusion Body Fibromatosis; Juvenile Granulosa Cell Tumor; Neuroblastoma and Ganglioneuroblastoma; Primitive Neuroectodermal Tumor; Rhabdomyosarcoma; Synovial Sarcoma; Teratomas; Thymoma
CD117	C-kit, tyrosine-protein kinase activity	C-19 (C-KIT), 104D2, 2E4, C-KIT, A4502, H300, CMA-767	Acute Myeloid Leukemia; Calcifying Fibrous Tumor; Choroid Plexus Tumor; Childhood Myelodysplastic Syndrome; Dysgerminoma; Gastrointestinal Stromal Tumor; Gonadoblastoma; Infantile Fibromatosis; Inflammatory Myofibroblastic Tumor; Mastocytosis; Myeloid Proliferations Related to Down Syndrome; Pleomorphic Adenoma; Secretory Carcinoma; Thymoma
CD138	syndecan; a useful marker for plasma cells	B-B4, AM411-10M, MI15	Anaplastic Large Cell Lymphoma, ALK+; Burkitt Lymphoma; Diffuse Large B-Cell Lymphoma
CD163	macrophage hemoglobin scavenging system	10D6	Acute Myeloid Leukemia

ANTIBODY INDEX

CD271	nerve growth factor receptor	ME 20.4, MS-394-P1, P75NGFR, NGFR5, P75NTR	Giant Cell Fibroblastoma/ Dermatofibrosarcoma Protuberans
CD303	monoclonal antibody directed toward immature plasmacytoid dendritic cells	BDCA-2	Myeloid Sarcoma
CEA-M	carcinoembryonic antigen, monoclonal	CEA-B18, CEA-D14, CEA-GOLD 1, T84.6, CEA-GOLD 2, CEA 11, CEA-GOLD 3, CEA 27, CEA-GOLD 4, CEA 41, CEA-GOLD 5, T84.1, CEA-M, A5B7, CEJ065, IL-7, T84.66, TF3H8-1, 0062, D14, alpha-7, PARLAM 1, ZC23, CEM010, A115, COL-1, AF4, 12.140.10, 11-7, M773, CEA-M431_31, CEJO65, mCEA	Follicular Adenoma; Medullary Thyroid Carcinoma
CEA-P	carcinoembryonic antigen, polyclonal		Hepatocellular Carcinoma; Medullary Thyroid Carcinoma; Yolk Sac Tumor
Chromogranin-A	pituitary secretory protein 1	PHE-5, PHE5, E001, DAK-A3	Medullary Thyroid Carcinoma; Follicular Adenoma; Islet Cell Adenoma; Medullary Thyroid Carcinoma; Neuroendocrine Tumors; Pancreatoblastoma
Chymase	serine protease found in mast cells and basophils; acts as a mediator of inflammation		Mastocytosis
Chymotrypsin	digestive enzyme synthesized in pancreas, involved in proteolysis		Pancreatoblastoma
CITED-1	melanocyte specific gene 1 antibody, CBP/P300-interacting transactivator 1	J72220K, MSG1	Follicular Adenoma; Papillary Thyroid Carcinoma
CK-PAN	cytokeratin-pan (AE1/AE3/LP34); cocktail of high and low molecular weight cytokeratins	keratin pan, MAK-6, K576, LU-5, KL-1, KC-8, MNF 116, pankeratin, pancytokeratin	Follicular Adenoma; Gingival Granular Cell Tumor of the Newborn; Mucoepidermoid Carcinoma; Myofibroma and Myofibromatosis; Pancreatoblastoma; Pleomorphic Adenoma; Sialoblastoma; Synovial Sarcoma; T Lymphoblastic Leukemia/Lymphoma; Thecoma-Fibroma; Yolk Sac Tumor
CK5/6	cytokeratin 5/6, high molecular weight cytokeratins	D5/16 B4	Mucoepidermoid Carcinoma
CK7	cytokeratin 7, low molecular weight cytokeratin	K72.7, KS7.18, OVTL 12/30, LDS-68, CK 07	Craniopharyngioma; MiTF/TFE Family Translocation-associated Carcinoma; Mucoepidermoid Carcinoma; Papillary Thyroid Carcinoma; Pleomorphic Adenoma; Sertoli-Leydig Cell Tumors; Synovial Sarcoma Wilms Tumor
CK8	cytokeratin 8	K8.8, 4.1.18, TS1, C-51, M20	Craniopharyngioma
CK10	cytokeratin 10	LHP1, DE-K10, RKSE60	Syringoma
CK14	cytokeratin 14, high molecular weight cytokeratin	LL002	Mucoepidermoid Carcinoma
CK8/18/CAM5.2	cytokeratin 8/18; simple epithelial-type cytokeratins	5D3, Zym5.2, CAM 5.2, KER 10.11, NCL-5D3, cytokeratin LMW	Follicular Adenoma; Islet Cell Adenoma; Neuroendocrine Tumors; Rhabdoid Tumor
CK17	cytokeratin 17	E3	Mucoepidermoid Carcinoma
CK18	cytokeratin 18	M9, DC-10, CY-90, KS18.04	MiTF/TFE Family Translocation-associated Carcinoma
CK19	cytokeratin 19, low molecular weight cytokeratin	BA17, RCK108, LP2K, B170, A53-BA2, KS19.1, 170.2.14	Follicular Adenoma; Follicular Carcinoma; Mucoepidermoid Carcinoma; Pancreatoblastoma; Papillary Thyroid Carcinoma; Sialoblastoma; Synovial Sarcoma; Thymoma
CK20	cytokeratin 20, low molecular weight cytokeratin	KS20.8	Craniopharyngioma; Mucoepidermoid Carcinoma; Papillary Thyroid Carcinoma; Pleomorphic Adenoma
Clusterin	clusterin, alpha chain specific	41D, E5	Anaplastic Large Cell Lymphoma, ALK+
Collagen II	major component of articular and hyaline cartilage	2B1.5	Chondromyxoid Fibroma
Collagen IV	major constituent of the basement membranes along with laminins, proteoglycans, and enactins	CIV22, COL4A [1-5], collagen α-1(IV) chain	Chondromyxoid Fibroma; Gastrointestinal Stromal Tumor; Giant Cell Fibroblastoma/ Dermatofibrosarcoma Protuberans; Glomus Tumor; Hemangiopericytoma; Medulloepithelioma; Neurofibroma
Cyclin-D1	protein with important cell cycle regulatory functions	bcl-1 (cyclin D1) A-12, PRAD1, AM29, DCS-6, SP4, 5D4, D1GM, P2D11F11, CCND1Cyl-1	Papillary Thyroid Carcinoma; Pediatric Follicular Lymphoma

ANTIBODY INDEX

Cytokeratin			Papillary Thyroid Carcinoma; Pediatric Follicular Lymphoma; Chondroblastoma; Clear Cell Sarcoma; Craniopharyngioma; Desmoplastic Small Round Cell Tumor; Ependymoma; Glioblastoma; Glomus Tumor; Juvenile Granulosa Cell Tumor; Malignant Melanoma; Medullary Thyroid Carcinoma Medulloblastoma; Medulloepithelioma; Neuroendocrine Tumors; Oligodendroglioma; Phyllodes Tumor; Pleomorphic Adenoma; Rhabdomyosarcoma; Secretory Carcinoma; Sialoblastoma; Synovial Sarcoma; T Lymphoblastic Leukemia/ Lymphoma; Thymoma; Wilms Tumor
Cytokeratin 14	high molecular weight cytokeratin	LL002	Pleomorphic Adenoma; Secretory Carcinoma
Cytokeratin 19	low molecular weight cytokeratin	BA17, RCK108, LP2K, B170, A53-BA2, KS19.1, 170.2.14	Papillary Thyroid Carcinoma
Cytokeratin 20	low molecular weight cytokeratin	KS20.8	T Lymphoblastic Leukemia/Lymphoma
Cytokeratin 5/6	high molecular weight cytokeratins	D5/16 B4	Secretory Carcinoma
Cytokeratin 8/18	simple epithelial-type cytokeratins	5D3, Zym5.2, CAM 5.2, KER 10.11, NCL-5D3, cytokeratin LMW	Secretory Carcinoma
D2-40	reacts with an O-linked sialoglycoprotein found on lymphatic endothelium	podoplanin, M2A, D2-40	Kaposiform Hemangioendothelioma
Desmin	class III intermediate filaments found in muscle cells	M760, DE-R-11, D33, DE5, DE-U-10, ZC18	Atypical Teratoid/Rhabdoid Tumor; Botryoid Rhabdomyosarcoma; Calcifying Fibrous Tumor; Clear Cell Sarcoma; Desmoid Fibromatosis; Desmoplastic Small Round Cell Tumor; Ewing Sarcoma; Fetal Rhabdomyoma; Fibroma; Fibrous Hamartoma of Infancy; Fibrous Histiocytoma; Fibrous Umbilical Polyp; Gastrointestinal Stromal Tumor; Gingival Granular Cell Tumor of the Newborn; Glomus Tumor; Hemangiopericytoma; Inclusion Body Fibromatosis; Infantile Fibromatosis; Infantile Fibrosarcoma; Inflammatory Myofibroblastic Tumor; Malignant Melanoma; Malignant Peripheral Nerve Sheath Tumor; Medulloblastoma; Mesoblastic Nephroma; Myeloid Sarcoma; Myofibroma and Myofibromatosis; Omental Mesenteric Hamartoma; Pleuropulmonary Blastoma; Primitive Neuroectodermal Tumor; Proliferative Fasciitis/Myositis; Rhabdoid Tumor; Rhabdomyoma; Rhabdomyosarcoma; Synovial Sarcoma; Thymoma; Wilms Tumor
DOG1	transmembrane protein 16A	DOG1 (TMEM16A), DOG 1.1	Gastrointestinal Stromal Tumor
DPC4	mothers against DPP homolog 4	MADR1 JV4-1, DPC4_SMAD4, SMAD4, B-8	Gastrointestinal Stromal Tumor
E-cadherin	epithelial calcium dependent adhesion molecule	36B5, ECH-6, ECCD-2, CDH1, 5H9, NCH 38, Clone 36, 4A2 C7, E9, 67A4, HECD-1, SC-8426	Giant Cell Fibroblastoma/ Dermatofibrosarcoma Protuberans; MiTF/ TFE Family Translocation-associated Carcinoma; Secretory Carcinoma
EBER	Epstein-Barr virus encoded RNA		Burkitt Lymphoma; Nodular Lymphocyte Predominant Hodgkin Lymphoma; Primary Mediastinal (Thymic) Large B-Cell Lymphoma
EBNA2	Epstein-Barr virus-associated nuclear antigen 2		Burkitt Lymphoma
EBV-LMP	Epstein-Barr virus latent membrane protein	LMP1, CS 1-4	Burkitt Lymphoma; Classical Hodgkin Lymphoma; Nodular Lymphocyte Predominant Hodgkin Lymphoma; Primary Mediastinal (Thymic) Large B-Cell Lymphoma
EGFR	v-erb b1 erythroblastic leukemia viral gene, epidermal growth factor receptor	2-18C9, EGFR1, EGFR PHRMDX, NCL-R1, H11, C-ERBB-1, E30, EGFR.113, 31G73C6, 2-18C9	Glioblastoma; Secretory Carcinoma
EMA	epithelial membrane antigen	GP1.4, 214D4, MC5, E29, MUC1, EMA/ MUC1	Adrenal Cortical Carcinoma; Anaplastic Large Cell Lymphoma, ALK+; Atypical

			Teratoid/Rhabdoid Tumor; Choroid Plexus Tumors; Classical Hodgkin Lymphoma; Diffuse Large B-Cell Lymphoma; Ependymoma; Ewing Sarcoma; Fibrous Umbilical Polyp; Glioblastoma; Glomus Tumor; Hemangiopericytoma; Medulloblastoma; Medulloepithelioma; Meningioangiomatosis; Neurofibroma; Neurothekeoma; Nodular Lymphocyte Predominant Hodgkin Lymphoma; Oligodendroglioma; Pineal Parenchymal Tumors; Primary Mediastinal (Thymic) Large B-Cell Lymphoma; Primitive Neuroectodermal Tumor; Rhabdomyosarcoma; Synovial Sarcoma; Syringoma
EMA/MUC1	epithelial membrane antigen	EMA, GP1.4, 214D4, MC5, E29, MUC1, LICR-LON-M8, BC3, DF3, VU3D1, MUSEII, RD-1, MA695, MA552, PS2P446, 115D8, MUC1, MAM6, CA15.3, MUC01	Anaplastic Large Cell Lymphoma, ALK +; Atypical Teratoid/Rhabdoid Tumor; Choroid Plexus Tumors; Dysgerminoma; MiTF/TFE Family Translocation-associated Carcinoma; Neurofibroma; Neurothekeoma; Rhabdoid Tumor; Sertoli-Leydig Cell Tumors; Synovial Sarcoma; Thecoma-Fibroma; Yolk Sac Tumor
EpCAM/BER-EP4/ CD326	epithelial cell adhesion molecule	AUA1, VU-1D9, EPCAM, C10, HEA125, BER-EP4	Choroid Plexus Tumors; Mucoepidermoid Carcinoma
Epithelial membrane antigen		EMA, GP1.4, 214D4, MC5, E29, MUC1, LICR-LON-M8, BC3, DF3, VU3D1, MUSEII, RD-1, MA695, MA552, PS2P446, 115D8, MUC1, MAM6, CA15.3, MUC01	Anaplastic Large Cell Lymphoma, ALK+; Chordoma; Ependymoma; Fibrolipomatous Hamartoma of Nerve; MiTF/TFE Family Translocation-associated Carcinoma; Sialoblastoma
Epstein-Barr virus encoded RNA		EBER	Autoimmune Lymphoproliferative Syndrome
ER	estrogen receptor protein	1D5, 6F11, SP1, 15D, H222, TE111, ERP, ER1D5, NCLER611, NCL-ER-LH2, PGP-1A6	Pleomorphic Xanthoastrocytoma; Gingival Granular Cell Tumor of the Newborn; Secretory Carcinoma
ERP	estrogen receptor protein	1D5, 6F11, SP1, 15D, H222, TE111, ER, ER1D5, NCLER611, NCL-ER-LH2, PGP-1A6	Secretory Carcinoma
Erythropoietin		EPO	Acute Myeloid Leukemia
Factor XIIIa	fibrin stabilizing factor	FXIIIA	Nodular Fasciitis
FAS	fatty acid synthase	CD95/fas	Autoimmune Lymphoproliferative Syndrome; Overview of Lymphoproliferative Disorders Associated with Primary Immune Deficiency
FASL	fatty acid synthase ligand	CD95L, G247-4, CD95-L, FAS-L, TNFSF6	Autoimmune Lymphoproliferative Syndrome
FAS ligand	fatty acid synthase ligand	CD95L, G247-4, CD95-L, FAS-L, TNFSF6, FASL	Autoimmune Lymphoproliferative Syndrome; Overview of Lymphoproliferative Disorders Associated with Primary Immune Deficiency
Fibrinogen	soluble plasma glycoprotein made by the liver and involved in blood coagulation		Hemaphagocytic Syndrome
FLI-1	Friend leukemia virus integration 1	EWSR2, GI146-222, SC356, FLK-1, FLT-1	Hemophagocytic Syndrome; Ewing Sarcoma; Kaposiform Hemangioendothelioma; Synovial Sarcoma
FVIIIRAg	factor VIII-related-antigen	FVIIIRAG, F8/86, von Willebrand factor	Clear Cell Sarcoma; Hemangioendothelioma; Hemangioma of Infancy
G-CSF	granulocyte colony stimulating factor	AB-1	Acute Myeloid Leukemia
Galectin-3		NCL-GAL3, B2C10, 9C4	Follicular Adenoma; Papillary Thyroid Carcinoma
Gastrin	hormone released by G cells in stomach, duodenum, and pancreas that stimulates secretion of gastric acid (HCl) by parietal cells of stomach		Islet Cell Adenoma
GCDFP-15	gross cystic fluid protein 15	SABP, GPIP4, Gp17, 23A3, BRST-2, D6 (GROSS CYSTIC DISEASE FLUID PROTEIN)	Secretory Carcinoma
GFAP	intermediate filament expressed by numerous cells of the CNS	6F2, M761, GA-51, GFP-8A	Anaplastic Astrocytoma; Atypical Teratoid/Rhabdoid Tumor; Choroid Plexus Tumors; Diffuse Astrocytoma

ANTIBODY INDEX

			(Low Grade); Ependymoma; Ganglion Cell Tumors; Glioblastoma; Heterotopic Neuroglial Tissue; Medulloblastoma; Mucoepidermoid Carcinoma; Neurofibroma; Neurothekeoma; Oligodendroglioma; Pilocytic Astrocytoma; Pleomorphic Adenoma; Pleomorphic Xanthoastrocytoma; Primitive Neuroectodermal Tumor; Retinoblastoma; Subependymal Giant Cell Tumor; Teratomas
GH	growth hormone	HGH, hGH	Craniopharyngioma; Follicular Carcinoma Pyogenic GranulomaChordoma
Glial fibrillary acidic protein	intermediate filament expressed by numerous cells of the CNS	GFAP, 6F2, M761, GA-51, GFP-8A	Ependymoma; Pleomorphic Adenoma; Sertoli-Leydig Cell Tumors
Glucagon	hormone secreted by the pancreas; functions to increase blood glucose levels		Islet Cell Adenoma; Nesidioblastosis; Pancreatoblastoma
Glypican-3	heparan sulfate proteoglycan with elevated expression in hepatocellular carcinoma	1G12, GPC3	Hepatocellular Carcinoma
GM-CSF	granulocyte macrophage colony stimulating factor	3209.1	Juvenile Myelomonocytic Leukemia
Granulocyte colony stimulating factor	granulocyte macrophage colony stimulating factor	3209.1, GM-CSF	Acute Myeloid Leukemia
Granzyme B	neutral serine protease	GZM-B, 11F1, GR-B7	Anaplastic Large Cell Lymphoma, ALK+
Growth hormone		GH, HGH, hGH	Craniopharyngioma; Pyogenic Granuloma
H-caldesmon		High molecular weight caldesmon, H-CD	Chrondromyxoid Fibroma; Synovial Sarcoma
HBME-1	mesothelioma antibody		Follicular Adenoma; Follicular Carcinoma; Papillary Thyroid Carcinoma
HCAD	H-caldesmon (high molecular weight caldesmon)	H-CD	Hemangiopericytoma; Synovial Sarcoma
HCG	human chorionic gonadotropin		Craniopharyngioma; Dysgerminoma; Gynecomastia; Pineal Parenchymal Tumors
Hep-Par1	hepatocyte paraffin 1	OCH1E5.2.10, HEPPAR1	Hepatocellular Carcinoma
HER2	v-erb-b2 erythroblastic leukemia viral gene protein, human epidermal growth factor receptor 2	c-erb-B2, HER2/neu, NEU, HER-2, NCL-CBE1, 10A7, 9G6.10, SP3, 4B5, epidermal growth factor receptor 2, P185, 9G6.20, A0485, C-ERBB-2, CB11, ERBB-2, 3B5, TAB250, HERCEPTEST, E2-4001, HER-2_NEU	Mucoepidermoid Carcinoma; Secretory Carcinoma
HMB-45	monoclonal antibody that reacts against an antigen present in melanocytic tumors		Blue Nevus; Glomus Tumor; Malignant Melanoma; Malignant Peripheral Nerve Sheath Tumor; Medulloblastoma; Melanotic Neuroectodermal Tumor of Infancy; MiTF/TFE Family Translocation-associated Carcinoma Schwannoma
Human chorionic gonadotropin		HCG, hCG	Craniopharyngioma; Dysgerminoma; Gynecomastia; Teratomas
IgA	immunoglobin A		Anaplastic Large Cell Lymphoma, ALK +; Autoimmune Lymphoproliferative Syndrome
IgD	immunoglobulin D		Nodular Lymphocyte Predominant Hodgkin Lymphoma
IGF-1	insulin growth factor-like 1	I-5C9	Craniopharyngioma; Medulloepithelioma
IGF-2	insulin growth factor-like 2	W2-H1	Adrenal Cortical Carcinoma
IgG	immunoglobulin G	IGG	Autoimmune Lymphoproliferative Syndrome
IgM	immunoglobulin M	IGM	Autoimmune Lymphoproliferative Syndrome; Burkitt Lymphoma; Overview of Lymphoproliferative Disorders Associated with Primary Immune Deficiency
IL-7	stimulates differentiation of pluripotent hematopoietic stem cells into lymphoid progenitor cells; important for T-cell development	Interleukin 7, Il7	Classical Hodgkin Lymphoma

ANTIBODY INDEX

IL-13	interleukin 13		Classical Hodgkin Lymphoma; Primary Mediastinal (Thymic) Large B-Cell Lymphoma
Immunoglobulin A		IgA, IGA	Autoimmune Lymphoproliferative Syndrome; Overview of Lymphoproliferative Disorders Associated with Primary Immune Deficiency
Inhibin	hormone released from testes or ovaries that down-regulates FSH synthesis and secretion	R1, beta A subunit, INHIBIN	Adrenal Cortical Carcinoma; Gonadoblastoma; Juvenile Granulosa Cell Tumor; Sertoli-Leydig Cell Tumors; Thecoma-Fibroma
Inhibin-α	produced by ovarina granulosa cells; inhibits production or secretion of pituitary gonadotropins, a sensitive marker for majority of sex cord-stromal tumors		Adrenal Cortical Carcinoma
INI1	member of SWI/SNF chromatin remodeling complex	BAF47/SNF5, SNF5	Atypical Teratoid/Rhabdoid Tumor; Choroid Plexus Tumors; Mesoblastic Nephroma; Rhabdoid Tumor
Intermediate filament	neurofilament triplet protein		Medulloblastoma
IRF-4	interferon regulatory factor 4	MUM1P, clone MUM1, MUM1-IRF.4, MUM1, M17	Burkitt Lymphoma; Classical Hodgkin Lymphoma; Primary Mediastinal (Thymic) Large B-Cell Lymphoma
JC virus	type of human polyomavirus genetically similar to BK virus and SV-40	John Cunningham virus	Diffuse Astrocytoma (Low Grade)
Keratin-Pan	cytokeratin-pan (AE1/AE3/LP34); cocktail of high and low molecular weight cytokeratins	keratin pan, MAK-6, K576, LU-5, KL-1, KC-8, MNF 116, pankeratin, pancytokeratin, CK-PAN	Pleomorphic Adenoma; Synovial Sarcoma
Kappa light chain		KAPPA, κ light chain	Autoimmune Lymphoproliferative Syndrome
Ki-67	Ki-67 (MIB-1); marker of cell proliferation	MMI, KI88, IVAK-2, MIB1	Adrenal Cortical Adenoma; Adrenal Cortical Carcinoma; Anaplastic Astrocytoma; Anaplastic Large Cell Lymphoma, ALK+; Atypical Teratoid/ Rhabdoid Tumor; Autoimmune Lymphoproliferative Syndrome; Burkitt Lymphoma; Choroid Plexus Tumors; Clear Cell Sarcoma; Craniopharyngioma; Diffuse Astrocytoma (Low Grade); Diffuse Large B-Cell Lymphoma; Ganglion Cell Tumors; Glioblastoma; Infantile Fibrosarcoma; Laryngotracheal Papillomatosis; Medulloblastoma; Mucoepidermoid Carcinoma; Nodular Lymphocyte Predominant Hodgkin Lymphoma; Oligodendroglioma; Pediatric Follicular Lymphoma; Pineal Parenchymal Tumors; Primitive Neuroectodermal Tumor; Synovial Sarcoma; T Lymphoblastic Leukemia/ Lymphoma
KI-M1P	marker of monocytes/macrophages		Fibrous Histiocytoma; Giant Cell Fibroblastoma/Dermatofibrosarcoma Protuberans
KP-1	cytoplasmic granule protein of monocytes, macrophages	CD68, PG-M1	Oligodendroglioma
Lambda light chain		λ light chain, LAMBDA	Autoimmune Lymphoproliferative Syndrome
Laminin	major protein in basal lamina	LAMININ-4C7, 4C12.8, LAM-89	Ganglion Cell Tumors; Gastrointestinal Stromal Tumor; Gingival Granular Cell Tumor of the Newborn; Glomus Tumor
LCA	leukocyte common antigen	PD7/26, 1.22/4.14, T29/33, CD45RB, RP2/18, CD45, PD7, 2D1, 2B11+PD7/26	Glioblastoma; Rhabdomyosarcoma
Leptin		LEP	Gynecomastia
LEU-7	β-1,3-glucuronyltransferase 1 (glucuronosyltransferase P)	CD57, NK1, HNK-1, TB01, B3GAT1	Oligodendroglioma
Leukocyte common antigen		LCA, PD7/26, 1.22/4.14, T29/33, CD45RB, RP2/18, CD45, PD7, 2D1, 2B11+PD7/26	Dysgerminoma
Lewis-Y	Lewis blood group antigen Y	BR-96, LEWIS-Y, BG8, 77/180, F3	Kaposiform Hemangioendothelioma

ANTIBODY INDEX

LH	lutenizing hormone	beta-LH	Mucoepidermoid Carcinoma
Lipase	pancreatic lipase		Islet Cell Adenoma
LMP1	Epstein-Barr virus latent membrane protein	EBV-LMP, CS 1-4	Burkitt Lymphoma
Lutenizing hormone		beta-LH	Craniopharyngioma
Lysozyme	1,4-beta N-acetylmuramidase C	Lyz, Lzm, Ec3.2.1.17	Juvenile Myelomonocytic Leukemia; Myeloid Sarcoma; T Lymphoblastic Leukemia/Lymphoma
Mart-1	mart-1 clone of Melan A		Gastrointestinal Stromal Tumor; Malignant Melanoma
MDM2	murine double minute oncogene (mdm2)	HDM2, IF2, 2A10, 1B10, SMP14, murine double minute 2	Ependymoma; Osteosarcoma
Melan-A	melanoma antigen recognized by T cells 1 (MART-1); protein found on melanocytes; melanocyte differentiation antigen	M2-7C10, CK-MM	Blue Nevus; Glomus Tumor; Malignant Melanoma; Malignant Peripheral Nerve Sheath Tumor; Neuroendocrine Tumors
met	met proto-oncogene	8F11, C-28, C-MET	Giant Cell Tumor; Mastocytosis; Medullary Thyroid Carcinoma
MIB1	Ki-67 (MIB1); marker of cell proliferation	MMI, KI88, IVAK-2, MIB1	Ganglion Cell Tumors
MIC2	cell surface glycoprotein for migration, T cell adhesion, MIC2	CD99, CD99-MEMB, MIC2, 12E7, HBA71, O13, P30/32MIC2, M3601	Primitive Neuroectodermal Tumor
MK	neurite growth promoting factor 2	MIDKINE, MK1	Pleuropulmonary Blastoma
MMP-2	Matrix metalloproteinase 1	41-1E5, F-67, 3B6	Giant Cell Fibroblastoma/ Dermatofibrosarcoma Protuberans
MPO	myeloperoxidase		Acute Myeloid Leukemia; Myeloid Sarcoma
MSA	actin, smooth muscle	actin-sm, ASM-1, CGA7, 1A4, HUC1-1	Myofibroma and Myofibromatosis
MSG1	melanocyte specific gene 1 antibody	CITED-1, J72220K	Papillary Thyroid Carcinoma
MT	metallothionein	CLONE E9	Follicular Carcinoma; Gingival Granular Cell Tumor of the Newborn; Juvenile Granulosa Cell Tumor; Medulloblastoma
MUC1	epithelial membrane antigen	LICR-LON-M8, BC3, DF3, VU3D1, MUSEII, RD-1, MA695, MA552, PS2P446, 115D8	Anaplastic Large Cell Lymphoma, ALK+
MUM1	Interferon regulatory factor 4	IRF-4, MUM1P, clone MUM1, MUM1-IRF.4, M17	Anaplastic Large Cell Lymphoma, ALK+; Diffuse Large B-Cell Lymphoma
Myeloperoxidase		MPO	Acute Myeloid Leukemia; Childhood Myelodysplastic Syndrome; Mastocytosis; Myeloid Sarcoma
MYOD1	myogenic differentiation 1	5.8A, 5.2F	Botryoid Rhabdomyosarcoma; Fetal Rhabdomyoma; Infantile Fibrosarcoma; Myeloid Sarcoma; Rhabdomyosarcoma; Wilms Tumor
Myogenin		F5D, MYF3, MYF4, MYOGENIN, LO26	Botryoid Rhabdomyosarcoma; Desmoplastic Small Round Cell Tumor; Ewing Sarcoma; Fetal Rhabdomyoma; Fibroma; Infantile Fibrosarcoma; Inflammatory Myofibroblastic Tumor; Malignant Peripheral Nerve Sheath Tumor; Medulloblastoma; Pleuropulmonary Blastoma; Rhabdoid Tumor; Rhabdomyosarcoma; Synovial Sarcoma; Wilms Tumor
Myoglobin	iron and oxygen-building protein found in muscle tissue	MG-1	Botryoid Rhabdomyosarcoma; Gingival Granular Cell Tumor of the Newborn; Inflammatory Myofibroblastic Tumor; Rhabdomyoma; Rhabdomyosarcoma
Myosin	motor protein responsible for actin-based motility		Pseudoangiomatous Stromal Hyperplasia; Rhabdomyosarcoma
N-myc	protooncogene and member of the MYC family of transcription factors		Neuroblastoma and Ganglioneuroblastoma
Nerve growth factor		NGF	Neuroblastoma and Ganglioneuroblastoma
Nestin	neural stem cell marker	10C2	Ependymoblastoma
NeuN	neuronal nuclear antigen	A60	Ganglion Cell Tumors

ANTIBODY INDEX

Neurofilament protein	neurofilament H/M phosphorylated protein	TPNFP-1A3, SMI31, SMI33, NFP, SMI32, TA-51, 2F11	Atypical Teratoid/Rhabdoid Tumor; Diffuse Astrocytoma (Low Grade); Neurofibroma
NFP	neurofilament H/M phosphorylated protein	TPNFP-1A3, SMI31, SMI33, NFP, SMI32, TA-51, 2F11	Atypical Teratoid/Rhabdoid Tumor; Diffuse Astrocytoma (Low Grade); Medulloblastoma; Neurofibroma
NGFR	nerve growth factor receptor		Teratomas
NOTCH1	translocation-associated notch protein		T Lymphoblastic Leukemia/Lymphoma
NSE	neuron specific enolase	BSS/H14	Adrenal Cortical Carcinoma; Burkitt Lymphoma; Ewing Sarcoma; Gingival Granular Cell Tumor of the Newborn; Infantile Fibrosarcoma; Medulloblastoma; Melanotic Neuroectodermal Tumor of Infancy; Neuroblastoma and Ganglioneuroblastoma; Neuroendocrine Tumors; Neurothekeoma; Pineal Parenchymal Tumors; Rhabdoid Tumor; Subependymal Giant Cell Tumor; Teratomas
Nuclear p53	p53 tumor suppressor gene protein	D07, 21N, BP53-12-1, AB6, CM1, PAB1801, DO1, BP53-11, PAP240, RSP53, MU195, P53	Choroid Plexus Tumors
O13	CD 99 (cell surface glycoprotein for migration, T-cell adhesion, MIC2)	CD99-MEMB, CD 99, MIC2, 12E7, HBA71, P30/32MIC2, M3601	Ewing Sarcoma
OCT2	octamer binding transcription factor 2	SC233	Classical Hodgkin Lymphoma; Primary Mediastinal (Thymic) Large B-Cell Lymphoma
OCT4	octamer-binding transcription factor-3	OCT3, POU5F1 (OCT3/4), C-10	Gonadoblastoma
p16	cyclin dependent kinase 4 inhibitor A	Cyclin dependent kinase inhibitor p16 antibody, INK4, INK4a, MLM, MTS1, multiple tumor suppressor 1 antibody, p12, p14, p16 γ, p16 INK4, p16 INK4a, INK4 p19, TP16, P16_INK4A, E6H4, sc1661, JC8, ZJ11, G175-405, F-12, DCS-50, 6H12, 16P07, 16P04	Glioblastoma; Malignant Melanoma
p53	p53 tumor suppressor gene protein	DO7, 21N, BP53-12-1, AB6, CM1, PAB1801, DO1, BP53-11, PAB240, RSP53, MU195, PAB1801, nuclear p53, P53	Adrenal Cortical Carcinoma; Choroid Plexus Tumors; Clear Cell Sarcoma; Diffuse Astrocytoma (Low Grade); Glioblastoma; Inflammatory Myofibroblastic Tumor; Medulloblastoma; Neurofibroma; Oligodendroglioma; Pediatric Follicular Lymphoma; Pleomorphic Adenoma; Sialoblastoma; Wilms Tumor
p63	tumor protein p63	P63-P53 HOMOLOGOUS NULCEAR PROTEIN;DELTA-NP63, 4A4, P63, H-137, 7JUL	Fibroadenoma; Mucoepidermoid Carcinoma; Pleomorphic Adenoma; Secretory Carcinoma; Sialoblastoma; Thymoma; Trichoepithelioma
p73	tumor protein p73	AB7824	Burkitt Lymphoma
PAP	Prostatic acid phosphatase	PASE/4LJ, PAP-P	Medullary Thyroid Carcinoma
pax-2	paired box gene 2	Z-RX2, PAX-2	Wilms Tumor
pax-5	paired box gene 5	PAX5 (BSAP)	Burkitt Lymphoma;; Classical Hodgkin Lymphoma Diffuse Large B-Cell Lymphoma; Nodular Lymphocyte Predominant Hodgkin Lymphoma; Primary Mediastinal (Thymic) Large B-Cell Lymphoma
PD-1	programmed cell death protein 1	EH12, NAT105, programmed death 1	Diffuse Large B-Cell Lymphoma
Perforin		P1-8, PE-41-PU, 5B10	Anaplastic Large Cell Lymphoma, ALK +; Autoimmune Lymphoproliferative Syndrome; Hemophagocytic Syndrome
PG-M1	cytoplasmic granule protein of monocytes, macrophages	CD-68, KP-1, LN5	Myeloid Sarcoma
PGP9.5	protein gene product 9.5	31A3,13C4	Neurothekeoma; Pineal Parenchymal Tumors
PLAP	placental alkaline phosphatase	228M, 8A9, 88B	Choroid Plexus Tumors; Dysgerminoma
Podoplanin	transmembrane mucoprotein (38 kd) recognized by the D2-40 monoclonal antibody	D2-40, M2A	Fibrous Histiocytoma; Giant Cell Fibroblastoma/Dermatofibrosarcoma Protuberans; Kaposiform Hemangioendothelioma
POU5F1	octamer-binding transcription factor-3	OCT3, OCT4, C-10	Gonadoblastoma

ANTIBODY INDEX

PR	progesterone receptor protein	PRP, 10A9, PGR-1A6, KD68, PGR-ICA, PRP-P, PRI, 1A6, 1AR, HPRA3, PGR-636, 636, PR88, NCL-PGR	Gingival Granular Cell Tumor of the Newborn; Secretory Carcinoma
Prealbumin	carrier protein of thyroxin and retinol; rich in a beta sheet structure	Transthyretin	Choroid Plexus Tumors
Prolactin		PRL	Chordoma; Juvenile (Virginal) Hypertrophy
Protein gene product 9.5		31A3,13C4	Neuroblastoma and Ganglioneuroblastoma
Protein Kinase C Theta		PKC-θ, CLONE 27, PKC-THETA	Gastrointestinal Stromal Tumor
PROX1	critical regulator of lymphangiogenesis		Lymphatic Malformation
PRP	progesterone receptor protein	PR, 10A9, PGR-1A6, KD68, PGR-ICA, PRP-P, PRI, 1A6, 1AR, HPRA3, PGR-636, 636, PR88, NCL-PGR	Craniopharyngioma
PTEN	phosphatase and tensin homolog	PN37	Anaplastic Astrocytoma; Fibrolipomatous Hamartoma of Nerve; Follicular Adenoma; Follicular Carcinoma; Glioblastoma; Papillary Thyroid Carcinoma
PTH	parathyroid hormone		Medullary Thyroid Carcinoma
PU.1	transcription factor PU.1	PTX1	Primary Mediastinal (Thymic) Large B-Cell Lymphoma
Renin	participates in renin-angiotensisn system	Angiotensinase	Adrenal Cortical Adenoma; Mesoblastic Nephroma
ret	Multiple endocrine neoplasia and medullary thyroid carcinoma 1	3F8	Medullary Thyroid Carcinoma; Papillary Thyroid Carcinoma
Retinal S antigen	localized to the photoreceptor cell layer of the retina		Medulloblastoma Primitive Neuroectodermal Tumor
Rhodopsin	photoreceptor that mediates dim-light vision		Medulloblastoma; Pineal Parenchymal Tumors; Primitive Neuroectodermal Tumor
S100	Low molecular weight protein normally present in cells derived from neural crest (Schwann cells, melanocytes, and glial cells), chondrocytes, adipocytes, myoepithelial cells, macrophages, Langerhans cells, dendritic cells, and keratinocytes	S-100, A6, 15E2E2, Z311, 4C4.9, S100 protein	Adrenal Cortical Adenoma; Adrenal Cortical Carcinoma; Atypical Teratoid/ Rhabdoid Tumor; Blue Nevus; Burkitt Lymphoma; Calcifying Fibrous Tumor; Chondroblastoma; Chondrosarcoma; Chordoma; Choroid Plexus Tumors; Clear Cell Sarcoma; Desmoplastic Small Round Cell Tumor; Diffuse Astrocytoma (Low Grade); Ependymoma; Ewing Sarcoma; Fibrous Umbilical Polyp; Gastrointestinal Stromal Tumor; Giant Cell Fibroblastoma/Dermatofibrosarcoma Protuberans; Gingival Granular Cell Tumor of the Newborn; Glioblastoma; Infantile Fibrosarcoma; Inflammatory Myofibroblastic Tumor; Inflammatory Polyps; Juvenile Xanthogranuloma; Langerhans Cell Histiocytosis; Malignant Melanoma; Malignant Peripheral Nerve Sheath Tumor; Medullary Thyroid Carcinoma; Melanocytic Nevus; Meningioangiomatosis; Mucoepidermoid Carcinoma; Myofibroma and Myofibromatosis; Neuroblastoma and Ganglioneuroblastoma; Neuroendocrine Tumors; Neurofibroma; Neurothekeoma; Oligodendroglioma; Pleomorphic Adenoma; Pleomorphic Xanthoastrocytoma; Schwannoma; Secretory Carcinoma; Sialoblastoma; Subependymal Giant Cell Tumor; Synovial Sarcoma
S100P	S100 placental	S100-pla	Teratomas
SMAD4	Similar to Mothers Against Decapentaplegic (MAD); mothers against DPP homolog 4	MADR1 JV4-1, DPC4_SMAD4, B-8	Cronkite-Canada Syndrome; Juvenile Polyps; Pancreatoblastoma
SMHC	myosin heavy chain smooth muscle	ID8, SM_MYOSIN_H, HSM-V, SMMS-1	Pleomorphic Adenoma; Pseudoangiomatous Stromal Hyperplasia
Smooth muscle myosin	myosin heavy chain smooth muscle	ID8, SM_MYOSIN_H, HSM-V, SMMS-1	Pseudoangiomatous Stromal Hyperplasia

SNF5	member of SWI/SNF chromatin remodeling complex	BAF47/SNF5, INI1	Atypical Teratoid/Rhabdoid Tumor; Rhabdoid Tumor
Sodium iodine symporter		Na-I symporter	Papillary Thyroid Carcinoma
Somatostatin			Craniopharyngioma
SOX9	SRY (sex-determining region Y)-box 9 protein	CMD1, CMPD1	Chondromyxoid Fibroma
SOX10	SRY (sex-determining region Y)-box 10 protein		Malignant Melanoma
Stem cell factor		SCF	Mastocytosis
Survivin	inhibitor of apoptosis	AB469, SURVIVIN, FL-142, D8, 8E12	Medulloblastoma
SV40	simian virus 40		Choroid Plexus Tumors; Ependymoma; Medulloblastoma
Synaptophysin	major synaptic vesicle protein p38 antibody	SVP38, SY38, SNP-88, SYP, SYPH, Sypl, Syn p38	Adrenal Cortical Adenoma; Adrenal Cortical Carcinoma; Atypical Teratoid/Rhabdoid Tumor; Desmoplastic Small Round Cell Tumor; Diffuse Large B-Cell Lymphoma; Ependymoma; Ewing Sarcoma; Follicular Adenoma; Follicular Carcinoma; Ganglion Cell Tumors; Islet Cell Adenoma; Medullary Thyroid Carcinoma; Medulloblastoma; Melanotic Neuroectodermal Tumor of Infancy; Neuroblastoma and Ganglioneuroblastoma; Neuroendocrine Tumors; Pancreatoblastoma; Pineal Parenchymal Tumors; Pleomorphic Xanthoastrocytoma; Primitive Neuroectodermal Tumor; Sertoli-Leydig Cell Tumors; T Lymphoblastic Leukemia/Lymphoma; Teratomas; Thymoma
SYT	SYT homolog 1		Calcifying Aponeuronic Fibroma; Ewing Sarcoma
TAU	microtubule-associated protein of axons	AT8	Ganglion Cell Tumors; Pineal Parenchymal Tumors
TCR	T-cell receptor antigen	T_Cell_AG_R, Beta-F1, 8A3, BF1	Autoimmune Lymphoproliferative Syndrome; Overview of Lymphoproliferative Disorders Associated with Primary Immune Deficiency; Primary Mediastinal (Thymic) Large B-Cell Lymphoma; T Lymphoblastic Leukemia/Lymphoma
TdT	terminal deoxynucleotidyl transferase	SEN28	Autoimmune Lymphoproliferative Syndrome; B Lymphoblastic Leukemia/Lymphoma; Burkitt Lymphoma; Desmoplastic Small Round Cell Tumor; Diffuse Large B-Cell Lymphoma; Primary Mediastinal (Thymic) Large B-Cell Lymphoma; T Lymphoblastic Leukemia/Lymphoma; Thymoma
Terminal deoxyneucleotidyl transferase		SEN28, TdT	B Lymphoblastic Leukemia/Lymphoma; Myeloid Sarcoma
TFE3	transcription factor E3		MiTF/TFE Family Translocation-associated Carcinoma
TFEB	transcription factor EB		MiTF/TFE Family Translocation-associated Carcinoma
Thyroglobulin	dimetric protein specific to thyroid gland	DAK-TG6	Follicular Adenoma; Follicular Carcinoma; Medullary Thyroid Carcinoma
TIA	T-cell intracellular antigen 1	NS/1-AG4, 2G9, TIA-1	Anaplastic Large Cell Lymphoma, ALK+
TIA-1	T-cell intracellular antigen 1	NS/1-AG4, 2G9, TIA	Anaplastic Large Cell Lymphoma, ALK+
TLE1	transducer like enhancer 1		Malignant Peripheral Nerve Sheath Tumor; Synovial Sarcoma
TNF-α	cytokine involved in systemic inflammation, stimulates the acute phase reaction	Gamma catenin, γ-catenin, G-catenin, alpha alpha, TNF, cachexin, cachectin	Classical Hodgkin Lymphoma
TRAF1	tumor necrosis factor receptor 1		Primary Mediastinal (Thymic) Large B-Cell Lymphoma

ANTIBODY INDEX

Transcription factor EB		TFEB	MiTF/TFE Family Translocation-associated Carcinoma
Tryptase	serine proteinase contained in mast cells		Mastocytosis
TSH	thyroid stimulating hormone	beta-TSH	Follicular Carcinoma
TTF-1	transcription termination factor	8G7G3/1, SPT-24, SC-13040	Follicular Adenoma; Follicular Carcinoma; Medullary Thyroid Carcinoma; Papillary Thyroid Carcinoma; Teratomas
Tuberin		Tuberous sclerosis protein 2, TSC2	Subependymal Giant Cell Tumor
TUJ1	beta tubulin	B-tubulin, β-tubulin	Subependymal Giant Cell Tumor
Tyrosinase	catalyzes production of melanin	NCL-TYROS, T311	Malignant Melanoma
Ubiquitin	Small regulatory protein that binds proteins and labels them for destruction		Ganglion Cell Tumors; Juvenile Myelomonocytic Leukemia; Pilocytic Astrocytoma; Rhabdomyoma
Vascular endothelial growth factor		VEGF, JH121, 26503.11, VPF, VPF/VEGF, VEGFA, VEGF-C, RP 077, VEGFR-1, RP 076, VEGFR-2, 9D9, VEGFR-3, FLT-4	Lymphatic Malformation
VEGF	vascular endothelial growth factor	JH121, 26503.11, VPF, VPF/VEGF, VEGFA, VEGF-C, RP 077, VEGFR-1, RP 076, VEGFR-2, 9D9, VEGFR-3, FLT-4	Adrenal Cortical Carcinoma; Hemangioma of Infancy; Pilocytic Astrocytoma
Vimentin	major subunit protein of the intermediate filaments of mesenchymal cells	43BE8, 3B4, V10, V9, VIM-3B4, VIM	Adrenal Cortical Carcinoma; Anaplastic Astrocytoma; Atypical Teratoid/ Rhabdoid Tumor; Chondroblastoma; Chondrosarcoma; Chordoma; Choroid Plexus Tumors; Clear Cell Sarcoma; Desmoid Fibromatosis; Desmoplastic Small Round Cell Tumor; Ependymoblastoma; Ependymoma; Ewing Sarcoma; Fibroma; Fibrous Hamartoma of Infancy; Gastrointestinal Stromal Tumor; Gingival Granular Cell Tumor of the Newborn; Glioblastoma; Glomus Tumor; Inclusion Body Fibromatosis; Infantile Fibromatosis; Infantile Fibrosarcoma; Inflammatory Myofibroblastic Tumor; Medulloblastoma; Mesoblastic Nephroma; MiTF/TFE Family Translocation-associated Carcinoma; Myofibroma and Myofibromatosis; Neurofibroma; Oligodendroglioma; Omental Mesenteric Hamartoma; Pancreatoblastoma; Pleomorphic Adenoma; Pleuropulmonary Blastoma; Rhabdoid Tumor; Synovial Sarcoma; Wilms Tumor
VIP	vasoactive intestinal peptide		Islet Cell Adenoma
WT1	Wilms tumor gene 1	6F-H2, C-19	Acute Myeloid Leukemia; Desmoplastic Small Round Cell Tumor; Myeloid Sarcoma; Rhabdomyosarcoma; Wilms Tumor

Molecular Factors Discussed

Molecular Factor	Chromosomal Location	Definition/Alternative Names	Chapters
β-catenin	3p21	catenin (cadherin-associated protein), beta 1; beta-catenin; CTNNB1	Adrenal Cortical Adenoma; Adrenal Cortical Carcinoma; Calcifying Fibrous Tumor; Craniopharyngioma; Desmoid Fibromatosis; Familial Adenomatous Polyposis; Fibroma; Fibromatosis Colli; Gardner Fibroma; Gastrointestinal Stromal Tumor; Hepatoblastoma; Infantile Fibrosarcoma; Infantile/Juvenile Hyaline Fibromatosis; Inflammatory Myofibroblastic Tumor; Medulloblastoma; Myofibroma and Myofibromatosis; Nodular Fasciitis; Pancreatoblastoma; Papillary Thyroid Carcinoma; Pilomatricoma; Rhabdoid Tumor; Wilms Tumor
κ light chain	2p11	immunoglobulin kappa light chain region	Burkitt Lymphoma
λ light chain	22q11	immunoglobulin lambda light chain region	Burkitt Lymphoma
1, chromosome	1		MiTF/TFE Family Translocation-associated Carcinoma; Nodular Lymphocyte Predominant Hodgkin Lymphoma
2, chromosome	2		Nodular Fasciitis
3, chromosome	3		Acute Myeloid Leukemia; Choroid Plexus Tumors; Nodular Lymphocyte Predominant Hodgkin Lymphoma
5, chromosome	5		Choroid Plexus Tumors
6, chromosome	6		Chondromyxoid Fibroma; Nodular Lymphocyte Predominant Hodgkin Lymphoma
7, chromosome	7		Choroid Plexus Tumors
8, chromosome	8		Infantile Fibrosarcoma; Pleuropulmonary Blastoma
9, chromosome	9		Choroid Plexus Tumors; Pleomorphic Xanthoastrocytoma
10, chromosome	10		Anaplastic Astrocytoma
11, chromosome	11		Adrenal Cortical Carcinoma; Desmoplastic Small Round Cell Tumor; Dysplastic Nevus; Ewing Sarcoma; Infantile Fibrosarcoma; Pineal Parenchymal Tumors
12, chromosome	12		Choroid Plexus Tumors; Hemangiopericytoma; Pineal Parenchymal Tumors
13, chromosome	13		Adrenal Cortical Carcinoma; Nodular Fasciitis
15, chromosome	15		Nodular Fasciitis
17, chromosome	17		Adrenal Cortical Carcinoma; Giant Cell Fibroblastoma/Dermatofibrosarcoma Protuberans; Infantile Fibrosarcoma; Nodular Lymphocyte Predominant Hodgkin Lymphoma; Osteoid Osteoma; Primitive Neuroectodermal Tumor
18, chromosome	18		Pediatric Follicular Lymphoma; Synovial Sarcoma
20, chromosome	20		Infantile Fibrosarcoma
21, chromosome	21		Ewing Sarcoma
22, chromosome	22		Atypical Teratoid/Rhabdoid Tumor; Ependymoma; Ewing Sarcoma; Giant Cell Fibroblastoma/Dermatofibrosarcoma Protuberans; Osteoid Osteoma; Pineal

			Parenchymal Tumors; Rhabdoid Tumor; Rhabdomyosarcoma
11, trisomy	11		Myeloid Sarcoma
11p	11p		Hepatoblastoma; Malignant Melanoma
11p11-12	11p11-12	EXT2	Osteochondroma
11p15	11p15		Adrenal Cortical Carcinoma; Nesidioblastosis; Wilms Tumor
11p15.5	11p15.5		Adrenal Cortical Carcinoma; Pancreatoblastoma; Rhabdomyosarcoma
11q	11q		Malignant Melanoma; Neuroblastoma and Ganglioneuroblastoma; Nodular Lymphocyte Predominant Hodgkin Lymphoma
11q11-12	11q11-12		Pigmented Villonodular Tenosynovitis
11q12	11q12		MiTF/TFE Family Translocation-associated Carcinoma
11q13	11q13	CCND1; cyclin D1	Adrenal Cortical Carcinoma; Malignant Melanoma
11q21	11q21		Mucoepidermoid Carcinoma
11q23	11q23	HRX; ALL1	Acute Myeloid Leukemia; Malignant Melanoma; Neuroblastoma and Ganglioneuroblastoma; Nodular Lymphocyte Predominant Hodgkin Lymphoma
12, trisomy	12		Juvenile Granulosa Cell Tumor
12q	12q		Chondromyxoid Fibroma; Nodular Lymphocyte Predominant Hodgkin Lymphoma
12q13-15	12q13-15		Pleomorphic Adenoma
13q	13q		Chondromyxoid Fibroma; Primary Mediastinal (Thymic) Large B-Cell Lymphoma
13q14	13q14		Primitive Neuroectodermal Tumor; Retinoblastoma
14q32	14q32		Burkitt Lymphoma
15q	15q		Primary Mediastinal (Thymic) Large B-Cell Lymphoma
16, monosomy	16		Myeloid Sarcoma
16p	16p		Chondromyxoid Fibroma; Subependymal Giant Cell Tumor
16q	16q		Trichoepithelioma; Wilms Tumor
16q, deletion	16q		Myeloid Sarcoma
17p	17p		Chondromyxoid Fibroma; Glioblastoma; Medulloblastoma; Primary Mediastinal (Thymic) Large B-Cell Lymphoma
17p13	17p13		Aneurysmal Bone Cyst; Dysplastic Nevus; Secretory Carcinoma
17p21	17p21		Nodular Lymphocyte Predominant Hodgkin Lymphoma
17q	17q		Malignant Melanoma; Medulloblastoma; Pilocytic Astrocytoma
17q11	17q11		Malignant Peripheral Nerve Sheath Tumor
17q11.2	17q11.2		Malignant Peripheral Nerve Sheath Tumor; Neurofibroma
17q13	17q13		Malignant Peripheral Nerve Sheath Tumor
17q23	17q23		MiTF/TFE Family Translocation-associated Carcinoma

MOLECULAR FACTORS INDEX

MOLECULAR FACTORS INDEX

MOLECULAR FACTORS INDEX

9p	9p		Malignant Melanoma
9q	9q		Malignant Melanoma
9q22	9q22		Nodular Lymphocyte Predominant Hodgkin Lymphoma
ABCC8	11p15.1	ATP-binding cassette, sub-family C (CFTR/MRP), member 8	Nesidioblastosis
ACVR1/ALK2			Fibrodysplasia Ossificans Progressiva
AF4	4q21	ALL1-fused gene from chromosome 4 protein	B Lymphoblastic Leukemia/ Lymphoma
AF9	9p22	ALL1-fused gene from chromosome 9 protein	B Lymphoblastic Leukemia/ Lymphoma
AKT	14q32.32	v-akt murine thymoma viral oncogene homolog 1	Adrenal Cortical Adenoma; Craniopharyngioma; Ganglion Cell Tumors; Myeloid Proliferations Related to Down Syndrome
ALK	2p23	anaplastic lymphoma receptor tyrosine kinase	Anaplastic Large Cell Lymphoma, ALK+; Calcifying Fibrous Tumor; Classical Hodgkin Lymphoma; Diffuse Large B-Cell Lymphoma; Inflammatory Myofibroblastic Tumor; Myeloid Sarcoma; Omental Mesenteric Hamartoma; Protocol for Non-Hodgkin Lymphoma Specimens
ALO17	17q25	ALK lymphoma oligomerization partner on chromosome 17	Anaplastic Large Cell Lymphoma, ALK+;
ANTXR2	4q21.21	anthrax toxin receptor 2	Infantile/Juvenile Hyaline Fibromatosis
APC	5q21-q22	adenomatosis polyposis coli	Desmoid Fibromatosis; Familial Adenomatous Polyposis; Gardner Fibroma; Gastrointestinal Stromal Tumor; Hepatoblastoma; Inflammatory Myofibroblastic Tumor; Medulloblastoma; Myofibroma and Myofibromatosis; Papillary Thyroid Carcinoma
APO1	10q24.1	apoptosis antigen 1; Fas (TNF receptor superfamily, member 6)	Autoimmune Lymphoproliferative Syndrome
ASPL	17q25.3	alveolar soft part sarcoma chromosome region, candidate 1 (ASPSCR1)	MiTF/TFE Family Translocation-associated Carcinoma
ASPL-TFE3	t(X;17)(p11.2;q25)		MiTF/TFE Family Translocation-associated Carcinoma
ASPSCR1	17q25.3	alveolar soft part sarcoma chromosome region, candidate 1 (ASPSCR1)	MiTF/TFE Family Translocation-associated Carcinoma
ATIC	2q35	5-aminoimidazole-4-carboxamide ribonucleotide formyltransferase/IMP cyclohydrolase	Anaplastic Large Cell Lymphoma, ALK+
ATM	11q22-23	ataxia telangiectasia mutated	Overview of Lymphoproliferative Disorders Associated with Primary Immune Deficiency
Basal-like			Secretory Carcinoma
BAX	19q13.3	BCL2-associated X protein	Burkitt Lymphoma
BCL2	18q21.3	B-cell CLL/lymphoma 2	Burkitt Lymphoma; Diffuse Large B-Cell Lymphoma; Pediatric Follicular Lymphoma; Primary Mediastinal (Thymic) Large B-Cell Lymphoma
BCL2-IGH	t(14;18)(q32;q21)		Pediatric Follicular Lymphoma
BCL6	3q27	B-cell CLL/lymphoma 6	Burkitt Lymphoma; Diffuse Large B-Cell Lymphoma; Nodular Lymphocyte Predominant Hodgkin Lymphoma; Pediatric Follicular Lymphoma; Primary Mediastinal (Thymic) Large B-Cell Lymphoma
BCR-ABL1	t(9;22)(q34;q11)	Philadelphia chromosome	B Lymphoblastic Leukemia/ Lymphoma; Juvenile Myelomonocytic Leukemia; Myeloid Sarcoma; Protocol for Bone Marrow Specimens; Protocol for Non-

MOLECULAR FACTORS INDEX

			Hodgkin Lymphoma Specimens; T Lymphoblastic Leukemia/Lymphoma
beta-catenin	3p21	catenin (cadherin-associated protein), beta 1; CTNNB1	Adrenal Cortical Adenoma; Craniopharyngioma
BMP4	14q22-23	bone morphogenetic protein 4	Juvenile Myelomonocytic Leukemia
BMPR1A	10q22.3	bone morphogenetic protein receptor type-1A	Cronkite-Canada Syndrome; Juvenile Polyps; Peutz-Jeghers Polyps
BRAF	7q34	v-raf murine sarcoma viral oncogene homolog B1	Follicular Adenoma; Papillary Thyroid Carcinoma
CALCA	11p15.2	calcitonin-related polypeptide alpha	Juvenile Myelomonocytic Leukemia
CASP10	2q33-q34	caspase 10, apoptosis-related cysteine peptidase	Autoimmune Lymphoproliferative Syndrome
CASP8	2q33-q34	caspase 8, apoptosis-related cysteine peptidase	Autoimmune Lymphoproliferative Syndrome
CBFβ-MYH11	inv(16)(q22p13)		Acute Myeloid Leukemia; Childhood Myelodysplastic Syndrome; Myeloid Sarcoma; Protocol for Bone Marrow Specimens
CCND1	11q13	cyclin D1	Primary Mediastinal (Thymic) Large B-Cell Lymphoma
CD40	20q12-13.2	CD40 molecule, TNF receptor superfamily member	Classical Hodgkin Lymphoma; Overview of Lymphoproliferative Disorders Associated with Primary Immune Deficiency
CD40LG	Xq26	CD40 ligand	Overview of Lymphoproliferative Disorders Associated with Primary Immune Deficiency
CD68	17p13	CD68 molecule	Fibrous Histiocytoma; Juvenile Xanthogranuloma; Myeloid Sarcoma; Oligodendroglioma; Proliferative Fasciitis/Myositis
CD95	10q24.1	Fas (TNF receptor superfamily, member 6)	Autoimmune Lymphoproliferative Syndrome
CDH11-USP6	t(16;17)(q21;p13)		Aneurysmal Bone Cyst
CDK4	12q14	cyclin-dependent kinase 4	T Lymphoblastic Leukemia/ Lymphoma
CDKN2A	9p21	cyclin-dependent kinase inhibitor 2A; p16	Malignant Melanoma; T Lymphoblastic Leukemia/Lymphoma
CDKN2B	9p21	cyclin-dependent kinase inhibitor 2B; p15	Juvenile Myelomonocytic Leukemia
CDNK2A	9p21	cyclin-dependent kinase inhibitor 2A	Glioblastoma
CEBPA	19q13.1	CCAAT/enhancer binding protein (C/EBP), alpha	Acute Myeloid Leukemia; Myeloid Sarcoma
CHS1/LYST	1q42.1-q42.2	Chediak-Higashi syndrome 1/ lysosomal trafficking regulator	Hemophagocytic Syndrome
CK19	17q21.2	keratin 19	Follicular Carcinoma; Pancreatoblastoma
c-KIT (see KIT)			
CLTC	17q11	clathrin, heavy chain (Hc)	MiTF/TFE Family Translocation-associated Carcinoma
CLTCL	22q11.2	clathrin, heavy chain-like 1	Anaplastic Large Cell Lymphoma, ALK+
c-myc (see MYC)			
COL1A1	17q21.33	collagen, type I, alpha 1	Giant Cell Fibroblastoma/ Dermatofibrosarcoma Protuberans
CSF1	1p21-p13	colony stimulating factor 1 (macrophage)	Pigmented Villonodular Tenosynovitis
CSF1R	5q32	colony stimulating factor 1 receptor	Pigmented Villonodular Tenosynovitis
CTNNB1	3p21	beta-catenin	Adrenal Cortical Carcinoma; Wilms Tumor
CYLD	16q12.1	cylindromatosis (turban tumor syndrome)	Trichoepithelioma
DICER1	14q32.13	dicer 1, ribonuclease type III	Pleuropulmonary Blastoma

MOLECULAR FACTORS INDEX

E2A-PBX1	t(1;19)(q23;p13.3)		B Lymphoblastic Leukemia/ Lymphoma; Protocol for Bone Marrow Specimens; Protocol for Non-Hodgkin Lymphoma Specimens
EBV		Epstein-barr virus	Acute Myeloid Leukemia; Autoimmune Lymphoproliferative Syndrome; Burkitt Lymphoma; Classical Hodgkin Lymphoma; Diffuse Large B-Cell Lymphoma; Hemophagocytic Syndrome; Juvenile Myelomonocytic Leukemia; Nodular Lymphocyte Predominant Hodgkin Lymphoma; Overview of Lymphoproliferative Disorders Associated with Primary Immune Deficiency; Protocol for Non-Hodgkin Lymphoma Specimens
E-cadherin	16q22.1	CDH1	Giant Cell Fibroblastoma/ Dermatofibrosarcoma Protuberans
EGFR	7p12	Epidermal growth factor receptor; ERBB1; HER1	Anaplastic Astrocytoma; Glioblastoma
ENL	19p13	MLLT1	B Lymphoblastic Leukemia/ Lymphoma
Epstein-Barr virus		EBV	Autoimmune Lymphoproliferative Syndrome; Burkitt Lymphoma; Overview of Lymphoproliferative Disorders Associated with Primary Immune Deficiency; Protocol for Bone Marrow Specimens; Protocol for Non-Hodgkin Lymphoma Specimens
ER	6q25.1	estrogen receptor	Pleomorphic Xanthoastrocytoma; Secretory Carcinoma
ERG	21q22.3	v-ets erythroblastosis virus E26 oncogene homolog	Ewing Sarcoma
ETV6	12p13	ets variant 6	Secretory Carcinoma
ETV6-NTRK3	t(12;15)(p13;q25)		Infantile Fibromatosis; Infantile Fibrosarcoma; Mesoblastic Nephroma; Secretory Carcinoma
EVER1/TMC6	17q25.3	epidermodysplasia verruciformis 1/ transmembrane channel-like	Epidermodysplasia Veruciformis
EVER2/TMC8	17q25.3	epidermodysplasia verruciformis 2/ transmembrane channel-like	Epidermodysplasia Veruciformis
EWS	22q12.2	Ewing sarcoma (EWS) breakpoint region 1 (EWSR1)	Desmoplastic Small Round Cell Tumor; Ewing Sarcoma; Myeloid Sarcoma; Synovial Sarcoma; T Lymphoblastic Leukemia/Lymphoma
EWS-CREB1	t(2;22)(q34;q12)		Malignant Peripheral Nerve Sheath Tumor
EWS-E1AF	t(17;22)(q12;q12)		Ewing Sarcoma
EWS-E1AF	t(17;22)(q12;q12)		Ewing Sarcoma
EWS-ERG	t(21;22)(q22;q12)		Desmoplastic Small Round Cell Tumor; Ewing Sarcoma; Malignant Peripheral Nerve Sheath Tumor
EWS-ETV1	t(7;22)(p22;q12)		Ewing Sarcoma
EWS-FEV	t(2;22)(q33;q12)		Ewing Sarcoma
EWS-FLI1	t(11;22)(q24;q12)		Ewing Sarcoma; Malignant Peripheral Nerve Sheath Tumor
EWSR1	22q12.2	Ewing sarcoma (EWS) breakpoint region 1 (EWSR1)	Malignant Peripheral Nerve Sheath Tumor
EWS-WT1	t(11;22)(p13;q12)		Desmoplastic Small Round Cell Tumor; Rhabdomyosarcoma
EWS-ZSG	t(1;22)(p36;q12)		Ewing Sarcoma
EXT1	8q24.1	exostosin 1	Osteochondroma
EXT2	11p11-12	exostosin 2	Osteochondroma
EXT3	19p	exostoses (multiple) 3	Osteochondroma
FAS	10q24.1	Fas (TNF receptor superfamily, member 6)	Autoimmune Lymphoproliferative Syndrome; Fibroadenoma; Follicular Adenoma; Overview of

MOLECULAR FACTORS INDEX

			Lymphoproliferative Disorders Associated with Primary Immune Deficiency
FASLG	1q23	Fas ligand (TNF superfamily, member 6)	Autoimmune Lymphoproliferative Syndrome; Overview of Lymphoproliferative Disorders Associated with Primary Immune Deficiency
FGFR1	8p12	fibroblast growth factor receptor 1	Protocol for Bone Marrow Specimens; T Lymphoblastic Leukemia/ Lymphoma
FIP1L1-PDGFRA	4q12		Mastocytosis
FLI1	11q24.1-q24.3	Friend leukemia virus integration 1	Desmoplastic Small Round Cell Tumor; Ewing Sarcoma; Myeloid Sarcoma
FLI-1	11q24.1-q24.3	Friend leukemia virus integration 1	Diffuse Large B-Cell Lymphoma
FLI1-EWS	t(11;22)(q24;q12)		Synovial Sarcoma
FLT3	13q12	fms-related tyrosine kinase	Acute Myeloid Leukemia; Mastocytosis; Medullary Thyroid Carcinoma; Myeloid Sarcoma
FOXC2	16q24.1	forkhead box C2	Lymphatic Malformation
G proteins			Fibrous Dysplasia
GATA1	Xp11.23	GATA binding protein 1	Myeloid Proliferations Related to Down Syndrome
GBY	Y		Gonadoblastoma
GNAS1	20q13.3	GNAS complex locus	Follicular Carcinoma
GPC3	Xq26.1	glypican 3	Hepatocellular Carcinoma
H19	11p15.5	imprinted maternally expressed transcript (non-protein coding)	Adrenal Cortical Carcinoma; Wilms Tumor
HER2	17q12	c-erbB-2	Secretory Carcinoma
HIV		human immunodeficiency virus	Burkitt Lymphoma; Childhood Myelodysplastic Syndrome; Classical Hodgkin Lymphoma; Diffuse Lipomatosis; Hemophagocytic Syndrome
HMGA2	12q15	high mobility group AT-hook 2; HMGIC	Pleomorphic Adenoma
HMGIC	12q15	high-mobility group (nonhistone chromosomal) protein isoform I-C; HMGA2	Pleomorphic Adenoma
HOX11	10q24	homeobox-11; TLX1	T Lymphoblastic Leukemia/ Lymphoma
HOX11L2	5q35.1	homeobox 11-like 2; TLX3	T Lymphoblastic Leukemia/ Lymphoma
HPV		human papilloma virus	Epidermodysplasia Veruciformis; Laryngotracheal Papillomatosis
HRAS	11p15.5	v-Ha-ras Harvey rat sarcoma viral oncogene homolo	Follicular Adenoma; Follicular Carcinoma
hSNF5/INI1 (see INI1)			
i17q	17q	isochromosome 17q	Medulloblastoma; Pediatric Follicular Lymphoma
IDH1	2q33.3	isocitrate dehydrogenase 1	Acute Myeloid Leukemia
IDH2	15q26.1	isocitrate dehydrogenase 2	Acute Myeloid Leukemia
IGF2	11p15.5	insulin-like growth factor 2	Wilms Tumor
IGH	14q32.33	immunoglobulin heavy chain complex	B Lymphoblastic Leukemia/ Lymphoma; Burkitt Lymphoma; Myeloid Sarcoma; Nodular Lymphocyte Predominant Hodgkin Lymphoma; Overview of Lymphoproliferative Disorders Associated with Primary Immune Deficiency; Pediatric Follicular Lymphoma; Primary Mediastinal (Thymic) Large B-Cell Lymphoma; T Lymphoblastic Leukemia/Lymphoma

MOLECULAR FACTORS INDEX

IGH/MALT1	t(14;18)(q32;q21)		Diffuse Large B-Cell Lymphoma; Pediatric Follicular Lymphoma
IGH-MYC	t(8;14)(q24;q32)		Burkitt Lymphoma; Diffuse Large B-Cell Lymphoma
IGK/MYC	t(2;8)(p12;q24)		Burkitt Lymphoma
IgVH		Immunoglobulin heavy chain gene, variable region	Classical Hodgkin Lymphoma
IL18R1	2q12	interleukin 18 receptor 1	Histiocytoid Cardiomyopathy
IL18RAP	2q12	interleukin 18 receptor accessory protein	Histiocytoid Cardiomyopathy
IL1RL1	2q12	interleukin 1 receptor-like 1	Histiocytoid Cardiomyopathy
IL3-IGH	t(5;14)(q31;q32)		B Lymphoblastic Leukemia/ Lymphoma; Protocol for Bone Marrow Specimens; Protocol for Non-Hodgkin Lymphoma Specimens
Immunoglobulin heavy chain gene	14q32.33	IGH	Overview of Lymphoproliferative Disorders Associated with Primary Immune Deficiency
INI1	22q11	integrase interactor 1; hSNF5; SMARCB1; BAF47	Atypical Teratoid/Rhabdoid Tumor; Choroid Plexus Tumors; Medulloblastoma; Mesoblastic Nephroma; Primitive Neuroectodermal Tumor; Rhabdoid Tumor
inv(16)	16		Myeloid Sarcoma
inv(16)/t(16;16)(p13.1q22)	inv(16)/t(16;16)(p13.1q22)	CBFβ-MYH11	Myeloid Sarcoma
inv(xp11;q12)			MiTF/TFE Family Translocation-associated Carcinoma
JAK2	9p24	Janus kinase 2	Acute Myeloid Leukemia; Myeloid Sarcoma; Primary Mediastinal (Thymic) Large B-Cell Lymphoma
KCNJ11	11p15.1	potassium inwardly-rectifying channel, subfamily J, member 11; kir6.2	Nesidioblastosis
Kir6.2	11p15.1	potassium inwardly-rectifying channel, subfamily J, member 11; KCNJ11	Nesidioblastosis
KIT	4q11-q12	v-kit Hardy-Zuckerman 4 feline sarcoma viral oncogene homolog;c-Kit;CD117	Acute Myeloid Leukemia; Desmoid Fibromatosis; Gastrointestinal Stromal Tumor; Inflammatory Myofibroblastic Tumor; Inflammatory Polyps; Mastocytosis; Protocol for Gastrointestinal Stromal Tumors; Desmoid Fibromatosis
KRAS	12p12.1	v-Ki-ras2 Kirsten rat sarcoma viral oncogene homolog; KRAS2	Juvenile Myelomonocytic Leukemia
KRAS2	12p12.1	v-Ki-ras2 Kirsten rat sarcoma viral oncogene homolog; KRAS	Juvenile Myelomonocytic Leukemia
LKB1	19p13.3	liver kinase B1; STK11	Peutz-Jeghers Polyps
LOH 10	10	loss of heterozygosity 10	Glioblastoma
LYL1	19p13.2	lymphoblastic leukemia derived sequence 1	T Lymphoblastic Leukemia/ Lymphoma
MALT	18q21	mucosa associated lymphoid tissue lymphoma translocation gene 1	Overview of Lymphoproliferative Disorders Associated with Primary Immune Deficiency; Protocol for Bone Marrow Specimens; Protocol for Non-Hodgkin Lymphoma Specimens
MAML2	11q21	mastermind-like gene family	Mucoepidermoid Carcinoma
MAML2-MECT1	t(11;19)(q21-22;p13)		Mucoepidermoid Carcinoma
MDM2	12q14.3-q15	mdm2 p53 binding protein homolog	Ependymoma
MECT1	19p13	mucoepidermoid carcinoma translocated 1	Mucoepidermoid Carcinoma
MEN2A	10q11.2	RET	Medullary Thyroid Carcinoma
MERRF		myoclonic epilepsy and ragged red muscle fibers	Histiocytoid Cardiomyopathy

MOLECULAR FACTORS INDEX

MET	7q31	met proto-oncogene	Giant Cell Tumor; Mastocytosis; Medullary Thyroid Carcinoma
Mitochondrial cytochrome b	Mitochondrion	CYTB	Histiocytoid Cardiomyopathy
MLL	11q23	HRX; ALL1	Acute Myeloid Leukemia; B Lymphoblastic Leukemia/Lymphoma; Myeloid Sarcoma; Protocol for Bone Marrow Specimens; Protocol for Non-Hodgkin Lymphoma Specimens; T Lymphoblastic Leukemia/Lymphoma
MLL-AF4	t(4;11)(q21;q23)		B Lymphoblastic Leukemia/ Lymphoma
MSI		microsatelite instability	Glioblastoma
MSN	Xq11.1	moesin	Anaplastic Large Cell Lymphoma, ALK+
MUM1	19p13.3	melanoma associated antigen (mutated) 1	Diffuse Large B-Cell Lymphoma
MutYH	1p34.1	mutY homolog	Familial Adenomatous Polyposis
MYC	8q24.21	v-myc myelocytomatosis viral oncogene homolog	Burkitt Lymphoma; Diffuse Large B-Cell Lymphoma; Medulloblastoma; Myeloid Sarcoma; Primary Mediastinal (Thymic) Large B-Cell Lymphoma; T Lymphoblastic Leukemia/Lymphoma
MYH			Familial Adenomatous Polyposis
MYH9	22q13.1	myosin, heavy chain 9, non-muscle	Anaplastic Large Cell Lymphoma, ALK+
MYO5A	15q21	myosin VA (heavy chain 12, myoxin)	Hemophagocytic Syndrome
NBS1			Overview of Lymphoproliferative Disorders Associated with Primary Immune Deficiency
NF1	17q11.2	neurofibromin 1	B Lymphoblastic Leukemia/ Lymphoma; Gastrointestinal Stromal Tumor; Glioblastoma; Juvenile Myelomonocytic Leukemia; Juvenile Xanthogranuloma; Malignant Peripheral Nerve Sheath Tumor; Neuroendocrine Tumors; Neurofibroma; Pilocytic Astrocytoma; Schwannoma
NF2	22q12.2	neurofibromin 2	Ependymoma; Gastrointestinal Stromal Tumor; Meningioangiomatosis; Schwannoma
NF-κB	4q24	nuclear factor of kappa light polypeptide gene enhancer in B-cells 1	Histiocytoid Cardiomyopathy; Primary Mediastinal (Thymic) Large B-Cell Lymphoma
N-Myc	2p24.3	v-myc myelocytomatosis viral related oncogene, neuroblastoma derived	Ganglioneuroma; Medulloblastoma; Neuroblastoma and Ganglioneuroblastoma; Primitive Neuroectodermal Tumor
Notch/CXRC1		survivin	Medulloblastoma
NOTCH1	9q34.3		Classical Hodgkin Lymphoma; T Lymphoblastic Leukemia/Lymphoma
NPM	5q35.1	nucleophosmin	Anaplastic Large Cell Lymphoma, ALK+
NPM1	5q35.1	nucleophosmin 1	Acute Myeloid Leukemia; Anaplastic Large Cell Lymphoma, ALK+; Myeloid Sarcoma
NPM-ALK	t(2;5)(p23;q35)		Anaplastic Large Cell Lymphoma, ALK+
NRAS	1p13.2	neuroblastoma RAS viral (v-ras) oncogene homolog	Autoimmune Lymphoproliferative Syndrome; Follicular Adenoma; Juvenile Myelomonocytic Leukemia
NTRK3	15q25	neurotrophic tyrosine kinase, receptor, type 3	Juvenile Myelomonocytic Leukemia
NTRK3-ETV6	t(12;15)(p13;q25)		Infantile Fibrosarcoma; Secretory Carcinoma
Nucleophosmin	5q35.1	NPM	Acute Myeloid Leukemia; Rhabdomyosarcoma

MOLECULAR FACTORS INDEX

p130/Rb2	16q12.2	retinoblastoma-like 2 (p130)	T Lymphoblastic Leukemia/ Lymphoma
p16	9p21	CDKN2A; p16-INK4A; ARF; MLM; P14; P16; P19; CMM2; INK4; MTS1; TP16; CDK4I; CDKN2; INK4A; MTS-1; P14ARF; P19ARF; P16INK4; P16INK4A	Burkitt Lymphoma; Glioblastoma; Malignant Melanoma; T Lymphoblastic Leukemia/Lymphoma
P53	17p13.1	TP53	Adrenal Cortical Carcinoma; Anaplastic Astrocytoma; Burkitt Lymphoma; Chondroblastoma; Choroid Plexus Tumors; Diffuse Astrocytoma (Low Grade); Ependymoma; Familial Adenomatous Polyposis; Follicular Carcinoma; Glioblastoma; Inflammatory Myofibroblastic Tumor; Malignant Peripheral Nerve Sheath Tumor; Medulloblastoma; Neurofibroma; Oligodendroglioma; Pediatric Follicular Lymphoma; Pilocytic Astrocytoma; Pleomorphic Xanthoastrocytoma; Primitive Neuroectodermal Tumor; Secretory Carcinoma; Wilms Tumor
p73	1p36.3	tumor protein p73	Burkitt Lymphoma
PAX3	2q35	paired-box 3	Rhabdomyosarcoma
PAX3-FKHR	t(2;13)(q35;q14)		Rhabdomyosarcoma; Synovial Sarcoma
PAX5	9p13	paired box 5	Classical Hodgkin Lymphoma
PAX7-FKHR	t(1;13)(p36;q14)		Rhabdomyosarcoma; Synovial Sarcoma
PAX8	2q13	paired box 8	Follicular Carcinoma
PAX8-PPARγ	t(2;3)(q13;p25)		Follicular Carcinoma
PDGFRA	4q12	platelet-derived growth factor receptor, alpha polypeptide; PDGFR-α	Gastrointestinal Stromal Tumor; Inflammatory Myofibroblastic Tumor; Inflammatory Polyps; Protocol for Bone Marrow Specimens; Protocol for Gastrointestinal Stromal Tumors
PDGFRB	5q33.1	platelet-derived growth factor receptor, beta polypeptide; PDGFR-β	Protocol for Bone Marrow Specimens
PDGF-β	5q33.1	platelet-derived growth factor receptor, beta polypeptide	Giant Cell Fibroblastoma/ Dermatofibrosarcoma Protuberans
PDS			Follicular Adenoma
Ph chromosome	t(9;22)(q34;q11)	Philadelphia chromosome; BCR-ABL1	Juvenile Myelomonocytic Leukemia
PI3KCA	3q26.3	PI3-kinase p110 subunit alpha; PIK3CA	Follicular Carcinoma
PIK3CA	3q26.3	phosphoinositide-3-kinase, catalytic, alpha polypeptide; PI3KCA	Follicular Carcinoma
PLAG1	8q12	pleiomorphic adenoma gene 1	Lipoblastoma; Pleomorphic Adenoma
Platelet-derived growth factor receptor α		PDGFR-α; PDGFRA	Inflammatory Polyps
PML-RARA	t(15;17)(q22;q12)	PML-RARA regulated adaptor molecule 1;PML-RARα	Acute Myeloid Leukemia; Childhood Myelodysplastic Syndrome; Protocol for Bone Marrow Specimens
PML-RARα	t(15;17)(q22;q12)	PML-RARA regulated adaptor molecule 1;PML-RARA	Myeloid Sarcoma
PPARγ	3p25	peroxisome proliferator-activated receptor gamma	Follicular Carcinoma
PR	11q22-q23	progesterone receptor	Secretory Carcinoma
PRCC	1q21.1	papillary renal cell carcinoma (translocation-associated)	MiTF/TFE Family Translocation-associated Carcinoma
PRCC2	17q25.3	ASPSCR1; ASPL	MiTF/TFE Family Translocation-associated Carcinoma
PRCC-TFE3	t(X;1)(p11.2;q21)		MiTF/TFE Family Translocation-associated Carcinoma
PRF1	10q22	perforin 1	Hemophagocytic Syndrome
PRKAR1A	17q23-q24	protein kinase, cAMP-dependent, regulatory, type I, alpha; TSE1	Follicular Adenoma; Follicular Carcinoma

MOLECULAR FACTORS INDEX

PROX1	1q41	prospero homeobox 1	Lymphatic Malformation
PSF	1p34.3	splicing factor proline/glutamine-rich	MiTF/TFE Family Translocation-associated Carcinoma
PSF-TFE3	t(X;1)(p11.2;p34		MiTF/TFE Family Translocation-associated Carcinoma
PTCH	9q22.3	patched 1; PTCH1	Fetal Rhabdomyoma
PTCH1	9q22.3	patched 1; PTCH	Fibroma; Medulloblastoma
PTEN	10q23.3	phosphatase and tensin homolog	Anaplastic Astrocytoma; Fibrolipomatous Hamartoma of Nerve; Follicular Adenoma; Follicular Carcinoma; Ganglion Cell Tumors; Glioblastoma; Papillary Thyroid Carcinoma; T Lymphoblastic Leukemia/Lymphoma
PTPN11	12q24		Juvenile Myelomonocytic Leukemia
RAB27A	15q15-q21.1	member RAS oncogene family	Hemophagocytic Syndrome
RARB	3p24	retinoic acid receptor, beta; RARβ	Juvenile Myelomonocytic Leukemia
RAS		RAS oncogene family	Follicular Adenoma; Follicular Carcinoma; Malignant Peripheral Nerve Sheath Tumor; Myeloid Sarcoma; Neurofibroma
Rb	13q14.2	retinoblastoma; RB1	Osteosarcoma; Primitive Neuroectodermal Tumor; Retinoblastoma
RET	10q11.2	ret proto-oncogene; MEN2A	Follicular Adenoma; Medullary Thyroid Carcinoma; Papillary Thyroid Carcinoma
RUNX1	21q22.3	runt-related transcription factor 1	B Lymphoblastic Leukemia/Lymphoma
S100A12	1q21.3		Histiocytoid Cardiomyopathy
S100A8	1q21.3		Histiocytoid Cardiomyopathy
S100A9	1q21.3		Histiocytoid Cardiomyopathy
SH2D1A	Xq25	SH2 domain containing 1A	Autoimmune Lymphoproliferative Syndrome; Hemophagocytic Syndrome
SLC26A4	7q31	solute carrier family 26, member 4	Follicular Adenoma
SMAD4	18q21.1	SMAD family member 4;DPC4	Cronkite-Canada Syndrome; Juvenile Polyps; Pancreatoblastoma; Peutz-Jeghers Polyps
SNF5/INI1 (see INI1)			
SOCS1	16p13.13	suppressor of cytokine signaling 1	Primary Mediastinal (Thymic) Large B-Cell Lymphoma
SOX18	20q13.33	SRY (sex determining region Y)-box 18	Lymphatic Malformation
Sox6		SRY (sex determining region Y)-box 6	Histiocytoid Cardiomyopathy
SRY	Yp11.3	sex determining region Y	Sertoli-Leydig Cell Tumors
SS18	18q11.2	synovial sarcoma translocation, chromosome 18; SYT	Synovial Sarcoma
SSX	Xp11.22	synovial sarcoma, X	Synovial Sarcoma
SSX1	Xp11.23	synovial sarcoma, X breakpoint 1	Synovial Sarcoma
SSX2	Xp11.22	synovial sarcoma, X breakpoint 2	Synovial Sarcoma
SSX4	Xp11.23	synovial sarcoma, X breakpoint 4	Synovial Sarcoma
STAT1	2q32.2	signal transducer and activator of transcription 1	Primary Mediastinal (Thymic) Large B-Cell Lymphoma
STK11	19p13.3	serine/threonine kinase 11	Peutz-Jeghers Polyps
STX11	6q24.2	syntaxin 11	Hemophagocytic Syndrome
SUR1	11p15.1	ATP-binding cassette, sub-family C (CFTR/MRP), member 8	Nesidioblastosis
Survivin		Notch/CXRC1	Medulloblastoma
SYT	18q11.2	synovial sarcoma translocation, chromosome 18; SS18	Calcifying Aponeuronic Fibroma; Malignant Peripheral Nerve Sheath Tumor; Synovial Sarcoma

MOLECULAR FACTORS INDEX

MOLECULAR FACTORS INDEX

t(2;X)(p23;q11-12)	t(2;X)(p23;q11-12)		Anaplastic Large Cell Lymphoma, ALK+
t(21;22)	t(21;22)		Malignant Peripheral Nerve Sheath Tumor
t(21;22)(q22;q12)	t(21;22)(q22;q12)		Ewing Sarcoma; T Lymphoblastic Leukemia/Lymphoma
t(4;11)	t(4;11)		B Lymphoblastic Leukemia/ Lymphoma
t(5;14)	t(5;14)		B Lymphoblastic Leukemia/ Lymphoma
t(6;11)	t(6;11)		Acute Myeloid Leukemia; MiTF/ TFE Family Translocation-associated Carcinoma
t(7;22)	t(7;22)		Malignant Peripheral Nerve Sheath Tumor
t(7;22)(p22;q12)	t(7;22)(p22;q12)		Ewing Sarcoma
t(8;14)	t(8;14)		Burkitt Lymphoma; Diffuse Large B-Cell Lymphoma
t(8;21)	t(8;21)		Acute Myeloid Leukemia
t(8;21)(q22;q22)	t(8;21)(q22;q22)		Myeloid Sarcoma
t(9;11)	t(9;11)		Acute Myeloid Leukemia
t(9;22)	t(9;22)		Acute Myeloid Leukemia; B Lymphoblastic Leukemia/Lymphoma; Protocol for Bone Marrow Specimens
t(X;1)(p11.2;p34)	t(X;1)(p11.2;p34)		MiTF/TFE Family Translocation-associated Carcinoma
t(X;1)(p11.2;q21)	t(X;1)(p11.2;q21)		MiTF/TFE Family Translocation-associated Carcinoma
t(X;17)(p11.2;q23)	t(X;17)(p11.2;q23)		MiTF/TFE Family Translocation-associated Carcinoma
t(X;17)(p11.2;q25)	t(X;17)(p11.2;q25)		MiTF/TFE Family Translocation-associated Carcinoma
t(X;17)(p11.2;q25.3)	t(X;17)(p11.2;q25.3)		MiTF/TFE Family Translocation-associated Carcinoma
t(X;18)	t(X;18)		Calcifying Aponeuronic Fibroma; Pleuropulmonary Blastoma; Synovial Sarcoma
t(X;18)(p11;q11)	t(X;18)(p11;q11)	SYT-SSX	Synovial Sarcoma
t(X;3)(p11;q23)	t(X;3)(p11;q23)		MiTF/TFE Family Translocation-associated Carcinoma
t(X;7)(q21.2;q11.2)	t(X;7)(q21.2;q11.2)		Giant Cell Fibroblastoma/ Dermatofibrosarcoma Protuberans
TAL1	1p32	T-cell acute lymphocytic leukemia 1	T Lymphoblastic Leukemia/ Lymphoma
TCF3-PBX1 (see E2A-PBX1)			
TCL-1	14q32.1	T-cell leukemia/lymphoma 1A	Overview of Lymphoproliferative Disorders Associated with Primary Immune Deficiency
TCR			Autoimmune Lymphoproliferative Syndrome; B Lymphoblastic Leukemia/Lymphoma; Overview of Lymphoproliferative Disorders Associated with Primary Immune Deficiency; Primary Mediastinal (Thymic) Large B-Cell Lymphoma; T Lymphoblastic Leukemia/Lymphoma
TCR γ β and α			T Lymphoblastic Leukemia/ Lymphoma
TCRδ			T Lymphoblastic Leukemia/ Lymphoma
TEL	12p13	ETV6	Secretory Carcinoma
TEL-AML1	t(12;21)(p13;q22)	TV6-RUNX6	B Lymphoblastic Leukemia/ Lymphoma; Protocol for Bone Marrow Specimens; Protocol for Non-Hodgkin Lymphoma Specimens

TET2	4q24	tet methylcytosine dioxygenase 2	Mastocytosis
TFE3	Xp11.22	transcription factor binding to IGHM enhancer 3	MiTF/TFE Family Translocation-associated Carcinoma
TFEB	6p21	transcription factor EB	MiTF/TFE Family Translocation-associated Carcinoma
TFEC	7q31.2	transcription factor EC	MiTF/TFE Family Translocation-associated Carcinoma
TFG	3q12.2	TRK-fused gene	Anaplastic Large Cell Lymphoma, ALK+
TNFRSF6	10q24.1	Fas (TNF receptor superfamily, member 6)	Autoimmune Lymphoproliferative Syndrome
TOP2A	17q21-q22	topoisomerase (DNA) II alpha 170kDa	Myeloid Sarcoma
TP53 (see p53)			
TPM4	19p13.1	tropomyosin 4	Anaplastic Large Cell Lymphoma, ALK+
TSC1	9q34	tuberous sclerosis 1	Subependymal Giant Cell Tumor
TSC1/TSC2		tuberous sclerosis 1 and 2	Rhabdomyoma
TSC2	16p13.3	tuberous sclerosis 2	Ganglion Cell Tumors; Subependymal Giant Cell Tumor
TV6-RUNX1	t(12;21)(p13;q23)		B Lymphoblastic Leukemia/ Lymphoma
TV6-RUNX6	t(12;21)(p13;q22)		B Lymphoblastic Leukemia/ Lymphoma
UNC13D/MUNC13-4			Hemophagocytic Syndrome
VEGF	6p12	vascular endothelial growth factor A (VEGFA)	Adrenal Cortical Carcinoma; Glioblastoma; Pilocytic Astrocytoma
VEGFR3		vascular endothelial growth factor receptor 3; FLT4	Lymphatic Malformation
VEGFRC			Lymphatic Malformation
VHL	3p25.3	von Hippel-Lindau tumor suppressor	Neuroendocrine Tumors
WASP	Xp11.4-p11.21	Wiskott-Aldrich syndrome (eczema-thrombocytopenia)	Autoimmune Lymphoproliferative Syndrome; Hemophagocytic Syndrome
WT1	11p13	Wilms tumor 1	Acute Myeloid Leukemia; Desmoplastic Small Round Cell Tumor; Myeloid Sarcoma; Rhabdomyosarcoma; Wilms Tumor
X, chromosome	X		Nodular Lymphocyte Predominant Hodgkin Lymphoma
Xp11.2			MiTF/TFE Family Translocation-associated Carcinoma
Xp11.23			Myeloid Proliferations Related to Down Syndrome
Xq12			MiTF/TFE Family Translocation-associated Carcinoma
ZNF198/FGFR1	t(8;13)(p12;q11-12)		Protocol for Bone Marrow Specimens; T Lymphoblastic Leukemia/ Lymphoma

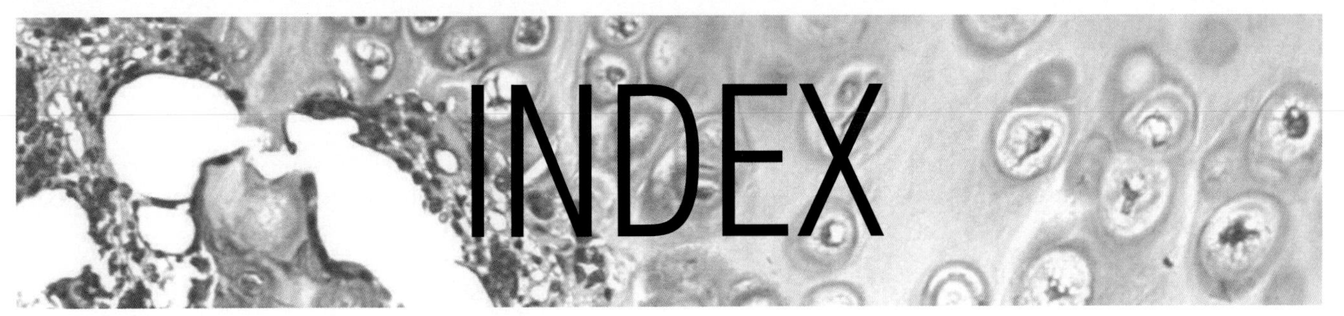

A

INDEX

INDEX

INDEX

C

INDEX

INDEX

INDEX

INDEX

D

INDEX

E

INDEX

INDEX

F

INDEX

INDEX

G

INDEX

INDEX

H

INDEX

INDEX

INDEX

I

INDEX

J

K

INDEX

L

INDEX

INDEX

M

INDEX

INDEX

INDEX

N

INDEX

O

INDEX

INDEX

INDEX

S

INDEX

INDEX

T

INDEX

INDEX

INDEX

X

Y